KARCH'S

Focus on Nursing Pharmacology

NINTH EDITION

KARCH'S

Focus on Nursing Pharmacology

NINTH EDITION

Rebecca G. Tucker, PhD, ACNPC, MEd, RN
Assistant Professor of Clinical Nursing
University of Rochester School of Nursing
Rochester, New York

With consultation from

Anne Schweighardt, PharmD, BCPS
Associate Professor
Wegmans School of Pharmacy
St. John Fisher College
Rochester, New York

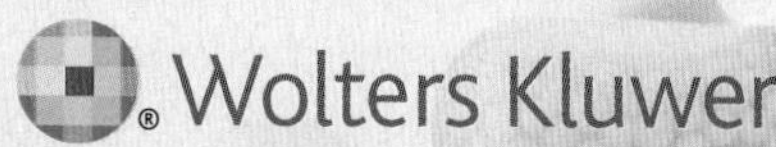

Philadelphia • Baltimore • New York • London
Buenos Aires • Hong Kong • Sydney • Tokyo

Vice President and Publisher: Julie K. Stegman
Executive Editor/Acquisitions Editor: Susan Hartman
Director, Content Management: Jamie Blum
Director of Product Development: Jennifer K. Forestieri
Development Editor: Chelsea Neve, Staci Wolfson
Editorial Coordinator: Julie Kostelnik and Varshaanaa Muralidharan
Editorial Assistant: Devika Kishore
Marketing Manager: Greta Swanson
Senior Production Project Manager: David Saltzberg
Manager, Graphic Arts & Design: Stephen Druding
Art Director, Illustration: Jennifer Clements
Manufacturing Coordinator: Margie Orzech-Zeranko
Prepress Vendor: Straive

Ninth Edition

9 8 7 6 5 4 3 2 1

Printed in Mexico

Cataloging in Publication data available on request from publisher

ISBN: 978-1-9751-8040-9

---

shop.lww.com

QUADM0722

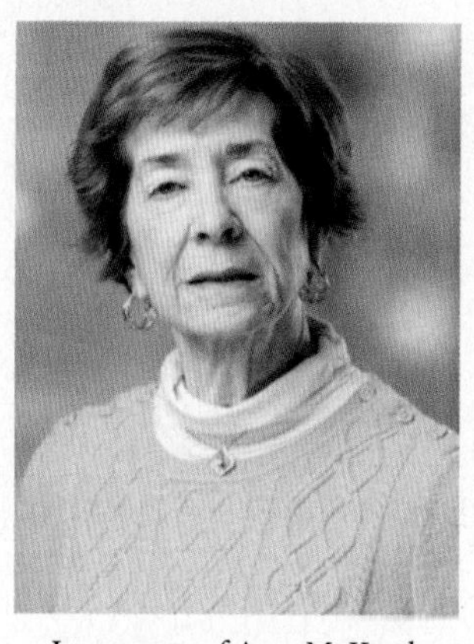

In memory of Amy M. Karch

Amy was a prolific and brilliant author who was dedicated to her dream of facilitating the learning of nurses who wanted to be the best for their patients/families. We (the faculty at the University of Rochester) were blessed to work with her generous and humorous soul. I was additionally fortunate to have her as a mentor and friend. Amy worked on eight editions, and I am extremely honored to be able to continue her work by authoring the ninth edition. This edition is dedicated to Amy Karch. She is missed dearly.

Rebecca G. Tucker
Assistant Professor, Clinical Nursing
University of Rochester School of Nursing
Rochester, New York

REVIEWERS

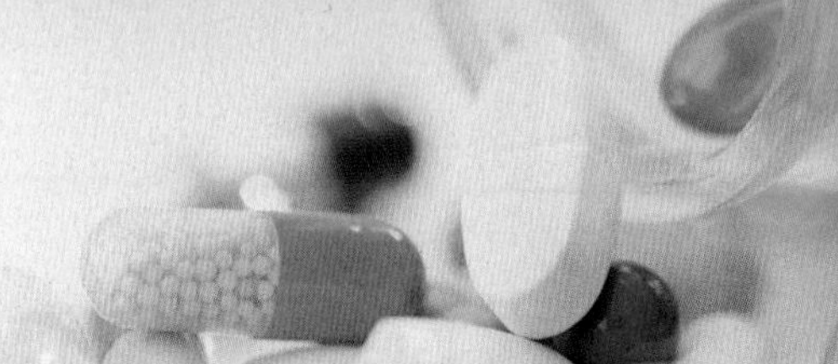

Stacey Amick, BSN, MN, ACNP
Nursing Instructor
Midlands Technical College
Columbia, South Carolina

Anna Boneberg, BSN, MSN, PNP-BC
Clinical Assistant Professor, Nursing
D'Youville University
Buffalo, New York

Lynette DeBellis, BSN, MA, EdD
Instructor of Nursing and Chair of the School of Nursing
Mount Saint Mary College
Newburgh, New York

Kenneth Faulkner, PhD, RN, ANP, FHFSA
Clinical Assistant Professor, Nursing
Stony Brook School of Nursing
Stony Brook, New York

Anita Fitzgerald, MS, PhD
Assistant Professor, Nursing
California State University, Long Beach
Long Beach, California

Margaret McCormick, MS, BSN
Clinical Associate Professor, Nursing
Towson University
Towson, Maryland

Nancy Petges, EdD, MSN, RN, CNE
Assistant Professor, Nursing
Northern Illinois University
DeKalb, Illinois

Jacqueline Sly, DNP, RN, FNP-C
Assistant Department Chair and Clinical Assistant Professor
Boston College Connell School of Nursing
Boston, Massachusetts

Billy Tart, MSN, RN
Nursing Department Chair
Wayne Community College
Goldsboro, North Carolina

Elizabeth Van Dyk, DNP, RN, FNP-C, ANP-C, ANP-BC
Associate Dean, Graduate Nursing
Felician University
Rutherford, New Jersey

PREFACE

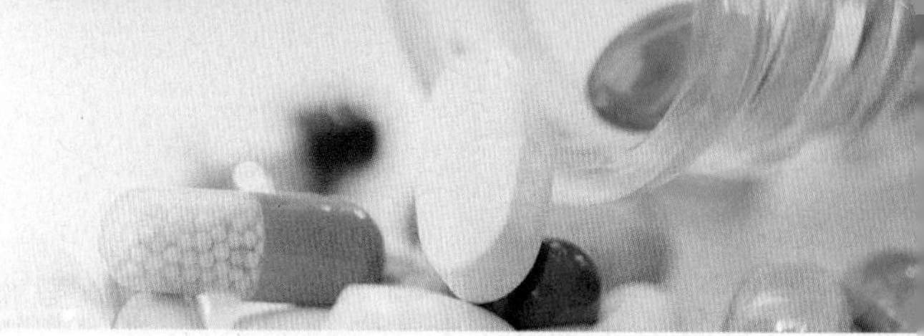

Pharmacology is a difficult course to teach in a standard nursing curriculum, whether it be a diploma, associate, baccalaureate, or graduate program. Instructors have the challenge to facilitate learning of material that is often in flux. New medications are approved, and others are discontinued. New side effects or prescribing warnings can be added as we learn more about how the substances effect people. Nurses and nurse practitioners need a foundational knowledge of medication classifications, yet also need the mental flexibility to build upon that foundation. Furthermore, it is imperative that all clinicians have the skills to evaluate research regarding pharmacology to be able to be knowledgeable in this evolving field.

Pharmacology should not be such a formidable obstacle in the nursing curriculum. The study of drug therapy incorporates physiology, pathophysiology, chemistry, and nursing fundamentals—subjects that are already taught in most schools. A textbook that approaches pharmacology as an understandable, teachable, and learnable subject would greatly facilitate the incorporation of this subject into nursing curricula. Yet many nursing pharmacology texts are large and burdensome, mainly because they need to cover not only the basic pharmacology but also the particulars included in each area considered.

The ninth edition of *Karch's Focus on Nursing Pharmacology* is based on the premise that students first need to have a solid and clearly focused concept of the principles of drug therapy before they can easily grasp the myriad details associated with individual drugs.

Armed with a fundamental knowledge of pharmacology, the student can appreciate and use the specific details that are so readily available in the many annually updated and published nursing drug guides, such as the *Lippincott Nursing Drug Guide*.

With this goal in mind, *Karch's Focus on Nursing Pharmacology* provides a concise, user-friendly, and uncluttered text for the modern student. This difficult subject is presented in a streamlined, understandable, teachable, and learnable manner. Because this book is designed to be used in conjunction with a handbook of current drug information, it remains streamlined. This ninth edition of *Karch's Focus on Nursing Pharmacology* continues to emphasize "need-to-know" concepts and information that is tested on the National Council Licensure Examination (NCLEX) for nurses.

The text reviews and integrates previously learned knowledge of physiology, chemistry, and nursing fundamentals into chapters focused on helping students conceptualize what is important to know about each group of drugs. Illustrations, boxes, and tables sum up concepts to enhance learning. Special features further focus student learning on clinical application, critical thinking, patient safety, lifespan issues related to drug therapy, evidence-based practice, patient teaching, and case study–based critical thinking exercises that incorporate nursing process principles. The text incorporates study materials that conclude each chapter. Check Your Understanding sections provide both new- and old-format NCLEX-style review questions, as well as study guide review questions to help the student master the material and prepare for the national licensing exam.

Organization

Karch's Focus on Nursing Pharmacology is organized following a "simple-to-complex" approach, much like the syllabus for a basic nursing pharmacology course. Because students learn best "from the bottom up," the text is divided into distinct parts.

Part I begins with an overview of basic nursing pharmacology, including challenges the new nurse may encounter. Each of the other parts begins with a review of the physiology of the system affected by the specific drugs being discussed. This review refreshes the information for the student and provides a quick and easy reference when reading about drug actions.

Part II of the text introduces the drug classes, starting with the chemotherapeutic agents—both antimicrobial and antineoplastic drugs. Because the effectiveness of these drugs depends on their interference with the most basic element of body physiology—the cell—students can easily understand the pharmacology of this class. Mastering the pharmacotherapeutic effects of this drug class helps the student establish a firm grasp of the basic principles taught in Part I. Once the easiest pharmacological concepts are understood, the student is prepared to move on to the more challenging physiological and pharmacological concepts.

Part III focuses on drugs affecting the immune system because recent knowledge about the immune system has made it the cornerstone of modern therapy. All of the immune system drugs act in ways in which the immune system would act if it were able. Recent immunological research has contributed to a much greater understanding of this system, making it important to position information about drugs affecting this system close to the beginning of the text instead of at the end as has been the custom.

Parts IV and **V** of the text address drugs that affect the nervous system, the basic functioning system of the body. Following the discussion of the nervous system, and closely linked with it in **Part VI**, is the endocrine system. The sequence of these parts introduces students to the concept of control, teaches them about the interrelatedness of these two systems, and prepares them for understanding many aspects of shared physiological function and the inevitable linking of the two systems into one: the neuroendocrine system.

Parts VII, **VIII**, and **IX** discuss drugs affecting the reproductive, cardiovascular, and renal systems, respectively. The sequencing of cardiovascular and renal drugs is logical because most of the augmenting cardiovascular drugs (such as diuretics) affect the renal system.

Part X covers drugs that act on the respiratory system, which provides the link between the left and right ventricles of the heart.

Part XI addresses drugs acting on the gastrointestinal system. A new chapter has been added to this section titled "Vitamin, Minerals, and Complementary/Alternative Medications."

Text Features

The features in this text are skillfully designed to support the text discussion, encouraging the student to look at the whole patient and to focus on the essential information that is important to learn about each drug class. Important features in the ninth edition focus on incorporating basic nursing skills, patient safety, critical thinking, and application of the material learned to the clinical scenario, helping the student to understand the pharmacology material.

Focus on Teaching/Learning Activities

thePoint® (available at http://thepoint.lww.com/), a trademark of Wolters Kluwer Health, is a web-based course and content management system that provides every resource instructors and students need in one easy-to-use site, where teaching, learning, and technology click!

Student Resources

Students can visit thePoint® to access supplemental multimedia resources to enhance their learning experience, download content, and upload assignments. thePoint® offers a variety of free student resources, including Watch and Learn video clips, and free recently published journal articles related to topics discussed in the book. Also included are videos on preventing medication errors and three-dimensional animated depictions of pharmacology concepts.

This edition includes ***vSim** for Nursing* | Pharmacology, a new virtual simulation platform, available via thePoint®. Codeveloped by Laerdal Medical, ***vSim** for Nursing* | Pharmacology helps students develop clinical competence and decision-making skills as they interact with virtual patients in a safe, realistic environment. ***vSim** for Nursing* records and assesses student decisions throughout the simulation, then provides a personalized feedback log highlighting areas needing improvement. Also available via thePoint®, Lippincott DocuCare combines web-based electronic health record simulation software with clinical case scenarios that link directly to many of the skills presented in *Karch's Focus on Nursing Pharmacology*. Lippincott DocuCare's nonlinear solution works well in the classroom, simulation lab, and clinical practice.

Instructor Resources

Advanced technology and superior content combine at thePoint® to allow instructors to design and deliver online and offline courses, maintain grades and class rosters, and communicate with students. thePoint® also provides additional resources, including Pre-Lecture Quizzes, PowerPoints with Guided Lecture Notes, Discussion Topics, Assignments, and over 1,700 Test Generator questions!

Lippincott® CoursePoint+

The same trusted solution, innovation, and unmatched support that you have come to expect from *Lippincott CoursePoint+* is now enhanced with more engaging learning tools and deeper analytics to help prepare students for practice. This powerfully integrated, digital learning solution combines learning tools, case studies, virtual simulation, real-time data, and the most trusted nursing education content on the market to make curriculum-wide learning more efficient and to meet students where they're at in their learning. And now, it's easier than ever for instructors and students to use, giving them everything they need for course and curriculum success!

Lippincott CoursePoint+ includes the following:

- Engaging course content provides a variety of learning tools to engage students of all learning styles.
- A more personalized learning approach, including adaptive learning powered by PrepU, gives students the content and tools they need at the moment they need it,

giving them data for more focused remediation and helping to boost their confidence.
- Varying levels of case studies, virtual simulation, and access to Lippincott Advisor help students learn the critical thinking and clinical judgment skills to help them become practice-ready nurses.
- Unparalleled reporting provides in-depth dashboards with several data points to track student progress and help identify strengths and weaknesses.
- Unmatched support includes training coaches, product trainers, and nursing education consultants to help educators and students implement CoursePoint with ease.

Build Clinical Judgment Skills and Prepare With Lippincott®

The NCLEX will include new types of questions designed to assess how well students can apply what they have learned—a true test of clinical judgment skills. Wolters Kluwer is committed to helping students practice and prepare by integrating these new question types into CoursePoint+ and PassPoint.

Exposing students to the new types of NGN questions before they take the exam will help build familiarity with the actual exam. We are integrating them into our core nursing curriculum solutions to assist students in building the competence and confidence they need for success—on the NCLEX and in clinical practice.

With additional question types and tools, faculty can assess student readiness and pinpoint areas that need additional preparation—throughout the curriculum, not just as students are preparing for the NCLEX.

NGN new item types included in Lippincott® CoursePoint+ and PassPoint:

- Complete case studies
- Stand-alone items (bowtie and trend)
- Deconstructed case studies in CoursePoint+ provide additional exposure to new question types and are unique to Lippincott®
- Knowledge items and NGN-style questions
- Partial scoring for NGN questions in PassPoint simulated exams

Special Elements and Learning Aids

Each chapter opens with a list of learning objectives for that chapter, helping the student understand what the key learning points will be. A list of featured drugs and a glossary of key terms are also found on the opening chapter page. Key points appear periodically throughout each chapter to summarize important concepts. The text of each chapter ends with a summary of important concepts. This is followed by a series of review exercises, Check Your Understanding, which includes NCLEX-style questions to focus student learning on the seminal information presented in the chapter.

- In the *Drug List* at the beginning of each chapter, a special icon appears next to the drug that is considered the prototype drug of each class. In each chapter, *prototype summary* boxes spotlight need-to-know information for each prototype drug.
- *Drugs in Focus* tables clearly summarize and identify the drugs within a class, highlighting them by generic and trade names, usual dosage, and indications.
- *Focus on Safe Medication Administration* boxes present important safety information to help keep the patient safe, prevent medication errors, and increase the therapeutic effectiveness of the drugs.
- *Focus on the Evidence* boxes compile information based on research to identify the best nursing practices associated with specific drug therapy.
- *Focus on Herbal and Alternative Therapies* boxes highlight known interactions with specific herbs or alternative therapies that could affect the actions of the drugs being discussed.
- *Focus on Calculations* reviews are designed to help the student hone calculation and measurement skills while learning about the drugs for which doses might need to be calculated.
- *Focus on Drug Therapy Across the Lifespan* boxes concisely summarize points to consider when using the drugs of each class with children, adults, and the older adults.
- *Focus on Sex Differences* and *Focus on Cultural Considerations* boxes encourage the student to think about the patient as a unique individual with a special set of characteristics that not only influences variations in drug effectiveness but also could influence a patient's perspective on drug therapy.
- *Critical Thinking Scenarios* tie each chapter's content together by presenting clinical scenarios about a patient using a particular drug from the class being discussed. Included in the case study are hints to guide critical thinking about the case and a discussion of drug- and non–drug-related nursing considerations for that particular patient and situation. Most important, the case study provides a plan of nursing care specifically developed for that patient and specifically based on the nursing process. The care plan is followed by a checklist of patient teaching points designed for the patient presented in the case study. This approach helps the student to see how assessment and the collected data are applied in the clinical situation.
- *Check Your Understanding* sections present NCLEX-style questions, including alternate format questions, to help

the student prepare for that exam. Other questions and activities in this section are designed to help students test their knowledge of the information that has been learned in the chapter.

- *Unfolding Patient Stories*, written by the National League for Nursing, are an engaging way to begin meaningful conversations in the classroom. These vignettes, which unfold in two parts each and are interspersed throughout the text, feature patients from Wolters Kluwer's ***vSim** for Nursing* for Nursing | *Pharmacology* (codeveloped by Laerdal Medical) and DocuCare products; however, each Unfolding Patient Story in the book stands alone, not requiring purchase of these products.
- *Concept Mastery Alerts* highlight and clarify the most common misconceptions in nursing pharmacology, as identified by Lippincott's online adaptive learning platform. Our team reviewed data from thousands of nursing pharmacology students across North America to identify the points of confusion for most students to help you learn more effectively.

To the Student Using This Text

As you begin your study of pharmacology, don't be overwhelmed or confused by all of the details. The study of drugs fits perfectly into your study of the human body—anatomy, physiology, chemistry, nutrition, psychology, and sociology. Approach the study of pharmacology from two main perspectives. First, review the names of the medication classifications, how they work, what the common and dangerous side effects are, and pertinent teaching points for clients. Once you understand the classification, pick a few of the common medications in each classification as prototypes to know more details about. The second way to review pharmacology is starting from the "indication" or disease. It is imperative to know what medications are commonly used for each clinical problem. For example, what typical medications would be prescribed for a client with hypertension? Keep in mind that pharmacology is evolving as new research is performed and new substances are created. Therefore, the study of pharmacology is lifelong. Enjoy!

Rebecca G. Tucker, PhD, ACNPC, MEd, RN

ACKNOWLEDGMENTS

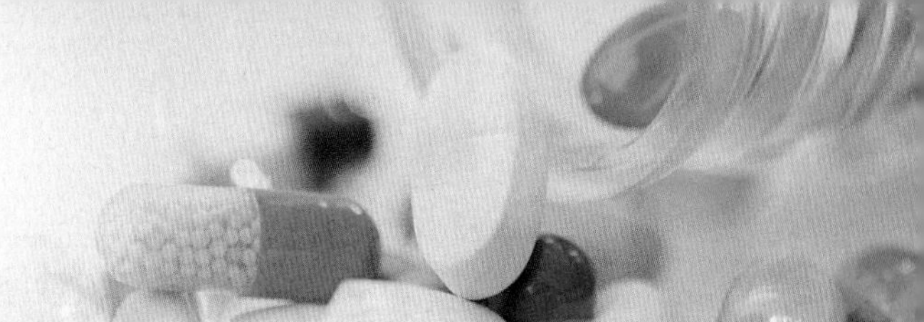

I would like to acknowledge that all previous editions were primarily authored by Amy M. Karch who dedicated her career to nursing education. I have been extremely blessed by her mentorship and miss her.

I would like to thank my coinstructors, Deans, and staff at the University of Rochester School of Nursing who are dedicated to facilitating learning in the context of supporting each other and students as family. Dean Kathy Rideout, Associate Dean Lydia Rotondo, Dr. Patrick Hopkins, Dr. Elizabeth Palermo, Dr. Craig Sellers, MariaLainea Chennell, and Joseph Gomulak-Cavicchio—these are only a few that I value and am so grateful for. I would like to acknowledge Dr. Anne Schweighardt who provided pharmaceutical expertise that is invaluable.

Thank you to the people at Wolters Kluwer who are so willing to facilitate a positive writing environment. I am especially appreciative of Staci Wolfson (Supervisory Development Editor) who was my "go to" if I had any questions/concerns throughout this process and to Julie Kostelnik and Varshaanaa Muralidharan who were responsible for the first round of content editing. Thank you to Jonathan Joyce and Susan Hartman who were the official leaders of this project.

I am very fortunate to be motivated by my patients and students. They drive me to continually learn and evolve to provide the best care and education possible. Furthermore, I am blessed to be loved by family and friends who support me through the best and worst of times. Without their support, this work would not be possible.

Rebecca G. Tucker, PhD, ACNPC, MEd, RN

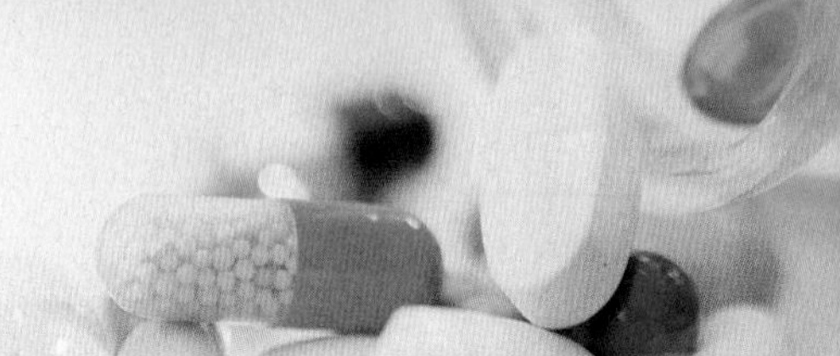

CONTENTS

PART 11 Drugs Acting on the Gastrointestinal System 1005

Appendices 1085

PART 1

Introduction to Nursing Pharmacology

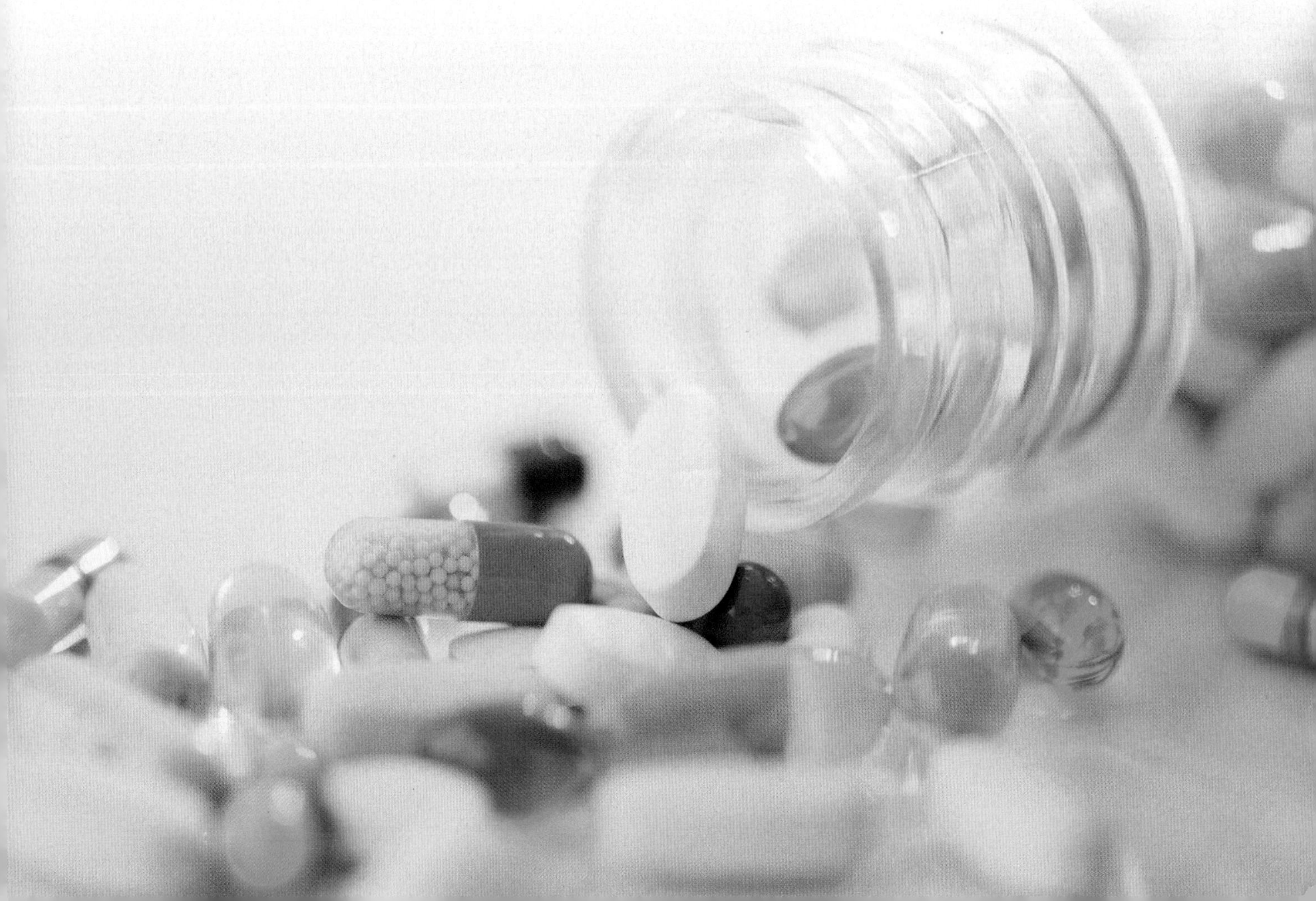

CHAPTER 1

Introduction to Drugs

Learning Objectives

Upon completion of this chapter, you will be able to:

1. Define the word pharmacology.
2. Outline the steps involved in developing and approving a new drug in the United States.
3. Describe the federal controls on drugs that have abuse potential.
4. Differentiate between generic and brand name drugs and over-the-counter and prescription drugs.
5. Explain the benefits and risks associated with the use of over-the-counter drugs.

Key Terms

adverse effects: drug effects, sometimes called side effects, that are not the desired therapeutic effects; may be unpleasant or even dangerous

brand name: name given to a drug by the pharmaceutical company that developed it; also called a trade name or proprietary name

chemical name: name that reflects the chemical structure of a drug

drugs: chemicals that are introduced into the body to bring about change

Food and Drug Administration (FDA): federal agency responsible for the regulation and enforcement of drug evaluation and distribution policies in the United States

generic drugs: drugs sold by their generic name; not brand name or trade name product

generic name: the original designation that a drug is given when the drug company that developed it applies for the approval process

genetic engineering: process of altering DNA, usually of bacteria, to produce a chemical to be used as a drug

off-label uses: uses of a drug that are not part of the stated therapeutic indications for which the drug was approved by the FDA; off-label uses may lead to new indications for a drug

orphan drugs: drugs that have been discovered but would not be profitable for a drug company to develop without outside financial incentives; usually drugs that would treat only a small number of people

over-the-counter (OTC) drugs: drugs that are available without a prescription for self-treatment of a variety of complaints; deemed to be safe when used as directed; often formerly only available by prescription

pharmacology: the study of the biological effects of chemicals

pharmacotherapeutics: clinical pharmacology—the branch of pharmacology that deals with drugs; chemicals that are used in medicine for the treatment, prevention, and diagnosis of disease in humans

phase I study: a pilot study of a potential drug using a small number of selected, usually healthy human volunteers

phase II study: a clinical study of a proposed drug by selected physicians using actual patients who have the disorder the drug is designed to treat

phase III study: use of a proposed drug on a larger sample of the population of patients who have the disease the drug is thought to treat

phase IV study: continuous evaluation of a drug after it has been released for marketing

preclinical trials: initial trials of a chemical thought to have therapeutic potential either with in vitro or in vivo techniques; not human subjects

teratogenic: having adverse effects on all phases of the development inside the womb (zygote, embryo, or fetus)

The human body works through a complicated series of chemical reactions and processes. **Pharmacology** is the study of the biological effects of chemicals. **Drugs** are chemicals that are introduced into the body to cause some sort of change. When drugs are administered, the body begins a sequence of processes designed to handle the new chemicals. These processes, which involve breaking down and eliminating the drugs, affect the body's complex series of chemical reactions. In clinical practice, health care providers focus on how chemicals act on people.

Nurses deal with **pharmacotherapeutics**, or clinical pharmacology, the branch of pharmacology that uses drugs to treat, prevent, and diagnose disease. Clinical pharmacology addresses two key concerns: the drug's effects on the body and the body's response to the drug.

For many reasons, understanding how drugs act on the body to cause changes and applying that knowledge in the clinical setting are important aspects of nursing practice. For instance, patients today often follow complicated drug regimens and receive potentially toxic drugs and/or drug combinations. Also, many patients need to manage their care at home. A drug can have many effects, and the nurse must know which ones may occur when a particular drug is administered. Some drug effects are therapeutic, or helpful, but others are undesirable or potentially dangerous. These negative effects are called **adverse effects**, or side effects, of the drug. (See Chapter 3 for a detailed discussion of adverse effects.)

The nurse is in a unique position regarding drug therapy because nursing responsibilities include the following:

- Administering drugs
- Assessing drug effects
- Intervening to make the drug regimen more tolerable
- Providing patient teaching about drugs and drug regimens
- Monitoring the overall patient care plan to prevent medication errors

Knowing how drugs work makes these tasks easier to handle, thus enhancing the effectiveness of drug therapy.

This text is designed to provide the pharmacological basis for understanding drug therapy. The physiology of a body system and the related actions of many drugs on that system are presented in a way that allows clear understanding of how drugs work and what to anticipate when giving a particular type of drug.

Thousands of drugs are available, and it is impossible to memorize all of the individual differences among drugs in a class. This text addresses *general* drug information. The nurse can refer to the most recent editions of the *Nursing Drug Handbook*, the *Lippincott Pocket Drug Guide for Nurses*, or to another drug guide to obtain the *specific* details required for safe and effective drug administration. Drug details are changing constantly. The practicing nurse must be knowledgeable about these changes and rely on an up-to-date and comprehensive drug guide in the clinical setting.

A section related to nursing considerations for patients receiving particular drugs will be found in each chapter of this book. This includes assessment points, nursing diagnoses to consider, planning for patient-centered care, implementation of particular interventions that should be considered, and evaluation points that will provide a guide for using the nursing process to effectively incorporate drug therapy into patient care. This information can be used to develop an individual nursing care plan for your patient (Table 1.1). The

Table 1.1 Sample Nursing Care Plan From *Nursing Drug Handbook* for a Patient Receiving Oral Linezolid

Assessment	Nursing Diagnosis	Implementation	Evaluation
History (contraindications/cautions) Hypertension Hyperthyroidism Blood dyscrasias Hepatic dysfunction Pheochromocytoma Phenylketonuria Carcinoid syndrome Pregnancy Lactation Known allergy to: linezolid **Medication History** (possible drug–drug interactions) Pseudoephedrine Selective serotonin reuptake inhibitors MAOIs Antiplatelet drugs **Diet History** (possible drug–food interactions) Foods high in tyramine **Physical Assessment** (screen for contraindications and to establish a baseline for evaluating effects and adverse effects) Local: culture site of infection CNS: affect, reflexes, orientation CV: P, BP, peripheral perfusion GI: bowel sounds, liver evaluation Skin: color, lesions Hematologic: CBC with differential, liver function tests	Malnutrition risk, less than body requirements, related to GI effects Acute pain related to GI effects, headache Altered tissue perfusion related to bone marrow effects Knowledge deficiency related to drug therapy	Safe and appropriate administration of drug: culture infection site to ensure appropriate use of drug Provision of safety and comfort measures: • Monitor BP periodically • Monitor platelet counts before and periodically during therapy • Alleviation of GI upset • Ready access to bathroom facilities • Nutritional consult • Safety provisions if dizziness and CNS effects occur • Avoidance of tyramine-rich foods Patient teaching regarding: Drug Side effects to anticipate Warnings Reactions to report Support and encouragement to cope with disease, high cost of therapy, and side effects Provision of emergency and life support measures in cases of acute hypersensitivity	Monitor for therapeutic effects of drug: resolution of infection If resolution does not occur, reculture site Monitor for adverse effects of drug: • GI upset—nausea, vomiting, diarrhea • Liver function changes • Pseudomembranous colitis • Blood dyscrasias—changes in platelet counts • Fever • Rash • Sweating • Photosensitivity • Acute hypersensitivity reactions Evaluate effectiveness of patient teaching program: patient can name drug, dose of drug, use of drug, adverse effects to expect, and reactions to report Evaluate effectiveness of comfort and safety measures Monitor for drug–drug and drug–food interactions as appropriate Evaluate effectiveness of life support measures if needed

MAOI, monoamine oxidase inhibitor; CNS, central nervous system; CV, cardiovascular; P, pulse; BP, blood pressure; GI, gastrointestinal; CBC, complete blood count.

monographs in the *Nursing Drug Handbook* (Fig. 1.1) or any other nursing drug guide can be used to provide the specific information that you need to plan care for each particular drug you might be giving. The various sections of each drug monograph can provide information to help in the development of patient teaching guides and drug cards for reference in the clinical setting. The Patient Drug Sheet: Oral Linezolid (Fig. 1.2) is an example of how this information can be used to develop a patient teaching guide.

The nurse can use this text as a resource for basic concepts of pharmacology and a nursing drug guide as an easy-to-use reference in the clinical setting.

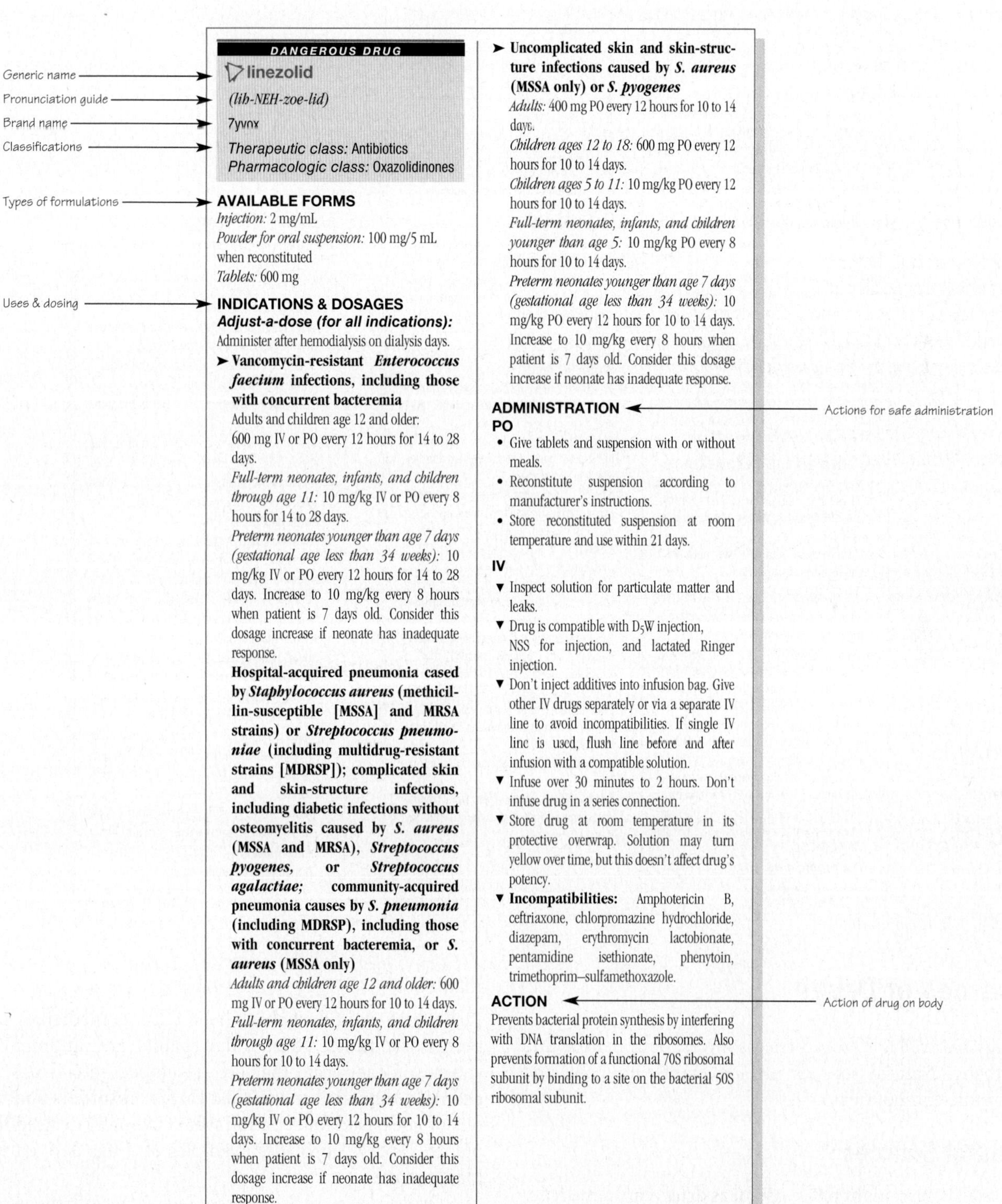

DANGEROUS DRUG

linezolid

(lih-NEH-zoe-lid)

Zyvox

Therapeutic class: Antibiotics
Pharmacologic class: Oxazolidinones

AVAILABLE FORMS

Injection: 2 mg/mL
Powder for oral suspension: 100 mg/5 mL when reconstituted
Tablets: 600 mg

INDICATIONS & DOSAGES

Adjust-a-dose (for all indications): Administer after hemodialysis on dialysis days.

➤ **Vancomycin-resistant *Enterococcus faecium* infections, including those with concurrent bacteremia**
Adults and children age 12 and older: 600 mg IV or PO every 12 hours for 14 to 28 days.
Full-term neonates, infants, and children through age 11: 10 mg/kg IV or PO every 8 hours for 14 to 28 days.
Preterm neonates younger than age 7 days (gestational age less than 34 weeks): 10 mg/kg IV or PO every 12 hours for 14 to 28 days. Increase to 10 mg/kg every 8 hours when patient is 7 days old. Consider this dosage increase if neonate has inadequate response.

Hospital-acquired pneumonia cased by *Staphylococcus aureus* (methicillin-susceptible [MSSA] and MRSA strains) or *Streptococcus pneumoniae* (including multidrug-resistant strains [MDRSP]); complicated skin and skin-structure infections, including diabetic infections without osteomyelitis caused by *S. aureus* (MSSA and MRSA), *Streptococcus pyogenes*, or *Streptococcus agalactiae*; community-acquired pneumonia causes by *S. pneumonia* (including MDRSP), including those with concurrent bacteremia, or *S. aureus* (MSSA only)
Adults and children age 12 and older: 600 mg IV or PO every 12 hours for 10 to 14 days.
Full-term neonates, infants, and children through age 11: 10 mg/kg IV or PO every 8 hours for 10 to 14 days.
Preterm neonates younger than age 7 days (gestational age less than 34 weeks): 10 mg/kg IV or PO every 12 hours for 10 to 14 days. Increase to 10 mg/kg every 8 hours when patient is 7 days old. Consider this dosage increase if neonate has inadequate response.

➤ **Uncomplicated skin and skin-structure infections caused by *S. aureus* (MSSA only) or *S. pyogenes***
Adults: 400 mg PO every 12 hours for 10 to 14 days.
Children ages 12 to 18: 600 mg PO every 12 hours for 10 to 14 days.
Children ages 5 to 11: 10 mg/kg PO every 12 hours for 10 to 14 days.
Full-term neonates, infants, and children younger than age 5: 10 mg/kg PO every 8 hours for 10 to 14 days.
Preterm neonates younger than age 7 days (gestational age less than 34 weeks): 10 mg/kg PO every 12 hours for 10 to 14 days. Increase to 10 mg/kg every 8 hours when patient is 7 days old. Consider this dosage increase if neonate has inadequate response.

ADMINISTRATION

PO

- Give tablets and suspension with or without meals.
- Reconstitute suspension according to manufacturer's instructions.
- Store reconstituted suspension at room temperature and use within 21 days.

IV

▼ Inspect solution for particulate matter and leaks.
▼ Drug is compatible with D_5W injection, NSS for injection, and lactated Ringer injection.
▼ Don't inject additives into infusion bag. Give other IV drugs separately or via a separate IV line to avoid incompatibilities. If single IV line is used, flush line before and after infusion with a compatible solution.
▼ Infuse over 30 minutes to 2 hours. Don't infuse drug in a series connection.
▼ Store drug at room temperature in its protective overwrap. Solution may turn yellow over time, but this doesn't affect drug's potency.
▼ **Incompatibilities:** Amphotericin B, ceftriaxone, chlorpromazine hydrochloride, diazepam, erythromycin lactobionate, pentamidine isethionate, phenytoin, trimethoprim–sulfamethoxazole.

ACTION

Prevents bacterial protein synthesis by interfering with DNA translation in the ribosomes. Also prevents formation of a functional 70S ribosomal subunit by binding to a site on the bacterial 50S ribosomal subunit.

FIGURE 1.1 Example of a drug monograph. (Created using an excerpt from (2020) *Nursing2021 drug handbook* (41st ed.). Wolters Kluwer.)

Pharmacokinetics →

Route	Onset	Peak	Duration
PO	Unknown	1–2 hr	Unknown
IV	Unknown	30 min	Unknown

Half-life: Adults, 4 to 5 hours; children age 1 week to 11 years, 1 1/2 to 3 hours.

Side effects or adverse reactions →

ADVERSE REACTIONS

CNS: headache, dizziness, fever, insomnia, vertigo (children). **GI:** diarrhea, nausea, altered taste, constipation, oral candidiasis, tongue discoloration, vomiting, abdominal pain. **GU:** vaginal candidiasis. **Hematologic:** *leukopenia, myelosuppression, neutropenia, thrombocytopenia,* anemia. **Skin:** rash. **Other:** fungal infection.

Clinically important interactions →

INTERACTIONS

Drug-drug. *Adrenergic drugs (dopamine, epinephrine, pseudoephedrine):* May cause HTN. Monitor BP and HR; start continuous infusions of dopamine and epinephrine at lower doses and titrate to response.

Insulin, oral antidiabetic agents: May cause symptomatic hypoglycemia. Monitor patient closely.

Serotonergic drugs: May cause serotonin syndrome, including confusion, delirium, restlessness, tremors, blushing diaphoresis, and hyperpyrexia. Notify prescriber immediately of signs and symptoms of serotonin syndrome.

Drug-food. *Foods and beverages high in tyramine (aged cheeses, air-dried meats, red wines, sauerkraut, soy sauce, tap beers):* May increase BP. Provide a list of foods containing tyramine and advise patient that tyramine content of meals shouldn't exceed 100 mg.

EFFECTS ON LAB TEST RESULTS

- May increase ALT, AST, bilirubin, alkaline phosphatase, BUN, creatinine, amylase, lipase, LDH, and BUN levels. May decrease Hb level.
- May decrease glucose level and WBC, neutrophil, and platelet counts.

Conditions limiting use →

CONTRAINDICATIONS & CAUTIONS

- Contraindicated in patients hypersensitive to drug or its components.

Alert: Concomitant use with psychiatric drugs or within 2 weeks of taking psychiatric drugs that work through the serotonin system of the brain (SSRIs, SSNRIs, TCAs, MAO inhibitors, and others) can cause serotonin syndrome (fever, mental status changes, muscle twitching, excessive sweating, shivering or shaking, diarrhea, and loss of coordination). Use linezolid with these drugs only for life-threatening or urgent conditions when the potential benefits outweigh the risks of toxicity.

Dialyzable drug: 30%

PREGNANCY-LACTATION-REPRODUCTION ← Reproduction information

- There are no adequate studies in pregnant women. Use during pregnancy only if potential benefit justifies potential risk to the fetus.
- Drug may appear in human milk. Use cautiously in breastfeeding women.

NURSING CONSIDERATIONS ← Nursing actions

- No dosage adjustment is needed when switching from IV to oral forms.

Alert: Before giving linezolid, stop any serotonergic drug and monitor patient for serotonin toxicity for 2 weeks (5 weeks if fluoxetine was taken) or until 24 hours after the last dose of linezolid, whichever comes first. May resume serotonergic psychiatric drugs 24 hours after last dose of linezolid.

Alert: Nausea and vomiting may be symptoms of lactic acidosis. Monitor patient for unexplained acidosis or low bicarbonate level, and notify prescriber immediately if these occur.

Alert: Drug may cause thrombocytopenia. In patients at increased risk for bleeding, those with existing thrombocytopenia, those taking other drugs that may cause thrombocytopenia, and those receiving this drug for longer than 14 days, monitor platelet count.

Alert: Drug may lead to myelosuppression. Monitor CBC weekly.

Alert: Prolonged use can cause superinfection, including CDAD, which can occur more than 2 months after treatment ends. Consider these diagnoses and take appropriate measures in patients with persistent diarrhea or secondary infections.

Alert: Drug may cause symptomatic hypoglycemia in patients taking insulin or oral antidiabetic agents. Monitor patient closely.

- Inappropriate use of antibiotics may lead to development of resistant organisms; carefully consider other drugs before starting therapy, especially in outpatient setting.
- Peripheral and optic neuropathies can occur, especially in patients treated for a longer-than-recommended duration. If these neuropathies occur, drug may need to be discontinued. Patients with vision changes should receive prompt ophthalmic evaluation.
- Use cautiously in patients with seizure disorder.
- ***Look alike-sound alike:*** Don't confuse Zyvox with Zovirax. Both come in a 400-mg strength.

PATIENT TEACHING ← Teaching points

- Tell patient that tablets and oral suspension may be taken with our without meals.
- Stress importance of completing entire course of therapy, even if patient feels better.
- Tell patient to report all adverse reactions promptly.
- Tell patient to alert prescriber if patient has high BP; is taking cough or cold preparations, insulin, or oral antidiabetic agents; or is being treated with SSRIs or other antidepressants.

Alert: Teach patient to recognize and immediately report signs and symptoms of serotonin toxicity (fever, mental status changes, muscle twitching,, excessive sweating, shivering or shaking, diarrhea, and loss of coordination).

- Advise patient taking prescribed psychiatric drugs that these drugs may need to be stopped during linezolid therapy but not to stop them without first speaking to prescriber.
- Teach patient to avoid eating large quantities of tyramine-containing foods (aged cheeses, soy sauce, tap beers, red wine) during therapy.
- Inform patient with phenylketonuria that each 5 mL of oral suspension contains 20 mg of phenylalanine. Tablets and injection don't contain phenylalanine.

FIGURE 1.1 *(Continued)*

Sources of Drugs

Drugs are available from varied sources, both natural and synthetic. Natural sources include plants, animals, and inorganic compounds.

Natural Sources

Chemicals that might prove useful as drugs can come from many natural sources, such as plants, animals, or inorganic compounds. To become a drug, a chemical must have a demonstrated therapeutic value or efficacy without severe toxicity or damaging properties.

Plants

Plants and plant parts have been used as medicines since prehistoric times. Even today, plants are an important source of chemicals that are developed into drugs. For example, digitalis used to treat cardiac disorders and various opiates used for sedation were originally derived from plants. Table 1.2 provides examples of drugs derived from plant sources.

Drugs also may be processed using a synthetic version of the active chemical found in a plant. An example of this type of drug is dronabinol (*Marinol*), which contains the active ingredient delta-9-tetrahydrocannabinol found in

Patient Drug Sheet: Oral Linezolid

Patient's Name: Mr. Kors
Prescriber's Name: J. Smith, ANP
Phone Number: 555-555-5555

Instructions:

1. The name of your drug is *linezolid*; the brand name is *Zyvox*. This drug is an antibiotic that is being used to treat your *pneumonia*. This drug is very specific in its action and is only indicated for your particular infection. Take the full course of your drug. Do not share this drug with other people or save tablets for future use.
2. The dose of the drug that has been prescribed for you is: *600 mg* (*1 tablet*).
3. The drug should be taken *once every 12 hours*. The best time for you to take this drug will be *8:00 in the morning and 8:00 in the evening*. Do not skip any doses. Do not take two doses at once if you forget a dose. If you miss a dose, take the dose as soon as you remember and then again in 12 hours.
4. The drug can be taken with food if GI upset is a problem. Avoid foods that are rich in tyramine (list is below) while you are taking this drug.
5. The following side effects may occur:
   Nausea, vomiting, abdominal pain (taking the drug with food and eating frequent small meals may help).
   Diarrhea (ensure ready access to bathroom facilities). Notify your healthcare provider if this becomes severe.
6. Do not take this drug with over-the-counter drugs or herbal remedies without first checking with your healthcare provider. Many of these agents can cause problems with your drug.
7. Tell any nurse, physician, or dentist who is taking care of you that you are on this drug.
8. Keep this and all medications out of the reach of children.

Notify your health care provider if any of the following occur:
Rash, severe GI problems, bloody or excessive diarrhea, weakness, tremors, increased bleeding or bruising, anxiety.

Foods high in tyramine to avoid: Aged cheeses, avocados, bananas, beer, bologna (polony), caffeinated beverages, chocolate, liver, over-ripe fruit, pepperoni, pickled fish, red wine, salami, smoked fish, yeast, yogurt.

FIGURE 1.2 Example of a patient teaching sheet. (Created using data from (2020) *Nursing2021 drug handbook* (41st ed.). Wolters Kluwer.)

marijuana. This drug helps to prevent nausea and vomiting in cancer patients and treats weight loss in clients with acquired immunodeficiency syndrome (AIDS) but does not have all the adverse effects that occur when the marijuana leaf is smoked. Marijuana leaf is a controlled substance with high abuse potential and is legal for medical use in some states but not approved for recreational use in many states. The synthetic version of the active ingredient allows for an accepted form to achieve the desired therapeutic effects.

Table 1.2 Drugs Derived From Plants

Plant	Product
Ricinus communis	Seed Oil Castor oil
Digitalis purpurea (foxglove)	Leaves Dried leaves Digitalis leaf
Papaver somniferum (poppy)	Unripe capsule Juice Opium (*Paregoric*) Morphine (*MS Contin*) Codeine Papaverine

Ingestion of a plant-derived food can sometimes lead to a drug effect. For instance, the ingredient in natural licorice (glycyrrhizine) inhibits the inactivation of cortisol. This increases the active cortisol and allows increased stimulation of renal mineralocorticoid receptors. This has a pseudoaldosterone effect. Aldosterone is a hormone found in the body that acts in the kidneys to increase fluid retention and decrease potassium levels. Therefore, when people ingest large amounts of licorice, they can retain fluid to cause high blood pressures and develop hypokalemia (low serum potassium levels). However, people seldom think of licorice as a drug. Black licorice candy does include the ingredient glycyrrhizine, but red licorice candy does not.

Finally, plants and plant by-products have become the main component of the growing herbal and alternative therapy movement. Chapters 6 and 60 discuss the alternative therapy movement and its impact on today's drug regimens.

Animal Products

Animal products are used to replace human chemicals that fail to be produced because of disease or genetic problems. Insulin for treating diabetes used to be obtained exclusively from the pancreas of cows and pigs. Now **genetic engineering**—the process of altering DNA—permits scientists to produce human insulin by altering *Escherichia coli* bacteria, making insulin a better product without some of the impurities that come with animal products.

Thyroid drugs and growth hormone preparations also may be obtained from animal thyroid and hypothalamic tissues. Many of these preparations are now created synthetically, however, and the synthetic preparations are considered purer and safer than preparations derived from animals.

Inorganic Compounds

Salts of various chemical elements can have therapeutic effects in the human body. Aluminum, fluoride, iron, and even gold are used to treat various conditions. The effects of these elements usually were discovered accidentally when a cause–effect relationship was observed. Table 1.3 shows examples of some elements used for their therapeutic benefit.

Table 1.3 Elements Used for Their Therapeutic Effects

Element	Therapeutic Use
Aluminum	Antacid to decrease gastric acidity Management of hyperphosphatemia Prevention of the formation of phosphate urinary stones
Fluorine (as fluoride)	Prevention of dental cavities Prevention of osteoporosis
Gold	Treatment of rheumatoid arthritis
Iron	Treatment of iron deficiency anemia

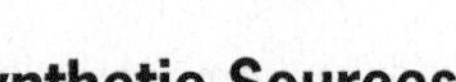

Synthetic Sources

Today, many drugs are developed synthetically after chemicals in plants, animals, or the environment have been tested and found to have therapeutic activity. Scientists use genetic engineering to alter bacteria to produce chemicals that are therapeutic and effective. Other technical advances allow scientists to alter a chemical with proven therapeutic effectiveness to make it better. Sometimes, a small change in a chemical's structure can make that chemical more useful as a drug—more potent, more stable, and less toxic. These technological advances have led to the development of groups of similar drugs, all of which are derived from an original prototype, but each of which has slightly different properties, making a particular drug more desirable in a specific situation.

Throughout this book, the icon P will be used to designate those drugs of a class that are considered the prototype of the class, the original drug in the class, or the drug that has emerged as the most effective. For example, the cephalosporins are a large group of antibiotics derived from the same chemical structure. Alterations in the chemical rings or attachments to that structure make it possible for some of these drugs to be absorbed orally, whereas others must be given parenterally. Some of these drugs cause severe toxic effects (e.g., renal toxicity), but others do not.

Key Points

- Clinical pharmacology is the study of drugs used to treat, diagnose, or prevent a disease.
- Drugs are chemicals that are introduced into the body and affect the body's chemical processes.
- Drugs can come from natural sources including plants, foods, animals, salts of inorganic compounds, or synthetic sources.

Drug Evaluation

After a chemical that might have therapeutic value is identified, it must undergo a series of scientific tests to evaluate its actual therapeutic and toxic effects. This process is tightly controlled by the U.S. **Food and Drug Administration (FDA)**, an agency of the U.S. Department of Health and Human Services that regulates the development and sale of drugs. FDA-regulated tests are designed to ensure the safety and reliability of any drug approved in this country. There are many more chemicals tested compared with the number of medications that are approved. Before receiving final FDA approval to be marketed to the public, drugs must pass through several stages of development to determine if the benefits outweigh the known and potential risks of the medication. These include preclinical trials and phase I, II, and III studies. The drugs listed in this book have been through rigorous testing and are approved for sale to the public, either with or without a prescription from a health care provider.

Preclinical Trials

In **preclinical trials**, chemicals that may have therapeutic value are tested either in vitro (outside of a living organism) or in vivo (inside or on a living organism) for two main purposes: (a) to determine whether they have the presumed effects in living tissue and (b) to evaluate any adverse effects. The trials do not include humans as participants. Preclinical trials with living organisms are important because unique biological differences can cause very different reactions to the chemical. These differences can be found only in living organisms, so computer-generated models alone are often inadequate.

At the end of the preclinical trials, some chemicals are discarded for the following reasons:

- The chemical lacks therapeutic activity when used with living organisms.
- The chemical is too toxic be worth the risk of developing into a drug.
- The chemical is highly **teratogenic** (causing adverse effects to a fetus).
- The safety margins are so small that the chemical would not be useful in the clinical setting.

Some chemicals, however, are found to have therapeutic effects and reasonable safety margins. This means that the chemicals are therapeutic at doses that are reasonably different from doses that cause toxic effects. Such chemicals will pass the preclinical trials and advance to phase I studies.

Phase I Studies

A **phase I study** uses human volunteers to test the drugs for safety and dosage information. These studies are more tightly controlled than preclinical trials and are performed by specially trained clinical investigators. The volunteers are fully informed of possible risks and may be paid for their participation. Usually, the studies would include 20 to 100 healthy volunteers or participants with the disease or condition that the medication is designed to help with. Volunteers who elect to participate in phase I studies have to be informed of the potential risks and must sign a consent form outlining the possible effects.

Some chemicals are therapeutic in other animals but have no effects in humans. Investigators in phase I studies scrutinize the drugs being tested for effects in humans. They also look for adverse effects and toxicity. At the end of phase I studies, about 70% of the drugs being tested move on to the next phase of testing. Many chemicals are dropped from the process for the following reasons:

- They cause unacceptable adverse effects.
- They are highly teratogenic.
- They are too toxic.
- They lack evidence of potential therapeutic effect in humans.

Some chemicals move to the next stage of testing despite undesirable effects. For example, the antihypertensive drug minoxidil was found to effectively treat hypertensive crisis, but it caused unusual hair growth on the palms and other body areas. However, because it was so much more effective for treating malignant hypertension at the time of its development than any other antihypertensive drug and because the undesired effects were not dangerous, it proceeded to phase II studies. (Now, its hair-growing effect has been channeled for therapeutic use into various topical hair-growth preparations such as *Rogaine*.)

Phase II Studies

A **phase II study** allows clinical investigators to evaluate the drug in more patients who have the disease that the drug is designed to treat. Patients are told about the possible benefits of the drug and are invited to participate in the study. Those who consent to participate are fully informed about possible risks and are monitored very closely, to evaluate the drug's effects. Usually, phase II studies are performed at various sites across the country—in hospitals, clinics, and doctors' offices—and are monitored by representatives of the pharmaceutical company studying the drug. At the end of phase II studies, a drug may be removed from further investigation for the following reasons:

- It is less effective than anticipated.
- It is too toxic when used with patients.
- It produces unacceptable adverse effects.
- It has a low benefit-to-risk ratio, meaning that the therapeutic benefit it provides does not outweigh the risk of potential adverse effects that it causes.
- It is no more effective than other drugs already on the market, making the cost of continued research and production less attractive to the drug company.

A drug that continues to show promise as a therapeutic agent receives additional scrutiny in phase III studies. About 33% of chemicals from phase II studies are able to move to phase III.

Phase III Studies

A **phase III study** involves use of the drug in a larger sample of the population. The purpose is to determine the treatment benefit and to monitor side effects that may not have been apparent in the earlier studies. Participants are informed of all the known reactions to the drug and precautions required for its safe use. Researchers observe patients very closely, monitoring them for any adverse effects. Often, participants are asked to keep journals and record any symptoms they experience. Researchers then evaluate the reported effects to determine whether they are caused by the disease or by the drug. Approximately 25% to 30% of the medications from phase III studies are able to move to the next phase. The medications that produce unacceptable side effects or unexpected responses will not be approved.

Food and Drug Administration Approval

Drugs that finish phase III studies are evaluated by the FDA, which relies on committees of experts familiar with the specialty area in which the drugs will be used. Only those drugs that receive FDA committee approval may be marketed. Figure 1.3 recaps the various phases of drug development discussed.

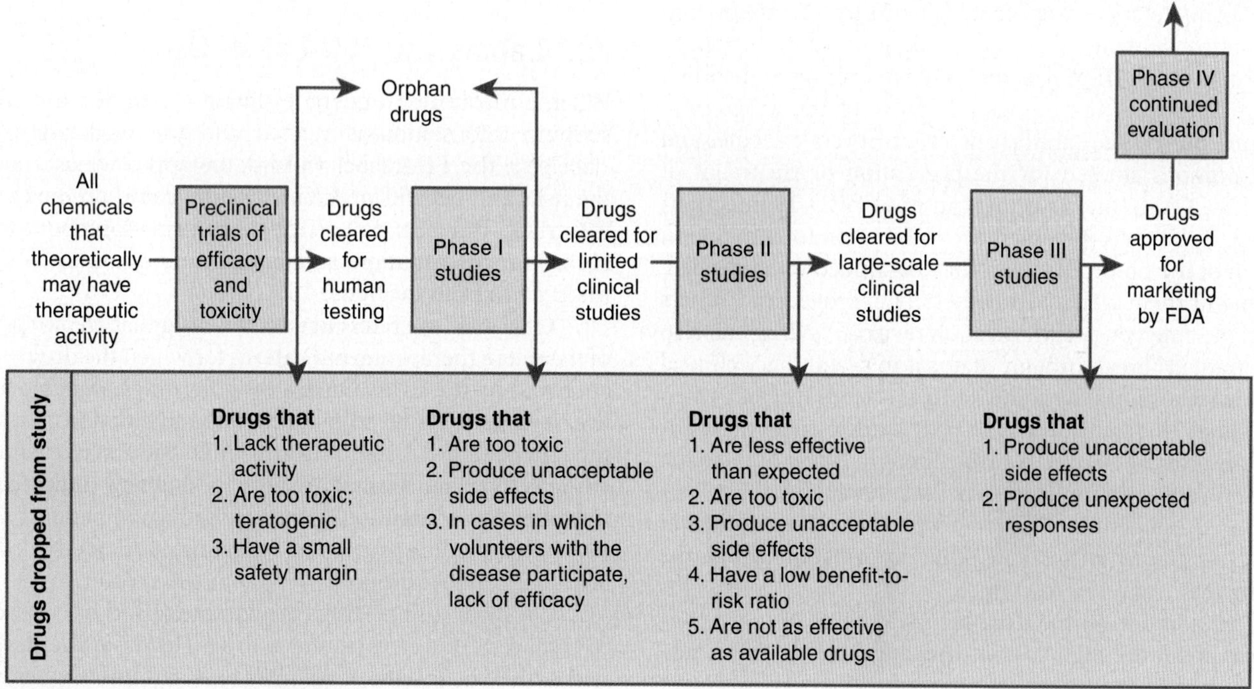

FIGURE 1.3 Phases of drug development.

Table 1.4 Comparison of Chemical, Generic, and Brand Names of Drugs

L-Thyroxine, T_4	←	Chemical name	→	Delta-9-tetrahydrocannabinol
Levothyroxine sodium	←	Generic name	→	Dronabinol
Levoxyl, Synthroid	←	Brand names	→	*Marinol*

An approved drug is given a **brand name** (trade name) by the pharmaceutical company that developed it. The **generic name** of a drug is the original designation that the drug was given when the drug company applied for the approval process. **Chemical names** are names that reflect the chemical structure of a drug. Some drugs are known by all three names. It can be confusing to study drugs when so many different names are used for the same compound. In this text, the generic and chemical names always appear in straight print, and the brand name is always capitalized and italicized (e.g., minoxidil [*Rogaine*]). Since there are times when multiple companies manufacture the medications, there can be multiple brand names for the same generic drug. Table 1.4 compares examples of drug names.

The entire drug development and approval process can take 5 to 6 years, resulting in a so-called drug lag in the United States. In some instances, a drug that is available in another country may not become available here for years. The FDA regards public safety as primary in drug approval, so the process remains strict; however, it can be accelerated in certain instances involving the treatment of deadly diseases. A drug can be "fast tracked" if it shows great promise and no other drug is available that gives those effects. For example, some drugs (e.g., delavirdine [*Rescriptor*] and efavirenz [*Sustiva*]) that were thought to offer a benefit to patients with AIDS, a potentially fatal immune disorder, were approved more quickly because of the progressive nature of AIDS and the lack of a cure. Several vaccines and medications studied for the prevention or treatment of SARS-COV-2 (the virus that causes COVID-19 infection) were authorized for emergency use prior to completion of all of the phase III trials. They continued to be studied. Some of them were eventually fully approved and others had the emergency authorization revoked. A drug can also be granted "breakthrough" status if in preliminary clinical evidence it shows the ability to treat serious diseases when no other therapy is available or it demonstrates substantial improvement over available therapy. Many of the most recent cancer therapies and enzyme therapies fall into this group. All literature associated with these drugs indicates that long-term effects and other information about the drug may not yet be known.

In addition to the drug lag issue, there also are concerns about the high cost of drug approval. A 2020 study published in the *Journal of American Medical Association (JAMA)* reported that the mean investment to bring a new medication to market was approximately $1.3 billion. Antineoplastic and immunomodulating agents generally cost even more to develop and market. Because of this kind of financial investment, pharmaceutical companies are unwilling to risk approval of a drug that might cause serious problems and prompt lawsuits.

Phase IV Studies

After a drug is approved for marketing, it enters a phase of continual evaluation, or **phase IV study**. Prescribers and all health care professionals are obligated to report to the FDA any untoward or unexpected adverse effects associated with drugs they are using, and the FDA continually evaluates this information. Some drugs cause unexpected effects that are not seen until wide distribution occurs. Sometimes, those effects are therapeutic. For example, patients taking the antiparkinsonism drug amantadine (*Symmetrel*) were found to have fewer cases of influenza than other patients, leading to the discovery that amantadine is an effective antiviral agent.

In other instances, the unexpected effects are dangerous. In 1997, the diet drug dexfenfluramine (*Redux*) was removed from the market only months after its release because patients taking it developed serious heart problems. In 2004, the drug company Merck withdrew its cyclooxygenase-2 (Cox-2)-specific nonsteroidal anti-inflammatory drug rofecoxib (*Vioxx*) from the market when postmarketing studies seemed to show a significant increase in cardiovascular mortality in patients who were taking the drug. These problems were not seen in any of the premarketing studies of the drug. The effects were only seen with a much wider use of the drug after it had been marketed.

FDA Labels and "Off-Label" Uses

When a medication undergoes Phase IV studies, the prescribing information is refined and the medication is "labeled". The FDA label will list the approved uses and the risks and benefits of the medication based on the clinical trials. The label will also have information about the absorption, distribution, metabolism, and excretion of the medication from the body.

"Off-label" use refers to uses of a drug that are not part of the stated therapeutic indications for which the drug was approved by the FDA. Once a drug becomes available for use, it may be found to be effective in a situation not on the approved list. Using it for this indication may eventually lead to an approval of the drug for that new indication. Off-label use is commonly done for groups of patients for which there is little premarketing testing, particularly pediatric and geriatric groups.

"Off-label" use of drugs is widespread and often leads to discovery of a new use for a drug. However, the nurse needs to be cognizant of off-label uses and know when to question the use of a drug before administering it. Liability issues surrounding many of these uses are unclear, and the nurse should be aware of the intended use, why the drug is being tried, and its potential for problems.

Key Points

- The FDA carefully regulates the testing and approval of all drugs in this country.
- To be approved for marketing by the FDA, a drug must pass through both preclinical and clinical trials.
- Off-label uses of drugs occur when a drug is used for an indication that is not on the FDA label.

Legal Regulation of Drugs

The FDA regulates the development and sale of drugs. Local laws further regulate the distribution and administration of drugs. In most cases, the strictest law is the one that prevails. Nurses should become familiar with the rules and regulations in the area in which they practice. These regulations can vary from state to state and even within a state.

Over the years, the FDA has become more powerful, usually in response to a drug disaster affecting many people. In the 1930s, the drug "elixir of sulfanilamide" was distributed in a vehicle of ethylene glycol that had never been tested in humans. It turned out that ethylene glycol is toxic to humans, and hundreds of people died and many others became very ill. This led to the Federal Food, Drug and Cosmetic Act of 1938, which gave the FDA power to enforce standards for testing drug toxicity and monitoring labeling.

In the 1960s, the drug thalidomide (*Thalomid*) was used as a sleeping aid during pregnancy, resulting in the birth of many babies with limb deformities. The public outcry resulted in the Kefauver-Harris Act of 1962, which gave the FDA regulatory control over the testing and evaluating of drugs and set standards for efficacy and safety.

Other laws have given the FDA control over monitoring of potentially addictive drugs, dietary supplements, and responsibility for monitoring the sale of drugs that are available without prescription. Table 1.5 provides a summary of some of these laws.

Table 1.5 Federal Legislation Affecting the Clinical Use of Drugs

Year Enacted	Law	Impact
1906	Pure Food and Drug Act	Prevented the marketing of adulterated drugs; required labeling to eliminate false or misleading claims
1938	Federal Food, Drug, and Cosmetic Act	Mandated tests for drug toxicity and provided means for recall of drugs; established procedures for introducing new drugs; gave FDA the power of enforcement
1951	Durham-Humphrey Amendment	Tightened control of certain drugs; specified drugs to be labeled "may not be distributed without a prescription"
1962	Kefauver-Harris Act	Tightened control over the quality of drugs; gave FDA regulatory power over the procedure of drug investigations; stated that efficacy as well as safety of drugs had to be established
1970	Comprehensive Drug Abuse Prevention and Control Act	Defined drug abuse and classified drugs as to their potential for abuse; provided strict controls over the distribution, storage, and use of these drugs
1983	Orphan Drug Act	Provided incentives for the development of orphan drugs for treatment of rare diseases
1988	Food and Drug Administration Act and Prescription Drug Marketing Act	FDA established at official agency of Department of Health and Human Services. Prescription drugs must go through legitimate commercial channels
1994	Dietary Supplement Health and Education Act	Established specific labeling requirements for dietary supplements and classified them as "foods"

Safety During Pregnancy

As part of the standards for testing and safety, in 1979 the FDA required that each new drug be assigned to a pregnancy category (Box 1.1). The categories indicated a drug's potential or actual teratogenic effects, thus offering guidelines for use of that particular drug in pregnancy. Research into the development of the human fetus, especially the nervous system, has led many health care providers to recommend that no drug should be used during pregnancy because of potential effects on the developing fetus. In cases in which a drug is needed, it is recommended that the drug of choice be one for which the benefit outweighs the potential risk. In 2014, the FDA established guidelines that led to categories related to the presence of the drug in human milk, indicating the possibility of effects on a baby who is fed human milk. This has been an ongoing issue, with increasing numbers of parents electing human milk feeding and no clinical studies or accurate information available for many drugs. In 2015, the FDA elected to change the pregnancy categories to risk levels (Box 1.1). As new med-

BOX 1.1

Food and Drug Administration Pregnancy Categories

The FDA established five categories to indicate the potential for a systemically absorbed drug to cause birth defects. The key differentiation among the categories rests on the degree (reliability) of documentation and the risk–benefit ratio. These labels have often been confusing, and in December 2014, the FDA passed a new rule, which phased out these categories. In their place, the prescribing information has more information under Section 8 in the prescribing information, "Use in Specific Populations." This area outlines the risk of using the drug during pregnancy and lactation with data to support the clinical information and information to help health care providers make prescribing and counseling decisions about the use of these drugs in pregnancy and lactation. The labels will also include information about how the medication affects male and female reproductive health. This change is occurring over time as new medications are approved and older medication labels are revised, and it is thought that it will provide safer use of drugs in these two groups. While the transition is occurring, the following categories will still appear and will eventually be phased out. During the transition, many will still refer to these categories, so understanding them is still important.

Category A: Adequate studies in pregnant people have not demonstrated a risk to the fetus in the first trimester of pregnancy, and there is no evidence of risk in later trimesters.

Category B: Animal studies have not demonstrated a risk to the fetus, but there are no adequate studies in pregnant people, *or* animal studies have shown an adverse effect, but adequate studies in pregnant people have not demonstrated a risk to the fetus during the first trimester of pregnancy, and there is no evidence of risk in later trimesters.

Category C: Animal studies have shown an adverse effect on the fetus, but there are no adequate studies in humans; the benefits from the use of the drug in pregnant people may be acceptable despite its potential risks, *or* there are no animal reproduction studies and no adequate studies in humans.

Category D: There is evidence of human fetal risk, but the potential benefits from the use of the drug in pregnant people may be acceptable despite its potential risks.

Category X: Studies in animals or humans demonstrate fetal abnormalities or adverse reactions; reports indicate evidence of fetal risk. The risk of use in a pregnant woman clearly outweighs any possible benefit.

Regardless of the designated pregnancy category or presumed safety, *no* drug should be administered during pregnancy unless it is clearly needed.

ications are approved and/or their prescribing labels are revised, the drugs will not have a pregnancy category listed but will have a risk level for effects on fertility, pregnancy, and when used while lactating. High risk for pregnancy would indicate that research has shown fetal toxicity. High risk for lactation would indicate that the drug is known to enter human milk and could cause problems for the infant. Low risk would indicate that research has not shown any problems thus far. The medications would also be evaluated regarding their impact on reproductive potential; some medications can change a person's reproductive potential and even cause infertility. By incorporating evidence-based data, it is thought that this will be a safer and clearer guide to the use of drugs in these special populations.

Controlled Substances

The Comprehensive Drug Abuse Prevention and Control Act of 1970 established categories for ranking the abuse potential of various drugs. This same act gave control over the coding of drugs and the enforcement of these codes to the FDA and the Drug Enforcement Agency (DEA), part of the U.S. Department of Justice. The FDA studies the drugs and determines their abuse potential; the DEA enforces their control. Drugs with abuse potential are called *controlled substances.* Box 1.2 contains descriptions of each category or schedule.

The prescription, distribution, storage, and use of controlled substance drugs are closely monitored by the DEA in an attempt to decrease substance abuse of prescribed medications. If a prescriber would like to prescribe a controlled substance, they must have a DEA number, which allows the DEA to monitor prescription patterns and possible abuse. A nurse should be familiar with not only the DEA guidelines for controlled substances but also the local policies and procedures, which might be even more rigorous.

Generic Drugs

When a drug receives approval for marketing from the FDA, the drug formula is given a time-limited patent, in much the same way as an invention is patented. The length of time for which the patent is good depends on the type of chemical involved. When the patent runs out on a brand name drug, the drug can be produced by other manufacturers. **Generic drugs** are chemicals that are produced by companies involved solely in the manufacturing of drugs. The FDA monitors the development of generic medications. The generic medication is compared with the brand name medication and must have the same strength of the active ingredient, use the same dosage form (tablet, capsule, or liquid), the same route of administration (oral, topical, or injectable), contain safe inactive ingredients, and safe packaging/storage. Generic medications are bioequivalent to brand name medications; in other words, they work in the body the same way, and the substances should have the same amount of active ingredient. Due to the margins of error allowed and the fact that inactive ingredients are not required to be the same, a generic medication can affect some people differently than the brand name. However, for most people, generic medications are safe, effective, cost-effective alternatives to brand name medications.

BOX 1.2

Drug Enforcement Agency Schedules of Controlled Substances

The Comprehensive Drug Abuse Prevention and Control Act of 1970 regulates the manufacturing, distribution, and dispensing of drugs that are known to have abuse potential. The DEA is responsible for the enforcement of these regulations. The controlled drugs are divided into five DEA schedules based on their potential for abuse and physical and psychological dependence:

Schedule I *(C-I):* High abuse potential and no accepted medical use (heroin, LSD)

Schedule II *(C-II):* High abuse potential with severe dependence liability (narcotics, amphetamines, and barbiturates)

Schedule III *(C-III):* Less abuse potential than schedule II drugs and moderate dependence liability (nonbarbiturate sedatives, nonamphetamine stimulants, limited amounts of certain narcotics)

Schedule IV *(C-IV):* Less abuse potential than schedule III and limited dependence liability (some sedatives, antianxiety agents, and nonnarcotic analgesics)

Schedule V *(C-V):* Limited abuse potential. Primarily small amounts of narcotics (codeine) used as antitussives or antidiarrheals. Under federal law, limited quantities of certain schedule V drugs may be purchased without a prescription directly from a pharmacist. The purchaser must be at least 18 years of age and must furnish suitable identification. All such transactions must be recorded by the dispensing pharmacist.

Prescribing physicians and dispensing pharmacists must be registered with the DEA, which also provides forms for the transfer of schedule I and II substances and establishes criteria for the inventory and prescribing of controlled substances. State and local laws are often more stringent than federal law. In any given situation, the more stringent law applies.

Many states require that a drug be dispensed in the generic form if one is available. This requirement helps to keep down the cost of drugs and health care. Some prescribers, however, specify that a drug prescription be "dispensed as written" (DAW) (i.e., that the brand name product be used). By doing so, the prescriber ensures the quality control and the action and effect expected with that drug. These elements may be most important in drugs that have narrow safety margins, such as digoxin (*Lanoxin*), a heart drug, and warfarin (*Coumadin*), an anticoagulant. The initial cost may be higher, because some insurance companies will not pay for these brand name drugs when the generic is available, but some prescribers believe that, in the long run, the cost to the patient will be less.

Concept Mastery Alert

Generic Drugs

Generic medications are bioequivalent to brand name drugs and are equally safe, more cost-effective, and have identical therapeutic uses when compared to the brand name medications.

Orphan Drugs

Orphan drugs are drugs that have been discovered but are not financially viable and, therefore, have not been "adopted" by any drug company. Orphan drugs may be useful in treating a rare disease, or they may have potentially dangerous adverse effects. Orphan drugs are often abandoned after preclinical trials or phase I studies. The Orphan Drug Act of 1983 provided tremendous financial incentives to drug companies to adopt these drugs and develop them. These incentives help the drug company put the drug through the rest of the testing process, even though the market for the drug in the long run may be very small (as in the case of a drug to treat a rare neurological disease that affects only a small number of people). Some drugs in this book have orphan drug uses listed.

Over-the-Counter Drugs

Over-the-counter (OTC) drugs are products that are available without prescription for self-treatment of a variety of complaints. Some of these agents were approved as prescription drugs but later were found to be very safe and useful for patients without the need of a prescription. Some were not rigorously screened and tested by the current drug evaluation protocols because they were developed and marketed before the current laws were put into effect. Many of these drugs were "grandfathered" into use because they had been used for so long. The FDA is currently testing the effectiveness of many of these products and, in time, will evaluate all of them. Although OTC drugs have been found to be safe when taken as directed, nurses should consider several problems related to OTC drug use:

- Taking these drugs could mask the signs and symptoms of underlying disease, making diagnosis difficult.
- Taking these drugs with prescription medications could result in drug interactions and interfere with drug therapy.
- Inactive ingredients (dyes, alcohol, or preservatives) can cause adverse reactions.
- Not taking these drugs as directed could result in serious overdoses.

Many patients do not consider OTC drugs to be medications and, therefore, do not report their use. Nurses must always include specific questions about OTC drug use when taking a drug history and should provide information in all drug teaching protocols about avoiding OTC use while taking prescription drugs or checking with the health care provider first if the patient feels a need for one of these drugs.

Behind-the-Counter Drugs

Behind-the-counter (BTC) drugs do not require a prescription, but have more restrictions than OTC medications. BTC medications must be kept in a secure location in the store (such as in a locked cabinet or within the pharmacy). Customers may buy the medications without a prescription, but there are limits to the quantities that an individual may purchase in a certain day or month. Sales are tracked by the retail agent.

In some states, pseudoephedrine is a BTC medication. Pseudoephedrine is an ingredient in some products for decreasing nasal or sinus congestion. It was designated for BTC status because it can also be used illegally to make methamphetamine. However, there are other states that require a prescription for these same products.

Key Points

- Legal regulation of medications has evolved and become more specific since the early 1900s. The FDA is the agency that regulates approval and distribution of medication in the United States.
- There are additional regulations of medications that are deemed "controlled substances," and enforcement of the regulations is monitored by the Drug Enforcement Agency (DEA).
- When brand name medications are no longer protected by a patent, companies can make generic drugs under the supervision of the FDA.
- OTC drugs are available without a prescription and are deemed safe when used as directed.
- Orphan drugs are drugs that have been discovered but that are not financially viable because they have a limited market or a narrow margin of safety. These drugs may have then been adopted for development by a drug company in exchange for tax incentives.

Sources of Drug Information

The fields of pharmacology and drug therapy change so quickly that it is important to have access to sources of information about drug doses, therapeutic and adverse effects, and nursing-related implications. Textbooks provide valuable background and basic information to help in the understanding of pharmacology, but in clinical practice, it is important to have access to up-to-the-minute information. Several sources of drug information are readily available. Nurses often need to consult more than one source. Nurses work with clinicians like pharmacists, nurse practitioners, physician assistants and physicians who often are able to provide valuable information. The following are descriptions of sources of information.

Drug Labels

Drug labels have specific information that identifies a specific drug. For example, a drug label identifies the brand and generic names for the drug, the drug dosage, the expiration date, and special drug warnings. Some labels also indicate the route and dose for administration. Figure 1.4 illustrates an example of a drug label.

Understanding how to read a drug label is essential. Nurses need to become familiar with each aspect of the label.

Package Inserts

All drugs come with a package insert prepared by the manufacturer according to strict FDA regulations. The package insert, or full prescribing information, contains all of the chemical and study information that led to the drug's approval. Package inserts sometimes are difficult to understand and are almost always in very small print, making them difficult to read; however, they are also one of the most accurate sources since they are continually updated. In 2006, the FDA revised the format for all the required package insert information to make it more readily useable. New and revised package inserts contain a highlights section at the beginning of the insert that highlights the most essential information for the health care provider. The FDA website is periodically revised to make it more user friendly, so information is much easier to access. The FDA website, www.fda.gov, is a good resource for finding the full prescribing information for most drugs.

Reference Books

A wide variety of reference books are available for drug information. The *Physician's Desk Reference* (*PDR*) is a compilation of the package insert information from drugs used in the United States, along with some drug advertising. Because this information comes directly from the manufacturers and is not refereed in any way, it may not be the best source for obtaining accurate information about a drug. This information is heavily cross-referenced. The book may be difficult to use.

Drug Facts and Comparisons provides a wide range of drug information, including comparisons of drug costs, patient information sections, and preparation and administration guidelines. This book is organized by drug class and can be more user friendly than the *PDR*. However, it is cumbersome and very expensive.

AMA Drug Evaluations contains detailed monographs in an unbiased format and includes many new drugs and drugs still in the research stage.

Nursing Drug Handbook has drug monographs organized alphabetically and includes nursing implications and patient teaching points.

Numerous other drug handbooks are also on the market and readily available for nurses to use.

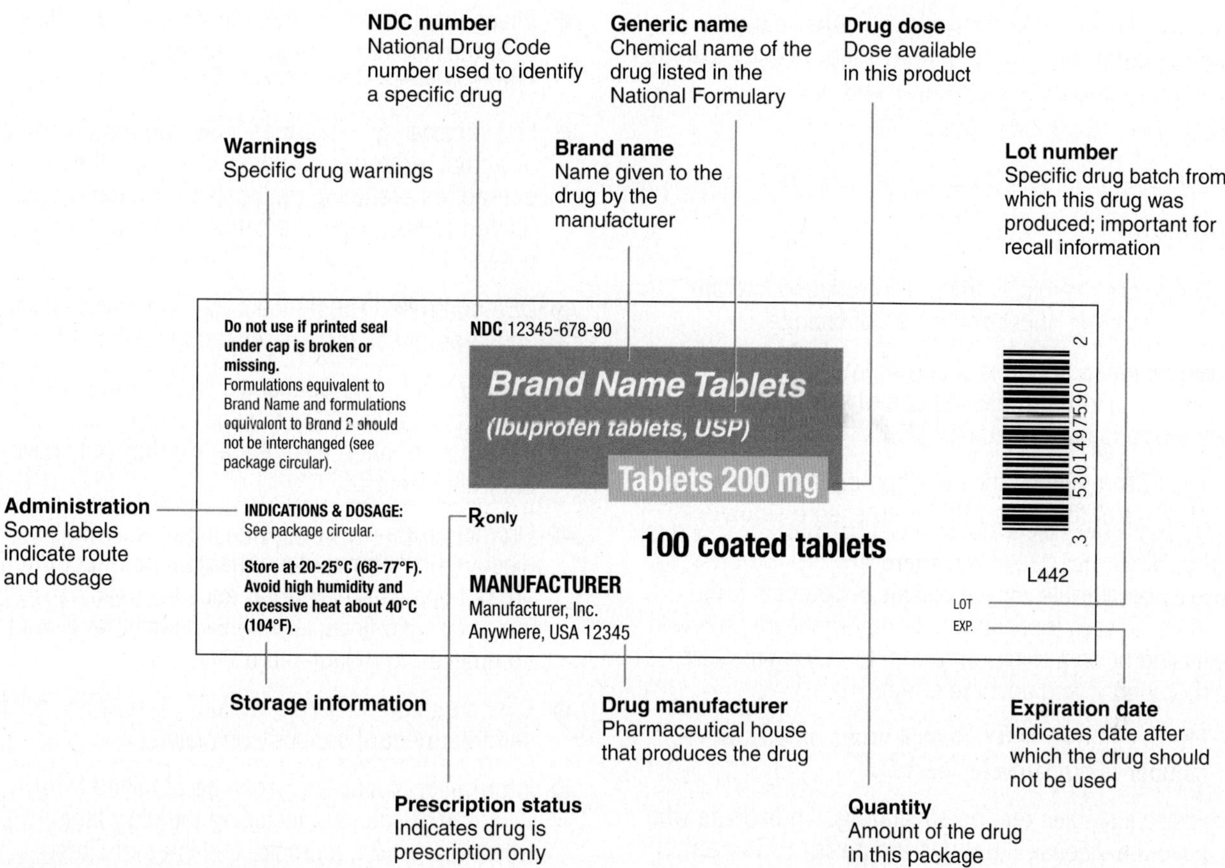

FIGURE 1.4 A sample drug label.

Journals

Various journals can be used to obtain drug information. For example, the *Medical Letter* is a monthly review of new drugs, drug classes, and specific treatment protocols. The *American Journal of Nursing* offers information on new drugs, drug errors, and nursing implications.

Internet Information

Many patients now use the internet as a source of medical information and advice. Box 1.3 lists some informative internet sites for obtaining drug information, patient information, or therapeutic information related to specific disease states. Nurses need to become familiar with

BOX 1.3

Sources of Internet Information

Evaluate sites with drug information on the internet

Government Sites

Agency for Health Care Research and Quality: https://www.ahrq.gov/
CancerNet (National Cancer Institute): http://www.cancer.gov
Centers for Disease Control and Prevention: http://www.cdc.gov
Food and Drug Administration: http://www.fda.gov
Healthfinder: http://www.healthfinder.gov
National Center for Complementary and Integrative Health: https://nccih.nih.gov/
National Institutes of Health: http://www.nih.gov
National Institute for Occupational Safety and Health: http://www.cdc.gov/niosh
National Library of Medicine: http://www.nlm.nih.gov
Office of Disease Prevention and Health Promotion: https://health.gov/

Nursing and Health Care Sites

American Diabetes Association: http://www.diabetes.org
American Nurses Association: https://www.nursingworld.org/
Cumulative Index to Nursing and Allied Health Literature: http://www.cinahl.com
International Council of Nurses: http://www.icn.ch
Joint Commission on Accreditation of Healthcare Organizations: https://www.jointcommission.org/
Journal of American Medical Association: https://jamanetwork.com/journals/jama
Lippincott's Nursing Center: http://www.nursingcenter.com
MayoClinic: https://www.mayoclinic.org/
Medscape: http://www.medscape.com
Merck & Co. (search the Merck Manual): https://www.merckmanuals.com/professional
New England Journal of Medicine: http://www.nejm.org
RxList: http://www.rxlist.com

what is available on the internet and what patients may be referencing. Educating patients about safe use of internet sites can be a very important aspect of patient care.

SUMMARY

- Drugs are chemicals that are introduced into the body to bring about some sort of change.
- Drugs can come from many sources: plants, animals, inorganic elements, and synthetic preparations.
- The FDA regulates the development and marketing of drugs in the United States to ensure safety and efficacy.
- Preclinical trials involve testing of potential drugs either in vitro (outside of a living organism) or in vivo (inside or on a living organism) to determine their therapeutic and adverse effects.
- Phase I studies test potential drugs on a small number of human volunteers.
- Phase II studies test potential drugs on patients who have the disease the drugs are designed to treat.
- Phase III studies test drugs in the clinical setting to determine any unanticipated effects or lack of effectiveness.
- FDA pregnancy categories indicated the potential or actual teratogenic effects of a drug; these categories are being replaced by risk categories related to pregnancy, lactation, and reproductive potential.
- DEA controlled substance categories indicate the abuse potential and associated regulation of a drug.
- Generic drugs are sold under their generic names, not brand names; they may be cheaper and are usually safe, but for some people they may have different effects.
- Orphan drugs are chemicals that have been discovered to have some therapeutic effect but that are not financially advantageous for development into drugs, so financial incentives may be given to companies to manufacture them.
- OTC drugs are available without prescription for the self-treatment of various complaints.
- Information about drugs can be obtained from a variety of sources, including the drug label, reference books, journals, and internet sites.

Unfolding Patient Stories: Danielle Young Bear • Part 1

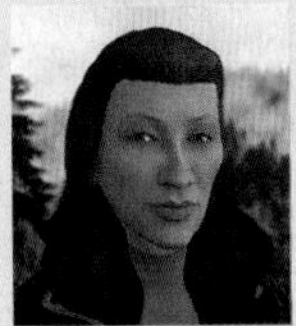

Danielle Young Bear is a 32-year-old construction worker who made a clinic appointment because she is experiencing a persistent cough and fatigue. She has a history of chronic lower back pain, and she visited the clinic 1 year ago with spasms caused by an injury. Danielle has followed guidance from a traditional Native American healer using herbal medicine. During that visit, she was given a prescription for pain medicine. Upon review of her current medications, you find that Danielle takes cyclobenzaprine, ibuprofen, and willow bark. While the nurse is providing education on the medications, the patient states that she is pregnant. What drug exposure risks during pregnancy should the nurse consider? (Danielle Young Bear's story continues in Chap. 16.)

Care for Danielle and other patients in a realistic virtual environment: ***vSim** for Nursing* (thepoint.lww.com/vSimPharm). Practice documenting these patients' care in DocuCare (thepoint.lww.com/DocuCareEHR).

CHECK YOUR UNDERSTANDING

Answers to the questions in this chapter can be found in Answers to Check Your Understanding Questions on thePoint®.

MULTIPLE CHOICE

Select the best answer.

1. Clinical pharmacology is the study of
   a. the biological effects of chemicals.
   b. drugs used to treat, prevent, or diagnose disease
   c. plant components that can be used as medicines.
   d. binders and other vehicles for delivering medication.

2. Phase I drug studies involve
   a. testing chemicals either in vitro or in vivo.
   b. patients with the disease the drug is designed to treat.
   c. mass marketing surveys of drug effects in large numbers of people.
   d. healthy human volunteers who are often paid for their participation.

3. The generic name of a drug is
   a. the name assigned to the drug by the pharmaceutical company developing it.
   b. the chemical name of the drug based on its chemical structure.
   c. the original name assigned to the drug at the beginning of the evaluation process.
   d. the name that is often used in advertising campaigns.

4. An orphan drug is a drug that
   a. has failed to go through the approval process.
   b. is available in a foreign country but not in this country.
   c. has been tested but is not considered to be financially viable without financial incentives.
   d. is available without a prescription.

5. The FDA pregnancy categories were used
   a. to indicate a drug's potential or actual teratogenic effects.
   b. for research purposes only.
   c. to list drugs that are more likely to have addicting properties.
   d. to follow regulations set by the DEA.

6. The storing, prescribing, and distributing of controlled substances—drugs that are more apt to be addictive—are monitored by
   a. the Food and Drug Administration.
   b. the Department of Commerce.
   c. the Federal Bureau of Investigation.
   d. the Drug Enforcement Agency.

7. Which of the following are not regulated by the FDA?
   a. over-the-counter medications.
   b. prescription medications from Canada.
   c. dietary supplements.
   d. none of the above.

8. A patient has been taking fluoxetine (*Prozac*) for several years, but when picking up the prescription this month found that the tablets looked different and became concerned. The nurse, checking with the pharmacist, found that fluoxetine had just become available in the generic form and the prescription had been filled with the generic product. The nurse should tell the patient
   a. that for most people the generic form will work similarly to the brand name medication.
   b. that generic drugs are available without a prescription and they are just as safe as the brand name medication.
   c. that the law requires that prescriptions be filled with the generic form if available to cut down the cost of medications unless a prescriber writes the insurance company.
   d. that the pharmacist filled the prescription with the wrong drug and it should be returned to the pharmacy for a refund.

MULTIPLE RESPONSE

Select all that apply.

1. When teaching a patient about OTC drugs, which points should the nurse include?
   a. These drugs are very safe and can be used freely to relieve your complaints.
   b. These compounds are called drugs, but they aren't really drugs.
   c. Many of these drugs were once prescription drugs but are now thought to be safe for use without a prescription when used as directed.
   d. Reading the label of these drugs is very important; the name of the active ingredient is prominent; you should always check the ingredient name.
   e. It is important to read the label and to see what the recommended dose of the drug is; some of these drugs can cause serious problems if too much of the drug is taken.
   f. It is important to report the use of any OTC drug to your health care provider because many of them can interact with drugs that might be prescribed for you.

2. A patient asks what generic drugs are and if they should be using them to treat his infection. Which of the following statements should be included in the nurse's explanation?
   a. A generic drug is a drug that is sold by the name of the ingredient, not the brand name.
   b. Generic drugs are always the best drugs to use because they are never any different from the familiar brand names.
   c. Generic drugs are not available until the patent expires on a specific drug.
   d. Generic drugs are usually cheaper than the well-known brand names, and some insurance companies require that you receive the generic drug if one is available.
   e. Generic drugs are forms of a drug that are available over the counter and do not require a prescription.
   f. Your physician may want you to have the brand name of a drug, not the generic form, and DAW will be on your prescription form.
   g. Generic drugs are less likely to cause adverse effects than brand name drugs.

REFERENCES

Barton, J. H., & Emanuel, E. J. (2005). The patient-based pharmaceutical development process: Rationale, problems and potential reforms. *Journal of the American Medical Association, 294*, 2075–2082. http://doi:10.1001/jama.294.16.2075

Brunton, L., Hilal-Dandan, R., & Knollman, B. (2018). *Goodman & Gilman's the pharmacological basis of therapeutics* (13th ed.). McGraw-Hill.

Centers for Disease Control and Prevention. (2017). V*ital signs: Changes in opioid prescribing in the US: 2001–2015*. https://www.cdc.gov/mmwr/volumes/66/wr/mm6626a4.htm

Creigle, V. (2007). MedWatch: The FDA safety information and adverse event reporting program. *Journal of the Medical Library Association, 95*(2), 224–225. http://doi:10.3163/1536-5050.95.2.224

Ebadi, M. (2007). *Pharmacodynamic basis of herbal medications* (2nd ed.). CRC Press.

Koo, M. M., Krass, I., & Aslani, P. (2003). Factors influencing consumer use of written drug information. *Annals of Pharmacotherapy, 37*(2), 259–267. https://doi.10.1345/aph.1C328

Sontia, B., Mooney, J., Gaudet, L., & Touyz, R.M. (2008). Pseudohyperaldosteronism, liquorice, and hypertension. *The journal of clinical hypertension, 10* (2), 153-157. https://doi.org/10.1111/j.1751-7176.2008.07470.x

Sun, S. X., Lee, K. Y., Bertram, C. T., & Goldstein, J. L. (2007). Withdrawal of COX-2 selective inhibitors rofecoxib and valdecoxib: Impact on NSAID and gastroprotective drug prescribing and utilization. *Current Medical Research and Opinion, 23*(8), 1859–1866. https://doi.org 10.1185/030079907X210561

US Food and Drug Administration. (2017a). *Overview and basics*. https://www.fda.gov/drugs/generic-drugs/overview-basics

US Food and Drug Administration. (2017b). *Legal requirements for the sale and purchase of drug products containing pseudoephedrine, ephedrine, and phenylpropanolamine*. https://www.fda.gov/drugs/information-drug-class/legal-requirements-sale-and-purchase-drug-products-containing-pseudoephedrine-ephedrine-and

US Food and Drug Administration. (2018a). *The drug development process*. https://www.fda.gov/patients/learn-about-drug-and-device-approvals/drug-development-process

US Food and Drug Administration. (2018b). *Milestones in U.S. food and drug law history*. https://www.fda.gov/about-fda/fdas-evolving-regulatory-powers/milestones-us-food-and-drug-law-history

US Food and Drug Administration. (2019). *Development and approval process: Drugs*. https://www.fda.gov/drugs/development-approval-process-drugs#Developing

Wouters, O. J., McKee, M., & Luyten, J. (2020). Estimated research and development investment needed to bring a new medicine to market, 2009–2018. *JAMA, 323*(9), 844–853. https://doi:10.1001/jama.2020.1166

CHAPTER 2

Drugs and the Body

Learning Objectives

Upon completion of this chapter, you will be able to:

1. Describe how body cells respond to the presence of drugs that are capable of altering their function.
2. Outline the process of dynamic equilibrium that determines the actual concentration of a drug in the body.
3. Explain the meaning of half-life of a drug and calculate the half-life of given drugs.
4. List at least six factors that can influence the actual effectiveness of drugs in the body.
5. Define drug–drug, drug–alternative therapy, drug–food, and drug–laboratory test interactions.

Key Terms

absorption: what happens to a drug from the time it enters the body until it enters the circulating fluid

active transport: the movement of substances across a cell membrane; this process requires the use of energy

chemotherapeutic agents: synthetic chemicals used to interfere with the functioning of foreign cell populations, causing cell death; this term is frequently used to refer to the drug therapy of neoplasms, but it also refers to drug therapy affecting any foreign cell

critical concentration: the concentration a drug must reach in the tissues that respond to the particular drug to cause the desired therapeutic effect

distribution: movement of a drug to body tissues; the places where a drug may be distributed depend on the drug's solubility, perfusion of the area, cardiac output, and binding of the drug to plasma proteins

enzyme induction: process by which the presence of a chemical causes increased activity of an enzyme system

excretion: removal of a drug from the body; routes include the kidneys, skin, lungs, bile, and feces

first-pass effect: a phenomenon in which drugs given orally are carried directly to the liver after absorption, where they may be largely inactivated by liver enzymes before they can enter the general circulation

glomerular filtration: the passage of water and water-soluble components from the plasma into the renal tubule

half-life: the time it takes for the amount of drug in the body to decrease to one half of the peak level it achieved

hepatic microsomal system: liver enzymes tightly packed together in the hepatic intracellular structure, responsible for the biotransformation of chemicals, including drugs

loading dose: a dose higher than what is usually used for treatment, administered to allow the drug to reach the critical concentration sooner

passive diffusion: movement of substances across a semipermeable membrane with the concentration gradient; this process does not require energy

pharmacodynamics: the study of the interactions between the chemical components of living systems and the foreign chemicals, including drugs, that enter living organisms; the way a drug affects a body

pharmacogenomics: the study of genetically determined variations in the response to drugs

pharmacokinetics: the way a medication travels through the body, including absorption, distribution, biotransformation, and excretion; how the body acts on a drug

placebo effect: documented effect of the mind on drug therapy; if a person perceives that a drug will be effective, the drug is much more likely to actually be effective

receptor sites: specific areas on cell membranes that react with certain chemicals to cause an effect within the cell

selective toxicity: property of a chemotherapeutic agent that affects only systems found in foreign cells without affecting healthy human cells (e.g., specific antibiotics can affect certain proteins or enzyme systems used by bacteria but not those used by human cells)

therapeutic index: ratio comparing the blood concentration at which a drug becomes toxic with the concentration at which the drug is effective

To understand what happens when a drug is administered, the nurse must understand pharmacodynamics—how the drug affects the body—and pharmacokinetics—how the body acts on the drug. These processes form the basis for the guidelines that have been established regarding drug administration—for example, determining why certain agents are given intramuscularly (IM) and not intravenously (IV), why some drugs are taken with food and others are not, and the standard dose that should be used to achieve the desired effect. Knowing the basic principles of pharmacodynamics and pharmacokinetics helps the nurse to anticipate therapeutic and adverse drug effects and to intervene in ways that ensure the most effective drug regimen for the patient.

Pharmacodynamics

Pharmacodynamics is the study of the interactions between the chemical components of living systems and the foreign chemicals, including drugs, that enter those systems. All living organisms function by a series of complicated, continuous chemical reactions.

When a new chemical enters the system, multiple changes to and interferences with cell functioning may occur. To avoid problematic changes, drug development works to provide the most effective and least toxic chemicals for therapeutic use.

Drugs usually work in one of four ways:

1. To replace or act as substitutes for missing chemicals
2. To increase or stimulate certain cellular activities
3. To depress or slow cellular activities
4. To interfere with the functioning of foreign cells, such as invading microorganisms or neoplasms that cause cell death (drugs that act in this way are called **chemotherapeutic agents**)

Drugs can act in several different ways to achieve these results.

Receptor Sites

Many drugs are thought to act at **receptor sites**, specific areas on cell membranes that react with certain chemicals to cause an effect within the cell. In many situations, nearby enzymes break down the reacting chemicals and open the receptor site for further stimulation.

To better understand this process, think of how a key works in a lock. The specific chemical (the key) approaches a cell membrane and finds a perfect fit (the lock) at a receptor site (see Fig. 2.1). The interaction between the chemical and the receptor site affects enzyme systems within the cell. The activated enzyme systems then produce certain effects, such as increased or decreased cellular activity, changes in cell membrane permeability, or alterations in cellular metabolism.

Some drugs interact directly with receptor sites to cause the same activity that natural chemicals would cause at that site. These drugs are called *agonists* (Fig. 2.1A). For example, insulin reacts with specific insulin-receptor sites to change cell membrane permeability, thus promoting the movement of glucose into the cell.

Other drugs act to prevent the breakdown of natural chemicals that are stimulating the receptor site. For example, monoamine oxidase (MAO) inhibitors block the breakdown of norepinephrine by the enzyme MAO. (Normally, MAO breaks down norepinephrine, removes it from the receptor site, and recycles the components to form new norepinephrine.) The blocking action of MAO inhibitors allows norepinephrine to stay on the receptor site, stimulating the cell longer and leading to prolonged norepinephrine effects. Those effects can be therapeutic (e.g., relieving depression) or adverse (e.g., increasing heart rate and blood pressure). Selective serotonin reuptake inhibitors work similarly to MAO inhibitors in that they also exert a blocking action. Specifically, they block removal of serotonin from the nerve synapse, allowing it to remain in the synapse longer, leading to further stimulation of receptor sites. This action leads to prolonged stimulation of certain brain cells, which is thought to provide relief from depression.

Some drugs react with receptor sites to block normal stimulation and, therefore, prevent the effect of that stimulation. For example, curare (a drug used on the tips of spears by inhabitants of the Amazon basin to paralyze prey and cause death) occupies receptor sites for acetylcholine, which is necessary for muscle contraction and movement. By blocking the action of acetylcholine at this receptor site, curare prevents muscle stimulation, causing paralysis. Curare is said to be a *competitive antagonist* of acetylcholine (Fig. 2.1B).

Still other drugs react with specific receptor sites on a cell and, by reacting there, prevent the reaction of another chemical with a different receptor site on that cell. Such drugs are called *noncompetitive antagonists* (Fig. 2.1C). For some drugs, the actual mechanisms of action are unknown. Speculation exists, however, that many drugs use receptor site mechanisms to bring about their effects.

Another category is *partial agonists.* These substances act both as agonists and antagonists. The action of a partial agonist is dependent on the specific receptor site at which it reacts. For example, nalbuphine is an agonist at kappa opioid receptors and an antagonist at mu opioid receptors. This allows for the medication to work at an analgesic with less potential for causing respiratory depression.

Drug–Enzyme Interactions

Drugs also can cause their effects by interfering with the enzyme systems that act as catalysts for various chemical reactions. Enzyme systems work in a cascade fashion, with one enzyme activating another, and then that enzyme activating another, until a cellular reaction eventually occurs. If a single step in an enzyme system is blocked, normal

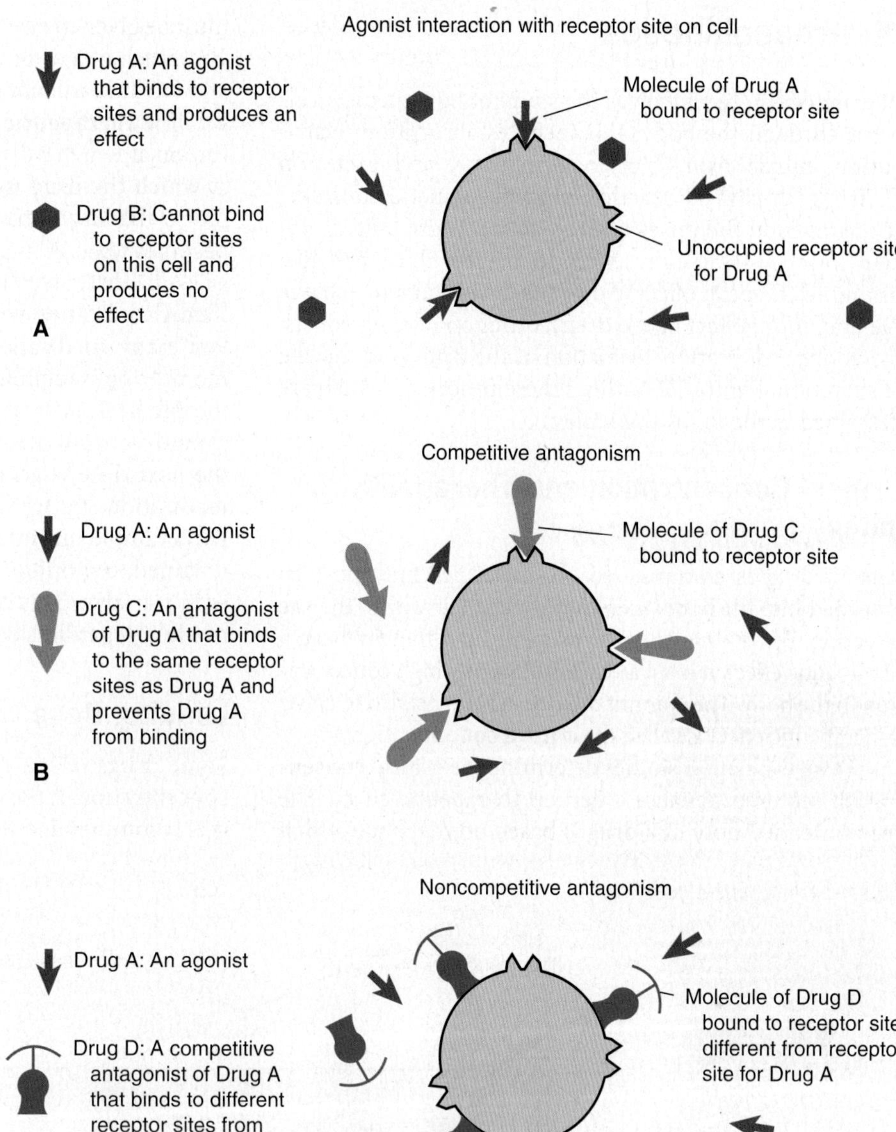
Agonist interaction with receptor site on cell
Drug A: An agonist that binds to receptor sites and produces an effect
Drug B: Cannot bind to receptor sites on this cell and produces no effect
Molecule of Drug A bound to receptor site
Unoccupied receptor site for Drug A
A
Competitive antagonism
Drug A: An agonist
Drug C: An antagonist of Drug A that binds to the same receptor sites as Drug A and prevents Drug A from binding
Molecule of Drug C bound to receptor site
B
Noncompetitive antagonism
Drug A: An agonist
Drug D: A competitive antagonist of Drug A that binds to different receptor sites from Drug A but still prevents Drug A from binding
Molecule of Drug D bound to receptor site different from receptor site for Drug A
C

FIGURE 2.1 Receptor theory of drug action. **A.** Agonist interaction with receptor site on cell. Molecules of drug A react with specific receptor sites on cells of effector organs and change the cells' activity. **B.** Competitive antagonism. Drug A and drug C have an affinity for the same receptor sites and compete for these sites; drug C has a greater affinity, occupies more of the sites, and antagonizes drug A. **C.** Noncompetitive antagonism. Drug D reacts with a receptor site that is different from the receptor site for drug A but still somehow prevents drug A from binding with its receptor sites. Drugs that act by inhibiting enzymes can be pictured as acting similarly to the receptor site antagonists illustrated in panels (**B**) and (**C**). Enzyme inhibitors block the binding of molecules of normal substrate to active sites on the enzyme.

cell function is disrupted. Acetazolamide (*Diamox*) is a diuretic that blocks the enzyme carbonic anhydrase, which subsequently causes alterations in the hydrogen ion and water exchange system in the kidney, as well as in the eye.

Selective Toxicity

Ideally, all chemotherapeutic agents would act only on enzyme systems that are essential for the life of a pathogen or neoplastic cell and would not affect healthy cells. The ability of a drug to attack only those systems found in foreign cells is known as **selective toxicity**. Penicillin, an antibiotic used to treat bacterial infections, has selective toxicity. It affects an enzyme system unique to bacteria, causing bacterial cell death without disrupting normal human cell functioning.

Unfortunately, most cancer chemotherapeutic agents also destroy normal human cells, causing many of the adverse effects associated with antipathogen and antineoplastic chemotherapy. Cells that reproduce or are replaced rapidly (e.g., bone marrow cells, gastrointestinal [GI] cells, hair follicles) are more easily affected by these agents. Consequently, the goal of many chemotherapeutic regimens is to deliver a dose that will be toxic to the invading cells yet cause the least amount of toxicity to the host.

Key Points

- Pharmacodynamics is the process by which a drug works within or affects the body.
- Drugs may work by replacing a missing body chemical, by stimulating or depressing cellular activity, or by interfering with the functioning of foreign cells.
- Drugs are thought to work by reacting with specific receptor sites or by interfering with enzyme systems in the body.

Pharmacokinetics

Pharmacokinetics involves the study of how medications travel through the body; this includes absorption, distribution, metabolism (biotransformation), and excretion of drugs. In clinical practice, pharmacokinetic considerations include the onset of drug action (how long it will take for the therapeutic effect to begin), drug half-life, timing of the peak effect (how long it will take to achieve the maximum effect of the drug), duration of drug effects, metabolism or biotransformation of the drug, and the site of excretion. Figure 2.2 outlines these processes, which are described in the following sections.

Critical Concentration and Therapeutic Index

After a drug is administered, its molecules first must be absorbed into the body; then they make their way to the site of action. For a drug to work properly, and thereby have a therapeutic effect, it must attain a sufficiently high concentration in the body. The amount of a drug that is needed to cause a therapeutic effect is called the **critical concentration.**

Drug evaluation studies determine the critical concentration required to cause a desired therapeutic effect. The recommended dose of a drug is based on the amount that must be given to eventually reach the critical concentration. Too much of a drug will produce toxic (poisonous) effects, and too little will not produce the desired therapeutic effect.

The **therapeutic index** is a ratio of the blood concentration at which a drug becomes toxic to the concentration at which the drug is effective. The higher the therapeutic index, the larger the safety margin before the medication becomes toxic. A medication with a high therapeutic index is less likely to need medication concentration monitoring than a medication with a low or narrow therapeutic index. For many medications, when medication concentration monitoring is required, a peak level should be drawn when the medication is at the highest level and a trough level should be drawn at its lowest level (usually right before the next dose is administered). However, there are some medications for which random monitoring is appropriate. For example, an international normalized ratio (INR) is obtained to monitor if a person is anticoagulated properly with warfarin. This can be drawn any time during the day or night regardless of when the person took the last dose.

Loading Dose

Some drugs take a prolonged period to reach the critical concentration. If the effect of such a drug is needed quickly, it is recommended to use a **loading dose.** This is a higher

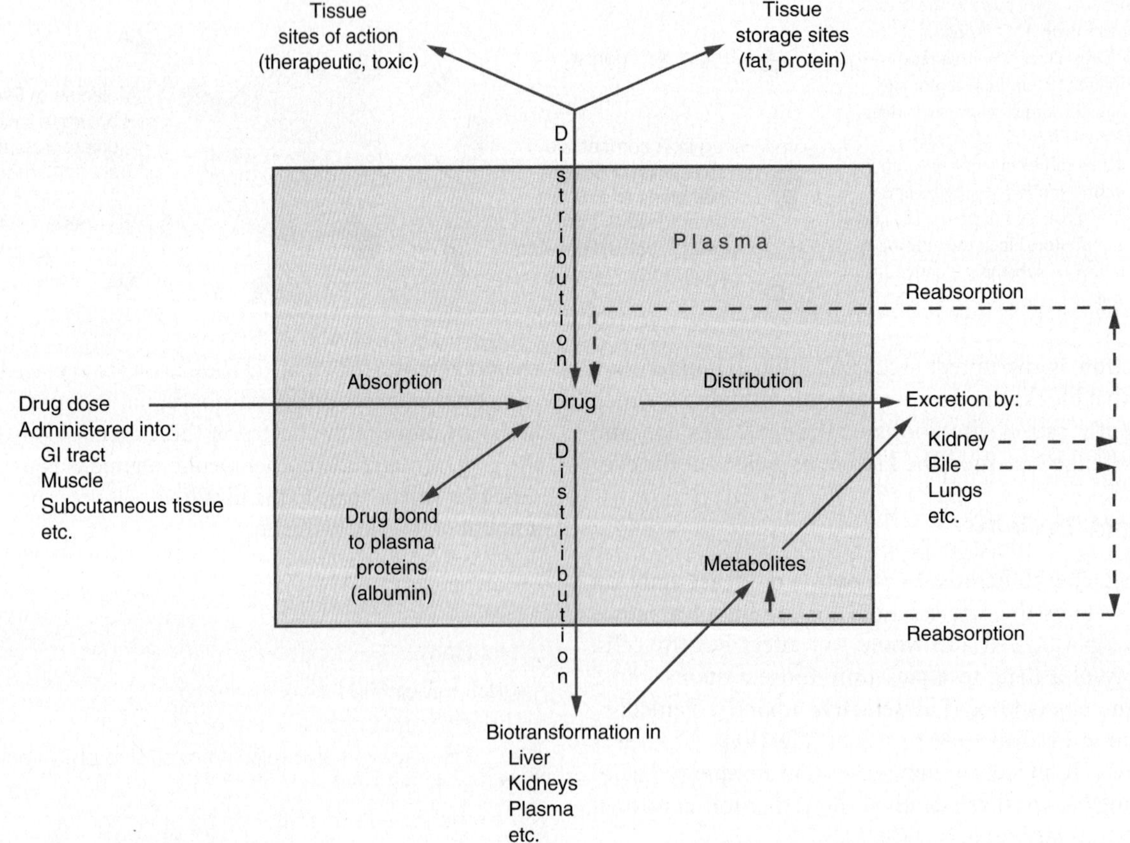

FIGURE 2.2 The processes by which a drug is handled by the body. *Dashed lines* indicate that some portion of a drug and its metabolites may be reabsorbed from the excretory organs. The dynamic equilibrium of pharmacokinetics is shown.

dose than is usually used for treatment, allowing the drug to reach the critical concentration sooner. Digoxin (*Lanoxin*), a drug used to increase the strength of heart contractions, and vancomycin, a broad-spectrum antibiotic that treats gram positive pathogens, are often started with a loading dose. The critical concentration is then maintained by using the recommended dosing schedule.

Dynamic Equilibrium

The actual concentration that a drug reaches in the body results from a dynamic equilibrium involving the rate of several processes:

- Absorption from the site of entry
- Distribution to the active site
- Biotransformation (metabolism)
- Excretion from the body

These processes are key elements in determining the amount of drug (dose) and the frequency of dose repetition (scheduling) required to achieve the critical concentration for the desired length of time. When administering a drug, the nurse needs to consider the phases of pharmacokinetics so that the drug regimen can be as effective as possible.

Absorption

To reach reactive tissues, a drug must first make its way into the circulating fluids of the body. **Absorption** refers to what happens to a drug from the time it is introduced to the body until it reaches the circulating fluids and tissues. Drugs can be absorbed from many different areas in the body: through the GI tract either orally or rectally, through mucous membranes, through the skin, through the lung, or through muscle or subcutaneous tissues (see Fig. 2.2). The rate of absorption impacts how soon the medication will take effect. The amount of medication absorbed affects the intensity of the medication's effects, and the route affects both rate and amount absorbed.

Routes of Administration

The route of administration influences the absorption of a drug. Generally, drugs given by the oral route are absorbed more slowly than those given parenterally. If a medication is administered directly into the blood stream, absorption is immediate. Medication administered via intramuscular (IM) injection will usually be absorbed faster than a subcutaneous injection due to there being more capillaries in the muscle tissue.

The oral route is the most frequently used drug administration route in clinical practice. Oral administration is not invasive and, as a rule, oral administration is less expensive than drug administration by other routes. Patients can easily continue their drug regimens at home when they are taking oral medications.

Oral administration subjects the drug to a number of barriers aimed at destroying ingested foreign chemicals. The acidic environment of the stomach is one of the first barriers to foreign chemicals. The acid breaks down many compounds and inactivates others. This is taken into account by pharmaceutical companies when preparing drugs in capsule or tablet form. The binders that are used are designed to break down in a certain acidity and release the active drug to be absorbed.

When food is present, stomach acidity is higher and the stomach empties more slowly, exposing the drug to the acidic environment for a longer period. Certain foods that increase stomach acidity, such as milk products, alcohol, and protein, also speed the breakdown of many drugs. Other foods may chemically bind drugs or block their absorption. When medications are administered orally, it is important to be aware if they are best absorbed on an empty stomach or in the presence of food. For oral absorption to occur, the medication must pass through the layer of epithelial cells in the GI tract lining.

Some drugs that are chemically unstable or are not absorbed in sufficient quantity when given orally are administered via injection directly into the body. Drugs that are injected intravenously bypass the barriers of oral absorption. These drugs have a rapid onset and are fully absorbed at administration because they directly enter the blood stream.

Drugs administered with IM injection are absorbed directly into the capillaries in the muscle and circulated in the blood stream. This takes time because the drug must be absorbed by the capillary and reach the target tissue. People assigned male at birth typically have more vascular muscles than people assigned female at birth do. As a result, drugs administered to assigned males via the IM route may reach a peak level faster than they do in assigned females.

Subcutaneous injections deposit the drug just under the skin, where it is slowly absorbed into circulation. Timing of absorption varies with subcutaneous injection, depending on the fat content of the injection site, adequacy of circulation, and drug characteristics. Highly soluble medications absorb more quickly into plasma compared to poorly soluble medications. Table 2.1 outlines the various factors that affect drug absorption for different routes of administration.

Absorption Processes

Drugs can be absorbed into cells through various processes, including passive diffusion, active transport, and filtration. **Passive diffusion** is the major process through which drugs are absorbed into the body. Passive diffusion occurs across a concentration gradient. When there is a greater concentration of drug on one side of a cell membrane, the drug will move through the membrane to the area of lower concentration. This process does not require any cellular energy. It occurs more quickly if the drug molecule is small, is soluble in water and in lipids (cell membranes are made of lipids and proteins—see Chapter 7), and has no electrical charge that could repel it from the cell membrane.

Table 2.1 Factors That Affect Absorption of Drugs

Route	Factors Affecting Absorption
Intravenous (IV)	None: direct entry into the venous system
Intramuscular (IM)	Perfusion or blood flow to the muscle Solubility of medication in water: absorption is more rapid with high solubility Temperature of the muscle: cold causes vasoconstriction and decreases absorption; heat causes vasodilation and increases absorption
Subcutaneous	Perfusion or blood flow to the tissue Fat content of the tissue Temperature of the tissue: cold causes vasoconstriction and decreases absorption; heat causes vasodilation and increases absorption
Oral (PO)	Acidity of stomach Length of time in stomach Health of gastrointestinal tract Blood flow to gastrointestinal tract Presence of interacting foods or drugs
Rectal (PR) or vaginal	Perfusion or blood flow to the rectum/vaginal canal Lesions in tissue or stool in the rectum Length of time retained for absorption
Mucous membranes (sublingual, buccal)	Perfusion or blood flow to the area Integrity of the mucous membranes Presence of food or smoking Length of time retained in area and correct placement of medication
Topical or intradermal (skin)	Perfusion or blood flow to the area Integrity of skin and ability for the medication to adhere to skin Adequacy of subcutaneous tissue
Inhalation	Perfusion or blood flow to the area Integrity of lung lining Ability to administer drug properly; inspiratory effort

Unlike passive diffusion, **active transport** is a process that uses energy to actively move a molecule across a cell membrane. The molecule may be large, or it may be moving against a concentration gradient. This process is not very important in the absorption of most drugs, but it is often a very important process in drug excretion in the kidney.

Filtration involves movement through pores in the cell membrane, either down a concentration gradient or as a result of the pull of plasma proteins (when pushed by hydrostatic, blood, or osmotic pressure). Filtration is another process the body commonly uses in drug excretion.

Distribution

Distribution involves the movement of a drug to the body's tissues (see Fig. 2.2). As with absorption, there are multiple factors that can affect distribution including the drug's lipid solubility and ionization and the perfusion of the reactive tissue. Specifically, circulation (conditions that change blood flow or perfusion), permeability of the cell membrane, and plasma protein binding all contribute to the distribution of the medication.

For example, tissue perfusion is a factor in treating a patient with diabetes who has a lower-leg infection and needs antibiotics to destroy the bacteria in the area. For this patient, systemic drugs may not be effective because part of the disease process involves changes in the vasculature and decreased blood flow to some areas, particularly the lower limbs. If there is inadequate blood flow to the area, little antibiotic can be delivered to the tissues, and little antibiotic effect will be seen.

Similarly, patients receiving therapeutic hypothermia may have constricted blood vessels (vasoconstriction) in their extremities, which prevents blood flow to those areas. The circulating blood would be unable to deliver drugs to those areas, and the patient would receive little therapeutic effect from drugs intended to react with those tissues.

Many drugs are bound to proteins and are not lipid soluble. These drugs are less likely to be distributed to the central nervous system (CNS) because of the effective blood–brain barrier (see later discussion), which is highly selective in allowing lipid-soluble substances to pass into the CNS.

Protein Binding

Most drugs are bound to some extent to proteins in the blood to be carried into circulation. The more bound to the protein, the more difficult it can be for the medication to be released and to cross membranes to get to the tissue cells. The drug must be freed from the protein's binding site to act on the tissues.

Some drugs are tightly bound and are released very slowly. These drugs have a very long duration of action because they are not free to be broken down or excreted. Therefore, they are released very slowly into the reactive tissue. Some drugs are loosely bound; they tend to act quickly and to be excreted quickly. Some drugs compete with each other for protein-binding sites, altering effectiveness or causing toxicity when the two drugs are given together.

Blood–Brain Barrier

The blood–brain barrier is a protective system of cellular activity that keeps many things (e.g., foreign invaders, poisons) away from the CNS. Drugs that are highly lipid soluble are more likely to pass through the blood–brain barrier and reach the CNS. Drugs that are not lipid soluble are not able to pass the blood–brain barrier. This is clinically significant in treating a brain infection with antibiotics. Almost all antibiotics are not lipid soluble and cannot cross the blood–brain barrier. Effective antibiotic treatment can occur only when the infection is severe enough to alter the blood–brain barrier and allow antibiotics to cross.

Although many drugs can cause adverse CNS effects, these are often the result of indirect drug effects and not the actual reaction of the drug with CNS tissue. For example, alterations in glucose levels and electrolyte changes can interfere with nerve functioning and produce CNS effects such as dizziness, confusion, or changes in thinking ability.

Placenta and Human Milk

Many drugs readily pass through the placenta and affect the developing fetus in people who are pregnant. It is best to evaluate all drugs before administering any to individuals who are pregnant because of the possible risk to the fetus. Drugs should be given only when the benefit clearly outweighs any risk. Many other drugs are secreted into human milk and, therefore, have the potential to affect the neonate. Because of this possibility, the nurse must always check the ability of a drug to pass into human milk when giving a drug to a person who is lactating. Prescribing information states the level of risk of drugs passing into human milk.

Biotransformation (Metabolism)

The body is well prepared to deal with a myriad of foreign chemicals. Enzymes in the liver, in the lining of the GI tract, and even circulating in the body detoxify foreign chemicals to protect the fragile homeostasis that keeps the body functioning (see Fig. 2.2). Almost all of the chemical reactions that the body uses to convert drugs and other chemicals into nontoxic substances are based on a few processes that work to make the chemical less active and more easily excreted from the body.

The liver is the most important site of drug metabolism, or biotransformation, the process by which drugs are changed into new chemicals. Think of the liver as a sewage treatment plant. Everything that is absorbed from the GI tract first enters the liver to be "treated." The liver detoxifies many chemicals and uses others to produce needed enzymes and structures. Through biotransformation, most medications are changed to be less active and more easily excreted. However, there are some types of medications that are activated by biotransformation and some medications that have active metabolites, even after biotransformation.

First-Pass Effect

Drugs that are taken orally are usually absorbed from the small intestine directly into the portal venous system (the blood vessels that flow through the liver on their way back to the heart). Aspirin and alcohol are two drugs that are known to be absorbed from the lower end of the stomach. The portal veins deliver these absorbed molecules into the liver, where a series of liver enzymes immediately transforms most of the chemicals. The enzymes break the drug into metabolites, some of which are active and cause effects in the body, and some of which are deactivated and can be readily excreted from the body. As a result, there is a potential for a large percentage of the oral dose to be destroyed at this point without reaching the targeted tissues. This phenomenon is known as the **first-pass effect**. The portion of the drug that gets through the first-pass effect is delivered to the circulatory system for transport throughout the body. Some medications have high bioavailability and most of the medication reaches the tissues, while some medications have lower bioavailability.

Injected drugs and drugs absorbed from sites other than the GI tract undergo similar biotransformation when they pass through the liver. Because some of the active drug already has had a chance to reach the reactive tissues before reaching the liver, an injected drug is often more effective at a lower dose than is its oral equivalent. With the first-pass effect taken into account, the recommended dose for oral drugs can be considerably higher than the recommended dose for parenteral drugs.

Hepatic Enzyme System

The intracellular structures of the hepatic cells are lined with enzymes packed together in what is called the **hepatic microsomal system**. Because orally administered drugs enter the liver first, the enzyme systems immediately work on the absorbed drug to biotransform it. As explained earlier, this first-pass effect is responsible for neutralizing some of the drugs that are taken. Phase I biotransformation involves oxidation, reduction, or hydrolysis of the drug via the cytochrome P450 system of enzymes. These enzymes are found in most cells but are especially abundant in the liver. Table 2.2 gives some examples of drugs that induce or inhibit the cytochrome P450 system. Phase II biotransformation usually involves a conjugation reaction that makes the drug more water soluble and more readily excreted by the kidneys.

The presence of a chemical that is metabolized by a particular enzyme system can increase the activity of enzyme systems. This process is referred to as **enzyme induction**. Only a few basic enzyme systems are responsible for metabolizing most of the chemicals that pass through the liver. Increased activity in an enzyme system speeds the metabolism of the drug that caused the enzyme induction, as well as any other drug that is

Table 2.2 Examples of Drugs That Alter the Effects of the Cytochrome P-450 Hepatic Enzyme System

Drugs That Induce or Increase Activity	Drugs That Inhibit or Decrease Activity
Nicotine (cigarette smoking)	Ketoconazole (*Nizoral*)
Alcohol (drinking)	Amiodarone (generic)
Glucocorticoids (cortisone, others)	Fluconazole (*Diflucan*)

metabolized via that same enzyme system. This explains why some drugs cannot be taken together effectively. The presence of one drug may speed the metabolism of others, preventing them from reaching their therapeutic levels. Some drugs inhibit an enzyme system, making it less effective. As a consequence, any drug that is metabolized by that system will not be broken down for **excretion**, or the removal of the drug from the body, and the blood level of that drug will increase, often to toxic levels. These actions also explain why liver disease is often a contraindication or a reason to use caution when administering certain drugs. If the liver is not functioning effectively, the drug will not be metabolized as it should be and could reach a toxic level rather quickly.

Excretion

The skin, saliva, lungs, bile, and feces are some of the routes by which drugs are excreted. The kidneys play the most important role in drug excretion (see Fig. 2.2). The blood urea nitrogen (BUN) and creatinine (Cr) levels are often monitored to evaluate kidney function if there is a concern regarding medication excretion.

Drugs that have been made water soluble in the liver are often readily excreted from the kidney by **glomerular filtration**—the passage of water and water-soluble components from the plasma into the renal tubule. Other drugs are secreted or reabsorbed through the renal tubule by active transport systems. The active transport systems that move the drug into the tubule often do so by exchanging it for acid or bicarbonate molecules. Therefore, the acidity of urine can play an important role in drug excretion. This concept is important to remember when trying to clear a drug rapidly from the system or trying to understand why a drug being given at the usual dose is reaching toxic levels in the system. One should always consider the patient's kidney function and urine acidity before administering a drug. Kidney dysfunction can lead to a toxic level of a drug in the body because the drug cannot be excreted (Box 2.1). Figure 2.3 outlines the pharmacokinetic processes that occur when a drug is administered orally.

Box 2.1 Focus on Safe Medication Administration

The liver is very important in metabolizing drugs in the body, and the kidneys are responsible for a large part of the excretion of drugs from the body. One should get into the habit of always checking a patient's liver and renal function before a patient starts a drug regimen. If the liver is not functioning properly, the drug may not be metabolized correctly and may reach toxic levels in the body. If the kidneys are not functioning properly, the drug may not be excreted properly and could accumulate in the body. Dose adjustment needs to be considered if a patient has problems with either the liver or the kidneys.

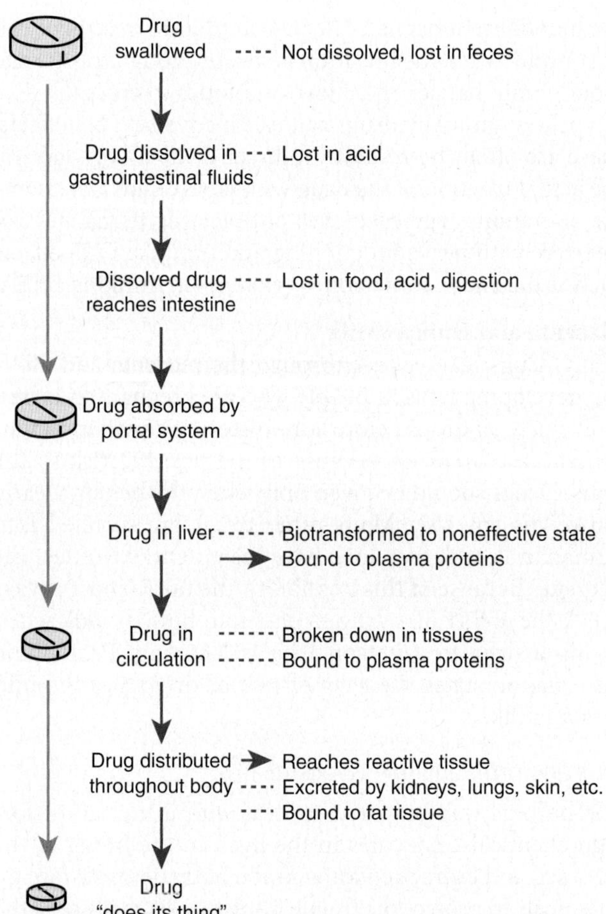

FIGURE 2.3 Pharmacokinetics affects the amount of a drug that reaches reactive tissues. Very little of an oral dose of a drug actually reaches reactive sites.

Half-Life

The **half-life** of a drug is the time it takes for the amount of drug in the body to decrease to one half of its peak level. For instance, if a patient takes 20 mg of a drug with a half-life of 2 hours, 10 mg of the drug will remain 2 hours after administration. Two hours later, 5 mg will be left (one half of the previous level); in 2 more hours, 2.5 mg will remain. This information is important in determining appropriate dose scheduling or the duration of a drug's effect on the body (Box 2.2). When a medication has a shorter half-life, the medication leaves the body more quickly and will need more frequent dosing to maintain a therapeutic level. Medications with longer half-lives stay in the body longer, requiring less frequent dosing, and have greater risk of medication accumulation causing toxicity.

The absorption rate, the distribution to the tissues, the speed of biotransformation, and how fast a drug is excreted are all taken into consideration when determining the half-life of the drug. The half-life that is indicated in any drug monograph is the mean half-life for a healthy person. Using this information, one can estimate the half-life of a drug for a patient with kidney or liver dysfunction (which could prolong biotransformation and the time

Box 2.2 Focus on Calculations

DETERMINING THE IMPACT OF HALF-LIFE ON DRUG LEVELS

A patient is taking a drug that has a half-life of 12 hours. You are trying to determine when a 50-mg dose of the drug will be gone from the body:

- In 12 hours, half of the 50 mg (25 mg) would be in the body.
- In another 12 hours (24 hours), half of 25 mg (12.5 mg) would remain in the body.
- After 36 hours, half of 12.5 mg (6.25 mg) would remain.
- After 48 hours, half of 6.25 mg (3.125 mg) would remain.
- After 60 hours, half of 3.125 (1.56 mg) would remain.
- After 72 hours, half of 1.56 (0.78 mg) would remain.
- After 84 hours, half of 0.78 (0.39 mg) would remain.
- Twelve more hours (for a total of 96 hours) would reduce the drug amount to 0.195 mg.
- Finally, 12 more hours (108 hours) would reduce the amount of the drug in the body to 0.097 mg, which would be quite negligible.
- Therefore, it would take about 9 half-lives or about 4.5 days to clear the medication.

required for excretion of a drug), allowing the prescriber to make changes in the dosing schedule.

The timing of drug administration is important for achieving the most effective drug therapy. Nurses can use their knowledge of drug half-life to explain to patients the importance of following a schedule of drug administration in the hospital or at home. Figure 2.4 shows the effects of drug administration on the critical concentration of a drug.

Key Points

- Pharmacokinetics is the study of how medication travels through the body.
- The concentration of a drug in the body is determined by the balance of absorption, distribution, metabolism (biotransformation), and excretion of the drug.
- In determining the amount, route, and appropriate timing of a drug dose, the pharmacokinetics of that drug must be considered.

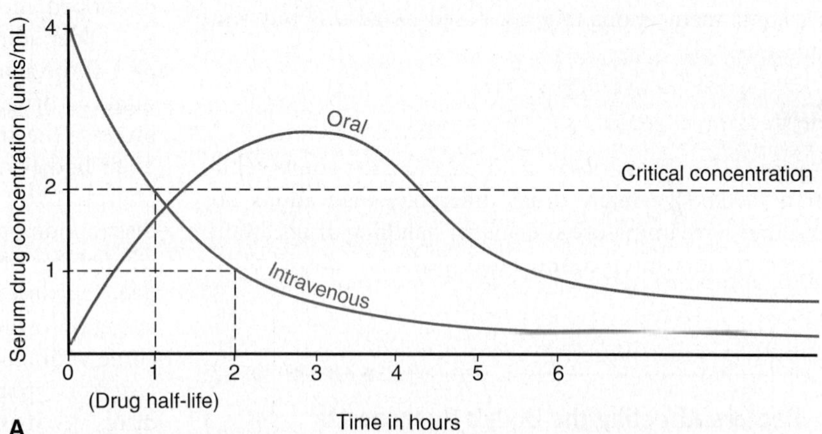

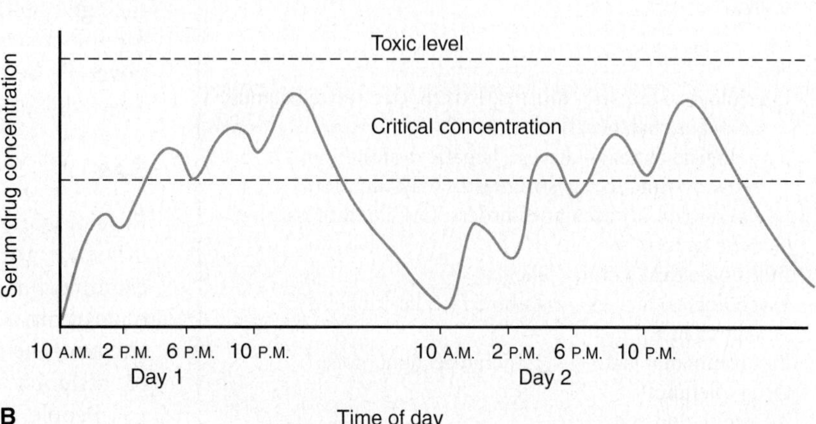

FIGURE 2.4 Influence of biological half-life, route of administration, and dosing regimen on serum drug levels. **A.** Influence of route of administration on the time course of drug levels after administration of a single dose of a drug. The *dashed lines* indicate how the biological half-life of the drug may be determined from the curve of drug concentration after an intravenous dose. At time 0, immediately after the injection, there were 4 units of the drug in each milliliter of serum. The drug concentration fell to half of this amount, 2 units/mL, after 1 hour, the drug's biological half-life. **B.** Influence of dosing regimen on serum drug levels (drug given four times daily, at 10 A.M. and at 2, 6, and 10 P.M.). The drug accumulates as successive doses are given throughout each day; the drug is being given at a rate greater than the patient's body can eliminate it. This dosing regimen has been chosen so that the patient will have a therapeutic level of the drug for a significant portion of the day yet never have a toxic level of the drug.

Factors Influencing Drug Effects

When administering a drug to a patient, the nurse must be aware that the human factor has a tremendous influence on what actually happens to a drug when it enters the body. No two people react in exactly the same way to any given drug. Even though textbooks and drug guides explain the pharmacodynamics and pharmacokinetics of a drug, it must be remembered that much of that information is based on controlled studies of both healthy adults and patients. Circumstances may be very different in the clinical setting. Consequently, before administering any drug, the nurse must consider a number of factors. These are discussed in detail in the following sections and summarized in Box 2.3.

Weight

The recommended dose of a drug is based on drug evaluation studies and is targeted at a 150-lb person. People who are much heavier may require larger doses to get a therapeutic effect from a drug because they have increased tissues to perfuse and increased receptor sites in some reactive tissue. People who weigh less than the norm may require smaller doses of a drug. Toxic effects may occur at the recommended dose if the person is very small. There are some medications that are dosed based on body surface area.

Age

Age is a factor primarily in children and older adults. Children metabolize many drugs differently than adults do, and they have immature systems for handling drugs. Many drugs come with recommended pediatric doses; those without recommended doses can be converted to pediatric doses using either body weight or body surface area (see Box 2.4). There are pharmacokinetic factors that are specific to children. For example, children have decreased gastric acid production and slower gastric emptying time as well as decreased first-pass medication metabolism. They may absorb topical medication faster due to thinner skin and higher blood flow to the skin. Their bodies have a higher proportion of water content that may dilute water-soluble medications. Until their blood–brain barrier is fully developed, medications may have more effect on the CNS.

Older adults undergo many physical changes that are a part of the aging process. They are more likely to be taking multiple drugs for various conditions. Polypharmacy can increase the risk of medication interactions and toxicities. Their bodies may respond very differently in all aspects of pharmacokinetics—less effective absorption, less efficient distribution because of fewer plasma proteins and less efficient perfusion, altered biotransformation or metabolism of drugs because of age-related liver changes, and less effective excretion owing to less efficient kidneys. Many drugs now come with recommended doses for patients who are older based on reports of their use to the FDA. The doses of other drugs also may need to be decreased for the older adult.

When administering drugs to a patient at either end of the age spectrum, one should monitor the patient closely for the desired effects. If the effects are not what would normally be expected, one should consider the need for a dose adjustment.

Sex

Physiological differences between males and females can influence a drug's effect. When giving IM injections, for example, it is important to remember that people assigned male at birth typically have more vascular muscles, so the effects of the drug will be seen sooner in them than in people assigned female at birth.

People assigned female typically have more fat cells than people assigned male do, so drugs that deposit in fat may be slowly released and cause effects for a prolonged

Box 2.4  **Focus on Calculations**

PEDIATRIC DOSES

Children often require different doses of drugs than adults because children's bodies often handle drugs very differently from adults' bodies. The medications that are approved by the FDA will have both adult and pediatric doses or dose ranges listed. Some of the medications will be dosed by age, body weight, or body surface area.

The body surface area can be calculated as follows:

$$\text{BSA}\left(\text{m}^2\right) = \text{square root of}\left\{\text{height (cm)} \times \text{weight (kg)}\right\} / 3{,}600$$

BOX 2.3

Factors Affecting the Body's Response to a Drug

Weight
Age
Sex
Physiological factors—diurnal rhythm, electrolyte balance, acid–base balance, hydration
Pathological factors—disease, hepatic dysfunction, renal dysfunction, gastrointestinal dysfunction, malnutrition, vascular disorders, low blood pressure
Genetic factors
Immunological factors—allergy
Psychological factors—placebo effect, health beliefs, compliance
Environmental factors—temperature, light, noise
Drug tolerance
Accumulation effects
Interactions

period. For example, gas anesthetics have an affinity for depositing in fat and can cause drowsiness and sedation sometimes weeks after surgery. People who can become pregnant who are given any drug should always be questioned about the possibility of pregnancy because, as stated previously, the use of drugs for individuals who are pregnant is not recommended unless the benefit clearly outweighs the potential risk to the fetus.

Physiological Factors

Physiological differences such as diurnal rhythm of the nervous and endocrine systems, acid–base balance, hydration, and electrolyte balance can affect the way that a drug works on the body and the way that the body handles the drug. If a drug does not produce the desired effect, one should review the patient's acid–base and electrolyte profiles and the timing of the drug.

Pathological Factors

Drugs are usually used to treat disease or pathology. However, the disease that the drug is intended to treat can change the functioning of the chemical reactions within the body and thus change the response to the drug.

Other pathological conditions can change the basic pharmacokinetics of a drug. For example, GI disorders can affect the absorption of many oral drugs. Vascular diseases and low blood pressure alter the distribution of a drug, preventing it from being delivered to the reactive tissue, thus rendering the drug nontherapeutic. Inadequate nutrition and low blood protein levels may change the distribution of the medication if it requires a protein carrier in the plasma. Liver or kidney diseases affect the way that a drug is biotransformed and excreted and can lead to toxic reactions when the usual dose is given.

Genetic Factors

Genetic differences can sometimes explain patients' varied responses to a given drug. Some people lack certain enzyme systems necessary for metabolizing a drug, whereas others have overactive enzyme systems that cause drugs to be broken down more quickly. Still others have differing metabolisms or slightly different enzymatic makeups that alter their chemical reactions and the effects of a given drug.

Predictable differences in the pharmacokinetics and pharmacodynamic effects of drugs can be anticipated based on an individual's genetic makeup. **Pharmacogenomics** is an area of study that explores the unique differences in response to drugs that each individual possesses based on genetic makeup. The mapping of the human genome has accelerated research in this area. Some drug regimens can be individually designed based on each person's unique genetic makeup. Trastuzumab (*Herceptin*) (see Chapter 17) is a drug that was developed to treat breast cancer when the tumor expresses human epidermal growth factor receptor 2—a genetic defect seen in some tumors. The drug has no effect on tumors that do not express that genetic defect. This drug was developed as a personalized or targeted medicine based on genetic factors. Such differences are highlighted throughout this book. Another example is that prior to prescribing abacavir (*Ziagen*), an antiviral medication, patients are screened for a specific genetic variant that makes them more likely to have an adverse reaction to the medication.

Immunological Factors

People can develop allergies to drugs. After exposure to a drug's proteins, a person can develop antibodies to that drug. With future exposure to the drug, that person may experience a full-blown allergic reaction. Sensitivity to a drug can range from mild (e.g., dermatological reactions such as a rash) to more severe (e.g., anaphylaxis, shock, and death). Drug allergies are discussed in detail in Chapter 3. Medications may lose efficacy in patients who have antibodies to those medications. This is most common with biologic medications.

Psychological Factors

The patient's attitude about a drug has been shown to have an effect on how that drug works. A drug is more likely to be effective if the patient thinks it will work than if the patient believes it will not work. This is called the **placebo effect**.

The patient's personality also influences adherence to the drug regimen. Some people who believe that they can influence their health actively seek health care and willingly follow a prescribed regimen. These people usually trust the medical system and believe that their efforts will lead to better health. Other people do not trust the medical system. They may believe that they have no control over their health and may be unwilling to adhere to any prescribed therapy. Knowing a patient's health-seeking history and feelings about health care is important in planning an educational program that will work for that patient. It is also important to know this information when arranging for necessary follow-up procedures and evaluations.

As the caregiver most often involved in drug administration, the nurse is in a position to influence the patient's attitude about drug effectiveness. Frequently, the nurse's positive attitude, combined with additional comfort measures, can improve the patient's response to a medication.

Environmental Factors

The environment can affect the success of drug therapy. Some drug effects are enhanced by a quiet, cool, nonstimulating environment. For example, sedating drugs are given to help a patient relax or to decrease tension. Reducing external stimuli to decrease tension and stimulation can help such drugs be more effective. Other drug effects may be influenced by temperature. For example, antihypertensives that work well during cold, winter months may become too effective in warmer environments. This is not due to a change in the medication, but due to people's blood pressure being higher in cold environments. In warm weather, blood vessels are more dilated, which can lower systemic blood pressure. If a patient's response to a medication is not as expected, look for possible changes in environmental conditions.

Tolerance

The body may develop a tolerance to some drugs over time. Tolerance may arise because of increased biotransformation of the drug, increased resistance to its effects, or other pharmacokinetic factors. When tolerance occurs, the drug no longer causes the same reaction. Therefore, increasingly larger doses are needed to achieve a therapeutic effect. An example is morphine, an opiate used for pain relief. The longer morphine is taken, the more tolerant the body becomes to the drug, so that larger and larger doses are needed to relieve pain. Clinically, this situation can be avoided by giving the drug in smaller doses or in combination with other drugs that may also relieve pain. Cross-tolerance—or resistance to drugs in the same class or in similar classes—may also occur in some situations.

Accumulation

If a drug is taken in successive doses at intervals that are shorter than recommended, or if the body is unable to eliminate a drug properly, the drug can accumulate in the body, leading to toxic levels and adverse effects. This can be avoided by following the drug regimen precisely. In reality, with many people managing their therapy at home, strict adherence to a drug regimen seldom occurs. Some people take all of their medications first thing in the morning, so that they won't forget to take the pills later in the day. Others realize that they forgot a dose and then take two to make up for it. Many interruptions of everyday life can interfere with strict adherence to a drug regimen. If a drug is causing serious adverse effects, review the drug regimen with the patient to find out how the drug is being taken, and then educate the patient appropriately.

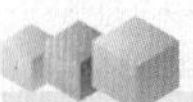
Concept Mastery Alert

Adverse Effects of Medication

When taken in excess, drugs may have adverse effects that are extensions of the primary actions, such as an antihypertensive medication causing low blood pressure. Secondary actions of the drug are those adverse effects that are additional to, not in correlation with, the desired effects.

Interactions

When two or more drugs or substances are taken together, there is a possibility that an interaction can occur, causing unanticipated effects in the body. Alternative therapies, such as herbal products, act as drugs in the body and can cause these same interactions. Certain foods can interact with drugs in much the same way. Usually, this is an increase or decrease in the desired therapeutic effect of one or all of the drugs or an increase in adverse effects.

Drug–Drug or Drug–Alternative Therapy Interactions

Clinically significant drug–drug interactions can produce serious adverse effects. Drug–drug interactions can occur in the following situations:

- *At the site of absorption:* One drug prevents or accelerates absorption of the other drug. For example, the antibiotic tetracycline is poorly absorbed from the GI tract if calcium or calcium products (milk) are present in the stomach. The calcium binds with the tetracycline.
- *During distribution:* One drug competes for the protein-binding site of another drug, so the second drug cannot be transported to the reactive tissue. For example, aspirin competes with the drug methotrexate (*Rheumatrex*) for protein-binding sites. Because aspirin is more competitive for the sites, the methotrexate is bumped off, resulting in increased release of methotrexate and increased toxicity to the tissues.
- *During biotransformation:* One drug stimulates or blocks the metabolism of the other drug. For example, warfarin (*Coumadin*), an oral anticoagulant, is biotransformed more quickly if it is taken at the same time as barbiturates, rifampin, or many other drugs. Because the warfarin is biotransformed to an inactive state more quickly, higher doses will be needed to achieve the desired effect. Patients who use St. John's wort may experience altered effectiveness of several drugs that are affected by that herb's effects on the liver. Digoxin, theophylline, oral contraceptives, anticancer drugs, drugs used to treat HIV, and antidepressants are all reported to have serious interactions with St. John's wort.
- *During excretion:* One drug competes for excretion with the other drug, leading to accumulation and toxic effects of one of the drugs. For example, there is evidence that when amoxicillin and methotrexate are administered together, amoxicillin can decrease the renal clearance of methotrexate. Probenecid administered with penicillin or cephalosporin can decrease their renal clearance as well.
- *At the site of action:* One drug may be an antagonist of the other drug or may cause effects that oppose those of the other drug, leading to no therapeutic effect. This is seen, for example, when an antihypertensive drug is taken with an antiallergy drug that also increases blood pressure. The effects on blood pressure are negated,

and there is a loss of the antihypertensive effectiveness of the drug. If a patient is taking antidiabetic medication and also takes the herb ginseng, which lowers blood glucose levels, they may experience episodes of hypoglycemia and loss of blood glucose control.

Whenever two or more drugs are being given together, first consult a drug guide for a listing of clinically significant drug–drug interactions. Sometimes problems can be avoided by staggering the administration of the drugs or adjusting their doses. (See Box 2.5 and the Critical Thinking Scenario.)

CRITICAL THINKING SCENARIO
Drug Interactions

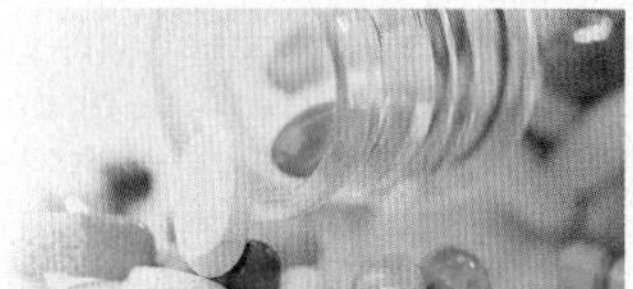

THE SITUATION

R.D. is a 68-year-old patient from Wisconsin, who has now lived in their Florida home for 6 months. R.D. has a history of hyperlipidemia and was started on treatment with atorvastatin (*Lipitor*), combined with a diet and exercise regimen 6 weeks ago. R.D. has lowered their lipid levels to the upper level of normal. R.D. comes into the clinic complaining of low-grade fever and severe muscle pain.

Critical Thinking

What are the important nursing implications in this case?
What are the effects of this drug and what issues should be considered?
What specific issues should be discussed?
What teaching points need to be clarified?

DISCUSSION

When a person presents with new signs and symptoms, it is important to do a complete history and physical and to do a thorough drug history. Dealing with the chief complaint is the patient's highest priority and should be the initial focus when dealing with the patient. Ensure the patient's comfort and arrange for any additional tests that might be needed. In this situation, looking up the drug shows that rhabdomyolysis is a potentially serious adverse effect associated with the use of atorvastatin, a lipid lowering drug known as a hydroxymethylglutaryl (HMG) coenzyme A inhibitor. Rhabdomyolysis is a disease of muscle breakdown and presents with low-grade fever and acute muscle pain. In severe cases, it can lead to renal failure and even death. Could this have happened after 6 weeks, or could something else be involved? Further reading about this drug shows that it cannot be combined with many other prescription drugs (which R.D. denies using) or with large amounts of grapefruit juice, which will block the biotransformation of the drug and lead to potentially toxic atorvastatin levels. R.D.'s blood tests reveal high creatine kinase levels, consistent with the diagnosis of rhabdomyolysis.

Discussing the drug therapy with R.D. needs to include an explanation of what seems to have happened to them. Encourage R.D. to present when they experience these signs and symptoms. Reviewing the need to avoid grapefruit juice reveals that they did not understand the previous instructions. R.D. has been drinking a lot of grapefruit juice, but never takes the drug with grapefruit juice. R.D. always takes the pill with water and then has the grapefruit juice later. This is a common misunderstanding when telling patients not to take a drug with grapefruit juice. The nurse should explain that the misunderstanding is common and that it takes 48 hours to clear the chemical in grapefruit juice that interferes with atorvastatin. The nurse can explain that drinking small amounts of grapefruit juice is not a problem. Drinking less than a liter per day has been shown to be safe, so it is possible that R.D. can drink a small amount of the grapefruit juice. However, it should be limited to decrease risk of rhabdomyolysis. By listening to the patient's needs and priorities, the health care team begins a plan to help R.D. lower their lipids safely while still allowing them to enjoy a favorite Florida beverage.

NURSING CARE GUIDE FOR R.D.

Assessment: History and Examination

Allergies to any drugs
Use of any over-the-counter (OTC) drugs or herbal therapies
CNS: affect, reflexes
Musculoskeletal: ROM (range of motion)
CV: P, BP
Hematological: lipid levels, creatine kinase

Nursing Conclusions

Acute pain related to muscle breakdown effects
Deficient knowledge related to drug therapy

Planning

When leaving the clinic, the patient will have a good understanding of their drug therapy and will have means of adjusting their lifestyle to keep their lipids lowered.

Interventions

Provide patient teaching regarding drug effects, safe use of the drug, and ways to avoid adverse effects.
Provide referral for evaluation of other drugs available to help keep lipids lowered.

(continues on page 32)

Evaluation

Monitor for adverse effects related to drug therapy.
Monitor effectiveness of referral for alternate therapy.

Patient Teaching

- Atorvastatin has been prescribed to help keep your lipid levels in a normal range. This drug must be combined with diet and exercise to be most effective.
- Common adverse effects you might experience include muscle pain, diarrhea or nasopharyngitis.
- Serious adverse effects that may occur include liver damage (report changes in color of urine or stool, extreme fatigue) and rhabdomyolysis (report acute muscle pain with fever).
- This drug cannot be combined with many other drugs. Always report the addition of any other drug to your drug regimen. This includes OTC drugs and herbal therapies.
- This drug cannot be combined with high amounts of grapefruit juice (greater than 1.2 L). The chemical in grapefruit juice that affects atorvastatin stays in the body for 48 hours.
- We will be arranging for a referral to discuss changing your lipid lowering plans so that you will be able to enjoy your grapefruit juice. Please continue your current therapy and avoid all grapefruit juice until that appointment.

Drug–Food Interactions

For the most part, a drug–food interaction occurs when the drug and the food are in direct contact in the stomach. Some foods increase acid production, speeding the breakdown of the drug molecule and preventing absorption and distribution of the drug. Some foods chemically react with certain drugs and prevent their absorption into the body. For this reason, the antibiotic tetracycline cannot be taken with iron products. Tetracycline also binds with calcium to some extent and should not be taken with foods or other drugs containing calcium. Grapefruit juice has been found to affect liver enzyme systems for up to 48 hours after it has been ingested. This can result in increased or decreased serum levels of certain drugs. Many drugs come with the warning that they should not be combined with grapefruit juice. This drug–food interaction does not take place in the stomach, so grapefruit juice needs to be avoided the entire time the drug is being used, not just while the drug is in the stomach.

In most cases, oral drugs are absorbed fastest when taken on an empty stomach; however, for many medications, the absorption speed is not clinically relevant so people can eat and drink normally when taking the medication. Sometimes nausea is a side effect of a medication and taking the drug with small meals might help decrease the side effect. If the patient cannot tolerate the drug on an empty stomach, the food selected for ingestion with the drug should be known not to interact with it. Drug labels will list important drug–food interactions and give guidelines for avoiding problems and optimizing the drug's therapeutic effects.

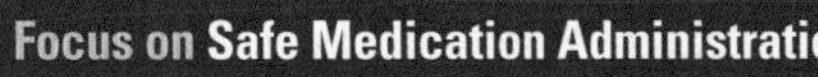
Box 2.5 Focus on Safe Medication Administration

Always check the monograph of any drug that is being given to monitor for clinically important drug–drug, drug–alternative therapy, or drug–food interactions.

Drug–Laboratory Test Interactions

As explained previously, the body works through a series of chemical reactions. Because of this, administration of a particular drug may alter results of tests that are done on various chemical levels or reactions as part of a diagnostic study. This drug–laboratory test interaction is caused by the drug being given and not necessarily by a change in the body's responses or actions. Keep these interactions in mind when evaluating a patient's diagnostic tests. If one test result is altered and does not fit in with the clinical picture or other test results, consider the possibility of a drug–laboratory test interference. For example, dalteparin (*Fragmin*), a low molecular weight heparin used to prevent deep vein thrombosis after abdominal surgery, may cause increased levels of the liver enzymes aspartate aminotransferase and alanine aminotransferase with no injury to liver cells or hepatitis.

Optimal Therapeutic Effect

As overwhelming as all of this information may seem, most patients can follow a drug regimen to achieve optimal therapeutic effects without serious adverse effects. Avoiding problems is the best way to treat adverse or ineffective drug effects. There are certain times when a medication is contraindicated (should not be used) based on the client's information. For example, your client may have an allergy to the medication. One should incorporate basic history and physical assessment factors into any plan of care so that obvious problems can be spotted and handled promptly. In the patient-centered approach to care, the nurse needs to also consider cultural, emotional, psychological, and environmental factors. If a drug does not have the expected effect, further examine the factors that are known to influence drug effects (see Box 2.3). Frequently, the drug regimen can be modified to deal with that influence. Rarely is it necessary to completely stop a needed drug regimen because of adverse or intolerable effects. In many cases, the nurse is the caregiver in the best position to assess problems and intervene early.

SUMMARY

- Pharmacodynamics is the study of the way that drugs affect the body.
- Most drugs work by replacing natural chemicals, by stimulating normal cell activity, or by depressing normal cell activity.
- Chemotherapeutic agents work by interfering with normal cell functioning, causing cell death. The most desirable chemotherapeutic agents are those with selective toxicity to foreign cells and foreign cell activities.
- Drugs frequently act at specific receptor sites on cell membranes to stimulate enzyme systems within the cell and to alter the cell's activities.
- Pharmacokinetics—the study of the way the body deals with drugs—includes absorption, distribution, biotransformation, and excretion of drugs.
- The goal of established dosing schedules is to achieve a critical concentration of the drug in the body. This critical concentration is the amount of the drug necessary to achieve the drug's therapeutic effects.
- Arriving at a critical concentration involves a dynamic equilibrium among the processes of drug absorption, distribution, metabolism or biotransformation, and excretion.
- Absorption involves moving a drug into the body for circulation. Oral drugs are absorbed from the small intestine, undergo many changes, and are affected by many things in the process. IV drugs are injected directly into the circulation and do not need additional absorption.
- Drugs are distributed to various tissues throughout the body depending on their solubility and ionization. Most drugs are bound to plasma proteins for transport to reactive tissues.
- Drugs are metabolized or biotransformed into less toxic chemicals by various enzyme systems in the body. The liver is the primary site of drug metabolism or biotransformation. The liver uses the cytochrome P-450 enzyme system to alter the drug and start its biotransformation.
- The first-pass effect is the breakdown of oral drugs in the liver immediately after absorption. Drugs given by other routes often reach reactive tissues before passing through the liver for biotransformation.
- Drug excretion is removal of the drug from the body. This occurs mainly through the kidneys.
- The half-life of a drug is the period of time it takes for an amount of drug in the body to decrease to one half of the peak level it previously achieved. The half-life is affected by all aspects of pharmacokinetics. Knowing the half-life of a drug helps in predicting dosing schedules and duration of effects.
- The actual effects of a drug are determined by its pharmacokinetics, its pharmacodynamics, and many human factors that can change the drug's effectiveness.
- To provide the safest and most effective drug therapy, the nurse must consider all of the possible factors that influence drug concentration and effectiveness.

Unfolding Patient Stories: Harry Hadley • Part 1

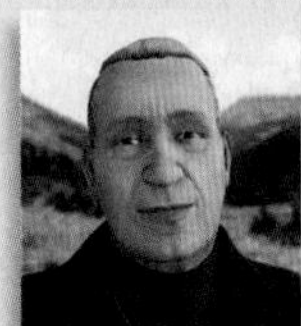

Harry Hadley was diagnosed 3 days ago with cellulitis in his right lower leg caused by a feral cat bite. A wound culture was obtained and oral augmentin was started. His infection has worsened, and he is admitted to the hospital for treatment with intravenous vancomycin. Culture results are positive for MRSA. How would the nurse respond when Harry questions why he was prescribed the augmentin 3 days ago instead of vancomycin? What are the spectra of organism coverage for augmentin and vancomycin? What drug resistance concerns should the nurse consider? Describe how the nurse evaluates wound culture and sensitivity findings and how the test determines the most effective anti-infective medication. (Harry Hadley's story continues in Chap. 9.)

Care for Harry and other patients in a realistic virtual environment: ***vSim** for Nursing* (thepoint.lww.com/vSimPharm). Practice documenting these patients' care in DocuCare (thepoint.lww.com/DocuCareEHR)

CHECK YOUR UNDERSTANDING

Answers to the questions in this chapter can be found in Answers to Check Your Understanding Questions on thePoint®.

MULTIPLE CHOICE

Select the best answer.

1. Chemotherapeutic agents are drugs that
   a. are used only to treat cancers.
   b. replace normal body chemicals that are missing because of disease.
   c. interfere with foreign cell functioning causing cell death, such as invading microorganisms or neoplasms.
   d. stimulate the normal functioning of a cell.
2. Receptor sites
   a. are a normal part of enzyme substrates.
   b. are protein areas on cell membranes that react with specific chemicals.
   c. can usually be stimulated by many different chemicals.
   d. are responsible for all drug effects in the body.
3. Selective toxicity is the ability of a drug to
   a. seek out a specific bacterial species or microorganism.
   b. cause only specific adverse effects.
   c. cause fetal damage.
   d. attack only those systems found in foreign or abnormal cells.
4. When trying to determine why the desired therapeutic effect is not being seen with an oral drug, the nurse should consider
   a. the blood flow to muscle beds.
   b. food altering the makeup of gastric juices.
   c. the weight of the patient.
   d. the temperature of the peripheral environment.
5. Much of the biotransformation that occurs when a drug is taken occurs as part of the
   a. protein-binding effect of the drug.
   b. functioning of the renal system.
   c. first-pass effect through the liver.
   d. distribution of the drug to the reactive tissues.
6. The half-life of a drug
   a. is determined by a balance of all pharmacokinetic processes.
   b. is a constant factor for all drugs taken by a patient.
   c. is only influenced by the fat distribution of the patient.
   d. can be calculated with the use of a body surface nomogram.
7. J.B. has Parkinson disease that has been controlled for several years with levodopa. After they begin a health food regimen with lots of vitamin B_6, their tremors return, and they develop a rapid heart rate, hypertension, and anxiety. The nurse investigating the problem discovers that vitamin B_6 can speed the conversion of levodopa to dopamine in the periphery, leading to these problems. The nurse would consider this problem
   a. a drug–laboratory test interaction.
   b. a drug–drug interaction.
   c. an accumulation effect.
   d. a sensitivity reaction.

MULTIPLE RESPONSE

Select all that apply.

1. When reviewing a drug to be given, the nurse notes that the drug is excreted in the urine. What points should be included in the nurse's assessment of the patient?
   a. The patient's liver function tests
   b. The patient's bladder tone
   c. The patient's renal function tests
   d. The patient's fluid intake
   e. Other drugs being taken that could affect the kidney
   f. The patient's intake and output for the day
2. When considering the pharmacokinetics of a drug, what points would the nurse need to consider?
   a. How the drug will be absorbed
   b. The way the drug affects the body
   c. Receptor site activation and suppression
   d. How the drug will be excreted
   e. How the drug will be metabolized
   f. The half-life of the drug
3. Drug–drug interactions are important considerations in clinical practice. When evaluating a patient for potential drug–drug interactions, what would the nurse expect to address?
   a. Bizarre drug effects on the body
   b. The need to adjust drug dose or timing of administration
   c. The need for more drugs to balance the effects of the drugs being given
   d. A new therapeutic effect not encountered with either drug alone
   e. Increased adverse effects
   f. The use of herbal or alternative therapies

REFERENCES

Agency for Health Care Research and Quality. (2018). *Twenty tips to help prevent medical errors.* http://www.ahrq.gov/patients-consumers/care-planning/errors/20tips/index.html

Barat, I., Anreassen, F., & Damsgaard, E. M. S. (2001). Drug therapy in the elderly: What doctors believe and what patients actually do. *British Journal of Clinical Pharmacology, 51*(6), 615–622. https://bpspubs.onlinelibrary.wiley.com/doi/full/10.1046/j.0306-5251.2001.01401.x

Brunton, L., Hilal-Dandan, R., & Knollman, B. (2018). *Goodman and Gilman's the pharmacological basis of therapeutics* (13th ed.). McGraw-Hill.

Gray, C., & Gandher, C. (2009). Adverse drug events in the elderly: An ongoing problem. *Journal of Managed Care Pharmacy, 15*(7), 568–571. https://journals.sagepub.com/doi/10.1177/2042098615615472

King, R. L. (2004). Nurses' perceptions of their pharmacology educational needs. *Journal of Advanced Nursing, 45*(4), 392–400. https://onlinelibrary.wiley.com/doi/abs/10.1046/j.1365-2648.2003.02922.x

Kudzma, E., & Carey, E. (2009). Pharmacogenomics: Personalizing drug therapy. *American Journal of Nursing, 109*(10), 50–57. 10.1097/01.NAJ.0000361493.75589.06

Mangoni, A. A., & Jackson, S. H. D. (2004). Age related changes in pharmacokinetics and pharmacodynamics: Basic principle and practical applications. *British Journal of Clinical Pharmacology, 57*(1), 6–14. https://bpspubs.onlinelibrary.wiley.com/doi/full/10.1046/j.1365-2125.2003.02007.x

Milos, P. M., & Seymour, A. B. (2004). Emerging strategies and applications of pharmacogenomics. *Human Genomics, 1*(6), 444–445. https://humgenomics.biomedcentral.com/articles/10.1186/1479-7364-1-6-444

Murphy, J. (2012). *Clinical pharmacokinetics.* American Society of Health-System Pharmacists.

National Human Genome Research Institute. (2020). *Pharmacogenomics FAQ.* https://www.genome.gov/FAQ/Pharmacogenomics

Palleria, C., DiPaolo, A., Giofre, C., Caglioti, C., Leuzzi, G., Siniscalchi, A., DeSarro, G., & Gallelli, L. (2013). Pharmacokinetic drug-drug interaction and their implication in clinical management. *Journal of Research and Medical Science, 18*(7), 601–610. https://www.ncbi.nlm.nih.gov/pmc/articles/PMC3897029/

Ray, W. A. (2003). Population based studies of adverse effects. *New England Journal of Medicine, 349*, 1592–1594. 10.1056/NEJMp038145

US Food and Drug Administration. (2019). *Nubain—(nalbuphine hydrochloride) injection, for intramuscular, subcutaneous, or intravenous use.* https://www.accessdata.fda.gov/drugsatfda_docs/label/2019/018024s042lbl.pdf

Wessling, S. (2013). *Ethnopharmacology: What nurses need to know.* https://minoritynurse.com/ethnopharmacology-what-nurses-need-to-know/

Zhou, S. F. (2008). Potential strategies for minimizing mechanism based inhibition or CP450-3A4. *Current Pharmaceutical Design, 14*(10), 990–1000. https://www.eurekaselect.com/66758/article

CHAPTER 3

Toxic Effects of Drugs

Learning Objectives

Upon completion of this chapter, you will be able to:

1. Define the term adverse drug reaction and explain the clinical significance of this reaction.
2. List four types of allergic responses to drug therapy.
3. Discuss five common examples of drug-induced tissue damage.
4. Define the term poison.
5. Outline the important factors to consider when applying the nursing process to selected situations of drug toxicity.

Key Terms

blood dyscrasia: bone marrow suppression caused by drug effects on the rapidly multiplying cells of the bone marrow; lower-than-normal levels of blood components can be seen

dermatological reactions: skin reactions commonly seen as adverse effects of drugs; can range from simple rash to potentially fatal exfoliative dermatitis

drug allergy or hypersensitivity: usually involves the formation of antibodies to a drug or drug protein; causes an immune response when the person is next exposed to that drug

poisoning: overdose of a drug that causes damage to multiple body systems and has the potential for fatal reactions

stomatitis: inflammation of the mucous membranes related to drug effects; can lead to alterations in nutrition and dental problems

superinfections: infections caused by the destruction of normal flora bacteria by certain drugs, which allow other bacteria to grow out of control and cause infection; may occur during antibiotic therapy

All drugs are potentially dangerous. Even though chemicals are carefully screened and tested in vivo or in vitro prior to human studies, drug products often cause unexpected or unacceptable reactions when administered. Drugs are chemicals, and the human body operates by a vast series of chemical reactions. Consequently, many effects can be seen when just one chemical factor is altered. Today's potent drugs can cause a variety of reactions, many of which are more extreme than seen previously.

Adverse Effects

Adverse effects are undesired effects that may be unpleasant or even dangerous. They can occur for many reasons, including the following:

- The drug may have other effects on the body besides the therapeutic effect.
- The patient may be sensitive to the drug being given.
- The drug's action on the body may cause other undesirable or unpleasant responses.
- The patient may be taking too much or too little of the drug, leading to adverse effects.

The nurse, as the caregiver who most frequently administers medications, must be constantly alert for signs of drug reactions of various types. Patients and their families need to be taught what to look for when taking drugs at home. Some adverse effects can be countered with specific comfort measures or precautions. Knowing these effects may occur and what actions to take to prevent or cope with them may be the most critical factor in helping the patient comply with drug therapy. Adverse drug effects can be one of several types: primary actions, secondary actions, and hypersensitivity reactions (Box 3.1).

Box 3.1 Focus on Safe Medication Administration

Before administering any drug to a patient, it is important to review the contraindications and cautions associated with that drug, as well as the anticipated adverse effects of the drug. This information will direct your assessment of the patient, helping you to focus on particular signs and symptoms that would alert you to contraindications or to proceed cautiously, and helping you to establish a baseline for that patient so that you will be able to identify the adverse effects that occur. When teaching the patient about a drug, you should list the adverse effects that can most often be anticipated, but not every adverse effect listed for that drug, along with the appropriate actions that the patient can take to alleviate any discomfort associated with these effects. Being alert to adverse effects—what to assess and how to intervene appropriately—can increase the effectiveness of a drug regimen, provide for patient safety, and improve patient compliance to the drug regimen.

Primary Actions

One of the most common occurrences in drug therapy is the development of adverse effects from simple overdose. In such cases, the patient suffers from effects that are merely an extension of the desired effect. For example, an anticoagulant may act so effectively that the patient experiences excessive and spontaneous bleeding. This type of adverse effect can be avoided by monitoring the patient carefully and adjusting the prescribed dose to fit that particular patient's needs.

In the same way, a patient taking an antihypertensive drug may become dizzy, weak, or faint when taking the standard recommended dose but will be able to tolerate the drug therapy with a reduced dose. These effects can be caused by individual response to the drug, high or low body weight, age, or underlying pathology that alters the effects of the drug.

A patient who has kidney impairment may not be able to excrete the drug and may accumulate the drug in the body, causing toxic effects. The patient will exhibit exaggerated adverse effects from a standard dose of the medication because of the accumulation of the drug.

Secondary Actions

Drugs can produce a wide variety of effects in addition to the desired pharmacological effect. Sometimes the drug dose can be adjusted to achieve the desired effect without producing undesired secondary reactions. Sometimes this is not possible, however, and the adverse effects are almost inevitable. In such cases, the patient needs to be informed that these effects may occur and counseled about ways to cope with them. For example, many antihistamines are very effective in drying up secretions and helping breathing, but they also cause drowsiness. The patient who is taking antihistamines needs to know that driving a car or operating power tools or machinery should be avoided because the drowsiness could be dangerous. A patient taking an oral antibiotic needs to know that frequently the effects of the antibiotic on the gastrointestinal (GI) tract result in diarrhea, nausea, and sometimes vomiting. The patient should be advised to eat small, frequent meals to help alleviate this problem.

In some cases, individuals exhibit increased therapeutic and adverse effects with no definite pathological condition. Each person has slightly different receptors and cellular responses. Frequently, older people will react to narcotics with increased stimulation and hyperactivity, not with the sedation that is expected. It is thought that this response is related to a change in receptors with age leading to an increased sensitivity to a drug's effects.

Drug Allergy or Hypersensitivity

Many **drug allergies**, or **hypersensitivities**, occur when the body forms antibodies to a particular drug, causing an immune response when the person is reexposed to the drug. A patient cannot be allergic to a drug they have never taken, although patients can have cross-allergies to drugs within the same drug class as one formerly taken. Many people state that they have a drug allergy because of the effects of a drug. For example, one patient stated that they were allergic to the diuretic furosemide (*Lasix*). On further questioning, the nurse discovered that the patient considered themselves to be "allergic" to the drug because it made them urinate frequently—the desired drug effect, but one that the patient thought was a reaction to the drug. Ask additional questions of patients who state that they have a drug allergy to ascertain the exact nature of the response and whether it is a true drug allergy or not.

Some allergic reactions are rapid and some take days or weeks to develop. Some are severe and life-threatening reactions, while others can be mild or merely irritating reactions.

Drug allergies fall into four main classifications: type I immediate hypersensitivity disorders, type II antibody-mediated disorders, type III immune complex–mediated disorders, and type IV cell-mediated hypersensitivity disorders (Table 3.1). The nurse, as the primary caregiver involved in administering drugs, must constantly assess for potential drug allergies and must be prepared to intervene appropriately.

Table 3.1 Interventions for Types of Drug Allergies

Allergy Type	Signs/Symptoms	Interventions
Type I immediate hypersensitivity disorders		
This allergy involves an antibody (IgE) that reacts with type 2 helper T cell that leads to plasma cell production of IgE and mast cell sensitization, which will cause the release of inflammatory chemicals (histamine and others). The T cells also recruit eosinophils, which can cause a secondary or later inflammatory response.	Hives, rash, difficulty breathing, labile blood pressure, dilated pupils, diaphoresis, "panic" feeling, increased heart rate, respiratory arrest, anaphylaxis.	Anaphylaxis: withdraw allergen, administer epinephrine, maintain airway and blood pressure. Local and/or less severe: withdraw allergen, over-the-counter antihistamines and/or decongestants. Prevention is the best treatment. Counsel patients with known allergies to wear Medic-Alert identification and, if appropriate, to carry an emergency epinephrine kit.
Type II antibody-mediated disorders		
This allergy involves antibodies (IgG or IgM) that circulate in the blood and attack antigens on cell sites, causing death of that cell. This reaction is not immediate but may be seen over a few days.	Signs and symptoms will be dependent on the cells/tissues that are attacked. Can range from renal dysfunction or liver dysfunction to symptoms of hyperthyroidism or myasthenia gravis (an autoimmune disease attacking the skeletal muscle receptors).	Notify the prescriber and/or primary caregiver and discontinue the drug. Support the patient to prevent infection and conserve energy until the allergic response is over.
Type III immune complex–mediated disorders		
This allergy involves antibodies (IgG and IgM) that circulate in the blood and cause damage to various tissues by depositing in blood vessels. This reaction may occur up to 1 week or more after exposure to the drug.	Itchy rash, high fever, swollen lymph nodes, swollen and painful joints, edema of the face and limbs. If systemic symptoms, the reaction is often called "serum sickness" since the antibody–antigen reaction is happening in the blood and damaging blood vessels.	Notify the prescriber and/or primary caregiver and discontinue the drug. Provide comfort measures to help the patient cope with the signs and symptoms (cool environment, skin care, positioning, ice to joints, administer antipyretics or anti-inflammatory agents, as appropriate).
Type IV cell-mediated hypersensitivity disorders		
This reaction can occur several hours to days after exposure and involves T cells being activated by the antigen and causing direct cell death or delayed reaction with cytokines that increase inflammation.	Itchy rash, hives, swollen joints if a contact dermatitis. If in the lungs, difficulty breathing, dry cough are common. If reaction attacks liver cells, can have signs of liver impairment due to hepatitis.	Notify the prescriber and/or primary caregiver and discontinue drug. If skin reaction, provide skin care and comfort measures that may include antihistamines or topical corticosteroids. Systemic reactions may require more advanced care.

Key Points

- All drugs have effects other than the desired therapeutic effect.
- Primary actions of the drug can be extensions of the desired effect.
- Secondary actions of the drug are effects that the drug causes in the body that are not related to the therapeutic effect.
- Drug allergies or hypersensitivity reactions can often occur when a patient develops antibodies to a drug after exposure to the drug.

Drug-Induced Tissue and Organ Damage

Drugs can act directly or indirectly to cause many types of adverse effects in various tissues, structures, and organs (Fig. 3.1). These drug effects account for many of the cautions noted before drug administration begins. The possibility that these effects can occur also accounts for the contraindications for the use of some drugs in patients with a particular history or underlying pathology. The specific contraindications and cautions for the administration of a given drug are noted with each drug type discussed

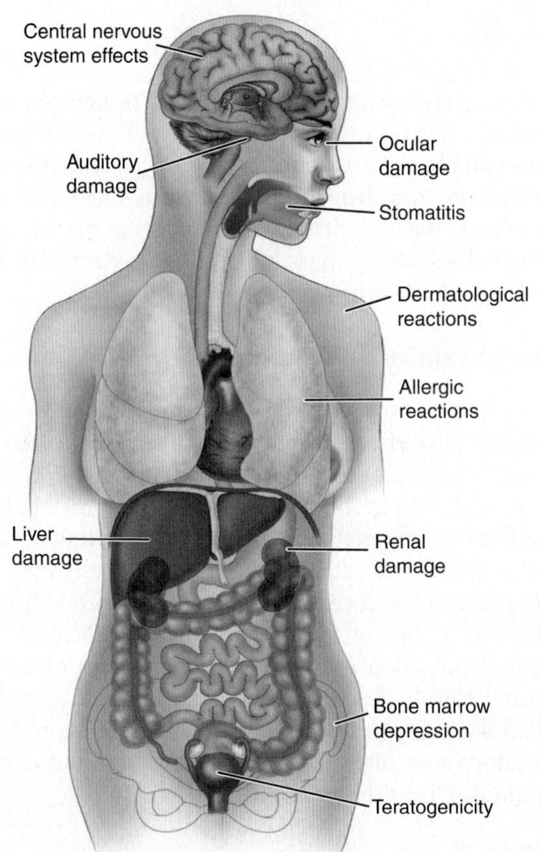

FIGURE 3.1 Variety of adverse effects and toxicities associated with drug use.

in this book and in the individual monographs found in various drug guides. These effects occur frequently enough that the nurse should be knowledgeable about the presentation of drug-induced damage and about appropriate interventions to use should it occur.

Dermatological Reactions

Dermatological reactions are adverse reactions involving the skin. These can range from a simple rash to potentially fatal exfoliative dermatitis. Many adverse reactions involve the skin because many drugs can deposit there or cause direct irritation to the tissue.

Rashes, Hives

Many drugs are known to cause skin reactions. Sulfamethoxazole and trimethoprim (*Bactrim*), a drug used to treat urinary tract infections and other infections caused by susceptible pathogens, can cause an itchy, red rash and in some patients has caused a serious and potentially fatal skin reaction, Stevens-Johnson syndrome. Although many patients will report that they are allergic to a drug because they develop a skin rash when taking the drug, it is important to determine whether a rash is a commonly associated adverse effect of the drug.

Assessment
Hives, rashes, and other dermatological lesions may be seen. Severe reactions may include exfoliative dermatitis, which is characterized by rash and scaling, fever, enlarged lymph nodes, enlarged liver, and the potentially fatal erythema multiforme exudativum (Stevens-Johnson syndrome), which is characterized by dark red papules appearing on the extremities with no pain or itching, often in rings or disk-shaped patches.

Interventions
In mild cases, or when the benefit of the drug outweighs the discomfort of the skin lesion, provide frequent skin care; instruct the patient to avoid rubbing, wearing tight or rough clothing, and using harsh soaps or perfumed lotions; and administer antihistamines, as appropriate. In severe cases, discontinue the drug and notify the prescriber and/or primary caregiver. Be aware that, in addition to these interventions, topical corticosteroids, antihistamines, and emollients are often used.

Stomatitis

Stomatitis, or inflammation of the mucous membranes, can occur because of a direct toxic reaction to the drug or because the drug deposits in the end capillaries in the mucous membranes, leading to inflammation. Many drugs are known to cause stomatitis. Antineoplastic drugs commonly cause these problems because they are toxic to rapidly turning-over cells such as those found in the GI tract. Patients receiving antineoplastic drugs are usually given instructions for proper mouth care when the drugs are started.

Assessment
Symptoms can include swollen gums, inflamed gums (gingivitis), and swollen and red tongue (glossitis). Other symptoms include difficulty swallowing, bad breath, and pain in the mouth and throat.

Interventions
Provide frequent mouth care with a nonirritating solution. Offer nutrition evaluation and development of a tolerated diet, which usually involves frequent, small meals. If necessary, arrange for a dental consultation. Note that antifungal agents and/or local anesthetics are sometimes used.

Gastrointestinal Irritation

Some medications may cause local irritation of the GI tract. For example, nonsteroidal anti-inflammatory drugs (NSAIDs) can decrease the mucosal membrane in the GI tract and increase risk of heartburn and mucosal damage. Other medications may stimulate nausea and vomiting and/or constipation. Opioid medications are known to slow peristalsis and increase risk of constipation.

Assessment

Symptoms can include nausea, vomiting, diarrhea, constipation, heart burn, and abdominal bloating.

Interventions

Some GI irritation may be decreased if the medications are taken with food. The constipation caused by some medications can be prevented with motility stimulants.

Superinfections

One of the body's protective mechanisms is provided by the wide variety of bacteria that live within or on the surface of the body and in the GI tract. This bacterial growth is called the *normal flora*. The normal flora protect the body from invasion by other bacteria, viruses, fungi, and so on. Several kinds of drugs (especially antibiotics) destroy the normal flora, leading to the development of **superinfections**, or infections caused by organisms that are usually controlled by the normal flora.

Assessment

Symptoms can include fever, diarrhea, black or hairy tongue, inflamed and swollen tongue (glossitis), mucous membrane lesions, and vaginal discharge with or without itching.

Interventions

Provide supportive measures (frequent mouth care, skin care, access to bathroom facilities, small and frequent meals). Administer antifungal therapy as appropriate. In severe cases, discontinue the drug responsible for the superinfection.

Blood Dyscrasia

Blood dyscrasia is bone marrow suppression caused by drug effects. This occurs when drugs that can cause cell death (e.g., antineoplastics, antibiotics) are used. Bone marrow cells multiply rapidly; they are said to be rapidly turning over. Because they go through cell division and multiply so often, they are highly susceptible to any agent that disrupts cell function.

Assessment

Symptoms include fever, chills, sore throat, weakness, back pain, dark urine, decreased hematocrit (anemia), low platelet count (thrombocytopenia), low white blood cell count (leukopenia), and a reduction of all cellular elements of the complete blood count (pancytopenia).

Interventions

Monitor blood counts. Provide supportive measures (rest, protection from exposure to infections, protection from injury, avoidance of activities that might result in injury or bleeding). In severe cases, discontinue the drug or stop administration until the bone marrow recovers to a safe level.

Key Points

- Adverse drug effects can include skin irritation ranging from rashes and hives to potentially fatal Stevens-Johnson syndrome.
- Superinfections, or infections caused by destruction of protective normal flora bacteria; blood dyscrasias caused by bone marrow suppression of blood-forming cells; and stomatitis or mucous membrane eruptions are common adverse drug effects.

Toxicity

Introducing chemicals into the body can sometimes affect the body in a very noxious or toxic way. These effects are not acceptable adverse effects but are potentially serious reactions to a drug. When a drug is known to have toxic effects, the benefit of the drug to the patient must be weighed against the possibility of toxic effects that may cause the patient harm.

Hepatotoxicity

Oral drugs are absorbed and passed directly into the liver in the first-pass effect. This exposes liver cells to the full impact of the drug before it is broken down for circulation throughout the body. Most drugs are metabolized in the liver, so any metabolites that are irritating or toxic will also affect liver integrity. Medication levels may rise to dangerous levels if the liver is unable to metabolize the medication. If two or more hepatotoxic medications are combined, the risk of liver injury increases. Liver function tests can be evaluated to monitor liver function if there is a risk of damage due to medication administration. Some medications may alter the liver enzymes without clinical indications of liver dysfunction.

Assessment

Symptoms may include fever, malaise, nausea, vomiting, jaundice, change in color of urine or stools, abdominal pain or colic, elevated liver enzymes (e.g., aspartate aminotransferase, alanine aminotransferase), alterations in bilirubin levels, and changes in clotting factors (e.g., partial thromboplastin time).

Interventions

Notify the prescriber and/or primary caregiver and discontinue the drug if needed. Offer supportive measures (small and frequent meals, skin care, a cool environment, and rest periods).

Nephrotoxicity

Medications can cause nephrotoxicity via multiple mechanisms including renal vasoconstriction, direct tubular damage, intratubular obstruction, or a combination of multiple mechanisms. Some medications are excreted from the kidney unchanged from their active form, and others are modified to be metabolites. Both the active form and the metabolites have the potential to cause damage to the nephron. Gentamicin (generic), an aminoglycoside antibiotic, is frequently associated with renal toxicity.

Assessment

Elevated blood urea nitrogen (BUN), elevated creatinine (Cr) concentration, decreased urine output, electrolyte imbalances, fatigue, malaise, edema, irritability, and skin rash may be seen.

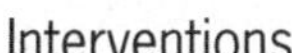

Interventions

Notify the prescriber and/or primary caregiver and discontinue the drug as needed. Offer supportive measures (positioning, diet and fluid restrictions, skin care, electrolyte therapy, rest periods, and a controlled environment). In severe cases, be aware that dialysis may be required for survival.

Poisoning

Poisoning occurs when an overdose of a drug damages multiple body systems, leading to the potential for fatal reactions. Assessment parameters vary with the particular drug. Treatment of drug poisoning also varies, depending on the drug. Throughout this book, specific antidotes or treatments for poisoning are identified, if known. Emergency and life support measures often are needed in severe cases.

Alterations in Glucose Metabolism

All cells need glucose for energy; the cells of the central nervous system (CNS) are especially dependent on constant glucose levels to function properly. The control of glucose in the body is an integrated process that involves a series of hormones and enzymes that use the liver as the place for glucose storage or release. Many drugs have an impact on glucose levels because of their effects on the liver or the endocrine system.

Hypoglycemia

Some drugs affect metabolism and the use of glucose, causing a low serum blood glucose concentration, or hypoglycemia. Glipizide (*Glucotrol*) and glyburide (*DiaBeta*) are antidiabetic agents that have the desired action of lowering the blood glucose level but can lower blood glucose too far, causing hypoglycemia.

Assessment

Symptoms may include fatigue; drowsiness; hunger; anxiety; headache; cold, clammy skin; shaking and lack of coordination (tremulousness); increased heart rate; increased blood pressure; numbness and tingling of the mouth, tongue, and/or lips; confusion; and rapid and shallow respirations. In severe cases, seizures and/or coma may occur.

Interventions

Restore glucose—orally (preferably) or intravenously. Provide supportive measures (skin care, environmental control of light and temperature, rest). Institute safety measures to prevent injury or falls. Monitor blood glucose levels to help stabilize the situation. Offer reassurance to help the patient cope with the experience.

Hyperglycemia

Some drugs stimulate the breakdown of glycogen or alter metabolism in such a way as to cause high serum glucose levels, or hyperglycemia. Prednisone, a corticosteroid that can be used to decrease inflammatory effects, can cause an elevation of blood glucose by increasing the resistance to insulin in the liver.

Assessment

Fatigue, increased urination (polyuria), increased thirst (polydipsia), deep respirations (Kussmaul respirations), restlessness, increased hunger (polyphagia), nausea, hot or flushed skin, and fruity odor to breath may be observed.

Interventions

Administer insulin therapy to decrease blood glucose as appropriate, while carefully monitoring glucose levels. Provide support to help the patient deal with signs and symptoms (e.g., provide access to bathroom facilities, control the temperature of the room, decrease stimulation while the patient is in crisis, offer reassurance, provide mouth care—the patient will experience dry mouth and bad breath with the ensuing acidosis, and mouth care will help to make this more tolerable).

Electrolyte Imbalances

Because they are chemicals acting in a body that works by chemical reactions, drugs can have an effect on various electrolyte levels in the body. The electrolyte that can cause the most serious effects when it is altered, even a little, is potassium.

Hypokalemia

Some drugs affecting the kidney can cause low serum potassium levels (hypokalemia) by altering the renal exchange system. For example, loop diuretics function by causing the loss of potassium, as well as of sodium and water. Potassium is essential for the normal functioning of nerves and muscles.

Assessment

Symptoms include a serum potassium concentration ($[K^+]$) lower than 3.5 mEq/L, weakness, numbness and tingling in the extremities, muscle cramps, nausea, vomiting, diarrhea, decreased bowel sounds, irregular pulse, weak pulse, orthostatic hypotension, and disorientation. In severe cases, paralytic ileus (absent bowel sounds, abdominal distention, and acute abdomen) may occur.

Interventions

Replace serum potassium and carefully monitor serum levels and patient response; achieving the desired level can take time, and the patient may experience high potassium levels in the process. Provide supportive therapy (e.g., safety precautions to prevent injury or falls, reorientation of the patient, comfort measures for pain and discomfort). Cardiac monitoring may be needed to evaluate the effect of the fluctuating potassium levels on heart rhythm.

Hyperkalemia

Some drugs that affect the kidney, such as the potassium-sparing diuretics, can lead to potassium retention and a resultant increase in serum potassium levels (hyperkalemia). Other drugs that cause cell death or injury, such as many antineoplastic agents, also can cause the cells to release potassium, leading to hyperkalemia.

Assessment

Symptoms include a serum potassium level higher than 5 mEq/L, weakness, muscle cramps, diarrhea, numbness and tingling, slow heart rate, low blood pressure, decreased urine output, and difficulty breathing.

Interventions

Institute measures to decrease the serum potassium concentration, including use of patiromer (*Veltassa*). When trying to stabilize the potassium level, it is possible that the patient may experience low potassium levels. Careful monitoring is important until the patient's potassium levels are stable. Offer supportive measures to cope with discomfort. Institute safety measures to prevent injury or falls. Monitor for cardiac irregularities because potassium is an important electrolyte in the action potential, which is needed for cell membrane stability. When potassium levels are too high, the cells of the heart become very irritable and rhythm disturbances can occur. Be prepared for a possible cardiac emergency. In severe cases, be aware that dialysis may be needed.

Sensory Effects

Drugs can affect the special senses, including the eyes and ears. Alterations in seeing and hearing can pose safety problems for patients.

Ocular Damage

The blood vessels in the retina are very tiny and are called "end arteries," that is, they stop and do not interconnect with other arteries feeding the same cells. Some drugs are deposited into these tiny arteries, causing inflammation and tissue damage. Chloroquine (*Aralen*), a drug used to treat some rheumatoid diseases, can cause retinal damage and even blindness.

Assessment

Blurring of vision, color vision changes, corneal damage, and blindness may be noted.

Interventions

Monitor the patient's vision carefully when the patient is receiving known oculotoxic drugs. Consult with the prescriber and/or primary caregiver and discontinue the drug as appropriate. Provide supportive measures, especially if vision loss is not reversible. Monitor lighting and exposure to sunlight.

Auditory Damage

Tiny vessels and nerves in the eighth cranial nerve are easily irritated and damaged by certain drugs. The macrolide antibiotics, if given in high doses, and the aminoglycosides, can cause severe auditory nerve damage. Aspirin, one of the most used drugs, is often linked to auditory ringing (tinnitus) and eighth cranial nerve effects.

Assessment

Dizziness, tinnitus, loss of balance, and loss of hearing may be assessed.

Interventions

Monitor the patient's perceptual losses or changes. Provide protective measures to prevent falling or injury. Consult with the prescriber to decrease dose or discontinue the drug. Provide supportive measures to cope with drug effects.

Neurological Effects

Many drugs can affect the functioning of the nerves in the periphery and the CNS. Nerves function by using a constant source of energy to maintain the resting membrane potential and allow excitation. This requires glucose, oxygen, and a balance of electrolytes.

General Central Nervous System Effects

Although the brain is fairly well protected from many drug effects by the blood–brain barrier, some drugs do affect neurological functioning, either directly or by altering electrolyte or glucose levels. Some medications may act as CNS stimulants and others may cause CNS depression. Corticosteroids have been shown to have varying effects on the CNS, causing changes in behavior including irritability, restlessness, and insomnia.

Assessment

Symptoms may include confusion, delirium, insomnia, drowsiness, hyperreflexia or hyporeflexia, bizarre dreams, hallucinations, numbness, tingling, seizures, and paresthesias.

Interventions

Provide safety measures to prevent injury. Caution the patient to avoid dangerous situations such as driving a car or operating dangerous machinery. Orient the patient and provide support. Consult with the prescriber to decrease drug dose or discontinue the drug.

Anticholinergic Effects

Some drugs block the effects of the parasympathetic nervous system by directly or indirectly blocking cholinergic receptors. Atropine, a drug used preoperatively to dry up secretions and any other indications, is the prototype anticholinergic drug. Many cold remedies and antihistamines also cause anticholinergic effects.

Assessment

Dry mouth altered taste perception, dysphagia, heartburn, constipation, bloating, paralytic ileus, urinary hesitancy and retention, impotence, blurred vision, cycloplegia (loss of ability to focus on near objects due to paralysis of the ciliary muscle of the eye), photophobia, headache, mental confusion, nasal congestion, palpitations, tachycardia, decreased sweating, and dry skin may be noted.

Interventions

Provide sugarless lozenges and mouth care to help mouth dryness. Arrange for bowel program as appropriate. Provide safety measures if vision changes occur and sunglasses to decrease photophobia. Arrange for medication for headache and nasal congestion as appropriate. Voiding prior to medication administration may reduce urinary retention. Advise patients to hydrate well to prevent dehydration and warn them of increased risk of overheating due to decreased ability to sweat.

Extrapyramidal Symptoms

Drugs that directly or indirectly affect dopamine levels in the brain can cause a syndrome resembling Parkinson's disease. Many of the antipsychotic and neuroleptic drugs can cause this effect. Haloperidol (*Haldol*) is an example of an antipsychotic medication that can cause tremor, tardive dyskinesia, dystonia, and akathisia. In most cases, the effects go away when the drug is withdrawn. These symptoms are known as extrapyramidal symptoms.

Assessment

Lack of activity, akinesia, muscular tremors, drooling, changes in gait, rigidity, extreme restlessness, or "jitters" (akathisia), or spasms (dyskinesia) may be observed.

Interventions

Discontinue the drug, if necessary. Know that treatment with anticholinergics or anti-Parkinson drugs may be recommended if the benefit of the drug outweighs the discomfort of its adverse effects. Provide small, frequent meals if swallowing becomes difficult. Provide safety measures if ambulation becomes a problem.

Neuroleptic Malignant Syndrome

General anesthetics and other drugs that have direct CNS effects can cause neuroleptic malignant syndrome (NMS), a generalized syndrome that includes high fever; if not treated quickly, NMS can be fatal. Metoclopramide (*Reglan*) is a medication that can be used for treatment of symptoms of gastroesophageal reflux and acts as a dopamine antagonist. Metoclopramide has been known to cause both tardive dyskinesia, other extrapyramidal symptoms, and NMS.

Assessment

Neurological symptoms, including slowed reflexes, rigidity, involuntary movements; hyperthermia; and autonomic disturbances, such as hypertension, fast heart rate, and fever, may be noted.

Interventions

Discontinue the drug and reduce the client's body temperature. Most common treatment is bromocriptine mesylate (a dopamine agonist) and dantrolene sodium (a muscle relaxant). This is a medical emergency.

Teratogenicity

Many drugs that reach the developing fetus or embryo can cause death or congenital defects, including skeletal and limb abnormalities, CNS alterations, and heart defects. The exact effects of a drug on the fetus may not be known. In some cases, a predictable syndrome occurs when a drug is given to an individual who is pregnant. In any situation, inform any pregnant patient who requires drug therapy about the possible effects on the baby. Before a drug is administered to a pregnant patient, the actual benefits should be weighed against the potential risks. People who are pregnant should be advised not to self-medicate during pregnancy. Emotional and physical support is needed to assist in coping with the possibility of fetal death or birth defects.

Box 3.2 summarizes all the adverse effects described throughout this chapter.

BOX 3.2

Summary of Adverse Drug Effects

- Extension of primary action
- Occurrence of secondary action
- Allergic reactions
  - Anaphylactic reactions
  - Cytotoxic reactions
  - Serum sickness reactions
  - Delayed allergic reactions
- Tissue and organ damage
  - Dermatological reactions
  - Stomatitis
  - Gastrointestinal irritation
  - Superinfections
  - Blood dyscrasia
- Toxicity
  - Hepatotoxicity
  - Nephrotoxicity
  - Poisoning
- Alterations in glucose metabolism
  - Hypoglycemia
  - Hyperglycemia
- Electrolyte imbalances
  - Hypokalemia
  - Hyperkalemia
- Sensory effects
  - Ocular toxicity
  - Auditory damage
- Neurological effects
  - General CNS effects
  - Atropinelike (cholinergic) effects
  - Extrapyramidal symptoms
  - Neuroleptic malignant syndrome
- Teratogenicity

SUMMARY

- No drug does only what is desired of it. All drugs have adverse effects associated with them.
- Adverse drug effects can range from allergic reactions to tissue and cellular damage. The nurse, as the health care provider most associated with drug administration, needs to assess each situation for potential adverse effects and intervene appropriately to minimize those effects.
- Adverse effects can be extensions of the primary action of a drug or secondary effects that are not necessarily desirable but are unavoidable.
- Allergic reactions can occur when a person's body makes antibodies to a drug or drug protein. If the person is exposed to that drug at another time, an immune response may occur. Allergic reactions can be of various types. The exact response should be noted to avoid future confusion in patient care.
- Tissue damage can include skin problems, mucous membrane inflammation, blood dyscrasias, superinfections, liver or renal toxicity, poisoning, hypoglycemia or hyperglycemia, electrolyte disturbances, various CNS problems (ocular damage, auditory damage, anticholinergic effects, extrapyramidal symptoms, NMS), and teratogenicity.

Unfolding Patient Stories: Toua Xiong • Part 1

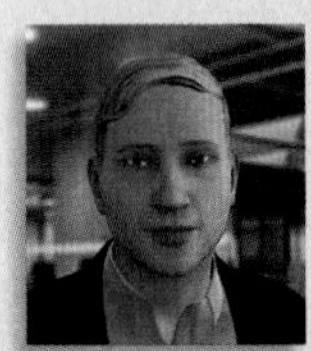

Toua Xiong has a 45-year history of smoking and is diagnosed with emphysema. The provider orders albuterol and ipratropium via metered-dose inhalers. What patient education would the nurse provide on the action and side effects of the medications? How would the nurse explain the use of an inhaler with a spacer and the sequence of medication delivery when the inhalers are ordered for the same time? (Toua Xiong's story continues in Chapter 55.)

Care for Toua and other patients in a realistic virtual environment: ***vSim** for Nursing* (thepoint.lww.com/vSimPharm). Practice documenting these patients' care in DocuCare (thepoint.lww.com/DocuCareEHR).

CHECK YOUR UNDERSTANDING

Answers to the questions in this chapter can be found in Answers to Check Your Understanding Questions on thePoint®.

MULTIPLE CHOICE

Select the best answer.

1. An example of a drug allergy is
   a. dry mouth occurring with use of an antihistamine.
   b. increased urination occurring with use of a thiazide diuretic.
   c. breathing difficulty after an injection of penicillin.
   d. urinary retention associated with atropine use.

2. A patient taking glyburide (an antidiabetic drug) has their morning dose and then does not have a chance to eat for several hours. An adverse effect that might be expected from this would be
   a. a teratogenic effect.
   b. a skin rash.
   c. an anticholinergic effect.
   d. hypoglycemia.

3. A patient with a severe infection is given gentamicin, the only antibiotic shown to be effective in culture and sensitivity tests. A few hours after the drug is started intravenously, the patient becomes very restless and develops edema. Blood tests reveal abnormal electrolytes and elevated blood urea nitrogen. This reaction was most likely caused by
   a. an anaphylactic reaction.
   b. renal toxicity associated with gentamicin.
   c. superinfection related to the antibiotic.
   d. hypoglycemia.

4. Patients receiving antineoplastic drugs that disrupt cell function often have adverse effects involving cells that turn over rapidly in the body. These cells include
   a. ovarian cells.
   b. liver cells.
   c. cardiac cells.
   d. bone marrow cells.

5. A patient has had repeated bouts of bronchitis throughout the fall and has been taking antibiotics. They call the clinic with complaints of vaginal pain and itching. When they are seen, it is discovered that they have developed a yeast infection. You understand that
   a. the patient's bronchitis has moved to the vaginal area.
   b. the patient has developed a superinfection, because the antibiotics kill bacteria that normally provide protection.
   c. the patient probably has developed a sexually transmitted disease.
   d. the patient will need to take even more antibiotics to treat this new infection.

6. Knowing that a patient is taking a loop diuretic and is at risk for developing hypokalemia, the nurse would assess the patient for
   a. hypertension, headache, and cold and clammy skin.
   b. decreased urinary output and yellowing of the sclera.
   c. weak pulse, low blood pressure, and muscle cramping.
   d. diarrhea and flatulence.

MULTIPLE RESPONSE

Select all that apply.

1. A patient is taking a drug that is known to be toxic to the liver. The patient is being discharged to home. What teaching points related to liver toxicity and the drug should the nurse teach the patient to report to the physician?
   a. Fever; changes in the color of urine
   b. Changes in the color of stool; malaise
   c. Rapid, deep respirations; increased sweating
   d. Dizziness; drowsiness; dry mouth
   e. Rash; black or hairy tongue; white spots in the mouth or throat
   f. Yellowing of the skin or the whites of the eyes

2. People who are pregnant should be advised of the potential risk to the fetus any time they take a drug during pregnancy. What fetal problems can be related to drug exposure in utero?
   a. Fetal death
   b. Nervous system disruption
   c. Skeletal and limb abnormalities
   d. Cardiac defects
   e. Low-set ears
   f. Deafness

3. A client is experiencing a reaction to the penicillin injection that the nurse administered approximately ½ hour ago. The nurse is concerned that it might be an anaphylactic reaction. What signs and symptoms would validate the nurse's suspicion?
   a. Rapid heart rate
   b. Diaphoresis
   c. Constricted pupils
   d. Hypotension
   e. Rash
   f. Client report of a panicky feeling

4. A client is experiencing a serum sickness reaction (type III allergy) to a recent rubella vaccination. Which of the following interventions would be appropriate when caring for this client?
   a. Administration of epinephrine
   b. Cool environment
   c. Positioning to provide comfort
   d. Ice to joints as needed
   e. Administration of anti-inflammatory agents
   f. Administration of topical corticosteroids

REFERENCES

Alqenae, F. A., Steinke, D., & Keers, R. N. (2020). Prevalence and nature of medication errors and medication-related harm following discharge from hospital to community settings: A systematic review. *Drug Safety, 43*(6), 517–537. https://www.ncbi.nlm.nih.gov/pmc/articles/PMC7235049/

Armitage, G., & Knapman, H. (2003). Adverse events in drug administration: A literature review. *Journal of Nursing Management, 11*(2), 130–140. https://onlinelibrary.wiley.com/doi/full/10.1046/j.1365-2834.2003.00359.x

Benkirane, R. R., R-Abouqal, R., Haimeur, C. C., S Ech Chefif El Kettani, S. S., Salma, S., Azzouzi, A. A., M'daghri Alaoui, A. A., Thimou, A. A., Nejmi, M. M., Maazouzi, W. W., Madani, N. N., R-Edwards, I., & Soulaymani, R. R. (2009). Incidence of adverse drug events and medication errors in intensive care units: A prospective multicenter study. *Journal of Patient Safety, 5*(1), 16–22. https://doi.org/10.1097/PTS.0b013e3181990d51

Bennett, C. L., Nebekar, J. R., Lyons, E. A., Samore, M. H., Feldman, M. D., McKoy, J. M., Carson, K. R., Belknap, S. M., Trifilio, S. M., Schumock, G. T., Yarnold, P. R., Davidson, C. J., Evens, A. M., Kuzel, T. M., Parada, J. P., Cournoyer, D., West, D. P., Sartor, O., Tallman, M. S., & Raisch, D. W. (2005). The research on adverse drug events and reports (RADAR) project. *Journal of the American Medical Association, 293*(17), 2131–2140. https://jamanetwork.com/journals/jama/fullarticle/200826

Brunton, L. L., Hilal-Dandan, R., & Knollman, B. C. (2018). *Goodman & Gilman's the pharmacological basis of therapeutics* (13th ed.). McGraw-Hill.

Budnitz, D. S., Pollack, D. A., Weidenbach, K. N., Mendelsohn, A. B., Schroeder, T. J., & Annest, J. L. (2006). National surveillance of emergency department visits for outpatient adverse drug events. *Journal of the American Medical Association, 296*(15), 1858–1866. https://jamanetwork.com/journals/jama/fullarticle/203690

Ciriaco, M., Ventrice, P., Russo, G., Scicchitano, M., Mazzitello, G., Scicchitano, F., & Russo, E. (2013). Corticosteroid-related central nervous system side effects. *Journal of Pharmacology and Pharmacotherapeutics, 4*(5), 94–98. https://doi.org/10.4103/0976-500X.120975

Lewis, P. J., Dornan, T., Taylor, D., Tully, M. P., Wass, V., & Ashcroft, D. M. (2009). Prevalence, incidence and nature of prescribing errors in hospital inpatients: A systematic review. *Drug Safety, 32*(5), 379–389. https://pubmed.ncbi.nlm.nih.gov/19419233/

Norris, T. L., & Lalchandani, R. (2018). *Porth's pathophysiology: Concepts of altered health states* (10th ed.). Wolters Kluwer.

Pierson, S., Hansen, R., Greene, S., Williams, C., Akers, R., Jonsson, M., & Carey, T. (2007). Preventing medication errors in long-term care: Results and evaluation of a large scale web-based error reporting system. *Quality and Safety in Health Care, 16*(4), 297–302. https://www.ncbi.nlm.nih.gov/pmc/articles/PMC2464957/

Stefanacci, R. G., & Riddle, A. (2016). Preventing medication errors. *Geriatric Nursing, 37*(4), 307–310. https://doi.org/10.1016/j.gerinurse.2016.06.005

Thomsen, L. A., Winterstein, A. G., Søndergaard, B., Haugbølle, L. S., & Melander, A. (2007). Systematic review of the incidence and characteristics of preventable adverse drug events in ambulatory care. *Annals of Pharmacotherapy, 41*(9), 1411–1426. https://journals.sagepub.com/doi/10.1345/aph.1H658

Tucker, R. (2021). *2022 pocket drug guide for nurses* (10th ed.). Wolters Kluwer.

U. S. Food and Drug Administration. (2021). *MedWatch: The FDA safety information and adverse event reporting program.* https://www.fda.gov/safety/medwatch-fda-safety-information-and-adverse-event-reporting-program

Wecker, L., Taylor, D. A., & Theobald Jr., R. J. (2018). *Brody's human pharmacology: Mechanism-based therapeutics* (6th ed.). Elsevier.

CHAPTER 4

The Nursing Process in Drug Therapy and Patient Safety

Learning Objectives

Upon completion of this chapter, you will be able to:

1. List the responsibilities of the nurse in drug therapy.
2. Explain each step of the nursing process as it relates to drug therapy.
3. Describe key points to incorporate into the assessment of a patient receiving drug therapy.
4. Describe types of nursing interventions involved in drug therapy.
5. Outline the important points to assess and consider before administering a drug, combining knowledge about the drug with knowledge of the patient and environment.
6. Describe the role of the nurse and the patient in preventing medication errors.

Key Terms

assessment: information gathering regarding the current status of a particular patient, including evaluation of past history and physical examination; provides a baseline of information and clues to effectiveness of therapy

evaluation: part of the nursing process; determining the effects of the interventions that were instituted for the patient and leading to further assessment and intervention

interventions: actions undertaken to meet a patient's needs, such as administration of drugs, comfort measures, or patient teaching

nursing: the art of nurturing and administering to the sick, combined with the scientific application of chemistry, anatomy, physiology, biology, nutrition, psychology, and pharmacology to the particular clinical situation

nursing conclusion: statement of an actual or potential concern, based on the assessment of a particular clinical situation, which directs needed nursing interventions

nursing process: the problem-solving process used to provide efficient nursing care; it involves gathering information, formulating a nursing conclusion, prioritizing the concerns for the patient/family, developing goals and desired outcomes for the patient/family, carrying out interventions, and evaluating the process

planning: the process of prioritizing the information gathered in assessment and, using the nursing conclusions, develop goals and desired outcomes for the patient/family

The delivery of medical care today is in a constant state of change, at times reaching crisis levels. The population is aging, resulting in an increased incidence and prevalence of chronic disease and more complex care issues. The population also is more transient, with individuals and families more mobile, often resulting in unstable support systems and fewer at-home care providers and helpers. At the same time, health care is undergoing a technological boom, including greater use of more sophisticated diagnostic methods and treatments; new, specialized drugs, including experimental drugs. Moreover, patients are being discharged earlier from acute care facilities or are not being admitted at all for procedures that used to be treated in-hospital with follow-up support and monitoring. Patients also are becoming more responsible for their care and for adhering to complicated medical regimens at home. The wide use of the internet and an emphasis in the media on the need to question all aspects of health care have led to more knowledgeable and challenging patients. Patients may no longer accept a drug regimen or therapy without question and often feel confident in adjusting it on their own because of information that they have found on the internet—information that might not be very accurate or even relevant to their particular situation.

Nursing: Art and Science

Nursing is a unique and complex science, as well as a nurturing and caring art. In the traditional sense, nursing has been viewed as ministering to and soothing the sick. In the current state of medical changes, nursing also has become increasingly technical and scientific. Nurses are assuming increasing responsibilities that involve not only nurturing and caring but also assessing and intervening to treat, prevent, and educate as they assist patients and families in coping with various health states. It is expected for the nurse to have knowledge of the laws governing prescribing and dispensing medications. Pharmacology is a field that changes quickly, so it is important that nurses have reliable and up-to-date resources to refer to for medication information, including indications for use, mechanisms of action, routes of administration, safe dosage range, adverse effects, precautions, contraindications, and interactions.

The nurse deals with the whole person, including physical, emotional, intellectual, social, cultural, and spiritual aspects. Nurses must consider how a person responds to disease and its treatment, including the changes in lifestyle that may be required. Therefore, a nurse is a key health care professional in a position to assess the whole patient, to administer therapy as well as medications, to teach the patient how best to cope with the therapy so as to ensure the most favorable outcome, and to evaluate the effectiveness of the therapy. Nurses collaborate with providers who legally write medication prescriptions and with pharmacists who dispense the medications.

The nurse is a key component in developing and implementing patient-centered care. Nurses accomplish these tasks by integrating knowledge of the basic sciences (anatomy, physiology, nutrition, chemistry, pharmacology), the social sciences (sociology, psychology), education, and many other disciplines and by applying the nursing process.

The Nursing Process

Nurses use the **nursing process**—a decision-making, problem-solving process—to provide efficient and effective care. Although not all nursing theorists completely agree on this process that defines the practice of nursing, most do include certain key elements: assessment, nursing conclusions, planning, intervention, and evaluation. Application of the nursing process with drug therapy ensures that the patient receives the best, safest, most efficient, scientifically based, holistic care. Box 4.1 outlines the steps of the nursing process, which are discussed in detail in the following paragraphs.

Assessment

Assessment (gathering information) is the first step of the nursing process. This involves systematic, organized collection of data about the patient. Because the nurse is responsible for holistic care, data must include information about

BOX 4.1 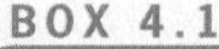

The Steps of the Nursing Process

Nursing Process

↓

ASSESSMENT

Past History

- Chronic conditions
- Drug use, including prescription, OTC, herbal, and street drugs
- Allergies
- Level of education
- Level of understanding of disease and therapy
- Social supports
- Financial supports
- Pattern of health care

Physical Examination

- Weight
- Age
- Physical parameters related to the disease state or known drug effects

↓

NURSING CONCLUSION

↓

PLANNING

↓

INTERVENTION

Proper Drug Administration

- Patient
- Drug
- Storage
- Route
- Dose
- Preparation
- Timing
- Recording

Comfort Measures

- Placebo effect
- Managing side effects
- Lifestyle adjustments

Patient/Family Education

↓

EVALUATION

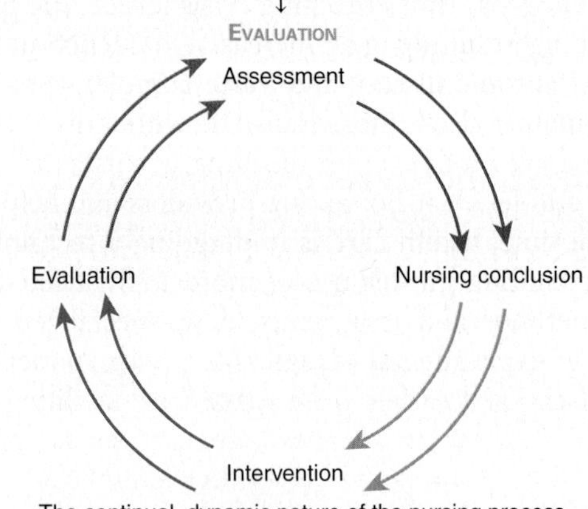

The continual, dynamic nature of the nursing process.

physical, intellectual, emotional, social, cultural, and environmental factors. When viewed together, this information provides the nurse with the facts needed to plan educational and discharge programs, arrange for appropriate consultations, and monitor the physical response to treatment or to disease.

Each nurse develops a unique approach to the organization of the assessment, one that is functional and useful in the clinical setting and that makes sense to that nurse and in the particular clinical situation. Regardless of the approach, the process of assessment never ends because the patient is in a dynamic state, continuously adjusting to physical, emotional, and environmental influences.

Drug therapy is a complex and important part of health care, and the principles of drug therapy must be incorporated into every patient assessment plan. The particular information that is needed varies with each drug, but the concepts involved are similar. Two major aspects associated with assessment are the patient's history (past illnesses and the current problem) and examination of their physical status.

History

The patient's history is an important element of assessment related to drug therapy because their past experiences and illnesses can influence a drug's effect. Knowledge of this important information before beginning drug therapy will help to promote safe and effective use of the drug and prevent adverse effects, clinically important drug–drug, drug–food, or drug–alternative therapy interactions, and medication errors. Relevant aspects of the patient's history specifically related to drug therapy are discussed next.

Chronic Conditions

Chronic conditions can affect the pharmacokinetics and pharmacodynamics of a drug. For example, certain conditions (e.g., renal disease, heart disease, diabetes, chronic lung disease) may be contraindications to the use of a drug. In addition, these conditions may require cautious use or dose adjustment when administering a certain drug. For example, a patient with renal disease may require a decreased dose of a drug owing to the way the drug is eliminated. If renal disease is mentioned in the patient history, the nurse should consider this factor to evaluate the dose of the drug that is prescribed.

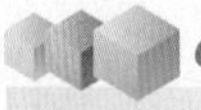

Concept Mastery Alert

Nursing Care of the Diabetic Client

Clients with diabetes who are prescribed new antihyperglycemic medication should be assessed for any other chronic conditions. The client's history is an important element of assessment related to drug therapy because prior and comorbid illnesses and current medications can influence a drug's effect. Once the presence of any other condition is established, the nurse can educate the client on adverse effects and how to take their medication.

Drug Use

Medication reconciliation is the process in which a list of every medication that the client is taking is documented, including the specific dosage, route, and last time it was taken. Medication reconciliation is required for each patient when they are being admitted and discharged from the hospital and/or being transferred between units or facilities. Medication reconciliation should also be completed for the patient at every outpatient visit as well.

Prescription drugs, over-the-counter (OTC) drugs, street drugs, alcohol, nicotine, alternative therapies, and caffeine may have an impact on a drug's effect. Patients often neglect to mention OTC drugs or alternative therapies because they do not consider them to be actual drugs, or they may be unwilling to admit their use to the health care provider. Ask patients specifically about OTC drugs (e.g., Do you buy any drugs to help you with cold symptoms, headaches, etc.?) or alternative therapy use (e.g., Do you use any herbs or other products to help control symptoms?). Patients also might forget to mention prescription drugs that they routinely take (such as oral contraceptives). Always ask specifically about all types of medications that the patient might use.

Allergies

A patient's history of allergies can affect drug therapy. Past exposure to a drug or other allergens can provoke a future reaction or necessitate the need for cautious use of the drug, food, or animal product. Obtain specific information about the patient's allergic reaction to determine whether the patient has experienced a true drug allergy or was experiencing an actual effect or adverse effect of the drug.

Level of Education and Understanding

Information about the patient's level of education provides a baseline from which the nurse can determine the appropriate types of teaching information to use with the patient. Gathering information about the patient's level of understanding about their condition, illness, or drug therapy helps the nurse determine where the patient is in terms of their status and the level of explanation that will be required. It also provides additional baseline information for developing a patient education program. It is important not to assume anything about the patient's ability to understand based on their reported education level. Stress, disease, and environmental factors can all affect a patient's learning readiness and ability. Direct assessment of actual learning abilities is critical for good patient education.

Social Supports

Patients are being discharged from health care facilities faster than ever before, often with continuing care needs. In addition, faster discharges leave minimal time for teaching. Often patients need help at home with care and drug therapy. A key aspect of discharge planning involves determining what support, if any, is available to the patient at home. In many situations, it also involves referral to appropriate community resources.

Financial Supports

The high cost of health care in general and of medications in particular must be considered when initiating drug therapy and promoting patient compliance. Financial constraints may cause a patient not to follow through with a prescribed drug regimen. For example, the drug may be too expensive or the patient may lack the means to get to a pharmacy to obtain the drug. In some situations, a less expensive drug might be appropriate in place of a very expensive drug. In addition, the nurse may need to refer the patient to appropriate resources that might offer financial assistance.

Pattern of Health Care

Knowing how a patient seeks health care provides the nurse with valuable information to include when preparing the patient's teaching plan. Does this patient routinely seek follow-up care, or do they wait for emergency situations? Does the patient tend to self-treat many complaints, or is every problem brought to a health care provider? Information about patterns of health care also provides insight into conditions that the patient may have but has not reported or medication use that has not been stated.

Physical Examination

It is important to assess the patient's physical status before beginning drug therapy. This assessment helps determine if any conditions exist that would be contraindications or cautions for using the drug and helps develop a baseline for evaluating the effectiveness of the drug and the occurrence of any adverse effects (Box 4.2). Relevant aspects of the patient's physical examination specifically related to drug therapy are discussed in the following text.

Weight

A patient's weight helps to determine whether the recommended drug dose is appropriate. Because the recommended dose typically is based on a 150-lb adult man, patients who are much lighter or much heavier often need a dose adjustment.

Age

Patients at the extremes of the age spectrum—children and older adults—often require dose adjustments based on the functional level of the liver and kidneys and the responsiveness of other organs. The child's age and developmental level will also alert the nurse to possible problems with drug delivery, such as the ability to swallow pills or follow directions related to other delivery methods. The child's developmental age will also influence pharmacokinetics and pharmacodynamics; the immature liver may not metabolize drugs in the same way as in the adult, or the kidneys may not be as efficient as those of an adult. As patients age, the body undergoes many normal changes that can affect drug therapy, such as decreased blood volume, decreased gastrointestinal absorption, reduced blood flow to muscles or skin, and changes in receptor site responsiveness. Older adults may often have a variety of chronic medical conditions and could be receiving a number of medications that need to be evaluated for possible interactions. Older adults with various central nervous system disorders, like Alzheimer's disease or Parkinson's disease, may develop difficulty swallowing and might require liquid forms of medication. Throughout this book, "Drug Therapy across the Lifespan" features will present information related to the drug class being discussed as it pertains specifically to children, adults, and the older population. These boxes highlight points that the nurse should consider to ensure safe and effective therapy in each age group.

Box 4.2 Focus on Safe Medication Administration

Review the monographs in a drug guide or handbook for specific parameters to be assessed in relation to the particular drug being discussed. This assessment provides not only the baseline information needed before giving that drug but also the data required to evaluate the effects of that drug on the patient. This information should supplement the overall nursing assessment of the patient, which includes social, intellectual, financial, environmental, and other factors.

Physical Parameters Related to Disease or Drug Effects

The specific parameters that need to be assessed depend on the disease process being treated and the expected therapeutic and adverse effects of the drug therapy. Assessing these factors before drug therapy begins provides a baseline level with which future assessments can be compared to determine the effects of drug therapy. For example, if a patient is being treated for chronic pulmonary disease, their respiratory status and reserve need to be assessed, especially if a drug known to affect the respiratory tract is being given. In contrast, a thorough respiratory evaluation would not be warranted in a patient with no known pulmonary disease who is taking a drug with little or no known effects on the respiratory system. Because the nurse has the greatest direct and continued contact with the patient, the nurse is in the best position to detect subtle changes that ultimately determine the course of drug therapy—therapeutic success or discontinuation because of adverse or unacceptable responses (see Box 4.2).

Nursing Conclusion

A **nursing conclusion** is simply a statement of the patient's status from a nursing perspective. The nurse analyzes the information gathered during assessment to describe an actual or potential concern that leads to a particular goal and set of interventions. A nursing conclusion shows actual or potential alterations in patient function based on assessment of the clinical situation. Because drug therapy is only a small part of the overall patient situation, nursing conclusions related to drug therapy must be incorporated into a total picture of the patient.

In the nursing considerations sections of this book, the nursing conclusions listed are those that reflect potential alteration of function based only on the particular drug's actions (i.e., therapeutic and adverse effects). No consideration is given to environmental or disease-related problems.

Planning

Nursing **planning** involves taking and prioritizing the information gathered and synthesized in the nursing conclusions to plan the patient care. This process includes setting goals and desired patient outcomes to ensure safe and effective drug therapy. These outcomes usually involve ensuring effective response to drug therapy, minimizing adverse effects, and understanding the drug regimen.

Intervention

Nursing **interventions** aim at achieving the goals of outcomes determined in the planning phase. Three types of nursing interventions are frequently involved in drug therapy: drug administration, provision of comfort measures, and patient/family education.

Proper Drug Administration

Proper drug administration begins with evaluation of the prescription. The components of a medication prescription include the client's first and last name, date and time, name of medication, dose of medication, route of administration, time and frequency of administration, quantity to dispense or duration if being prescribed in the hospital, number of refills (if any), and the signature of the prescribing provider.

The nurse must consider eight points, or "rights," to ensure safe and effective drug administration. These are right drug and patient, right storage of drug, right and most effective route, right dose, right preparation, right timing, and right recording of administration. See the later section on the prevention of medication errors for a detailed explanation of the nurse's role in implementing these rights. Remembering to review each point before administering a drug will help to prevent medication errors and improve patient outcomes.

Comfort Measures

Nurses are in a unique position to help the patient cope with the effects of drug therapy. A patient is more likely to be compliant with a drug regimen if the effects of the regimen are not too uncomfortable or overwhelming.

Placebo Effect

The anticipation that a drug will be helpful (placebo effect) has proven to have tremendous impact on the actual success of drug therapy. Therefore, the nurse's attitude and support can be a critical part of drug therapy. For example, a back rub, a kind word, and a positive approach may be as beneficial as the drug itself.

Managing Adverse Effects

Interventions can be directed at promoting patient safety and decreasing the impact of the anticipated adverse effects of a drug. Such interventions include environmental control (e.g., temperature, light), safety measures (e.g., avoiding driving, avoiding the sun, using side rails), and physical comfort measures (e.g., skin care, laxatives, frequent meals).

Lifestyle Adjustment

Some medications and their effects require that a patient make changes in their lifestyle. For example, patients taking diuretics may have to rearrange their day to be near toilet facilities when the drug action peaks. Patients taking bisphosphonates will need to plan their morning so they can take the drug on an empty stomach, stay upright for at least half an hour, and plan their first food of the day at least half an hour after taking the drug. Many drugs come with similar guidelines for ensuring effectiveness and decreasing adverse effects. Patients taking monoamine oxidase inhibitors must adjust their diet to prevent serious adverse effects due to potential drug–food interactions. In some cases, the change in lifestyle that is needed can have a tremendous impact on the patient and can affect their ability to cope and comply with any medical regimen. Lifestyle changes are quite difficult for patients to accomplish, and therefore, adherence with drug therapy requires a great deal of support, education, and encouragement (Box 4.3).

Patient and Family Education

With patients becoming increasingly responsible for their own care, it is essential that they have all the information necessary to ensure safe and effective drug therapy at home. In fact, many states now require that patients be given written information. Box 4.4 includes key elements for any drug education program. Also see the later section on prevention of medication errors for patient teaching tips related to the patient's role in preventing medication errors.

Evaluation

Evaluation is part of the continuing process of patient care that leads to changes in assessment, conclusion, planning, and intervention. The patient is continually evaluated for therapeutic response, the occurrence of adverse drug effects, and the occurrence of drug–drug, drug–food,

Box 4.3 Focus on Safe Medication Administration

Special points regarding drug administration and related comfort measures are noted with each drug class discussed in this book. Refer to the individual drug monographs in a drug guide or handbook for more detailed interventions regarding a specific drug.

Box 4.4 Focus on Patient and Family Teaching

INCLUDE THE FOLLOWING KEY ELEMENTS IN ANY DRUG EDUCATION PROGRAM

1. *Name, dose, and action of drug:* Ensure that patients know this information. Many patients see more than one health care provider; this knowledge is crucial to ensuring safe and effective drug therapy and avoiding drug–drug interactions. Urge patients to keep a written and/or electronic list of the drugs that they are taking to show to any health care provider taking care of them and in case of an emergency when they are not able to report their drug history.
2. *Timing of administration:* Teach patients when to take the drug with respect to frequency, other drugs, and meals.
3. *Special storage and preparation instructions:* Inform patients about any special handling or storing required. Some drugs may require refrigeration; others may need to be mixed with a specific liquid such as water or fruit juice. Be sure that patients know how to carry out these requirements.
4. *Specific OTC drugs or alternative therapies to avoid:* Prevent possible interactions between prescribed drugs and other drugs or remedies the patient may be using or taking. Many patients do not consider OTC drugs or herbal or alternative therapies to be actual drugs and may inadvertently take them along with their prescribed medications, causing unwanted or even dangerous drug–drug interactions. Prevent these situations by explaining which drugs or therapies should be avoided. Encourage patients to always report all of the drugs or therapies that they are using to health care providers to reduce the risk of possible inadvertent adverse effects.
5. *Special comfort measures:* Teach patients how to cope with anticipated adverse effects to ease anxiety and avoid noncompliance with drug therapy. If a patient knows that a diuretic is going to lead to increased urination, the day can be scheduled so that bathrooms are nearby when they might be needed. Also educate patients about the importance of follow-up tests or evaluation.
6. *Safety measures:* Instruct all patients to keep drugs out of the reach of children. Remind all patients to inform any health care provider they see about the drugs they are taking; this can prevent drug–drug interactions and misdiagnoses based on drug effects. Also alert patients to possible safety issues that could arise as a result of drug therapy. For example, teach patients to avoid driving or performing hazardous tasks if they are taking drugs that can make them dizzy or alter their thinking or response time.
7. *Specific points about drug toxicity:* Give patients a list of warning signs of drug toxicity. Advise patients to notify their health care provider if any of these effects occur.
8. *Specific warnings about drug discontinuation:* Remember that some drugs with a small margin of safety and drugs with particular systemic effects cannot be stopped abruptly without dangerous effects. Alert patients who are taking these types of drugs to this problem and encourage them to call their health care provider immediately if they cannot take their medication for any reason (e.g., illness, financial constraints).

drug–alternative therapy, or drug–laboratory test interactions. Some drug therapy requires evaluation of specific therapeutic drug levels. In addition, the efficacy of the nursing interventions and the education program also are evaluated. In some situations, the nurse evaluates the patient simply by reapplying the beginning steps of the nursing process and then analyzing for changes, either positive or negative. The process of evaluation may lead to changes in the nursing interventions being used to provide better and safer patient care.

Key Points

- Nurses use the nursing process to provide a framework for organizing the information that is needed to provide safe and effective patient care.
- The steps of the nursing process (assessment, nursing conclusion, planning, intervention, and evaluation) are constantly being repeated to meet the ever-changing needs of the patient/family.
- The nursing process provides an effective method for handling all of the scientific and technical information, as well as the unique emotional, social, and physical factors that each patient brings to a given situation.

Medication Errors

With the increase in the older adult patient population, the increase in the number of available drugs and OTC and alternative therapy preparations, and the reduced length of hospital stays for patients, the risk for medication errors is ever increasing. In 2000, the Institute of Medicine published a large-scale study of medication errors in the United States, entitled *To Err Is Human: Building a Safer Health System.* It reported that 44,000 reported deaths in hospitals each year occurred from medication errors and that the number could probably be closer to 98,000. Reports since this initial call to action estimate that the number of errors is now much higher, with fewer patients staying in the hospital and estimate that the annual cost to the health care system is over $21 billion each year. The study brought to light the many places in the system where a medication error could occur and suggested methods for improving the problem.

The drug regimen process, which includes prescribing, dispensing, and administering a drug to a patient, has a series of checks along the way to help catch errors before they occur. These include the physician or nurse practitioner who prescribes a drug, the pharmacist who dispenses the drug, and the nurse who administers the drug. Each serves as a check within the system to catch errors—the wrong drug, the wrong patient, the wrong dose, the wrong route, the wrong time, the wrong storage, or the wrong documentation. Often the nurse is the final check in the process because the nurse is the one who administers the drug and is the one responsible for patient education before the patient is discharged.

Nurse's Role

The monumental task of ensuring medication safety with all the potential problems that could confront the patient can best be managed by consistently using the "rights" of medication administration (Box 4.5).

Box 4.5 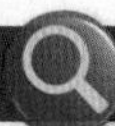 **Focus on Safe Medication Administration**

1. *Right patient.* It is always important to make sure that you are giving the drug to the correct patient. Checking the patient's wrist band and asking the patient to repeat their name and often birth date are good policies to make sure it is the patient you think it is. Avoid the error of asking a patient, "Are you Mr. Jones?" The patient could respond yes without thinking or may not have heard you correctly. Rely on the patient telling you their name and read it from the identification band. It is also important to make sure that the patient does not have allergies to the drug being given and that the patient is not taking interacting drugs, food, or alternative therapies.
2. *Right drug.* To prevent medication errors, always check to make sure that the drug you are going to administer is the one that was prescribed. Many drugs may look alike and/or have sound-alike names. Ask for the generic as well as the brand name if you are unsure. Never assume the computer is correct; always double-check. Avoid abbreviations, and if you are not sure about abbreviations that were used, ask. Make sure that the drug makes sense for the patient for whom it is ordered.
3. *Right storage.* Be aware that some drugs require specific storage environments (e.g., refrigeration, protection from light). Check to make sure that general guidelines have been followed.
4. *Right route.* Determine the best route of administration; this is frequently established by the formulation of the drug. Nurses can often have an impact in modifying the route to arrive at the most efficient, comfortable method for the patient based on the patient's specific situation. For example, perhaps a patient is having trouble swallowing, and a large capsule would be very difficult for the patient to handle. The nurse could check and see if the drug is available in a liquid form and bring this information to the attention of the person prescribing the drug. When establishing the prescribed route, check the proper method of administering a drug by that route. Review drug administration methods periodically to make sure that you have not forgotten important techniques. If you have instructed a patient in the proper administration of a drug, be sure to have the patient explain it back to you and demonstrate the proper technique. This should be done not only when the patient first learns this technique but also periodically to make sure that they have not forgotten any important points. Throughout this book, "Focus on Safe Medication Administration" boxes will provide review of proper medication administration technique.
5. *Right dose.* Always double-check calculations, and always do the calculations if the drug is not available in the dose ordered. Calculate the drug dose appropriately, based on the available drug form, the patient's body weight or surface area, or the patient's kidney function. Do not assume that the computer program or preparation of the medication by the pharmacist is always right; you are one more check in the system. Do not cut tablets to get to a correct dose without checking to make sure that the tablet can be cut, crushed, or chewed. Many tablets cannot be altered this way. Be very cautious if you see an order that starts with a decimal point; these orders are often the cause of medication errors. You should never see .5 mg as an order because it could be interpreted as 5 mg, 10 times the ordered dose. The proper dose would be 0.5 mg. If you see an order for 5.0 mg, be cautious; it could be interpreted as 50 mg. If a dose seems too big, question it. Throughout this book, "Focus on Calculations" boxes will provide review for calculating dose properly.
6. *Right preparation.* Know the specific preparation required before administering any drug. For example, oral drugs may need to be crushed or shaken; parenteral drugs may need to be reconstituted or diluted with specific solutions; and topical drugs may require specific handling, such as the use of gloves during administration or shaving of a body area before application. Many current oral drugs cannot be cut, crushed, or chewed. Checking that information can help to prevent serious adverse effects. If a drug needs to be diluted or reconstituted, check the manufacturer's instructions to make sure that this is done correctly.
7. *Right time.* When drugs are studied and evaluated, a suggested timing of administration is established. This timing takes into account all aspects of pharmacokinetics to determine a dosing schedule that will provide the needed therapeutic level of the drug. Recognize that the administration of one drug may require coordination with the administration of other drugs, foods, or physical parameters. In a busy hospital setting, getting the drug to the patient at the prescribed time can be a real challenge. As the caregiver most frequently involved in administering drugs, the nurse must be aware of and manage all of these factors, as well as educate the patient to do this on their own. Organizing the day and the drug regimen to make it the least intrusive on a patient's lifestyle can help to prevent errors and improve compliance. Providing written instructions regarding timing can be crucial in some situations.
8. *Right recording.* Always document drug administration. If it isn't written, it didn't happen. Document the information in accordance with the local requirements for recording medication administration after assessing the patient, making the appropriate nursing diagnoses, and delivering the correct drug, by the correct route, in the correct dose, and at the correct time. Accurately record the drug given and the time given only once you have given the drug to avoid inadvertent overdoses or missing doses, which would lead to a lack of therapeutic effect. Encourage patients to keep track of their drugs at home, what they take, and when they take it, especially if they could be confused.

The Patient's Role

With so many patients managing their drug regimens at home, one other very important check in the system also exists: the patient. Only the patient really knows what is being taken and when, and only the patient can report the actual as opposed to the prescribed drug regimen being followed. Patient and family education plays a vital role in the prevention of medication errors. Encourage patients to be their own advocates and to speak up and ask questions. Doing so helps prevent medication errors. The following teaching points help reduce the risk of medication errors in the home setting:

- *Keep a written and/or electronic list of all medications you are taking, including prescription, OTC, and herbal medications.* Keep this list with you at all times in case of an emergency in which health care providers may not have the current information. This list can be essential if you are traveling and need to refill a prescription while away from home.
- *Know what each of your drugs is being used to treat.* If you know why you are taking each drug, you will have a better understanding of what to report, what to watch for, and when to report to your health care provider if the drug is not working.
- *Read the labels and follow the directions.* It is easy to make up your own schedule or to just take everything all at once in the morning. Always check the labels to see if there are specific times you should be taking your drugs. Make a calendar or use an electronic organizer/app to help remind you to take your medications at correct times. A weekly pillbox may also help organize the medications.
- *Store drugs in a dry place, away from children and pets.* Humid and hot storage areas (like the bathroom) tend to cause drugs to break down faster. Storing drugs away from children and pets can prevent possible toxic effects if these drugs are inadvertently ingested by children or your family pet.
- *Speak up.* You are the most important member of the health care team, and you have information to share that no one else knows. Don't be shy about reporting the use of OTC or herbal therapies; these are your choices and are important to you. Sharing information about the use of these products will help your health care provider incorporate them into your total drug regimen in a safe and effective way.

Children present unique challenges related to medication errors. Children often cannot speak for themselves and rely on a caregiver or caregivers to manage their drug regimen. Because their bodies are still developing and respond differently than those of adults to many drugs, the risk of serious adverse reactions is greater with children. The margin of safety with many drugs is very small when dealing with a child. When teaching parents about their children's drug regimens, be sure to include the following instructions:

- *Keep a list of all medications you are giving your child, including prescription, OTC, and herbal medications.* Share this list with any health care provider who cares for your child. Never assume that a health care provider already knows what your child is taking.
- *Never use adult medications to treat a child.* The body organs and systems of children, primarily their livers and kidneys, are very different from those of an adult. As a result, children respond differently to drugs.
- *Read all labels before giving your child a drug.* Many OTC drugs contain the same ingredients, and you could accidentally overdose your child if you are not careful. In addition, some OTC drugs are not to be used with children younger than a certain age. Doses also may differ for children.
- *Measure liquid medications using appropriate measuring devices.* Never use your flatware teaspoon or tablespoon to measure your child's drugs. Always use a measured dosing device or the spoon from a measuring set.
- *Keep medication out of reach from children and do not attempt to increase cooperation from the child by telling them that the medication is "candy" or a "treat."* The goal is to prohibit the child from taking more doses than prescribed, which could cause severe toxicity.
- *Call your health care provider immediately if your child seems to get worse or seems to be having trouble with a drug.* Do not hesitate; many drugs can cause serious or life-threatening problems with children, and you should act immediately.
- *When in doubt, do not hesitate to ask questions.* You are your child's best advocate.

Reporting of Medication Errors

Medication errors must be reported on a national level as well as an institutional level. National reporting programs are coordinated by the U.S. Pharmacopeia, and they help gather information about errors to prevent their recurrence at other health care sites and by other health care providers. These reports might prompt the issuing of health care provider warnings, which point out potential or actual medication errors and suggest ways to avoid these errors in the future. For example, in 2007, the name of the drug *Omacor* (omega-3 fatty acid) was changed to *Lovaza* after many reports of confusion between *Omacor* and *Amicar* (aminocaproic acid). Other reports have led to public warnings about look-alike or sound-alike drug names and common dosing errors and transcribing issues.

Institutions also have their own policies for reporting medication errors that protect patients and staff and identify particular areas in which education or system changes may be needed. Always be aware of the policies of your employing institution or agency. If you see or participate in a medication error, report it to your institution and then report it to the national reporting program. Box 4.6 provides information about reporting medication errors.

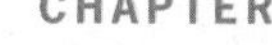

BOX 4.6

Reporting Medication Errors

1. Institute for Safe Medication Practices (ISMP) Medication Error Reporting Program—https://www.ismp.org/
2. FDA MedWatch Program—www.fda.gov/Safety/MedWatch/default.htm

Your report will be shared with all the appropriate agencies—the U.S. Food and Drug Administration, the drug manufacturer, and the Institute for Safe Medication Practices. Health care providers working together and sharing information can make a big impact in decreasing the occurrence of medication errors.

SUMMARY

- Nursing is a complex art and science that provides for nurturing and care of the sick, as well as prevention and education services.
- Components of the nursing assessment (history of past illnesses and the current complaint, as well as a physical examination) provide a database of baseline information to ensure safe administration of a drug and to evaluate the drug's effectiveness and adverse effects.
- Nursing assessment must include information on the history of past illnesses and the current complaint as well as a complete drug history and a physical examination; this provides a database of baseline information to ensure safe administration of a drug and to evaluate the drug's effectiveness and adverse effects.
- Nursing conclusions are developed from the information gathered during the assessment phase of the nursing process. A nursing conclusion is a statement of an actual or potential concern for the patient/family.
- Planning uses the information gathered and the resultant nursing conclusions to determine the desired patient outcomes, setting goals for safe and effective drug administration. The plan will lead to the necessary nursing interventions.
- Nursing interventions related to drug therapy include safely administering the drug, providing comfort measures to help the patient cope with the therapeutic or adverse effects of a drug, and providing patient and family education to ensure safe and effective drug therapy.
- Evaluation is part of the continuing process of patient care that leads to changes in assessment, conclusions, and interventions. The patient is continually evaluated for therapeutic response, the occurrence of adverse drug effects, and the occurrence of drug–drug, drug–food, drug–alternative therapy, or drug–laboratory test interactions.
- A nursing care guide and patient education materials can be prepared for each drug being given, using information about a drug's therapeutic effects, adverse effects, and special considerations.
- Prevention of medication errors is a complicated task that involves the prescriber, the pharmacist, the nurse administering the drugs, and the patient. The nurse needs to be vigilant in administering drugs to check the "rights" of drug administration. The patient needs to be educated to be their own advocate and to take steps to avoid medication errors.

Unfolding Patient Stories: Junetta Cooper • Part 1

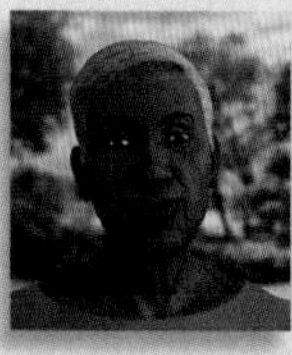

Junetta Cooper, a 75-year-old woman with chronic stable (exertional) angina pectoris secondary to coronary artery disease (CAD), is hospitalized. Junetta has had hypertension for 20 years that is well controlled with antihypertensives. Her morning medications include four oral medications, a transdermal patch, and an IV push medication. What measures can the nurse implement to prevent medication errors and ensure patient safety when preparing and administering these six medications? (Junetta Cooper's story continues in Chapter 43.)

Care for Junetta and other patients in a realistic virtual environment: ***vSim*** *for Nursing* (thepoint.lww.com/vSimPharm). Practice documenting these patients' care in DocuCare (thepoint.lww.com/DocuCareEHR).

CHECK YOUR UNDERSTANDING

Answers to the questions in this chapter can be found in Answers to Check Your Understanding Questions on thePoint*.

MULTIPLE CHOICE

Select the best answer.

1. A patient reports that they have a drug allergy. In exploring the allergic reaction with the patient, which of the following might indicate an allergic response?
   a. Increased urination
   b. Dry mouth
   c. Rash
   d. Drowsiness
2. The nurse obtains a medical history from a patient before beginning drug therapy based on an understanding of which of the following?
   a. Medical conditions can alter a drug's pharmacokinetics and pharmacodynamics.
   b. A medical history is a key component of any nursing protocol.
   c. A baseline of information is necessary to evaluate a drug's effects.
   d. The medical history is the first step in the nursing process.
3. The nurse writes a nursing conclusion for which reason?
   a. Direct medical care
   b. Help to increase patient compliance
   c. Identify actual or potential concerns in patient health
   d. Determine insurance reimbursement in most cases
4. A patient receiving an antihistamine complains of dry mouth and nose. An appropriate comfort measure for this patient would be to
   a. suggest that the patient use a humidifier.
   b. encourage voiding before taking the drug.
   c. have the patient avoid sun exposure.
   d. give the patient a back rub.
5. When establishing the nursing interventions appropriate for a given patient
   a. the patient should not be actively involved.
   b. the patient support systems should be included only at discharge.
   c. teaching should be done when the patient states they are ready to learn.
   d. an evaluation of all the data accumulated should be incorporated to achieve an effective care plan.
6. The evaluation step of the nursing process
   a. is often used as a last resort.
   b. is important primarily in the acute setting.
   c. is a continuous process.
   d. includes making nursing conclusions.
7. After teaching a patient about digoxin (*Lanoxin*)—a drug used to increase the effectiveness of the heart's contractions—which statement indicates that the teaching was effective?
   a. "I need to take my pulse every morning before I take my pill."
   b. "If I forget my pills, I usually make up the missed dose once I remember."
   c. "This pill might help my hay fever when it becomes a problem."
   d. "I don't remember the name of it, but it is the white one."

MULTIPLE RESPONSE

Select all that apply.

1. A client is being started on a laxative regimen. Before administering the medication, the nurse should perform which of the following processes?
   a. Assessing for allergies
   b. Evaluating the medication effectiveness
   c. Evaluating the route of administration
   d. Diagnosing the patient with ischemic colitis
   e. Asking the patient for name and birth date record when the medication was dispensed from the pharmacy
2. The nursing care of a patient receiving drug therapy should include measures to decrease the anticipated adverse effects of the drug. Which of the following measures would a nurse consider?
   a. A positive approach
   b. Environmental temperature control
   c. Safety measures
   d. Skin care
   e. Refrigeration of the drug
   f. Involvement of the family
3. A nurse is preparing to administer a drug to a patient for the first time. What questions should the nurse consider before actually administering the drug?
   a. Is this the right patient?
   b. Is this the right drug?
   c. Is there a generic drug available?
   d. Is this the right route for this patient?
   e. Is this the right dose, as ordered?
   f. Did I record this properly?

REFERENCES

Bickley, L. S. (2017). *Bates' guide to physical examination and history taking* (12th ed.). Wolters Kluwer.

Buchanan, L. M. (1994). Therapeutic nursing intervention knowledge development and outcome measures for advanced practice. *Nursing and Health Care, 15*(4), 190–195. https://pubmed.ncbi.nlm.nih.gov/7970251/

Butcher, H. K., Bulechek, G. M., Dochterman, J. M., & Wagner, C. M. (2019). *Nursing interventions classification (NIC)* (7th ed.). Elsevier.

Carpenito, L. J. (2016). *Handbook of nursing diagnoses* (15th ed.). Lippincott Williams & Wilkins.

Carpenito, L. J. (2016). *Nursing diagnosis: Application to clinical practice* (15th ed.). Lippincott Williams & Wilkins.

Carpenito, L. J. (2017). *Nursing care plans: Transitional patient & family centered care* (7th ed.). Lippincott Williams & Wilkins.

Jones, J. H., & Treiber, L. (2010). When the 5 rights go wrong: Medication errors from the nursing perspective. *Journal of Nursing Care Quality, 25*(3), 240–247. https://journals.lww.com/jncqjournal/Fulltext/2010/07000/When_the_5_Rights_Go_Wrong__Medication_Errors_From.8.aspx

Karch, A. M. (2003). *Lippincott's guide to preventing medication errors.* Lippincott Williams & Wilkins.

Kohn, L. T., Corrigan, J. M., & Donaldson, M. S. (Eds.). (2000). *To err is human: Building a safer health system.* National Academies Press. https://doi.org/10.17226/9728

Redman, B. (2007). *The practice of patient education: A case study approach* (10th ed.). Elsevier/Mosby.

Spath, P. L. (2011). *Error reduction in health care: A systems approach to improving patient safety* (2nd ed.). Jossey-Bass.

CHAPTER 5

Dosage Calculations

Learning Objectives

Upon completion of this chapter, you will be able to:

1. Describe different measuring systems that have been used for drug therapy.
2. Convert between different measuring systems when given drug orders and available forms of the drugs.
3. Calculate the correct dose of a drug using one of the three acceptable methods for dosage calculations.
4. Discuss why children require different dosages of drugs than adults.

Key Terms

conversion: finding the equivalent values between two systems of measure

metric system: the most widely used system of measure, based on the decimal system; all units in the system are determined as multiples of 10

ratio and proportion: an equation in which a ratio containing two known equivalent amounts is on one side and a ratio containing the amount desired to convert and its unknown equivalent is on the other side

To determine the correct dose of a particular drug for a patient, we consider the patient's sex, weight, age, physical condition, and the other drugs that the patient is taking. Frequently, the dose that is needed for a patient is not the dose that is available, and it is necessary to convert the dose form available into the prescribed dose. Doing the necessary mathematical calculations to determine what should be given is the responsibility of the prescriber who orders the drug, the pharmacist who dispenses the drug, and the nurse who administers the drug. This allows the necessary checks on the dose being given before the patient actually receives the drug. Another check to help prevent medication errors is that in many institutions, drugs arrive at the patient care area in unit dose form, prepackaged for each individual patient. The nurse administering the drugs may come to rely on this prepackaged system, forgoing any recalculation or rechecking of a dose to match the written order. The electronic medical record in many health care institutions has decreased the number of manual calculations. However, it is still important for clinicians to be able to perform and check the calculations. Unfortunately, despite the electronic medical record and multiple clinical personnel who are checking the doses, medication dosing errors still happen. Nurses are the people administering drugs, so they will be partially legally and professionally responsible for any errors that might occur. Practicing nurses must know how to convert drug-dosing orders into appropriate doses of available forms of a drug to ensure that the right patient is getting the right dose of a drug.

Measuring Systems

There have been different measuring systems used in drug preparation and delivery. Table 5.1 compares the basic units of measure of three of the measuring systems. With the growing number of drugs available and increasing awareness of medication errors that occur in daily practice, efforts have been made to decrease the dependence on so many different systems. In 1995, the U.S. Pharmacopeia Convention established standards requiring that all prescriptions, regardless of the system that was used in the drug dosing, include the metric measure for the quantity and strength of drug. It was also established that drugs may be dispensed only in the metric form. While the metric system is the predominant measuring system, nurses are expected to know several standard factors for **conversion**, or finding the equivalent values between two systems of measure (see Table 5.2).

Table 5.1 Comparing Basic Units of Measure by Measuring Systems

System	Solid Measure	Liquid Measure
Metric	gram (g) 1 gram (g) = 1,000 milligram (mg) 1 milligram (mg) = 1,000 microgram (mcg) 1 kilogram (kg) = 1,000 g	liter (L) 1 milliliter (mL) = 0.001 L 1 mL = 1 cubic centimeter = 1 cc
Apothecary	grain (gr) 60 gr = 1 dram (dr) 8 dr = 1 ounce (oz)	minim (min) 60 min = 1 fluidram (fl dr) 8 fl dr = 1 fluid ounce (fl oz)
Household	pound (lb) 1 lb = 16 ounces (oz)	pint (pt) 2 pt = 1 quart (qt) 4 qt = 1 gallon (gal) 16 oz = 1 pt = 2 cups (c) 32 tablespoons (tbsp) = 1 pt 3 teaspoons (tsp) = 1 tbsp 60 drops (gtt) = 1 tsp

Concept Mastery Alert

U.S. Pharmacopeia Convention

While the FDA is involved with tracking medication errors and ensuring proper labeling of drugs, food, and cosmetics, it is the U.S. Pharmacopeia Convention that publishes an annual catalog of medicinal drugs and their uses, side effects, and metric system measurements.

Metric System

The **metric system** is the most widely used system of measure. It is based on the decimal system, so all units are determined as multiples of 10. This system is used worldwide and makes the sharing of knowledge and research information easier. The metric system uses the gram as the basic unit of solid measure and the liter as the basic unit of liquid measure (see Table 5.1). For correct medication dosing, be sure to have the patient's weight documented in kilograms. Using weight in pounds leads to errors, as pounds are not a metric unit of measurement.

Table 5.2 Commonly Accepted Conversions Between Systems of Measurement

Metric System	Apothecary System	Household System
Solid Measure		
1 kg		2.2 lb
454 g		1 lb
1 g = 1,000 mg	~15 gr	
60 mg	~1 gr	
30 mg	~½ gr	
Liquid Measure		
1 L = 1,000 mL	~34 fl oz	~1 qt
240 mL	~8 fl oz	1 c
30 mL	~1 fl oz	2 tbsp
15 mL	4 fl dr	1 tbsp = 3 tsp
8 mL	2 fl dr 1 fl dr	~2 tsp
5 mL		1 tsp = 60 gtt

Apothecary System

The apothecary system is a very old system of measurement that was specifically developed for use by apothecaries or pharmacists. The apothecary system uses the minim as the basic unit of liquid measure and the grain as the basic unit of solid measure (see Table 5.1). This system is much harder to use than the metric system and is rarely seen in clinical settings. Occasionally, a prescriber will write an order in this system, and the dose will have to be converted to an available form. An interesting feature of this system is that it uses Roman numerals placed after the unit of measure to denote amount. For example, 15 grains would be written "gr xv."

Household System

The household system is the measuring system that is found in recipe books. This system uses the pint as the basic unit of fluid measure and the pound as the basic unit of solid measure (see Table 5.1). Although efforts have been made in recent years to standardize these measuring devices, wide variations have been noted in the capacity of some of them. Patients need to be advised that flatware teaspoons and drinking cups vary tremendously in the volume that they contain. A flatware teaspoon could hold up to two measuring teaspoons of quantity. When a patient is using a liquid medication at home, it is important to clarify that the measures indicated in the instructions refer to a standardized measuring device.

Avoirdupois System

The avoirdupois system is another older system that was very popular when pharmacists routinely had to compound medications. This system uses ounces and grains, but they measure differently than those of the apothecary and household systems. The avoirdupois system is seldom used by prescribers but may be used for bulk medications that come directly from the manufacturer.

Other Systems

Some drugs are measured in units other than those already discussed. These measures may reflect chemical activity or biological equivalence. One of these measures is the unit. A unit usually reflects the biological activity of the drug in 1 mL of solution. The unit is unique for the drug it measures; a unit of heparin is not comparable with a unit of insulin. Milliequivalents (mEq) are used to measure electrolytes (e.g., potassium, sodium, calcium, fluoride). The milliequivalent refers to the ionic activity of the drug in question; the order is usually written for a number of milliequivalents instead of a volume of drug. International units are sometimes used to measure certain vitamins or enzymes. These are also unique to each drug and cannot be converted to another measuring form.

Key Points

- At least four different systems have been used in drug preparation and delivery. These are the metric system, the apothecary system, the household system, and the avoirdupois system.
- The metric system is the most widely used system of measure. The U.S. Pharmacopeia Convention established standards requiring that all prescriptions, regardless of the system that was used in drug dosing, include the metric measure for the quantity and strength of drug. All drugs are dispensed in the metric system.

Conversion Between Systems

The simplest way to convert measurements from one system to another is to set up a **ratio and proportion** equation. The ratio containing two known equivalent amounts is placed on one side of an equation, and the ratio containing the amount you wish to convert and its unknown equivalent is placed on the other side. To do this, it is necessary to first check a table of conversions to determine the equivalent measure in the two systems you are using. Table 5.2 presents some accepted conversion equivalents between systems of measurement. It is a good idea to post a conversion guide in the medication room or on the medication cart for easy access. When conversions are used frequently, it is easy to remember them. When conversions are not used frequently, it is best to look them up.

Try the following conversion using Table 5.2. Convert 6 fl oz (apothecary system) to the metric system of measure. According to Table 5.2, 1 fl oz is equivalent to 30 mL. Use this information to set up a ratio:

$$\frac{1\ \text{fl oz}}{30\ \text{mL}} = \frac{6\ \text{fl oz}}{X}$$

The known ratio—1 fl oz (apothecary system) is equivalent to 30 mL (metric system)—is on one side of the equation. The other side of the equation contains 6 fl oz, the amount (apothecary system) that you want to convert, and its unknown (metric system) equivalent, X. Because the fluid ounce measurement is in the numerator (top number) on the left side of the equation, it must also be in the numerator on the right side of the equation. This equation would read as follows: 1 fl oz is to 30 mL as 6 fl oz is to how many milliliters?

The first step in the conversion is to cross-multiply (multiply the numerator from one side of the equation by the denominator from the other side, and vice versa):

$$\frac{1\ \text{fl oz}}{30\ \text{mL}} = \frac{6\ \text{fl oz}}{X}$$

$$1\ \text{fl oz} \times X = 6\ \text{fl oz} \times 30\ \text{mL}$$

This could also be written as

$$(1\ \text{fl oz})(X) = (6\ \text{fl oz})(30\ \text{mL})$$

After multiplying the numbers, you have

$$1(\text{fl oz})X = 180\ (\text{fl oz})(\text{mL})$$

Next, rearrange the terms to let the unknown quantity stand alone on one side of the equation:

$$X = \frac{180(\text{mL})(\text{fl oz})}{1\ \text{fl oz}}$$

Whenever possible, cancel out numbers, as well as units of measure. In this example, canceling out leaves $X = 180$ mL.

By canceling out, you are left with the appropriate amount and unit of measure. The answer to the problem is that 6 fl oz is equivalent to 180 mL. Once you have completed the math equation, check your answer to see if it is plausible. Ask yourself if the answer makes sense based on what you know from the conversion guide. In this scenario, you are converting 6 oz. The conversion guide is based on 1 oz, so you know that your final number should be about 6 times larger than the original equivalent amount. Indeed, 180 is 6 times 30. Performing checks like this can help you avoid errors.

Try another conversion. Convert 32 gr (apothecary system) to its equivalent in the metric system, expressing the answer in milligrams. First, find the conversion in Table 5.2: 1 gr is equal to 60 mg. Set up the ratio.

$$\frac{1\text{ gr}}{60\text{ mg}} = \frac{32\text{ gr}}{X}$$

Cross-multiply:

$$(1\text{ gr})(X) = (32\text{ gr})(60\text{ mg})$$
$$1(\text{gr})X = 1{,}920(\text{gr})(\text{mg})$$

Rearrange:

$$X = \frac{1{,}920\,(\text{gr})(\text{mg})}{1\text{ gr}}$$

Finally, cancel out like units and numbers:

$$X = 1{,}920\text{ mg}$$

Therefore, 32 gr is equivalent to 1,920 mg.

This answer is plausible since 1,920 mg is much larger than the 60 mg that was equal to 1 gr.

Calculating Dose

There are several systems of measurement available that might be used when a drug is ordered. Because drugs are made available only in certain forms or doses, it may be necessary to calculate what the patient should be receiving. The following methods can be used for dosage calculations: ratio and proportion, formula (desired over have), and dimensional analysis. Examples of these methods will be shown for different types of medication calculations.

Oral Drugs

Frequently, tablets or capsules for oral administration are not available in the exact dose that has been ordered. In these situations, the nurse who is administering the drug must calculate the number of tablets or capsules to give for the ordered dose.

Here is an example: An order is written for 324 mg of aspirin to be administered orally. The tablets that are available are 81 mg tablets. How many tablets should the nurse give?

Ratio and Proportion Method

One method to calculate the number of tablets needed is the ratio and proportion method. The ratio containing the two known equivalent amounts is put on one side of the equation, and the ratio containing the unknown value is put on the other side. The known equivalent is the amount of drug available in one tablet or capsule; the unknown is the number of tablets or capsules that are needed for the prescribed dose:

$$\frac{\text{amount of drug available}}{\text{one tablet or capsule}} = \frac{\text{amount of drug prescribed}}{\text{number of tablets or capsules to give}}$$

The phrase "amount of drug" serves as the unit, so this information must be in the numerator of each ratio.

$$\frac{81\text{ mg}}{1\text{ tablet}} = \frac{324\text{ mg}}{X\text{ tablets}}$$

Cross-multiply the ratio:

$$(81\text{ mg})(X\text{ tablets}) = (324\text{ mg})\,(1\text{ tablet})$$

Solve for X:

$$X\text{ tablets} = \frac{(324\text{ mg})(1\text{ tablet})}{(81\text{ mg})}$$

$$X\text{ tablets} = 4$$

Therefore, the nurse would administer four tablets.

Desired Over Have Method

Try another example using the desired over have method of calculation. An order is written for 0.05 g spironolactone (Aldactone) to be given orally (per os, PO). Aldactone is available in 25-mg tablets. How many tablets would you have to give?

First, determine the unit of measurement you need to calculate. In this case, you need to calculate number of tablets. Then determine the dose that you need to administer. The prescribed dose is 0.05 g. Now determine the dose available: 25-mg tablets. The available dose is in milligrams and the order is for grams, so a conversion is needed.

$$\frac{1\text{ g}}{1{,}000\text{ mg}} = \frac{0.05\text{ g}}{X}$$

Cross-multiply:

$$1(\text{g})\,X = (0.05 \times 1{,}000)(\text{g})(\text{mg})$$

Simplify:

$$X = \frac{50(\text{g})(\text{mg})}{1(\text{g})}$$

Cancel out like units to simplify further: $X = 50$ mg

So 0.05 g of Aldactone is equal to 50 mg of Aldactone.

Set up the equation: X = desired dose × quantity of tablets/dose that the nurse has

$$X = \frac{50\text{ mg} \times 1\text{ tablet}}{25\text{ mg}}$$
$$X = 2\text{ tablets}$$

Before administering the tablets to a patient, think about if your calculation is reasonable. It would be common for a patient to be prescribed 1 or 2 tablets. However, it would be much less common to have a patient take more than 3 tablets of the same medication in a single dose.

Dimensional Analysis Method

This method is slightly different than the ratio and proportion or desired over have methods. Use the same order for 0.05 g spironolactone (Aldactone) to be given orally (per os, PO), with the available dose being 25-mg tablets. Solve for the number of tablets using dimensional analysis.

First, determine the unit of measurement needed to calculate; put this on the left side of the equation. In this example, the unit of measurement is tablets. Then determine the ratio that contains the same unit as the unit being calculated and place this on the right side of the equation. The numerator on the right side should match the unit being calculated on the left side.

$$X \text{ tablets} = \frac{1 \text{ tablet}}{25 \text{ mg}}$$

Then, place any other ratios relevant to the item on the right side and cancel out other unwanted units of measurement.

$$X \text{ tablets} = \frac{1 \text{ tablet}}{25 \text{ mg}} \times \frac{1{,}000 \text{ mg}}{1 \text{ g}} \times \frac{0.05 \text{ g}}{1}$$

$$X \text{ tablets} - 2 \text{ tablets}$$

No matter what method you use to calculate the dose, be sure to evaluate if the number makes sense based on the patient and the medication. Rounding up or down may be necessary at times.

Sometimes the desired dose will be a fraction of a tablet or capsule, 1/2 or 1/4. Some tablets come with scored markings that allow them to be cut. Pill cutters are readily available in most pharmacies. One must use caution when advising a patient to cut a tablet. Many tablets come in a matrix system that allows for slow and steady release of the active drug. These drugs cannot be cut, crushed, or chewed. Always consult a drug reference before cutting a tablet. As a quick reference, any tablet that is designated as having delayed, controlled, or sustained release may very well be one that cannot be cut. Capsules can be very difficult to divide precisely, and some of them also come with warnings that they cannot be cut, crushed, or chewed. If the only way to deliver the correct dose to a patient is by cutting one of these preparations, a different formulation of the drug, a different drug, or a different approach to treating the patient should be tried.

Other oral drugs come in liquid preparations. Many of the drugs used in pediatrics and for adults who might have difficulty swallowing a pill or tablet are prepared in a liquid form. Some drugs that do not come in a standard liquid form can be prepared as a liquid by the pharmacist. If the patient is not able to swallow a tablet or capsule, check for other available forms and consult with the pharmacist about the possibility of preparing the drug in a liquid as a suspension or a solution. The same methods used to determine the number of tablets needed for the prescribed dose can be used to determine the volume of liquid that will be required to administer the prescribed dose.

Calculating Oral Drug Dosage Three Ways

Try this example: An order has been written for 250 mg of amoxicillin. The bottle states that the solution contains 125 mg/5 mL. How much of the liquid should you give?

Ratio and Proportion Method

The ratio on the left of the equation shows the known equivalents, and the ratio on the right side contains the unknown. The phrase "amount of drug" must appear in the numerator of both ratios, and the volume to administer is the unknown (*X*). Cross-multiply:

$$125(\text{mg})\,X = (250 \times 5)(\text{mg})(\text{mL})$$

Simplify:

$$X = \frac{1{,}250 \text{ (mg)(mL)}}{125(\text{mg})}$$

The desired dose is $X = 10$ mL.

Desired Over Have Method

First, determine the unit of measurement you need to calculate. For the above example, you need to know how many mL to administer. The order is for 250 mg. The available dose is 125 mg/5 mL. Now you can set up your equation:

$$X \text{ mL} = 250 \text{ mg} \times \frac{5 \text{ mL}}{125 \text{ mg}}$$

Solve the equation:

$$X \text{ mL} = 10 \text{ mL}$$

Dimensional Analysis Method

You can solve the same problem using dimensional analysis. Put the unit you need to calculate on the left of the equation. The ratios on the right should be set up so that the numerator matches the unit being calculated.

$$X \text{ mL} = \frac{5 \text{ mL}}{125 \text{ mg}} \times \frac{250 \text{ mg}}{1}$$

Solve the equation.

$$X \text{ mL} = 10 \text{ mL}$$

Even if you are working in an institution that provides unit-dose medications, practice your calculation skills occasionally to keep them sharp. Power can be lost, computers can go down, and the ability to determine conversions is a skill that anyone who administers drugs should have in reserve. Periodically throughout this text, you will find a box to help you refresh your dose calculation skills as they apply to the drugs being discussed.

Injectable Dosage

All drugs administered via injections must be administered in liquid form. The person administering the drug needs to calculate the volume of the liquid that must be given to administer the prescribed dose. The same methods used for determining the dose of an oral liquid drug can be used to determine the dose of an injectable drug.

Try this example: An order has been written for 7.5 mg of midazolam to be given intramuscularly. The vial states that 1 mL = 5 mg. How much should you give?

Ratio and Proportion Method

$$\frac{\text{amount of drug available}}{\text{volume available}} = \frac{\text{amount of prescribed}}{\text{volume to administer}}$$

$$\frac{5\text{ mg}}{1\text{ mL}} = \frac{7.5\text{ mg}}{X}$$

$$(5\text{ mg})\ (X) = (1\text{ mL})\ (7.5\text{ mL})$$

Thus, $X = 1.5$ mL.

Desired Over Have Method

The unit of measurement that you need to calculate is mL, and the dose that you need to administer is 7.5 mg. The dose that is available is 5 mg in 1 mL. The next step is to set up the equation.

$$X\text{ mL} = \text{desired} \times \frac{\text{quantity}}{\text{have}}$$

$$X\text{ mL} = 7.5\text{ mg} \times \frac{1\text{ mL}}{5\text{ mg}}$$

$$X\text{ mL} = 1.5\text{ mL}$$

Dimensional Analysis Method

The left side of the equation should have the unit of measurement that you need to calculate (mL). The ratios on the right should be set up so that the numerator matches the unit being calculated. Place as many ratios as are relevant and that are needed to cancel out unwanted units of measurements.

$$X\text{ mL} = \frac{1\text{ mL}}{5\text{ mg}} \times \frac{7.5\text{ mg}}{1}$$

$$X\text{ mL} = 1.5\text{ mL}$$

Intravenous Solutions

Intravenous (IV) solutions are used to deliver a prescribed amount of fluid, electrolytes, vitamins, nutrients, or drugs directly into the bloodstream. Although most institutions now use electronically monitored delivery systems, it is still important to be able to use standard calculations to determine the amount of an IV solution that should be given. Most IV delivery systems come with a standard control called a microdrip, by which each milliliter delivered contains 60 drops. Macrodrip systems, which usually deliver 15 drops/mL, are also available; they are usually used when a large volume must be delivered quickly. Always check the packaging of the IV tubing to see how many drops/mL are delivered by that particular device.

Two examples of calculating dosing for IV solutions will be described below. The first is when there is an electronic infusion pump and the second is for a manual IV infusion.

Calculating for an Electronic Infusion Pump

You are preparing to administer 1 gram of cefotaxime as an IV bolus over 45 minutes. The cefotaxime is available in 100 mL of 0.9% sodium chloride. How many mL/h should you set the IV infusion pump to deliver? Round to the nearest whole number.

Ratio and Proportion and Desired Over Have Methods

$$X\text{ mL/h} = \frac{\text{volume (mL)}}{\text{time (h)}}$$

Put in the numbers that are known from the example and solve for X.

$$X\text{ mL/h} = 100\text{ mL}/0.75\text{ h}$$

$$X\text{ mL/h} = 133.333\text{ mL/h}$$

This rounds to 133 mL/h.

Dimensional Analysis Method

$$X\text{ mL/h} = \frac{100\text{ mL}}{45\text{ min}} \times \frac{60\text{ min}}{1\text{ h}}$$

$$X\text{ mL/h} = 133.3333\text{ mL/h}$$

This rounds to 133 mL/h.

Calculating for a Manual IV Infusion

An order has been written for a patient to receive 400 mL of 5% dextrose in water (D5W) over a period of 4 hours in a standard microdrip system (i.e., 60 drops/mL). Calculate the correct setting (drops per minute). The number of drops per minute, or the rate that you will set by adjusting the valve on the IV tubing, is equal to the amount of solution that has been prescribed per hour times the number of drops delivered per milliliter (mL), divided by 60 minutes in an hour.

Ratio and Proportion and Desired Over Have Methods

$$X = \frac{(400\text{ mL}/4\text{ h})\ (60\text{ drops/min})}{(60\text{ min})/(1\text{ h})}$$

Simplify:

$$X = \frac{(100\text{ mL/h})\ (60\text{ drops/min})}{(60\text{ min})/(1\text{ h})}$$

$$X = \frac{6{,}000\text{ drops/h}}{(60\text{ min})/(1\text{ h})}$$

Therefore, $X = 100$ drops/min.

Now calculate the same order for an IV set that delivers 15 drops/mL:

$$X = \frac{(400\text{ mL}/4\text{ h})\ (15\text{ drops/min})}{(60\text{ min})/(1\text{ h})}$$

$$X = \frac{(100\text{ mL/h})\ (15\text{ drops/min})}{(60\text{ min})/(1\text{ h})}$$

$$X = \frac{1{,}500\text{ drops/h}}{(60\text{ min})/(1\text{ h})}$$

Therefore, $X = 25$ drops/min.

If a patient has an order for an IV drug, the same principle can be used to calculate the speed of the delivery. For example, an order is written for a patient to receive 50 mL of an antibiotic over 30 minutes. The IV set used dispenses 60 drops/mL, which allows greater control. Calculate how fast the delivery should be.

$$X = \frac{(50\text{ mL}/0.5\text{ h})(60\text{ drops}/\text{min})}{(60\text{ min})/(1\text{ h})}$$

$$X = \frac{(100\text{ mL}/\text{h})(60\text{ drops}/\text{min})}{(60\text{ min})/(1\text{ h})}$$

$$X = \frac{6{,}000\text{ drops}/\text{h}}{(60\text{ min})/(1\text{ h})}$$

Therefore, $X = 100$ drops/min.

Dimensional Analysis Method

Place the unit of measure to be calculated on the left side of the equation. Place the ratio that contains the same unit that needs to be calculated on the right side. Then use conversion factors to cancel out unwanted units of measurements.

$$X\text{ drops/min} = 60\text{ drops/mL} \times 400\text{ mL}/4\text{ hours} \times 1\text{ hour}/60\text{ min}$$

$$X\text{ drops/min} = 100\text{ drops}/\text{min}$$

There are multiple methods that can be used to calculate the correct dosages. No matter what mathematical method you use, be sure to review your answer to see if the number makes sense in the scope of the medication delivery system. It is important to have someone else check your work before administering the medication to the patient.

Body Weight Versus Body Surface Area

There are many times when a dose is calculated for an individual based on their body weight measured in kilograms. Body weight is different than body surface area (BSA). BSA is the measured or calculated area of the surface of the entire human body. One medication that is dosed by BSA is doxorubicin (*Doxil*), which is an antineoplastic antibiotic that can be used to treat multiple myeloma, ovarian cancer, and AIDS-related Kaposi sarcoma. It is common for cancer chemotherapy to be dosed by BSA to individualize the therapy to optimize treatment and reduce adverse side effects. An equation to calculate BSA is the Mosteller formula:

$$\text{BSA}\left(\text{m}^2\right) = \text{square root of}\left[\text{height}\left(\text{cm}\right) \times \text{weight}\left(\text{kg}\right)\right]/3{,}600$$

There are also websites that can be used to calculate BSA. One website for this calculation is: http://www.med-calc.com/body.html

Pediatric Considerations

For most drugs, children require doses different from those given to adults. A child's body may handle a drug differently in all areas of pharmacokinetics—absorption, distribution, metabolism, and excretion. In addition, the responses of the child's organs to the effects of the drug also may vary because of the immaturity of the organs. Most of the time a child requires a smaller dose of a drug to achieve the critical concentration comparable to that for an adult. On rare occasions, a child may require a higher dose of a drug. The drug guide that you have selected to use in the clinical setting will have the pediatric dose listed if this information is available, but there are many times when the pediatric doses are calculated based on weight or on height and weight.

For example, if a child with postoperative nausea is to be treated with chlorpromazine (generic), the recommended dose is 0.55 mg/kg by intramuscular injection. If the child weighs 22 kg, the dose for this child would be 0.55 mg/kg times 22 kg, or 12.1 mg, rounded down to 12 mg. If a child weighed only 6 kg, the recommended dose would be 0.55 mg/kg times 6 kg or 3.3 mg, rounded down to 3 mg. The established guidelines allow the drug to be used safely for a large range of children. Some adult doses will also be written in this way. This is usually found in drugs with a small margin of safety or high potential for toxic effects, such as antineoplastic drugs. Be sure to note the difference between mg/kg/dose versus mg/kg/day. If the amount is listed as mg/kg/day, the nurse will need to divide the amount by the number of doses required each day.

SUMMARY

- At least four different measuring systems have been used in drug preparation and delivery. These are the metric system, the apothecary system, the household system, and the avoirdupois system.
- The metric system is the most widely used system of measure. The U.S. Pharmacopeia Convention established standards requiring that all prescriptions, regardless of the system that was used in drug dosing, include the metric measure for the quantity and strength of drug. All drugs are dispensed in the metric system.
- It is important to know how to convert doses from one system to another. The method of ratio and proportion, which uses basic principles of algebra to find an unknown, is a method of converting doses within and between systems.
- Dosage calculations can be completed using several different methods: ratio and proportion, desired over have, or dimensional analysis.
- For most drugs, children require doses different from those for adults due to the way their bodies handle drugs and the way that drugs affect their tissues and organs.
- Some medications are dosed by weight. This is most common for pediatric doses, but also applies to some adult medication dosing.

CHECK YOUR UNDERSTANDING

Answers to the questions in this chapter can be found in Answers to Check Your Understanding Questions on thePoint®.

MULTIPLE CHOICE

Select the best answer.

1. A dose of 0.125 mg of digoxin was ordered for a patient who has been having trouble swallowing. The bottle of digoxin elixir reads 0.05 mg/mL. How much would you give?
   a. 5 mL
   b. 0.5 mL
   c. 2.5 mL
   d. 2 mL

2. A client being treated for multiple myeloma has been prescribed doxorubicin hydrochloride liposome (Doxil) 30 mg/m^2 IV. If the client is 180 cm tall and weighs 90 kg, what is the correct dose to administer?
   a. 1 mg
   b. 7 mg
   c. 14 mg
   d. 21 mg

3. An order is written for 700 mg of ampicillin PO. The drug is supplied in liquid form as 1 g/3.5 mL. How much of the liquid should be given?
   a. 5.25 mL
   b. 2.55 mL
   c. 6.25 mL
   d. 2.45 mL

4. An order is written for 1,000 mL of normal saline to be administered IV over 10 hours. The drop factor on the IV tubing states 15 drops/mL. What is the IV flow rate?
   a. 50 mL/h at 50 drops/min
   b. 100 mL/h at 25 drops/min
   c. 100 mL/h at 100 drops/min
   d. 100 mL/h at 15 drops/min

5. A 5-year-old child has been prescribed midazolam hydrochloride 0.25 mg/kg/dose PO. The child weighs 23 kg. If the order allows for up to 4 doses/day, what is the maximum amount of the medication administered per day?
   a. 47 mg
   b. 5 mg
   c. 23 mg
   d. 0.5 mg

6. A patient needs to take 0.75 g of tetracycline PO. The drug comes in 250-mg tablets. How many tablets should the patient take?
   a. 2 tablets
   b. 3 tablets
   c. 4 tablets
   d. 30 tablets

7. Aminophylline is supplied in a 500 mg/2.5 mL solution. How much would be given if an order were written for 100 mg of aminophylline IV?
   a. 5 mL
   b. 1.5 mL
   c. 2.5 mL
   d. 0.5 mL

8. Heparin 800 units is ordered for a patient. The heparin is supplied in a multidose vial that is labeled 10,000 units/mL. How many milliliters of heparin would be needed to treat this patient?
   a. 0.8 mL
   b. 0.08 mL
   c. 8 mL
   d. 0.4 mL

COMPLETE THE FOLLOWING PROBLEMS

1. Change to equivalents within the system:
   a. 100 mg =______ g
   b. 1,500 g =______ kg
   c. 0.1 L =______ mL
   d. 500 mL =______ L

2. Convert to units in the metric system:
   a. 150 gr = ______ g
   b. gr = ______ mg
   c. 45 min = ______ mL
   d. 2 qt = ______ L

3. Convert to units in the household system:
   a. 5 mL = ______ tsp
   b. 30 mL = ______ tbsp

4. Convert the weights in the following problems:
   a. A patient weighs 170 lb. What is the patient's weight in kilograms?
   b. 200 lb = _______ kg
   c. A patient weighs 3,200 g. What is the patient's weight in pounds?
   d. 4,000 g = _______ lb
5. *Robitussin* cough syrup 225 mg PO is ordered. The bottle reads 600 mg in 1 oz. How much cough syrup should be given? _______ mL
6. A postoperative order is written for 15 gr of codeine every 4 hours as needed (*pro re nata*, p.r.n.) for pain. Each dose given will contain how many milligrams of codeine? _______ mg
7. Ordered: 6.5 mg. Available: 10 mg/mL. Proper dose: _______ mL.
8. Ordered: 0.35 mg. Available: 1.2 mg/2 mL. Proper dose: _______ mL.
9. Ordered: 80 mg. Available: 50 mg/mL. Proper dose: _______ mL.
10. Ordered: 150,000 units. Available: 400,000 units/5 mL. Proper dose: _______ mL.

REFERENCES

Brunton, L., Hilal-Dandan, R., & Knollman, B. (2018). *Goodman and Gilman's the pharmacological basis of therapeutics* (13th ed.). McGraw-Hill.

Craig, G. (2011). *Clinical calculations made easy*. Lippincott Williams & Wilkins.

DeCastillo, S., & Werner-McCullough, M. (2012). *Calculating drug dosages: An interactive approach* (3rd ed.). Davis.

Harvey, M. (Ed.) (2016). *Dosage calculations made incredibly easy* (5th ed.). Wolters Kluwer.

Kaestner, S. A., & Sewell, G. J. (2007). Chemotherapy dosing part 1: Scientific basis for current practice and use of body surface area. *Clinical Oncology, 19*(1), 23–37. 10.1016/j.clon.2006.10.010

Karch, A. (2003). *Lippincott's guide to preventing medication errors*. Lippincott Williams & Wilkins.

Mosteller, R. D. (1987). Simplified calculation of body surface area. *New England Journal of Medicine, 317*(17), 1098. 10.1056/NEJM198710223171717

Ogden, S. (2015). *Calculation of drug dosages* (10th ed.). Mosby.

Snyder, R., & Schoeborn, B. (2011). *Medical dosage and calculations for dummies*. Wiley Publishing.

Tyreman, C. (2013). *How to master nursing calculations* (2nd ed.). Kogan Page Limited.

CHAPTER 6

Challenges to Effective Drug Therapy

Learning Objectives

Upon completion of this chapter, you will be able to:

1. Discuss the impact of the media, the internet, and direct-to-consumer advertising on consumers and health care professionals.
2. Explain the growing use of over-the-counter drugs and the impact it has on safe medical care.
3. Discuss the lack of controls on herbal or alternative therapies and the impact this has on safe drug therapy.
4. Describe measures being taken to protect the public in cases of bioterrorism, during the opioid crisis, and during the COVID-19 pandemic.
5. Discuss the health care ramifications of the COVID-19 pandemic.

Key Terms

alternative therapy: includes herbs and other "natural" products as often found in ancient records; since they are considered dietary supplements, these products are not controlled or tested by the U.S. Food and Drug Administration in the same way that medications are controlled; however, they are sometimes the basis for discovery of an active ingredient that is later developed into an FDA-regulated medication

biological weapons: so-called germ warfare; the use of bacteria, viruses, and parasites on a large scale to incapacitate or destroy a population

cost comparison: a comparison of the relative cost of the same drug provided by different pharmacies or manufacturers to determine the costs to the consumer

self-care: patients self-diagnosing and determining their own treatment needs

street drugs: nonprescription drugs with no known therapeutic use; used to enhance mood or increase pleasure

The 21st century arrived with myriad new considerations and pressures in the health care industry. For the first time, consumers have access to medical and pharmacological information from many sources and are requesting specific treatments and considerations. Alternative therapies are being offered and advertised at a record pace, causing people to rethink their approach to medical care and the medical system. At the same time, financial pressures have led to early discharge of patients from health care facilities and to provision of outpatient care for patients who, in the past, would have been hospitalized and monitored closely. Health care providers are being pushed to make decisions about patient care and prescriptions based on finances in addition to medical judgment. The events of 9/11 and the increased perceived threat of terrorism led to serious ongoing concerns about dealing with exposure to biological or chemical weapons. Illicit drug use is at an all-time high, causing increased health risks and safety concerns. The opioid crisis has led to many changes in prescribing and safety measures for patients on prescription drugs. Concerns about the environment and the need to protect it from contamination are increasing. Furthermore, the COVID-19 pandemic and the need for social distancing introduced new challenges to person- and family-centered health care. The use of technology for family and patient visits became more common during the pandemic. The nurse is caught in the middle of all this change. Patients are more demanding of information but may not fully understand it when they have it. Patient teaching and home care provisions are vital to the success of any health regimen. The nurse is frequently in the best position to learn, teach, and explain information to the patient and to facilitate the care of the patient in the health system. In the push for patient-centered care, where each individual's unique concerns, culture, and needs are incorporated into the overall health regimen, the nurse is most often the one to provide support, incentive, and advocacy to the patient and patient's family.

Consumer Awareness

Access to information has become so broad that consumers are often overwhelmed with details, facts, and choices that affect their health care. Gone is the era when the health care provider was seen as omniscient and always right. The patient often comes into the health care system influenced by advertising, the internet, and the alternative therapy industry. Many patients no longer unquestioningly accept whatever medication is selected for them. They often come to appointments with requests and demands, and they often partake of a complex array of over-the-counter (OTC) and alternative medicines that can further complicate the safety and efficacy of standard drug therapy.

Media Influence

The last 30 years have seen an explosion of drug advertising in the mass media. In the 1990s, it became legal to advertise prescription drugs directly to the public, and it is now rare to watch television, listen to the radio, flip through a magazine, or browse the internet without encountering numerous direct-to-consumer drug advertisements.

Federal guidelines determine what can be said in an advertisement, but in some cases, this results in confusion for many consumers. If a drug advertisement states what the drug is used for, it must also state contraindications, adverse effects, and precautions. Because listing the possible adverse effects is not a good selling point, many advertisements dramatically downplay that information. Moreover, if the use of a drug is not stated, the advertisement can use any images and suggestions to sell the drug. When it comes to health care, consumers can lose sight of the fact that advertisements are business ploys intended to motivate a person to request a particular drug from their health care provider (even if it is unclear what the drug is used for). It is not unusual to see an ad featuring a smiling, healthy-looking person romping through a field of beautiful flowers on a sunny day with a cute baby or puppy in tow. The ad might simply state how wonderful it is to be outside on a day like today—"contact your health care provider if you, too, would like to feel this way." Although most people now know what the erectile dysfunction drug sildenafil (*Viagra*) is used for, some of the ads for this drug simply show a happy older couple smiling and dancing the night away and then encourage viewers to ask their health care providers about *Viagra*. What older person wouldn't want a drug that makes them feel young, happy, and energetic?

Parenting magazines, which are often found in pediatricians' offices, are full of advertisements for antibiotics and asthma medications. These ads feature smiling, cute children and encourage readers to check with their pediatricians about the use of the drugs. If the drug's indication is mentioned, the second page of the ad may well have the U.S. Food and Drug Administration (FDA)-approved drug insert printed in medical jargon in extremely tiny print. Many readers have trouble reading the words on these required pages. Even if the words are legible, they frequently don't have any meaning for the reader. The pediatrician or nurse may spend a great deal of time explaining why a particular drug is not indicated for a particular child and may actually experience resistance on the part of the parent who wants the drug for their child. As the marketing power for prescription drugs continues to grow, the health care provider must be constantly aware of what patients are seeing, what the ads are promising, and the real data behind the indications and contraindications for these popular drugs. Staying up-to-date and knowledgeable about drug therapy is an ongoing challenge.

The media also look for headlines in current medical research or reports. It is not unusual for the media to create articles and news segments based solely on the title or surface understanding of the contents of medical research and reports. Sometimes the interpretation of a medical report is not accurate or does not offer all of the pertinent details; this can influence a patient to seek out a new therapy or approach their health care provider with new requests or questions. Many television talk shows include a medical segment that presents a small amount of information, sometimes out of context, that opens a whole new area of interest for the viewer. Some health care providers have learned to deal with the "disease of the week" as seen on these shows; others can be unprepared to deal with what was presented and may lose credibility when they are unable to address a patient's questions about the popular new topic.

The Internet

The internet is readily accessible to most consumers. Though inequities in internet access persist, many people who do not have internet access at home can often find it at the local library, at school, at work, or in public places with free Wi-Fi. An increasing number of people have constant internet access through the widespread use of smartphones, tablets, and other handheld devices. The information available over the internet is overwhelming to many people. A person can spend hours looking up information on a drug from various online sources—including pharmaceutical company sites, chat rooms with people who are taking the drug, online pharmacies, lists of government regulations, and research reports about the drug and its effectiveness. Many people do not know how to evaluate the information that they access, including whether the information is accurate or anecdotal. This is especially challenging with the pervasiveness of direct-to-consumer advertising, as patients typically receive from these ads only the most optimistic perspective on the

BOX 6.1

Evaluating Internet Sites

Address Identification

- *.com:* commercial, advertising, selling, business site
- *.edu:* education site—school system, university, college
- *.gov:* government site
- *.net:* part of a linked network system, may include any of the above
- *.org:* sponsored by an organization, including professional, charitable, and educational groups

Site Evaluation

- *Navigation*: Is the site easy to access and navigate?
- *Contributors*: Who created the site? Is it reviewed? Is it purely commercial? What are the qualifications of the person(s) maintaining the site? Is there a mechanism for feedback or interaction with the site?
- *Dates*: Is the site updated frequently? When was the site last updated?
- *Accuracy/reliability*: Is the information supported by other sites? Is the information accurate and in agreement with other sources you have reviewed? Does the site list other links that are reasonable and reliable? Are potential conflicts of interest declared? Is funding transparent?
- *References*: Does the site provide references for stated facts?

drugs being marketed. Patients often come into the health care system with pages of information that they think pertains to their particular situation. The nurse or physician can spend a tremendous amount of time interpreting the information and explaining it to the patient. Some tips that might be helpful in determining the usefulness or accuracy of information found on the internet are given in Box 6.1.

Key Points

- An overwhelming amount of readily accessible information is available to consumers. This information has changed the way people approach the health care system.
- Direct-to-consumer advertising of prescription drugs, mass media health reports and suggestions, and the internet influence some patients to request specific treatments, to question therapy, and to challenge the health care provider, opening up dialogue for a discussion about treatments between the patient and the health care provider.

Over-the-Counter Drugs

OTC medications allow people to take care of simple medical problems without seeking advice from health care providers. Although OTC drugs have been deemed safe when used as directed, many of these medications were "grandfathered in" as drugs when stringent testing and evaluation systems became law. As a result, they have not been tested or evaluated to the extent that new drugs are today. Aspirin, one of the nonprescription standbys for many years, falls into this category. Slowly, the FDA is looking at all of these drugs to determine their effectiveness and safety. Ipecac, a former standard OTC drug, was used for many years by parents to induce vomiting in children in cases of suspected poisoning or suspected drug overdose. The drug was finally tested, and in 2003, the FDA announced that it was not found to be effective for its intended use. New guidelines have since been established for parents regarding possible poisoning, and parents were advised to dispose of any ipecac that they had at home. Some well-known approved OTC drugs are acetaminophen (*Tylenol*) for decreasing fever and pain, various vaginal antifungal medications (*Mycelex, Gyne-Lotrimin*) for treating yeast infections, and omeprazole (*Prilosec*) and famotidine (*Pepcid*) for managing heartburn.

Each year, several prescription drugs are reviewed for possible OTC status. One factor involved in the review process is the ability of the patient to engage in **self-care**, which is the act of self-diagnosing and determining one's treatment needs. In 2009 and again in 2010, lovastatin, an antihyperlipidemic drug, was considered for OTC status. The FDA eventually decided that the public would have a hard time self-prescribing this drug because high lipid levels, which present no signs and symptoms, can be determined only with a blood test, so the drug's OTC status was not approved. OTC drugs can mask the signs and symptoms of an underlying problem, making it difficult to arrive at an accurate diagnosis if the condition persists. These drugs are safe when used as directed, but many times, consumers do not follow or even read the directions. Moreover, many people are not aware of what drugs are contained in these preparations and can inadvertently overdose when taking one preparation for each symptom they have. Table 6.1 gives examples of the ingredients that are found in some common cold and allergy preparations. Patients who take doses of different preparations to cover their various symptoms could easily wind up with an unintended overdose or toxic reaction.

Because many OTC drugs interact with prescription drugs, with possibly serious adverse or toxic effects for the patient, it is important that the health care provider specifically ask when taking a drug history if the patient is taking any OTC drugs or other medications. Many patients do not consider OTC drugs to be "real" drugs and do not mention their use when reporting a drug history to the health care provider. Specifically asking a patient about the use of any products for headache, colds, constipation, etc., can often prompt a patient to remember and report the use of these products. Every patient drug-teaching session should include information on which particular OTC drugs must be avoided and the advice to check with the health care provider before taking any other medications or OTC products.

Table 6.1 Ingredients Found in Some Common Cold and Flu Over-the-Counter Preparations[a]

Drug Name	Ingredients	Use
Vicks NyQuil Severe Cold & Flu Nighttime	acetaminophen, dextromethorphan, phenylephrine, doxylamine	Runny nose, cough, headache, sore throat, aches and pains, sinus pressure, fever, sneezing
Vicks DayQuil Severe Cold & Flu	acetaminophen, phenylephrine, dextromethorphan, guaifenesin	Nasal congestion, fever, sore throat, aches, cough
Theraflu Nighttime Severe Cold & Cough	acetaminophen, diphenhydramine, phenylephrine	Nasal congestion, sore throat, cough, sneezing
Theraflu Daytime Severe Cold & Cough	acetaminophen, phenylephrine, dextromethorphan	Nasal congestion, sore throat, cough, headache
Theraflu Multi-Symptom Severe Cold	acetaminophen, phenylephrine, dextromethorphan	Stuffy head, nasal congestion, sore throat, cough, headache, body aches, fever

[a]Safety precautions: A patient might take one preparation for cough, a second for sinus pressure, a third for aches and pains, and a fourth to stay awake or fall asleep. When the total amounts of the drugs contained in these products are combined, a serious overdose of acetaminophen, phenylephrine, or dextromethorphan could easily occur.

Concept Mastery Alert

Self-Prescribing Over-the-Counter Medications

Patients who report taking multiple over-the-counter combination medications to treat a cold should be assessed for indications of overdose. Taking doses of different medications to cover symptoms can lead to unintended overdose or toxic reaction.

Alternative Therapies and Herbal Medicine

Another aspect of the self-care movement is the market of herbal medicines and other **alternative therapies.** Alternative therapies are often found in ancient records, and some have been the basis for the discovery of an active ingredient that is later developed into an FDA-regulated medication. Today, alternative therapies can also include nondrug measures, such as imagery, massage, acupuncture, and relaxation. Herbal or alternative therapies are considered by the FDA to be dietary supplements and are not as strictly regulated by the FDA as compared to medications. Dietary supplements are substances that contain some dietary ingredient(s). Some examples are vitamins, minerals, amino acids, and herbs. Even though they are not categorized as drugs or medications, herbal medicines are not benign. They can produce unexpected effects and toxic reactions, interact with prescription or OTC drugs, and contain various unknown ingredients that alter their effectiveness and toxicity. The challenge for the clinician is to balance the therapies that the patient wishes to use with the medical regimen that is prescribed. This may involve altering doses or timing of various drugs. Chapter 60 has more information regarding common alternative and complementary herbal therapies.

Key Points

- OTC drugs have been deemed safe by the FDA when used as directed and do not require a prescription or advice from a health care provider.
- OTC drugs can mask the signs and symptoms of disease, can interact with prescription drugs, and can be taken in greater than the recommended dose, leading to toxicity.
- Herbal or alternative therapies are considered to be dietary supplements and are not tightly regulated by the FDA.
- Herbal medicines can produce unexpected effects and toxic reactions, can interact with prescription drugs, and can contain various unknown ingredients that alter their effectiveness and toxicity.

Costs of Health Care and the Importance of Patient Teaching

The health care crisis in the United States has caused the cost of medical care and drugs to skyrocket. This is partly due to the demand to have the best possible, most up-to-date, and safest care and drug therapies. The research and equipment requirements to meet these demands are huge. At the same time, the rising cost of insurance to pay for health care is a major complaint for employers and consumers. As a result, health maintenance organizations (HMOs) have surged in popularity. These groups treat the medical care system like a business, with financial aspects becoming the overriding concern. Decisions are often made by nonmedical personnel with a keen eye on the bottom line. To save costs, patients are being discharged from hospitals far earlier than ever before, and many are not even admitted to hospitals for surgical or invasive procedures that used to require several days of hospitalization and monitoring. There is therefore less monitoring of the patient, and more responsibility for care falls on the patient or the patient's significant others. Teaching the patient about self-care, drug therapies, and what to expect during treatment or recovery is crucial. The nurse is the one who most often is responsible for this teaching. The Affordable Care Act was designed to help relieve rising health care costs and ensure access to care for more people, but the full impact of this act on the health care system won't be known for many years, and the impact of efforts to change the act further complicate the understanding of effects it may have.

Health Maintenance Organizations and Regulations

HMOs maintain a centralized control system to provide patient medical care within a budget. In many communities, the HMO provides a group of participating physicians and services housed in a local area. Consumers are often provided with all of their health care by this group of providers at a lower price than what would be charged by out-of-network providers. The tradeoff is a loss of choice. The health care providers in the organization are the only ones who can be consulted unless the patient is willing to pay higher costs. The HMO may regulate access to emergency facilities, types and timing of tests allowed, and procedures covered. Accessibility to prescription drugs is also controlled. The formulary for each HMO differs. Sometimes only generic products are covered, and newer drugs must be paid for by the patient; in other instances, a tier system exists, and the patient may urge the provider to choose a drug from a lower tier, at a lower cost. Many health care providers believe that their ability to make decisions is limited by such regulations and that decisions are often made by nonmedical personnel who have no contact with the patient.

Home Care

The home care industry is one of the more rapidly growing responses to the changes in costs and medical care delivery. Patients go home directly from surgery with the responsibility for changing dressings, assessing wounds, administering medications, and monitoring their recovery. Patients are being discharged earlier from hospitals because the hospital days allowed for particular diagnoses have been reduced. These patients may be responsible for their own monitoring, rehabilitation, and drug regimens. At the same time, the population is aging and may be less accepting of or less equipped to handle this responsibility. Home health aides, visiting nurses, and home care programs are taking over some of the responsibilities that used to be handled in the hospital, particularly for patients who are aging and have additional issues that go with the changes in the aging body. The *Beer's List* is a good resource of high-risk medications that are potentially inappropriate in older adults.

The responsibility of meeting the tremendous increase in teaching needs of patients frequently resides with the nurse. Patients need to know exactly what medications they are taking (generic and brand names), the dose of each medication, and what each is supposed to do. Patients also need to know what they can do to alleviate some of the adverse effects that are expected with each drug (e.g., eating small meals if gastrointestinal upset is common, using a humidifier if secretions will be dried and make breathing difficult); which OTC drugs or alternative therapies they need to avoid while taking their prescribed drugs; what to watch for that would indicate a need to call the health care provider; and how to properly store drugs (e.g., humidity and heat in bathrooms is not good for drug storage, controlled substances need to be secured, particular drugs may need to refrigerated). With patients who are taking multiple drugs at the same time, this information should be provided in writing in plain, clear language. Many pharmacies provide written information with each drug that is dispensed, but organizing these sheets of information into a usable and understandable form is difficult for many patients. The nurse is often the one who needs to sort through the provided information to organize, simplify, and make sense of it for the patient. The cost of dealing with toxic or adverse effects is often much higher, in the long run, than the cost of the time spent teaching the patient.

The projections for trends in health care indicate even greater expansion of the home health care system, with hospitals being used for only the most critically ill patients. The role of the nurse in this home health system is crucial—as teacher, assessor, diagnostician, and patient advocate.

Cost Considerations

Despite the insurance coverage a patient may have for prescription medications, it is often necessary for the health care provider to choose a drug therapy based on the costs of the drugs available. With more and more of the population reaching retirement age and depending on a fixed income, costs are an area of great concern. Patients may be forced into deciding whether to "treat or eat." Sometimes patients do not tell the health care provider that they are not filling a prescription because of cost and are therefore losing the therapeutic benefit of the drug. Sometimes cost concerns mean not selecting a first-choice drug but instead settling for one that, while still effective, may have drawbacks. Patients may be tempted to stop taking an antibiotic in order to save the remaining pills for the next time they feel sick and to save the costs of another health care visit and a new prescription. This practice has contributed to the problem of resistant bacteria, which is becoming more dangerous all the time. Patients must be reminded to take the full course and not to stop the drug when they feel better.

Patients also need to be advised not to split tablets in half unless specifically advised to do so. Some drugs can be split; it can be cheaper to order the higher strength tablets and have the patient cut them for the correct dose. Some patients think that by cutting any drug in half, they will have coverage for twice the time allowed by the prescription and will not be as dependent on the drug. With the new matrix delivery systems used for many medications, however, splitting a drug can cause it to become toxic or ineffective. Patients should be specifically alerted to avoid cutting drugs when it could be dangerous, especially if they are being advised to cut other tablets to be economical. The cost of treating the toxic reactions may far exceed the cost of the original drug.

Generic drug availability in many cases reduces the cost of medication. Generic drugs are preparations that are off-patent and therefore can be sold by their generic name, without the cost associated with brand name products. Generic drugs are tested for bioequivalence with the brand name product; resulting information is available to prescribers. When a drug has a small margin of safety (a small difference between the therapeutic and the toxic dose), a prescriber may feel more comfortable ordering the drug by brand name to ensure that the dose and binders are what the prescriber expects. When "DAW" (dispense as written) is on a prescription, the prescription is filled with the brand name drug—such as Lanoxin instead of digoxin or Coumadin instead of warfarin. In some situations, the generic drug is not less expensive than the brand name drug, so using a generic drug does not guarantee that the patient is getting the least expensive preparation. Many pharmacies post the costs of commonly used drugs, and patients may do **cost comparisons** to compare the relative cost of the same drug among various pharmacies or among manufacturers of drugs and then request that a different drug be prescribed. There are several websites (e.g., RxSaver and GoodRx) that can be used by consumers to compare costs of both brand name and generic medications that are sold at multiple pharmacies. Table 6.2 presents an example of a cost comparison between some generic and trade name medications. The nurse is often the person who is called upon to explain the reason for a drug choice or request that the prescriber consider an alternative treatment.

In recent years, with the cost of drugs becoming a political as well as a social issue, many people have begun ordering drugs on the internet, often from other countries. These drugs may be cheaper, do not require the patient to see a health care provider (many of these sites simply have customers fill out a questionnaire that is reviewed by a doctor), and are delivered right to the patient's door. The FDA has begun checking these drugs as they arrive in the United States and have found many discrepancies between what was ordered and what is in the product, as well as problems in the storage of these products. Some foreign brand names are the same as brand names in the United States but are associated with different generic drugs. The FDA has issued many warnings to consumers about the risk of taking some of these drugs without medical supervision, reminding consumers that they are not protected by U.S. laws or regulations when they purchase drugs from other countries. The FDA website, https://www.fda.gov/drugs/drug-information-consumers/imported-drugs-raise-safety-concerns, provides important information and guidelines for people who elect to use the internet to purchase cheaper drugs.

Table 6.2 Generic or Trade Name Drugs? What Do They Cost?

Drug Name	Daily Dose (mg)	Approximate Cost of a 30-Day Supply
metoprolol tartrate (generic)	200	$4.00
Lopressor		$231.00
divalproex sodium (generic)	1,000	$150.00
Depakote		$400.00
topiramate (generic)	100	$11.00
Topamax		$574.60
sumatriptan	150	$11.70
Imitrex		$605.00

This table shows several prescription migraine drug prices in October 2020. It is presented to illustrate the wide price range between generic and trade name drugs. Prices may vary based on pharmacy and coupon availability.

Emergency Preparedness for Bioterrorism and Pandemics

The events of 9/11 diminished the sense of security and safety that generally prevailed in the United States. Now there are terrorist alerts, long lines for security at airports, and increased inspection of bags at sporting events and theme parks. One of the potential threats being addressed by the Centers for Disease Control and Prevention (CDC) and the Office of Homeland Security is the risk of exposure to biological and chemical weapons. The threat of exposure to **biological weapons**, so-called germ warfare, or the use of bacteria, viruses, and parasites on a large scale to incapacitate or destroy a population, is somewhat theoretical but very concerning, as seen in the anthrax mail scares in Washington, DC; Pennsylvania; and New York in 2001. The CDC has worked diligently to establish guidelines for treating possible exposure to biological weapons. For complete information on presenting signs and symptoms, diagnoses, and current research in this area, go to www.cdc.gov and click on "Emergency Preparedness," then click on "Bioterrorism" in the drop-down menu. Education of health care providers and the public is one of the central points in coping effectively with any biological assault.

The CDC website also has up-to-date information about pandemics in the Emergency Preparedness tab section. A pandemic is defined as the rapid spreading of a disease worldwide. Some of the information on the website is about past pandemics and the influenza virus that evolves every year. The CDC website also contains information about the COVID-19 pandemic, including information on symptoms, testing, and treatments for the infection. Some information is written for health care workers and professionals. This is a website that can be used as a resource for nurses who need current information about detection, diagnosis, prevention, and management of past or current epidemics or pandemics. The nurse is often called upon to answer questions, reassure the public, offer educational programs, and serve on emergency preparedness committees.

Drug Misuse and the Opioid Crisis

Illicit drug use in the United States is a growing problem. People in communities across the country use **street drugs**—nonprescription drugs with no known therapeutic use—to enhance their moods and increase pleasure. Alcohol and nicotine are two common drugs that can cause serious problems for people who use them. These drugs can interact with various medications and alter a patient's response to a prescribed drug; these interactions are often not seen as drug addiction issues. Parents are often very concerned that their children will use street drugs, and many communities in the United States have found themselves facing an opioid crisis. The CDC reports that nearly 70% of the deaths due to drug overdose in 2018 involved an opioid. This is particularly concerning since opioids are often legally prescribed for pain control. Some people misuse and become addicted to prescription drugs following an injury, when confronted with chronic pain, when their occupation puts them in contact with readily available drugs, or when someone else in the home is using a prescription drug. The opioid crisis includes deaths from prescribed opioids, heroin, and synthetic opioids that are illicitly manufactured. It is estimated that more than 128 Americans die every day from opioid overdose, and two third of these deaths are caused by synthetic opioids. The regulations regarding prescriptions are stricter, so deaths from prescription medications have decreased, but deaths caused by use of illicit opioids have increased. Steps to deal with this crisis have included tightening the controlled substance class of the opioids, making reversal agents readily available to first responders and the public, research into safer delivery of these opioids, research into better ways to treat chronic pain, and research into more effective and more readily available rehabilitation. The financial burden and loss of life makes this a crucial teaching point for health care professionals and patients. More information regarding opioids and medications to support withdrawal and/or abstinence from opioids is provided in Chapter 26.

Many of the drugs used illicitly are also addictive and can change a person's entire life, with drug-seeking behavior becoming a major factor. Researchers have identified changes in the brain and neurotransmitter patterns of people who are addicted to such drugs. Trying to reverse these changes and return the person to a nonaddicted state is a physiological, as well as a psychological, challenge. The use of these drugs can have severe consequences on health, can mask underlying signs and symptoms of medical problems, and can interact with other medications that the person may need (see Table 6.3).

Being informed about drugs available in the community, current trends among teenagers or young adults, and community resources available to help patients can guide parents and health care professionals. Education provides a crucial defense against drug misuse and helps the public and health care professionals recognize it and address it when it occurs. The National Institutes of Health has a division called the National Institute on Drug Abuse. Go to http://www.nida.nih.gov to find educational programs for teens, parents, and health care professionals; the latest information on trends in illicit drug use; research on dealing with drug use problems; and links to sites for identifying unknown drugs, community resources, and laws.

Protecting the Environment

In March 2008, many news services across the United States reported studies showing that many prescription drugs had been found in the drinking water of various large cities. These studies showed contamination of ground water and watershed with many pharmaceutical products. The levels of these drugs were small, but the question was raised about what this would mean for the future and how the presence of these drugs would affect people, animals, and crops. More recent studies have found that wastewater treatment systems are able to remove enough of the substances from water, so that levels are low enough for people to drink the water safely. However, urban planning for water treatment facilities is imperative to keep these levels low. Drugs end up in the water for many reasons. Patients may get a prescription and then get switched to a different drug. Some patients end up with extra pills at the end of a prescription because they did not follow the dosing guidelines exactly. Many people store these extra pills and end up with a medicine cabinet full of prescription drugs. In the past, people would often just flush these drugs down the toilet, where the drugs would enter the water system.

Table 6.3 Frequently Misused Substances and Their Potential Health Consequences

Drug or Classification	Street Names	Classification or Action on CNS	Health Consequences
Amphetamines	Uppers, whites, dexies, speed	CNS stimulant	Hypertension, tachycardia, insomnia, restlessness
Amyl nitrate	Poppers, pearls, amies	CNS stimulant	Tachycardia, restlessness, hypotension, vertigo
Anabolic steroids	Roids, muscle builders, pumpers	Steroid	Hypertension, hyperlipidemia, acne, cancer, cardiomyopathy
Barbiturates	Downers, reds, barbs	CNS depressant	Bradycardia, hypotension, laryngospasm, ataxia, impaired thinking
Benzodiazepines	Benzos, downers, chill pills, zannies	CNS depressant	Confusion, fatigue, impaired memory, impaired coordination, respiratory depression
Cannabis/THC With formaldehyde or phencyclidine With cocaine	Flower, trees, weed, green; fry; chase, cocktail	Mixed CNS	Drowsiness, elation, dizziness, memory lapse, hallucinations
Cocaine	Snow, blow, crack, dust	CNS stimulant	Tachycardia, hypertension, hallucinations, confused thinking
Fentanyl	Jackpot, China white	Opioid	Sedation, arrhythmias, shock, cardiac arrest, decreased respirations, constipation
Gamma-hydroxybutyrate (*Xyrem*)	G, gina, liquid X, liquid E, date rape drug	CNS depressant	Memory loss, hypotension, somnolence
Heroin	Black, dope, junk, smack, white horse	Opioid	Sedation, arrhythmias, shock, cardiac arrest, decreased respirations, constipation
Ketamine	Cat valium, super acid, special K	CNS depressant	Paralysis, loss of sensation, disorientation, psychic changes
LSD	Acid, yellow sunshine, blotter, dots	Hallucinogen	Hallucinations, hypotension, changes in thinking, loss of social control
MDMA	Ecstasy, e-bomb, molly, Scooby snacks, vitamin E	Hallucinogen	Hallucinations, psychic change, loss of memory, hypotension, cardiac arrest
Methamphetamine	Crystal, glass, speed, crystal meth, dunk, go fast	CNS stimulant	Hypertension, tachycardia, restlessness, changes in thinking
Methylphenidate	Ritalin, kiddie coke	CNS stimulant	Agitation, tachycardia, hypertension, hyperreflexia, fever
Morphine	Morpho, Miss Emma, M	Opioid	Sedation, arrhythmias, shock, cardiac arrest, decreased respirations, constipation
Oxycodone (Xtampza ER); oxycodone hydrochloride (OxyContin)	Oxy, Oxycotton, hillbilly heroin, ozone, berries	Opioid	Sedation, arrhythmias, shock, cardiac arrest, decreased respirations, constipation
PCP	Angel dust, zombie	Hallucinogen	Acute psychosis, heart failure, death, seizures, memory loss
Peyote	Black button, green button, shaman, cactus	Hallucinogen	Acute psychosis, tremor, altered perception, death
Flunitrazepam (*Rohypnol*)	Roofies, circles, mind eraser, date rape drug	Benzodiazepine—CNS depressant	Date rape drug, loss of memory, immobility

CNS, central nervous system; ED, erectile dysfunction; LSD, lysergic acid diethylamide; MDMA, methylenedioxymethamphetamine; PCP, phencyclidine; THC, tetrahydrocannabinol.

Box 6.2 Focus on Patient and Family Teaching

PROPER DISPOSAL OF UNUSED, UNNEEDED, OR EXPIRED MEDICATIONS

If you do not have access to a take-back location:

- Take unused, unneeded, or expired prescription drugs out of their original containers.
- Mix the prescription drugs with an undesirable substance, such as used coffee grounds or kitty litter, and put them in impermeable, nondescript containers, such as empty cans or sealable bags, further ensuring that the drugs are not diverted or accidentally ingested by children or pets.
- Throw these closed containers in the trash.
- Flush prescription drugs down the toilet *only* if the accompanying patient information *specifically instructs* that this is safe to do.
- Be sure to scratch off or mark out any personal information on the prescription bottles/containers.

The safest route is to return unused, unneeded, or expired prescription drugs to a pharmaceutical take-back location that allows the public to bring unused drugs to a central location for safe disposal. Many hospitals have these locations. Many local governments have regular take-back days or drop-off sites. Check with your local hospital, health department, or police department. The following websites have information about home disposal methods and disposal locations:

https://www.deadiversion.usdoj.gov/drug_disposal/takeback/index.html https://apps2.deadiversion.usdoj.gov/pubdispsearch/spring/main;jsessionid=8CBScJnDSa2hAm3wTAM8KXrv7clZhUE9A25Cz_U_.web2?execution=e1s1

Some people just threw them out, where the drugs would eventually enter the ground of various landfills or would be diverted for illicit use by people looking for drugs at garbage sites. With these issues in mind and the push to protect the environment, the FDA released specific guidelines for the proper disposal of prescription drugs. See Box 6.2 for the guidelines for drug disposal. It is important to teach patients how to dispose of drugs properly. Encourage patients to clean out their medicine cabinet at least yearly and to properly dispose of the drugs that they are no longer using. Many local governments now have drug take-back events to promote the safe disposal of drugs.

COVID-19 and the Health Care System

The COVID-19 pandemic has changed aspects of people's lives all over the world. It has certainly prompted changes in health care and resources. Many people in the United States have medical and prescription insurance linked to employment. Due to the pandemic, millions of Americans were without work or were furloughed from their work. There is concern that state and federal laws and regulations have not yet fully solved the issue of securing medical and prescription insurance for unemployed people, and the surge of uninsured people during and after the pandemic may negatively impact population health.

Another significant change to the health care system since the beginning of the COVID-19 pandemic has been the transition to telehealth for many outpatient visits. The telemedicine movement has allowed communication between a person and their provider without either needing to go to a health care office. The visit is conducted over the phone or video media. It is unclear how this structural change for many outpatient visits will affect long-term population health. For example, are health care providers able to assess and diagnose as accurately as they can in person? How do patients feel about interacting with health care providers in these ways?

There is still uncertainty regarding how the COVID-19 pandemic will affect medication resources in the long term. The pharmaceutical supply chain includes manufacturers, distributors, pharmacies (physical and mail order), and tens of thousands of workers to distribute about 6 billion prescriptions in the United States each year. The original concerns were regarding overseas manufacturing and whether there would be medication shortages. However, it is also thought that there may be a need for expansion of mail-order and home delivery of medications due to recommendations for social distancing and quarantining and to reduced availability of retail pharmacies. The implications of COVID-19 and our responses to the pandemic are still evolving.

SUMMARY

- In the 21st century, drugs pose new challenges for patients and health care providers, including information overload, demands for specific treatments, increased access to self-care systems, and financial pressures to provide cost-effective care.
- The mass media bombards consumers with medical reviews, research updates, and direct-to-consumer advertising for prescription drugs. If the use of a drug is stated, the adverse effects and cautions also must be stated. If the use is not stated, the drug advertisement is free to use any images and suggestions to sell the drug.
- The internet provides consumer access to drug information, advertising, and even purchasing without a mediator of this information. Determining the reliability of an internet site is a challenge for the consumer and the health care provider.
- OTC drugs and herbal and alternative therapies allow patients to make medical decisions and self-treat many common signs and symptoms. Problems arise when they are used inappropriately, when they

interact with prescription drugs, or when they mask signs and symptoms, making diagnosis difficult.

- Increasing costs of drugs and health care led to the emergence of HMOs and tight regulations on medical therapy and drug therapy alternatives. The choice of a drug to be used may be determined by the HMO formulary or insurance company database or by cost comparison with other drugs in the same or a similar class. Cost comparison is a major consideration in the use of many drugs.
- Home care has become a significant portion of the health care system. Patients are increasingly more responsible for managing their medical regimens from home with dependence on home health providers and teaching and support from knowledgeable nurses.
- Emergency preparedness in the post-9/11 era includes awareness of risks associated with biological or chemical weapon exposure and medical management for the victims.
- Illicit drug use and abuse of prescription drugs can lead to dependence on the drug and physiological changes, causing health problems and changing the body's response to prescribed drugs.
- Proper disposal of unused or expired medications can help to protect the environment and may decrease drug-searching behaviors in some situations.
- COVID-19 and our responses to the infection have changed the health care system and decreased many people's health care resources.

CHECK YOUR UNDERSTANDING

Answers to the questions in this chapter can be found in Answers to Check Your Understanding Questions on thePoint®.

MULTIPLE CHOICE

Select the best answer.

1. Drugs can be advertised in the mass media only if
   a. the FDA indication is clearly stated.
   b. the actual use is never stated.
   c. adverse effects and precautions are stated if the use is stated.
   d. all adverse effects are clearly stated.

2. Herbal treatments and alternative therapies
   a. are considered drugs and regulated by the FDA.
   b. are considered dietary supplements and are not strictly regulated by the FDA.
   c. have no restrictions on claims and advertising.
   d. contain no drugs, only natural substances.

3. Over-the-counter drugs are drugs that are
   a. deemed to be safe when used as directed.
   b. harmless to the public.
   c. too old to be tested.
   d. cheaper to use than prescription drugs.

4. The home health care industry has grown because
   a. there is a shortage of hospital beds.
   b. patients feel safer at home and prefer to be cared for at home.
   c. patients are going home from the hospital and becoming responsible for their own care sooner than in the past.
   d. the nursing shortage makes it difficult to care for patients in hospitals.

5. The cost of drug therapy is a major consideration in most areas because
   a. generic drugs are always cheaper.
   b. the high cost of drugs combined with more fixed-income consumers puts constraints on drug use.
   c. pharmacies usually carry only one drug from each class.
   d. patients like to shop around and get the best drug for their money.

6. Which is a strategy that can help to reduce mortality from opioid overdose?
   a. Ensuring access to reversal agents when opioids are prescribed
   b. Increasing toxicology screening at every patient visit
   c. Increasing availability of opioids by making them over-the-counter medications
   d. Teaching patients about how to dispose of opioid medications

MULTIPLE RESPONSE

Select all that apply.

1. When taking a health history, the nurse should include specific questions about the use of OTC drugs and alternative therapies. This is an important aspect of the health history because
   a. many insurance policies cover these drugs.
   b. patients should be reprimanded about the use of these products.
   c. patients often do not consider them to be drugs and do not report their use.
   d. patients should never use these products when taking prescription drugs.
   e. these products can mask or alter presenting signs and symptoms.
   f. many of these products interact with prescription drugs.

2. A nurse is caring for a patient who prefers to take herbal medications instead of prescription medications. Which statement would be correct to tell the patient?
   a. "Herbal medications do not interact with prescription medications."
   b. "The Food and Drug Administration does not regulate herbal medications as strictly as prescription medications."
   c. "Herbal supplements have fewer side effects than prescription medications."
   d. "Herbal supplements may have benefits that come from the placebo effect."
   e. "Herbal supplements are regulated like over-the-counter medications."

REFERENCES

Alexander, G. C., & Qato, D. M. (2020). Ensuring access to medication in the US during the COVID-19 pandemic. *JAMA, 324*(1), 31–32. 10.1001/jama.2020.6016

American Geriatrics Society. (2019). American Geriatrics Society 2019 updated AGS Beers Criteria for potentially inappropriate medication use in older adults. *Journal of American Geriatric Society, 67*, 674–694. 10.1111/jgs.15767

Barton, J. H., & Emmanuel, E. J. (2005). The patient-based pharmaceutical development process: Rationale, problems and potential reforms. *Journal of the American Medical Association, 294*, 2075–2082. 10.1001/jama.294.16.2075

Blumenthal, D., Fowler, E. J., Abrans, M., & Collins, S. R. (2020). Covid-19—Implications for the health care system. *The New England Journal of Medicine, 383*, 1483–1488. https://www.nejm.org/doi/full/10.1056/nejmsb2021088

Brunton, L., Hilal-Dandan, R., & Knollman, B. (2018). *Goodman and Gilman's the pharmacological basis of therapeutics* (13th ed.). McGraw-Hill.

Centers for Disease Control and Prevention. (2020). *Opioid overdose.* https://www.cdc.gov/drugoverdose/index.html#:~:text=Drug%20overdose%20remains%20a%20leading,of%20128%20people%20every%20day

Centers for Disease Control and prevention. (2020). *Understanding the epidemic.* https://www.cdc.gov/drugoverdose/epidemic/index.html

Centers for Disease Control and Prevention. (2020). *Using telehealth to expand access to essential health services during the COVID-19 pandemic.* https://www.cdc.gov/coronavirus/2019-ncov/hcp/telehealth.html

Cruipi, R. S., Asnis, D. S., Lee, C. C., Santucci, T., Marino, M. J., & Flanz, B. J. (2003). Meeting the challenge of bioterrorism: Lessons learned from the West Nile virus and anthrax. *American Journal of Emergency Medicine, 21*(1), 77–79. 10.1053/ajem.2003.50015

Davoli, E., Zuccato, E., & Castiglioni, S. (2019). Illicit drugs in drinking water. *Current Opinion in Environmental Science and Health, 7*, 92–97. https://doi.org/10.1016/j.coesh.2018.12.004

DerMarderosian, A., & Beutler, J. A. (Eds.). (2014). *The review of natural products* (8th ed.). Facts and Comparisons.

Ebadi, M. (2006). *Pharmacodynamic basis of herbal medicine* (2nd ed.). Taylor & Francis.

Hendler, C. B. (Ed.) (2021). *Nursing 2021 drug handbook.* Wolters Kluwer.

Koo, M. M., Krass, I., & Aslani, P. (2003). Factors influencing consumer use of written drug information. *Annals of Pharmacotherapy, 37*(2), 259–267. 10.1177/106002800303700218

National Institute on Drug Abuse. (2020). *Opioid overdose crisis.* https://www.drugabuse.gov/drugs-abuse/opioids/opioid-crisis

Pizzorno, J. E., & Murray, M. T. (2012). *Textbook of natural medicine* (4th ed.). Elsevier.

Pizzorno, J. E., Murray, M. T., & Joiner-Bey, H. (2015). *The clinician's handbook of natural medicine* (3rd ed.). Churchill-Livingstone.

Smith, K., Richie, D., & Henyon, N. (2010). *Handbook of critical drug data* (11th ed.). McGraw Hill Medical.

Stargrove, M. B., Treasure, J., & McKee, D. L. (2007). *Herb, nutrient and drug interactions: Clinical implications and therapeutic strategies.* Mosby.

U.S. Food and Drug Administration. (2020). *Where and how to dispose of unused medicines.* https://www.fda.gov/consumers/consumer-updates/where-and-how-dispose-unused-medicines

PART 2

Chemotherapeutic Agents

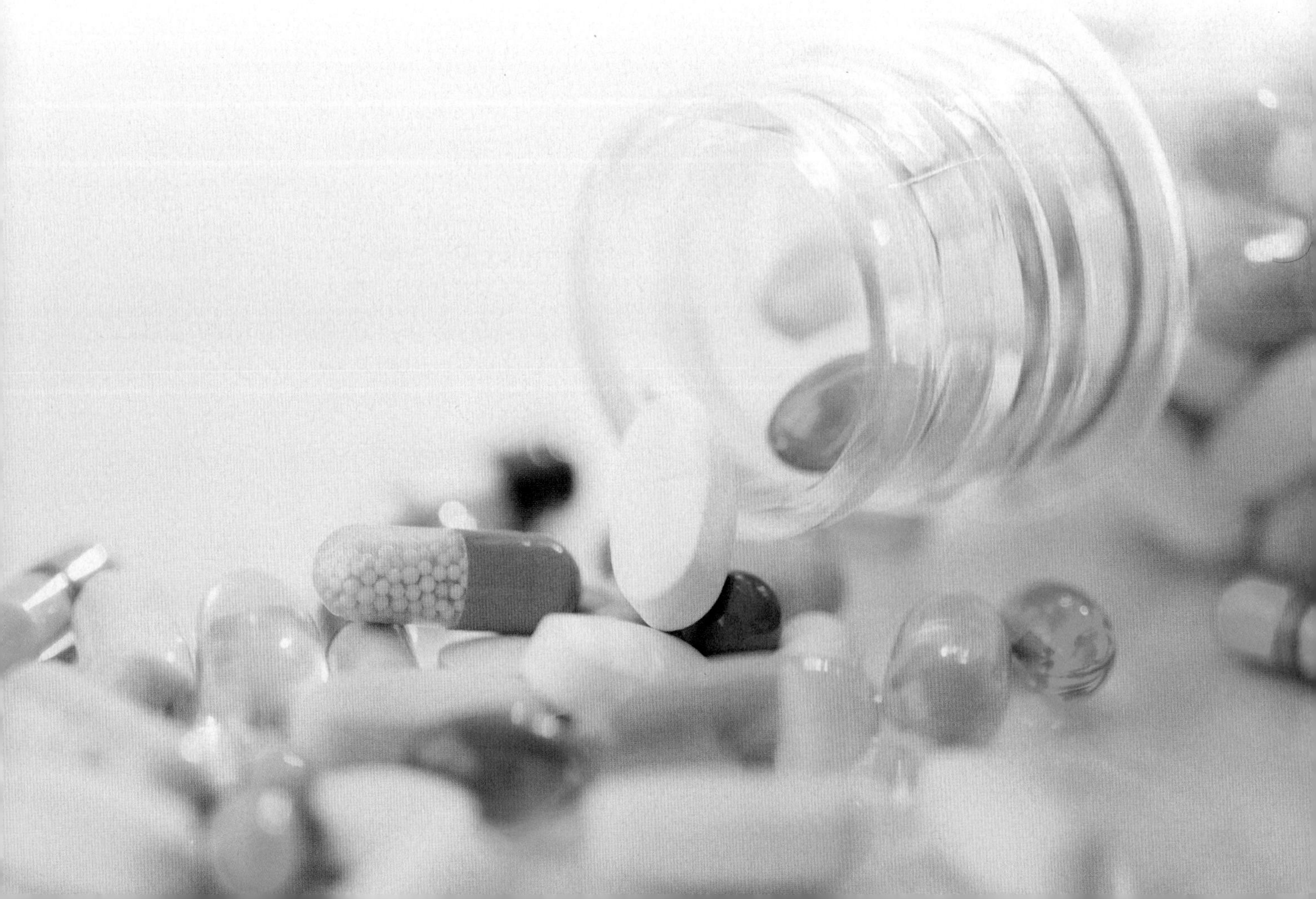

CHAPTER 7

Introduction to Cell Physiology

Learning Objectives

Upon completion of this chapter, you will be able to:

1. Identify the parts of the human cell.
2. Describe the role of each organelle found within the cell cytoplasm.
3. Explain the unique properties of the cell membrane.
4. Describe processes used by the cell to move things across the cell membrane.
5. Outline the cell cycle, including the activities occurring within the cell in each phase.

Key Terms

cell cycle: life cycle of a cell, which includes the phases G_0, G_1, S, G_2, and M

cell membrane: lipoprotein structure that separates the interior of a cell from the external environment; regulates what can enter and leave a cell

cytoplasm: lies within the cell membrane; contains organelles

diffusion: movement of solutes from an area of high concentration to an area of low concentration across a concentration gradient

endocytosis: the process of engulfing substances and moving them into a cell by extending the cell membrane around the substance; pinocytosis and phagocytosis are two kinds of endocytosis

endoplasmic reticulum: fine network of interconnected channels known as cisternae found in the cytoplasm; site of chemical reactions within the cell

exocytosis: removal of substances from a cell by pushing them through the cell membrane

genes: make up the physical and functional units of heredity; stored in deoxyribonucleic acid (DNA) and control basic cell functions, determine physical appearance, and can play a role in susceptibility to disease and reaction to medication

Golgi apparatus: a series of flattened sacs in the cytoplasm that prepare hormones or other substances for secretion and may produce lysosomes and store other synthesized proteins

histocompatibility antigens: proteins found on the surface of the cell membrane; they are determined by the genetic code and provide cellular identity as a self-cell (i.e., a cell belonging to that individual)

lipoprotein: structure composed of proteins and lipids; the bipolar arrangement of the lipids monitors substances passing in and out of the cell

lysosomes: encapsulated digestive enzymes found within a cell; they digest old or damaged areas of the cell and are responsible for destroying the cell when the membrane ruptures and the cell dies

mitochondria: rod-shaped organelles that produce energy within the cell in the form of adenosine triphosphate (ATP)

mitosis: cell division resulting in two identical daughter cells; referred to as the M phase in the cell cycle

nucleus: the part of a cell that contains the DNA and genetic material; regulates cellular protein production and cellular properties

organelles: distinct structures found within the cell cytoplasm

osmosis: movement of water from an area of low solute concentration to an area of high solute concentration in an attempt to equalize the concentrations

ribosomes: membranous structures that are the sites of protein production within a cell

Chemotherapeutic drugs are used to destroy both organisms that invade the body (e.g., bacteria, viruses, parasites, protozoa, fungi) and abnormal cells within the body (e.g., neoplasms, cancers). These drugs affect cells by altering cellular function or disrupting cellular integrity and causing cell death, or by preventing cellular reproduction, eventually leading to cell death. Because most chemotherapeutic agents do not possess complete selective toxicity, they also affect the normal cells of patients. To understand the actions and adverse effects caused by chemotherapeutic agents and to determine interventions that increase therapeutic effectiveness, it is important to understand the various properties and the basic structure and function of the cell.

The Cell

The cell is the basic structural unit of the body. The cells that make up living organisms, which are arranged into tissues and organs, all have the same basic structure. Each cell has a nucleus, a cell membrane, and cytoplasm, which contains a variety of organelles (Fig. 7.1).

Cell Nucleus

Each cell is "programmed" by the **genes**, which are contained in sequences of double-stranded deoxyribonucleic acid (DNA). DNA has components called nucleotides that are made up of deoxyribose (5 carbon sugar) with one of the four nitrogenous bases (thymine, cytosine, adenine, or guanine). The nitrogenous bases contain the genetic material that directs the production of specific proteins that allow the cell to carry out its functions, maintain cell homeostasis or stability, and serve as units of inheritance. The **nucleus** is the part of a cell that contains all genetic material necessary for cell reproduction and for the regulation of cellular production of proteins. The nucleus is encapsulated in its own membrane and remains distinct from the rest of the cytoplasm. A small spherical mass, called the nucleolus, is located within the nucleus. Within this mass are dense fibers and proteins that will eventually become **ribosomes**, the sites of protein synthesis within the cell. Ribonucleic acid (RNA) is made within the nucleus and is similar to DNA except it is single stranded, contains ribose for the sugar instead of deoxyribose, and contains uracil as its nitrogenous base instead of thymine. DNA contains the instructions for protein synthesis, and RNA actually makes the proteins. During the process of transcription, DNA is used to generate messenger RNA, which is the template for protein synthesis. The messenger RNA will leave the nucleus, go to the cytoplasm, and make proteins in the ribosomes.

Cell Membrane

The cell is surrounded by a thin barrier called the **cell membrane**, which separates intracellular fluid from extracellular fluid. The membrane is essential for cellular integrity and is equipped with many mechanisms for maintaining cell homeostasis.

Lipoproteins

The cell membrane is a **lipoprotein** structure, meaning that it is mainly composed of proteins and lipids—phospholipids, glycolipids, and cholesterol. The bipolar arrangement of the lipids monitors substances passing in and out of the cell. The phospholipids, which are bipolar in nature, line up with their polar regions pointing toward the interior or exterior of the cell and their nonpolar region lying within

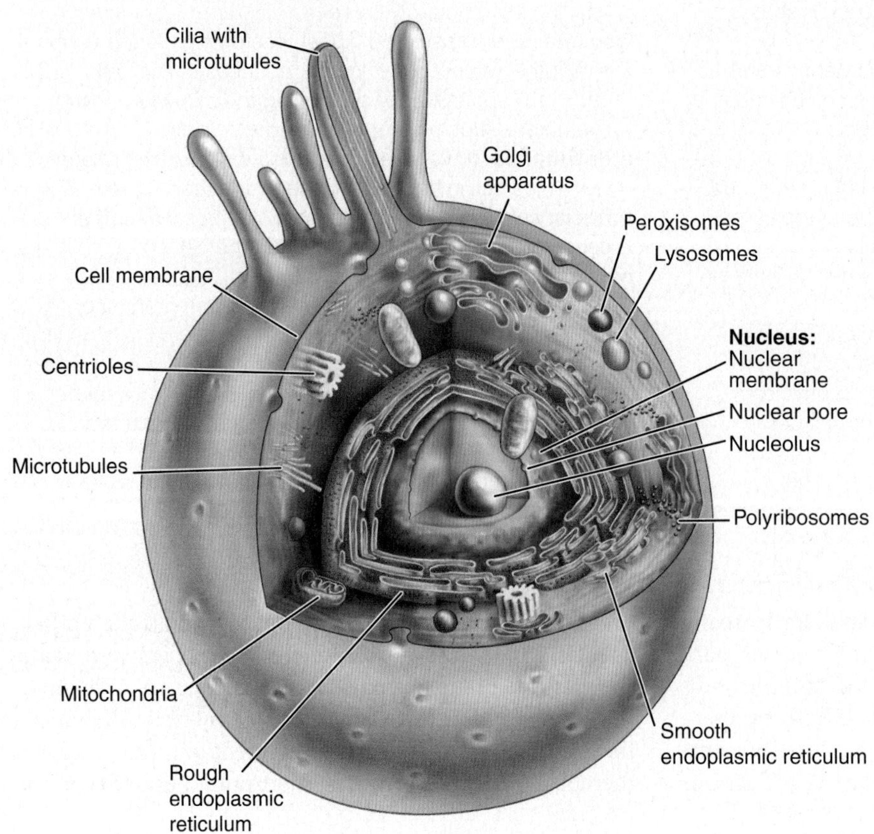

FIGURE 7.1 General structure of a cell and the location of its organelles.

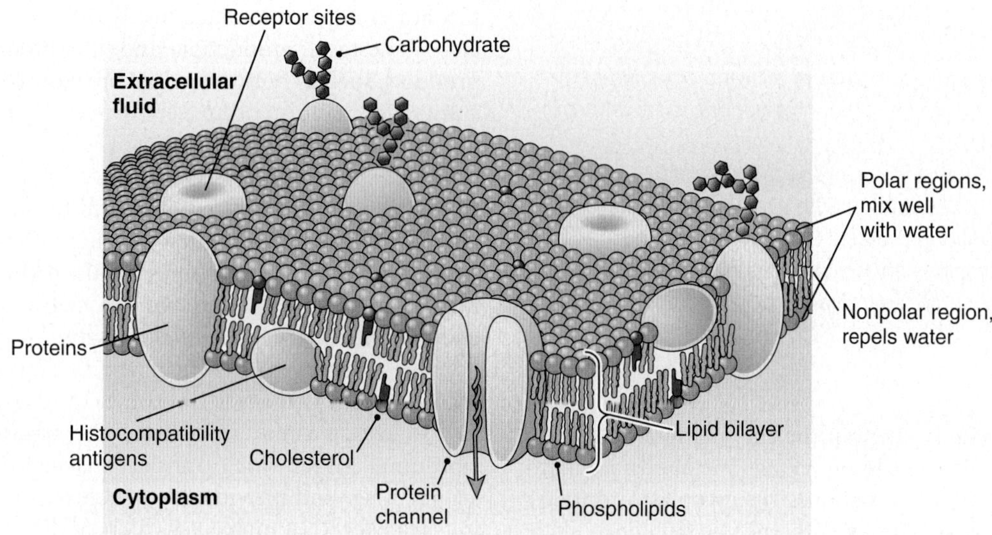

FIGURE 7.2 Structure of the lipid bilayer of the cell membrane.

the cell membrane. The polar regions mix well with water, and the nonpolar region repels water. These properties allow the membrane to act as a barrier to regulate what can enter the cell (Fig. 7.2). The freely moving nature of the membrane allows it to adjust to the changing shape of the cell so that areas of the membrane can move together to repair the membrane should it become torn or injured. Some of the outward-facing phospholipids have a sugar group attached to them called glycolipids. Cholesterol is found in large quantities in the membrane, and it works to keep the phospholipids in place and the cell membrane stable.

Receptor Sites

Embedded in the cell membrane are a series of peripheral proteins with several functions. As discussed in Chapter 2, one type of protein located on the cell membrane is known as a receptor site. This protein reacts with specific chemicals outside the cell to stimulate a reaction within the cell. For example, the receptor site for insulin reacts with the hormone insulin to cause activation of specific enzymes within the cell to change the cell membrane's permeability and allow more glucose into the cell, in addition to other metabolic cellular changes. Receptor sites are very important in the functioning of neurons, muscle cells, endocrine glands, and other cell types, and they play a very important role in clinical pharmacology.

Identifying Markers

Other surface proteins are surface antigens, or genetically determined identifying markers. These proteins are called **histocompatibility antigens** or human leukocyte antigens, which the body uses to identify a cell as a self-cell (i.e., a cell belonging to that individual). The body's immune system recognizes these proteins and acts to protect self-cells and to destroy nonself-cells. When an organ is transplanted from one person to another, a great effort is made to match as many histocompatibility antigens as possible to reduce the chance that the "new" body will reject the transplanted organ.

Histocompatibility antigens can be changed in several ways: by cell injury, with viral invasion of a cell, with age, and so on. If the markers are altered, the body's immune system reacts to the change and can ignore it, allowing neoplasms to grow and develop. The immune system may also attack the cell, leading to many of the problems associated with autoimmune disorders and chronic inflammatory conditions.

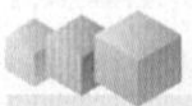
Concept Mastery Alert

Receptor Sites and Diabetes

Protein receptors are embedded in the cell membrane to carry out a specific function. Specific chemicals react with the protein receptors outside the cell to stimulate a reaction within the cell. For example, the receptor site for insulin reacts with the hormone insulin to cause activation of specific enzymes within the cell to change the cell membrane's permeability and allow more glucose into the cell, in addition to other metabolic cellular changes.

Channels

Channels (also called pores) within the cell membrane are made by proteins in the cell wall that allow the passage of small substances in or out of the cell. Specific channels have been identified for sodium, potassium, calcium, chloride, bicarbonate, and water; other channels may also exist. Some drugs are designed to affect certain channels specifically. For example, calcium channel blockers like amlodipine prevent the movement of calcium into a cell through calcium channels.

Key Points

- The cell is the basic structure of all living organisms.
- The cell nucleus is the location of genetic material held in DNA molecules.
- The cell membrane features specific receptor sites that allow interaction with various chemicals, histocompatibility proteins that allow for self-identification, and channels or pores that allow for the passage of substances into and out of the cell.

Cytoplasm

The cell **cytoplasm** lies within the cell membrane outside the nucleus and is the site of cellular metabolism activities and special cellular functions. The cytoplasm contains many **organelles**, structures with specific functions such as producing proteins and energy. The organelles within the cytoplasm include the mitochondria, the endoplasmic reticulum, free ribosomes, the Golgi apparatus, and the lysosomes.

Mitochondria

Mitochondria are rod-shaped double membraned organelle within each cell that produce energy in the form of adenosine triphosphate (ATP), which allows the cell to function. They act like power plants within each cell. Mitochondria, which can reproduce when a cell is very active, are always very abundant in cells that consume energy. For example, cardiac muscle cells, which must work continually to keep the heart contracting, contain a great number of mitochondria. Milk-producing cells in breast tissue, which are normally quite dormant, contain very few mitochondria. If a person is lactating, however, the mitochondria become more abundant to meet the demands of the milk-producing cells. The mitochondria can take carbohydrates, fats, and proteins from the cytoplasm and make ATP via the citric acid cycle or Krebs cycle, followed by a process of oxidation of hydrogen, which depends on oxygen being available. When there is not enough oxygen available, less ATP can be generated. Cells use the ATP to maintain homeostasis, produce proteins, and carry out specific functions. If oxygen is not available, lactic acid builds up as a by-product of cellular respiration. Lactic acid leaves the cell and is transported to the liver for conversion to glycogen and carbon dioxide.

Endoplasmic Reticulum

Much of the cytoplasm of a cell is made up of a fine network of interconnected channels known as cisternae, which form the **endoplasmic reticulum**. The undulating surface of the endoplasmic reticulum provides a large surface for chemical reactions within the cell. Many granules that contain enzymes and ribosomes, which produce protein, are scattered over the surface of the rough endoplasmic reticulum. Production of proteins, phospholipids, and cholesterol takes place in the rough endoplasmic reticulum. The smooth endoplasmic reticulum is the site of further lipid and cholesterol production and the production of cell products, such as hormones. The breakdown of many toxic substances may also occur here in particular cells.

Free Ribosomes

Other ribosomes that are not bound to the surface of the endoplasmic reticulum exist throughout the cytoplasm. These free-floating ribosomes produce proteins that are important to the structure of the cell and some of the enzymes necessary for cellular activity.

The messenger RNA from the nucleus can diffuse to the cytoplasm to the free ribosomes or ribosomes attached to the endoplasmic reticulum. The ribosomes contain ribosomal RNA, which translate instructions from messenger RNA and provide the structure for protein building. Transfer RNA molecules will read the instructions and deliver the correct amino acids to the ribosome that will be used to make the protein.

Golgi Apparatus

The **Golgi apparatus** is a series of flattened sacs that may be part of the endoplasmic reticulum. These structures prepare hormones or other substances for secretion by processing them and packaging them in vesicles to be moved to the cell membrane for excretion from the cell. In addition, the Golgi apparatus may produce lysosomes and store other synthesized proteins and enzymes until they are needed.

Lysosomes

Lysosomes are membrane-covered organelles containing specific digestive enzymes that can break down proteins, nucleic acids, carbohydrates, and lipids. Lysosomes are responsible for digesting worn or damaged sections of a cell when the membrane ruptures and the cell dies. Lysosomes form a membrane around any substance that needs to be digested and secrete the digestive enzymes directly into the isolated area, protecting the rest of the cytoplasm from injury. This phenomenon can be seen with old lettuce in the refrigerator. The side of the lettuce head that has been "lying down" for a prolonged period becomes brown and wet as the lettuce cells die and self-digest when their lysosomes are released. If the lettuce is not used, the released lysosomes begin to digest any healthy lettuce that remains, with eventual destruction of the entire head. Lysosomes are important in ecology. Dead trees, animals, and other organisms self-digest. Lysosomes become very important clinically when cell death (from disease or a drug effect) leads to the death of neighboring cells. When lysosomes are released from the dead cell, they have a potential to lyse or digest the proteins and membrane of neighboring cells. This can cause more cell death and more lysosomes to be released. A decubitus ulcer is a good example of cell death leading to the death of neighboring cells and becoming a potentially very difficult wound to heal. Debridement of dead cells may help the healing process by removing the lysosomes and facilitating growth of healthy tissue.

Key Points

- The cytoplasm of the cell contains various organelles that are important for cellular function.
- The mitochondria produce energy for the cell; the endoplasmic reticulum contains ribosomes that produce proteins; the Golgi apparatus packages proteins; and lysosomes contain protein-dissolving enzymes that are important for digestion and the recycling of organisms in nature.

Cell Properties

Cells have certain properties that allow them to survive. **Endocytosis** involves incorporation of material into the cell by extending the cell membrane around the substance. Pinocytosis, a form of endocytosis, refers to the engulfing of specific substances that have reacted with a receptor site on the cell membrane. This process allows cells to absorb nutrients, enzymes, and other materials. Phagocytosis is a similar process; it allows the cell, usually a neutrophil or macrophage, to engulf a bacterium or a foreign protein and destroy it within the cell by secreting digestive enzymes into the area. **Exocytosis** is the opposite of endocytosis and involves removing substances from a cell by pushing them through the cell membrane. Hormones, neurotransmitters, enzymes, and other substances produced within a cell are excreted into the body by this process (Fig. 7.3).

Homeostasis

The main goal of a cell is to maintain homeostasis, which means keeping the cytoplasm stable within the cell membrane. Each cell uses a series of active and passive transport systems to achieve homeostasis; the exact system used depends on the type of cell and its reactions with the immediate environment. For a cell to produce the energy needed to carry out cellular metabolism and other processes, the cell must have a means to obtain necessary elements from the outside environment. In addition, it must have a way to dispose of waste products that could be toxic to its cytoplasm. To dispose of waste, the cell moves substances across the cell membrane, either by passive transport or by active (energy-requiring) transport (Fig. 7.4).

Passive Transport

Passive transport happens without the expenditure of energy and can occur across any semipermeable membrane. There are essentially three types of passive transport: diffusion, osmosis, and facilitated diffusion.

Diffusion

Diffusion is the movement of a substance from a region of higher concentration to a region of lower concentration. The difference between the concentrations of the substance in the two regions is called the *concentration gradient* of the substance; usually, the greater the concentration gradient, the faster the substance moves. Movement into and out of a cell is regulated by the cell membrane. Some substances move through channels or pores in the cell membrane. Small substances and materials with no ionic charge move most freely through the channels. Substances with a negative charge move more freely than substances with a positive charge. Substances that move into and out of a cell by diffusion include carbon dioxide, oxygen, and water.

When a cell is very active and using energy and oxygen, the concentration of oxygen within the cell decreases. The concentration of oxygen outside the cell remains relatively high, so oxygen moves across the cell membrane (down the concentration gradient) to supply needed oxygen to the inside of the cell. Cells use this process to maintain homeostasis during many activities that occur during their life.

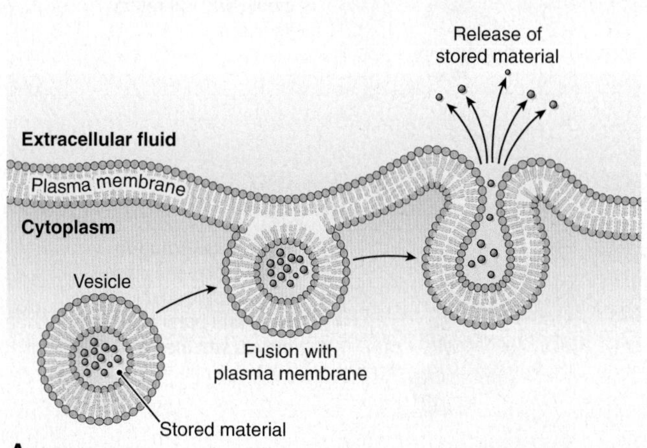

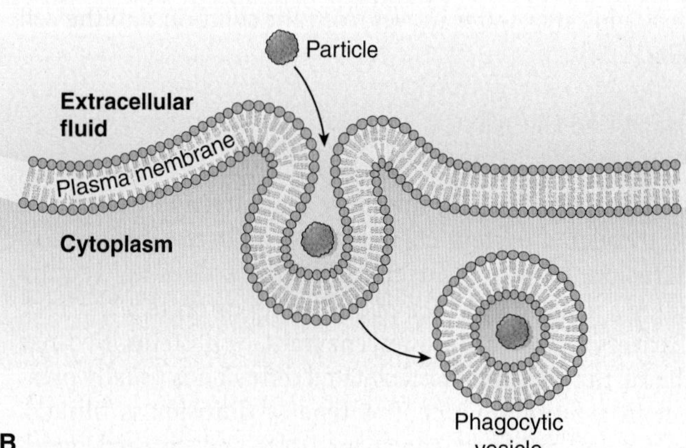

FIGURE 7.3 Schematic representation of endocytosis and exocytosis. **A.** Exocytosis is the movement of substances (waste products, hormones, neurotransmitters) out of the cell. **B.** Endocytosis involves the destruction of engulfed proteins or bacteria.

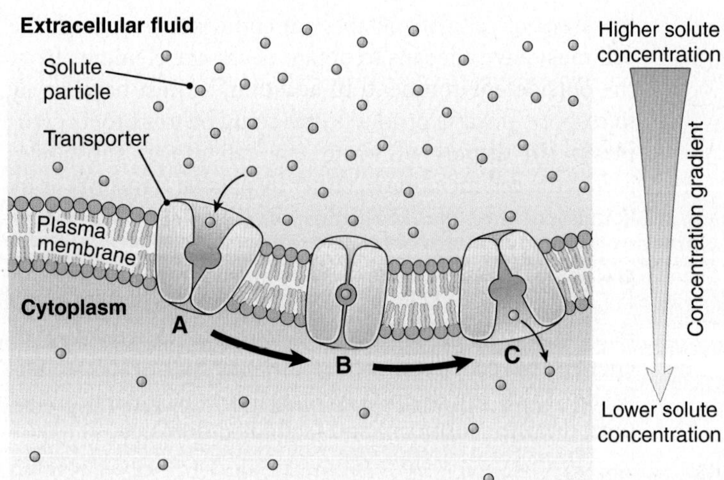

FIGURE 7.4 Schematic representation of passive pore diffusion of solute through a protein channel.

Osmosis

Osmosis, a special form of diffusion, is the movement of water across a semipermeable membrane from an area that is low in dissolved solutes to one that is high in dissolved solutes. The water is attempting to equalize the dilution of the solutes. This diffusion of water across a cell membrane from an area of high concentration (of water) to an area of low concentration creates pressure on the cell membrane called *osmotic pressure.* The greater the concentration of solutes in the solution to which the water is flowing, the higher the osmotic pressure.

A fluid that contains the same concentration of solutes as human plasma is called an *isotonic* solution. A fluid that contains a higher concentration of solutes than human plasma is a *hypertonic* solution, and it draws water from cells. A fluid that contains a lower concentration of solutes than human plasma is *hypotonic,* and it loses water to cells. If a human red blood cell, which has a cytoplasm that is isotonic with human plasma, is placed into a hypertonic solution, it shrinks and shrivels because the water inside the cell diffuses out of the cell into the solution. If the same cell is placed into a hypotonic solution, the cell swells and bursts because water moves from the solution into the cell (Fig. 7.5).

Facilitated Diffusion

Sometimes a substance cannot move freely on its own in or out of a cell. Such a substance may attach to a carrier or go through a protein channel to be diffused. This form of diffusion, known as *facilitated diffusion,* does not require energy, just the presence of the carrier or protein channel. Carriers may be hormones, enzymes, or proteins. Because the carrier required for facilitated diffusion is usually present in a finite amount, this type of diffusion is limited. Facilitated diffusion allows for polar and charged molecules (like carbohydrates, amino acids, and ions) to cross the cell membrane.

Active Transport

Sometimes a cell requires a substance in greater concentration than is found in the environment or needs to maintain its cytoplasm in a situation that would normally allow chemicals to leave the cell. When this happens, the cell

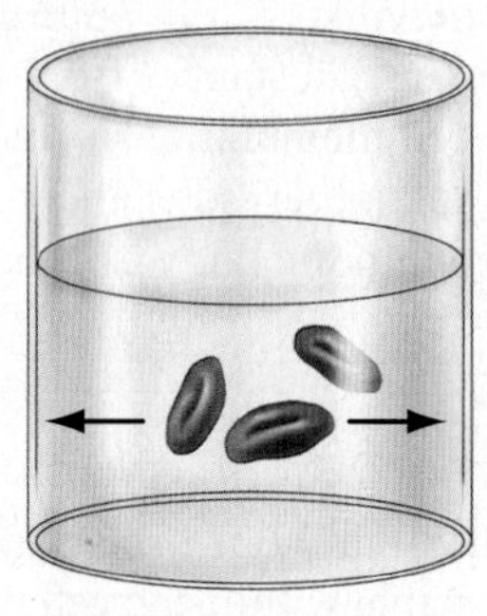

Hypertonic solution
A red blood cell placed in hypertonic solution will shrink and shrivel up as water moves out of the cell

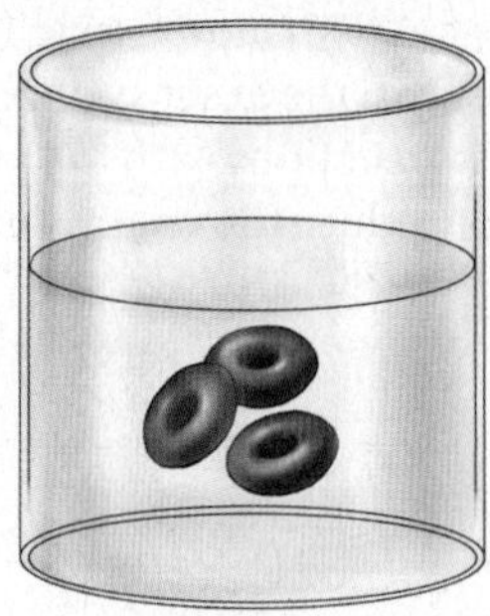

Isotonic solution
A red blood cell placed in isotonic solution is stable and will retain its shape

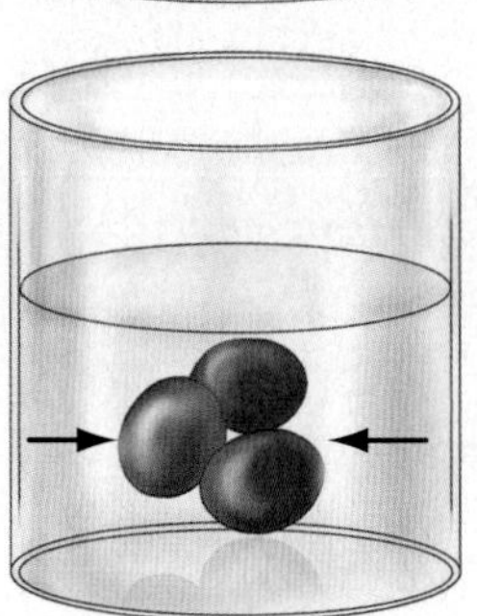

Hypotonic solution
A red blood cell placed in hypotonic solution will swell and burst as water moves into the cell

FIGURE 7.5 Red blood cell, showing the cell's response to hypertonic, isotonic, and hypotonic solutions.

must move substances against the concentration gradient using active transport, which requires energy. When a cell is deprived of oxygen because of a blood supply problem or insufficient oxygenation of the blood, systems of active transport begin to malfunction, placing the cell's integrity in jeopardy.

One of the best-known systems of active transport is the sodium–potassium pump. Cells use active transport to maintain a cytoplasm with a higher level of potassium and a lower level of sodium than the extracellular fluid contains. This allows the cell to maintain an electrical charge on the cell membrane, which gives many cells the electrical properties of excitation (the ability to generate a movement of electrons) and conduction (the ability to send this stimulus to other areas of the membrane). Some drugs use energy to move into cells by active transport. Drugs frequently bond with a carrier when move into the cell. Cells in the kidney use active transport to excrete drugs from the body, as well as to maintain electrolyte and acid–base balances.

Cell Cycle

Many cells have the ability to reproduce themselves through the process of **mitosis**. The genetic makeup of a particular cell determines the rate at which that cell can multiply. Some cells reproduce very quickly (e.g., the cells lining the gastrointestinal tract have a generation time of 72 hours), and some reproduce very slowly (e.g., the cells found in breast tissue have a generation time of a few months). In some cases, certain factors influence cell reproduction. Erythropoietin, a hormone produced by the kidney, can stimulate the production of new red blood cells. Active leukocytes release chemicals that stimulate the production of white blood cells when the body needs new ones. Regardless of the rate of reproduction, each cell has approximately the same life cycle. The life cycle of a cell, called the **cell cycle**, consists of four active phases and a resting phase (Fig. 7.6).

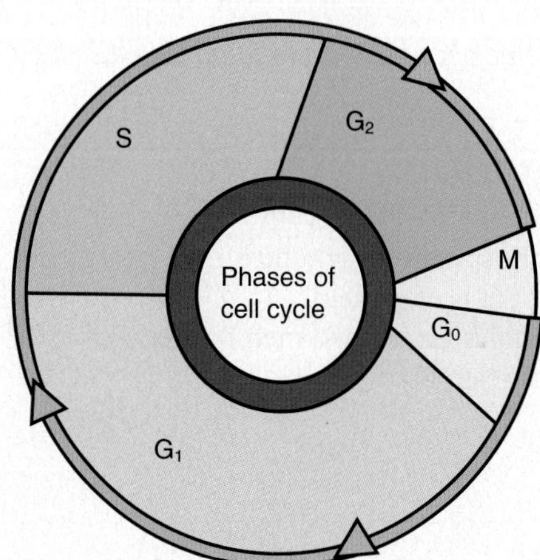

FIGURE 7.6 Diagram of the cell cycle, showing G_0, G_1, S, G_2, and M phases.

G_0 Phase

During the G_0 phase, or resting phase, the cell is stable. It is not making any proteins associated with cell division and is basically dormant as far as reproduction goes. These cells are just functioning to do whatever they are supposed to do. Cells in the G_0 phase cause a problem in the treatment of some cancers. Cancer chemotherapy usually works on active, dividing cells, leaving resting cells fairly untouched. When the resting cells are stimulated to become active and regenerate, the cancer can return, which is why cancer chemotherapeutic regimens are complicated and extended over time, and why a 5-year cancer-free period is usually the basic guide for considering a cancer to be cured.

G_1 Phase

When a cell is stimulated to emerge from its resting phase, it enters what is called the G_1 phase or gap phase, which lasts from the time of stimulation from the resting phase until the formation of DNA. During this period, the cell synthesizes substances needed for DNA formation. The cell is actively collecting materials to make these substances and producing the building blocks for DNA.

S Phase

The next phase, called the S phase or synthesis phase, involves the actual synthesis of DNA, which is an energy-consuming activity. The cell remains in this phase until the amount of cellular DNA has doubled.

G_2 Phase

After the cellular DNA has doubled in preparation for replication, the G_2 phase begins, another gap phase. During this phase, the cell produces all the substances required for the manufacture of the mitotic spindles.

M Phase

After the cell has produced all the substances necessary for formation of a new cell, or daughter cell, it undergoes cell division or mitosis. This occurs during the M phase of the cell cycle. During this phase, the cell splits to form two identical daughter cells.

Key Points

- Many cells progress through a cell cycle, which allows them to reproduce.
- The cell cycle includes a resting phase (G_0) a gap phase (G_1), when the components needed for cell division are collected by the cell; a synthesizing phase (S), when DNA and other components are produced; a final gap phase (G_2), when the last substances needed for division are collected and produced; and an M phase, when actual cell division occurs, producing two identical daughter cells.

SUMMARY

- The cell is composed of a nucleus, which contains genetic material and controls the production of proteins by the cell; a cell membrane, which separates the inside of the cell from the outside environment; and a cytoplasm, which contains various organelles important to cell function.
- The cell membrane functions as a fluid barrier made of lipids and proteins. The arrangement of the lipoprotein membrane controls what enters and leaves the cell.
- Proteins on the cell membrane surface can act either as receptor sites for specific substances or as histocompatibility markers that identify the cell as a self-cell (i.e., a cell belonging to that individual).
- Channels or pores in the cell membrane allow for easier movement of specific substances needed by the cell for normal functioning.
- Mitochondria are rod-shaped organelles that produce energy in the form of ATP for use by cells.
- Ribosomes are sites of protein production within the cell cytoplasm. The specific proteins produced by a cell are determined by the genetic material within the cell nucleus.
- The Golgi apparatus packages particular substances for removal from the cell (e.g., neurotransmitters, hormones).
- Lysosomes are packets of digestive enzymes located in the cell cytoplasm. These enzymes are responsible for destroying injured or nonfunctioning parts of the cell and for promoting cellular disintegration when the cell dies.
- Endocytosis is the process of moving substances into a cell by extending the cell membrane around the substance and engulfing it. Pinocytosis refers to the engulfing of necessary materials, and phagocytosis refers to the engulfing and destroying of bacteria or other proteins by white blood cells.
- Exocytosis is the process of removing substances from a cell by moving them toward the cell membrane and then changing the cell membrane to allow passage of the substance out of the cell.
- Cells maintain homeostasis by regulating the movement of solutes and water into and out of the cell.
- Diffusion, which does not require energy, is the movement of solutes from a region of high concentration to a region of lower concentration across a concentration gradient.
- Osmosis, which like diffusion does not require energy, is the movement of water from an area low in solutes to an area high in solutes. Osmosis exerts a pressure against the cell membrane that is called osmotic pressure.
- Active transport, an energy-requiring process, is the movement of particular substances against a concentration gradient. Active transport is important in maintaining cell homeostasis.
- Cells replicate at differing rates, depending on the genetic programming of the cell. Many cells go through a life cycle consisting of the following phases: G_0, the resting phase; G_1, which involves the production of proteins for DNA synthesis; S, which involves the synthesis of DNA; G_2, which involves manufacture of the materials needed for mitotic spindle production; and M, the mitotic phase, in which the cell splits to form two identical daughter cells.

CHECK YOUR UNDERSTANDING

Answers to the questions in this chapter can be found in Answers to Check Your Understanding Questions on thePoint®.

MULTIPLE CHOICE

Select the best answer.

1. The basic unit of human structure is
   a. the mitochondria.
   b. the nucleus.
   c. the nucleolus.
   d. the cell.

2. The cell membrane is composed of
   a. a phospholipid structure.
   b. channels of protein.
   c. a cholesterol-based membrane.
   d. Golgi apparatus.

3. The saying, "One rotten apple can spoil the whole barrel," can be used to refer to the cell-degrading properties of
   a. calcium channels.
   b. lysosomes.
   c. histocompatibility receptors.
   d. nuclear spindles.

4. The ribosomes are important sites for
   a. digestion of nutrients.
   b. excretion of waste products.
   c. production of proteins.
   d. hormone receptors.

5. A human cell placed in salty seawater will
   a. burst from water entering the cell.
   b. shrivel and die from water leaving the cell.
   c. not be affected in any way.
   d. break apart from the salt effect.

6. The sodium–potassium pump maintains a negative charge on the cell membrane by
   a. osmosis.
   b. diffusion.
   c. active transport.
   d. facilitated diffusion.

7. Most cells progress through basically the same cell cycle, including
   a. two phases.
   b. four active phases and a resting phase.
   c. three periods of rest and a splitting phase.
   d. four active phases.

MULTIPLE RESPONSE

Select all that apply.

1. The amount of time that a cell takes to progress through the cell cycle is determined by which of the following?
   a. The acidity of the environment
   b. The genetic makeup of the cell
   c. The location of the cell in the body
   d. The number of ribosomes in the cell
   e. The cell response to contact inhibition
   f. The availability of nutrients and oxygen

2. Some substances will pass into the human cell by simple diffusion. Which of the following substances diffuse into the cell?
   a. Calcium
   b. Nitrogen
   c. Sodium
   d. Carbon dioxide
   e. Oxygen
   f. Potassium

3. Some substances require a channel or pore to enter a cell membrane. Which of the following substances use a channel to enter the cell?
   a. Calcium
   b. Urea
   c. Fat-soluble vitamins
   d. Sodium
   e. Oxygen
   f. Potassium

REFERENCES

Alberts, B., Johnson, A., Lewis, J., Morgan, D., Raff, M., Roberts, K., & Walter, P. (Eds.). (2015). *Molecular biology of the cell* (6th ed.). Garland Science.

Barrett, K., Barman, S., Boitano, S., & Brooks, H. (2016). *Ganong's review of medical physiology* (25th ed.). McGraw-Hill.

Brunton, L. L., Hilal-Dandan, R., & Knollman, B. C. (2018). *Goodman and Gilman's the pharmacological basis of therapeutics* (13th ed.). McGraw-Hill.

Cooper, G. M., & Hausman, R. E. (2015). *The cell: A molecular approach* (7th ed.). ASM Press/Sinauer Associates.

Hall, J. E. (2016). *Guyton and Hall textbook of medical physiology* (13th ed.). Elsevier.

Landowne, D. (2006). *Cell physiology*. McGraw-Hill.

Lodish, H. F., Berk, A., Kaiser, C. A., Krieger, M., Bretscher, A., Ploegh, H. L., Amon, A., & Martin, K. C. (2016). *Molecular cell biology* (8th ed.). W. H. Freeman.

Morgan, D. O. (2014). *The cell cycle: Principles of control* (2nd ed.). New Science Press.

Norris, T. L., & Lalchandani, R. (2018). *Porth's pathophysiology: Concepts of altered health states* (10th ed.). Wolters Kluwer.

Sherwood, L. (2013). *Human physiology: From cells to systems* (8th ed.). Brooks/Cole, Cengage Learning.

CHAPTER 8

Anti-Infective Agents

Learning Objectives

Upon completion of this chapter, you will be able to:

1. Explain selective toxicity and discuss its importance in anti-infective therapies.
2. Differentiate broad-spectrum and narrow-spectrum drugs.
3. Define resistance to anti-infectives and discuss the emergence of resistant strains.
4. Explain ways to minimize resistance.
5. Explain how anti-infective agents are used for both treatment and prophylaxis.
6. Describe at least three common adverse reactions associated with the use of anti-infectives.

Key Terms

bactericidal: substance that causes the death of bacteria, usually by interfering with cell membrane stability or with proteins or enzymes necessary to maintain the cellular integrity of the bacteria

bacteriostatic: substance that prevents or slows the replication of bacteria, usually by interfering with proteins or enzyme systems necessary for reproduction of the bacteria

culture: sample of the bacteria (e.g., from sputum, cell scrapings, urine) to be grown in a laboratory to determine the species of bacteria causing a particular infection

prophylaxis: treatment to prevent an infection before it occurs or to prevent a second infection, as in the use of antibiotics to prevent bacterial endocarditis in high-risk patients or antiprotozoals to prevent malaria

resistance: ability of pathogens over time to adapt to an anti-infective to produce cells that are no longer affected by a particular drug

selective toxicity: the ability to affect certain proteins or enzyme systems that are used by the infecting organism but not by human cells

sensitivity testing: evaluation of pathogens obtained in a culture to determine which anti-infectives will be effective against the organisms causing a particular infection

spectrum: range of bacteria against which an antibiotic is effective (e.g., broad-spectrum antibiotics are effective against a wide range of bacteria; narrow-spectrum antibiotics are effective only against very selective bacteria)

superinfection: infections that occur when opportunistic pathogens have the opportunity to invade tissues and cause infections because the normal flora bacteria that kept them in check have been destroyed by antibiotic therapy

Drug List

gentamicin

meropenem

vancomycin

Anti-infective agents are drugs designed to target foreign organisms that have invaded and infected the body of a human host. For centuries, people have used various naturally occurring chemicals in an effort to treat disease. Often treatment arose from a random act that proved useful. For instance, ancient Chinese people found that applying moldy soybean curds to boils and infected wounds helped prevent infection or hastened cure. Their finding was, perhaps, a forerunner of the penicillins used today.

The use of drugs to treat systemic infections is a relatively new concept, beginning with Paul Ehrlich in the 1920s. Ehrlich's research to develop a synthetic chemical that would be effective only against infection-causing cells,

Box 8.1 Focus on Drug Therapy Across the Lifespan

This box presents general principles of use of anti-infectives across the lifespan. Specifics for each type of anti-infective agent are discussed in their respective chapters within this unit.

ANTI-INFECTIVE AGENTS

Children

Use anti-infectives with caution; early exposure can lead to early sensitivity.

Controversy is widespread regarding the use of antibiotics to treat ear infections, a common pediatric problem. Some believe that the habitual use of antibiotics for what might well be a viral infection has contributed greatly to the development of resistant strains.

Because children can have increased susceptibility to anti-infectives' effects on the gastrointestinal (GI) and nervous systems, carefully monitor their hydration and nutritional status.

Adults

Adults often demand anti-infectives for a "quick cure" of various signs and symptoms. Drug allergies and the emergence of resistant strains can be a challenge with this group.

Extreme caution must be exercised in the use of anti-infectives in people who are pregnant or lactating. Many anti-infectives can affect the fetus and cross into human milk, leading to toxic effects in the neonate.

Older Adults

Older patients often do not present with the same signs and symptoms of infection that are seen in younger people.

The older patient is susceptible to severe adverse GI, renal, and neurological effects and must be monitored for nutritional status and hydration during drug therapy.

Anti-infectives that adversely affect the liver and kidneys must be used with caution in older patients, who may have decreased organ function.

not human cells, led the way for the scientific investigation of anti-infective agents. In the late 1920s, scientists discovered penicillin in a mold sample; in 1935, sulfonamides were introduced. Since then, the number of available anti-infectives has grown tremendously. However, many of the organisms these drugs were designed to treat are rapidly adapting to repel the effects of anti-infectives. Therefore, much work remains to deal with these emergent or resistant strains.

Although anti-infective agents target foreign organisms infecting the body of a human host, they do not possess total **selective toxicity**, which is the ability to affect particular proteins or enzyme systems used only by the infecting organism but not by human cells. Because all living cells are somewhat similar, developing an anti-infective drug that does not affect the host remains a challenge.

This chapter focuses on the principles involved in the use of anti-infective therapy and presents some anti-infectives as examples of these principles. The following chapters discuss specific anti-infectives used to treat particular infections: antibiotics for bacterial infections; antivirals; antifungals; antiprotozoals for infections caused by specific protozoa, including malaria; and anthelmintics for infections caused by worms. The final chapter in this section discusses antineoplastics, which are drugs used to treat diseases caused by abnormal human cells such as cancers. Antineoplastics specifically affect human cells to cause cell death or prevent cell growth and reproduction. The effects of anti-infectives on various age groups are discussed in Box 8.1.

Therapeutic Actions

Anti-infective agents act on the cells of invading organisms in several different ways. The goal of anti-infective use is interference with the normal function of the invading organism to prevent it from reproducing and to cause cell death without affecting host cells. Various mechanisms of action are briefly described here and shown in Figure 8.1. The specific mechanism of action for each drug class is discussed in the chapters that follow.

- Some anti-infectives interfere with biosynthesis of the pathogen cell wall. Because bacterial cells have a slightly different composition than human cells, this is an effective way to destroy the bacteria without interfering with the host. The penicillins are one classification of antibiotics that work in this way.
- Some anti-infectives prevent the cells of the invading organism from using substances essential to their growth and development, leading to an inability to divide and eventually to cell death. The sulfonamides, some antimycobacterial drugs, and trimethoprim–sulfamethoxazole (a combination drug frequently used to treat urinary tract infections) work in this way.
- Many anti-infectives interfere with the steps involved in protein synthesis, a function necessary to maintain the cell and allow for cell division. The aminoglycosides and the macrolides (see the information on adverse effects of gentamicin in Box 8.4) work in this way.
- Some anti-infectives interfere with DNA synthesis in the cell, leading to inability to divide and cell death. The fluoroquinolones work in this way.
- Other anti-infectives alter the permeability of the cell membrane to allow essential cellular components to leak out, causing cell death. Some antibiotics, antifungals, and antiprotozoal drugs work in this manner.

Anti-Infective Activity

The anti-infectives used today vary in their **spectrum** of activity; that is, they vary in their effectiveness against

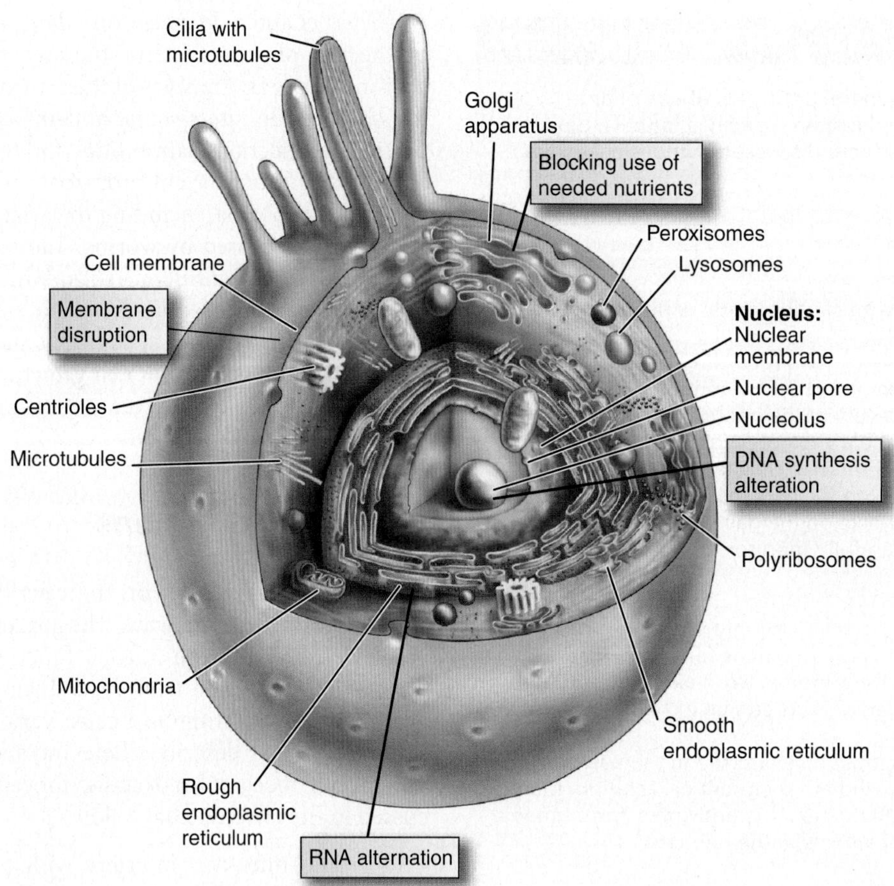

FIGURE 8.1 Anti-infectives can affect cells by disrupting the cell membrane, interfering with DNA synthesis, altering RNA, or blocking the use of essential nutrients.

invading organisms. Some anti-infectives are so selective in their action that they are effective against only a few microorganisms with a very specific metabolic pathway or enzyme. These drugs are said to have a narrow spectrum of activity. Other drugs interfere with biochemical reactions in many different kinds of microorganisms, making them useful in the treatment of a wide variety of infections. Such drugs are said to have a broad spectrum of activity.

Some anti-infectives are so active against the infective microorganisms that they actually cause the death of the cells they affect. These drugs are said to be **bactericidal** or fungicidal, depending upon the nature of the infective microorganism. Some anti-infectives are not as aggressive against invading organisms; they interfere with the ability of the cells to reproduce or divide, thereby preventing or slowing cell replication. These drugs are said to be **bacteriostatic** or fungistatic. Several drugs are both "cidal" and "static," often depending on the concentration of the drug that is present. Many of the adverse effects noted with the use of anti-infectives are associated with the aggressive properties of the drugs and their effect on the cells of the host in addition to those of the pathogen.

There are times when anti-infective medications are not able to treat the infection due to the site of infection. Infections in the central nervous system can be more difficult to treat since medication needs to cross the blood–brain barrier to be effective. Bacterial infections within the heart (endocarditis) and purulent abscesses in the body with decreased blood supply are also difficult to treat with anti-infective medications. Surgical removal of purulent infection can often facilitate the treatment of the infection. Foreign materials implanted in the body (e.g., pacemakers, surgical mesh, joint prostheses) can increase risk of infection when immune cells around the foreign material are less able to destroy the microorganisms.

Human Immune Response

The goal of anti-infective therapy is reduction of the population of the invading organism to a point at which the human immune response can eliminate the infection. If a drug were aggressive enough to eliminate all traces of an invading pathogen, it also might be toxic to the host. The immune response (see Chapter 15) involves complex interactions among chemical mediators, leukocytes, lymphocytes, antibodies, and locally released enzymes and chemicals. When this response is completely functional and all the necessary proteins, cells, and chemicals are being produced by the body, it can isolate and eliminate foreign proteins, including bacteria, fungi, and viruses. However, if a person is immunocompromised for any reason (e.g., malnutrition, age, acquired immune deficiency syndrome, use of immunosuppressant drugs), the immune system may be incapable of dealing effectively with the invading organisms. It is difficult to treat any infections in such patients for two reasons: (a) anti-infective drugs cannot totally eliminate the pathogen without causing severe toxicity in the host and (b) these patients do not have the inflammatory or immune response in place to deal with even a few invading organisms. Immunocompromised patients present a significant challenge to health care providers. In helping people cope with infections, prevention of infection and proper nutrition are often as important as drug therapy.

Anti-infective medications are not effective on all pathogens that cause illness in humans. Therefore, the principles of preventing infection are important for the nurse to practice and teach to patients and families. Examples of preventative measures to decrease the spread of infection include the following:

1. Washing hands frequently, especially before and after caring for a patient in the health care setting
2. Removing invasive catheters (urinary and/or IV) as soon as it is safe to do so because their presence increases risk of infection
3. Maintaining up-to-date immunization status, for example, getting the influenza vaccine every year
4. Following transmission-based precautions to prevent spread of resistant micro organisms, for example, using face masks to prevent the spread of COVID-19 as recommended by the Centers for Disease Control and Prevention

Resistance

Resistance can be natural or acquired and refers to the ability of microorganisms to adapt over time to an anti-infective drug and produce cells that are no longer affected by a particular drug. Because anti-infectives act on specific enzyme systems or biological processes, many microorganisms that do not use that system or process are not affected by a particular anti-infective drug and are said to have a natural or intrinsic resistance. When prescribing a drug for treatment of an infection, this innate resistance should be anticipated. The selected drug should be one that is known to affect the specific microorganism causing the infection.

Since the advent of anti-infective drugs, microorganisms that were once very sensitive to the effects of particular drugs have begun to develop acquired resistance to the agents (see Box 8.2). This can result in a serious clinical problem. The emergence of resistant strains of bacteria and other organisms poses a threat: Anti-infective drugs may no longer control potentially life-threatening diseases, and uncontrollable epidemics may occur.

BOX 8.2

Bacterial Resistance to an Anti-Infective Drug

Vancomycin (IV: *Vancocin*, Oral: *Firvanq*) is an antibiotic that interferes with cell wall synthesis in susceptible bacteria. It was developed to address the need for a drug that could be used both to treat patients who are intolerant to or allergic to penicillin and/or cephalosporins and to treat patients with staphylococcal infections that no longer respond to penicillin or cephalosporins. This drug was the first drug in a class called lipoglycopeptides (Chapter 9). This anti-infective drug can be used intravenously to treat life-threatening infections when less toxic drugs cannot be used. However, for *Clostridium difficile*–associated diarrhea and staphylococcal enterocolitis, vancomycin must be dosed orally.

Because intravenous vancomycin may be highly toxic, its use is reserved for very serious and severe infections. It can cause renal failure; ototoxicity; superinfections; and sudden and severe hypotension, fever, chills, paresthesias, and erythema or redness of the neck and back. Administering the medication slowly can decrease the risk of adverse effects. Due to the risk of renal toxicity, renal function should be monitored with therapy, especially in patients 65 years and older. IV dosing should be adjusted if there is chronic renal impairment, and peak and trough levels of the medication are frequently assessed to assist with dosing adjustments.

Despite the adverse effects of vancomycin, when it is the only antibiotic that is effective against a specific bacterium, the benefits may outweigh the risks. Unfortunately, there are now vancomycin-resistant bacteria that can cause infections the drug is not able to treat.

Concept Mastery Alert

Adverse Effects of Vancomycin

Vancomycin's use is reserved for serious and severe infections as it may be highly toxic and can cause renal failure, ototoxicity, and superinfections. Renal failure is a primary concern and should be reported immediately to the health care provider. When infused quickly, there is a higher risk of adverse reactions including anaphylactoid reactions, erythema, and hypotension.

Acquiring Resistance

Microorganisms develop resistance in a number of ways, including the following:

- They can produce an enzyme that deactivates the antimicrobial drug. For example, some strains of bacteria that were once controlled by penicillin now produce an enzyme called penicillinase, which inactivates penicillin before it can affect the bacteria. This has led to the development of new drugs that are resistant to penicillinase.

- Cellular permeability can change to prevent the drug from entering the cell, or transport systems can be altered to exclude the drug from active transport into the cell.
- The microorganism can alter binding sites on the membranes or ribosomes, which will then no longer accept the drug.
- They can produce a chemical that acts as an antagonist to the drug.

Most commonly, the development of resistance depends on the degree to which the drug acts to eliminate the invading microorganisms that are most sensitive to its effects. The cells that remain may be somewhat resistant to the effects of the drug; with time, these cells form the majority in the population. These cells differ from the general population of the species because of slight variations in their biochemicals or biochemical processes. The drug does not cause a mutation of these cells; it simply allows the somewhat different cells to become the majority or dominant group after elimination of the sensitive cells. Other microbes may develop resistance through actual genetic mutation. A mutated cell survives the effects of an anti-infective agent and divides, forming a new colony of resistant microbes with a genetic composition that provides resistance to the anti-infective agent.

Preventing Resistance

Because the emergence of resistant strains of microbes is a serious public health problem that continues to grow, health care providers must work together to prevent the emergence of resistant pathogens. Exposure of a pathogen to an antimicrobial agent leads to the development of resistance, so it is important to limit the use of antimicrobial agents to the treatment of specific pathogens known to be sensitive to the drug being used.

Drug dosing is important in preventing resistance. Doses should be high enough, and the duration of drug therapy should be long enough to treat the infection while minimizing adverse effects. The recommended dosage for a specific anti-infective agent takes this issue into account. Around-the-clock dosing reduces the peaks and valleys in drug concentration and helps to maintain a constant therapeutic level to prevent the emergence of resistant microbes during times of low concentration. The duration of drug use is critical to ensure that the microbes are completely, not partially, eliminated and are not given the chance to grow and develop resistant strains. It can be difficult to convince patients who are taking anti-infective drugs that the timing of doses and the length of time they continue to take the drug are important. Many people stop taking a drug once they start to feel better and then keep the remaining pills to treat future illness. This practice favors the emergence of resistant strains. Box 8.3 gives tips on patient teaching.

Health care providers should also be cautious about the indiscriminate use of anti-infectives. Antibiotics are not effective in treating viral infections or illnesses such as common cold. However, many patients demand prescriptions for these drugs when they visit practitioners because they are convinced that they need to take something to feel better. Health care providers who prescribe anti-infectives without knowing the causative organism and which drugs might be appropriate may be promoting the emergence of resistant strains of microbes. With many serious illnesses, including cases of pneumonia in which a bacterial organism is suspected, antibiotic therapy may be started as soon as a **culture**, or sample of the bacteria, is taken and before the results are known. However, it is best to refrain from prescribing antibiotics if there is more evidence that the infection is viral.

Box 8.3 Focus on Patient and Family Teaching

USING ANTI-INFECTIVE AGENTS

When teaching patients who are prescribed an anti-infective agent, it is important to always include some general points:

- This drug is prescribed for treating the particular infection that you have now. Do not use this drug to treat other infections.
- This drug needs to be taken as prescribed the correct number of times each day and for the full number of days. Do not stop taking the drug if you start feeling better. You need to take the drug for the full number of treatment days to ensure that the infection has been treated.

Key Points

- The goal of anti-infective therapy is the reduction of the invading organisms to a point at which the human immune response can eliminate the infection.
- Anti-infectives can act to destroy an infective pathogen (-cidal) or to prevent the pathogen from reproducing (-static).
- Anti-infectives can be effective against a small group of pathogens (narrow spectrum), or they can be effective against many pathogens (broad spectrum).

Using Anti-Infective Agents

Anti-infective agents are used to treat both systemic and local infections. They are sometimes used as a means of **prophylaxis** (treatment to prevent an infection before it occurs or to prevent a second infection).

Treatment of Systemic Infections

Many infections that once led to lengthy, organ-damaging, or even fatal illnesses are now managed quickly and efficiently with the use of systemic anti-infective agents. Before the introduction of penicillin to treat streptococcal infections, many people developed rheumatic fever with serious cardiac complications. Today, rheumatic fever and the resultant cardiac valve defects are seldom seen. Several factors should be considered before beginning a systemic anti-infective regimen to ensure that the patient obtains the greatest benefit possible with the fewest adverse effects. These factors include identification of the correct pathogen and selection of a drug that is most likely to (a) cause the fewest complications for that patient and (b) be most effective against the pathogen involved.

Identification of the Pathogen

Identification of the infecting pathogen is done by culturing a tissue sample from the infected area. Cultures are performed in a laboratory, in which a swab of infected tissue is allowed to grow on an agar plate. Staining techniques and microscopic examination are used to identify the offending pathogen. When investigators search for parasitic sources of infection, they may examine stool for ova and parasites. Microscopic examination of other samples is also used to detect fungal and protozoal infections. The correct identification of the organism causing the infection is an important first step in determining which anti-infective drug should be used.

Sensitivity of the Pathogen

In many situations, health care providers use a broad-spectrum anti-infective agent that has been shown to be most effective in treating an infection with certain presenting signs and symptoms. In other cases of severe infection, a broad-spectrum antibiotic is started after a culture is taken but before the exact causative organism has been identified. Again, experience influences selection of the drug, based on the presenting signs and symptoms. In many cases, it is necessary to perform **sensitivity testing** on the cultured microbes to evaluate bacteria and determine which drugs are capable of controlling the particular microorganism. This testing is especially important with microorganisms that have known resistant strains. In these cases, culture and sensitivity testing identify the causal pathogen and the most appropriate drug for treating the infection.

Combination Therapy

In some situations, a combination of two or more types of drugs will effectively treat the infection. When the offending pathogen is known, combination drugs may be effective in interfering with its cellular structure in different areas or developmental phases. Unfortunately, using combination therapy may be more expensive and may lead to more adverse effects.

Combination therapy may be used for several reasons:

- Some drugs are synergistic, which means that they are more powerful when given in combination.
- Many microbial infections are caused by more than one pathogen, and each pathogen may react to a different anti-infective agent.
- Sometimes, the combined effects of the different drugs delay the emergence of resistant strains. This is important in the treatment of tuberculosis (a mycobacterial infection), malaria (a protozoal infection), HIV infection (a viral infection), and some bacterial infections. Resistant strains may be more likely to emerge when fixed combinations are used over time; however, this may be prevented by individualizing the combination.

Prophylaxis

Sometimes it is clinically useful to use anti-infectives as a means of prophylaxis to prevent infections before they occur. For example, when patients anticipate traveling to an area where malaria is endemic, they may begin taking antimalarial drugs before the journey and continue taking them periodically during the trip. Patients who are undergoing gastrointestinal (GI) or genitourinary surgery, which might introduce bacteria from those areas into the system, often receive antibiotics during or immediately after the surgery and periodically thereafter, as appropriate, to prevent infection. Patients with known cardiac valve disease, valve replacements, and other conditions are especially prone to the development of subacute bacterial endocarditis because of the vulnerability of their heart valves. When these patients are at high risk for developing one of these infections, they may use prophylactic antibiotic therapy as a precaution when undergoing certain invasive procedures, including dental work.

Key Points

- Resistance of a pathogen to an anti-infective agent can be natural (the pathogen does not use the process on which the anti-infective works) or acquired (the pathogen develops a process to oppose the anti-infective agent).
- The emergence of resistant strains is a serious public health problem. Health care providers need to be alert to preventing the emergence of resistant strains by not using antibiotics inappropriately, ensuring that the anti-infective is taken at a high enough dose for a long enough period of time, and avoiding the use of newer, powerful anti-infectives if other drugs would be just as effective.

Adverse Reactions to Anti-Infective Therapy

Because anti-infective agents affect cells, it is always possible that the host cells will also be damaged (see Box 8.4). No anti-infective agent has been developed that is completely free of adverse effects. The most common adverse effects associated with the use of anti-infective agents are direct toxic effects on the kidney, GI tract, and nervous system. Hypersensitivity reactions and superinfections also can occur.

Kidney Damage

Kidney damage occurs most frequently with drugs that are metabolized by the kidney or eliminated in the urine. Such drugs, which have a direct toxic effect on the fragile cells in the kidney, can cause conditions ranging from renal dysfunction to full-blown renal failure. When patients are taking these drugs (e.g., aminoglycosides), they should be monitored closely for any sign of renal dysfunction. To prevent any accumulation of the drug in the kidney, patients should be well hydrated throughout the course of the drug therapy.

Gastrointestinal Toxicity

GI toxicity is very common with many anti-infectives. Many of these agents have direct toxic effects on the cells lining the GI tract, causing nausea, vomiting, stomach upset, or diarrhea; such effects are sometimes severe (see Box 8.5). There is also some evidence that the death of the microorganisms releases chemicals and toxins into the body, which can stimulate the chemoreceptor trigger zone in the medulla and induce nausea and vomiting.

BOX 8.4

Serious Adverse Effects of Antibiotic Treatment

Gentamicin (generic), an aminoglycoside antibiotic, inhibits protein synthesis in susceptible strains of gram-negative bacteria. This disrupts the functional integrity of the cell wall, leading to cell death. Because of the potential toxic effects of this drug, its use is limited to serious infections for which no other antibiotic is effective. Gentamicin can cause severe renal damage and ototoxicity. In addition, the drug may cause bone marrow depression. Despite the risk of renal failure and other toxicities, it has stayed on the market because it is used to treat serious infections caused by bacteria that are not sensitive to any other antibiotic. It is now available in parenteral, topical, and ophthalmic forms. When administered systemically, dosing should be adjusted if there is acute or chronic renal impairment.

BOX 8.5

Severe Gastrointestinal Toxicity Resulting From Anti-Infective Treatment

Meropenem (*Merrem IV*), an IV antibiotic from the carbapenem class of antibiotics (see Chapter 9), inhibits the synthesis of cell walls in susceptible bacteria. Carbapenems are beta lactam antibiotics like the penicillin, cephalosporin, and monobactam classifications. Meropenem is used to treat polymicrobial and drug resistant infections. Meropenem can cause very uncomfortable GI effects; in fact, use of this drug has been associated with potentially fatal pseudomembranous colitis. The GI effects of all the beta lactam antibiotics can range from mild discomfort to severe and fatal effects. Use of meropenem can also result in headache, dizziness, rash, and superinfections. Meropenem is a very broad-spectrum antibiotic, so is reserved for resistant infections. Dosing is adjusted for patients with renal impairment and for pediatric patients.

Some anti-infectives are toxic to the liver. These drugs can cause hepatitis and even liver failure. When a patient is taking a drug known to be toxic to the liver (e.g., many of the cephalosporins), they should be monitored closely, and the drug should be stopped at any sign of liver dysfunction.

Neurotoxicity

Some anti-infectives can damage or interfere with the function of nerve tissue, usually in areas where drugs tend to accumulate in high concentrations. For example, the aminoglycoside antibiotics collect in the eighth cranial nerve and can cause dizziness, vertigo, and loss of hearing. Chloroquine, which is used to treat malaria and some other rheumatoid disorders, can accumulate in the retina and optic nerve and cause blindness. Other anti-infectives can cause dizziness, drowsiness, lethargy, changes in reflexes, and even hallucinations when they irritate specific nerve tissues.

Hypersensitivity Reactions

Allergic or hypersensitivity reactions occur with many antimicrobial agents. Most of these agents, which are protein bound for transfer through the cardiovascular system, are able to induce antibody formation in susceptible people. With the next exposure to the drug, immediate or delayed allergic responses may occur. In severe cases, anaphylaxis can occur, which can be life threatening. Some of these drugs have demonstrated cross-sensitivity (e.g., penicillins, cephalosporins); care must be taken to obtain a complete patient history before administering one of these drugs. It is important to determine what the allergic reaction was (what actually happened that made the patient think an allergy existed) and when the patient experienced it (e.g., after first use of the drug or after years of use). Some patients report having a drug allergy, but closer investigation indicates that their reaction actually constituted an anticipated effect or a known adverse effect of the drug such as nausea or diarrhea. Proper interpretation of this information is important to allow treatment of a patient with a drug to which the patient reported a supposed allergic reaction but that would be very effective against a known pathogen.

Superinfections

One effect of the use of anti-infectives, especially broad-spectrum anti-infectives, is destruction of the normal flora. **Superinfections** are infections that occur when opportunistic pathogens that were kept in check by "normal" flora bacteria have the opportunity to invade tissues. Common superinfections include vaginal or GI yeast infections, which are associated with antibiotic therapy and caused by *Candida*. In recent years, the emergence of *Clostridium difficile* infections has been associated with the use of specific antibiotics. If patients receive drugs that are known to induce superinfections, they should be monitored closely for any signs of a new infection—sore white patches in the mouth, vaginal itching and/or discharge, diarrhea—and the appropriate treatment for any superinfection should be started as soon as possible.

SUMMARY

- Anti-infectives are drugs designed to act with selective toxicity on foreign organisms that have invaded and infected the human host, which means that they affect biological systems or structures found in the invading organisms but not in the host.
- Anti-infectives include antibiotics, antivirals, antifungals, antiprotozoals, and anthelmintic agents.
- The goal of anti-infective therapy is interference with the normal function of invading organisms to prevent them from reproducing and promotion of cell death without negative effects on the host cells. The infection should be eradicated with the least toxicity to the host and the least likelihood for development of resistance.
- Anti-infectives can work by altering the cell membrane of the pathogen, by interfering with protein synthesis, or by interfering with the ability of the pathogen to obtain needed nutrients.
- Anti-infectives also work to kill invading organisms or to prevent them from reproducing, thus depleting the size of the invasion to one that can be eliminated by the human immune system.
- Pathogens can develop resistance to the effects of anti-infectives over time when (a) mutated organisms that do not respond to the anti-infective become the majority of the pathogen population or (b) the pathogen develops enzymes to block the anti-infectives or develops alternative routes to obtain nutrients or maintain the cell membrane.
- An important aspect of clinical care involving anti-infective agents is preventing or delaying the development of resistance. This can be done by ensuring that the particular anti-infective agent is the drug of choice for the specific pathogen involved and that it is given in high enough doses for sufficiently long periods to rid the body of the pathogen.
- Culturing and sensitivity testing of a suspected infection ensures that the correct drug is being used to treat the infection effectively. In many cases, culturing and sensitivity testing should be performed before an anti-infective agent is prescribed.
- Anti-infectives can have several adverse effects on the human host, including renal toxicity, multiple GI effects, neurotoxicity, hypersensitivity reactions, and superinfections.
- Some anti-infectives are used as a means of prophylaxis when patients expect to be in situations that will expose them to a known pathogen, such as travel to an area where malaria is endemic, or before oral or invasive GI surgery if the patient is a high-risk person who is susceptible to subacute bacterial endocarditis.

CHECK YOUR UNDERSTANDING

Answers to the questions in this chapter can be found in Answers to Check Your Understanding Questions on thePoint®.

MULTIPLE CHOICE

Select the best answer.

1. The spectrum of activity of an anti-infective indicates the
   a. acidity of the environment in which it is most effective.
   b. cell membrane type that the anti-infective affects.
   c. anti-infective's effectiveness against different invading organisms.
   d. resistance factor that bacteria have developed to this anti-infective.
2. The emergence of resistant strains of microbes is a serious public health problem. Health care providers can work to prevent the emergence of resistant strains by
   a. recommending the patient to stop the antibiotic as soon as the symptoms are resolved to prevent overexposure to the drug.
   b. encouraging the use of antibiotics when patients feel they will help.
   c. limiting the use of antimicrobial agents to the treatment of specific pathogens known to be sensitive to the drug being used.
   d. using the most recent powerful drug available to treat an infection to ensure eradication of the microbe.
3. Sensitivity testing of a culture shows
   a. drugs that are capable of controlling that particular microorganism.
   b. the patient's potential for allergic reactions to a drug.
   c. the offending microorganism.
   d. an immune reaction to the infecting organism.
4. Combination therapy is often used in treating infections. An important consideration for using combination therapy is that
   a. it is cheaper to use two drugs in one tablet than one drug alone.
   b. most infections are caused by multiple organisms.
   c. the combination of drugs can delay the emergence of resistant strains.
   d. combining anti-infectives will prevent adverse effects from occurring.
5. Superinfections can occur when anti-infective agents destroy the normal flora of the body. *Candida* infections are commonly associated with antibiotic use. A patient with this type of superinfection would exhibit
   a. difficulty breathing.
   b. vaginal discharge or white patches in the mouth.
   c. elevated blood urea nitrogen.
   d. dark lesions on the skin.
6. Which is an example of an anti-infective used as a means of prophylaxis?
   a. Penicillin used for tonsillitis
   b. Penicillin used to treat an abscess
   c. Amoxicillin used before dental surgery
   d. Co-trimoxazole used for a bladder infection
7. A broad-spectrum antibiotic would be the drug of choice when
   a. the patient has many known allergies.
   b. the provider is waiting for culture and sensitivity results.
   c. the infection is caused by one specific bacterium.
   d. treatment is being given for an upper respiratory infection of unknown cause.

MULTIPLE RESPONSE

Select all that apply.

1. Bacterial resistance to an anti-infective could be the result of which of the following?
   a. Natural or intrinsic properties of the bacteria
   b. Changes in cellular permeability or cellular transport systems
   c. Production of chemicals that antagonize the drug
   d. Initial exposure to the anti-infective
   e. Combination of too many antibiotics for one infection
   f. Narrow spectrum of activity
2. Anti-infective drugs destroy cells that have invaded the body. They do not specifically destroy only the cell of the invader, and because of this, many adverse effects can be anticipated when an anti-infective is used. Which of the following adverse effects are often associated with anti-infective use?
   a. Superinfections
   b. Hypotension
   c. Renal toxicity
   d. Diarrhea
   e. Loss of hearing
   f. Constipation

REFERENCES

Bassler, B., & Winans, S. C. (2008). *Chemical communication among bacteria.* John Wiley & Sons.

Brunton, L., Hilal-Dandan, R., & Knollman, B. (2018). *Goodman and Gilman's the pharmacological basis of therapeutics* (13th ed.). McGraw-Hill.

Centers for Disease Control and Prevention. (2020). *CDC calls on Americans to wear masks to prevent COVID-19 spread.* https://www.cdc.gov/media/releases/2020/p0714-americans-to-wear-masks.html

Chopra, I., O'Neill, A. J., & Miller, K. (2003). The role of mutators in the emergence of antibiotic-resistant bacteria. *Drug Resistance Updates, 6*, 137–145. https://doi.org/10.1016/S1368-7646(03)00041-4

Donadio, S., Maffioli, S., Monciardini, P., Sosio, M., & Jabes, D. (2010). Antibiotic discovery in the twenty-first century: Current trends and future perspectives. *Journal of Antibiotics, 63*, 423–430. https://www.nature.com/articles/ja201062

Hendler, C. B. (Ed.) (2021). *Nursing 2021 drug handbook.* Wolters Kluwer.

Norris, T. L. (2019). *Porth's pathophysiology concepts of altered health states* (10th ed.). Wolters Kluwer.

Shnayerson, M., & Plotkin, M. (2003). *The killers within: The deadly rise of drug-resistant bacteria.* Little, Brown and Company.

Stephenson, J. (2008). Drug-resistant bacteria. *Journal of the American Medical Association, 299*(7), 755. https://jamanetwork.com/journals/jama/article-abstract/181496

CHAPTER 9

Antibiotics

Learning Objectives

Upon completion of this chapter, you will be able to:

1. Explain how an antibiotic is selected for use in a particular clinical situation.
2. Describe therapeutic actions, indications, pharmacokinetics, contraindications, most common adverse reactions, and important drug–drug interactions associated with each of the classes of antibiotics.
3. Discuss the use of antibiotics across the lifespan.
4. Compare and contrast prototype drugs for each class of antibiotics with other drugs in that class.
5. Outline nursing considerations for patients receiving each class of antibiotic.

Key Terms

aerobic: bacteria that depend on oxygen for survival

anaerobic: bacteria that survive without oxygen, which are often found in chronic infections and in the GI tract

antibiotic: chemical that inhibits the growth of specific bacteria or causes the death of susceptible bacteria

gram-negative: bacteria that have only a thin layer of peptidoglycan, making them less likely to absorb stain or become decolorized by alcohol; these bacteria are frequently associated with infections of the genitourinary or gastrointestinal (GI) tract

gram-positive: bacteria that have cell walls with more peptidoglycan layers, which absorb more stain or resist decolorization with alcohol during preliminary identification; these bacteria are frequently associated with infections of the respiratory tract and soft tissues

Gram staining: a process used to identify between types of bacteria based on differences of components in their cell walls

synergistic: drugs that work together to increase drug effectiveness

Drug List

AMINOGLYCOSIDES
amikacin
(P) gentamicin
neomycin
plazomicin
streptomycin
tobramycin

CARBAPENEMS
doripenem
(P) ertapenem
imipenem–cilastatin
imipenem–cilastatin–relebactam
meropenem
meropenem–vaborbactam

CEPHALOSPORINS

First Generation
cefadroxil
cefazolin
cephalexin

Second Generation
(P) cefaclor
cefotetan
cefoxitin
cefprozil
cefuroxime

Third Generation
cefdinir
cefixime
cefotaxime
cefpodoxime
ceftazidime
ceftriaxone

Fourth Generation
cefepime

Other cephalosporins
cefiderocol
ceftaroline
ceftazidime–avibactam
ceftolozane–tazobactam

FLUOROQUINOLONES
(P) ciprofloxacin
delafloxacin
gemifloxacin
levofloxacin
moxifloxacin
ofloxacin

PENICILLINS AND PENICILLINASE-RESISTANT ANTIBIOTICS

Natural Penicillins
penicillin G benzathine
penicillin G potassium
penicillin G procaine
penicillin V

Aminopenicillins
(P) amoxicillin
amoxicillin–clavulanate
ampicillin
ampicillin–sulbactam

Penicillinase-Resistant (Antistaphylococcal) Penicillins
dicloxacillin
nafcillin
oxacillin

Antipseudomonal Penicillins
piperacillin
piperacillin–tazobactam

SULFONAMIDES
sulfadiazine
(P) trimethoprim–sulfamethoxazole or cotrimoxazole

TETRACYCLINES
demeclocycline
doxycycline
eravacycline
minocycline
omadacycline
sarecycline
(P) tetracycline

ANTIMYCOBACTERIALS

Antituberculosis Drugs
bedaquiline
capreomycin
cycloserine
ethambutol
ethionamide
(P) isoniazid
pyrazinamide
rifabutin
rifampin
rifapentine

Leprostatic Drugs
dapsone

OTHER ANTIBIOTICS

Lincosamides
(P) clindamycin
lincomycin

Lipoglycopeptide
dalbavancin
oritavancin
telavancin
(P) vancomycin

Macrolides
azithromycin
clarithromycin
(P) erythromycin
fidaxomicin

Oxazolidinones
(P) linezolid
tedizolid

Monobactams
(P) aztreonam

MISCELLANEOUS ANTIBIOTICS AND ADJUNCTS
daptomycin
quinupristin–dalfopristin
rifaximin
tigecycline

Adjuncts to Antibiotic Therapy
avibactam
clavulanic acid
sulbactam
tazobactam
thalidomide
vaborbactam

Many new bacteria appear each year, and researchers are challenged to develop new **antibiotics**—chemicals that inhibit specific bacteria—to deal with each new threat. Antibiotics are made in three ways: by living microorganisms, by synthetic manufacture, and in some cases through genetic engineering. Antibiotics may either be bacteriostatic (inhibiting the growth of bacteria) or bactericidal (killing bacteria directly), although several antibiotics are both bactericidal and bacteriostatic, depending on the concentration of the particular drug and the bacteria it is treating.

This chapter discusses the major classes of antibiotics: aminoglycosides, carbapenems, cephalosporins, fluoroquinolones, penicillins and penicillinase-resistant drugs, sulfonamides, tetracyclines, and the disease-specific antimycobacterials, including the antitubercular and leprostatic drugs. Antibiotics that do not fit into the large antibiotic classes include lincosamides, lipoglycopeptides, macrolides, monobactams, and oxazolidinones. Figures 9.1 and 9.2 show sites of cellular action of these classes of antibiotics.

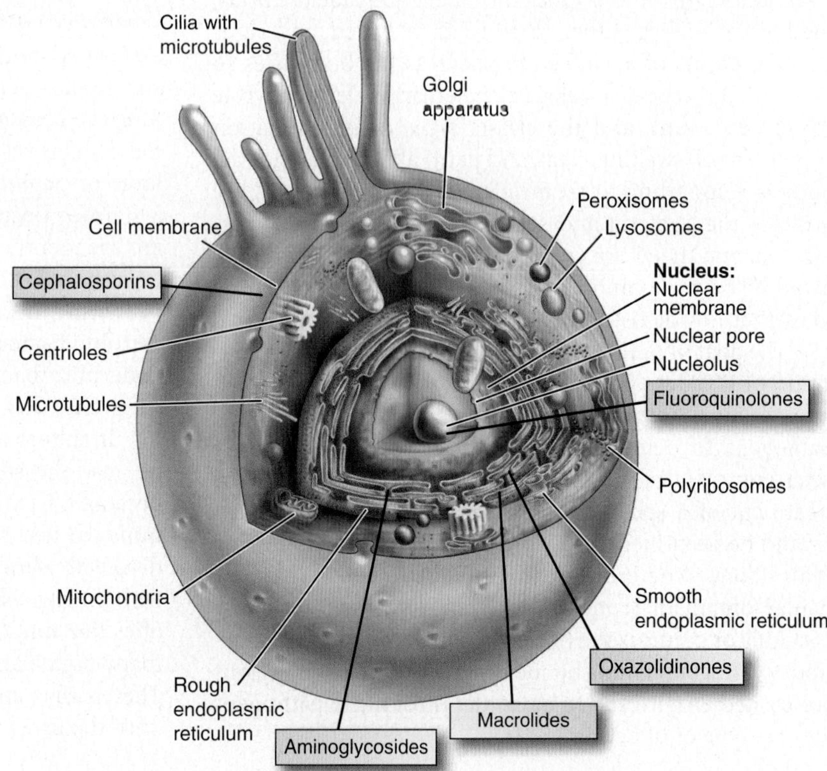

FIGURE 9.1 Sites of cellular action of aminoglycosides, cephalosporins, fluoroquinolones, oxazolidinones, and macrolides. Cephalosporins cause bacteria to build weak cell walls when dividing. Fluoroquinolones interfere with the DNA enzymes needed for growth and reproduction. Aminoglycosides, macrolides, and oxazolidinones change protein synthesis by binding to ribosome within the cell to cause cell death or prevent cell division.

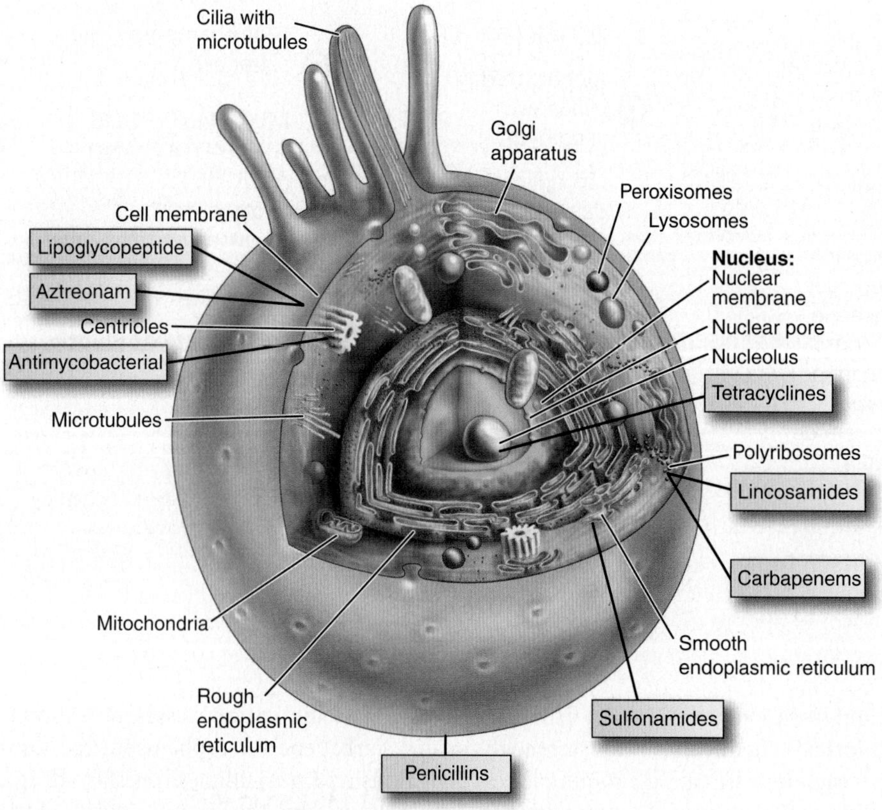

FIGURE 9.2 Sites of cellular action of carbapenems, lincosamides, lipoglycopeptides, aztreonam, penicillins, sulfonamides, tetracyclines, and antimycobacterials. Carbapenems and lincosamides change protein function and prevent cell division or cause cell death. Aztreonam and lipoglycopeptides alter cell membranes to allow leakage of intracellular substances and cause cell death. Penicillins prevent bacteria from building their cells during division. Sulfonamides inhibit folic acid synthesis for RNA and DNA production. Tetracyclines inhibit protein synthesis, thereby preventing reproduction. Antimycobacterial drugs affect mycobacteria in three ways: they (a) affect the mycotic coat of the bacteria, (b) alter DNA and RNA, and (c) prevent cell division.

Bacteria and Antibiotics

Bacteria can invade the human body through many routes including the respiratory tract, the gastrointestinal (GI) tract, and many others. Once the bacteria invade the body, the human inflammatory response is activated, and signs and symptoms of an infection occur as the body tries to rid itself of the foreign cells. Fever, lethargy, elevated white blood cell count, and the classic signs of inflammation (e.g., redness, swelling, heat, and pain) all indicate that the body is responding to an invader. The body becomes the host for the bacteria and supplies proteins and enzymes the bacteria need for reproduction. Unchallenged, the invading bacteria can multiply and send out other bacteria to further invade tissue.

The goal of antibiotic therapy is to decrease the population of invading bacteria to a point at which the human inflammatory/immune system can effectively deal with the pathogen. To determine which antibiotic will effectively interfere with the specific proteins or enzyme systems for treatment of a specific infection, the causative organism should be identified through a culture. Sensitivity testing is also done to determine the antibiotic to which that particular organism is most sensitive (i.e., which antibiotic best kills or controls the bacteria). Often the specific infectious pathogen cannot be identified, and these infections are treated empirically to cover the most likely pathogens for that type of infection.

Gram staining is a technique that can be used to categorize types of bacteria based on their types of cell wall. **Gram-positive** bacteria have cell walls with more peptidoglycan layers, which retain more dye, or Gram stain, and resist decolorization with alcohol during culture and sensitivity testing. Gram-positive bacteria are commonly associated with infections of the respiratory tract and soft tissues. An example of a gram-positive bacterium is *Streptococcus pneumoniae*, a common cause of pneumonia. In contrast, **gram-negative** bacteria have only a thin layer of peptidoglycan, making them more likely to lose a stain or become decolorized by alcohol. These bacteria are frequently associated with infections of the genitourinary (GU) or GI tract. An example of a gram-negative bacterium is *Escherichia coli*, a common cause of cystitis. **Aerobic** bacteria depend on oxygen for survival, whereas **anaerobic** bacteria (e.g., those bacteria associated with gangrene) do not use oxygen.

If culture and sensitivity testing is not possible, either because the source of the infection is not identifiable or because the patient is too sick to wait for test results to determine the best treatment, clinicians attempt to administer a drug with a broad spectrum of activity against the organisms with the highest probability of causing the infection. Antibiotics that interfere with a biochemical reaction common to many organisms are known as broad-spectrum antibiotics. These drugs are often given at the beginning of treatment until the exact organism and sensitivity can be established.

Human cells have many of the same properties as bacterial cells and can be affected in much the same way, so damage may occur to the human cells, as well as to the bacterial cells.

Because there is no perfect antibiotic that is without effect on the human host, clinicians try to select an antibiotic with selective toxicity, or the ability to strike foreign cells with little or no effect on human cells. Certain antibiotics may be contraindicated in some patients because of known adverse effects. See Box 9.1 for effects of antibiotics across the lifespan. The antibiotic of choice is one that is most efficacious against causative organism and leads to the fewest adverse effects for the patient.

In some cases, antibiotics are given in combination because they are **synergistic**, meaning their combined effect is greater, or they are able to treat a more severe infection, when given together than when given individually (Box 9.2).

In some situations, antibiotics are used as a means of prophylaxis, or prevention of potential infection.

Patients who will soon be in a situation that commonly results in a specific infection (e.g., patients undergoing GI surgical procedures, which may introduce GI bacteria into the bloodstream or peritoneum; patients traveling to other countries with endemic bacteria that are not in their home area) may be given antibiotics before they are exposed to the bacteria.

BOX 9.2

Using Combination Drugs to Fight Resistant Bacteria

Clavulanic acid protects certain beta-lactam antibiotics from breakdown in the presence of penicillinase enzymes.

A combination of amoxicillin and clavulanic acid (*Augmentin*) is commonly used to allow the amoxicillin to remain effective against certain strains of resistant bacteria (usual dosage, 250 to 500 mg PO q8h for adults or 20 to 40 mg/kg/d PO in divided doses for children).

Zosyn (piperacillin and tazobactam) is a combination antibiotic that includes a penicillin and a beta-lactamase inhibitor. It can be used to treat a wide variety of infections including gram-positive bacteria (*Staphylococcus aureus*), several types of gram-negative bacteria, and anaerobic bacteria. Zosyn is administered by intravenous infusion to adults and pediatric patients.

Box 9.1  Focus on **Drug Therapy Across the Lifespan**

ANTIBIOTICS

Children

Children are very sensitive to the GI and central nervous system (CNS) effects of most antibiotics, and more severe reactions can be expected when these drugs are used in children. It is important to monitor the hydration and nutritional status of children who are adversely affected by drug-induced diarrhea, anorexia, nausea, and vomiting. Superinfections can be a problem for small children as well. For example, thrush (oral candidiasis) is a common superinfection that makes eating and drinking difficult.

Many antibiotics do not have proven safety and efficacy in pediatric use, and extreme caution should be used when giving them to children. The fluoroquinolones, for instance, are associated with damage to developing cartilage and are not recommended for growing children. Tetracyclines are not indicated for children because of effects on growing bones and teeth.

Pediatric dosages of antibiotics should be double-checked to make sure that the child is receiving the correct dose, thereby improving the chance of eradicating the infection and decreasing the risk of adverse effects. Medications for pediatrics are usually ordered based on the patient weight. Use caution to ensure that there is no confusion between mg/kg/day versus mg/kg/dose.

Antibiotic treatment of ear infections, a common pediatric problem, is controversial. Ongoing research suggests that judicious use of decongestants and anti-inflammatories may be just as successful as the use of antibiotics without the risk of development of resistant bacterial strains.

Parents, not wanting to see their child sick, may demand antibiotics as a cure-all whenever their child is fussy or feverish. Parent education is very important in helping to cut down the unnecessary use of antibiotics in children.

Adults

Many adults believe that antibiotics are a cure-all for any discomfort and fever. It is very important to explain that antibiotics are useful against only specific bacteria and actually can cause problems when used unnecessarily for viral infections, such as the common cold.

Adults need to be cautioned to take the entire course of the medication as prescribed and not to store unused pills for future infections or share antibiotics with symptomatic friends.

People who are pregnant or lactating should not take antibiotics unless the benefit clearly outweighs the potential risk to the fetus or neonate. Tetracyclines, for example, are associated with pitting of enamel in developing teeth and with calcium deposits in growing bones. These drugs can cause serious problems for neonates. People who can become pregnant should be advised to use barrier contraceptives if any of these drugs are used.

Older Adults

In many instances, older adults do not present with the same signs and symptoms of infections as other patients. For example, a urinary tract infection may cause confusion without urinary frequency or discomfort in an older adult. Therefore, assessing the problem and obtaining appropriate specimens for culture is especially important with this population.

Older patients may be more susceptible to the adverse effects associated with antibiotic therapy. Their hydration and nutritional status should be monitored closely, as should the need for safety precautions if CNS effects occur. Hepatic or renal dysfunction may be a higher risk in older patients; the dose may need to be lowered, and the patient should be monitored more frequently.

Older patients also need to be cautioned to complete the full course of drug therapy, even when they feel better, and not to save pills for self-medication at a future time.

Bacteria and Resistance to Antibiotics

Bacteria have survived for hundreds of years because they can adapt to their environment. They do this by altering their cell wall or enzyme systems to become resistant to (e.g., protect themselves from) unfavorable conditions or situations. Many species of bacteria have developed resistance to certain antibiotics. For example, bacteria that were once sensitive to penicillin have developed an enzyme called penicillinase, which inactivates many of the penicillin-type drugs. New drugs had to be developed to effectively treat infections involving these bacteria. It is important to use these drugs only when the identity and sensitivity of the offending bacterium have been established or if a wide variety of pathogens could be causing the infection. Indiscriminate use of these new drugs can lead to the development of more resistant strains for which there is no effective antibiotic.

The longer an antibiotic has been in use, the greater the chance that the bacteria will develop resistance. Efforts to control the emergence of resistant strains involve intensive educational programs that advocate the use of antibiotics only when necessary and effective and not for the treatment of viral infections such as the common cold (Box 9.3).

In addition, the use of antibiotics may result in the development of superinfections or overgrowth of resistant pathogens, such as bacteria, fungi, or yeasts, because antibiotics (particularly broad-spectrum agents) destroy bacteria in the flora that normally work to keep these opportunistic invaders in check (Fig. 9.3). When "normal"

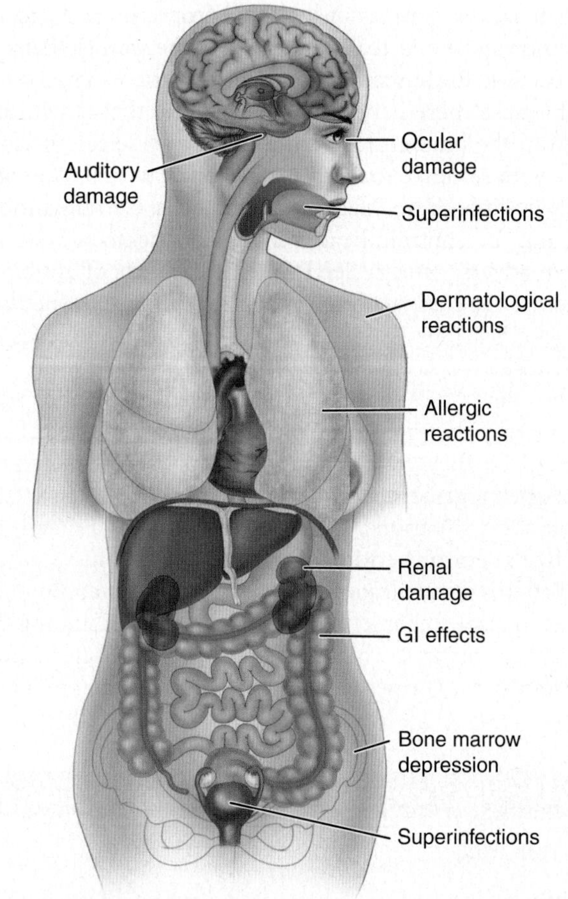

FIGURE 9.3 Common adverse effects associated with antibiotics.

Box 9.3 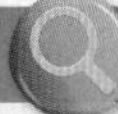 **Focus on The Evidence**

USING ANTIBIOTICS PROPERLY

The Food and Drug Administration (FDA) and Centers for Disease Control and Prevention (CDC) have joined efforts to educate the public and health care providers about the dangers of inappropriate use of antibiotics. The evidence-based practice guidelines combine data from many studies to outline the most efficacious use of antibiotics. To review some of the studies, look at the references listed in the "Bibliography and References" section. Nurses should include some of the following points about the risks and dangers of antibiotic abuse in the patient education plan:

- Explain clearly that a particular antibiotic is effective against only certain bacteria and that a culture may need to be taken to identify the bacteria.
- Explain that bacteria can develop resistant strains that will not be affected by antibiotics in the future, so use of antibiotics now may make them less effective in situations in which they are really necessary.
- Ensure that patients understand the importance of taking the full course of medication as prescribed, even if they feel better. Stopping an antibiotic midway through a regimen often leads to the development of resistant bacteria. Using all of the medication will also prevent patients from saving unused medication to self-treat future infections or to share with other family members.
- Tell patients that allergies may develop with repeated exposures to certain antibiotics. In addition, exposure to antibiotic early in life increases the risk of allergic disease later in life.
- Offer other medications, such as antihistamines, decongestants, or even chicken soup, to patients who request antibiotics; this may satisfy their need for something to take. Explaining that viral infections do not respond to antibiotics usually offers little consolation to patients who are suffering from a cold or the flu.

The publicity that many emergent, resistant strains of bacteria have received in recent years may help to get the message across to patients about the need to take the full course of an antibiotic and to use antibiotics only when they are appropriate. To view the educational program developed by the FDA and the CDC for use with patients and the data behind these efforts, go to https://www.cdc.gov/antibiotic-use/index.html.

bacteria are destroyed or greatly reduced in number, there is nothing to prevent the invaders from occupying the host. In most cases, the superinfection is an irritating adverse effect (e.g., vaginal yeast infection, thrush, diarrhea), but in some cases, the superinfection can be more severe than the infection that was originally being treated. Treatment of the superinfection leads to new adverse effects and the potential for different superinfections. A vicious cycle of treatment and resistance is the result.

Key Points

- The goal of antibiotic therapy is to reduce the population of invading bacteria to a size that the human immune response can deal with.
- Bacteria can be classified as gram-positive or gram-negative. They can also be classified as anaerobic (not needing oxygen) or aerobic (dependent on oxygen).
- Culture and sensitivity testing can facilitate choosing an antibiotic that is most likely to treat a specific pathogen. This may help decrease the number of emerging resistant-strain bacteria.

Aminoglycosides

The aminoglycosides (Table 9.1) are a group of antibiotics used to treat infections caused by primarily aerobic gram-negative bacilli. Because most of these drugs have potentially serious adverse effects, newer, less-toxic drugs have replaced aminoglycosides in the treatment of some infections. Aminoglycosides include amikacin (generic), gentamicin (generic), neomycin (generic), streptomycin (generic), plazomicin (*Zemdri*), and tobramycin (*Bethkis, TOBI, Tobrex Ophthalmic*). Paromomycin is also an aminoglycoside, but it will be discussed in Chapter 12 since it is used to treat intestinal amebiasis.

Therapeutic Actions and Indications

The aminoglycosides are bactericidal. They inhibit protein synthesis in susceptible strains of aerobic gram-negative bacteria, including *E. coli*, *Klebsiella pneumoniae*, *Proteus mirabilis*, and *Pseudomonas aeruginosa*. They irreversibly bind to a unit of the bacteria ribosomes, leading to misreading of the genetic code and cell death (see Fig. 9.1). See Table 9.1 for usual indications for each of these drugs.

Pharmacokinetics

The aminoglycosides are poorly absorbed from the GI tract but rapidly absorbed after intramuscular (IM) injection, reaching peak levels within 1 hour. These drugs have an average half-life of 2 to 3 hours. They are widely distributed throughout the body, cross the placenta and enter human milk, and are excreted unchanged in the urine (see "Contraindications and Cautions").

Amikacin is available for short-term IM or intravenous (IV) use.

Table 9.1 *Drugs in Focus*: Aminoglycosides

Drug Name	Dosage/Route	Usual Indications
amikacin (*Amikin*)	15 mg/kg/d IM or IV divided into two or three equal doses; reduce dose in renal dysfunction	Treatment of serious gram-negative infections
gentamicin (*Garamycin*)	*Adult*: 3–5 mg/kg/d IM or IV in three equal doses q8h; reduce dose in renal dysfunction *Pediatric*: 2–2.5 mg/kg/d q8h IV or IM	Treatment of serious gram-negative infections
neomycin (*Mycifradin*)	*Adult*: 4–12 g/d in divided doses PO for 5–6 d *Pediatric*: 50–100 mg/kg/d in divided doses PO for hepatic coma	Suppression of GI normal flora preoperatively; treatment of hepatic encephalopathy; topical treatment of skin wounds
plazomicin (*Zemdri*)	*Adult:* 15 mg/kg/d IV infusion over 30 min if creatinine clearance 90 mL/min or greater. Dose reduction indicated if renal impairment	Treatment of complicated UTI and pyelonephritis
streptomycin (generic)	*Adult*: 1–2 g/d IM in divided doses q6–12h *Pediatric*: 20–40 mg/kg/d IM in divided doses q6–12h	Fourth drug in combination therapy regimen for treatment of tuberculosis; treatment of severe infections if the organism has been shown to be sensitive to streptomycin and no less-toxic drugs can be used
tobramycin (*Bethkis, TOBI, Tobrex*)	*Adult*: 3–5 mg/kg/d in three equal doses IM or IV q8h; reduce dose in renal dysfunction; 300 mg b.i.d. by nebulizer *Pediatric*: 6–7.5 mg/kg/d IM or IV in three to four equally divided doses; 300 mg b.i.d. by nebulizer	Short-term IV or IM treatment of serious infections; ocular infections caused by susceptible bacteria; nebulizer management of cystic fibrosis and *Pseudomonas aeruginosa* infections

Gentamicin is available in many forms: Ophthalmic, topical, IV, IM, intrathecal.
Neomycin is available in topical and oral forms.
Plazomicin is available for IV use only.
Streptomycin is only available for IM use.
Tobramycin is used for short-term IM or IV treatment and is also available in an ophthalmic form and as a nebulizer solution.

Contraindications and Cautions

The risks and benefits of aminoglycosides must be carefully weighed in the following conditions: known allergy to any of the aminoglycosides; renal disease that could be exacerbated by toxic aminoglycoside effects and could interfere with drug metabolism and excretion, leading to higher toxicity; preexisting hearing loss, which could be intensified by toxic drug effects on the auditory nerve; and myasthenia gravis or parkinsonism, which can be exacerbated by the effects of aminoglycosides on the nervous system.

Caution is necessary when these agents are administered during pregnancy because aminoglycosides cross the placenta and may have potential adverse effects on the fetus. Streptomycin has been associated with deafness in newborns when administered to people who are pregnant. It is necessary to test renal function and drug levels frequently and use lower doses with patients that have renal impairment when these drugs are used because they depend on the kidney for excretion and are toxic to the kidney.

The potential for nephrotoxicity and ototoxicity with aminoglycosides is high, so these drugs are used for resistant infections and only for as long as necessary. Streptomycin, once a commonly used drug, is reserved for use in special situations because it is very toxic to the eighth cranial nerve and kidney. It can be used in severe infections if the organism has been shown to be sensitive to streptomycin and no less-toxic drugs can be used. It is effective in resistant tuberculosis.

Adverse Effects

The serious adverse effects associated with aminoglycosides limit their usefulness. The drugs come with a boxed warning alerting health care professionals to the serious risk of ototoxicity and nephrotoxicity. Central nervous system (CNS) effects include ototoxicity, possibly leading to irreversible deafness; vestibular paralysis resulting from drug effects on the auditory nerve; confusion; depression; disorientation; and numbness, tingling, and weakness related to drug effects on other nerves.

Renal toxicity, which may progress to renal failure, is caused by direct drug toxicity in the glomerulus and nephron tubule, meaning that the drug molecules cause damage directly to the kidney nephrons. In contrast to ototoxicity, the renal toxicity is usually reversible. Bone marrow depression may result from direct drug effects on the rapidly dividing cells in the bone marrow, leading, for example, to immune suppression and resultant infections.

GI effects include nausea, vomiting, diarrhea, weight loss, and stomatitis. These effects are a result of direct GI irritation, loss of bacteria of the normal flora with resultant superinfections, and toxic effects in the mucous membranes.

Cardiac effects can include palpitations, hypotension, and hypertension. Hypersensitivity reactions include purpura, rash, urticaria, and exfoliative dermatitis.

Clinically Important Drug–Drug Interactions

Most aminoglycosides have a synergistic bactericidal effect when given with penicillins or cephalosporins. In certain conditions, this synergism is used therapeutically to increase the effectiveness of treatment. Avoid combining aminoglycosides with loop diuretics; this increases the incidence of ototoxicity. Caution should be used with coadministering aminoglycosides with other nephrotoxic medications such as vancomycin as it may lead to cumulative nephrotoxicity. If these antibiotics are given with anesthetics, nondepolarizing neuromuscular blockers, succinylcholine, or citrate anticoagulated blood, increased neuromuscular blockade with paralysis is possible. If a patient who has been receiving an aminoglycoside requires surgery and will be receiving any of these drugs, indicate prominently on the patient's chart the fact that the aminoglycoside has been given. Provide extended monitoring and support after surgery.

Prototype Summary: Gentamicin

Indications: Treatment of serious infections caused by susceptible bacteria.

Actions: Inhibits protein synthesis in susceptible strains of gram-negative bacteria, disrupting functional integrity of the cell membrane and causing cell death.

Pharmacokinetics:

Route	Onset	Peak
IM, IV	Rapid	30–90 min

$T_{1/2}$: 2 to 3 hours; excreted in the urine.

Adverse Effects: Hypersensitivity, sinusitis, dizziness, rash, fever, risk of nephrotoxicity, and ototoxicity.

Carbapenems

The carbapenems (Table 9.2) are a class of broad-spectrum beta-lactam antibiotics effective against gram-positive and gram-negative bacteria. Carbapenems discussed here include doripenem (*Doribax*), ertapenem (*Invanz*), imipenem–cilastatin (*Primaxin*), imipenem–cilastatin–relebactam (*Recarbrio*), meropenem (*Merrem IV*), and meropenem–vaborbactam (*Vabomere*), the newest form that combines meropenem with a beta-lactamase inhibitor.

Nursing Considerations for Patients Receiving Aminoglycosides

Assessment: History and Examination

- Assess for possible contraindications or cautions: known allergy to any aminoglycoside (obtain specific information about the nature and occurrence of allergic reactions), history of renal, preexisting hearing loss, myasthenia gravis, parkinsonism, infant botulism, and current pregnancy or lactation status.
- Perform a physical assessment to establish baseline data for assessing the effectiveness of the drug and the occurrence of any adverse effects associated with drug therapy.
- Perform culture and sensitivity tests at the site of infection to ensure appropriate use of the drug.
- Conduct orientation and reflex assessment, as well as auditory testing, to evaluate any CNS effects of the drug.
- Assess vital signs: respiratory rate and adventitious sounds to monitor for signs of infection or hypersensitivity reactions; temperature to assess for signs and symptoms of infection; and blood pressure to monitor for cardiovascular effects of the drug.
- Perform renal and hepatic function tests to determine baseline function of these organs and, possibly, the need to adjust dose.

Nursing Conclusions

Nursing conclusions related to drug therapy might include the following:

- Impaired comfort related to GI or CNS effects of drug
- Hearing impairment related to CNS effects of drug
- Infection risk related to bone marrow suppression
- Fluid overload risk related to nephrotoxicity
- Knowledge deficiency regarding drug therapy

Planning

- The patient will receive the best therapeutic effect from the drug therapy.
- The patient will have limited adverse effects from the drug therapy.
- The patient will have an understanding of the drug therapy, adverse effects to anticipate and measures to relieve discomfort and improve safety.

Intervention With Rationale

- Check culture and sensitivity reports to ensure that this is the drug of choice for this patient.
- Ensure that the patient receives a full course of aminoglycoside as prescribed to facilitate complete treatment of infection.
- Monitor the infection site and presenting signs and symptoms (e.g., fever, lethargy) throughout the course of drug therapy. Failure of these signs and symptoms to resolve may indicate the need to reculture the site
- Monitor the patient regularly for signs of hypersensitivity, nephrotoxicity, neurotoxicity, and bone marrow suppression to effectively arrange for discontinuation of drug or decreased dose, as appropriate, if any of these toxicities occurs.
- Provide safety measures to protect the patient if CNS effects, such as confusion, disorientation, or numbness and tingling, occur.
- Provide small, frequent meals as tolerated; frequent mouth care; and ice chips or sugarless candy to suck if stomatitis and sore mouth are problems, to relieve discomfort.
- Instruct the patient about the appropriate dosage regimen and possible adverse effects to enhance patient knowledge about drug therapy and to promote adherence.
- Provide the following patient teaching:
  - Take safety precautions, such as changing position slowly and avoiding driving and hazardous tasks, if CNS effects occur.
  - Try to drink an adequate amount of fluids and maintain nutrition even though nausea, vomiting, and diarrhea may occur.
  - Report difficulty breathing, rash, itching, severe headache, loss of hearing or ringing in the ears, or changes in urine output.

Evaluation

- Monitor patient response to the drug (resolution of bacterial infection).
- Monitor for adverse effects (orientation and affect, hearing changes, bone marrow suppression, renal toxicity, GI effects).
- Evaluate effectiveness of the teaching plan (patient can name drug, dosage, possible adverse effects to watch for, and specific measures to help avoid adverse effects).
- Monitor effectiveness of comfort and safety measures and adherence to the therapeutic regimen.

Key Points

- Aminoglycosides inhibit protein synthesis in susceptible strains of aerobic gram-negative bacteria.
- These drugs are reserved for use in serious infections because of potentially serious adverse effects. Monitor for hypersensitivity, ototoxicity, renal toxicity, GI disturbances, bone marrow depression, and superinfections.

Therapeutic Actions and Indications

The carbapenems are bactericidal. They inhibit cell membrane synthesis in susceptible bacteria, leading to cell death (see Fig. 9.2). These drugs are used to treat serious infections caused by susceptible strains of *S. pneumoniae*, *Haemophilus influenzae*, *Moraxella catarrhalis*, *S. aureus*, *Streptococcus pyogenes*, *E. coli*, *Peptostreptococcus* spp., *K. pneumoniae*, *Clostridium clostridioforme*, *Eubacterium lentum*, *Bacteroides fragilis*, *Bacteroides distasonis*, *Bacteroides ovatus*, *Bacteroides thetaiotaomicron*, *Bacteroides uniformis*, *P. mirabilis*, *Proteus aeruginosa*, *Acinetobacter baumannii*, *Streptococcus agalactiae*, *Porphyromonas asaccharolytica*, *Prevotella bivia*, and other susceptible bacteria. They are indicated for treating serious intra-abdominal, urinary tract, skin and skin structure, bone and joint, and gynecological infections. See Table 9.2 for usual indications for each of these drugs.

Pharmacokinetics

These drugs are rapidly absorbed if given IM and reach peak levels at the end of the infusion if given IV. They are widely distributed throughout the body. The ability of carbapenems to cross the placenta or to enter human milk varies by individual drug (see "Contraindications and Cautions"). Carbapenems are excreted unchanged in the urine and have an average half-life of 1 to 4 hours.

Doripenem is given IV every 8 hours by a 1-hour IV infusion.

Ertapenem can be given IV or IM.

Imipenem–cilastatin is a combination of imipenem, which interferes with cell wall synthesis and causes bacterial cell death, and cilastatin, which decreases renal metabolism of imipenem by inhibiting the enzyme dehydropeptidase, so imipenem is active in the body for a longer period of time. It can be given IM or IV and is approved for use in children. Imipenem–cilastatin–relebactam is a combination medication that has a beta-lactamase inhibitor added in order to reduce destruction of imipenem by certain beta-lactamases. This medication is only available IV.

Meropenem is given IV over 1 hour, every 8 hours; when combined with vaborbactam, and it is given IV over 3 hours every 8 hours.

Contraindications and Cautions

Carbapenems are contraindicated when there is a known allergy to any of the carbapenems or beta-lactams.

Use caution during pregnancy and lactation because the benefits of the drug must be carefully weighed against potential adverse effects on the fetus or infant. Test renal function regularly when these drugs are used because they depend on the kidney for excretion and may be toxic to the kidney.

Meropenem–vaborbactam is not recommended for use in patients younger than 18 years of age.

Adverse Effects

Toxic effects on the GI tract can limit the use of carbapenems in some patients. Pseudomembranous colitis, *Clostridium difficile* diarrhea, and nausea and vomiting can lead to serious dehydration and electrolyte imbalances, as well as to new serious infections.

Table 9.2 *Drugs in Focus*: Carbapenems

Drug Name	Dosage/Route	Usual Indications
doripenem (*Doribax*)	500 mg IV, over 1 h q8h, reduce dose in renal dysfunction	Treatment of complicated intra-abdominal infections or complicated UTIs, including pyelonephritis, caused by susceptible bacteria
ertapenem (*Invanz*)	*Adult*: 1 g/d IV or IM, reduce dose in renal dysfunction *Pediatric*: 15 mg/kg b.i.d. IV or IM max 1 g/d	Treatment of community-acquired pneumonia, complicated GU infections, acute pelvic infections, complicated intra-abdominal infections, skin and skin structure infections
imipenem–cilastatin (*Primaxin*)	500–1,000 mg IV q6h–q8h, reduce dose in renal dysfunction	Treatment of serious respiratory, intra-abdominal, urinary tract, gynecological, bone and joint, skin and skin structure infections; septicemia, endocarditis, bone and joint infections, and polymicrobic infections
imipenem–cilastatin–relebactam (*Recarbrio*)	*Adult:* 1.25 g IV every 6 h over 30 min if creatinine clearance 90 mL/min or greater; reduce dose in renal dysfunction	Treatment of hospital-acquired bacterial pneumonia and ventilator-associated bacterial pneumonia, complicated UTI, including pyelonephritis, and complicated intra-abdominal infections for patients without other treatment options
meropenem (*Merrem IV*)	*Adult*: 500–1,000 mg IV q8h, reduce dose in renal dysfunction	Treatment of bacterial meningitis, complicated skin and skin structure infections, intra-abdominal infections
meropenem–vaborbactam (*Vabomere*)	4 g IV q8h over 3 h, dose reduce in renal dysfunction	Treatment of adults with complicated urinary tract infections, including pyelonephritis

Superinfections can occur with any of the carbapenems. Closely monitor patients to deal with the new infection before it becomes overwhelming.

CNS effects can include headache, dizziness, and altered mental state. Seizures have been reported when carbapenems are combined with other drugs. Monitor patients to provide safety measures if any of these occur.

Clinically Important Drug–Drug Interactions

Consider an alternative antibiotic treatment if a patient is on valproic acid. Combination of these drugs can cause serum valproic acid levels to fall and increase the risk of seizures. Avoid concurrent use of imipenem with ganciclovir because this combination may also cause seizures.

Prototype Summary: Ertapenem

Indications: Treatment of community-acquired pneumonia, complicated GU infections, complicated intra-abdominal infections, skin and skin structure infections, and acute pelvic infections caused by susceptible bacteria.

Actions: Inhibits protein synthesis in susceptible strains of gram-negative bacteria, disrupting functional integrity of the cell membrane and causing cell death.

Pharmacokinetics:

Route	Onset	Peak
IM, IV	Rapid	30–120 min

$T_{1/2}$: 4 hours; excreted unchanged in the urine.

Adverse Effects: Headache, dizziness, nausea, vomiting, pseudomembranous colitis, rash, pain at injection site.

Nursing Considerations for Patients Receiving Carbapenems

Assessment: History and Examination

- Assess for possible contraindications or cautions: known allergy to any carbapenem or beta-lactam (obtain specific information about the nature and occurrence of allergic reactions), history of renal disease, history of seizures, and current pregnancy or lactation status.
- Perform physical assessment to establish baseline data for assessing the effectiveness of the drug and the occurrence of any adverse effects associated with drug therapy.
- Perform culture and sensitivity tests at the site of infection to ensure appropriate use of the drug.
- Conduct orientation and reflex assessment to evaluate any CNS effects of the drug.
- Assess respiratory rate and adventitious sounds to monitor for signs of infection or hypersensitivity reactions.
- Assess temperature to monitor for signs and symptoms of infection.
- Perform renal function tests to determine baseline function of the kidneys and, possibly, the need to adjust dose.

Nursing Conclusions

Nursing conclusions related to drug therapy might include the following:

- Impaired comfort related to GI or CNS effects of the drug
- Suprainfection risk related to loss of normal flora
- Knowledge deficit regarding drug therapy

Planning

- The patient will receive the best therapeutic effect from the drug therapy.
- The patient will have limited adverse effects from the drug therapy.
- The patient will have an understanding of the drug therapy, adverse effects to anticipate, and measures to relieve discomfort and improve safety.

Intervention With Rationale

- Check culture and sensitivity reports to ensure that this is the drug of choice for this patient.
- Ensure that the patient receives the full course of the carbapenem as prescribed to increase effectiveness and decrease the risk for the development of resistant strains of bacteria.
- Monitor the site of infection and presenting signs and symptoms (e.g., fever, lethargy) throughout the course of drug therapy. Failure of these signs and symptoms to resolve may indicate the need to reculture the site.
- Monitor the patient regularly for signs of pseudomembranous colitis, severe diarrhea, or superinfections to effectively arrange for discontinuation of drug or decreased dose, as appropriate, if any of these toxicities occur.
- Provide safety measures to protect the patient if CNS effects, such as confusion, dizziness, or seizures, occur.
- Provide small, frequent meals as tolerated to relieve GI discomfort. Also provide adequate fluids to replace fluid lost with diarrhea, if appropriate.
- Instruct the patient about the appropriate dosage regimen and possible adverse effects to enhance patient knowledge about drug therapy and to promote adherence.
- Provide the following patient teaching:
  - Take safety precautions, such as changing position slowly and avoiding driving and hazardous tasks, if CNS effects occur.

(continues on page 110)

- Try to drink an adequate amount of fluids and to maintain nutrition even though nausea, vomiting, and diarrhea may occur.
- Report difficulty breathing, severe headache, severe diarrhea, fever, and signs of infection.

Evaluation

- Monitor patient response to the drug (resolution of bacterial infection).
- Monitor for adverse effects (orientation and affect, superinfections, GI toxicity, severe diarrhea effects).
- Evaluate effectiveness of the teaching plan (patient can name drug, dosage, possible adverse effects to watch for, and specific measures to help avoid adverse effects).
- Monitor effectiveness of comfort and safety measures and adherence to the therapeutic regimen.

Key Points

- Carbapenems are beta-lactam antibiotics used to treat serious infections caused by a wide range of bacteria.
- Monitor for hypersensitivity, GI effects, serious diarrhea, dizziness, and superinfections.

Cephalosporins

The cephalosporins (Table 9.3) are a type of beta-lactam antibiotic that were first introduced in the 1960s. These drugs are similar to the penicillins in structure and activity. Over time, multiple generations of cephalosporins have been introduced, each group with its own spectrum of activity.

First-generation cephalosporins are largely effective against the same gram-positive bacteria that are affected by penicillin G, as well as the gram-negative bacteria *P. mirabilis*, *E. coli*, and *K. pneumoniae* (use the letters *PEcK* as a mnemonic device to remember which bacteria are susceptible to the first-generation cephalosporins). First-generation drugs include cefazolin (generic), cefadroxil (generic), and cephalexin (*Keflex*).

Second-generation cephalosporins are effective against the previously mentioned strains, as well as *H. influenzae*, *Enterobacter aerogenes*, and *Neisseria* spp. (remember *HENPeCK*). Second-generation drugs are less effective against some gram-positive bacteria. These include cefaclor (*Ceclor*), cefotetan (generic), cefoxitin (generic), cefprozil (generic), and cefuroxime (*Zinacef*).

Third-generation cephalosporins, which are effective against all of the previously mentioned strains, have less activity against gram-positive bacteria but are more active

Table 9.3 *Drugs in Focus*: Cephalosporins

Drug Name	Dosage/Route	Usual Indications
First-Generation Cephalosporins		
cefadroxil (generic)	*Adult*: 1–2 g PO in a single or two divided doses; reduce dose in renal impairment *Pediatric*: 30 mg/kg/d PO in single or divided doses q12h	Treatment of UTIs, pharyngitis, and tonsillitis caused by group A beta-hemolytic streptococci, as well as skin infections
cefazolin (generic)	*Adult:* 500 mg–1.5 g every 6–12 h depending on indication. Routes can be PO, IM or IV. Dose reduction *Pediatric:* Dosed by weight	Treatment of respiratory tract, urinary tract, skin and skin structure, biliary tract, bone and joint, and genital infections. Treatment of septicemia and endocarditis. Prophylaxis for perioperative patient
cephalexin (*Keflex*)	*Adult*: 250–500 mg PO q6h–q12h, reduce dose in renal impairment *Pediatric*: 25–50 mg/kg/d PO in 2–4 divided doses	Treatment of respiratory, skin, bone, and GU infections; used for otitis media in children
Second-Generation Cephalosporins		
cefaclor (*Ceclor*)	*Adult*: 250–500 mg PO q8h *Pediatric*: 20 mg/kg/d PO in divided doses q8h; do not exceed 1 g/d	Treatment of respiratory tract infections, skin infections, UTIs, otitis media, typhoid fever, anthrax exposure
cefotetan (generic)	*Adult:* 1–6 g/d IV depending on type and severity of infection. Reduce dose for renal impairment	Treatment of UTI, lower respiratory tract, skin and skin structure, gynecologic, intra-abdominal, bone, and joint infections. Prophylaxis to prevent postoperative infection
cefoxitin (generic)	*Adult*: 3–8 g/d IM or IV in divided doses q6–8h; reduce dose with renal impairment *Pediatric*: 80–160 mg/kg/d IM or IV in divided doses q4–6h	Treatment of severe infections; preoperative prophylaxis for cesarean section and abdominal, vaginal, biliary, or colorectal surgery; more effective in gynecological and intra-abdominal infections than some other agents

Table 9.3 *Drugs in Focus*: Cephalosporins *(Continued)*

Drug Name	Dosage/Route	Usual Indications
cefprozil (generic)	*Adult*: 250–500 mg PO q12h–q24h reduce dose with renal impairment *Pediatric*: 7.5–20 mg/kg PO q12h–24h	Treatment of pharyngitis, tonsillitis, otitis media, sinusitis, secondary bronchial infections, and skin infections
cefuroxime (*Zinacef*)	*Adult*: 250–500 mg PO b.i.d.; 750 mg to 1.5 g IM q8h; reduce dose with renal impairment *Pediatric*: 20–30 mg/kg PO b.i.d.; 50–240 mg/kg/d IM or IV in divided doses q6–8h	Treatment of a wide range of infections, as listed for other second-generation drugs; Lyme disease; preferred treatment in situations involving an anticipated switch from parenteral to oral drug use
Third-Generation Cephalosporins		
cefdinir (generic; a suspension form is available for children)	*Adult*: 300 mg PO q12h or 600 mg/d PO; reduce dose with renal impairment *Pediatric*: 7 mg/kg PO q12h or 14 mg/d	Treatment of respiratory infections, otitis media, sinusitis, laryngitis, bronchitis, skin infections
cefixime (*Suprax*)	*Adult*: 400 mg/d PO *Pediatric (6 months and older)*: 8 mg/kg/d PO	Treatment of UTI, otitis media, pharyngitis and tonsillitis, acute exacerbations of chronic bronchitis, and uncomplicated gonorrhea
cefotaxime (*Claforan*)	*Adult*: 2–12 g/d IM or IV in divided doses q4–8h; reduce dose with renal impairment *Pediatric*: 50–180 mg/kg/d IM or IV in divided doses q4–6h	Treatment of moderate to severe skin, urinary tract, and respiratory tract infections; pelvic inflammatory disease; intra-abdominal infections; peritonitis; septicemia; bone infections; CNS infections; preoperative prophylaxis
cefpodoxime (generic)	*Adult*: 100–400 mg PO q12h; reduce dose with renal impairment *Pediatric*: 5 mg/kg/dose PO q12h	Treatment of respiratory infections, UTIs, gonorrhea, skin infections, and otitis media
ceftazidime (*Tazicef*)	*Adult*: 250 mg–2 g q8–12h IM or IV; reduce dose with renal impairment *Pediatric*: 30–50 mg/kg q8–12h IM or IV	Treatment of moderate to severe skin, urinary tract, and respiratory tract infections; intra-abdominal infections; septicemia; bone infections; CNS infections
ceftriaxone (generic)	*Adult*: 1–2 g IM or IV in divided doses q12–24h *Pediatric*: 50–100 mg/kg/d IV or IM in divided doses q12h or given once daily	Treatment of moderate to severe skin, urinary tract, and respiratory tract infections; pelvic inflammatory disease; intra-abdominal infections; peritonitis; septicemia; bone infections; CNS infections; preoperative prophylaxis
Fourth-Generation Cephalosporin		
cefepime (*Maxipime*)	*Adult*: 0.5–2 g IM or IV q8–12h; reduce dose with renal impairment *Pediatric*: 50 mg/kg/dose q8–12h IV or IM	Treatment of moderate to severe skin, urinary tract, and respiratory tract infections
Other Cephalosporins		
cefiderocol (*Fetroja*)	*Adult:* 2 g IV every 8 hours administered over 3 hours if creatinine clearance between 60 and 119 mL/min. Dose adjustments required if renal creatinine clearance lower than 60 or higher than 119 mL/min	Treatment of gram-negative microorganisms causing complicated UTI, including pyelonephritis, hospital-acquired bacterial pneumonia and ventilator-associated bacterial pneumonia
ceftaroline (*Teflaro*)	600 mg IV over 1 h q12h	Treatment of skin and skin structure infections; community-acquired pneumonia
ceftazidime–avibactam (*Avycaz*)	*Adult with creatinine clearance >50 mL/min:* 2.5 g IV every 8 h infused over 2 h. Dose adjustment needed for pediatric patients and patients with renal impairment	Treatment of complicated intra-abdominal, UTI (including pyelonephritis), and hospital-acquired bacterial pneumonia and ventilator-associated bacterial pneumonia infections caused by gram-negative microorganisms
ceftolozane–tazobactam (*Zerbaxa*)	1.5 g IV q8h over 1 h, reduce dose with renal impairment	Treatment of complicated intra-abdominal or complicated urinary tract infections

against the gram-negative bacilli, as well as against *Serratia marcescens* (remember *HENPeCKS*). Third-generation drugs include cefdinir (*Omnicef*), cefotaxime (*Claforan*), cefpodoxime (generic), ceftazidime (*Ceptaz, Tazicef*), and ceftriaxone (*Rocephin*).

Cefepime (*Maxipime*) is the fourth-generation cephalosporin. Cefepime (*Maxipime*) is active against gram-negative and gram-positive organisms, including *P. aeruginosa.* Ceftolozane–tazobactam (*Zerbaxa*) and ceftazidime–avibactam (*Avycaz*) are cephalosporins combined with two different beta-lactamase inhibitors. Ceftaroline (*Teflaro*) is effective against some methicillin-resistant organisms and is indicated for treatment of community-acquired pneumonia and some skin and skin structure infections. Cefiderocol (*Fetroja*) was approved to treat complicated urinary tract infections and hospital-acquired or ventilator-associated bacterial pneumonia. In general, as the generation number increases, the medication is more likely to reach cerebrospinal fluid, be less susceptible to beta-lactamase destruction, and be more effective against gram-negative organisms.

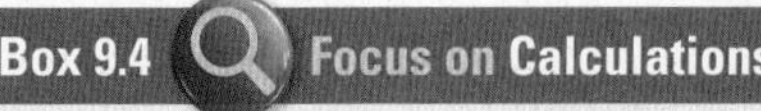

Your patient is a 20-kg child with a severe case of tonsillitis. An order is written for cefdinir (14 mg/kg/d PO for 10 days). Take one dose per day. The drug comes in an oral suspension 125 mg/mL. What should you administer at each dose?

The order is for 14 mg/kg, so 14 mg/kg × 20 kg = 280 mg. The available form is 125 mg/mL. Use the following formula:

$$\frac{\text{amount of drug available}}{\text{volume available}} = \frac{\text{amount of drug prescribed}}{\text{volume to administer}}$$

$$\frac{125\text{ mg}}{1\text{ mL}} = \frac{280\text{ mg}}{X}$$

$$125\text{ mg}/(X) = 280\text{ mg/mL}$$

$$X = \frac{280\text{ mg/mL}}{125\text{ mg}}$$

$$X = 2.24\text{ mL}$$

Round to 2.0 mL

Therapeutic Actions and Indications

The cephalosporins are both bactericidal and bacteriostatic, depending on the dose used and the specific drug involved. In susceptible species, these agents interfere with the cell wall–building ability of bacteria when they divide; that is, they prevent the bacteria from biosynthesizing the framework of their cell walls. The bacteria with weakened cell walls swell and burst as a result of the osmotic pressure within the cell (see Fig. 9.1).

Cephalosporins are indicated for the treatment of infections caused by susceptible bacteria. See Table 9.3 for usual indications for each of these agents. Selection of an antibiotic from this class depends on the sensitivity of the involved organism, the route of administration, and sometimes the cost involved. Before therapy begins, a culture and sensitivity test should be performed to evaluate the causative organism and appropriate sensitivity to the antibiotic being used.

Pharmacokinetics

Most cephalosporins are primarily excreted unchanged in the urine. Lower doses may be prescribed for those with renal impairment. However, ceftriaxone is eliminated primarily by the liver. These drugs cross the placenta and enter human milk (see "Contraindications and Cautions"). Box 9.4 provides calculation practice using cefdinir.

Contraindications and Cautions

Use caution when a cephalosporin is prescribed in patients with known allergies to cephalosporins or penicillins, as cross-sensitivity may occur. Use with caution in patients with hepatic or renal impairment because these drugs are toxic to the kidneys and could interfere with the metabolism and excretion of the drug. In addition, use with caution in pregnant or lactating patients; use only if the benefits clearly outweigh the potential risk of toxicity to the fetus or infant.

Reserve cephalosporins for appropriate situations because cephalosporin-resistant bacteria are appearing in increasing numbers. Before therapy begins, perform a culture and sensitivity test to evaluate the causative organism and appropriate sensitivity to the antibiotic being used.

Adverse Effects

The most common adverse effects of the cephalosporins involve the GI tract and include nausea, vomiting, diarrhea, anorexia, abdominal pain, and flatulence. Pseudomembranous colitis—a potentially dangerous disorder—has also been reported with some cephalosporins. Antibiotics should be held and a provider consulted if a patient complains of diarrhea, fever, or abdominal pain. With *C. difficile*–associated diarrhea, it may benefit the patient to continue the antibiotic and treat the *C. difficile* infection. However, there are other times when a different antibiotic can be chosen or antibiotic use can be stopped.

CNS symptoms include headache, dizziness, lethargy, and paresthesia. Nephrotoxicity is also associated with the use of some cephalosporins, particularly in patients who have a predisposing renal insufficiency. Other adverse effects include superinfections, which occur due to the death of the normal flora. Monitor patients receiving parenteral cephalosporins for the possibility of phlebitis with IV administration or local abscess at the site of an IM injection.

Clinically Important Drug–Drug Interactions

Concurrent administration of cephalosporins with aminoglycosides increases the risk for nephrotoxicity. Frequently monitor patients receiving this combination and evaluate serum urea nitrogen (BUN) and creatinine levels.

Patients who receive warfarin in addition to cephalosporins may experience increased bleeding. Teach these patients how to monitor for blood loss (e.g., bleeding gums, easy bruising) and to be aware that the dose of warfarin may need to be reduced.

Prototype Summary: Cefaclor

Indications: Treatment of respiratory, dermatological, urinary tract, and middle ear infections caused by susceptible strains of bacteria.

Actions: Inhibits the synthesis of bacterial cell walls, causing cell death in susceptible bacteria.

Pharmacokinetics:

Route	Peak	Duration
Oral	30–60 min	8–10 h

$T_{1/2}$: 30 to 60 minutes; excreted unchanged in the urine.

Adverse Effects: Nausea, vomiting, diarrhea, rash, superinfection, bone marrow depression, risk for pseudomembranous colitis.

Nursing Considerations for Patients Receiving Cephalosporins

Assessment: History and Examination

- Assess for possible contraindications or cautions: known allergy to any cephalosporin, penicillin, or any other allergens because cross-sensitivity may occur (obtain specific information about the nature and occurrence of the allergic reactions); history of renal disease, which could exacerbate nephrotoxicity related to the cephalosporin; and current pregnancy or lactation status.
- Perform physical assessment to establish baseline data for assessing the effectiveness of the drug and the occurrence of any adverse effects associated with drug therapy.
- Examine the skin for any rash or lesions; examine injection sites for abscess formation; and note respiratory status—including rate, depth, and adventitious sounds—to provide a baseline for determining adverse reactions.
- Perform culture and sensitivity tests at the site of infection to ensure appropriate use of the drug.
- Check renal function test results, including BUN and creatinine clearance, to assess the status of renal functioning and to detect the possible need to alter dose.

Nursing Conclusions

Nursing conclusions related to drug therapy might include the following:

- Impaired comfort related to GI or CNS effects of drug
- Infection risk related to repeated IV injections
- Dehydration and malnutrition risk related to diarrhea
- Knowledge deficit regarding drug therapy

Planning

- The patient will receive the best therapeutic effect from the drug therapy.
- The patient will have limited adverse effects from the drug therapy.
- The patient will have an understanding of the drug therapy, adverse effects to anticipate, and measures to relieve discomfort and improve safety.

Intervention With Rationale

- Check culture and sensitivity reports to ensure that this is the drug of choice for this patient.
- Monitor renal function test values before and periodically during therapy to arrange for appropriate dose reduction as needed.
- Ensure that patient receives the full course of the cephalosporin as prescribed, divided around the clock to increase effectiveness and to decrease the risk of development of resistant strains.
- Monitor the infection site and presenting signs and symptoms (e.g., fever, lethargy) throughout the course of drug therapy. Failure of these signs and symptoms to resolve may indicate the need to reculture the site.
- Provide small, frequent meals as tolerated, frequent mouth care, and ice chips or sugarless candy to suck if stomatitis and sore mouth are problems to relieve discomfort and provide nutrition.
- Provide adequate fluids to replace fluid lost with diarrhea.
- Monitor the patient for any signs of superinfection to arrange for treatment if superinfection occurs.
- Monitor injection sites regularly, and provide warm compresses and gentle massage to injection sites if they are painful or swollen. If signs of phlebitis occur, remove the IV line and reinsert in a different vein.
- Initiate safety measures, including adequate lighting, side rails on the bed, and assistance with ambulation to protect the patient from injury if CNS effects occur.
- Instruct the patient about the appropriate dosage schedule and about possible side effects to enhance

(continues on page 114)

patient knowledge about drug therapy and to promote compliance.

- Provide the following patient teaching:
  - Take safety precautions, including changing position slowly and avoiding driving and hazardous tasks, if CNS effects occur.
  - Try to drink an adequate amount of fluids and to maintain nutrition even though nausea, vomiting, and diarrhea may occur.
  - Report difficulty breathing, severe headache, severe diarrhea, dizziness, or weakness.

Evaluation

- Monitor patient response to the drug (resolution of bacterial infection).
- Monitor for adverse effects (orientation and affect; renal toxicity; hepatic dysfunction; GI effects; and local irritation, including phlebitis at injection and IV sites).
- Evaluate effectiveness of the teaching plan (patient can name drug, dosage, possible adverse effects to expect, and specific measures to help avoid adverse effects).
- Monitor effectiveness of comfort and safety measures and the patient's adherence to the regimen.

Key Points

- Cephalosporins are beta-lactam antibiotics that have multiple generations of medications effective against a wide range of bacteria.
- Monitor for GI upset and diarrhea, pseudomembranous colitis, headache, dizziness, renal function, and superinfections.

Fluoroquinolones

The fluoroquinolones (Table 9.4) are a synthetic class of bactericidal antibiotics with a broad spectrum of activity. Systemic fluoroquinolones include ciprofloxacin (*Cipro*), delafloxacin (*Baxdela*), levofloxacin (*Levaquin*), moxifloxacin (*Avelox*), and ofloxacin (generic). Many fluoroquinolones are also available as topical preparations. Topical agents are discussed in Appendix B.

Therapeutic Actions and Indications

The fluoroquinolones enter the bacterial cell by passive diffusion through channels in the cell membrane. Once inside, they interfere with the action of DNA enzymes necessary for the growth and reproduction of the bacteria (see Fig. 9.1). This leads to cell death because the bacterial DNA is damaged and the cell cannot be maintained. The fluoroquinolones have the advantage of a unique way of disrupting bacterial activity. There is little cross-resistance with other classes of antibiotics. However, misuse of these drugs in the short time the class has been available has led to the existence of resistant strains of bacteria (see "Contraindications and Cautions").

The fluoroquinolones are indicated for treating infections caused by susceptible strains of gram-positive and gram-negative bacteria, including *E. coli*, *P. mirabilis*, *K. pneumoniae*, *Enterobacter cloacae*, *Proteus vulgaris*, *Proteus rettgeri*, *Morganella morganii*, *M. catarrhalis*, *H. influenzae*, *Haemophilus parainfluenzae*, *P. aeruginosa*, *Citrobacter freundii*, *S. aureus*, *Staphylococcus epidermidis*, some *Neisseria gonorrhoeae*, and group D streptococci. These infections frequently include urinary tract, respiratory tract, and skin infections. Some of the fluoroquinolones are able to prevent or treat postexposure of anthrax infection. See Table 9.4 for usual indications for each of these agents.

Table 9.4 ***Drugs in Focus*: Fluoroquinolones**

Drug Name	Dosage/Route	Usual Indications
ciprofloxacin (*Cipro*)	*Adult*: 2,500–7,500 mg q8–12h. PO; reduce dose in renal dysfunction	Treatment of infections caused by a wide spectrum of gram-negative bacteria
delafloxacin (*Baxdela*)	300 mg IV over 60 min q12h or 450 mg PO q12h, reduce dose in renal dysfunction	Treatment of acute bacterial skin and skin structure infections caused by susceptible bacteria
gemifloxacin (*Factive*)	*Adult*: 320 mg/d PO for 5–7 d	Treatment of acute exacerbations of chronic bronchitis, community-acquired pneumonia
levofloxacin (*Levaquin*)	*Adult*: 250–750 mg/d PO or IV; reduce dose in renal impairment	Treatment of respiratory, urinary tract, skin, and sinus infections caused by susceptible gram-negative bacteria in adults; treatment after exposure to anthrax, plague
moxifloxacin (*Avelox*)	*Adult*: 400 mg/d PO or IV	Treatment of adults with sinusitis, bronchitis, or community-acquired pneumonia
ofloxacin (*Ocuflox*)	*Adult*: 200–400 mg q12h PO; reduce dose in renal impairment	Treatment of respiratory, skin, and urinary tract infections; pelvic inflammatory disease; ocular infections; otic form available for otitis media

Pharmacokinetics

The fluoroquinolones are absorbed from the GI tract, metabolized in the liver, and excreted in the urine and feces. These drugs are widely distributed in the body and cross the placenta and enter human milk (see "Contraindications and Cautions").

Ciprofloxacin and ofloxacin are available in injectable, oral, and topical forms. Moxifloxacin, delafloxacin and levofloxacin are available in oral and IV forms.

Contraindications and Cautions

Systemic fluoroquinolones have multiple boxed warnings related to potential serious adverse effects that could occur: tendinitis, tendon rupture, peripheral neuropathy, CNS effects, and exacerbation of muscle weakness in patients with myasthenia gravis. Because of these issues, these drugs are no longer recommended for treating uncomplicated infections except when no other drug treatment is possible. They are also contraindicated in patients with a known allergy to any fluoroquinolone. The use of fluoroquinolones is not recommended in pregnant or lactating patients except in specific circumstances. Most infections in patients who are pregnant should be treated with an alternative class of antibiotics. Use with caution in the presence of renal dysfunction, which could interfere with the excretion of the drug, and seizures, which could be exacerbated by the drugs' effects on cell membrane channels.

Because so many resistant strains are emerging, always perform culture and sensitivity tests of infected tissue to determine the exact bacterial cause and sensitivity. Because these drugs have been associated with damage to developing cartilage, they are not recommended for systemic use in patients younger than 18 years of age.

Adverse Effects

The most serious adverse effects of these drugs are tendinitis, tendon rupture, peripheral neuropathy, CNS effects, prolonged QT interval, *C. difficile* diarrhea, and liver toxicity. The most common adverse effects are headache, dizziness, insomnia, and depression related to possible effects on the CNS membranes. GI effects include nausea, vomiting, diarrhea, and dry mouth, related to direct drug effect on the GI tract and possibly to stimulation of the chemoreceptor trigger zone in the CNS.

Immunological effects include bone marrow depression, which may be related to drug effects on the cells of the bone marrow that rapidly turn over. Other adverse effects include fever, rash, and photosensitivity, a potentially serious adverse effect that can cause severe skin reactions. Advise patients to avoid sun and ultraviolet light exposure and to use protective clothing and sunscreens.

Clinically Important Drug–Drug Interactions

When oral fluoroquinolones are taken concurrently with iron salts, sucralfate, multivitamins, calcium or magnesium supplements, or antacids, the therapeutic effect of the fluoroquinolone is decreased. If this drug combination is necessary, administration of the two agents should be separated by at least 4 hours.

If fluoroquinolones are taken with drugs that increase the QTc interval or cause torsades de pointes (i.e., amiodarone, sotalol, erythromycin, tricyclics, phenothiazines), severe-to-fatal cardiac reactions are possible. These combinations should be avoided, but if they must be used, patients should be carefully monitored.

Combining fluoroquinolones with theophylline leads to increased levels of theophylline due to similar metabolic pathways. Warfarin levels may also increase with concurrent use with fluoroquinolones, so INR needs to be monitored closely. In addition, when fluoroquinolones are combined with nonsteroidal anti-inflammatory drugs, an increased risk of CNS stimulation is possible. If this combination is used, closely monitor patients, especially those who have a history of seizures, dizziness, or headaches. Combining a fluoroquinolone with corticosteroids can lead to an increased risk of tendonitis and tendon rupture. If this combination must be used, instruct the patient to report any tendon pain or weakness.

Prototype Summary: Ciprofloxacin (IR)

Indications: Treatment of respiratory, dermatological, urinary tract, ear, eye, bone, and joint infections; treatment after anthrax exposure, typhoid fever, plague.

Actions: Interferes with DNA replication in susceptible gram-positive and gram-negative bacteria, preventing cell reproduction.

Pharmacokinetics:

Route	Onset	Peak	Half-life
Oral	Varies	60–120 min	4–5 h
IV	10 min	Immediate	4–5 h

$T_{1/2}$: 3.5 to 4 hours; metabolized in the liver, excreted in bile and urine.

Adverse Effects: Headache, dizziness, hypotension, nausea, vomiting, diarrhea, fever, rash.

Nursing Considerations for Patients Receiving Fluoroquinolones

Assessment: History and Examination

- Assess for possible contraindications or cautions: known allergy to any fluoroquinolone (obtain specific information about the nature and occurrence of allergic

(continues on page 116)

reactions); history of myasthenia gravis; history of renal disease, which could interfere with excretion of the drug; and current pregnancy or lactation status because of potential adverse effects on the fetus or infant.
- Perform physical assessment to establish baseline data for assessing the effectiveness of the drug and the occurrence of any adverse effects associated with drug therapy.
- Examine the skin for any rash or lesions to provide a baseline for possible adverse effects.
- Perform culture and sensitivity tests at the site of infection to ensure appropriate use of the drug.
- Conduct assessment of orientation, affect, and reflexes to establish a baseline for any CNS effects of the drug.
- Perform renal function tests, including BUN and creatinine clearance, to evaluate the status of renal function and to assess necessary changes in dose.

Nursing Conclusions

Nursing conclusions related to drug therapy might include the following:
- Impaired comfort related to GI, CNS, or skin effects of the drug
- Fluid deficit and malnutrition risk related to GI effects of the drug
- Knowledge deficit regarding drug therapy

Planning

- The patient will receive the best therapeutic effect from the drug therapy.
- The patient will have limited adverse effects from the drug therapy.
- The patient will have an understanding of the drug therapy, adverse effects to anticipate, and measures to relieve discomfort and improve safety.

Intervention With Rationale

- Check culture and sensitivity reports to ensure that this is the drug of choice for this patient.
- Monitor renal function tests before initiating therapy to appropriately arrange for dose reduction if necessary.
- Ensure that the patient receives the full course of the fluoroquinolone as prescribed to eradicate the infection and to help prevent the emergence of resistant strains.
- Monitor the site of infection and presenting signs and symptoms (e.g., fever, lethargy) throughout the course of drug therapy. Failure of these signs and symptoms to resolve may indicate the need to reculture the site.
- Provide small, frequent meals as tolerated, frequent mouth care, and ice chips or sugarless candy to suck if dry mouth is a problem to relieve discomfort and provide nutrition, and provide adequate fluids to replace those lost with diarrhea.
- Implement safety measures, including adequate lighting, use of side rails, and assistance with ambulation to protect the patient from injury if CNS effects occur.
- Instruct the patient about the appropriate dosage schedule and possible adverse effects to enhance patient knowledge about drug therapy and to promote adherence.
- Provide the following patient teaching:
  - Take safety precautions, including changing position slowly and avoiding driving and hazardous tasks, if CNS effects occur.
  - Try to drink an adequate amount of fluids and to maintain nutrition, although nausea, vomiting, and diarrhea may occur.
  - Avoid ultraviolet light and sun exposure, using protective clothing and sunscreens.
  - Report difficulty breathing, severe headache, severe diarrhea, severe skin rash, fainting spells, and heart palpitations, tendon pain, or weakness.

Evaluation

- Monitor patient response to the drug (resolution of bacterial infection).
- Monitor for adverse effects (orientation and affect, GI effects, photosensitivity).
- Evaluate effectiveness of the teaching plan (patient can name drug, dosage, possible adverse effects to expect, and specific measures to help avoid adverse effects).
- Monitor effectiveness of comfort and safety measures and adherence to the therapeutic regimen.

Key Points

- Fluoroquinolones inhibit the action of DNA enzymes in susceptible gram-positive and gram-negative bacteria. They are used to treat a wide range of infections.
- Monitor the patient for headache, dizziness, GI upset, and bone marrow depression, and caution the patient about the risk of photosensitivity reactions. Be aware that the patient may be at increased risk for tendonitis and tendon rupture.

Penicillins and Penicillinase-Resistant Antibiotics

Penicillin (Table 9.5) was the first antibiotic introduced for clinical use. Sir Alexander Fleming used *Penicillium* molds to produce the original penicillin in the 1920s. Subsequent versions of penicillin were developed to decrease the adverse effects of the drug and to modify it to act on resistant bacteria. The natural penicillins include penicillin G benzathine (*Bicillin L.A., Permapen*), penicillin G potassium (*Pfizerpen*), penicillin G procaine (generic), and penicillin V (*Penicillin-VK*). The aminopenicillins include

Table 9.5 ***Drugs in Focus*: Penicillins and Penicillinase-Resistant Antibiotics**

Drug Name	Dosage/Route	Usual Indications
Natural Penicillins		
penicillin G benzathine (*Bicillin, Permapen*)	*Adult*: 600,000 units to 2.4 million units IM	Severe infections caused by sensitive organisms; treatment of syphilis and erysipeloid infections
penicillin G potassium (*Pfizerpen*)	*Adult*: 1–24 million units/d IM or IV, depending on condition, reduce dose in renal impairment *Pediatric*: 100,000–1 million units/d IM or IV	Treatment of infections
penicillin G procaine (generic)	*Adult*: 1.2–2.4 million units IM *Pediatric*: 600,000–2.4 million units IM	Treatment of moderately severe infections daily for 8–12 d
penicillin V (*Penicillin-VK*)	*Adult*: 125–500 mg q6–8h PO *Pediatric*: 15–62.5 mg/kg/d PO in divided doses q6–8h	Used for prophylaxis for bacterial endocarditis, Lyme disease, UTIs
Aminopenicillins		
amoxicillin (*Amoxil*)	*Adult*: 250–1,000 mg PO q8–12h, reduce dose in renal impairment	Broad spectrum of uses for adults and children
amoxicillin–clavulanate	*Adults and pediatric >40 kg*: 250–875 mg every 8–12 h PO *Pediatric <40 kg*: weight and age-based dosing	Treatment of lower respiratory tract, acute bacterial otitis media, sinusitis, skin and skin structure, and urinary tract infections
ampicillin (generic)	*Adult*: 250–500 mg IM or IV q6h, or 250—500 mg PO q6h when oral use is feasible	Broad spectrum of activity; useful form if switch from parenteral to oral is anticipated; monitor for nephritis
ampicillin-sulbactam (*Unasyn*)	*Adult*: 1.5–3 g IV or IM every 6 h; dose reduction if renal impairment *Pediatric: weight-based dosing*	Treatment of skin and skin structure, intra-abdominal and gynecological infections
Penicillinase-Resistant (Antistaphylococcal) Antibiotics		
dicloxacillin (generic)	*Adult:* 125–250 mg PO every 6 hours *Pediatric:* weight-based dosing	Treatment of infections caused by penicillinase-producing staphylococci
nafcillin (generic)	*Adult*: 500–1,000 mg IV q4h	Infections by penicillinase-producing staphylococci as well as group A hemolytic streptococci, plus *Streptococcus viridans*; drug of choice if switch to oral form is anticipated
oxacillin (generic)	250–1,000 mg IV q4–6h, reduce dose in renal dysfunction	Infections by penicillinase-producing staphylococci; streptococci; drug of choice if switch to oral form is anticipated
Antipseudomonal Penicillins		
piperacillin (generic)	*Adult*: 3–4 g every 6 h IV; doses reduced with renal impairment	Treatment of infections caused by intra-abdominal, urinary tract, gynecologic, lower respiratory, skin and skin structure, and bone and joint infections. Treatment of septicemia and uncomplicated gonococcal urethritis. Prophylaxis against infection from surgical procedures
piperacillin-tazobactam (*Zosyn*)	*Adult*: 3.375–4.5 g every 6 h IV, dose reduction with renal impairment *Pediatric*: weight and age based	Treatment of intra-abdominal, nosocomial pneumonia, skin and skin structure, female pelvic and community-acquired pneumonia infections

amoxicillin (*Amoxil*), ampicillin (generic), and the combination medications amoxicillin–clavulanate (*Augmentin*), and ampicillin–sulbactam (*Unasyn*).

With the prolonged use of penicillin, more and more bacterial species have synthesized the enzyme penicillinase to counteract the effects of penicillin. Researchers have developed a group of drugs with a resistance to penicillinase, which allows them to remain effective against bacteria that are now resistant to the penicillins. Penicillinase-resistant (antistaphylococcal) antibiotics include dicloxacillin (generic), nafcillin (generic), and oxacillin (generic). The antipseudomonal penicillins are piperacillin (generic) and piperacillin–tazobactam (*Zosyn*). The actual drug chosen depends on the sensitivity of the bacteria causing the infection, the desired and available routes, and the personal experience of the clinician with the particular agent.

Therapeutic Actions and Indications

The natural penicillins and penicillinase-resistant antibiotics produce bactericidal effects by interfering with the ability of susceptible bacteria to build their cell walls when they are dividing (see Fig. 9.2). These drugs prevent the bacteria from biosynthesizing the framework of the cell wall, and the bacteria with weakened cell walls swell and then burst from osmotic pressure within the cell. Because human cells do not use the biochemical process that the bacteria use to form the cell wall, this effect is a selective toxicity.

The natural penicillins and penicillinase resistant are indicated for the treatment of streptococcal infections, including pharyngitis, tonsillitis, scarlet fever, and endocarditis; pneumococcal infections; staphylococcal infections; fusospirochetal infections; rat-bite fever; diphtheria; anthrax; syphilis; and uncomplicated gonococcal infections. At high doses, these drugs are also used to treat meningococcal meningitis. The aminopenicillins have enhanced ability to treat more gram-negative infections than the natural penicillins. The antipseudomonal penicillins have the widest spectrum of activity and are effective against both some gram-positive and gram-negative organisms. See Table 9.5 for usual indications for each agent. (See the "Critical Thinking Scenario.")

CRITICAL THINKING SCENARIO
Antibiotics and Adverse Effects

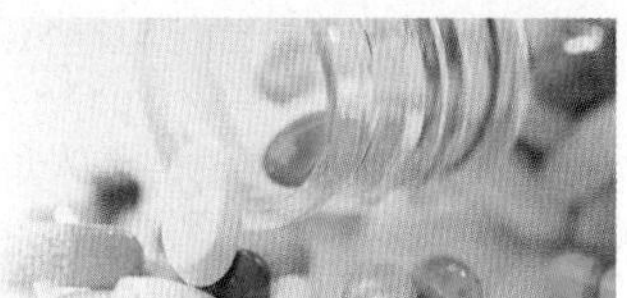

THE SITUATION

N.S., an 18-month-old child, was diagnosed with acute otitis media when their parent brought them to the clinic following a sleepless night of inconsolable crying, low-grade fever, and inability to take a bottle. A prescription was given for amoxicillin, and the parent was told to return in 10 days for a follow-up appointment.

In talking with the parent, you discover that this is their first child and this is the first time the child has been sick.

Critical Thinking

How does amoxicillin affect a child with an ear infection?
What adverse effects and safety issues need to be considered?
What nursing interventions are appropriate for N.S. and their parent?
What teaching points should be stressed with the parent?
What potential medication errors should you consider?
What points do you need to include to help the parent safely administer the drug and evaluate its effectiveness?

DISCUSSION

Amoxicillin is an antibiotic that interferes with the bacterial cell wall to cause bacterial cell death. It needs to be taken for duration prescribed. The adverse effects most frequently seen with this antibiotic are nausea, diarrhea, rash, and superinfections. The pain and discomfort of the ear infection may persist for a day or 2 after starting the drug, and the toddler may require additional comfort measures.

The parent in this case will need clear, concise written information. This is their first child and the first time the child has been sick, so the parent may also need support and encouragement to get through the experience. The medication will be prepared in a suspension form, so the child can swallow it safely. Measuring out the dosage should be emphasized. A pharmacist should supply a measuring device, often a dosing syringe, to ensure that the correct dose is given. It is not recommended to use home measuring systems. Proper storage of the drug may require refrigeration. The bottle will need to be shaken before each use. It will be important to explain that the toddler needs to receive the full prescribed dose, giving the drug for the prescribed duration. The parent needs to understand that the toddler may seem to feel just fine, but the bacteria may still be present, and the full dose needs to be given.

N.S.'s parent will need to understand that some adverse effects are possible. Diarrhea is very common when this drug is used in this age group. The parent will need to be encouraged to watch for any signs of dehydration, to encourage lots of fluid intake, and to take special care in frequently changing the diaper and cleansing with each diaper change because diarrhea can be very irritating to the skin. They may also notice white patches in the mouth if a superinfection should occur. This may first present with the toddler unable to suck a bottle and unable to eat without crying. A mild rash may also occur; the parent might want to have this evaluated if they are concerned. The child may need further comfort measures until the infection resolves; N.S. could have a standby order for ibuprofen or acetaminophen in proper dosage for this age group. Warm compresses on the affected ear(s) and holding the child against the parent's body to provide warmth to the ear are appropriate comfort measures. The parent should be taught that over-the-counter (OTC) cold medicines are not approved for this age group and should be discouraged from using them. They could offer the child yogurt with live cultures to help balance any diarrhea that might occur. Encourage the parent to call if unable to control the discomfort their child is experiencing.

The parent should be encouraged to monitor the toddler's reactions. Is the child still feverish, are they now playing and eating, can they sleep soundly again? If there is any indication that things might be getting worse (continued high fever, persistent crying, drainage from the ears), the parent should be encouraged to call or bring the toddler back into the clinic. They should be praised for bringing the child to the clinic and encouraged to call with reports of the child's progress.

This first encounter with the health care system with a sick child is a unique opportunity for the nurse to do preventative and safety teaching around the experience, drug administration, use of OTC products, and safety measures when giving drugs. Current standards no longer call for immediate antibiotic use with an otitis media in a child. It is now recommended to do the following for a few days to see if the infection will resolve without antibiotics: give support, nasal saline, fluids, humidifiers, avoid exposure to smoke, and offer NSAIDs for fever reduction and pain relief. This cuts down on the use of antibiotics and the development of resistant strains. Most will resolve, but if symptoms become worse or fever climbs, medical follow-up is recommended. This approach is often very hard on new parents who want to do something to make the child feel better.

NURSING CARE GUIDE FOR N.S.: AMOXICILLIN

Assessment: History and Examination

Allergy to any amoxicillin
Concurrent use of any other drugs
General: Site of infection, culture, and sensitivity
Skin: Color, lesions
Respiratory: Respiration, adventitious sounds
GI: Bowel sounds, usual output
Laboratory data: Liver and renal function tests if warranted

Nursing Conclusions

Malnutrition risk related to GI effects
Injury risk related to possible dehydration
Knowledge deficit regarding drug therapy

Planning

- The patient will receive the best therapeutic effect from the drug therapy.
- The patient will have limited adverse effects from the drug therapy.
- The patient's family will have an understanding of the drug therapy, adverse effects to anticipate, and measures to relieve discomfort and improve safety.

Intervention

Perform culture and sensitivity tests before beginning therapy.
Store suspension in refrigerator; shake before each use; use appropriate measuring device.
Monitor for and provide hygiene measures and treatment if superinfections occur.
Monitor nutritional status and fluid intake if diarrhea occurs.
Provide appropriate perianal cleansing and care if diarrhea is a problem.
Provide comfort measures to deal with ear pain; warm compresses, analgesic as appropriate.
Provide patient's family with teaching regarding drug name, dosage, storage, measuring, adverse effects, possible adverse effects, warnings to report.

Evaluation

Evaluate drug effects: resolution of bacterial infections.
Monitor for adverse effects: diarrhea, superinfections.
Evaluate effectiveness of patient teaching program.
Evaluate effectiveness of comfort and safety measures.

Patient Teaching the Parent of N.S.

- Amoxicillin is an antibiotic that is specific for your child's ear infection. You need to store the drug in the refrigerator; shake the bottle before each use. Use the measuring device provided, not a flatware teaspoon to administer the drug.
- Make sure you give your child the full course of this antibiotic. Do not stop giving it if the child seems better. It is very important to give the full course of the drug to prevent another infection or the development of resistant bacteria.
- Your child may experience stomach upset or diarrhea. If diarrhea occurs, make sure you change the diaper often and cleanse the diaper area well. Monitor your child for any signs of dehydration and try to encourage fluid intake.
- Your child may develop other infections in the mouth or vagina. You may notice that it is difficult for your child to suck a nipple or to swallow, or you may notice white patches in the mouth or vaginal area. If this occurs, consult your provider for appropriate treatment; do not stop taking the drug.
- Your child may still experience pain for the first few days; a prescription for an analgesic may be given to you; warm compresses on the ear may help; holding the child close to your body will also provide warmth and may help ease the ear pain.
- Report any of the following to your health care provider if your child experiences: worsening pain, higher fever, inability to swallow, lethargy, dry skin, or severe diaper rash.

Pharmacokinetics

Most of the penicillins are rapidly absorbed from the GI tract, reaching peak levels in 1 hour. They are sensitive to gastric acid levels in the stomach and should be taken on an empty stomach to ensure adequate absorption. Penicillins are excreted unchanged in the urine, making renal function an important factor in safe use of the drug. Penicillins enter human milk and can cause adverse reactions (see "Contraindications and Cautions").

Contraindications and Cautions

These drugs are contraindicated in patients with allergies to penicillin or other allergens. Penicillin sensitivity tests are available if the patient's history of allergy is unclear, and penicillin is the drug of choice. Use with caution in patients with renal disease (lowered doses are necessary because excretion is reduced). Use in patients who are pregnant or lactating should be limited to situations in which the patient clearly would benefit from the drug, because diarrhea and superinfections in the infant may occur.

Perform culture and sensitivity tests to ensure that the causative organism is sensitive to the penicillin selected for use. With the emergence of many resistant strains of bacteria, this has become increasingly important.

Adverse Effects

The major adverse effects of penicillin therapy involve the GI tract. Common adverse effects include nausea, vomiting, diarrhea, abdominal pain, glossitis, stomatitis, gastritis, sore mouth, and furry tongue. These effects are primarily related to the loss of bacteria from the normal flora and the subsequent opportunistic infections that occur. Superinfections, including yeast infections, are also very common and are again associated with the loss of bacteria from the normal flora. Pain and inflammation at the injection site can occur with injectable forms of the drugs. Hypersensitivity reactions may include rash, fever, wheezing, and with repeated exposure anaphylaxis that can progress to anaphylactic shock and death.

Clinically Important Drug–Drug Interactions

In addition, when the parenteral forms of penicillins and penicillinase-resistant drugs are administered in combination with any of the parenteral aminoglycosides, inactivation of the aminoglycosides occurs. These combinations should also be avoided.

Prototype Summary: Amoxicillin

Indications: Treatment of infections caused by susceptible strains of bacteria, and treatment of *Helicobacter* infections as part of combination therapy. Off label uses include postexposure prophylaxis for anthrax and prophylaxis for endocarditis.

Actions: Inhibits synthesis of the cell wall in susceptible bacteria, causing cell death.

Pharmacokinetics:

Route	Onset	Peak	Duration
Oral	Varies	1 h	6–8 h

$T_{1/2}$: 1 to 1.4 hours; excreted unchanged in the urine.

Adverse Effects: Nausea, vomiting, diarrhea, glossitis, stomatitis, bone marrow suppression, rash, fever, superinfections, lethargy.

Nursing Considerations for Patients Receiving Penicillins and Penicillinase-Resistant Antibiotics

Assessment: History and Examination

- Assess for possible contraindications or cautions: known allergy to any cephalosporins, penicillins, or other allergens because cross-sensitivity can occur (obtain specific information about the nature and occurrence of allergic reactions); history of renal disease that could interfere with excretion of the drug; and current pregnancy or lactation status.
- Perform a physical assessment to establish baseline data for evaluating the effectiveness of the drug and the occurrence of any adverse effects associated with drug therapy.
- Examine skin and mucous membranes for any rashes or lesions and injection sites for abscess formation to provide a baseline for possible adverse effects.
- Perform culture and sensitivity tests at the site of infection to ensure that this is the drug of choice for this patient.
- Note respiratory status to provide a baseline for the occurrence of hypersensitivity reactions.
- Examine the abdomen to monitor for adverse effects. Evaluate renal function test findings, including UN and creatinine clearance, to assess the status of renal functioning and to determine any needed alteration in dose.

Nursing Conclusions

Nursing conclusions related to drug therapy might include the following:

- Impaired comfort related to GI effects of drug
- Dehydration and malnutrition risk related to multiple GI effects of the drug or to superinfections
- Knowledge deficit regarding drug therapy

Planning

- The patient will receive the best therapeutic effect from the drug therapy.
- The patient will have limited adverse effects from the drug therapy.
- The patient will have an understanding of the drug therapy, adverse effects to anticipate, and measures to relieve discomfort and improve safety.

Intervention With Rationale

- Check culture and sensitivity reports to ensure that this is the drug of choice for this patient.
- Monitor renal function tests before and periodically during therapy to arrange for dose reduction as needed.
- Ensure that the patient receives the full course of the medication as prescribed, in doses around the clock, to increase effectiveness.
- Explain storage requirements for suspensions and the importance of completing the prescribed therapeutic course even if signs and symptoms have disappeared to increase the effectiveness of the drug and decrease the risk of developing resistant strains.
- Monitor the site of infection and presenting signs and symptoms (e.g., fever, lethargy) throughout the course of drug therapy. Failure of these signs and symptoms to resolve may indicate the need to reculture the site.
- Provide small, frequent meals as tolerated, ensure frequent mouth care, and offer ice chips or sugarless candy to suck if stomatitis and sore mouth are problems to relieve discomfort and ensure nutrition.
- Provide adequate fluids to replace fluid lost with diarrhea.
- Monitor the patient for any signs of superinfection to arrange for treatment if superinfections occur.
- Monitor injection sites regularly, and provide warm compresses and gentle massage to injection sites if they are painful or swollen. If signs of phlebitis occur, remove the IV line, and reinsert it in a different vein to continue the drug regimen.
- Instruct the patient regarding the appropriate dosage regimen and possible adverse effects to enhance the patient's knowledge about drug therapy and promote compliance.
- Provide the following patient teaching:
  - Try to drink an adequate amount of fluids and to maintain nutrition even though nausea, vomiting, and diarrhea may occur.
  - Report difficulty breathing, severe headache, severe diarrhea, dizziness, weakness, mouth sores, and vaginal itching or sores to a health care provider. Box 9.5 contains a teaching checklist for penicillins.

Evaluation

- Monitor patient response to the drug (resolution of bacterial infection).
- Monitor for adverse effects (GI effects; local irritation, phlebitis at injection and IV sites; superinfections).
- Evaluate the effectiveness of the teaching plan (patient can name the drug, dosage, possible adverse effects to expect, and specific measures to help avoid adverse effects).
- Monitor the effectiveness of comfort and safety measures and adherence to the regimen.

Box 9.5 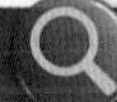 **Focus on Patient and Family Teaching**

PENICILLINS

- The penicillins are used to help destroy specific bacteria that are causing infections in the body. They are effective against only certain bacteria; they are not effective against viruses (such as cold germs) or fungi. To clear up a bacterial infection, the penicillins must act on the bacteria over a period of time, so it is very important to complete the full course of this penicillin to avoid recurrence of the infection.
- The drug should be taken on an empty stomach with a full 8-oz glass of water—1 hour before meals or 2 to 3 hours after meals is best. Do not use fruit juice, soft drinks, or milk to take your drug, because these foods may interfere with its effectiveness. (This does not apply to amoxicillin and penicillin V; these can be taken with meals.)
- Common effects of these drugs include stomach upset, diarrhea, changes in taste, and change in the color of the tongue. Small, frequent meals may help. It is important to try to maintain good nutrition. These effects should go away when the drug is stopped.
- Report any of the following to your health care provider: hives, rash, fever, difficulty breathing, and severe diarrhea.
- Tell any doctor, nurse, or other health care provider that you are taking this drug.
- Keep this drug and all medications out of the reach of children and pets.
- Do not share this drug with other people, and do not use this medication to self-treat other infections.

Key Points

- The penicillins are one of the oldest classes of antibiotics, and many resistant strains have evolved. The penicillinase-resistant antibiotics were created to combat bacteria that produce an enzyme to destroy the penicillin. Penicillins are used to treat many different infections, including respiratory tract infections and sexually transmitted infections.
- Monitor the patient on penicillin for nausea, vomiting, diarrhea, superinfections, and the possibility of hypersensitivity reactions.

Sulfonamides

The sulfonamides, or sulfa drugs (Table 9.6), are drugs that inhibit folic acid synthesis. Sulfonamides include sulfadiazine (generic) and cotrimoxazole or trimethoprim–sulfamethoxazole (*Septra, Bactrim*).

Therapeutic Actions and Indications

Folic acid is necessary for the synthesis of purines and pyrimidines, which are precursors of RNA and DNA. For cells to grow and reproduce, they require folic acid. Humans cannot synthesize folic acid and depend on the folate in their diet to obtain this essential substance. Bacteria are impermeable to folic acid and must synthesize it inside the cell. The sulfonamides competitively block *para*-aminobenzoic acid to prevent the synthesis of folic acid in susceptible bacteria that synthesize their own folates for the production of RNA and DNA (see Fig. 9.2). This includes gram-negative and gram-positive bacteria such as *Chlamydia trachomatis* and *Nocardia* and some strains of *H. influenzae*, *E. coli*, and *P. mirabilis*.

Because of the emergence of resistant bacterial strains and the development of newer antibiotics, the sulfa drugs are not used as frequently. However, they remain an inexpensive and effective treatment for UTIs and trachoma, especially in developing countries and when cost is an issue. These drugs are used to treat trachoma (a leading cause of blindness from *C. trachomatis* infection), nocardiosis (which causes pneumonias, as well as brain abscesses and inflammation), and UTIs. See Table 9.6 for usual indications for each of these agents.

Pharmacokinetics

The sulfonamides are teratogenic; they are distributed into human milk (see "Contraindications and Cautions"). These drugs, given orally, are absorbed from the GI tract, metabolized in the liver, and excreted in the urine. The time to peak level and the half-life of the individual drug vary.

Cotrimoxazole is a combination drug that contains sulfamethoxazole and trimethoprim, another antibacterial drug. It is rapidly absorbed from the GI tract, reaching peak levels in 2 hours. After being metabolized in the liver, it is excreted in the urine with a half-life of 7 to 12 hours.

Contraindications and Cautions

The sulfonamides are contraindicated with any known allergy to any sulfonamide, to sulfonylureas, or to thiazide or loop diuretics because cross-sensitivities may occur. These medications should be not routinely be used during pregnancy because the drugs can cause birth defects, as well as kernicterus, and during lactation because of a risk of kernicterus, diarrhea, and rash in the infant. They should be used with caution in patients with renal disease or a history of kidney stones because of the possibility of development of kidney stones especially if not well hydrated. They should be used with caution in older adults because of the increased incidence of thrombocytopenia, hyperkalemia, and folate deficiency.

Adverse Effects

Adverse effects associated with sulfonamides include GI effects, such as nausea, vomiting, diarrhea, abdominal pain, anorexia, stomatitis, and hepatic injury, which are all related to direct irritation of the GI tract and the death of normal bacteria. Renal effects are related to the filtration of the drug in the glomerulus and include crystalluria, hematuria, hyperkalemia, and proteinuria, which can progress to a nephrotic syndrome and possible toxic nephrosis. CNS effects include headache, dizziness, vertigo, ataxia, convulsions, and depression. Bone marrow depression may occur and is related to drug effects on the cells that turn over rapidly in the bone marrow.

Dermatological effects include photosensitivity and Stevens-Johnson syndrome, which is a rare but severe skin and mucus membrane reaction. A wide range of hypersensitivity reactions may also occur.

Clinically Important Drug–Drug Interactions

If sulfonamides are taken with the antidiabetic agents, glyburide, glipizide, or the risk of hypoglycemia increases. If this combination is needed, the patient should be

Table 9.6 *Drugs in Focus*: Sulfonamides

Drug Name	Dosage/Route	Usual Indications
sulfadiazine (generic)	*Adult*: 2–4 g/d PO in three to six divided doses	Treatment of a broad spectrum of infections
cotrimoxazole; trimethoprim-sulfamethoxazole (*Septra, Bactrim*)	*Adult*: 1–2 tablets PO q12h; reduce dose with renal impairment *Pediatric*: 8 mg/kg/d trimethoprim plus 40 mg sulfamethoxazole PO q12h	Treatment of otitis media, bronchitis, urinary tract infections, and pneumonitis caused by *Pneumocystis jirovecii*

monitored and a dose adjustment of the antidiabetic agent should be made. An increase in dose will then be needed when sulfonamide therapy stops.

There is increased risk of hyperkalemia when these medications are combined with other medications that have the same risk, like ace inhibitors, and potassium sparing diuretics.

When sulfonamides are taken with cyclosporine, the risk of nephrotoxicity rises. If this combination is essential, the patient should be monitored closely and the sulfonamide stopped at any sign of renal dysfunction.

Prototype Summary: Trimethoprim–sulfamethoxazole/cotrimoxazole

Indications: Treatment of urinary tract infection, acute otitis media in children, exacerbations of chronic bronchitis in adults, traveler's diarrhea in adults, and *Pneumocystis jirovecii* pneumonia when caused by susceptible strains of bacteria.

Actions: Blocks two consecutive steps in protein and nucleic acid production, leading to inability for cells to multiply.

Pharmacokinetics:

Route	Onset	Peak
Oral	Rapid	1–4 h

$T_{1/2}$: 8 to 10 hours; excreted in the urine.

Adverse Effects: Nausea, vomiting, diarrhea, hepatocellular necrosis, hematuria, hyperkalemia, bone marrow suppression, Stevens-Johnson syndrome, rash, urticaria, photophobia, fever, chills.

Nursing Considerations for Patients Receiving Sulfonamides

Assessment: History and Examination

- Assess for possible contraindications or cautions: known allergy to any sulfonamide, sulfonylureas, or thiazide or loop diuretic because cross-sensitivity often results (obtain specific information about the nature and occurrence of allergic reactions); history of renal disease that could interfere with excretion of the drug and lead to increased toxicity; and current pregnancy or lactation status because of potential adverse effects on the fetus or baby.
- Perform a physical assessment to establish baseline data for assessing the effectiveness of the drug and the occurrence of any adverse effects associated with drug therapy.
- Examine skin and mucous membranes for any rash or lesions to provide a baseline for possible adverse effects.
- Obtain specimens for culture and sensitivity tests at the site of infection to ensure that this is the appropriate drug for this patient.
- Note respiratory status to provide a baseline for the occurrence of hypersensitivity reactions.
- Conduct assessment of orientation, affect, and reflexes to monitor for adverse drug effects and examination of the abdomen to monitor for adverse effects.
- Monitor renal function test findings, including UN and creatinine clearance, to evaluate the status of renal function and to determine any needed alteration in dosage. Also perform a complete blood count (CBC) to establish a baseline to monitor for adverse effects.

Nursing Conclusions

Nursing conclusions related to drug therapy might include the following:

- Impaired comfort related to GI, CNS, or skin effects of the drug
- Altered sensory perception related to CNS effects
- Malnutrition risk related to multiple GI effects of the drug
- Knowledge deficit risk regarding drug therapy

Planning

- The patient will receive the best therapeutic effect from the drug therapy.
- The patient will have limited adverse effects from the drug therapy.
- The patient will have an understanding of the drug therapy, adverse effects to anticipate, and measures to relieve discomfort and improve safety.

Intervention With Rationale

- Check culture and sensitivity reports to ensure that this is the drug of choice for this patient, and repeat cultures if response is not as anticipated.
- Monitor renal function tests before and periodically during therapy to arrange for a dose reduction as necessary.
- Ensure that the patient receives the full course of the sulfonamide as prescribed to increase therapeutic effects and decrease the risk for development of resistant strains.
- Administer orally with or without food and with a full glass of water to reduce risk of crystalluria.
- Discontinue immediately if hypersensitivity reactions occur to prevent potentially fatal reactions.
- Provide small, frequent meals and adequate fluids as tolerated; encourage frequent mouth care; and offer ice chips or sugarless candy to suck if stomatitis and sore mouth are problems to relieve discomfort, ensure nutrition, and replace fluid lost with diarrhea.
- Monitor CBC and urinalysis test results before and periodically during therapy to check for adverse effects.

(continues on page 124)

- Instruct the patient about the appropriate dosage regimen, the proper way to take the drug (with a full glass of water), and possible adverse effects, to enhance patient knowledge about drug therapy and to promote adherence.
- Provide the following patient teaching:
  - Avoid driving or operating dangerous machinery because dizziness, lethargy, and ataxia may occur.
  - Try to drink an adequate amount of fluids and to maintain nutrition, even though nausea, vomiting, and diarrhea may occur.
  - Report difficulty in breathing, rash, ringing in the ears, fever, sore throat, or change in urine.

Evaluation

- Monitor patient response to the drug (resolution of bacterial infection).
- Monitor for adverse effects (GI effects, CNS effects, rash, and crystalluria).
- Evaluate the effectiveness of the teaching plan (patient can name the drug, dosage, possible adverse effects to expect, and specific measures to help avoid adverse effects).
- Monitor the effectiveness of comfort and safety measures and adherence to the regimen.

Key Points

- Sulfonamides are older drugs; many bacterial strains have developed resistance to the sulfonamides, so their use can be limited.
- Monitor the patient for rash, CNS toxicity, nausea, vomiting, diarrhea, liver injury, renal toxicity, and bone marrow depression.

Tetracyclines

The tetracyclines (Table 9.7) were developed as semisynthetic antibiotics based on the structure of a common soil mold. They are composed of four rings, which is how they got their name. Researchers have developed newer tetracyclines to increase absorption and tissue penetration. Tetracyclines include tetracycline (generic), demeclocycline (generic), doxycycline (*Doryx, Acticlate*), eravacycline (*Xerava*), omadacycline (*Nuzyra*), minocycline (*Arestin, Minocin*), and sarecycline (*Seysara*).

Therapeutic Actions and Indications

The tetracyclines are bacteriostatic and work by inhibiting protein synthesis in a wide range of bacteria, leading to the inability of the bacteria to multiply (see Fig. 9.2). Because the affected protein is similar to a protein found in human cells, these drugs can be toxic to humans at high concentrations.

Tetracyclines are indicated for treatment of infections caused by *Rickettsia* spp., *Mycoplasma pneumoniae, Borrelia recurrentis, H. influenzae, Haemophilus ducreyi, Pasteurella pestis, Pasteurella tularensis, Bartonella bacilliformis, Bacteroides* spp., *Vibrio comma, Vibrio fetus, Brucella* spp., *E. coli, E. aerogenes, Shigella* spp., *Acinetobacter calcoaceticus, Klebsiella* spp., *Diplococcus pneumoniae*, and *S. aureus*; against agents that cause psittacosis/ornithosis, lymphogranuloma venereum, and granuloma inguinale; when penicillin is contraindicated in susceptible infections; and for treatment of acne and uncomplicated GU infections caused by *C. trachomatis*. Some of the tetracyclines are also used as adjuncts in the treatment of certain protozoal infections. See Table 9.7 for usual indications for each agent.

Pharmacokinetics

Tetracyclines are absorbed adequately, but not completely, from the GI tract. Their absorption is affected by food, iron, calcium, and other drugs in the stomach. Tetracycline is concentrated in the liver and excreted unchanged in the urine. However, other medications in the class have alternate metabolic pathways and are only partially excreted in the urine. The tetracyclines have half-lives that range from 12 to 25 hours. These drugs cross the placenta and pass into human milk, but only in low concentrations (see "Contraindications and Cautions").

Tetracycline, demeclocycline, and sarecycline are available in oral form. Doxycycline and omadacycline are available orally and IV, and minocycline are available in topical, IV, and oral forms. Eravacycline is available in IV form.

Contraindications and Cautions

Tetracyclines are contraindicated in patients with known allergy to tetracyclines and during pregnancy and lactation because of effects on developing bones and teeth (see "Critical Thinking Scenario").

Tetracyclines should be used with caution in children younger than 8 years of age because they can potentially damage developing bones and teeth.

Adverse Effects

The major adverse effects of tetracycline therapy involve direct irritation of the GI tract and include nausea,

Table 9.7 *Drugs in Focus*: Tetracyclines

Drug Name	Dosage/Route	Usual Indications
demeclocycline (generic)	*Adult*: 150 mg PO four times daily *or* 300 mg PO b.i.d. *Pediatric (>8 y)*: 6–13 mg/kg/d PO in two to four divided doses	Treatment of a wide variety of infections when penicillin cannot be used
doxycycline (*Doryx, Vibramycin*)	*Adult*: 200 mg/d IV in two infusions of 1–4 h each *or* 200 mg q12h PO *Pediatric (>8 y)*: 4.4 mg/kg/d PO in divided doses	Treatment of a wide variety of infections, including traveler's diarrhea and sexually transmitted diseases; periodontal disease, Lyme disease
eravacycline (*Xerava*)	*Adults*: 1 mg/kg every 12 h IV for 4–14 d; dose adjustment for severe hepatic impairment and concomitant use of strong cytochromo P450 isoenzymes inducer	Treatment of complicated intra-abdominal infections
minocycline (*Arestin, Minocin, Ximino*)	*Adult*: 200 mg IV or PO, followed by 100 mg IV or PO q12h *or* 200 mg PO, then 100 mg PO q12h *Pediatric (>8 y)*: 4 mg/kg IV or PO followed by 2 mg/kg IV or PO q12h	Treatment of meningococcal carriers and of various uncomplicated genitourinary and gynecological infections, periodontal disease
omadacycline (*Nuzyra*)	*Adult loading dose*: 200 mg/d IV as single or two doses on day 1 or 450 mg/d PO *Adult maintenance dose for 6–13 days*: 100 mg/d IV or 300 mg/d PO	Treatment of community-acquired bacterial pneumonia (IV formulation only for loading dose), and acute bacterial skin and skin structure infections
sarecycline (*Seysara*)	*Adult and pediatric 9 years and older*: 60 mg/d PO (if weight 33–54 kg); 100 mg/d PO (if weight 55–84 kg); 150 mg/d PO (if weight 85–136 kg)	Treatment of moderate to severe acne vulgaris. Efficacy beyond 12 weeks and safety beyond 12 months have not been established
tetracycline (generic)	*Adult*: 1–2 g/d PO in divided doses; topical applied generously to affected area *Pediatric (>8 y)*: 25–50 mg/kg/d PO in four divided doses	Treatment of a wide variety of infections when penicillin is contraindicated, including acne vulgaris and minor skin infections caused by susceptible organisms; as an ophthalmic agent to treat superficial ocular lesions caused by susceptible microorganisms; as a prophylactic agent for ophthalmia neonatorum caused by *Neisseria gonorrhoeae* and *Chlamydia trachomatis*

vomiting, diarrhea, abdominal pain, glossitis, and dysphagia. Fatal hepatotoxicity related to the drug's irritating effect on the liver has also been reported. Skeletal effects involve damage to the teeth and bones. Because tetracyclines have an affinity for teeth and bones, they accumulate there, weakening the structure and causing staining and pitting of teeth and bones. Dermatological effects include photosensitivity and rash. Superinfections, including yeast infections, occur when bacteria of the normal flora are destroyed. Local effects, such as pain and stinging with topical application, are fairly common. Hematological effects are less frequent, such as hemolytic anemia and bone marrow depression secondary to the effects on bone marrow cells that turn over rapidly. Hypersensitivity reactions reportedly range from urticaria to anaphylaxis and also include intracranial hypertension.

Clinically Important Drug–Drug Interactions

Digoxin toxicity rises when tetracyclines are taken concurrently. Digoxin levels should be monitored and the dose adjusted appropriately during treatment and after tetracycline therapy is discontinued. Finally, decreased absorption of tetracyclines results from oral combinations with calcium salts, magnesium salts, zinc salts, aluminum salts, bismuth salts, and iron.

Clinically Important Drug–Food Interactions

Because oral tetracyclines are not absorbed effectively if taken with food or dairy products, they should be administered on an empty stomach with water 1 hour before or 2 to 3 hours after any meal or other medication. However, if gastric distress occurs, clients may take with small amounts of food even though this decreases absorption.

CRITICAL THINKING SCENARIO
Antibiotics and Pregnancy

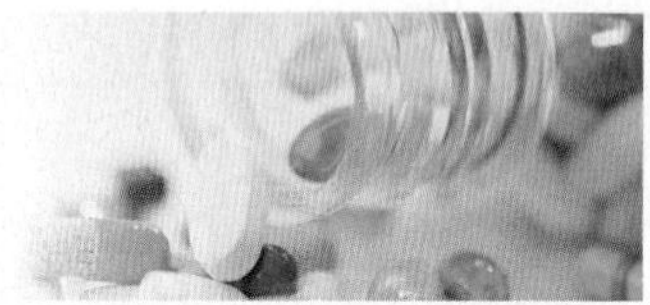

THE SITUATION

G.S. is a 27-year-old graduate student seen in the student health clinic a few weeks into the fall semester. They developed a severe sinusitis and complains of head pressure, difficulty sleeping, fever, and muscle aches and pains. A culture is done, and the next day the culture and sensitivity report identifies the infecting organism as a strain of *Klebsiella* that is sensitive to tetracycline. G.S. returns to the clinic to get the prescription for tetracycline.

G.S. tells you that they plan to become pregnant and start a family in 2 years, after completing their graduate program. They are a very organized person and have carefully planned their rigorous course work and nonacademic activities so that almost every hour is scheduled. They state that they are sexually active with their partner, but they are careful to not engage in sex during the time of their cycle when they believe they are ovulating.

Critical Thinking

Would it be best to test G.S. for possible pregnancy at this time? Why or why not?
What are the possible ramifications of continuing to take oral contraceptives during a pregnancy?
What nursing interventions are appropriate for G.S.?
What teaching points should be stressed with G.S.? Think about the nature of the patient's personality and the problems that an unplanned pregnancy might cause.
How can you help G.S. to cope with the infection, drug regimen, and their rigorous schedule?

DISCUSSION

Several antibiotics, including tetracycline, are known to cross the placenta and can affect the developing fetus. The medication can accumulate in both teeth and bones and even cause permanent discoloring of teeth, especially when there is lengthy or repeated exposure to the medication. In addition to the risk to the fetus, there is risk to the person who is pregnant. There may be higher risk of liver toxicity, especially if they have kidney disease. Due to the risk to the fetus and the patient who is pregnant, use of tetracyclines is avoided if possible to treat infection with another agent.

G.S. will need a pregnancy test prior to starting the antibiotic and also a clear explanation and follow-up in written form about the risks of pregnancy while receiving tetracycline therapy. They should be encouraged to use a form of birth control during the course of antibiotic use.

G.S. also may need a great deal of support and encouragement at this time. The sinus infection may increase stress by interfering with their ability to stick to their rigid schedule. Discussing the possibility of an unplanned pregnancy may cause even more stress. The health clinic visit could be used as an opportunity to allow G.S. to talk, to vent any frustrations and stress, and then to encourage them to make time for self-care. The nurse should stress the importance of a good diet, which will ensure that the body has the components needed to fight this infection and to heal and to ward off other infections, as well as the importance of adequate rest and exercise. The nurse should also make sure that G.S. is receiving annual gynecological exams and has been advised not to smoke.

All health care professionals who are involved with G.S. should consider the impact that an unplanned pregnancy could have on this very organized person and use this as an example of the importance of clear, concise patient teaching in the administration of drug therapy.

NURSING CARE GUIDE FOR G.S.: TETRACYCLINE

Assessment: History and Examination

Allergy to any tetracycline
Hepatic or renal dysfunction
Pregnancy or lactation
Concurrent use of antacids, iron products, digoxin, or penicillins
General: Site of infection, culture, and sensitivity
Skin: Color, lesions
Respiratory: Respiration, adventitious sounds
GI: Liver evaluation, bowel sounds, usual output
Laboratory data: Liver and renal function tests, urinalysis

Nursing Conclusions

Impaired comfort related to GI effects, superinfections
Malnutrition risk related to GI effects
Injury risk related to CNS effects
Knowledge deficit regarding drug therapy

Planning

- The patient will receive the best therapeutic effect from the drug therapy.
- The patient will have limited adverse effects from the drug therapy.
- The patient will have an understanding of the drug therapy, adverse effects to anticipate, and measures to relieve discomfort and improve safety.

Intervention

Perform culture and sensitivity tests before beginning therapy.
Administer drug on an empty stomach, 1 hour before or 2 to 3 hours after meals. Do not give with antacids, milk, or iron products.
Do not use outdated drug because of the risk of nephrotoxicity.
Monitor for and provide hygiene measures and treatment if superinfections occur.

Monitor nutritional status and fluid intake.
Provide ready access to bathroom facilities if diarrhea is a problem.
Provide support and reassurance for dealing with the drug effects and infection.
Provide patient teaching regarding drug name, dosage, adverse effects, precautions, warnings to report, and drugs that might cause a drug–drug interaction.

Evaluation

Evaluate drug effects: resolution of bacterial infections.
Monitor for adverse effects: GI effects, superinfections, CNS effects.
Monitor for drug–drug interactions: lack of antibacterial effect with antacids or iron.
Evaluate effectiveness of patient teaching program.
Evaluate effectiveness of comfort and safety measures.

Patient Teaching for G.S.

- Tetracycline is an antibiotic that is specific for your infection. You should take it throughout the day for best results.
- It is best to take this drug on an empty stomach, 1 hour before or 2 to 3 hours after meals, with a full glass of water. However, taking it with a small meal may decrease gastric discomfort.
- Do not take this drug with dairy products, iron preparations, or antacids.
- Take the full course of this antibiotic. Do not stop taking it if you feel better.
- Do not save tetracycline; outdated products can be very toxic to your kidneys.
- You may experience stomach upset or diarrhea.
- You may develop other infections in your mouth or vagina. (If this occurs, consult with your health care provider for appropriate treatment.)
- Tell any health care provider who is caring for you that you are taking this drug.
- Keep this, and all medications, out of the reach of children and pets.
- Report any of the following to your health care provider: changes in color of urine or stool, severe cramps, difficulty breathing, rash or itching, or yellowing of the skin or eyes.

Prototype Summary: Tetracycline

Indications: Treatment of various infections caused by susceptible strains of bacteria; acne; when penicillin is contraindicated for eradication of susceptible organisms.

Actions: Inhibits protein synthesis in susceptible bacteria, preventing cell replication.

Pharmacokinetics:

Route	Onset	Peak
Oral	Varies	2–4 h

$T_{1/2}$: 6 to 12 hours; excreted unchanged in the urine.

Adverse Effects: Nausea, vomiting, diarrhea, glossitis, discoloring and inadequate calcification of primary teeth of fetus when used in people who are pregnant or of secondary teeth when used in children, bone marrow suppression, photosensitivity, superinfections, rash, local irritation with topical forms.

Nursing Considerations for Patients Receiving Tetracyclines

Assessment: History and Examination

- Assess for possible contraindications or cautions: known allergy to any tetracycline (obtain specific information about the nature and occurrence of allergic reactions), any history of renal or hepatic disease that could interfere with metabolism and excretion of the drug and lead to increased toxicity, current pregnancy or lactation status because of the potential for adverse effects to the fetus or infant, and age because of the risk of damage to bones and teeth.
- Perform a physical examination to establish baseline data for assessing the effectiveness of the drug and the occurrence of any adverse effects associated with drug therapy.
- Examine the skin for any rash or lesions to provide a baseline for possible adverse effects.
- Perform culture and sensitivity tests at the site of infection to ensure that this is the appropriate drug for this patient.
- Note respiratory status to provide a baseline for the occurrence of hypersensitivity reactions.
- Evaluate renal and liver function test reports, including BUN and creatinine clearance, to assess the status of renal and liver functioning, which helps to determine any needed changes in dose.

Nursing Conclusions

Nursing conclusions related to drug therapy might include the following:

- Impaired comfort related to drug effects on GI tract
- Malnutrition risk related to GI effects, alteration in taste, and superinfections
- Altered skin integrity risk related to rash and photosensitivity
- Knowledge deficit risk regarding drug therapy

Planning

- The patient will receive the best therapeutic effect from the drug therapy.

(continues on page 128)

- The patient will have limited adverse effects from the drug therapy.
- The patient will have an understanding of the drug therapy, adverse effects to anticipate, and measures to relieve discomfort and improve safety.

Intervention With Rationale

- Check culture and sensitivity reports to ensure that this is the drug of choice for this patient. Arrange for repeated cultures if response is not as anticipated.
- Monitor renal and liver function test results before and periodically during therapy to arrange for a dose reduction as needed.
- Ensure that the patient receives the full course of the tetracycline as prescribed. The oral drug should be taken on an empty stomach 1 hour before or 2 hours after meals with a full 8-oz glass of water. Concomitant use of antacids or magnesium or calcium salts should be avoided because they interfere with drug absorption. These precautions will increase drug effectiveness and decrease the development of resistant strains of bacteria.
- Discontinue the drug immediately if hypersensitivity reactions occur to avoid the possibility of severe reactions.
- Provide small, frequent meals as tolerated, frequent mouth care, and ice chips or sugarless candy to suck if stomatitis and sore mouth are problems to relieve discomfort and ensure nutrition. Also provide adequate fluids to replace fluid lost with diarrhea.
- Monitor for signs of superinfections to arrange for treatment as appropriate.
- Encourage the patient to apply sunscreen and wear clothing to protect exposed skin from skin rashes and sunburn associated with photosensitivity reactions.
- Instruct the patient about the appropriate dosage regimen, how to take the oral drug, and possible side effects to enhance patient knowledge about drug therapy and to promote compliance.
- Provide the following patient teaching:
  - Try to drink fluids and to maintain nutrition even though nausea, vomiting, and diarrhea may occur.
  - Know that superinfections may occur. Appropriate treatment can be arranged through the health care provider.
  - Use sunscreens and protective clothing if sensitivity to the sun occurs.
  - Know when to report dangerous adverse effects, such as difficulty breathing, rash, itching, watery diarrhea, cramps, or changes in color of urine or stool.

Evaluation

- Monitor the patient's response to the drug (resolution of bacterial infection).
- Monitor for adverse effects (GI effects, rash, and superinfections).
- Evaluate the effectiveness of the teaching plan (patient can name the drug, dosage, possible adverse effects to expect, and specific measures to help avoid adverse effects).
- Monitor the effectiveness of comfort and safety measures and adherence to the regimen.

Key Points

- Tetracyclines are bacteriostatic; they inhibit protein synthesis and prevent bacteria from multiplying.
- Tetracyclines can cause damage to developing teeth and bones and should not be used with people who are pregnant or children younger than 8 years of age.
- Monitor the patient for GI effects, bone marrow depression, rash, and superinfections.

Antimycobacterials

Mycobacteria—the group of bacteria that contains the pathogens that cause tuberculosis and leprosy—are classified on the basis of their ability to hold a stain even in the presence of a "destaining" agent such as acid. Because of this property, they are called "acid-fast" bacteria. The mycobacteria have an outer coat of mycolic acid that protects them from many disinfectants and allows them to survive for long periods in the environment. It may be necessary to treat these slow-growing bacteria for several years before they can be eradicated.

Mycobacteria cause serious infectious diseases. The bacterium *Mycobacterium tuberculosis* causes tuberculosis, the leading cause of death from infectious disease in the world. For several years, the disease was thought to be under control, but with the increasing number of people with compromised immune systems and the emergence of resistant bacterial strains, tuberculosis is once again on the rise.

Mycobacterium leprae causes leprosy, also known as Hansen disease, which is characterized by disfiguring skin lesions and destructive effects on the respiratory tract. Leprosy is also a worldwide health problem; it is infectious when the mycobacteria invade the skin or respiratory tract of susceptible individuals. *Mycobacterium avium-intracellulare*, which causes mycobacterium avium complex, is seen in patients with AIDS or in other patients who are severely immunocompromised.

Antituberculosis Drugs

Tuberculosis can lead to serious damage in the lungs, the GU tract, bones, and the meninges. Because *Mycobacterium tuberculosis* is so slow growing, the treatment must be continued for 6 months to 2 years. Using the drugs in combination helps to decrease the emergence of resistant strains and to affect the bacteria at various phases during their long and slow life cycle (Table 9.8).

First-line drugs for treating tuberculosis are used in combinations of two or more agents until bacterial conversion occurs or maximum improvement is seen. The first-line drugs for treating tuberculosis are isoniazid (generic), rifampin (*Rifadin*), pyrazinamide (generic), ethambutol (*Myambutol*), rifabutin (*Mycobutin*), and rifapentine (*Priftin*).

If the patient cannot take one or more of the first-line drugs, or if the disease continues to progress because of the emergence of a resistant strain, second-line drugs can be

Table 9.8 *Drugs in Focus*: Antimycobacterials

Drug Name	Dosage/Route	Usual Indications
Antituberculosis Drugs		
First Line Drugs		
ethambutol (*Myambutol*)	*Adult*: 15–25 mg/kg/d PO as a single dose	Treatment of *Mycobacterium tuberculosis*
isoniazid (generic)	*Adult*: 5 mg/kg/d PO *Pediatric*: 10–15 mg/kg/d PO *Prevention*: *Adult*: 300 mg/d PO *Pediatric*: 10 mg/kg/d PO	Treatment/prevention of *M. tuberculosis*
pyrazinamide (generic)	*Adult and pediatric*: 15–30 mg/kg/d PO	Treatment of *M. tuberculosis*
rifabutin (*Mycobutin*)	*Adult*: 300 mg PO daily *Pediatric*: 5 mg/kg/d PO	Second-line treatment of *M. tuberculosis*
rifampin (*Rifadin, Rimactane*)	*Adult*: 600 mg PO or IV as a single daily dose *Pediatric*: 10 mg/kg/d PO or IV	Treatment of *M. tuberculosis*
rifapentine (*Priftin*)	*Adult*: 600 mg PO two times a week for 2 mo *Pediatric (<12 y)*: Safety not established	Treatment of *M. tuberculosis*
Second-Line Drugs		
bedaquiline (*Sirturo*)	*Adult*: 400 mg/d PO for 2 wk, then 200 mg PO three times a week for 22 wk *Pediatric*: Safety not established	Second-line treatment of resistant *M. tuberculosis*; not for use in extrapulmonary, latent, or drug-sensitive TB
capreomycin (*Capastat*)	*Adult*: 1 g/d IM or IV for 60–120 d, followed by 1 g IM two to three times a week for 18–24 mo; reduce dose with renal impairment *Pediatric*: 15 mg/kg/d IM	Second-line drug for treatment of *M. tuberculosis*
cycloserine (*Seromycin*)	*Adult*: 250 mg PO b.i.d. for 2 wk, then 500 mg to 1 g/d PO in divided doses *Pediatric*: Safety not established	Second-line treatment of *M. tuberculosis*
ethionamide (*Trecator-SC*)	*Adult*: 15–20 mg/kg/d PO in divided doses with pyridoxine *Pediatric*: 10–20 mg/kg/d PO in divided doses with pyridoxine	Second-line treatment of *M. tuberculosis*
streptomycin (generic)	*Adult*: 15 mg/kg/d IM *or* 25–30 mg/kg IM given two to three times a week *Pediatric*: 20–40 mg/kg/d IM or 25–30 mg/kg IM given two to three times a week	Treatment of *M. tuberculosis*, tularemia, plague, subacute bacterial endocarditis
Leprostatic Drug		
dapsone (generic)	*Adult/pediatric*: 50–100 mg/d PO	Treatment of leprosy, *Pneumocystis jirovecii* pneumonia in AIDS patients, and a variety of infections caused by susceptible bacteria and brown recluse spider bites

used. The second-line drugs include ethionamide (*Trecator-SC*), capreomycin (*Capastat*), and cycloserine (*Seromycin*), and Bedaquiline (*Sirturo*) had accelerated approval from the FDA to treat adult and pediatric patients diagnosed with pulmonary multidrug-resistant tuberculosis in combination with other medications.

In addition, drugs from other antibiotic classes have been found to be effective in second-line treatment, such as levofloxacin (*Levaquin*), moxifloxacin (*Avelox*), and streptomycin.

Leprostatic Drugs

The antibiotic used to treat leprosy is dapsone (generic), which has been the mainstay of leprosy treatment for many years, although resistant strains are emerging (Table 9.8). Similar to the sulfonamides, dapsone inhibits folate synthesis in susceptible bacteria. In addition to its use in leprosy, dapsone is used to treat *Pneumocystis jirovecii* pneumonia in AIDS patients and for a variety of infections caused by susceptible bacteria, as well as for brown recluse spider bites. The topical form can be used to treat acne.

The immunomodulatory drug thalidomide (*Thalomid*) was approved for use to treat cutaneous reactions due to leprosy. The condition called erythema nodosum leprosum is a complication of leprosy that can cause inflammatory skin nodules in addition to systemic symptoms like fever, malaise, and neuritis (Box 9.6).

BOX 9.6

Indication for Thalidomide

In the 1950s, the drug thalidomide became internationally known because it caused serious abnormalities (e.g., lack of limbs, defective limbs) in the fetuses of many patients who received the drug during pregnancy to help them sleep and to decrease stress. This tragedy led to the recall of thalidomide in the United States and the establishment of more stringent standards for drug testing and labeling. In 1998, the FDA approved the use of this controversial drug for the treatment of erythema nodosum leprosum, which is a painful inflammatory condition related to an immune reaction to dead bacteria that occurs after treatment for leprosy. It is also approved for use in the treatment of multiple myeloma with dexamethasone. To take thalidomide, a patient must have a monthly negative pregnancy test with results posted in their medical record, receive instruction in using birth control, and sign a release stating that they understand the risks associated with the drug. The medication is only available via a restricted distribution program run by the FDA.

Thalidomide (*Thalomid*) is typically given in doses of 100 to 300 mg/d PO for treatment of erythema nodosum leprosum, but doses up to 400 mg/d can be administered.

Therapeutic Actions and Indications

Most of the antimycobacterial agents act on the DNA and/or RNA of the bacteria, leading to a lack of growth and eventually to bacterial death (see Fig. 9.2). Isoniazid (INH) specifically affects the mycolic acid coat around the bacterium. Rifampin (*Rifadin, Rimactane*) inhibits protein synthesis and is bactericidal. It is mostly active against mycobacteria, but resistance to rifampin develops quickly if used as monotherapy. Streptomycin is an aminoglycoside, which are also bactericidal by inhibiting protein synthesis. Although many of the antimycobacterial agents are effective against other species of susceptible bacteria, their primary indications are in the treatment of tuberculosis or leprosy (as previously indicated). The antituberculosis drugs are always used in combination to affect the bacteria at various stages and to help to decrease the emergence of resistant strains (see Table 9.8). The combination drug *Rifater* provides isoniazid, pyrazinamide, and rifampin in one tablet to help patients maintain adherence to the drug regimen.

Pharmacokinetics

The antimycobacterial agents are generally well absorbed from the GI tract. These drugs, given orally, are metabolized in the liver and excreted in the urine; they cross the placenta and enter human milk, placing the fetus or child at risk for adverse reactions (see "Contraindications and Cautions").

Contraindications and Cautions

Antimycobacterials are contraindicated for patients with any known allergy to these agents and in patients with severe renal or hepatic failure, which could interfere with the metabolism or excretion of the drug. If an antituberculosis regimen is necessary during pregnancy, the combination of isoniazid, ethambutol, and rifampin is considered the safest.

Adverse Effects

CNS effects, such as neuritis, dizziness, headache, malaise, drowsiness, and hallucinations, are often reported and are related to direct effects of the drugs on neurons. These drugs also are irritating to the GI tract, causing nausea, vomiting, anorexia, stomach upset, abdominal pain, and, rarely, pseudomembranous colitis. Rifampin, rifabutin, and rifapentine cause discoloration of body fluids from urine to sweat and tears. Alert patients that in many instances orange-tinged urine, sweat, and tears may stain clothing and permanently stain contact lenses. This can be frightening if the patient is not alerted to the possibility that it will happen. As with other antibiotics, there is always a possibility of hypersensitivity reactions. Monitor the patient on a regular basis. The newest drug in this group, bedaquiline, has a boxed warning that an increased risk of death has been reported when this drug is used so it should be reserved for use when no other drug is effective. Bedaquiline also has a boxed warning that QTc intervals may be increased when using the drugs; a baseline ECG should be done as well as periodic checks of the QTc interval during treatment.

Clinically Important Drug–Drug Interactions

Concurrent use of isoniazid, rifampin, and/or pyrazinamide increases the risk of hepatotoxicity. Eating foods with tyramine and taking isoniazid can cause a histamine reaction causing headache, diaphoresis, or flushing. Taking isoniazid with alcohol use can also increase risk of liver damage. Patients should be monitored closely.

Rifampin accelerates metabolism of warfarin, oral contraceptives, protease inhibitors, and non-nucleoside reverse transcriptase inhibitors, which can lead to decreased effectiveness of medication treatment. Isoniazid inhibits metabolism of phenytoin, which can increase risk of phenytoin toxicity causing ataxia and decrease motor coordination. Patients taking bedaquiline should avoid any other drugs that prolong the QTc interval. Patients who are taking these drug combinations should be monitored closely and dose adjustments made as needed.

Prototype Summary: Isoniazid

Indications: Treatment of tuberculosis as part of combination therapy; prophylactic treatment of household members of recently diagnosed tuberculosis.

Actions: Interferes with lipid and nucleic acid synthesis in actively growing tubercle bacilli.

Pharmacokinetics:

Route	Onset	Peak	Duration
Oral	Varies	1–2 h	24 h

$T_{1/2}$: 1 to 4 hours; metabolized in the liver, excreted in the urine.

Adverse Effects: Peripheral neuropathies, nausea, vomiting, hepatitis, bone marrow suppression, fever, local irritation at injection sites, gynecomastia, lupus syndrome.

Nursing Considerations for Patients Receiving Antimycobacterials

Assessment: History and Examination

- Assess for possible contraindications or cautions: known allergy to any antimycobacterial drug (obtain specific information about the nature and occurrence of allergic reactions); history of renal or hepatic disease, which could interfere with metabolism and excretion of the drug and lead to toxicity; and current pregnancy status to ensure appropriate drug selection to prevent adverse effects on the fetus.
- Perform a physical examination to establish baseline data for assessing the effectiveness of the drug and the occurrence of any adverse effects associated with drug therapy.
- Examine the skin for any rash or lesions to provide a baseline for possible adverse effects.
- Obtain specimens for culture and sensitivity testing to establish the sensitivity of the organism being treated.
- Evaluate CNS for orientation, affect, and reflexes to establish a baseline and to monitor for adverse effects.
- Note respiratory status to provide a baseline for the occurrence of hypersensitivity reactions.
- Evaluate renal and liver function tests, including BUN and creatinine clearance, to assess the status of renal and liver functioning to determine any needed alteration in dose.

Nursing Conclusions

Nursing conclusions related to drug therapy might include the following:

- Malnutrition risk related to GI effects
- Altered sensory perception (kinesthetic) risk related to CNS effects of the drug
- Impaired comfort related to GI effects of the drug
- Knowledge deficit risk regarding drug therapy

Planning

- The patient will receive the best therapeutic effect from the drug therapy.
- The patient will have limited adverse effects from the drug therapy.
- The patient will have an understanding of the drug therapy, adverse effects to anticipate, and measures to relieve discomfort and improve safety.

Intervention With Rationale

- Check culture and sensitivity reports to ensure that this is the drug of choice for this patient, and arrange repeated cultures if response is not as anticipated.
- Monitor renal and liver function test results before and periodically during therapy to arrange for dose reduction as needed.
- Ensure that the patient receives the full course of the drugs to improve effectiveness and decrease the risk of development of resistant bacterial strains. These drugs are often taken for years and usually in combination. Periodic medical evaluation and reteaching are often essential to ensure compliance. A technique of directly observed therapy is recommended, in which a trained

(continues on page 132)

health care worker may be hired to administer all of the medications and ensure that the medication is ingested.
- Discontinue drug immediately if hypersensitivity reactions occur to avert potentially serious reactions.
- Encourage the patient to eat small, frequent meals as tolerated, perform frequent mouth care, and drink adequate fluids to ensure adequate nutrition and hydration. Monitor nutrition if GI effects become a problem.
- Instruct the patient about the appropriate dosage regimen, use of drug combinations, and possible adverse effects to enhance patient knowledge about drug therapy and to promote adherence.
- Provide the following patient teaching:
  - Try to drink fluids and to maintain hydration even though nausea, vomiting, and diarrhea may occur.
  - Use barrier contraceptives and understand that hormonal contraceptives may not be effective if antimycobacterials are being used.
  - Understand that normally some of these drugs impart an orange stain to urine or tears. If this occurs, the fluids may stain clothing and tears may stain contact lenses or fabric.
  - Report difficulty breathing, hallucinations, numbness, and tingling, worsening of condition, fever and chills, or changes in color of urine or stool.

Evaluation

- Monitor patient response to the drug (resolution of mycobacterial infection).
- Monitor for adverse effects (GI effects, CNS changes, and hypersensitivity reactions).
- Evaluate the effectiveness of the teaching plan (patient can name the drug, dosage, possible adverse effects to expect, and specific measures to help avoid adverse effects).
- Monitor the effectiveness of comfort and safety measures and adherence to the regimen.

Key Points

- The mycobacteria have an outer coat of mycolic acid that protects them from many disinfectants and allows them to survive for long periods in the environment. These slow-growing bacteria may need to be treated for several months or years before they can be eradicated. They cause tuberculosis and leprosy.
- Antituberculosis drugs are used in combination to increase effectiveness and decrease the emergence of resistant strains. These drugs are divided into first-line and second-line drugs. Adverse effects include rashes, an orange tint to body fluids, liver impairment, peripheral neuropathy, and GI reactions.
- Dapsone can be used to treat leprosy or Hansen disease. Thalidomide can be used to treat a complication of leprosy called erythema nodosum leprosum.

Other Antibiotics

There are other antibiotics that do not fit into the large antibiotic classes. These drugs—the lincosamides, lipoglycopeptides, macrolides, oxazolidinones, and monobactams—work in unique ways and are effective against specific bacteria (Table 9.9).

Lincosamides

The lincosamides (Table 9.9) are similar to the macrolides. They are bacteriostatic and interfere with protein synthesis of gram-positive bacteria. These drugs include clindamycin (*Cleocin*) and lincomycin (*Lincocin*).

Therapeutic Actions and Indications

The lincosamides react at almost the same site in bacterial protein synthesis and are effective against the same strains of bacteria (see Fig. 9.2). They can be used to treat infections caused by gram-positive and some anaerobic bacteria.

Pharmacokinetics

The lincosamides are rapidly absorbed from the GI tract or from IM injections but are typically administered IV. They are metabolized in the liver and excreted in the urine and feces. These drugs cross the placenta and enter human milk (see "Contraindications and Cautions").

Clindamycin has a half-life of 2 to 3 hours. It is available in parenteral and oral forms, as well as in topical and vaginal forms for the treatment of local infections.

Lincomycin has a half-life of 5 hours. It can be given IM or IV.

Contraindications and Cautions

Use lincosamides with caution in patients with hepatic impairment, which could interfere with the metabolism and excretion of the drug. Liver function may need to be monitored frequently. Dose adjustment is recommended for lincomycin if severe renal impairment is present. Use during pregnancy and lactation only if the benefit clearly outweighs the risk to the fetus or neonate.

Adverse Effects

Severe GI reactions, including fatal pseudomembranous colitis, have occurred, limiting the usefulness of lincosamides. However, for a serious infection caused by a susceptible bacterium, a lincosamide may be the drug of choice. Some other toxic effects that limit usefulness are

Table 9.9 *Drugs in Focus*: Other Antibiotics

Drug Name	Dosage/Route	Usual Indications
Lincosamides		
clindamycin (*Cleocin*)	*Adult*: 150–450 mg PO q6h *or* 600–2,700 mg/d IV in two to four equal doses *Pediatric*: 8–20 mg/kg/d PO *or* 15–40 mg/kg/d IM or IV in three to four divided doses	Treatment of severe infections when penicillin or other, less toxic antibiotics cannot be used
lincomycin (*Lincocin*)	*Adult*: 600 mg IM q12–24h *or* 600 mg to 1 g IV q8–12h; reduce dose with renal impairment *Pediatric*: 10 mg/kg IM q12–24h *or* 10–20 mg/kg/d IV in divided doses	Treatment of severe infections when penicillin or other less toxic antibiotics cannot be used
Lipoglycopeptides		
dalbavancin (*Dalvance*)	*Adult*: 1,500 mg IV as a single dose or 1,000 mg IV over 30 min as a single dose followed by 500 mg IV over 30 min 1 wk later, reduce dose in renal dysfunction	Treatment of complicated skin and skin structure infections caused by susceptible strains of gram-positive bacteria
oritavancin (*Orbactiv*)	*Adult*: Single dose of 1,200 mg IV over 3 h	Treatment of complicated skin and skin structure infections caused by susceptible strains of gram-positive organisms
telavancin (*Vibativ*)	*Adult*: 10 mg/kg IV over 60 min, reduce dose in renal dysfunction	Treatment of complicated skin and skin structure infections caused by susceptible strains of gram-positive organisms including methicillin-resistant strains
vancomycin (*Vancocin*)	*Adult*: 500 mg to 2 g/d PO in divided doses *or* 15–20 mg/kg q8h, reduce dose in renal dysfunction *Pediatric*: 40 mg/kg/d PO in divided doses *or* 10 mg/kg/dose IV q6h	Treatment of severe infections caused by susceptible strains, treatment of *C. difficile* pseudomembranous colitis
Oxazolidinones		
linezolid (*Zyvox*)	*Adult/pediatric (12>)*: 400–600 mg PO or IV *Pediatric (5–11 y)*: 10 mg/kg PO or IV q8–12h	Treatment of pneumonia, skin, and skin structure infections caused by susceptible strains, including resistant strains; diabetic foot ulcers
tedizolid (*Sivextro*)	*Adult*: 200 mg/d PO or IV over 1 h	Treatment of acute skin and skin structure infections by susceptible strains
Macrolides		
azithromycin (*Zithromax*)	*Adult*: 500 mg PO as a single dose on day 1, then 250 mg/d PO to a total dose of 1.5 g or 1–2 g as a single dose *Pediatric*: 10 mg/kg PO as a single dose on day 1, then 5 mg/kg PO on day 2–5 or 30 mg/kg PO as a single dose	Treatment of mild to moderate respiratory infections and urethritis in adults and otitis media and pharyngitis/tonsillitis in children
clarithromycin (*Biaxin*)	*Adult*: 250–500 mg q12h PO; reduce dose with renal impairment *Pediatric*: 15 mg/kg/d PO given q12h	Treatment of various respiratory, skin, sinus, and maxillary infections; *H. pylori* infections, effective against mycobacteria
erythromycin (*Ery-Tab, Eryc*)	*Adult*: 15–20 mg/kg/d IV or 250–500 mg PO q6–12h *Pediatric*: 30–50 mg/kg/d PO in divided doses	Treatment of infections in patients allergic to penicillin; drug of choice for treatment of Legionnaire disease, infections caused by *Corynebacterium diphtheriae*, *Ureaplasma* spp., syphilis, *Mycoplasma pneumonia*, and chlamydial infections
fidaxomicin (*Dificid*)	200 mg PO b.i.d. for 10 d	Treatment of *C. difficile*–associated diarrhea
Monobactam		
aztreonam (*Azactam*)	*Adult*: 500 mg to 1 g q6–12h IM or IV; reduce dose in renal and impairment *Pediatric*: 30 mg/kg IM or IV q6–8h	Treatment of gram-negative enterobacterial infections; safe alternative for treating infections caused by susceptible bacteria in patients who may be allergic to penicillins or cephalosporins

abdominal discomfort, skin reactions, and bone marrow depression.

Prototype Summary: Clindamycin

Indications: Treatment of serious infections caused by susceptible strains of bacteria, including some anaerobes; useful in septicemia and chronic bone and joint infections.

Actions: Inhibits protein synthesis in susceptible bacteria (bacteriostatic).

Pharmacokinetics:

Route	Onset	Peak	Duration
Oral	Varies	1–2 h	8–12 h
IM	20–30 min	1–3 h	8–12 h
IV	Immediate	Minutes	8–12 h
Topical	Minimal absorption		

$T_{1/2}$: 2 to 3 hours; metabolized in the liver, excreted in the urine and feces.

Adverse Effects: Nausea, vomiting, diarrhea, pseudomembranous colitis, bone marrow suppression.

Lipoglycopeptides

The lipoglycopeptides class of antibiotics was first introduced in 2010. Drugs in this class include telavancin (*Vibativ*), dalbavancin (*Dalvance*), oritavancin (*Orbactiv*), and the original drug in the class vancomycin (*Vancocin, Firvanq*).

Therapeutic Actions and Indications

Lipoglycopeptides are semisynthetic derivatives of the original drug in this class, vancomycin (see Chapter 8). They inhibit bacterial cell wall synthesis by interfering with the polymerization and cross-linking of peptidoglycans. They bind to the bacterial membrane and disrupt the membrane barrier function, causing bacterial cell death. The lipoglycopeptides are effective against susceptible strains of the gram-positive organisms: *S. aureus* (including methicillin-susceptible and methicillin-resistant isolates), *S. pyogenes, S. agalactiae, Streptococcus anginosus, Enterococcus faecalis, Enterococcus faecium, Streptococcus intermedius*, and *Streptococcus constellatus.*

The most common approved use for the newer lipoglycopeptides drugs is treating complicated skin and skin structure infections in adults (see Table 9.9). Vancomycin is used in the oral form to treat *C. difficile* diarrhea and *S. aureus*–induced enterocolitis, including methicillin-resistant strains, and in the parenteral form, it is used to treat serious infections responsive to the drug. Dalbavancin and Oritavancin have a single IV dose option, making them a good choice if follow-up or adherence is an issue.

Pharmacokinetics

Lipoglycopeptides are available as IV drugs; only vancomycin has an oral form. However, oral vancomycin is poorly absorbed and is not used to treat systemic infections. The lipoglycopeptides reach peak levels at the end of the infusion. These drugs are widely distributed, may cross the placenta, and may pass into human milk. The site of metabolism varies by drug and many lipoglycopeptides are not significantly metabolized; half-life ranges vary significantly based on drug. They are excreted in the urine and feces.

Contraindications and Cautions

These drugs are contraindicated with known allergy to any component of the drug to avoid hypersensitivity reactions, and they should be used with caution in pregnant and lactating patients because of the potential for toxic effects on the fetus or infant. Telavancin has a boxed warning regarding serious fetal risk and is not recommended for people who are pregnant or who might become pregnant. Use of contraceptive measures is urged.

Perform culture and sensitivity testing to ensure that the drug is used appropriately.

Adverse Effects

The adverse effects associated with the lipoglycopeptides are largely secondary to toxic effects on the GI tract: nausea, vomiting, taste alterations, diarrhea, loss of appetite, and risk of *C. difficile* diarrhea. Vancomycin and some of the other lipoglycopeptides cause nephrotoxicity. Telavancin may cause patients to experience foamy urine, something they should be alerted to when the drug is started. There is a risk of prolonged QTc interval with telavancin. A transfusion reaction with flushing, sweating, and hypotension can occur with rapid infusion. Infusion site reactions with pain and redness have also been reported.

Clinically Important Drug–Drug Interactions

There is an increased risk of prolonged QT interval and resultant arrhythmias if telavancin is combined with other drugs known to prolong the QT interval; if this combination is used, the patient's ECG should be monitored. There is increased risk of nephrotoxicity with telavancin and vancomycin if combined with other nephrotoxic drugs; if this combination must be used, the patient's renal function should be monitored.

Prototype Summary: Vancomycin

Indications: Treatment of complicated septicemia, infective endocarditis, skin and skin structure infections, bone infections, and lower respiratory tract infections caused by susceptible bacteria. The oral form is only indicated for treatment of *Clostridioides difficile*–associated diarrhea and enterocolitis caused by *S. aureus*.

Actions: Affects bacterial cell wall synthesis leading to disruption of cell membrane function and bacterial cell death. Also alters bacterial cell membrane permeability and RNA synthesis.

Pharmacokinetics:

Route	Onset	Peak
IV	Rapid	End of infusion

PO Not absorbed

$T_{1/2}$: 4–6 hours; no known metabolism; excreted in the urine (IV) or feces (oral).

Adverse Effects: Abdominal pain, nausea, nephrotoxicity, hypokalemia, ototoxicity (PO or IV), *C. diff* diarrhea, phlebitis, flushing, sweating, hypotension (IV).

Macrolides

The macrolides (see Table 9.9) are antibiotics that bind to the subunit of the ribosome within the bacterial cell and interfere with protein synthesis in susceptible bacteria. Macrolides include erythromycin (*Ery-Tab, Eryc,* and others), azithromycin (*Zithromax* and others), clarithromycin (*Biaxin*), and, the newest drug in the class, fidaxomicin (*Dificid*).

Therapeutic Actions and Indications

The macrolides, which may be bactericidal at high doses or bacteriostatic, exert their effect by binding to the ribosomes within the cell and changing protein synthesis (see Fig. 9.1). This action can prevent the cell from dividing or cause cell death, depending on the sensitivity of the bacteria and the concentration of the drug.

Azithromycin, clarithromycin, and erythromycin are indicated for treatment of the following conditions: acute infections caused by susceptible strains of *S. pneumoniae, M. pneumoniae, Listeria monocytogenes,* and *Legionella pneumophila*; infections caused by group A beta-hemolytic streptococci; pelvic inflammatory disease caused by *N. gonorrhoeae*; upper respiratory tract infections caused by *H. influenzae* (with sulfonamides); infections caused by *Corynebacterium diphtheriae* and *Corynebacterium minutissimum* (with antitoxin); intestinal amebiasis; and infections caused by *C. trachomatis*. Fidaxomicin works locally in the GI tract and is used to treat *C. difficile*–associated diarrhea. See Table 9.9 for usual indications for each of these agents.

In addition, macrolides may be used as prophylaxis for endocarditis before dental procedures in high-risk patients with valvular heart disease who are allergic to penicillin. Topical macrolides are indicated for the treatment of ocular infections caused by susceptible organisms and for acne vulgaris.

Pharmacokinetics

Most of the macrolides are widely distributed throughout the body; they cross the placenta and enter human milk (see "Contraindications and Cautions"). These drugs are absorbed in the GI tract.

Erythromycin and azithromycin are primarily metabolized in the liver, with excretion mainly in the bile to feces. The half-life of erythromycin is 1.6 hours.

Clarithromycin is partially excreted unchanged in the urine. The half-life of azithromycin is 68 hours, making it useful for patients who have trouble remembering to take pills because it can be given once a day. The half-life of clarithromycin is 3 to 7 hours.

Fidaxomicin is minimally absorbed systemically and acts in the GI tract. It is metabolized in the GI tract and excreted in the feces, with a half-life of 9 hours.

Contraindications and Cautions

Macrolides are contraindicated in patients with a known allergy to any macrolide because cross-sensitivity occurs. Use with caution in patients with hepatic dysfunction, which could alter the metabolism of the drug. Also use with caution in patients who are lactating because macrolides secreted in human milk can cause diarrhea and superinfections in the infant, and in patients who are pregnant because of potential adverse effects on the developing fetus; use only if the benefit clearly outweighs the risk to the fetus or the infant. Fidaxomicin is low risk in this group because it is not absorbed systemically.

Adverse Effects

The most frequent adverse effects involve the GI tract, including abdominal cramping, anorexia, diarrhea, vomiting, and pseudomembranous colitis. Other effects include neurological symptoms such as confusion, abnormal thinking, and uncontrollable emotions, which could be related to drug effects on the CNS membranes; hypersensitivity reactions ranging from rash to anaphylaxis; and superinfections related to the loss of normal flora. High doses may result in ototoxicity and QT interval prolongation in some people.

Clinically Important Drug–Drug Interactions

Increased serum levels of digoxin occur when digoxin is taken concurrently with macrolides. Patients who receive both drugs should have their digoxin levels monitored and dose adjusted during and after treatment with the macrolide.

In addition, when oral anticoagulants, carbamazepine, are administered concurrently with macrolides, the effects of these drugs reportedly increase as a result of metabolic changes in the liver. Patients who take any of these combinations may require reduced dose of the particular drug and careful monitoring.

Clinically Important Drug–Food Interactions

Food in the stomach decreases absorption of oral macrolides, except for azithromycin. Therefore, the antibiotic should be taken on an empty stomach with a full, 8-oz glass of water 1 hour before or at least 2 to 3 hours after meals.

Prototype Summary: Erythromycin

Indications: Treatment of respiratory, dermatological, urinary tract, and gastrointestinal infections caused by susceptible strains of bacteria.

Actions: Binds to ribosomes within the bacterial cell, causing a change in protein synthesis and cell death; can be bacteriostatic or bactericidal with high doses.

Pharmacokinetics:

Route	Onset	Peak
Oral	1–2 h	1–4 h
IV	Rapid	Immediate after infusion

$T_{1/2}$: 3 to 5 hours; metabolized in the liver, excreted in bile and urine.

Adverse Effects: Abdominal cramping, vomiting, diarrhea, rash, superinfection, liver toxicity, risk for pseudomembranous colitis, potential for hearing loss with high doses and prolonged QT interval.

Oxazolidinones

There are currently two antibiotics available in this class: tedizolid (*Sivextro*) and linezolid (*Zyvox*).

Therapeutic Actions and Indications

The oxazolidinones interfere with protein synthesis on the bacterial ribosome, within the bacterial cell. They also act as MAO (monoamine oxidase) inhibitors. They are effective against vancomycin-resistant strains of enterococci (VRE), *Staphylococcus* and methicillin-resistant *Staphylococcus aureus* (MRSA), and penicillin-resistant pneumococci. Tedizolid is FDA approved for skin and skin structure infections caused by susceptible organisms. Linezolid is used in pneumonia and skin and skin structure infections caused by susceptible strains as well as diabetic foot infections without osteomyelitis.

Pharmacokinetics

Tedizolid is available for oral or IV use. It is rapidly absorbed, has a half-life of 12 hours, is metabolized in the liver, and is excreted in urine and feces. Linezolid is also available for IV or oral use. It is rapidly absorbed, has a half-life of 5 hours, is metabolized in the liver, and is excreted in the urine.

Contraindications and Cautions

These drugs are contraindicated for patients with any known allergy to the drug or drug components; patients with phenylketonuria (with the oral suspension of linezolid) because medication contains phenylalanine that can build up in their body and cause muscle pains, decreased pigment, seizures, and intellectual disability; and patients taking MAO inhibitors because these drugs can act as reversible MAO inhibitors. Caution should be used with patients who are pregnant or lactating, especially with tedizolid, because the drug enters human milk and can be toxic to the child. Oxazolidinones should be used with caution with hepatic impairment, pheochromocytoma, hypertension, hyperthyroidism, and bone marrow suppression because the effects of the drugs could exacerbate these conditions.

Adverse Effects

Adverse effects of the oxazolidinones include CNS effects of headache, insomnia, dizziness; GI effects of dry mouth, nausea, vomiting, and diarrhea with the potential for pseudomembranous colitis; optic neuritis, thrombocytopenia, bone marrow suppression, and hypertension.

Drug–Drug Interactions

Oxazolidinones have a risk of hypertension and related adverse effects if combined with other drugs that increase blood pressure. An increased risk of bleeding and further thrombocytopenia occurs if oxazolidinones are combined with drugs that affect bleeding, including nonsteroidal anti-inflammatory drugs (NSAIDs) and platelet inhibitors. Potentially serious serotonin syndrome can occur if used with other serotonergic drugs; this combination should be avoided unless these drugs are needed for the treatment of resistant strains.

Prototype Summary: Linezolid

Indications: Treatment of infections caused by resistant strains, pneumonias, skin and skin structure infections, diabetic foot infections.

Actions: Binds to ribosomes within the bacterial cell, causing a change in protein function and cell death in susceptible strains of bacteria.

Pharmacokinetics:

Route	Onset	Peak
Oral	Rapid	1–2 h
IV	Rapid	End of infusion

$T_{1/2}$: 5 hours; excreted in urine.

Adverse Effects: Headache, dizziness, vomiting, diarrhea, thrombocytopenia, risk for pseudomembranous colitis.

Drug–Food Interactions

Potential for serious to life-threatening hypertension is combined with large amounts of tyramine-containing foods. These should be avoided.

Monobactam Antibiotic

The only monobactam antibiotic currently available for use is aztreonam (*Azactam*) (Table 9.9).

Therapeutic Actions and Indications

Among the antibiotics, aztreonam's structure is unique, and little cross-resistance occurs. It is effective against gram-negative enterobacteria and has no effect on gram-positive or anaerobic bacteria. Aztreonam disrupts bacterial cell wall synthesis, which promotes leakage of cellular contents and cell death in susceptible bacteria (see Fig. 9.2). The drug is indicated for the treatment of urinary tract, skin, intra-abdominal, and gynecological infections, as well as septicemia caused by susceptible bacteria, including *E. coli*, *Enterobacter* spp., *Serratia* spp., *Proteus* spp., *Salmonella* spp., *Providencia* spp., *Pseudomonas* spp., *Citrobacter* spp., *Haemophilus* spp., *Neisseria* spp., and *Klebsiella* spp.

Pharmacokinetics

Aztreonam is available for IV and IM use only and reaches peak effect levels immediately if the route of administration is IV but slower if it is IM. Its half-life is 1.5 to 2 hours. The drug is excreted unchanged in the urine. It crosses the placenta and enters human milk (see "Contraindications and Cautions").

Contraindications and Cautions

Aztreonam is contraindicated with any known allergy to aztreonam. Use with caution in patients with a history of acute allergic reaction to penicillins or cephalosporins because of the possibility of cross-reactivity; in patients with renal dysfunction that could interfere with the clearance and excretion of the drug; and in pregnant and lactating patients because of potential adverse effects on the fetus or neonate.

Adverse Effects

The adverse effects associated with the use of aztreonam are relatively mild. Local GI effects include nausea, GI upset, vomiting, and diarrhea. Hepatic enzyme elevations related to direct drug effects on the liver may also occur. Other effects include inflammation, phlebitis, and discomfort at injection sites, as well as the potential for allergic response, including anaphylaxis.

Clinically Important Drug–Drug Interactions

Aztreonam and aminoglycosides may have synergistic effect when used together to treat certain organisms.

Prototype Summary: Aztreonam

Indications: Treatment of lower respiratory, dermatological, urinary tract, intra-abdominal, and gynecological infections caused by susceptible strains of gram-negative bacteria.

Actions: Interferes with bacterial cell wall synthesis, causing cell death in susceptible gram-negative bacteria; is not effective against gram-positive or anaerobic bacteria.

Pharmacokinetics:

Route	Onset	Peak	Duration
IM	Varies	60–90 min	6–8 h
IV	Immediate	Immediate after infusion	6–8 h

$T_{1/2}$: 1.5 to 2 hours; excreted unchanged in the urine.

Adverse Effects: Nausea, vomiting, diarrhea, rash, superinfection, anaphylaxis, local discomfort at injection sites.

Nursing Considerations for Patients Receiving Other Antibiotics

Assessment: History and Examination

- Assess for possible contraindications or precautions: known allergy to lincosamides, lipoglycopeptides, macrolides, oxazolidinones, and monobactams (obtain specific information about the nature and occurrence of allergic reactions); history of liver disease that could interfere with metabolism of the drug; history of renal disease, which could be aggravated by the drug; and current pregnancy or lactation status because of potential adverse effects on the fetus or infant.
- Perform a physical assessment to establish baseline data for assessing the effectiveness of the drug and the occurrence of any adverse effects associated with drug therapy.
- Examine the skin for any rash or lesions to provide a baseline for possible adverse effects.
- Obtain specimens for culture and sensitivity testing from the site of infection to ensure appropriate use of the drug.
- Monitor temperature to detect infection.
- Conduct assessment of orientation, affect, and reflexes to establish a baseline for any CNS effects of the drug.
- Assess renal function test values to determine the status of renal and liver functioning and to determine any needed alteration in dosage.
- Obtain baseline electrocardiogram to rule out conditions that could put the patient at risk for serious arrhythmias.

Nursing Conclusions

Nursing conclusions related to drug therapy might include the following:

- Impaired comfort related to GI or CNS effects of the drug
- Infection risk related to potential for superinfections
- Knowledge deficit risk regarding drug therapy

Planning

- The patient will receive the best therapeutic effect from the drug therapy.
- The patient will have limited adverse effects from the drug therapy.
- The patient will have an understanding of the drug therapy, adverse effects to anticipate, and measures to relieve discomfort and improve safety.

Intervention With Rationale

- Check culture and sensitivity reports to ensure that this is the drug of choice for this patient.
- Monitor hepatic and renal function test values before therapy begins to arrange to reduce dose as needed.
- Ensure that the patient receives the full course of the medication as prescribed to eradicate the infection and to help prevent the emergence of resistant strains.
- Monitor the site of infection and presenting signs and symptoms (e.g., fever, lethargy, urinary tract signs and symptoms) throughout the course of drug therapy. Failure of these signs and symptoms to resolve may indicate the need to reculture the site.
- Provide small, frequent meals as tolerated to ensure adequate nutrition with GI upset; frequent mouth care and ice chips or sugarless candy to suck to provide relief of discomfort if dry mouth is a problem; and adequate fluids to replace fluid lost with diarrhea.
- Ensure ready access to bathroom facilities to assist patients with problems associated with diarrhea.
- Institute safety measures to protect patient from injury if CNS effects occur.
- Arrange for appropriate treatment of superinfections as needed to decrease the severity of infection and complications.
- Instruct the patient about the appropriate dosage regimen and possible adverse effects to enhance patient knowledge about drug therapy and to promote compliance. The monobactam agent aztreonam and telavancin can be given only IV or IM, so the patient will not be responsible for administering the drug.
- For lincosamides, take additional precautions that include careful monitoring of GI activity and fluid balance and stopping the drug at the first sign of severe or bloody diarrhea.
- For lipoglycopeptides, take additional precautions to obtain a baseline QT interval on the ECG; alert the patient to the possibility of foamy urine; and ensure that the patient is not pregnant or planning to become pregnant when on the drug.
- Provide the following patient teaching:
  - Take safety precautions, including changing position slowly and avoiding driving and hazardous tasks, if CNS effects occur.
  - Try to drink fluids and to maintain nutrition even though nausea, vomiting, and diarrhea may occur.
  - Report difficulty breathing, severe headache, severe diarrhea, severe skin rash, and mouth or vaginal sores.

Evaluation

- Monitor patient response to the drug (resolution of bacterial infection).
- Monitor for adverse effects (orientation and affect, GI effects, superinfections).
- Evaluate the effectiveness of the teaching plan (patient can name the drug, dosage, possible adverse effects to expect, and specific measures to help avoid adverse effects).
- Monitor the effectiveness of comfort and safety measures and adherence to the regimen.

Key Points

- Lincosamides are similar to macrolides. They are used to treat severe infections. Monitor the patient for pseudomembranous colitis, bone marrow depression, pain, and CNS effects.
- Lipoglycopeptides, including vancomycin, telavancin, oritavancin, and dalbavancin, prevent the synthesis of the bacterial cell wall, which leads to cell death. Some are associated with high risk to the fetus. Monitor patients for prolonged QT interval, changes in renal function, GI effects, and foamy urine.
- Macrolides are in a class of older antibiotics that can be bactericidal or bacteriostatic. They are used to treat upper respiratory infections (URIs), bacterial endocarditis, Legionnaires' disease, pertussis, acute diphtheria, and chlamydial infections, and are often used when patients are allergic to penicillin. Monitor the patient for nausea, vomiting, diarrhea, dizziness, and other CNS effects. Monitor liver function if indicated for long-term use.
- Oxazolidinones are newer drugs that are especially effective against various resistant strains. They are used for skin and skin structure infections, pneumonias, or any infection caused by a resistant bacterium that is sensitive to the drug. These drugs are also MAO inhibitors, and caution must be used to prevent serotonin syndrome and hypertension-related effects.
- The monobactam antibiotic aztreonam is effective against only gram-negative bacteria; it is safely used when patients are allergic to penicillin or cephalosporins. Monitor the patient taking aztreonam for GI problems, liver toxicity, and pain at the injection site.

Miscellaneous Antibiotics

Research is constantly being done to develop new antibiotics to affect the emerging resistant strains of bacteria, and some antibiotics do not fit exactly into any of the classifications described in this chapter. The following miscellaneous antibiotics will be discussed: daptomycin (*Cubicin*), tigecycline (*Tygacil*), quinupristin and dalfopristin (*Synercid*), and rifaximin (*Xifaxan*).

Adjuncts to antibiotic therapy include clavulanic acid, sulbactam, avibactam, and tazobactam (see Box 9.2) and thalidomide (see Box 9.6).

- Daptomycin was introduced in the fall of 2003 as the first in a class of drugs called cyclic lipopeptide antibiotics. This class of drugs binds to bacterial cell membranes, causing a rapid depolarization of membrane potential. The loss of membrane potential leads to the inhibition of protein and DNA and RNA synthesis, which results in bacterial cell death. Daptomycin is approved for treating complicated skin and skin structure infections caused by susceptible gram-positive bacteria, including methicillin-resistant strains of *S. aureus*. It is also approved to treat *S. aureus* blood stream infections (bacteremia) in adults and children and endocarditis. It must be given IV over 30 minutes of by a 2-minute IV injection, once each day. Patients should be monitored for pseudomembranous colitis and myopathies.
- Tigecycline (*Tygacil*) is the first drug of a new class of antibiotics called glycylcyclines, similar to tetracycline. This antibiotic inhibits protein translation on ribosomes of certain bacteria, leading to their inability to maintain their integrity and culminating in the death of the bacterium. It is approved for use in the treatment of complicated skin and skin structure infections and intra-abdominal infections caused by susceptible bacteria and in the treatment of community-acquired pneumonia. Caution should be used with a known allergy to tetracycline antibiotics because cross-sensitivity may occur. People able to become pregnant should be advised to use a barrier form of contraceptive when on this drug. Patients should be monitored for pseudomembranous colitis, rash, and superinfections. The drug has a boxed warning noting the all-cause mortality was higher in patients on this drug, so the drug should be reserved for use when alternative treatment is not available. Tigecycline is given as 100 mg IV followed by 50 mg IV every 12 hours, infused over 30 to 60 minutes.
- Streptogramins became available in 1999 and include quinupristin and dalfopristin, which are available only in a combination form called *Synercid*. Together, they work synergistically and have been effective in treating VRE, resistant *S. aureus*, and resistant *S. epidermidis*. The drug is approved for VRE and methicillin-sensitive *S. aureus* infections. The drug also seems to be active against penicillin-resistant pneumococcus. The usual dosage of this drug for patients of 16 years old and older is 7.5 mg/kg IV every 12 hours for 7 days. The drug should not be used unless the bacterium is clearly identified as being resistant to other antibiotics and sensitive to this one. Indiscriminate use of this new drug can lead to the development of even more invasive and resistant bacteria.
- Rifaximin (*Xifaxan*) was approved specifically for the treatment of traveler's diarrhea. It is similar to rifampin and blocks bacterial RNA synthesis, which leads to bacterial death; 97% of the drug passes through the GI tract unchanged, and it directly affects *E. coli* bacteria, which cause traveler's diarrhea. It is also approved for treating hepatic encephalopathy, lowering ammonia levels because of its local effect on the GI bacteria and for the treatment of irritable bowel syndrome with diarrhea. The usual dose is 200 mg, orally, three times a day for traveler's diarrhea; 550 mg orally twice a day or 400 mg three times a day for hepatic encephalopathy; and 550 mg three times a day for irritable bowel syndrome. It should not be used if diarrhea is bloody and accompanied by fever, which might indicate that another pathogen is involved.

SUMMARY

- Antibiotics work by disrupting protein or enzyme systems within a bacterium, causing cell death (bactericidal) or preventing multiplication (bacteriostatic).
- The proteins or enzyme systems affected by antibiotics are more likely to be found or used in bacteria than in human cells.
- The primary therapeutic use of each antibiotic is determined by the bacterial species that are sensitive to that drug, the clinical condition of the patient receiving the drug, and the benefit-to-risk ratio for the patient.
- The longer an antibiotic has been available, the more likely that resistant bacterial strains will have developed.
- The most common adverse effects of antibiotic therapy involve the GI tract (nausea, vomiting, diarrhea, anorexia, abdominal pain) and superinfections (invasion of the body by normally occurring microorganisms that are usually kept in check by the normal flora).
- To prevent or contain the growing threat of drug-resistant strains of bacteria, it is very important to use antibiotics cautiously, to complete the full course of an antibiotic prescription, and to avoid saving antibiotics for self-medication in the future. A patient- and family-teaching program should address these issues, as well as the proper dosing procedure for the drug (even if the patient feels better) and the importance of keeping a record of any reactions to antibiotics.

Unfolding Patient Stories: Harry Hadley • Part 2

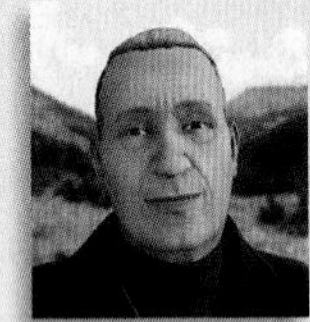

Recall Harry Hadley from Chapter 2, who is being treated for cellulitis of his right lower leg caused by a feral cat bite. Oral augmentin was changed to intravenous vancomycin when culture results identified MRSA. How would the nurse explain why the oral route was preferred over topical antibiotic application for the initial treatment of the feral cat bite and why the route of medication was subsequently changed from oral augmentin to intravenous vancomycin administration?

Care for Harry and other patients in a realistic virtual environment: ***vSim** for Nursing* (thepoint.lww.com/vSimPharm). Practice documenting these patients' care in DocuCare (thepoint.lww.com/DocuCareEHR).

CHECK YOUR UNDERSTANDING

Answers to the questions in this chapter can be found in Answers to Check Your Understanding Questions on thePoint®.

MULTIPLE CHOICE

Select the best answer.

1. A bacteriostatic substance is one that
   a. directly kills any bacteria in which it comes into contact.
   b. directly kills any bacteria that are sensitive to the substance.
   c. prevents the growth of any bacteria.
   d. prevents the growth of specific bacteria that are sensitive to the substance.

2. Where are gram-negative bacteria most likely to cause infection?
   a. Respiratory tract
   b. Soft tissues in the legs
   c. GI and GU tracts
   d. Brain tissue

3. Antibiotics that are used together to increase their effectiveness and limit the associated adverse effects are said to be
   a. broad spectrum.
   b. synergistic.
   c. bactericidal.
   d. anaerobic.

4. An aminoglycoside antibiotic might be the drug of choice in treating
   a. serious infections caused by susceptible strains of gram-negative bacteria.
   b. otitis media in an infant.
   c. cystitis in a patient who is 4 months pregnant.
   d. suspected pneumonia before the culture results are available.

5. Which of the following is not a caution for the use of cephalosporins?
   a. Allergy to penicillin
   b. Renal failure
   c. Allergy to aspirin
   d. Concurrent treatment with aminoglycosides

6. The fluoroquinolones
   a. are found freely in nature.
   b. are associated with Achilles tendon rupture.
   c. are widely used to only treat gram-positive infections.
   d. are broad-spectrum antibiotics with few associated adverse effects.

7. Ciprofloxacin is an example of
   a. a penicillin.
   b. a fluoroquinolone.
   c. an aminoglycoside.
   d. a macrolide antibiotic.

8. A patient receiving a fluoroquinolone should be cautioned to anticipate
   a. increased salivation.
   b. constipation.
   c. photosensitivity.
   d. cough.

9. The goal of antibiotic therapy is
   a. to eradicate all bacteria from the system.
   b. to suppress resistant strains of bacteria.
   c. to reduce the number of invading bacteria so that the immune system can deal with the infection.
   d. to stop the drug as soon as the patient feels better.

10. The penicillins
    a. are bacteriostatic.
    b. are bactericidal, interfering with bacteria cell walls.
    c. are effective only if given intravenously.
    d. do not produce cross-sensitivity within their class.

MULTIPLE RESPONSE

Select all that apply.

1. A young patient is found to have a soft tissue infection that is most responsive to tetracycline. Your teaching plan for this patient, who is able to become pregnant, should include which of the following points?
   a. Tetracycline can cause gray baby syndrome.
   b. Do not use this drug if you are pregnant because it can cause tooth and bone defects in the fetus.
   c. Tetracycline can cause severe acne.
   d. You should use a second form of contraception if you are using oral contraceptives because tetracycline can make them ineffective.
   e. This drug should be taken in the middle of a meal to decrease GI upset.
   f. You may experience a vaginal yeast infection as a result of this drug therapy.

2. In general, all patients receiving antibiotics should receive teaching that includes which of the following points?
   a. The need to complete the full course of drug therapy
   b. The possibility of oral contraceptive failure
   c. When to take the drug related to food and other drugs
   d. The need for assessment of blood tests
   e. Advisability of saving any leftover medication for future use
   f. How to detect superinfections and what to do if they occur

REFERENCES

Bancroft, E. (2007). Antimicrobial resistance: It's not just for hospitals. *Journal of the American Medical Association, 298*(15), 1803–1804. https://doi.org/10.1001/jama.298.15.1803

Brunton, L. L., Hilal-Dandan, R., & Knollman, B. C. (2018). *Goodman and Gilman's the pharmacological basis of therapeutics* (13th ed.). McGraw-Hill.

Centers for Disease Control and Prevention. (2021). *Antibiotic prescribing and use.* https://www.cdc.gov/antibiotic-use/index.html

Kim, D. H., Han, K., & Kim S. W. (2018). Effects of antibiotics on the development of asthma and other allergic diseases in children and adolescents. *Allergy, Asthma and Immunology Research, 10*(5), 457–465. https://doi.org/10.4168/aair.2018.10.5.457

Klevens, R. M., Morrison, M. A., Nadle, J., Petit, S., Gershman, K., Ray, S., Harrison, L. H., Lynfield, R., Dumyati, G., Townes, J. M., Craig, A. S., Zell, E. R., Fosheim, G. E., McDougal, L. K., Carey, R. B., & Fridkin, S. K. (2007). Invasive methicillin-resistant *Staphylococcus aureus* infections in the United States. *Journal of the American Medical Association, 298*(15), 1763–1771. https://doi.org/10.1001/jama.298.15.1763

Nahid, P., Dorman, S. E., Alipanah, N., Barry, P. M., Brozek, J. L., Cattamanchi, A., Chaisson, L. H., Chaisson, R. E., Daley, C. L., Grzemska, M., Higashi, J. M., Ho, C. S., Hopewell, P. C., Keshavjee, S. A., Lienhardt, C., Menzies, R., Merrifield, C., Narita, M., O'Brien, R., … Vernon, A. (2016). Official American Thoracic Society/Centers for Disease Control and Prevention/Infectious Diseases Society of America clinical practice guidelines: Treatment of drug-susceptible tuberculosis. *Clinical Infectious Diseases, 63*(7), 853–867. https://doi.org/10.1093/cid/ciw376

Norris, T. L., & Lalchandani, R. (2018). *Porth's pathophysiology: Concepts of altered health states* (10th ed.). Wolters Kluwer.

Workowski, K. A., Berman, S. M., & Douglas, J. M. (2008). Emerging antimicrobial resistance in *Neisseria gonorrhoeae*: Urgent need to strengthen prevention strategies. *Annals of Internal Medicine, 148*(8), 606–613. https://doi.org/10.7326/0003-4819-148-8-200804150-00005

CHAPTER 10

Antiviral Agents

Learning Objectives

Upon completion of this chapter, you will be able to:

1. Discuss the problems with treating viral infections in humans and the use of antivirals across the life span.
2. Describe the characteristics of common viruses and the resultant clinical presentations of common viral infections.
3. Describe the therapeutic actions, indications, pharmacokinetics, contraindications, most common adverse reactions, and important drug–drug interactions associated with each of the types of antivirals discussed in the chapter.
4. Compare and contrast the prototype drugs for each type of antiviral with the other drugs within that group.
5. Outline the nursing considerations for patients receiving each class of antiviral agent.

Key Terms

acquired immunodeficiency syndrome (AIDS): collection of opportunistic infections and cancers that occurs when the immune system is severely depressed by a decrease in the number of functioning helper T cells; caused by infection with human immunodeficiency virus (HIV)

AIDS-related complex (ARC): collection of less serious opportunistic infections with HIV infection; the decrease in the number of helper T cells is less severe than in fully developed AIDS

CCR5 coreceptor antagonist: drug that blocks the receptor site on the T-cell membrane that the HIV virus needs to interact with in order to enter the cell

coronavirus: variety of types of RNA viruses that can cause several types of primarily respiratory illnesses; one of the coronaviruses causes COVID-19

cytomegalovirus (CMV): DNA virus that accounts for many respiratory, ophthalmic, and liver infections

fusion inhibitor: a drug that prevents the fusion of the HIV-1 virus with the human cellular membrane, preventing it from entering the cell

helper T cell: human lymphocyte that helps to initiate immune reactions in response to tissue invasion

hepatitis B virus: virus that causes a serious to potentially fatal infection of the liver, transmitted by body fluids (usually blood)

hepatitis C virus: virus that causes a usually mild infection of the liver that can progress to chronic inflammation with eventual need for liver transplantation

herpes: DNA virus that accounts for many diseases, including varicella-zoster, cold sores, genital infections, and encephalitis

human immunodeficiency virus (HIV): retrovirus that attacks helper T cells, leading to a decrease in immune function and AIDS or ARC

influenza A: RNA virus that invades tissues of the respiratory tract, causing the signs and symptoms of the common cold or "flu"

integrase strand transfer inhibitors: drug that inhibits the activity of the virus-specific enzyme integrase, an encoded enzyme needed for viral replication; blocking this enzyme prevents the formation of the HIV-1 provirus

interferon: tissue hormone that is released in response to viral invasion; blocks viral replication

nonnucleoside reverse transcriptase inhibitors: drugs that bind to sites on the reverse transcriptase within the cell cytoplasm, preventing RNA- and DNA-dependent DNA polymerase activities needed to carry out viral DNA synthesis; prevents the transfer of information that allows the virus to replicate and survive

nucleoside reverse transcriptase inhibitors: drugs that prevent the growth of the viral DNA chain, preventing it from inserting into the host DNA, so viral replication cannot occur

protease inhibitors: drugs that block the activity of the enzyme protease in HIV; protease is essential for the maturation of infectious virus, and its absence leads to the formation of an immature and noninfective HIV particle

virus: particle of DNA or RNA surrounded by a protein coat that survives by invading a cell to alter its functioning

Agent List

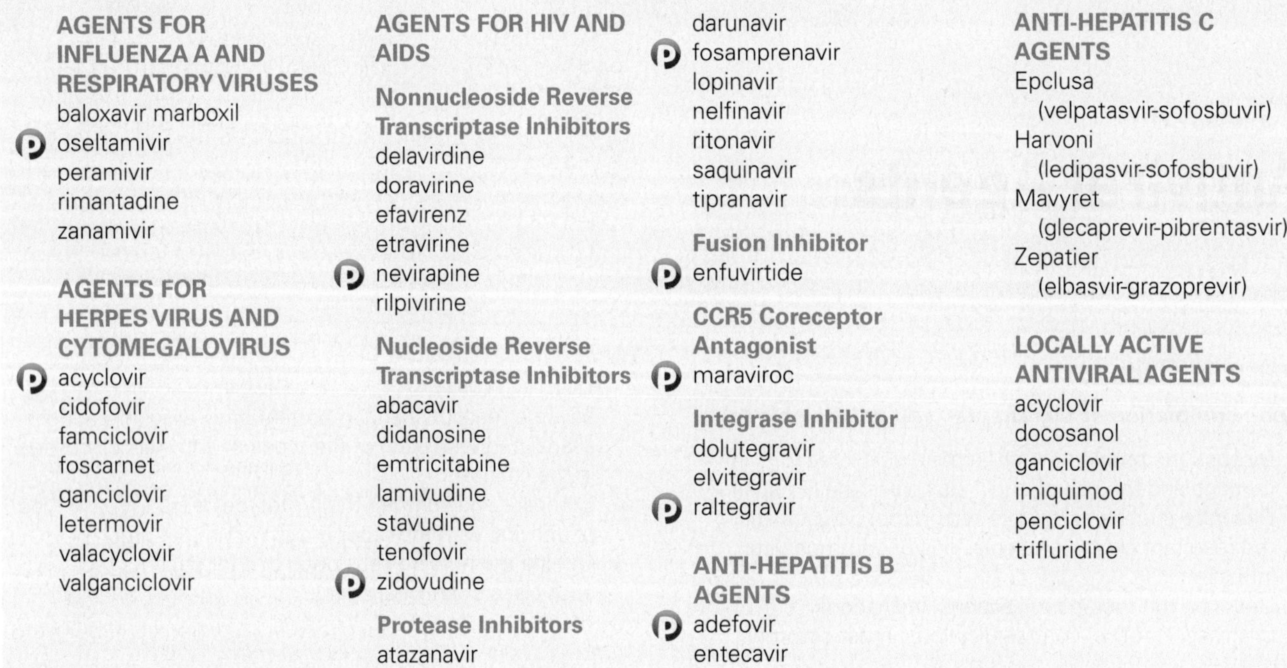

AGENTS FOR INFLUENZA A AND RESPIRATORY VIRUSES

baloxavir marboxil
oseltamivir
peramivir
rimantadine
zanamivir

AGENTS FOR HERPES VIRUS AND CYTOMEGALOVIRUS

acyclovir
cidofovir
famciclovir
foscarnet
ganciclovir
letermovir
valacyclovir
valganciclovir

AGENTS FOR HIV AND AIDS

Nonnucleoside Reverse Transcriptase Inhibitors

delavirdine
doravirine
efavirenz
etravirine
nevirapine
rilpivirine

Nucleoside Reverse Transcriptase Inhibitors

abacavir
didanosine
emtricitabine
lamivudine
stavudine
tenofovir
zidovudine

Protease Inhibitors

atazanavir
darunavir
fosamprenavir
lopinavir
nelfinavir
ritonavir
saquinavir
tipranavir

Fusion Inhibitor

enfuvirtide

CCR5 Coreceptor Antagonist

maraviroc

Integrase Inhibitor

dolutegravir
elvitegravir
raltegravir

ANTI-HEPATITIS B AGENTS

adefovir
entecavir

ANTI-HEPATITIS C AGENTS

Epclusa (velpatasvir-sofosbuvir)
Harvoni (ledipasvir-sofosbuvir)
Mavyret (glecaprevir-pibrentasvir)
Zepatier (elbasvir-grazoprevir)

LOCALLY ACTIVE ANTIVIRAL AGENTS

acyclovir
docosanol
ganciclovir
imiquimod
penciclovir
trifluridine

Viruses cause a variety of conditions, ranging from warts to the common cold and influenza to diseases such as chickenpox, measles, and AIDS. A single **virus** particle is composed of a piece of either DNA or RNA inside a protein coat. To carry on any metabolic processes, including replication, a virus must enter a host cell. Once a virus has fused with a cell wall and injected its DNA or RNA into the host cell, that cell is altered (i.e., it is "programmed" to control the metabolic processes that the virus needs to survive). The virus, including the protein coat, replicates in the host cell (see Fig. 10.1). When the host cell can no longer carry out its own metabolic functions because of the viral invader, the host cell dies and releases the new viruses into the body to invade other cells.

Because viruses are contained inside human cells while they are in the body, researchers have difficulty developing effective drugs that destroy a virus without harming the human host. **Interferons** (see Chapter 15) are released by the host in response to viral invasion of a cell and act to prevent the replication of that particular virus.

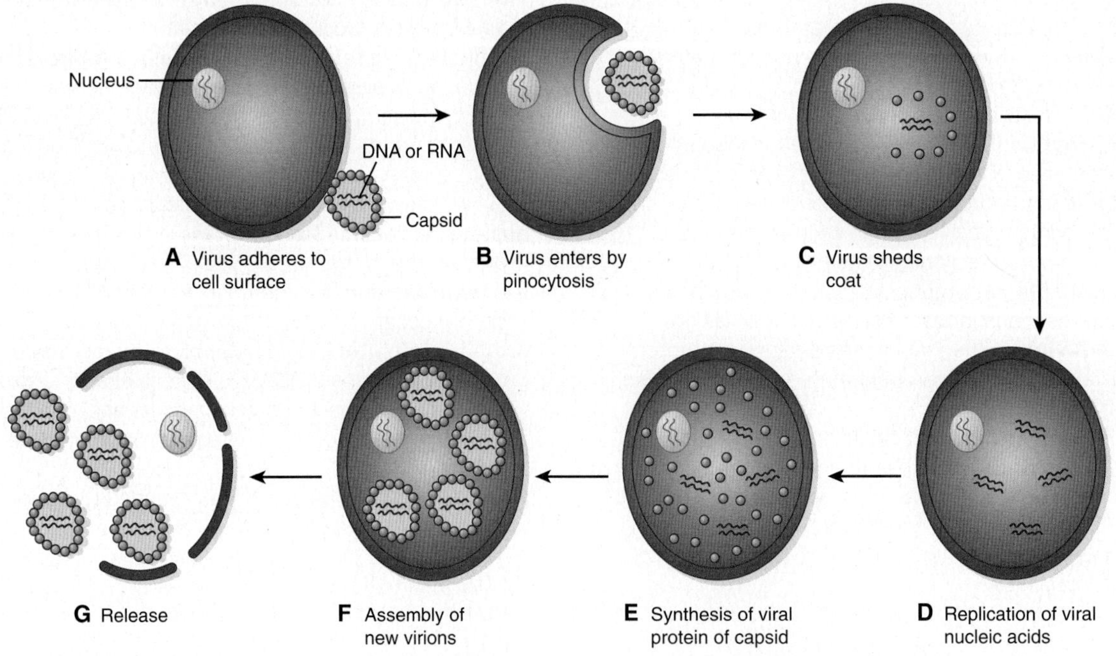

FIGURE 10.1 The stages in the replication cycle of a virus.

Box 10.1 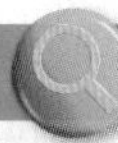 Focus on The Evidence

CORONAVIRUS 2019 DISEASE (COVID-19) AND THERAPIES

A novel coronavirus that causes severe acute respiratory syndrome was identified in late 2019. The virus was designated as severe acute respiratory syndrome coronavirus 2 (SARS-CoV-2), and the disease was later named COVID-19. The virus spread globally very quickly, and the World Health Organization (WHO) declared a public health emergency and characterized it as a pandemic on March 11, 2020. The virus seemed to spread person-to-person primarily via respiratory droplets, although some transmission could be via airborne particles and/or contaminated surfaces.

Initially, there were no FDA-approved treatments or vaccines for COVID-19. People were instructed by the Centers for Disease Control and Prevention (CDC) and other regulatory bodies to take preventative precautions by washing hands frequently, avoiding touching one's face with unwashed hands, wearing face masks over the nose and mouth in public, and avoiding close proximity with people who were outside one's household (social distancing; maintaining at least 6-feet distance). More detailed guidance is available on the CDC website: https://www.cdc.gov/coronavirus/2019-ncov/prevent-getting-sick/prevention.html

Clinicians and researchers around the world worked quickly and diligently to find ways to help people who were infected. Many research studies were conducted to see what types of medications would be helpful for treating the virus and/or eliminating symptoms. The FDA granted emergency approval for several substances during the year 2020 including: remdesivir, favipiravir, interferons, hydroxychloroquine, and convalescent plasma. Steroid treatments were investigated to see if they would help to decrease the lung inflammation caused by COVID-19.

Currently, the only FDA-approved antiviral treatment for COVID-19 is remdesivir *(Veklury)*. Remdesivir inhibits the SARS-CoV-2 RNA-dependent RNA polymerase enzyme that is used for viral RNA synthesis. It has been approved for adults and pediatric patients (12 years and older and weighing at least 40 kg) who have been hospitalized due to COVID-19. A loading dose of 200 mg IV is administered, followed by daily doses of 100 mg IV for 5 to 10 days.

There is still much to be learned about the prevention and treatment of COVID-19. Individuals are still being encouraged to practice social distancing to prevent the person-to-person spread of the virus. Several vaccines are approved by the FDA for prevention of COVID-19.

Some interferons that affect particular viruses can now be genetically engineered to treat particular viral infections. Other drugs that are used in treating viral infections are not natural substances and have been effective against only a limited number of viruses.

Viruses that respond to some antiviral therapy include influenza A and some respiratory viruses, herpes viruses, cytomegalovirus (CMV), HIV that causes AIDS, hepatitis B, hepatitis C, and some viruses that cause warts and certain eye infections. **Coronaviruses** are a variety of types of RNA viruses that can cause several types of primarily respiratory illnesses. One of the coronaviruses causes COVID-19. This is an illness for which the treatments and prevention techniques are evolving (see Box 10.1). Box 10.2 discusses the

Box 10.2 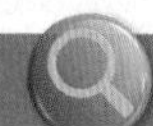 Focus on Drug Therapy Across the Life Span

ANTIVIRALS

Children

Children are very sensitive to the effects of most antiviral drugs, and more severe reactions can be expected when these drugs are used in children.

Many antiviral drugs do not have proven safety and efficacy in children, and extreme caution should be used.

Most of the drugs for prevention and treatment of influenza virus infections can be used in smaller doses for children.

Acyclovir is the drug of choice for children with herpes virus or CMV infections.

The drugs used in the treatment of AIDS are frequently used in children. Many of these drugs now have recommended pediatric dosing, but others may be used without the evidence of safety because of the seriousness of the disease. The dose should be calculated according to body weight, and children must be monitored very closely for adverse effects on the kidneys, bone marrow, and the liver.

Adults

Adults need to know that antiviral drugs are specifically for the treatment of viral infections. The use of antibiotics to treat such infections can lead to the development of resistant strains and superinfections that can complicate care for the entire population.

Patients with HIV infection who are taking antiviral medications need to be taught that these drugs do not cure the disease, that opportunistic infections can still occur, and that precautions to prevent transmission of the disease need to be taken.

Antiviral therapy can have significant adverse effects on fetal development. Patients who are pregnant or can become pregnant should be informed about the risks and benefits of all of the indicated therapies. Patients who can become pregnant should be advised to use barrier contraceptives if they take any of these drugs. Some antiviral medications have safer use in pregnant patients than others, so be sure to review the individual medication labels.

The Centers for Disease Control and Prevention advises that patients with HIV infection should not breast or chestfeed to protect the neonate from the virus.

Older Adults

Older patients may be more susceptible to the adverse effects associated with antiviral drugs; they should be monitored closely.

Patients with hepatic dysfunction are at increased risk for worsening hepatic problems and toxic effects of those drugs that are metabolized in the liver. Drugs that are excreted unchanged in the urine may accumulate in patients who have renal dysfunction. If hepatic or renal dysfunction is expected (due to extreme age, alcohol abuse, or use of other hepatotoxic or nephrotoxic drugs), the dose may need to be lowered and the patient should be monitored more frequently.

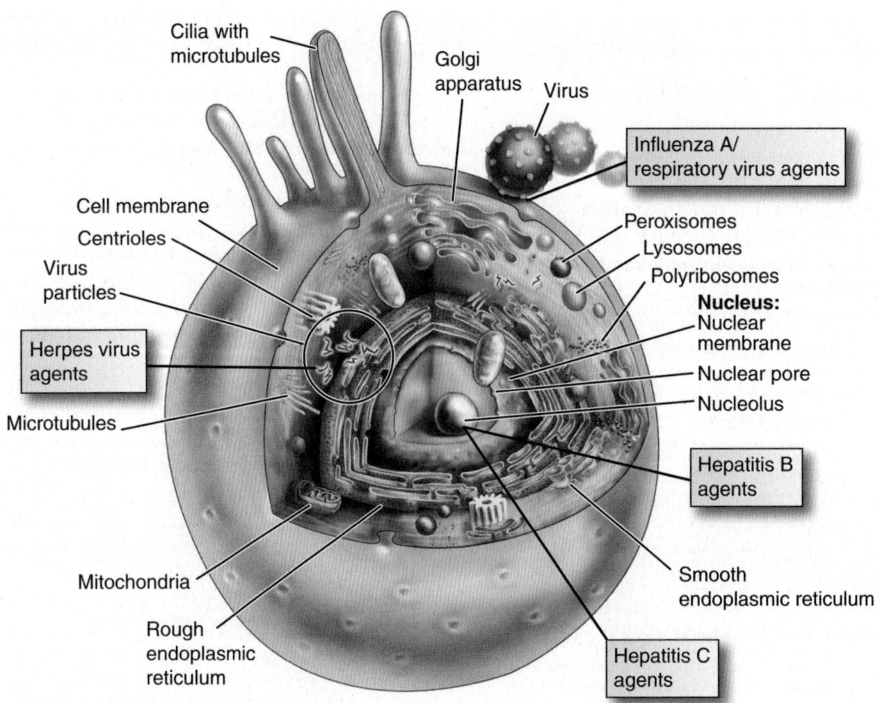

FIGURE 10.2 Agents for treating influenza A and respiratory viruses prevent shedding of the protein coat and entry of virus into the cell. Herpes virus agents alter viral DNA production. Anti-hepatitis B and C agents block DNA formation, preventing the formation of new viruses.

use of antivirals across the life span. Figures 10.2 and 10.3 show sites of action for these agents.

Agents for Influenza A and Respiratory Viruses

Influenza A and other respiratory viruses, including influenza B and respiratory syncytial virus (RSV), invade the respiratory tract and cause the signs and symptoms of respiratory "flu." Vaccines have been developed (see Chapter 18) to stimulate immunity against influenza A and RSV. Preventing viral infection is the best option, but if patients do develop a viral infection, some drug therapies are available. Agents for influenza A and respiratory viruses include baloxavir marboxil (*Xofluza*), oseltamivir (*Tamiflu*), peramivir (*Rapivab*), rimantadine (*Flumadine*), and zanamivir (*Relenza*). These drugs are described in detail in Table 10.1.

Therapeutic Actions and Indications

The mechanism of action for oseltamivir, peramivir, and zanamivir is to inhibit neuraminidase, a viral enzyme that helps with the release of viral particles that can spread to uninfected cells. This inhibition in turn slows the spread of the virus from infected cells to uninfected cells. Baloxavir is an endonuclease inhibitor that prevents viral replication by inhibiting an enzyme (endonuclease) that is used for viral gene transcription (see Fig. 10.2). This action prevents viral replication, causing viral death. These agents for influenza A and respiratory viruses are especially important for health care workers and other high-risk individuals and for reducing the severity of infection if it occurs. See Table 10.1 for usual indications specific to each antiviral drug. Oseltamivir is the only antiviral agent that has been shown to be effective in treating H1N1 and avian flu.

Pharmacokinetics

Oseltamivir is readily absorbed from the GI tract, extensively metabolized in the urine, and excreted in the urine with a half-life of 6 to 10 hours.

Peramivir is given intravenously (IV) as a single dose, reaches peak level at the end of the infusion, and has a half-life of 20 hours.

Zanamivir must be delivered by a Diskhaler device, which comes with every prescription of zanamivir. It has minimal systemic absorption through the respiratory tract, is excreted unchanged in the urine and feces, and has a half-life of 2.5 to 5.1 hours.

Baloxavir is administered as a single oral dose, peaks approximately 4 hours after ingestion, and has a half-life of approximately 80 hours. It is eliminated primarily in the feces.

Contraindications and Cautions

Patients with renal dysfunction who are taking oseltamivir require reduced doses and close monitoring to avoid altered metabolism and excretion of the drug.

Peramivir is not considered a first-line therapy during pregnancy, due to limited experience with the drug. These drugs should not be used by patients who are breast or chestfeeding, as limited data are available.

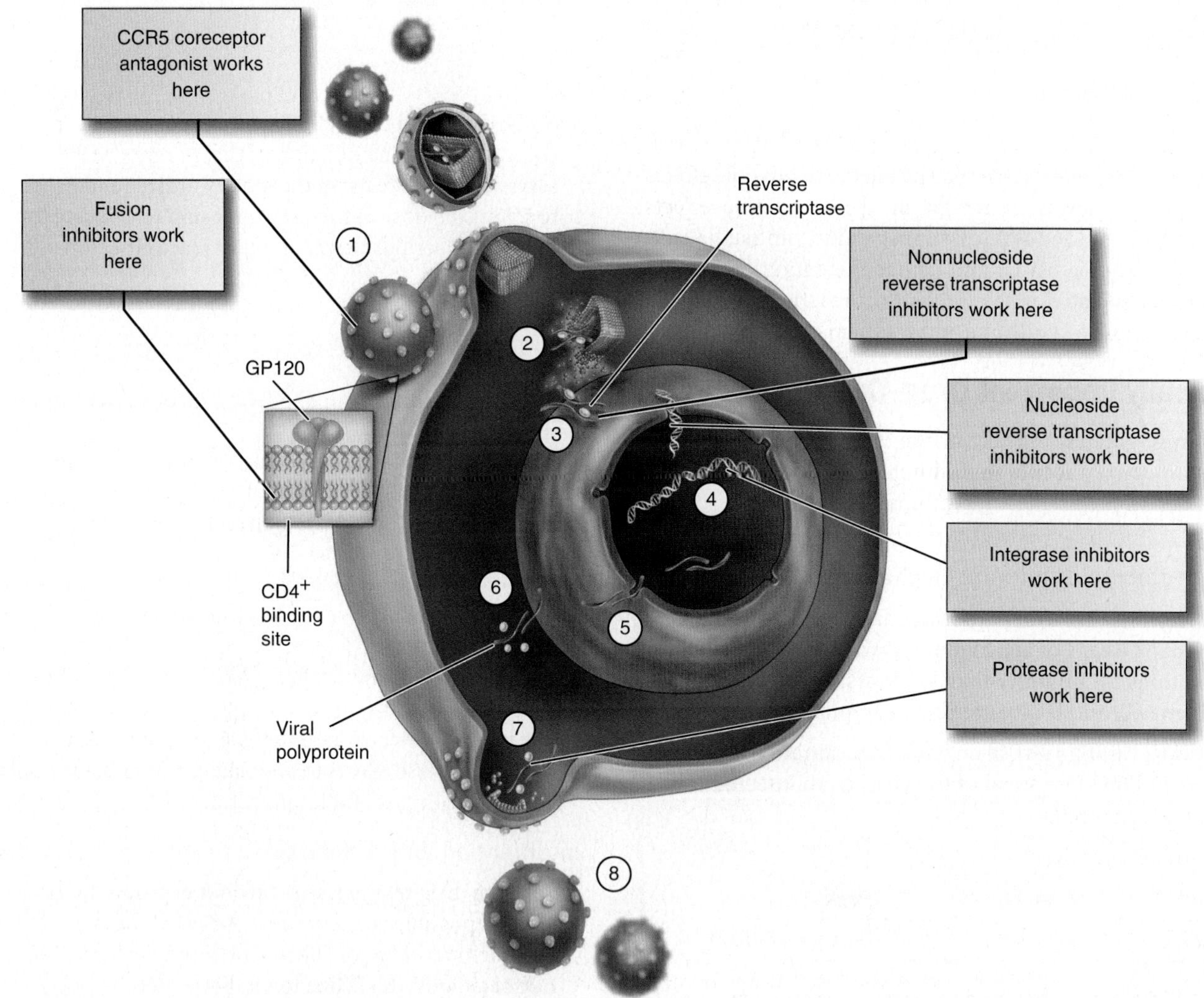

FIGURE 10.3 Stages of HIV replication. *1.* Virus reacts with receptor site on CD4 cell, fuses, and enters cell. *2.* Reverse transcriptase enzyme used to copy RNA of the virus into DNA strand. *3.* Viral DNA able to enter CD4 cell nucleus due to integrase enzyme. *4.* Viral proteins replicated. *5.* Viral protein chains leave the host cell nucleus. *6* and *7.* Chains of long proteins cleaved into smaller chains via protease enzyme and packaged for release from the host CD4 cell. *8.* HIV virus leaves host CD4 cell and is able to enter other CD4 cells. Agents that attempt to control HIV and AIDS work in the following ways: Interference with HIV replication by blocking synthesis of viral DNA (nonnucleoside and nucleoside reverse transcriptase inhibitors); blockage of protease within the virus, leading to immature, noninfective virus particles (protease inhibitors); prevention of virus from fusing with the cellular membrane, thereby preventing the HIV-1 virus from entering the cell (fusion inhibitors); blockage of HIV virus reaction with the receptor site that would allow it to enter the cell (CCR5 coreceptor antagonists); and prevention of necessary encoded enzyme action for viral reproduction (integrase inhibitors).

Table 10.1 *Drugs in Focus*: Agents for Influenza A and Respiratory Viruses

Drug Name	Dosage/Route	Usual Indications
baloxavir marboxil (*Xofluza*)	*Adult and pediatric (12 y and older)*: 40 mg dose once PO (weight <80 kg) or 80 mg dose once PO (weight at least 80 kg)	Treatment of influenza in patients who have been symptomatic for <2 d; postexposure prophylaxis of influenza
oseltamivir (*Tamiflu*)	*Adult*: 75 mg PO b.i.d. for 5 d (treatment); 75 mg/d PO for at least 10 d (prevention) *Pediatric*: Weight-based dosing	Treatment and prevention of uncomplicated influenza for patients who are symptomatic for <2 d; only antiviral agent effective in treatment of avian flu
peramivir (*Rapivab*)	*Adult*: 600 mg IV over 15 min	Treatment of acute uncomplicated influenza in patients who have been symptomatic no more than 2 d
rimantadine (*Flumadine*)	*Adult*: 100 mg PO b.i.d. *Pediatric (≥10 y)*: 5 mg/kg PO daily	Treatment and prevention of influenza A infections
zanamivir (*Relenza*)	*Adult and children ≥7 y*: Two inhalations b.i.d. (12 h apart) for 5 d; prevention of influenza in patients >5 y; two inhalations per day for 10 d (household) to 28 d (community)	Treatment and prevention of uncomplicated influenza infections in adults and in children >7 y of age who have had symptoms for <2 d

RSV, respiratory syncytial virus.

Adverse Effects

Use of these antiviral agents is frequently associated with various adverse effects that may be related to possible effects on dopamine levels in the brain. These adverse effects include light-headedness, dizziness, and insomnia; nausea; orthostatic hypotension; and urinary retention. Peramivir has been associated with serious skin reactions, including Stevens–Johnson syndrome and erythema multiforme.

Clinically Important Drug–Drug Interactions

To ensure greatest efficacy of the vaccine, live attenuated nasal influenza vaccine should not be used within 2 weeks before or 48 hours after neuraminidase inhibitors.

Prototype Summary: Oseltamivir

Indications: Treatment of influenza A and B in patients 2 weeks of age and older who have had symptoms for no more than 48 hours. Prophylaxis of influenza A and B in patients 1 year and older.

Actions: Inhibits a viral enzyme (neuraminidase) in order to slow the spread of the virus from infected cells to uninfected cells.

Pharmacokinetics:

Route	Onset	Peak
Oral	Unknown	Post metabolism

$T_{1/2}$: 1–3 hours, converted to active metabolite by esterase in liver, eliminated renally.

Adverse Effects: Headache, nausea, rash, vomiting.

Nursing Considerations for Patients Receiving Agents for Influenza A and Respiratory Viruses

Assessment: History and Examination

- Assess for contraindications or cautions. This includes assessing known history of allergy to antivirals to avoid hypersensitivity reactions, history of liver or renal dysfunction that might interfere with drug metabolism and excretion, and current status related to pregnancy or lactation to prevent adverse effects on the fetus or nursing baby.
- Perform a physical assessment to establish baseline data for evaluating the effectiveness of the drug and the occurrence of any adverse effects associated with drug therapy.
- Assess for orientation and reflexes to evaluate any CNS effects of the drug; vital signs (temperature, respiratory rate, breath sounds for adventitious sounds) to assess for signs and symptoms of the viral infection; blood pressure to monitor for orthostatic hypotension; urinary output to monitor genitourinary (GU) effects of the drug; and renal and hepatic function tests to determine baseline function of these organs and to assess adverse effects on the kidney or liver and need to adjust the dose of the drug; and skin to evaluate for potentially serious dermatological reactions.

Nursing Conclusions

Nursing conclusions related to drug therapy might include the following:

- Impaired comfort related to GI, CNS, or GU effects of the drug
- Altered sensory perception (kinesthetic) related to CNS effects of the drug
- Knowledge deficit regarding drug therapy

Planning

- The patient will receive the best therapeutic effect from the drug therapy.
- The patient will have limited adverse effects from the drug therapy.
- The patient will have an understanding of the drug therapy, adverse effects to anticipate, and measures to relieve discomfort and improve safety.

Intervention With Rationale

- Start the drug regimen as soon after exposure to the virus as possible, ideally within 2 days of the start of symptoms to enhance effectiveness and decrease the risk of complications due to viral infection.
- Administer influenza A vaccine before the flu season begins, if at all possible, to decrease the risk of contracting the flu and the risk of complications.
- Administer the full course of the drug to obtain full beneficial effects.
- Provide safety provisions if CNS effects occur to protect the patient from injury.
- Instruct the patient about the appropriate dose scheduling; safety precautions, including changing position slowly and avoiding driving and hazardous tasks, that should be taken if CNS effects occur; and the need to report any adverse effects such as difficulty walking or talking to enhance patient knowledge about drug therapy and to promote adherence.

Evaluation

- Monitor patient response to the drug (prevention of respiratory flulike symptoms, alleviation of flulike symptoms).
- Monitor for adverse effects (changes in orientation and affect, blood pressure, urinary output, skin changes, and/or liver or renal function test changes).
- Determine the effectiveness of the teaching plan. The patient should be able to name the drug, dosage, possible adverse effects to watch for, and specific measures to help to avoid or minimize adverse effects.
- Monitor the effectiveness of comfort and safety measures and adherence to the regimen.

Key Points

- Viruses are segments of RNA or DNA enclosed in a protein coat.
- A virus must enter a human cell to survive, making it difficult to treat without serious toxic effects for the host.
- Antiviral drugs that prevent the viral replication of respiratory viruses can be used to prevent or treat influenza A or other respiratory viruses.

Agents for Herpes and Cytomegalovirus

Herpes viruses account for a broad range of conditions, including cold sores, encephalitis, varicella-zoster, and genital infections. **Cytomegalovirus (CMV)**, although slightly different from the herpes virus, is a DNA virus that can affect the eye, respiratory tract, and liver and reacts to many of the same drugs. Antiviral drugs used to combat these infections include acyclovir (*Sitavig, Zovirax*), cidofovir (generic), famciclovir (generic), foscarnet (*Foscavir*), ganciclovir (*Cytovene*), letermovir (*Prevymis*), valacyclovir (*Valtrex*), and valganciclovir (*Valcyte*) (see Table 10.2).

Therapeutic Actions and Indications

Drugs that combat herpes and CMV inhibit viral DNA replication by competing with viral substrates to form shorter, noneffective DNA chains (see Fig. 10.2). This action prevents replication of the virus, but it has little effect on the host cells of humans because human cell DNA uses different substrates. These antiviral agents are indicated for treatment of the DNA viruses herpes simplex, varicella-zoster viruses, and CMV. Research has shown that they are very effective in immunocompromised individuals, such as patients with AIDS, those taking immunosuppressants, older adults, and those with multiple infections. See Table 10.2 for usual indications for each of these agents.

Pharmacokinetics

Acyclovir, which can be given orally, buccally, or parenterally or applied topically, reaches peak level within 1 hour and has a half-life of 2.5 to 5 hours. It is excreted unchanged in the urine. It crosses into human milk.

Cidofovir, which is given by IV infusion, reaches peak level at the end of the infusion. It is excreted unchanged in the urine and must be given with probenecid to decrease nephrotoxicity by reducing the uptake of cidofovir by specific cells in the kidney. The dose must be decreased

Table 10.2 *Drugs in Focus*: Agents for Herpes Virus and Cytomegalovirus

Drug Name	Dosage/Route	Usual Indications
acyclovir (*Sitavig, Zovirax*)	*Adult*: 5–10 mg/kg q8h IV q8h or 200–800 mg q4h PO *Pediatric*: 10 mg/kg IV q8h or 20 mg/kg four times a day PO for 5 d	Treatment of herpes simplex and varicella-zoster virus infections
cidofovir (generic)	5 mg/kg IV (over 1 h) once weekly for 2 wk, then every other week	Treatment of CMV retinitis in patients with AIDS
famciclovir (generic)	500 mg PO q8h for 7 d *Suppression of recurrent herpes*: 250 mg PO b.i.d. for up to 1 y	Treatment of herpes virus infections such as varicella-zoster infections and for recurrent episodes of genital herpes
foscarnet (*Foscavir*)	*Adult*: 40–90 mg/kg q8–12h IV given as a 2-h infusion *Pediatric*: Safety and efficacy not established	Treatment of CMV and acyclovir-resistant mucocutaneous herpes simplex infections in immunocompromised patients
ganciclovir (*Cytovene*)	*Adult*: 5 m/kg q12h IV given over 1 h for 14–21 d, then over 1 h daily 7 d/wk or 6 mg/kg/d for 5 d/wk for prophylaxis	Long-term treatment and prevention of CMV infection
letermovir (*Prevymis*)	*Adult:* 480 mg/d PO or IV through 100 d posttransfusion	Prophylaxis of cytomegalovirus (CMV) infection and disease in CMV-seropositive recipients of an allogeneic hematopoietic stem cell transplant
valacyclovir (*Valtrex*)	*Adult:* 1–2 g b.i.d. or t.i.d. based on indication *Chickenpox*: *Pediatric (2–18 y)*: 20 mg/kg PO t.i.d. for 5 d	Treatment of varicella-zoster infections and recurrent genital herpes; cold sores (herpes labialis), chicken pox
valganciclovir (*Valcyte*)	*Adult:* 900 mg PO b.i.d. for 21 d, then 900 mg PO once a day for maintenance; reduce dose with renal impairment	Treatment of CMV retinitis in patients with AIDS

CMV, cytomegalovirus.

according to renal function and creatinine clearance; renal function tests must be done before each dose, with the dose then planned accordingly.

Famciclovir, an oral drug, is well absorbed from the GI tract, reaching peak level in approximately 1 hour. Famciclovir is metabolized in the liver and excreted in the urine and feces. It has a half-life of 2 hours.

Foscarnet is available in IV form only. It reaches peak level at the end of the infusion and has a half-life of about 2 hours. About 90% of foscarnet is excreted unchanged in the urine, and it is toxic to the kidneys. Use caution and at a reduced dose in patients with renal impairment.

Ganciclovir is available in IV and oral forms. The oral form is valganciclovir; it is the prodrug of ganciclovir. A prodrug is an agent that is converted by the body into a drug. It has a slow onset and reaches peak level immediately post infusion if given IV and 1 to 3 hours if given orally. This drug is primarily excreted unchanged in the feces with some urinary excretion and has a half-life of 2 to 4 hours.

Valacyclovir is a prodrug that is rapidly absorbed from the GI tract and metabolized in the liver to acyclovir. Excretion occurs through the urine, so caution should be used in patients with renal impairment.

Contraindications and Cautions

Some drugs indicated for the treatment of herpes and CMV are highly toxic and should only be used during pregnancy or lactation if the benefits clearly outweigh the potential risks to the fetus or infant. Avoid use in patients with known allergies to antiviral agents to prevent serious hypersensitivity reactions; in patients with renal disease, which could interfere with excretion of the drug; and in patients with severe CNS disorders because the drug can affect the CNS, causing headache, neuropathy, paresthesia, confusion, and hallucinations.

Cidofovir has been proven to be embryotoxic in animals and should not be used during pregnancy.

For famciclovir, safety of use in children younger than 18 years of age has not been established.

Foscarnet deposits in the bone of children to a greater extent than in adult patients. It is unknown if this has an effect on bone growth or development. Foscarnet should not be used in children unless the benefit clearly outweighs the risk and the child is monitored very closely.

Adverse Effects

The adverse effects more commonly associated with these antivirals include nausea and vomiting, headache, depression, paresthesia, neuropathy, rash, and hair loss (see Fig. 10.4). Rash, inflammation, and burning often occur at sites of IV injection and topical application. Renal dysfunction and renal failure also have been reported. Cidofovir is associated with severe renal toxicity and granulocytopenia. Ganciclovir and valganciclovir have been associated with bone marrow suppression. Foscarnet has been associated with seizures, especially in patients with electrolyte imbalance.

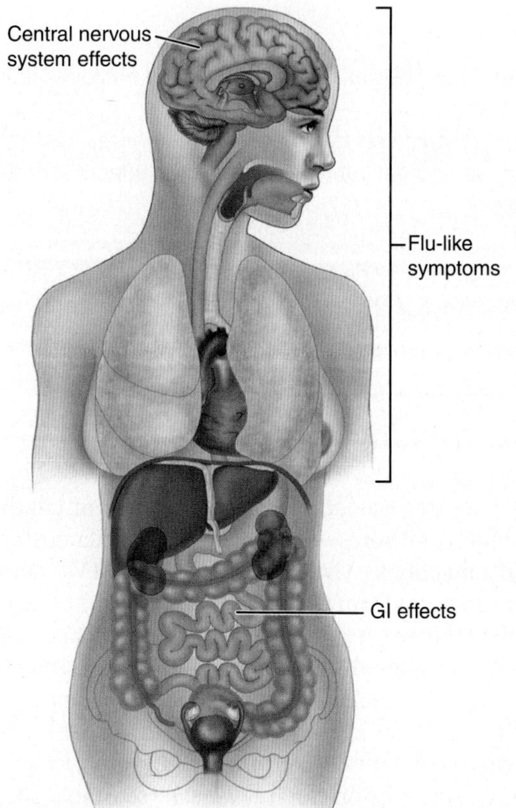

FIGURE 10.4 Common adverse effects associated with antivirals.

Clinically Important Drug–Drug Interactions

The risk of nephrotoxicity increases when agents indicated for the treatment of herpes and CMV are used in combination with other nephrotoxic drugs, such as the aminoglycoside antibiotics.

The risk of drowsiness also rises when these antiviral agents are taken with zidovudine, an antiretroviral agent.

Prototype Summary: Acyclovir

Indications: Treatment of herpes simplex virus (HSV) 1 and 2 infections; treatment of severe genital HSV infections; treatment of HSV encephalitis; acute treatment of varicella-zoster viruses; ointment for the treatment of genital herpes infections; cream for the treatment of cold sores (herpes labialis).

Actions: Inhibits viral DNA replication.

Pharmacokinetics:

Route	Onset	Peak	Duration
Oral	Varies	1.5–2 h	Not known
IV	Immediate	1 h	Not known
Topical	Not generally absorbed systemically		

$T_{1/2}$: 2.5 to 5 hours; excreted unchanged in the urine.

Adverse Effects: Headache, vertigo, tremors, nausea, vomiting, rash, nephrotoxicity.

Nursing Considerations for Patients Receiving Agents for Herpes Virus and Cytomegalovirus

Assessment: History and Examination

- Assess patients receiving DNA-active antiviral agents for contraindications or cautions, including any history of allergy to antivirals to avoid hypersensitivity reactions, renal dysfunction that might interfere with the metabolism and excretion of the drug and increase the risk of renal toxicity, severe CNS disorders that could be aggravated, and pregnancy or lactation to prevent adverse effects on the fetus or nursing baby.
- Perform a physical assessment to establish baseline data for assessing the effectiveness of the antiviral drug and the occurrence of any adverse effects associated with drug therapy.
- Assess orientation and reflexes to monitor CNS baseline and adverse effects of the drug.
- Examine skin (color, temperature, and lesions) to monitor adverse effects such as rashes.
- Evaluate renal function tests to determine baseline function of the kidneys and to assess adverse effects on the kidney and need to adjust the dose of the drug.

Nursing Conclusions

Nursing conclusions related to drug therapy might include the following:

- Impaired comfort related to GI, CNS, or local effects of the drug
- Impaired sensory (kinesthetic) perception related to CNS effects of the drug
- Knowledge deficit regarding drug therapy

Planning

- The patient will receive the best therapeutic effect from the drug therapy.
- The patient will have limited adverse effects from the drug therapy.
- The patient will have an understanding of the drug therapy, adverse effects to anticipate, and measures to relieve discomfort and improve safety.

Intervention With Rationale

- Administer the drug as soon as possible after the diagnosis has been made to improve effectiveness of the antiviral activity.
- Ensure good hydration to decrease the toxic effects on the kidneys.
- Ensure that the patient takes the complete course of the drug regimen to improve effectiveness and decrease the risk of the emergence of resistant viruses.
- Wear protective gloves when applying the drug topically to decrease the risk of exposure to the drug and inadvertent absorption.
- If CNS effects occur, provide safety measures (e.g., use of side rails, appropriate lighting, orientation, assistance) to protect the patient from injury.
- To prevent undue anxiety and increase awareness of the importance of nutrition, warn the patient that GI upset, nausea, and vomiting can occur.
- Monitor renal function periodically during treatment to ensure prompt detection of and early intervention for renal toxicity.
- Instruct the patient about the drug to enhance patient knowledge about drug therapy and to promote adherence.
- Provide the following patient teaching:
  - Avoid sexual intercourse if active genital herpes is being treated because these drugs do not cure the disease.
  - Wear protective gloves when applying topical agents.
  - If dizziness or drowsiness occurs, avoid driving and hazardous tasks.

Evaluation

- Monitor patient response to the drug (alleviation of signs and symptoms of herpes or CMV infection).
- Monitor for adverse effects (orientation and affect, GI upset, and renal function).
- Evaluate the effectiveness of the teaching plan. The patient should be able to name the drug, dosage, possible adverse effects to watch for, and specific measures to help avoid adverse effects.
- Monitor the effectiveness of comfort and safety measures and adherence to the regimen.

Key Points

- Drugs that interfere with viral DNA replication are used to treat herpes infections and CMV infections.
- These antiviral drugs are associated with GI upset and nausea, confusion, insomnia, nephrotoxicity, and dizziness.

Agents for HIV and AIDS

Human immunodeficiency virus (HIV) is a retrovirus that attacks the **helper T cells** (CD4 [cluster of differentiation 4] cells) within the immune system, leading to a decrease in immune function and AIDS or ARC. A helper T cell is a human lymphocyte that helps to initiate immune reactions in response to tissue invasion. This virus (an RNA strand) reacts with a receptor site on the CD4 cell, fuses with the membrane, and then enters the helper T cell, where it uses reverse transcriptase to copy the RNA and produce a double-stranded viral DNA. The virus uses various nucleosides found in the cell to synthesize this DNA strand. The virus uses the enzyme integrase to insert the viral DNA into the host nuclear DNA. This will change the host cell for the remainder of its life span. The cell changes into a virus-producing cell. As a result, the cell loses its ability to perform normal immune functions. The newly produced viruses migrate to the cytoplasm and assemble into immature HIV particles. Protease enzymes cleave the long polyprotein HIV chains into mature smaller, functional HIV proteins that are infectious once released from the CD4 cell. Upon release, they find a new cell to invade, and the process begins again. Eventually, as more and more viruses are released and invade more CD4 cells, the immune system loses an important mechanism responsible for propelling the immune reaction into full force when the body is invaded.

Loss of helper T-cell function causes **acquired immunodeficiency syndrome (AIDS)** and **AIDS-related complex (ARC)**, diseases that are characterized by the emergence of a variety of opportunistic infections and cancers that occur when the immune system is depressed and unable to function properly. HIV mutates over time, presenting a slightly different configuration with each new generation. Treatment of AIDS and ARC has been difficult due to: (a) the length of time the virus can remain dormant within the T cells (months to years); (b) the adverse effects of many potent drugs, which may include further depression of the immune system; and (c) the ability of the virus to mutate, causing resistance to medications. Usually, a combination of at least three different antiviral drugs is used to attack the virus at various points in its life cycle to achieve maximum effectiveness with the least amount of toxicity. The types of antiviral agents that are used to treat HIV infections are the nonnucleoside reverse transcriptase inhibitors (NNRTIs), the nucleoside reverse transcriptase inhibitors (NRTIs), the protease inhibitors, a fusion inhibitor, a CCR5 (C–C chemokine receptor type 5) coreceptor antagonist, and integrase inhibitors (see Table 10.3). Collectively, these drugs are known as antiretroviral agents.

Table 10.3 *Drugs in Focus*: Agents for HIV and AIDS

Drug Name	Dosage/Route	Usual Indications
Nonnucleoside Reverse Transcriptase Inhibitors		
delavirdine (*Rescriptor*)	*Adult*: 400 mg PO t.i.d.	Part of combination therapy regimens for treatment of HIV in adults
efavirenz (*Sustiva*)	*Adult*: 600 mg/d PO *Pediatric*: Dose determined by age and weight	Treatment of adults and children with HIV in combination with other antiretroviral agents
etravirine (*Intelence*)	*Adult*: 200 mg PO b.i.d. after a meal	Treatment of HIV in adults with treatment experience who have evidence of viral replication and HIV strains resistant to standard therapy
nevirapine (*Viramune*)	*Adult*: 200 mg/d PO for 14 d, then 200 mg PO b.i.d. *Pediatric*: 150 mg/m^2 PO for 14 d, then 150 mg/m^2 PO b.i.d.	Treatment of adults and children with HIV in combination with other antiretroviral agents
rilpivirine (*Edurant*)	*Adult*: 25 mg/d PO with food	Combination treatment of adults with HIV-1 infection
Nucleoside Reverse Transcriptase Inhibitors		
abacavir (*Ziagen*)	*Adult*: 300 mg PO b.i.d. or 600 mg/d PO *Pediatric*: 8 mg/kg PO b.i.d. or 16 mg/kg PO once a day	Combination therapy for the treatment of adults and children with HIV
didanosine (*Videx*)	*Adult*: 250–400 mg/d PO or 125–250 mg PO b.i.d. *Pediatric*: 100–120 mg/m^2 PO b.i.d.	Treatment of advanced infections in adults and children with HIV as part of combination therapy
emtricitabine (*Emtriva*)	*Adult*: 200 mg/d PO or 240 mg oral solution/d *Pediatric (3 mo to 17 y)*: 6 mg/kg/d PO to a maximum 240 mg oral solution	Part of combination therapy for treatment of HIV-1 infection
lamivudine (*Epivir*)	*Adult*: 150 mg PO b.i.d. or 300 mg/d PO *Pediatric:* Weight-based dosing	With other antiretroviral agents for the treatment of adults and children with HIV; as an oral solution for the treatment of chronic HBV

Table 10.3 *Drugs in Focus*: Agents for HIV and AIDS *(Continued)*

Drug Name	Dosage/Route	Usual Indications
stavudine (*Zerit*)	*Adult, pediatric (≥60 kg)*: 40 mg PO q12h *Adult, pediatric (30–60 kg)*: 30 mg PO q12h *Pediatric*: Other doses based on weight	Treatment of patients with HIV in combination with other antiretroviral agents
tenofovir (*Viread*)	*Adult*: 300 mg/d PO *Pediatric (2–11 y)*: 8 mg/kg/d PO (for HIV, not recommended for HBV)	Treatment of adults and children with HIV infection in combination with other antiretroviral drugs; treatment of chronic HBV
zidovudine	*Adult*: 600/d mg PO divided *Pediatric:* Weight-based dosing *Maternal*: 100 mg PO five times per day from 14-wk gestation until start of labor	Treatment of symptomatic HIV in adults and children as part of combination therapy; prevention of maternal transmission of HIV
Protease Inhibitors		
atazanavir (*Reyataz*)	*Adult*: 300 mg/d PO with ritonavir *Pediatric*: Weight-based dosing	Treatment of adults and children with HIV as part of combination therapy
darunavir (*Prezista*)	*Adult*: 600 mg PO b.i.d. with ritonavir 100 mg PO b.i.d. or 800 mg PO daily *Pediatric*: Dose based on weight and surface area	Treatment of adults and children with advanced HIV with progression following standard treatment, used as part of combination therapy that must contain ritonavir
fosamprenavir (*Lexiva*)	*Adult*: 1,400 mg PO daily with 100–200 mg/d ritonavir PO or 700 mg PO b.i.d. with ritonavir 100 mg PO b.i.d. *Pediatric*: Weight-based dosing	Part of combination therapy for the treatment of HIV
lopinavir/ritonavir (*Kaletra*)	*Adult*: Dose varies based on indication and other antivirals; 400/100 mg–800/200 mg daily or b.i.d. PO *Pediatric (14 d to 12 y)*: Weight-based dosing	Treatment of adults and children with HIV in combination with other antiretroviral agents
nelfinavir (*Viracept*)	*Adult*: 750 mg PO t.i.d. or 1,250 mg PO b.i.d. *Pediatric (2–13 y)*: 45–55 mg/kg PO b.i.d. or 25–35 mg/kg PO t.i.d.	Combination therapy for the treatment of adults and children with HIV
ritonavir (*Norvir*)	*Adult*: 600 mg PO b.i.d. *Pediatric*: 250 mg/m^2 PO b.i.d. to a max 600 mg b.i.d.	Part of combination therapy for the treatment of adults and children with HIV
saquinavir (*Invirase*)	*Adult*: 1,000 mg PO b.i.d. with ritonavir 100 mg PO b.i.d.	Treatment of adults with HIV as part of combination therapy
tipranavir (*Aptivus*)	*Adult*: 500 mg/d PO b.i.d. with 200 mg ritonavir *Pediatric*: 14 mg/kg PO b.i.d. with ritonavir	Treatment of adults and children with HIV in combination with ritonavir
Fusion Inhibitor		
enfuvirtide (*Fuzeon*)	*Adult*: 90 mg b.i.d. by subcutaneous injection *Pediatric (6–16 y)*: 2 mg/kg b.i.d. by subcutaneous injection	Part of combination therapy in treatment of patients with HIV with evidence of HIV replication despite antiretroviral therapy
CCR5 Coreceptor Antagonist		
maraviroc (*Selzentry*)	*Adult*: 300 mg PO b.i.d.; dosage may need to be adjusted based on other drugs in the regimen	Part of combination therapy for treatment of HIV-1 infections
Integrase Inhibitor		
dolutegravir (*Tivicay*)	*Adult, pediatric (≥40 kg)*: 50 mg/d PO in combination with other antiretrovirals	Part of combination therapy for treatment of HIV-1 infections
raltegravir (*Isentress*)	*Adult, pediatric 12 y and older*: 400 mg PO b.i.d. *Pediatric*: Weight-based dosing	Part of combination therapy for treatment of HIV-1 infections

AZT, zidovudine.

The HIV virus poses a serious health risk. The patient and their family will need support and teaching to cope with the disease and its treatment.

Because therapy for HIV infection involves the use of several different antiviral drugs, many are now available as combination drugs, which reduces the number of tablets a patient has to take each day. Box 10.3 discusses combination drugs.

Nonnucleoside Reverse Transcriptase Inhibitors

Nonnucleoside reverse transcriptase inhibitors (NNRTIs) have direct effects on the HIV virus's activities within the cell. The NNRTIs available include delavirdine (*Rescriptor*), efavirenz (*Sustiva*), etravirine (*Intelence*), nevirapine (*Viramune*), and rilpivirine (*Edurant*).

Therapeutic Actions and Indications

NNRTIs bind directly to HIV reverse transcriptase, blocking both RNA- and DNA-dependent DNA polymerase activities. They prevent the transfer of information that would allow the virus to carry on the formation of viral DNA. As a result, the virus is unable to take over the cell and reproduce. These antiviral agents are indicated for the treatment of patients with documented AIDS or ARC who have decreased numbers of helper T cells and evidence of increased opportunistic infections. They are used in combination with other antiviral drugs (see Table 10.3).

Pharmacokinetics

Delavirdine is rapidly absorbed from the GI tract, with peak level occurring within 1 hour. Delavirdine is extensively metabolized by the cytochrome P-450 system in the liver and is excreted through the urine and feces.

Efavirenz is absorbed rapidly from the GI tract, reaching peak level in 3 to 5 hours. Efavirenz is metabolized in the liver by the cytochrome P-450 system and is excreted in the urine and feces. It has a half-life of 52 to 76 hours.

Etravirine is rapidly absorbed from the GI tract, reaching peak level in 2.5 to 4 hours. Etravirine is metabolized in the liver by the cytochrome P-450 system, is excreted in feces, and has a half-life of 21 to 61 hours.

Nevirapine is recommended for use in adults and children older than 2 months. After rapid GI absorption with peak effect occurring at 4 hours, nevirapine is metabolized by the cytochrome P-450 system in the liver. Excretion is through the urine, and it has a half-life of 45 hours.

Rilpivirine (*Edurant*) is the newest drug in this class. It is rapidly absorbed from the GI tract, reaching peak level in 4 to 5 hours. It is metabolized in the liver and excreted in feces. It has a half-life of 50 hours.

BOX 10.3

Fixed-Combination Antiretroviral Medications

Antiretroviral medications are often used in combination tablets, capsules, or other formulations. Such combinations of multiple medications best help to decrease HIV viral load and decrease the risk of viral resistance. Having multiple medications in one dose can simplify the treatment regimen as well. Many of the combination medications can be administered once or twice daily, but the FDA has also approved a monthly injection medication.

Cabenuva is a combination of cabotegravir (an integrase inhibitor) and rilpivirine (a nonnucleoside reverse transcriptase inhibitor). It is indicated as a complete regimen for treatment of HIV-1 infection in adults to replace a previous antiretroviral regimen in those who are virologically suppressed and have not had previous treatment failure. The monthly intramuscular injection can be started after a month of oral dosing with both cabotegravir and rilpivirine to assess tolerability.

There are a few cautions about combination tablets and capsules. First, they can be expensive. Also, if a patient has an adverse reaction, it may be more difficult to evaluate which substance caused the side effect. In addition, due to fixed doses, it may be difficult to reduce doses for renal impairment or adverse effects that decrease medication tolerance. The following are some examples of fixed-dose oral combinations. When possible, a specialist practitioner should prescribe and monitor antiretroviral therapy.

Combivir, a combination of 150 mg lamivudine and 300 mg zidovudine (both nucleoside analogue reverse transcriptase inhibitors), is taken as one tablet twice a day.

Trizivir combines 300 mg abacavir, 150 mg lamivudine, and 300 mg zidovudine and is taken as one tablet twice a day. Patients taking this combination should be warned at the time the prescription is filled about the potentially serious hypersensitivity reactions associated with abacavir and should be given a written list of warning signs to watch for.

Epzicom (600 mg abacavir with 300 mg lamivudine) is taken as one tablet once a day. *Truvada* (200 mg emtricitabine with 300 mg tenofovir) is also a once-a-day tablet and is not only indicated for treatment of HIV infection but also for HIV preexposure prophylaxis. Atripla (600 mg efavirenz, 200 mg emtricitabine, and 300 mg tenofovir) is recommended for patients 18 years old and older who have already been stabilized on each antiviral individually. *Complera* combines 200 mg emtricitabine, 25 mg rilpivirine, and 300 mg tenofovir. *Triumeq* combines 50 mg dolutegravir, 600 mg abacavir, and 300 mg lamivudine and is recommended for adults who experience success with each of the drugs alone. *Odefsey* contains 200 mg emtricitabine, 25 mg rilpivirine, and 25 mg tenofovir and is not recommended for patients with renal impairment. *Stribild* contains 150 mg elvitegravir, 200 mg emtricitabine, and 300 mg tenofovir combined with cobicistat, which makes the drugs more effective. *Genvoya* combines cobicistat with 150 mg elvitegravir, 200 mg emtricitabine, and 10 mg tenofovir alafenamide. *Descovy* combines 200 mg emtricitabine with 25 mg tenofovir alafenamide.

Contraindications and Cautions

There are no NNRTIs that are the preferred regimen in pregnancy, so use should be limited to situations in which the benefits clearly outweigh any risks. It is suggested that people not breast or chestfeed if they are infected with HIV. Safety for the use of delavirdine in children has not been established.

Adverse Effects

The adverse effects most commonly experienced with these drugs are GI related—dry mouth, constipation or diarrhea, nausea, abdominal pain, and dyspepsia. Dizziness, blurred vision, and headache have also been reported. A flulike syndrome of fever, muscle aches and pains, fatigue, and loss of appetite often occurs with the anti-HIV drugs, but these signs and symptoms may also be related to the underlying disease. A rare but serious rash due to Stevens–Johnson syndrome can occur.

Clinically Important Drug–Drug Interactions

Life-threatening effects can occur if delavirdine is combined with antiarrhythmics, clarithromycin, sildenafil, antituberculosis drugs, calcium channel blockers, warfarin, quinidine, indinavir, saquinavir, or dapsone. These combinations should be avoided if at all possible. There is a risk of serious adverse effects if efavirenz is combined with midazolam, rifabutin, triazolam, or ergot derivatives; these combinations should be avoided. There may be a lack of effectiveness if nevirapine is combined with hormonal contraceptives or protease inhibitors. St. John's wort should not be used with these drugs; a decrease in antiviral effects can occur. There are many more clinically significant drug–drug interactions than are listed here. It is best to check for medication interactions whenever changing the medication regimen.

Prototype Summary: Nevirapine

Indications: Treatment of HIV-1–infected patients who have experienced clinical or immunological deterioration, in combination with other antiretrovirals.

Actions: Binds to HIV-1 reverse transcriptase and blocks replication of the HIV by changing the structure of the HIV enzyme.

Pharmacokinetics:

Route	Onset	Peak
Oral	Rapid	4 h

$T_{1/2}$: 45 hours for single dose, then 25 to 30 hours when administered chronically; metabolized in the liver and excreted in the urine.

Adverse Effects: Headache, nausea, vomiting, diarrhea, rash, liver dysfunction, chills, fever.

Nucleoside Reverse Transcriptase Inhibitors

The **nucleoside reverse transcriptase inhibitors** (NRTIs) (see Table 10.3) were the first class of drugs developed to treat HIV infections. They are often prescribed in pairs as the "backbone" of antiviral therapy. These are drugs that compete with the naturally occurring nucleosides within a human cell that the virus would need to develop. The NRTIs include the following agents: abacavir (*Ziagen*), didanosine (*Videx*), emtricitabine (*Emtriva*), lamivudine (*Epivir*), stavudine (*Zerit*), tenofovir (*Viread*, *Vemlidy*), and zidovudine (*Retrovir*).

Therapeutic Actions and Indications

NRTIs compete with the naturally occurring nucleosides within the cell that the virus uses to build the DNA chain. These nucleosides, however, lack a substance needed to extend the DNA chain. As a result, the DNA chain cannot lengthen and cannot insert itself into the host DNA. Thus, the virus cannot reproduce. NRTIs are used as part of combination therapy for the treatment of HIV infection. See Table 10.3 for usual indications for each of these agents.

Pharmacokinetics

Abacavir is an oral drug that is rapidly absorbed from the GI tract. It is metabolized in the liver and excreted in feces and urine and has a half-life of 1 to 2 hours.

Didanosine is rapidly destroyed in an acidic environment and therefore must be taken in a buffered form. It reaches peak level in 15 to 75 minutes. Didanosine undergoes intracellular metabolism and has a half-life of 8 to 24 hours. It is excreted in the urine.

Emtricitabine has the advantage of being a one-capsule-a-day therapy. Emtricitabine has a rapid onset and peaks in 1 to 2 hours. It has a half-life of 10 hours. After being metabolized in the liver, it is excreted in the urine and feces. The dose needs to be reduced in patients with renal impairment. It has been associated with severe and even fatal hepatomegaly with steatosis, a fatty degeneration of the liver.

Lamivudine is rapidly absorbed from the GI tract and is excreted primarily unchanged in the urine. It peaks within 4 hours and has a half-life of 5 to 7 hours. Because excretion depends on renal function, dose reduction is recommended in the presence of renal impairment. The drug is available as an oral solution, *Epivir-HBV*; it is also recommended for the treatment of chronic hepatitis B.

Stavudine is rapidly absorbed from the GI tract, reaching peak level in 1 hour. Most of the drug is excreted unchanged in the urine, making it important to reduce dose and monitor patients carefully in the presence of renal dysfunction. It can be used for adults and children and is only available in an extended release form, allowing for once-a-day dosing.

Tenofovir is a newer drug that affects the virus at a slightly different point in replication—a nucleotide that becomes a nucleoside. It is rapidly absorbed from the GI tract, reaching peak level in 45 to 75 minutes. Its metabolism is not known, but it is excreted in the urine.

Zidovudine was one of the first drugs found to be effective in the treatment of AIDS. It is rapidly absorbed from the GI tract, with peak level occurring in 30 to 75 minutes. Zidovudine is metabolized in the liver and excreted in the urine. It has a half-life of 1 hour.

Contraindications and Cautions

Several of the NRTIs are components of preferred treatment regimens during pregnancy. Patients infected with HIV are urged not to breast or chestfeed. Tenofovir, zidovudine, and emtricitabine should be used with caution in the presence of hepatic dysfunction or severe renal impairment because of their effects on the liver and kidneys. Zidovudine should also be used with caution with any bone marrow suppression because it could aggravate the suppression.

Adverse Effects

Serious-to-fatal hypersensitivity reactions have occurred with abacavir, and it must be stopped immediately at any sign of a hypersensitivity reaction (fever, chills, rash, fatigue, GI upset, flulike symptoms).

Serious pancreatitis, hepatomegaly, and neurological problems have been reported with didanosine, which is why its use is limited to the treatment of advanced infections.

Emtricitabine has been associated with severe and even fatal hepatomegaly with steatosis.

Severe hepatomegaly with steatosis has been reported with tenofovir, so it must be used with extreme caution in any patient with hepatic impairment or lactic acidosis. Patients also need to be alerted that the drug may cause changes in body fat distribution, with loss of fat from arms, legs, and face and deposition of fat in the trunk, neck, and breasts.

Severe bone marrow suppression has occurred with zidovudine. Anemia, agranulocytosis, and thrombocytopenia can result from the bone marrow suppression.

Clinically Significant Drug–Drug Interactions

Tenofovir can cause large increases in the serum level of didanosine. If both of these drugs are given, tenofovir should be given 2 hours before or 1 hour after didanosine. Lamivudine and zalcitabine inhibit the effects of each other and should not be used together. Severe toxicity can occur if abacavir is combined with alcohol; therefore, this combination should be avoided. Didanosine can cause decreased effects of several antibiotics and antifungals; any antibiotic or antifungal started with didanosine should be evaluated carefully. There is an increased risk of potentially fatal pancreatitis if stavudine is combined with didanosine and increased risk of severe hepatomegaly if it is combined with other nonnucleoside antivirals; these combinations are often used, and the patient needs to be monitored very closely. There have been reports of severe drowsiness and lethargy when zidovudine is combined with cyclosporine; warn the patient to take appropriate safety precautions.

Prototype Summary: Zidovudine

Indications: Management of adults with symptomatic HIV infection in combination with other antiretrovirals; prevention of maternal–fetal HIV transmission.

Actions: A thymidine analogue that is activated to a triphosphate form, which inhibits the replication of various retroviruses, including HIV.

Pharmacokinetics:

Route	Onset	Peak
Oral	Varies	30–90 min
IV	Rapid	End of infusion

$T_{1/2}$: 30 to 60 minutes; metabolized in the liver and excreted in the urine.

Adverse Effects: Headache, insomnia, dizziness, nausea, diarrhea, fever, rash, bone marrow suppression.

Protease Inhibitors

The **protease inhibitors** block protease activity within the HIV virus. The protease inhibitors that are available for use include atazanavir (*Reyataz*), darunavir (*Prezista*), fosamprenavir (*Lexiva*), lopinavir/ritonavir (*Kaletra*), nelfinavir (*Viracept*), ritonavir (*Norvir*), saquinavir (*Invirase*), and tipranavir (*Aptivus*).

Therapeutic Actions and Indications

Protease is essential for the maturation of an infectious virus; without it, an HIV particle is immature and noninfective, unable to fuse with, and inject itself into a cell. All of these drugs are used as part of combination therapy for the treatment of HIV infection (see Table 10.3).

Pharmacokinetics

Atazanavir is rapidly absorbed from the GI tract and can be taken with food. After metabolism in the liver, it is excreted in the urine and feces with a half-life of 6.5 to 7.9 hours. It is not recommended for patients with severe hepatic impairment; for those with moderate hepatic impairment, the dose should be reduced.

Darunavir is well absorbed from the GI tract, reaching peak level in 2.5 to 4 hours. It is metabolized in the liver and excreted in the urine and feces. It has a half-life of 15 hours. It is not recommended for patients with severe hepatic impairment.

Fosamprenavir is rapidly absorbed after oral administration, reaching peak level in 1.5 to 4 hours. It is metabolized in the liver and excreted in the urine and feces.

Lopinavir is used as a fixed combination drug that combines lopinavir and ritonavir. The ritonavir inhibits the metabolism of lopinavir, leading to increased lopinavir serum levels and effectiveness. (Box 10.4 reviews the dose calculation with lopinavir.) It is readily absorbed from the GI tract, reaching peak level in 3 to 4 hours, and undergoes extensive hepatic metabolism by the cytochrome P-450 system. Lopinavir is excreted in urine and feces.

Tipranavir is used in combination with 200 mg of ritonavir for the treatment of HIV infection in adults. It is taken orally with food, two 250-mg capsules each day with the ritonavir. It is slowly absorbed, reaching peak level in 2.9 hours. It is metabolized in the liver and has a half-life of 4.8 to 6 hours; excretion is through urine and feces.

Nelfinavir is well absorbed from the GI tract, reaching peak levels in 2 to 4 hours. Nelfinavir is metabolized in the liver using the cytochrome P-450 CY3A system, and caution must be used in patients with any hepatic dysfunction. It is primarily excreted in the feces, with a half-life of 3.5 to 5 hours. Because there is little renal excretion, this is considered a good drug for patients with renal impairment.

Ritonavir is rapidly absorbed from the GI tract, reaching peak level in 2 to 4 hours. Ritonavir undergoes extensive metabolism in the liver and is excreted in the feces and urine.

Saquinavir is slowly absorbed from the GI tract and is metabolized in the liver by the cytochrome P-450 3A4, so it must be used cautiously in the presence of hepatic dysfunction. It is primarily excreted in the feces and has a short half-life.

Box 10.4 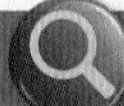 **Focus on Calculations**

The health care provider prescribes lopinavir/ritonavir (*Kaletra*), 10 mg/kg, PO b.i.d. for a 14-year-old child weighing 50 kg. The drug comes in 200/50-mg tablets. How many tablets should the child receive at each dose?

To figure out the ordered dose, perform the following calculation:

$$10 \text{ mg/kg} \times 50 \text{ kg} = 500 \text{ mg/dose}$$

Then use

$$200 \text{ mg } (X) = 500 \text{ mg (tablet)}$$

$$X = \frac{500 \text{ mg (tablet)}}{200 \text{ mg}}$$

$$X = 2.5 \text{ mg (tablet)}$$

You would give 2.5 of the 200-mg tablets.

You notice that it is also available in an 80-mg/mL solution. How much solution would you give?

$$\frac{500 \text{ mg}}{\text{dose}} = \frac{80 \text{ mg}}{\text{mL}}$$

$$80 \text{ mg(dose)} = 500 \text{ mg(mL)}$$

$$\text{dose} = \frac{500 \text{ mg/(mL)}}{80 \text{ mg}}$$

$$\text{dose} = 6.25 \text{ mL}$$

You would give 6.25 mL of the 80-mg/mL solution.

Contraindications and Cautions

There are several protease inhibitors that are considered preferred therapy during pregnancy. It is suggested that patients not breast or chestfeed if they are infected with HIV.

Patients with hepatic dysfunction should receive a lower dose of fosamprenavir. Patients with severe hepatic dysfunction should not receive darunavir, as it has not been studied in this population. Patients receiving tipranavir must have their liver function monitored regularly because of the possibility of potentially fatal liver dysfunction. Saquinavir must also be used cautiously in the presence of hepatic dysfunction.

Patients receiving darunavir may also be at risk for developing diabetes mellitus or hyperglycemia and may require dosage adjustments if being treated with antidiabetic drugs. Darunavir is also associated with mild to severe dermatologic reactions including Stevens–Johnson syndrome, and the drug should be stopped if a severe reaction develops.

Darunavir should not be used in children younger than 3 years of age because of the potential for toxic effects.

Adverse Effects

As with the other antivirals, patients taking these drugs often experience GI effects, including nausea, vomiting, diarrhea, anorexia, and changes in liver function. Elevated cholesterol and triglyceride levels may occur. There is often a redistribution of fat to the face, back of the neck, and upper back, with thinning of arms and legs. Rashes, pruritus, and the potentially fatal Stevens–Johnson syndrome have also occurred.

Clinically Significant Drug–Drug Interactions

Tipranavir, darunavir, and fosamprenavir have been shown to interact with many other drugs. Before administering these drugs, it is important to check a drug guide to assess for potential interactions with other drugs being given.

Many potentially serious toxic effects can occur when ritonavir is taken with nonsedating antihistamines, sedatives/hypnotics, or antiarrhythmics because of the activity of ritonavir in the liver. Patients with hepatic dysfunction are at increased risk for serious effects when taking ritonavir and require a reduced dose and close monitoring. Ritonavir decreases levels of estradiol in oral contraceptives.

Protease inhibitors can be reduced with concurrent use of phenobarbital, phenytoin, carbamazepine, and St. John's wort. Grapefruit juice can decrease protease inhibitors' metabolism.

Prototype Summary: Fosamprenavir

Indications: Management of symptomatic HIV infection in adults in combination with other antiretrovirals.

Actions: Inhibits protease activity, leading to the formation of immature, noninfectious virus particles.

Pharmacokinetics:

Route	Onset	Peak
Oral	Varies	1.5–4 h

$T_{1/2}$: 7.7 hours; metabolized in the liver and excreted in the feces and urine.

Adverse Effects: Headache, mood changes, nausea, diarrhea, fatigue, rash, Stevens–Johnson syndrome, redistribution of body fat (increase of fat to the face, back of the neck, and upper back; thinning of arms and legs).

Fusion Inhibitor

The **fusion inhibitor** prevents the fusion of the virus with the human cellular membrane, which prevents the HIV-1 virus from entering the cell (Table 10.3). Enfuvirtide (*Fuzeon*) is used in combination with other antiretroviral agents to treat adults and children older than 6 years who have evidence of HIV-1 replication despite ongoing antiretroviral therapy.

Enfuvirtide is given by subcutaneous injection twice a day and peaks in effect in 3 to 12 hours. After metabolism in the liver, it is recycled in the tissues and not excreted. The half-life of enfuvirtide is 3.2 to 4.4 hours. Enfuvirtide is contraindicated with hypersensitivity to any component of the drug and in patients who are breast or chestfeeding. It should be used with caution in the presence of lung disease or pregnancy. The drug has been associated with insomnia, depression, peripheral neuropathy, nausea, diarrhea, pneumonia, and injection site reactions. There are no reported drug interactions, but caution should be used when it is combined with any other drug.

Prototype Summary: Enfuvirtide

Indications: Treatment of patients with HIV-1 who have experienced clinical or immunological deterioration after treatment with other agents, in combination with other antiretrovirals.

Actions: Prevents the entry of the HIV-1 virus into cells by inhibiting the fusion of the virus membrane with the cellular membrane.

Pharmacokinetics:

Route	Onset	Peak
Subcutaneous	Slow	4–8 h

$T_{1/2}$: 3.2 to 4.4 hours; metabolized in the liver, tissues recycle the amino acids, not excreted.

Adverse Effects: Headache, nausea, vomiting, diarrhea, rash, anorexia, pneumonia, chills, injection site reactions.

CCR5 Coreceptor Antagonist

Maraviroc (*Selzentry*) is a **CCR5 coreceptor antagonist**, which means it blocks the receptor site on the T-cell membrane with which the HIV virus needs to interact to enter the cell. It is indicated for the treatment of HIV in adults as part of combination therapy with other antivirals. Maraviroc is rapidly absorbed from the GI tract, metabolized in the liver, and excreted primarily through the feces. It has a half-life of 14 to 18 hours. Maraviroc should not be used with known hypersensitivity to any component of the drug or by patients who are breast or chestfeeding. The safety and efficacy of maraviroc in children has not been established. Caution should be used in the presence of liver disease or coinfection with hepatitis B because of the risk of serious hepatic toxicity. Patients at increased risk for cardiovascular events or with hypotension should be monitored very closely if this is the drug of choice for them. As with other antivirals, it should be used in pregnancy only if the benefit outweighs the potential risk to the fetus.

Severe hepatotoxicity has been reported with this drug, often preceded by a systemic allergic reaction with eosinophilia and rash. Maraviroc has a boxed warning regarding the risk for serious hepatotoxicity. Regular monitoring of liver function should be routine when using this drug. CNS effects include dizziness, orthostatic hypotension, and paresthesia; patients experiencing these should be cautioned to take measures to assure safety. Patients may also be at increased risk of upper respiratory tract infections because of the way the drug affects the cell membrane of the CD4 cells. Appropriate precautions are necessary.

There is a risk of increased serum levels and toxicity when combined with cytochrome P-450 CYP3A inhibitors (ketoconazole, lopinavir/ritonavir, ritonavir, saquinavir, atazanavir, delavirdine), and the maraviroc dose should be adjusted accordingly. Decreased serum levels and loss of effectiveness may occur if maraviroc is combined with CYP3A inducers (nevirapine, rifampin, efavirenz), and the maraviroc dose should be adjusted accordingly. Patients should not use St. John's wort while on this drug because there is a loss of antiviral effects when the two are combined.

Prototype Summary: Maraviroc

Indications: Combination antiretroviral treatment of adults infected with CCR5-tropic HIV-1 who have evidence of viral replication and HIV-1 strains resistant to multiple antiretroviral agents.

Actions: Selectively binds to the human chemokine receptor CCR5 on the cell membrane, preventing interaction of HIV-1 and CCR5, which is necessary for the HIV to enter the cell; therefore, HIV cannot enter the cell and cannot multiply.

Pharmacokinetics:

Route	Onset	Peak
Oral	Slow	0.5–4 h

$T_{1/2}$: 14 to 28 hours; metabolized in the liver, excreted in the feces and urine.

Adverse Effects: Dizziness, paresthesia, nausea, vomiting, diarrhea, cough, upper respiratory infection (URI), fever, musculoskeletal symptoms, hepatotoxicity.

Integrase Strand Transfer Inhibitors

Integrase strand transfer inhibitors (INSTIs) inhibit the activity of the virus-specific enzyme integrase, an encoded enzyme needed for viral replication. Blocking this enzyme prevents the formation of the HIV-1 provirus and leads to a decrease in viral load and an increase in active CD4 cells. These medications are often used in combination with two nucleoside analogues. Raltegravir (*Isentress*) is rapidly absorbed from the GI tract and metabolized in the liver. It has a half-life of 9 hours and is excreted in the urine and feces. Dolutegravir (*Tivicay*) is rapidly absorbed, reaching peak level in 2 to 3 hours. It is metabolized in the liver, excreted in the urine and feces, and has a half-life of 14 hours.

Integrase inhibitors are contraindicated with known hypersensitivity to any component of the drug. Monitor for rash that can develop into Stevens–Johnson syndrome. Caution should be used if the patient is at risk for rhabdomyolysis or myopathy and during pregnancy. Liver failure and/or renal impairment can occur. Suicidal ideation has been reported occasionally in patients taking these medications. Common adverse effects include headache, insomnia, weight gain, dizziness, and an increased risk for the development of rhabdomyolysis and myopathy. There is a risk of decreased serum levels if combined with rifampin; the patient should be monitored and the dose adjusted if this combination must be used. Patients should avoid the use of St. John's wort, which can interfere with the effectiveness of INSTIs.

Prototype Summary: Raltegravir

Indications: In combination with other antiviral agents for the treatment of HIV-1 infection in treatment-experienced adult patients who have evidence of viral replication and HIV-1 strains resistant to multiple antiretroviral agents.

Actions: Inhibits the activity of the virus-specific enzyme integrase, an encoded enzyme needed for viral replication. Blocking this enzyme prevents the formation of the HIV-1 provirus and leads to a decrease in viral load and an increase in active CD4 cells.

Pharmacokinetics:

Route	Onset	Peak
Oral	Rapid	3 h

$T_{1/2}$: 9 hours; metabolized in the liver, excreted in the feces and urine.

Adverse Effects: Headache, dizziness, nausea, vomiting, diarrhea, fever, rhabdomyolysis.

Nursing Considerations for Patients Receiving Agents for HIV and AIDS

Assessment: History and Examination

- Assess for contraindications and cautions for the use of these drugs: any history of allergy to antivirals to avoid hypersensitivity reactions, renal or hepatic dysfunction that might interfere with the metabolism and excretion of the drug, any medication or herbal substances that may decrease the effectiveness of the medication, and pregnancy or lactation because of possible adverse effects on the fetus or infant.
- Perform a physical assessment to establish baseline data for assessing the effectiveness of the drug and the occurrence of any adverse effects associated with drug therapy.
- Assess level of orientation and reflexes to evaluate any CNS effects of the drug.

(continues on page 160)

- Examine the skin (color, temperature, and lesions) to monitor for adverse effects of the drug.
- Check temperature to monitor for infections.
- Evaluate hepatic and renal function tests to determine baseline function of the kidneys and liver. Check results of a complete blood count with differential to monitor bone marrow activity and helper T-cell number to determine the severity of the disease and indicate the effectiveness of the drugs.

Nursing Conclusions

Nursing conclusions related to drug therapy might include the following:

- Impaired comfort related to GI, CNS, or dermatological effects of the drugs
- Altered sensory (kinesthetic) perception related to CNS effects of the drugs
- Malnutrition related to GI effects of the drugs
- Injury related to CNS effects of the drugs
- Knowledge deficit regarding drug therapy

Planning

- The patient will receive the best therapeutic effect from the drug therapy.
- The patient will have limited adverse effects from the drug therapy.
- The patient will have an understanding of the drug therapy, adverse effects to anticipate, and measures to relieve discomfort and improve safety.

Intervention With Rationale

- Monitor renal and hepatic function before and periodically during therapy to detect changes requiring dose adjustments or additional treatment as needed.
- Ensure that the patient consistently takes the drug regimen and takes all drugs included in a particular combination to improve the effectiveness of the drug and decrease the risk of emergence of resistant viral strains.
- Administer the drug around the clock, if indicated, to provide the critical concentration needed for the drug to be effective.
- Monitor nutritional status if GI effects are severe, and take appropriate action to maintain balanced nutrition, including small, frequent meals to provide protein and other nutrients.
- Stop use of the drug if severe rash occurs, especially if accompanied by blisters, fever, and other signs, to avert potentially serious reactions.
- If CNS effects occur, provide safety precautions (e.g., the use of side rails, appropriate lighting, orientation, assistance) to protect patient from injury.
- Teach the patient about the drugs prescribed to enhance patient knowledge about drug therapy and to promote adherence. Include as a teaching point the fact that these drugs do not cure the disease, so appropriate precautions should still be taken to prevent transmission.
- Provide the following patient teaching:
  - Have regular medical care.
  - Set up a regular schedule for taking all of your drugs at the correct time during the day.
  - Have periodic blood tests for renal and hepatic function and a complete blood count (CBC), which are necessary to monitor the effectiveness and toxicity of the drug.
  - Realize that GI upset, nausea, and vomiting may occur but that efforts must be taken to maintain adequate nutrition.
  - If dizziness or drowsiness occurs, avoid driving and hazardous tasks.
  - Report extreme fatigue, severe headache, difficulty breathing, or severe rash to a health care provider.

See the "Critical Thinking Scenario" for a case study and focused follow-up for the antiviral agents used for HIV and AIDS. See Box 10.5 for information on an antidiarrheal medication available to help patients with diarrhea caused by antiretroviral drugs.

BOX 10.5

An Antidiarrheal Drug for Patients on Antiretroviral Agents

One of the potentially serious adverse effects of antiretroviral drugs is diarrhea, which can lead to dehydration, skin breakdown, and infection. Crofelemer (*Mytesi*) is an antidiarrheal agent that works in the GI tract to stimulate chloride ion channels and calcium channels. This blocks chloride secretion and high-volume water loss in diarrhea and helps to normalize the flow of chloride and water in the GI tract. The drug is approved for symptomatic diarrhea in adults on antiretroviral therapy. It is very important to make sure that the diarrhea is not being caused by an infectious process. The oral tablets (125-mg extended release) must be swallowed whole and are taken twice a day. The drug is not recommended for use in pregnancy, so patients who can become pregnant should be encouraged to use contraceptive measures. Patients who are breast or chestfeeding need to be advised to find another method of feeding the baby.

CRITICAL THINKING SCENARIO
Antiviral Agents for HIV and AIDS

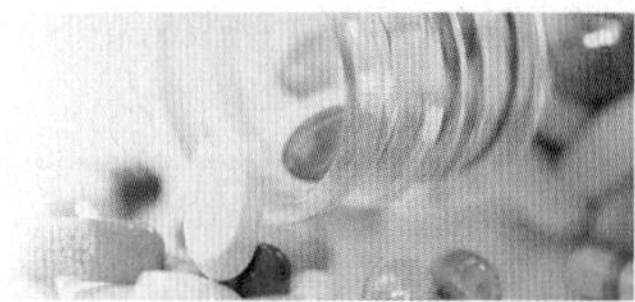

THE SITUATION

H.P. is a 34-year-old attorney who was diagnosed with AIDS, having had a positive HIV test 10 years ago. Although their helper T-cell count had been stabilized with treatment with zidovudine and efavirenz, it recently dropped remarkably. H.P. presents with numerous opportunistic infections and Kaposi sarcoma. H.P. admits that they have been under tremendous stress at work and at home in the last few weeks. They begin a combination regimen of abacavir/dolutegravir/lamivudine.

Critical Thinking

What are the important nursing implications in this case?
What role would stress play in the progress of this disease?
What specific issues should be discussed?
What other clinical implications should be considered?

DISCUSSION

Combination therapy with antivirals has been found to be effective in decreasing some of the morbidity and mortality associated with HIV and AIDS. However, this treatment does not cure the disease. H.P. needs to understand that opportunistic infections can still occur and that regular medical help should be sought. They also need to understand that these drugs may help to decrease the risk of transmitting HIV by sexual contact or through blood contamination if the drugs decrease the viral load to nondetectable levels.

It is important to make a dosing schedule for H.P., or even to prepare a weekly drug box, to ensure that H.P. takes all medications as indicated. It is helpful that the newer combination medications have more convenient dosing, once or twice a day. H.P. should also receive interventions to help them decrease stress because activation of the sympathetic nervous system during periods of stress depresses the immune system. Further depression of H.P.'s immune system could accelerate the development of opportunistic infections and decrease the effectiveness of the antiviral drugs. Measures that could be used to decrease stress should be discussed and tried with H.P.

Discussing the adverse effects that H.P. may experience is important because GI upset, diarrhea, and discomfort may occur while they are taking antiretroviral medications. Small, frequent meals may help alleviate the discomfort. It is important that every effort be made to maintain H.P.'s nutritional state, and a nutritional consultation may be necessary if GI effects are severe. H.P. also may experience headaches, dizziness, fatigue, and confusion, which could cause more problems for them at work and may necessitate changes in their workload. There is a boxed warning for *Triumeq* regarding multiorgan hypersensitivity reactions to abacavir. Before starting the medication, patients should be screened for the HLA-B*5701 allele, since people who carry this allele are at higher risk of severe hypersensitivity reactions. In addition, there is a warning regarding severe exacerbation of hepatitis B in patients who have a hepatitis B coinfection and have discontinued lamivudine. These patients need their liver function monitored frequently and, when indicated, anti-hepatitis B treatment. It is important that a health care provider work consistently with H.P. to help them to manage their disease and treatment as effectively as possible.

NURSING CARE GUIDE FOR H.P.: ANTIVIRAL AGENTS FOR HIV AND AIDS

Assessment: History and Examination

- Allergies to any of these drugs
- Bone marrow depression
- Renal or liver dysfunction
- Skin: color, lesions, texture
- CNS: affect, reflexes, orientation
- GI: abdominal and liver evaluation
- Hematological: complete blood count (CBC) and differential; viral load; T-cell levels; renal and hepatic function tests

Nursing Conclusions

- Impaired comfort related to GI, skin, CNS effects
- Altered sensory perception (kinesthetic) related to CNS effects
- Malnutrition related to GI effects
- Knowledge deficit regarding drug therapy

Planning

- The patient will receive the best therapeutic effect from the drug therapy.
- The patient will have limited adverse effects from the drug therapy.
- The patient will have an understanding of the drug therapy, adverse effects to anticipate, and measures to relieve discomfort and improve safety.

Intervention

- Screen for HLA-B*5701 allele before starting medication.
- Monitor liver function.
- Monitor CD4 count and HIV viral load.
- Provide comfort and implement safety measures: assistance, temperature control, lighting control, mouth care, back rubs.
- Provide small, frequent meals, and monitor nutritional status.

(continues on page 162)

- Monitor for opportunistic infections and arrange treatment as indicated.
- Provide support and reassurance for managing drug effects and discomfort.
- Provide patient teaching regarding drug name, dosage, adverse effects, warnings, precautions, use of OTC or herbal remedies, and signs to report.

Evaluation

- Evaluate drug effects, including relief of signs and symptoms of AIDS and ARC stabilization of helper T-cell levels.
- Monitor for adverse effects, including GI alterations, rash, dizziness, confusion, headache, and fever.
- Monitor for drug–drug interactions as indicated for each drug.
- Evaluate effectiveness of patient teaching plan.
- Evaluate effectiveness of comfort and safety measures.

PATIENT TEACHING FOR H.P.

A combination of antiviral drugs has been prescribed to treat your HIV infection. These drugs work in combination to stop the replication of HIV, to control AIDS, and to maintain the functioning of your immune system. The combination of medications is in one tablet to be taken daily with or without food. These drugs are not a cure for HIV, AIDS, or ARC. Opportunistic infections may occur, and regular medical follow-up should be sought to manage the disease.

These drugs do not eliminate the risk of transmission of HIV to others by sexual contact or by blood contamination; use appropriate precautions.

Common effects of these drugs include the following:

- Dizziness, weakness, and loss of feeling: Change positions slowly. If you feel drowsy, avoid driving and dangerous activities.
- Headache, fever, and muscle aches: Analgesics may be ordered to alleviate this discomfort. Consult with your health care provider.
- Nausea, loss of appetite, and change in taste: Small, frequent meals may help. It is important to try to maintain good nutrition. Consult your health care provider if this becomes a problem.
- Report any of the following to your health care provider: excessive fatigue, lethargy, severe headache, difficulty breathing, or skin rash.
- Avoid OTC medications and herbal therapies. Many of them interact with your drugs and may make them ineffective. If you feel that you need one of these, check with your health care provider first.
- Schedule regular medical evaluations, including blood tests, which are needed to monitor the effects of these drugs on your body so we may adjust doses as needed.
- Tell any doctor, nurse, or other health care provider that you are taking these drugs.
- Keep all medications out of the reach of children. Do not share these drugs with other people.

EVALUATION

- Monitor patient response to the drug (alleviation or reduction of signs and symptoms of AIDS or ARC and maintenance of helper T-cell levels).
- Monitor for adverse effects, including level of orientation and affect, GI upset, renal and hepatic function, skin, and levels of blood components.
- Evaluate the effectiveness of the teaching plan. The patient should be able to name the drug, dosage, possible adverse effects to watch for, and specific measures to help avoid adverse effects.
- Monitor the effectiveness of comfort and safety measures and adherence to the regimen.

Key Points

- The HIV virus infects helper T cells, leading to a loss of immune function and the development of opportunistic infections.
- Drugs used to treat HIV usually are given in combination to affect the virus at various points in the body: NNRTIs, and NRTIs block RNA and DNA activity in the cell; protease inhibitors prevent maturation of the virus; fusion inhibitors prevent the entry of the virus into the cell; CCR5 coreceptor antagonists prevent the virus from reacting with the receptor on the cell membrane, preventing its entry into the cell; and integrase strand transfer inhibitors block an enzyme essential for formation of the provirus within the cell, leading to a decrease in the number of virus particles.
- Patients taking drugs to treat HIV need to take all of the medications continuously as prescribed and take precautions to prevent the spread of the disease to others.

Anti-Hepatitis B Agents

Hepatitis B virus (HBV) is a serious to potentially fatal viral infection of the liver. HBV can be spread by blood or blood products, sexual contact, or contaminated needles or instruments. Health care workers are at especially high risk for contracting HBV due to needle sticks. HBV has a higher mortality than other types of hepatitis. Individuals who are infected may also develop a chronic condition or become a carrier. HBV can be treated with interferons (see Chapter 17) or antiviral medications. In 2004 and 2005, adefovir (*Hepsera*) and entecavir (*Baraclude*) were the first drugs approved specifically for treating chronic HBV. Tenofovir alafenamide (*Vemlidy*) is a NRTI indicated for HBV treatment (see Table 10.4). Lamivudine and tenofovir disoproxil are NRTIs that have dual indications for treating both HIV and HBV (see Table 10.3).

Therapeutic Actions and Indications

All of these antiviral drugs are indicated for the treatment of adults with chronic HBV who have evidence of active viral replication and either evidence of persistent elevations in serum aminotransferases or histologically active disease. The drugs inhibit reverse transcriptase in HBV and cause DNA chain termination, leading to blocked viral replication and decreased viral load (see Table 10.4).

Pharmacokinetics

These drugs are rapidly absorbed from the GI tract, with the peak effect occurring in 0.5 to 1.5 hours for entecavir and tenofovir alafenamide and in 0.5 to 4 hours for adefovir. Entecavir, tenofovir alafenamide, and adefovir are metabolized in the liver and excreted in the urine. Adefovir has a half-life of 7.5 hours; entecavir has a half-life of 128 to 149 hours; and tenofovir alafenamide has a half-life of about 0.5 hours. It is not known whether these drugs cross the placenta or enter human milk.

Contraindications and Cautions

These drugs are contraindicated with any known allergy to the drugs to prevent hypersensitivity reactions and with lactation because of potential toxicity to the infant. Use caution when administering these drugs to patients with renal impairment and severe liver disease because of increased toxicity with these drugs and to patients who are pregnant because the effects on the fetus are not known. Tenofovir alafenamide should not be used with patients who have HIV infection or CrCl < 15 mL/min unless they are on hemodialysis.

Table 10.4 *Drugs in Focus*: Anti-Hepatitis B Agents

Drug Name	Dosage/Route	Usual Indications
adefovir (*Hepsera*)	*Adult, pediatric 12 y and older:* 10 mg/d PO Reduce dose with renal impairment	Treatment of HBV with evidence of active viral replication and persistent elevation of liver enzymes
entecavir (*Baraclude*)	*Adult, pediatric (≥16 y):* 0.5 mg/d PO *If also receiving lamivudine:* 1 mg/d PO Reduce dose with renal impairment	Treatment of chronic HBV in adults with evidence of active viral replication and persistent liver enzyme elevation
tenofovir alafenamide (*Vemlidy*)	*Adult:* 25 mg/d PO; not recommended if CrCl < 15 mL/min if not on hemodialysis	Treatment of chronic HBV infection in adults with compensated liver disease

Adverse Effects

The adverse effects most frequently seen with these drugs are headache, dizziness, nausea, diarrhea, and elevated liver enzymes. Severe hepatomegaly with steatosis, sometimes fatal, has been reported with adefovir use. Lactic acidosis and renal impairment have been reported with entecavir, tenofovir alafenamide, and adefovir. A potential risk for HBV exacerbation could occur when the drugs are stopped. Therefore, teach patients the importance of not running out of their drugs and use extreme caution when discontinuing these drugs.

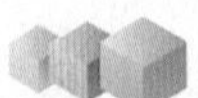
Concept Mastery Alert

Treatment of Hepatitis B

Not all people with HBV are treated with antiviral medications. The medications are primarily indicated for patients with cirrhosis and/or elevated alanine transaminase (ALT) levels that can be a sign of liver damage. It is best if HBV treatment is guided by a liver specialist. Premature discontinuation of antiviral treatment for HBV can cause severe acute exacerbations of HBV. Liver function should be monitored closely in all patients.

Prototype Summary: Adefovir

Indications: Treatment of chronic HBV in adults with evidence of active viral replication and either evidence of persistent elevations in alanine aminotransferase and aspartate aminotransferase or histologically active disease.

Actions: Inhibits HBV reverse transcriptase, causes DNA chain termination, and blocks viral replication.

Pharmacokinetics:

Route	Onset	Peak	Duration
Oral	Rapid	0.6–4 h	Unknown

$T_{1/2}$: 7.5 hours; excreted in the urine.

Adverse Effects: Headache, asthenia, nausea, severe to fatal hepatomegaly with steatosis, nephrotoxicity, lactic acidosis, exacerbation of HBV when discontinued.

Clinically Important Drug–Drug Interactions

There is an increased risk of renal toxicity if these drugs are taken with other nephrotoxic drugs. If such a combination is used, monitor the patient closely. An evaluation of risks versus benefits may be necessary if renal function begins to deteriorate.

Nursing Considerations for Patients Receiving Anti-Hepatitis B Agents

Assessment: History and Examination

- Assess for contraindications or cautions: any history of allergy to the antiviral agents to avoid hypersensitivity reactions; renal dysfunction, which could be exacerbated by the nephrotoxic effects of these drugs; severe liver impairment, which could affect the metabolism and exacerbate the liver toxicity of these drugs; and pregnancy and lactation because the potential effects of these drugs on the fetus or baby are not known.
- Perform a physical assessment to establish baseline data for assessing the effectiveness of these drugs and the occurrence of any adverse effects associated with drug toxicity.
- Assess body temperature to monitor underlying disease.
- Assess level of orientation and reflexes to assess for CNS changes.
- Evaluate renal and liver function tests to monitor for developing toxicity and to determine drug effectiveness.

Nursing Conclusions

Nursing conclusions related to drug therapy might include the following:

- Impaired comfort related to the CNS and GI effects of the drug
- Malnutrition related to the GI effects of the drug
- Knowledge deficit regarding drug therapy

Planning

- The patient will receive the best therapeutic effect from the drug therapy.
- The patient will have limited adverse effects from the drug therapy.
- The patient will have an understanding of the drug therapy, adverse effects to anticipate, and measures to relieve discomfort and improve safety.

Intervention With Rationale

- Monitor renal and hepatic function prior to and periodically during therapy to detect renal or hepatic function changes and determine the need for possible dose reduction; institute treatment as needed.
- Withdraw the drug and monitor the patient if they develop signs of lactic acidosis or hepatotoxicity because these adverse effects can be life threatening.
- Caution the patient to not stop the medication without discussion with their health care provider because acute exacerbation of HBV can occur when the drug is stopped.
- Advise patients who can become pregnant to use barrier contraceptives because the potential adverse effects of this drug on the fetus are not known.
- Advise patients who are breast or chestfeeding to find another method of feeding the baby while using the drug because the potential toxic effects on the baby are not known.
- Advise patients that these drugs do not always eliminate the virus, and there is still a risk of transferring the virus, so the patient should continue to take appropriate steps to prevent transmission of HBV.
- Instruct the patient about the drug prescribed to enhance patient knowledge about drug therapy and to promote adherence.
- Provide the following patient teaching:
  - Have regular blood tests and medical follow-up.
  - Take precautions to avoid running out of the drug because it must be taken continually.
  - Realize that GI upset, nausea, and diarrhea are common with this drug.
  - Report severe weakness, muscle pain, palpitations, yellowing of the eyes or skin, or trouble breathing.

Evaluation

- Monitor patient response to the drug (decreased viral load of HBV).
- Monitor for adverse effects, including liver or renal dysfunction, headache, nausea, and diarrhea.
- Evaluate the effectiveness of the teaching plan. The patient should be able to name the drug, dosage, possible adverse effects to watch for, and specific measures to avoid adverse effects.
- Monitor the effectiveness of comfort and safety measures and adherence to the drug regimen.

Key Points

- HBV is a serious, potentially fatal, viral infection of the liver spread by blood or blood products, sexual contact, or contaminated needles or instruments. HBV has a higher mortality than other types of hepatitis.
- Prevention of infection through use of HBV vaccines, and avoiding exposure is essential in stopping the spread of this disease.
- HBV used to be treated only with interferons and rest. There are several antiviral medications now available for the treatment of HBV.

Anti-Hepatitis C Agents

Hepatitis C virus (HCV), which usually causes a mild viral infection of the liver, can cause both acute and chronic infection. After initial infection with HCV, most people develop chronic hepatitis C. Some will develop cirrhosis of the liver over many years. People can get HCV in a number of ways including exposure to blood that is infected with the virus, being birthed by a person with HCV, sharing a needle, having sex with an infected person, sharing personal items such as a razor or toothbrush with someone who is infected with the virus, or from unsterilized tattoo or piercing tools.

The goal of antiviral treatment for HCV is to eliminate the HCV RNA. The HCV RNA should be undetectable 12 weeks after finishing the antiviral treatment course. There has been good success with treatment for HCV with current antiviral therapies. Eradication of the virus is associated with lower mortality, no need for liver transplant, absence of liver cancer, and fewer complications of liver fibrosis. Antiviral therapy regimens can vary due to genotype, presence of cirrhosis, and patient treatment history. Some patients are treated with interferon (see Chapter 17) with ribavirin instead of or before antiviral treatments discussed in this chapter. While not required, it can be beneficial to consult a liver specialist regarding management of patients with HCV.

Therapeutic Effects and Indications

Combination dosing is recommended for all genotypes for the most effective elimination of HCV. The more commonly recommended treatment regimens will be discussed, but the following list is not inclusive of all medications available.

Harvoni combines ledipasvir with sofosbuvir for treatment of patients 3 years and older with genotypes 1, 4, 5, or 6. Ledipasvir inhibits a protein within HCV that is required for viral replication. Sofosbuvir inhibits a viral enzyme that is required for viral replication.

Zepatier combines elbasvir with grazoprevir for treatment of adults with genotype 1 or 4. It is indicated to be used with ribavirin in certain patient populations. Similar to ledipasvir, elbasvir inhibits a protein to decrease viral replication. Grazoprevir is an HCV protease inhibitor that decreases the viral ability to cleave polyprotein into mature proteins.

Epclusa (combination of sofosbuvir with velpatasvir) is used for all genotypes of chronic HCV in patients 6 years of age and older weighing at least 17 kg. Velpatasvir is similar to ledipasvir and elbasvir in mechanism of action.

Mavyret combines glecaprevir with pibrentasvir and is indicated for all genotypes in patients 12 years and older weighing at least 45 kg. Pibrentasvir inhibits an HCV viral protein required for replication.

Pharmacokinetics

These are oral drugs that are readily absorbed from the GI tract, metabolized in the liver, and excreted in the urine and/or feces. Half-lives range from 4 to 47 hours.

Contraindications and Cautions

These drugs are contraindicated with any known allergy to the drugs to prevent hypersensitivity reactions and with lactation and pregnancy if they are given with ribavirin, which has known toxicity to the infant. There is lack of adequate data regarding reproductive harm with these medications in humans. Use caution when administering these drugs to patients with severe liver disease because of increased toxicity. Special care must be taken when treating patients who have coinfection of HIV and HCV due to multiple dangerous medication interactions. In addition, patients being treated for HCV should be assessed for coinfection of HBV and if indicated started on appropriate treatment for HBV. HBV reactivation infections have been reported in patients being treated for HCV. The financial burden of these drugs was problematic when they were introduced. See Box 10.6 for a discussion of the impact of very costly new drugs on the health care system.

BOX 10.6

High Cost of Hepatitis C Drugs

The introduction of drugs to treat HCV opened a new therapeutic option for patients with the disease. It is estimated that most of the people awaiting liver transplant are in need of a transplant because of HCV. Most people with the disease, however, do not experience serious liver problems and would do fine without treatment, which is very costly. For example, the brand-name version of sofosbuvir, *Sovaldi*, costs about $1,000 per pill, or $84,000 for a bottle. The wholesale list price for a 4-week supply of *Mavyret*, which combines glecaprevir and pibrentasvir, is $13,200. The newest combination drug *Harvoni* (a combination of ledipasvir and sofosbuvir) is $1,125 per pill or approximately $94,500 for a 12-week supply. Drug companies argue that in the long run, the cost of a liver transplant would be higher. To help manage the financial burden, there are sometimes co-pay cards that dramatically lower the cost for the patient. Some insurance plans will assist with more of the cost than others. Some experts have suggested, based on studies, that these drugs should be reserved for use in those with more advanced liver scarring and higher risk. However, multimedia advertisements have marketed the drug to all people who have known chronic HCV, which has raised demand considerably. Insurance companies are very concerned about the ability to cover the cost of these drugs. Medicaid, the Veterans Affairs (VA) system, and other insurance providers will have to make significant decisions regarding the possibilities of cutting off health care to some consumers to cover these enormous costs. This may impact the number of patients who would be able to afford treatment. The ability to treat this disease that once had no pharmacological options has caused a heated debate and raised much needed discussion about the cost of developing drugs and the price of this development on the whole health care system in the United States.

Adverse Effects

The most common adverse effects are headache, fatigue, nausea, diarrhea, and rash. Severe skin reactions can occur.

Clinically Important Drug Interactions

Toxic effects or loss of therapeutic effect could occur if combined with other protease inhibitors and many other medications. If initiating or discontinuing any other medications for a patient on HCV medications, check a drug reference to make sure dosage is adjusted as needed. St. John's wort should be avoided, as it leads to loss of effectiveness.

Nursing Considerations for Patients Receiving Anti-Hepatitis C Agents

Assessment: History and Examination

- Assess for contraindications or cautions: any history of allergy to drug or drug components to avoid hypersensitivity reactions; severe liver impairment, which could affect the metabolism and exacerbate the liver toxicity of these drugs; coinfection with HBV or HIV, which would require HBV treatment and careful monitoring of HIV regimens; and pregnancy and lactation because the potential effects of these drugs on the fetus or baby are not known.
- Perform a physical assessment to establish baseline data for assessing the effectiveness of these drugs and the occurrence of any adverse effects associated with drug toxicity.
- Assess body temperature to monitor underlying disease.
- Assess level of orientation and reflexes to assess for CNS changes.
- Evaluate liver function to monitor for developing toxicity and to determine drug effectiveness.

Nursing Conclusions

Nursing conclusions related to drug therapy might include the following:

- Impaired comfort related to the CNS and GI effects of the drug
- Malnutrition related to the GI effects of the drug
- Knowledge deficit regarding drug therapy

Planning

- The patient will receive the best therapeutic effect from the drug therapy.
- The patient will have limited adverse effects from the drug therapy.
- The patient will have an understanding of the drug therapy, adverse effects to anticipate, and measures to relieve discomfort and improve safety.

Intervention With Rationale

- Monitor hepatic function prior to and periodically during therapy to detect hepatic function changes and determine the need for possible dose reduction or institute treatment as needed.
- Advise patients who can become pregnant to use barrier contraceptives because the potential adverse effects of this drug on the fetus are not known.
- Advise patients who are breast or chestfeeding to find another method of feeding the baby while using the drug because the potential toxic effects on the baby are not known.
- Advise patients that there is still a risk of transferring the disease and that viral cure is assessed weeks after treatment is ended, so the patient should continue to take appropriate steps to prevent transmission of HCV.
- Instruct the patient about the drug prescribed to enhance patient knowledge about drug therapy and to promote adherence.
- Provide the following patient teaching:
  - Have regular blood tests of hepatic function and viral load and medical follow-up.
  - Realize that headache and fatigue are the most common side effects with these medications.
  - Report severe changes in color of urine or stool, rash, or lethargy.

Evaluation

- Monitor patient response to the drug (decreased viral load of hepatitis C).
- Monitor for adverse effects, including liver dysfunction, headache, nausea, diarrhea, and rash.
- Evaluate the effectiveness of the teaching plan. The patient should be able to name the drug, dosage, possible adverse effects to watch for, and specific measures to avoid adverse effects.
- Monitor the effectiveness of comfort and safety measures and adherence to the drug regimen.

Locally Active Antiviral Agents

Some antiviral agents are given locally to treat local viral infections, including warts and eye infections. These agents include acyclovir (*Zovirax*), docosanol (*Abreva*), ganciclovir (*Zirgan*), imiquimod (*Aldara*), penciclovir (*Denavir*), and trifluridine (*Viroptic*).

Therapeutic Actions and Indications

These antiviral agents act on viruses by interfering with normal viral replication and metabolic processes. They are indicated for specific, local viral infections (see Table 10.5).

Table 10.5 *Drugs in Focus*: Locally Active Antiviral Agents

Drug Name	Usual Indications
acyclovir (*Zovirax*)	Treatment of recurrent herpes labialis (cold sores)
docosánol (*Abreva*)	Local treatment of oral and facial herpes simplex cold sores and fever blisters
ganciclovir (*Zirgan*)	Topical ophthalmic gel for herpetic keratitis
imiquimod (*Aldara*)	Local treatment of genital and perianal warts
penciclovir (*Denavir*)	Local treatment of herpes labialis (cold sores) on the face and lips
trifluridine (*Viroptic*)	Ophthalmic ointment to treat herpes simplex infections in the eye

CMV, cytomegalovirus.

Contraindications and Cautions

Locally active antiviral drugs are not absorbed systemically, but caution must be used in patients with known allergic reactions to any topical drugs. They should not be applied to open wounds.

Adverse Effects

Because these drugs are not absorbed systemically, the adverse effects most commonly reported are local burning, stinging, and discomfort. These effects usually occur at the time of administration and pass with time.

Nursing Considerations for Patients Receiving Locally Active Antiviral Agents

Assessment: History and Examination

- Assess for history of allergy to antivirals to avoid allergic response to these drugs.
- Perform a physical assessment to establish baseline data for evaluating the effectiveness of the drug and the occurrence of any adverse effects associated with drug therapy.
- Assess the infected area, including location, size, and character of lesions to provide baseline information and evaluation of drug effects.
- Evaluate for signs of inflammation at the site of infection to ensure safe use of the drug.

Nursing Conclusions

Nursing conclusions related to drug therapy might include the following:

- Impaired comfort related to local effects of the drug
- Knowledge deficit regarding drug therapy

Planning

- The patient will receive the best therapeutic effect from the drug therapy.
- The patient will have limited adverse effects from the drug therapy.
- The patient will have an understanding of the drug therapy, adverse effects to anticipate, and measures to relieve discomfort and improve safety.

Intervention With Rationale

- Ensure proper administration of the drug to improve effectiveness and decrease risk of adverse effects.
- Stop the drug if severe local reaction occurs or if open lesions occur near the site of administration to prevent systemic absorption and adverse effects.
- Instruct the patient about the drug being used to enhance patient knowledge about drug therapy and to promote adherence.
- Include as a teaching point the fact that these drugs do not cure the disease but should alleviate discomfort and prevent damage to healthy tissues.
- Encourage the patient to report severe local reaction or discomfort.

Evaluation

- Monitor patient response to the drug (alleviation of signs and symptoms of viral infection).
- Monitor for adverse effects, including local irritation and discomfort.
- Evaluate the effectiveness of the teaching plan. The patient should be able to name the drug, the dosage, proper administration technique, and adverse effects to watch for and report to a health care provider.
- Monitor the effectiveness of comfort and safety measures and adherence to the regimen.

Key Points

- Medications used to treat HBC are most frequently administered as fixed combinations. They can be combined with ribavirin and peginterferon.
- Some antivirals are available only for the local treatment of viral infections, including warts and eye infections.
- Topical antivirals should not be applied to open wounds; local reactions can occur with administration.

SUMMARY

- Viruses are particles of DNA or RNA surrounded by a protein coat that survive by injecting their own DNA or RNA into a healthy cell and taking over its functioning.
- Because viruses are contained within human cells, it has been difficult to develop drugs that are effective antivirals and yet do not destroy human cells. Antiviral agents are available that are effective against only a few types of viruses.
- Influenza A and respiratory viruses cause the signs and symptoms of the common cold or "flu." The drugs that are available to prevent the replication of these viruses are used for prophylaxis against these diseases during peak seasons and to treat disease when it occurs.
- Herpes viruses and CMV are DNA viruses that cause a multitude of illnesses, including cold sores, encephalitis, infections of the eye and liver, and genital herpes.
- Helper T cells are essential for maintaining a vigilant, effective immune system. When these cells are decreased in number or effectiveness, opportunistic infections occur. AIDS and ARC are syndromes of opportunistic infections that occur when the immune system is depressed.
- HIV, which specifically attacks helper T cells, may remain dormant in these cells for long periods and has been known to mutate easily.
- Antiviral agents that are effective against HIV and AIDS include NNRTIs and NRTIs, protease inhibitors, fusion inhibitors, CCR5 coreceptor antagonists, and integrase inhibitors, all of which affect the way the virus communicates, replicates, or matures within the cell. These drugs are known as antiretroviral agents. They are given in combination to most effectively destroy the HIV virus and prevent mutation.
- There are several medications that are approved for treating HBV infection.
- HBC is often treated with combination antiviral therapy.
- Some antivirals are available for the local treatment of viral infections, including warts and eye infections. These drugs are not absorbed systemically.

CHECK YOUR UNDERSTANDING

Answers to the questions in this chapter can be found in Answers to Check Your Understanding Questions on thePoint®.

MULTIPLE CHOICE

Select the best answer.

1. In assessing a patient, a viral cause might be suspected if the patient is diagnosed with
   a. tuberculosis.
   b. leprosy.
   c. the common cold.
   d. gonorrhea.
2. Viral infections are difficult to treat because they
   a. have a protein coat.
   b. inject themselves into human cells to survive and to reproduce.
   c. are bits of RNA or DNA.
   d. easily resist drug therapy.
3. Naturally occurring substances that are released in the body in response to viral invasion are called
   a. antibodies.
   b. immunoglobulins.
   c. interferons.
   d. interleukins.
4. Herpes viruses cause a broad range of conditions but have not been identified as the causative agent in
   a. cold sores.
   b. varicella-zoster.
   c. genital infections.
   d. leprosy.
5. Which of the following is an important teaching point for the patient receiving an agent to treat herpes virus or CMV?
   a. Stop taking the drug as soon as the lesions have disappeared.
   b. Sexual intercourse is fine because as long as you are taking the drug, you are not contagious.
   c. Drink plenty of fluids to decrease the drug's toxic effects on the kidneys.
   d. There are few associated GI adverse effects.

6. HIV selectively enters which of the following cells?
   a. B clones
   b. Helper T cells
   c. Suppressor T cells
   d. Cytotoxic T cells

7. Nursing interventions for the patient receiving antiviral drugs for the treatment of HIV probably would include
   a. monitoring renal and hepatic function periodically during therapy.
   b. administering the drugs just once a day to increase drug effectiveness.
   c. encouraging the patient to avoid eating if GI upset is severe.
   d. stopping the drugs and notifying the prescriber if severe rash occurs.

8. Locally active antiviral agents can be used to treat
   a. HIV infection.
   b. warts.
   c. RSV.
   d. CMV systemic infections.

MULTIPLE RESPONSE

Select all that apply.

1. When explaining to a patient the reasoning behind using combination therapy in the treatment of HIV, the nurse would include which of the following points?
   a. The virus can remain dormant within the T cell for a very long time; it can mutate while in the T cell.
   b. Adverse effects of many of the drugs used to treat this virus include immunosuppression, so the disease could become worse.
   c. The drugs are cheaper if used in combination.
   d. The virus slowly mutates with each generation.
   e. Attacking the virus at many points in its life cycle has been shown to be most effective.
   f. Research has shown that using only one type of drug that targeted only one point in the virus life cycle led to more mutations and more difficulty in controlling the disease.

2. Appropriate nursing conclusions related to drug therapy for a patient receiving combination antiviral therapy for the treatment of HIV infection would include the following:
   a. Disturbed sensory (kinesthetic) perception related to the CNS effects of the drugs
   b. Altered nutrition: Higher than body requirements related to appetite stimulation
   c. Heart failure related to cardiac effects of the drugs
   d. Adrenal insufficiency related to endocrine effects of the drugs
   e. Acute pain related to GI, CNS, or dermatological effects of the drugs
   f. Deficient knowledge regarding drug therapy

REFERENCES

AASLD/IDSA/IAS–USA. (2020). *HCV guidance: Recommendations for testing, managing, and treating hepatitis C.* https://www.hcvguidelines.org/unique-populations/hiv-hcv

AASLD/IDSA/IAS–USA. (2020). *HCV testing and linkage to care. Recommendations for testing, managing, and treating hepatitis C.* http://www.hcvguidelines.org/full-report/hcv-testing-and-linkage-care

American Association for the Study of Liver Disease. (2018). Update on prevention, diagnosis, and treatment of chronic hepatitis B: AASLD 2018 hepatitis B guidance. *Hepatology, 67*(4), 1560–1599. https://doi.org/10.1002/hep.29800

Brunton, L., Hilal-Dandan, R., & Knollman, B. (2018). *Goodman and Gilman's the pharmacological basis of therapeutics* (13th ed.). McGraw-Hill.

Centers for Disease Control and Prevention. (2019). *Guidelines for management of AIDS.* http://www.cdc.gov/hiv/guidelines/index.html

Centers for Disease Control and Prevention. (2020). *Evidence of HIV treatment and viral suppression in preventing the sexual transmission of HIC.* https://www.cdc.gov/hiv/pdf/risk/art/cdc-hiv-art-viral-suppression.pdf

Centers for Disease Control and Prevention. (2020). *How to protect yourself and others.* https://www.cdc.gov/coronavirus/2019-ncov/prevent-getting-sick/prevention.html

Chopra, S., & Muir, A. J. (2019). Treatment regimens for chronic hepatitis C virus genotype 1 infection in adults. *UpToDate.* https://www.uptodate.com/contents/treatment-regimens-for-chronic-hepatitis-c-virus-genotype-1-infection-in-adults?search=hepatitis%20c%20treatment&topicRef=3673&source=see_link

Chopra, S., & Pockros, P. J. (2020). Overview of the management of chronic hepatitis C virus infection. *UpToDate.* https://www.uptodate.com/contents/overview-of-the-management-of-chronic-hepatitis-c-virus-infection?search=hepatitis c&source=search_result&selectedTitle=1~150&usage_type=default&display_rank=1

Fletcher, C. V. (2020). Overview of antiretroviral agents used to treat HIV. *UpToDate.* https://www.accessdata.fda.gov/drugsatfda_docs/label/2020/214787Orig1s000lbl.pdf

Henry, B. (2018). Drug pricing and challenges to hepatitis C treatment access. *Journal of Health and Biomedical Law, 14*, 265–283. https://www.ncbi.nlm.nih.gov/pmc/articles/PMC6152913/

Hepatitis B Foundation. (2020). *Approved drugs for adults.* https://www.hepb.org/treatment-and-management/treatment/approved-drugs-for-adults/

HBV Primary Care Workgroup. (2020). *Hepatitis B management: Guidance for the primary care provider.* https://www.hepatitisb.uw.edu/page/primary-care-workgroup/guidance

Infectious Diseases Society of America. (2018). Clinical practice guidelines by the infectious diseases society of America: 2018 update on diagnosis, treatment, chemoprophylaxis, and institutional outbreak management of seasonal influenza. *Clinical Infectious Diseases, 68*(6), 895–902. https://doi.org/10.1093/cid/ciy874

Kaiser, L., Wat, C., Mills, T., Mahoney, P., Ward, P., & Hayden, F. (2003). Impact of oseltamivir treatment on influenza-related lower respiratory tract complications and hospitalizations. *Archives of Internal Medicine, 163*, 1667–1672. http://dx.doi.org/10.1001/archinte.163.14.1667

Kim, A. Y., & Gandhi, R. T. (2020). Coronavirus disease 2019 (COVID-19): Management in hospitalized adults. *UpToDate.* https://www.uptodate.com/contents/coronavirus-disease-2019-covid-19-management-in-hospitalized-adults?search=coronavirus%20disease%202019%20hospital&source=search_result&selectedTitle=1~150&usage_type=default&display_rank=1

Mandell, G., Bennett, J., & Dolin, R. (Eds.). (2014). *Mandell, Douglas and Bennett's principles and practice of infectious diseases* (8th ed.). Elsevier.

McIntosh, K., Hirsch, M. S., & Bloom, A. (2020). Coronavirus disease 2019 (COVID-19): Epidemiology, virology and prevention. *UpToDate.* https://www.uptodate.com/contents/coronavirus-disease-2019-covid-19-epidemiology-virology-and-prevention/print?search=covid%2019%20pathophysiology&source=search_result&selectedTitle=1~150&usage_type=default&display_rank=1

Norris, T. L. (2029). *Porth's pathophysiology concepts of altered health states.* Wolters Kluwer.

Panel of Antiretroviral Guidelines for Adults and Adolescents. (2019). *Guidelines for the use of antiretroviral agents in adults and adolescents with HIV.* https://clinicalinfo.hiv.gov/sites/default/files/guidelines/documents/AdultandAdolescentGL.pdf

Pasternak, B., & Hvid, A. (2010). Use of acyclovir, valacyclovir and famciclovir in the first trimester of pregnancy and the risk of birth defects. *Journal of the American Medical Association, 304*(8), 859–866. http://dx.doi.org/10.1001/jama.2010.1206

U.S. Food and Drug Administration. (2019). *Abacavir, dolutegravir, and lamivudine (Triumeq).* https://apps.who.int/iris/bitstream/handle/10665/325892/WHO-CDS-HIV-19.15-eng.pdf?ua=1

U.S. Food and Drug Administration. (2020). *Veklury (remdesivir).* https://www.accessdata.fda.gov/drugsatfda_docs/label/2020/214787Orig1s000lbl.pdf

World Health Organization. (2019). *Update of recommendations on first- and second-line antiretroviral regimens.* https://apps.who.int/iris/bitstream/handle/10665/325892/WHO-CDS-HIV-19.15-eng.pdf?ua=1

CHAPTER 11

Antifungal Agents

Learning Objectives

Upon completion of this chapter, you will be able to:

1. Describe the characteristics of a fungus and a fungal infection.
2. Discuss the therapeutic actions, indications, pharmacokinetics, contraindications, proper administration, most common adverse reactions, and important drug–drug interactions associated with systemic and topical antifungals.
3. Compare and contrast the prototype drugs for systemic and topical antifungals with the other drugs in each class.
4. Discuss the impact of using antifungals across the lifespan.
5. Outline the nursing considerations for patients receiving a systemic or topical antifungal.

Key Terms

azoles: a group of drugs used to treat fungal infections

***Candida*:** fungus that is normally found on mucous membranes; can cause yeast infections or thrush of the gastrointestinal (GI) tract and vagina in immunosuppressed patients; can cause serious systemic infection that can affect multiple organs in the body

ergosterol: steroid-type protein found in the cell membrane of fungi; similar in configuration to adrenal hormones and testosterone

fungus: a cellular organism with a hard cell wall that contains chitin and many polysaccharides, as well as a cell membrane that contains ergosterols

mycosis: disease caused by a fungus

***Pneumocystis jirovecii* pneumonia:** opportunistic infection that occurs when the immune system is depressed; *Pneumocystis jirovecii* is a common fungus that spreads through the air; a frequent cause of pneumonia in patients with AIDS and in those who are receiving immunosuppressive therapy

Tinea: fungus called ringworm that causes such infections as athlete's foot, jock itch, and others

Drug List

SYSTEMIC ANTIFUNGALS

AZOLE ANTIFUNGALS

(P) fluconazole
isavuconazonium
itraconazole
ketoconazole
posaconazole
voriconazole

ECHINOCANDIN ANTIFUNGALS

anidulafungin
caspofungin
micafungin

OTHER ANTIFUNGALS

amphotericin B
flucytosine
griseofulvin
nystatin
terbinafine

TOPICAL ANTIFUNGALS

AZOLE TOPICAL ANTIFUNGALS

butoconazole
(P) clotrimazole
econazole
efinaconazole
ketoconazole
luliconazole
miconazole
oxiconazole
sertaconazole
sulconazole
terbinafine
terconazole
tioconazole

OTHER TOPICAL ANTIFUNGALS

butenafine
ciclopirox
gentian violet
naftifine
tolnaftate
undecylenic acid

Fungal infections in humans range from uncomfortable but minor conditions such as "athlete's foot" to potentially fatal systemic infections. An infection caused by a **fungus** is called a **mycosis**. Fungi differ from bacteria in that a fungus has a rigid cell wall that is made up of chitin and various polysaccharides and a cell membrane that contains **ergosterol**, which is a steroid-type protein similar in configuration to adrenal hormones and testosterone. The composition of the protective layers of the fungal cell makes the organism resistant to antibiotics. Conversely, because of their cellular makeup, bacteria are resistant to antifungal drugs.

The incidence of fungal infections has increased with the rising number of immunocompromised individuals—patients with AIDS and AIDS-related complex; those taking immunosuppressant drugs; people who have undergone transplantation surgery or cancer treatment; and members of the increasing older adults population, whose bodies have diminished protection from the many fungi that are found throughout the environment (see Box 11.1 for information on treatment across the lifespan). For example, ***Candida***, a fungus that is normally found on mucous membranes, can cause yeast infections or "thrush" in the gastrointestinal (GI) tract and yeast infections or "vaginitis" in the vagina. *Candida* can also cause serious systemic infections affecting multiple organs in the body.

Pneumocystis jirovecii is an endemic fungus that does not usually cause illness in humans. However, when an individual's immune system becomes suppressed because of AIDS or AIDS-related complex, the use of immunosuppressant drugs, or advanced age, this fungus is able to invade the lungs, leading to severe inflammation and ***Pneumocystis jirovecii* pneumonia**. This disease is the most common opportunistic respiratory infection in patients with AIDS. It is commonly prevented or treated with the antimicrobial medication trimethoprim/sulfamethoxazole (TMP/SMX), which is described in Chapter 9.

Systemic Antifungals

The drugs used to treat systemic fungal infections (see Table 11.1) can be toxic to the host and are not to be used indiscriminately. It is important to get a culture of the fungus causing the infection to ensure that the right drug is being used so that the patient is not put at additional risk from the toxic adverse effects associated with antifungal drugs. Systemic antifungal drugs are classified in the following groups: azoles, echinocandins, and other antifungal agents.

Azole Antifungals

The **azoles** are a large group of antifungals used to treat systemic and topical fungal infections (see Table 11.1). The azoles include fluconazole (*Diflucan*), itraconazole (*Sporanox*), ketoconazole (*Nizoral*), posaconazole (*Noxafil*), voriconazole (*Vfend*), and isavuconazonium (*Cresemba*). Although azoles are considered less toxic than some other antifungals, such as amphotericin B, they may also be less effective in very severe and progressive infections.

Box 11.1 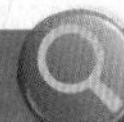 **Focus on Drug Therapy Across the Lifespan**

ANTIFUNGAL AGENTS

Children

Many of these drugs do not have proven safety and efficacy in children, and extreme caution should be exercised when using them. Fluconazole, ketoconazole, terbinafine, and griseofulvin have established pediatric doses and are drugs of choice if appropriate for a particular infection.

Topical agents should not be used over open or draining areas that would increase the risk of systemic absorption and toxicity. Occlusive dressings, including tight diapers, should be avoided over the affected areas.

Adults

These drugs can be very toxic to the body, and their use should be reserved for situations in which the causative organism has been identified. Over-the-counter topical preparations are widely used, and patients should be cautioned to follow the instructions and to report continued problems to their health care provider.

Pregnant and nursing patients should not use these drugs unless the benefit clearly outweighs the potential risk to the fetus or neonate. Patients who can become pregnant should be advised to use barrier contraceptives if any of these drugs are used. A severe fungal infection may threaten the life of the patient and/or fetus; in these situations, the potential risk of treatment should be carefully explained.

Topical agents should not be used over open or draining areas, which would increase the risk of systemic absorption.

Older Adults

Older patients may be more susceptible to the adverse effects associated with these drugs and should be monitored closely.

Patients with hepatic dysfunction are at increased risk for worsening hepatic problems and toxic effects of many of these drugs (ketoconazole, itraconazole, griseofulvin). If hepatic dysfunction is expected (extreme age, alcohol abuse, use of other hepatotoxic drugs), the dose may need to be lowered and the patient monitored more frequently.

Other agents are associated with renal toxicity (amphotericin B, flucytosine, griseofulvin); these should be used cautiously in the presence of renal impairment. Patients at risk for renal toxicity should be monitored carefully. With fluconazole, the dose should be reduced in the presence of renal dysfunction to prevent adverse effects related to accumulation of the medication.

Table 11.1 *Drugs in Focus:* Systemic Antifungals

Drug Name	Dosage/Route	Usual Indications
Azole Antifungals		
fluconazole (*Diflucan*)	*Adult:* 200–400 mg PO or IV on day 1, followed by 200 mg/d for 2–3 wk. Treatment of vaginal *Candida*: 150 mg PO as a single dose *Pediatric:* 3–12 mg/kg PO or IV; do not exceed 12 mg/kg	Treatment of candidiasis, cryptococcal meningitis, other systemic fungal infections; prophylaxis for reducing the incidence of candidiasis in bone marrow transplant recipients
isavuconazonium (*Cresemba*)	372 mg IV or PO q8h for 6 doses; then 372 mg/d PO or IV 12–24 hours post last loading dose	Treatment of invasive aspergillosis and invasive mucormycosis
itraconazole (*Sporanox*)	*Adult:* 100–400 mg/d PO *Pediatric:* Safety and efficacy not established	Treatment of blastomycosis, histoplasmosis, and aspergillosis
ketoconazole (generic)	*Adult:* 200 mg/d PO, up to 400 mg/d PO in severe cases *Pediatric (≥2 y):* 3.3–6.6 mg/kg/d PO *Pediatric (<2 y):* Safety not established *Topical:* As a shampoo and cream for skin	Treatment of aspergillosis, leishmaniasis, cryptococcosis, blastomycosis, moniliasis, coccidioidomycosis, histoplasmosis, and mucormycosis; topical treatment of mycoses (cream) and to reduce the scaling of dandruff (shampoo)
posaconazole (*Noxafil*)	*Adult and pediatric (≥13 y):* 100–600 mg PO or IV per day depending on type of infection and loading vs. maintenance dose	Prophylaxis of invasive *Aspergillus* and *Candida* infections in adults and children >13 y who are immunosuppressed secondary to antineoplastic, chemotherapy, graft versus host disease following transplants or hematological malignancies
voriconazole (*Vfend*)	*Adult:* 6 mg/kg IV q12h for two doses, then 4 mg/kg IV q12h; switch to oral dose as soon as possible: *>40 kg:* 200 mg PO q12h *<40 kg:* 100 mg PO q12h *Pediatric (<11 y):* 9 mg/kg IV or PO	Treatment of invasive aspergillosis; treatment of serious fungal infections caused by *Scedosporium apiospermum* or *Fusarium* spp. when the patient is intolerant to or not responding to other therapy
Echinocandin Antifungals		
anidulafungin (*Eraxis*)	100–200 mg IV on day 1, then 50–100 mg/d IV for 14 d; dose varies with infection being treated	Treatment of candidemia (infection of the bloodstream) and other forms of *Candida* infection, intra-abdominal infections, and esophageal candidiasis
caspofungin acetate (*Cancidas*)	*Adult:* 70 mg/d IV loading dose, then 50 mg/d IV infusion; dose should be reduced to 35 mg/d IV infusion with hepatic impairment *Pediatric (3 mo–17 y):* 70 mg/m^2 IV loading dose then 50 mg/m^2 IV daily for 14 d	Treatment of invasive aspergillosis in patients who do not respond or are intolerant to other therapies
micafungin (*Mycamine*)	*Adult:* 150 mg/d IV over 1 h for 6–30 d *Adult prophylaxis:* 50 mg/d IV over 1 h for about 19 d *Pediatric:* 2.5–3 mg/kg/d IV *Pediatric prophylaxis:* 1 mg/kg/d IV	Treatment of patients with esophageal candidiasis; prophylaxis of *Candida* infections in patients with hematopoietic stem cell transplant
Other Antifungals		
amphotericin B (*Abelcet, AmBisome*)	0.3–5 mg/kg/d IV based on the infection being treated; each brand name has different dosages	Treatment of aspergillosis, leishmaniasis, cryptococcosis, blastomycosis, moniliasis, coccidioidomycosis, histoplasmosis, and mucormycosis; use is reserved for progressive, potential fatal infections due to many associated adverse effects
flucytosine (*Ancobon*)	50–150 mg/kg/d PO in divided doses at 6-h intervals	Treatment of systemic infections caused by *Candida* or *Cryptococcus*

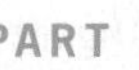

Table 11.1 *Drugs in Focus:* Systemic Antifungals *(Continued)*

Drug Name	Dosage/Route	Usual Indications
griseofulvin (generic)	*Tinea corporis, tinea cruris, and tinea capitis:* *Adult:* 500 mg (microsize) or 330–375 mg/d (ultramicrosize) PO *Pediatric:* Dosage varies by weight *Tinea pedis and tinea unguium:* *Adult:* 0.75–1 g (microsize) or 660–750 mg (ultramicrosize) PO daily *Pediatric (>2 y):* 11 mg/kg/d (microsize) or 7.3 mg (ultramicrosize) PO daily (not recommended for children ≤2 y)	Treatment of variety of ringworm or tinea infections caused by susceptible *Trichophyton* spp., including tinea corporis, tinea pedis, tinea cruris, tinea barbae, tinea capitis, and tinea unguium
nystatin (generic)	*Adult and pediatric:* 500,000–1,000,000 units 4 times/d PO; continue for 48 h after resolution to prevent relapse; also used topically	Treatment of candidiasis (oral form); treatment of local candidiasis, vaginal candidiasis, and cutaneous and mucocutaneous infections caused by *Candida* spp.
terbinafine (*Lamisil*)	*Adult:* 250 mg/d PO for 6 wk (fingernail) or 12 wk (toenail) *Pediatric:* 125–250 mg/d PO for 6 wk (sprinkle capsules)	Treatment of onychomycosis of the fingernail or toenail caused by dermatophytes; approved in late 2007 for treatment of tinea capitis (ringworm of the scalp) in children ≥4 y

Therapeutic Actions and Indications

These drugs bind to sterols and can cause cell death (a fungicidal effect) or interfere with cell replication (a fungistatic effect), depending on the type of fungus being affected and the concentration of the drug (see Fig. 11.1).

Ketoconazole, fluconazole, and itraconazole work by blocking the activity of a sterol in the fungal wall. In addition, they may block the activity of human steroids, including testosterone and cortisol (see Table 11.1 for usual indications).

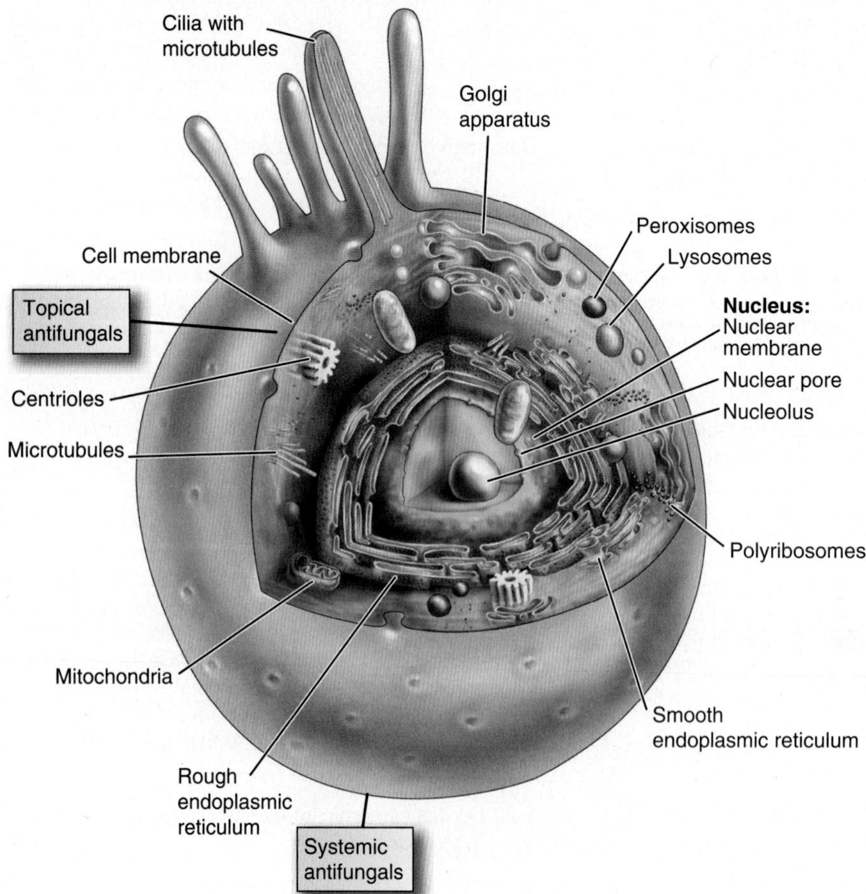

FIGURE 11.1 Sites of action of antifungal agents. Both systemic and topical antifungals alter fungal cell permeability, preventing replication and leading to cell death.

Posaconazole (see Table 11.1 for uses), voriconazole, and isavuconazonium are triazole antifungals that inhibit the synthesis of ergosterol, which leads to the inability of the fungus to form a cell wall, resulting in cell death. Isavuconazonium is slightly different than the other two medications, since it is actually a prodrug that is changed into the active ingredient isavuconazole.

Pharmacokinetics

Ketoconazole and itraconazole are administered orally. Ketoconazole is also available as a shampoo and a cream for topical treatment.

Fluconazole, isavuconazonium, posaconazole, and voriconazole are available in oral and IV preparations, making it possible to start the drug intravenously for a serious infection and then switch to an oral form when the patient's condition improves and they are able to take oral medications.

Ketoconazole is absorbed rapidly from the GI tract, with peak level occurring in 1 to 3 hours. It is extensively metabolized in the liver and excreted through the feces. Fluconazole reaches peak level 1 to 2 hours after administration. Most of the drug is excreted unchanged in the urine; dosages need to be reduced in the presence of renal dysfunction. Itraconazole is slowly absorbed from the GI tract and is metabolized in the liver by the CYP450 system. It is excreted in the urine and feces. When posaconazole is given orally, it has a rapid onset of action and peaks in 3 to 5 hours. It is metabolized in the liver and excreted in the feces. Voriconazole reaches peak level in 1 to 2 hours if given orally and at the onset of the infusion if given IV. It is metabolized in the liver with a half-life of 24 hours and is excreted in the urine. Isavuconazonium reaches peak level in 2 to 3 hours when taken orally and within an hour when given IV. It is metabolized in the liver, excreted in urine and stool, and has a half-life of 130 hours.

Contraindications and Cautions

The azoles have been associated with severe hepatic toxicity and should be avoided in patients with hepatic dysfunction to prevent serious hepatic toxicity. In addition, ketoconazole is not the drug of choice for patients with endocrine or fertility problems because of its effects on sex hormones. Male patients may have gynecomastia, decreased libido, and/or erectile dysfunction. Female patients may have irregular menstrual flow. Although fluconazole should be used with caution in the presence of liver or renal impairment because it could cause liver toxicity, fluconazole is not associated with the endocrine problems seen with ketoconazole.

It is not known whether posaconazole crosses the placenta or enters human milk, so it should not be used during pregnancy or lactation unless the benefits clearly outweigh the potential risks. Caution should be used if posaconazole is used in the presence of liver impairment because it can cause liver toxicity. Carefully monitor patients for bone marrow suppression and GI and liver toxicity if using this drug.

Box 11.2 Focus on Herbal and Alternative Therapies

Patients being treated with voriconazole or posaconazole should be cautioned about the risk of ergotism if they combine this drug with ergot, an herb frequently used to treat migraine headache and menstrual problems. If the patient is using either of these drugs, it should be suggested that ergot not be used until the antifungal therapy is finished.

Adverse Effects

All azoles are associated with liver toxicity and can cause severe effects on a fetus or a nursing baby.

Clinically Important Drug–Drug Interactions

The azoles strongly inhibit the CYP450 enzyme system in the liver and are associated with many drug–drug interactions, including increased serum levels of the following agents: cyclosporine, digoxin, oral hypoglycemics, warfarin, oral anticoagulants, and phenytoin. If these combinations cannot be avoided, closely monitor the patient and anticipate the need for dose adjustments. A drug guide should be consulted any time one of these drugs is added to or removed from a drug regimen. Itraconazole has a boxed warning regarding the potential for serious cardiovascular effects if it is given with lovastatin, simvastatin, triazolam, midazolam, pimozide, or dofetilide. These combinations should be avoided. Voriconazole, isavuconazonium, and posaconazole should not be used with any other drugs that prolong the QTc interval. Additionally, they can cause ergotism if taken with ergot alkaloids. Box 11.2 highlights important information about hazardous interactions between voriconazole and posaconazole and the herb ergot.

Prototype Summary: Fluconazole

Indications: Treatment of oropharyngeal, esophageal, and vaginal candidiasis; cryptococcal meningitis; systemic fungal infections; prophylaxis to decrease the incidence of candidiasis in bone marrow transplants.

Actions: Binds to sterols in the fungal cell membrane, changing membrane permeability; fungicidal or fungistatic, depending on the concentration of drug and the organism.

Pharmacokinetics:

Route	Onset	Peak	Duration
Oral	Slow	1–2 h	2–4 d
IV	Rapid	End of infusion	2–4 d

$T_{1/2}$: 30 hours; metabolized in the liver and excreted in the urine.

Adverse Effects: Headache, nausea, vomiting, diarrhea, abdominal pain, rash.

Echinocandin Antifungals

The echinocandin antifungals are another group of antifungals. Drugs in this class include anidulafungin (*Eraxis*), caspofungin (*Cancidas*), and micafungin (*Mycamine*).

Therapeutic Actions and Indications

The echinocandins work by inhibiting glucan synthesis. Glucan is an enzyme that is present in the fungal cell wall but not in human cell walls. If this enzyme is inhibited, the fungal cell wall cannot form, leading to death of the cell wall. See Table 11.1 for usual indications for each of these agents.

Pharmacokinetics

Anidulafungin is given as a daily IV infusion. It has a rapid onset of action, is metabolized by degradation, and has a half-life of 40 to 50 hours. This drug is excreted in the feces.

Caspofungin is available for IV use. This drug is slowly metabolized in the liver, with half-lives of 9 to 11 hours, then 6 to 48 hours, and then 40 to 50 hours. It is bound to protein and widely distributed throughout the body. It is excreted through the urine.

Micafungin is an IV drug. It has a rapid onset, has a half-life of 14 to 17 hours, and is excreted in the urine.

Contraindications and Cautions

Anidulafungin may cross the placenta and enter human milk and should not be used by pregnant or lactating patients. Both anidulafungin and caspofungin can be toxic to the liver; therefore, caution must be taken and reduced doses used if a patient has known hepatic impairment. Caspofungin is embryotoxic in animal studies and is known to enter human milk; therefore, it should be used with great caution during pregnancy and lactation. Micafungin should be used during pregnancy and lactation only if the benefits clearly outweigh the risks because of the potential for adverse reactions in the fetus or the neonate.

Adverse Effects

Anidulafungin and caspofungin are associated with hepatic toxicity, and liver function should be monitored closely when using these drugs. Potentially serious hypersensitivity reactions have occurred with micafungin. In addition, bone marrow suppression can occur; monitor patients closely.

Clinically Important Drug–Drug Interactions

Concurrent use of cyclosporine with caspofungin is contraindicated unless the benefit clearly outweighs the risk of hepatic injury.

Other Antifungal Agents

Other antifungal drugs that are available do not fit into either of these classes. These include amphotericin B (*Abelcet, AmBisome*), flucytosine (*Ancobon*), griseofulvin (*Gris-Peg*), nystatin, and terbinafine (*Lamisil*).

Therapeutic Actions and Indications

Other antifungal agents work to cause fungal cell death or to prevent fungal cell reproduction. Amphotericin B is a very potent drug with many adverse effects (see "Adverse Effects" section). The drug binds to the sterols in the fungus cell wall, changing the cell wall permeability. This change can lead to cell death (fungicidal effect) or prevent the fungal cells from reproducing (fungistatic effect; see Table 11.1 for usual indications). Because of the many adverse effects associated with this agent, its use is reserved for progressive, potentially fatal infections.

Flucytosine is a less toxic drug that alters the cell membrane of susceptible fungi, causing cell death (see Table 11.1 for usual indications).

Griseofulvin is an older antifungal that acts in much the same way, changing cell membrane permeability and causing cell death.

Nystatin binds to sterols in the cell wall, changing membrane permeability and allowing leaking of the cellular components, resulting in cell death.

Terbinafine is a nonazole antifungal that blocks the formation of ergosterol. See Box 11.3 for a caution about potential confusion with a brand name of terbinafine.

Pharmacokinetics

Amphotericin B is available in IV form in two formulations that have reduced adverse effects and in the original deoxycholate formulation. All formulations are excreted in the urine, with a plasma half-life of 24 hours and an elimination 15-day half-life. Their metabolism is not fully understood. Flucytosine is well absorbed from the GI tract, with peak level occurring in 2 hours. Most of the drug is excreted unchanged in the urine and a small amount in the feces, with a half-life of 2.4 to 4.8 hours. Griseofulvin is administered orally and reaches peak level in around 4 hours. It is metabolized in the liver and excreted in the urine with a half-life of 24 hours. Nystatin is not absorbed from the GI tract and passes unchanged in the stool. Terbinafine is

Box 11.3 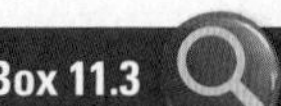 **Focus on Safe Medication Administration**

Name confusion has occurred between the brand names *Lamisil* (terbinafine) and *Lamictal* (lamotrigine, an antiepileptic agent). Use extreme caution if your patient is receiving either of these drugs to make sure that the correct drug is being used.

available in a sprinkle formulation for children. It is rapidly absorbed from the GI tract, extensively metabolized in the liver, and excreted in the urine with a half-life of 36 hours.

Contraindications and Cautions

Amphotericin B is available in several formulations; caution must be used to differentiate the formulation used as the dosages vary. Amphotericin B has been used successfully during pregnancy, but it should be used cautiously. It crosses into human milk and should not be used during lactation because of the potential risk to the neonate. Because flucytosine is excreted primarily in the urine, extreme caution is needed in the presence of renal impairment because drug accumulation and toxicity can occur. Toxicity is associated with serum levels higher than 100 mcg/mL. Because of the potential for adverse reactions in the fetus or neonate, flucytosine should be used during pregnancy and lactation only if the benefits clearly outweigh the risks. It is not known whether nystatin crosses the placenta or enters human milk, so it should not be used systemically during pregnancy or lactation unless the benefits clearly outweigh the potential risks; however, it is typically used topically.

Adverse Effects

The adverse effects of these drugs are related to their toxic effects on the liver and kidneys. Patients should be monitored closely for any changes in liver or kidney function. Bone marrow suppression has also been reported with the use of these drugs. Rash and dermatological changes have been reported with these antifungals. Amphotericin B is associated with severe renal impairment; bone marrow suppression; GI irritation with nausea, vomiting, and potentially severe diarrhea; anorexia and weight loss; and pain at the injection site with the possibility of phlebitis or thrombophlebitis. The adverse effects of griseofulvin are relatively mild, with headache and central nervous system (CNS) changes occurring most frequently (see Fig. 11.2).

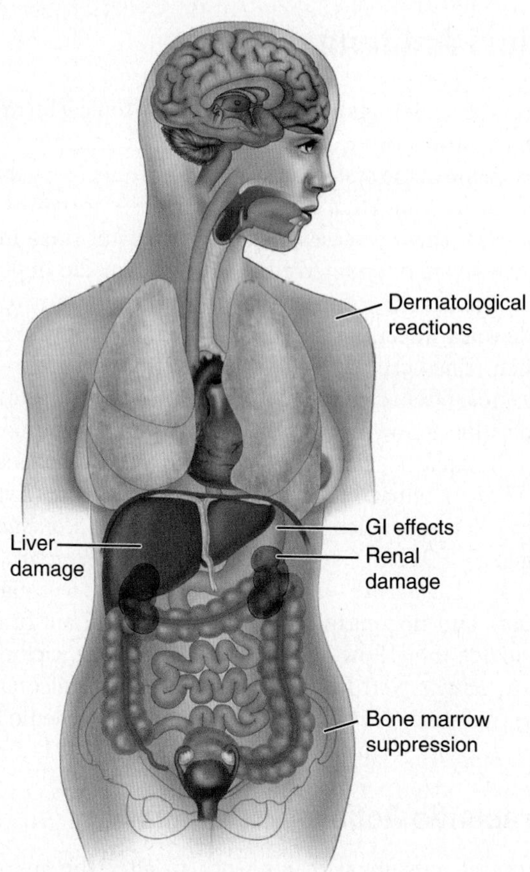

FIGURE 11.2 Common adverse effects associated with antifungals.

Clinically Important Drug–Drug Interactions

Because of the increased risk of severe renal toxicity, patients who receive amphotericin B should not take other nephrotoxic drugs such as nephrotoxic antibiotics, antineoplastics, or cyclosporine unless absolutely necessary.

Nursing Considerations for Patients Receiving Systemic Antifungals

Assessment: History and Examination

- Assess the patient for contraindications or cautions: history of allergy to antifungals to prevent potential hypersensitivity reactions, history of liver or renal dysfunction that might interfere with metabolism and excretion of the drug, and pregnancy or lactation because of potential adverse effects to the fetus or infant.
- Perform a physical assessment to establish baseline data for assessing the effectiveness of the drug and the occurrence of any adverse effects associated with drug therapy; test orientation and reflexes to evaluate any CNS effects; and examine skin for color and lesions to monitor for any dermatological effects.
- Obtain a culture of the infected area to make an accurate determination of the type and responsiveness of the fungus.
- Evaluate renal and hepatic function tests and complete blood count to determine baseline function of these organs and to assess possible toxicity during drug therapy.

Nursing Conclusions

Nursing conclusions related to drug therapy might include the following:

- Impaired comfort related to GI, CNS, and local effects of the drug
- Altered sensory (kinesthetic) perception related to CNS effects
- Knowledge deficit regarding drug therapy

Planning

- The patient will receive the best therapeutic effect from the drug therapy.

(continues on page 178)

- The patient will have limited adverse effects to the drug therapy.
- The patient will have an understanding of the drug therapy, adverse effects to anticipate, and measures to relieve discomfort and improve safety.

Intervention With Rationale

- Arrange for appropriate culture and sensitivity tests before beginning therapy to ensure that the appropriate drug is being used. However, in some cases, treatment can begin before test results are known because of the seriousness of the systemic infections.
- Administer the entire course of the drug to get the full beneficial effects; this may take as long as 6 months for some chronic infections.
- Monitor IV sites to ensure that phlebitis or infiltration does not occur. Treat appropriately, and restart the IV at another site if phlebitis occurs. Be sure to use a large vein for infusions.
- Monitor for infusion reactions including fever, chills, rigors, and headache. Pretreat with diphenhydramine and acetaminophen if indicated. Notify the provider immediately if the patient exhibits rigors.
- Monitor renal and hepatic function before and periodically during treatment to assess for possible dysfunction, and arrange to stop the drug if signs of renal or hepatic failure occur.
- If CNS effects occur, provide comfort and safety provisions (e.g., side rails and assistance with ambulation for dizziness and weakness, analgesics for headache, antipyretics for fever and chills, and temperature regulation for fever) to protect the patient from injury.
- Provide small, frequent, nutritious meals if GI upset is severe. Monitor nutritional status and arrange a dietary consultation as needed to ensure nutritional status. GI upset may be decreased by taking an oral drug with food.
- Instruct the patient to enhance patient knowledge about drug therapy and to promote adherence.
- Provide the following patient teaching:
  - Follow the appropriate dosage regimen.
  - If CNS effects occur, take safety precautions, including changing position slowly and avoiding driving and hazardous tasks.
  - Take an oral drug with meals and try small, frequent meals if GI upset is a problem.
  - Report to a health care provider any of the following: sore throat, unusual bruising and bleeding, or yellowing of the eyes or skin, all of which could indicate hepatic toxicity, or severe nausea and vomiting, which could interfere with nutritional state and slow recovery.

Evaluation

- Monitor patient response to the drug (resolution of fungal infection).
- Monitor for adverse effects (orientation and affect, nutritional state, skin color and lesions, and/or renal and hepatic function).
- Evaluate the effectiveness of the teaching plan. The patient should be able to name the drug, dosage, possible adverse effects to watch for, and specific measures to help avoid adverse effects.
- Monitor the effectiveness of comfort and safety measures and adherence to the regimen.

Key Points

- Fungi can cause many different infections in humans.
- Fungi differ from bacteria in that a fungus has a rigid cell wall that is made up of chitin and various polysaccharides and a cell membrane that contains ergosterol.
- Systemic antifungal drugs can be very toxic; extreme care should be taken to ensure that the right drug is used to treat an infection and that the patient is monitored closely to prevent severe toxicity.
- Systemic azole antifungals are associated with many drug–drug interactions because of their effects on the liver. Monitor the patient closely when adding or removing a drug from a drug regimen if the patient is receiving a systemic azole antifungal.

Topical Antifungals

Some antifungal drugs are available only in topical forms for treating a variety of mycoses of the skin and mucous membranes. Some of the systemic antifungals are also available in topical forms. Fungi that cause these mycoses are called *dermatophytes.* These diseases include a variety of **tinea** infections, which are often referred to as ringworm, although the causal organism is a fungus, not a worm. These mycoses include tinea infections such as athlete's foot (tinea pedis), jock itch (tinea cruris), and yeast infections of the mouth and vagina often caused by *Candida.* Topical antifungals include the following azole-type antifungals: butoconazole (*Gynazole-1*), clotrimazole (*Lotrimin, Mycelex*), econazole (*Ecoza*), efinaconazole (*Jublia*), ketoconazole (*Extina, Nizoral, Xolegel*), miconazole (*Lotrimin AF, Monistat-3*), oxiconazole (*Oxistat*), sertaconazole nitrate (*Ertaczo*), sulconazole (*Exelderm*), terbinafine (*Lamisil*), terconazole (*Terazol*), and tioconazole (*Vagistat-1*). Topical antifungals also include the following: butenafine (*Mentax*), ciclopirox (*Loprox, Penlac Nail Lacquer*), gentian violet, luliconazole (*Luzu*), naftifine (*Naftin*), tolnaftate, and undecylenic acid (*Cruex, Desenex, Pedi-Dri, Fungoid AF*) (see Table 11.2).

Therapeutic Actions and Indications

The topical antifungal drugs work to alter the cell permeability of the fungus, preventing replication and caus-

Table 11.2 *Drugs in Focus:* Topical Antifungals

Drug Name	Application/Available Form	Usual Indications
Azole Topical Antifungals		
butoconazole (*Gynazole I*)	Vaginal cream; applied once daily for 4 wk	Available OTC for treatment of vaginal *Candida* infections
clotrimazole (*Lotrimin, Mycelex*)	Available OTC as a cream, lotion, or solution; applied as a thin layer twice daily for 2–4 wk	Available OTC for treatment of oral and vaginal *Candida* infections; tinea infections
econazole (*Spectazole*)	Available OTC as a cream; applied as a thin layer once or twice daily for 2 wk	Treatment of tinea
efinaconazole (*Jublia*)	Topical solution, applied with flow-through brush to affected toenails daily for 48 wk, must completely cover all aspects of the involved toe(s)	Treatment of onychomycosis of the toenails due to *Trichophyton rubrum, Trichophyton mentagrophytes*
ketoconazole (*Extina, Xolegel*)	Available in cream, gel, foam, and shampoo; applied once or twice daily for 2–4 wk	Treatment of seborrheic dermatitis, tinea corporis, tinea cruris, tinea pedis
luliconazole (*Luzu*)	Available as a cream; applied to affected and surrounding area once daily for 1–2 wk	Treatment of interdigital tinea pedis, tinea cruris, tinea corporis
miconazole (*Monistat*-3)	Available OTC as a vaginal suppository, cream, powder, solution, ointment, gel, and spray; dosing recommendation varies per formulation	Treatment of local, topical mycoses, including bladder and vaginal infections and athlete's foot
oxiconazole (*Oxistat*)	Available as a cream or lotion; applied once or twice daily as needed	Short-term (up to 4 wk) treatment of topical mycosis
sertaconazole nitrate (*Ertaczo*)	Available as a topical cream; applied between toes affected by tinea pedis and to the surrounding healthy tissue two times a day for 4 wk	Treatment of tinea pedis infections (up to 4 wk)
sulconazole (*Exelderm*)	Available as a cream for athlete's foot and a solution for other tinea injections; applied once or twice daily for 4–6 wk	Treatment of tinea infections
terbinafine (*Lamisil*)	Available as a cream or gel; used for 1–4 wk; applied twice daily	Short-term (1–4 wk) treatment of topical mycosis; treatment of tinea infections
terconazole (*Terazol*)	Available as a suppository or a vaginal cream; one vaginal applicator applied daily for 3–7 consecutive days; topical cream may be applied twice daily for 1–4 wk	Local treatment of *Candida* infections
tioconazole (*Vagistat-1*)	Vaginal ointment, meant for one-dose treatment only; one applicator full of ointment is inserted vaginally at bedtime	Treatment of recurrent vaginal *Candida* infections
Other Topical Antifungals		
butenafine (*Mentax*)	Topical cream; applied in a thin layer once or twice daily for up to 4 wk	Treatment of tinea infections
ciclopirox (*Loprox, Penlac Nail Lacquer*)	Available as a gel, cream, lotion, suspension, solution, and shampoo; applied twice daily for up to 4 wk	Treatment of topical tinea infections; solution for treatment of toenail and fingernail tinea infections caused by *Trichophyton rubrum*
gentian violet (generic)	Available as a topical solution; applied twice daily to affected area	Treatment of topical mycosis
naftifine (*Naftin*)	Available as a cream or gel; applied twice daily for up to 4 wk	Short-term treatment of severe topical mycosis (up to 4 wk)
tavaborole (*Kerydin*)	Available as topical solution; applied to toenails once daily for up to 48 wk	Treatment of onychomycosis of the toenails
tolnaftate (generic)	Available as a cream, solution, gel, powder, and spray; applied twice daily for 2–4 wk	Available OTC for treatment of athlete's foot
undecylenic acid (*Cruex, Desenex*)	Available as a powder, cream, and ointment; used as needed	Available OTC for treatment of athlete's foot, jock itch, diaper rash, burning, and chafing in the groin area

OTC, over-the-counter.

ing fungal death (see Fig. 11.1). They are indicated only for local treatment of mycoses, including tinea infections. See Table 11.2 for usual indications (also see the "Critical Thinking Scenario" related to drug therapy).

Pharmacokinetics

These drugs are not absorbed systemically and do not undergo metabolism or excretion in the body.

Contraindications and Cautions

Because these drugs are not absorbed systemically, contraindications are limited to known allergy to any of these drugs and to open lesions. Econazole can cause intense, local burning and irritation and should be discontinued if these conditions become severe. Gentian violet stains skin and clothing bright purple; more importantly, it is very toxic when absorbed, so it cannot be used near active lesions. Naftifine, oxiconazole, and sertaconazole nitrate should not be used for longer than 4 weeks due to the risk of adverse effects and possible emergence of resistant strains of fungi. Sulconazole should not be used for longer than 6 weeks due to the risk of adverse effects and possible emergence of resistant strains of fungi. Terbinafine should not be used for longer than 4 weeks. This drug should be stopped when the fungal condition appears to be improved or if local irritation and pain become too great to avoid toxic effects. Efinaconazole must be applied with the supplied flow-through brush applicator.

Adverse Effects

When these drugs are applied locally as a cream, lotion, or spray, local effects include irritation, burning, rash, and swelling. When they are taken as a suppository or troche, adverse effects include nausea, vomiting, and hepatic dysfunction (related to absorption of some of the drug by the GI tract) or urinary frequency, burning, and change in sexual activity (related to local absorption in the vagina).

Prototype Summary: Clotrimazole

Indications: Treatment of oropharyngeal candidiasis (troche); prevention of oropharyngeal candidiasis in patients receiving radiation or chemotherapy; local treatment of vulvovaginal candidiasis (vaginal preparations); topical treatment of tinea pedis, tinea cruris, and tinea corporis.

Actions: Binds to sterols in the fungal cell membrane, changing membrane permeability and allowing leakage of intracellular components, causing cell death.

Pharmacokinetics: Not absorbed systemically; pharmacokinetics is unknown.

Adverse Effects: Troche: nausea, vomiting, abnormal liver function tests. Topical: stinging, redness, urticaria, edema. Vaginal: lower abdominal pain, urinary frequency, burning or irritation in sexual partner.

Nursing Considerations for Patients Receiving Topical Antifungals

Assessment: History and Examination

- Assess for known allergy to any topical antifungal agent to prevent hypersensitivity reactions.
- Perform a physical assessment to establish baseline data for evaluation of the effectiveness of the drug and the occurrence of any adverse effects associated with drug therapy.
- Perform culture and sensitivity testing of the affected area to determine the causative fungus and appropriate medication.
- Inspect the area of application for color, temperature, and evidence of lesions to establish a baseline to monitor the effectiveness of the drug and to monitor for local adverse effects of the drug.

Nursing Conclusions

Nursing conclusions related to drug therapy might include the following:

- Impaired comfort related to local effects of the drug
- Knowledge deficit regarding drug therapy
- Altered skin integrity

Planning

- The patient will receive the best therapeutic effect from the drug therapy.
- The patient will have limited adverse effects to the drug therapy.
- The patient will have an understanding of the drug therapy, adverse effects to anticipate, and measures to relieve discomfort and improve safety.

Intervention With Rationale

- Ensure that the patient takes the complete course of the drug regimen to achieve maximal results.
- Instruct the patient in the correct method of administration, depending on the route, to improve effectiveness and decrease the risk of adverse effects:
  - Troches should be dissolved slowly in the mouth.
  - Vaginal suppositories, creams, and tablets should be inserted high into the vagina with the patient remaining recumbent for at least 10 to 15 minutes after insertion.
  - Topical creams and lotions should be gently rubbed into the affected area after it has been cleansed with soap and water and patted dry. Occlusive bandages should be avoided.
- Advise the patient to stop the drug if a severe rash occurs, especially if it is accompanied by blisters or if local irritation and pain are very severe. This development may indicate sensitivity to the drug or worsening of the condition being treated.

- Provide patient instruction to enhance patient knowledge about drug therapy and to promote adherence.
- Provide the following patient teaching:
  - The correct method of drug administration; demonstrate proper application
  - The length of time necessary to treat the infection adequately
  - Use of clean, dry socks when treating athlete's foot, to help eradicate the infection
  - The need to keep the infected area clean, washing with mild soap and water, and patting dry; keeping the area dry
  - The need to avoid scratching the infected area, including advising use of cool compresses to decrease itching
  - The need to avoid occlusive dressings because of the risk of increasing systemic absorption
  - The importance of not applying drugs near open wounds or active lesions because these agents are not intended to be absorbed systemically
  - The need to report severe local irritation, burning, or worsening of the infection to a health care provider

Evaluation

- Monitor patient response to the drug (alleviation of signs and symptoms of the fungal infection).
- Monitor for adverse effects (rash, local irritation, and burning).
- Evaluate the effectiveness of the teaching plan. The patient should be able to name the drug, dosage, possible adverse effects to watch for, and specific measures to help avoid adverse effects.
- Monitor the effectiveness of comfort and safety measures and adherence to the regimen.

CRITICAL THINKING SCENARIO
Poor Nutrition and Opportunistic Infection

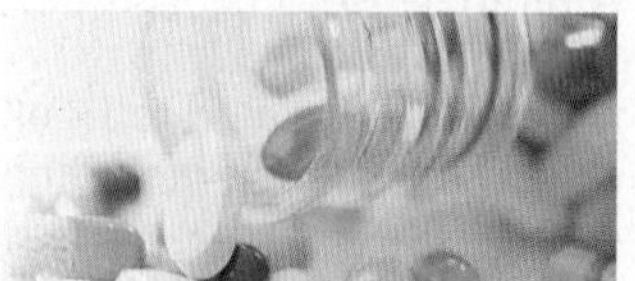

THE SITUATION

P.P., a 19-year-old aspiring model, complains of abdominal pain, difficulty swallowing, and a very sore throat. The strict diets P.P. has followed for long periods have sometimes amounted to a starvation regimen. In the last 18 months, P.P. has received treatment for a variety of bacterial infections (e.g., pneumonia, cystitis) with a series of antibiotics.

P.P. appears to be very thin and extremely pale and looks older than their stated age. P.P.'s mouth is moist, and small, white colonies that extend down the pharynx cover the mucosa. A vaginal examination reveals similar colonies. Cultures are performed, and it is determined that P.P. has mucocutaneous candidiasis. Fluconazole (*Diflucan*) is prescribed, and P.P. is asked to return in 10 days for follow-up.

CRITICAL THINKING

What are the effects of taking a variety of antibiotics on the normal flora? Think about the possible cause of the mycosis.

What happens to the immune system and to the skin and mucous membranes when a person's nutritional status deteriorates?

How is P.P.'s chosen profession affecting their health?

What are the possible ramifications of suggesting that P.P. change their profession or lifestyle?

What are the important nursing implications for P.P.?

Think about how the nurse can work with P.P. to ensure adherence to therapy and a return to a healthy state.

DISCUSSION

Because of P.P.'s appearance, a complete physical examination should be performed before drug therapy is initiated. It is necessary to know baseline functioning to evaluate any underlying problems that may exist. Poor nutrition and total starvation result in suppression of the protective inflammation and immune responses. In this case, the fact that liver changes often occur with poor nutrition is particularly important; such hepatic dysfunction may cause deficient drug metabolism and lead to toxicity.

An intensive program of teaching and support should be started for P.P., who should have an opportunity to vent their feelings and fears. P.P. needs help accepting the diagnosis and adapting to the drug therapy and nutritional changes that are necessary for the effective treatment of this infection. P.P. should understand the possible causes of their infection (poor nutrition and the loss of normal flora secondary to antibiotic therapy); the specifics of their drug therapy, including timing and administration; and adverse effects and warning signs that should be reported. P.P. should be monitored closely for adverse effects and should return for follow-up regularly while taking the ketoconazole. Nutritional counseling or referral to a dietitian for thorough nutritional teaching may prove beneficial.

The actual resolution of the fungal infection may occur only after a combination of prolonged drug and nutritional therapy. Because the required therapy will affect P.P.'s lifestyle tremendously, they will need a great deal of support and encouragement to make the

(continues on page 182)

necessary changes and to maintain adherence. A health care provider, such as a nurse who P.P. trusts and with whom they can regularly discuss concerns, may be an essential element in helping to eradicate the fungal infection.

NURSING CARE GUIDE FOR P.P.: ANTIFUNGAL AGENTS

Assessment: History and Examination

Assess history of allergy to any antifungal drug.
Also check history of renal or hepatic dysfunction and pregnancy or lactation status.
Focus the physical examination on the following:
Local: Culture of infected site
Skin: Color, lesions, texture
GU: Urinary output
GI: Abdominal, liver evaluation
Hematological: Renal and hepatic function tests

Nursing Conclusions

Impaired comfort related to GI, local, CNS effects
Altered sensory (kinesthetic) perception related to CNS effects
Malnutrition related to GI effects
Knowledge deficit regarding drug therapy

Planning

The patient will receive the best therapeutic effect from the drug therapy.
The patient will have limited adverse effects to the drug therapy.
The patient will have an understanding of the drug therapy, adverse effects to anticipate, and measures to relieve discomfort and improve safety.

Intervention

Obtain a culture of the infection before beginning therapy.
Perform baseline and routine liver function studies.
Provide comfort, and implement safety measures (e.g., provide assistance and raise side rails).
Ensure temperature control, lighting control, mouth care, and skin care.
Provide small, frequent meals, and monitor nutritional status.
Provide support and reassurance for dealing with drug effects and discomfort.
Provide patient teaching regarding drug name, dosage, adverse effects, precautions, and warning signs to report.

Evaluation

Evaluate drug effects: relief of signs and symptoms of fungal infection.
Monitor for adverse effects: GI alterations, dizziness, confusion, headache, fever, renal or hepatic dysfunction, menstrual irregularities, local pain, and discomfort.
Monitor for drug–drug interactions as indicated for each drug.
Evaluate effectiveness of patient teaching program and of comfort and safety measures.

PATIENT TEACHING FOR P.P.

- Fluconazole is an antifungal drug that works to destroy the fungi that have invaded the body. This medication will need to be taken for 7 to14 days.
- It is very important to take all of the prescribed medication.
- Fluconazole is generally well tolerated. Common adverse effects of this drug include the following: nausea, headache, skin rash, abdominal pain, vomiting, and diarrhea.
  - Headache: An analgesic may be taken to help alleviate the headache.
  - Stomach upset, nausea, and vomiting: Small, frequent meals may help. Take the drug with food if appropriate because this may decrease the GI upset associated with these drugs. Try to maintain adequate nutrition.
- There have been rare occurrences of allergy reactions and severe skin reactions. Report any of the following to your health care provider: severe vomiting, abdominal pain, fever or chills, yellowing of the skin or eyes, dark urine or pale stools, facial edema, or skin rash.
- Avoid over-the-counter medications. If you feel that you need one of these, check with your health care provider first.
- Take the full course of your prescription. Never use this drug to self-treat any other infection, and never give this drug to any other person.
- Tell any doctor, nurse, or other health care provider involved in your care that you are taking this drug.
- Keep this drug and all medications out of the reach of children.

Key Points

- Local fungal infections include vaginal and oral yeast infections (*Candida*) and a variety of tinea infections, including athlete's foot and jock itch.
- Topical antifungals are agents that are not designed to be used systemically but are effective in the treatment of local fungal infections.
- Proper administration of topical antifungals improves their effectiveness. They should not be used near open wounds or lesions.
- Topical antifungals can cause serious local irritation, burning, and pain. The drug should be stopped if these conditions occur.

SUMMARY

- A fungus is a cellular organism with a hard cell wall that contains chitin and polysaccharides and a cell membrane that contains ergosterols.
- Any infection with a fungus is called a mycosis. Systemic fungal infections, which can be life threatening, are increasing with the rise in the number of immunocompromised patients.
- Systemic antifungals alter cell permeability, leading to leakage of cellular components. This prevents cell replication and causes cell death.
- Because systemic antifungals can be very toxic, patients should be monitored closely while receiving them. Adverse effects may include hepatic and renal failure.
- Local fungal infections include vaginal and oral yeast infections (*Candida*) and a variety of tinea infections, including athlete's foot and jock itch.
- Topical antifungals are agents that are designed to work on skin and mucosal membranes to treat local fungal infections.
- Proper administration of topical antifungals improves their effectiveness. They should not be used near open wounds or lesions.
- Topical antifungals can cause serious local irritation, burning, and pain. The drug should be stopped if these conditions occur.

CHECK YOUR UNDERSTANDING

Answers to the questions in this chapter can be found in Answers to Check Your Understanding Questions on thePoint®.

MULTIPLE CHOICE

Select the best answer.

1. How are fungal cells different from bacterial cells?
   a. A fungal cell wall has fewer but more selective protective layers.
   b. The composition of the fungal cell wall is highly rigid and protective.
   c. A fungus does not reproduce by the usual methods of cell division.
   d. Fungal cells are not able to survive on mucosal surfaces.
2. What is the mechanism of action of systemic antifungal medications?
   a. Breaking apart the fungus nucleus
   b. Interfering with fungus DNA production
   c. Altering cell permeability of the fungus, leading to cell death
   d. Preventing the fungus from absorbing needed nutrients
3. After assessing a patient, the nurse would question an order for amphotericin B to prevent the possibility of serious nephrotoxicity if the patient was also receiving which of the following?
   a. Digoxin
   b. Oral anticoagulants
   c. Phenytoin
   d. Loop diuretic
4. The nurse is describing fungi that cause infections of the skin and mucous membranes, appropriately calling these which of the following?
   a. Mycoses
   b. Meningeal fungi
   c. Dermatophytes
   d. Worms

5. After teaching a group of students about topical fungal infections, the instructor determines that the students need additional instruction when they identify which of the following as an example?
   a. Athlete's foot
   b. Rocky Mountain spotted fever
   c. Jock itch
   d. Vaginal yeast infections

6. Which of the following would the nurse recommend that a patient with repeated vaginal yeast infections keep on hand?
   a. Tolnaftate
   b. Butenafine
   c. Clotrimazole
   d. Naftifine

7. A nurse is infusing IV amphotericin B to a patient with a systemic fungal infection. Based on the adverse effects of the medication, which blood work would NOT need to be evaluated?
   a. Complete blood count
   b. Albumin level
   c. Blood glucose level
   d. Renal function

8. A patient with a severe case of athlete's foot is seen with lesions between the toes; the lesions are oozing blood and serum. After teaching the patient, the nurse determines that the instruction was effective when the patient states which of the following?
   a. "I have to wear black socks and must be careful not to change them very often because it could pull more skin off of my feet."
   b. "I need to apply a thick layer of the antifungal cream between my toes, making sure that all of the lesions are full of cream."
   c. "I should wear white socks and keep my feet clean and dry. I shouldn't use the antifungal cream in areas where I have open lesions."
   d. "After I apply the cream to my feet, I should cover my feet in plastic wrap for several hours to make sure the drug is absorbed."

MULTIPLE RESPONSE

Select all that apply.

1. When administering a systemic antifungal, the nurse would include which of the following in the patient's plan of care?
   a. Ensuring that a culture of the affected area had been done
   b. Having the patient swallow the troche used for oral *Candida* infections
   c. Ensuring that the patient stays flat for at least 1 hour if receiving a vaginal suppository
   d. Monitoring the IV site to prevent phlebitis
   e. Keeping the patient NPO (nothing by mouth) if GI upset occurs to prevent vomiting
   f. Providing antipyretics if fever occurs with IV antifungals

2. The nurse would include which of the following in a teaching plan for a patient who is receiving an oral antifungal drug?
   a. It is important that you complete the full course of your drug therapy.
   b. You can share this drug with other family members if they develop the same symptoms.
   c. If you feel drowsy or dizzy, you should avoid driving or operating dangerous machinery.
   d. If GI upset occurs, avoid eating and drinking so you don't vomit and lose the drug.
   e. Use over-the-counter drugs to counteract any adverse effects like headache, fever, or rash.
   f. Notify your health care provider if you experience yellowing of the skin or eyes, dark urine or light-colored stools, or fever and chills.

REFERENCES

Brunton, L., Hilal-Dandan, R., & Knollman, B. (2018). *Goodman and Gilman's the pharmacological basis of therapeutics* (13th ed.). McGraw-Hill.

Eschenauer, G., Lam, S., & Carver, P. (2009). Antifungal prophylaxis in liver transplant recipients. *Liver Transplantation, 15*(8), 842–858. https://doi.org/10.1002/lt.21826

Gupta, A., & Cooper, E. (2008). Update in antifungal therapy of dermatophytosis. *Mycopathologia, 116*(5/6), 353–367. 10.1007/s11046-008-9109-0

Hendler, C. B. (2021). *Nursing 2021 drug handbook.* Wolters Kluwer.

Herbrecht, R., Maertens, J., Baila, L., Aoun, M., Heinz, W., Martino, R., Schwartz, S., Ullmann, A. J., Meert, L., Paesmans, M., Marchetti, O., Akan, H., Ameye, L., Shivaprakash, M., & Viscoli, C. (2010). Caspofungin first-line therapy for invasive aspergillosis in allogeneic hematopoietic stem cell transplant patients. *Bone Marrow Transplantation, 45*(7), 1227–1233. 10.1038/bmt.2009.334

Juang, P. (2007). Update on new antifungal therapy. *AACN Advanced Critical Care, 18*(3), 253–260. 10.1097/01.AACN.0000284425.71083.30

Kuse, E., Chetchotisakd, P., Arns da Cunha, C., Ruhnke, M., Barrios, C., Raghunadharao, D., Sekhon, J. S., Freire, A., Ramasubramanian, V., Demeyer, I., Nucci, M., Leelarasamee,

A., Jacobs, F., Decruyenaere, J., Rittet, D., Ullmann, A. J., Ostrosky-Zeichner, L., Lortholary, O., Koblinger, S., … Cornely, O. A. (2007). Micafungin versus liposomal amphotericin B for candidemia and invasive candidosis: A phase III randomized double-blind trial. *The Lancet, 369*(9572), 1519–1527. 10.1016/S0140-6736(07)60605-9

Norris, T. L. (2019). *Porth's pathophysiology concepts of altered health states* (13th ed.). Wolters Kluwer.

Pappas, P. G., Kauffman, C. A., Andes, D. R., Clancy, C. J., Marr, K. A., Ostrosky-Zeichner, L., Reboli, A. C., Schuster, M. G., Vazquez, J. A., Walsh, T. J., Zaoutis, T. E., & Sobel, J. D. (2016). Clinical practice guideline for the management of Candidiasis: 2016 update by the infectious diseases society of America. *Clinical Infectious Disease*, *62*(4), e1–e50. doi:10.1093/cid/civ933

CHAPTER 12

Antiprotozoal Agents

Learning Objectives

Upon completion of this chapter, you will be able to:

1. Outline the life cycle of the protozoan that causes malaria.
2. Describe the therapeutic actions, indications, pharmacokinetics, contraindications, proper administration, most common adverse reactions, and important drug–drug interactions associated with drugs used to treat malaria.
3. Describe other common protozoal infections, including cause and clinical presentation.
4. Compare and contrast the antimalarials with other drugs used to treat protozoal infections.
5. Outline the nursing considerations for patients receiving an antiprotozoal agent across the lifespan.

Key Terms

amebiasis: amebic dysentery, which is caused by intestinal invasion of the trophozoite stage of the protozoan *Entamoeba histolytica*

***Anopheles* mosquito:** type of mosquito that is essential to the life cycle of *Plasmodium*; injects the protozoa into humans for further maturation

cinchonism: syndrome of quinine toxicity characterized by nausea, vomiting, tinnitus, and vertigo

giardiasis: protozoal intestinal infection that causes severe diarrhea and epigastric distress; may lead to serious malnutrition

leishmaniasis: infection of the skin, mucous membrane, or viscera caused by a protozoan passed to humans by the bites of sand flies

malaria: protozoal infection with *Plasmodium*, characterized by cyclic fever and chills as the parasite is released from ruptured red blood cells; causes serious liver, central nervous system (CNS), heart, and lung damage

***Plasmodium*:** a protozoan that causes malaria in humans; its life cycle includes the *Anopheles* mosquito, which injects protozoa into humans

protozoa: single-celled organisms that pass through several stages in their life cycle, including at least one phase as a human parasite; found in areas with poor sanitation and hygiene and crowded living conditions

trichomoniasis: infestation with a protozoan that causes vaginitis in females but no signs or symptoms in males

trophozoite: a developing stage of a parasite, which uses the host for essential nutrients needed for growth

trypanosomiasis: African sleeping sickness, which is caused by a protozoan that inflames the CNS and is spread to humans by the bite of the tsetse fly; also, Chagas disease, which causes a serious cardiomyopathy after the bite of the housefly

Drug List

ANTIMALARIALS
- (P) chloroquine
- hydroxychloroquine sulfate
- mefloquine
- primaquine
- pyrimethamine
- quinine
- tafenoquine

OTHER ANTIPROTOZOALS
- atovaquone
- benznidazole
- (P) metronidazole
- nitazoxanide
- pentamidine
- tinidazole

Infections caused by **protozoa**—single-celled organisms that pass through several stages in their life cycles, including at least one phase as a human parasite—are very common in several parts of the world. In tropical areas, where protozoal infections are most prevalent, many people suffer multiple infestations at the same time. These illnesses are relatively rare in the United States, but it is not unusual to find an individual who returns home from a trip to Africa, Asia, or South America with a fully developed protozoal infection. Protozoa thrive in tropical climates, but they may also survive and reproduce in any area where people live in very crowded or unsanitary conditions. This chapter focuses on agents used for protozoal infections that are caused by insect bites (malaria, trypanosomiasis, and leishmaniasis) and those that result from ingestion or contact with the causal organism (amebiasis, giardiasis, and trichomoniasis). Box 12.1 discusses the use of antiprotozoals across the lifespan. Figure 12.1 shows sites of action for these agents.

Malaria

Malaria is a parasitic disease that has killed hundreds of millions of people and has even changed the course of history. The progress of several battles in Africa and the building of the Panama Canal were altered by outbreaks of malaria. Even with the introduction of drugs for the treatment of this disease, it remains endemic in many parts of the world. The only known method of transmission of malaria is through the bite of a female ***Anopheles* mosquito**, an insect that harbors the protozoal parasite and carries it to humans.

Four protozoal parasites, all in the genus ***Plasmodium***, have been identified as causes of malaria:

- *Plasmodium falciparum* is considered to be the most dangerous type of protozoan. Infection with this protozoan results in an acute, rapidly fulminating disease with high fever, severe hypotension, swelling and reddening of the limbs, loss of red blood cells, and even death.
- *Plasmodium vivax* causes a milder form of the disease, which seldom results in death.
- *Plasmodium malariae* is endemic in many tropical countries and causes very mild signs and symptoms in the local population. It can cause more acute disease in travelers to endemic areas.
- *Plasmodium ovale* can be caused by two different species (*curtisi* and *wallikeri*), which are both most prevalent in Africa.

A major problem with controlling malaria is that the mosquito that is responsible for transmitting the disease has developed a resistance to the insecticides designed to eradicate it. In the past, widespread efforts at mosquito control were successful, with fewer cases of malaria being seen each year. However, the rise of insecticide-resistant mosquitoes has allowed malaria to flourish, increasing the incidence of the disease. In addition, the protozoa that cause malaria have developed strains resistant to the usual antimalarial drugs. This combination of factors has led to a worldwide public health challenge.

Life Cycle of Plasmodium

The parasites that cause human malaria spend part of their life in the *Anopheles* mosquito and part in the human host (see Fig. 12.2). When a mosquito bites a human who is infected with malaria, it sucks blood infested with

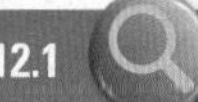

Box 12.1 Focus on Drug Therapy Across the Lifespan

ANTIPROTOZOAL AGENTS

Children

Many of these drugs do not have proven safety and efficacy in children, and extreme caution should be used. The dangers of infection resulting from travel to areas endemic with many of these diseases are often much more severe than the potential risks associated with cautious use of these drugs.

If a child needs to travel to an area with endemic protozoal infections, the CDC or local health department should be consulted about the safest possible preventative measures.

Adults

Adults should be well advised about the need for prophylaxis against various protozoal infections and the need for immediate treatment if the disease is contracted. It is very helpful to mark calendars as reminders of the days before, during, and after exposure on which the drugs should be taken.

Pregnant and nursing patients should not use these drugs unless the benefit clearly outweighs the potential risk to the fetus or neonate. Patients who can become pregnant should be advised to use barrier contraceptives if some of these drugs are used. A pregnant person traveling to an area endemic with protozoal infections should be advised of the serious risks to the fetus associated with both preventive therapy and treatment of acute attacks and of the risks associated with contracting the disease.

Older Adults

Older patients may be more susceptible to the adverse effects associated with these drugs. They should be monitored closely.

Patients with hepatic dysfunction are at increased risk for worsening hepatic problems and toxic effects of many of these drugs. If hepatic dysfunction is expected due to extreme age, alcohol abuse, or use of other hepatotoxic drugs, the dose may need to be lowered and the patient monitored more frequently.

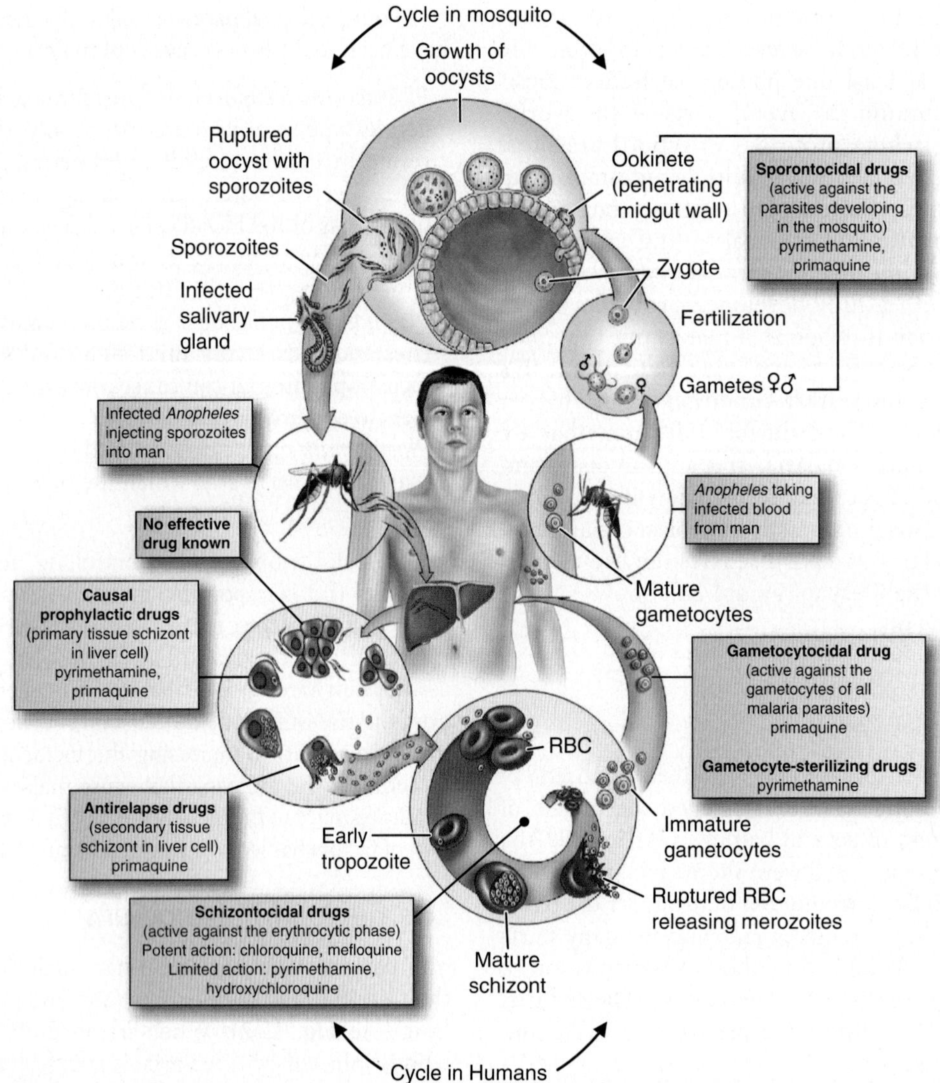

FIGURE 12.1 Sites of action of antimalarials and other antiprotozoals. Antimalarials block protein synthesis and cause cell death. Other antiprotozoals block DNA synthesis, prevent cell reproduction, and lead to cell death. RBC, red blood cell.

gametocytes, which are male and female forms of the *Plasmodium*. These gametocytes mate in the stomach of the mosquito and produce a zygote that goes through several phases before forming sporozoites (spore animals) that make their way to the mosquito's salivary glands. The next person who is bitten by that mosquito is injected with thousands of sporozoites. These organisms travel through the bloodstream, where they quickly become lodged in the human liver and other tissues and invade the cells.

Inside human cells, the organisms undergo asexual cell division and reproduction. Over the next 7 to 10 days, these primary tissue organisms called schizonts grow and multiply within their invaded cells, using the cell for needed nutrients (as trophozoites). Merozoites are then formed from the primary schizonts and burst from invaded cells when those cells rupture because of overexpansion. These merozoites enter the circulation and invade red blood cells. Here they continue to divide until the blood cells also burst, sending more merozoites into the circulation to invade yet more red blood cells.

Eventually, there are a large number of merozoites in the body, as well as many ruptured and invaded red blood cells. At this point, the acute malarial attack occurs. The rupture of the red blood cells causes a massive inflammatory reaction with chills and fever related to the pyrogenic effects of the protozoa and the toxic effects of the red blood cell components on the system. This cycle of chills and fever usually occurs about every 72 hours. These cycles typically resolve in about 2 weeks.

With *P. vivax* and *P. malariae* malaria, this cycle may continue for a longer period of time. Many of the tissue schizonts lay dormant until they eventually find their way to the liver, where they multiply and then invade more red blood cells, again causing the acute cycle. This cycle of emerging from dormancy to cause a resurgence of the acute phase may occur for years in an untreated patient.

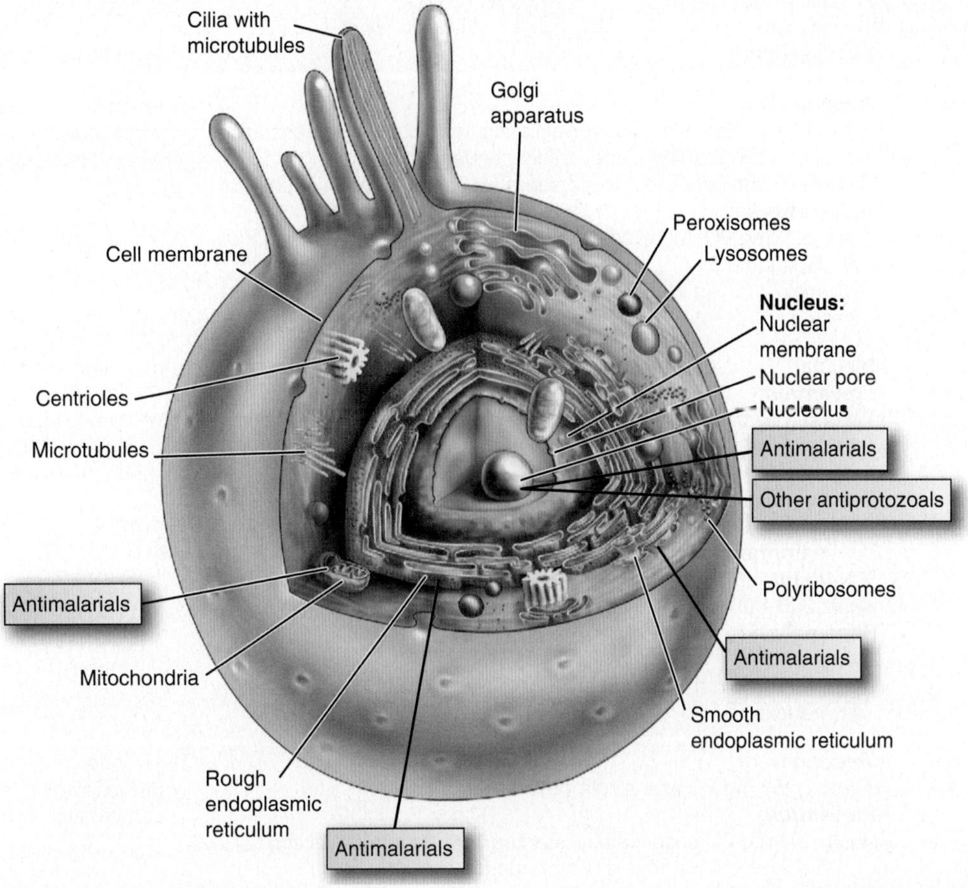

FIGURE 12.2 Antimalarial and other antiprotozoal drugs work in a variety of ways on the cells due to needing to target the protozoa in different life stages.

With *P. falciparum* malaria, there are no extrahepatic sites for the schizonts. If the patient survives an acute attack, no prolonged periods of relapse occur. The first attack of this type of malaria can destroy so many red blood cells that the patient's capillaries become clogged and the circulation to vital organs is interrupted, leading to death.

Antimalarials

Choice of antimalarial drugs (Table 12.1) is based on the type of malaria, whether the infection was acquired in an area of chloroquine resistance, severity of the symptoms, and whether the person was taking prophylactic antimalarial medication. Antimalarial drugs can be schizonticidal (acting against the red blood cell phase of the life cycle), gametocytocidal (acting against the gametocytes), sporontocidal (acting against the parasites that are developing in the mosquito), or they can work against tissue schizonts as prophylactic or antirelapse agents. Quinine (*Qualaquin*) was the first drug found to be effective in the treatment of malaria; it was absent from the market for a while but is now available for the treatment of uncomplicated malaria. Other antimalarials used today include chloroquine (*Aralen*), hydroxychloroquine sulfate (*Plaquenil*), mefloquine (generic), primaquine (generic), and tafenoquine (*Arakoda, Krintafel*). Fixed dose combination drugs for malaria prevention and treatment are discussed in Box 12.2.

Therapeutic Actions and Indications

Chloroquine or hydroxychloroquine are first-line therapy, even for patients who are pregnant, unless the infection was acquired in a chloroquine-resistant area or the patient is ill enough to require IV medication. These medications may hinder the parasite by inhibiting the combining of heme molecules. They are weak bases and may affect the acid vesicles of the parasite. They can also interact with the DNA and inhibit parasite enzymes (see Fig. 12.1). Because some strains of the parasite are developing resistance to chloroquine, the Centers for Disease Control and Prevention (CDC) often recommend the use of certain antibiotics as part of combination therapy for treatment of malaria caused by these resistant strains. Box 12.3 lists the antibiotics used to treat malaria. See Table 12.1 for usual indications. The drugs have different mechanisms of action.

Mefloquine increases the acidity of plasmodial food vacuoles, causing cell rupture and death. In combination therapy, mefloquine is used in malarial prevention and in treatment.

Table 12.1 *Drugs in Focus*: Antimalarials

Drug Name	Dosage/Route	Usual Indications
chloroquine (*Aralen*)	***Suppression:*** *Adult*: 300 mg PO every week beginning 1–2 wk before exposure and continuing for 4 wk after leaving endemic area *Pediatric*: 5 mg/kg/wk PO, using same schedule as for an adult ***Acute attacks:*** *Adult*: 600 mg PO, followed by 300 mg PO in 6 h; then 300 mg PO on days 2 and 3 *Pediatric*: 10 mg/kg PO, followed by 5 mg/kg PO in 6 h and on days 2 and 3	Prevention and treatment of *Plasmodium* malaria; treatment of extraintestinal amebiasis
hydroxychloroquine sulfate (*Plaquenil*)	**Malaria:** ***Prevention:*** *Adult and pediatric:* 6.5 mg/kg not to exceed 400 mg or *(adult only)* 400 mg once per week 2 wk prior to travel and continued for 4 wk after leaving endemic area ***Treatment:*** *Adult and pediatric:* Weight-based dosing or scheduled dosing over 48 h **Lupus Erythematosus** ***Treatment:*** *Adult:* 200–400 mg PO daily or twice a day **Rheumatoid Arthritis** ***Treatment:*** *Adult:* 400–600 mg PO once or twice daily; with good response may be reduced	Prevention and treatment of *Plasmodium* malaria; treatment of chronic lupus erythematosus; treatment of acute and chronic rheumatoid arthritis in adults
mefloquine (*Lariam*)	***Treatment:*** *Adult*: 1,250 mg PO as a single dose ***Prevention:*** *Adult*: 250 mg PO once weekly, starting 1 wk before travel and continuing for 4 wk after leaving endemic area *Pediatric*: 15–19 kg, 1/4 tablet; 20–30 kg, 1/2 tablet; 31–45 kg, 3/4 tablet; >45 kg, 1 tablet; once a week, starting 1 wk before travel and continuing until 4 wk after leaving area	Prevention and treatment of *Plasmodium* malaria in combination with other drugs
primaquine (generic)	*Adult*: 26.3 mg/d PO for 14 d *Pediatric*: 0.5 mg/kg/d PO for 14 d; begin therapy during last 2 wk of (or after) therapy with chloroquine or other drugs	Prevention of relapses of *Plasmodium vivax* and *Plasmodium malariae* infections; radical cure of *P. vivax* malaria
quinine (*Qualaquin*)	*Adult*: 648 mg PO q8h for 7 days	Treatment of uncomplicated malaria caused by *Plasmodium falciparum*

BOX 12.2

Combination Drugs Used for Malaria Prevention and Treatment

There are fixed-combination drugs available for use in the prevention and treatment of malaria. Combining two different preparations in one drug may increase adherence by reducing the number of pills a patient has to take, and it conforms to the treatment protocol of taking drugs that affect the protozoa at different stages on their life cycle.

Malarone and *Malarone Pediatric* combine atovaquone and proguanil. They are indicated for the prevention of *Plasmodium falciparum* malaria when chloroquine resistance has been reported. The combination is used for the treatment of uncomplicated *P. falciparum* malaria when chloroquine, halofantrine, and mefloquine have not proved successful, most likely because of resistance. This combination should be used in pregnancy and lactation only if the benefit clearly outweighs the potential risk to the fetus or neonate.

A newer combination drug is *Coartem*, a combination of artemether and lumefantrine, antimalarials only available in this combination. This drug is approved for the treatment of acute, uncomplicated malaria caused by *P. falciparum* in patients weighing 5 kg or more. It should only be used with extreme caution in patients with severe hepatic impairment. It should be taken with food to improve absorption. This drug combination is known to prolong the QT interval and should be avoided in patients with known prolonged QT interval and should not be used in combination with other drugs known to prolong the QT interval.

BOX 12.3

Antibiotics Used to Treat Malaria

With the emergence of chloroquine-resistant strains of *Plasmodium*, the CDC has recommended several different options for treatment. One option is the use of quinine and one of the following antibiotics as a combination therapy for the treatment of uncomplicated or severe malaria caused by chloroquine-resistant strains or uncomplicated malaria caused by strains with unknown resistance:

Doxycycline: 100 mg/d PO for 7 days for adults; 2.2 mg/kg PO q12h for 7 days for children

Tetracycline: 250 mg PO for 7 days for adults; 25 mg/kg/d PO in divided doses q.i.d. for 7 days for children

Clindamycin: 20 mg base/kg/d PO in divided doses t.i.d. for 7 days for adults and children

In severe cases, the antibiotics can be started IV and then switched to oral forms as soon as the patient is able to take oral drugs.

See Chapter 9 for a full discussion of these drugs.

Other options for treating the chloroquine-resistant strains are to administer one of the following combination medications: atovaquone–proguanil or artemether–lumefantrine (see Box 12.2 for more detail).

Primaquine, another very old drug for treating malaria, similar to quinine, disrupts the mitochondria of the *Plasmodium*. It also causes death of gametocytes and exoerythrocytic (outside of the red blood cell) forms and prevents other forms from reproducing.

Quinine inhibits nucleic acid synthesis, protein synthesis, and glycolysis in *P. falciparum*. It is used to treat uncomplicated malaria and is used effectively in regions where chloroquine resistance has been documented. Quinine (with clindamycin) is one of the preferred therapies for patients who are pregnant and have chloroquine-resistant malaria. The other preferred therapy, specifically for pregnant patients in their 2nd and 3rd trimesters, is *Coartem*, a combination of artemether and lumefantrine (see Box 12.2).

Tafenoquine (*Arakoda*) is indicated for antimalarial prophylaxis in adults, and tafenoquine (*Krintafel*) is indicated for prevention of relapse of patients with *P. vivax* malaria who are being treated with chloroquine for *P. vivax* infection. It is contraindicated in pregnancy.

Pharmacokinetics

Chloroquine is readily absorbed from the gastrointestinal (GI) tract, with peak serum level occurring in 1 to 6 hours. It is concentrated in the liver, spleen, kidney, and brain and is excreted very slowly in the urine, primarily as unchanged drug.

Hydroxychloroquine is absorbed from the GI tract, and peak blood concentration is reached in about 3 hours. The terminal half-life range is very long (40 to 50 days). It is excreted slowly in the urine due to extensive tissue uptake of the medication.

Mefloquine is a mixture of molecules that are absorbed, metabolized, and excreted at different rates. The terminal half-life is 13 to 24 days. Metabolism occurs in the liver; caution should be used in patients with hepatic dysfunction.

Primaquine is readily absorbed and metabolized in the liver. Excretion occurs primarily in the urine. This medication is contraindicated in pregnancy and breast or chestfeeding.

Quinine is rapidly absorbed from the GI tract, with peak serum level occurring in 1 to 3 hours. It is metabolized in the liver, has a half-life of 4 to 6 hours, and is excreted in the urine.

Tafenoquine is absorbed from the GI tract, and peak serum level occurs in 12 to 15 hours. The terminal half-life is 15 to 16.5 days. Very little seems to be metabolized, and the full excretion profile is unknown.

Contraindications and Cautions

Antimalarials are contraindicated in the presence of known patient allergy to any of these drugs. They should be used with caution in patients with liver disease or alcoholism, both because of the parasitic invasion of the liver and because of the need for the hepatic metabolism to prevent toxicity, and during lactation because the drugs can enter human milk and could be toxic to the infant. Another method of feeding the baby should be used if treatment is necessary. There are specific medications that are preferred for use during pregnancy (see individual medication descriptions). With mefloquine, which was found to be teratogenic in preclinical studies, pregnancy should be avoided during and for 2 months after completion of therapy. Use caution in patients with retinal disease or damage because many of these drugs can affect vision and the retina, and the likelihood of problems increases if the retina is already damaged; use caution in patients with psoriasis or porphyria because of skin damage. There have been some genetic enzyme differences identified in various groups that predispose them to adverse effects associated with these drugs. See Box 12.4 for cultural considerations of the use of some antimalarials in regard to the potential for hemolytic crisis in patients with glucose-6-phospahte dehydrogenase (G6PD) deficiency.

Adverse Effects

A number of adverse effects may be encountered with the use of these antimalarial agents (see Fig. 12.3). Central nervous system (CNS) effects include headache and dizziness. Immune reaction effects related to the release

Box 12.4 Focus on Cultural Considerations

POTENTIAL FOR HEMOLYTIC CRISIS

Patients with glucose-6-phosphate dehydrogenase (G6PD) deficiency, which is more likely to occur in people from Africa, the Middle East, and South Asia, may experience a hemolytic crisis if they are taking the antimalarial agent chloroquine or primaquine.

This enzyme deficiency results from a mutation on the X-chromosome so the disease can present differently in female patients versus male patients. The World Health Organization classifies the deficiency on a spectrum of severity. For people of high risk, if no history is known, testing should be done prior to prescribing these medications. The patient should be monitored very closely and informed about the potential need for hospitalization and emergency services.

of merozoites include fever, shaking, chills, and malaise. Nausea, vomiting, dyspepsia, and anorexia are associated with direct effects of the drug on the GI tract and the effects on CNS control of vomiting caused by the products of cell death and protein changes. Hepatic dysfunction is associated with the toxic effects of the drug on the liver in addition to the effects of the disease on the liver. Dermatological effects include rash, pruritus, and loss of hair associated with changes in protein synthesis of the hair follicles. Visual changes, including possible blindness related to retinal damage from the drug, and ototoxicity related to other nerve damage may occur. **Cinchonism**, a syndrome of toxicity characterized by nausea, vomiting, tinnitus, and vertigo, may occur with high levels of quinine or primaquine. Chloroquine and hydroxychloroquine have been associated with cardiomyopathy and fatal cardiac arrhythmias including heart block and prolonged QT interval that can lead to torsades de pointes. Despite these risks, some people have touted use of these drugs for COVID-19. See Box 12.5 for a focus on the evidence regarding use of antimalarial medication to treat COVID-19.

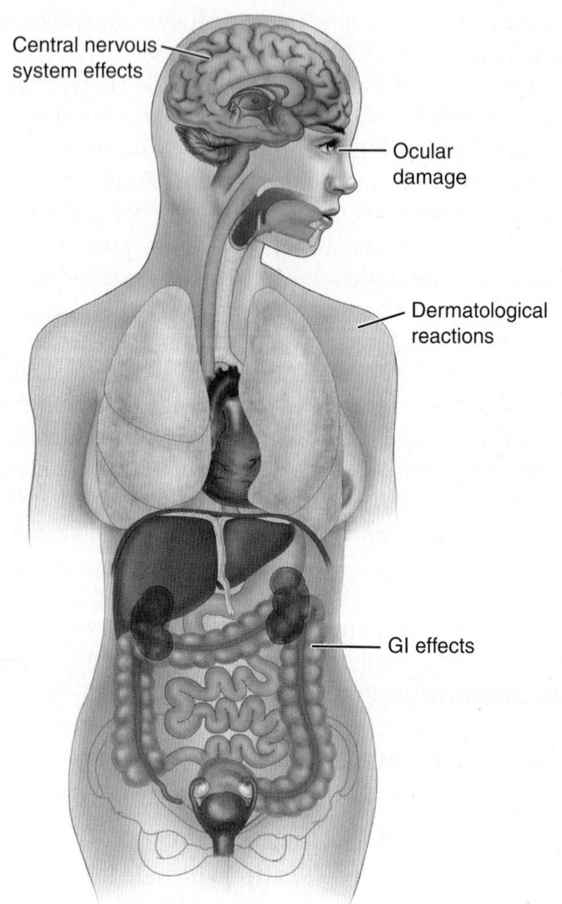

FIGURE 12.3 Common adverse effects associated with antiprotozoals.

Clinically Important Drug–Drug Interactions

The patient who is receiving combinations of the quinine derivatives and quinine is at increased risk for cardiac toxicity and convulsions. Therefore, monitor the patient closely, checking drug levels and anticipating dose adjustments as needed.

Increased bone marrow suppression may occur if antifolate drugs (methotrexate, sulfonamides, etc.) are combined with pyrimethamine; discontinue pyrimethamine if signs of folate deficiency develop (diarrhea, fatigue, weight loss, anemia).

Hydroxychloroquine can lower seizure threshold and should, therefore, be used with caution with other medications that are known to also lower seizure threshold. Antiepileptic medications may be less efficacious if coadministered with hydroxychloroquine. Antacids may reduce the absorption of chloroquine and hydroxychloroquine. Ampicillin may have reduced bioavailability when used with these medications.

Prototype Summary: Chloroquine

Indications: Treatment and prophylaxis of acute attacks of malaria caused by susceptible strains of *Plasmodium*; treatment of extraintestinal amebiasis.

Actions: Inhibits protozoal reproduction and protein synthesis.

Pharmacokinetics:

Route	Onset	Peak	Duration
Oral	Varies	1–2 h	1 wk

$T_{1/2}$: 70 to 120 hours; metabolized in the liver and excreted in the urine.

Adverse Effects: Visual and auditory disturbances, retinal changes, hypotension, nausea, vomiting, diarrhea.

Nursing Considerations for Patients Receiving Antimalarial Agents

Assessment: History and Examination

- Assess for contraindications or cautions: history of allergy to any of the antimalarials to prevent hypersensitivity reactions; liver dysfunction or alcoholism that might interfere with the metabolism and excretion of the drug; porphyria or psoriasis, which could be exacerbated by the drug effects; retinal disease that could increase the visual disturbances associated with these drugs; and pregnancy and lactation because these drugs could affect the fetus and could enter human milk and be toxic to the infant.
- Perform a physical assessment to establish baseline data for assessment of the effectiveness of the drug and the occurrence of any adverse effects associated with drug therapy. Assess the CNS (reflexes and muscle strength).
- Perform ophthalmic and retinal examinations and auditory screening to determine the need for cautious administration and to evaluate changes that occur as a result of drug therapy.
- Assess the patient's liver function to determine appropriateness of therapy and to monitor for toxicity.
- Obtain blood culture to identify the causative *Plasmodium* spp. and ensure appropriate use of the drug.
- Inspect the skin closely for color, temperature, texture, and evidence of lesions to monitor for adverse effects.

Nursing Conclusions

Nursing conclusions related to drug therapy might include the following:

- Impaired comfort related to GI, CNS, and skin effects of the drug
- Altered sensory (kinesthetic, visual) perception related to CNS effects
- Injury risk related to CNS changes
- Knowledge deficit regarding drug therapy

Planning

- The patient will receive the best therapeutic effect from the drug therapy.
- The patient will have limited adverse effects to the drug therapy.
- The patient will have an understanding of the drug therapy, adverse effects to anticipate, and measures to relieve discomfort and improve safety.

Intervention With Rationale

- Arrange for appropriate culture and sensitivity tests before beginning therapy to ensure the proper drug for susceptible *Plasmodium* spp. Treatment may begin before test results are known.
- Administer a complete course of the drug to get the full beneficial effects. Mark a calendar for prophylactic doses. Use combination therapy as indicated.
- Monitor hepatic function and perform ophthalmological examination before and periodically during treatment to ensure early detection and prompt intervention with cessation of drug if signs of failure or deteriorating vision occur.
- If CNS effects occur, provide comfort and safety measures (e.g., side rails and assistance with ambulation if dizziness and weakness are present) to prevent patient injury. Provide oral hygiene and ready access to bathroom facilities as needed to cope with GI effects.
- Provide small, frequent, nutritious meals if GI upset is severe to ensure adequate nutrition. Monitor nutritional status, and arrange a dietary consultation as needed. Taking the drug with food may also decrease GI upset.
- Instruct the patient concerning the appropriate dosage regimen and the importance of adhering to the drug schedule to enhance patient knowledge about drug therapy and to promote adherence.
- Provide the following patient teaching:
  - If CNS effects occur, take safety precautions, including changing position slowly and avoiding driving and hazardous tasks.
  - If GI upset is a problem, take the drug with meals, and try small, frequent meals.
  - Report blurring of vision, which could indicate retinal damage; loss of hearing or ringing in the ears, which could indicate CNS toxicity; and fever or worsening of condition, which could indicate a resistant strain or noneffective therapy.

Evaluation

- Monitor patient response to the drug (resolution of malaria or prevention of malaria).
- Monitor for adverse effects (orientation and affect, nutritional state, skin color and lesions, hepatic function, and visual and auditory changes).
- Evaluate the effectiveness of the teaching plan. The patient should be able to name the drug, dosage, possible adverse effects to watch for, and specific measures to help avoid adverse effects.
- Monitor the effectiveness of comfort and safety measures and adherence to the regimen.

Key Points

- A protozoan is a parasitic cellular organism. Its life cycle includes a parasitic phase inside human tissues or cells.
- Malaria is the most common protozoal infection and is spread to humans by the bite of an *Anopheles* mosquito. The signs and symptoms of malaria are related to the destruction of red blood cells and toxicity to the liver.
- Antimalarial agents attack the parasite at the various stages of its development inside and outside the human body.

Box 12.5 Focus on the Evidence

HYDROXYCHLOROQUINE AND COVID-19

Hydroxychloroquine sulfate has been approved by the FDA to prevent and treat malaria as well as for treatment of lupus erythematosus and rheumatoid arthritis. Its mechanism of action for modulating inflammation and immune response and for acting against the *Plasmodium* causing malaria is not completely understood. Due to its effectiveness for the above indications, some people believed that hydroxychloroquine and/or the similar medication chloroquine would be helpful for treatment of coronavirus 2019 disease (COVID-19). During the early months of 2020, there was a lack of any FDA-approved treatment for COVID-19, so multiple medications were used "off-label" in attempt to decrease mortality and/or treatment time of the disease. As clinicians were desperately trying to find treatments that would be helpful, researchers were attempting to gather the data necessary to guide the best possible medical treatment. After many "off-label" uses in both animal and human studies, hydroxychloroquine and chloroquine were not found to reduce mortality of hospitalized patients with COVID-19. In fact, they were associated with more harm, especially in high doses and when used with other anti-infective medications, due to risk of QT prolongation and cardiac arrhythmias. This is an example in which evidence for which medications to use for treatment evolved very quickly due to an emergent situation.

Other Protozoal Infections

Other protozoal infections that are encountered in clinical practice include amebiasis, leishmaniasis, trypanosomiasis, trichomoniasis, and giardiasis. These infections, which are caused by single-celled protozoa, are usually associated with unsanitary, crowded conditions and use of poor hygienic practices. Patients traveling outside the United States may encounter these infections, cases of which are also increasing in the United States.

Amebiasis

Amebiasis, an intestinal infection caused by *Entamoeba histolytica*, is often known as amebic dysentery. *E. histolytica* has a two-stage life cycle: (a) a cystic, dormant stage, in which the protozoan can live for long periods outside the body or in the human intestine, and (b) a **trophozoite** stage in its ideal environment, the human large intestine. See Figure 12.4.

The disease is transmitted while the protozoan is in the cystic stage in fecal matter, from which it can enter water and the ground. It can be passed to other humans who drink this water or eat food that has been grown in this ground. The cysts are swallowed and pass, unaffected by gastric acid, into the intestine. Some of these cysts are passed in fecal matter, and some of them become trophozoites that grow and reproduce. The trophozoites migrate into the mucosa of the colon, where they penetrate into the intestinal wall, forming erosions. These forms of *Entamoeba* release a chemical that dissolves mucosal cells, and eventually they eat away tissue until they reach the vascular system, which carries them throughout the body. The trophozoites lodge in the liver, lungs, heart, and brain.

Early signs of amebiasis include mild to fulminate diarrhea. In the worst cases, if the protozoan is able to invade extraintestinal tissue, it can dissolve the tissue and eventually cause the death of the host. Some individuals can become carriers of the disease without having any overt signs or symptoms. These people seem to be resistant to the intestinal invasion but pass the cysts in the stool.

Leishmaniasis

Leishmaniasis is a disease caused by a protozoan that is passed from sand flies to humans. The sand fly injects an asexual form of this flagellated protozoan, called a promastigote, into the body of a human, where it is rapidly attacked and digested by human macrophages. Inside the macrophages, the promastigote divides, developing many new forms called amastigotes, which keep dividing and eventually kill the macrophage, releasing the amastigotes into the system to be devoured by more macrophages. Thus, a cyclic pattern of infection is established. These amastigotes can cause serious lesions in the skin, the viscera, or the mucous membranes of the host.

Trypanosomiasis

Trypanosomiasis is caused by infection with *Trypanosoma*. Two parasitic protozoal species cause very serious and often fatal diseases in humans:

- African sleeping sickness, which is caused by *Trypanosoma brucei gambiense*, is transmitted by the tsetse fly. After the pathogenic organism has lived and grown in human blood, it eventually invades the CNS, leading to acute inflammation that results in lethargy, prolonged sleep, and even death.
- Chagas disease, which is caused by *Trypanosoma cruzi*, is almost endemic in many South American countries. It is passed to humans by the common housefly. This protozoan results in severe cardiomyopathy that accounts for numerous deaths and disabilities in certain regions.

Trichomoniasis

Trichomoniasis, which is caused by another flagellated protozoan, *Trichomonas vaginalis*, is a common cause of vaginitis. This infection is usually spread during sexual intercourse by males who have no signs and symptoms of infection. In females, this protozoan causes reddened, inflamed vaginal mucosa, itching, burning, and a yellowish-green discharge.

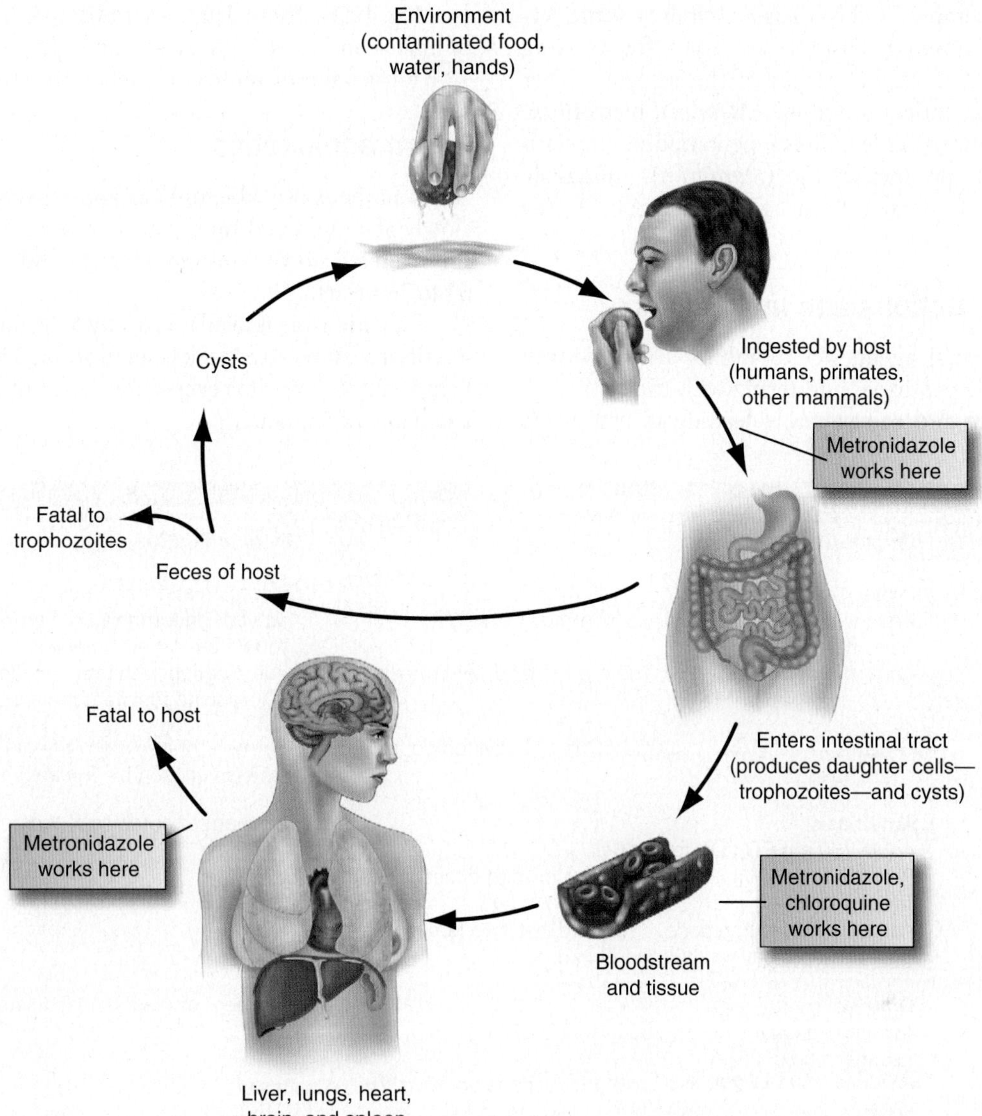

FIGURE 12.4 Life cycle of *Entamoeba histolytica* and the sites of action of metronidazole and chloroquine, which are used to treat amebiasis. Cysts ingested by the host enter the intestinal tract and produce trophozoites. Trophozoites enter the bloodstream to reach tissue. Trophozoites enter the liver, lungs, heart, brain, and spleen; this can be fatal to the host. Trophozoites are excreted in the stool and die. Cysts excreted in the stool contaminate water and can be ingested by the host.

Giardiasis

Giardiasis, which is caused by *Giardia lamblia*, is the most commonly diagnosed intestinal parasite in the United States. This protozoan forms cysts, which survive outside the body and allow transmission through contaminated water or food, and trophozoites, which break out of the cysts in the upper small intestine and eventually cause signs and symptoms of disease. Diarrhea, rotten egg–smelling stool, and pale and mucus-filled stool are commonly seen. Some patients experience epigastric distress, weight loss, and malnutrition as a result of the invasion of the mucosa.

Toxoplasmosis

Toxoplasmosis is an infection caused by the gondii parasite. The infection can be transmitted by eating contaminated undercooked meat, being exposed from infected cat feces, or to a fetus during pregnancy. Many people with an adequate immune system do not require treatment, but if a person is immunocompromised and/or pregnant, the medication commonly used to treat toxoplasmosis is pyrimethamine (*Daraprim*). It acts by blocking the use of folic acid in protein synthesis by the *Plasmodium*, eventually leading to inability to reproduce and cell death.

Other Antiprotozoal Agents

Drugs that are available specifically for the treatment of these various protozoan infections include many of the malarial drugs. Chloroquine is effective against extraintestinal amebiasis, and pyrimethamine is also effective in treating toxoplasmosis. Other drugs, including some tetracyclines and aminoglycosides, are used for treating these conditions at various stages of the disease. Other antiprotozoals include atovaquone (*Mepron*), metronidazole (*Flagyl*), nitazoxanide (*Alinia*), pentamidine (*Pentam 300, NebuPent*), pyrimethamine (*Daraprim*), tinidazole (*Tindamax*), and the newest drug benznidazole 9 (see Table 12.2).

Therapeutic Actions and Indications

These antiprotozoal agents act to inhibit DNA synthesis in susceptible protozoa, interfering with the cell's ability to reproduce and subsequently leading to cell death (see Fig. 12.1). These drugs are indicated for the treatment of infections caused by susceptible protozoa. See Table 12.2 for usual indications for each of these agents.

Pharmacokinetics

Atovaquone is available only as an oral suspension and is slowly absorbed and highly protein bound in circulation. It is excreted slowly through the feces and has a half-life of 67 to 76 hours.

Benznidazole is available orally for children with Chagas disease. It reaches peak level in about 3 hours. Metabolism is not known. It is excreted in urine and feces and has a half-life of 13 hours.

Table 12.2 *Drugs in Focus*: Other Antiprotozoals

Drug Name	Dosage/Route	Usual Indications
atovaquone (*Mepron*)	***Prevention:*** *Adult and pediatric (>13 y)*: 1,500 mg/d PO ***Treatment:*** *Adult and pediatric (>13 y)*: 750 mg PO b.i.d. with meals	Prevention and treatment of *Pneumocystis jirovecii* pneumonia who are not able to tolerate other therapies; used in combination with proguanil for treatment of chloroquine-resistant malaria
benznidazole (generic)	*Pediatric (2–12 y)*: 5–8 mg/kg/d PO in two divided doses 12 h apart for 60 d	Treatment of pediatric patients with Chagas disease caused by *Trypanosoma cruzi*
metronidazole (*Flagyl, MetroGel, Noritate*)	**Amebiasis:** *Adult*: 750 mg PO t.i.d. for 5–10 d *Pediatric*: 35–50 mg/kg/d PO in three divided doses for 10 d **Trichomoniasis:** *Adult*: 2 g PO as one dose, or divided into two doses given on the same day *or* 250 mg PO t.i.d. for 7 d	Treatment of amebiasis, trichomoniasis, giardiasis
nitazoxanide (*Alinia*)	***Giardia*:** *Adult and pediatric (>12 y)*: 500 mg PO q12h or 25 mL suspension q12h *Pediatric (4–11 y)*: 200 mg as 10 mL suspension PO q12h *Pediatric (1–3 y)*: 100 mg as 5 mL suspension PO q12h ***Cryptosporidium parvum*:** *Pediatric*: same as that for *Giardia*	Treatment of diarrhea associated with *Cryptosporidium parvum* or *Giardia lamblia*
pentamidine (*Pentam, NebuPent*)	***Adult and pediatric:*** *Inhalation*: 300 mg once q4wk *Injection*: 4 mg/kg/d IM or IV for 14 d	As inhalation treatment of *Pneumocystis jirovecii* pneumonia; as a systemic agent in the treatment of trypanosomiasis and leishmaniasis
pyrimethamine (*Daraprim*)	***Treatment:*** *Adult*: 50–75 mg PO daily with sulfonamide for 1–3 weeks (toxoplasmosis); 50 mg PO for 2 d (treatment of malaria); 25 mg PO weekly (prevention of malaria) *Pediatric:* 1 mg/kg/d PO divided into two equal daily doses with sulfonamide; after 2 to 4 d this dose may be reduced to one half and continued for ~1 mo (toxoplasmosis; 25 mg PO daily for 2 d (treatment of malaria); weight-based dosing (prevention of malaria)	Treatment of toxoplasmosis when used with sulfonamide; treatment and prevention of malaria
tinidazole (*Tindamax*)	**Trichomoniasis, giardiasis:** *Adult*: 2 g PO as a single dose with food *Pediatric (≥3 y)*: 50 mg/kg PO as a single dose with food **Amebiasis:** *Adult*: 2 g/d PO with food for 3 d *Pediatric (≥3 y)*: 50 mg/kg/d PO with food, do not exceed 2 g/d	Treatment of trichomoniasis, giardiasis, amebiasis

Metronidazole is well absorbed orally, reaching peak level in 1 to 2 hours. It is metabolized in the liver and has a half-life of 8 to 15 hours. Excretion occurs primarily through the urine.

Nitazoxanide is rapidly absorbed after oral administration, reaching peak level in 1 to 4 hours. Nitazoxanide is metabolized in the liver and excreted in the urine and feces; it has a half-life of 8 to 12 hours.

Pentamidine is readily absorbed through the lungs when inhaled. It is also available to be administered intravenously. Excretion occurs in the urine, with traces found in the urine for up to 6 weeks.

Pyrimethamine is readily absorbed from the GI tract, with its peak level occurring in 2 to 6 hours. It is metabolized in the liver and has a half-life of 4 days. It usually maintains suppressive concentrations in the body for about 2 weeks.

Tinidazole is rapidly absorbed after oral administration, reaching peak level in 60 to 90 minutes. It is excreted in the urine and has a half-life of 12 to 14 hours.

Contraindications and Cautions

Contraindications include the presence of any known allergy or hypersensitivity to any of these drugs to prevent hypersensitivity reactions. These drugs should be used with caution in pregnancy because they may affect developing fetal DNA and proteins can cause fetal abnormalities and even death. Use caution when administering these drugs to patients with CNS disease because of possible disease exacerbation due to drug effects on the CNS; hepatic disease because of possible exacerbation when hepatic drug effects occur; and with patients who are lactating because these drugs may pass into human milk and could have severe adverse effects on the infant. The safety and efficacy of pentamidine in children have not been established. Tinidazole should never be combined with alcohol and should be used with caution in patients with renal dysfunction, which could interfere with excretion of the drug.

Adverse Effects

Adverse effects of these antiprotozoal agents include CNS effects such as headache, dizziness, ataxia, loss of coordination, and peripheral neuropathy related to drug effects on the neurons. GI effects include nausea, vomiting, diarrhea, unpleasant taste, cramps, and changes in liver function. Superinfections also can occur when the normal flora are disrupted.

Clinically Important Drug–Drug Interactions

Tinidazole, benznidazole, and metronidazole should not be combined with alcohol, which could cause severe adverse effects; patients are advised to avoid alcohol for at least 3 days after treatment has ended. Metronidazole and tinidazole combined with warfarin can lead to increased risk of bleeding; patients should be monitored closely and dose adjustments made to the warfarin during therapy and for up to 8 days after stopping therapy. Psychotic reactions have been reported when tinidazole or metronidazole is combined with disulfiram; this combination should be avoided, and 2 weeks should elapse between benznidazole or tinidazole therapy and starting treatment with disulfiram.

Prototype Summary: Metronidazole

Indications: Acute intestinal amebiasis, amebic liver abscess, trichomoniasis, acute infections caused by susceptible strains of anaerobic bacteria, and preoperative and postoperative prophylaxis for patients undergoing several surgical procedures.

Actions: Inhibits DNA synthesis of specific anaerobes, causing cell death; mechanism of action as an antiprotozoal and amebicidal is not known.

Pharmacokinetics:

Route	Onset	Peak
Oral	Varies	1–2 h
IV	Rapid	Immediately post-infusion

$T_{1/2}$: 6 to 8 hours; metabolized in the liver and excreted in the urine and feces.

Adverse Effects: Headache, dizziness, ataxia, seizures, nausea, vomiting, metallic taste, diarrhea, darkening of the urine (note that this is a harmless effect).

Nursing Considerations for Patients Receiving Antiprotozoal Agents

Assessment: History and Examination

- Assess for contraindications and cautions: history of allergy to any of the antiprotozoals to prevent hypersensitivity reactions; liver dysfunction that might interfere with metabolism and excretion of the drug or be exacerbated by the drug; pregnancy, which is a contraindication, and lactation because these drugs could enter human milk and be toxic to the infant; CNS disease that could be exacerbated by the drug; and candidiasis that could become severe as a result of the effects of these drugs on the normal flora.
- Perform a physical assessment to establish baseline data for determining the effectiveness of the drug and the

(continues on page 198)

occurrence of any adverse effects associated with drug therapy.
- Evaluate the CNS to check reflexes and muscle strength to identify the need for cautious drug use and to evaluate changes that occur as a result of drug therapy.
- Examine the skin and mucous membranes to check for lesions, color, temperature, and texture to monitor for adverse effects and superinfections.
- Evaluate liver function to determine the appropriateness of therapy and to monitor for toxicity.
- Obtain cultures to determine the exact protozoal species causing the disease.

Nursing Conclusions

Nursing conclusions related to drug therapy might include the following:
- Impaired comfort related to GI and CNS effects of the drug
- Malnutrition related to severe GI effects of the drug
- Altered sensory (kinesthetic, visual) perception related to CNS effects
- Knowledge deficit regarding drug therapy

Planning

- The patient will receive the best therapeutic effect from the drug therapy.
- The patient will have limited adverse effects to the drug therapy.
- The patient will have an understanding of the drug therapy, adverse effects to anticipate, and measures to relieve discomfort and improve safety.

Intervention With Rationale

- Arrange for appropriate culture and sensitivity tests before beginning therapy to ensure proper drug for susceptible organisms. Treatment may begin before test results are known.
- Administer a complete course of the drug to get the full beneficial effects. Use combination therapy as indicated.
- Monitor hepatic function before and periodically during treatment to arrange to effectively stop the drug if signs of failure or worsening liver function occur.
- If CNS effects occur, provide comfort and safety measures, such as side rails and assistance with ambulation if dizziness and weakness are present, to prevent injury to the patient.
- Provide oral hygiene and ready access to bathroom facilities as needed to cope with GI effects.
- Arrange for the treatment of superinfections as appropriate to prevent severe infections.
- If GI upset is severe, provide small, frequent, nutritious meals to ensure proper nutrition. Monitor nutritional status, and arrange a dietary consultation as needed. Taking the drug with food may also decrease GI upset.
- Instruct the patient about the appropriate dosage regimen to enhance patient knowledge about drug therapy and to promote adherence.
- Provide the following patient teaching:
  - If CNS effects occur, take safety precautions, including changing position slowly and avoiding driving and hazardous tasks.
  - If GI upset is a problem, take the drug with meals, and try small, frequent meals.
  - Follow drug dosing guidelines carefully.
  - Report severe GI problems and interference with nutrition; fever and chills, which may indicate the presence of a superinfection; and dizziness, unusual fatigue, or weakness, which may indicate CNS effects.

Evaluation

- Monitor patient response to the drug (resolution of infection and negative cultures for parasite).
- Monitor for adverse effects (orientation and affect, nutritional state, skin color and lesions, hepatic function, and occurrence of superinfections).
- Evaluate the effectiveness of the teaching plan. The patient should be able to name the drug, dosage, possible adverse effects to watch for, and specific measures to help avoid adverse effects.
- Monitor the effectiveness of comfort and safety measures and adherence to the regimen.

See the "Critical Thinking Scenario" for additional information related to coping with amebiasis and the use of metronidazole.

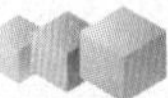

Concept Mastery Alert

Patient Education

Headaches, dizziness, a metallic taste, and nausea are common adverse effects for metronidazole. Vision changes are not associated with use of metronidazole.

CRITICAL THINKING SCENARIO
Coping With Amebiasis

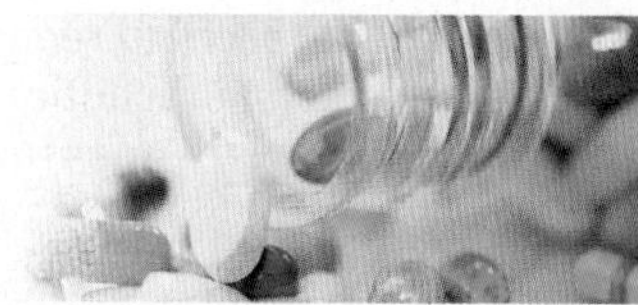

THE SITUATION

J.C., a 20-year-old college student, reported to the university health center complaining of severe diarrhea, abdominal pain, and, most recently, blood in their stool. J.C. had a mild fever and appeared to be dehydrated and very tired. J.C. denied travel outside the country and reported eating most meals at the local bar where they worked in the kitchen each night making pizza.

A stool sample for ova and parasites (O&P) was obtained, and a diagnosis of amebiasis was made. Metronidazole was prescribed. A public health referral was sent to find the source of the infection, which was the kitchen of the bar where J.C. worked. The kitchen was shut down until all the food, utensils, and environment passed state health inspection. Although a potential epidemic was averted (only three other cases of amebiasis were reported), the action of the public health officials added new stress to J.C.'s life because they were unemployed for several months.

CRITICAL THINKING

What are the important nursing implications for J.C.? Think about the usual nutritional state of a college student who eats most of their meals at a bar.

What are the implications for recovery when a patient is malnourished and then has a disease that causes severe diarrhea, dehydration, and potential malnourishment? Consider how difficult it will be for J.C. to be a full-time student while trying to cope with the signs and symptoms of the disease, as well as the adverse effects associated with the drug therapy and the need to maintain adequate nutrition to allow healing and recovery.

What potential problems could the added stress of being out of work have for J.C.? Consider the physiological impact of stress, as well as the psychological problems of trying to cope with one more stressor.

DISCUSSION

J.C. needed a great deal of reassurance and an explanation of their disease. J.C. learned that oral hygiene and small, frequent meals would help alleviate some of their discomfort until the metronidazole could control the amebiasis and that good hygiene and strict hand washing when the disease is active would help to prevent transmission. J.C. was advised to watch for the occurrence of specific adverse drug effects, such as a possible severe reaction to alcohol. J.C. was advised to avoid alcoholic beverages while taking this drug. They were also advised to watch for GI upset and a strange metallic taste (the importance of good nutrition to promote healing of the GI tract was stressed), dizziness or light-headedness, and signs of superinfections.

J.C. was scheduled for a follow-up examination for stool O&P and nutritional status. Metronidazole was continued until the stool sample came back negative. J.C. needed and received a great deal of support and encouragement because they were far from home and the disease and the drug effects were sometimes difficult to cope with. The effects of stress—decreasing blood flow to the GI tract, for example—can make it more difficult for patients such as J.C. to recover from this disease. Support and encouragement can be major factors in their eventual recovery. J.C. was given a telephone number to call if they needed information or support and a complete set of written instructions regarding the disease and the drug therapy.

NURSING CARE GUIDE FOR J.C.: METRONIDAZOLE

Assessment: History and Examination

Allergies to metronidazole, renal or liver dysfunction

Concurrent use of barbiturates, oral anticoagulants, alcohol

Local: Culture of stool for accurate diagnosis of infection

CNS: Orientation, affect, vision, reflexes

Skin: Color, lesions, texture

GI: Abdominal, liver evaluation

Hematological: CBC, liver function tests

Nursing Conclusions

Impaired comfort related to GI, superinfection effects

Altered sensory (kinesthetic, visual) perception related to CNS effects

Malnutrition related to GI effects

Knowledge deficit regarding drug therapy

Planning

The patient will receive the best therapeutic effect from the drug therapy.

The patient will have limited adverse effects to the drug therapy.

The patient will have an understanding of the drug therapy, adverse effects to anticipate, and measures to relieve discomfort and improve safety.

Intervention

Obtain a culture of the infection before beginning therapy.

Provide comfort and safety measures: oral hygiene, safety precautions, treatment of superinfections, and maintenance of nutrition.

Provide small, frequent meals and monitor nutritional status.

Provide support and reassurance for dealing with drug effects and discomfort.

(continues on page 200)

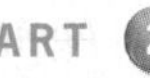

Provide patient teaching regarding drug name, dosage, adverse effects, precautions, and warning signs to report and hygiene measures to observe.

Evaluation

Evaluate drug effects including resolution of protozoal infection.

Monitor for adverse effects: GI alterations, dizziness, confusion, CNS changes, vision loss, hepatic function, superinfections.

Monitor for drug–drug interactions with oral anticoagulants, alcohol, or barbiturates.

Evaluate effectiveness of patient teaching program.

Evaluate effectiveness of comfort and safety measures.

PATIENT TEACHING FOR J.C.

You have been prescribed metronidazole to treat your amebic infection. This antiprotozoal drug acts to destroy certain protozoa that have invaded your body. Because it affects specific phases of the protozoal life cycle, it must be taken over a period of time to be effective. It is very important to take all the drug that has been ordered for you.

- This drug frequently causes stomach upset. If it causes you to have nausea, heartburn, or vomiting, take the drug with meals or a light snack.
- Common effects of this drug include the following:
  - Nausea, vomiting, and loss of appetite: Take the drug with food and have small, frequent meals.
  - Superinfections of the mouth or skin: These go away when the course of the drug has been completed. If they become uncomfortable, notify your health care provider for an appropriate solution.
  - Dry mouth, strange metallic taste: Frequent mouth care and sucking sugarless lozenges may help. This effect will also go away when the course of the drug is finished.
  - Intolerance of alcohol (nausea, vomiting, flushing, headache, and stomach pain): Avoid alcoholic beverages or products containing alcohol while taking this drug.
- Report any of the following to your health care provider: sore throat, fever, or chills; skin rash or redness; severe GI upset; and unusual fatigue, clumsiness, or weakness.
- Take the full course of your prescription. Never use this drug to self-treat any other infection or give it to any other person.
- Tell any doctor, nurse, or other health care provider that you are taking this drug.
- Keep this drug and all medications out of the reach of children.

Key Points

- Other protozoal infections include amebiasis, leishmaniasis, trypanosomiasis, trichomoniasis, and giardiasis.
- Patients receiving antiprotozoal agents should be monitored regularly to detect any serious adverse effects.

SUMMARY

- A protozoan is a parasitic cellular organism. Its life cycle includes a parasitic phase inside human tissues or cells.
- Malaria is caused by *Plasmodium* protozoa, which must go through a cycle in the *Anopheles* mosquito before being passed to humans via the mosquito bite. Once inside a human, the protozoa invade red blood cells.
- The characteristic cyclic chills and fever of malaria occur when red blood cells burst, releasing more protozoa into the bloodstream.
- Malaria is often treated with a combination of drugs that attack the protozoan at various stages in its life cycle.
- Amebiasis is caused by the protozoan *Entamoeba histolytica*, which invades human intestinal tissue after being passed to humans through unsanitary food or water. It is best treated with metronidazole or tinidazole.
- Leishmaniasis, a protozoan-caused disease, can result in serious lesions in the mucosa, viscera, and skin. It is treated with systemic pentamidine.
- Trypanosomiasis, which is caused by infection with a *Trypanosoma* parasite, may assume two forms. African sleeping sickness leads to inflammation of the CNS, and Chagas disease results in serious cardiomyopathy. These diseases can be treated with systemic pentamidine, and children with Chagas disease can be treated with benznidazole.
- Trichomoniasis is caused by *Trichomonas vaginalis*. This common cause of vaginitis results in no signs or symptoms in males but results in serious vaginal inflammation in females. It is treated with metronidazole and tinidazole.
- Giardiasis, which is caused by *Giardia lamblia*, is the most commonly diagnosed intestinal parasite in the United States. This disease may lead to serious malnutrition when the pathogen invades intestinal mucosa. It is treated with nitazoxanide, metronidazole, and tinidazole.
- Patients receiving antiprotozoal agents should be monitored regularly to detect any serious adverse effects.

CHECK YOUR UNDERSTANDING

Answers to the questions in this chapter can be found in the Answers to Check Your Understanding Questions on thePoint®.

MULTIPLE CHOICE

Select the best answer.

1. After students are taught about protozoal infections, which infection, if a student states is caused by an insect bite, would indicate the need for additional teaching?
   a. Malaria
   b. Trypanosomiasis
   c. Leishmaniasis
   d. Giardiasis

2. When describing the development of malaria caused by the *Plasmodium* protozoan, the instructor would explain that the organism depends on
   a. a snail to act as intermediary in the life cycle of the protozoan.
   b. a mosquito and a red blood cell for maturation.
   c. a human liver cell for cell division and reproduction.
   d. stagnant water for maturation.

3. A patient who is receiving a combination drug to treat malaria asks the nurse why. The nurse responds to the patient based on the understanding that combination drugs are
   a. associated with a much lower degree of toxicity than single-drug treatments.
   b. absorbed more completely than single-drug treatments when administered.
   c. more effective in preventing mosquitoes from biting the individual.
   d. effective at various stages in the life cycle of the protozoan.

4. A patient traveling to an area of the world where malaria is known to be endemic should be taught to
   a. avoid drinking the water.
   b. begin and complete the antimalarial therapy as prescribed.
   c. pack a supply of antimalarial drugs in case they get a mosquito bite.
   d. change the dates of their trip to when there is less risk of infection.

5. Amebiasis or amebic dysentery
   a. is seen only in tropical countries.
   b. is caused by a protozoan that enters the body through an insect bite.
   c. is caused by a protozoan that can enter the body in the cyst stage in water or food.
   d. usually has no signs and symptoms.

6. Giardiasis is the most common intestinal parasite seen in the United States, and it
   a. does not respond to drug therapy.
   b. can invade the liver and cause death.
   c. is seen only in areas with poor sanitation.
   d. is associated with rotten egg–smelling stool, diarrhea, and mucus-filled stool.

7. Trypanosomiasis may assume which of the following two different forms?
   a. African sleeping sickness and Chagas disease
   b. Elephantiasis and malaria
   c. Dysentery and African sleeping sickness
   d. Malaria and Chagas disease

8. A nurse would note that a patient had a good understanding of their antimalarial drug regimen if the patient reported,
   a. "I keep these pills with me at all times while I'm away and take them only when I have been bitten by a mosquito."
   b. "I will need to start these pills now and then continue to take them every day for the rest of my life."
   c. "I'll start the pills before my trip and will keep taking them during the trip and for a period of time after I'm home."
   d. "I will start taking these pills as soon as I arrive at my vacation destination, before I get off the plane."

MULTIPLE RESPONSE

Select all that apply.

1. A parent calls in concerned that their child, a college freshman, has been diagnosed with giardiasis. The nurse would respond to the parent's concerns by telling them which of the following?
   a. You should have your child come home immediately so that they can be treated appropriately.
   b. This is a very rare disorder; it is not usually seen in this country.

c. This is the most common protozoal infection seen in this country and is usually transmitted through food or water.
d. This infection can be treated with oral drugs, and your child should be able to get the drugs where the infection was diagnosed.
e. This is an infection that has to be treated quickly with IV medications.
f. Encourage your child to get the medicine and to try very hard to eat nutritious food.

2. Your 32-year-old HIV-positive patient is being treated for *Pneumocystis jirovecii* pneumonia; they did well on a course of atovaquone and are now being discharged on pentamidine to prevent a recurrence of the infection. In preparing a teaching plan, you would need to include which of the following?
    a. Pentamidine is an inhaled drug used once every 4 weeks.
    b. Pentamidine is an oral drug that will need to be taken daily for a very long time.
    c. Pentamidine requires very special handling to prevent toxicity.
    d. Pentamidine must be inhaled using the Respigard inhaler.
    e. The patient may also need to be put on an antihypertensive drug while using pentamidine.
    f. Periodic renal, hepatic, and complete blood count (CBC) blood tests will be needed while using this drug.

REFERENCES

Ambachew, M., Yohannes, A., Bergqvist, Y., & Ringwald, P. (2011). Confirmed vivax resistance to chloroquine and effectiveness of artemether-lumefantrine for the treatment of vivax malaria in Ethiopia. *American Journal of Tropical Medicine and Hygiene, 84*(1), 137–140. 10.4269/ajtmh.2011.09-0723

Andrews, M., & Boyle, J. (2011). *Transcultural concepts in nursing care* (6th ed.). Lippincott Williams & Wilkins.

Brunton, L., Hilal-Dandan, R., & Knollman, B. (2018). *Goodman and Gilman's the pharmacological basis of therapeutics* (13th ed.). McGraw-Hill.

Centers for Disease Control. (2018). *Malaria risk assessment for travelers*. http://www.cdc.gov/malaria/travelers/risk_assessment.html

Centers for Disease Control and Prevention. (2020). *Malaria treatment (United States)*. https://www.cdc.gov/malaria/diagnosis_treatment/trea

Cortegiani, A., Ippolito, M., Ingoglia, G., Iozzo, P., Giarratano, A., & Einav, S. (2020). Update I. A systemic review on the efficacy and safety of chloroquine/hydroxychloroquine for COVID-19. *Journal of Critical Care, 59*, 176–190 https://doi.org/10.1016/j.jcrc.2020.06.019

Kovacs, J., & Masur, H. (2009). Evolving health effects of *Pneumocystis*: One hundred years of progress in diagnosis and treatment. *Journal of the American Medical Association, 301*(24), 2578–2585. 10.1001/jama.2009.880

Mahittikorn, A., Masangkay, F. R., Kotepui, K. U., Milanez, G. D., & Kotepui, M. (2021). Comparison of *Plasmodium ovale curtisi* and *Plasmodium ovale wallikeri* infections by a meta-analysis approach. *Scientific Reports, 11*, 6409. https://doi.org/10.1038/s41598-021-85398-w

Morilla, C. A., Marin-Neto, J., Avezum, A., Sosa-Estani, S., Rassi, A., Rosas, F., Villena, E., Quiroz, R., Bonilla, R., Britto, C., Guhl, F, Velazquez, E., Bonilla, L., Meeks, B., Rao-Melacini, P., Pogue, J., Mattos, A., Lazdins, J., Rassi, A., …BENEFIT Investigators. (2015). Randomized trial of benznidazole for chronic Chagas' cardiomyopathy. *The New England Journal of Medicine, 373*, 1295–1306. https://www.nejm.org/doi/full/10.1056/nejmoa1507574

Norris, T. L. (2019). *Porth's pathophysiology concepts of altered health states* (13th ed.). Wolters Kluwer.

Ryan, K., & Tekwani B. L. (2021). Current investigations on clinical pharmacology and therapeutics of Glucose-6-phosphate dehydrogenase deficiency. *Pharmacology and Therapeutics, 222*, 107788. https://doi.org/10.1016/j.pharmthera.2020.107788

World Health Organization. (2020). *Caronavirus disease (COVID-19): Hydroxychloroquine*. https://www.who.int/news-room/q-a-detail/q-a-hydroxychloroquine-and-covid-19?gclid=EAIaIQobChMI14DSwc_i7AIVV-DICh0_xQDaEAAYASAAEgLiSPD_BwE

CHAPTER 13

Anthelmintic Agents

Learning Objectives

Upon completion of this chapter, you will be able to:

1. List the common worms that cause disease in humans.
2. Describe the therapeutic actions, indications, pharmacokinetics, contraindications, most common adverse reactions, and important drug–drug interactions associated with the anthelmintics.
3. Discuss the use of anthelmintics across the lifespan.
4. Compare and contrast the prototype drug mebendazole with other anthelmintics.
5. Outline the nursing considerations, including important teaching points to stress, for patients receiving an anthelmintic.

Key Terms

Ascaris: parasitic worm that causes the most prevalent helminthic infection; ingested fertilized roundworm eggs hatch in the small intestine and then make their way to the lungs, where they may cause cough, fever, and other signs of a pulmonary infiltrate

cestode: tapeworm with a head and segmented body parts; capable of growing to several yards in the human intestine

filariasis: infection of the blood and tissues of healthy individuals by worm embryos or filariae

helminth: worm that can cause disease by invading the human body

hookworm: worm that attaches itself to the small intestine of an infected individual, where it sucks blood from the walls of the intestine, damaging the intestinal wall and leading to severe anemia with lethargy, weakness, and fatigue

nematode: a roundworm such as the commonly encountered pinworm, whipworm, threadworm, *Ascaris*, or hookworm; causes a common helminthic infection in humans; can cause intestinal obstruction as the adult worms clog the intestinal lumen or severe pneumonia when the larvae migrate to the lungs and form a pulmonary infiltrate

pinworm: nematode that causes a common helminthic infection in humans; lives in the intestine and causes anal and possible vaginal irritation and itching

platyhelminth: a flatworm, including the cestode and tapeworm; a worm that can live in the human intestine or can invade other human tissues (flukes)

schistosomiasis: infection with a blood fluke that is carried by a snail; it poses a common problem in tropical countries, where the snail is the intermediary in the life cycle of the worm; larvae burrow into the skin in fresh water and migrate throughout the human body, causing a rash, diarrhea, and liver and brain inflammation

threadworm: pervasive nematode that can send larvae into the lungs, liver, and central nervous system (CNS); can cause severe pneumonia or liver abscess

trichinosis: disease that results from ingestion of encysted roundworm larvae in undercooked pork; larvae migrate throughout the body to invade muscles, nerves, and other tissues; can cause pneumonia, heart failure, and encephalitis

whipworm: worm that attaches itself to the intestinal mucosa and sucks blood; may cause severe anemia and disintegration of the intestinal mucosa

Drug List

ANTHELMINTICS
albendazole
ivermectin
(P) mebendazole
praziquantel
pyrantel

Helminthic infections are infections in the gastrointestinal (GI) tract or other tissues due to infestation of the human body by a **helminth**, a worm that can cause disease. Helminthic infections affect about 1 billion people, making these types of infections among the most common of all diseases. These infestations are very common in tropical areas, but they are also often found in other regions, including the United States and Canada. With so many people traveling to many parts of the world, it is not uncommon for a traveler to contract a helminthic infection in one country and inadvertently bring it home, where the worms then can infect other individuals (see Box 13.1). The helminths that most commonly infect humans are of two types: the **nematodes** (or roundworms) and the **platyhelminths** (or flatworms) that cause intestine-invading worm infections and can be tissue-invading worms.

Frequently, patients have a very difficult time dealing with a diagnosis of worm infestation. It is very important for the nurse to understand the disease process and to explain the disease and treatment carefully to help the patient to cope with both the diagnosis and the treatment.

Box 13.1 Focus on Cultural Considerations

TRAVELERS AND HELMINTHS

People who come from or travel to areas of the world where schistosomiasis is endemic should always be assessed for the possibility of infection with such a disease when seen for health care. Areas of the world where this disease is endemic are mainly tropical and include Puerto Rico, islands of the West Indies, Africa, parts of South America, the Philippines, China, Japan, and Southeast Asia. People traveling to these areas should be warned about wading, swimming, or bathing in freshwater streams, ponds, or lakes. For example, swimming in the Nile River is a popular attraction on Egyptian vacation tours; however, this activity may result in a lasting (unhappy) memory when the traveler returns home and is diagnosed with schistosomiasis. The nurse can suggest to patients who are planning a visit to one of these areas that they contact the CDC for health and safety guidelines, as well as what signs and symptoms to watch for after returning home. Travel information from the CDC can be found at http://www.cdc.gov/travel.

Intestine-Invading Worm Infections

Many of the worms that infect humans live only in the intestinal tract. Proper diagnosis of a helminthic infection requires a stool examination for ova (eggs) and parasites. Treatment of a helminthic infection requires the use of an anthelmintic drug. Another important part of therapy for helminthic infections involves the prevention of reinfection or spread of an existing infection. Measures such as thorough hand washing after use of the toilet; frequent laundering of bed linens and underwear in very hot, chlorine-treated water; disinfection of toilets and bathroom areas after each use; and good personal hygiene to wash away ova are important to prevent the spread of the disease. See Table 13.1 for a summary of worms that cause intestinal infections.

Infections by Nematodes

Nematodes, or roundworms, include the commonly encountered pinworms, whipworms, threadworms, *Ascaris*, and hookworms. These worms cause diseases that range in severity from mild to potentially fatal.

Pinworm Infections

Pinworms are usually transmitted when the worm eggs are ingested, either by transfer by touching the eggs when they are shed to clothing, toys, or bedding or by the inhalation of eggs that become airborne and are then swallowed. Pinworms, which remain in the intestine, cause little discomfort except for perianal itching or occasionally vaginal itching. Infection with pinworms is the most common helminthic infection among school-aged children. (See the "Critical Thinking Scenario" for a case study of a child exposed to pinworms.)

Table 13.1 Helminthic Infections

Intestine-Invading Worm	Mechanism of Disease	Manifestations
Pinworms	Remain in intestine	Perianal itching; occasionally, vaginal itching
Whipworms	Attach to wall of colon	Bloody diarrhea (with large numbers of worms)
Threadworms	Burrow into the intestine; can enter the lungs, liver, and other tissue	Pneumonia, liver abscess
Ascaris	Burrow into the intestine; enter the blood and infect lungs	Cough, fever, pulmonary infiltrates; abdominal distention and pain
Hookworms	Attach to the wall of the intestine	Anemia, fatigue, malabsorption
Cestodes	Live in the intestine, ingesting nutrients from the host	Weight loss, abdominal distention

CRITICAL THINKING SCENARIO
Treating Pinworm Infections

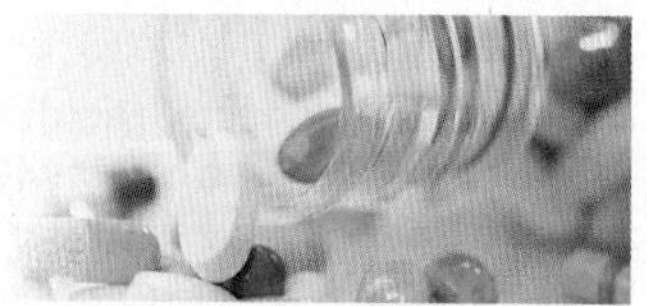

THE SITUATION

J.K. is a 4-year-old child who attends prekindergarten classes 5 days a week at a local childhood development center. J.K. brought a note home from the director of the school explaining that pinworm infections had been diagnosed in two of J.K.'s classmates. The director outlined steps that the school was taking to prevent spread of the disease. Since pinworm infections are very contagious, the director also advised all families to contact their health care provider and mentioned that treatment with mebendazole had been suggested. J.K.'s parents became very upset and immediately called the clinic to make an appointment. At the clinic, J.K. was diagnosed with a pinworm infection.

CRITICAL THINKING

What are the important nursing implications for J.K. and their family? Think about the impact a diagnosis of a worm infection in a child would have on a young parent. Think about how contagious this disease is and how the whole family needs to be involved in the treatment regimen.

What drug therapy will most likely be suggested, and who will need to take the drug?

What nondrug interventions are crucial in the treatment and prevention of further spread of this disease?

Is there any risk of spreading this disease in the clinic?

What steps should be taken to ensure the safety of other children who might come into the clinic? Think about the way that pinworms spread and how the spread can be prevented.

DISCUSSION

Pinworm infections are the most common helminth infection in young children. Hearing that your child has "worms" can be very upsetting to a parent. It will be important to explain what a pinworm infection is, how easy it is to spread, and how easy it is to treat. Assure the parents that it happens all the time and that a pinworm infection in their young child is not a reflection on their family. It will be important to discuss the need for the whole family to be treated, just in case. It will be crucial to cover all of the hygiene measures needed to eradicate the infection: strict hand washing; showering the child every morning; cleaning bedding and undergarments in hot water, with chlorine if possible; and cleaning the toilet area daily. Assure J.K.'s parents that it will be a 3-day drug treatment course and few, if any, adverse effects are expected from the drug. Keeping the child and family calm will be a major part of this visit. Many recommend that the whole family be treated if pinworms have been in one member's system. The 3-day drug treatment is easy, and very few adverse effects are experienced. The parents might feel better knowing that since the possibility of cross infection exists something is being done to take care of the issue. Since pinworms are very contagious, it is important to know if the child used the toilet facilities at the clinic and, if they have, to have the area properly cleaned. Toys or other objects the child might have played with also need to be sanitized; if the child has long fingernails or had not washed their hands, the worms could be spread. It would be a good exercise to help them wash their hands at the clinic. Singing the "Happy Birthday" song is often a guideline for how long should be spent washing the hands, and the child might relax and enjoy the activity while you are talking to J.K.'s parents.

NURSING CARE GUIDE FOR J.K. PINWORM TREATMENT

Assessment: History and Examination

Allergies to this drug, any history of liver or renal issues

Local: Culture of infection, stool for ova and parasites

Skin: Color, lesions, texture; perianal inspection

GI: Abdominal evaluation

Nursing Conclusions

Impaired comfort related to GI or central nervous system (CNS) effects

Altered body image perception related to diagnosis and treatment

Knowledge deficit regarding drug therapy

Planning

The patient will receive the best therapeutic effect from the drug therapy.

The patient will have limited adverse effects to the drug therapy.

The patient will have an understanding of the drug therapy, adverse effects to anticipate, and measures to relieve discomfort and improve safety.

Intervention

Obtain a culture for ova and parasites before beginning therapy.

Provide support and reassurance to deal with drug effects, discomfort, and diagnosis.

Provide parent/patient teaching regarding drug name, dosage regimen, adverse effects, precautions to report, and hygiene measures to observe.

Stress the importance of hygiene measures in eradicating the infection.

(continues on page 206)

Evaluation

Evaluate drug effects (resolution of helminth infection).
Monitor for adverse effects (GI alterations).
Evaluate effectiveness of parent/patient teaching program.
Evaluate effectiveness of comfort and safety measures.

PARENT/PATIENT TEACHING FOR J.K.

- This drug is called an anthelmintic. It works by destroying certain helminths, or worms, that have invaded the body.
- It is important that you take/give the full course of the drug. Chew the tablets thoroughly and take one tablet twice a day for 3 days.
- Other measures will be very important to eradicate the infection. Trim fingernails, encourage hand washing, shower in the morning, wash bedding and underwear every day in hot water (with chlorine if possible), and clean the toilet and toilet area daily.
- Common effects of this drug include nausea and loss of appetite. Eating small, frequent meals may help.
- Report any of the following conditions to your health care provider: diarrhea, abdominal pain.
- Never use this drug to self-treat any other infection or give it to any other person.
- Tell any doctor, nurse, or other health care provider that you/your child are/is taking this drug.
- Keep this drug and all medications out of the reach of children.

Whipworm Infections

Whipworms are transmitted when eggs found in the soil are ingested. Whipworms attach to the intestinal mucosa and suck blood. In large numbers, they cause colic and bloody diarrhea. In severe cases, whipworm infestation may result in prolapse of the intestinal wall and anemia related to blood loss.

Threadworm Infestation

Threadworms can cause more damage to humans than most of the other helminths. Threadworms are transmitted as larvae found in the soil and inadvertently ingested. The larvae mature into worms, and female worms lay eggs after burrowing into the wall of the small intestine. These eggs hatch into larvae that invade many body tissues, including the lungs, liver, and heart. In very severe cases, death may occur from pneumonia or from lung or liver abscesses that result from larval invasion.

Ascaris

Worldwide, *Ascaris* infection is the most prevalent helminthic infection. It may occur wherever sanitation is poor. Eggs from the soil are ingested with vegetables or other improperly washed foods. Many individuals are unaware that they have this infestation unless they see a worm in their stool. However, others become quite ill.

Initially, the individual ingests fertilized roundworm eggs, which hatch in the small intestine and then make their way to the lungs, where they may cause cough, fever, and other signs of a pulmonary infiltrate. The larvae then migrate back to the intestine, where they grow to adult size (i.e., about as long and as big around as an earthworm), causing abdominal distention and pain. In the most severe cases, intestinal obstruction by masses of worms can occur.

Hookworm Infections

Hookworm eggs are found in the soil, where they hatch into larvae that molt and become infective to humans. The larvae penetrate the skin and then enter the blood and within about a week reach the intestine. Hookworms attach to the small intestine of infected individuals. The worms suck blood from the walls of the intestine, damaging the intestinal wall and leading to severe anemia with lethargy, weakness, and fatigue. Malabsorption problems may occur as the small intestinal mucosa is altered. Treatment for anemia and fluid and electrolyte disturbances is an important part of the therapy for this infection.

Infections Caused by Platyhelminths

The platyhelminths (flatworms) include the cestodes (tapeworms) that live in the human intestine and the schistosomes (flukes) that live in the intestine and also invade other tissues as part of their life cycle. Because schistosomes invade tissues, they are discussed in the following section on tissue-invading worm infections.

Cestodes

Cestodes are segmented flatworms with a head, or scolex, and a variable number of segments that grow from the head. Cestodes enter the body as larvae found in undercooked meat or fish; they sometimes form worms that are several yards long. A person with a tapeworm may experience abdominal discomfort and distention, as well as weight loss because the worm eats ingested nutrients. Many infected patients require a great deal of psychological support when they excrete parts of the tapeworm or when the worm occasionally exits through the mouth or nose.

Tissue-Invading Worm Infections

Some of the worms that invade the body exist outside of the intestinal tract and can seriously damage the tissues they invade. Because of their location within healthy tissue, they can also be more difficult to treat.

Trichinosis

Trichinosis is the disease caused by ingestion of the encysted larvae of the roundworm, *Trichinella spiralis*, in undercooked pork. Once ingested, the larvae are deposited in the intestinal mucosa, pass into the bloodstream, and are carried throughout the body. They can penetrate skeletal muscle and can cause an inflammatory reaction in cardiac muscle and in the brain. Fatal pneumonia, heart failure, and encephalitis may occur.

The best treatment for trichinosis is prevention. Because the larvae are ingested by humans in undercooked pork, instructing individuals about freezing pork meat, monitoring the food eaten by pigs, and properly cooking pork can be most beneficial.

Filariasis

Filariasis refers to infection of the blood and tissues of healthy individuals by worm embryos, which enter the body via insect bites. These threadlike embryos, or filariae, can overwhelm the lymphatic system and cause massive inflammatory reactions. This may lead to severe swelling of the hands, feet, legs, arms, scrotum, or breast—a condition called elephantiasis.

Schistosomiasis

Schistosomiasis (see Fig. 13.1) is a platyhelminthic infection by a fluke that is carried by a snail. This disease is a common problem in parts of Africa, Asia, and certain South American and Caribbean countries that have climates and snails conducive to the life cycle of schistosomes.

Eggs that are excreted in the urine and feces of infected individuals hatch in fresh water into a form that infects a certain snail. In the snail, larvae called cercariae develop. The snail sheds the cercariae back into the freshwater pond or lake. People become infected when they come in contact with the infested water. The larvae attach to the skin and quickly burrow into the bloodstream and lymphatic tissue. Then they move into the lungs, and later to the liver, where they mature into adult worms that mate and migrate

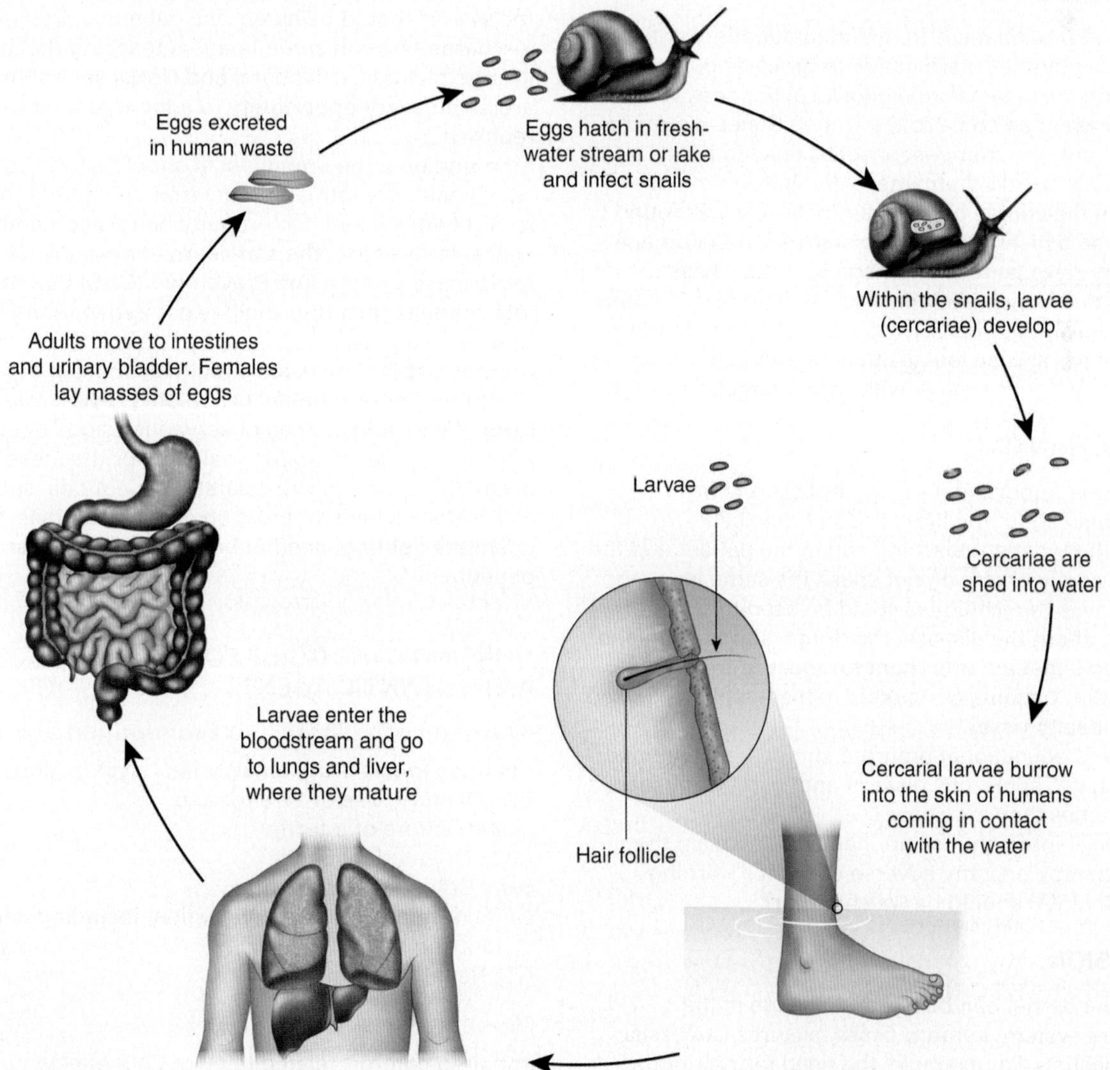
Eggs excreted in human waste
Eggs hatch in fresh-water stream or lake and infect snails
Within the snails, larvae (cercariae) develop
Cercariae are shed into water
Larvae
Cercarial larvae burrow into the skin of humans coming in contact with the water
Hair follicle
Larvae enter the bloodstream and go to lungs and liver, where they mature
Adults move to intestines and urinary bladder. Females lay masses of eggs

FIGURE 13.1 Life cycle of schistosomes.

to the intestines and urinary bladder. The female worms then lay large numbers of eggs, which are expelled in the feces and urine, and the cycle begins again.

Signs and symptoms may include a pruritic rash, often called swimmer's itch, where the larva attaches to the skin. About 1 or 2 months later, affected individuals may experience several weeks of fever, chills, headache, and other symptoms. Chronic or severe infestation may lead to abdominal pain and diarrhea, as well as blockage of blood flow to areas of the liver, lungs, and CNS. These blockages can lead to liver and spleen enlargement and to signs of CNS and cardiac ischemia. (See the "Critical Thinking Scenario" for a case study of a patient diagnosed with chronic schistosomiasis.)

Key Points

- Helminths are worms that cause disease by invading the human body. Some helminths invade body tissues and can seriously damage the lymphatic tissue, lungs, CNS, heart, or liver.
- Pinworms are the most frequent cause of helminth infection in the United States, and roundworms called *Ascaris* are the most frequent cause of helminth infections throughout the world.
- Patient teaching is important for decreasing the stress and anxiety that may occur when individuals are diagnosed with a worm infestation.

CRITICAL THINKING SCENARIO Anthelmintics

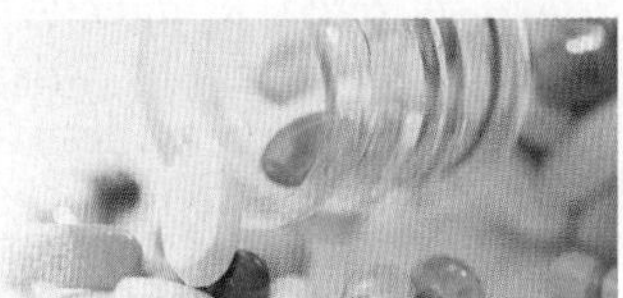

THE SITUATION

V.Y., a 33-year-old patient from Vietnam, underwent a complete physical examination in preparation for a training job in custodial work at a local hospital. V.Y. was a refugee who had come to the United States 6 months earlier as part of a church-sponsored resettlement program. V.Y. speaks Vietnamese and has limited use of English. In the course of the examination, it was found that V.Y. had a history of chronic diarrhea, hepatomegaly, pulmonary rales, and splenomegaly. Further tests indicated that they had chronic schistosomiasis. V.Y. was hospitalized so that their disease, which was unfamiliar to most of the associated health care providers, could be monitored. V.Y. was treated with praziquantel.

CRITICAL THINKING

What are the important nursing implications for V.Y.? Think about the limitations of medical care, particularly patient teaching, when the patient and the health care workers do not speak the same language.

What innovative techniques could be used to teach this patient about the disease, the drugs, and the hygiene measures that are important for them to follow?

Are the other patients or workers in the hospital exposed to any health risks?

What sort of educational program should be developed to teach V.Y. about this disease and to allay any fears or anxieties they may have?

What special interventions are needed to explain the drug therapy and any adverse effects or warning signs that V.Y. should be watching for?

DISCUSSION

A language barrier can be a real challenge in the health care system. In many cases, pictures can assist communication. For example, the need for nutritious food is conveyed by using appropriate pictures of foods that should be eaten. The patient is prepared for discharge through careful patient teaching that may involve pictures, calendars, and clocks so that they are given every opportunity to adhere to their medical regimen.

In addition, the nursing staff should contact the local health department to determine whether the local sewer system can properly handle contaminated waste. In this case, the staff learned from the Centers for Disease Control and Prevention (CDC) that the fluke's intermediate host (the snail) is not native to the United States, so the hazards posed by this waste are small, and normal disposal of waste should be appropriate.

Although praziquantel is a relatively well-tolerated drug, V.Y. should also be observed for signs of adverse effects. Drug fever, abdominal pain, or dizziness may occur. If dizziness occurs, safety precautions, such as assistance with ambulation, use of side rails, and adequate lighting, need to be taken without alarming the patient.

NURSING CARE GUIDE FOR V.Y.: ANTHELMINTIC AGENTS

Assessment: History and Examination

Allergies to this drug, renal or liver dysfunction
Drug history: Use of albendazole
Local: Culture of infection
CNS: Orientation, affect
Skin: Color, lesions, texture
GI: Abdominal and liver evaluation, including hepatic function tests
GU: Renal function tests

Nursing Conclusions

Impaired comfort related to GI or CNS effects

Altered body image perception related to diagnosis and treatment
Fear related to communication problems, health issues
Knowledge deficit regarding drug therapy

PLANNING

The patient will receive the best therapeutic effect from the drug therapy.
The patient will have limited adverse effects to the drug therapy.
The patient will have an understanding of the drug therapy, adverse effects to anticipate, and measures to relieve discomfort and improve safety.

Intervention

Obtain a culture for ova and parasites before beginning therapy.
Provide comfort and safety measures: small, frequent meals; safety precautions; hygiene measures; maintenance of nutrition.
Monitor nutritional status as needed.
Provide support and reassurance to deal with drug effects, discomfort, and diagnosis.
Provide patient teaching regarding drug name, dosage regimen, adverse effects, precautions to report, and hygiene measures to observe.

Evaluation

Evaluate drug effects (resolution of helminth infection).
Monitor for adverse effects (GI alterations, CNS changes, dizziness and confusion, renal and hepatic function).
Monitor for drug–drug interactions (concurrent use of albendazole).
Evaluate effectiveness of patient teaching program.
Evaluate effectiveness of comfort and safety measures.

PATIENT TEACHING FOR V.Y.

- This drug is called an anthelmintic. It works by destroying certain helminths, or worms, that have invaded your body.
- It is important that you take the full course of the drug. You will take three doses the first day, then we will retest before repeating this course if needed to ensure that all of the worms, in all phases of their life cycle, have disappeared from your body.
- You may take this drug with water and meals or with a light snack to help decrease any stomach upset that you may experience. Swallow the tablets whole and avoid holding them in your mouth for any length of time because a very unpleasant taste may occur.
- Common effects of this drug include the following:
  - Nausea, vomiting, and loss of appetite: Take the drug with food, and eat small, frequent meals.
  - Dizziness and drowsiness: If this occurs, avoid driving a car or operating dangerous machinery. Change positions slowly to avoid falling or injury.
- Report to your health care provider any of the following conditions: fever, chills, rash, headache, weakness, or tremors.
- Take all of the drug that has been prescribed. Never use this drug to self-treat any other infection or give it to any other person.
- Tell any doctor, nurse, or other health care provider that you are taking this drug.
- Keep this drug and all medications out of the reach of children.

Anthelmintics

The anthelmintic drugs (see Table 13.2) act on metabolic pathways that are present in the invading worm but are absent from or significantly different in the human host. Anthelmintic drugs include albendazole (*Albenza*), ivermectin (*Stromectol*), mebendazole (*Emverm*, *Vermox*), praziquantel (*Biltricide*), and pyrantel (*Antiminth*, *Pin-Rid*, *Pin-X*, *Reese's Pinworm*). Box 13.2 includes information about use of these drugs across the lifespan. See the "Critical Thinking Scenario" for a case study of a patient receiving anthelmintics.

Therapeutic Actions and Indications

Anthelmintic agents are indicated for the treatment of infections by certain susceptible worms and are specific to the worms that they affect; they are not interchangeable for treating various worm infections. See Table 13.2 for usual indications for each of these agents. Anthelmintics interfere with metabolic processes in particular worms. Figure 13.2 shows sites of action for these drugs.

Pharmacokinetics

Mebendazole is available in the form of a chewable tablet. Very little of the mebendazole is absorbed systemically, so adverse effects are few. The drug is metabolized by the liver, and most of it is excreted unchanged in the feces. A small amount may be excreted in the urine.

Albendazole is poorly absorbed from the GI tract, reaching peak plasma level in about 5 hours. It is metabolized in the liver and primarily excreted in feces.

Ivermectin is readily absorbed from the GI tract and reaches peak plasma level in 4 hours. It is completely metabolized in the liver with a half-life of 18 hours; excretion is through the feces.

Praziquantel is taken in a series of three oral doses at 4- to 6-hour intervals. It is rapidly absorbed from the GI tract and reaches peak plasma level in 1 to 3 hours. It is metabolized in the liver and has a half-life of 0.8 to 1.5 hours. Excretion of praziquantel occurs primarily through the urine.

Pyrantel is poorly absorbed, and most of the drug is excreted unchanged in the feces, although a small amount may be found in the urine.

Table 13.2 *Drugs in Focus:* Anthelmintics

Drug Name	Dosage/Route	Usual Indications
albendazole (*Albenza*)	***Hydatid disease:*** *≥60 kg:* 400 mg b.i.d. *<60 kg:* 15 mg/kg/d PO in divided doses, b.i.d., on a 28-d cycle, followed by 14 d of rest, for a total of three cycles ***Neurocysticercosis:*** *≥60 kg:* 400 mg b.i.d. *<60 kg:* 15/mg/kg/d PO in divided doses, b.i.d., for 8–30 d of treatment	Treatment of active lesions caused by pork tapeworm and cystic disease of the liver, lungs, and peritoneum caused by dog tapeworm
ivermectin (*Stromectol*)	150–200 mcg/kg PO as a single dose	Treatment of threadworm disease or strongyloidiasis; onchocerciasis or river blindness, which is found in tropical areas of Africa, Mexico, and South America
mebendazole (*Emverm, Vermox*)	100 mg PO morning and evening on 3 consecutive days ***Enterobiasis:*** 100 mg PO as a single dose (Emverm brand) 500 mg PO as a single dose (Vermox brand)	Treatment of diseases caused by pinworms, roundworms, whipworms, and hookworms
praziquantel (*Biltricide*)	Three doses of 20–25 mg/kg PO as a 1-d treatment	Treatment of a wide number of schistosomes or flukes
pyrantel (*Antiminth, Pin-Rid, Pin-X, Reese's Pinworm*)	*Adult and child (>4 y):* Dosage is based on weight, type of infection, and response to treatment. Max single dose 1 g	Treatment of diseases caused by pinworms and roundworms; because may be administered in single dose, may be preferred for patients who could have trouble remembering to take medication or following drug regimens

Contraindications and Cautions

Overall contraindications for the use of anthelmintic drugs include the presence of known allergy to any of these drugs to prevent hypersensitivity reactions; lactation because the drugs can enter human milk and could be toxic to the infant, so patients are advised to refrain from breast or chestfeeding when using these drugs; and pregnancy (in some cases) because of reported associated fetal abnormalities or death. Patients who can become pregnant should be advised to use barrier contraceptives while taking these drugs. Pyrantel has not been established as safe for use in children younger than 2 years. Albendazole should be used only after the causative worm has been identified because it can cause adverse effects on the liver, which could be problematic if the patient has liver involvement.

Use caution in the presence of renal or hepatic disease that interferes with the metabolism or excretion of drugs

Box 13.2 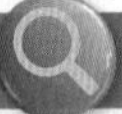 **Focus on Drug Therapy Across the Lifespan**

ANTHELMINTIC AGENTS

Children

Obtaining a culture of the suspected worm is important before beginning any drug therapy.

The more toxic drugs—albendazole, ivermectin, and praziquantel—should be avoided in children.

The most commonly used anthelmintic, mebendazole, comes in a chewable tablet that is convenient for use in children.

Nutritional status and hydration are major concerns with children who develop serious GI effects while taking these drugs.

Adults

Adults may be somewhat repulsed by the idea that they have a worm infestation, and they may be reluctant to discuss the necessary lifestyle adjustments and treatment plans.

Pregnant and nursing patients should not use these drugs unless the benefit clearly outweighs the potential risk to the fetus or neonate. If a severe helminth infestation threatens a pregnant or nursing patient, some of the drugs can be used as long as the patient is informed of the potential risk.

Older Adults

Older patients may be more susceptible to the CNS and GI effects of some of these drugs. Therefore, dose adjustment is needed for these agents. Monitor hydration and nutritional status carefully.

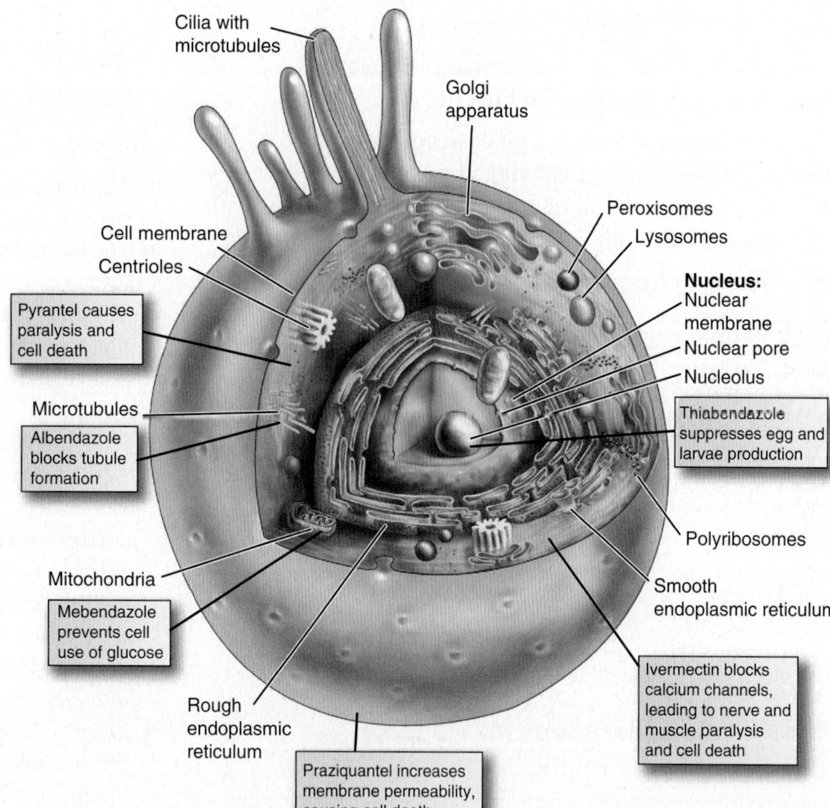

FIGURE 13.2 General structure of a cell, showing the sites of action of anthelmintic agents. Mebendazole interferes with the ability to use glucose, leading to an inability to reproduce and cell death. Albendazole blocks tubule formation, resulting in cell death. Ivermectin blocks calcium channels, leading to nerve and muscle paralysis and cell death. Pyrantel is a neuromuscular polarizing agent that causes paralysis and cell death. Praziquantel increases membrane permeability, leading to a loss of intracellular calcium and muscular paralysis; it may also result in disintegration of the integument.

that are absorbed systemically and in cases of severe diarrhea and malnourishment, which could alter the effects of the drug on the intestine and any preexisting helminths.

Adverse Effects

Adverse effects frequently encountered with the use of anthelmintic agents are related to their absorption or direct action in the intestine. Mebendazole and pyrantel, which are not absorbed systemically, may cause abdominal discomfort, diarrhea, or pain but have very few other effects and are well tolerated. Anthelmintics that are absorbed systemically may cause the following effects: headache and dizziness; fever, shaking, chills, and malaise associated with an immune reaction to the death of the worms; rash; pruritus; and loss of hair.

Renal failure and severe bone marrow depression are associated with albendazole, which is toxic to some human tissues. Patients taking this drug require careful monitoring (see Fig. 13.3).

Clinically Important Drug–Drug Interactions

The effects of albendazole, which are already severe, may increase if the drug is combined with dexamethasone, praziquantel, or cimetidine. These combinations should be avoided if at all possible; if they are necessary, patients should be monitored closely for adverse effects.

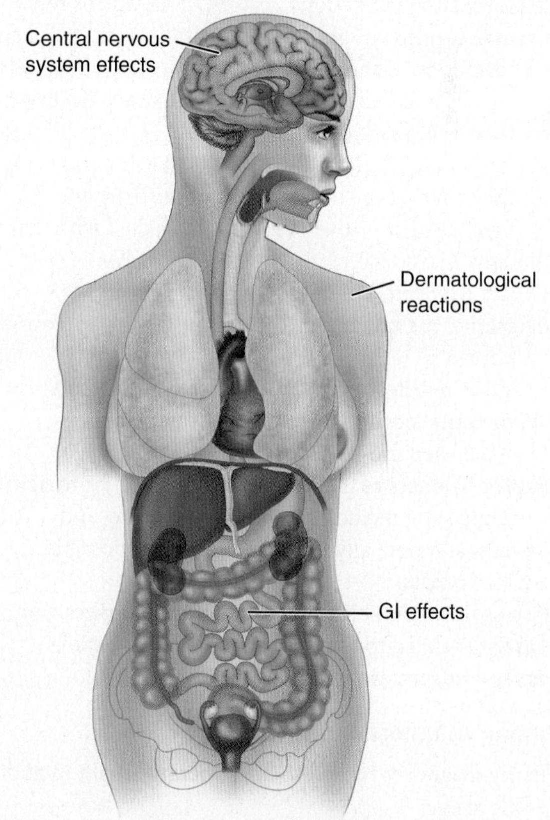

FIGURE 13.3 Common adverse effects associated with anthelmintics.

Prototype Summary: Mebendazole

Indications: Treatment of whipworm, pinworm, roundworm, and hookworm infections.

Actions: Irreversibly blocks glucose uptake by susceptible helminths, depleting glycogen stores needed for survival and reproduction, causing the death of the helminth.

Pharmacokinetics:

Route	Onset	Peak
Oral	Slow	2–4 h

$T_{1/2}$: 2.5 to 9 hours; metabolized in the liver and excreted in the feces.

Adverse Effects: Transient abdominal pain, diarrhea, fever.

Nursing Considerations for Patients Receiving Anthelmintics

Assessment: History and Examination

- Assess for possible contraindications or cautions: history of allergy to any of the anthelmintics to avoid hypersensitivity reactions; history of hepatic or renal dysfunction that might interfere with drug metabolism and excretion of the drug; and current status related to pregnancy and lactation, which are contraindications for the use of these drugs.
- Perform a physical assessment to establish baseline data for determining the effectiveness of the drug and the occurrence of any adverse effects associated with drug therapy.
- Obtain a culture of stool for ova and parasites to determine the infecting worm and establish appropriate treatment.
- Examine reflexes and muscle strength to evaluate changes that occur as a result of drug therapy.
- Evaluate liver and renal function to determine appropriateness of therapy and to monitor for toxicity.
- Examine skin, including color, temperature, and texture, and note any lesions to assess for possible adverse effects.
- Assess the abdomen to evaluate for any changes from baseline related to the infection, identify possible adverse effects, and monitor for improvement.

Nursing Diagnoses

Nursing diagnoses related to drug therapy might include the following:

- Impaired comfort related to GI, CNS, or skin effects of drug
- Altered body image perception related to diagnosis and treatment
- Knowledge deficit regarding drug therapy

Planning

- The patient will receive the best therapeutic effect from the drug therapy.
- The patient will have limited adverse effects to the drug therapy.
- The patient will have an understanding of the drug therapy, adverse effects to anticipate, and measures to relieve discomfort and improve safety.

Intervention With Rationale

- Arrange for appropriate culture and sensitivity tests before beginning therapy to ensure identification of the correct cause and use of the appropriate drug.
- Administer the complete course of the drug to obtain the full beneficial effects. Ensure that chewable tablets are chewed. Give the drug with food if necessary, but avoid giving the drug with high-fat meals, which might interfere with drug effectiveness.
- Monitor hepatic and renal function before and periodically during treatment to allow for early identification and prompt intervention if signs of failure due to albendazole administration occur.
- If CNS effects occur, provide comfort and safety measures (e.g., side rails and assistance with ambulation in the presence of dizziness and weakness) to protect the patient from injury. Provide oral hygiene and ready access to bathroom facilities as needed to cope with GI effects.
- If GI upset is severe, provide small, frequent, nutritious meals to ensure adequate nutrition. Monitor nutritional status and arrange a dietary consultation as needed. Taking the drug with food may also decrease GI upset.
- Instruct the patient about the appropriate dosage regimen and other measures to enhance patient knowledge about drug therapy and to promote adherence.
- Provide the following patient teaching:
  - If CNS effects occur, take safety precautions, including changing position slowly and avoiding driving and hazardous tasks.
  - Take the drug with meals and try small, frequent meals if GI upset is a problem.
  - Identify the importance of strict hand washing and hygiene measures, including daily laundering of underwear and bed linens, daily disinfection of toilet facilities, and periodic disinfection of bathroom floors (see Box 13.3).
  - Report to a health care provider any fever, severe diarrhea, or aggravation of condition, which could indicate a resistant strain or noneffective therapy.

Evaluation

- Monitor patient response to the drug (resolution of helminth infestation and improvement in signs and symptoms).

- Monitor for adverse effects (changes in orientation and affect, nutritional state, skin color and evidence of lesions, hepatic and renal function, and reports of abdominal discomfort and pain).
- Evaluate the effectiveness of the teaching plan. The patient should be able to name the drug, dosage, possible adverse effects to watch for, and specific measures to help avoid adverse effects).
- Monitor the effectiveness of comfort and safety measures and adherence to the regimen.

Key Points

- Anthelmintic drugs affect metabolic processes that are either different in worms than in human hosts or are not found in humans. These agents all cause death of the worm by interfering with normal functioning.
- Proper hygiene and sanitation processes are an important part of preventing the spread of helminths; this includes good hand hygiene and proper preparation and storage of food.

Box 13.3  Focus on Patient and Family Teaching

MANAGING PINWORM INFECTIONS

Some worm infestations are not that uncommon in the United States, especially infestation with pinworms.

Pinworms can spread very rapidly among children in schools, summer camps, and other institutions. Once the infestation starts, careful hygiene measures and drug therapy are required to eradicate the disease. After the diagnosis has been made and appropriate drug therapy started, proper hygiene measures are essential. Some suggested hygiene measures that might help to control the infection include the following:

- Keep the child's nails cut short and hands well scrubbed because reinfection results from the worm's eggs being carried back to the mouth after becoming lodged under the fingernails when the child scratches the pruritic perianal area.
- Give the child a shower in the morning to wash away any ova deposited in the anal area during the night.
- Change and launder undergarments, bed linens, and pajamas every day.
- Disinfect toilet seats daily and the floors of bathrooms and bedrooms periodically.
- Encourage the child to wash their hands vigorously after using the toilet.

In some areas of the United States, parents are asked to check for worm ova by pressing sticky tape against the anal area in the morning before bathing. The sticky tape is then pressed against a slide that can be taken or sent to a clinical laboratory for evaluation. It may take 5 to 6 weeks to get a clear reading with this method of testing. Some health care providers believe that the psychological trauma involved in doing this type of follow-up, especially with a school-aged child, makes this task too onerous to ask parents to do. Instead, many believe that the ease of treating this relatively harmless disease makes it more prudent to continue to treat as prescribed and to forgo this follow-up testing.

Infestation with worms can be a frightening and traumatic experience for most people. Seeing the worm can be an especially difficult experience. It is important to reassure patients and families that these types of infections do not necessarily reflect negatively on their hygiene or lifestyle. It takes a coordinated effort among medical personnel, families, and patients to control a pinworm infestation.

SUMMARY

- Helminths are worms that cause disease by invading the human body. Helminths that affect humans include nematodes (round-shaped worms), such as pinworms, hookworms, threadworms, whipworms, and roundworms, and platyhelminths (flatworms), which include tapeworms and flukes.
- Pinworms are the most frequent cause of helminth infection in the United States, and roundworms called *Ascaris* are the most frequent cause of helminth infections throughout the world.
- Some helminths invade body tissues and can seriously damage the lymphatic tissue, lungs, CNS, heart, liver, and so on. These helminths include trichinosis-causing tapeworms, which are found in undercooked pork; filariae, which occur when threadlike worm embryos clog vascular spaces; and schistosomiasis-causing flukes. Schistosomiasis is a common problem in many tropical areas where the snail that is necessary in the life cycle of the fluke lives.
- Anthelmintic drugs affect metabolic processes that are either different in worms than in human hosts or are not found in humans. These agents all cause death of the worm by interfering with normal functioning.
- Prevention is a very important part of the treatment of helminths. Thorough hand washing; laundering of bed linens, pajamas, and underwear to destroy ova that are shed during the night; and disinfection of toilet facilities at least daily and of bathroom floors periodically help to stop the spread of these diseases. In addition, proper sanitation and hygiene in food preparation and storage is essential for reducing the incidence of these infestations.
- Patient teaching is important for decreasing the stress and anxiety that may occur when individuals are diagnosed with a worm infestation.

CHECK YOUR UNDERSTANDING

Answers to the questions in this chapter can be found in Answers to Check Your Understanding Questions on thePoint®.

MULTIPLE CHOICE

Select the best answer.

1. To ensure effective treatment of pinworm infections, which instruction would be most important to emphasize to the patient and family?
   a. Keeping nails long so cutting will not introduce more infection
   b. Laundering undergarments, bed linens, and pajamas every day
   c. Boiling all drinking water
   d. Maintaining a clear liquid diet for at least 7 to 10 days
2. Which of the following would the nurse expect to assess in a patient who is suspected of having an *Ascaris* infection?
   a. Cough and signs of pulmonary infestation
   b. Cardiac arrhythmias and low blood pressure
   c. Seizures and disorientation
   d. Bloody diarrhea and excessive vomiting
3. The nurse describes schistosomiasis to a group of students as an infection caused by
   a. a protozoan carried by a mosquito.
   b. improperly cooked pork.
   c. a fluke carried by a snail.
   d. eating food contaminated by fecal material.
4. A patient has traveled to Egypt and come home with schistosomiasis. The family is very concerned about spreading the disease. Which information would be most helpful to teach the family?
   a. Strict hand washing will stop the spread of the disease.
   b. Isolating the patient will be necessary to stop the spread of the disease.
   c. Carefully cooking all of the patient's food will help to stop the spread of the disease.
   d. The snail needed for the life cycle of this worm does not live in this climate.
5. A patient is prescribed mebendazole. The nurse knows that this is the most commonly used anthelmintic, being the drug of choice for treating
   a. pinworms, roundworms, whipworms, and hookworms.
   b. trichinosis, flukes, cestodes, and hookworms.
   c. pork tapeworm, threadworms, cestodes, and whipworms.
   d. all stages of schistosomal infections.
6. Patient teaching regarding the use of anthelmintics should include counseling about
   a. the use of oral contraceptives.
   b. maintenance of nutrition during therapy.
   c. the use of oral anticoagulants.
   d. cardiac drug effects.
7. Patients may experience anxiety about the diagnosis and treatment of helminthic infections. Teaching may help to alleviate this anxiety and should include
   a. what they may experience if the worms are passed from the body.
   b. emphasis of the cleanliness of the home.
   c. measures to isolate the organism in the home.
   d. criticism of their personal hygiene practices.

MULTIPLE RESPONSE

Select all that apply.

1. An adult patient is being treated with mebendazole for a pinworm infection. Appropriate nursing diagnoses that might apply to this patient would include which of the following?
   a. Disturbed personal identity related to treatment
   b. Abdominal distention related to worm infestation
   c. Acute pain related to GI effects
   d. Risk for social isolation related to quarantine conditions
   e. Impaired physical mobility related to muscle infestation
   f. Deficient knowledge related to drug therapy

REFERENCES

Andrews, M., & Boyle, J. (2011). *Transcultural concepts in nursing care* (6th ed.). Lippincott Williams & Wilkins.

Brunton, L., Hilal-Dandan, R., & Knollman, B. (2018). *Goodman and Gilman's the pharmacological basis of therapeutics* (13th ed.). McGraw-Hill.

Falcone, F., & Pritchard, D. (2005). Parasite reversal: Worms on trial. *Trends in Parasitology, 21*, 157–160. 10.1016/j.pt.2005.02.002

Hotez, P. J., Brooker, S., Bethony, J., Bottazzi, M. E., Loukas, A., & Xiao, S. (2004). Hookworm infection. *New England Journal of Medicine, 351*, 799–807. 10.1056/NEJMra032492

James, D. T., Breman, J. G., & Measham, A. (Eds.). (2006). *Disease control priorities in developing countries* (2nd ed.). World Bank Publications.

Keiser, J., & Utzinger, J. (2008). Efficacy of current drugs against soil transmitted helminth infections: Systematic review. *Journal of American Medical Association, 299*, 1937–1948. 10.1001/jama.299.16.1937

Petri, W. (2008). *Diagnostic medical parasitology* (5th ed.). ASM Press.

CHAPTER 14

Antineoplastic Agents

Learning Objectives

Upon completion of this chapter, you will be able to:

1. Describe the nature of cancer and the changes it makes to the body.
2. Describe the therapeutic actions, indications, pharmacokinetics, contraindications, most common adverse reactions, and important drug–drug interactions associated with each class of antineoplastic agents and with their adjunctive therapy use.
3. Discuss the use of antineoplastic drugs across the lifespan.
4. Compare and contrast the prototype drugs for each class of antineoplastic agents with the other drugs in that class.
5. Outline the nursing considerations and teaching needs for patients receiving each class of antineoplastic agents.

Key Terms

alopecia: hair loss; a common adverse effect of many antineoplastic drugs, which are more effective against rapidly multiplying cells, such as those of hair follicles

anaplasia: a loss of cellular differentiation and organization, which leads to a loss of normal cellular function; a property of cancer cells

angiogenesis: the generation of new blood vessels; cancer cells release an enzyme that causes the growth of new blood vessels (angiogenesis) to feed the cancer cells

antineoplastic agent: drug used to combat cancer or the growth of neoplasms

autonomy: loss of the normal controls and reactions that inhibit growth and spreading; a property of cancer cells

bone marrow suppression: inhibition of the blood-forming components of the bone marrow; a common adverse effect of many antineoplastic drugs, which are more effective against rapidly multiplying cells, such as those in bone marrow; seen as anemia, thrombocytopenia, and leukopenia

carcinoma: tumor that originates in epithelial cells

metastasis: ability to enter the circulatory or lymphatic system and travel to other areas of the body that are conducive to growth and survival; a property of cancer cells

neoplasm: new or cancerous growth; occurs when abnormal cells have the opportunity to multiply and grow

sarcoma: tumor that originates in the mesenchyme and is made up of embryonic connective tissue cells

Drug List

ALKYLATING AGENTS
altretamine
bendamustine
busulfan
carboplatin
carmustine
(P) chlorambucil
cisplatin
cyclophosphamide
ifosfamide
lomustine
mechlorethamine
melphalan
oxaliplatin
procarbazine
streptozocin
temozolomide
thiotepa
trabectedin

ANTIMETABOLITES
capecitabine
cladribine
clofarabine
cytarabine
dacarbazine
floxuridine
fludarabine
fluorouracil
gemcitabine
hydroxyurea
mercaptopurine
(P) methotrexate
pemetrexed
pentostatin
pralatrexate
thioguanine

ANTINEOPLASTIC ANTIBIOTICS
bleomycin
dactinomycin
daunorubicin
(P) doxorubicin
epirubicin
idarubicin
mitomycin
mitoxantrone
valrubicin

MITOTIC INHIBITORS
cabazitaxel
docetaxel
eribulin
etoposide
ixabepilone
paclitaxel
vinblastine
(P) vincristine
vinorelbine

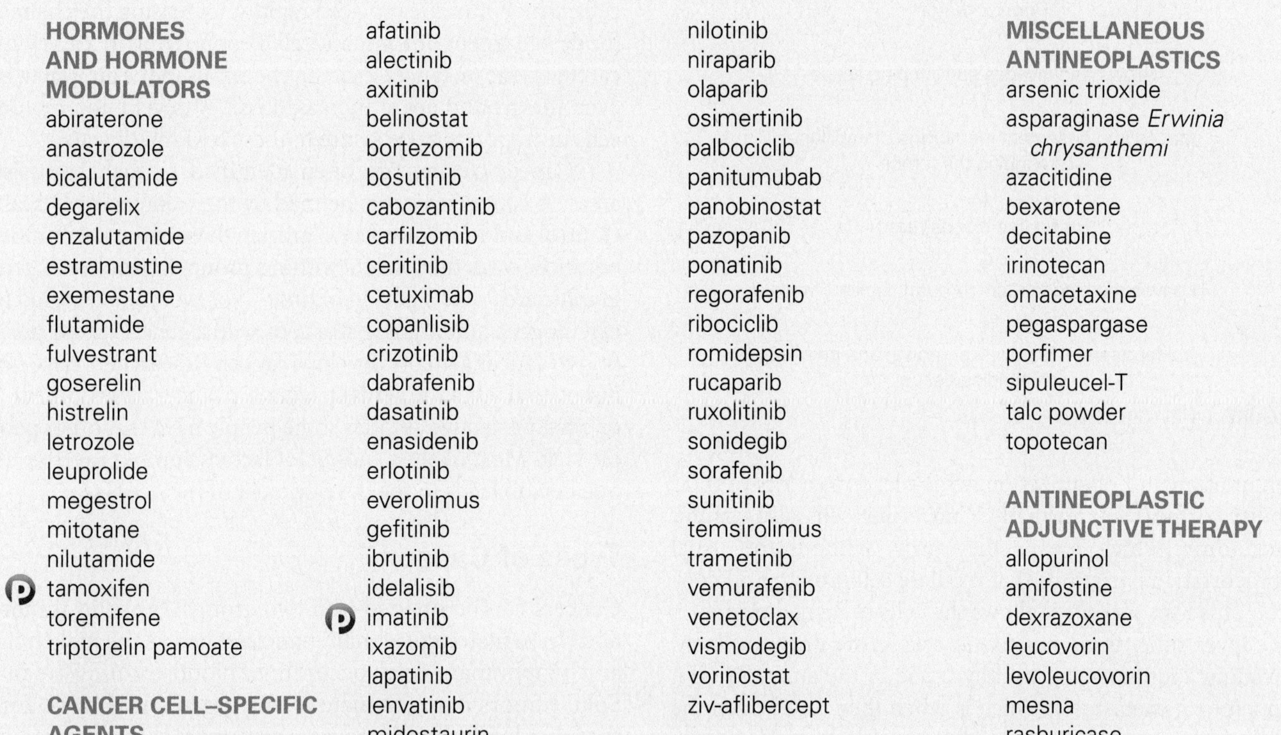

HORMONES AND HORMONE MODULATORS
abiraterone
anastrozole
bicalutamide
degarelix
enzalutamide
estramustine
exemestane
flutamide
fulvestrant
goserelin
histrelin
letrozole
leuprolide
megestrol
mitotane
nilutamide
Ⓟ tamoxifen
toremifene
triptorelin pamoate

CANCER CELL–SPECIFIC AGENTS
abemaciclib
afatinib
alectinib
axitinib
belinostat
bortezomib
bosutinib
cabozantinib
carfilzomib
ceritinib
cetuximab
copanlisib
crizotinib
dabrafenib
dasatinib
enasidenib
erlotinib
everolimus
gefitinib
ibrutinib
idelalisib
Ⓟ imatinib
ixazomib
lapatinib
lenvatinib
midostaurin
neratinib
nilotinib
niraparib
olaparib
osimertinib
palbociclib
panitumubab
panobinostat
pazopanib
ponatinib
regorafenib
ribociclib
romidepsin
rucaparib
ruxolitinib
sonidegib
sorafenib
sunitinib
temsirolimus
trametinib
vemurafenib
venetoclax
vismodegib
vorinostat
ziv-aflibercept

MISCELLANEOUS ANTINEOPLASTICS
arsenic trioxide
asparaginase *Erwinia chrysanthemi*
azacitidine
bexarotene
decitabine
irinotecan
omacetaxine
pegaspargase
porfimer
sipuleucel-T
talc powder
topotecan

ANTINEOPLASTIC ADJUNCTIVE THERAPY
allopurinol
amifostine
dexrazoxane
leucovorin
levoleucovorin
mesna
rasburicase

To most people, the term chemotherapy implies cancer treatment. However, only one branch of chemotherapy involves drugs developed to act on and kill or alter human cells—the **antineoplastic agents**, which are designed to fight **neoplasms**, or cancers.

Antineoplastic drugs alter human cells in a variety of ways. Their intended action is to target the abnormal cells that compose the neoplasm, or cancer, and impact abnormal cells more than normal cells. Unfortunately, normal cells also are affected by antineoplastic agents.

This area of pharmacology, which has grown tremendously in recent years, now includes many drugs that act on or are part of the immune system. These substances fight the cancerous cells using components of the immune system instead of directly destroying cells (see Chapter 17). This chapter discusses the classic antineoplastic agents, drugs that are used in cancer chemotherapy.

Cancer

Cancer is a disease that can strike a person at any age. It remains second only to coronary disease as the leading cause of death in the United States. Treatment of cancer can be prolonged and often debilitating. The patient can experience numerous and wide-ranging complications and effects.

All cancers start with a single cell that is genetically different from the other cells in the surrounding tissue. This cell divides, passing along its abnormalities to daughter cells, eventually producing a tumor or neoplasm that has characteristics quite different from those of the original tissue (see Fig. 14.1). It is thought that all cells contain genes, called oncogenes, that allow cells to become cancerous. Oncogenes are responsible for the characteristics seen in cancer cells. In healthy cells, these characteristics are not expressed. As abnormal cells continue to divide, they lose more and more of their original cell characteristics. The cancerous cells exhibit **anaplasia**—a loss of cellular dif-

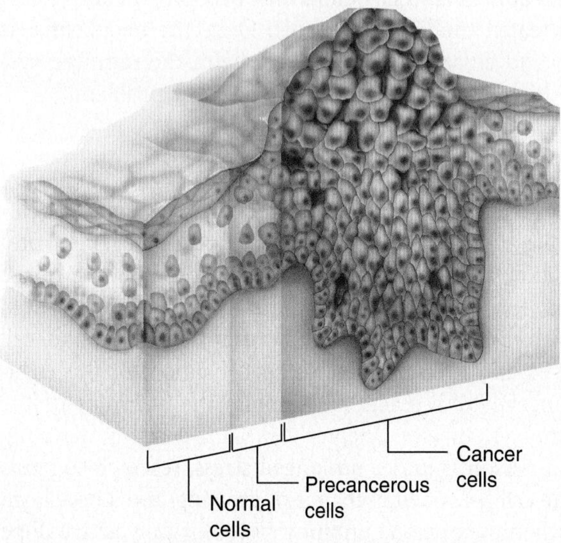

FIGURE 14.1 Malignant tumors develop from one cell, with somatic mutations occurring during cell division as the tumor grows.

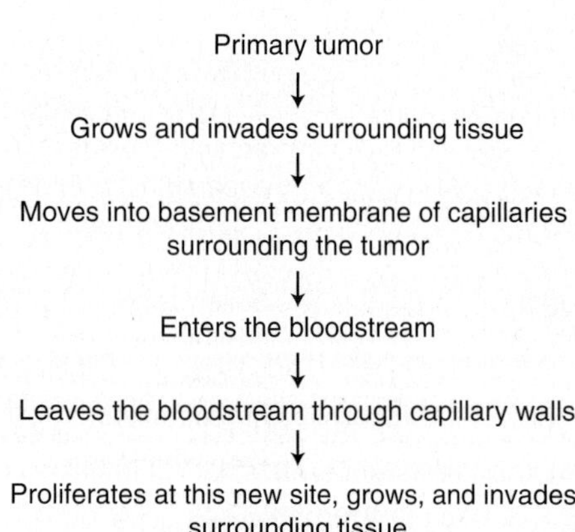
Primary tumor
Grows and invades surrounding tissue
Moves into basement membrane of capillaries surrounding the tumor
Enters the bloodstream
Leaves the bloodstream through capillary walls
Proliferates at this new site, grows, and invades surrounding tissue

FIGURE 14.2 Metastasis of cancer cells.

ferentiation and organization, which leads to a loss of their ability to function normally. Cancerous cells also exhibit **autonomy**, which means they grow without the usual homeostatic restrictions that regulate cell growth and control. This loss of control allows the cells to form a tumor.

Over time, these neoplastic cells grow uncontrollably, invading and damaging healthy tissue in the area and even undergoing **metastasis**, which is when they travel from the place of origin to other areas of the body where conditions are favorable for cell growth and develop new tumors (see Fig. 14.2). The abnormal cells release enzymes that generate blood vessels, a process known as **angiogenesis**, in the area to supply both oxygen and nutrients to the cells, thus contributing to their growth. Overall, as the result of pressure and intrusion on normal cells, the cancerous cells rob the host cells of energy and nutrients and block normal lymph and vascular vessels, leading to a loss of normal cellular function.

The body's immune system can damage or destroy some neoplastic cells. T cells, which recognize the abnormal cells and destroy them; antibodies, which form in response to parts of the abnormal cell protein; interferons; and tissue necrosis factor all play a role in the body's attempt to eliminate the abnormal cells before they become uncontrollable and threaten the life of the host. Once the neoplasm has grown and enlarged, it may overwhelm the immune system, which is no longer able to manage the problem.

Causes of Cancer

What causes the cells to mutate and become genetically different is not clearly understood. In some cases, a genetic predisposition to such a mutation can be found. Some breast cancers, for example, seem to have a definite genetic link. In other cases, viral infection, constant irritation and cell turnover, and even stress have been blamed for the ensuing cancer. Stress reactions suppress the activities of the immune system (see Chapter 29), so if a cell is mutating while a person is under prolonged stress, research suggests that the cell has a better chance of growing into a neoplasm than when the person's immune system is fully active. Pipe smokers are at increased risk for development of tongue and mouth cancers because the heat of the pipe and chemicals in the pipe tobaccos and smoke continuously destroy normal cells, which must be replaced rapidly, increasing the chances for development of a mutant cell. People living in areas with carcinogenic or cancer-causing chemicals in the air, water, or even the ground are at increased risk of developing mutant cells in response to exposure to these toxic chemicals.

Cancer clusters are often identified in such high-risk areas. A cancer cluster is defined by the Centers for Disease Control and Prevention as a "greater-than-expected number of cancer cases that occurs within a group of people in a geographic area over a period of time." Not everyone exposed to carcinogens, undergoing stress, or with a genetic predisposition to cancer actually develops cancer. Researchers have not discovered what the actual trigger for cancer development is or what protective abilities some people have that other people lack. Most likely, a mosaic of factors coming together in one person leads to the development of the neoplasm.

Types of Cancer

Cancers can be divided into two groups: (a) solid tumors and (b) hematological malignancies, such as the leukemias and lymphomas, which occur in the blood-forming organs. Solid tumors may originate in any organ and may be further divided into **carcinomas**, or tumors that originate in epithelial cells, and **sarcomas**, or tumors that originate in the mesenchyme and are made up of embryonic connective tissue cells. Examples of carcinomas include granular cell tumors of the breast, bronchogenic tumors arising in cells that line the bronchial tubes, and squamous and basal tumors of the skin. Sarcomas include osteogenic tumors, which form in the primitive cells of the bone, and rhabdomyosarcomas, which occur in striated muscles. Hematological malignancies involve the blood-forming organs of the body, the bone marrow, and the lymphatic system. These malignancies alter the body's ability to produce and regulate the cells found in the blood.

Key Points

- Cancers arise from a single abnormal cell that multiplies and grows.
- Cancer cells lose their normal function (anaplasia), develop characteristics that allow them to grow in an uninhibited way (autonomy), and have the ability to travel to other sites in the body that are conducive to their growth (metastasis). They also have the ability to grow new blood vessels to feed the tumor (angiogenesis).
- The goal of cancer chemotherapy is to decrease the size of the neoplasm so that the human immune system can eliminate the abnormal cells.

Antineoplastic Drugs

Antineoplastic drugs can work by affecting cell survival or by boosting the immune system in its efforts to combat the abnormal cells (see Fig. 14.3). Chapter 17 discusses the immune agents that are used to combat cancer. The

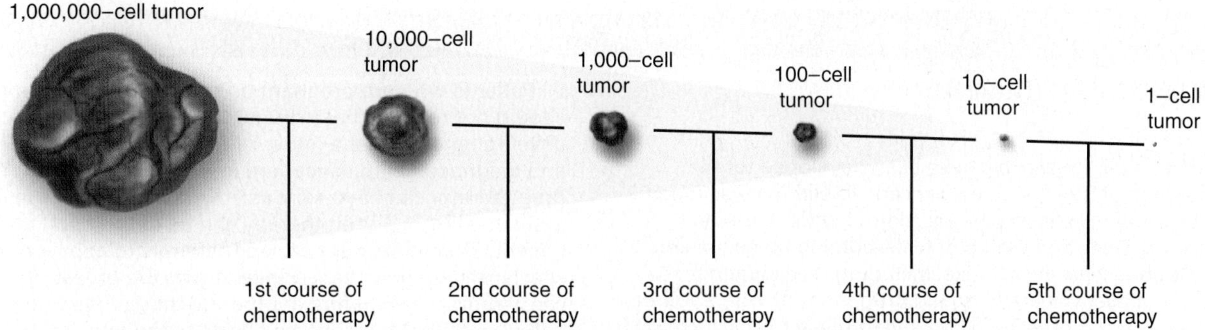

FIGURE 14.3 Cell kill theory. A set percentage of cells is killed after each dose of chemotherapy. The percentage killed is dependent upon the drug therapy. In this example, each course of chemotherapy kills 90% of cells in a cancerous tumor. After the fifth course of chemotherapy in this example, a single cell tumor remains; the patient's immune system would destroy this malignant cell.

present chapter focuses on those drugs that affect cell survival. Antineoplastic drugs commonly used today include alkylating agents, antimetabolites, antineoplastic antibiotics, mitotic inhibitors, hormones and hormone modulators, cancer cell–specific agents including protein tyrosine kinase inhibitors (which target enzymes specific to the cancer cells), and a group of antineoplastic agents that cannot be classified elsewhere. Other drugs are used as adjunctive therapy to combat the serious adverse effects associated with the antineoplastic drugs. Figure 14.4 shows sites of action of antineoplastic agents. Box 14.1 discusses their use across the lifespan.

As discussed in Chapter 7, all cells progress through a cell cycle. Different types of cells progress at different

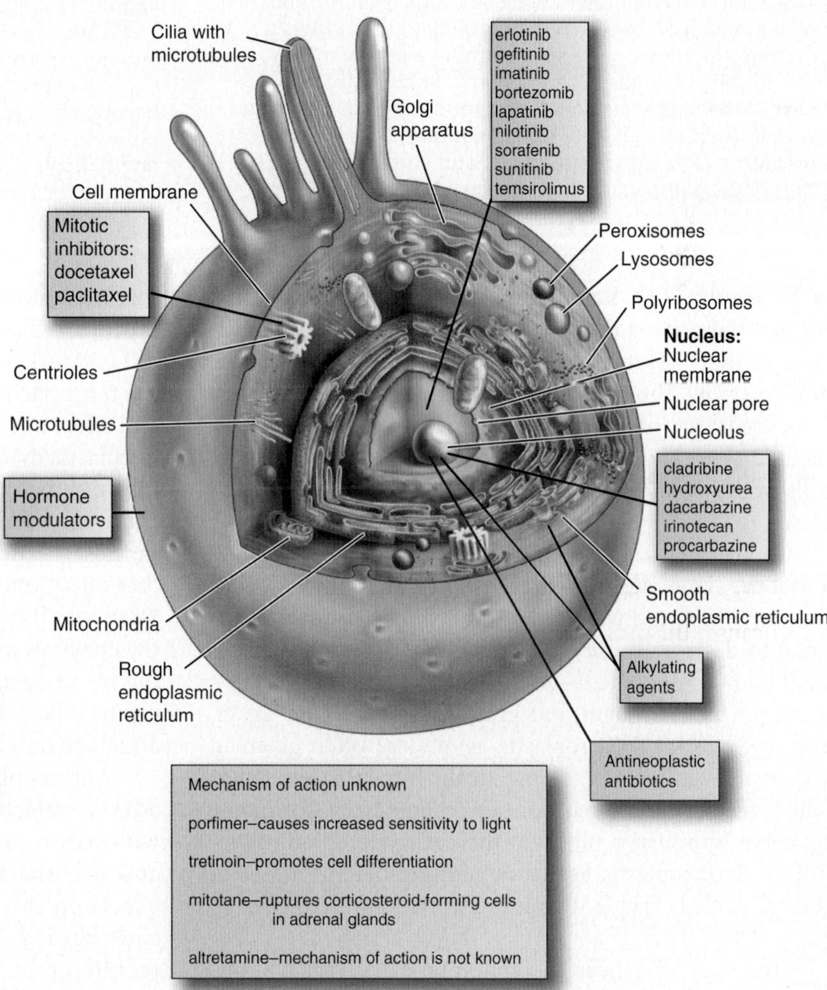

FIGURE 14.4 Sites of action of non–cell cycle–specific antineoplastic agents. Alkylating agents interfere with RNA, DNA, or other cellular proteins. For example, dacarbazine blocks DNA and RNA synthesis, whereas procarbazine blocks DNA, RNA, and protein synthesis. Hormone modulators react with specific receptor sites to block cell growth and activity. Mitotic inhibitors such as docetaxel and paclitaxel inhibit microtubular reorganization. The antimetabolite cladribine and miscellaneous agent hydroxyurea block DNA synthesis. The miscellaneous agent irinotecan disrupts DNA strands. Cell-specific agents inhibit protein tyrosine kinases or other cell-specific systems.

Box 14.1 Focus on Drug Therapy Across the Lifespan

ANTINEOPLASTIC AGENTS

Children

Antineoplastic protocols have been developed for the treatment of most pediatric cancers. To eliminate as many of the mutant cells as possible, combination therapy is stressed. Dose and timing of these combinations are crucial.

Double-checking of dose, including recalculating desired dose and verifying the drug amount with another nurse, is good practice when giving these toxic drugs to children.

Children need to be monitored closely for hydration and nutritional status. The nutritional needs of a child are greater than those of an adult, and this needs to be considered when formulating a care plan.

These children need support and comfort, and they also need to be allowed to explore and learn like any other children. Body image problems, lack of energy, and the need to protect the child from exposure to infection can isolate a child receiving antineoplastic agents. The total care plan of the child needs to include social, emotional, and intellectual stimulation.

Monitor bone marrow activity very carefully and adjust the dose accordingly.

Adults

The adult receiving antineoplastic drugs is confronted with many dilemmas that the nurse needs to address. Changes in body image are common, along with loss of hair, skin changes, GI complaints, and weight loss. Fear of the diagnosis and the treatment is also common with these patients. Networking support systems and providing teaching, reassurance, and comfort can have a tremendous impact on the success of the drug therapy.

Patients who are pregnant or breast or chestfeeding should not receive these drugs, which are toxic to the developing cells of the fetus. Patients who are pregnant and diagnosed with cancer are in a difficult situation: The drug therapy can have serious adverse effects on the fetus, and not using the drug therapy can be detrimental to the patient. Education, support, and referrals to appropriate specialists are important. Patients who are breast or chestfeeding should find another method of feeding the baby to prevent the adverse effects to the fetus that occur when these drugs cross into human milk. Use of barrier contraceptives is urged when these drugs are being used by patients who can become pregnant.

Older Adults

Older adults may be more susceptible to the CNS and GI effects of some of these drugs. Older patients should be monitored for hydration and nutritional status regularly. Safety precautions should be instituted if CNS effects occur, including increased lighting, assistance with ambulation, and use of supports.

Many older patients have decreased renal and/or hepatic function. Many of these drugs depend on the liver and kidney for metabolism and excretion. Renal and liver function tests should be done before (baseline) and periodically during the use of these drugs, and dose should be adjusted accordingly.

Protecting these patients from exposure to infection and injury is a very important aspect of their nursing care. Older patients are naturally somewhat immunosuppressed because of age, and giving drugs that further depress the immune system can lead to infections that are serious and difficult to treat. Monitor blood counts carefully and arrange for rest or reduced dose as indicated.

rates (see Fig. 7.6). Rapidly multiplying cells, or cells that replace themselves quickly, include those lining the gastrointestinal (GI) tract and those in hair follicles, skin, and bone marrow. These cells complete the cell cycle every few days. Cells that proceed very slowly through the cell cycle include those in the breasts, testicles, and ovaries. Some cells take weeks, months, or even years to complete the cycle.

Cancer cells tend to move through the cell cycle at about the same rate as their cells of origin. Malignant cells that remain in a dormant phase for long periods are difficult to destroy. These cells can emerge long after cancer treatment has finished—weeks, months, or years later—to begin their division and growth cycle all over again. For this reason, antineoplastic agents are often given in sequence over periods of time, in the hope that the drugs will affect the cancer cells as they emerge from dormancy or move into a new phase of the cell cycle. A combination of antineoplastic agents targeting different phases of the cell cycle is frequently most effective in treating many cancers.

The goal of cancer therapy, much like that of anti-infective therapy, is to limit the offending cells to the degree that the immune system can respond without causing too much toxicity to the host. However, this is a particularly difficult task when using antineoplastic drugs because, for the most part, these agents are not specific to mutant cells and affect normal human cells as well. In most cases, antineoplastic drugs primarily affect human cells that are rapidly multiplying, with many cells in many phases of the cell cycle (e.g., those in the hair follicles, GI tract, and bone marrow). Much research is being done to develop drugs that affect only the abnormal cells. Imatinib, released in 2001, was the first of a growing number of drugs to target the enzymes used by very specific abnormal cells. A growing list of agents that affect only the mechanisms of cancer cells have been marketed. Many more such drugs are anticipated in the future.

Antineoplastic drugs are associated with many adverse effects, with specific adverse effects occurring with particular drugs. These effects are often unpleasant and debilitating. Some antineoplastic drugs exert toxic effects on ova and sperm production, affecting the person's fertility. These agents are also usually selective for rapidly growing cells, posing a danger to the developing fetus during pregnancy. Consequently, pregnancy is a contraindication to the use of antineoplastic drugs. These agents also jeopardize the immune system by causing **bone marrow suppression**, inhibiting the blood-forming components of the bone marrow and interfering with the body's normal protective actions against abnormal cells. The patient's hematological profile must always be assessed for toxic effects. Patients also need to understand the importance of returning every few weeks to go through the chemotherapy, despite its adverse effects, over and over again. Many patients experience nausea and vomiting, direct effects of the toxic drug as well as the body's response to the elements of cell death circulating in the bloodstream. Patients may also experience hair and/or skin effects as hair follicles and skin cells rapidly turn over and may be especially susceptible to the effects of the antineoplastic drugs.

Many antineoplastic drugs often result in another adverse effect, cancer itself. Cell death due to these agents increases the need for cellular growth, placing the person at increased risk for mutant cell development. Bone marrow is suppressed by the drug therapy, making the immune system very weak and less effective, which might allow mutant cells to progress.

Most patients who have cancer are not considered to be "cured" until they have been cancer free for a period of 5 years, due to the possibility that cancer cells will emerge from dormancy to cause new tumors or problems. Some experts now consider cancer a chronic disease, with the possibility of dormant cells emerging and becoming active again always present. No cells have yet been identified that can remain dormant for longer than 5 years, so the chance of the emergence of one after that time is rather slim.

Sometimes, a cancerous mass may be so large that no therapy can arrest its growth without killing the host. In such cases, antineoplastic agents are used as palliative therapy to shrink the size of the tumor and alleviate some of the signs and symptoms of the cancer, decreasing pain and increasing function. Here, the goal of drug therapy is not to cure the disease but to try to improve the patient's quality of life in a situation in which there is no cure. Antineoplastic medications may also be hazardous to health care providers. The Occupational Safety and Health Administration and Centers for Disease Control and prevention provide information pertaining to risks of these agents and instructions regarding safe medication administration (Box 14.2). A novel strategy for cancer treatment is introduced in Box 14.3.

Box 14.2 Focus on Safe Medication Administration

OSHA (Occupational Safety and Health Administration) and the CDC (Centers for Disease Control and Prevention) warn health care providers about the risk of exposure to antineoplastic agents. The list of hazardous drugs was updated in 2016 and includes drugs that could cause cancer, fetal death, reproductive toxicity, organ toxicity at low doses, and genotoxicity. Antineoplastics generally fall into this category. Special care needs to be taken when administering these drugs. Some of these drugs must be prepared in a special setting using a hood that cuts down lung exposure. The nurse should avoid any skin, eye, or mucous membrane contact with these drugs that involves always wearing gloves when exposed to the drug, oral or injected, and may involve using protective goggles, and a mask or respirator to protect the lungs, depending on the drug being used. Protecting other people is also an issue. Placing used syringes in a yellow box for biohazard disposal; double flushing patient wastes; and if the patient is taking the drug at home, the proper disposal of the drug and administration materials all need to be stressed. Nurses working in cancer centers that do a great deal of antineoplastic drug administration receive special training to reduce the risk of exposure and to protect the health care providers and others from the potentially dangerous effects of these drugs.

Box 14.3 Focus on The Evidence

NEW APPROACHES IN THE BATTLE AGAINST CANCER

Clustered regularly interspaced short palindromic repeats (CRISPER-Cas9) is a genome engineering tool that is able to identify and modulate specific genes. Cancer is a disease that involves multiple genetic mutations that often lead to resistance to conventional treatment. Therefore, understanding tumor-specific genes can enhance cancer therapy. One example of how CRISPER-Cas9 has been used is with lung cancer treatment.

It is important to identify specific genetic mutations when treating non–small cell lung cancer, particularly adenocarcinoma. Some of the genetic aberrations have treatment options; however, the treatments are limited by specific molecular targets and medication resistance. CRISPER-Cas9 has been used to identify the mutant gene on the cancer cells, so that the cancerous cells are selectively eliminated in preclinical trials. Other researchers are investigating how to use CRISPER-Cas9 to assist with breast, brain, liver, and colorectal cancers. There are still some problems to overcome before CRISPER-associated nucleases can be used in the clinical setting; however, being able to identify the specific target for treatment is extremely important in developing better treatments.

Alkylating Agents

Because alkylating agents can even affect cells in the resting phase, these drugs are said to be non–cell cycle specific (see Fig. 14.4). Alkylating agents (Table 14.1) include the following drugs: altretamine (*Hexalen*), bendamustine (*Bendeka, Treanda*), busulfan (*Busulfex, Myleran*), carboplatin (generic), carmustine (*BiCNU, Gliadel*), chlorambucil (*Leukeran*), cisplatin (generic), cyclophosphamide (generic), ifosfamide (*Ifex*), lomustine (generic), mechlorethamine (*Mustargen*), melphalan (*Alkeran*), oxaliplatin (*Eloxatin*), procarbazine (*Matulane*), streptozocin (*Zanosar*), and temozolomide (*Temodar*), thiotepa (*Tepadina*), trabectedin (*Yondelis*).

Table 14.1 *Drugs in Focus:* Alkylating Agents

Drug Name	Dosage/Route	Usual Indications
altretamine (*Hexalen*)	260 mg/m²/d PO for 14–21 consecutive days of a 28-d cycle	Palliative treatment of persistent or recurrent ovarian cancer after failure of first-line therapy *Special considerations:* Premedicate with antiemetic; monitor blood counts and central nervous system status regularly
bendamustine (*Bendeka, Treanda*)	CLL: 100 mg/m² IV over 30 min (*Treanda*) or 10 min (*Bendeka*) on days 1 and 2 of a 28-d cycle for up to 6 cycles Non–B-cell lymphoma: 120 mg/m² IV over 60 min (*Treanda*) or 10 min (*Bendeka*) on days 1 and 2 of a 21-d cycle for up to 8 cycles	Treatment of chronic lymphocytic leukemia, indolent non–B-cell Hodgkin lymphoma *Special considerations:* Dosing may need to be adjusted based on blood counts; monitor for infection, skin reactions; note that infusion rates vary by brand name
busulfan (*Busulfex, Myleran*)	*Induction:* 4–8 mg/d PO *Maintenance:* 1–3 mg/d PO *Injection:* 0.8 mg/kg as a 2-h IV infusion q6h for 4 d via a central venous catheter for a total of 16 doses	Palliative treatment of chronic myelogenous leukemia, other myeloproliferative disorders *Special considerations:* Dosing is monitored by effects on bone marrow; always push fluids to decrease toxic renal effects; alopecia is common
carboplatin (generic)	360 mg/m² IV over at least 15 min on day 1 every 4 wk; reduce dose as needed based on blood counts and with renal impairment	Palliative or initial treatment of ovarian cancer; may be useful in several other cancers *Special considerations:* Dose and timing are determined by bone marrow response; alopecia is common
carmustine (*BiCNU, Gliadel*)	150–200 mg/m² IV every 6 wk as a single dose or divided daily injections; wafers implanted into brain at time of surgery	Treatment of brain tumors, Hodgkin disease, and multiple myelomas; available in implantable wafer form for treatment of glioblastoma *Special considerations:* Dose determined by bone marrow toxicity; do not repeat for 6 wk because of delayed toxicity may cause pulmonary fibrosis, liver and kidney toxicity
chlorambucil (*Leukeran*)	0.1–0.2 mg/kg/d PO for 3–6 wk; or 0.4 mg/kg PO every 2 wk *PO maintenance:* 0.03–0.1 mg/kg/d PO	Palliative treatment of lymphomas and leukemias including Hodgkin disease and CLL *Special considerations:* Toxic to liver and bone marrow; dosing based on bone marrow response; carcinogenic, avoid use in pregnancy
cisplatin (generic)	20–50 mg/m²/d IV, once every 3 wk used in combination with other antineoplastic agents	Combination therapy for metastatic testicular or ovarian tumors, advanced bladder cancers *Special considerations:* Neurotoxic, nephrotoxic, and can cause serious hypersensitivity reactions; highly emetogenic
cyclophosphamide (generic)	*Induction:* 40–50 mg/kg/d IV over 2–5 d *or* 1–5 mg/kg/d *PO maintenance:* 1–5 mg/kg/d PO, or 10–15 mg/kg IV q7–10d	Treatment of lymphoma, myelomas, leukemias, and other cancers in combination with other drugs *Special considerations:* Hemorrhagic cystitis is a potentially fatal side effect; may cause sterility; alopecia is common
ifosfamide (*Ifex*)	1.2 g/m²/d IV over 30 min for 5 consecutive days; repeat every 3 wk	Combination therapy as a third-line agent in treating germ cell testicular cancers, bone and soft tissue sarcomas *Special considerations:* Alopecia is common; monitor for bone marrow depression; push fluids to help prevent bladder toxicity
lomustine (generic)	130 mg/m² PO as a single dose every 6 wk; adjust dose based on blood counts	Palliative combination therapy for Hodgkin disease and primary and metastatic brain tumors *Special considerations:* Immune suppression and GI effects are common
mechlorethamine (*Mustargen*)	0.4 mg/kg IV for each course; usually repeated every 3–6 wk; intracavity 0.2–0.4 mg/kg; apply thin film to affected skin area	Nitrogen mustard; palliative treatment in Hodgkin disease, leukemia, bronchial carcinoma, other cancers; injected for treatment of effusions secondary to cancer metastases; topical treatment of mycosis fungoides–type T-cell lymphoma after skin treatment *Special considerations:* GI toxicity, bone marrow suppression, and impaired fertility are common; handle with precautions; monitor for extravasation

Table 14.1 *Drugs in Focus:* Alkylating Agents *(Continued)*

Drug Name	Dosage/Route	Usual Indications
melphalan (*Alkeran*)	*Multiple myeloma:* 6 mg/d PO for 2–3 wk, then a rest period, or 16 mg/m² IV at 2-wk intervals for four doses, then at 4-wk intervals *Ovarian cancer:* 0.2 mg/kg/d PO for 5 d; repeat course every 4–5 wk	Nitrogen mustard; treatment for multiple myeloma, ovarian cancers *Special considerations:* Oral route is preferred; pulmonary fibrosis, bone marrow suppression, and alopecia are common
oxaliplatin (*Eloxatin*)	85 mg/m² IV with leucovorin, followed by fluorouracil (5-FU) at 2-wk cycles, or 1,000 mg/m² IV at weekly intervals	Treatment of metastatic carcinoma of the colon or rectum when disease progresses after standard therapy; used in combination therapy *Special considerations:* Premedicate with antiemetics and dexamethasone; monitor for potentially dangerous anaphylactic reactions
procarbazine (*Matulane*)	*Adult:* 2–6 mg/kg/d PO; base the dose on bone marrow response	Used in combination therapy for treatment of stages III and IV of Hodgkin disease *Special considerations:* Bone marrow toxicity; GI toxicity and skin lesions also limit use in some patients; severity of adverse effects regulates the dose of the drug
streptozocin (*Zanosar*)	500 mg/m² IV for 5 consecutive days, usually given every week, or 1,000 mg/m³ IV at weekly intervals	Treatment of metastatic islet cell carcinoma of the pancreas *Special considerations:* GI and renal toxicity are common; causes infertility; wear rubber gloves to avoid drug contact with the skin—if contact occurs, wash with soap and water
temozolomide (*Temodar*)	*Astroma:* 150 mg/m²/d PO or IV for 5 consecutive days in a 28-d cycle *Glioblastoma:* 75 mg/m²/d PO or IV for 42 d with radiation	Treatment of refractory astrocytoma or glioblastoma in patients refractory to other treatments *Special considerations:* Monitor bone marrow closely; especially toxic in female patients and older adults
thiotepa (*Tepadina*)	0.3–0.4 mg/kg IV; 0.6–0.8 mg/kg intracavity	Treatment of adenocarcinoma of breast, ovary; superficial papillary carcinoma of urinary bladder; intracavity effusions *Special considerations:* Monitor for severe bone marrow suppression; may be carcinogenic, monitor patient closely
trabectedin (*Yondelis*)	1.5 mg/m² as a 24-h infusion every 3 wk	Treatment of unresectable or metastatic liposarcoma or leiomyosarcoma after anthracycline-containing therapy *Special considerations:* Premedicate with dexamethasone; reduce dose with hepatic impairment

CLL, chronic lymphocytic leukemia.

Therapeutic Actions and Indications

Alkylating agents produce their cytotoxic effects by reacting chemically with portions of the RNA, DNA, or other cellular proteins, being most potent when they bind with cellular DNA. The oldest drugs in this class are the nitrogen mustards, and modifications of the structure of these drugs have led to the development of the nitrosoureas and platinum compounds. They are nonspecific to a cell cycle phase, but more toxic to dividing cells.

These drugs are most useful in the treatment of slow-growing cancers, such as various lymphomas, leukemias, myelomas; some ovarian, testicular, and breast cancers; and some pancreatic cancers. See Table 14.1 for usual indications for each of the alkylating agents. These agents are not used interchangeably.

Pharmacokinetics

The alkylating agents vary in their degree of absorption, and little is known about their distribution in the tissues. They are metabolized and sometimes activated in the liver, with many of these agents using the cytochrome P450 systems. They are excreted in the urine.

Contraindications and Cautions

Alkylating agents are contraindicated during pregnancy and lactation due to their potential for severe effects on the fetus and neonate. Caution is necessary when giving alkylating agents to any individual with a known allergy to any of them; with bone marrow suppression, which is often the index for redosing and dosing levels; or with suppressed renal or hepatic function, which may interfere with metabolism or excretion of these drugs and often indicates a need to change the dose.

Adverse Effects

Adverse effects frequently encountered with the use of these alkylating agents are listed below; see Table 14.1 for a list of special considerations and/or adverse effects specific to each agent. Amifostine (*Ethyol*) and mesna (*Mesnex*) are cytoprotective (cell-protecting) drugs that may be given to limit certain effects of cisplatin and ifosfamide, respectively (Box 14.4).

Hematological effects include bone marrow suppression, with leukopenia, thrombocytopenia, anemia, and pancytopenia, secondary to the effects of the drugs on the rapidly multiplying cells of the bone marrow. GI effects include nausea, vomiting, anorexia, diarrhea, and mucous membrane deterioration, all of which are related to the drugs' effects on the rapidly multiplying cells of the GI tract. Hepatic toxicity and renal toxicity may occur, depending on the exact mechanism of action. **Alopecia**, or hair loss, related to effects on the hair follicles, may also occur. All drugs that cause cell death can cause a potentially toxic increase in uric acid levels. Allopurinol has been used to help alleviate this problem, and in 2004, a new drug, rasburicase (*Elitek*), was introduced to manage uric acid levels in patients receiving antineoplastics resulting in tumor lysis and elevated uric acid levels (Box 14.5).

BOX 14.4

Drugs That Are Used as Adjuncts in Antineoplastic Chemotherapy

Amifostine (*Ethyol*) is a cytoprotective (cell-protecting) drug that preserves healthy cells from the toxic effects of cisplatin. It is thought to react to the specific acidity and vascularity of nontumor cells to protect them, and it may also act as a scavenger of free radicals released by cells that have been exposed to cisplatin. Amifostine is given at a dose of 910 mg/m^2 four times a day as a 15-minute IV infusion starting within 30 minutes after starting cisplatin therapy; timing is very important to its effectiveness. It is FDA approved for use to prevent the renal toxicity associated with the use of cisplatin in patients with advanced ovarian cancer and for reduction of development of xerostomia in clients undergoing radiation treatment for head and neck cancer when the treatment includes the parotid glands. Because amifostine is associated with severe nausea and vomiting, concurrent administration of an antiemetic is recommended. It also can cause hypotension, and patients should be monitored closely for this condition.

Mesna (*Mesnex*) is a cytoprotective agent that is used to reduce the incidence of hemorrhagic cystitis caused by ifosfamide or cyclophosphamide. Mesna, which is known to react chemically with urotoxic metabolites of ifosfamide, is given intravenously or orally at the time of the ifosfamide injection. Because mesna has been associated with nausea and vomiting, an antiemetic may be useful. There is risk of dermatologic toxicity, so patients need to be monitored for changes in the skin.

Dexrazoxane (*Totect, Zinecard*) is approved for the treatment of extravasation resulting from IV antineoplastic antibiotic chemotherapy (*Totect* only) or reducing cardiomyopathy associated with doxorubicin in patients being treated for breast cancer. The mechanism of action that allows this drug to protect cells from damage related to extravasation is not understood, but it may block certain enzymes affected by the drugs. Dose should be reduced in patients with renal failure.

BOX 14.5

Drugs to Manage Rising Uric Acid Levels Associated With Tumor Lysis

Allopurinol (*Aloprim, Zyloprim*) inhibits the enzyme that allows the conversion of purines to uric acid, which is toxic to the body. It is used to help manage patients with leukemia, lymphoma, or other malignancies that result in elevated levels of serum and urinary uric acid levels. It lowers the level of uric acid to protect the kidneys and tissues. It is given orally at doses of 600 to 800 mg a day for 2 to 3 days with high fluid intake, and maintenance doses are then determined based on the patient's response and serum uric acid levels.

Rasburicase (*Elitek*) is approved for the management of plasma uric acid levels in patients with leukemia, lymphoma, and solid tumor malignancies who are receiving antineoplastic therapy associated with tumor lysis and subsequent elevated serum uric acid levels. It is administered as a single daily IV infusion of 0.15 to 0.2 mg/kg over 30 minutes for 5 days. Chemotherapy should be started 4 to 24 hours after the first dose of rasburicase. Uric acid levels should be monitored frequently, using prechilled, heparinized vials that are kept in an ice-water bath. This analysis should be done within 4 hours of each rasburicase dose.

Clinically Important Drug–Drug Interactions

Alkylating agents that are known to cause hepatic or renal toxicity should be used cautiously with any other drugs that have similar effects. In addition, drugs that are toxic to the liver may adversely affect drugs that are metabolized in the liver or that act in the liver (e.g., oral anticoagulants). Using cyclophosphamide concurrently with succinylcholine can increase neuromuscular blockage. Using carmustine with cimetidine can increase bone marrow suppression. Cisplatin with aminoglycoside may increase renal toxicity risk; with furosemide use, it may cause hearing loss. Always check for specific drug–drug interactions for each agent in a nursing drug guide.

Prototype Summary: Chlorambucil

Indications: Palliative treatment of chronic lymphocytic leukemia, malignant lymphomas, and Hodgkin disease.

Actions: Alkylates cellular DNA, interfering with the replication of susceptible cells.

Pharmacokinetics:

Route	Onset	Peak	Duration
Oral	Varies	1 h	15–20 h

$T_{1/2}$: 60 to 90 minutes, metabolized in the liver and excreted in the urine.

Adverse Effects: Tremors, muscle twitching, confusion, nausea, vomiting, hepatotoxicity, bone marrow suppression, sterility, cancer.

Nursing Considerations for Patients Receiving Alkylating Agents

Assessment: History and Examination

- Assess for contraindications or cautions: history of allergy to any of the alkylating agents to avoid hypersensitivity reactions, bone marrow suppression to prevent further suppression, renal or hepatic dysfunction that might interfere with drug metabolism and excretion, and current status related to pregnancy or lactation to prevent potentially serious adverse effects on the fetus or nursing baby.
- Perform a physical assessment to establish baseline data for determining the effectiveness of the drug and the occurrence of any adverse effects associated with drug therapy.
- Assess orientation and reflexes to evaluate any central nervous system (CNS) effects; respiratory rate and adventitious sounds to monitor the disease and to evaluate for respiratory or hypersensitivity effects; pulse, rhythm, and auscultation to monitor for systemic or cardiovascular effects; and bowel sounds and mucous membrane status to monitor for GI effects.
- Monitor the results of laboratory tests, such as complete blood count with differential to identify possible bone marrow suppression and toxic drug effects and establish appropriate dosing for the drug. Monitor renal and liver function tests to determine the need for possible dose adjustment and identify toxic drug effects.

Nursing Conclusions

Nursing conclusions related to drug therapy might include the following:

- Impaired comfort related to GI, CNS, and skin effects of the drug
- Altered body image perception related to alopecia, skin effects, impaired fertility
- Malnutrition risk due to GI side effects
- Infection risk due to bone marrow suppression effects on immune system
- Acute or chronic anxiety or fear related to diagnosis and treatment
- Knowledge deficit risk regarding drug therapy

Planning

- The patient will receive the best therapeutic effect from the drug therapy.
- The patient will have limited adverse effects to the drug therapy.
- The patient will have an understanding of the drug therapy, adverse effects to anticipate, and measures to relieve discomfort and improve safety.

Intervention With Rationale

- Arrange for blood tests before, periodically during, and for at least 3 weeks after therapy to monitor bone marrow function to aid in determining the need for a change in dose or discontinuation of the drug (see Box 14.6).
- Administer medication according to scheduled protocol and in combination with other drugs as indicated to improve effectiveness.
- Ensure that the patient is well hydrated to decrease risk of renal toxicity. Monitor for blood in urine; mesna may be indicated.
- Protect the patient from exposure to infection; limit invasive procedures when bone marrow suppression limits the patient's immune/inflammatory responses.
- Provide small, frequent meals, frequent mouth care, and dietary consultation as appropriate to maintain nutrition when GI effects are severe. Anticipate the need for antiemetics if necessary (see Box 14.7).
- Arrange for proper head coverings at extremes of temperature if alopecia occurs; a wig, scarf, or hat is important for maintaining body temperature.
- Provide patient teaching about the following:
  - Follow the appropriate dosage regimen, including dates to return for further doses.
  - Cover the head at extremes of temperature.
  - Maintain nutrition if GI effects are severe.
  - Avoid exposure to infection.
  - Plan for appropriate rest periods because fatigue and weakness are common effects of the drugs.
  - Consult with a health care provider, if appropriate, related to the possibility of impaired fertility.
  - Use barrier contraceptives to reduce the risk of pregnancy during therapy.

Evaluation

- Monitor patient response to the drug (alleviation of cancer being treated, palliation of signs and symptoms of cancer).
- Monitor for adverse effects (bone marrow suppression, GI toxicity, neurotoxicity, alopecia, renal or hepatic dysfunction, bleeding, infection).
- Evaluate the effectiveness of the teaching plan (patient can name the drug, dosage, possible adverse effects to watch for, and specific measures to help avoid adverse effects).

BOX 14.6

Dealing With Bone Marrow Suppression

Bone marrow suppression is a frequently encountered adverse effect of antineoplastic chemotherapy. The cells in the bone marrow are rapidly turning over cells, constantly stimulated to produce blood components, and so they are more likely to be affected by drugs that kill cells. The patient may experience a low red blood cell (RBC) count (anemia), low platelet counts, and low white blood cell (WBC) counts. The nurse is in the position to help the patient cope with these effects and prevent serious complications that occur. Drugs often used to help stimulate the bone marrow are also available.

Decreased Red Blood Cells

The patient with a low RBC count will experience fatigue. The patient should be counseled to space activities during the day and incorporate rest periods into their daily schedule. Sometimes just knowing that this is a normal response is helpful to the patient. Epoetin alfa (*Epogen*, *Procrit*) or darbepoetin (*Aranesp*) (see Chapter 49) is often used to stimulate RBC production. These drugs act like endogenous erythropoietin to directly stimulate the cells in the bone marrow to make RBCs. Caution must be used to closely monitor the patient's hemoglobin level as levels over 10 g/dL have been associated with more rapid cancer growth and cardiac events. These drugs must be injected, and the patient's lab values must be followed closely.

Decreased Platelets

Platelet aggregation is the first step in preventing blood loss when a blood vessel is injured (see Chapter 48). When platelet levels are low, the patient is at increased risk of blood loss. Patients should be alert for increased bruising, bleeding while brushing their teeth, or increased bleeding with any injury. Protection is the best approach for these patients. Using a soft bristled toothbrush, using an electric razor, and avoiding sports or activities that could lead to injury are key teaching points.

Decreased White Blood Cells

The neutrophils are the first WBCs stimulated with any injury or infection. They are phagocytes that are called to an injured area to remove damage and prevent further injury. A patient with low WBC counts is at high risk for infection and even cancer development. Protection is a key teaching point for these patients: They should be advised to avoid crowded areas, sick friends or hospitals, people who are known to be ill, activities that could cause injury, and digging in dirt without protective gloves (many pathogens live in the soil). Drugs called colony-stimulating agents may be used to stimulate WBC production when it falls dangerously low. Filgrastim (*Neupogen*), which comes in prefilled syringes for patients to use at home; pegfilgrastim (*Neulasta*); and tbo-filgrastim (*Granix*) (see Chapter 17) are administered by subcutaneous injection, with the patient's blood counts followed closely to determine dosing and duration of treatment.

BOX 14.7

Antiemetics and Cancer Chemotherapy

Antineoplastic drugs can directly stimulate the chemoreceptor trigger zone (CTZ) in the medulla to induce nausea and vomiting. These drugs also cause cell death, which releases many toxins into the system, which in turn stimulate the CTZ. Because patients expect nausea and vomiting with the administration of antineoplastic agents, the higher cortical centers of the brain can stimulate the CTZ to induce vomiting just at the thought of the chemotherapy.

A variety of antiemetic agents have been used in the course of antineoplastic therapy. Sometimes a combination of drugs is most helpful. It should also be remembered that an accepting environment, plenty of comfort measures (e.g., environmental control, mouth care, ice chips), and support for the patient can help to decrease the discomfort associated with the emetic effects of these drugs. Antihistamines to decrease secretions and corticosteroids to relieve inflammation are useful as adjunctive therapies.

Drugs that are known to help in treating antineoplastic chemotherapy–induced nausea and vomiting include the following:

- Dronabinol (*Marinol*) and nabilone (*Cesamet*) are synthetic derivatives of delta-9-tetrahydrocannabinol, the active ingredient in marijuana; this is not usually a first-line drug because of associated CNS effects.
- Ondansetron (*Zofran*), granisetron (*Kytril*), and palonosetron (*Aloxi*) block serotonin receptors in the CTZ and are among the most effective antiemetics, especially if combined with a corticosteroid such as dexamethasone. A combination oral product with netupitant (a human substance P/neurokinin receptor blocker) and palonosetron (*Akynzeo*) is available for added effects.
- Aprepitant (*Emend*) blocks human substance P/neurokinin 1 receptors in the CNS, blocking the nausea and vomiting caused by severely emetogenic antineoplastic drugs without effects on dopamine, serotonin, or norepinephrine.
- Two benzodiazepines—alprazolam (*Xanax*) and lorazepam (*Ativan*)—seem to be effective in directly blocking the CTZ to relieve nausea and vomiting caused by cancer chemotherapy; they are especially effective when combined with a corticosteroid.
- Haloperidol (*Haldol*) is a dopaminergic blocker that also is believed to have direct CTZ effects.
- Metoclopramide (*Reglan*) calms the activity of the GI tract; it is especially effective if combined with a corticosteroid, an antihistamine, and a centrally acting blocker such as haloperidol or lorazepam.
- Prochlorperazine (generic) is a phenothiazine that has been found to have strong antiemetic action in the CNS; it can be given by a variety of routes.

Nausea and vomiting are unavoidable aspects of many chemotherapeutic regimens. However, treating the patient as the chemotherapy begins, using combination regimens, and providing plenty of supportive and comforting nursing care can help to alleviate some of the distress associated with these adverse effects.

Key Points

- Alkylating agents affect cellular RNA, DNA, or other cellular proteins. They are cell cycle phase nonspecific but are especially toxic to rapidly growing cells.
- Patients receiving alkylating agents may experience alopecia, nausea, and vomiting and need to be monitored for bone marrow suppression and CNS toxicity.

Antimetabolites

Antimetabolites (see Table 14.2) are drugs that have chemical structures similar to those of various natural metabolites that are necessary for the growth and division of rapidly growing neoplastic cells and normal cells. Antimetabolites include capecitabine (*Xeloda*), cladribine (generic), clofarabine (*Clolar*), cytarabine (*DepoCyt, Tarabine PFS*), dacarbazine (generic), floxuridine (generic), fludarabine (generic), fluorouracil (*Carac, Efudex, Fluoroplex*), gemcitabine (*Gemzar*), hydroxyurea (*Droxia, Hydrea, Siklos*), mercaptopurine (*Purixan*), methotrexate (*Rheumatrex, Trexall*), pemetrexed (*Alimta*), pentostatin (*Nipent*), pralatrexate (*Folotyn*), and thioguanine (generic).

Therapeutic Actions and Indications

Antimetabolites inhibit DNA production in cells that depend on certain natural metabolites to produce their DNA. They replace these needed metabolites and thereby prevent normal cellular function. Many of these agents inhibit thymidylate synthetase, DNA polymerase, or folic acid reductase, all of which are needed for DNA synthesis. They are considered to be S phase specific in the cell cycle (see Fig. 14.5). They are most effective in rapidly dividing cells, preventing cell replication, and leading to cell death. The antimetabolites are indicated for the treatment of various leukemias and some GI and basal cell cancers (see Table 14.2 for usual indications for each agent). Use of these

Table 14.2 *Drugs in Focus:* Antimetabolites

Drug Name	Dosage/Route	Usual Indications
capecitabine (*Xeloda*)	2,500 mg/m²/d PO in two divided doses for 2 wk, then 1 wk of rest, for 3 cycles	Treatment of metastatic breast cancer with resistance to paclitaxel or anthracyclines; treatment of metastatic colorectal cancer as first-line therapy treatment of breast cancer with docetaxel in patients with metastatic disease; postsurgery Dukes C colon cancer *Special considerations:* Severe diarrhea can occur—monitor hydration and nutrition; monitor for bone marrow suppression; risk of severe to fatal bleeding if combined with warfarin
cladribine (generic)	0.09–0.1 mg/kg/d IV for 7 consecutive days	Treatment of active hairy cell leukemia *Special considerations:* Severe bone marrow depression can occur—monitor patient closely and reduce dose as needed; fever is common, especially early in treatment
clofarabine (*Clolar*)	52 mg/m² by IV infusion over 2 h daily for 5 d; repeat every 2–6 wk, based on baseline function	Treatment of patients 1–21 y of age with ALL after at least two relapses on other regimens *Special considerations:* GI toxicity, bone marrow suppression, and infection are common
cytarabine (*Tarabine PFS*)	*Induction:* 100 mg/m²/d by continuous IV infusion days 1–7 *Meningeal leukemia*: 5–75 mg/m²/d for 3 d; intrathecal use, 50 mg every 14 d for 3 doses	Treatment of meningeal and myelocytic leukemias; used in combination with other agents; lymphomatous meningitis *Special considerations:* GI toxicity and cytarabine syndrome (fever, myalgia, bone pain, chest pain, rash, conjunctivitis, and malaise) are common—this syndrome sometimes responds to corticosteroids; alopecia may occur; monitor for bone marrow suppression
dacarbazine (generic)	*Adult and pediatric:* 2–4.5 mg/kg/d IV for 10 d, repeat at 4-wk intervals, or 250 mg/m²/d IV for 5 d in combination with other drugs	Treatment of metastatic malignant melanoma and as second-line therapy with other drugs for the treatment of Hodgkin disease *Special considerations:* Bone marrow depression, GI toxicity, severe photosensitivity are common; extravasation can cause tissue necrosis or cellulitis—use extreme care, and monitor injection sites regularly
floxuridine (generic)	0.1–0.6 mg/kg/d via intra-arterial line	Palliative management of GI adenocarcinoma metastatic to the liver in patients who are not candidates for surgery *Special considerations:* Administer by intra-arterial line only; bone marrow suppression, GI toxicity, neurotoxicity, and alopecia are common
fludarabine (generic)	40 mg/m² PO or 25 mg/m²/d IV over 30 min for 5 d; repeat every 28 d	Treatment of CLL; unresponsive B-cell CLL with no progress with at least one other treatment *Special considerations:* CNS toxicity can be severe; GI toxicity, respiratory complications, renal failure, and tumor lysis syndrome are common

(continues on page 228)

Table 14.2 *Drugs in Focus:* Antimetabolites *(Continued)*

Drug Name	Dosage/Route	Usual Indications
fluorouracil (*Carac, Efudex, Fluoroplex*)	12 mg/kg/d IV on days 1–4, then 6 mg/kg IV on days 6, 8, 10, and 12; topical treatment, apply twice daily to cover lesions	Palliative treatment of various GI cancers, breast cancer, pancreatic cancer; topical treatment of basal cell carcinoma and actinic and solar keratoses *Special considerations:* GI toxicity, bone marrow suppression, alopecia, and skin rash are common; avoid occlusive dressings with topical forms; wash hands thoroughly after contact with drug
gemcitabine (*Gemzar*)	1,000–1,250 mg/m² IV over 30 min once a week; timing based on other therapies and patient response	Treatment of locally advanced or metastatic adenocarcinoma of the pancreas; given with cisplatin for the treatment of inoperable non–small cell lung cancer; metastatic breast cancer, ovarian cancer after failure of a platinum-based therapy *Special considerations:* Can cause severe bone marrow depression, GI toxicity, pain, alopecia, and interstitial pneumonitis
hydroxyurea (*Droxia, Hydrea, Siklos*)	Dosing individualized based on tumor type, disease state, response to treatment, patient risk factors, and clinical practice standards *Sickle cell*: 15–35 mg/kg/d PO	Treatment of melanoma, ovarian cancer, CML; in combination therapy for primary squamous cell cancers of the head and neck; also used in the treatment of sickle cell anemia to reduce painful crises and need for blood transfusions *Special considerations:* Reduce dose for renal impairment. Can cause bone marrow depression, headache, rash, GI toxicity, and renal dysfunction
mercaptopurine (*Purixan*)	1.5–2.5 mg/kg/d PO for 4 wk; then reevaluate	Remission induction and maintenance therapy in acute leukemias *Special considerations:* Bone marrow toxicity and GI toxicity are common; hyperuricemia is a true concern—ensure that the patient is well hydrated during therapy
methotrexate (*Rheumatrex, Trexall*)	Dose varies with route and disease being treated; commonly 15–30 mg PO or IM	Treatment of gestational choriocarcinoma; chorioadenoma destruens; hydatidiform, meningeal leukemia; breast cancer, head and neck cancers, some lymphomas, and lung cancers, symptomatic control of severe psoriasis; rheumatoid arthritis; juvenile rheumatoid arthritis *Special considerations:* Hypersensitivity reactions can be severe; liver toxicity and GI complications are common; monitor for bone marrow suppression and increased susceptibility to infections; dose pack is available for the oral treatment of psoriasis and rheumatoid arthritis
pemetrexed (*Alimta*)	500 mg/m² IV over 10 min on day 1 with 75 mg/m² cisplatin IV over 2 h; repeat cycle every 21 d	Treatment of malignant mesothelioma in patients whose disease is unresectable or who are not candidates for surgery; locally advanced or metastatic non–small cell lung cancer as a single agent after other chemotherapy *Special considerations:* Pretreat with corticosteroids, folic acid, and vitamin B_{12}; monitor for bone marrow suppression and GI effects
pentostatin (*Nipent*)	4 mg/m² IV every other week	Hairy cell leukemia in adults if refractory to interferon-alpha therapy *Special considerations:* Associated with severe renal, hepatic, CNS, and pulmonary toxicities—monitor patient closely and reduce dose accordingly; 3–6 mo of interferon-alpha therapy should be tried before using pentostatin
pralatrexate (*Folotyn*)	30 mg/m² IV push over 2–5 min once weekly for 6 wk in a 7-wk cycle	Treatment of relapsed or refractory peripheral T-cell lymphoma *Special considerations:* Bone marrow suppression common; severe mucositis can occur—patient should receive vitamin B_{12} 1 mg IM every 8–10 wk and folic acid 1–1.25 mg/d PO
thioguanine (generic)	*Adult and pediatric (>3 y):* 2 mg/kg/d PO for 4 wk; may increase dose if tolerated well	Remission induction and maintenance of acute leukemias alone or as part of combination therapy *Special considerations:* Bone marrow suppression, GI toxicity, miscarriage, and birth defects have been reported; monitor bone marrow status to determine dose and redosing; ensure that the patient is well hydrated during therapy to minimize hyperuricemia—patient may respond to allopurinol and urine alkalinization

ALL, acute lymphocytic leukemia; CLL, chronic lymphocytic leukemia.

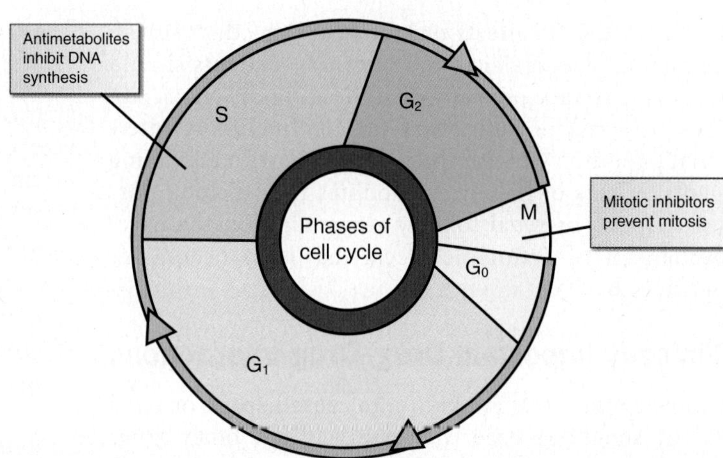

FIGURE 14.5 Sites of action of cell cycle–specific antineoplastic agents.

drugs has been somewhat limited because neoplastic cells rapidly develop resistance to these agents. For this reason, these drugs are usually administered as part of a combination therapy. Aside from the treatment of cancer, methotrexate has added indications for treatment of arthritis and is thought to slow joint degeneration and progression of rheumatoid arthritis. Some of the formulations for hydroxyurea are indicated for treatment of sickle cell anemia, with the goal of reducing sickle cell crises and the need for blood transfusions. The exact mechanism of action for providing benefit for sickle cell anemia is not entirely clear, but it could be due to increasing hemoglobin F levels in red blood cells, decreasing neutrophils, increasing deformability of sickled cells, and changing the adhesion of red blood cells to the vessel wall.

Pharmacokinetics

Methotrexate is absorbed well from the GI tract and is excreted unchanged in the urine. Patients with renal impairment may require a reduced dose and increased monitoring when taking methotrexate. Methotrexate readily crosses the blood–brain barrier. Hydroxyuria is also absorbed well from the GI tract, but over half is metabolized. Doses need to be reduced if a patient has renal impairment. Cytarabine, clofarabine, floxuridine, fluorouracil, gemcitabine, pemetrexed, and pralatrexate are not absorbed well from the GI tract and need to be administered parenterally. They are metabolized in the liver and excreted in the urine, necessitating close monitoring of patients with hepatic or renal impairment who are receiving these drugs. Mercaptopurine and thioguanine are absorbed slowly from the GI tract and are metabolized in the liver and excreted in the urine.

Contraindications and Cautions

Antimetabolites are contraindicated for use during pregnancy and lactation because of the potential for severe effects on the fetus and neonate. Caution is necessary when administering antimetabolites to any individual with a known allergy to any of them to prevent hypersensitivity reactions; with bone marrow suppression, which is often the index for redosing and dosing levels; and with renal or hepatic dysfunction, which might interfere with the metabolism or excretion of these drugs and often indicates a need to change the dose.

Adverse Effects

Adverse effects frequently encountered with the use of the antimetabolites are listed below. To counteract the effects of treatment with one antimetabolite—methotrexate—the drug leucovorin or its isomer levoleucovorin is sometimes given (Box 14.8).

Hematological effects include bone marrow suppression, with leukopenia, thrombocytopenia, anemia, and pancytopenia, secondary to the effects of the drugs on the rapidly multiplying cells of the bone marrow. Toxic GI effects include nausea, vomiting, anorexia, diarrhea, and mucous membrane deterioration, all of which are related to drug effects on the rapidly multiplying cells of

BOX 14.8

Drugs that Protect Against an Antimetabolite

Leucovorin (generic) is an active form of folic acid that is used to "rescue" normal cells from the adverse effects of methotrexate therapy in the treatment of osteosarcoma. This drug is also used to treat folic acid deficiency conditions such as sprue, nutritional deficiency, pregnancy, and lactation. Leucovorin is given orally or intravenously starting at the time of methotrexate therapy. Use of this drug has been associated with pain at the injection site.

In 2008, levoleucovorin (*Fusilev*), an isomer of leucovorin, was also approved to diminish the toxicity and counteract the effects of impaired methotrexate elimination and of inadvertent overdose of folic acid antagonists after high-dose methotrexate therapy in osteosarcoma. The drug is given IV for up to 4 days, and dose is determined by the serum methotrexate level of the patient. There are high calcium levels in the solution, and the drug needs to be given slowly.

the GI tract. CNS effects include headache, drowsiness, aphasia, fatigue, malaise, and dizziness. Patients should be advised to take precautions if these conditions occur. There is a risk of pulmonary toxicity, including interstitial pneumonitis with these drugs. As with alkylating agents, effects of the antimetabolites may include possible hepatic or renal toxicity, depending on the exact mechanism of action. Alopecia may also occur. See Figure 14.6.

Clinically Important Drug–Drug Interactions

Antimetabolites that are known to cause hepatic or renal toxicity should be used with care with any other drugs known to have the same effect. In addition, drugs that are toxic to the liver may adversely affect drugs that are metabolized in the liver or that act in the liver (e.g., oral anticoagulants). There is an increased risk of toxic effects when methotrexate is used concurrently with salicylates, other NSAIDs, and some antibiotics. Folic acid supplements decrease the action of methotrexate. If taken concurrently with medications that affect coagulation, cytarabine may reduce the absorption of digoxin, decrease the effectiveness of live vaccines, and increase bleeding risk. Check for specific drug–drug interactions for each agent in a nursing drug guide.

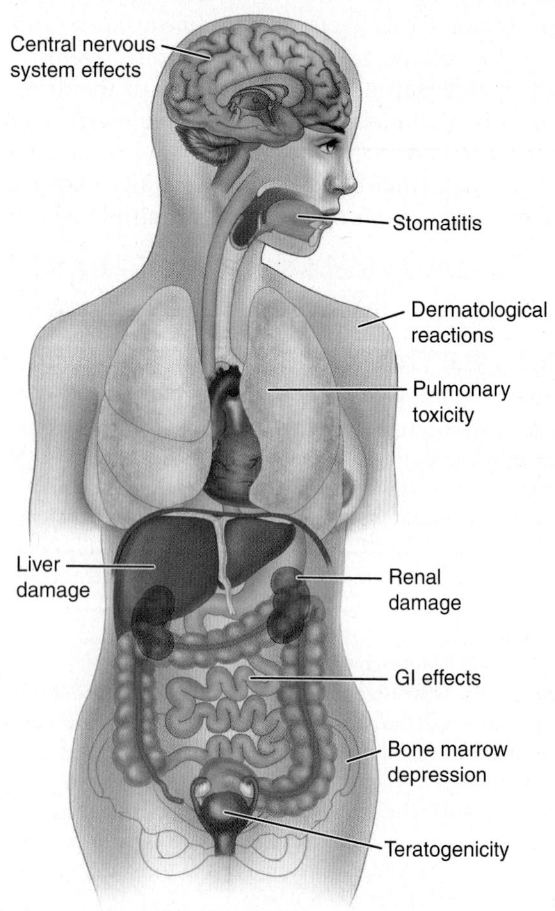

FIGURE 14.6 Common adverse effects associated with antineoplastic agents.

Prototype Summary: Methotrexate

Indications: Treatment of gestational choriocarcinoma; chorioadenoma destruens; hydatidiform, meningeal leukemia; breast cancer, head and neck cancers, some lymphomas, and lung cancers; symptomatic control of severe psoriasis; rheumatoid arthritis; juvenile rheumatoid arthritis.

Actions: Inhibits folic acid reductase, leading to inhibition of DNA synthesis and inhibition of cellular replication; affects the most rapidly dividing cells.

Pharmacokinetics:

Route	Onset	Peak
Oral	Varies	1–4 h
Intravenous	Rapid	0.5–2 h

$T_{1/2}$: 2 to 4 hours, excreted unchanged in the urine.

Adverse Effects: Fatigue, malaise, rashes, alopecia, ulcerative stomatitis, hepatic toxicity, severe bone marrow suppression, nausea, vomiting, interstitial pneumonitis, chills, fever, anaphylaxis, reproductive toxicity, hyperuricemia, renal toxicity.

Nursing Considerations for Patients Receiving Antimetabolites

Assessment: History and Examination

- Assess for contraindications and cautions: history of allergy to the specific antimetabolite, to avoid hypersensitivity reactions; bone marrow suppression, to prevent further suppression; renal or hepatic dysfunction that might interfere with drug metabolism and excretion; current status related to pregnancy or lactation, to prevent potentially serious effects to the fetus or nursing baby; and a history of GI ulcerative disease, which could be exacerbated with the use of these drugs.
- Perform a physical assessment to establish baseline data for determining the effectiveness of the drug and the occurrence of any adverse effects associated with drug therapy.
- Assess orientation and reflexes to evaluate any CNS effects; respiratory rate and adventitious sounds to monitor the disease and to evaluate for respiratory or hypersensitivity effects; pulse, rhythm, and cardiac auscultation to monitor for systemic or cardiovascular effects; and bowel sounds and mucous membrane status to monitor for GI effects.
- Monitor the results of laboratory tests, such as complete blood count with differential to identify possible bone marrow suppression and toxic drug effects. Monitor renal and liver function tests to determine the need for possible dose adjustment and toxic drug effects.

Nursing Conclusions

Nursing conclusions related to drug therapy might include the following:

- Impaired comfort related to GI, CNS, or skin effects of the drug
- Altered body image perception related to alopecia, skin effects, impaired fertility
- Malnutrition risk related to GI effects
- Infection risk due to bone marrow suppression
- Acute or chronic anxiety or fear related to diagnosis and treatment
- Knowledge deficit risk regarding drug therapy

Planning

- The patient will receive the best therapeutic effect from the drug therapy.
- The patient will have limited adverse effects to the drug therapy.
- The patient will have an understanding of the drug therapy, adverse effects to anticipate, and measures to relieve discomfort and improve safety.

Intervention With Rationale

- Arrange for blood tests to monitor bone marrow function before, periodically during, and for at least 3 weeks after therapy to arrange to discontinue the drug or reduce the dose as needed (see Box 14.5).
- Administer medication according to the scheduled protocol and in combination with other drugs as indicated to improve the effectiveness and safety of drug therapy.
- Ensure that the patient is well hydrated to decrease the risk of renal toxicity. Anticipate reduced dosing if renal impairment is present.
- Provide small, frequent meals, frequent mouth care, and dietary consultation as appropriate to maintain nutrition when GI effects are severe. Anticipate the use of antiemetics as necessary (see Box 14.4).
- Arrange for proper head coverings at extremes of temperature if alopecia occurs; a wig, scarf, or hat is important for maintaining body temperature. If alopecia is an anticipated effect of drug therapy, advise the patient to obtain a wig or head covering before the condition occurs.
- Protect the patient from exposure to infections because bone marrow suppression will limit immune/inflammatory responses.
- Provide support and encouragement to help the patient cope with the diagnosis and the effects of drug therapy.
- Provide the following patient teaching:
  - Follow the appropriate dosage regimen, including dates to return for further doses. Patients need to be reminded to report all other drugs and alternative therapies that they might be using.
  - Maintain nutrition if GI effects are severe.
  - Cover the head at extremes of temperature if alopecia is anticipated.
  - Plan for appropriate rest periods because fatigue and weakness are common effects of the drugs.
  - Avoid situations that might lead to infection, including crowded places, sick people, and working in soil.
  - Use safety measures such as not driving or using dangerous equipment, due to possible dizziness, headache, and drowsiness.
  - Think about consulting with a health care provider, if appropriate, due to the possibility of impaired fertility.
  - Use barrier contraceptives to reduce the risk of pregnancy during therapy.

Evaluation

- Monitor patient response to the drug (alleviation of cancer being treated, palliation of signs and symptoms of cancer, palliation of rheumatoid arthritis or psoriasis).
- Monitor for adverse effects (bone marrow suppression, GI toxicity, neurotoxicity, alopecia, renal or hepatic dysfunction).
- Evaluate the effectiveness of the teaching plan (patient can name the drug, dosage, possible adverse effects to watch for, and specific measures to help avoid adverse effects).
- Monitor the effectiveness of comfort and safety measures and compliance with the regimen.

Key Points

- Antimetabolites inhibit DNA production by inhibiting metabolites needed for the synthesis of DNA in susceptible cells.
- Antimetabolites are S phase cell cycle specific and are used for a wide variety of types of cancers.
- Bone marrow suppression, alopecia, renal/hepatic impairment, and toxic GI effects are adverse effects of antimetabolites. They are known to have teratogenic effects on fetal development.

Antineoplastic Antibiotics

Antineoplastic antibiotics (see Table 14.3), although selective for bacterial cells, are also toxic to human cells. Because these drugs tend to be more toxic to cells that are multiplying rapidly, they are more useful in the treatment of certain cancers. Antineoplastic antibiotics include bleomycin (generic), dactinomycin (*Cosmegen*), daunorubicin (*Cerubidine*), doxorubicin (*Doxil*), epirubicin (*Ellence*), idarubicin (*Idamycin PFS*), mitomycin (generic), mitoxantrone (generic), and valrubicin (*Valstar*).

Table 14.3 *Drugs in Focus:* Antineoplastic Antibiotics

Drug Name	Dosage/Route	Usual Indications
bleomycin (generic)	0.25–0.5 units/kg IM, IV, or subcutaneous once or twice weekly *Pleural effusion:* 60 units dissolved in 50–100 mL normal sterile saline per thoracotomy tube	Palliative treatment of squamous cell carcinomas, testicular cancers, and lymphomas; used to treat malignant pleural effusion *Special considerations:* GI toxicity, severe skin reactions, and hypersensitivity reactions may occur; pulmonary fibrosis can be a serious problem—baseline and periodic chest radiographs and pulmonary function tests are necessary
dactinomycin (*Cosmegen*)	*Adult:* 1,000 mcg/m² IV on day 1 as part of combination therapy or daily for 5 d *Pediatric:* 15 mcg/kg/d IV for up to 5 d	Part of combination drug regimen in the treatment of a variety of sarcomas and carcinomas; potentiates the effects of radiation therapy *Special considerations:* Bone marrow suppression and GI toxicity, which may be severe, limiting the dose; effects may not appear for 1–2 wk; local extravasation can cause necrosis and should be treated with injectable corticosteroids, ice to the area, and restarting of the IV line in a different vein
daunorubicin (*Cerubidine*)	40 mg/m² IV, infused over 1 h; repeat every 2 wk	First-line treatment of advanced HIV infection and associated Kaposi sarcoma *Special considerations:* Complete alopecia is common; GI toxicity and bone marrow suppression may also occur; severe necrosis may occur at sites of local extravasation—immediate treatment with corticosteroids, normal saline, and ice may help; if ulcerations occur, a plastic surgeon should be called
doxorubicin (*Doxil*)	60–75 mg/m² as a single IV dose; repeat every 21 d *Liposomal form:* 30 mg/m² IV over 1 h once every 2–4 wk	Treatment of a number of leukemias and cancers; used to induce regression; available in a liposomal form for treatment of AIDS-associated Kaposi sarcoma *Special considerations:* Complete alopecia is common; GI toxicity and bone suppression may occur; severe necrosis may occur at sites of local extravasation—immediate treatment with corticosteroids, normal saline, and ice may help; if ulcerations occur, a plastic surgeon should be called; toxicity is dose related—an accurate record of each dose received is important in determining dose; severe pulmonary toxicity, cardiotoxicity, alopecia, and injection site and GI toxicity occur
epirubicin (*Ellence*)	100–120 mg/m² IV given in repeated 3- to 4-wk cycles all on day 1 or divided on days 1 and 8	Adjunctive therapy in patients with evidence of axillary node tumor involvement after resection of primary breast cancer *Special considerations:* May cause cardiotoxicity and delayed cardiomyopathy; monitor for myelosuppression and hyperuricemia; severe local cellulitis and tissue necrosis can occur with extravasation
idarubicin (*Idamycin PFS*)	12 mg/m²/d IV for 3 d with cytarabine	Combination therapy for treatment of acute myeloid leukemia in adults *Special considerations:* May cause severe bone marrow suppression, which regulates dose; associated with cardiac toxicity, which can be severe; GI toxicity and local necrosis with extravasation are also common; severe necrosis may occur at sites of local extravasation—immediate treatment with corticosteroids, normal saline, and ice may help; if ulcerations occur, a plastic surgeon should be called; it is essential to monitor heart and bone marrow function to protect the patient from potentially fatal adverse effects
mitomycin (generic)	20 mg/m² IV as a single dose at 6- to 8-wk intervals	Palliative treatment of disseminated adenocarcinoma of the stomach and pancreas with other drugs *Special considerations:* Severe pulmonary toxicity, alopecia, and injection site and GI toxicity occur
mitoxantrone (generic)	12 mg/m²/d IV for 1–3 d *Multiple sclerosis:* 12 mg/m² IV as a short infusion every 3 mo	Part of combination therapy in the treatment of adult leukemias; treatment of bone pain in advanced prostatic cancer; reduction of neurological disability and frequency of relapses in chronic, progressive, relapsing multiple sclerosis *Special considerations:* Severe bone marrow suppression may occur and limits dose; alopecia, GI toxicity, and congestive heart failure often occur; avoid direct skin contact with the drug—use gloves and goggles; monitor bone marrow activity and cardiac activity to adjust dose or discontinue drug as needed
valrubicin (*Valstar*)	800 mg intravesically once a week for 6 wk	Intravesical therapy for carcinoma in situ of the bladder if refractory to bacillus Calmette-Guérin therapy (orphan drug) *Special considerations:* Use goggles and gloves when handling; avoid contact with eyes; severe bladder spasms have occurred; use caution with history of irritable bowel syndrome; do not clamp bladder catheter in place

Therapeutic Actions and Indications

Some antineoplastic antibiotics break up DNA links, and others prevent DNA or RNA synthesis and/or repair. These medications are cell cycle phase nonspecific.

The antineoplastic antibiotics are cytotoxic and often interfere with cellular DNA synthesis by inserting themselves between base pairs in the DNA chain. This, in turn, causes a mutant DNA molecule, leading to cell death (see Fig. 14.4). See Table 14.3 for usual indications for each antineoplastic antibiotic. Like other antineoplastics, the main adverse effects of these drugs are seen in cells that multiply rapidly, such as those in the bone marrow, GI tract, and skin. The potentially serious adverse effects of antineoplastic antibiotics may limit their usefulness in patients with preexisting diseases and in those who are debilitated and, therefore, more susceptible to these effects.

Pharmacokinetics

The antineoplastic antibiotics are not absorbed well from the GI tract. They are given IV or injected into specific sites. They are metabolized in the liver and excreted in the urine at various rates. Many of them have very long half-lives (e.g., 45 hours for idarubicin, more than 5 days for mitoxantrone). Daunorubicin and doxorubicin do not cross the blood–brain barrier, but they are widely distributed in the body and are taken up by the heart, lungs, kidneys, and spleen. This can lead to toxic effects in these organs.

Contraindications and Cautions

All of these agents are contraindicated for use during pregnancy and lactation because of the potential risk to the fetus and neonate. Use caution when giving antineoplastic antibiotics to an individual with a known allergy to the antibiotic or related antibiotics, to prevent hypersensitivity reactions. Care is necessary when administering these agents to patients with the following conditions: bone marrow suppression, which is often the index for redosing and dosing levels; suppressed renal or hepatic function, which might interfere with the metabolism or excretion of these drugs and often indicates a need to change the dose; known GI ulcerations or ulcerative diseases, which may be exacerbated by the effects of these drugs; pulmonary problems with bleomycin or mitomycin; or cardiac problems with doxorubicin, idarubicin, or mitoxantrone, which are specifically toxic to these organ systems.

Adverse Effects

Adverse effects frequently encountered with the use of these antibiotics include bone marrow suppression, with leukopenia, thrombocytopenia, anemia, and pancytopenia, secondary to the effects of the drugs on the rapidly multiplying cells of the bone marrow. Toxic GI effects include nausea, vomiting, anorexia, diarrhea, and mucous membrane deterioration, all of which are related to drug effects on the rapidly multiplying cells of the GI tract. As with the alkylating agents and antimetabolites, effects of antineoplastic antibiotics may include renal or hepatic toxicity, depending on the exact mechanism of action. Alopecia may also occur. Specific antineoplastic antibiotics are toxic to the heart and lungs. Dexrazoxane (*Totect*, *Zinecard*) is approved for reducing cardiomyopathy associated with doxorubicin in patients being treated for breast cancer (see Box 14.3). *Totect* is also approved for the treatment of extravasation resulting from IV antineoplastic antibiotic chemotherapy.

Clinically Important Drug–Drug Interactions

Antimetabolites that are known to cause hepatic or renal toxicity should be used with care with any other drugs known to have the same effect. Drugs that result in toxicity to the heart or lungs should be used with caution with any other drugs that produce that particular toxicity. ACE inhibitors with doxorubicin may be cardioprotective, but calcium channel blockers may increase cardiotoxicity. There is a higher risk of doxorubicin toxicity with phenobarbital or paclitaxel. Concurrent use of doxorubicin and live vaccines increase risk of adverse reactions and decreased antibody response. Check for specific drug–drug interactions for each agent in a nursing drug guide.

Prototype Summary: Doxorubicin

Indications: To produce regression in acute lymphoblastic lymphoma, acute myeloblastic leukemia, Wilms' tumor, neuroblastoma, soft tissue and bone sarcoma, breast carcinoma, ovarian carcinoma, thyroid carcinoma, Hodgkin and non-Hodgkin lymphomas, bronchogenic carcinoma; also to treat AIDS-related Kaposi sarcoma.

Actions: Binds to DNA and inhibits DNA synthesis in susceptible cells, causing cell death. Liposomal doxorubicin has increased uptake to cancer cells.

Pharmacokinetics:

Route	Onset	Peak	Duration
IV	Rapid	2 h	24–36 h

$T_{1/2}$: 12 minutes, then 3.3 hours, then 29.6 hours; metabolized in the liver and excreted in the bile, feces, and urine.

Adverse Effects: Cardiac toxicity, complete but reversible alopecia, nausea, vomiting, mucositis, red urine, myelosuppression, fever, chills, rash.

Nursing Considerations for Patients Receiving Antineoplastic Antibiotics

Assessment: History and Examination

- Assess for contraindications and cautions: history of allergy to the antibiotic in use, to avoid hypersensitivity reactions; bone marrow suppression to prevent further suppression; renal or hepatic dysfunction that might interfere with drug metabolism and excretion; respiratory or cardiac disease that could be further aggravated by the toxic effects of these drugs; current status related to pregnancy or lactation to prevent potentially serious adverse effects to the fetus or nursing baby; and GI ulcerative disease, which could be exacerbated by these drugs.
- Perform a physical assessment to establish baseline data for determining the effectiveness of the drug and the occurrence of any adverse effects associated with drug therapy.
- Assess orientation and reflexes to evaluate any CNS effects; respiratory rate and adventitious sounds to monitor the disease and evaluate for respiratory or hypersensitivity effects; pulse, rhythm, cardiac auscultation, and baseline electrocardiogram to monitor for systemic or cardiovascular effects; and bowel sounds and mucous membrane status to monitor for GI effects.
- Monitor the results of laboratory tests, such as complete blood count with differential to identify possible bone marrow suppression and toxic drug effects. Monitor renal and liver function tests, to determine the need for possible dose adjustment.

Nursing Conclusions

Nursing conclusions related to drug therapy might include the following:

- Impaired comfort related to GI, CNS, or local effects of the drug
- Altered body image perception related to alopecia or skin effects
- Malnutrition risk due to GI side effects.
- Infection risk due to bone marrow suppression.
- Acute or chronic anxiety or fear related to diagnosis and treatment
- Knowledge deficit risk regarding drug therapy

Planning

- The patient will receive the best therapeutic effect from the drug therapy.
- The patient will have limited adverse effects to the drug therapy.
- The patient will have an understanding of the drug therapy, adverse effects to anticipate, and measures to relieve discomfort and improve safety.

Intervention With Rationale

- Arrange for blood tests to monitor bone marrow function before, periodically during, and for at least 3 weeks after therapy to arrange to discontinue the drug or reduce the dose as needed (see Box 14.5).
- Monitor cardiac and respiratory function, as well as clotting times as appropriate for the drug being used, to arrange to discontinue the drug or reduce the dose as needed.
- Protect the patient from exposure to infection because bone marrow suppression will decrease immune/inflammatory reactions.
- Administer medication according to scheduled protocol and in combination with other drugs as indicated to improve the effectiveness of drug therapy.
- Ensure that the patient is well hydrated to decrease the risk of renal toxicity.
- Provide small, frequent meals, frequent mouth care, and dietary consultation as appropriate to maintain nutrition when GI effects are severe. Anticipate the need for antiemetics as necessary (see Box 14.4).
- Arrange for proper head coverings at extremes of temperature if alopecia occurs; a wig, scarf, or hat is important for maintaining body temperature. If alopecia is an anticipated effect of drug therapy, advise the patient to obtain a wig or head covering before the condition occurs to promote self-esteem and a positive body image.
- Provide the following patient teaching:
  - Follow the appropriate dosage regimen, including dates to return for further doses.
  - Maintain nutrition if GI effects are severe.
  - Cover the head at extremes of temperature if alopecia is anticipated.
  - Plan for appropriate rest periods because fatigue and weakness are common effects of the drugs.
  - Avoid exposure to possible infection, including avoiding crowded places, sick people, and working in soil.
  - Use safety measures such as avoiding driving or using dangerous equipment to prevent injury due to possible dizziness, headache, and drowsiness.
  - Consult with a health care provider, if appropriate, regarding possibility of impaired fertility.
  - Use barrier contraceptives to reduce the risk of pregnancy during therapy.

Evaluation

- Monitor patient response to the drug (alleviation of cancer being treated and palliation of signs and symptoms of cancer).
- Monitor for adverse effects (bone marrow suppression, GI toxicity, neurotoxicity, alopecia, renal or hepatic dysfunction, and cardiac or respiratory dysfunction).
- Evaluate the effectiveness of the teaching plan (patient can name the drug, dosage, possible adverse effects to watch for, and specific measures to help avoid adverse effects).

Key Points

- Antineoplastic antibiotics are toxic to rapidly dividing cells, are nonspecific to a cell cycle phase, and break DNA strands and/or inhibit DNA synthesis.
- Bone marrow suppression, alopecia, reproductive toxicity, and toxic GI effects are common adverse effects of antineoplastic antibiotics.
- Doxorubicin has been known to cause cardiotoxicity in addition to nonharmful red coloration of urine and sweat.

Mitotic Inhibitors

Mitotic inhibitors (see Table 14.4) are drugs that kill cells as the process of mitosis begins (see Fig. 14.5). These cell cycle–specific agents inhibit DNA synthesis. Like other antineoplastics, the main adverse effects of the mitotic inhibitors occur with cells that rapidly multiply: those in the bone marrow, GI tract, and skin. Mitotic inhibitors include cabazitaxel (*Jevtana*), docetaxel (*Taxotere*), eribulin (*Halaven*), etoposide (generic), ixabepilone (*Ixempra*), paclitaxel (*Abraxane*), vinblastine (generic), vincristine (*Marqibo*), and vinorelbine (*Navelbine*).

Table 14.4 ***Drugs in Focus:*** **Mitotic Inhibitors**

Drug Name	Dosage/Route	Usual Indications
cabazitaxel (*Jevtana*)	25 mg/m² IV as a 1-h infusion every 3 wk	In combination with oral prednisone for the treatment of patients with hormone refractory metastatic prostate cancer previously treated with a docetaxel-containing regimen *Special considerations:* Serious to life-threatening hypersensitivity reactions have occurred; serious to life-threatening neutropenia can occur; monitor neutrophil count and withhold drug as needed; patient may experience GI disturbances or renal or hepatic failure; older adults are more susceptible to adverse effects—monitor accordingly
docetaxel (*Taxotere*)	60–100 mg/m² IV over 1 h every 3 wk	Treatment of breast cancer and non–small cell lung cancer; androgen-dependent prostate cancer; gastric adenocarcinoma *Special considerations:* Monitor patient closely—deaths have occurred during use; severe fluid retention can occur—premedicate with corticosteroids and monitor for weight gain; skin rash and nail disorders are usually reversible; monitor patients and bone marrow function closely during use
eribulin (*Halaven*)	1.4 mg/m² IV over 2–5 min on days 1 and 8 of 21-d course	Treatment of metastatic breast cancer in patients with at least two previous chemotherapy regimens *Special considerations:* Risk of prolonged QT interval—monitor ECG; risk of bone marrow suppression; peripheral neuropathy; alopecia may occur
etoposide (generic)	35–100 mg/m²/d IV for 4–5 d	Treatment of testicular cancers refractory to other agents; non–small cell lung carcinomas *Special considerations:* Fatigue, GI toxicity, bone marrow depression, and alopecia are common side effects; avoid direct skin contact with the drug; use protective clothing and goggles; monitor bone marrow function to adjust dose; rapid fall in blood pressure can occur during IV infusion—monitor patient carefully
ixabepilone (*Ixempra*)	40 mg/m² IV over 3 h every 3 wk	In combination with capecitabine for the treatment of patients with metastatic or locally advanced breast cancer *Special considerations:* Peripheral neuropathies are common; monitor for bone marrow suppression and hepatic impairment; dose will need to be adjusted based on these tests
nelarabine (*Arranon*)	*Adult:* 1, 500 mg/m² IV over 2 h on days 1, 3, and 5 of a 21-d cycle *Pediatric:* 650 mg/m² IV over 1 h for 5 consecutive days every 21 d	Treatment of T-cell acute lymphoblastic leukemia and T-cell lymphoblastic lymphoma that has relapsed after at least two other chemotherapies *Special considerations:* Severe neurological events have been reported, many not reversible; closely monitor patient and stop drug at any sign of neurologic events; adjust dose based on bone marrow suppression; take measures to prevent hyperuricemia
paclitaxel (*Abraxane, Taxol*)	*Breast cancer:* 260 mg/m²/d IV over 3 h every 3 wk *Non–small cell lung cancer:* 100 mg/m² IV over 30 min on days 1, 8, and 15 of a 21-d cycle	Treatment of metastatic breast cancer, non–small cell lung cancer, and AIDS-related Kaposi sarcoma *Special considerations:* Anaphylaxis and severe hypersensitivity reactions have occurred—monitor very closely during administration; monitor for bone marrow suppression; cardiovascular toxicity and neuropathies have occurred

(continues on page 236)

Table 14.4 *Drugs in Focus:* Mitotic Inhibitors *(Continued)*

Drug Name	Dosage/Route	Usual Indications
vinblastine (generic)	*Adult:* 3.7 mg/m² IV once weekly *Pediatric:* 2.5 mg/m² IV once weekly; dose may then be increased based on leukocyte count and patient response	Palliative treatment of various lymphomas and sarcomas; advanced Hodgkin disease; alone or as part of combination therapy for the treatment of advanced testicular germ cell cancers *Special considerations:* GI toxicity, CNS effects, and total loss of hair are common; antiemetics may help; avoid contact with drug; monitor injection sites for reactions
vincristine (*Marqibo*)	*Adult:* 1.4 mg/m² IV every 7 days *Pediatric:* 1.5–2 mg/m² IV once weekly *Relapsed ALL:* 2.25 mg/m² IV over 1 h for 7 d (*Marqibo only*)	Treatment of acute leukemia, various lymphomas, and sarcomas; treatment of adults with Philadelphia chromosome–negative acute ALL who have relapsed (*Marqibo* only) *Special considerations:* Extensive CNS effects are common; GI toxicity, local irritation at injection IV site, and hair loss commonly occur; syndrome of inappropriate secretion of antidiuretic hormone has been reported—monitor urine output and arrange for fluid restriction and diuretics as needed
vinorelbine (*Navelbine*)	30 mg/m² IV once weekly, based on granulocyte count	First-line treatment of unresectable advanced non–small cell lung cancer, stage IV non–small cell lung cancer, and stage III non–small cell lung cancer with cisplatin *Special considerations:* GI and CNS toxicity are common; total loss of hair, local reaction at injection site, and bone marrow depression also occur; prepare a calendar with return dates for the series of injections; avoid extravasation but arrange for hyaluronidase infusion if it occurs; antiemetics may be helpful if reaction is severe

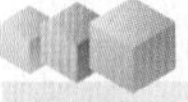
Concept Mastery Alert

Route of Administration

The drug cabazitaxel (prescribed for the treatment of prostate cancer) is given via IV, not PO.

Therapeutic Actions and Indications

The mitotic inhibitors interfere with the ability of a cell to divide; they block or alter DNA synthesis, thus causing cell death. They work in the M phase of the cell cycle. These drugs are used for the treatment of a variety of tumors and leukemias. See Table 14.4 for usual indications for each of these agents.

Pharmacokinetics

Generally, these drugs are given intravenously because they are not well absorbed from the GI tract. They are metabolized in the liver and excreted primarily in the feces, making them safer for use in patients with renal impairment than the antineoplastics that are cleared through the kidney.

Contraindications and Cautions

These drugs should not be used during pregnancy or lactation because of the potential risk to the fetus or neonate. Use caution when giving these drugs to anyone with a known allergy to the drug or related drugs to decrease the risk of serious hypersensitivity reactions. Care is necessary for patients with the following conditions: bone marrow suppression (with some medications), which is often the index for redosing and dosing levels; renal or hepatic dysfunction, which could interfere with the metabolism or excretion of these drugs and often indicates a need to change the dose; known GI ulcerations or ulcerative diseases, which may be exacerbated by the effects of these drugs; and prolonged QT interval when using eribulin, which may prolong the QT interval leading to potentially serious arrhythmias.

Adverse Effects

Adverse effects frequently encountered with the use of mitotic inhibitors include bone marrow suppression (with some medications), with leukopenia, thrombocytopenia, anemia, and pancytopenia, secondary to the effects of the drugs on the rapidly multiplying cells of the bone marrow. GI effects include nausea, vomiting, anorexia, diarrhea, and mucous membrane deterioration. Eribulin is associated with prolonged QT intervals. Vincristine and paclitaxel have been associated with nerve injury, causing changes in bowel and urinary function, as well as peripheral neuropathy. As with the other antineoplastic agents, effects of the mitotic inhibitors may include possible hepatic or renal toxicity, depending on the exact mechanism of action. Alopecia is often a side effect. These drugs also cause necrosis and cellulitis if extravasation occurs, so it is necessary to regularly monitor injection sites and take appropriate action as needed (Box 14.9).

Clinically Important Drug–Drug Interactions

Mitotic inhibitors that are known to be toxic to the liver or the CNS should be used with care with any other drugs

Box 14.9 Focus on Safe Medication Administration

PREVENTING AND TREATING EXTRAVASATION

When an IV antineoplastic drug extravasates, or infiltrates into the surrounding tissue, serious tissue damage can occur. These drugs are toxic to cells, and the resulting tissue injury can result in severe pain, scarring, nerve and muscle damage, infection, and in very severe cases even amputation of the limb.

Prevention is the best way to deal with extravasation. Interventions that can help to prevent extravasation include the following: Use a distal vein, and avoid small veins on the wrist or digits; never use an existing line unless it is clearly open and running well; start the infusion with plain 5% dextrose in water (D5W) and monitor for any sign of extravasation; check the site frequently, and ask the patient to report any discomfort in the area; and, if at all possible, do not use an infusion pump to administer one of these drugs because it will continue to deliver the drug under pressure and can cause severe extravasation.

If extravasation occurs, there are specific antidotes to use with some antineoplastic drugs. Hyaluronidase and sodium thiosulfate are two examples of antidotes. The antidote is usually administered through the IV line to allow it to infiltrate the same tissue, but if the line has been pulled, a tuberculin syringe can be used to inject the antidote subcutaneously into the tissue surrounding the infiltrated area.

known to have the same adverse effect. Avoid concurrent use with live virus vaccines due to an increased risk of adverse reactions and decreased antibody response. Check specific drug–drug interactions for each agent in a nursing drug guide.

Prototype Summary: Vincristine

Indications: Acute leukemia, Hodgkin disease, non-Hodgkin lymphoma, rhabdomyosarcoma, neuroblastoma, Wilms' tumor.

Actions: Arrests mitotic division at the stage of metaphase; the exact mechanism of action is not understood.

Pharmacokinetics:

Route	Onset	Peak
IV	Varies	15–30 min

$T_{1/2}$: 5 minutes, then 2.3 hours, then 85 hours; metabolized in the liver and excreted in the feces and urine.

Adverse Effects: Ataxia, cranial nerve manifestations, neuritic pain, muscle wasting, constipation, leukopenia, weight loss, loss of hair, death. Severe tissue damage if extravasation occurs.

Nursing Considerations for Patients Receiving Mitotic Inhibitors

Assessment: History and Examination

- Assess for contraindications or cautions: history of allergy to the drug used (or related drugs) to avoid hypersensitivity reactions; bone marrow suppression to prevent further suppression; renal or hepatic dysfunction that might interfere with drug metabolism and excretion; current status of pregnancy or lactation to prevent potentially serious adverse effects on the fetus or nursing baby; GI ulcerative disease, which could be exacerbated by these drugs; and QT prolongation with eribulin, which could further prolong QT intervals.
- Perform a physical assessment to establish baseline data for determining the effectiveness of the drug and the occurrence of any adverse effects associated with drug therapy.
- Assess orientation and reflexes to evaluate any CNS effects; skin to evaluate for lesions; hair and hair distribution to monitor for adverse effects; respiratory rate and adventitious sounds to monitor the disease and to evaluate for respiratory or hypersensitivity effects; bowel sounds and mucous membrane status to monitor for GI effects; and baseline ECG with eribulin to monitor QT interval.
- Monitor the results of laboratory tests, such as complete blood count with differential to identify possible bone marrow suppression and toxic drug effects. Monitor renal and liver function tests to determine the need for possible dose adjustment as needed and to evaluate toxic drug effects.
- Regularly inspect IV insertion sites for signs of extravasation or inflammation, which need to be treated quickly.

Nursing Conclusions

Nursing conclusions related to drug therapy might include the following:

- Impaired comfort related to GI, CNS, or local effects of the drug
- Altered body image perception risk related to alopecia, skin effects
- Injury risk based on CNS effects
- Acute or chronic anxiety/fear related to diagnosis and treatment
- Knowledge deficit risk regarding drug therapy

Planning

- The patient will receive the best therapeutic effect from the drug therapy.
- The patient will have limited adverse effects to the drug therapy.
- The patient will have an understanding of the drug therapy, adverse effects to anticipate, and measures to relieve discomfort and improve safety.

(continues on page 238)

Intervention With Rationale

- Arrange for blood tests to monitor bone marrow function before, periodically during, and for at least 3 weeks after therapy to arrange to discontinue the drug or reduce the dose as needed (see Box 14.5). Arrange for baseline and periodic ECG if using eribulin to monitor the QT interval, which could become prolonged.
- Avoid direct skin or eye contact with the drug. Wear protective clothing and goggles while preparing and administering the drug to prevent toxic reaction to the drug.
- Administer medication according to scheduled protocol and in combination with other drugs as indicated to improve the effectiveness of drug therapy.
- Ensure that the patient is well hydrated to decrease the risk of renal toxicity.
- Monitor injection sites to arrange appropriate treatment for extravasation, local inflammation, or cellulitis.
- Protect the patient from exposure to infection because bone marrow suppression will decrease immune/inflammatory responses.
- Provide small, frequent meals, frequent mouth care, and dietary consultation as appropriate to maintain nutrition if GI effects are severe. Anticipate the need for antiemetics as necessary (see Box 14.4).
- Arrange for proper head coverings at extremes of temperature if alopecia or epilation occurs; a wig, scarf, or hat is important for maintaining body temperature. If alopecia is an anticipated effect of drug therapy, advise the patient to obtain a wig or head covering before the condition occurs to promote self-esteem and a positive body image.
- Provide the following patient teaching:
  - Follow the appropriate dosage regimen, including dates to return for further doses.
  - Maintain nutrition if GI effects are severe.
  - Cover the head at extremes of temperature if alopecia is anticipated.
  - Plan for appropriate rest periods because fatigue and weakness are common effects of the drugs.
  - Avoid situations that might lead to infection, including crowded areas, sick people, and working in soil.
  - Use safety measures such as avoiding driving or using dangerous equipment, due to possible dizziness, headache, decreased reflexes, weakness, paresthesia, and sensory loss and drowsiness.
  - Consult with a health care provider, as appropriate, related to the possibility of impaired fertility.
  - Use barrier contraceptives to reduce the risk of pregnancy during therapy.

Evaluation

- Monitor patient response to the drug (alleviation of cancer being treated and palliation of signs and symptoms of cancer).
- Monitor for adverse effects (bone marrow suppression, GI toxicity, neurotoxicity, alopecia, renal or hepatic dysfunction, prolonged QT interval, and local reactions at the injection site).
- Evaluate the effectiveness of the teaching plan (patient can name the drug, dosage, possible adverse effects to watch for, and specific measures to help avoid adverse effects).

Key Points

- Mitotic inhibitors kill cells during the M phase and are used to treat a variety of cancers.
- These drugs are usually given intravenously. Extravasation could be a serious problem.
- Bone marrow suppression, alopecia, neurotoxicity, and toxic GI effects are common adverse effects of mitotic inhibitors.

Hormones and Hormone Modulators

Some cancers, particularly those involving the breast tissue, ovaries, uterus, prostate, and testes, are sensitive to estrogen stimulation. Estrogen receptor sites on the tumor react with circulating estrogen, and this reaction stimulates the tumor cells to grow and divide. Several antineoplastic agents are used to block or interfere with these receptor sites to prevent cancer growth, and in some situations, to cause cell death. Some hormones are used to block the release of gonadotropic hormones, which can cause some types of tumors to grow in the prostate or breast tissue. Others may block androgen receptor sites directly and are useful in the treatment of advanced prostate cancers. Hormones and hormone modulators include abiraterone (*Zytiga*), anastrozole (*Arimidex*), bicalutamide (*Casodex*), degarelix (*Firmagon*), enzalutamide (*Xtandi*), estramustine (*Emcyt*), exemestane (*Aromasin*), flutamide (generic), fulvestrant (*Faslodex*), goserelin (*Zoladex*), histrelin (*Vantas*), letrozole (*Femara*), leuprolide (*Eligard*, *Lupron*), megestrol (*Megace*), mitotane (*Lysodren*), nilutamide (*Nilandron*), tamoxifen (*Soltamox*), toremifene (*Fareston*), and triptorelin pamoate (*Trelstar*) (Table 14.5). Additional estrogen receptor modulators are discussed in Chapter 40.

Therapeutic Actions and Indications

The hormones and hormone modulators used as antineoplastics are receptor site specific or hormone specific to block the stimulation of growing cancer cells that are sensitive to the presence of that hormone (see Fig. 14.4). These drugs

Table 14.5 *Drugs in Focus:* Hormones and Hormone Modulators

Drug Name	Dosage/Route	Usual Indications
abiraterone (*Zytiga*)	1,000 mg/d PO with 5-mg prednisone PO twice daily	Treatment of metastatic, castration-resistant prostate cancer in male patients who have received prior chemotherapy *Actions:* Androgen biosynthesis inhibitor *Special considerations:* Risk of mineral corticoid excess and cardiovascular events; liver toxicity; must be taken on an empty stomach; GI effects are common
anastrozole (*Arimidex*)	1 mg/d PO	Treatment of advanced breast cancer in postmenopausal patients after tamoxifen therapy; first-line and adjunctive treatment of postmenopausal patients with locally advanced breast cancer *Actions:* Antiestrogen drug; blocks estradiol production without effects on adrenal hormones *Special considerations:* GI effects; signs and symptoms of menopause (hot flashes, mood swings, edema, vaginal dryness and itching); bone pain and back pain may occur—treat with analgesics; monitor lipid concentrations in patients at risk for high cholesterol level
bicalutamide (*Casodex*)	50 mg/d PO	In combination with a luteinizing hormone for the treatment of advanced prostate cancer *Actions:* Antiandrogen drug that competitively binds androgen receptor sites *Special considerations:* Gynecomastia and breast tenderness occur in 33% of patients; GI complaints are common; pregnancy category X
degarelix (*Firmagon*)	240 mg by subcutaneous injection given in two 120-mg injections *Maintenance*: 80 mg subcutaneous every 28 d	Treatment of patients with advanced prostate cancer *Actions:* Gonadotropin-releasing hormone receptor site antagonist, leads to decreased follicle-stimulating hormone and luteinizing hormone and decreased testosterone levels *Special considerations:* Pregnancy category X; risk of prolonged QT interval; injection site reactions, hot flashes, increased weight are common
enzalutamide (*Xtandi*)	160 mg/d PO	Treatment of metastatic, castration-resistant prostate cancer in male patients who have received prior chemotherapy *Actions:* Androgen receptor inhibitor *Special considerations:* Swallow capsules whole; pregnancy category X; GI effects, spinal cord compression, hypertension, anxiety, dizziness are common; reacts with many drugs, check drug regimen carefully
estramustine (*Emcyt*)	10–16 mg/kg/d PO in 3–4 divided doses for 30–90 d, then reevaluate	Palliative for treatment of metastatic and progressive prostate cancer *Actions:* Binds to estrogen steroid receptors, causing cell death *Special considerations:* GI toxicity, rash, bone marrow depression, breast tenderness, and cardiovascular toxicity are common; 30–90 d of therapy may be required before effects are seen; monitor cardiovascular, liver, and bone marrow function
exemestane (*Aromasin*)	25 mg/d PO with meals	Treatment of advanced, metastatic breast cancer in postmenopausal patients whose disease has progressed after tamoxifen therapy; adjunct treatment of postmenopausal patients who have receptor-positive early breast cancer and who have received tamoxifen for 2–3 y to finish 5-y course *Actions:* Inactivates steroid aromatase, lowering circulating estrogen levels and preventing the conversion of androgens to estrogen *Special considerations:* Avoid use in premenopausal patients or in patients with liver or renal dysfunction; hot flashes, headache, GI upset, anxiety, and depression are common
flutamide (generic)	250 mg PO t.i.d. given 8 h apart	With a luteinizing hormone for treatment of locally confined and metastatic prostate cancer *Actions:* Antiestrogenic drug, inhibits androgen uptake and binding on target cells *Special considerations:* May cause liver toxicity—monitor liver function regularly; associated with impaired fertility and cancer development; urine may become greenish; photosensitivity is common—protect patient from exposure to the sun
fulvestrant (*Faslodex*)	500 mg IM on days 1, 15, 29 then monthly	Treatment of hormone receptor–positive metastatic breast cancer in postmenopausal patients with disease progression after antiestrogen therapy *Actions:* Competitively binds to estrogen receptors, down-regulating the estrogen receptor protein in breast cancer cells *Special considerations:* Pregnancy category X; hot flashes, depression, headache, and GI upset are common; mark calendar with monthly injection dates; injection site reactions may occur

(continues on page 240)

Table 14.5 *Drugs in Focus:* Hormones and Hormone Modulators *(Continued)*		
Drug Name	**Dosage/Route**	**Usual Indications**
goserelin (*Zoladex*)	3.6 mg implant, subcutaneous, every 28 d to 12 wk, varies with diagnosis	Treatment of advanced prostatic and breast cancers; management of endometriosis *Actions:* Synthetic luteinizing hormone that inhibits pituitary release of gonadotropic hormones *Special considerations:* A 3.6-mg dose is effective in decreasing the signs and symptoms of endometriosis; associated with hypercalcemia and bone density loss—monitor serum calcium levels regularly; impairs fertility and is carcinogenic; monitor male patients for possible ureteral obstruction, especially during month 1
histrelin (*Vantas*)	50-mg implant subcutaneously every 12 mo	Palliative treatment of advanced prostate cancer *Actions:* Inhibits gonadotropic secretion; decreases follicle-stimulating hormone and luteinizing hormone levels and testosterone levels *Special considerations:* Must be surgically implanted and removed; hot flashes very common; monitor implantation site
letrozole (*Femara*)	2.5 mg/d PO	Treatment of advanced breast cancer in postmenopausal patients with disease after antiestrogen therapy; postsurgery adjunct for postmenopausal patients with early hormone receptor–positive breast cancer who have had 5 y of tamoxifen *Actions:* Prevents the conversion of precursors to estrogens in all tissues *Special considerations:* GI toxicity, bone marrow depression, alopecia, hot flashes, and CNS depression are common; discontinue drug at any sign that the cancer is progressing
leuprolide (*Lupron, Eligard*)	1 mg/d subcutaneously or depot or 7.5–45 mg by injection, implant, or depot every 1–4 mo, depending on preparation used	Treatment of advanced prostate cancer; also used to treat precocious puberty and endometriosis; depot form for uterine leiomyomata *Actions:* A natural luteinizing hormone that blocks the release of gonadotropic hormones *Special considerations:* Monitor patient's prostate-specific antigen levels periodically; monitor bone density and serum calcium levels; warn patient that they may have difficulty voiding the first few weeks and may experience bone pain, hot flashes, and pain at injection site
megestrol (*Megace*)	*Breast cancer:* 160 mg/d PO *Endometrial cancer:* 40–320 mg/d PO *Appetite stimulant:* 400–800 mg/d suspension PO	Palliative treatment of advanced breast or endometrial cancer; appetite stimulant for HIV patients *Actions:* Blocks luteinizing hormone release; efficacy not understood *Special considerations:* Monitor for thromboembolic events and weight gain; not for use during pregnancy
mitotane (*Lysodren*)	2–6 g PO in divided doses t.i.d. to q.i.d.; maximum dose 9–10 g/d	Treatment of inoperable adrenocortical carcinoma *Actions:* Cytotoxic to corticosteroid-forming cells of the adrenal gland *Special considerations:* Can cause GI toxicity, CNS toxicity with vision and behavioral changes, adrenal insufficiency; monitor adrenal function, and arrange for replacement therapy as indicated
nilutamide (*Nilandron*)	300 mg/d PO for 30 d, then 150 mg/d PO	With surgical castration for treatment of metastatic prostate cancer *Actions:* Antiandrogenic drug, inhibits androgen uptake and binding on target cells *Special considerations:* May cause liver toxicity—monitor liver function test results regularly; associated with interstitial pneumonitis—obtain baseline and periodic chest radiographs and discontinue drug at first sign of dyspnea
tamoxifen (*Soltamox*)	*Treatment:* 20–40 mg/d PO *Prevention:* 20 mg/d PO for 6 y	In combination therapy with surgery to treat breast cancer; treatment of advanced breast cancer; first drug approved for the prevention of breast cancer in patients at high risk for breast cancer *Actions:* Antiestrogen, competes with estrogen for receptor sites in target tissues *Special considerations:* Signs and symptoms of menopause are common; CNS depression, bone marrow depression, and GI toxicity are also common; can change visual acuity and cause corneal opacities and retinopathy—pretherapy and periodic ophthalmic examinations are indicated
toremifene (*Fareston*)	60 mg/d PO	Treatment of advanced breast cancer in patients with estrogen receptor–positive disease *Actions:* Binds to estrogen receptors and prevents growth of breast cancer cells *Special considerations:* Signs and symptoms of menopause, CNS depression, and GI toxicity are all common
triptorelin pamoate (*Trelstar*)	3.75 mg IM depot monthly, or 11.25 mg IM depot every 12 wk, or 22.5 mg IM depot every 24 wk	Palliative treatment of advanced prostatic cancer *Actions:* Analogue of luteinizing hormone–releasing hormone; causes a decrease in follicle-stimulating hormone and luteinizing hormone levels, leading to a suppression of testosterone production *Special considerations:* Monitor prostate-specific antigen and testosterone levels regularly; sexual dysfunction, urinary tract symptoms, bone pain, and hot flashes are common; schedule depot injections and mark calendars for patient

are indicated for the treatment of breast cancer in patients who are postmenopausal or in other female patients without ovarian function whose tumors show responsiveness to these hormones. In 2017, the first combination pack of oral agents became available with letrozole (*Femara*) and ribociclib (*Kisqali*), called *Kisqali Femara Co-Pack*. It was approved for the treatment of postmenopausal patients with hormone receptor–positive, human epidermal growth factor receptor 2–negative advanced, or metastatic breast cancer.

Some hormone modulators are indicated for the treatment of prostatic cancers that are sensitive to hormone manipulation. The gonadotropin-releasing hormone (GnRH) agonists and antagonists work by preventing release of luteinizing and follicle-stimulating hormones to decrease testosterone production in the testicles. These medications are also discussed in Chapter 35. The androgen receptor blockers, like flutamide, are used in conjunction with the GnRH agonists for prostate cancer suppression by blocking the testosterone effects at the receptor site. Table 14.5 shows usual indications for each of the hormones and hormone modulators.

Pharmacokinetics

These drugs are readily absorbed from the GI tract, metabolized in the liver, and excreted in the urine. Caution must be used with any patient who has hepatic or renal impairment. These drugs cross the placenta and enter into human milk.

Contraindications and Cautions

These drugs are contraindicated during pregnancy and lactation because of toxic effects on the fetus and neonate. Hypercalcemia is a contraindication to the use of toremifene, which is known to increase calcium levels. Use caution when giving hormones and hormone modulators to anyone with a known allergy to any of these drugs to prevent hypersensitivity reactions.

Adverse Effects

Adverse effects frequently encountered with the use of these drugs include those seen when estrogen is blocked or inhibited. Menopause-associated effects include hot flashes, vaginal spotting, vaginal dryness, moodiness, and depression. Other effects include bone marrow suppression and GI toxicity, including hepatic dysfunction. Hypercalcemia is also encountered as the calcium is pulled out of the bones without estrogen activity to promote calcium deposition. Many of these drugs increase the risk for thromboembolic events because of their effects on the body. Abiraterone can increase the risk of adrenocortical insufficiency.

Clinically Important Drug–Drug Interactions

If hormones and hormone modulators are taken with oral anticoagulants, there is often an increased risk of bleeding. Care is also necessary when administering these agents with any drugs that might increase serum lipid levels.

Prototype Summary: Tamoxifen

Indications: Treatment of metastatic breast cancer, reduction of risk of invasive breast cancer in female patients with ductal carcinoma in situ, reduction in occurrence of contralateral breast cancer in patients receiving adjuvant tamoxifen therapy, reduction in incidence of breast cancer in patients at high risk for breast cancer, treatment of McCune-Albright syndrome, and treatment of precocious puberty in female patients 2 to 10 years of age.

Actions: Competes with estrogen for binding sites in target tissues, such as the breast; a potent antiestrogenic agent.

Pharmacokinetics:

Route	Onset	Peak
Oral	Varies	4–7 h

$T_{1/2}$: 7 to 14 days; metabolized in the liver and excreted in the feces.

Adverse Effects: Hot flashes, rash, nausea, vomiting, vaginal bleeding, menstrual irregularities, edema, pain, thromboembolic events.

Nursing Considerations for Patients Receiving Hormones and Hormone Modulators

Assessment: History and Examination

- Assess for contraindications or cautions: history of allergy to the drug in use or any related drugs to avoid hypersensitivity reactions, renal or hepatic dysfunction that might interfere with drug metabolism and excretion, current status of pregnancy or lactation to prevent potentially serious adverse effects on the fetus or nursing baby, and history of hypercalcemia and hypercholesterolemia to avoid further increases in levels.
- Perform a physical assessment and tumor responsiveness to establish baseline data for determining the effectiveness of the drug and the occurrence of any adverse effects associated with drug therapy.
- Monitor bone density and blood calcium levels due to risk of decreased bone density and hypercalcemia; blood pressure, pulse, and perfusion to evaluate the status of the cardiovascular system and monitor for adverse drug effects; and bowel sounds and mucous membrane status to monitor for GI effects.
- Assess for hot flashes, decreased libido, gynecomastia, erectile dysfunction, or irregular menstruation due to effects on reproductive hormones.

See the "Critical Thinking Scenario" for a full discussion of assessing and evaluating antineoplastic therapy for a patient with breast cancer.

(continues on page 242)

Nursing Conclusions

Nursing conclusions related to drug therapy might include the following:

- Impaired comfort related to GI, CNS, or menopausal effects of the drug
- Altered body image perception related to antiestrogen effects, virilization
- Acute or chronic anxiety or fear related to diagnosis and treatment
- Knowledge deficit risk regarding drug therapy

Planning

- The patient will receive the best therapeutic effect from the drug therapy.
- The patient will have limited adverse effects to the drug therapy.
- The patient will have an understanding of the drug therapy, adverse effects to anticipate, and measures to relieve discomfort and improve safety.

Intervention With Rationale

- Monitor bone density and plasma calcium levels due to risk of decreased bone density. Encourage calcium and vitamin D intake.
- Provide comfort measures such as hygiene measures, temperature control, and stress reduction to help the patient cope with changes in reproductive health (decreased libido/erectile dysfunction) or menopausal signs and symptoms. Expect to reduce the dose if these effects become severe or intolerable.
- Provide the following patient teaching:
  - Follow the appropriate dosage regimen, including dates to return for further doses.
  - Maintain nutrition even if GI effects are severe.
  - Use barrier contraceptives to prevent pregnancy during therapy.
  - Try using comfort measures such as staying in a cool environment.
  - Perform hygiene and skin care and use measures to reduce stress to help cope with menopausal effects.
  - You may need to have periodic blood tests to monitor the effects of this drug on your body.

Evaluation

- Monitor patient response to the drug (alleviation of cancer being treated and palliation of signs and symptoms of cancer being treated).
- Monitor for adverse effects (GI or liver toxicity, menopausal signs and symptoms, decreased reproductive health, hypercalcemia, and thromboembolic events).
- Evaluate the effectiveness of the teaching plan (patient can name the drug, dosage, possible adverse effects to watch for, and specific measures to help avoid adverse effects).

Key Points

- Hormones and hormonal agents are used to treat specific cancers that respond to hormone stimulation such as breast cancer or prostate cancer.
- The adverse effects of hormones and hormonal agents used to treat cancers are often associated with increased or decreased effects of the hormones on the body.

Cancer Cell–Specific Agents

The goal of much of the current antineoplastic drug research is directed at finding cancer cell–specific drugs. These drugs would not have the same devastating effects on healthy cells in the body and would be more effective against particular cancer cells. Drugs available for cancer cell–specific actions include protein tyrosine kinase inhibitors, an epidermal growth factor inhibitor, proteasome inhibitors, and other specific enzyme blockers (see Table 14.6). Many monoclonal antibodies have also been developed for specific cancers. These drugs are discussed in Chapter 17.

Protein Tyrosine Kinase Inhibitors

The protein kinase inhibitors (see Table 14.6) act on specific enzymes that are needed by specific tumor cells for protein building. Blocking these enzymes inhibits tumor cell growth and division.

Each drug that has been developed inhibits a very specific protein kinase and acts on very specific tumors. They do not affect healthy human cells, so the patient experiences fewer of the adverse effects associated with antineoplastic chemotherapy. Imatinib (*Gleevec*), the first drug approved in this class, is given orally and is approved to treat chronic myelocytic leukemia (CML), several GI stromal tumors, various myeloproliferative disorders, aggressive systemic mastocytosis, and unresectable dermatofibrosarcoma protuberans. When the drug was first introduced in 2001, patients who had CML and who had been switched to imatinib after traditional chemotherapy reported feeling significantly better and that they had recovered from the numerous adverse effects of the traditional chemotherapy. However, long-term effects include development of new cancers, cardiac toxicity, and bone marrow suppression. Unfortunately, this drug is expensive. It was estimated that 1 year of treatment with the drug (which needs to be taken continually) cost the patient between $30,000 and $35,000. Now that there are generic options, there are better deals and prices. However, even with GoodRx coupons, 30-day supplies are over $200 for uninsured patients. Patients prescribed this drug and others like it may need support and assistance in obtaining financial help. Because they are relatively new to the market, all of the kinase inhibitors are relatively expensive. The protein tyrosine kinase inhibitors that are available include abemaciclib (*Verzenio*), afatinib (*Gilotrif*), alectinib (*Alecensa*), axitinib

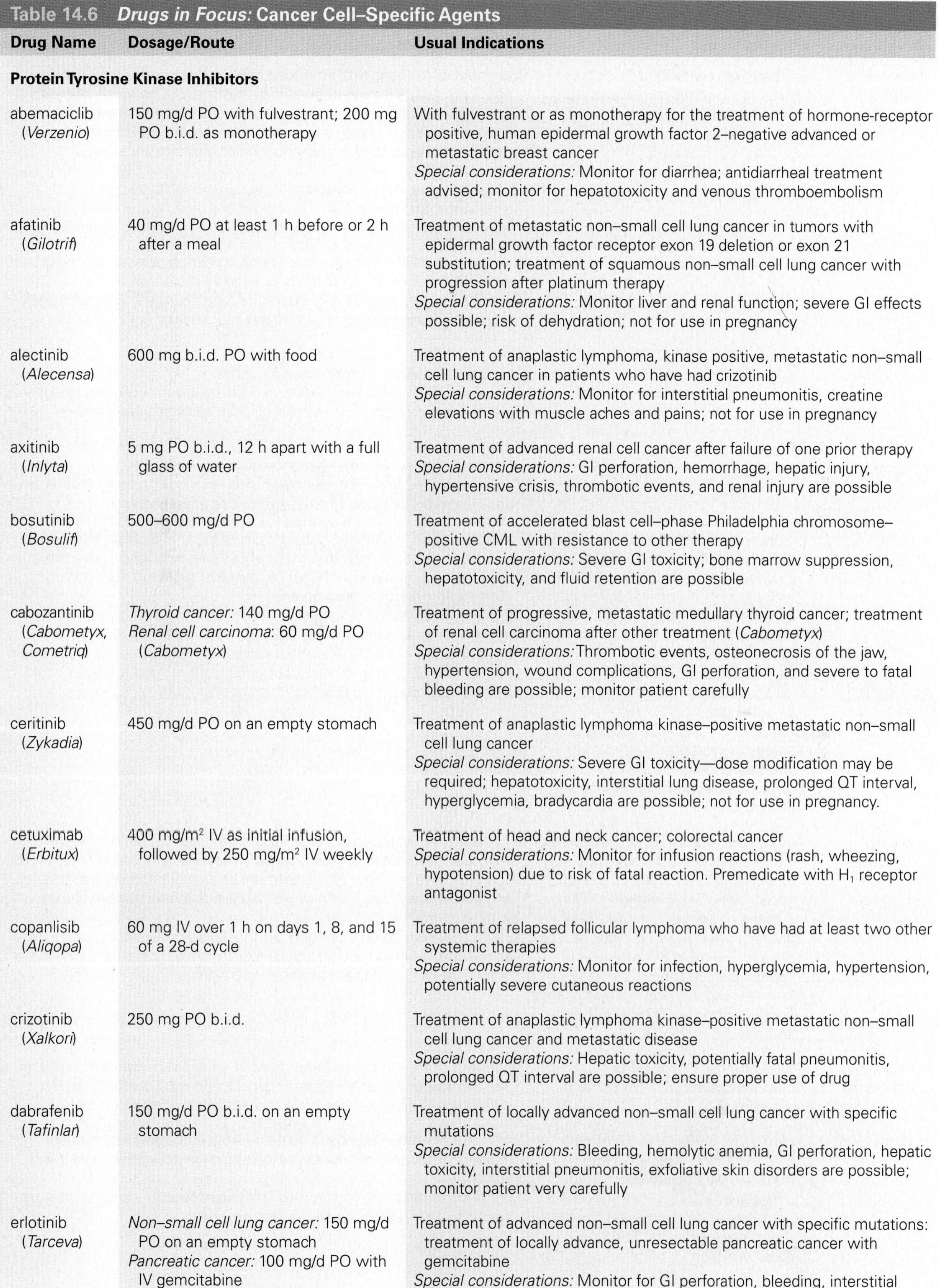

Table 14.6 *Drugs in Focus:* Cancer Cell–Specific Agents

Drug Name	Dosage/Route	Usual Indications
Protein Tyrosine Kinase Inhibitors		
abemaciclib (*Verzenio*)	150 mg/d PO with fulvestrant; 200 mg PO b.i.d. as monotherapy	With fulvestrant or as monotherapy for the treatment of hormone-receptor positive, human epidermal growth factor 2–negative advanced or metastatic breast cancer *Special considerations:* Monitor for diarrhea; antidiarrheal treatment advised; monitor for hepatotoxicity and venous thromboembolism
afatinib (*Gilotrif*)	40 mg/d PO at least 1 h before or 2 h after a meal	Treatment of metastatic non–small cell lung cancer in tumors with epidermal growth factor receptor exon 19 deletion or exon 21 substitution; treatment of squamous non–small cell lung cancer with progression after platinum therapy *Special considerations:* Monitor liver and renal function; severe GI effects possible; risk of dehydration; not for use in pregnancy
alectinib (*Alecensa*)	600 mg b.i.d. PO with food	Treatment of anaplastic lymphoma, kinase positive, metastatic non–small cell lung cancer in patients who have had crizotinib *Special considerations:* Monitor for interstitial pneumonitis, creatine elevations with muscle aches and pains; not for use in pregnancy
axitinib (*Inlyta*)	5 mg PO b.i.d., 12 h apart with a full glass of water	Treatment of advanced renal cell cancer after failure of one prior therapy *Special considerations:* GI perforation, hemorrhage, hepatic injury, hypertensive crisis, thrombotic events, and renal injury are possible
bosutinib (*Bosulif*)	500–600 mg/d PO	Treatment of accelerated blast cell–phase Philadelphia chromosome–positive CML with resistance to other therapy *Special considerations:* Severe GI toxicity; bone marrow suppression, hepatotoxicity, and fluid retention are possible
cabozantinib (*Cabometyx*, *Cometriq*)	*Thyroid cancer:* 140 mg/d PO *Renal cell carcinoma*: 60 mg/d PO (*Cabometyx*)	Treatment of progressive, metastatic medullary thyroid cancer; treatment of renal cell carcinoma after other treatment (*Cabometyx*) *Special considerations:* Thrombotic events, osteonecrosis of the jaw, hypertension, wound complications, GI perforation, and severe to fatal bleeding are possible; monitor patient carefully
ceritinib (*Zykadia*)	450 mg/d PO on an empty stomach	Treatment of anaplastic lymphoma kinase–positive metastatic non–small cell lung cancer *Special considerations:* Severe GI toxicity—dose modification may be required; hepatotoxicity, interstitial lung disease, prolonged QT interval, hyperglycemia, bradycardia are possible; not for use in pregnancy.
cetuximab (*Erbitux*)	400 mg/m^2 IV as initial infusion, followed by 250 mg/m^2 IV weekly	Treatment of head and neck cancer; colorectal cancer *Special considerations:* Monitor for infusion reactions (rash, wheezing, hypotension) due to risk of fatal reaction. Premedicate with H_1 receptor antagonist
copanlisib (*Aliqopa*)	60 mg IV over 1 h on days 1, 8, and 15 of a 28-d cycle	Treatment of relapsed follicular lymphoma who have had at least two other systemic therapies *Special considerations:* Monitor for infection, hyperglycemia, hypertension, potentially severe cutaneous reactions
crizotinib (*Xalkori*)	250 mg PO b.i.d.	Treatment of anaplastic lymphoma kinase–positive metastatic non–small cell lung cancer and metastatic disease *Special considerations:* Hepatic toxicity, potentially fatal pneumonitis, prolonged QT interval are possible; ensure proper use of drug
dabrafenib (*Tafinlar*)	150 mg/d PO b.i.d. on an empty stomach	Treatment of locally advanced non–small cell lung cancer with specific mutations *Special considerations:* Bleeding, hemolytic anemia, GI perforation, hepatic toxicity, interstitial pneumonitis, exfoliative skin disorders are possible; monitor patient very carefully
erlotinib (*Tarceva*)	*Non–small cell lung cancer:* 150 mg/d PO on an empty stomach *Pancreatic cancer:* 100 mg/d PO with IV gemcitabine	Treatment of advanced non–small cell lung cancer with specific mutations: treatment of locally advance, unresectable pancreatic cancer with gemcitabine *Special considerations:* Monitor for GI perforation, bleeding, interstitial pneumonitis, and serious skin disorders

(continues on page 244)

Table 14.6 *Drugs in Focus:* Cancer Cell–Specific Agents *(Continued)*

Drug Name	Dosage/Route	Usual Indications
everolimus (*Afinitor*)	5–10 mg/d PO with food *Adult, child with tuberous sclerosis:* 4.5 mg/m²/d PO	Treatment of patients with advanced renal cell carcinoma after failure of treatment with sunitinib or sorafenib; treatment of tuberous sclerosis complex with brain tumor; treatment of advanced postmenopausal hormone receptor–positive, growth factor–negative breast cancer; treatment of advanced neuroendocrine pancreatic cancer, renal angiomyolipoma *Special considerations:* Pneumonitis, serious to fatal infections, oral ulcerations, and elevations in blood glucose, lipid, and creatinine levels may occur; monitor patient very closely; do not use in pregnancy
gefitinib (*Iressa*)	250 mg/d PO	Treatment of metastatic non–small cell lung cancer with epidermal growth factor receptor exon 19 deletions or exon 21 mutations *Special considerations:* Risk of interstitial lung disease and hepatotoxicity; monitor for respiratory symptoms and liver impairment
ibrutinib (*Imbruvica*)	*Lymphoma:* 560 mg/d PO *Leukemia:* 420 mg/d PO	Treatment of mantle cell lymphoma after at least one other regimen; treatment of chronic lymphocytic leukemia *Special considerations:* Bone marrow suppression and secondary malignancy are possible; monitor bone marrow function and screen for cancers
idelalisib (*Zydelig*)	150 mg PO b.i.d.	Treatment of relapsed CLL, relapsed follicular B-cell non-Hodgkin lymphoma, relapsed small lymphocytic lymphoma *Special considerations:* Serious cutaneous reactions and anaphylaxis are possible; monitor blood counts; not for use in pregnancy
imatinib (*Gleevec*)	*Chronic-phase CML: Adult:* 400 mg/d PO, may be increased to 600 mg/d if needed *Pediatric:* 260 mg/m²/d PO with neutropenic or liver dysfunction patients; 340 mg/m²/d for general pediatric patients *Blast-crisis CML:* 600 mg/d PO; may be increased to 400 mg PO b.i.d. *First-line CML treatment: Pediatric (>2 y):* 340 mg/m²/d PO *GI stromal tumors:* 400–600 mg/d PO *Aggressive systemic mastocytosis:* 400 mg/d PO *Dermatofibrosarcoma protuberans:* 800 mg/d PO	Treatment of CML patients in blast crisis or in chronic phase after interferon-alpha therapy; treatment of patients with Kit-positive malignant GIST; first-line treatment of CML; aggressive systemic mastocytosis; dermatofibrosarcoma protuberans *Special considerations:* Administer with a meal and a full glass of water; arrange for small, frequent meals if GI upset is a problem; provide analgesics for headache and muscle pain; monitor complete blood count and for edema to arrange for dose reduction if needed; patient should receive consultation to deal with high cost of drug
lapatinib (*Tykerb*)	*Advanced or metastatic breast cancer:* 1,250 mg (5 tablets) orally once daily on days 1–21, in combination with capecitabine 2,000 mg/m²/d PO in 2 doses ~12 h apart on days 1–14; give in a repeating 21-d cycle; reduce dose to 750 mg/d PO with severe hepatic dysfunction *Hormone receptor–positive metastatic breast cancer:* 1,500 mg/d PO with letrozole 2.5 mg/d PO	In combination with capecitabine for the treatment of patients with advanced or metastatic breast cancer whose tumors overexpress HER2 and who have received prior treatment including anthracycline, taxane, and trastuzumab; treatment of HER2-positive metastatic breast cancer with letrozole *Special considerations:* Monitor heart function closely and decrease dose as needed; monitor for rash and GI toxicity; avoid grapefruit juice; many drug–drug interactions are possible, use caution
lenvatinib (*Lenvima*)	*Thyroid cancer:* 24 mg/d PO *Renal cell cancer:* 18 mg/d PO with everolimus	Treatment of thyroid cancer; treatment of renal cell cancer with everolimus *Special considerations:* Monitor for hepatic and renal dysfunction; GI perforation is possible; use of contraceptives is advised.
midostaurin (*Rydapt*)	*Acute myeloid leukemia*: 50 mg PO b.i.d. with food, days 8–20 and in combo with daunorubicin and cytarabine *Aggressive systemic mastocytosis, mast cell leukemias:* 100 mg PO b.i.d. with food	Treatment of newly diagnosed acute myeloid leukemia with mutation markers; treatment of aggressive systemic mastocytosis, mast cell leukemia *Special considerations:* Monitor for pulmonary toxicity; contraceptive use advised; many drug interactions, use caution.

Table 14.6 *Drugs in Focus:* Cancer Cell–Specific Agents *(Continued)*

Drug Name	Dosage/Route	Usual Indications
neratinib (*Nerlynx*)	240 mg/d PO for 1 y	Extended adjunctive treatment of early-stage HER2-overexpressed breast cancer after trastuzumab therapy *Special considerations:* Severe diarrhea, provide supportive care; monitor for liver toxicity; many drug interactions, use caution
nilotinib (*Tasigna*)	400 mg PO b.i.d., ~12 h apart without food	Treatment of newly diagnosed, chronic-phase and accelerated-phase Philadelphia chromosome–positive chronic myelogenous leukemia in adult patients resistant or intolerant to prior therapy that included imatinib *Special considerations:* Monitor for prolonged QT interval, bone marrow suppression, and possible liver toxicity. Capsules must be swallowed whole with water
osimertinib (*Tagrisso*)	80 mg/d PO	Treatment of metastatic epidermal growth factor receptor T790M mutation positive non–small cell lung cancer after progression following other therapy *Special considerations:* Ensure presence of mutation before use; monitor for interstitial lung disease, prolonged QT interval, and cardiomyopathy; refer to ophthalmologist at signs of keratitis
palbociclib (*Ibrance*)	125 mg/d PO for 21 d with food, followed by 7 d of rest; cycle repeated every 28 d, but dosing may be adjusted or halted due to toxicities	Treatment of postmenopausal, ER-positive, HER2-negative advanced breast cancer with aromatase inhibitor *Special considerations:* Monitor for infections and bone marrow suppression; not for use in pregnancy; interacts with many drugs, use caution
panitumumab (*Vectibix*)	6 mg/kg every 14 days IV	Treatment of some types of metastatic colorectal cancer *Special considerations:* Dermatologic toxicity common (90%) and severe in 15% of patients; monitor for pulmonary complications and ocular toxicities
pazopanib (*Votrient*)	800 mg/d PO without food; reduce dose with hepatic impairment	Treatment of advanced renal cell carcinoma; treatment of soft tissue sarcoma after progression following other therapy *Special considerations:* Monitor for prolonged QT interval; fatal hemorrhagic events have been reported; GI perforation and fistulas, hypertension, hypothyroidism have been reported; common effects include diarrhea, depigmentation of hair, and GI upset
ponatinib (*Iclusig*)	45 mg/d PO with food, adjust dose based on toxicity	Treatment of T3151-positive CML, T3151-positive ALL *Special considerations:* Hepatotoxicity, heart failure possible; monitor closely; not for use in pregnancy or lactation.
regorafenib (*Stivarga*)	160 mg/d PO for first 21 d of 28-d cycle with low-fat meal	Treatment of previously treated metastatic colorectal cancer; treatment of unresectable GI stromal tumors *Special considerations:* Risk of GI perforation, hepatotoxicity, MI, arrhythmias, dermatological toxicity; reacts with many drugs and grapefruit juice; stop 24 h before any surgery; not for use in pregnancy or lactation
ribociclib (*Kisqali*)	600 mg/d PO for 21 consecutive days followed by 7 d of rest	Treatment of postmenopausal hormone receptor–positive, epidermal growth factor receptor 2–negative advanced, or metastatic breast cancer *Special considerations:* Dosage adjustment or interruption may be necessary based on toxicity; monitor for QT prolongation, hepatobiliary toxicity, and bone marrow suppression; many drug interactions, use caution
ruxolitinib (*Jakafi*)	5–20 mg PO b.i.d.	Treatment of intermittent, high-risk myelofibrosis *Special considerations:* Stop after 6 mo if no sign of spleen reduction; monitor for infections; take safety precautions if dizziness is an issue
sorafenib (*Nexavar*)	400 mg PO b.i.d. on an empty stomach	Treatment of patients with advanced renal cell carcinoma, unresectable hepatocellular carcinoma, advanced thyroid cancer refractive to radioactive iodine therapy *Special considerations:* Monitor for skin reactions, hand–foot syndrome, hypertension, and QT prolongation
sunitinib (*Sutent*)	50 mg/d PO for 4 wk, followed by 2 wk of rest; repeat cycle *Pancreatic tumors:* 37.5 mg/d PO continuously	Treatment of GIST, advanced renal cell cancer, progressive neuroendocrine cancerous pancreatic tumors *Special considerations:* Monitor for GI disturbances and bone marrow suppression; adjust dose as needed

(continues on page 246)

Table 14.6 *Drugs in Focus:* Cancer Cell–Specific Agents *(Continued)*

Drug Name	Dosage/Route	Usual Indications
temsirolimus (*Torisel*)	25 mg IV, infused over 30–60 min once per wk, given 30 min after diphenhydramine 25–50 mg IV	Treatment of advanced renal cell carcinoma *Special considerations:* Monitor lung function, blood glucose, renal function; may experience slowed healing; avoid grapefruit juice and St. John's wort
trametinib (*Mekinist*)	2 mg/d PO, 1 h before or 2 h after a meal	Treatment of unresectable or metastatic melanoma with BRAF V600E or V600K mutations *Special considerations:* Ensure regular ophthalmic exams; serious vision changes or blindness are possible; monitor LV function at least every 3 mo, as serious cardiomyopathy can occur; interstitial pneumonitis is possible; risk of serious to fatal dermatological reactions
vemurafenib (*Zelboraf*)	960 mg PO b.i.d., 12 h apart	Treatment of unresectable or metastatic melanoma with appropriate BRAF mutations *Special considerations:* Ensure mutation is present; serious ophthalmologic damage, dermatologic toxicity with risk of Stevens-Johnson syndrome, new malignant melanoma, squamous cell carcinoma, liver toxicity and prolonged QT interval are all possible; assure proper use; monitor patient closely
ziv-aflibercept (*Zaltrap*)	4 mg/kg IV over 1 h every 2 wk	Treatment of metastatic colon cancer resistant to oxaliplatin as part of combo therapy *Special considerations:* GI toxicity, hemorrhage, thrombotic events, proteinuria, bone marrow suppression are all possible; do not use within 4 wk of surgery; advise contraceptive use during and for 3 mo after therapy
Other Cancer Cell–Specific Agents		
belinostat (*Beleodaq*)	1,000 mg/m²/d IV over 30 min on days 1–5 of a 21-d cycle	Histone deacetylase inhibitor for the treatment of relapsed/refractory peripheral T-cell lymphoma *Special considerations:* Monitor bone marrow and liver function; tumor lysis syndrome is possible
bortezomib (*Velcade*)	1.3 mg/m² as a 3–5-s IV bolus or subcutaneously for nine 6-d cycles on days 1, 4, 8, 11, then 10 d of rest, 22, 25, 29, and 32	Proteasome inhibitor for treatment of mantle cell lymphoma in patients with disease progression after at least one other therapy *Special considerations:* Monitor for neurologic changes and bone marrow suppression; not for use in pregnancy or lactation
carfilzomib (*Kyprolis*)	20 mg/m²/d IV over 10 min for 2 consecutive days, each week for 3 wk, days 1, 2, 8, 9, 15, 16 followed by a 12-d rest period then 27 mg/m²/d IV over 10 min	Proteasome inhibitor for the treatment of relapsed multiple myeloma as monotherapy or with other drugs *Special considerations:* Monitor for heart failure, pulmonary toxicity, liver dysfunction, and tumor lysis syndrome. Premedicate with dexamethasone
ixazomib (*Ninlaro*)	4 mg/d PO on days 1, 8, and 15 of a 28-d cycle	Proteasome inhibitor for the treatment of relapsed multiple myeloma *Special considerations:* Monitor bone marrow and liver function; many drug interactions, use caution
niraparib (*Zejula*)	300 mg/d PO with food	Poly polymerase inhibitor for the maintenance treatment of recurrent epithelial ovarian fallopian tube or primary peritoneal cancer with progression after platinum-based therapy *Special considerations:* Monitor for severe bone marrow depression, development of myelodysplastic syndrome, acute myeloid leukemia, and cardiovascular effects
olaparib (*Lynparza*)	300 mg/d PO b.i.d.	Poly polymerase inhibitor for the maintenance treatment of recurrent epithelial ovarian fallopian tube or primary peritoneal cancer with progression after platinum-based therapy; treatment of deleterious germline BRCA-mutated advanced ovarian cancer after failure of three of more other therapies *Special considerations:* Monitor for myelodysplastic syndrome, acute myeloid leukemia, and pneumonitis; many drug interactions, use caution.
panobinostat (*Farydak*)	20 mg PO once every other day for 3 doses per week, days 1, 3, 5, 8, 10, and 12 of weeks 1 and 2 of each 21-d cycle for 8 cycles	Histone deacetylase inhibitor for the treatment of multiple myeloma after at least 2 other regimens, given with dexamethasone and bortezomib *Special considerations:* Risk of severe diarrhea, severe to fatal cardiac events, liver toxicity, and hemorrhage; many drug interactions, use caution

Table 14.6 *Drugs in Focus:* Cancer Cell–Specific Agents *(Continued)*

Drug Name	Dosage/Route	Usual Indications
romidepsin (*Istodax*)	14 mg/m² IV over 4 h on days 1, 8, 15 of a 28-d cycle; repeat every 28 d	Histone deacetylase inhibitor for the treatment of cutaneous, peripheral T-cell lymphoma progressing after other therapy *Special considerations:* Risk of severe bone marrow depression, QT prolongation, and tumor lysis syndrome; mark calendar for treatment days; monitor patient closely
rucaparib (*Rubraca*)	600 mg PO b.i.d.	Poly polymerase inhibitor for the treatment of deleterious BRCA mutation advanced ovarian cancer after failure of two or more other regimens *Special considerations:* Ensure presence of the mutation; risk of myelodysplastic syndrome and development of acute myeloid leukemia
sonidegib (*Odomzo*)	200 mg/d PO on an empty stomach	Hedgehog pathway inhibitor for the treatment of locally advanced basal cell carcinoma *Special considerations:* Rule out pregnancy; male patients should not procreate during and for 8 mo following treatment; many drug interactions, use caution
venetoclax (*Venclexta*)	20 mg/d PO for 7 d, then increase to recommended dose of 400 mg/d	BCL-2 inhibitor for the treatment of CLL with 17p depletion after at least one other therapy *Special considerations:* Tablets cannot be cut, crushed, or chewed; tumor lysis syndrome possible; monitor bone marrow; do not give immunizations
vismodegib (*Erivedge*)	150 mg/d PO	Hedgehog pathway inhibitor for the treatment of metastatic or locally advanced basal cell carcinoma *Special considerations:* Alopecia common; rule out pregnancy; blood cannot be donated during or for 24 mo after treatment; should not nurse a baby during or for 24 mo after treatment; barrier contraceptives advised
vorinostat (*Zolinza*)	400 mg/d PO with food	Histone deacetylase inhibitor for the treatment of cutaneous manifestations in patients with cutaneous T-cell lymphoma *Special considerations:* Monitor for increased bleeding; excessive nausea and vomiting may occur; encourage fluid intake to prevent dehydration

CML, chronic myelocytic leukemia; CLL, chronic lymphocytic leukemia; GIST, gastrointestinal stromal tumor; HER2, human epidermal receptor 2; ALL, acute lymphocytic leukemia; MI, myocardial infarction; BRAF, a gene on chromosome 7q34.

(*Inlyta*), bosutinib (*Bosulif*), cabozantinib (*Cometriq*), ceritinib (*Zykadia*), cetuximab (*Erbitux*), copanlisib (*Aliqopa*), crizotinib (*Xalkori*), dabrafenib (*Tafinlar*), dasatinib (*Sprycel*), everolimus (*Afinitor*), gefitinib (*Iressa*), ibrutinib (*Imbruvica*), idelalisib (*Zydeliq*), imatinib (*Gleevec*), lapatinib (*Tykerb*), lenvatinib (*Lenvima*), midostaurin (*Rydapt*), neratinib (*Nerlynx*), nilotinib (*Tasigna*), osimertinib (*Tagrisso*), palbociclib (*Ibrance*), panitumumab (*Vectibix*), pazopanib (*Votrient*), ponatinib (*Iclusig*), regorafenib (*Stivarga*), ribociclib (*Kisqali*), ruxolitinib (*Jakafi*), sorafenib (*Nexavar*), sunitinib (*Sutent*), temsirolimus (*Torisel*), trametinib (*Mekinist*), vemurafenib (*Zelboraf*), and ziv-aflibercept (*Zaltrap*).

CRITICAL THINKING SCENARIO
Antineoplastic Therapy and Breast Cancer

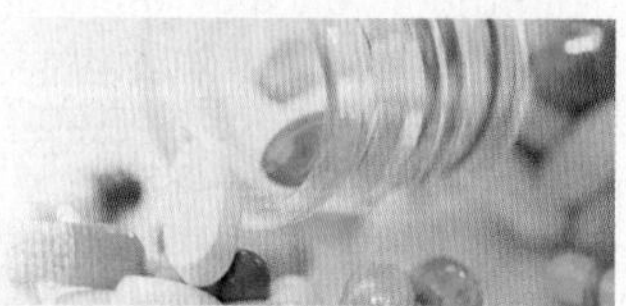

THE SITUATION

B.P., a 34-year-old female patient, is a schoolteacher with two young children assigned female at birth. The patient noticed a slightly painful lump under their arm when showering. About 2 weeks later, the patient found a mass in the right breast. Initial patient assessment found that they had no other underlying medical problems, had no allergies, and took no medications. Family history was significant for multiple family members having cancer—their mother, two grandmothers, three aunts, two older siblings, and one younger sibling died of breast cancer when they were in their early 30s. All data from the initial examination, including an evaluation of the lump in the upper outer quadrant of the breast and the presence of a fixed axillary node, were recorded as baseline data for further drug therapy and treatment. B.P. underwent a radical mastectomy with biopsy report for grade IV infiltrating ductal carcinoma (28 of 35 lymph nodes were positive for tumor) and then radiation therapy. Then, the patient began a 1-year course of doxorubicin, cyclophosphamide, and paclitaxel (AC/paclitaxel/sequential).

(continues on page 248)

CRITICAL THINKING

What are the important nursing implications for B.P.? Think about the outlook for B.P. based on biopsy results and family history.

What are the effects of high levels of stress on the immune system and the body's ability to fight cancer?

What impact will this disease have on B.P.'s job and family? Think about the adverse drug effects that can be anticipated.

How can good patient teaching help B.P. to anticipate and cope with these many changes and unpleasant effects?

What future concerns should be addressed or at least approached at this point in the treatment of B.P.'s disease?

What are the implications for B.P.'s two children?

How may a coordinated health team work to help the children cope with their parent's disease, as well as the prospects for their future?

DISCUSSION

The extent of B.P.'s disease, as evidenced by the biopsy results, does not signify a very hopeful prognosis. In this case, the overall nursing care plan should take into account not only the acute needs related to surgery and drug therapy but also future needs related to potential debilitation and even the prospect of death. Immediate needs include comfort and teaching measures to help B.P. deal with the mastectomy and recovery from the surgery. B.P. should be given an opportunity to vent their feelings and thoughts in a protected environment. Efforts should be made to help organize their life and plans around radiation therapy and chemotherapy.

The adverse effects associated with the antineoplastic agents B.P. will be given should be explained and possible ways to cope should be discussed. These effects include the following:

Alopecia. B.P. should be reassured that hair will grow back, but they will need to cover their head in extremes of temperature. Purchasing a wig before the hair loss begins may be a good alternative to trying to remember later what their hair was like.

Nausea and vomiting. These effects will most often occur immediately after the drugs are given. Antiemetics may be ordered, but they are frequently not very effective.

Bone marrow suppression. This will make B.P. more susceptible to disease, which could be a problem for a teacher and a parent with young children. Ways to avoid contact and infection, as well as warning signs to report immediately, should be discussed.

Mouth sores. Stomatitis and mucositis are common problems. Frequent mouth care is important. The patient should be encouraged to maintain fluid intake and nutrition.

Because the antineoplastic therapy will be a long-term regimen, it might help to prepare a calendar of drug dates for use in planning other activities and events. All of B.P.'s treatment should be incorporated into a team approach that helps B.P. and the family deal with the impact of this disease and its therapy, as well as with the potential risk to their daughters. B.P.'s children are in a very high risk group for this disease, so the importance of frequent examinations as they grow up needs to be stressed. It may be recommended that B.P.'s children be screened for gene mutations that would increase their risk for developing cancer. In some areas of the country, health care providers are encouraging prophylactic mastectomies for patients in this very high risk group.

NURSING CARE GUIDE FOR B.P.: ANTINEOPLASTIC AGENTS

Assessment: History and Examination

Allergies to any of these drugs, renal or hepatic dysfunction, pregnancy or lactation, bone marrow suppression, or GI ulceration

Concurrent use of ketoconazole, diazepam, verapamil, quinidine, dexamethasone, cisplatin, cyclosporine, etoposide, vincristine, testosterone, digoxin, which could interact with these drugs

Local: Evaluation of injection site

CNS: Orientation, affect, reflexes

Skin: Color, lesions, texture

GI: Abdominal, liver evaluation

Laboratory tests: Complete blood count with differential; renal and hepatic function tests

Nursing Conclusions

Impaired comfort related to GI, CNS, or skin effects

Malnutrition risk related to GI effects

Altered body image perception related to diagnosis, therapy, adverse effects

Knowledge deficit risk regarding drug therapy

Infection risk due to potential of bone marrow suppression

Acute and/or chronic anxiety or fear related to diagnosis and effects of drug treatment

Planning

The patient will receive the best therapeutic effect from the drug therapy.

The patient will have limited adverse effects to the drug therapy.

The patient will have an understanding of the drug therapy, adverse effects to anticipate, and measures to relieve discomfort and improve safety.

Intervention

Ensure safe administration of the drug.

Provide comfort and safety measures: mouth and skin care, rest periods, safety precautions, antiemetics as needed, maintenance of nutrition, and head covering.

Provide support and reassurance to deal with drug effects, body image changes, discomfort, and diagnosis.

Provide patient teaching regarding drug name, dosage, adverse effects, precautions to take, signs and symptoms to report, and comfort measures to observe.

Evaluation

Evaluate drug effects: resolution of cancer.

Monitor for adverse effects: GI toxicity, bone marrow suppression, CNS changes, renal and hepatic damage, alopecia, extravasation of drug.

Monitor for drug–drug interactions as listed.

Evaluate effectiveness of patient teaching program.

Evaluate effectiveness of comfort and safety measures.

PATIENT TEACHING FOR B.P.

Antineoplastic agents work to destroy cells at various phases of their life cycle. The drugs are given in combination to affect the cells at these various stages. These drugs are prescribed to kill cancer cells that are growing in the body. Because these drugs also affect normal cells, they sometimes cause many adverse effects. Your drug combination includes doxorubicin, cyclophosphamide, and paclitaxel.

- These drugs are given in a 21-day cycle, followed by a rest period. You will need to mark your calendar with the treatment days and rest days. You will need to have regular blood tests to follow the effects of these drugs on your blood cells.
- Common adverse effects of these drugs include the following:
  - *Nausea and vomiting.* Antiemetic drugs and sedatives may help. Your health care provider will be with you to help if these effects occur.
  - *Loss of appetite.* It is very important to keep up your strength. Tell people if there is something that you would be interested in eating—anything that appeals to you. Alert someone if you feel hungry, regardless of the time of day.
  - *Loss of hair.* Your hair will grow back, although its color or consistency may be different from what it was originally. It may help to purchase a wig before you lose your hair so that you can match appearance if you would like to. Hats and scarves may also be worn. It is very important to keep your head covered in extremes of temperature and to protect yourself from sun, heat, and cold. Because much of the body's heat can be lost through the head, not protecting yourself could cause serious problems.
  - *Mouth sores.* Frequent mouth care is very helpful. Try to avoid very hot or spicy foods.
  - *Fatigue, malaise.* Frequent rest periods and careful planning of your day's activities can be very helpful.
  - *Bleeding.* You may bruise more easily than you normally do, and your gums may bleed while you are brushing your teeth. Special care should be taken when shaving or brushing your teeth. Avoid activities that might cause an injury, and avoid medications that contain aspirin.
  - *Susceptibility to infection.* Avoid people with infections or colds, and avoid crowded, public places. In some cases, the people who are caring for you may wear gowns and masks to protect you from their germs. Avoid working in your garden because soil is full of bacteria.
- Report any of the following to your health care provider: bruising and bleeding, fever, chills, sore throat, difficulty breathing, flank pain, and swelling in your ankles or fingers.
- Take the full course of your prescription. It is very important to take the complete regimen that has been ordered for you. Cancer cells grow at different rates, and they go through rest periods during which they are not susceptible to the drugs. The disease must be attacked over time to eradicate the problem.
- Tell any doctor, nurse, or other health care provider that you are taking this drug.
- Try to maintain a balanced diet and keep hydrated while you are taking this drug.
- For the time that these drugs are being taken, you are urged to use a barrier contraceptive. These drugs can cause serious effects to a developing fetus, and precautions must be taken to avoid pregnancy. If you think that you are pregnant, consult your health care provider immediately.
- You need to have periodic blood tests and examinations while you are taking this drug. These tests help to guard against serious adverse effects and may be needed to determine the next dose of your drug.

Proteasome Inhibitors and Other Cancer Cell–Specific Inhibitors

In 2003, the FDA approved bortezomib (*Velcade*) for the treatment of multiple myeloma in patients whose disease had progressed after two other standard therapies. This drug inhibits proteasome in human cells, a large protein complex that works to maintain cell homeostasis and protein production. Without it, the cell loses homeostasis and dies. This drug was shown to delay growth in selected tumors. Other proteasome inhibitors include carfilzomib (*Kyprolis*) and ixazomib (*Ninlaro*), used in treating multiple myeloma. Drugs that alter the hedgehog pathway, a signaling pathway needed for cell development, include sonidegib (*Odomzo*) and vismodegib (*Erivedge*), both used to treat basal cell carcinoma. Drugs that affect other specific systems in the cell are being released regularly as more becomes known about these cells and how to alter them. Belinostat (*Beleodaq*), panobinostat (*Farydak*), romidepsin (*Istodax*), and vorinostat (*Zolinza*) are histone deacetylase inhibitors used to treat T cell lymphoma and multiple myeloma, respectively. Other relatively new specific inhibitors include venetoclax (*Venclexta*), a BCL-2 inhibitor for CLL, and three poly polymerase inhibitors, olaparib (*Lynparza*), used to treat mutated advanced ovarian cancer; niraparib (*Zejula*), used to treat recurrent ovarian, fallopian tube and peritoneal cancers; and rucaparib (*Rubraca*), used to treat relapsed mutated ovarian cancer.

Therapeutic Actions and Indications

Imatinib is an oral antineoplastic drug, a protein tyrosine kinase inhibitor that selectively inhibits the BCR-ABL tyrosine kinase created by the Philadelphia chromosome abnormality in CML. Blocking this enzyme inhibits proliferation and induces cell division in BCR-ABL–positive cell lines, as well as in new leukemic cells, thereby inhibiting tumor growth in CML patients in blast crisis. It also inhibits a specific receptor site in patients with GI stromal tumors. Because of its specific effects on these tumor cells, it is not associated with adverse effects on normal human cells.

There are several epidural growth factor receptor (EGFR) tyrosine kinase inhibitors, including cetuximab (*Erbitux*), panitumumab (*Vectibix*), gefitinib (*Iressa*), erlotinib (*Tarceva*), and afatinib (*Gilotrif*). EGFR is a glycoprotein that is normally expressed in epithelial tissue (including skin and hair follicles). It can be overexpressed in certain cancers. The EGFR tyrosine kinase inhibitors can be indicated in specific head, neck, and colorectal cancers. Testing of the tumor must be completed prior to therapy to see if it will respond to these treatments.

Table 14.6 shows usual indications for all protein tyrosine kinase inhibitors and other cell-specific inhibitors.

Pharmacokinetics

Imatinib is slowly absorbed from the GI tract, reaching peak levels in 2 to 4 hours. It is extensively metabolized in the liver, with a half-life of 18 and then 40 hours. Each of the many kinase inhibitors is metabolized in the liver; the absorption and pharmacokinetics vary with kinase inhibitor.

Erlotinib is well absorbed orally from the GI tract, reaching peak level in 4 hours. It is metabolized in the liver with a half-life of 36 hours.

Bortezomib, given IV, reaches peak effect at the end of the infusion. It is metabolized in the liver and has a half-life of 40 to 193 hours.

Contraindications and Cautions

All of these drugs are high risk in pregnancy. For the time that these drugs are being taken, patients able to become pregnant should be advised to use barrier contraceptives. It can enter human milk, and it should be used during lactation only if the benefits to the parent clearly outweigh the risks to the baby. Several of the drugs are contraindicated with patients who have or who are at risk for prolonged QT intervals (hypokalemia, hypomagnesemia, or taking another drug that prolongs the QT interval) because they prolong the QT interval, and sudden death could occur. These drugs should not be given to anyone who has a history of hypersensitivity to any component of the drug being given. Severe infusion reactions and skin toxicity are common for some of the medications that are administered intravenously.

Adverse Effects

The adverse effects associated with imatinib include GI upset, muscle cramps, heart failure, fluid retention, and skin rash. The severe bone marrow suppression, alopecia, and severe GI effects associated with more traditional antineoplastic therapy do not occur. Several of these drugs prolong the QT interval and need to be used with caution in patients with cardiac problems. Erlotinib and bortezomib are associated with cardiovascular events and pulmonary toxicity. Bortezomib has also been associated with peripheral neuropathy and liver and kidney impairment. Cetuximab is associated with severe infusion reactions, pulmonary toxicity, and skin toxicity that can be worsened by sun exposure.

Clinically Important Drug–Drug Interactions

Use caution when administering these drugs with other drugs affected by the cytochrome P450 enzyme system. In addition, St. John's wort decreases the effectiveness of many of these drugs and should be avoided. It is also important to avoid any other drugs that are known to prolong the QT interval.

Prototype Summary: Imatinib

Indications: Treatment of adults with CML who are in blast crisis, accelerated phase, or chronic phase after failure with interferon-alpha therapy. It has since also been approved for use in the treatment of patients with CD117-positive unresectable or metastatic gastrointestinal stromal tumor (GIST), various myeloproliferative disorders, aggressive systemic mastocytosis, and unresectable dermatofibrosarcoma protuberans.

Actions: Tyrosine kinase inhibitor that selectively inhibits the BCR-ABL tyrosine kinase created by the Philadelphia chromosome abnormality in CML and certain tumor cells present in GIST; blocking this enzyme inhibits proliferation and induces cell division.

Pharmacokinetics:

Route	Onset	Peak
Oral	Slow	2–4 h

$T_{1/2}$: 18 to 40 hours; metabolized in the liver and excreted in the feces.

Adverse Effects: Nausea, vomiting, heart failure, headache, hepatotoxicity, GI bleeds, renal toxicity, dizziness, edema, rash.

Nursing Considerations for Patients Receiving Cancer Cell–Specific Agents

These are similar to nursing care considerations for patients receiving alkylating agents.

Key Points

- Cancer cell–specific drugs have been developed to target processes that occur in cancer cells but not in healthy cells. This specificity results in fewer toxic effects than with traditional antineoplastic therapy.
- Protein tyrosine kinase inhibitors, epidermal growth factor inhibitors, proteasome inhibitors hedgehog pathway inhibitors, polymerase inhibitors, histone deacetylase inhibitors, and other specific inhibitors have been developed to target cancer cells specifically.

Miscellaneous Antineoplastics

Many other agents that do not fit into one of the previously discussed groups are used as antineoplastics to cause cell death. These drugs are used for treating a wide variety of cancers.

Topotecan (*Hycamtin*) is a topoisomerase inhibitor that breaks DNA strands during DNA synthesis. This medication is indicated for treatment of metastatic ovarian cancer, small cell lung cancer, and persistent cervical cancer. Side effects include severe bone marrow suppression, alopecia, and GI discomfort. Doses may need to be reduced for people with renal impairment.

Asparaginase *Erwinia chrysanthemi* (*Elspar, Erwinaze*) is a medication that can be used to treat acute lymphocytic leukemia. This medication acts as an enzyme to decrease the levels of asparagine needed for leukemic cells to survive. Complications include hypersensitivity reactions; GI discomfort; liver, renal, and pancreas toxicity; and CNS effects including tremor, confusion, and coma.

Table 14.7 lists several of the unclassified antineoplastic drugs, their indications, and any special considerations associated with the drug. Specific information about each drug may be obtained in a nursing drug guide. See Figure 14.4 for sites of action of miscellaneous antineoplastic agents.

Table 14.7 ***Drugs in Focus:*** **Miscellaneous Antineoplastics**

Drug Name	Dosage/Route	Usual Indications
arsenic trioxide (*Trisenox*)	*Induction:* 0.15 mg/kg/d IV until remission *Consolidation:* Continue 3–6 wk after inducting	Induction and consolidation in patients with APL who are refractory to or relapsed from standard therapy *Actions:* Causes damage to fusion proteins and DNA failure, leading to cell death *Special considerations:* Monitor for cardiac toxicity; do not use during pregnancy
asparaginase *Erwinia chrysanthemi* (*Erwinaze*)	25,000 units/m² IM as part of a specific combination regimen	As part of combination therapy in treatment of ALL in patients with sensitivity to asparaginase or pegaspargase *Actions:* An enzyme that hydrolyzes the amino acid asparagine, which is needed by malignant cells for protein synthesis; inhibits cell proliferation; most effective in G_1 phase of the cell cycle *Special considerations:* Coagulation disorders, hyperglycemia, and hypersensitivity reactions to this drug are common, and patients should be tested and desensitized, if necessary, before using the drug; monitor blood tests regularly
azacitidine (*Vidaza*)	75 mg/m²/d IV or subcutaneous for 7 d q4wk	Treatment of patients with myelodysplastic syndrome *Action:* Causes demethylation of DNA *Special considerations:* Premedicate for nausea; monitor for bone marrow suppression; patient should avoid pregnancy or procreation while on drug
bexarotene (*Targretin*)	100–300 mg/m² PO daily	Treatment of cutaneous manifestations of cutaneous T-cell lymphoma in patients refractory to at least one other systemic therapy *Actions:* Binds and activates retinoid receptors *Special considerations:* Risk of serious pancreatitis, hepatic toxicity and photosensitivity
decitabine (*Dacogen*)	15 mg/m² IV over 3 h q8h for 3 d; repeat q6wk for at least 4 cycles	Treatment of patients with myelodysplastic syndromes *Actions:* Affects DNA and inhibits DNA transfer *Special considerations:* Premedicate with antiemetics; monitor for bone marrow suppression
irinotecan (*Camptosar*)	125 mg/m² IV over 90 min, once a week for 4 wk, followed by 2 wk of rest; repeat every 6 wk	Treatment of metastatic colon or rectal cancer with 5-FU *Actions:* Disrupts DNA strands during DNA synthesis, causing cell death *Special considerations:* Can cause severe bone marrow depression, which regulates dose of the drug; causes GI toxicity, dyspnea, and alopecia
omacetaxine (*Synribo*)	1.25 mg/m² subcutaneously b.i.d. for 14 consecutive days of a 28-d cycle, then 1.25 mg/m² subcutaneously for 7 consecutive days of a 28-d cycle	Treatment of accelerated, resistant CML *Actions:* Inhibits protein synthesis, causing cell death *Special considerations:* Monitor for severe bone marrow suppression or bleeding

(continues on page 252)

Table 14.7 *Drugs in Focus:* Miscellaneous Antineoplastics *(Continued)*

Drug Name	Dosage/Route	Usual Indications
pegaspargase (*Oncaspar*)	2,500 IU/m^2 IM or IV q14d	Treatment of ALL *Actions:* An enzyme that hydrolyzes the amino acid asparaginase, which is needed by malignant cells for protein synthesis; inhibits cell proliferation; most effective in G_1 phase of the cell cycle *Special considerations:* Can cause potentially fatal hyperthermia, bone marrow depression, renal toxicity, and pancreatitis; monitor patient regularly, arrange decreased dose as appropriate if toxic effects occur
porfimer (*Photofrin*)	2 mg/kg IV over 3–5 min; laser treatment must follow in 40–50 h and again in 96–120 h	Photosensitizing agent that is used with laser light to decrease tumor size in patients with obstructive esophageal cancers not responsive to laser treatment alone; transitional cell carcinoma in situ of urinary bladder; endobronchial non–small cell lung cancer; high-grade dysplasia or Barrett esophagus *Actions:* Taken up by cells, causing radical reactions when cells are exposed to laser light, causing cell death *Special considerations:* Has been associated with pleural effusion and fistula; associated with GI and cardiac toxicity; must be given in conjunction with scheduled laser treatment, with at least 30 d between treatments; protect patient from exposure to light with protective clothing for 30 d after treatment (sunscreens are not effective); avoid direct contact with the drug—protective clothing and goggles are suggested
sipuleucel-T (*Provenge*)	3 doses IV over 60 min, administer over 3 wk	Autologous cellular immunotherapy used to induce an immune response to antigens found in most prostate cancers; treatment of asymptomatic or minimally symptomatic metastatic hormone refractory prostate cancer *Special considerations:* Premedicate with oral acetaminophen and an antihistamine; universal precautions are required; severe infusion reactions are possible; monitor closely during administration; patient may experience fever, headache, nausea, and joint pain.
talc powder (*Sclerosol*)	5 g injected through open thoracotomy or during thoracoscopy	Prevention of recurrence of malignant pleural effusion *Actions:* Induces the inflammatory response, promoting adhesion of the pleura and preventing accumulation of fluid *Special considerations:* Monitor for cardiac and respiratory effects; no actual antineoplastic actions; change patient position every 2 h
topotecan (*Hycamtin*)	1.5 mg/m^2/d IV over 30 min for 5 d as part of a 21-d course; minimum of four courses	Treatment of patients with metastatic ovarian cancer, small cell lung cancer, persistent cervical cancer *Actions:* Damages DNA strand, causing cell death during cell division *Special considerations:* Can cause severe bone marrow depression, which regulates the dose of the drug; total alopecia, GI toxicity, and CNS effects may also limit the use of the drug; analgesics may be helpful
vorinostat (*Zolinza*)	400 mg/d PO with food	Treatment of cutaneous manifestations in patients with cutaneous T-cell lymphoma *Action:* Histone deacetylase inhibitor *Special considerations:* Monitor for increased bleeding; excessive nausea and vomiting may occur; encourage fluid intake to prevent dehydration

APL, acute promyelocytic leukemia; ALL, acute lymphocytic leukemia; CML, chronic myelocytic leukemia; 5-FU, fluorouracil.

SUMMARY

- Cancers arise from a single abnormal cell that multiplies and grows.
- Cancers can manifest as diseases of the blood and lymph tissue or as growth of tumors arising from epithelial cells (carcinomas) or from mesenchymal cells and connective tissue (sarcomas).
- Cancer cells lose their normal function (anaplasia), develop characteristics that allow them to grow in an uninhibited way (autonomy), have the ability to travel to other sites in the body that are conducive to their growth (metastasis), and can stimulate the production of blood vessels to bring nutrients to the growing tumor (angiogenesis).
- Antineoplastic drugs affect both normal cells and cancer cells by disrupting cell function and division at various points in the cell cycle; new drugs, such as protein kinase inhibitors, are being developed to target cancer cell–specific functions.
- Cancer drugs are usually most effective against cells that multiply rapidly (i.e., proceed through the cell cycle quickly). These cells include most neoplasms, bone marrow cells, cells in the GI tract, and cells in the skin or hair follicles.

- The goal of cancer chemotherapy is to decrease the size of the neoplasm so that the human immune system can deal with it.
- Antineoplastic drugs are often given in combination so that they can affect cells in various stages of the cell cycle, including cells that are emerging from rest or moving to a phase of the cycle that is disrupted by these drugs.
- Adverse effects associated with antineoplastic therapy include effects caused by damage to the rapidly multiplying cells, such as bone marrow suppression, which may limit the drug use; GI toxicity, with nausea, vomiting, mouth sores, and diarrhea; and alopecia (hair loss).
- Chemotherapeutic agents should not be used during pregnancy or lactation because they may result in potentially serious adverse effects on the rapidly multiplying cells of the fetus and neonate.
- The newest drugs developed as antineoplastic agents target very specific enzyme systems or processes used by the cancer cells but not by healthy human cells. These drugs are not as toxic to the patient as traditional antineoplastic drugs.

CHECK YOUR UNDERSTANDING

Answers to the questions in this chapter can be found in Answers to Check Your Understanding Questions on thePoint®.

MULTIPLE CHOICE

Select the best answer.

1. Some properties of neoplastic cells are the same as the properties of normal cells, including
   a. anaplasia.
   b. metastasis.
   c. mitosis.
   d. autonomy.

2. Carcinomas are tumors that originate in
   a. mesenchyme.
   b. bone marrow.
   c. striated muscle.
   d. epithelial cells.

3. The goal of traditional antineoplastic drug therapy is to
   a. reduce the size of abnormal cell mass for immune system destruction.
   b. eradicate all of the abnormal cells that have developed.
   c. destroy all cells of the originating type.
   d. stimulate the immune system to destroy the neoplastic cells.

4. Cancer can be a difficult disease to treat because
   a. cells no longer progress through the normal cell cycle.
   b. cells can fail to develop resistance to drug therapy.
   c. cells remain dormant, emerging months to years later.
   d. the exact cause of cancer is not known.

5. Antineoplastic drugs destroy human cells. They are most likely to cause cell death among healthy cells that
   a. have poor cell membranes.
   b. are rapidly turning over.
   c. are in dormant tissues.
   d. are across the blood–brain barrier.

6. Cancer treatment usually occurs in several different treatment phases. In assessing the appropriateness of another round of chemotherapy for a particular patient, the nurse would evaluate which as most important?
   a. Hair loss
   b. Bone marrow function
   c. Anorexia
   d. Heart rate

7. It is important to explain to patients that chemotherapeutic agents should not be used during pregnancy because
   a. the tendency to cause nausea and vomiting will be increased.
   b. of potential serious adverse effects on the rapidly multiplying cells of the fetus.
   c. bone marrow toxicity could alter hormone levels.
   d. patients may be weakened by the drug regimen.

8. Cancer drugs are given in combination and over a period of time because it is difficult to affect
   a. slowly growing cells.
   b. cells in the dormant phase of the cell cycle.
   c. cells that multiply rapidly and go through the cell cycle quickly.
   d. cells that have moved from their normal site in the body.

MULTIPLE RESPONSE

Select all that apply.

1. Which of the following points would be most important for the nurse to stress when developing a patient teaching plan for a patient receiving antineoplastic therapy?
   a. The importance of keeping the head covered at extremes of temperature.
   b. The need to use barrier contraceptives because of the risk of serious fetal effects.
   c. The importance of avoiding exposure to infection because the ability to heal or to fight infection is impaired.
   d. The importance of avoiding food if nausea or vomiting is a problem.
   e. The importance of avoiding digging in the dirt without protective coverings because of the many pathogens that live in the dirt that could cause infection.
   f. The importance of taking periodic rest periods during the day because you will feel tired when your red blood cell count falls.
2. Hair loss, or alopecia, is an adverse effect of many antineoplastic agents. If a client is receiving a drug that usually causes alopecia, it is important that the nurse do which of the following?
   a. Warn the patient that alopecia will occur.
   b. Encourage the patient to arrange for an appropriate head covering at extremes of temperature.
   c. Advise the patient to lie with the legs elevated and head low to promote circulation and prevent hair loss.
   d. Encourage the patient to arrange for a wig or other head covering before the hair loss occurs.
   e. Advise the patient that people will stare and can be rude when hair loss occurs.
   f. Make arrangements for the patient to attend a support group before hair loss happens.

REFERENCES

Brunton, L. L., Hilal-Dandan, R., & Knollman, B. C. (2018). *Goodman and Gilman's the pharmacological basis of therapeutics* (13th ed.). McGraw-Hill.

Centers for Disease Control and Prevention. (2019). *Cancer cluster guidelines update.* https://www.cdc.gov/nceh/clusters/default.htm

Centers for Disease Control and Prevention. (2016). *NIOSH list of antineoplastic and other hazardous drugs in healthcare settings, 2016.* https://www.cdc.gov/niosh/docs/2016-161/default.html

Chabner, B. A., & Roberts, T. G. (2005). Chemotherapy and the war on cancer. *Nature Reviews Cancer, 5*, 65–72. https://doi.org/10.1038/nrc1529

DeVita, V. T., Lawrence, T. S., & Rosenberg, S. A. (2015). *Cancer: Principles and practice of oncology* (10th ed.). Wolters Kluwer Health.

Grochow, L. B., & Ames, M. M. (1998). *A clinician's guide to chemotherapy, pharmacokinetics, and pharmacodynamics.* Williams & Wilkins.

Kaushik, I., Ramachandran, S., & Srivastava, S. K. (2019). CRISPR-Cas9: A multifaceted therapeutic strategy for cancer treatment. *Seminars in Cell and Developmental Biology, 96*, 4–12. https://doi.org/10.1016/j.semcdb.2019.04.018

Liu, B., Saber, A., & Haisma, H. J. (2019). CRSPR/Cas9: A powerful tool for identification of new targets for cancer treatment. *Drug Discovery Today, 24*(4), 955–970. https://doi.org/10.1016/j.drudis.2019.02.011

Meric-Bernstam, F., & Hung, M. (2006). Advances in targeting human epidermal growth factor receptor-2 signaling for cancer therapy. *Clinical Cancer Research, 12*(21), 6326–6334. https://doi.org/10.1158/1078-0432.CCR-06-1732

Nelson, R. (2019, December 19). Prices drop at last for transformative cancer drug. *Medscape Medical News.* https://www.medscape.com/viewarticle/922912#vp_3

Norris, T. L., & Lalchandani, R. (2018). *Porth's pathophysiology: Concepts of altered health states* (10th ed.). Wolters Kluwer.

Schulmeister, L. (2009). Vesicant chemotherapy—The management of extravasation. *Cancer Nursing Practice, 8*(3), 34–37. https://doi.org/10.7748/cnp2009.04.8.3.34.c6979

Torimura, T., Iwamoto, H., Nakamura, T., Koga, H., Ueno, T., Kerbel, R. S., & Sata, M. (2013). Metronomic chemotherapy: Possible clinical application to advanced hepatocellular carcinoma. *Translational Oncology, 6*(5), 511–519. https://doi.org/10.1593/tlo.13481

PART 3

Drugs Acting on the Immune System

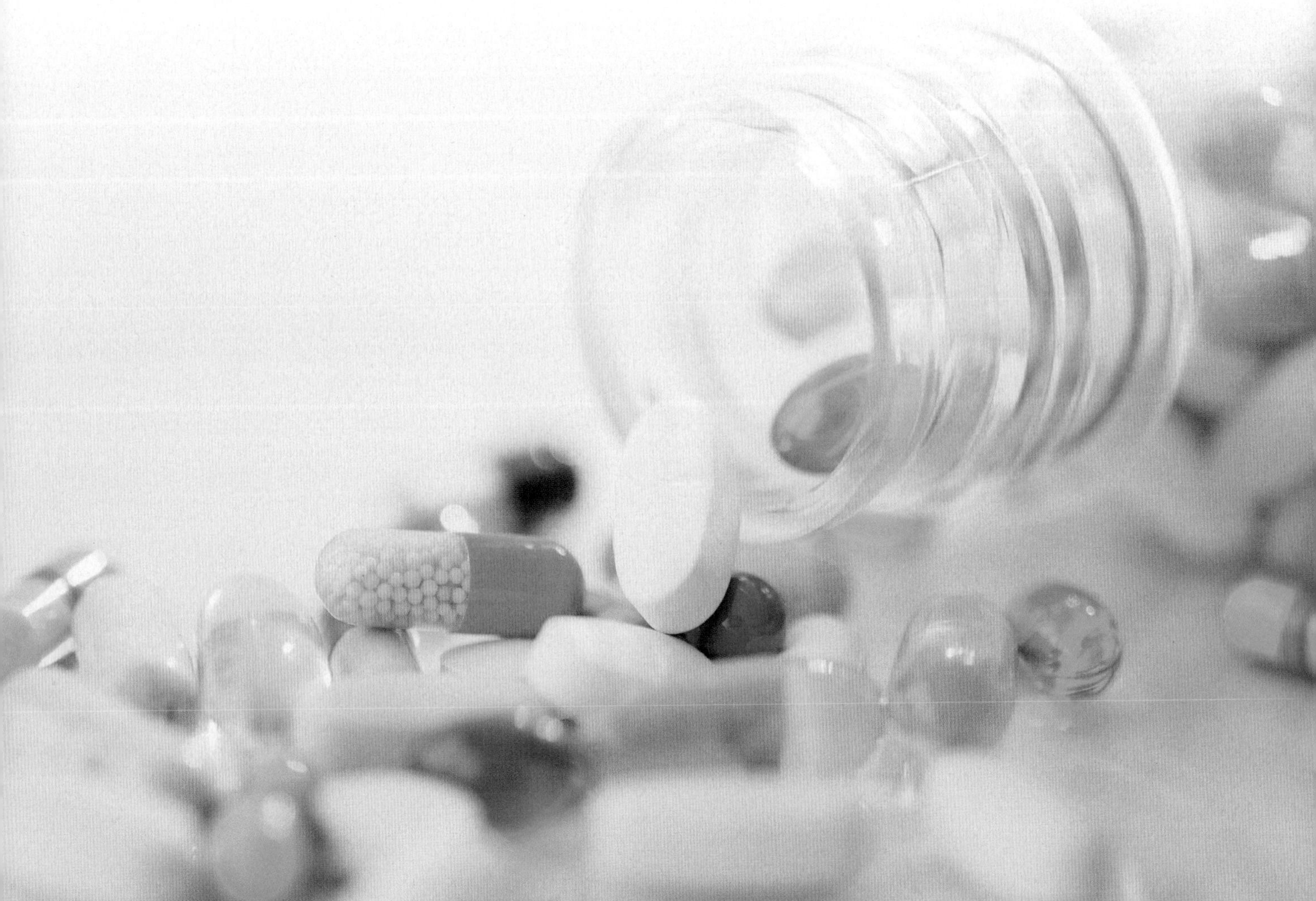

CHAPTER 15

Introduction to the Immune Response and Inflammation

Learning Objectives

Upon completion of this chapter, you will be able to:

1. List four natural body defenses against infection.
2. Describe the cells associated with the body's fight against infection and their basic functions.
3. Outline the sequence of events in the inflammatory response.
4. Correlate the events in the inflammatory response with the clinical picture of inflammation.
5. Outline the sequence of events in an antibody-related immune reaction and correlate these events with the clinical presentation of such a reaction.

Key Terms

antibodies: immunoglobulins; produced by B-cell plasma cells and memory cells in response to a specific protein; react with that protein to cause its destruction directly or through activation of the inflammatory response

antigen: composed of proteins, peptides, and polysaccharides; portions of cell walls; proteins that have potential of facilitating an immune response

arachidonic acid: released from injured cells to stimulate the inflammatory response through activation of various chemical substances

autoimmune disease: a disorder that occurs when the body responds to specific self-antigens to produce antibodies or cell-mediated responses against its own cells

B cells: lymphocytes programmed to recognize specific proteins; when activated, these cells cause the production of antibodies to react with that protein

calor: heat, one of the four cardinal signs of inflammation; caused by activation of the inflammatory response

chemotaxis: property of drawing neutrophils to an area

complement proteins: series of cascading proteins that react with the antigen–antibody complex to destroy the protein or stimulate an inflammatory reaction

dolor: pain, one of the four cardinal signs of inflammation; caused by activation of the inflammatory response

Hageman factor: first factor activated when a blood vessel or cell is injured; starts the cascading reaction of the clotting factors, activates the conversion of plasminogen to plasmin to dissolve clots, and activates the kinin system responsible for activation of the inflammatory response

interferon: type of cytokine that is released in response to viral invasion; blocks viral replication and helps to modulate inflammation

interleukins: chemicals released by white blood cells (WBCs) to communicate with other WBCs and to support the inflammatory and immune reactions

kinin system: system activated by Hageman factor as part of the inflammatory response; includes bradykinin

leukocytes: white blood cells; can be neutrophils, basophils, or eosinophils

lymphocytes: white blood cells with large, varied nuclei; can be T cells, B cells, or natural killer cells

macrophages: mature leukocytes that are capable of phagocytizing an antigen (foreign protein); also called monocytes or mononuclear phagocytes

major histocompatibility complex: the genetic identification code carried on a chromosome; produces several proteins or antigens that allow the body to recognize cells as being self-cells

mast cells: fixed basophils, found in the respiratory and gastrointestinal tracts and in the skin, which release chemical mediators of the inflammatory and immune responses when they are stimulated by local irritation

myelocytes: leukocyte-producing cells in the bone marrow that can develop into neutrophils, basophils, eosinophils, monocytes, or macrophages

phagocytes: neutrophils and macrophages that are able to engulf and digest foreign material

phagocytosis: the process of engulfing and digesting foreign organic materials

pyrogen: fever-causing substance

rubor: redness, one of the four cardinal signs of inflammation; caused by activation of the inflammatory response

T cells: lymphocytes programmed in the thymus gland to recognize self-cells; may be effector T cells, helper T cells, or suppressor T cells

tumor: swelling, one of the four cardinal signs of inflammation; caused by activation of the inflammatory response

The body has many defense systems in place to keep it intact and to protect it from external stressors. These stressors can include bacteria, viruses, other foreign pathogens or nonself-cells, trauma, and exposure to extremes of environmental conditions. The same defense systems that protect the body also help to repair it after cellular trauma or damage. Understanding the basic mechanisms involved in these defense systems helps to explain the actions of the drugs that affect the immune system and inflammation.

Body Defenses

The body's defenses include barrier defenses, cellular defenses, the inflammatory response, and the immune response. Each of these defenses plays a major role in maintaining homeostasis and preventing disease.

Barrier Defenses

Certain anatomical barriers exist to prevent the entry of foreign pathogens and to serve as important lines of defense in protecting the body. These barriers include the skin and mucous membranes, gastric acid, and the major histocompatibility complex (MHC).

Skin

The skin is the first line of defense. The skin acts as a physical barrier to protect the internal tissues and organs of the body. Glands in the skin secrete chemicals that destroy or repel many pathogens. The top layer of the skin falls off daily, which makes it difficult for any pathogen to colonize on the skin. In addition, the normal bacterial flora of the skin helps to destroy many disease-causing pathogens.

Mucous Membranes

Mucous membranes line the areas of the body that are exposed to external influences but do not have the benefit of skin protection. These body areas include the respiratory tract, which is exposed to air; the gastrointestinal (GI) tract, which is exposed to anything ingested by the mouth; and the genitourinary (GU) tract, which is exposed to many pathogens from the perineal and rectal area. Like the skin, the mucous membrane acts as a physical barrier to invasion. It also secretes a sticky mucus capable of trapping and inactivating invaders for later destruction and removal by the body.

In the conducting airways of the respiratory tract, the mucous membrane is lined with tiny, hairlike processes called cilia. The cilia sweep any captured pathogens or foreign materials upward toward the mouth, where they will be swallowed. The cilia also can move the captured material to an area causing irritation, which leads to removal by coughing or sneezing.

In the GI tract, the mucous membrane serves as a protective coating, preventing erosion of GI cells by the acidic environment of the stomach, the digestive enzymes of the small intestine, and the waste products that accumulate in the large intestine. The mucous membrane also secretes mucus that serves as a lubricant throughout the GI tract to facilitate movement of the food bolus and of waste products. The mucous membrane acts as a thick barrier to prevent foreign pathogens from penetrating the GI tract and entering the body.

In the GU tract, the mucous membrane provides direct protection against injury and trauma and traps any pathogens in the area for destruction by the body.

Gastric Acid

The stomach secretes acid in response to many stimuli. The acidity of the stomach not only aids digestion but also destroys many pathogens that are either ingested or swallowed after removal from the respiratory tract. Normal flora that live in this acidic environment also help to destroy many of these ingested pathogens.

Major Histocompatibility Complex

The body's last barrier of defense is the ability to distinguish between self-cells and foreign cells. All of the cells and tissues of each person are marked for identification as part of that individual's genetic code. No two people have exactly the same code. In humans, the genetic identification code is carried on a chromosome and is called the **major histocompatibility complex** (MHC). The MHC produces several proteins called histocompatibility antigens or human leukocyte antigens (HLAs). These **antigens** (proteins) are located on the cell membrane and allow the body to recognize cells as being self-cells. Cells that do not have these proteins are identified as foreign and are targeted for destruction by the body.

Cellular Defenses

Any pathogen that manages to get past the barrier defenses will encounter the human inflammatory and immune systems or the mononuclear phagocyte system (MPS). Previously called the reticuloendothelial system, the MPS is composed primarily of leukocytes, lymphocytes, lymphoid tissues, and numerous chemical mediators.

Stem cells in the bone marrow produce two types of white blood cells or **leukocytes**: lymphocytes and myelocytes. The lymphocytes are the key components of the immune system and consist of T cells, B cells, and natural killer cells (see later discussion of the immune response). The **myelocytes** can develop into a number of different cell types that are important in both the basic inflammatory response and the immune response. Myelocytes include neutrophils, basophils, eosinophils, and monocytes or macrophages (see Fig. 15.1).

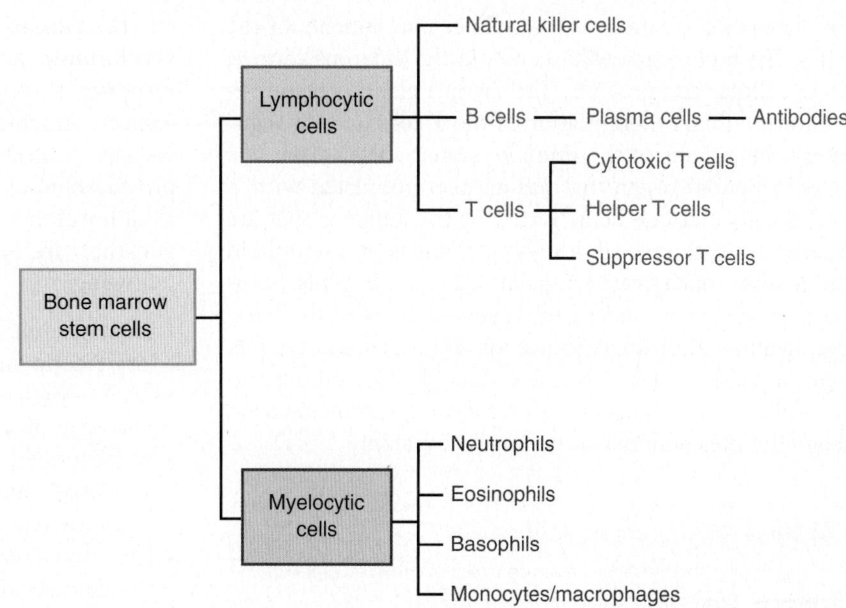

FIGURE 15.1 Types of white blood cells, or leukocytes, produced by the body.

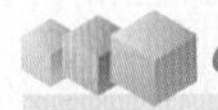
Concept Mastery Alert

Immune System

Lymphocytes are the key components of the immune system. They consist of T cells, B cells, and natural killer cells. Leukocytes are the basis of two types of cells: lymphocytes and myelocytes.

Neutrophils

Neutrophils are polymorphonuclear leukocytes that are capable of moving outside of the bloodstream (diapedesis) and engulfing and digesting foreign material (**phagocytosis**). When the body is injured or invaded by a pathogen, neutrophils are rapidly produced and move to the site of the insult, a property called **chemotaxis**, to attack the foreign substance. Because neutrophils are able to engulf and digest foreign material, they are called **phagocytes**. Phagocytes are able to identify nonself-cells by use of the MHC, and they can engulf these cells or mark them for destruction by cytotoxic T lymphocytes.

Basophils

Basophils are myelocytic leukocytes that are not capable of phagocytosis. They contain chemical substances or mediators that are important for initiating and maintaining an immune or inflammatory response. These substances include histamine, heparin, and other chemicals used in the inflammatory response.

Basophils that are fixed and do not circulate are called **mast cells**. They are found in the respiratory and GI tracts and in the skin. They release many of the chemical mediators of the inflammatory and immune responses when they are stimulated by local irritation.

Eosinophils

Eosinophils are circulating myelocytic leukocytes similar to neutrophils. They are often more numerous during allergic reactions and parasitic infections.

Monocytes/Macrophages

Monocytes or mononuclear phagocytes are also called **macrophages**. These are mature leukocytes that are capable of phagocytizing an antigen. Macrophages help to remove foreign material from the body, including pathogens, debris from dead cells, and necrotic tissue from injury sites, so that the body can heal. They also can process antigens and present them to active lymphocytes for destruction.

Macrophages can circulate in the bloodstream or they can be fixed in specific tissues, such as the Kupffer cells in the liver, the cells in the alveoli of the respiratory tract, and the microglia in the central nervous system (CNS), GI, circulatory, and lymph tissues. As active phagocytes, macrophages release chemicals that are necessary to elicit a strong inflammatory reaction. These cells also respond to chemical mediators released by other cells that are active in the inflammatory and immune responses to increase the intensity of a response and to facilitate the body's reaction.

Lymphoid Tissues

Lymphoid tissues that play an important part in the cellular defense system include the lymph nodes, spleen, thymus gland (a bipolar gland that is located in the middle of the chest and becomes smaller with age), bone marrow, and lymphoid tissue throughout the respiratory and GI tracts. The bone marrow and the thymus gland are important for creation of the cellular components of the MPS. The bone marrow has a role in the differentiation of these cellular components. The thymus gland is responsible for the final differentiation of the T cells and for regulating the actions of the immune system. The spleen is a large lymphoid organ that has an area populated with T and B cells that can be activated by the antigens that are filtered from the blood. The lymph nodes and lymphoid tissue store concentrated populations of neutrophils, basophils, eosinophils, and lymphocytes in areas of the body that facilitate their surveillance for and destruction of foreign proteins. Other cells travel through the cardiovascular and lymph systems to search for foreign proteins or to reach the sites of injury or pathogen invasion.

Key Points

- The body has several defense mechanisms in place to protect it from injury or foreign invasion.
- Barrier defenses include the skin, mucous membranes, normal flora, and gastric acid.
- Cellular defenses include blood cells such as the lymphocytes (T and B cells) and the myelocytes (neutrophils, eosinophils, basophils, and macrophages).

The Inflammatory Response

The inflammatory response is the local reaction of the body to invasion or injury. Any insult to the body that injures cells or tissues sets off a series of events and chemical reactions. Acute inflammation involves both a vascular and a cellular response.

Cell injury causes the activation of a chemical in the plasma called factor XII or **Hageman factor**. Hageman factor is responsible for activating at least three systems in the body: the kinin system, which is discussed here; the clotting cascade, which initiates blood clotting; and the plasminogen system, which initiates the dissolution of blood clots. The last two systems are discussed in Part 8: Drugs Acting on the Cardiovascular System. Hageman factor is an important inflammatory mediator that enhances the vascular phase of inflammation.

Kinin System

The **kinin system** is activated when Hageman factor activates kallikrein, a substance found in the local tissues, which causes the precursor substance kininogen to be converted to bradykinin and other kinins. Bradykinin was the first kinin identified and remains the one that is best understood.

Bradykinin causes local vasodilation and changes in capillary permeability, which brings more blood to the injured area and allows white blood cells to escape into the tissues. It also stimulates nerve endings to cause pain, which alerts the body to the injury.

Bradykinin also causes the cell membrane to release **arachidonic acid**, which stimulates the inflammatory response through activation of various chemical substances. Arachidonic acid is the precursor to many substances called autocoids, including cyclooxygenase, prostacyclin, and thromboxane. These substances act like local hormones that cause an effect in the immediate area and then are broken down. These autocoids include the following:

- Prostaglandins, some of which augment the inflammatory reaction and some of which block it
- Cyclooxygenase, which is involved in inflammation and various protective actions in the body
- Leukotrienes, some of which can cause vasodilation and increased capillary permeability and some of which can block the reactions
- Thromboxanes, which cause local vasoconstriction and facilitate platelet aggregation and blood coagulation

Histamine Release

While this series of Hageman factor–initiated events is proceeding, another locally mediated response is occurring. Injury to a cell membrane causes the local release of histamine. Histamine causes vasodilation, which brings more blood and blood components to the area. It also alters capillary permeability, making it easier for neutrophils and blood chemicals to leave the bloodstream and enter the injured area. In addition, histamine stimulates pain perception. The vasodilation and changes in capillary permeability bring neutrophils to the area to engulf and get rid of the invader or to remove the cell that has been injured.

Chemotaxis and Cellular Phase of Inflammation

Some leukotrienes activated by arachidonic acid have a property called chemotaxis, which is the ability to attract neutrophils and to stimulate them and other macrophages in the area to be very aggressive. The leukocytes are attracted to the capillaries that are permeable, and the cells are able to leave circulation to act on the exact site of tissue injury. Activation of the neutrophils and release of other chemicals in the area can lead to cell injury and destruction. When destroyed, the cell releases various lysosomal enzymes that dissolve or destroy cell membranes and cellular proteins. The lysosomal enzymes are an important part of biological recycling and the breakdown of once-living tissues after death. In the case of an inflammatory reaction, they can cause local cellular breakdown and further inflammation, which can develop into a vicious cycle leading to cell death.

Acute inflammation is a response to cellular injury that can last from minutes to a few days. It is protective and part of the process of tissue healing. Unlike acute inflammation, chronic inflammation may last weeks, months, or even years. It can be harmful by stimulating more cellular damage and even causing healthy tissue to become scarred and/or fibrotic.

Many inflammatory diseases, such as rheumatoid arthritis and systemic lupus erythematosus, are examples of these uncontrolled cycles. The prostaglandins and leukotrienes are important to the inflammatory response because they act to moderate the reaction, thus preventing this destructive cycle from happening on a regular basis. Many of the drugs used to affect the inflammatory and immune systems modify or interfere with these inflammatory reactions.

Clinical Presentation

Activation of the acute inflammatory response produces a characteristic clinical picture. The Latin words *calor*, *tumor*, *rubor*, and *dolor* describe a typical inflammatory reaction. **Calor**, or heat, occurs because of the increased blood flow to the area. **Tumor**, or swelling, occurs because of the fluid that leaks into the tissues as a result of the change in capillary permeability. **Rubor**, or redness, is also related to the increase in blood flow caused by the vasodilation. **Dolor**, or pain, comes from the activation of pain fibers by histamine and the kinin system. These signs and symptoms occur any time a cell is injured (see Fig. 15.2). For example, if you scratch the top of your hand and wait for about a minute, the direct line of the scratch will be red (rubor) and raised (tumor). If you feel it gently, it will be warmer than the surrounding area (calor). You should also experience a burning sensation or discomfort at the site of the scratch (dolor). These same signs occur all over the body. For example, invasion of the lungs by bacteria can produce pneumonia. If the lungs could be examined closely, they would show the four signs of inflammation. They would be red from increased blood flow; fluid would start to leak out of the capillaries (often this can be heard as rales); the patient would complain of chest discomfort; and the increased blood flow to the area of infection would make it appear hot or very active on a scan. No matter what the cause of the insult, the body's local response is the same.

Once the inflammatory response is under way and neutrophils become active, engulfing and digesting injured cells or the invader, they release a chemical that is a natural **pyrogen**, or fever-causing substance. This pyrogen resets specific neurons in the hypothalamus to maintain a higher body temperature, seen clinically as a fever. The higher temperature acts as a catalyst for many of the body's chemical reactions, making the inflammatory and

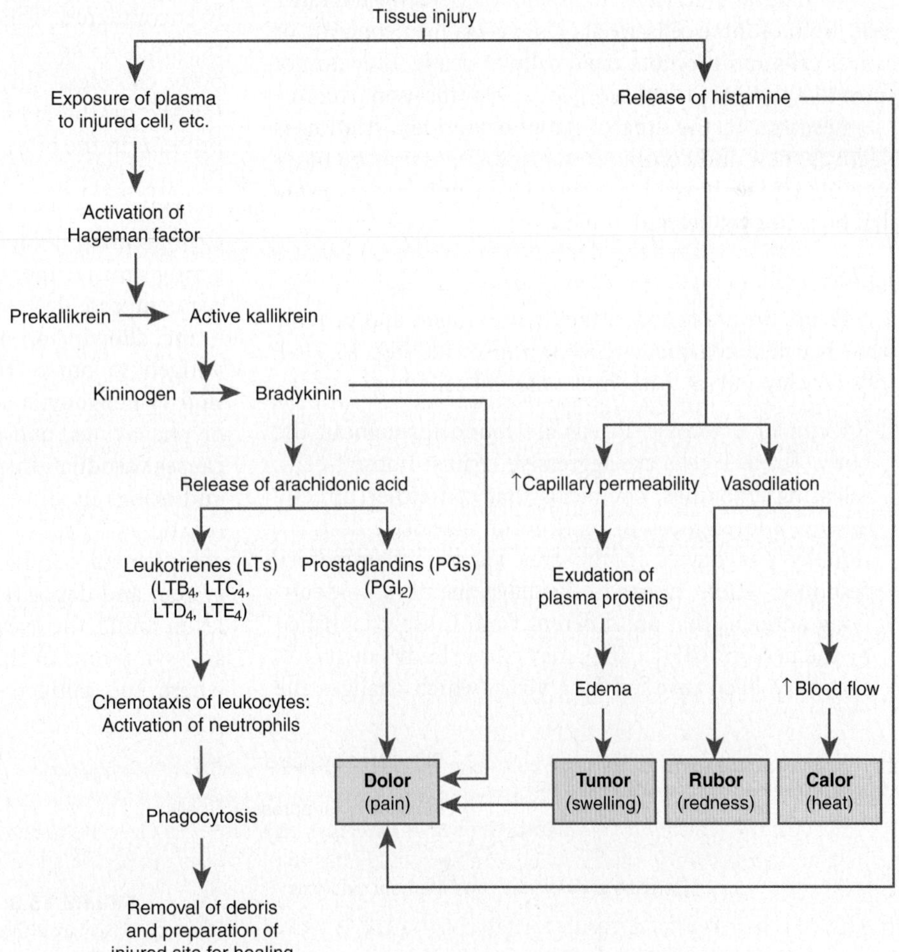

FIGURE 15.2 The inflammatory response in relation to the four cardinal signs of inflammation.

immune responses more effective. Treating fevers remains a controversial subject because lowering a fever decreases the efficiency of the immune and inflammatory responses.

The leukotrienes (autocoids activated through the kinin system) affect the brain to induce slow-wave sleep, which is believed to be an important energy conservation measure for fighting the invader. They also cause myalgia and arthralgia (muscle and joint pain)—common signs and symptoms of various inflammatory diseases—which also encourage reduced activity and save energy. All of these chemical responses make up the total clinical picture of an inflammatory reaction. When a patient has an infection, you will see these signs and symptoms.

The Immune Response

More specific invasion can stimulate a more specific response through the immune system. As mentioned previously, stem cells in the bone marrow produce lymphocytes that can develop into T lymphocytes (so named because they migrate from the bone marrow to the thymus gland for activation and maturation) or B lymphocytes (so named because they are activated in the bursa of Fabricius in the chicken, although the specific point of activation in humans has not been identified). Other identified lymphocytes include natural killer cells and lymphokine-activated killer cells. Both of these cells are aggressive against neoplastic or cancer cells and promote rapid cellular death. They do not seem to be programmed for specific identification of cells.

Research in the area of lymphocyte identification is relatively new and continues to grow. There may be other lymphocytes with particular roles in the immune response that have not yet been identified.

T Cells

T cells are programmed in the thymus gland and provide what is called cell-mediated immunity (see Fig. 15.3). T cells develop into at least three different cell types:

1. Effector or cytotoxic T cells are found throughout the body. These T cells are aggressive against nonself-cells, releasing cytokines, chemicals that can either directly destroy a foreign cell or mark it for aggressive destruction by phagocytes in the area via an inflammatory response. These nonself-cells have membrane-identifying antigens that are different from those established by the person's MHC. They may be the body's own cells that have been invaded by a virus, which changes the cell membrane, neoplastic cancer cells, or transplanted foreign cells.
2. Helper T cells, also called CD4 cells, respond to the chemical indicators of immune activity and stimulate other lymphocytes, including B cells, to be more aggressive and responsive.
3. Suppressor T cells, also called CD8 cells, respond to rising levels of chemicals associated with an immune response to suppress or slow the reaction. The balance of the helper and suppressor T cells allows for a rapid response to body injury or invasion by pathogens, which may destroy foreign antigens immediately and then be followed by a slowing reaction if the invasion continues. This slowing allows the body to conserve energy and the components of the immune and inflammatory reaction necessary for basic protection and to prevent cellular destruction from a continued inflammatory reaction.

B Cells

B cells are found throughout the MPS in groups called clones. B cells are programmed to identify specific proteins or antigens. They provide what is called humoral immunity (see Fig. 15.4). When a B cell reacts with its specific antigen, it changes to become a plasma cell. Plasma cells produce **antibodies**, or immunoglobulins, which circulate in the body and react with this specific antigen when it is encountered. This is a direct chemical reaction. When the antigen and antibody react, they form an antigen–antibody complex. This new structure reveals a new receptor site on the antibody that activates a series of plasma proteins in the body called complement proteins.

Complement Proteins

Complement proteins react in a cascade fashion to form a ring around the antigen–antibody complex. The complement can destroy the antigen by altering the membrane, allowing an osmotic inflow of fluid that causes the antigen to burst. They also induce chemotaxis (attraction of phagocytic cells to the area), increase the activity of phagocytes, and release histamine. Histamine release causes vasodilation, which increases blood flow to the area and brings in all of the components of the inflammatory reaction to destroy the antigen. The antigen–antibody–complement complex precipitates out of the circulatory system and deposits in various sites, including end arteries in joints, the eyes, the kidneys, and the skin. The signs and symptoms of the inflammatory response can be seen where the antigen–antibody complexes are deposited.

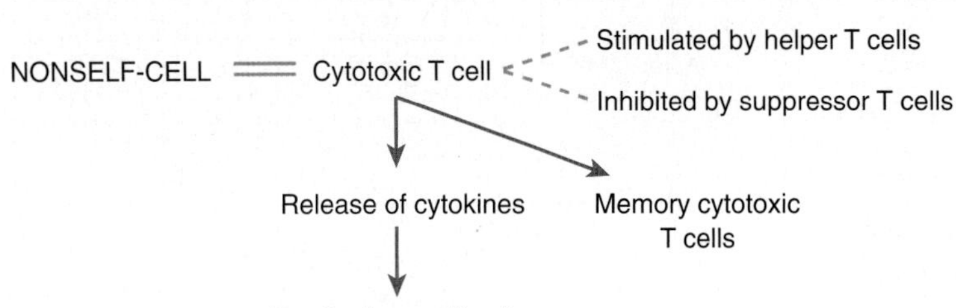

FIGURE 15.3 Cell-mediated immune response. Cytotoxic T cells are activated when recognizing a nonself-cell. Memory T cells are formed. Cytokines are released to destroy the nonself-cell.

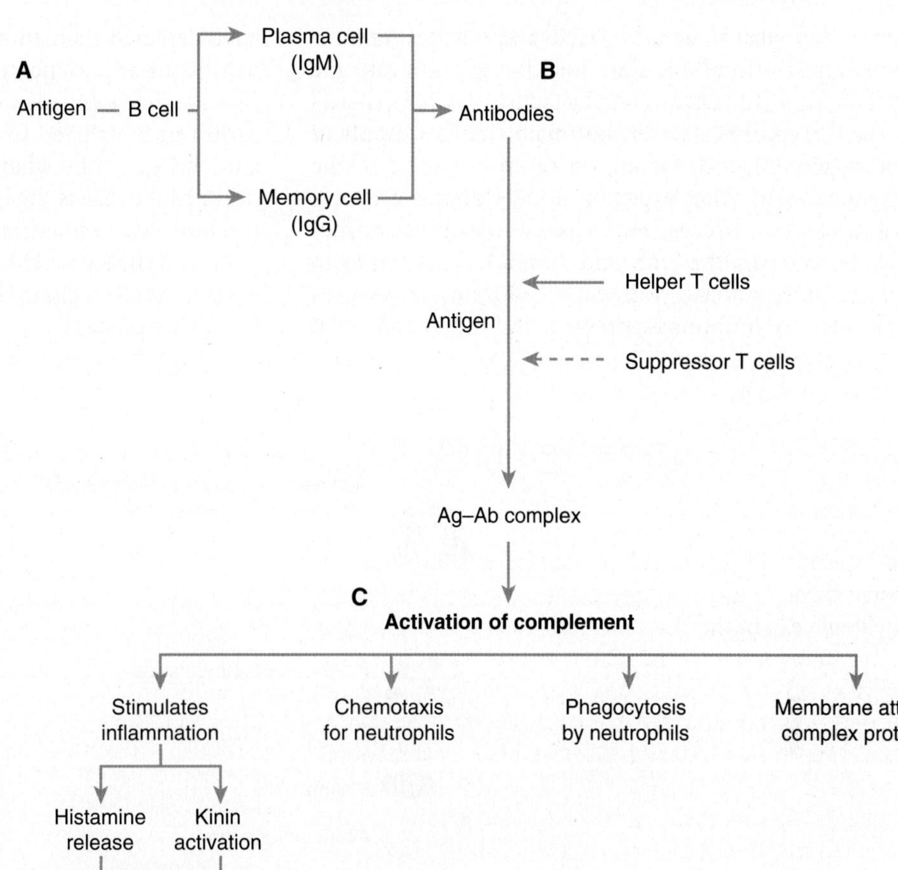

FIGURE 15.4 The humoral immune response. **A.** A B cell reacts with a specific antigen to form plasma cells and memory cells, which produce antibodies. **B.** Circulating antibodies react with the antigen to form an antigen–antibody (Ag–Ab) complex. This process is facilitated by helper T cells and suppressed by suppressor T cells. **C.** The Ag–Ab complex activates circulating complement proteins, which facilitates an aggressive inflammatory reactions, increases chemotaxis and phagocytosis of neutrophils, and forms a membrane attack complex protein. **D.** All of the actions of complement enhance antigen lysis.

Chickenpox eruptions are an example of an antigen–antibody–complement complex that deposits in the skin and causes a local inflammatory reaction.

Antibody Formation

The initial formation of antibodies, or primary response, takes several days. Once activated, the B cells form memory cells that will produce antibodies for immediate release in the future if the antigen is encountered. The antibodies are released in the form of immunoglobulins. Five different types of immunoglobulins have been identified:

- The first immunoglobulin released is M (IgM), which contains the antibodies produced at first exposure to the antigen.
- IgG contains antibodies made by the memory cells that circulate and enter the tissue; most of the immunoglobulin found in the serum is IgG.
- IgA is found in tears, saliva, sweat, mucus, and bile. It is secreted by plasma cells in the GI and respiratory tracts and in epithelial cells. These antibodies react with specific pathogens that are encountered in exposed areas of the body.
- IgE is present in small amounts and seems to be related to allergic responses and to the activation of mast cells.
- IgD is another identified immunoglobulin whose role has not been determined. However, it is found primarily on B lymphocyte cell membranes so it may function in B-cell differentiation.

This process of antibody formation, called acquired or active immunity, is a lifelong reaction. For example, a person exposed to chickenpox will have a mild respiratory reaction when the virus (varicella) first enters the respiratory tract. There will then be a 2- to 3-week incubation period as the body is forming IgM antibodies and preparing to attack any chickenpox virus that appears. The chickenpox virus enters a cell and multiplies. The cell eventually ruptures and ejects more viruses into the system. When this happens, the body responds with the immediate release of antibodies, and a full-scale antigen–antibody response is seen throughout the body. Fever, myalgia, arthralgia, and skin lesions are all part of the immune response to the virus. Once all of the invading chickenpox viruses have been destroyed or have entered the CNS to safely hibernate away from the antibodies, the clinical signs and symptoms resolve. (Varicella can enter the CNS and stay dormant for many years. The antibodies are not able to cross into the CNS, and the virus remains unaffected while it stays there.)

The B memory cells will continue to make a supply of immunoglobulin, IgG, for use on future exposure to the chickenpox virus. That exposure usually does not evolve into a clinical case because the viruses are destroyed immediately on entering the body and do not have a chance to multiply. Older patients with weakened immune systems, people who are immunosuppressed, and individuals who have depleted their immune system fighting an infection or who are experiencing a prolonged stress reaction are at risk for development of shingles if they had chickenpox earlier in their lives. The dormant virus, which has aged and changed somewhat, is able to leave the CNS along a nerve root because the immunosuppressed body is slow to respond. The antibodies do eventually respond to the varicella, and the signs and symptoms of shingles occur as the virus is attacked along the nerve root. Figure 15.5 outlines this entire process.

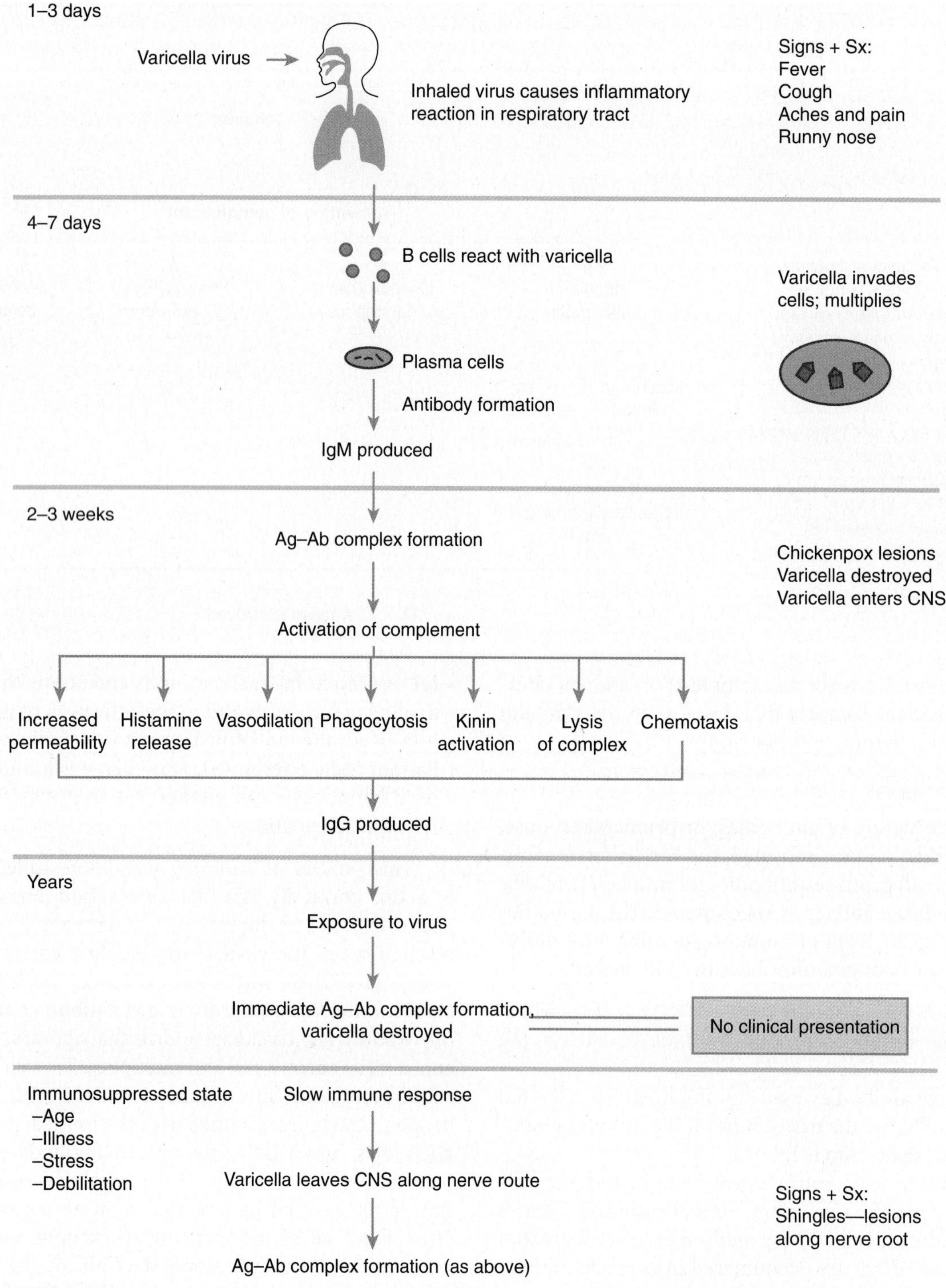

FIGURE 15.5 Process of response to varicella exposure in humans. Ag–Ab, antigen–antibody complex; Ig, immunoglobulin.

B clones cluster in areas where they are most likely to encounter the specific antigen that they have been programmed to recognize. For example, pathogens or antigens that are introduced into the body via the respiratory tract will encounter the B cells in the tonsils and upper respiratory tract; antigens that enter the body through the GI tract will meet their B cells situated in the esophagus and GI tract. Theorists believe that the B cells are programmed genetically and are formed by the time of birth. Clones of B cells contain similar cells. The introduction of an antigen to which there are no preprogrammed B cells could result in widespread disease because the body would have no way of responding. A major concern about space travel has always been the introduction of a completely new antigen to Earth; for this reason, long decontamination processes are used after rocks or debris are brought back to Earth. Germ warfare research is ongoing in some countries to develop an antigen that has not been seen before and to which people would have no response.

Other Mediators

Several other factors also play an important role in the immune reaction. **Interferons** are chemicals (types of cytokines) that are secreted by cells that have been invaded by viruses and possibly by other stimuli. The interferons prevent viral replication and also suppress malignant cell replication and tumor growth.

Interleukins are chemicals secreted by active leukocytes to influence other leukocytes. Interleukin-1 (IL-1) stimulates T and B cells to initiate an immune response. IL-2 is released from active T cells to stimulate the production of more T cells and to increase the activity of B cells, cytotoxic cells, and natural killer cells. Interleukins also cause fever, arthralgia, and myalgia and induce slow-wave sleep—all things that help the body to conserve energy for use in fighting off the invader. Several other factors released by lymphocytes and basophils have been identified. These include interleukins such as B-cell growth factor, macrophage-activating factor, macrophage-inhibiting factor, platelet-activating factor, eosinophil chemotactic factor, and neutrophil chemotactic factor.

The thymus gland also releases a number of hormones that aid in the maturation of T cells and that circulate in the body to stimulate and communicate with T cells. Thymosin, a thymus hormone that has been replicated, is important in the maturation of T cells and cell-mediated immunity. Research is ongoing on the use of thymosin in certain leukemias and melanomas to stimulate the immune response.

Tumor necrosis factor (TNF), a cytokine, is a chemical released by macrophages that inhibits tumor growth and can actually cause tumor regression. It also works with other chemicals to make the inflammatory and immune responses more aggressive and efficient. Research is ongoing to determine the therapeutic effectiveness of TNF. TNF receptor sites are now available for injection into patients with acute rheumatoid arthritis. These receptor sites react with TNF released by the macrophages in this inflammatory disease. All of these chemicals act as communication factors within the immune system, allowing coordination of the immune response.

Interrelationship of the Immune and Inflammatory Responses

The immune and inflammatory responses work together to protect the body and to maintain a level of homeostasis within the body. Both Hageman factor and histamine help to increase capillary permeability so that neutrophils are able to leave the capillaries to go to damaged tissue and engulf pathogens. Helper T cells stimulate the activity of B cells and effector T cells. Suppressor T cells monitor the chemical activity in the body and act to suppress B-cell and T-cell activity when the foreign antigen is under control. Both B cells and T cells ultimately depend on an effective inflammatory reaction to achieve the end goal of destruction of the foreign protein or cell (see Fig. 15.6).

Key Points

- The response to the inflammatory stimuli involves local vasodilation, increased capillary permeability, and the stimulation of pain fibers. These reactions alert the person to the injury and increase blood flow to the area.
- The immune response provides a specific reaction to foreign cells or proteins.
- T cells can be cytotoxic, destroying nonself-cells; helper, augmenting an immune reaction; or suppressor, dampening the immune response to save energy and prevent cell damage.
- B cells produce antibodies in response to exposure to specific antigens or proteins. Antibodies react with the specific antigen to produce an antigen–antibody complex that activates complement proteins and will result in destruction of the antigen.
- Other mediators that affect the immune and inflammatory responses include interferons, tumor necrosis factor, and interleukins.
- The immune and inflammatory responses work together to protect the body from injury or foreign pathogens.

Pathophysiology Involving the Immune System

Several conditions can arise that cause problems involving the immune system. These conditions, many of which are treated by drugs that stimulate or suppress the immune system, include neoplasms, viral invasion, autoimmune disease, and transplant rejection.

Neoplasms

Neoplasms occur when mutant cells escape the normal surveillance of the immune system and begin to grow and multiply. This can happen in many ways. For example, aging causes a decreased efficiency of the immune

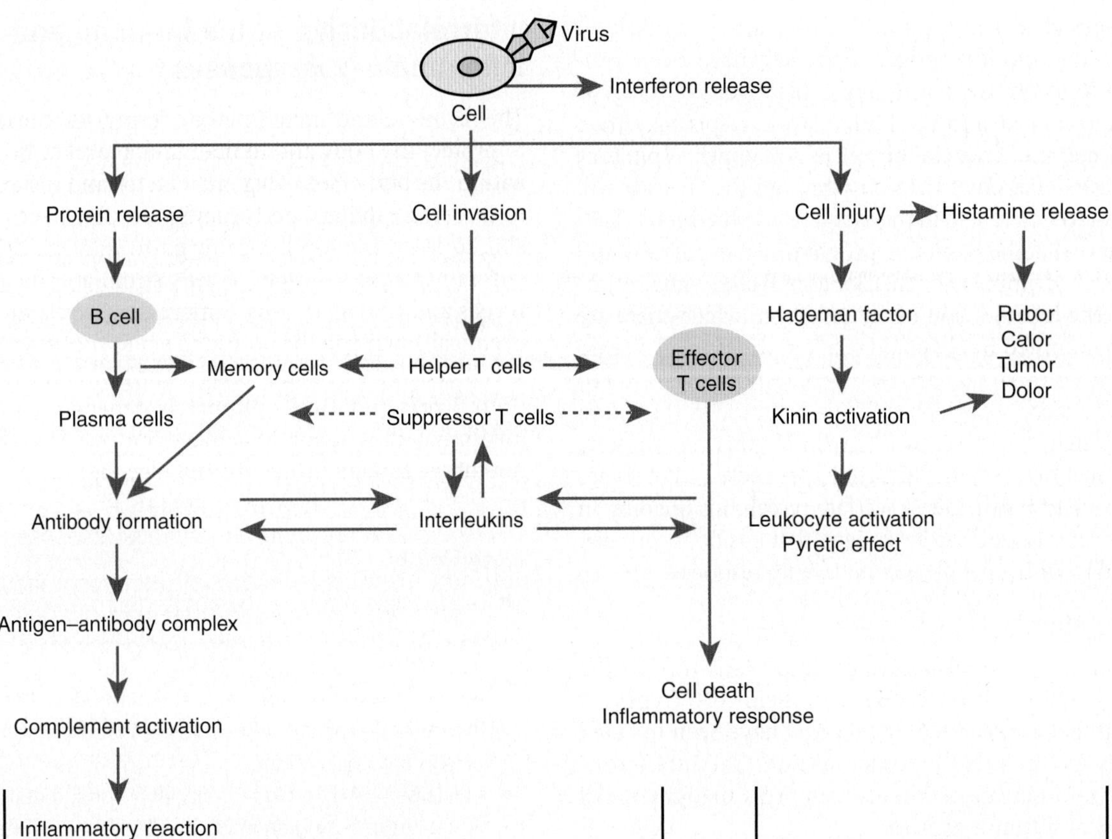

FIGURE 15.6 Interrelationship of immune and inflammatory reactions.

system, allowing some cells to escape detection. Location of the mutant cells can make it difficult for lymphocytes to get to an area to respond. Mutant cells in breast tissue, for example, are not well perfused with blood and may escape detection until they are quite abundant. Sometimes cells are able to avoid detection by the T cells until the growing mass of cells is so large that the immune system cannot deal with it. Tumors also can produce blocking antibodies that cover the antigen receptor sites on the tumor and prevent recognition by cytotoxic T cells. In addition, a weakly antigenic tumor may develop; such a tumor elicits a mild response from the immune system and somehow tricks the T cells into allowing it to survive.

Viral Invasion of Cells

Viruses are parasites that can survive only by invading a host cell that provides the nourishment necessary for viral replication. Invasion of a cell alters the cell membrane and the antigenic presentation of the cell (the MHC). This change can activate cellular immunity, or it can be so subtle that the immune system's response to the cell is mild or absent. In some cases, the response activates a cellular immune reaction to normal cells similar to the one that was invaded. This is one theory for the development of autoimmune disease.

Autoimmune Disease

Autoimmune disease occurs when the body responds to specific self-antigens to produce antibodies or cell-mediated immune responses against its own cells. The cause of autoimmune disease is not known, but theories speculate that (a) it could be a result of response to a cell that was invaded by a virus, leading to production of antibodies for similar cells; (b) production of autoantibodies is a normal process that goes on all the time, but in a state of immunosuppression, the suppressor T cells do not suppress autoantibody production; or (c) there is a genetic predisposition to develop autoantibodies.

Transplant Rejection

With the growing field of organ transplantation, more is being learned about the reaction to foreign cells that are introduced into the body. Typically, self-transplantation, or autotransplantation, results in no immune response. All other transplants produce an immune reaction. Therefore, matching a donor's HLA markers as closely as possible to those of the recipient for histocompatibility is essential. The more closely the foreign cells can be matched, the less aggressive the immune reaction to the donated tissue will be.

SUMMARY

- The body has several defense mechanisms in place to protect it from injury or foreign invasion: the skin, mucous membranes, normal flora, gastric acid, and the inflammatory and immune responses.
- The inflammatory response is a general response to any cell injury and involves activation of various chemicals and neutrophil activity, particularly the activation of Hageman factor to stimulate the kinin system and release of histamine from injured cells to generate local inflammatory responses.
- The clinical presentation of an inflammatory reaction is heat (calor), redness (rubor), swelling (tumor), and pain (dolor).
- The immune response is specific to an antigen or protein that has entered the body and involves B cells, antibodies, and T cells.
- Several types of T cells exist: effector or cytotoxic T cells, helper T cells, and suppressor T cells. Effector or cytotoxic T cells immediately destroy foreign cells. Helper T cells stimulate the immune and inflammatory reactions. Suppressor T cells dampen the immune and inflammatory responses to conserve energy and prevent cellular damage.
- B cells are programmed to recognize specific proteins or foreign antigens. Once in contact with a specific protein, the B cell produces antibodies (immunoglobulins) that react directly with the protein.
- Reaction of an antibody with the specific receptor site on the protein activates the complement cascade of proteins and lyses the associated protein or precipitates an aggressive inflammatory reaction around it.
- Other chemicals are involved in communication among parts of the immune system and in local response to invasion. Any of these chemicals has the potential to alter the immune response.
- The T cells, B cells, and inflammatory reaction work together to protect the body from invasion, limit the response to that invasion, and return the body to a state of homeostasis.
- Patient problems that occur within the immune system include the development of neoplasms, viral invasions of cells that trigger immune responses, autoimmune diseases, and rejection of transplanted organs.

CHECK YOUR UNDERSTANDING

Answers to the questions in this chapter can be found in Answers to Check Your Understanding Questions on thePoint®.

MULTIPLE CHOICE

Select the best answer.

1. Antibodies
   a. are carbohydrates.
   b. are secreted by activated T cells.
   c. are not found in circulating gamma globulins.
   d. are effective only against specific antigens.

2. B and T cells are similar in that they both
   a. secrete antibodies.
   b. play important roles in the immune response.
   c. are activated in the thymus gland.
   d. release cytotoxins to destroy cells.

3. Which of the following is not a cytokine?
   a. Interleukin-2
   b. Antibody
   c. Tumor necrosis factor
   d. Interferon

4. As part of the nonspecific defense against infection,
   a. blood flow and vascular permeability to proteins increase throughout the circulatory system.
   b. particles in the respiratory tract are engulfed by phagocytes.
   c. B cells are released from the bone marrow.
   d. neutrophils release lysosomes, heparin, and kininogen into the extracellular fluid.

5. B cells respond to an initial antigen challenge by
   a. reducing in size.
   b. immediately producing antigen-specific antibodies.
   c. producing a large number of cells that are unlike the original B cell.
   d. producing new cells that become plasma cells and memory cells.

6. Treating fevers remains a controversial subject because higher temperatures
   a. make people feel ill.
   b. act as catalysts to many of the body's chemical reactions.
   c. can suppress the body's normal metabolism.
   d. alter the body's hormone levels, particularly that of progesterone.

7. After describing the function of T cells, the nurse would identify the need for additional teaching if the patient stated that T cells become which type of cells?
   a. Cytotoxic T cells
   b. Helper T cells
   c. Suppressor T cells
   d. Antibody-secreting T cells

8. Interleukins are
   a. chemicals released when a virus enters a cell.
   b. chemicals secreted by activated leukocytes.
   c. part of the kinin system.
   d. activated by arachidonic acid.

MULTIPLE RESPONSE

Select all that apply.

1. Which of the following statements could be used to describe a neutrophil?
   a. They possess the property of phagocytosis.
   b. When activated, they release a pyrogen that causes fever.
   c. When the body is injured, they are produced rapidly and in large numbers.
   d. They are not capable of movement outside the circulatory system.
   e. They are most often seen in response to an allergic reaction.
   f. They float around in the blood and release chemicals in response to injury.

2. The inflammatory response is activated whenever cell injury occurs. An inflammatory response would involve which activities?
   a. Activation of Hageman factor
   b. Vasodilation in the area of the injury
   c. Generalized edema and tumor development
   d. Changes in capillary permeability to allow proteins to leak out of the capillaries
   e. Activation of complement proteins
   f. Production of interferon

REFERENCES

Abbas, A., & Lichtman, A. (2015). *Basic immunology* (5th ed.). W.B. Saunders.

Brunton, L., Hilal-Dandan, R., & Knollman, B. (2018). *Goodman and Gilman's the pharmacological basis of therapeutics* (13th ed.). McGraw-Hill.

Doan, T., Melvold, R., Viselli, S., & Waltenbaugh, C. (2007). *Lippincott's illustrated reviews: Immunology*. Lippincott Williams & Wilkins.

Ganong, W. (2017). *Review of medical physiology* (25th ed.). Appleton & Lange.

Guyton, A., & Hall, J. (2015). *Textbook of medical physiology* (13th ed.). W.B. Saunders.

Norris, T. L. (2019). *Porth's pathophysiology concepts of altered health states*. Wolters Kluwer.

Peakman, M., & Vergani, D. (2009). *Basic and clinical immunology* (2nd ed.). Churchill-Livingstone.

Sompayrac, L. (2015). *How the immune system works* (5th ed.). Blackwell Science.

CHAPTER 16

Antiinflammatory, Antiarthritis, and Related Agents

Learning Objectives

Upon completion of this chapter, you will be able to:

1. Describe the sites of action of the various antiinflammatory agents.
2. Describe the therapeutic actions, indications, pharmacokinetics, contraindications, most common adverse reactions, and important drug–drug interactions associated with each class of antiinflammatory agents.
3. Discuss the use of antiinflammatory drugs across the lifespan.
4. Compare and contrast the prototype drugs for each class of antiinflammatory drugs with the other drugs in that class.
5. Outline the nursing considerations and teaching needs for patients receiving each class of antiinflammatory agents.

Key Terms

analgesic: compound with pain-blocking properties, capable of producing analgesia

antiinflammatory agents: drugs that block the effects of the inflammatory response

antipyretic: fever-blocking property; often achieved by direct effects on the thermoregulatory center in the hypothalamus or by blockade of prostaglandin mediators

chrysotherapy: treatment with gold salts in which gold is taken up by macrophages, which then inhibit phagocytosis; it can be very toxic and is reserved for use in patients who are unresponsive to conventional therapy

disease-modifying antirheumatic drugs (DMARDs): class of medications that are designed to treat inflammatory arthritis disease processes; they can also help to treat some connective tissue disorders, inflammatory bowel disease, and some cancers

gout: disorders that are related to increased blood uric acid and urate crystal deposits in joints and kidneys

inflammatory bowel disease: two disorders (Crohn's disease and ulcerative colitis) that both are characterized by chronic inflammation of the gastrointestinal tract; they are related but also have unique characteristics

inflammatory response: the body's nonspecific response to cell injury, resulting in pain, swelling, heat, and redness in the affected area

nonsteroidal antiinflammatory drugs (NSAIDs): drugs that block prostaglandin synthesis and reduce inflammation, as well as have antipyretic and analgesic properties

salicylates: salicylic acid compounds, used as antiinflammatory, antipyretic, and analgesic agents; they block the prostaglandin system

salicylism: syndrome associated with high levels of salicylates—dizziness, ringing in the ears, difficulty hearing, nausea, vomiting, diarrhea, mental confusion, and lassitude

Drug List

SALICYLATES
(P) aspirin
balsalazide
choline magnesium trisalicylate
diflunisal
mesalamine
olsalazine
salsalate
sulfasalazine

NONSTEROIDAL ANTI-INFLAMMATORY AND RELATED AGENTS

Nonsteroidal Anti-inflammatory Agents (NSAIDs)

Propionic Acids
fenoprofen
flurbiprofen
(P) ibuprofen
ketoprofen
naproxen
oxaprozin

Acetic Acids
diclofenac

etodolac
indomethacin
ketorolac
nabumetone
sulindac
tolmetin
Fenamates
meclofenamate
mefenamic acid
Oxicam Derivatives
meloxicam
piroxicam

Cyclooxygenase-2 Inhibitor
Celecoxib

Related Agent
(P) acetaminophen

ANTIARTHRITIS AGENTS

Gold Compound
(P) auranofin

Tumor Necrosis Factor Blockers
adalimumab
certolizumab
(P) etanercept
golimumab
infliximab

OTHER ANTIARTHRITIS DRUGS
anakinra
hyaluronidase derivatives
leflunomide
penicillamine
sarilumab
sodium hyaluronate
tofacitinib

ANTIGOUT/ HYPERURICEMIA AGENTS
allopurinol
(P) colchicine
febuxostat
pegloticase
probenecid

The **inflammatory response** is designed to protect the body from injury and pathogens. It employs a variety of potent chemical mediators to produce the reaction that helps to destroy pathogens and promote healing. As the body reacts to these chemicals, it produces signs and symptoms of disease, such as swelling, fever, aches, and pains. Occasionally, the inflammatory response becomes a chronic condition and can result in damage to the body, leading to increased inflammatory reactions. **Inflammatory bowel disease** (Crohn's disease and ulcerative colitis) is an example of how chronic inflammation (in this case, of the gastrointestinal tract) can damage tissues and cause significant distress to individuals. Another example is **gout**, which refers to a group of disorders that are characterized by hyperuricemia and urate crystal deposits in joints and kidneys. Often people with gout suffer from gouty arthritis attacks that may be alleviated by antiinflammatory medications. **Antiinflammatory agents** generally block or alter the chemical reactions associated with the inflammatory response to stop one or more of the signs and symptoms of inflammation.

Antiinflammatory, Antiarthritis, and Related Agents

Several different types of drugs are used as antiinflammatory agents. Corticosteroids (discussed in Chapter 36) are used systemically to block the inflammatory and immune systems. Blocking these important protective processes may produce many adverse effects, including decreased resistance to infection and neoplasms. Corticosteroids also are used topically to produce a local antiinflammatory effect without as many adverse effects. Antihistamines (discussed in Chapter 54) are used to block the action of histamine in the initiation of the inflammatory response. Many of the immune-modulating agents are used to block or decrease the effects of inflammation in chronic disorders such as rheumatoid arthritis and Crohn's disease (discussed in Chapter 17). In this chapter, discussion of antiinflammatory agents primarily focuses on drugs that have a direct effect on the inflammatory response, including salicylates, nonsteroidal antiinflammatory and related agents, and antiarthritis drugs.

Because many antiinflammatory drugs are available over the counter (OTC), there is a potential for misuse and overdosing. In addition, patients may take these drugs and block the signs and symptoms of a present illness, thus potentially leading to a misdiagnosis of a problem. Patients also may combine these drugs and unknowingly induce toxicity. All of these drugs have adverse effects that can be dangerous if toxic levels of drug circulate in the body. See Box 16.1 for information on using these drugs with various age groups.

Salicylates

Salicylates (Table 16.1) are antiinflammatory agents not only because of their ability to block the inflammatory response but also because of their **antipyretic** (fever-blocking) and **analgesic** (pain-blocking) properties. Salicylates are some of the oldest antiinflammatory drugs used. They were extracted from willow bark, poplar trees, and other plants by ancient peoples to treat fever, pain, and what we now call inflammation. They are generally available without prescription and are relatively nontoxic when used as directed. Aspirin (*Bayer*, *Empirin*, and others) is available OTC. Additional synthetic salicylates include balsalazide (*Colazal*, *Glazo*), choline magnesium trisalicylate (*Tricosal*), diflunisal (generic), mesalamine (*Pentasa* and others), olsalazine (*Dipentum*), salsalate (*Amigesic*), and sulfasalazine (*Azulfidine*). A person who does not respond to one salicylate may respond to a different one.

Box 16.1  **Focus on Drug Therapy Across the Lifespan**

ANTIINFLAMMATORY AGENTS

Children

Care must be taken to make sure that the child receives the correct dose of any antiinflammatory agent. This can be a problem because many of these drugs are available in over the counter (OTC) pain, cold, flu, and combination products. Parents need to be taught to read the label to find out the ingredients and the dose they are giving the child.

Choline magnesium trisalicylate and aspirin (though not as the first choice) are the only salicylates recommended for children. They should not be used when any risk of Reye's syndrome exists; this includes when the child has had a viral infection (influenza, chickenpox, etc.), who becomes febrile or lethargic, or who has personality changes.

Ibuprofen, naproxen, tolmetin, meloxicam, and, in some cases, indomethacin are the NSAIDs approved for use in children.

Acetaminophen is the most used analgesic/antipyretic drug for children. Care must be taken to avoid overdose, which can cause severe hepatotoxicity. Dosages available in OTC products have been reduced; parents need to be cautioned about combining products.

Children with arthritis may receive treatment with gold salts or etanercept; they must be monitored very closely for toxic effects.

Adults

To avoid serious toxic effects, adults need to be cautioned about the presence of these drugs in many OTC products and taught to be aware of exactly what they are taking. They should also be cautioned to report OTC drug use to their health care provider when they are receiving any other prescription drug to avoid possible drug–drug interactions and the masking of signs and symptoms of disease.

Patients who are pregnant or breast or chestfeeding should not use these drugs unless the benefit clearly outweighs the potential risk to the fetus or neonate. Salicylates, NSAIDs, and gold products have potentially severe adverse effects on the neonate and possibly the parent. Acetaminophen can be used cautiously if a pain preparation or antipyretic is needed. Nondrug measures should be taken when at all possible to decrease the potential risk. Patients who are pregnant or breast or chestfeeding also need to be urged to avoid OTC drugs unless they are suggested by their health care providers.

Older Adults

Older adult patients may be more susceptible to the CNS and GI effects of some of these drugs. Dose adjustment is not needed for many of these agents. Geriatric warnings have been associated with naproxen, ketorolac, and ketoprofen because of reports of increased toxicity when they are used by older adult patients. These NSAIDs should be avoided if possible.

Table 16.1 ***Drugs in Focus:*** **Salicylates**

Drug Name	Dosage/Route	Usual Indications
aspirin (*Bayer*, *Empirin*, others)	*Adult:* 325–650 mg PO or PR q4h *MI:* 81 mg PO *Pediatric:* 65–100 mg/kg/d PO or PR in four to six divided doses; if <2 y of age, consult with prescriber	Treatment of fever, pain, inflammatory conditions; at low dose to prevent the risk of death and MI in patients with history of MI; prevention of transient ischemic attacks
balsalazide (*Colazal*)	Three 750-mg capsules PO t.i.d.	Treatment of mildly to moderately acute ulcerative colitis in adults
choline magnesium trisalicylate (*Tricosal*)	*Adult:* 1.5–3 g/d PO in two to three divided doses *Pediatric:* 50 mg/kg/d PO in two divided doses	Relief of mild pain, fevers; treatment of arthritis
diflunisal (generic)	500–1,000 mg/d PO in two divided doses	Treatment of moderate pain, arthritis in adults
mesalamine (*Pentasa*, others)	800 mg PO t.i.d. for 6 wk or 4 g/60 mL rectal suspension daily at bedtime or 500 mg suppository PR, retained for 1–3 h b.i.d.	Treatment of ulcerative colitis and other inflammatory bowel disease in adults
olsalazine (*Dipentum*)	1 g/d PO in two divided doses	Treatment of ulcerative colitis and other inflammatory bowel disease in adults
salsalate (*Disalcid*)	3,000 mg/d PO in divided doses	Treatment of pain, fever, inflammation in adults
sulfasalazine (*Azulfidine*)	*Initial:* 3–4 g/d PO in divided doses *Maintenance:* 2 g/d	Treatment of ulcerative colitis

MI, myocardial infarction.

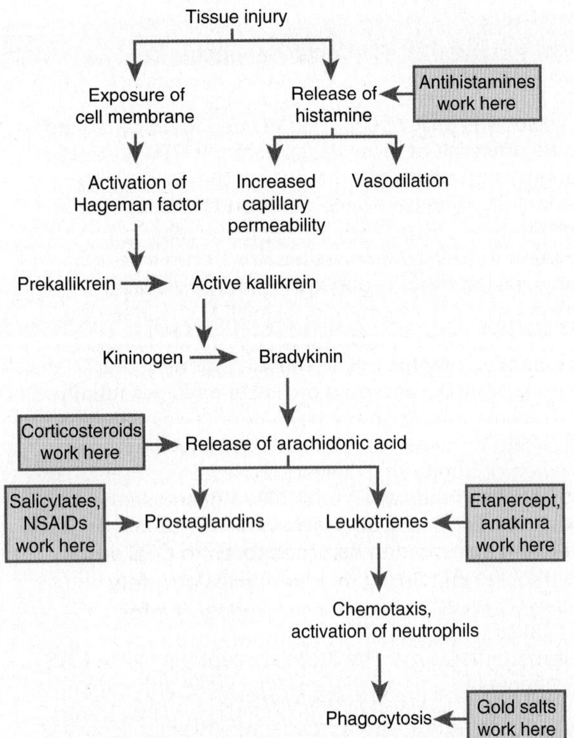

FIGURE 16.1 Sites of action of antiinflammatory agents.

BOX 16.2

Pathophysiology of Rheumatoid Arthritis

Rheumatoid arthritis is a chronic, systemic, autoimmune disease that affects people of all ages. Patients with rheumatoid arthritis have high levels of rheumatoid factor (RF), an antibody to immunoglobulin G (IgG). RF interacts with circulating IgG to form immune complexes, which tend to deposit in the synovial fluid of joints, as well as in the eye and other small vessels. The formation of the immune complex activates complement and precipitates an inflammatory reaction and release of tumor necrosis factor (TNF). During the immune reaction, lysosomal enzymes are released that destroy the tissues surrounding the joint. This destruction of normal tissue causes a further inflammatory reaction, and a cycle of destruction and inflammation ensues. Over time, the joint becomes severely damaged and the synovial space fills with scar tissue. Several pharmaceutical interventions help to manage symptoms and slow the progression of disease. Categories of these medications used for rheumatoid arthritis include disease-modifying antirheumatic medications (DMARDs), glucocorticoids, immunosuppressants, and nonsteroidal anti-inflammatory drugs (NSAIDs).

Therapeutic Actions and Indications

Salicylates inhibit the synthesis of prostaglandin, an important mediator of the inflammatory reaction (see Fig. 16.1). The antipyretic effect of salicylates may be related to blocking of a prostaglandin mediator of pyrogens (chemicals that cause an increase in body temperature and that are released by active white blood cells) at the thermoregulatory center of the hypothalamus. At low levels, aspirin also affects platelet aggregation by inhibiting the synthesis of thromboxane A_2, a potent vasoconstrictor that normally increases platelet aggregation and blood clot formation. At higher levels, aspirin inhibits the synthesis of prostacyclin, a vasodilator that inhibits platelet aggregation.

Salicylates are indicated for the treatment of mild to moderate pain, fever, and numerous inflammatory conditions, including inflammatory bowel disease, rheumatoid arthritis, and osteoarthritis. (See Box 16.2 and the "Critical Thinking Scenario" for more on rheumatoid arthritis.) See Table 16.1 for usual indications for each type of salicylate.

CRITICAL THINKING SCENARIO
Treatment of Rheumatoid Arthritis

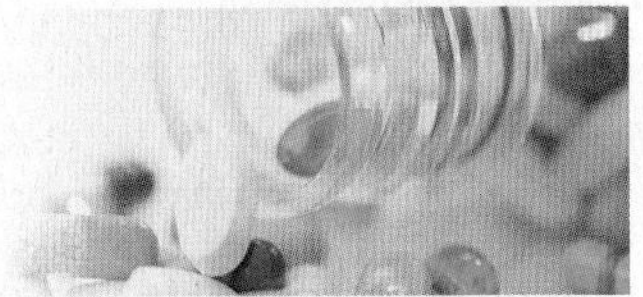

THE SITUATION

G.T. is an 82-year-old patient on a fixed income with a 14-year history of rheumatoid arthritis. G.T. is seen in the clinic for evaluation of their arthritis and to address their complaint that medications are not helping. On examination, it is found that G.T.'s range of motion (ROM), physical examination of joints, and overall presentation have not changed since their last visit. G.T. states that they had been taking aspirin instead of their prescribed medication. G.T. was originally prescribed leflunomide, but about 9 months prior to their current clinic visit, it became too expensive due to a change in insurance coverage. The aspirin was cheaper, and a friend said that it worked for arthritis. However, G.T. read that aspirin can cause severe stomach problems, so they wanted to ask about this during their clinic visit.

CRITICAL THINKING

Think about the pathophysiology of rheumatoid arthritis and how the drugs ordered act on the inflammatory process:

How can the nurse best explain the disease and the drug regimen to this patient?
What could be contributing to G.T.'s perception that their condition has worsened?
What nursing interventions would be appropriate to help G.T. cope with the disease and need for medication?

DISCUSSION

G.T. should be offered encouragement and support for managing their progressive disease and the drug regimen required. The fact that G.T.'s physical status has not changed but they perceive that the disease is worse may reflect other underlying problems that are making it more difficult to cope with chronic pain and limitations. The nurse should explore the patient's social situation, any changes in living situation, and support services. An examination should be done to determine whether other physical problems have emerged that could be adding to G.T.'s sense that things are getting worse. The provider and the nurse can also evaluate if there is a cost-effective way to obtain leflunomide for patient G.T., since they felt better when taking this medication. The differences of how leflunomide and aspirin work on the arthritic process should be reviewed in basic terms, with emphasis on the importance of preventing further damage and maintaining a safe, therapeutic and cost-effective medication regimen. Pictures of the process involved in rheumatoid arthritis may help—the simpler the better in most cases.

If G.T. has been having gastrointestinal (GI) complaints due to taking the aspirin, they should be evaluated for peptic ulcer disease before taking aspirin and/or NSAID. A discussion with the provider is necessary before G.T. resumes aspirin therapy since this was not the medication recommended for treatment of the rheumatoid arthritis. With support and encouragement, G.T. can be helped to follow the prescribed drug regimen and delay further damage from arthritis.

NURSING CARE GUIDE FOR G.T.: RHEUMATOID ARTHRITIS

Assessment: History and Examination

Allergies to medications; renal or hepatic impairment; ulcerative GI disease, peptic ulcer, hearing impairment, blood dyscrasias
Concurrent use of anticoagulants, steroids, ascorbic acid, alcohol, furosemide, acetazolamide, antacids, methotrexate, valproic acid, sulfonylureas, insulin, beta-adrenergic blockers, probenecid, spironolactone, nitroglycerin
Neurologic: Orientation, reflexes, affect
Musculoskeletal system: ROM, joint assessment
Skin: Color, lesions
Cardiovascular: Pulse, cardiac auscultation, blood pressure, perfusion
GI: Liver evaluation, bowel sounds
Lab tests: Complete blood count, liver and renal function tests

Nursing Conclusions

Acute pain related to GI effects, headache
Altered sensory perception (auditory, kinesthetic) related to central nervous system (CNS) effects
Knowledge deficit regarding drug therapy

Planning

The patient will receive the best therapeutic effect from the drug therapy.
The patient will have limited adverse effects to the drug therapy.
The patient will have an understanding of the drug therapy, adverse effects to anticipate, and measures to relieve discomfort and improve safety.

Intervention

Ensure proper administration of the drug.
Administer with food if GI upset occurs.
Provide support and comfort measures to deal with adverse effects: Small, frequent meals; safety measures if CNS effects occur; measures for headache; bowel training as needed.
Provide patient teaching regarding drug name, dosage, side effects, precautions, and warnings to report; supplementary measures to help decrease arthritis pain.

Evaluation

Evaluate drug effects: Decrease in signs and symptoms of inflammation.
Monitor for adverse effects: CNS changes, rash, GI upset, GI bleeding.
Monitor for drug–drug interactions as listed.
Evaluate effectiveness of patient teaching program.
Evaluate effectiveness of comfort/safety measures.

PATIENT TEACHING FOR G.T.

- Your provider did not prescribe aspirin, but it was used as over-the-counter (OTC) medication to help relieve the signs and symptoms of your rheumatoid arthritis. Aspirin works as an antiinflammatory drug. It works in the body to decrease inflammation and to relieve the signs and symptoms of inflammation, such as pain, swelling, heat, tenderness, and redness. It does not cure your arthritis, but it will help you to live with it more comfortably. It may not be the best treatment option for rheumatoid arthritis; there are other medications that can better limit the progression, and there may be a way to get an affordable prescription medication.
- Take your medication exactly as prescribed. Do not take over-the-counter drugs as substitutes unless you have discussed them with your provider.
- Some of the following adverse effects may occur with aspirin:
  - Nausea, vomiting, abdominal discomfort: Taking the drug with food or eating small, frequent meals may help. If these effects persist, consult with your health care provider.

(continues on page 274)

- Diarrhea, constipation: These effects may decrease over time; ensure ready access to bathroom facilities and consult with your health care provider for possible treatment.
- Drowsiness, dizziness, blurred vision: If you experience any of these problems, avoid driving or performing tasks that require alertness.
- Headache: If this becomes a problem, consult with your health care provider. Do not self-treat with more aspirin or other analgesics.
- Salicylism (signs of overdose/toxicity): tinnitus (ringing in ears), sweating, headache, dizziness, and fever. Stop medication immediately and notify provider. This is a serious adverse effect that can progress to be very dangerous and/or life threatening.
- Tell any health care provider who is taking care of you that you are taking this drug.
- Avoid using other OTC preparations while you are taking this drug. If you feel that you need one of these drugs, consult with your health care provider for the most appropriate choice. Many of these drugs may also contain aspirin and could cause an overdose.
- Report any of the following to your health care provider: fever, rash, GI pain, nausea, itching, or black or tarry stools.
- Keep this drug and all medications out of the reach of children.

Pharmacokinetics

Salicylates are readily absorbed directly from the stomach, reaching peak levels within 5 to 30 minutes. They are metabolized in the liver and excreted in the urine, with a half-life of 15 minutes to 12 hours, depending on the salicylate. Salicylates cross the placenta and enter human milk; they are not indicated for use during pregnancy or lactation because of the potential adverse effects on the neonate and associated bleeding risks for the patient.

Contraindications and Cautions

Salicylates are contraindicated in the presence of known allergy to salicylates, other nonsteroidal antiinflammatory drugs (NSAIDs) (more common with a history of nasal polyps, asthma, or chronic urticaria), or tartrazine (a dye that has a cross-sensitivity with aspirin) because of the risk of allergic reaction; bleeding abnormalities because of the changes in platelet aggregation associated with these drugs; impaired renal function because the drug is excreted in the urine; chickenpox or influenza because of the risk of Reye's syndrome in children and teenagers; surgery or other invasive procedures scheduled within 1 week because of the risk of increased bleeding; and pregnancy or lactation because of the potential adverse effects on the neonate or patient.

Adverse Effects

The adverse effects associated with salicylates may be the result of direct drug effects on the stomach (nausea, dyspepsia, heartburn, epigastric discomfort) and on clotting systems (blood loss, bleeding abnormalities). **Salicylism** can occur with high levels of aspirin. Dizziness, ringing in the ears, difficulty hearing, nausea, vomiting, diarrhea, mental confusion, fever, and lassitude can occur. Acute salicylate toxicity may occur at doses of 20 to 25 g in adults or 4 g in children. Signs of salicylate toxicity include hyperpnea, tachypnea, hemorrhage, dehydration, excitement, confusion, pulmonary edema, convulsions, tetany, metabolic acidosis, electrolyte imbalances, fever, coma, and cardiovascular (CV), renal, and respiratory collapse.

Clinically Important Drug–Drug Interactions

The salicylates interact with many other drugs, primarily because of alterations in absorption, effects on the liver, or extension of the therapeutic effects of the salicylate or the interacting drug (or both). The list of interacting drugs in each drug monograph in a nursing drug guide should be consulted along with the prescriber before adding or removing a salicylate from any drug regimen.

Prototype Summary: Aspirin

Indications: Treatment of mild to moderate pain, fever, inflammatory conditions; reduction of risk of transient ischemic attack or stroke; reduction of risk of myocardial infarction.

Actions: Inhibits the synthesis of prostaglandins; blocks the effects of pyrogens at the hypothalamus; inhibits platelet aggregation by blocking thromboxane A_2.

Pharmacokinetics:

Route	Onset	Peak	Duration
Oral	5–30 min	0.25–2 h	3–6 h
Rectal	1–2 h	4–5 h	6–8 h

$T_{1/2}$: 15 minutes to 12 hours; metabolized in the liver and excreted in the urine.

Adverse Effects: Nausea, vomiting, heartburn, epigastric discomfort, occult blood loss, dizziness, tinnitus, acidosis; salicylism toxicity; Reye's syndrome in children and adolescents with viral illness.

Nursing Considerations for Patients Receiving Salicylates

Assessment: History and Examination

- Assess for contraindications or cautions: history of allergy to any salicylate or tartrazine to avoid hypersensitivity reactions; renal disease because these drugs are excreted through the urine; bleeding disorders because of the drug effects on blood clotting; chickenpox or influenza in children to avoid the risk of Reye's syndrome; and pregnancy or lactation to avoid adverse effects on the fetus or infant and risk of bleeding in the patient.
- Perform physical assessment to establish baseline status before beginning therapy and to monitor for any potential adverse effects.
- Assess for the presence of any skin lesions to monitor for dermatological effects.
- Monitor temperature to evaluate the drug's effectiveness in lowering temperature.
- Evaluate CNS status—orientation, reflexes, eighth cranial nerve function, and affect—to assess CNS effects of the drug.
- Monitor pulse, blood pressure, and perfusion to assess for bleeding effects or cardiovascular effects of the drug.
- Evaluate respirations and adventitious sounds to detect hypersensitivity reactions.
- Perform a liver evaluation and monitor bowel sounds to detect hypersensitivity reactions, bleeding, and GI effects of the drug.
- Monitor laboratory tests for complete blood count (CBC), liver and renal function tests, urinalysis, stool guaiac, and clotting times to detect bleeding or other adverse effects of the drug and changes in function that could interfere with drug metabolism and excretion.

Nursing Conclusions

Nursing conclusions related to drug therapy might include the following:

- Impaired comfort related to CNS and GI effects
- Altered breathing pattern risk, if there is toxicity
- Altered sensory perception (auditory, kinesthetic) risk, if there is toxicity
- Knowledge deficit risk regarding drug therapy

Planning

- The patient will receive the best therapeutic effect from the drug therapy.
- The patient will have limited adverse effects to the drug therapy.
- The patient will have an understanding of the drug therapy, adverse effects to anticipate, and measures to relieve discomfort and improve safety.

Implementation with Rationale

- Administer with food if GI upset is severe; provide small, frequent meals to alleviate GI effects.
- Administer drug as indicated; check all drugs being taken for possible salicylate ingredients; monitor dose to avoid toxic levels.
- Monitor for severe reactions to avoid problems and provide emergency procedures (gastric lavage, induction of vomiting, administration of charcoal) if they occur.
- Arrange for supportive care and comfort measures (rest, environmental control) to decrease body temperature or to alleviate inflammation.
- Ensure that the patient is well hydrated during therapy to decrease the risk of toxicity.
- Provide thorough patient teaching, including measures to avoid adverse effects and warning signs of problems, as well as proper administration, to increase knowledge about drug therapy and to increase compliance with the drug regimen.
- Offer support and encouragement for managing the drug regimen.

Evaluation

- Monitor patient response to the drug (improvement in condition being treated, relief of signs and symptoms of inflammation).
- Monitor for adverse effects (GI upset, CNS changes, bleeding).
- Evaluate the effectiveness of the teaching plan (patient can name drug, dosage, adverse effects to watch for, specific measures to avoid adverse effects).
- Monitor the effectiveness of comfort measures and compliance with the drug regimen.

Key Points

- Salicylates block prostaglandin activity, which decreases the inflammatory response and relieves the signs and symptoms of inflammation.
- Salicylates can cause GI irritation, eighth cranial nerve stimulation, and salicylism—ringing in the ears, acidosis, nausea, vomiting, diarrhea, fever, mental confusion, and lassitude.

Nonsteroidal Antiinflammatory and Related Agents

Nonsteroidal antiinflammatory drugs (**NSAIDs**) provide strong antiinflammatory and analgesic effects without the adverse effects associated with the corticosteroids (see Table 16.2). Acetaminophen (*Tylenol*) is not an NSAID

Table 16.2 *Drugs in Focus:* Nonsteroidal Antiinflammatory Drugs (NSAIDs) and Related Agents

Drug Name	Dosage/Route	Usual Indications
NSAID Propionic Acids		
fenoprofen (*Nalfon*)	200–600 mg PO t.i.d. or q.i.d.	Treatment of pain, arthritis in adults
flurbiprofen (*Ansaid*)	200–300 mg PO in divided doses; ophthalmic solution: 1 drop (gtt) q30min beginning 2 h after surgery	Long-term management of arthritis; topically to manage pain after eye surgery in adults
ibuprofen (*Motrin, Advil, Caldolor* IV, others)	*Adult:* 400–800 PO t.i.d. to q.i.d. 400–800 mg IV over 30 min q6h for pain; 400 mg IV over 30 min for fever followed by 400 mg q4–6h or 100–200 mg q4h to control fever *Pediatric:* 30–40 mg/kg/d PO in three to four divided doses for arthritis; 5–10 mg/kg PO q6–8 h for fever	Treatment of pain, arthritis, dysmenorrhea, juvenile arthritis
ketoprofen (*Orudis*)	25–75 mg PO t.i.d. to q.i.d.; reduce dose with hepatic or renal impairment; ER form: 200 mg/d PO	Short-term management of pain; long-term management of arthritis (ER form)
naproxen (*Naprosyn*)	*Adult:* 250–500 mg PO b.i.d.; do not give >200 mg q12h for geriatric patients *Pediatric:* 10 mg/kg/d PO in two divided doses for juvenile arthritis; do not give OTC versions to children <12 y without consulting health care provider	Treatment of pain, arthritis, dysmenorrhea, juvenile arthritis
oxaprozin (*Daypro*)	1,200 mg PO daily	Treatment of arthritis in adults
Acetic Acids		
diclofenac (*Voltaren, Cataflam, Flector*)	100–200 mg/d PO; 25–50 mg b.i.d. to q.i.d. PO *Topical:* Apply one patch b.i.d. to most painful area	Treatment of acute and chronic pain associated with inflammatory conditions in adults
etodolac (*Lodine*)	800–1,200 mg/d PO in divided doses; 200–400 mg q6–8h PO for pain management	Treatment of arthritis pain in adults; management of chronic pain (extended-release formulation)
indomethacin (*Indocin*)	*Adult:* 75–150 mg/d PO in three to four divided doses *Pediatric (>2 y):* In special circumstances, 2 mg/kg/d PO in divided doses	Relief of moderate to severe pain in PO, topical, and PR forms; closure of patent ductus arteriosus in premature infants (given IV)
ketorolac (*Toradol*)	10 mg PO q4–6h or 30–60 mg IM, switching to oral form as soon as possible, or 30 mg IV as a single dose *Ophthalmic:* 1 gtt to affected eye q.i.d.; reduce dose with renal impairment and in patients >65 y	Short-term management (5 d or fewer) of pain in adults; topically to relieve ocular itching
nabumetone (*Relafen*)	1,000 mg/d PO as a single dose	Treatment of acute and chronic arthritis pain in adults
sulindac (*Clinoril*)	150–200 mg PO b.i.d.	Treatment of various inflammatory conditions in adults
tolmetin (*Tolectin*)	*Adult:* 400 mg PO t.i.d.; 600–800 mg/d in three to four doses for maintenance *Pediatric:* 20 mg/kg/d PO in three to four divided doses	Treatment of acute flares of rheumatoid and juvenile arthritis
Fenamates		
meclofenamate (generic)	100–400 mg/d PO	Treatment of mild to moderate pain, primary dysmenorrhea, rheumatoid arthritis, osteoarthritis
mefenamic acid (*Ponstel*)	500 mg PO, then 250 mg PO q6h as needed	Short-term treatment of pain in adults and children >14 y; primary dysmenorrhea

Table 16.2 *Drugs in Focus:* Nonsteroidal Antiinflammatory Drugs (NSAIDs) and Related Agents *(Continued)*		
Drug Name	**Dosage/Route**	**Usual Indications**
Oxicam Derivative		
meloxicam (*Mobic*)	*Adult:* 7.5 mg/d PO to a maximum of 15 mg/d *Pediatric:* 0.125 mg/kg/d PO to a maximum of 7.5 mg/d	Treatment of osteoarthritis, rheumatoid arthritis, and juvenile arthritis
piroxicam (*Feldene*)	20 mg/d PO as a single dose	Treatment of acute and chronic arthritis in adults
Cyclooxygenase-2 Inhibitor		
celecoxib (*Celebrex*)	Initially 100–200 mg PO b.i.d.; acute pain 400 mg PO; then 200 mg PO b.i.d. for FAP	Treatment of acute and chronic arthritis in adults; acute pain; primary dysmenorrhea; reduction of the number of colorectal polyps in FAP; ankylosing spondylitis
Related Agent		
acetaminophen (*Tylenol, Ofirmev*)	*Adult:* 1,000 mg PO t.i.d. to q.i.d. or 325–650 mg PR q4–6h or 1,000 mg IV q6h or 650 mg IV q4h max. 1,000 mg/dose or 4,000 mg/d *Pediatric:* Adjust dose based on age and weight	Relief of pain and fever in a variety of situations

ER, extended release; OTC, over the counter; FAP, familial adenomatous polyposis.

but is a widely used analgesic. It has antipyretic and analgesic properties but does not have the antiinflammatory effects of the salicylates or the NSAIDs. It is discussed in this chapter because it is used for many of the same reasons that NSAIDs are used, and the nurse needs to understand the similarities and differences of these drugs.

Nonsteroidal Antiinflammatory Drugs

The NSAIDs are a drug class that has become one of the most commonly used drug types in the United States. Following unanticipated study results linking drugs in this class to an increased risk of CV events and death as well as increased bleeding in the GI tract, a boxed warning was added to all of these drugs pointing out the CV and GI risks associated with taking them.

This group of drugs includes propionic acids, acetic acids, fenamates, oxicam derivatives, and cyclooxygenase-2 (COX-2) inhibitors. The classes are defined by chemical structural differences, but clinically, the NSAIDs are all-inclusive. See Table 16.2 for a list of these drugs by group, as well as their specific indications. The choice of NSAID depends on personal experience and the patient's response to the drug. A patient may have little response to one NSAID but respond to another. It may take several trials to determine the drug of choice for any particular patient. See Box 16.3 for more information about emerging research involving NSAID use for patients with COVID-19.

Therapeutic Actions and Indications

The antiinflammatory, analgesic, and antipyretic effects of the NSAIDs are largely related to inhibition of prostaglandin synthesis (see Fig. 16.1). The NSAIDs block two enzymes, known as COX-1 and COX-2. COX-1 is present in all tissues and seems to be involved in many body functions, including blood clotting, protecting the stomach lining, and maintaining sodium and water balance in the kidney. COX-1 turns arachidonic acid into prostaglandins as needed in a variety of tissues. COX-2 is active at sites of trauma or injury when more prostaglandins are needed, but it is less involved in other tissue functions. By interfering with this part of the inflammatory reaction, NSAIDs block inflammation before all of the signs and symptoms can develop. Most NSAIDs, which block both COX-1 and COX-2, also block various other functions of the prostaglandins, including protection of the stomach lining, regulation of blood clotting, and water and salt balance in the kidney. NSAIDs with predominantly COX-1 effects may have more GI adverse effects; NSAIDs with more COX-2 selectivity may have more cardiovascular adverse effects.

The adverse effects associated with most NSAIDs are related to the blocking of both of these enzymes and changes in the functions that they influence—GI integrity, blood clotting, and sodium and water balance. The COX-2 inhibitors are designed to primarily affect the activity of COX-2, the enzyme that becomes active in response to trauma and injury. They interfere less with COX-1, which is needed for normal functioning of these systems. Consequently, these drugs should have fewer of the associated adverse effects seen when both COX-1 and COX-2 are inhibited. Patients taking more selective COX-2 inhibitors may have effects on these other functions and should be evaluated for GI effects, changes in clotting, and water retention. Box 16.4 summarizes the actions and adverse effects of the COX-1 and COX-2 enzymes.

BOX 16.3 Focus on The Evidence

NONSTEROIDAL ANTIINFLAMMATORY DRUGS AND COVID-19

Nonsteroidal antiinflammatory drugs (NSAIDs) are often taken by clients to decrease pain and/or fever from inflammatory processes. The infection caused by SARS-CoV-2 virus (COVID-19) can often cause headache, fever, sore throat, and other symptoms of inflammation. There has been controversy whether the NSAIDs are helpful or harmful when treating COVID-19 symptoms. Some theorize that the use of NSAIDs may worsen the infection due to increased activity of the enzyme that SARS-CoV-2 binds to in order to enter human cells. However, others hypothesize that NSAIDs would be helpful in relieving inflammatory symptoms by inhibiting prostaglandin and proinflammatory cytokines, including interleukin-6 overproduction. This interleukin is thought to be related to the cytokine release syndrome that some patients suffer from when they have COVID-19. The studies completed through 2021 have some contradictory information regarding the risks and benefits, and more studies are underway. At this time, the World Health Organization has recommended that patients who are prescribed NSAIDs continue their therapy. In addition, people suffering from symptoms from COVID-19 may take either acetaminophen or NSAIDs to relieve symptoms.

The NSAIDs are indicated for relief of the signs and symptoms of rheumatoid arthritis and osteoarthritis, for relief of mild to moderate pain, for treatment of primary dysmenorrhea, and for fever reduction.

BOX 16.4

Comparison of Cyclooxygenase (COX) Receptors

COX-1	COX-2
Site of action	**Site of action**
Found in many tissues, important for homeostasis	Induced by inflammatory stimuli at the site of inflammation
Effects	**Effects**
• Converts arachidonic acid to inflammatory prostaglandins • Maintains renal function • Provides for gastric mucosa integrity • Promotes vascular hemostasis, increases bleeding • Autocrine effects causing fever	• Increases pain, inflammation • Vasodilates • Blocks platelet clumping
Effects of blocking	**Effects of blocking**
• Decreases swelling, pain, inflammation • Sodium retention, edema, increased blood pressure • GI erosion, bleeding • Decreases fever	• Decreases pain, inflammation • Prevents protective vasodilation, allows platelet clumping, which can lead to MI, cerebrovascular accident • Myriad of skin reactions, including Stevens-Johnson syndrome

Pharmacokinetics

The NSAIDs are rapidly absorbed from the GI tract, reaching peak levels in 1 to 3 hours. They are metabolized in the liver and excreted in the urine. NSAIDs cross the placenta and cross into human milk. Therefore, they are not recommended during pregnancy and lactation because of the potential adverse effects on the fetus or neonate.

Contraindications and Cautions

The NSAIDs are contraindicated in the presence of allergy to any NSAID or salicylate, and celecoxib is also contraindicated in the presence of allergy to sulfonamides. Additional precautions are CV dysfunction or hypertension because of the varying effects of the prostaglandins and increased risk of heart attack and stroke; peptic ulcer or known GI bleeding because of the potential to exacerbate the GI bleeding; and pregnancy or lactation because of potential adverse effects on the neonate or mother. Caution should be used with renal or hepatic dysfunction, which could alter the metabolism and excretion of these drugs, and with any other known allergies, which indicate increased sensitivity.

Adverse Effects

Patients receiving NSAIDs often experience nausea, dyspepsia, GI pain, constipation, diarrhea, or flatulence caused by direct GI effects of the drug. The potential for GI bleeding often is a cause of discontinuation of the drug. Headache, dizziness, somnolence, and fatigue also occur frequently and could be related to prostaglandin activity in the CNS. Bleeding, platelet inhibition, hypertension, and even bone marrow depression have been reported with chronic use and are probably related to the blocking of prostaglandin activity. Rash and mouth sores may occur, and anaphylactoid reactions ranging up to fatal anaphylactic shock have been reported in cases of severe hypersensitivity. All NSAIDs can contribute to acute kidney insufficiency. However, renal impairment is especially at risk with use of ketorolac, so this medication should not be used if a patient has advanced renal disease and it should only be used short-term (5 days or fewer).

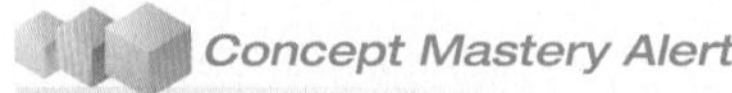

NSAIDs and Client Education

Heartburn, GI bleeding, and peptic ulcer disease are possible adverse effects of taking NSAIDs. While nausea is a possible adverse effect of taking NSAIDs, vomiting is not typically seen. Risk is increased in older adults and patients who smoke or use alcohol.

Clinically Important Drug–Drug Interactions

There is often a decreased diuretic effect when these drugs are taken with loop diuretics; there is a potential for decreased antihypertensive effect of beta-blockers if these drugs are combined; and there have been reports of lithium toxicity, especially when combined with ibuprofen. Concurrent use with anticoagulants, alcohol, or glucocorticoids can increase risk of bleeding. Use of ibuprofen with low-dose aspirin decreases the antiplatelet effects of the aspirin. Supplements like ginkgo biloba, garlic, and ginger can also increase risk of bleeding. Patients who receive these combinations should be monitored closely, and appropriate dose adjustments should be made by the prescriber.

Prototype Summary: Ibuprofen

Indications: Relief of the signs and symptoms of rheumatoid arthritis and osteoarthritis; relief of mild to moderate pain; treatment of primary dysmenorrhea; fever reduction.

Actions: Inhibits prostaglandin synthesis by blocking COX-1 and COX-2 receptor sites, leading to an antiinflammatory effect, analgesia, and antipyretic effects.

Pharmacokinetics:

Route	Onset	Peak	Duration
Oral	30 min	1–2 h	4–6 h
IV	Start of infusion	Minutes	4–6 h

$T_{1/2}$: 1.8 to 2.5 hours; metabolized in the liver and excreted in the urine.

Adverse Effects: Headache, dizziness, somnolence, fatigue, rash, nausea, dyspepsia, bleeding, constipation, bone marrow suppression, myocardial infarction, stroke.

Acetaminophen

Acetaminophen (*Tylenol, Ofirmev*) is used to treat moderate to mild pain and fever and often is used in place of the NSAIDs or salicylates. It has been the most frequently used drug for managing pain and fever in children. It is widely available OTC and is found in many combination products. It can be extremely toxic at high doses. It causes severe liver toxicity that can lead to death. Maximum daily dose for most clients is 4 g/d, but for some with alcohol use or hepatic injury, a lower maximum daily dose should be used. Every year children die from inadvertent acetaminophen overdose when parents give their child more than one OTC drug containing acetaminophen or administer a high dose of acetaminophen. The U.S. Food and Drug Administration and drug manufacturers have joined forces to produce mass media ads warning parents about this possibility and to limit the amount of acetaminophen that can be used in each OTC product.

Therapeutic Actions and Indications

Acetaminophen acts directly on the thermoregulatory cells in the hypothalamus to cause sweating and vasodilation; this in turn causes the release of heat and lowers fever. The mechanism of action related to the analgesic effects of acetaminophen has not been identified.

Acetaminophen is indicated for the treatment of pain and fever associated with a variety of conditions, including influenza; for the prophylaxis of children receiving diphtheria–pertussis–tetanus immunizations (aspirin may mask Reye's syndrome in children); and for the relief of musculoskeletal pain associated with arthritis (see Table 16.2).

Pharmacokinetics

Acetaminophen is rapidly absorbed from the GI tract, reaching peak level in 0.5 to 2 hours. It is extensively metabolized in the liver and excreted in the urine, with a half-life of about 2 hours. It is also available for IV use in adults and children 2 and over if oral use of the drug is not possible. Caution should be used in patients with hepatic or renal impairment, which could interfere with metabolism and excretion of the drug, leading to toxic levels. Acetaminophen crosses the placenta and enters human milk; it should be used cautiously during pregnancy or lactation because of the potential adverse effects on the fetus or neonate.

Contraindications and Cautions

Acetaminophen is contraindicated in the presence of allergy to acetaminophen because of the risk of hypersensitivity reactions. It should be used cautiously in pregnancy or lactation because of the potential for adverse effects on the fetus or infant and in hepatic dysfunction or chronic alcoholism because of associated toxic effects on the liver.

Adverse Effects

Adverse effects associated with acetaminophen use include headache, hemolytic anemia, renal dysfunction, skin rash, and fever. Hepatotoxicity is a potentially fatal adverse effect that is usually associated with chronic use and overdose and is related to direct toxic effects on the liver. The dose that could prove toxic varies with the age of the patient, other drugs that the patient might be taking, and the underlying hepatic function of that patient. When overdose occurs, acetylcysteine can be used as an antidote. It acts by restoring glutathione levels so that there is more of it to bind with the toxic metabolite from acetaminophen, which allows for safe excretion of the medication. Life support measures may also be necessary.

Clinically Important Drug–Drug Interactions

There is an increased risk of bleeding with oral anticoagulants because of effects on the liver; of toxicity with chronic ethanol ingestion because of toxic effects on the liver; and of hepatotoxicity with barbiturates, carbamazepine, hydantoins, or rifampin. These combinations should be avoided, but if they must be used, appropriate dose adjustment should be made, and the patient should be monitored closely.

Prototype Summary: Acetaminophen

Indications: Treatment of mild to moderate pain, fever, or signs and symptoms of the common cold or flu; musculoskeletal pain associated with arthritis and rheumatic disorders.

Actions: Acts directly on the hypothalamus to cause vasodilation and sweating, which will reduce fever; mechanism of action as an analgesic is not understood.

Pharmacokinetics:

Route	Onset	Peak	Duration
Oral	Varies	0.5–2 h	3–6 h
IV	Beginning of infusion	End of infusion	4–6 h

$T_{1/2}$: 1 to 3 hours; metabolized in the liver and excreted in the urine.

Adverse Effects: Rash, fever, chest pain, liver toxicity and failure, bone marrow suppression.

Nursing Considerations for Patients Receiving NSAIDs and Related Agents

Assessment: History and Examination

(Refer to Salicylates for nursing conclusions, planning, intervention with rationale, and evaluation.)

- Assess for contraindications or cautions: known allergies to any salicylates, NSAIDs, or tartrazine; pregnancy or lactation; hepatic or renal disease; CV dysfunction; hypertension; and GI bleeding or peptic ulcer.
- Assess for baseline status before beginning therapy and for any potential adverse effects: presence of any skin lesions; temperature; orientation, reflexes, and affect; pulse, blood pressure, and perfusion; respirations and adventitious sounds; liver evaluation; bowel sounds; and CBC, liver and renal function tests, urinalysis, stool guaiac, and serum electrolytes.

Key Points

- NSAIDs block prostaglandin synthesis at the COX-1 and COX-2 sites. This blocks inflammation but also blocks protection of the stomach lining, as well as the kidneys' regulation of water.
- There are many different NSAIDs. If one does not work for a particular patient, another one might.
- Acetaminophen causes vasodilation and heat release, lowering fever and working to relieve pain but does not have the direct antiinflammatory effects.
- Acetaminophen can cause liver failure. It is found in many OTC products. Teach patients to avoid toxic doses of acetaminophen.

Antiarthritis Agents

Other drugs that are used to block the inflammatory process include the antiarthritis drugs. Arthritis is a potentially debilitating inflammatory process in the joints that causes pain and bone deformities. Antiarthritis drugs include one gold compound, which is used to prevent and suppress arthritis in selected patients with rheumatoid arthritis. The other antiarthritis drugs are specifically used to block the inflammation and tissue damage of rheumatoid arthritis (see Table 16.3).

Gold Compound

Some patients with rheumatic inflammatory conditions do not respond to the usual antiinflammatory therapies, and their conditions worsen despite weeks or months of standard pharmacological treatment. Some of these patients respond to treatment with gold salts, also known as **chrysotherapy**, in which gold is taken up by macrophages, which then inhibit phagocytosis; it can be very toxic and is reserved for use in patients who are unresponsive to conventional therapy. The gold salt available for use is auranofin (*Ridaura*).

Therapeutic Actions and Indications

Chrysotherapy results in inhibition of phagocytosis (see Fig. 16.1). Because phagocytosis is blocked, the release of lysosomal enzymes is inhibited and tissue destruction is decreased. This action allows gold salts to suppress and prevent some arthritis and synovitis. Gold salts are indicated to treat selected cases of rheumatoid and juvenile rheumatoid arthritis in patients whose disease has been unresponsive to standard therapy (see Table 16.3 for usual indications). This drug does not repair damage; it may prevent further damage and so is most effective if used early in the disease.

Table 16.3 ***Drugs in Focus:* Antiarthritis Agents**

Drug Name	Dosage/Route	Usual Indications
Gold Compounds		
auranofin (*Ridaura*)	*Adult:* 6 mg/d PO; monitor geriatric patients carefully *Pediatric:* 0.1–0.15 mg/kg/d PO	Oral agent for long-term therapy of rheumatic disorders
Tumor Necrosis Factor Blockers		
adalimumab (*Humira*)	*Adult:* 40 mg subcutaneous every other week; 80 mg then 40 mg every other week with *Plaque psoriasis* *Pediatric:* 10–40 mg subcutaneous every other week	Reduction of signs and symptoms of rheumatoid arthritis, psoriatic arthritis, ankylosing spondylitis, plaque psoriasis, juvenile idiopathic arthritis, Crohn's disease, ulcerative colitis
certolizumab (*Cimzia*)	*Adult:* 400 mg/wk subcutaneous (Crohn's), 200 mg/wk subcutaneous (arthritis)	Reduction of signs and symptoms of rheumatoid arthritis, Crohn's disease
etanercept (*Enbrel*)	*Adult:* 25 mg subcutaneous two times per week or 50 mg subcutaneous once a week *Pediatric (4–17 y):* 0.4 mg/kg subcutaneous two times per week with 72–96 h between doses; not recommended for patients <4 y	Reduction of signs and symptoms of severe rheumatoid arthritis in patients whose disease is unresponsive to other therapy; prevention of damage early in the disease; ankylosing spondylosis; psoriatic arthritis
golimumab (*Simponi*)	*Adult:* 50 mg/mo subcutaneous or 2 mg/kg IV over 30 min at weeks 0, 4 then q8wk	Treatment of active rheumatoid arthritis, psoriatic arthritis, ankylosing spondylosis
infliximab (*Remicade*)	*Adult:* 3 mg IV at weeks 0, 2, 6, then q8wk (rheumatoid arthritis) *Adult and child:* 5 mg IV at weeks 0, 2, 6, then 5 mg/kg IV q8wk (Crohn's disease, ulcerative colitis, ankylosing spondylosis, psoriatic arthritis, plaque psoriasis)	Treatment of Crohn's disease, ulcerative colitis, ankylosing spondylosis, rheumatoid arthritis, psoriatic arthritis, plaque psoriasis
Other Antiarthritis Drugs		
anakinra (*Kineret*)	*Adult:* 100 mg/d subcutaneous *Pediatric neonatal disease:* 1–2 mg/kg/d subcutaneous	Reduction of signs and symptoms of rheumatoid arthritis in patients ≥18 y if one or more antiarthritis drugs have failed Treatment of neonatal-onset multisystem inflammatory disease
hyaluronidase derivatives (hylan G-F 20 [*Synvisc*])	2 mL once a week for 3 wk injected into the affected knee	Relief of pain in the knees of arthritis patients whose disease is unresponsive to conventional treatment
leflunomide (*Arava*)	100 mg PO daily for 3 d, then 20 mg PO daily	Treatment of active rheumatoid arthritis, to relieve signs and symptoms and to slow the progression of disease in adults
penicillamine (*Depen*)	125–250 mg PO daily	Treatment of severe, active rheumatoid arthritis in adults whose disease is unresponsive to conventional therapy
sarilumab (*Kevzara*)	200 mg subcutaneous q2wk	Treatment of adults with moderately to severely active rheumatoid arthritis who have inadequate response to one or more other agents
sodium hyaluronate (*Hyalgan*)	2 mg once a week for 5 wk injected into the affected knee	Relief of pain in the knees of arthritis patients whose disease is unresponsive to conventional treatment
tofacitinib (*Xeljanz*)	*Adult:* 5 mg PO b.i.d.	Treatment of adults with moderate to severe active arthritis intolerant to other therapies

Pharmacokinetics

The gold salts are absorbed at varying rates, depending on route of administration. They are widely distributed throughout the body but seem to concentrate in the hypothalamic–pituitary–adrenocortical system and in the adrenal and renal cortices. The gold salts are excreted in urine and feces. This drug crosses the placenta and crosses into human milk. It has been shown to be teratogenic in animal studies and should not be used during pregnancy or lactation. Barrier contraceptives should be recommended to those able to become pregnant, and another method of feeding the infant should be used if gold therapy is needed in a person who is lactating.

Contraindications and Cautions

Gold salts can be quite toxic and are contraindicated in the presence of any known allergy to gold, severe diabetes, congestive heart failure, severe debilitation, renal or hepatic impairment, hypertension, blood dyscrasias, recent radiation treatment, history of toxic levels of heavy metals, and pregnancy or lactation.

Adverse Effects

A variety of adverse effects is common with the use of gold salts, and they are probably related to their deposition in the tissues and effects at that local level: stomatitis, glossitis, gingivitis, pharyngitis, laryngitis, colitis, diarrhea, and other GI inflammation; gold bronchitis and interstitial pneumonitis; bone marrow depression; vaginitis and nephrotic syndrome; dermatitis, pruritus, and exfoliative dermatitis; allergic reactions ranging from flushing, fainting, and dizziness to anaphylactic shock; and renal toxicity causing proteinuria.

Clinically Important Drug–Drug Interactions

This drug should not be combined with penicillamine, antimalarials, cytotoxic drugs, or immunosuppressive agents other than low-dose corticosteroids because of the potential for severe toxicity.

P Prototype Summary: Auranofin

Indications: Treatment of selected adults with rheumatoid arthritis, who have insufficient response to or intolerance to NSAIDs.

Actions: Taken up by macrophages, which inhibits phagocytosis and release of lysosomal enzymes that cause damage associated with inflammation.

Pharmacokinetics:

Route	Onset	Peak
Oral	Slow	4–6 h

$T_{1/2}$: 3 to 7 days; excreted in the urine and feces.

Adverse Effects: Bone marrow suppression, renal toxicity, dermatitis, nausea, vomiting, stomatitis, hepatitis, rashes.

Disease-Modifying Antirheumatic Drugs

Other antiarthritis drugs, called **disease-modifying antirheumatic drugs (DMARDs)**, are available for treating arthritis and aggressively affect the process of inflammation. Many rheumatologists are selecting DMARDs early in the diagnosis, before damage to the joints has occurred, because they alter the course of the inflammatory process. DMARDs can be categorized as nonbiologic or biologic. Two types of DMARDs discussed include tumor necrosis factor (TNF) blockers, which are biologic, and other DMARDs. Several DMARDs are discussed in other chapters: methotrexate (Chapter 14), hydroxychloroquine (Chapter 12), and many immunosuppressant medications (Chapter 17). The adverse effects associated with these drugs (see the "Adverse Effects" section below) can be severe to life-threatening because they alter the ability of the body to initiate or carry on an inflammatory reaction.

Tumor Necrosis Factor Blockers

TNF blockers are often the first class used with progressing arthritis. These drugs are discussed in Chapter 17 with immune modulators, but because of their increasing use in treating the various forms of arthritis, they will also be discussed in depth here. These drugs include adalimumab (*Humira*), certolizumab (*Cimzia*), etanercept (*Enbrel*), golimumab (*Simponi*), and infliximab (*Remicade*).

Therapeutic Actions and Indications

TNF blockers act to decrease the local effects of TNF, a locally released cytokine that can cause the death of tumor cells and stimulate a wide range of proinflammatory activities. The actions of this cytokine when inflammation occurs within a joint capsule can lead to the destruction of bone and the malformation of joints that is associated with arthritis. Drugs that block that action of TNF slow the inflammatory response and the joint damage associated with it. These drugs are indicated for the treatment of rheumatoid arthritis, polyarticular juvenile arthritis, psoriatic arthritis, plaque psoriasis, and ankylosing spondylitis. Adalimumab, certolizumab, and infliximab are also used in Crohn's disease and ulcerative colitis. See the "Critical Thinking Scenario" for a case study about DMARDs and psoriatic arthritis.

Pharmacokinetics

TNF blockers must be given subcutaneously, with the exception of infliximab, which is given IV. They have a slow onset, usually peaking in 48 to 72 hours. They are primarily excreted in the tissues and have very long half-lives ranging from 115 hours to 2 weeks. They cross the placenta and may enter human milk, so use in pregnancy and breast or chestfeeding should be discouraged.

CRITICAL THINKING SCENARIO DMARDs and Psoriatic Arthritis

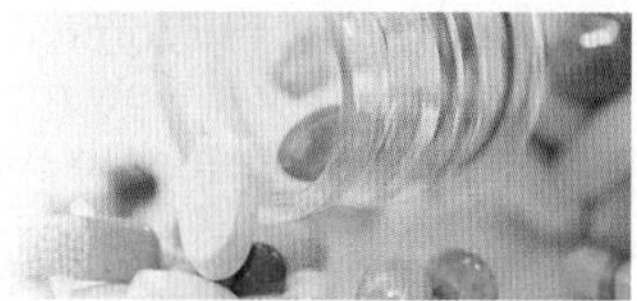

THE SITUATION

J.G. is a 46-year-old, former semi-pro baseball player. J.G. has had progressive difficulty walking, opening jars, and moving things, and has attributed it to years of athletic training and what they describe as "body abuse." J.G. is seen in the clinic for evaluation after severe joint pain and loss of ROM forced them to try to find some help. Examination reveals swollen red patches on the skin, and thick, silver scaly lesions on arms and legs, markedly decreased ROM—the worst being the right shoulder—swollen feet, a marked limp when walking, and complaints of severe joint pain, which is worse in the morning. Blood tests show an elevated sedimentation rate, no elevation in rheumatoid factor, and the presence of the HLA-B27 genetic marker. A bone scan reveals bone loss. The diagnosis is made of psoriatic arthritis. After consulting with family and discovering several cousins with the same diagnosis, J.G. asked for aggressive treatment. Numerous blood tests are ordered, including tests for HIV and hepatitis B, a tuberculin (TB) test, an order for a colonoscopy, and gluten sensitivity. When all the tests come in, J. G. is prescribed adalimumab (*Humira*).

CRITICAL THINKING

Think about the pathophysiology of psoriatic arthritis and how the drug ordered acts on the inflammatory process.

How can the nurse best explain the disease and the drug regimen to this patient?
How can the nurse explain the numerous tests required before using these drugs and the need for continued follow-up?
What nursing interventions would be appropriate to help J.G. deal with this disease?

DISCUSSION

Psoriatic arthritis is different than rheumatoid arthritis. It is an autoimmune disease that often runs in families and often expresses a particular genetic marker, the HLA-B27 allele. People with this often also have gluten sensitivity, and efforts are usually made to bring that under control with diet if it is a concurrent issue. The joints of these patients are slowly destroyed by the body's response to antigen–antibody deposits, and the fingers and toes are often more involved than in rheumatoid arthritis. Since J.G. has had this progressive arthritis for many years without seeking medical help, it was decided to start out with a DMARD. Adalimumab is a TNF inhibitor, which will slow the destruction of the joints and also help to alleviate the dermal reaction that causes the skin lesions. It is hoped that this will alleviate pain and slow the destruction and remodeling of the joint and improve J.G.'s quality of life. The nurse needs to explain this process and then educate J.G. about the overall role of TNF in the immune response and the risks involved when this protective mechanism is gone. J.G. will be at increased risk for infections and cancers. The many blood tests ordered will ensure that the patient doesn't have an infection already. The colonoscopy will screen for any GI cancers and establish a baseline that can be followed. J.G. will need to learn how to administer a subcutaneous injection and the proper disposal of needles and syringes, signs of infection to be aware of, dietary changes if they do have gluten sensitivity, and exercises that will be beneficial in keeping active and helping the joints.

NURSING CARE GUIDE FOR J.G.: DMARDs AND PSORIATIC ARTHRITIS

Assessment: History and Examination

Assess for tuberculosis, hepatitis B, HIV, travel exposure to fungal infections, cancers, active infection, heart failure, demyelinating diseases
Concurrent use of other tumor necrosis factor blockers, live vaccines
Neurologic: Orientation, reflexes, affect
Musculoskeletal system: ROM, joint assessment
Skin: Color, lesions
Cardiovascular: Pulse, cardiac auscultation, blood pressure, perfusion
GI: Liver evaluation
Lab tests: CBC, liver, and renal function tests, tests for HIV, hepatitis B, sedimentation rate

Nursing Conclusions

Acute pain related to injection site reactions, headache
Altered sensory perception (auditory, kinesthetic) related to CNS effects
Knowledge deficit risk regarding drug therapy

Planning

The patient will receive the best therapeutic effect from the drug therapy.
The patient will have limited adverse effects to the drug therapy.
The patient will have an understanding of the drug therapy, adverse effects to anticipate, and measures to relieve discomfort and improve safety.

Intervention

Ensure proper administration of the drug; teach patient proper administration of subcutaneous injections; proper disposal of needles and syringes; rotation of injection sites.

(continues on page 284)

Provide support and comfort measures to deal with adverse effects: safety measures if CNS effects occur; measures for headache; treatment of injection site reactions.

Provide patient teaching regarding drug name, dosage, proper administration, side effects, precautions, and warnings to report; supplementary measures to help decrease arthritis pain.

Evaluation

Evaluate drug effects: decrease in signs and symptoms of inflammation; stopping progression of joint deterioration.

Monitor for adverse effects: CNS changes, headache, infections, cancer.

Monitor for drug–drug interactions as listed.

Evaluate effectiveness of patient teaching program.

Evaluate effectiveness of comfort/safety measures.

PATIENT TEACHING FOR J.G.

- Your doctor has prescribed adalimumab to help relieve the signs and symptoms of your psoriatic arthritis. This drug works to block part of your body's normal response to injury. It works in the body to decrease inflammation and to relieve the signs and symptoms of inflammation, such as pain, swelling, heat, tenderness, and redness. It does not cure your arthritis but will help you to live with it more comfortably and will delay the damage to the joints that occurs with this disease.
- You must administer this drug by subcutaneous injection every other week. Mark your calendar with the days you will need the injection. You will learn the proper administration of a subcutaneous injection. You must properly dispose of the needle and syringes as we have discussed.
- Some of the following adverse effects may occur:
  - Drowsiness, dizziness, blurred vision: If you experience any of these problems, avoid driving or performing tasks that require alertness.
  - Headache: If this becomes a problem, consult with your health care provider. Do not self-treat with more aspirin or other analgesics.
  - Infections: You will be more susceptible to infections; you should avoid people with known illnesses, use a mask and gloves if digging in the dirt, and wash your hands frequently.
  - Cancer is more likely to occur: You should have all the routine cancer screening that is recommended: a skin evaluation, colonoscopy, and prostate examination. Early detection is the best response.
- Tell any health care provider who is taking care of you that you are taking this drug.
- Avoid using other OTC preparations while you are taking this drug. If you feel that you need one of these drugs, consult with your health care provider for the most appropriate choice.
- Report any of the following to your health care provider: fever, worsening rash, blurred vision, numbness or tingling in the extremities, and extreme fatigue.
- Keep this drug and all medications out of the reach of children.

Contraindications and Cautions

These drugs cannot be used in anyone with an acute infection, cancer, sepsis, tuberculosis, hepatitis, myelosuppression, or demyelinating disorders because they block the body's immune/inflammatory response and serious reactions could occur. Etanercept cannot be used with a history of allergy to Chinese hamster ovary *products because it is made from these products.* They should not be used in pregnancy or breast or chestfeeding because of the potential effects on the fetus or neonate. Caution should be used with renal or hepatic disorders, heart failure, and latex allergies to prevent adverse reactions.

Adverse Effects

TNF blockers come with boxed warnings about the risk of serious to fatal infections and the development of lymphomas and other cancers. Patients need to be screened and monitored accordingly. Demyelinating disorders have occurred, including multiple sclerosis and various neuritis conditions. Myocardial infarction (MI), heart failure, and hypotension are also reported with the use of these drugs. Irritation at the injection site can also occur.

Clinically Important Drug–Drug Interactions

Use of any other immune suppressant drugs with TNF blockers increases the risk of serious infections and cancer. Live vaccines should not be given while on these drugs.

Prototype Summary: Etanercept

Indications: Reduction of signs and symptoms, and improvement of function with rheumatoid arthritis, polyarticular juvenile idiopathic arthritis, psoriatic arthritis, ankylosing spondylitis, and plaque psoriasis.

Actions: Genetically engineered TNF receptors react with and deactivate TNF released by active leukocytes, keeping the inflammatory response in check.

Pharmacokinetics:

Route	Onset	Peak
Subcutaneous	Slow	72 h

$T_{1/2}$: 115 hours; metabolized in the tissues and excreted in the tissues.

Adverse Effects: Serious to fatal infections, lymphoma and other cancers, demyelinating disorders, MI, heart failure, injection site reactions.

Other Disease-Modifying Antirheumatic Drugs

Other DMARDs discussed in this chapter include drugs used when patients do not respond to conventional therapy—anakinra (*Kineret*), leflunomide (*Arava*), sarilumab (*Kevzara*), tofacitinib (*Xeljanz*) and penicillamine (*Depen*)—and drugs used to directly decrease pain in joints affected by arthritis, including hyaluronidase derivative (*Synvisc*) and sodium hyaluronate (*Hyalgan*). Additional drugs also used to modify the disease process in rheumatoid arthritis include the antineoplastic drug methotrexate (see Chapter 14), the T cell suppressor abatacept (*Orencia*) (see Chapter 17), certain antimalarial drugs (see Chapter 12), some additional antineoplastic drugs such as cyclophosphamide (see Chapter 14), and the immune modulators cyclosporine A and azathioprine (see Chapter 17).

Therapeutic Actions and Indications

Anakinra is a relatively new antiarthritis drug. This drug is an interleukin-1 receptor antagonist. It blocks the increased interleukin-1, which is responsible for the degradation of cartilage in rheumatoid arthritis. This drug must be given each day by subcutaneous injection and is often used in combination with other antiarthritis drugs. See Table 16.3 for usual indications.

Hyaluronidase derivatives, such as hylan G-F 20 and sodium hyaluronate, have elastic and viscous properties. These drugs are injected directly into the joints of patients with severe rheumatoid arthritis of the knee. They seem to cushion and lubricate the joint and relieve the pain associated with degenerative arthritis. They are given weekly for 3 to 5 weeks.

Leflunomide directly inhibits an enzyme, dihydroorotate dehydrogenase, that is active in the autoimmune process that leads to rheumatoid arthritis, relieving signs and symptoms of inflammation and blocking the structural damage this inflammation can cause, slowing disease progression.

Sarilumab is an interleukin-6 receptor antagonist. Blocking this causes a decrease in inflammatory processes systemically and locally within the joint, relieving signs and symptoms. It is reserved for patients who do not respond to other DMARDs.

Penicillamine lowers the immunoglobulin M rheumatoid factor levels in patients with acute rheumatoid arthritis, relieving the signs and symptoms of inflammation. It may take 2 to 3 months of therapy before a response is noted.

Tofacitinib is a kinase inhibitor that blocks signaling pathways within immune cells to prevent their activity. It is an oral agent and is reserved for patients who have not responded to traditional therapies.

Pharmacokinetics

Anakinra is slowly absorbed from the subcutaneous tissue, reaching peak level in 3 to 7 hours. It is metabolized in the tissues and excreted in the urine. It has a half-life of 4 to 6 hours. Sarilumab is slowly absorbed after subcutaneous injection, reaching peak level in 2 to 4 days; it has a half-life of 10 days. The hyaluronidase derivatives are not absorbed systemically. Leflunomide is slowly absorbed from the GI tract, reaching peak level in 6 to 12 hours. It undergoes hepatic metabolism and excretion in the urine. The half-life of leflunomide is 14 to 18 days.

Penicillamine is an oral drug that reaches peak level in 1 to 3 hours after administration. It is extensively metabolized in the liver and excreted in the urine with a half-life of 2 to 3 hours. Tofacitinib is absorbed quickly, reaching peak level in 0.5 to 1 hour; it is metabolized in the liver and excreted in the urine with a half-life of 3 hours.

Contraindications and Cautions

These drugs are contraindicated in the presence of allergy to the drugs or to the animal products from which they were derived (chicken products in hylan G-F 20 and sodium hyaluronate) to avoid hypersensitivity reactions; pregnancy or lactation because of the potential for adverse effects on the fetus or neonate; acute infection because of the blocking of normal inflammatory pathways; and liver or renal impairment, which could be exacerbated by these drugs.

Adverse Effects

A variety of adverse effects are common with the use of these drugs, including local irritation at injection sites (anakinra, sarilumab, etanercept, hyaluronidase derivatives, and sodium hyaluronate), pain with injection, and increased risk of infection. Leflunomide is associated with potentially fatal hepatic toxicity and rashes. Penicillamine is associated with a potentially fatal myasthenic syndrome, bone marrow depression, and assorted hypersensitivity reactions. Leflunomide has been associated with severe hepatic toxicity; hence, the patient's liver function needs to be monitored closely. Tofacitinib and sarilumab have boxed warnings outlining the risk of serious to fatal infections including tuberculosis and the development of lymphomas and other cancers.

Clinically Important Drug–Drug Interactions

Hyaluronidase derivatives such as sodium hyaluronate should not be injected at the same time as local anesthetics.

Because leflunomide can cause severe liver dysfunction if it is combined with other hepatotoxic drugs, this combination should be avoided.

The absorption of penicillamine is decreased if it is taken with iron salts or antacids; if these are both being given, they should be separated by at least 2 hours.

Anakinra and tofacitinib should not be used with other immune suppressants because of an increased risk of serious infections.

Nursing Considerations for Patients Receiving DMARDs

Patients receiving DMARDs have moderate to severe arthritis or other immune conditions. These drugs alter the disease process by altering the patient's immune response to slow or block inflammation and damage that occurs with chronic inflammatory states. Details related to each individual drug can be found in the specific drug monograph in your nursing drug guide.

Assessment: History and Examination

- Assess for contraindications or cautions: history of allergy to any components of the drug, Chinese hamster ovary products (etanercept), or chicken products (hyaluronidase) to avoid hypersensitivity reactions; active infections or cancers because these drugs alter the immune response and these conditions could worsen; pregnancy or lactation to avoid adverse effects on the fetus or infant.
- Perform physical assessment to establish baseline status before beginning therapy and to monitor for any potential adverse effects.
- Assess lesions, temperature, any sign of infection to monitor for adverse effects.
- Evaluate CNS status—orientation, reflexes, eighth cranial nerve function, and affect—to assess CNS effects of the drug.
- Arrange for required cancer screening to evaluate potential adverse effects of the drug.
- Monitor range of motion, movement, and pain levels to evaluate effectiveness of drug therapy.
- Evaluate respirations and adventitious sounds to detect signs of infection.
- Monitor laboratory tests for CBC, liver and renal function tests, and TB test to establish baseline and monitor for adverse effects of the drug.

Nursing Conclusions

Nursing diagnoses related to drug therapy might include the following:

- Acute pain related to CNS, disease process
- Infection risk related to drug effects
- Fear/anxiety risk related to disease process and drug effects
- Knowledge deficit risk regarding drug therapy

Planning

- The patient will receive the best therapeutic effect from the drug therapy.
- The patient will have limited adverse effects to the drug therapy.
- The patient will have an understanding of the drug therapy, adverse effects to anticipate, and measures to relieve discomfort and improve safety.

Intervention with Rationale

- Teach patient proper preparation, administration of subcutaneous injections, and safe disposal of needles and syringes to ensure therapeutic effectiveness and safety.
- Monitor for immune suppression reactions to avoid problems and provide emergency care as needed.
- Monitor for CNS toxicity to evaluate toxicity and provide appropriate interventions of drug discontinuation.
- Arrange for continuation of nondrug therapies to deal with arthritis to improve quality of life and enhance therapeutic effectiveness of drug therapy.
- Ensure that the patient has routine cancer screening and regular follow-up to avoid serious adverse effects and manage them quickly if they occur.
- Provide thorough patient teaching, including measures to avoid adverse effects and warning signs of problems, as well as proper administration, to increase knowledge about drug therapy, and to increase compliance with the drug regimen.
- Offer support and encouragement to deal with the drug regimen and diagnosis.

Evaluation

- Monitor patient response to the drug (improvement in condition being treated, relief of signs and symptoms of arthritis).
- Monitor for adverse effects (infections, cancer development, and CNS toxicity).
- Evaluate the effectiveness of the teaching plan (patient can name drug, dosage, administration, and adverse effects to watch for, specific measures to avoid adverse effects).
- Monitor the effectiveness of and adherence to the drug regimen.

Key Points

- Gold salts prevent macrophage phagocytosis, lysosomal release, and tissue damage because the gold salts are taken up by phagocytes, which then are not able to function in the normal way.
- Gold salts are deposited in the tissues and cause an assortment of inflammatory reactions, including stomatitis, glossitis, gingivitis, pharyngitis, laryngitis, colitis, diarrhea, and other GI inflammation; gold bronchitis and interstitial pneumonitis; bone marrow depression; vaginitis and nephrotic syndrome; dermatitis, pruritus, and exfoliative dermatitis; and allergic reactions ranging from flushing, fainting, and dizziness to anaphylactic shock.
- Drugs used to alter the inflammatory process involved in arthritis are called disease-modifying antirheumatic drugs (DMARDs) and can be associated with serious to potentially fatal infections. If used early in the disease, they can prevent or slow down the damage caused to the joints.
- TNF blockers prevent the actions of TNF in the inflammatory/immune process. This relieves the signs and symptoms of arthritis and helps to slow bone breakdown and damage but also makes the patient prone to serious infections and the development of cancers.
- The DMARDs can cause local irritation at the injection site, liver impairment, and a variety of CNS problems, including demyelinating disorders.

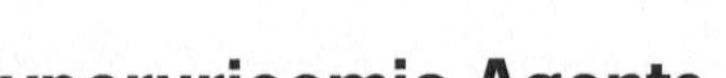

Antigout/Hyperuricemia Agents

Gout disorders are often characterized by elevated uric acid and urate crystal deposits in kidneys and joints. Gouty arthritis can be extremely painful due to the crystal deposits causing local acute inflammation. Antigout medications either attempt to decrease the inflammation or lower the blood uric acid levels. NSAIDs and glucocorticoids may be used for their antiinflammatory actions. Medications that are primarily used for gout treatment are colchicine, allopurinol, febuxostat, pegloticase, and probenecid (see Table 16.4).

Therapeutic Actions and Indications

Colchicine is indicated for treatment of acute gout arthritis flares and treatment of Familial Mediterranean fever. Its mechanism of action is theorized to be the prevention of actions of neutrophils that facilitate inflammation.

Allopurinol, febuxostat, and probenecid are designed to lower blood levels of uric acid in symptomatic clients. Allopurinol and febuxostat inhibit xanthine oxidase, which is an enzyme needed to convert xanthine to uric acid. Pegloticase is indicated for treatment of chronic gout. It works to lower uric acid by increasing its oxidation to the substance allantoin, which is easily eliminated via renal excretion. Probenecid inhibits tubular resorption of urate so that urinary excretion of uric acid increases; this process lowers the blood levels.

Pharmacokinetics

Colchicine is absorbed orally and takes effect in 1 to 2 hours. Administration with food does not have a clinically significant effect on absorption. Colchicine crosses the placenta and enters human milk. It is metabolized by the CYP3A4 enzymes in the liver and is excreted via the kidneys, enterohepatic recirculation, and bile.

Allopurinol is absorbed orally, reaches peak serum level in about 1.5 hours, and has a half-life of about 1 to 2 hours. It is excreted renally and via feces. Febuxostat is absorbed orally and reaches max plasma level in 1 to 1.5 hours. It is metabolized in the liver and has a half-life of 5 to 8 hours. It is excreted renally and hepatically.

Pegloticase is administered as intravenous infusion. Max concentration of the medication is influenced by dose amount. Formal studies have not been conducted for people with renal or hepatic impairment, but dosing does not need to be altered for renal impairment.

Contraindications and Cautions

Colchicine should be used with caution and requires dose reduction in patients with severe renal and hepatic disease due to increased risk of toxicity; fatal overdoses have occurred in both patient populations. Dose adjustments can be made for patients requiring hemodialysis; medication is not dialyzed out.

Allopurinol should be discontinued if a rash or other signs of allergic reaction are present. Hypersensitivity reactions may be higher in patients with renal insufficiency and patients receiving thiazide medications. When initiating treatment with allopurinol, there may be an increase in acute gouty attacks, so it can be administered with colchicine prophylactically.

A higher rate of cardiovascular death in patients taking febuxostat compared to allopurinol for gout has been reported, so febuxostat should only be given if allopurinol is not effective or if the patient is intolerant.

There is a boxed warning for pegloticase due to the risk of anaphylaxis and infusion reactions. Patients should be premedicated with antihistamines and corticosteroids, and the medication should be administered in a health care setting staffed by providers that can manage anaphylaxis and infusion reactions. People with G6PD deficiency have a higher risk of hemolysis and methemoglobinemia with pegloticase, so screening should be performed prior to dosing.

Table 16.4 ***Drugs in Focus*: Antigout/Hyperuricemia Agents**

Drug Name	Dosage/Route	Usual Indications
allopurinol (*Lopurin, Zyloprim*)	200–600 mg/day PO; doses of more than 300 mg should be in divided doses	Treatment of gout and symptomatic hyperuricemia
colchicine (*Colcrys*)	Gout: 1.2 mg PO followed by 0.6 mg PO FMF: *Adult* 1.2 to 2.4 mg/d PO	Treatment of gout flares and familial Mediterranean fever (FMF)
febuxostat (*Uloric*)	40–80 PO mg/d; titrate to goal for uric acid level <6 mg/dL after 2 wk	Management of hyperuricemia due to gout if not controlled with allopurinol
pegloticase (*Krystexxa*)	8 mg IV q2wk	Treatment of chronic gout in adults refractory to conventional therapy
probenecid (*Probalan*)	250 mg twice daily PO for a week, followed by 500 mg twice daily	Treatment of hyperuricemia due to gout

Probenecid may increase the risk of an acute gout attack, so it should not be given during, or recently after, an acute attack.

Adverse Effects

Colchicine can cause mild to severe GI distress. It is recommended to take with food, and antidiarrheal agents can help relieve the side effects of diarrhea. A provider needs to be notified if any severe reactions occur. Blood dyscrasias can occur due to suppressed bone marrow, so bleeding risk needs to be monitored. Rhabdomyolysis is also a side effect of colchicine, especially with long-term use.

During the first few months of therapy, allopurinol and febuxostat may cause hypersensitivity reactions (such as fever and rash), hepatic and renal dysfunction, nausea and vomiting, and transient increase in gout attacks.

Pegloticase may cause infusion reactions (including anaphylaxis), nausea, constipation, chest pain, vomiting, gout flares, ecchymosis, and nasopharyngitis.

There is a risk of renal calculi and renal injury with probenecid. This risk can be decreased with adequate hydration, usually 2 to 3 L of fluid a day. Hypersensitivity reactions are uncommon but can occur.

Clinically Important Drug–Drug Interactions

Concurrent use of P-gp and/or CYP3A4 inhibitors with colchicine can cause an overdose severe enough to cause mortality, so all drug interactions need to be evaluated prior to administration.

Allopurinol may slow the metabolism of warfarin and increase the risk of bleeding. PT/INR levels need to be monitored. Use of febuxostat with azathioprine or mercaptopurine can increase plasma concentrations to severe toxic levels. Salicylates can decrease the effectiveness of probenecid.

Prototype Summary: Colchicine

Indications: Treatment of gout flares and familial Mediterranean fever (FMF).

Actions: Prevention of actions of neutrophils that facilitate inflammation.

Pharmacokinetics:

Route	Onset	Peak
Oral	1 h	2 h

$T_{1/2}$: 26 to 31 hours.

Adverse Effects: GI disturbances: nausea, vomiting, diarrhea, abdominal pain; muscle pain and rhabdomyolysis; blood dyscrasias.

Key Points

- Gout is caused by elevated levels of uric acid in the blood. Gouty arthritis occurs when uric acid crystals are deposited in kidneys and joints, causing inflammation and pain.
- Colchicine is indicated to treat acute gout attacks.
- Allopurinol, febuxostat, and probenecid can be used to treat symptomatic hyperuricemia.

SUMMARY

- The inflammatory response, which is important for protecting the body from injury and invasion, produces many of the signs and symptoms associated with disease, including fever, aches and pains, and lethargy.
- Chronic or excessive activity by the inflammatory response can lead to the release of lysosomal enzymes and cause tissue destruction.
- Antiinflammatory drugs block various chemicals associated with the inflammatory reaction. Antiinflammatory drugs also may have antipyretic (fever-blocking) and analgesic (pain-blocking) activities.
- Salicylates block prostaglandin activity. NSAIDs block prostaglandin synthesis. Acetaminophen causes vasodilation and heat release, lowering fever and working to relieve pain. Gold salts prevent macrophage phagocytosis, lysosomal enzyme release, and tissue damage. DMARDs alter the course of the inflammatory process and treat arthritis by aggressively affecting the process of inflammation.
- Salicylates can cause acidosis and eighth cranial nerve damage. NSAIDs are most associated with GI irritation and bleeding. Acetaminophen can cause serious liver toxicity. The gold salts cause many systemic inflammatory reactions. Other antiarthritis drugs are associated with local injection site irritation and increased susceptibility to infection; leflunomide is associated with severe hepatic toxicity.
- Many antiinflammatory drugs are available OTC, and care must be taken to prevent abuse or overuse of these drugs.
- DMARDs affect the immune response to slow inflammation and joint damage. They are associated with serious to potentially fatal injections and the development of cancers.
- There are several medications that are indicated to treat and/or prevent gout attacks by treating inflammation or hyperuricemia.

Unfolding Patient Stories: Danielle Young Bear • Part 2

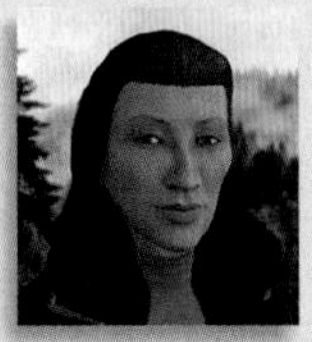

Recall Danielle Young Bear, the 32-year-old construction worker you met in Chapter 1, who is being seen at the clinic for persistent cough and fatigue who also has a history of chronic lower back pain and spasms. Danielle requests a nonnarcotic, inexpensive medication. Compare and contrast the actions and side effects of acetaminophen, aspirin, and ibuprofen for managing pain and inflammation. Which of these would you recommend? Why? If you don't recommend one of these, what do you recommend? Provide your rationale.

Care for Danielle and other patients in a realistic virtual environment: ***vSim** for Nursing* (thepoint.lww.com/vSimPharm). Practice documenting these patients' care in DocuCare (thepoint.lww.com/DocuCareEHR).

CHECK YOUR UNDERSTANDING

Answers to the questions in this chapter can be found in Answers to Check Your Understanding Questions on thePoint®.

MULTIPLE CHOICE

Select the best answer.

1. A drug could be classified as an analgesic if it
   a. reduces fever.
   b. reduces swelling.
   c. reduces redness.
   d. reduces pain.

2. An antipyretic is a drug that can
   a. block pain.
   b. block swelling.
   c. block fever.
   d. block inflammation.

3. A nurse might not see a salicylate used as an antiinflammatory if a drug was needed for its
   a. antipyretic properties.
   b. analgesic properties.
   c. OTC availability.
   d. parenteral availability.

4. The nonsteroidal NSAIDs affect the COX-1 and COX-2 enzymes. By blocking COX-2 enzymes, the NSAIDs block inflammation and the signs and symptoms of inflammation at the site of injury or trauma. By blocking COX-1 enzymes, these drugs block
   a. fever regulation.
   b. prostaglandins that protect the stomach lining.
   c. swelling in the periphery.
   d. liver function.

5. Your patient has been receiving ibuprofen for many years to relieve the pain of osteoarthritis. Assessment of the patient should include
   a. an electrocardiogram.
   b. CBC with differential.
   c. respiratory auscultation.
   d. renal evaluation.

6. Patients taking NSAIDs should be taught to avoid the use of OTC medications without checking with their prescriber because
   a. many of the OTC preparations contain NSAIDs, and inadvertent toxicity could occur.
   b. no one should take more than one type of pain reliever at a time.
   c. increased GI upset could occur.
   d. there is a risk of Reye's syndrome.

7. Chronic or excessive activity by the inflammatory response can lead to
   a. loss of white blood cells.
   b. coagulation problems.
   c. release of lysosomal enzymes and tissue destruction.
   d. adrenal suppression.

8. A patient with rheumatoid arthritis is being administered adalimumab. Based on how the medication is administered, what should the nurse be sure to assess?
   a. The vein for thrombophlebitis
   b. The rectum for lesions
   c. The eyes for redness
   d. The skin for redness

MULTIPLE RESPONSE

Select all that apply.

1. A client is being treated for gout with allopurinol. The nurse should teach the client to monitor for which of the following adverse effects?
   a. Stomatitis
   b. Insomnia
   c. Nausea
   d. Rash
   e. Increased gout pain
   f. Fever

2. The nurse notes an order for oxaprozin (*Daypro*) for the treatment of arthritis. Before administering the drug, the nurse would assess the patient for which problems that could be cautions or contraindications?
   a. Headaches
   b. Dysmenorrhea
   c. Active peptic ulcer disease
   d. Chronic obstructive pulmonary disease
   e. Renal impairment
   f. Bleeding disorders

REFERENCES

Bresalier, R. S., Sandler, R. E., Quan, H., Bolognese, J. A., Oxenius, B., Horgan, K., Lines, C., Riddell, C., Morton, D., Lana, A., Konstam, M. A., & Baron, J. A. (2005). Cardiovascular events associated with rofecoxib in a colorectal adenoma chemoprevention trial. *New England Journal of Medicine, 352*, 1092–1102. https://doi.org/10.1056/NEJMoa050493

Brunton, L. L., Hilal-Dandan, R., & Knollman, B. C. (2018). *Goodman and Gilman's the pharmacological basis of therapeutics* (13th ed.). McGraw-Hill.

Fitzgerald, G. A. (2004). Coxibs and cardiovascular disease. *New England Journal of Medicine, 351*, 1709–1711. https://doi.org/10.1056/NEJMp048288

Giollo, A., Adami, G., Gatti, D., Idolazzi, L., & Rossini, M. (2021). Coronavirus disease 19 (Covid-19) and nonsteroidal anti-inflammatory drugs (NSAID). *Annals of the Rheumatic Diseases, 80*(2), e12. https://pubmed.ncbi.nlm.nih.gov/32321720/

Heard, K., Bui, A., Mlynarchek, S. L., Green, J. L., Bond, G. R., Clark, R. F., Kozer, E., Koff, R.S., & Dart, R. C. (2014). Toxicity from repeated doses of acetaminophen in children: Assessment of causality and dose in reported cases. *American Journal of Therapeutics, 21*(3), 174–183. https://doi.org/10.1097/mjt.0b013e3182459c53

Hendler, C. B. (Ed.). (2021). *Nursing 2021 drug handbook.* Wolters Kluwer.

Her, M., & Kavanaugh, A. (2012). Patient-reported outcomes in rheumatoid arthritis. *Current Opinion in Rheumatology, 24*(3), 327–334. https://doi.org/10.1097/BOR.0b013e3283521c64

Jeong, H. E., Lee, H., Shin, H. J., Choe, Y. J., Filion, K. B., & Shin, J. Y. (2020). Association between nonsteroidal anti-inflammatory drug use and adverse clinical outcomes among adults hospitalized with coronoavirus 2019 in South Korea: A nationwide study. *Clinical Infectious Diseases,* ciaa1056. Advance online publication. https://doi.org/10.1093/cid/ciaa1056

Kuehn, B. M. (2009). New pain guidelines for older patients: Avoid NSAIDs, consider opioids. *Journal of the American Medical Association, 302*(1), 19. https://doi.org/10.1001/jama.2009.887

Lavonas, E. J., Reynolds, K. M., & Dart, R. C. (2010). Therapeutic acetaminophen is not associated with liver injury in children: A systematic review. *Pediatrics, 126*(6), e1430–e1444. https://doi.org/10.1542/peds.2009-3352

Norris, T. L., & Lalchandani, R. (2018). *Porth's pathophysiology: Concepts of altered health states* (10th ed.). Wolters Kluwer.

Rinott, E., Kozer, E., Shapira, Y., Bar-Haim, A., & Youngster, I. (2020). Ibuprofen use and clinical outcomes in COVID-19 patients. *Clinical Microbiology and Infection, 26*(9), 1259.e5–1259.e7. https://doi.org/10.1016/j.cmi.2020.06.003

Ruderman, E. M. (2012). Overview of safety of non-biologic and biologic DMARDs. *Rheumatology, 51*(Suppl 6), vi37–vi43. https://doi.org/10.1093/rheumatology/kes283

World Health Organization. (2020). *The use of non-steroidal anti-inflammatory drugs (NSAIDs) in patients with COVID-19.* https://www.who.int/news-room/commentaries/detail/the-use-of-non-steroidal-anti-inflammatory-drugs-(nsaids)-in-patients-with-covid-19

CHAPTER 17

Immune Modulators

Learning Objectives

Upon completion of this chapter, you will be able to:

1. Describe the sites of actions of the various immune modulators.
2. Describe the therapeutic actions, indications, pharmacokinetics, contraindications, most common adverse effects, and important drug–drug interactions associated with each class of immune stimulants and immune suppressants.
3. Discuss the use of immune modulators across the lifespan.
4. Compare and contrast the prototype drugs for each class of immune modulators with the other drugs in that class and with drugs in other classes.
5. Outline the nursing considerations and teaching needs for patients receiving each class of immune modulators.

Key Terms

immune stimulant: drug used to energize the immune system when it is exhausted from fighting prolonged invasion or needs help fighting a specific pathogen or cancer cell

immune suppressant: drug used to block or suppress the actions of the T cells and antibody production; used to prevent transplant rejection and to treat autoimmune diseases

monoclonal antibodies: specific antibodies produced by a single clone of B cells to react with a specific antigen

recombinant DNA technology: use of bacteria to produce chemicals normally produced by human cells

Drug List

IMMUNE STIMULANTS

Interferons

- (P) interferon alfa-2b
- interferon beta-1a
- interferon beta-1b
- interferon gamma-1b
- peginterferon alfa-2a
- peginterferon alfa-2b

Interleukins

- (P) aldesleukin
- oprelvekin

Colony-Stimulating Factors

- (P) filgrastim
- pegfilgrastim
- sargramostim
- tbo-filgrastim

IMMUNE SUPPRESSANTS

Immune Modulators

- apremilast
- dimethyl fumarate
- fingolimod
- lenalidomide
- pomalidomide
- teriflunomide
- (P) thalidomide

T- and B-Cell Suppressors

- abatacept
- alefacept
- azathioprine
- belatacept
- (P) cyclosporine
- glatiramer acetate
- mycophenolate
- pimecrolimus
- sirolimus
- tacrolimus

Interleukin Receptor Antagonist

- anakinra

Monoclonal Antibodies

- adalimumab
- ado-trastuzumab
- alemtuzumab
- avelumab
- basiliximab
- belimumab
- (P) bevacizumab
- blinatumomab
- brentuximab
- canakinumab
- certolizumab
- cetuximab
- daclizumab
- daratumumab
- denosumab
- eculizumab
- golimumab
- ibritumomab
- infliximab
- ipilimumab
- natalizumab
- nivolumab
- obinutuzumab
- ocrelizumab
- ofatumumab
- olaratumab
- omalizumab
- palivizumab
- pegaptanib
- pembrolizumab
- pertuzumab
- ramucirumab
- ranibizumab
- raxibacumab
- rituximab
- sarilumab
- siltuximab
- tocilizumab
- tositumomab
- trastuzumab
- ustekinumab
- vedolizumab

As the name implies, immune modulators are used to modify the actions of the immune system. **Immune stimulants** are used to energize the immune system when it is exhausted from fighting prolonged invasion or when the immune system needs help fighting a specific pathogen or cancer cell. **Immune suppressants** are used to block the normal effects of the immune system in cases of organ transplantation (in which nonself-cells are transplanted into the body and destroyed by the immune reaction), in autoimmune disorders (in which the body's defenses recognize self-cells as foreign and work to destroy them), and in some cancers. Each group acts at various sites within the immune response (see Fig. 17.1).

The knowledge base about the actions and components of the immune system is continually growing and changing. As new discoveries are made and the actions and interactions of the various components of the system become better understood, new applications will be found for modulating the immune system in a variety of disorders. Box 17.1 discusses the use of immune modulators across the lifespan. Box 17.2 discusses use of these agents during pregnancy.

Immune Stimulants

Immune stimulants (see Table 17.1) include the interferons, which are naturally released from human cells in response to viral invasion; interleukins, which are chemicals produced by T cells to communicate between leukocytes; and the colony-stimulating factors that are used to stimulate the bone marrow to produce more white blood cells in situations where the levels of these cells are very low and the patient is at serious risk for infection.

Interferons

Interferons are substances naturally produced and released by human cells that have been invaded by viruses. They may also be released from cells in response to other stimuli, such as cytotoxic T-cell activity. A number of interferons are available for use. Several are produced by **recombinant DNA technology**, including interferon alfa-2b (*Intron-A*), peginterferon alfa-2a (*Pegasys*), peginterferon alfa-2b (*Peg-Intron*), and interferon beta-1b (*Betaseron*). Interferon alfa-n3 (*Alferon N*) is produced by harvesting human leukocytes. Interferon beta-1a (*Avonex*) is produced from Chinese hamster ovary cells. Interferon gamma-1b (*Actimmune*) is produced by *Escherichia coli* bacteria. The interferon of choice depends on the condition being treated (see Table 17.1).

Therapeutic Actions and Indications

Interferons act to prevent virus particles from replicating inside cells. They also stimulate interferon receptor sites on noninvaded cells to produce antiviral proteins, which prevent viruses from entering the cell. In addition, interferons

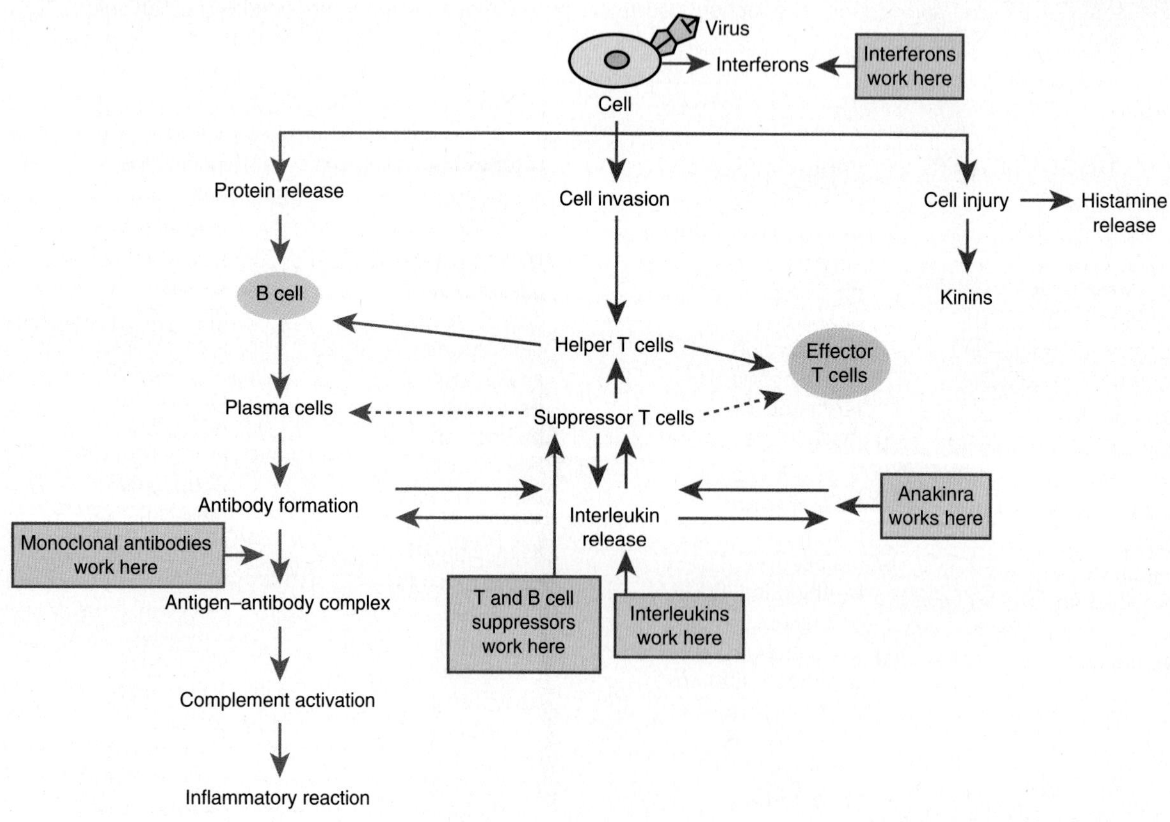

FIGURE 17.1 Sites of action of the immune modulators.

Box 17.1 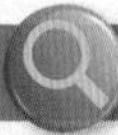 Focus on Drug Therapy Across the Lifespan

IMMUNE MODULATORS

Children

Most of the drugs that affect the immune system are not recommended for use in children or have not been tested in children. The exceptions—interferon alfa-2b, azathioprine, raxibacumab, cyclosporine, tacrolimus, and palivizumab—should be used cautiously, monitoring the child frequently for infection, GI, renal, hematological, or CNS effects.

The immune suppressants (azathioprine, cyclosporine, and tacrolimus) are usually needed in higher doses for children than for adults to achieve the same therapeutic effect.

Protecting the child from infection and injury is a very important part of the care of a child taking an immune modulator. This can be a great challenge with an active child.

Adults

Both the adult patient who is receiving a parenteral immune modulator and a friend, family member, or significant other who can assist with administering the medication if needed should learn the proper technique for injection, disposal of needles, and special storage precautions for the drug. It is important to stress ways to avoid exposure to infection and injury to prevent further complications. The patient should be encouraged to seek regular follow-up and medical care.

Immune modulators are contraindicated during pregnancy and lactation because of the potential for adverse effects on the fetus or neonate and complications for the parent. Patients able to become pregnant should be advised to use barrier contraceptives while taking these drugs and, if breast or chestfeeding, should be counseled to find another method of feeding the baby. Some of these drugs impair fertility, and the patient should be advised of this fact before taking the drug.

Older Adults

Older patients may be more susceptible to the effects of the immune modulators, partly because the aging immune system is less efficient and less responsive.

These patients need to be monitored closely for infection, GI, renal, hepatic, and CNS effects. Baseline renal and liver function tests can help to determine whether a decreased dosage will be needed before beginning therapy.

Because these patients are more susceptible to infection, they need to receive extensive teaching about ways to avoid infection and injury sites on noninvaded cells to produce antiviral proteins, which prevent viruses from entering the cell. In addition, interferons have been found to inhibit tumor growth and replication, to stimulate cytotoxic T-cell activity, and to enhance the inflammatory response. Of interest, interferon gamma-1b also acts like an interleukin, stimulating phagocytes to be more aggressive. See Table 17.1 for usual indications for each interferon.

have been found to inhibit tumor growth and replication, to stimulate cytotoxic T-cell activity, and to enhance the inflammatory response. Of interest, interferon gamma-1b also acts like an interleukin, stimulating phagocytes to be more aggressive (see Table 17.1 for usual indications of each interferon).

Box 17.2 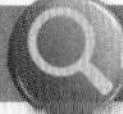 Focus on Sex Differences

IMMUNE MODULATORS AND PREGNANCY

Generally, immune modulators are contraindicated for use during pregnancy and lactation, largely because these drugs have been associated with fetal abnormalities, increased maternal and fetal infections, and suppressed immune responses in nursing babies. Patients able to become pregnant should be informed of the risk of using these drugs during pregnancy and receive counseling in the use of barrier contraceptives. (The use of barrier contraceptives is advised because the effects of oral contraceptives may be altered by liver changes or by changes in the body's immune response, potentially resulting in unexpected pregnancy.)

If a patient taking immune modulators becomes pregnant or decides that they want to become pregnant, they should discuss this with their health care provider and review the risks associated with use of the drug or drugs being taken. The monoclonal antibodies should be used with caution during pregnancy and lactation. Because long-term studies of most of these drugs are not yet available, it may be prudent to advise patients taking these drugs to avoid pregnancy if possible.

Pharmacokinetics

The interferons are generally well absorbed after subcutaneous or intramuscular injection. They have a rapid onset of action and peak within 3 to 8 hours, with a half-life ranging from 3 to 8 hours, with the exception of interferon beta-1a, which has an onset of action of 12 hours, reaches peak level in 48 hours, and has a half-life of 10 hours. Interferons are broken down in the liver and kidneys and seem to be excreted primarily through the kidneys.

Contraindications and Cautions

The use of interferons is contraindicated in the presence of known allergy to any interferon or product components to prevent hypersensitivity reactions. Many of the interferons are teratogenic in animals and, therefore, should not be used during pregnancy. Use of barrier contraceptives is advised for patients able to become pregnant. It is not known whether these drugs cross into human milk, but because of the potential adverse effects on the baby, it is advised that the drugs not be used during lactation unless the benefits to the parent clearly outweigh any risks to the baby. Caution should be used in the presence of known cardiac disease because hypertension and arrhythmias have been reported with the use of these drugs; with myelosuppression because

Table 17.1 *Drugs in Focus*: Immune Stimulants

Drug Name	Dosage/Route	Usual Indications
Interferons		
interferon alfa-2b (*Intron-A*)	*Adult*: Dose varies widely based on indication *Pediatric*: For hepatitis B, adjust adult dose to weight	Treatment of leukemias, Kaposi sarcoma, warts, hepatitis B, malignant melanoma, follicular lymphoma, chronic hepatitis C
interferon alfa-n3 (*Alferon N*)	250,000 IU intralesionally twice per week for 8 wk	Intralesional treatment of warts
interferon beta-1a (*Avonex*)	30 mcg IM once a week	Treatment of multiple sclerosis in adults
interferon beta-1b (*Betaseron, Extavia*)	0.0625–0.25 mg subcutaneous every other day (dose increased over a 6-wk period); discontinue if disease is unremitting >6 mo	Treatment of multiple sclerosis in adults
interferon gamma-1b (*Actimmune*)	50 mcg/m² subcutaneous three times per week	Treatment of serious, chronic granulomatous disease in adults; delaying time to disease progression in severe, malignant osteopetrosis
peginterferon alfa-2a (*Pegasys*)	*Hepatitis C: Adult*: 180 mcg subcutaneous weekly for 48 wk *Pediatric 5 and older*: 180 mcg/1.73 m² subcutaneous weekly *Hepatitis B: Adult and child over 45 kg*: 2 doses of 6 mg subcutaneously given a week apart	Treatment of hepatitis C; treatment of compensated chronic hepatitis B
peginterferon alfa-2b (*Peg-Intron*)	*Adult*: 1.5 mcg/kg subcutaneous once a week for 1 y in combination with Rebetol *Pediatric*: 60 mcg/m²/wk subcutaneous in combination with Rebetol	Treatment of chronic hepatitis C
Interleukins		
aldesleukin (*Proleukin*)	Two 5-d cycles of 600,000 IU/kg IV q8h given over 15 min for a total of 14 doses, then 9 d of rest and repeat. Maximum 28 doses per course	Treatment of metastatic renal carcinomas, metastatic melanoma in adults
oprelvekin (*Neumega*)	50 mcg/kg/d subcutaneously; decreased if renal impairment is present	Prevention and treatment of thrombocytopenia in adult clients being treated with myelosuppressive chemotherapy
Colony-Stimulating Factors		
filgrastim (*Neupogen*); filgrastim-sndz (*Zarxio*); tbo-filgrastim (*Granix*)	4–8 mcg/kg/d subcutaneously or IV as a single dose; dosing of Zarxio will vary per type of cancer; 5 mcg/kg/d subcutaneously at least 24 h after chemotherapy	Reduction of incidence of infection and reduction of time to neutrophil recovery in patients with severe neutropenia due to receiving antineoplastic chemotherapy for a variety of types of cancer
pegfilgrastim (*Neulasta*)	*Adult*: 6 mg subcutaneously as a single dose once per chemotherapy cycle *Pediatric*: Dose based on weight	Reduction of the incidence of infection in patients with nonmyeloid malignancies receiving bone marrow–suppressing antineoplastic drugs; increase survival after myelosuppressive doses of radiation
sargramostim (*Leukine*)	250 mcg/m²/d as a 2–4 h IV infusion	Myeloid reconstitution following bone marrow transplantation; treatment of neutropenia following bone marrow transplantation failure; induction chemotherapy with AML
tbo-filgrastim (*Granix*)	5 mcg/kg/d subcutaneously; administer first dose no earlier than 24 h after chemotherapy; do not administer within 24 h of chemotherapy	Reduction in the duration of severe neutropenia in nonmyeloid malignancies being treated with myelosuppressive anticancer drugs

AML, acute myeloid leukemia.

these drugs may further suppress the bone marrow; and with central nervous system (CNS) dysfunction of any kind because of the potential for CNS depression and personality changes that have been reported.

Adverse Effects

The adverse effects associated with the use of interferons are related to the immune or inflammatory reaction that is being stimulated (stimulating the immune and inflammatory response causes a flulike syndrome with lethargy, myalgia, arthralgia, anorexia, nausea). Other commonly seen adverse effects include headache, dizziness, bone marrow depression, depression and suicidal ideation, photosensitivity, and liver impairment.

Prototype Summary: Interferon Alfa-2b

Indications: Hairy cell leukemia, malignant melanoma, AIDS-related Kaposi sarcoma, chronic hepatitis B and C, follicular lymphoma, intralesional treatment of condylomata acuminata in patients 18 years of age or older.

Actions: Inhibits the growth of tumor cells and enhances the immune response.

Pharmacokinetics:

Route	Onset	Peak
IM, subcutaneous	Rapid	3–12 h
IV	Rapid	End of infusion

$T_{1/2}$: 2 to 3 hours; metabolized in the kidney; excretion is unknown.

Adverse Effects: Dizziness, confusion, rash, dry skin, anorexia, nausea, bone marrow suppression, flulike syndrome.

Clinically Important Drug–Drug Interactions

Concurrent use with theophylline can lead to theophylline toxicity. Use caution when using interferons with zidovudine or other myelosuppressive treatment due to potential increased risk of neutropenia or thrombocytopenia.

Interleukins

Interleukins are synthetic compounds much like the interferons; they communicate between lymphocytes, which stimulate cellular immunity and inhibit tumor growth. Interleukin-2 stimulates cellular immunity by increasing the activity of natural killer cells, platelets, and cytokines. Two interleukin preparations are available for use. Aldesleukin (*Proleukin*) is a human interleukin produced by recombinant DNA technology using *E. coli* bacteria. Oprelvekin (*Neumega*) is interleukin eleven, a thrombopoietic growth factor that stimulates the hematopoietic stem cells to mature into more platelets (see Table 17.1).

Therapeutic Actions and Indications

Natural interleukin-2 is produced by various lymphocytes to activate cellular immunity and inhibit tumor growth by increasing lymphocytes and their activity. When interleukins are administered, natural killer cells and lymphocytes, cytokine activity, and circulating platelets all increase. See Table 17.1 for usual indications. Oprelvekin acts as an interleukin and a colony-stimulating thrombopoietic growth factor.

Pharmacokinetics

The interleukins are rapidly distributed after injection. Aldesleukin, given IV, reaches peak level in 13 minutes and has a half-life of 85 minutes. Oprelvekin, which is given subcutaneously, reaches peak level in 3 to 5 hours and has a half-life of 7 to 8 hours. They are primarily cleared from the body by the kidneys.

Contraindications and Cautions

Interleukins are contraindicated in the presence of any allergy to an interleukin or *E. coli*–produced product to prevent hypersensitivity reactions. Because they were shown to be embryocidal and teratogenic in animal studies, they should not be used during pregnancy. Use of barrier contraceptives is recommended for patients able to become pregnant who require one of these drugs. It is not clear whether the drugs cross into human milk, but it is recommended that they not be used during lactation; if they must be used, another method of feeding the baby must be chosen because of the potential for adverse effects in the baby. Caution should be used with renal, liver, or cardiovascular impairment and/or arrhythmias because of the adverse effects of the drugs.

Adverse Effects

The adverse effects associated with the interleukins can be attributed to their effect on the body during inflammation (flulike effects: lethargy, myalgia, arthralgia, fatigue, fever). Respiratory difficulties, capillary leak syndrome, CNS changes that can progress to coma, and cardiac arrhythmias also have been reported, and the patient should be monitored for these effects and the drug stopped if they occur. Oprelvekin has been associated with severe hypersensitivity reactions, and patients should be closely watched when beginning therapy and encouraged to report any difficulty breathing or swallowing, chest tightness, or swelling. There is also risk of fluid retention, cardiac dysrhythmias, and inflammation of the eye and eyelid.

Clinical Important Drug–Drug Interactions

Concurrent use with medications that are either cardio or neurotoxic may exacerbate the adverse effects of the medication. There is higher risk of hypersensitivity if used with other antineoplastic medications.

Prototype Summary: Aldesleukin

Indications: Metastatic renal cell carcinoma in adults, treatment of metastatic melanomas.

Actions: Activates human cellular immunity and inhibits tumor growth through increases in lymphocytes, platelets, and cytokines.

Pharmacokinetics:

Route	Onset	Peak	Duration
IV	5 min	13 min	3–4 h

$T_{1/2}$: 85 minutes; metabolized in the kidney and excreted in the urine.

Adverse Effects: Mental status changes, dizziness, hypotension, sinus tachycardia, arrhythmias, pruritus, nausea, vomiting, diarrhea, anorexia, gastrointestinal bleed, bone marrow suppression, respiratory difficulties, fever, chills, pain.

Colony-Stimulating Factors

The colony-stimulating factors are produced by recombinant DNA technology. Filgrastim (*Neupogen*), pegfilgrastim (*Neulasta*), and tbo-filgrastim (*Granix*) increase the production of neutrophils in the bone marrow, with little effect on other hematopoietic cells. Sargramostim (*Leukine*) increases the proliferation and differentiation of hematopoietic progenitor cells and can activate mature granulocytes and monocytes. The colony-stimulating factor of choice will depend on the condition being treated (see Table 17.1).

Therapeutic Actions and Indications

By increasing the production of white cells, the colony-stimulating factors can be used to reduce the incidence of infection in patients with bone marrow suppression, decrease the neutropenia associated with bone marrow transplants and chemotherapy, and help in the treatment of various blood-related cancers. See Table 17.1 for usual indications.

Pharmacokinetics

Filgrastim can be given IV or by subcutaneous injection, reaching peak level in 2 hours IV or 8 hours subcutaneously. It has a half-life of about 220 minutes and a duration of 4 days; its metabolism and excretion are not known. Pegfilgrastim is only given by subcutaneous injection with a similar onset but it has a much longer half-life—15 to 80 hours—than filgrastim. Tbo-filgrastim is only given subcutaneously, reaches peak level in 4 to 6 hours and has a half-life of 3.5 hours. Sargramostim can be given IV or subcutaneously with a duration of 6 hours (IV) or 12 hours subcutaneously. It has a half-life of 1 to 3 hours; its metabolism and excretion are not known.

Contraindications and Cautions

Colony-stimulating factors are contraindicated in the presence of any allergy to any component of the drug or to *E. coli*–produced products to prevent hypersensitivity reactions. Sargramostim is contraindicated in neonates because of benzyl alcohol in the solution, and with excessive leukemic myeloid blasts in the bone marrow or peripheral blood, which could be worsened by the drug. These drugs should be used with caution in pregnancy and lactation because the potential effects on the fetus or neonate are not known. The drugs need to be used with caution for patients with bone marrow cancer or sickle cell disease due to the stimulation effect on the bone marrow. Sargramostim should also be used with caution in hepatic or renal failure, which could alter the pharmacokinetics of the drug, and during or immediately after radiation or chemotherapy because of a potential loss of effectiveness.

Adverse Effects

The adverse effects associated with colony-stimulating factors are gastrointestinal (GI) effects (nausea, vomiting, diarrhea, constipation, anorexia), headache, fatigue, generalized weakness, alopecia and dermatitis, and generalized pain and bone pain. The effects are thought to be associated with the drug effects on the bone marrow cells and their increased activity. There is also risk of splenomegaly or splenic rupture with filgrasim and pegfilgrastim. Leukocytosis can occur with these products and white blood cell counts should be monitored. Thrombocytosis is a complication of sargramostim.

Clinically Important Drug–Drug Interactions

The only reported drug–drug interactions associated with these drugs is an increase in the myeloproliferative effects of sargramostim when combined with lithium or corticosteroids; these combinations should be used with caution.

Prototype Summary: Filgrastim

Indications: Reduction of the incidence of infection and reduction in time to neutrophil recovery with myelosuppressive chemotherapy, leukemia, and bone marrow transplants.

Actions: Increases the production of neutrophils in the bone marrow.

Pharmacokinetics:

Route	Peak	Duration
IV	2 h	4 d
Subcutaneous	8 h	4 d

$T_{1/2}$: 210 to 231 minutes; metabolism and excretion unknown.

Adverse Effects: Headache, fatigue, alopecia, rash, nausea, vomiting, diarrhea, stomatitis, anorexia, bone pain, cough, generalized pain.

Nursing Considerations for Patients Receiving Immune Stimulants

Assessment: History and Examination

- Assess for contraindications and cautions: known allergies to any of these drugs or their components, to prevent hypersensitivity reactions; current status related to pregnancy or lactation, to avoid serious adverse effects on the fetus or baby; and conditions that could be exacerbated by the effects of these drugs including a history of hepatic, renal, or cardiac disease; bone marrow depression; leukemic states; and CNS disorders, including seizures.
- Perform a physical assessment before beginning therapy to determine baseline status and any potential adverse effects: inspect for the presence of any skin lesions to detect early dermatological effects; obtain weight to monitor for fluid retention; monitor temperature to detect any infection; check heart rate and rhythm and blood pressure to monitor for any cardiac effects of the drug; and assess level of orientation and reflexes to evaluate CNS effects of the drug.
- Obtain a baseline electrocardiogram if appropriate to evaluate cardiac function and monitor adverse effects of the drugs.
- Assess patient's renal and liver function, including renal and liver function tests, to determine the appropriateness of therapy and the need for possible dose adjustment and toxic drug effects.
- Monitor the results of laboratory tests such as complete blood count (CBC) to identify changes in bone marrow function.

Nursing Conclusions

Nursing conclusions related to drug therapy might include the following:

- Impaired comfort related to CNS, GI, and flulike effects
- Malnutrition risk related to flulike effects
- Acute or chronic fear or anxiety related to diagnosis and drug therapy
- Knowledge deficit risk regarding drug therapy

Planning

- The patient will receive the best therapeutic effect from the drug therapy.
- The patient will have limited adverse effects to the drug therapy.
- The patient will have an understanding of the drug therapy, adverse effects to anticipate, and measures to relieve discomfort and improve safety.

Intervention With Rationale

- Arrange for laboratory tests before and periodically during therapy, including CBC and differential, to monitor for drug effects and adverse effects.
- Administer drug as indicated; instruct the patient and a friend, family member, or significant other if injections are required to ensure that the drug will be given even if the patient is not able to administer it.
- Monitor for severe reactions, such as severe hypersensitivity reactions, and arrange to discontinue the drug immediately if they occur.
- Arrange for supportive care and comfort measures for flulike symptoms (e.g., rest, environmental control, acetaminophen) to help the patient cope with the drug effects. Ensure that the patient is well hydrated during therapy to prevent severe adverse effects.
- Instruct patients able to become pregnant in the use of barrier contraceptives to avoid pregnancy during therapy because of the potential for adverse effects on the fetus.
- Offer support and encouragement to deal with the diagnosis and the drug regimen.
- Provide patient teaching about measures to avoid adverse effects, warning signs of problems, and proper administration technique.

Evaluation

- Monitor patient response to the drug (improvement in condition being treated).
- Monitor for adverse effects (flulike symptoms, GI upset, CNS changes, bone marrow depression).
- Evaluate the effectiveness of the teaching plan (patient can name drug, dosage, adverse effects to watch for, specific measures to avoid adverse effects).
- Monitor the effectiveness of comfort measures and adherence to the regimen.

Key Points

- Immune stimulants assist the immune system to fight specific pathogens or cancer cells; in doing so, they cause flulike symptoms (lethargy, muscle and joint aches and pains, anorexia, nausea).
- Interferons are used to treat various cancers, hepatitis, and warts.
- Interleukins stimulate cellular immunity and inhibit tumor growth.
- Colony-stimulating factors increase the production of blood cells by working in the bone marrow.

Immune Suppressants

Immune suppressants (see Table 17.2) often are used in conjunction with corticosteroids, which block the inflammatory reaction and decrease initial damage to cells. They are especially beneficial in cases of organ transplantation and in the treatment of autoimmune diseases.

Table 17.2 *Drugs in Focus*: Immune Suppressants

Drug Name	Dosage/Route	Usual Indications
Immune Modulators		
fingolimod (*Gilenya*)	0.5 mg/d PO	Treatment of patients with relapsing forms of multiple sclerosis to reduce frequency of exacerbations and delay accumulation of physical disability
lenalidomide (*Revlimid*)	10–20 mg/d PO with water; 25 mg/d PO on days 1–21 of a 28-d cycle for multiple myeloma *Mantle cell lymphoma*: 25 mg/d PO on days 1–21 at repeated 28-d cycles	Treatment of patients with transfusion-dependent anemia, treatment of multiple myeloma in patients who have received at least one other therapy; treatment of mantle cell lymphoma after other therapy
thalidomide (*Thalomid*)	100–300 mg/d PO for at least 2 wk, taper	Treatment of erythema nodosum following treatment for leprosy; newly diagnosed multiple myeloma
T- and B-Cell Suppressors		
abatacept (*Orencia*)	*Adult*: *<60 kg*: 500 mg/d IV repeated at 2 and 4 wk, then every 4 wk; *60–100 kg*: 750 mg/d IV, repeated at 2 and 4 wk, then every 4 wk; *>100 kg*: 1 g/d IV, repeated at 2 and 4 wk, then every 4 wk *Pediatric*: 75 kg or more, adult dose; under 75 kg: 10 mg/kg/d IV	Reduction of the signs and symptoms and slowing structural damage in adults with rheumatoid arthritis who have inadequate response to other drugs; treatment of juvenile idiopathic arthritis in children 6 and over
azathioprine (*Azasan, Imuran*)	*Adult*: 3–5 mg/kg/d PO for prevention of rejection *Maintenance*: 1–3 mg/kg/d PO *Rheumatoid arthritis*: 1–2.5 mg/kg/d PO; reduce dose with renal impairment	Prevention of rejection in renal transplants, treatment of rheumatoid arthritis
belatacept (*Nulojix*)	*Initial:* 10 mg/kg IV day of transplant, day 5, end of week 2, 4, 8, and 12 *Maintenance:* 5 mg/kg IV end of week 16 and about every 4 weeks thereafter	Prophylaxis of organ rejection in adult patients with kidney transplant who are Epstein–Barr virus seropositive
cyclosporine (*Sandimmune*)	15 mg/kg PO as a single oral dose 4–12 h before transplantation, then 5–10 mg/kg/d PO *Pediatric*: Larger doses may be needed to achieve therapeutic levels	Suppression of rejection in a variety of transplant situations
cyclosporine (*Neoral*)	9–15 mg/kg PO as a single oral dose 4–12 h before transplantation, then 5–10 mg/kg/d PO—titrate down *Rheumatoid arthritis*: 2.5 mg/kg/d PO in 2 divided doses *Psoriasis*: 2.5 mg/kg PO b.i.d.	Treatment of rheumatoid arthritis, psoriasis; prophylaxis of organ rejection for variety of transplants
glatiramer acetate (*Copaxone*)	20 mg/d subcutaneously; 40 mg subcutaneously three times a week	Reduction of the number of relapses in multiple sclerosis in adults
mycophenolate (*CellCept*)	*Adult*:1–1.5 g PO b.i.d.; may be started IV during transplantation, with switch to oral route as soon as possible *Pediatric*: 600 mg/m^2 PO b.i.d.	Prevention of rejection after renal, hepatic, or heart transplantation in adults; not for use in pregnancy
pimecrolimus (*Elidel*)	Topical, apply a thin layer over affected area twice daily	Treatment of atopic dermatitis; limit length of use, may be associated with skin malignancies
sirolimus (*Rapamune*)	6 mg PO as soon after transplant as possible, then 2 mg/d PO *Pediatric (<13 y)*: 3 mg/m^2 PO loading dose, then 1 mg/m^2/d PO	Prevention of rejection after renal transplantation
tacrolimus (*Prograf*)	0.075–0.2 mg/kg/d PO divided every 12 h or 0.01–0.05 mg/kg/d IV as a continuous infusion; topical, apply thin layer to affected area b.i.d.	Prophylaxis for organ injection in liver, kidney, or heart transplants; topical treatment of atopic dermatitis

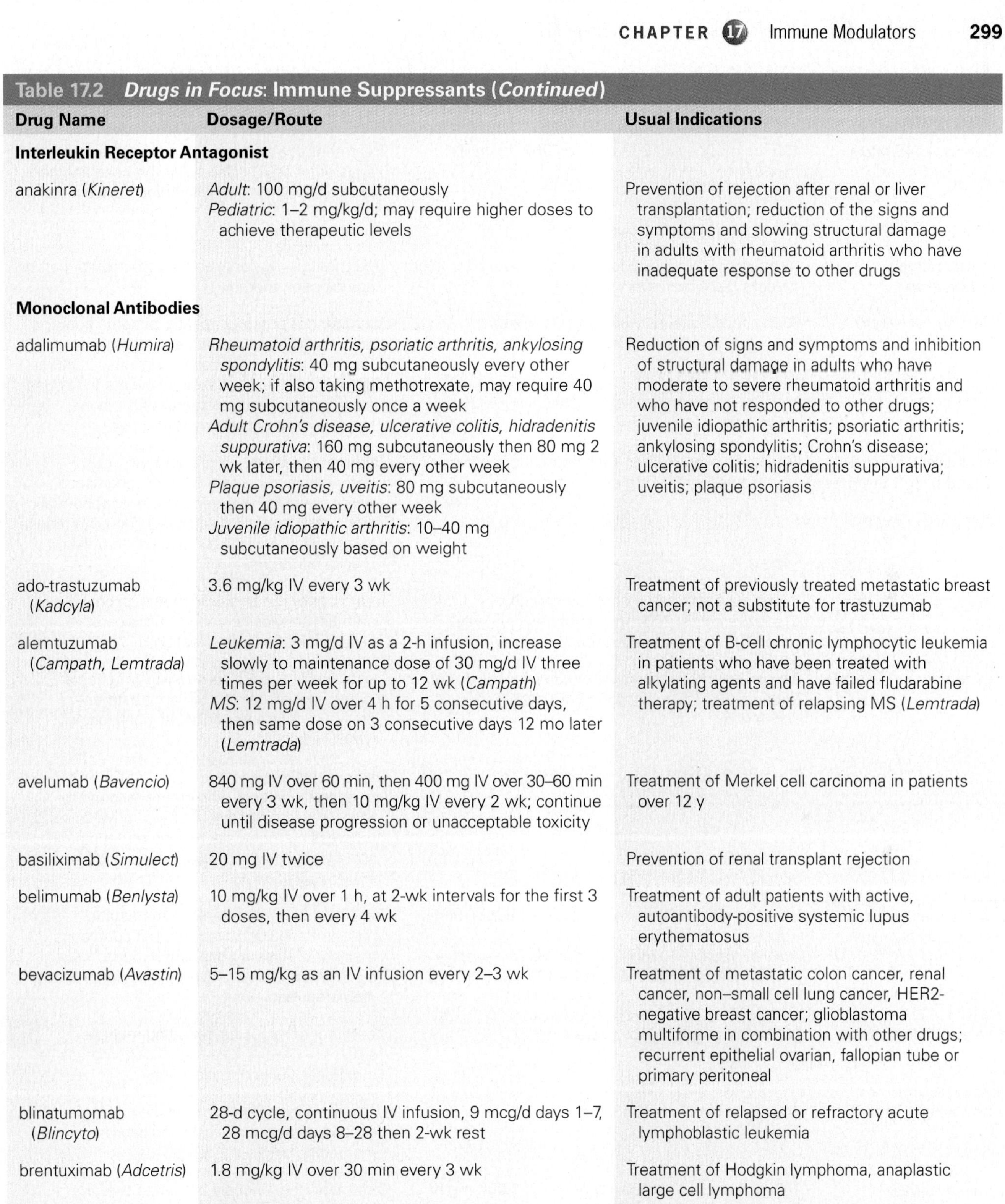

Table 17.2 *Drugs in Focus*: Immune Suppressants (*Continued*)

Drug Name	Dosage/Route	Usual Indications
Interleukin Receptor Antagonist		
anakinra (*Kineret*)	*Adult*: 100 mg/d subcutaneously *Pediatric*: 1–2 mg/kg/d; may require higher doses to achieve therapeutic levels	Prevention of rejection after renal or liver transplantation; reduction of the signs and symptoms and slowing structural damage in adults with rheumatoid arthritis who have inadequate response to other drugs
Monoclonal Antibodies		
adalimumab (*Humira*)	*Rheumatoid arthritis, psoriatic arthritis, ankylosing spondylitis*: 40 mg subcutaneously every other week; if also taking methotrexate, may require 40 mg subcutaneously once a week *Adult Crohn's disease, ulcerative colitis, hidradenitis suppurativa*: 160 mg subcutaneously then 80 mg 2 wk later, then 40 mg every other week *Plaque psoriasis, uveitis*: 80 mg subcutaneously then 40 mg every other week *Juvenile idiopathic arthritis*: 10–40 mg subcutaneously based on weight	Reduction of signs and symptoms and inhibition of structural damage in adults who have moderate to severe rheumatoid arthritis and who have not responded to other drugs; juvenile idiopathic arthritis; psoriatic arthritis; ankylosing spondylitis; Crohn's disease; ulcerative colitis; hidradenitis suppurativa; uveitis; plaque psoriasis
ado-trastuzumab (*Kadcyla*)	3.6 mg/kg IV every 3 wk	Treatment of previously treated metastatic breast cancer; not a substitute for trastuzumab
alemtuzumab (*Campath, Lemtrada*)	*Leukemia*: 3 mg/d IV as a 2-h infusion, increase slowly to maintenance dose of 30 mg/d IV three times per week for up to 12 wk (*Campath*) *MS*: 12 mg/d IV over 4 h for 5 consecutive days, then same dose on 3 consecutive days 12 mo later (*Lemtrada*)	Treatment of B-cell chronic lymphocytic leukemia in patients who have been treated with alkylating agents and have failed fludarabine therapy; treatment of relapsing MS (*Lemtrada*)
avelumab (*Bavencio*)	840 mg IV over 60 min, then 400 mg IV over 30–60 min every 3 wk, then 10 mg/kg IV every 2 wk; continue until disease progression or unacceptable toxicity	Treatment of Merkel cell carcinoma in patients over 12 y
basiliximab (*Simulect*)	20 mg IV twice	Prevention of renal transplant rejection
belimumab (*Benlysta*)	10 mg/kg IV over 1 h, at 2-wk intervals for the first 3 doses, then every 4 wk	Treatment of adult patients with active, autoantibody-positive systemic lupus erythematosus
bevacizumab (*Avastin*)	5–15 mg/kg as an IV infusion every 2–3 wk	Treatment of metastatic colon cancer, renal cancer, non–small cell lung cancer, HER2-negative breast cancer; glioblastoma multiforme in combination with other drugs; recurrent epithelial ovarian, fallopian tube or primary peritoneal
blinatumomab (*Blincyto*)	28-d cycle, continuous IV infusion, 9 mcg/d days 1–7, 28 mcg/d days 8–28 then 2-wk rest	Treatment of relapsed or refractory acute lymphoblastic leukemia
brentuximab (*Adcetris*)	1.8 mg/kg IV over 30 min every 3 wk	Treatment of Hodgkin lymphoma, anaplastic large cell lymphoma
canakinumab (*Ilaris*)	***Periodic syndrome:*** *Over 40 kg*: 150 mg subcutaneously every 4–8 wk *15–40 kg*: 2 mg/kg subcutaneously every 4 wk *Juvenile arthritis*: 150–300 mg subcutaneously every 4 wk	Treatment of cryopyrin-associated periodic syndromes, tumor necrosis factor–associated periodic syndrome, hyperimmunoglobulin D syndrome, familial Mediterranean fever; juvenile idiopathic arthritis in patients 2 y and older
certolizumab (*Cimzia*)	400 mg subcutaneously, repeated at weeks 2 and 4, then every 4 wk	Reduction of the signs and symptoms of Crohn's disease in adults with moderate to severe disease not controlled by standard therapy; treatment of adults with rheumatoid arthritis, psoriatic arthritis, ankylosing spondylitis

(continues on page 300)

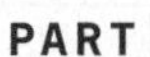

Table 17.2 ***Drugs in Focus*: Immune Suppressants (*Continued*)**

Drug Name	Dosage/Route	Usual Indications
cetuximab (*Erbitux*)	400 mg/m² IV over 120 min, then 250 mg/m² IV weekly	Treatment of advanced colon cancer; advanced squamous cell carcinoma of the head and neck; premedicate with antihistamine before infusion
daclizumab (*Zinbryta*)	150 mg/mo subcutaneously	Treatment of MS
daratumumab (*Darzalex*)	16 mg/kg/wk IV weekly for 8 wk then every 2 wk for weeks 9–24 then every 4 wk	Treatment of myeloma as monotherapy or part of combination therapy
denosumab (*Prolia*, *Xgeva*)	60 mg subcutaneously every 6 mo (*Prolia*) 120 mg subcutaneously every 4 wk (*Xgeva*)	Treatment of postmenopausal patients and patients with osteoporosis at high risk for fracture, to increase bone mass after fracture (*Prolia*). Treatment of skeletal events with bone metastases, giant cell tumor of the bone, hyperkalemia of malignancy (*Xgeva*)
eculizumab (*Soliris*)	600 mg IV every 7 d for 4 wk, then 900 mg every 7 d, followed by 900 mg every 14 d	Treatment of paroxysmal nocturnal hemoglobinuria, a rare genetic condition in which patients have generations of abnormal blood cells that are lysed by the body, to reduce hemolysis; treatment of atypical hemolytic uremia syndrome
golimumab (*Simponi*)	50 mg subcutaneously once per month *Ulcerative colitis*: 200 mg subcutaneously week 0 then 100 mg at week 2, then 100 mg every 4 wk	Treatment of rheumatoid arthritis; psoriatic arthritis; ankylosing spondylitis, ulcerative colitis; risk of severe infections
ibritumomab (*Zevalin*)	2 mg of antibody labeled with 0.3 or 0.4 mCi/kg of yttrium-90 IV in conjunction with rituximab	Treatment of B-cell non-Hodgkin lymphoma in conjunction with rituximab; treatment of previously untreated follicular non-Hodgkin lymphoma
infliximab (*Remicade*, *Inflectra*)	5 mg/kg IV over 2 h, may be repeated at 2 and 6 wk then every 8 wk	Decreases signs and symptoms of Crohn's disease in patients who do not respond to other therapy; treatment of ulcerative colitis; progressing moderate to severe rheumatoid arthritis; psoriatic arthritis; plaque psoriasis; ankylosing spondylitis
ipilimumab (*Yervoy*)	3 mg/kg IV over 90 min every 3 wk for a total of 4 doses *Adjunct therapy*: 10 mg/kg IV over 90 min every 3 wk for a total of 4 doses then every 12 wk for up to 3 y	Treatment of unresectable or metastatic melanoma; adjunct treatment of cutaneous melanoma with regional lymph node involvement; risk of severe to fatal immune-mediated reactions
natalizumab (*Tysabri*)	300 mg IV over 1 h once every 4 wk	Treatment of relapsing–remitting multiple sclerosis; Crohn's disease; risk of progressive multifocal leukoencephalopathy
nivolumab (*Opdivo*)	240 mg IV every 2 wk; 480 mg every 4 wk; or 3 mg/kg IV over 60 min every 2 wk	Unresectable metastatic multiple myeloma; squamous non–small cell lung cancer; metastatic colorectal cancer
obinutuzumab (*Gazyva*)	100 mg IV on day 1, 900 mg IV day 2, 1,000 mg IV on days 8 and 15 of a 28-d cycle, then 1,000 mg IV on day 1 of cycles 2–6	Treatment of previously untreated chronic lymphocytic leukemia with chlorambucil; treatment of follicular lymphoma with bendamustine
ocrelizumab (*Ocrevus*)	300 mg IV, then 300 mg IV 2 wk later, then 600 mg IV every 6 mo	Treatment of multiple sclerosis
ofatumumab (*Arzerra*)	300 mg IV, 1 wk later 1,000 mg IV on day 8, then 1,000 mg IV on day 1 of subsequent 28-d cycles	Treatment of chronic lymphocytic leukemia
olaratumab (*Lartruvo*)	15 mg/kg IV over 60 min on days 1, 8 of a 21-d cycle	Treatment of soft tissue sarcoma of a specific genotype, given with other drugs

Table 17.2 *Drugs in Focus*: Immune Suppressants (*Continued*)

Drug Name	Dosage/Route	Usual Indications
omalizumab (*Xolair*)	*Asthma*: 75–375 mg subcutaneously every 2–4 wk *Chronic urticaria*: 150–300 mg subcutaneously every 4 wk	Treatment of asthma with a very strong allergic component and seasonal allergic rhinitis not well controlled with traditional medications; treatment of chronic idiopathic urticaria
palivizumab (*Synagis*)	15 mg/kg IM as a single dose at the start of RSV season	Prevention of serious RSV infection in high-risk children
pegaptanib (*Macugen*)	0.3 mg injected into the intravitreal fluid of the eye once every 6 wk	Treatment of neovascular (wet) age-related macular degeneration
pembrolizumab (*Keytruda*)	200 mg IV over 30 min every 3 wk	Treatment of metastatic or unresectable multiple myeloma; non–small cell lung cancer; head and neck squamous cell cancer; Hodgkin lymphoma; urothelial carcinoma; metastatic microsatellite instability–high cancer; gastric cancer
pertuzumab (*Perjeta*)	840 mg IV over 60 min followed every 3 wk by 420 mg IV over 30–60 min	With other drugs for treatment of HER2-positive metastatic breast cancer or early-stage breast cancer
ramucirumab (*Cyramza*)	*Gastric cancer*: 8 mg/kg IV every 2 wk *Lung cancer*: 10 mg/kg IV on day 1 of a 21-d cycle *Colorectal cancer*: 8 mg/kg IV every 2 wk	Treatment of advanced gastric or gastroesophageal adenocarcinoma; treatment of small cell lung cancer; colorectal cancer
ranibizumab (*Lucentis*)	0.5 mg by intravitreal injection once a month *Diabetic macular edema, diabetic retinopathy*: 0.3 mg by intravitreal injection once a month	Treatment of macular degeneration (wet); treatment of macular edema following retinal vein occlusion; diabetic macular edema; diabetic retinopathy; myopic choroidal neovascularization
raxibacumab (generic)	*Over 50 kg*: 40 mg/kg IV over 2.25 h *15–50 kg*: 60 mg/kg IV over 1.25 h *15 kg or less*: 80 mg/kg IV over 1.25 h	Treatment of adults and children with inhalational anthrax exposure with appropriate antibiotic therapy
rituximab (*Rituxan*)	375 mg/m^2 IV once weekly for 4 doses *Rheumatoid arthritis*: two 1,000 mg IV infusions separated by 2 wk every 24 wk	Treatment of relapsed follicular B-cell non-Hodgkin lymphoma; chronic lymphocytic leukemia; rheumatoid arthritis; granulomatosis with polyangiitis
sarilumab (*Kevzara*)	200 mg subcutaneously every 2 wk	Treatment of adults with moderately to severely active rheumatoid arthritis
siltuximab (*Sylvant*)	11 mg/kg IV over 1 h every 3 wk	Treatment of multicentric Castleman's disease
tocilizumab (*Actemra*)	*Adult*: 4–8 mg/kg IV every 4 wk, with methotrexate or 162 mg subcutaneously every other week *Pediatric*: 8–12 mg/kg IV every 2–4 wk based on weight and diagnosis	Relief of signs and symptoms of moderate to severe rheumatoid arthritis in adults; giant cell arteritis; polyarticular and systemic juvenile idiopathic arthritis
trastuzumab (*Herceptin*)	*Breast cancer*: 4 mg/kg IV over 90 min, then 2 mg/kg IV once a week over at least 30 min *Gastric cancers*: 8 mg/kg IV over 90 min then 6 mg/kg IV over 30–90 min every 3 wk	Treatment of metastatic breast cancer and metastatic gastric or gastroesophageal junction adenocarcinoma with tumors that overexpress HER2
ustekinumab (*Stelara*)	45–90 mg by subcutaneously injection once a week, progressing to once a month, then once every 3 mo as determined by patient condition and response *Crohn's disease*: 260–520 mg IV as a single dose, then 90 mg subcutaneously every 8 wk for maintenance	Treatment of recalcitrant plaque psoriasis; psoriatic arthritis in adults and children 12 y and older not responsive to traditional therapy; active Crohn's disease
vedolizumab (*Entyvio*)	300 mg IV over 30 min weeks 0, 2, and 6, then every 8 wk	Treatment of ulcerative colitis and Crohn's disease in patients with lack of response to TNF blockers and corticosteroids

HER2, human epidermal growth factor receptor 2; RSV, respiratory syncytial virus; CD20, a protein expressed on the surface of B cells; TNF, tumor necrosis factor.

The immune suppressants include the immune modulators, T- and B-cell suppressors, an interleukin receptor antagonist, and **monoclonal antibodies**—antibodies produced by a single clone of B cells that react with specific antigens.

Immune Modulators

The immune modulators block the release of various cytokines involved in the inflammatory response and activation of lymphocytes, decreasing immune activity. The result of blocking these chemicals is immune suppression. The immune modulators are a relatively new class of drugs and include fingolimod (*Gilenya*), lenalidomide (*Revlimid*), thalidomide (*Thalomid*), apremilast (*Otezla*), dimethyl fumarate (*Tecfidera*), pomalidomide (*Pomalyst*), and teriflunomide (*Aubagio*).

Therapeutic Actions and Indications

The immune modulators have a number of effects on the inflammatory system. Lenalidomide and thalidomide inhibit the secretion of proinflammatory cytokines, increase the secretion of anti-inflammatory cytokines from monocytes, and have varying effects on cell proliferation. Fingolimod inhibits the release of lymphocytes from lymph nodes into the peripheral blood so they cannot migrate to activate immune and inflammatory reactions. Fingolimod is the first oral agent for the treatment of relapsing forms of multiple sclerosis. Lenalidomide is used in treating multiple myeloma and myelodysplastic syndromes. Thalidomide is also used for treating multiple myeloma and erythema nodosum leprosum. The newer agent apremilast is used for adults with psoriatic arthritis. Dimethyl fumarate and teriflunomide are used to treat multiple sclerosis. Pomalidomide is a thalidomide analog that is used in treating multiple myeloma.

Pharmacokinetics

Fingolimod is slowly absorbed from the GI tract, reaching peak level in 12 to 16 hours. It is metabolized in the liver, excreted through the kidneys, and has a half-life of 6 to 9 days. Lenalidomide is absorbed quickly from the GI tract, reaching peak level in 30 to 90 minutes. It is excreted unchanged in the urine and has a half-life of 3 hours. Thalidomide is very slowly absorbed from the GI tract, reaching peak level in 3 to 6 hours. The metabolism of thalidomide is not known; it is excreted in the urine and has a half-life of 12 to 24 hours. Pomalidomide is absorbed from the GI tract, reaching peak level in 2 to 3 hours. It is metabolized in the liver, excreted in the urine, and has a half-life of 7.5 to 9.5 hours. Apremilast is absorbed from the GI tract, reaching peak level in 2.5 hours. It is also metabolized in the liver, excreted in both urine and feces, and has a half-life of 6 to 9 hours. Dimethyl fumarate is absorbed from the GI tract with peak level occurring within 2 to 2.5 hours. It is metabolized by esterases throughout the body, with the main excretion occurring as CO_2 through the lungs. The half-life of this drug is about 1 hour. Oral teriflunomide reaches peak level in 1 to 4 hours; it is excreted unchanged in the bile. Most of the drug is eliminated from the body within 21 days.

Contraindications and Cautions

All of these drugs are contraindicated during pregnancy because their effects on cells can cause serious fetal harm; patients able to become pregnant should be advised to use barrier contraceptives when using this drug, and proof that the patient is not pregnant needs to be documented in the chart before beginning therapy and periodically during therapy. Teriflunomide is also contraindicated with severe hepatic impairment, which could become more severe due to the drug effects.

T- and B-Cell Suppressors

Several T- and B-cell immune suppressors are available for use. Agents include abatacept (*Orencia*), alefacept (*Amevive*), azathioprine (*Imuran*), belatacept (*Nulojix*), cyclosporine (*Sandimmune, Neoral*), glatiramer (*Copaxone, Glatopa*), mycophenolate (*CellCept*), pimecrolimus (*Elidel*), sirolimus (*Rapamune*), and tacrolimus (*Prograf*).

Therapeutic Actions and Indications

The exact mechanism of actions of the T- and B-cell suppressors varies. It has been shown that they block antibody production by B cells, inhibit suppressor and helper T cells, and modify the release of interleukins and of T-cell growth factor (see Fig. 17.1).

The T- and B-cell suppressors are indicated for the prevention and treatment of specific transplant rejections as well and treating some types of arthritis. See Table 17.2 for usual indications of each agent.

Pharmacokinetics

Cyclosporine is well absorbed from the GI tract, reaching peak level in 1 to 2 hours. It is extensively metabolized in the liver by the cytochrome P450 system and is primarily excreted in the bile. The half-life of the drug is about 19 hours for *Sandimmune* and 8.4 hours for *Neoral*. It is available as an oral solution that can be mixed with milk, chocolate milk, or orange juice for ease of administration. Abatacept must be given as a 30-minute infusion every 2 to 4 weeks, depending on the patient's response. Peak level is reached at the end of the infusion. Abatacept has a half-life of 12 to 23 days and usually reaches a steady state by 60 days of treatment. The drug is cleared from the body by the kidneys.

Alefacept is rapidly absorbed and can be given IM or IV. It reaches peak level in 4 to 6 hours and has a half-life of 270 hours.

Azathioprine is rapidly absorbed from the GI tract, reaching peak level in 1 to 2 hours. This drug is catabolized in the liver and red blood cells.

Belatacept is administered intravenously. The half-life is between 8 to 10 days.

Little is known about the pharmacokinetics of glatiramer. Some of it is immediately hydrolyzed on injection, some enters the lymph system, and some may actually reach the systemic circulation.

Mycophenolate mofetil is readily absorbed and immediately metabolized to its active metabolite, mycophenolic acid. Most of the metabolized drug is then excreted in the urine.

Sirolimus is rapidly absorbed from the GI tract, reaching peak level in 1 hour. It is extensively metabolized in the liver, partly by the cytochrome P450 system. The drug is then excreted primarily in the feces.

Tacrolimus is rapidly absorbed from the GI tract, reaching peak level in 1.5 to 3.5 hours. It is extensively metabolized in the liver by the cytochrome P450 system and is excreted in the urine.

Contraindications and Cautions

The use of T- and B-cell suppressors is contraindicated in the presence of any known allergy to the drug or its components to prevent hypersensitivity reactions and during pregnancy and lactation because of the potential serious adverse effects on the fetus or neonate. Caution should be used with renal or hepatic impairment, which could interfere with the metabolism or excretion of the drug, and in the presence of known neoplasms, which potentially could spread with immune system suppression.

Adverse Effects

Patients receiving these drugs are at increased risk for infection and for the development of neoplasms due to the drugs' blocking effect on the immune system. Other potentially dangerous adverse effects include hepatotoxicity, renal toxicity, renal dysfunction, and pulmonary edema. Patients may experience headache, tremors, secondary infections such as acne, GI upset, diarrhea, and hypertension. Cyclosporine is also known to cause reversable hirsutism and gingival hyperplasia.

Clinically Important Drug–Drug Interactions

There is an increased risk of toxicity if these drugs are combined with other drugs that are hepatotoxic or nephrotoxic. Extreme care should be used if such combinations are necessary. Other reported drug–drug interactions are drug specific; consult a drug guide or drug handbook.

Prototype Summary: Cyclosporine

Indications: Prophylaxis for organ rejection in kidney, liver, and heart transplants (used with corticosteroids); treatment of chronic rejection in patients previously treated with other immune suppressants; treatment of rheumatoid arthritis and recalcitrant psoriasis.

Actions: Reversibly inhibits immunocompetent lymphocytes; inhibits T helper cells and T suppressor cells, lymphokine production, and release of interleukin-2 and T-cell growth factor.

Pharmacokinetics:

Route	Onset	Peak
PO	Varies	3.5 h
IV	Rapid	1–2 h

$T_{1/2}$: 8 to 19 hours (varies per formulation); metabolized in the liver and excreted in the bile and urine.

Adverse Effects: Tremor, hypertension, gingival hyperplasia, renal dysfunction, diarrhea, hirsutism, acne, bone marrow suppression, interleukin receptor antagonist.

Interleukin Receptor Antagonist

An interleukin receptor antagonist works to block the activity of the interleukins that are released in an inflammatory or immune response. The only available interleukin-1 receptor antagonist is anakinra (*Kineret*). See Table 17.2 for additional information about this drug.

Therapeutic Actions and Indications

Anakinra specifically antagonizes human interleukin-1 receptors, blocking the activity of interleukin-1. Interleukin-1 levels are elevated in response to inflammation or immune reactions and are thought to be responsible for the degradation of cartilage that occurs in rheumatoid arthritis. Anakinra is used to reduce the signs and symptoms of moderately to severely active rheumatoid arthritis in patients 18 years of age or older who have not responded to the traditional antirheumatic drugs.

Pharmacokinetics

The recommended dosage is 100 mg/d by subcutaneous injection. Anakinra is absorbed slowly, reaching peak effects in 3 to 7 hours. It is metabolized in the tissues, excreted in the urine, and has a half-life of 4 to 6 hours.

Contraindications and Cautions

Anakinra is contraindicated with any known allergy to *E. coli*–produced products or to anakinra itself to prevent hypersensitivity reactions. It should be used with caution during pregnancy and lactation because the drug may cross the placenta and enter human milk. It is also used cautiously in patients with renal impairment, immunosuppression, or any active infection because these could be exacerbated by the effects of the drug. There is an increased risk of infection whenever this drug is used, and the patient needs to be protected from exposure to infections and monitored closely after any invasive procedures. Live vaccines should not be given while the patient is on this drug.

Adverse Effects

Headache, sinusitis, nausea, diarrhea, upper respiratory and other infections, and injection site reactions are among the most common adverse effects.

Clinically Important Drug–Drug Interactions

Patients who are also receiving etanercept (*Enbrel*) must be monitored very closely because severe and even life-threatening infections have occurred. Anakinra should not be combined with abatacept because of the potential for serious infections.

Monoclonal Antibodies

Antibodies that attach to specific receptor sites are being developed to respond to very specific situations. Every year, several new monoclonal antibodies are marketed, showing the rapid pace with which these agents are being developed and approved for clinical use. Monoclonal antibodies include adalimumab (*Humira*), ado-trastuzumab (*Kadcyla*), alemtuzumab (*Campath*), avelumab (*Bavencio*), basiliximab (*Simulect*), belimumab (*Benlysta*), bevacizumab (*Avastin*), blinatumomab (*Blincyto*), brentuximab (*Adcetris*), canakinumab (*Ilaris*), certolizumab (*Cimzia*), cetuximab (*Erbitux*), daclizumab (*Zinbryta*), daratumumab (*Darzalex*), denosumab (*Prolia*), eculizumab (*Soliris*), erlotinib (*Tarceva*), golimumab (*Simponi*), ibritumomab (*Zevalin*), infliximab (*Remicade*), ipilimumab (*Yervoy*), natalizumab (*Tysabri*), nivolumab (*Opdivo*), obinutuzumab (*Gazyva*), ocrelizumab (*Ocrevus*), ofatumumab (*Arzerra*), olaratumab (*Lartruvo*), omalizumab (*Xolair*), palivizumab (*Synagis*), pegaptanib (*Macugen*), pembrolizumab (*Keytruda*), pertuzumab (*Perjeta*), ramucirumab (*Cyramza*), ranibizumab (*Lucentis*), raxibacumab (generic), rituximab (*Rituxan*), siltuximab (Sylvant), tocilizumab (*Actemra*), tositumomab combined with iodine-131 tositumomab (*Bexxar*), trastuzumab (*Herceptin*), ustekinumab (*Stelara*), and vedolizumab (*Entyvio*).

Therapeutic Actions and Indications

Monoclonal antibodies are proteins designed to be attracted to a specific target. They may be designed to attach to a specific cell, virus, bacteria, or an antibody that was produced in the body (see Fig. 17.1). They have specific functions and have been designed to treat cancers, types of arthritis, multiple sclerosis, and other diseases.

Adalimumab, certolizumab, golimumab, and infliximab are antibodies specific for human tumor necrosis factor. They keep the inflammatory reaction in check by reacting with and deactivating the free-floating tumor necrosis factor released by active leukocytes. These drugs are used for treating various forms of arthritis, Crohn's disease, and ulcerative colitis. These drugs are discussed in Chapter 16.

Alemtuzumab is an antibody specific for lymphocyte receptor sites.

Basiliximab and daclizumab are specific to interleukin-2 receptor sites on activated T lymphocytes; they react with those sites and block cellular response to allograft transplants. Daclizumab is indicated for treatment of relapsing forms of multiple sclerosis. Canakinumab is a specific interleukin-6 blocker and is used for cryopyrin-associated periodic syndromes and juvenile arthritis.

Cetuximab and olaratumab are antibodies specific to epidermal growth factor receptor sites. Olaratumab, pertuzumab, ado-trastuzumab, and trastuzumab react with human epidermal growth factor receptor 2 (HER2), a genetic defect that is seen in certain metastatic breast cancers. It is used in the treatment of metastatic breast cancer in tumors that overexpress HER2.

Blinatumomab, brentuximab, and obinutuzumab are specific T-cell antibodies, altering their function.

Eculizumab binds to complement proteins and prevents the formation of the complement complex.

Ocrelizumab use in treating multiple sclerosis and daratumumab use in treating multiple myeloma are lymphocyte-specific antibodies.

Ranibizumab binds to sites of active forms of vascular endothelial growth factor, preventing new vascular growth in the area of injection. Ramucirumab and ranibizumab also inhibit endothelial growth receptors. Ramucirumab is effective in gastric and lung cancers. Ranibizumab is used for treating macular edema and macular degeneration. Bevacizumab is a vascular endothelial growth factor inhibitor indicated for treatment of metastatic colorectal cancer when used in combination with IV fluorouracil chemotherapy.

Erlotinib, pegaptanib, and tositumomab combined with iodine-131 tositumomab are effective against specific malignant receptor sites.

Ibritumomab, ofatumumab, and rituximab are antibodies specific to sites on activated B lymphocytes.

Natalizumab is an antibody specific to surface receptors on all leukocytes except neutrophils.

Avelumab, nivolumab, and pembrolizumab are antibodies that block the programmed death receptor-1 sites and are used for treating specific cancers. By blocking the death ligand-1, the T cells are able to be more active to fight certain cancers.

Omalizumab is an antibody to immunoglobulin E, an important factor in allergic reactions. It has not had a great deal of success because of related respiratory adverse effects but is now approved for chronic urticaria conditions.

Palivizumab is specific to the antigenic site on respiratory syncytial virus (RSV); it inactivates that virus. It is used to prevent RSV disease in high-risk children.

Tocilizumab, siltuximab, and ustekinumab are antibodies specific to interleukins.

Belimumab is a specific inhibitor of B-lymphocyte stimulator, which inhibits the survival of B lymphocytes and their differentiation into immunoglobulin-producing cells. It is used for adult patients with active, autoantibody-positive systemic lupus erythematosus who are receiving standard therapy.

Ipilimumab is a human cytotoxic T-cell antigen-4–blocking antibody. By blocking this site, T cells are activated and proliferate at a faster rate. It is used to treat patients with unresectable or metastatic melanoma. It is associated with potentially fatal immune-mediated reactions, and its use must be carefully evaluated.

Vedolizumab is an integrin blocker that inhibits the movement of T cells across the gastric mucosa. It is used for treating ulcerative colitis and Crohn's disease in patients who do not respond to traditional therapies.

Pharmacokinetics

With the exception of erlotinib (an oral agent), all of the monoclonal antibodies have to be injected. They may be given IV, IM, or subcutaneously, depending on the drug. Because antibodies are proteins, they are rapidly broken down in the GI tract. They are processed by the body like naturally occurring antibodies.

Contraindications and Cautions

Monoclonal antibodies are contraindicated in the presence of any known allergy to the drug or to murine products, to prevent hypersensitivity reactions, and in the presence of fluid overload, which could be exacerbated. They should be used cautiously with fever (treat the fever before beginning therapy) and in patients who have had previous administration of the monoclonal antibody (serious hypersensitivity reactions can occur with repeat administration). Because of the potential for adverse effects, monoclonal antibodies should not be used during pregnancy or lactation unless the benefit clearly outweighs the potential risk to the fetus or neonate.

Adverse Effects

The most serious adverse effects associated with the use of monoclonal antibodies are acute pulmonary edema (dyspnea, chest pain, wheezing), which is associated with severe fluid retention, and cytokine release syndrome (flu-like symptoms that can progress to third-spacing of fluids and shock). Other adverse effects that can be anticipated include fever, chills, malaise, myalgia, nausea, diarrhea, vomiting, and increased susceptibility to infection and cancer development (Fig. 17.2).

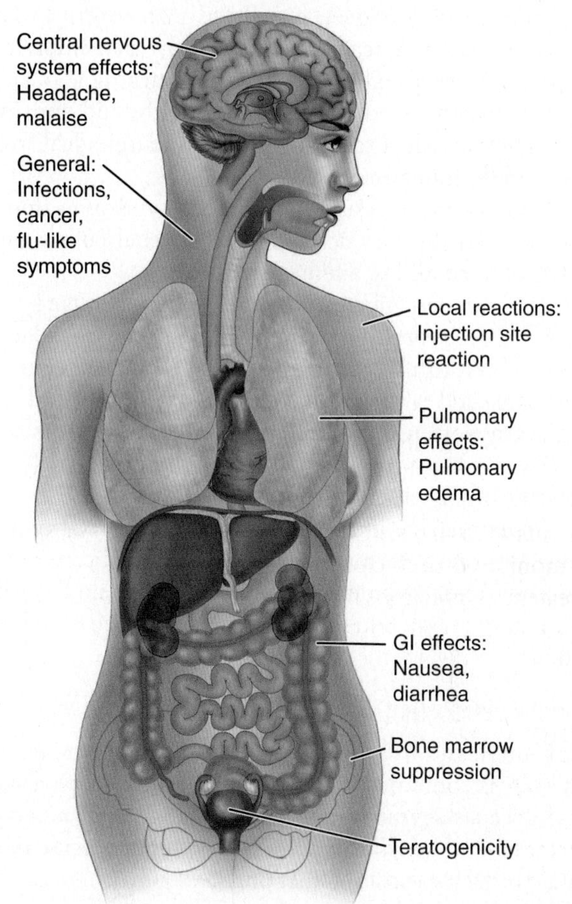

FIGURE 17.2 Variety of adverse effects and toxicities associated with immune modulators.

Eculizumab can lead to intravascular hemolysis with resultant fatigue, pain, dark urine, shortness of breath, and blood clots.

Bevacizumab is associated with GI perforation, hemorrhage, thromboembolism, hypertension, embryo–fetal toxicity, renal injury, heart failure, and impaired healing.

Erlotinib is reserved for patients whose disease has progressed after other therapies.

The manufacturer of natalizumab stopped marketing the drug weeks after its release because of reports of CNS complications. It was returned to the market in June 2006 with warnings about the potential for CNS complications.

Blinatumomab is associated with potentially life-threatening cytokine release syndrome and life-threatening neurological toxicities.

Brentuximab and obinutuzumab are associated with progressive multifocal leukoencephalopathy.

Ramucirumab is associated with potentially life-threatening hemorrhage.

Belimumab is associated with CNS effects including an increased risk for depression and suicidality. There is also a risk of hypersensitivity reactions during the IV infusion, and patients should be premedicated before each infusion.

Ipilimumab has been associated with severe to fatal immune-mediated reactions due to the activation and proliferation of T cells. It has a boxed warning about this possible reaction and suggests baseline thyroid and liver function tests and exams of the skin, neurological function, and GI function.

Rituximab can cause tumor lysis syndrome due to rapid cellular death which may lead to renal failure, electrolyte abnormalities, and hyperuricemia.

A higher percentage of patients will have flulike symptoms (nausea, vomiting, fever, weakness, pain, headache) after the first infusion of trastuzumab. This medication is also associated with cardiotoxicity, heart failure, and pulmonary hypertension, so use caution with patients with preexisting heart or lung disease. Monitor closely for hypersensitivity reactions.

Cetuximab has increased risk of client developing pulmonary toxicity, dermatologic toxicity, infusion reactions including rash, hypotension, and wheezing, and cardiopulmonary arrest. Sun exposure may increase risk of skin toxicity.

Clinically Important Drug–Drug Interactions

Use caution and arrange to reduce the dose if a monoclonal antibody is combined with any other immunosuppressant drug because severe immune suppression with increased infections and neoplasms can occur. Refer to specific medication label for exact interactions.

Prototype Summary: Bevacizumab

Indications: Treatment of metastatic colorectal cancer, non–squamous cell non–small cell lung cancer, glioblastoma, renal cell carcinoma, cervical cancer, ovarian cancer.

Actions: Monoclonal antibody that binds to and inhibits vascular endothelial growth factor leading to decreased angiogenesis and cell proliferation.

Pharmacokinetics:

Route	Onset	Peak	Duration
IV	Minutes	2–7 d	7–10 d

$T_{1/2}$: 20 days, metabolized in the tissues.

Adverse Effects: Headache, back pain, hypertension, GI perforation, hemorrhage, surgery and wound complications, thrombotic events.

Nursing Considerations for Patients Receiving Immune Suppressants

Assessment: History and Examination

- Assess for contraindications and cautions: any known allergies to any of these drugs or their components, to prevent hypersensitivity reactions; current status related to pregnancy or lactation, because of the potential risk to the fetus or baby; history of renal or hepatic impairment that might interfere with drug metabolism and excretion; and history of neoplasm, which could be exacerbated with the use of these drugs.
- Perform a physical assessment before beginning therapy to determine baseline status and any potential adverse effects: inspect the skin to detect the presence of any lesions; obtain weight to monitor for fluid retention; monitor temperature to determine potential for infection; monitor pulse and blood pressure to assess the cardiac effects of these drugs; and assess level of orientation and reflexes to monitor for any CNS changes associated with drug use.
- Obtain a baseline electrocardiogram to evaluate cardiac function.
- Assess the patient's renal and liver function, including renal and liver function tests, to determine the appropriateness of therapy and the need for possible dose adjustment and toxic drug effects.
- Monitor the results of laboratory tests such as CBC to identify changes in bone marrow function.

Nursing Conclusions

Nursing conclusions related to drug therapy might include the following:

- Impaired comfort related to CNS, GI, and flulike effects
- Infection risk related to immune suppression
- Malnutrition risk related to nausea and vomiting
- Knowledge deficit risk regarding drug therapy

Planning

- The patient will receive the best therapeutic effect from the drug therapy.
- The patient will have limited adverse effects to the drug therapy.
- The patient will have an understanding of the drug therapy, adverse effects to anticipate, and measures to relieve discomfort and improve safety.

Intervention With Rationale

- Arrange for laboratory tests before and periodically during therapy, including CBC, differential, and liver and renal function tests, to monitor for drug effects and adverse effects.
- Administer the drug as indicated; instruct the patient and a friend, family member, or significant other if injections are required to ensure proper administration of the drug.
- Protect the patient from exposure to infections and maintain a strict aseptic technique for any

invasive procedures, to prevent infections during immunosuppression.
- Arrange for supportive care and comfort measures for flulike symptoms (rest, environmental control, acetaminophen) to decrease patient discomfort and increase therapeutic compliance.
- Monitor nutritional status during therapy; provide small, frequent meals, mouth care, and nutritional consultation as necessary to ensure adequate nutrition.
- Instruct patients able to become pregnant in the use of barrier contraceptives to avoid pregnancy during therapy because of the risk of adverse effects to the fetus.
- Suggest another method of feeding the baby if a patient is breast or chestfeeding while on these drugs, because of the potential for adverse effects on the baby.
- Offer support and encouragement to help the patient deal with the diagnosis and the drug regimen.
- Provide thorough patient teaching, including measures to avoid adverse effects, warning signs of problems, and proper administration, to increase knowledge about drug therapy and adherence to the drug regimen.

Evaluation

- Monitor patient response to the drug (prevention of transplant rejection, improvement in autoimmune disease or cancer, prevention of RSV disease, improvement in signs and symptoms of Crohn's disease or rheumatoid arthritis).
- Monitor for adverse effects (flulike symptoms, GI upset, increased infections, neoplasms, fluid overload).
- Evaluate the effectiveness of the teaching plan (patient can name drug, dosage, adverse effects to watch for, specific measures to avoid adverse effects, proper administration technique).
- Monitor the effectiveness of comfort measures and adherence to the regimen (see "Critical Thinking Scenario").

CRITICAL THINKING SCENARIO
Holistic Care for a Heart Transplant Patient

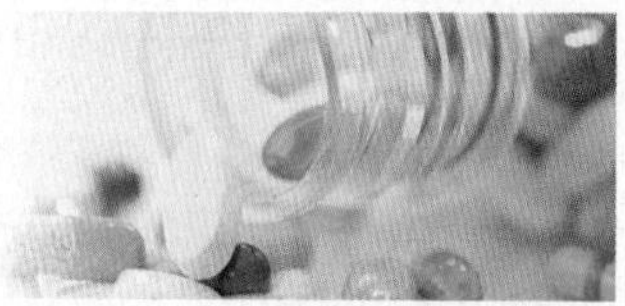

THE SITUATION

After waiting on a transplant list for 4 years, T.B. received a human heart transplant to replace their heart, which had been severely damaged by cardiomyopathy. Before getting the transplant, T.B. was bedridden, on oxygen, and near death. The transplant has given T.B. a "new lease on life," and they are determined to do everything possible to stay healthy and improve their activity and lifestyle. Currently, T.B. is being maintained on cyclosporine, mycophenolate, and corticosteroids.

CRITICAL THINKING

What important teaching facts would help T.B. to achieve their goal? Think about the psychological impact of the heart transplant and the "new lease on life."

What activity, dietary, and supportive guidelines should be outlined for T.B.?

What impact will T.B.'s drug regimen have on their plans?

How can all of the aspects of their condition and medical care be coordinated to give T.B. the best possible advantages for the future?

DISCUSSION

T.B.'s medical regimen will include a very complicated combination of rehabilitation, nutrition, drug therapy, and prevention. T.B. should know the risks of transplant rejection and the measures that will be used to prevent it. They should also know the names of their medications and when to take them, the signs and symptoms of rejection to watch for, and what to do if they occur. T.B. must understand the need to prevent exposure to infections and the precautions required, such as avoiding crowded areas and people with known diseases, avoiding injury, and taking steps to maintain cleanliness and avoid infection if an injury occurs.

The medications that T.B. is taking may cause them to experience flulike symptoms, which can be quite unpleasant. A restful, quiet environment may help to decrease stress. Acetaminophen may be ordered to help alleviate the fever, aches, and pains.

T.B. may also experience GI upset, nausea, and vomiting related to drug effects. A nutritional consultation may be requested to help T.B. maintain a good nutritional state. Frequent mouth care and small, frequent meals may help. Proper nutrition will help T.B. to recover, heal, and maintain their health.

T.B.'s primary health care provider will need to work with the transplantation surgeon, rehabilitation team, nutritionist, and cardiologist to coordinate a total program that will help T.B. avoid problems and make the most of their transplanted heart.

NURSING CARE GUIDE FOR T.B.: CYCLOSPORINE, MYCOPHENOLATE, AND CORTICOSTEROIDS

Assessment: History and Examination

- Assess for history of allergies to any immunosuppressant; renal or hepatic impairment; history of neoplasm; concurrent use of cholestyramine,

(continues on page 308)

theophylline, phenytoin, other nephrotoxic drugs, digoxin, lovastatin, diltiazem, metoclopramide, nicardipine, amiodarone, androgens, azole antifungals, or macrolides; grapefruit juice.

- Review physical examination findings, including orientation, reflexes, affect (neurological); temperature and weight (general); pulse, cardiac auscultation, blood pressure, edema, electrocardiogram (cardiovascular); liver evaluation (GI); and laboratory test results (CBC, liver and renal function tests, condition being treated).

Nursing Conclusions

Impaired comfort related to CNS, GI, flulike symptoms
Infection risk related to immune suppression
Malnutrition risk related to GI effects
Activity intolerance related to fatigue, drug effects
Knowledge deficit regarding drug therapy

Planning

The patient will receive the best therapeutic effect from the drug therapy.
The patient will have limited adverse effects to the drug therapy.
The patient will have an understanding of the drug therapy, adverse effects to anticipate, and measures to relieve discomfort and improve safety.

Intervention

Arrange for laboratory tests before and periodically during therapy.
Administer drug as indicated.
Protect patient from exposure to infection.
Provide supportive and comfort measures to deal with adverse effects.
Monitor nutritional status and intervene as needed.
Provide patient teaching regarding the drugs and their dosage, adverse effects, precautions, and warning signs to report to care provider.

EVALUATION

Evaluate drug effects: prevention of transplant rejection, improvement of autoimmune disease.
Monitor for adverse effects: infection, flulike symptoms, GI upset, fluid overload, neoplasm.
Monitor for drug–drug interactions and drug–food interactions.
Evaluate effectiveness of patient teaching program and of comfort and safety measures.

PATIENT TEACHING FOR T.B.: CYCLOSPORINE, MYCOPHENOLATE, AND CORTICOSTEROIDS

- You will need to take a combination of drugs to prevent your body from rejecting your new organ. These drugs include cyclosporine, mycophenolate, and corticosteroids. They suppress the activity of your immune system and prevent your body from rejecting any transplanted tissue.
- You should never stop taking your drugs without consulting your health care provider. If your prescription is low or you are unable to take the medication for *any* reason, notify your health care provider.
- You should not take your cyclosporine with grapefruit juice.
- Some of the following adverse effects may occur:
  - Nausea, vomiting: Taking the drug with food and eating small frequent meals may help. It is very important that you maintain good nutrition. A consult with a nutritionist may be needed to help you if these GI problems are severe.
  - Diarrhea: This may not decrease; ensure ready access to bathroom facilities.
  - Flulike symptoms: Rest and a cool, peaceful environment may help; acetaminophen may be ordered to help relieve discomfort.
  - Rash, mouth sores: Frequent skin and mouth care may ease these effects.
- You will be more susceptible to infection because your body's normal defenses will be decreased. You should avoid crowded places, people with known infections, and working in soil. If you notice any signs of illness or infection, notify your health care provider immediately.
- Tell any doctor, nurse, or other health care provider involved in your care that you are taking these drugs.
- You will need to schedule periodic blood tests and perhaps biopsies while you are being treated with these drugs.
- Report any of the following to your health care provider: unusual bleeding or bruising, fever, sore throat, mouth sores, fatigue, and any other signs of infection or injury.
- Keep your medications safely out of the reach of children and pets and do not share medications with anyone else.

Key Points

- Immune suppressants are used to depress the immune system when needed to prevent transplant rejection or severe tissue damage associated with autoimmune disease. Research is ongoing to extend the use of various immune suppressants to other situations, including various autoimmune disorders.
- Increased susceptibility to infection and increased risk of neoplasm are potentially dangerous effects associated with the use of immune suppressants. Patients need to be protected from infection, injury, and invasive procedures.

SUMMARY

- Immune stimulants boost the immune system when it is exhausted from fighting off prolonged invasion or needs help to fight a specific pathogen or cancer cell. They include interferons and interleukins.
- Interferons are naturally released from cells in response to viral invasion; they are used to treat various cancers and warts.
- Interleukins stimulate cellular immunity and inhibit tumor growth; they are used to treat very specific cancers.
- Adverse effects seen with immune stimulants are related to the immune response (flulike symptoms, including fever, myalgia, lethargy, arthralgia, and fatigue).
- Immune suppressants are used to depress the immune system when needed to prevent transplant rejection or severe tissue damage associated with autoimmune disease. Research is ongoing to extend the use of various immune suppressants to other situations, including various autoimmune disorders.
- Increased susceptibility to infection and increased risk of neoplasm are potentially dangerous effects associated with the use of immune suppressants. Patients need to be protected from infection, injury, and invasive procedures.

CHECK YOUR UNDERSTANDING

Answers to the questions in this chapter can be found in Answers to Check Your Understanding Questions on thePoint®.

MULTIPLE CHOICE

Select the best answer.

1. In which situation would the nurse least likely expect to administer an immune suppressant?
   a. Treatment of transplant rejection
   b. Treatment of autoimmune disease
   c. Reduction of number of relapses in multiple sclerosis
   d. Treatment of aggressive cancers
2. The nurse would expect to administer interferon alfa-n3 (*Alferon N*) as the drug of choice for
   a. treatment of leukemias.
   b. treatment of multiple sclerosis.
   c. intralesional treatment of warts.
   d. treatment of Kaposi sarcoma.
3. Patient teaching for a patient receiving an interferon would include
   a. proper use of oral contraceptives.
   b. use of aspirin to control adverse effects.
   c. importance of cardiovascular workouts.
   d. proper methods injecting the drug.
4. Patients who are receiving an immune stimulant may experience any of the clinical signs of immune response activity, including
   a. flulike symptoms.
   b. diarrhea.
   c. constipation.
   d. headache.
5. Organ transplants are often rejected by the body because the T cells recognize the transplanted cells as foreign and try to destroy them. Treatment with an immune suppressant would
   a. activate antibody production.
   b. stimulate interleukin release.
   c. stimulate thymus secretions.
   d. block the initial damage to the transplanted cells.

6. You might use a monoclonal antibody in treating
   a. warts.
   b. herpes zoster.
   c. tumors that overexpress HER2.
   d. Kaposi sarcoma.

MULTIPLE RESPONSE

Select all that apply.

1. The nurse is assigned to care for a client who is receiving immune suppressants. The nurse would continually assess the client for which of the following anticipated adverse effects?
   a. Development of cancers
   b. Increased risk of infection
   c. Cardiac standstill
   d. Development of secondary infections
   e. Increased bleeding tendencies
   f. Hepatomegaly

2. Teaching points that the nurse would incorporate into the care of a client receiving cyclosporine would include which information?
   a. Use barrier contraceptives to avoid pregnancy.
   b. If mouth sores occur, try to restrict eating as much as possible.
   c. Dilute the solution with milk, chocolate milk, or orange juice and drink immediately.
   d. Avoid drinking grapefruit juice when on this drug.
   e. Stop taking the drug if GI upset or fever occurs.
   f. Refrigerate the oral solution.

REFERENCES

Brunton, L. L., Hilal-Dandan, R., & Knollman, B. C. (2018). *Goodman and Gilman's the pharmacological basis of therapeutics* (13th ed.). McGraw-Hill.

Dimitrov, A. S. (Ed.). (2009). *Therapeutic antibodies; methods and protocols*. Humana Press.

Fox, D. A. (2010). *New insights into rheumatoid arthritis*. Saunders.

Hashkes, P. J., & Laxer, R. M. (2005). Medical treatment of juvenile idiopathic arthritis. *Journal of the American Medical Association, 294*(13), 1671–1684. https://doi.org/10.1001/jama.294.13.1671

Hendler, C. B. (Ed.). (2021). *Nursing 2021 drug handbook*. Wolters Kluwer.

Mitka, M. (2010). Targeted therapies take aim against lung cancer and melanoma. *Journal of the American Medical Association, 304*(6), 624–626. https://doi.org/10.1001/jama.2010.1055

Norris, T. L., & Lalchandani, R. (2018). *Porth's pathophysiology: Concepts of altered health states* (10th ed.). Wolters Kluwer.

Slomski, A. (2013). Monoclonal antibody may be helpful for inflammatory bowel disease. *Journal of the American Medical Association, 310*(16), 1665. https://doi.org/10.1001/jama.2013.281199

Weisman, M. H., Weinblatt, M. E., Louie, J. S., & van Vollenhoven, R. F. (2010). *Targeted treatment of the rheumatic diseases*. Saunders/Elsevier.

CHAPTER 18

Vaccines and Sera

Learning Objectives

Upon completion of this chapter, you will be able to:

1. Define the terms active immunity and passive immunity.
2. Describe the therapeutic actions, indications, pharmacokinetics, contraindications, most common adverse effects, and important drug–drug interactions associated with each vaccine, immune serum, antitoxin, and antivenin.
3. Discuss the use of vaccines and sera across the lifespan, including recommended immunization schedules.
4. Compare and contrast the prototype drugs for each class of vaccine and immune serum with others in that class.
5. Outline the nursing considerations and teaching needs for patients receiving a vaccine or immune serum.

Key Terms

active immunity: the formation of antibodies secondary to exposure to a specific antigen; leads to the formation of plasma cells, antibodies, and memory cells to immediately produce antibodies if exposed to that antigen in the future; imparts lifelong immunity

antitoxins: immune sera that contain antibodies to specific toxins produced by invaders; may prevent the toxin from adhering to body tissues and causing disease

antivenins: immune sera that contain antibodies to specific venins produced by poisonous snakes or spiders; may prevent the venom from causing cell death

biological: vaccines, immune sera, and antitoxins that are used to stimulate the production of antibodies, to provide preformed antibodies to facilitate an immune reaction, or to react specifically with the toxins produced by an invading pathogen

immune sera: preformed antibodies found in immune globulin from animals or humans who have had a specific disease and developed antibodies to it

immunization: the process of stimulating active immunity by exposing the body to weakened or less toxic proteins associated with specific disease-causing organisms; the goal is to stimulate immunity without causing the full course of a disease

passive immunity: the injection of preformed antibodies into a host at high risk for exposure to a specific disease or when a pregnant person passes antibodies to the fetus; immunity is limited by the amount of circulating antibody

serum sickness: reaction of a host to injected antibodies or foreign sera; host cells make antibodies to the foreign proteins, and a massive immune reaction can occur

vaccine: immunization containing weakened or altered protein antigens to stimulate a specific antibody formation against a specific disease; refers to a product used to stimulate active immunity

Drug List

VACCINES

Bacterial Vaccines

anthrax vaccine
bacille Calmette-Guérin (BCG)
cholera vaccine
Haemophilus influenzae b conjugate vaccine
Haemophilus influenzae b conjugate vaccine and hepatitis B surface antigen
meningococcal groups C and Y, *Haemophilus influenza* b tetanus toxoid conjugate
meningococcal polysaccharide vaccine
meningococcal vaccine, serotype B
pneumococcal vaccine, polyvalent
pneumococcal 13-valent conjugate vaccine
typhoid vaccine

Toxoids

diphtheria and tetanus toxoids, adsorbed
diphtheria and tetanus toxoids and acellular pertussis vaccine, adsorbed
diphtheria and tetanus toxoids and acellular pertussis and *Haemophilus influenzae b conjugate vaccines*
diphtheria and tetanus toxoids and acellular pertussis and inactivated poliovirus vaccine (recombinant) and inactivated poliovirus vaccines, combined

Viral Vaccines

H5N1 influenza vaccine
hepatitis A vaccine, inactivated
hepatitis A vaccine, inactivated, with hepatitis B recombinant vaccine
hepatitis B vaccine
human papillomavirus recombinant vaccine, bivalent types 16 and 18
human papillomavirus recombinant vaccine, quadrivalent
influenza A (H5N1) vaccine
influenza A (H5N1) vaccine adjuvanted
influenza virus vaccine
influenza virus vaccine, intranasal
Japanese encephalitis vaccine
measles, mumps, rubella vaccine, live
measles, mumps, rubella, varicella virus vaccine, live
poliovirus vaccine, inactivated
rabies vaccine
rotavirus vaccine, live, oral
varicella virus vaccine, live
yellow fever vaccine
zoster vaccine, live

IMMUNE SERA

antithymocyte immune globulin
botulism immune globulin
cytomegalovirus immune globulin
hepatitis B immune globulin
immune globulin, intramuscular
immune globulin, intravenous
immune globulin, subcutaneous
lymphocyte immune globulin
rabies immune globulin
RHO immune globulin
RHO immune globulin, microdose
tetanus immune globulin
vaccinia immune globulin IV
varicella-zoster immune globulin

ANTITOXINS AND ANTIVENINS

antivenin (*Micrurus fulvius*)
black widow spider antivenin (*Latrodectus mactans*)
botulism antitoxin
centruroides (scorpion) immune fab
crotalidae polyvalent immune fab

Vaccines and **immune sera**, including **antivenins** and **antitoxins**, are usually referred to as **biologicals**. They are used to stimulate the production of antibodies, to provide preformed antibodies to facilitate an immune reaction, or to react specifically with the toxins produced by invading pathogens or venins injected by poisonous snakes or spiders. Stimulating the production of antibodies to specific antigens with vaccines provides the person with immunity to that antigen. Vaccines are frequently called **immunizations** because they stimulate immunity. Many diseases that were once devastating or fatal can now be prevented by stimulating an immune response and the development of antibodies without the need for the patient to actually contract the disease. Prudent, preventative medical care requires the routine administration of certain vaccines to prevent diseases. The immune sera provide treatments for specific antigens, toxins, or venins and are used after exposure to antigens or toxins, or after bites from poisonous snakes or spiders, to prevent clinical problems from developing and make diseases less invasive and aggressive if they do develop. Box 18.1 discusses the use of biologicals among various age groups.

Immunity

Immunity is a state of relative resistance to a disease that develops after exposure to the specific disease-causing agent. People are not born with immunity to diseases, so they must acquire immunity by stimulating B-cell clones to form plasma cells and then antibodies.

Active immunity occurs when the body recognizes a foreign protein and begins producing antibodies to react with that specific protein or antigen. After plasma cells are formed to produce antibodies, specific memory cells that produce the same antibodies are created. If the specific foreign protein is introduced into the body again, these memory cells react immediately to release antibodies. This type of immunity was always thought to be lifelong, but it was discovered that patients who had been immunized against smallpox often had no antibodies to smallpox after many years. It is thought that the eradication of the disease has resulted in no stimulation of the memory cells, and after a prolonged period with no stimulation, perhaps the memory cells no longer produce antibodies. Active artificial immunity is when a person is administered an antigen, often in a vaccine, that is similar to a pathogen antigen that could harm the person and stimulates the body to develop antibodies. The expected outcome is that the antibodies that are developed will be able to help protect the person when exposed to the pathogen. Active natural immunity refers to when an antigen enters a person's body via natural exposure, and the antigen stimulates the body to make antibodies.

Unlike active immunity, **passive immunity** is limited. It lasts only as long as the circulating antibodies last because the body does not produce its own antibodies. Passive artificial immunity occurs when preformed antibodies are injected into the system and react with a specific antigen. These antibodies can be manufactured from animal plasma that has been infected with the disease or from humans who have had the disease and have developed antibodies. An example of this is when immune globulins are administered to a person to protect against a snake bite or rabies exposure. In some cases, the host human responds to the circulating injected antibodies, which are

Box 18.1 Focus on Drug Therapy Across the Lifespan

BIOLOGICALS

Children

Routine immunization for children has become a standard of care in the United States. The Centers for Disease Control and Prevention have recommended dosing schedules for children's vaccines. Parents should receive written records of immunizations given to their children to assure continuity of care. The parent should be asked to report adverse reactions to any immunization.

Simple comfort measures—warm soaks at the injection site, acetaminophen to reduce fever or aches and pains, and comfort from parents or caregivers—will help the child to deal with the immunization experience.

Parent education is a very important aspect of the immunization procedure. Parents may need reassurance and educational materials when concerns about the safety of immunizations arise.

Immune sera are used for specific exposures. Botulism immune globulin is specific for treatment of infants younger than 1 year of age with botulism.

Adults

There are a number of reasons adults should receive certain immunizations. For example, adults who are traveling to areas with high risk for particular diseases—and who may not have previously been exposed to those diseases—are advised to be immunized.

In addition, all adults are advised to be immunized yearly with an influenza vaccine. The influenza vaccine changes yearly, depending on predictions of which flu strain might be emergent in that year. Adults older than 19 years of age who are immunocompromised or have specific chronic diseases should be administered the pneumococcal vaccines prior to 65 years of age, and immunocompetent adults aged 65 years and older should also be administered the pneumococcal vaccine.

Tetanus shots also are recommended for adults every 10 years or with any injury that potentially could precipitate a tetanus infection and is currently given with a pertussis booster to help protect children from this exposure.

The varicella vaccine is indicated for adults who do not have evidence of immunity. The zoster vaccination is recommended for adults 50 years of age and older.

Immunization schedules from the CDC should be reviewed to assess the vaccines needed.

Immune sera are used for specific exposures.

Older Adults

Older adults are at greater risk for severe illness from influenza and pneumococcal infections. The yearly flu shot and the pneumococcal and pneumococcal 13-valent vaccines should be stressed for this group.

A tetanus booster every 10 years will also help to protect older adults from exposure to that illness. Ask the patient about any adverse reaction to previous tetanus boosters and weigh the risk against the possible exposure to tetanus. The zoster vaccination is recommended for adults 50 years of age and older.

If an older patient is traveling to an area where a particular disease is endemic and the risk of exposure is great, the Centers for Disease Control and Prevention (http://www.cdc.gov) should be contacted to determine whether the appropriate vaccine is acceptable for use in the older patient.

Immune sera are used for specific exposures. Older adults are at increased risk for severe reactions and should be monitored closely.

foreign proteins to the host's body, by producing its own antibodies to the injected antibodies. This results in **serum sickness**, a massive immune reaction manifested by fever, arthritis, flank pain, myalgia, and arthralgia.

Passive natural immunity is when a person who is pregnant or lactating passes antibodies to the fetus or infant via the placenta or human milk. The circulating antibodies act in the same manner as those produced from plasma cells, recognizing the foreign protein and attaching to it, rendering it harmless.

Immunization

Immunization is the process of artificially stimulating active immunity by exposing the body to weakened or less-toxic proteins associated with specific disease-causing organisms. The proteins could be a weakened bacterial cell membrane, the protein coat of a virus, or a virus (protein coat with the genetic fragment that makes up the virus) that has been chemically weakened so that it cannot cause disease. The goal is to cause an immune response without having the patient suffer the full course of a disease. Adults may require immunizations in certain situations: exposure; travel to an area endemic for a disease they have not had and have not been immunized against; and occupations that are considered high risk. Children are routinely immunized against many infections that were once quite devastating (Box 18.2). For example, smallpox was one of the first diseases against which children were immunized. Today, smallpox is considered to be eradicated worldwide. Concerns over biological terrorism led to renewed interest in this disease, and in the early 2000s, smallpox vaccine was made available to the U.S. military to provide help for people who might be at high risk for exposure to a potential attack by terrorists using smallpox. Every year in January, the Centers for Disease Control and Prevention (CDC) publishes the recommended immunization schedule for the coming year. The recommendations change based on experience, exposure, and new developments. Health care professionals should go to the CDC website to stay up to date on recommendations (https://www.cdc.gov/vaccines/schedules/index.html). Free downloads are available in many sizes such as pocket or poster sizes, which can be useful for teaching as well as patient and parent education.

BOX 18.2

Patient Teaching

Pediatric Immunization: It is well documented that by preventing potentially devastating diseases, society prevents unneeded suffering and death and saves valuable citizens for the future. Pediatric immunization has helped to greatly decrease the incidence of most childhood diseases and has prevented associated complications. In the United States, routine immunization is considered standard medical practice. The 2015 outbreak of measles stemming from the very popular theme park Disney World was a real reminder of the severity and danger of these diseases that one seldom sees when all children are vaccinated.

Ensuring that every child has the opportunity to receive the recommended immunizations has become a political as well as a social issue. The cost of becoming vaccinated can be a significant barrier to some individuals and families, and it can be difficult to gain support for it when most people have never experienced these diseases in today's society. Widespread campaigns to provide free immunizations and health screening to all children have addressed this problem but have not been fully successful.

In addition, periodic reports of severe or even fatal reactions to standard immunizations alarm many parents about the risks of immunizations. There has been controversy regarding whether the measles, mumps, and rubella (MMR) vaccine increase the risk for autism. The experts at the CDC and the American Academy of Pediatrics reviewed the evidence and have determined that the MMR vaccine is not responsible for children developing autism. Parents need facts regarding the true side effects of vaccines as well as reassurance about modern efforts to prevent and screen for these reactions.

Public education efforts should be directed at providing parents with information about pediatric immunization and encouraging them to act on that information. Nurses are often in the ideal position to provide this information during prenatal visits, while screening for other problems, or even standing in line at a grocery store. It is important for nurses to be well versed on the need for standard immunizations and screening to prevent severe reactions. The Centers for Disease Control and Prevention (http://www.cdc.gov) offer current information and updates for health care providers, as well as patient-teaching materials that can be printed for easy reference.

Diphtheria, pertussis, tetanus, *Haemophilus influenzae* b, hepatitis B, hepatitis A, varicella, poliovirus, meningitis, measles, mumps, rotavirus, pneumococcal, influenza, meningococcal, human papillomavirus, and rubella are all standard childhood immunizations today in the United States. The bacille Calmette-Guérin vaccine for tuberculosis is widely used throughout the world in countries with a high incidence of tuberculosis to limit the spread of the disease. However, it is not routinely used in the United States because the incidence of tuberculosis is relatively low and it can induce false-positive tuberculin skin test results.

The use of vaccines is not without controversy. Severe reactions, although rare, have occurred, resulting in concerns about the safety of vaccines and their administration, especially in children (Box 18.2). The central reporting of adverse effects or suspected adverse effects may help to clarify concerns about reactions to immunizations.

Antigens are also processed and injected to help some people who have severe allergic reactions. The purpose of allergy shots is to slowly increase the person's exposure to the antigenic proteins they are allergic to. As they are exposed in small doses, the body is stimulated to become more immune, so the person's allergy symptoms decrease. Many of these proteins are now available in a sublingual form, which avoids the need for repeated injections (Box 18.3).

Box 18.3 Focus on Safe Medication Administration

USE OF ALLERGENIC EXTRACTS

Many people receive "allergy shots" or injections of allergenic extracts. These extracts contain various antigens based on specific standardizations. The exact action of these extracts is not completely understood, but it has been shown that after injection, specific immunoglobulin G (IgG) antibodies appear in the serum. These antibodies compete with immunoglobulin E (IgE) for the receptor site on a specific antigen that is the cause of the allergy (IgE is the immunoglobulin that is associated with allergic reactions; these antibodies react with mast cells, causing the release of histamine and other inflammatory chemicals when they have combined with the antigen). After repeated exposure to the antigens, the levels of IgG antibodies increase and the circulating levels of IgE seem to decrease, leading to less allergic response. It may take 4 to 6 months of subcutaneous injections of the allergenic extract every 3 to 14 days to achieve relief from the symptoms of the allergic reaction. The IgG levels remain high for weeks or sometimes months, but the individual response varies widely. Many people are maintained with a weekly injection once the desired response has been achieved. Since 2014, four sublingual allergen extracts have been approved. These are thought to work in the same way that the injections work but avoid the need for injections and visits to the health care facility. Ragweed pollen extract (*Ragwitek*), Timothy grass pollen extract (*Grastek*), grass pollen extract (*Oralair*), and dust mite extract (*Odactra*) are administered sublingually and rapidly absorbed into the bloodstream. An extract for peanut allergies is in testing. The patient needs to be observed for at least 30 minutes following the first dose because of a risk of anaphylactic reaction. Once it is determined that the patient can tolerate the drug, it is taken daily, starting 12 to 16 weeks before the allergen season begins and continuing throughout the season. The patient should also be prescribed an EpiPen to have on hand in case a severe allergic response develops.

Vaccines

The word vaccine comes from the Latin word for smallpox, *vaccinia*. Vaccines are immunizations containing weakened or altered protein antigens that stimulate the formation of antibodies against a specific disease (see Fig. 18.1). They are used to promote active artificial immunity (see Table 18.1).

Since the late 20th century, there has been more concern around possible terrorist activities, and concern has risen about the use of various diseases as biological weapons as well. Box 18.4 discusses vaccines and the use of biological weapons.

Vaccines can be made from chemically inactivated microorganisms or from live or weakened viruses or bacteria. Toxoids are vaccines that are made from the toxins produced by the microorganism. The toxins are altered so that they are no longer poisonous but still have the recognizable protein antigen that will stimulate antibody production.

The particular vaccine that is used depends on the possible exposure a person will have to a particular disease and the age of the person. Some vaccines are used only in children, and some cannot be used in infants. Some vaccines require booster doses—doses that are given a few months after the initial dose to further stimulate antibody production. In many cases, antibody titers (levels of the antibody in the serum) can be used to evaluate a person's response to an immunization and determine the need for a booster dose. Since the SARS-CoV-2 (COVID-19) virus began to spread, there has been ongoing research to develop and market vaccines to protect people from severe illness (see Box 18.5).

Therapeutic Actions and Indications

Vaccines stimulate active immunity in people who are at high risk for development of a particular disease. The vaccine needed for a patient depends on the exposure that person will have to the pathogen. Exposure is usually determined by where the person lives, their travel plans, and work or family environment exposures. Vaccines are thought to provide long-term immunity to the disease against which the patient is being immunized. Table 18.1 lists the various vaccines available along with usual indications.

Pharmacokinetics

There is no pharmacokinetic information on these biologicals, which are treated like endogenous antibodies in the body.

Contraindications and Cautions

The use of vaccines is contraindicated in the presence of immune deficiency that prohibits the individual's

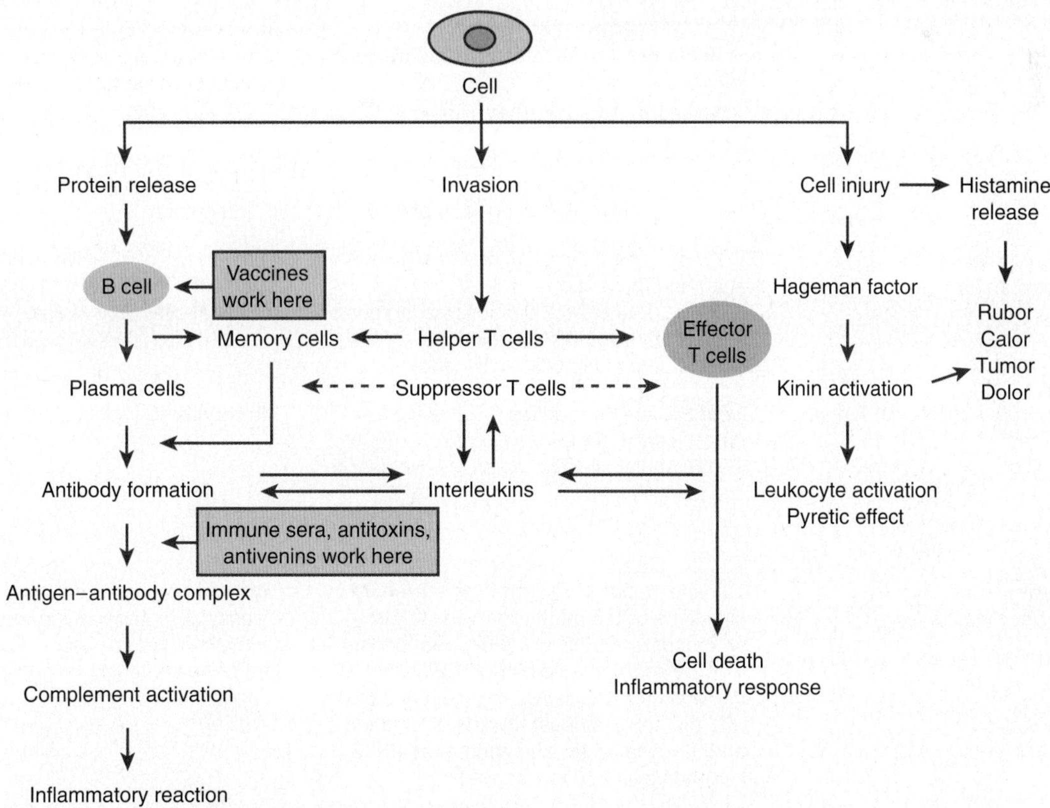

FIGURE 18.1 Sites of action of biologicals.

Table 18.1 *Drugs in Focus:* Vaccines

Drug Name	Dosage/Route	Usual Indications
Bacterial Vaccines		
anthrax vaccine, adsorbed (*BioThrax*)	*Preexposure:* 0.5 mL IM at 0, 1, and 6 mo; booster at 6 and 12 mo then at 12-mo intervals; or subcutaneously at 0.2 and 4 wk, booster at 6 and 12 mo then every 12 mo *Postexposure:* 0.5 mL subcutaneously at 1, 2, and 4 wk with antibiotics	Prevention and postexposure prophylaxis of inhalational anthrax infection in patients 18–65 y
bacille Calmette-Guérin (*TICE*)	0.2–0.3 mL percutaneously	Prevention of tuberculosis with high risk of exposure
cholera vaccine, live oral	One packet active agent, one packet buffer compound PO at least 10 d before travel	Prevention of cholera in adults 18–64 y expecting exposure to cholera; must be given in facility that can deal with medical wastes; shed in stool for 7 d, use caution near immunocompromised people
Haemophilus influenzae b conjugate vaccine (*Hiberix, Liquid PedvaxHIB, ActHIB*)	0.5 mL IM; ages vary with preparation	Active immunization against *H. influenzae* type b infection in infants and children
H. influenzae b conjugate vaccine and hepatitis B surface antigen (*Comvax*)	Three 0.5-mL IM injections at 2, 4, and 6 mo, with 0.5-mL booster at 15–18 mo	Immunization of children against *H. influenzae* type b and hepatitis B infections
meningococcal groups C and Y, *Haemophilus b* tetanus toxoid conjugate vaccine (*MenHibrix*)	Four doses of 0.5 mL IM at 2, 4, 6 mo and then as 12–15 mo	Immunization of children 6 wk to 18 mo against *H. influenza* type b and meningococcal infections
meningococcal polysaccharide vaccine (*Menomune-A/C/Y/W-135, Menactra, Menveo*)	0.5 mL IM	Immunization against meningococcal infections for patients 9 mo to 55 y of age
meningococcal vaccine serotype B (*Bexsero, Trumenba*)	Two 0.5-mL IM doses at least a month apart (*Bexsero*) Three 0.5-mL doses at months 0, 2, and 6 (*Trumenba*)	Immunization against meningococcal infections, serotype B in patients 10–25 y of age
pneumococcal vaccine, polyvalent (*Pneumovax 23*)	0.5 mL subcutaneously or IM, not recommended for children <2 y of age	Immunization against pneumococcal infections
pneumococcal 13-valent conjugate vaccine (*Prevnar 13*)	*7–11 mo:* Three 0.5-mL IM doses at least 4 wk apart and the last one at >1 y *12–23 mo:* Two 0.5-mL IM doses 2 mo apart *24 mo to 9 y:* One 0.5-mL IM dose *50 y and older:* One 0.5-mL IM dose	Prevention of invasive pneumococcal disease in infants and children and adults over 65 y of age
typhoid vaccine (*Vivotif Berna, Typhim VI*)	*Vivotif Berna*—Four doses PO every other day at least 1 wk prior to exposure; *Typhim VI* 0.5-mL IM injection at least 2 wk prior to exposure	Immunization against typhoid fever
Toxoids		
diphtheria and tetanus toxoids, adsorbed (*Decavac, Tenivac*)	*Adult and pediatric 7 y and older:* Three IM injections of 0.5 mL at intervals of 8 wk, with booster of 0.5 mL in 6–8 mo; booster at 11–12 y and then every 10 y (*Tenivac*) *Adult and pediatric:* Three IM injections of 0.5 mL, the first 2 at least 4 wk apart and the third 6 mo later, routine booster at 11–12 y and then every 10 y (*Decavac*)	Immunization of adults and children against diphtheria and tetanus

Table 18.1 *Drugs in Focus:* Vaccines (*Continued*)

Drug Name	Dosage/Route	Usual Indications
diphtheria and tetanus toxoids and acellular pertussis vaccine, adsorbed DTaP, adsorbed (*Tripedia, Infanrix, Adacel, Boostrix*)	Three IM doses of 0.5 mL at 4- to 6-wk intervals starting by 6–8 wk of age; fourth dose of 0.5 mL IM at 15–20 mo; then 0.5 mL at 4–6 y; booster at 10–18 y *Boostrix*: 0.5 mL IM; at 11–65 y and older *Adacel*: 0.5 mL IM	Immunization of children against diphtheria, tetanus, and pertussis as the fourth and fifth doses of the immunization series; booster for adolescents and adults
diphtheria and tetanus toxoids and acellular pertussis, adsorbed, and hepatitis B (recombinant) and inactivated poliovirus vaccine, combined (*PEDIARIX*)	0.5 mL IM, three doses at 8-wk intervals or completion of series in combined form, beginning at 2 mo of age	Active immunization against diphtheria, tetanus, pertussis (DTaP), hepatitis B, and poliovirus in infants with HBsAg-negative birthing parents
diphtheria and tetanus toxoids and acellular pertussis, adsorbed, and poliovirus vaccine (*Kinrix*)	0.5-mL IM, children 4–6 y, to complete the series started with *Infanrix* or *PEDIARIX*	Active immunization against DTaP and poliovirus in children needing to complete the series
Viral Vaccines		
H5N1 influenza vaccine	*Patients 18–64 y:* 1 mL IM, then 1 mL IM 21–35 d later	Active immunization of patients 18–64 y of age at increased risk for exposure to avian flu
hepatitis A vaccine, inactivated (*Havrix, Vaqta*)	*Adult:* 1 mL IM with a booster dose in 6–12 mo *Pediatric:* 0.5 mL IM with a repeat dose in 6–12 mo	Immunization of adults and children against hepatitis A infection
hepatitis A vaccine, inactivated, with hepatitis B recombinant vaccine (*Twinrix*)	1 mL IM followed by booster doses at 1 and 6 mo	Immunization against hepatitis A and hepatitis B infections in people ≥18 y of age
hepatitis B vaccine (*Engerix-B, Recombivax HB*)	0.5–1 mL IM, followed by 0.5–1 mL IM at 1 and 6 mo	Immunization against hepatitis B infections in susceptible people and in infants born to mothers with hepatitis B
HPV recombinant vaccine, bivalent types 16 and 18 (*Cervarix*)	Three doses of 0.5 mL IM given at 0, 1, and 6 mo	Prevention of diseases caused by oncogenic HPV types 16 and 18 in females ages 10–25 y
HPV, recombinant, quadrivalent (*GARDASIL*)	*9–45 y:* 0.5 mL IM, then 0.5 mL IM 2 mo later, followed by 0.5 mL IM 6 mo after the first dose	Active immunization against HPV responsible for causing genital warts and cervical cancer; prevention of genital warts in males; prevention of anal cancer and associated precancerous lesions in patients 9–26 y
influenza A (H5N1) vaccine	0.5 mL IM yearly	Active immunization against influenza virus in patients 6 mo and older
influenza virus types A and B vaccine (*Afluria, Fluarix, Fluzone, Fluvirin, Fluzone High-Dose*)	*Adult:* 0.5 mL IM *Pediatric:* 0.25–0.5 mL IM, repeated in 4 wk	Active immunization against influenza types A and B in all patients over 6 mo of age
influenza virus types A and B vaccine, intranasal (*FluMist*)	*9–49 y:* 0.5 mL intranasal once each flu season *5–8 y not previously vaccinated with FluMist:* Two doses of 0.5 mL each intranasally given 60 d apart *5–8 y previously vaccinated with FluMist:* 0.5 mL intranasally once per flu season *2–8 y not previously vaccinated:* Two doses given as 0.1 mL in each nostril at least 1 mo apart *2–8 y old previously vaccinated:* One dose of 0.1 mL in each nostril	Active immunization to prevent disease caused by influenza A and B viruses (live vaccine can be used for individuals between 2 and 49 years of age who are healthy and not pregnant)

(*continues on page 318*)

Table 18.1 *Drugs in Focus:* Vaccines (*Continued*)

Drug Name	Dosage/Route	Usual Indications
Japanese encephalitis vaccine (*Ixiaro*)	2 mo to <3 y old: two doses of 0.25 mL IM 28 d apart; 3 y old: two doses of 0.5 mL IM 28 d apart	Immunization of persons >1 y of age who reside in or will travel to endemic areas
measles, mumps, rubella vaccine (*M-M-R-II*)	0.5 mL subcutaneously	Immunization against measles, mumps, and rubella in adults and children >12 mo of age
measles, mumps, rubella, varicella virus vaccine (*ProQuad*)	0.5 mL subcutaneously	Simultaneous immunization against measles, mumps, rubella, and varicella in children aged 12 mo to 12 y
poliovirus vaccine, inactivated (*IPOL*)	0.5 mL subcutaneously at 2, 4, and 12–15 mo; booster when starting school *Adult:* 0.5 mL subcutaneously, two doses at intervals of 1–2 mo, with a third dose 6–12 mo later	Immunization against polio infections in adults and children
rabies vaccine (*Imovax Rabies, RabAvert*)	*Preexposure:* 1 mL IM on days 0, 7, and 21 or 28 (three doses) *Postexposure:* 1 mL IM on days 0, 3, 7, 21, and 28 (five doses)	Preexposure immunization against rabies for high-risk people; postexposure antirabies regimen with rabies immune globulin
rotavirus vaccine, live, oral pentavalent (*RotaTeq*)	Three doses of 2 mL PO starting at age 6–12 wk, with subsequent doses at 4- to 10-wk intervals (third dose should be given at 32 wk)	Prevention of rotavirus gastroenteritis in infants and children
varicella virus vaccine (*VARIVAX*)	0.5 mL subcutaneously, followed by 0.5 mL subcutaneously 4–8 wk later	Immunization against chicken pox infections in adults and children ≥12 mo of age
yellow fever vaccine (*YF-VAX*)	*Pediatric 1–12 y:* 0.5 mL subcutaneously; 0.5 mL subcutaneous booster every 10 y	Immunization of travelers to areas where yellow fever is endemic
zoster vaccine (*Zostavax*)	*Adults 50 y and older:* 0.65 mL by subcutaneous injection	Prevention of herpes zoster (shingles) in adults 50 y and older

DTaP, diphtheria and tetanus toxoids and acellular pertussis vaccine; HBsAg, hepatitis B surface antigen; HPV, human papillomavirus.

capability to make antibodies because the vaccine could cause disease and the body would not be able to respond as anticipated if it is in an immunodeficient state (this is primarily true of live vaccines); live vaccines during pregnancy because of potential effects on the fetus and on the success of the pregnancy; and for patients with known allergies to any of the components of the vaccine (refer to each individual vaccine for specifics, sometimes including eggs, where some pathogens are cultured). It is recommended to delay vaccination for patients who are receiving immune globulin or who have received blood or blood products as patients may not mount an appropriate immune response.

Caution should be used any time a vaccine is given to a child with a history of febrile convulsions or cerebral injury or in any condition in which a potential fever would be dangerous. Caution also should be used in the presence of any acute infection that is more severe than the common cold.

Adverse Effects

Adverse effects of vaccines are associated with the immune or inflammatory reaction that is being stimulated: moderate fever, rash, malaise, chills, fretfulness, drowsiness, anorexia, vomiting, and irritability. Pain, redness, swelling, and even nodule formation at the injection site are also common. In rare instances, severe hypersensitivity and central nervous system (seizures) reactions have been reported. Rotavirus has the rare adverse effect of intussusception.

Clinically Important Drug–Drug Interactions

Immunosuppressant drugs have the potential of altering how the body may respond to a vaccine. If the immunosuppressant drug suppresses the ability of the body to make antibodies, the vaccine will not be effective and, in the case of a live vaccine, could cause severe illness.

BOX 18.4

Vaccines and Biological Weapons

The events of September 11, 2001, and the subsequently declared "war on terror," heightened awareness of several diseases potentially in development as biological weapons. Anthrax, plague, tularemia, smallpox, botulism, and a variety of viral hemorrhagic fevers are all considered to be likely biological warfare weapons.

Anthrax

A vaccine is available in the United States made from inactivated cell-free filtrate of an avirulent strain of the anthrax bacillus. It is typically available before exposure when an individual is at high risk due to their occupation, but it is also available for postexposure emergency use. People who are pregnant and people with latex allergy should not be administered the vaccine. Ciprofloxacin and doxycycline are antibiotics that can be used to prevent anthrax. The monoclonal antibody, raxibacumab, is specific to the anthrax bacillus and is used for treatment postexposure, along with standard antibiotic therapy.

Smallpox

Smallpox was considered eradicated since no new cases had been seen in 20 years. Smallpox is highly transmissible and has a 30% mortality rate in unvaccinated people. Immunization against smallpox ended in the 1970s. There is now a vaccine, which is available to be given to some military personnel and people thought to be at high risk. It is currently thought that the vaccine is not effective after 3 years, so boosters are recommended if a person is at high risk.

Tularemia

Tularemia in an aerosolized form can cause systemic and respiratory illness with a 35% mortality rate. It is not passed from person to person. There is an investigational live attenuated vaccine that is being evaluated by the Food and Drug Administration. Doxycycline and ciprofloxacin can be used after exposure, and gentamicin has been effective after symptoms appear.

Botulism

Botulism, produced by *Clostridium botulinum*, can be aerosolized or used to contaminate food. The toxin it produces causes cranial nerve palsies that can result in muscle paralysis and respiratory failure. A botulinum toxoid is available through the Centers for Disease Control and Prevention for the military and high-risk workers. Antitoxin is also available for patients with specific exposures, and research is ongoing with an equine antitoxin effective against all seven serotypes of botulism that is thought to cause fewer hypersensitivity reactions than what is currently available.

Viral Hemorrhagic Fever

Lassa, Marburg, Junin, and Ebola viruses cause hemorrhagic fevers with mortality rates as high as 90%. No vaccines are currently available for most of these agents, although the U.S. Army has had success with a vaccine for Junin and the FDA has approved a vaccine for Ebola. Ribavirin has been effective in some cases of Lassa fever and has been effective orally for postexposure prophylaxis. It is being studied for effectiveness with these other viruses. Currently, there is no established treatment, and this area is one of the highest priorities for combating possible biological warfare. The outbreak of Ebola in Africa in 2014 and return of infected workers to the United States brought a great deal of attention to this problem. Many drug companies are working to find a treatment for these viral infections.

Box 18.5 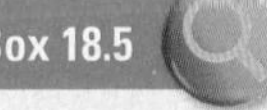 Focus on the Evidence

SARS-CoV-2 (COVID-19) VACCINE

Since the emergence of SARS-CoV-2 (COVID-19) at the end of 2019, researchers have been developing vaccines to prevent transmission and illness from this virus. At first, the FDA provided emergency authorization for several vaccines that showed promise in the phase 3 trials. The FDA also formed a Coronavirus Treatment Acceleration Program to facilitate fast tracking medications and vaccines that targeted COVID-19. Research quickly evolved and two mRNA-based vaccines were formally approved for use by the FDA. There was also a viral vector vaccine that was formally approved. The speed of the research and development of both vaccines and treatments that have been developed to fight the COVID-19 virus has been unprecedented.

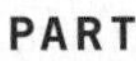

Nursing Considerations for Patients Receiving Vaccines

Assessment: History and Examination

- Assess for contraindications or cautions: known allergies to any vaccines or to the components of the one being used, to prevent hypersensitivity reactions; current status related to pregnancy, which is a contraindication to the use of live vaccines; recent administration of immune globulin or blood products, which could alter the response to the vaccine; history of immune deficiency, which could alter immune reactions; and evidence of acute infection, which could be exacerbated by the introduction of other antigens.
- Perform a physical assessment before beginning therapy to determine baseline status and any potential adverse effects: inspect for the presence of any skin lesions to monitor for hypersensitivity reactions; check temperature to monitor for possible infection; monitor pulse, respirations, and blood pressure; auscultate lungs for adventitious sounds; and assess level of orientation and affect to monitor for hypersensitivity reactions to the vaccine.
- Evaluate the range of motion of the extremity to be used for vaccine administration to assure adequate blood flow to deal with the antigen and inflammatory reaction.
- Assess tissue perfusion to establish a baseline to monitor for potential hypersensitivity reactions.

Nursing Conclusions

Nursing conclusions related to drug therapy might include the following:

- Impaired comfort related to injection, gastrointestinal (GI), and flulike effects
- Altered tissue perfusion if severe reaction occurs
- Knowledge deficit risk regarding drug therapy

Planning

- The patient will receive the best therapeutic effect from the drug therapy.
- The patient will have limited adverse effects to the drug therapy.
- The patient will have an understanding of the drug therapy, adverse effects to anticipate, and measures to relieve discomfort and improve safety.

Intervention With Rationale

- Do not use to treat acute infection; a vaccine is only used to prevent infection with future exposures.
- Do not administer if the patient exhibits signs of severe acute infection or immune deficiency because the vaccine can cause an inflammatory process and can exacerbate acute infections.
- Do not administer if the patient has received blood, blood products, or immune globulin recently because a severe immune reaction could occur.
- Arrange for proper preparation and administration of the vaccine; check on the timing and dose of each injection because dose, preparation, and timing vary with individual vaccines.
- Maintain emergency equipment on standby, including epinephrine, in case of severe hypersensitivity reaction.
- Arrange for supportive care and comfort measures for flulike symptoms (rest, environmental control, acetaminophen) and for injection discomfort (local heat application, anti-inflammatories, resting arm) to promote patient comfort.
- Do not administer aspirin to children for the treatment of discomfort associated with the immunization. Aspirin can provoke Reye's syndrome, a potentially serious disease.
- Provide thorough patient teaching, including measures to avoid adverse effects, warning signs of problems, and the need to keep a written record of immunizations, to increase knowledge about drug therapy and to increase adherence with the drug regimen.
- Provide a written record of the immunization, including the need to return for booster immunizations and timing of the boosters, if necessary, to increase patient adherence with medical regimens.

Evaluation

- Monitor patient response to the drug (prevention of disease, appropriate antibody titer levels).
- Monitor for adverse effects (flulike symptoms; GI upset; local pain, swelling, nodule formation at the injection site).
- Evaluate the effectiveness of the teaching plan (patient can name drug, dosage, adverse effects to watch for; has written record of immunizations; can state when to return for the next immunization or booster if needed).
- Monitor the effectiveness of comfort measures and adherence to the regimen.

See "Critical Thinking Scenario" for additional information on educating a parent about vaccines.

CRITICAL THINKING SCENARIO
Educating a Parent About Vaccines

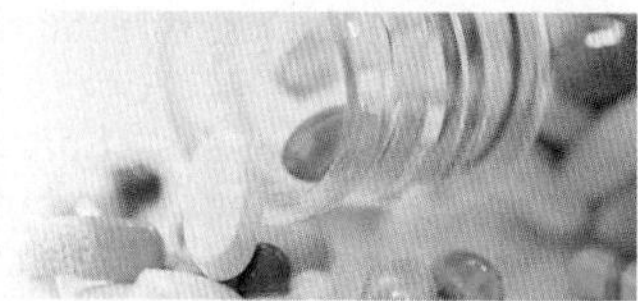

THE SITUATION

S.D. is a 25-year-old, first-time parent who has brought their 2-month-old infant to the well-baby clinic for a routine evaluation. The infant is found to be healthy, growing well, and within normal parameters for their age. At the end of the visit, the nurse prepares to give the infant the first of their routine immunizations. S.D. becomes concerned and expresses fears about paralysis and infant deaths associated with immunizations.

CRITICAL THINKING

What information should S.D. be given about immunizations?
What nursing interventions would be appropriate at this time? Think of ways to explain the importance of immunizations to S.D. while supporting their concerns for the welfare of their child.
How can this experience be incorporated into a teaching plan for S.D. and their child?

DISCUSSION

S.D. should be reassured before the infant is immunized. The nurse can explain that paralysis and infant deaths were reported in the past but that efforts continue to make the vaccines pure. Careful monitoring of the child and the child's response to each immunization can help avoid such problems. Reassure S.D. that the immunizations will prevent their child from contracting many, sometimes deadly, diseases. Praise S.D.'s efforts for researching information that might affect their child and for asking questions that could have an impact on their child and understanding of their care.

The recommended schedule of immunizations should be given to S.D. so that they are aware of what is planned and how the various vaccines are spaced and combined. They should be encouraged to monitor the infant after each injection for fever, chills, and flulike reactions. When they get home, they can medicate the infant with acetaminophen to avert many of these symptoms before they happen. (S.D. should be advised not to give the infant aspirin, which could provoke Reye's syndrome, a potentially serious disorder.) S.D. also should be told that the injection site might be sore, swollen, and red but that this will pass in a couple of days. S.D. can ease the infant's discomfort by applying warm soaks to the area for about 10 to 15 minutes every 2 hours.

S.D. should be encouraged to write down all of the immunizations that their child has had and to keep this information handy for easy reference. They should also be encouraged to record any adverse effects that occur after each immunization. If reactions are uncomfortable, it is possible to split doses of future immunizations.

The nurse should give S.D. a chance to vent their concerns and fears. First-time parents may be more anxious than experienced ones when dealing with issues involving a new child. To alleviate S.D.'s anxiety, the nurse should provide a telephone number that S.D. can call if the infant seems to be having a severe reaction or if S.D. wants to discuss any questions or concerns. They should feel that support is available for any concern that they may have. Because this interaction is likely to form the basis for future interactions with S.D., it is important to establish a sense of respect and trust.

NURSING CARE GUIDE FOR S.D.'S CHILD: VACCINES

Assessment: History and Examination

Allergies to the serum base, acute infection, immunosuppression
General: Temperature
Cardiovascular (CV): Pulse, cardiac auscultation, blood pressure, edema, perfusion
Respiratory: Respirations, adventitious sounds
Skin: Lesions
Joints: Range of motion

Nursing Conclusions

Impaired comfort related to inflammation and flulike symptoms
Altered tissue perfusion if severe reaction occurs
Knowledge deficit risk regarding drug therapy

Planning

The patient will receive the best therapeutic effect from the drug therapy.
The patient will have limited adverse effects to the drug therapy.
The patient will have an understanding of the drug therapy, adverse effects to anticipate, and measures to relieve discomfort and improve safety.

Implementation

Ensure proper preparation and administration of vaccine within appropriate time frame.
Provide supportive and comfort measures to deal with adverse effects: Anti-inflammatory/antipyretic, local heat application, small meals, rest, and a quiet environment.
Provide parent teaching regarding drug name, adverse effects and precautions, and warning signs to report.
Provide emergency life support if needed for acute reaction.

Evaluation

Evaluate drug effects: serum titers reflecting immunization (if appropriate).

(continues on page 322)

Monitor for adverse effects: pain, flulike symptoms, local discomfort.
Evaluate effectiveness of parent teaching program.
Evaluate effectiveness of comfort and safety measures.
Evaluate effectiveness of emergency measures if needed.

PATIENT TEACHING FOR S.D.

- This immunization will help your infant to develop antibodies to protect them against diphtheria, tetanus, and pertussis. The infant will develop antibodies to these diseases, and this will prevent them from contracting one of these potentially deadly diseases in the future.
- The injection site might be sore and painful. Heat applied to the area may help this discomfort and speed the infant's recovery.
- Adverse effects that the infant might experience include fever, muscle aches, joint aches, fatigue, malaise, crying, and fretfulness. Acetaminophen may help reduce symptoms; check with your health care provider for the correct dose to use for the infant. Rest, small meals, and a quiet environment may also help the infant to feel better.
- The adverse effects should pass within 2 to 3 days. If they seem to be causing undue discomfort or persist longer than a few days, notify your health care provider.
- Booster immunizations are required for this immunization. Your child should receive a booster immunization at your next checkup. Keep a written record of this immunization.
- Please contact your health care provider if you have any questions or concerns.

Prototype Summary: Measles, Mumps, and Rubella Vaccine

Indications: Active immunization against measles, mumps, and rubella (MMR) in children older than 15 months and adults.

Actions: Attenuated MMR viruses produce a modified infection and stimulate an active immune reaction with the production of antibodies to these viruses.

Pharmacokinetics:

Route	Onset	Peak
SQ	Rapid	3–12 h

$T_{1/2}$: Unknown; metabolized in the tissues; excretion is unknown.

Adverse Effects: Moderate fever, rash, or burning or stinging wheal or flare at the site of injection; rarely, febrile convulsions and high fever; vision and hearing impairment; numbness, pain, and tingling; altered balance.

Key Points

- Immunity is a state of relative resistance to a disease that develops only after exposure to the specific disease-causing antigen.
- Vaccines provide active artificial immunity by stimulating the production of antibodies to a specific protein, which may produce the signs and symptoms of a mild immune reaction but protects the person from the more devastating effects of disease.

Immune Sera

As explained earlier, passive artificial immunity can be achieved by providing preformed antibodies to a specific antigen. These antibodies are found in immune sera, which may contain antibodies to toxins, venins, bacteria, viruses, or even red blood cell antigenic factors. The term immune sera is usually used to refer to sera that contain antibodies to specific bacteria or viruses. The term antitoxin refers to immune sera that have antibodies to very specific toxins that might be released by invading pathogens. The term antivenin is used to refer to immune sera that have antibodies to venom that might be injected through spider or snake bites. These drugs are used to provide early treatment following exposure to known antigens. They are very specific for antigens to which they can respond (see Table 18.2).

Therapeutic Actions and Indications

Immune sera are used to provide passive immunity to a specific antigen, which could be a pathogen, venom, or toxin. They also may be used as prophylaxis against specific diseases after exposure in patients who are immunosuppressed. In addition, immune sera may be used to lessen the severity of a disease after known or suspected exposure (see Fig. 18.1 for sites of action of immune sera and antitoxins). Table 18.2 lists the various available immune sera, antitoxins, and antivenins, as well as usual indications.

Pharmacokinetics

No pharmacokinetic data are available for these biologicals.

Table 18.2 *Drugs in Focus:* Immune Sera

Drug Name	Dosage/Route	Usual Indications
Immune Sera		
antithymocyte immune globulin (*Thymoglobulin*)	1.5 mg/kg/d for 7–14 d as 6-h infusion for the first dose and ≥4 h for each subsequent dose	Treatment of renal transplant acute rejection in conjunction with immunosuppression
botulism immune globulin (*Baby BIG*)	*Pediatric (<1 y):* 50 mg/kg IV as an infusion	Treatment of patients <1 y with infant botulism caused by toxin type A or B
cytomegalovirus immune globulin (*CytoGam*)	50–150 mg/kg IV; doses vary per type of transplant; doses highest at first and titrated down	Attenuation of primary cytomegalovirus disease after renal, liver, pancreas, lung, and heart transplantation
hepatitis B immune globulin (*BayHep B, Nabi-HB*)	0.06 mL/kg IM, repeated at 1 mo	Postexposure prophylaxis against hepatitis B
immune globulin, intramuscular (*BayGam*, others)	Dose varies with exposure; check manufacturer's instructions	Prophylaxis after exposure to hepatitis A, measles, varicella, or rubella
immune globulin, intravenous (*Gamimune N*, *Octagam*, and others)	Dose varies with exposure; check manufacturer's instructions	Prophylaxis after exposure to hepatitis A, measles, varicella, or rubella; bone marrow and other transplants; Kawasaki's disease; chronic lymphocytic leukemia; treatment of patients with immunoglobulin deficiency
immune globulin, subcutaneous (*Gamunex-C, Hizentra, Vivaglobin*)	300–2,000 mg/kg IV or 1.37 times IV dose if given SQ; dosing varies per diagnosis	Treatment of idiopathic thrombocytopenic purpura, chronic inflammatory demyelinating polyneuropathy
lymphocyte immune globulin (*Atgam*)	*Adult:* 10–30 mg/kg/d IV *Pediatric:* 5–25 mg/kg/d IV for aplastic anemia	Management of allograft rejection in renal transplantation; treatment of aplastic anemia
rabies immune globulin (*HyperRAB S/D, Imogam Rabies*)	20 IU/kg IM	Protection against rabies in nonimmunized patients exposed to rabies
RHO immune globulin (*HyperRHO S/D Full Dose, RhoGAM*)	1 vial IM within 72 h after delivery	Prevention of sensitization to the Rh factor
RHO immune globulin, microdose (*HyperRHO S/D Mini-Dose, MICRhoGAM, Prophylac*)	1 vial IV within 72 h after delivery	Prevention of sensitization to the Rh factor
tetanus immune globulin (*BayTet*)	250 units IM	Passive immunization against tetanus at time of injury
vaccinia immune globulin IV (*VIGIV*)	2 mL/kg (100 mg/kg) IV 6,000 units/kg IV as soon as symptoms appear; doses may be increased if needed	Treatment and management of vaccinia infections
varicella zoster immune globulin (*VARIZIG*)	1.25 mL diluted IM *or* 2.5 mL diluted IV over 3–5 min	Reduction in the severity of chickenpox if used within 4 d of exposure
Antitoxins and Antivenins		
antivenin (*Micrurus fulvius*) (generic)	30–50 mL IV, flush with fluids after antivenin has infused	Neutralizes the venom of coral snakes
Black widow spider antivenin (generic)	25 mL IM or IV in 10–50 mL saline over 15 min	Treatment of symptoms of black widow spider bites
botulism antitoxin (*Botulism Antitoxin Heptavalent*)	IV, dose based on CDC protocol and exposure	Treatment of suspected or known exposure to all types of botulism neurotoxin, patients 1 y and older
centruroides immune fab (*Anascorp*)	3 vials IV over 10 min, then 1 vial at a time every 30–60 min until clinically stable	Treatment of scorpion stings
crotalidae polyvalent immune fab (*CroFab*)	*Initial dose*: 4–6 vials; may give additional 4–6 vials to control envenomation *Maintenance after gain control*: 2 vials every 6 h for total of 18 h	Treatment of rattlesnake bites

CDC, Centers for Disease Control and Prevention.

Contraindications and Cautions

Immune sera are contraindicated in patients with a history of severe reaction to any immune sera or to products similar to the components of the sera to prevent potential serious hypersensitivity reactions. They should be used with caution during pregnancy because of potential risk to the fetus, in patients with coagulation defects or thrombocytopenia, or in patients with a known history of previous exposure to the immune sera because increased risk of hypersensitivity reaction occurs with each use.

Adverse Effects

Adverse effects can be attributed either to the effect of immune sera on the immune system (rash, nausea, vomiting, chills, fever) or to allergic reactions (chest tightness, falling blood pressure, difficulty breathing). Local reactions, such as swelling, tenderness, pain, or muscle stiffness at the injection site, are very common (see Fig. 18.2).

Clinically Important Drug–Drug Interactions

Caution should be used if these drugs are combined with any immunosuppressant drugs, including corticosteroids. These can alter the body's response to the biologicals.

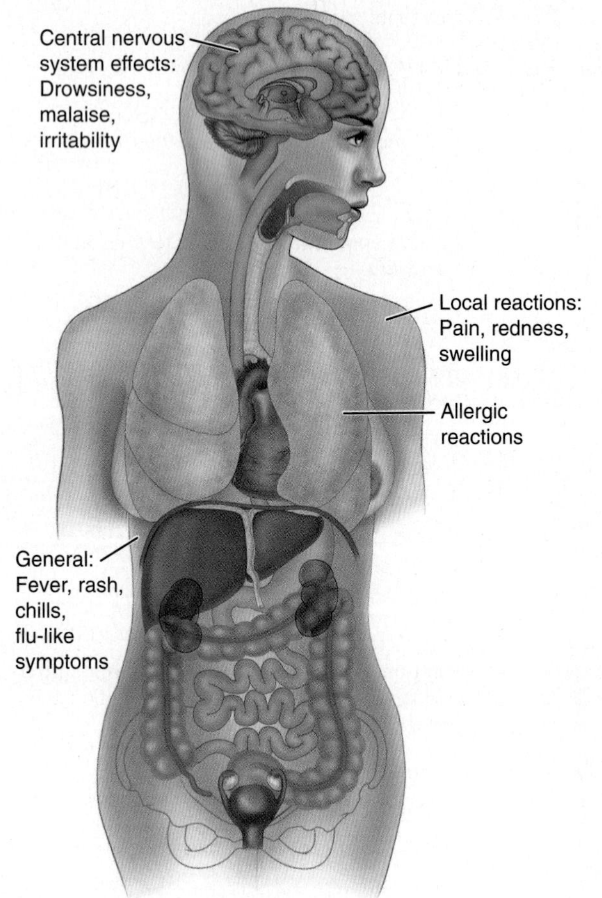

FIGURE 18.2 Variety of adverse effects and toxicities associated with vaccines and immune sera.

Prototype Summary: Immune Globulin, Intramuscular

Indications: Prophylaxis against hepatitis A, measles, varicella, rubella; prophylaxis for patients with immunoglobulin deficiency.

Actions: Provides preformed antibodies to hepatitis A, measles, varicella, rubella, and perhaps other antigens, providing a passive, short-term immunity.

Pharmacokinetics:

Route	Onset	Peak
IM	Slow	2–5 d

$T_{1/2}$: Unknown; metabolized in the tissues; excretion is unknown.

Adverse Effects: Tenderness, muscle stiffness at site of injection; urticaria, angioedema, nausea, vomiting, chills, fever, chest tightness.

Nursing Considerations for Patients Receiving Immune Sera

Assessment: History and Examination

- Assess for contraindications or cautions: any known allergies to any of these drugs or their components to prevent hypersensitivity reactions; current status related to pregnancy, which would be a contraindication for immune sera; previous exposure to the serum being used because hypersensitivity reactions become worse with repeated exposure; evidence of thrombocytopenia or coagulation disorders, which could be exacerbated by the effects of immune sera; and immunization history to determine the potential for hypersensitivity reactions.
- Perform a physical assessment before beginning therapy to determine baseline status and any potential adverse effects: inspect for the presence of any skin lesions to monitor for hypersensitivity reactions; check temperature to monitor for possible infection; monitor pulse, respirations, and blood pressure; auscultate lungs for adventitious sounds; and assess level of orientation and affect to monitor for hypersensitivity reactions to the vaccine.

Nursing Conclusions

Nursing conclusions related to drug therapy might include the following:

- Impaired comfort related to local, GI, and flulike effects
- Altered tissue perfusion related to possible severe reactions
- Knowledge deficit risk regarding drug therapy

Planning

- The patient will receive the best therapeutic effect from the drug therapy.
- The patient will have limited adverse effects to the drug therapy.
- The patient will have an understanding of the drug therapy, adverse effects to anticipate, and measures to relieve discomfort and improve safety.

Intervention With Rationale

- Do not administer to any patient with a history of severe reaction to immune globulins or to the components of the drug being used because severe immune reactions can occur.
- Administer the drug as indicated. Preparation varies with each product; always check the manufacturer's guidelines.
- Monitor for severe reactions and have emergency equipment ready to allow prompt intervention should a severe reaction occur.
- Arrange for supportive care and comfort measures for flulike symptoms (rest, environmental control, acetaminophen) and for the local reaction (heat to injection site, anti-inflammatories) to promote patient comfort.
- Provide thorough patient teaching, including measures to avoid adverse effects and warning signs of problems, to improve patient compliance.
- Provide a written record of immune sera use and encourage the patient or family to keep that information to ensure proper medical treatment and avert future reactions.

Evaluation

- Monitor the patient's response to the drug (improvement in disease signs and symptoms, prevention of severe disease).
- Monitor for adverse effects (flulike symptoms, GI upset, local inflammation, and pain).
- Evaluate the effectiveness of the teaching plan (patient can name drug, dosage, adverse effects to watch for, and specific measures to avoid adverse effects and to promote comfort and acknowledge the need to retain a written record of injection).
- Monitor the effectiveness of comfort measures and compliance with the regimen.

Key Points

- Immune sera provide preformed antibodies to specific proteins for people who have been exposed to them or are at high risk for exposure.
- The term immune sera typically refers to sera that contain antibodies to specific bacteria or viruses.

SUMMARY

- Immunity (relative resistance to a disease) may be active or passive. Active immunity results from the body making antibodies against specific proteins for immediate release if that protein reenters the body. Passive immunity results from preformed antibodies to a specific protein, which offers protection against the protein only for the life of the circulating antibodies.
- Immunizations are given to stimulate active immunity in a person who is at high risk for exposure to specific diseases. Immunizations are a standard part of preventive medicine.
- Vaccines can be made from chemically inactivated microorganisms or from live, weakened viruses or bacteria. Toxoids are vaccines that are made from the toxins produced by the microorganism that are altered so that they are no longer poisonous but still have the recognizable protein antigen that will stimulate antibody production.
- Immune sera provide preformed antibodies to specific proteins for people who have been exposed to them or are at high risk for exposure.
- The term immune sera typically refers to sera that contain antibodies to specific bacteria or viruses. Antitoxins are immune sera that have antibodies to very specific toxins that might be released by invading pathogens. Antivenins are immune sera that have antibodies to venom that might be injected through spider or snake bites.
- Serum sickness—a massive immune reaction—occurs more frequently with immune sera than with vaccines. Patients need to be monitored for any history of hypersensitivity reactions, and emergency equipment should be available.
- Patients/parents should be advised to keep a written record of all immunizations or immune sera used. Booster doses for various vaccines may be needed to further stimulate antibody production.

Unfolding Patient Stories: Juan Carlos • Part 2

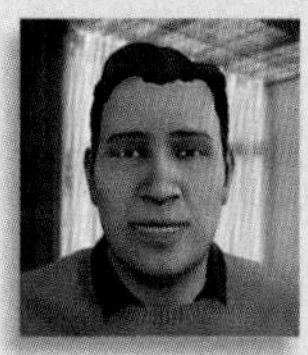

Juan Carlos, a 52-year-old male with diabetes type 2, hypertension, and hyperlipidemia, is seen at the clinic for his annual checkup. According to age and health status, what vaccinations are recommended for him? What factors should the nurse consider if Juan's immunizations are not up-to-date? How would the nurse intervene if cultural factors, past experiences, or apprehension cause a reluctance to receive vaccinations? (Juan Carlos' story continues in Chapter 38.)

Care for Juan and other patients in a realistic virtual environment: ***vSim** for Nursing* (thepoint.lww.com/vSimPharm). Practice documenting these patients' care in DocuCare (thepoint.lww.com/DocuCareEHR).

CHECK YOUR UNDERSTANDING

Answers to the questions in this chapter can be found in Answers to Check Your Understanding Questions on thePoint®.

MULTIPLE CHOICE

Select the best answer.

1. When preparing a presentation for a local parent group about vaccines, the nurse would describe vaccines as being used to stimulate
   a. passive immunity to a foreign protein.
   b. active immunity to a foreign protein.
   c. serum sickness.
   d. a mild disease in healthy people.

2. After teaching a parent about common adverse effects associated with routine immunizations, which of the following, if stated by the parent, would indicate the need for additional teaching?
   a. Difficulty breathing and fainting
   b. Fever and rash
   c. Drowsiness and fretfulness
   d. Swelling and nodule formation at the site of injection

3. Which vaccine would the nurse be least likely to recommend for a 6-month-old child?
   a. Diphtheria, tetanus, pertussis vaccine
   b. *Haemophilus influenzae* b vaccine
   c. Poliovirus vaccine
   d. Varicella vaccine

4. It is now recommended that all people over the age of 6 months should receive a flu vaccine every fall based on the understanding that the vaccine is repeated because
   a. the immunity wears off after a year.
   b. the strains of virus predicted to cause the flu change every year.
   c. a booster shot will activate the immune system.
   d. flu shots do not produce good antibodies.

5. The nurse reviews a patient's record to make sure that tetanus booster shots have been given
   a. only with exposure to anaerobic bacteria.
   b. every 2 years.
   c. every 5 years.
   d. every 10 years.

6. A nurse suffers a needlestick after injecting a patient with suspected hepatitis B. The nurse should
   a. have repeated titers to determine whether they were exposed to hepatitis B and if they have hepatitis immune globulin.
   b. immediately receive hepatitis immune globulin and begin hepatitis B vaccines if they have not already received them.
   c. start antibiotic therapy immediately.
   d. go on sick leave until all screening tests are negative.

7. A patient is to receive immune globulin after exposure to hepatitis A. The patient has a previous history of allergies to various drugs. Before giving the immune globulin, the nurse should
   a. have emergency equipment readily available.
   b. premedicate the patient with aspirin.
   c. make sure all of the patient's vaccinations are up to date.
   d. make sure the patient has a ride home.

MULTIPLE RESPONSE

Select all that apply.

1. A public education campaign to stress the importance of childhood immunizations should include which points?
   a. Prevention of potentially devastating diseases outweighs the discomfort and risks of immunization.
   b. Routine immunization is standard practice in the United States.
   c. The practice of routine immunizations has virtually wiped out many previously deadly or debilitating diseases.
   d. The risk of severe adverse reactions is on the rise and is not being addressed.
   e. If there is a family history of autism, that person should avoid immunizations.
   f. The temporary discomfort associated with the immunization can be treated with over-the-counter drugs.
2. A parent brings their child to an 18-month wellness visit. The nurse would not give the child their routine immunizations in which situations?
   a. The child cried at their last immunization.
   b. The child developed a fever or rash after their last immunization.
   c. The child currently has a fever and symptoms of a cold.
   d. The child is allergic to aspirin.
   e. The child is currently taking oral corticosteroids.
   f. The child's siblings are all currently being treated for a viral infection.
3. When assessing the medical record of an older adult to evaluate the status of their immunizations, the nurse would be looking for evidence of which immunizations?
   a. Yearly pneumococcal vaccination
   b. Yearly flu vaccination
   c. Tetanus booster every 10 years
   d. Tetanus booster every 5 years
   e. Measles, mumps, rubella vaccine if the patient was born after 1957
   f. Varicella vaccine only if there is evidence that the patient had chickenpox as a child

REFERENCES

Alta Charo, R. (2007). Politics, parents and prophylaxis: Mandating HPV vaccination in the United States. *New England Journal of Medicine, 356*, 1905–1908. https://doi.org/10.1056/NEJMp078054

Brunton, L. L., Hilal-Dandan, R., & Knollman, B. C. (2018). *Goodman and Gilman's the pharmacological basis of therapeutics* (13th ed.). McGraw Hill.

Centers for Disease Control and Prevention. (2013). Prevention and control of meningococcal disease: Recommendations of the advisory committee on immunization practices. *Morbidity and Mortality Weekly Report, 62*(RR02), 1–22. https://www.cdc.gov/mmwr/preview/mmwrhtml/rr6202a1.htm

Centers for Disease Control and Prevention. (2014). CDC grand rounds: Reducing the burden of HPV-associated cancer and disease. *Morbidity and Mortality Weekly Report, 63*(4), 69–72. http://www.cdc.gov/mmwr/preview/mmwrhtml/mm6304a1.htm

Centers for Disease Control and Prevention. (2021, November 24). *Understanding how COVID-19 vaccines work.* https://www.cdc.gov/coronavirus/2019-ncov/vaccines/about-vaccines/how-they-work.html

Guilano, A. R., Palefsky, J. M., Goldstone, S., Moreira, E. D., Penny, M. E., Aranda, C., Vardas, E., Moi, H., Jessen, H., Hillman, R., Chang, Y.-H., & Ferris, D. (2011). Efficacy of quadrivalent HPV vaccine against HPV infection and disease in males. *New England Journal of Medicine, 364*, 401–411. https://doi.org/10.1056/NEJMoa0909537

Hendler, C. B. (Ed.) (2021). *Nursing 2021 drug handbook.* Wolters Kluwer.

Institute of Medicine (US) Immunization Safety Review Committee. (2004). *Immunization safety review: Vaccines and autism.* National Academies Press.

Katz, S. L. (2005). A vaccine-preventable infectious disease kills half a million children a year. *Journal of Infectious Diseases, 192*(10), 1679–1680. https://doi.org/10.1086/497172

Moderna. (2020, November 16). *Moderna's COVID-19 vaccine candidate meets its primary efficacy endpoint in the first interim analysis of the phase 3 COVE study.* https://investors.modernatx.com/news-releases/news-release-details/modernas-covid-19-vaccine-candidate-meets-its-primary-efficacy

Norris, T. L. (2019). *Porth's pathophysiology concepts of altered health states.* Wolters Kluwer.

Pfizer. (2020, November 9). *Pfizer and BioNTech announce vaccine candidate against COVID-19 achieved success in first interim analysis from phase 3 study.* https://www.pfizer.com/news/press-release/press-release-detail/pfizer-and-biontech-announce-vaccine-candidate-against

U.S. Food and Drug Administration. (2021, November 15). *Coronavirus treatment acceleration program (CTAP).* https://www.fda.gov/drugs/coronavirus-covid-19-drugs/coronavirus-treatment-acceleration-program-ctap

PART 4

Drugs Acting on the Central and Peripheral Nervous Systems

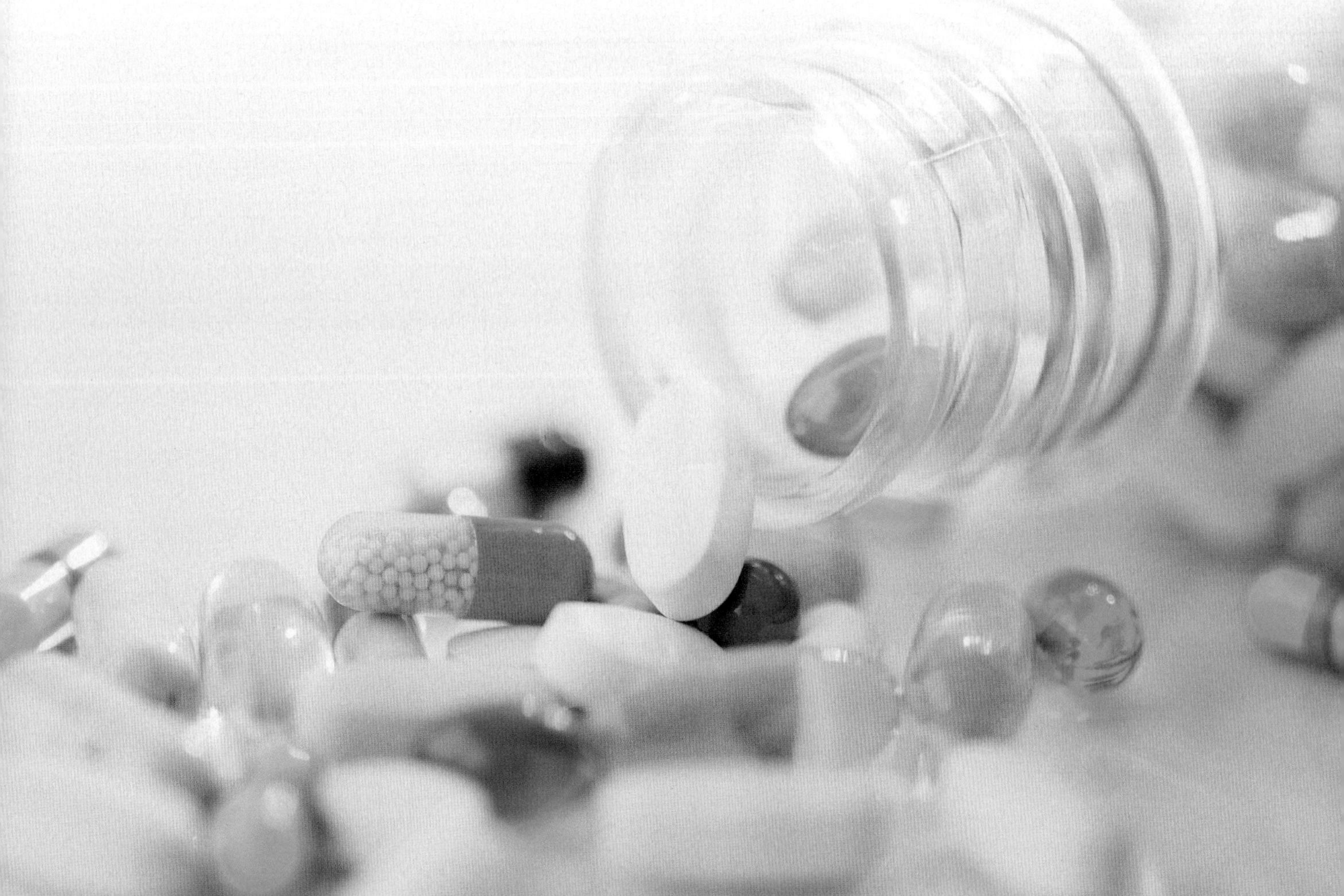

CHAPTER 19

Introduction to Nerves and the Nervous System

Learning Objectives

Upon completion of this chapter, you will be able to:

1. Label the parts of a neuron and describe the functions of each part.
2. Describe an action potential, including the roles of the various electrolytes involved in the action potential.
3. Explain what a neurotransmitter is, including its origins and functions at the synapse.
4. Describe the function of the cerebral cortex, cerebellum, hypothalamus, thalamus, midbrain, medulla, spinal cord, and reticular activating system.
5. Discuss what is known about learning and the impact of emotion on the learning process.

Key Terms

action potential: sudden change in electrical charge of a nerve cell membrane; the electrical signal by which neurons send information

afferent fibers: nerve axons that run from peripheral receptors into the central nervous system

axon: long projection from a neuron that carries information from one nerve to another nerve or effector

dendrite: short projection on a neuron that transmits information

depolarization: opening of the sodium channels in a nerve membrane to allow the influx of positive sodium ions, reversing the membrane charge so it is no longer polarized

effector cell: cell stimulated by a nerve; may be a muscle, a gland, or another nerve cell

efferent fibers: nerve axons that carry nerve impulses from the central nervous system to the periphery to stimulate muscles or glands

engram: short-term memory made up of a reverberating electrical circuit of action potentials

forebrain: upper level of the brain; consists of the two cerebral hemispheres, where thinking and coordination of sensory and motor activity occur, contains the hypothalamus and thalamus and the area of the limbic system

ganglia: groups of nerve bodies

hindbrain: most primitive area of the brain, the brainstem; consists of the pons and medulla, which control basic vital functions, and the cerebellum, which controls motor functions that regulate balance

limbic system: area in the forebrain that is rich in epinephrine, norepinephrine, and serotonin and seems to control emotions

midbrain: the middle area of the brain; it consists of many of the cranial nerves and areas related to arousal and sleep/wakefulness; sits just below the hypothalamus

neuron: structural unit of the nervous system

neurotransmitter: chemical produced by a nerve and released when the nerve is stimulated; reacts with a specific receptor site to cause a reaction

repolarization: return of a membrane to a resting state, with more sodium ions outside the membrane and a relatively negative charge inside the membrane

Schwann cell: insulating cell found on nerve axons; allows "leaping" electrical conduction to speed the transmission of information and prevent tiring of the neuron

soma: cell body of a neuron; contains the nucleus, cytoplasm, and various granules

synapse: junction between a nerve and an effector; consists of the presynaptic nerve ending, a space called the synaptic cleft, and the postsynaptic cell

The nervous system is responsible for controlling the functions of the human body, analyzing incoming stimuli, and integrating internal and external responses. The nervous system is composed of the central nervous system (CNS; the brain and spinal cord) and the peripheral nervous system (PNS). The PNS is composed of sensory receptors that bring information into the CNS and motor nerves that carry information away from the CNS to facilitate response to stimuli. The autonomic nervous system, which is discussed in Chapter 29, uses components of the CNS and PNS to regulate automatic or unconscious responses to stimuli.

The structural unit of the nervous system is the nerve cell or **neuron**. There are billions of nerve cells that make up the nervous system. Neurons are organized to facilitate movement, transmit sensations, respond to internal and external stimuli, support learning, and convey emotions. The mechanisms that are involved in all of these processes are not clearly understood. The actions of drugs that are used to affect nerve function and the responses that these drugs cause throughout the nervous system provide some of the current theories about the workings of the nervous system.

Physiology of the Nervous System

The nervous system operates through the use of electrical impulses and chemical messengers to transmit information throughout the body and to respond to internal and external stimuli. The properties and functions of the neuron provide the basis for all nervous system functions.

Neurons

The neuron is the structural unit of the nervous system. The human body contains about 14 billion neurons. About 10 billion of these are located in the brain, and the remainder makes up the spinal cord and PNS.

Neurons have several distinctive cellular features (Fig. 19.1). Each neuron is made up of a cell body, or **soma**, which contains the cell nucleus, cytoplasm, and various granules and other particles. Short, branchlike projections that cover most of the surface of a neuron are called **dendrites**. These structures, which provide increased surface area for the neuron, bring information into the neuron from other neurons.

One end of the nerve body extends into a long process that does not branch out until the very end of the process. This elongated process is called the nerve **axon**, and it emerges from the soma at the axon hillock, a slightly enlarged area of the soma. The axon of a nerve can be extremely tiny, or it can extend for several feet. The axon carries information from a nerve to be transmitted to **effector cells**—cells stimulated by a nerve, which may include a muscle, gland, or another nerve. This transmission occurs at the end of the axon, where the axon branches out into what is called the axon terminal.

The axons of many nerves are packed closely together in the nervous system and look like cable or fiber tracts. **Afferent fibers** are nerve axons that run from peripheral receptors into the CNS. In contrast, **efferent fibers** are nerve axons that carry nerve impulses from the CNS to the periphery to stimulate muscles or glands. (An easy way to remember the difference between afferent and efferent is to recall that efferent fibers exit from the CNS.)

It is currently thought that neurons are unable to reproduce; so, if nerves are destroyed, they are lost. If dendrites and axons are lost, nerves regenerate those structures; however, for this regeneration to occur, the soma and the axon hillock must remain intact. For a clinical example, consider a person who has closed a car door on their finger. Sensation and movement may be lost or limited for a certain period, but because the nerve bodies for most of the nerves in the hand are located in **ganglia** (groups of nerve bodies) in the wrist, they are able to regenerate the damaged axon or dendrites. Over time, sensation and full movement should return.

Research on possible ways to stimulate the reproduction of nerves is under way. Although scientists have used nerve growth factor with fetal cell implants to stimulate some nerve growth, it is currently assumed that nerves in normal situations are unable to reproduce.

Action Potential

Nerves send messages by conducting electrical impulses called **action potentials**.

Nerve membranes, which are capable of conducting action potentials along the entire membrane, send messages via this electrical communication system to nearby neurons or to effector cells that may be located inches to feet away. Like all cell membranes, nerve membranes have various channels or pores that control the movement of substances into and out of the cell. Some of these channels allow the movement of sodium, potassium, and calcium. When cells are at rest, their membranes are impermeable to sodium. However, the membranes are permeable to potassium ions.

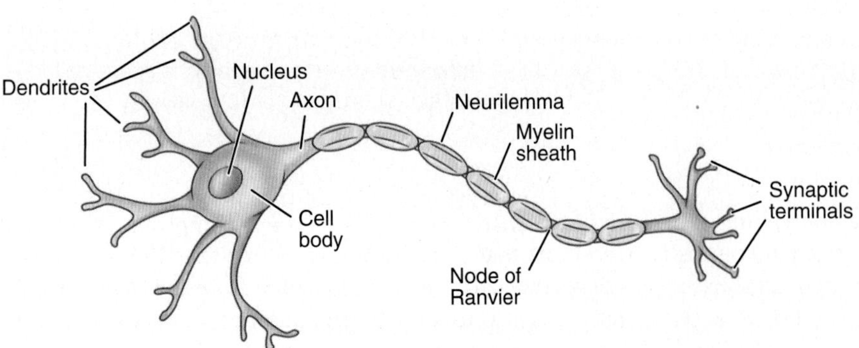

FIGURE 19.1 The neuron, functional unit of the nervous system.

The sodium–potassium pump that is active in the membranes of neurons is responsible for this property of the membrane. This system pumps sodium ions out of the cell and potassium ions into the cell. At rest, more sodium ions are outside the cell membrane, and more potassium ions are inside. Electrically, the inside of the cell is relatively negative compared with the outside of the membrane, which establishes an electrical potential along the nerve membrane. This membrane is polarized, with the positive pole outside the membrane and the negative pole inside the membrane. When nerves are at rest, this is referred to as the resting membrane potential of the nerve.

Stimulation of a neuron causes **depolarization** of the nerve, which means that the sodium channels open in response to the stimulus, and sodium ions rush into the cell, following the established concentration gradient. If an electrical monitoring device is attached to the nerve at this point, a positive rush of ions is recorded. The electrical charge on the inside of the membrane changes from relatively negative to relatively positive. The cell has become depolarized, losing the positive and negative poles. This sudden reversal of membrane potential, called the action potential (Fig. 19.2), lasts less than a microsecond. Using the sodium–potassium pump, the cell then returns that section of membrane to the resting membrane potential, a process called **repolarization**. The action potential generated at one point along a nerve membrane stimulates the generation of an action potential in adjacent portions of the cell membrane, and the stimulus travels the length of the cell membrane.

Nerves can respond to stimuli several hundred times per second, but for a given stimulus to cause an action potential, it must have sufficient strength and must occur when the nerve membrane is able to respond—that is, when it has repolarized. A nerve cannot be stimulated again while it is depolarized. The balance of sodium and potassium across the cell membrane must be reestablished.

Nerves require energy (i.e., oxygen and glucose) and the correct balance of the electrolytes sodium and potassium to maintain normal action potentials and transmit information into and out of the nervous system. If a person has anoxia or hypoglycemia, the nerves might not be able to maintain the sodium–potassium pump, and that person may become severely irritable or too stable (not responsive to stimuli).

Long nerves are myelinated: They have a myelin sheath that speeds electrical conduction and protects the nerves from the fatigue that results from frequent formation of action potentials. Even though many of the tightly packed nerves in the brain do not need to travel far to stimulate another nerve, some of them are myelinated. The effect of this myelination is not understood.

Myelinated nerves have neuroglial cells called **Schwann cells** (in the PNS) or oligodendrocytes (in the CNS), located at specific intervals along nerve axons, that are very resistant to electrical stimulation (see Fig. 19.1).

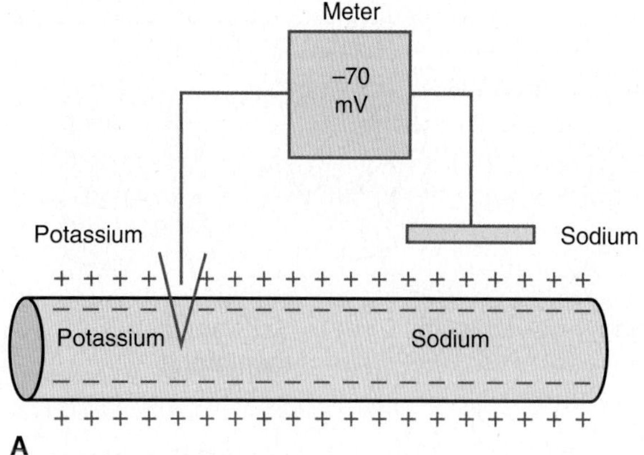

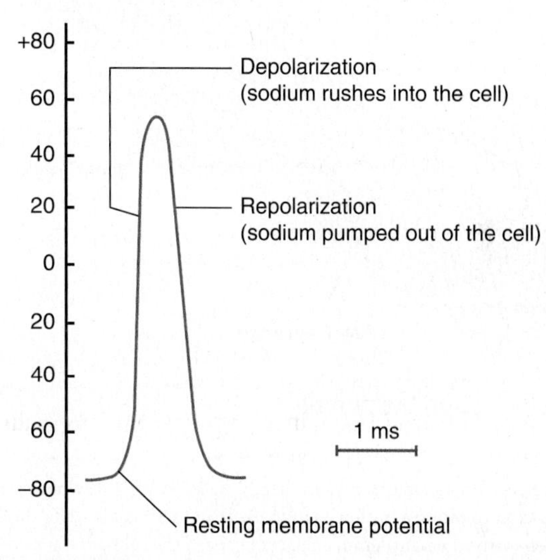

FIGURE 19.2 The action potential. **A.** Segment of an axon showing that, at rest, the inside of the membrane is relatively negatively charged and the outside is positively charged. A pair of electrodes placed as shown would record a potential difference of about –70 mV; this is the resting membrane potential. **B.** An action potential of about 1 ms that would be recorded if the axon shown in panel (**A**) were brought to threshold. At the peak of the action potential, the charge on the membrane reverses polarity.

The oligodendrocytes extend several processes and wrap myelin around several axons. The Schwann cells wrap themselves around the axon in a jelly roll fashion (Fig. 19.3). Between the Schwann cells are areas of uncovered nerve membrane called the nodes of Ranvier. So-called leaping nerve conduction occurs along these exposed nerve fibers. An action potential excites one section of the nerve membrane, and the electrical impulse then "skips" from one node to the next, generating an action potential. Because the membrane is forming fewer action potentials, the speed of conduction is much faster, and the nerve is protected from being exhausted or using up energy to form multiple action potentials. This node-to-node mode of conduction is termed saltatory, or leaping, conduction (see Fig. 19.1).

Segmental demyelination can occur when there is damage to the Schwann cell or the myelin sheath.

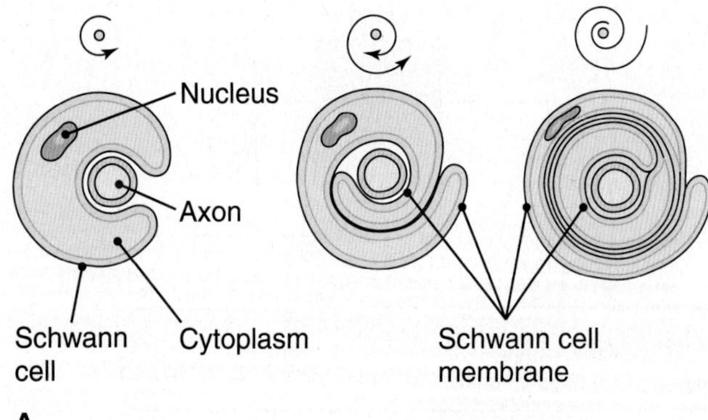

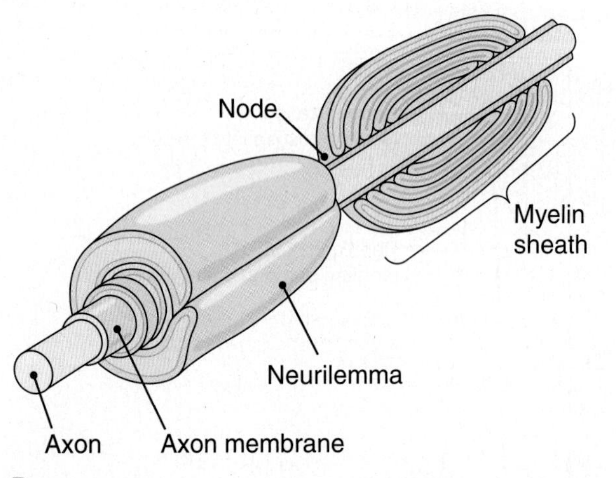

FIGURE 19.3 Formation of a myelin sheath. **A.** Schwann cells wrap around the axon, creating a myelin coating. **B.** The outermost layer of the Schwann cell forms the neurilemma. Spaces between the cells are the nodes of Ranvier.

Guillain-Barré syndrome is an example of damage to the peripheral neurons and demyelination of peripheral nerves causing rapidly progressive ascending symmetric limb weakness/paralysis and loss of deep tendon reflexes. Multiple sclerosis is an immune-mediated condition in which there is inflammation and breakdown of the CNS myelin. The myelin break down results in lesions called plaques. Acute plaques demonstrate signs of inflammation and immune response. Older lesions often show decreased numbers of oligodendrocytes, demyelination, and scar formation. This process can interrupt nerve conduction and cause a variety of symptoms including visual disturbances, speech and/or swallowing changes, muscle weakness, imbalance, nystagmus, and sensory impairments.

Nerve Synapse

When the electrical action potential reaches the end of an axon, the electrical impulse comes to a halt. At this point, the stimulus no longer travels at the speed of electricity. The transmission of information between two nerves or between a nerve and a gland or muscle is chemical. Nerves communicate with other nerves or effectors at the nerve **synapse** (Fig. 19.4). The synapse is made up of a presynaptic nerve, the synaptic cleft, and the postsynaptic effector cell. The nerve axon, called the presynaptic nerve, releases a chemical called a neurotransmitter into the synaptic cleft, and the neurotransmitter reacts with a very specific receptor site on the postsynaptic cell to cause a reaction.

Neurotransmitters

Neurotransmitters are chemicals produced by a nerve and released when the nerve is stimulated. Neurotransmitters stimulate postsynaptic cells either by exciting or by inhibiting them. The reaction that occurs when a neurotransmitter stimulates a receptor site depends on the specific neurotransmitter a nerve releases and the receptor site it activates. A nerve may produce only one type of neurotransmitter, using building blocks such as tyrosine or choline from the extracellular fluid, often absorbed from dietary sources. The neurotransmitter, packaged into vesicles, moves to the terminal membrane of the axon, and when the nerve is stimulated, the vesicles contract and push the neurotransmitter into the synaptic cleft. The calcium channels in the nerve membrane are open during the action potential, and the presence of calcium causes the contraction. When the cell repolarizes, calcium leaves the cell, and the contraction stops. Once released into the synaptic cleft, the neurotransmitter reacts with very specific receptor sites to cause a reaction.

To return the effector cell to a resting state so that, if needed, it can be stimulated again, neurotransmitters must be inactivated. Neurotransmitters may be either reabsorbed by the presynaptic nerve in a process called reuptake (a recycling effort by the nerve to reuse the materials and save resources) or broken down by enzymes in the area (e.g., monoamine oxidase breaks down the catecholamine neurotransmitters; the enzyme acetylcholinesterase breaks down the neurotransmitter acetylcholine).

Several neurotransmitters have been identified. As research continues, other neurotransmitters may be discovered, and the actions of known neurotransmitters will be better understood.

The following are selected neurotransmitters:

- Acetylcholine, which communicates between nerves and muscles, is also important as the preganglionic neurotransmitter throughout the autonomic nervous system and as the postganglionic neurotransmitter in the parasympathetic nervous system and in several pathways in the brain.
- Norepinephrine and epinephrine are catecholamines, which are released by nerves in the sympathetic branch of the autonomic nervous system and are classified as hormones when they are released from cells in the adrenal medulla. These neurotransmitters also occur in high levels in particular areas of the brain, such as the limbic system.

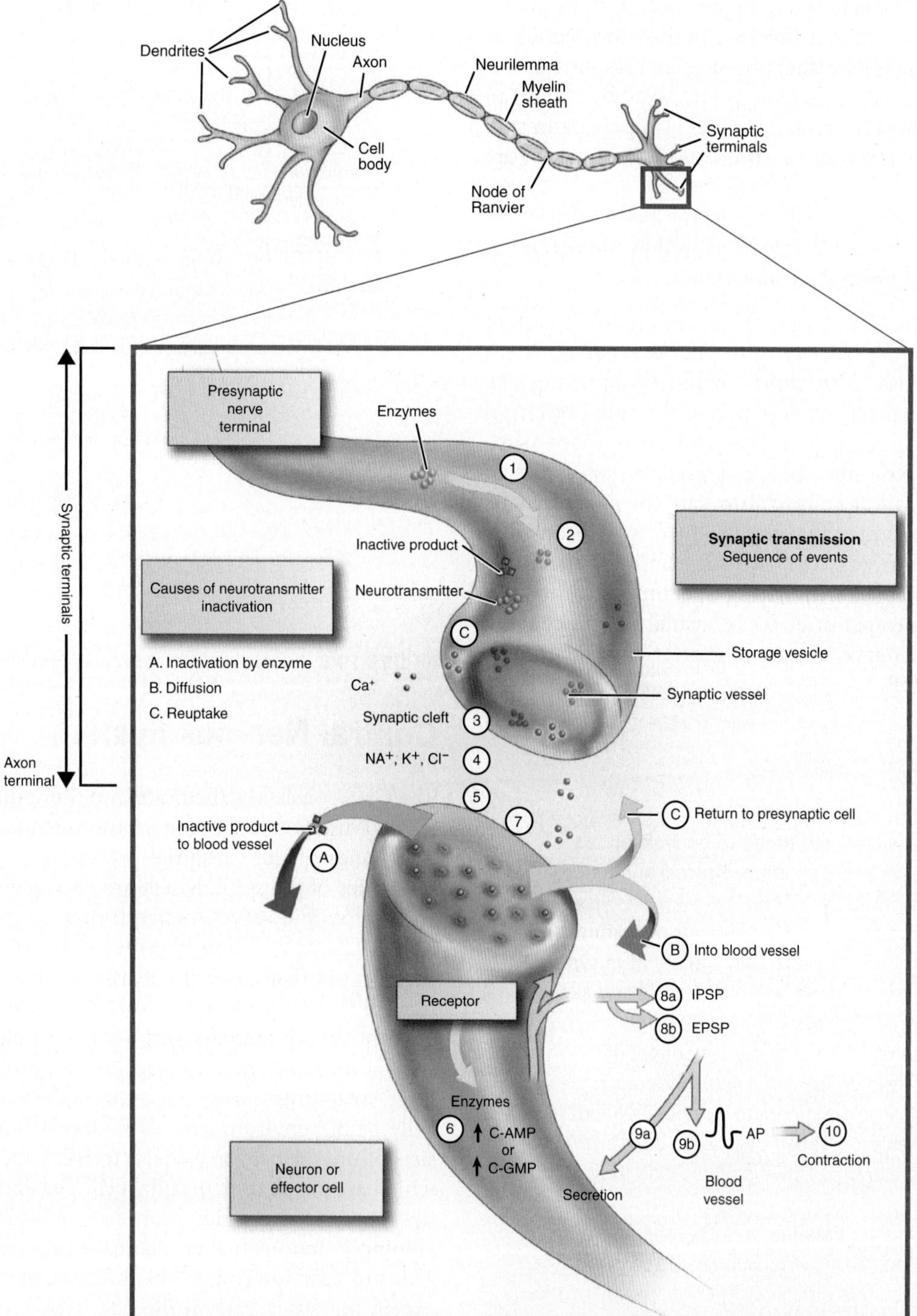

FIGURE 19.4 The sequence of events in synaptic transmission: (*1*) synthesis of the neurotransmitter, (*2*) uptake of the neurotransmitter into storage vesicles, (*3*) release of the neurotransmitter by an action potential in the presynaptic nerve, (*4*) diffusion of the neurotransmitter across the synaptic cleft, (*5*) combination of the neurotransmitter with a receptor, (*6*) a sequence of events leading to activation of second messengers within the postsynaptic nerve, and (*7*) change in permeability of the postsynaptic membrane to one or more ions, causing (*8a*) an inhibitory postsynaptic potential or (*8b*) an excitatory postsynaptic potential. Characteristic responses of the postsynaptic cell are as follows: (*9a*) the gland secretes hormones, (*9b*) the muscle cells have an action potential, and (*10*) the muscle contracts. The action of the neurotransmitter is terminated by one or more of the following processes: (*A*) inactivation by an enzyme, (*B*) diffusion out of the synaptic cleft and removal by the vascular system, and (*C*) reuptake into the presynaptic nerve followed by storage in a synaptic vesicle or deactivation by an enzyme.

- Dopamine, which is found in high concentrations in certain areas of the brain, is involved in the coordination of both motor and intellectual impulses and responses.
- Gamma-aminobutyric acid or GABA, which is found in the brain, inhibits nerve activity and is important in preventing overexcitability or stimulation such as seizure activity.
- Serotonin, which is also found in the limbic system, is important in arousal and sleep, as well as in preventing depression and promoting motivation.

Many of the drugs that affect the nervous system involve altering the activity of the nerve synapse. These drugs have several functions, including blocking the reuptake of neurotransmitters so that they are present in the synapse in greater quantities and cause more stimulation of receptor sites; blocking receptor sites so that the neurotransmitter cannot stimulate the receptor site; blocking the enzymes that break down neurotransmitters to cause an increase in neurotransmitter concentration in the synapse; stimulating specific receptor sites when the neurotransmitter is not available; and causing the presynaptic nerve to release greater amounts of the neurotransmitter.

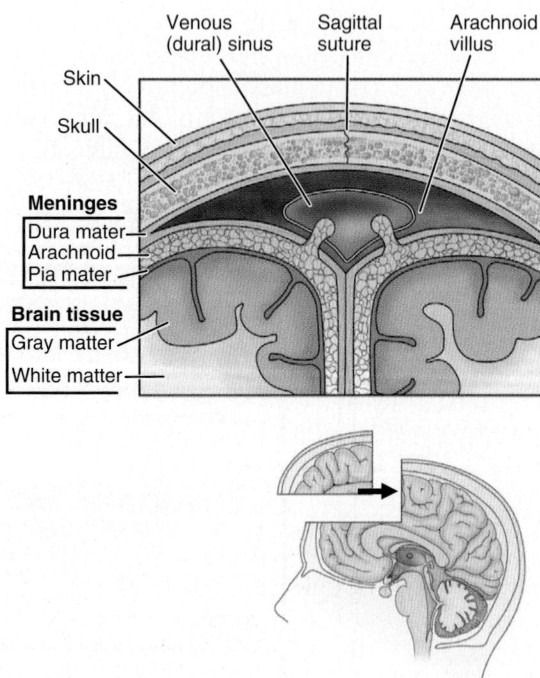

FIGURE 19.5 Bony and membranous protection of the brain.

Key Points

- The nervous system controls the body, analyzes external stimuli, and integrates internal and external responses to stimuli.
- The neuron, composed of a cell body, dendrites, and an axon, is the functional unit of the nervous system. Dendrites route information to the nerve, and axons take the information away.
- Nerves transmit information by way of action potentials. An action potential is a sudden change in membrane charge from negative to positive that is triggered when stimulation of a nerve opens sodium channels and allows positive sodium ions to flow into the cell.
- When sodium ions flow into a nerve, the nerve membrane depolarizes. Mechanically, this is recorded as a flow of positive electrical charges. Repolarization immediately follows, with the sodium–potassium pump in the cell membrane pumping sodium and potassium ions out of the cell, leaving the inside of the membrane relatively negative to the outside, returning the resting membrane potential.
- At the end of the axon, neurons communicate via chemicals called neurotransmitters, which are produced by the nerve. Neurotransmitters are released into the synapse when the nerve is stimulated; they react with very specific receptor sites to cause a reaction and are immediately broken down or removed from the synapse.

Central Nervous System

The CNS consists of the brain and the spinal cord, the two parts of the body that contain the vast majority of nerves. The bones of the vertebrae protect the spinal cord, and the bones of the skull, which are corrugated much like an egg carton and serve to absorb impact, protect the brain (Fig. 19.5). In addition, the meninges, which are stretchy membranes that cover the nerves in the brain and spine, furnish further protection.

The blood–brain barrier, a functioning boundary, also plays a defensive role. It keeps toxins, proteins, and other large structures out of the brain and facilitates a chemically stable environment. The blood–brain barrier consists of unique capillary characteristics and the astrocytes, which are a type of neuroglial cell. The endothelial cells in the capillaries supplying brain neurons have tight or overlapping junctions, which decrease capillary permeability. This can slow and control the diffusion of most substances, except for water, carbon dioxide, and oxygen. The astrocytes link the neurons and capillaries, are able to uptake potassium and neurotransmitters to protect the nerves, and can help repair scar formation in the brain.

The blood–brain barrier represents a therapeutic challenge to drug treatment of brain-related disorders because a large percentage of drugs are carried bound to plasma proteins and are unable to cross into the brain. When a patient is suffering from a brain infection, many antibiotics cannot cross into the brain until the infection is so severe that the blood–brain barrier is less functional and capillary permeability increases. Lipid-soluble substances (such as alcohol, nicotine, and heroin) are able to cross the blood–brain barrier more easily than water-soluble substances that often have a high ionic charge.

The brain has a unique blood supply to protect the neurons from lack of oxygen and glucose. The two carotid arteries branch off the aortic arch and go up into each side of the brain at the front of the head. The two vertebral arteries enter the back of the brain to become the basilar arteries. These arteries all deliver blood to a common vessel at the bottom of the brain called the circle of Willis, which distributes the blood to the brain as it is needed (Fig. 19.6). The role of the circle of Willis becomes apparent when a person has an occluded carotid artery. Although the passage of blood through one of the carotid arteries may be negligible, the areas of the brain on that side will still have a full blood supply because of the blood sent to those areas via the circle of Willis.

Anatomy of the Brain

The brain has three major divisions: the hindbrain, the midbrain, and the forebrain (Fig. 19.7).

The **hindbrain**, which runs from the top of the spinal cord into the midbrain, is the most primitive area of the brain. It contains the brainstem, where the pons and medulla oblongata are located. These areas of the brain control basic vital functions, such as the respiratory centers, which control breathing; the cardiovascular centers, which regulate blood pressure; the chemoreceptor trigger zone and emetic zone, which control vomiting; and the swallowing center, which coordinates the complex swallowing reflex.

The cerebellum—a part of the brain that looks like a skein of yarn and lies behind the other parts of the hindbrain—coordinates the motor function that regulates posture, balance, and voluntary muscle activity.

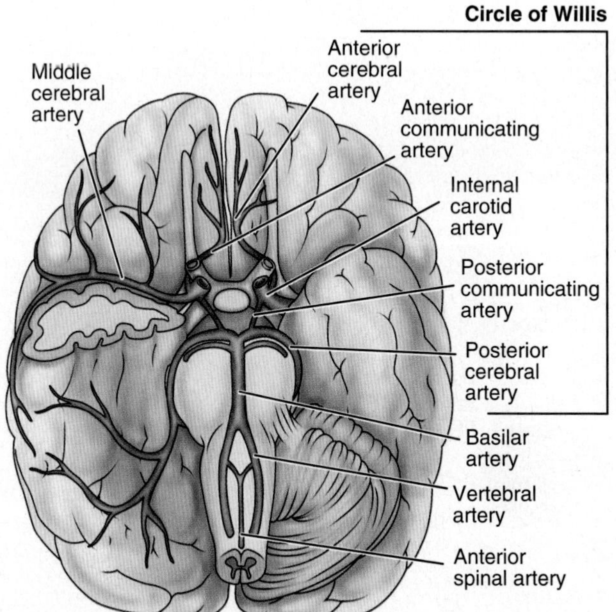

FIGURE 19.6 The protective blood supply of the brain: the carotid, vertebral, and basilar arteries join to form the circle of Willis.

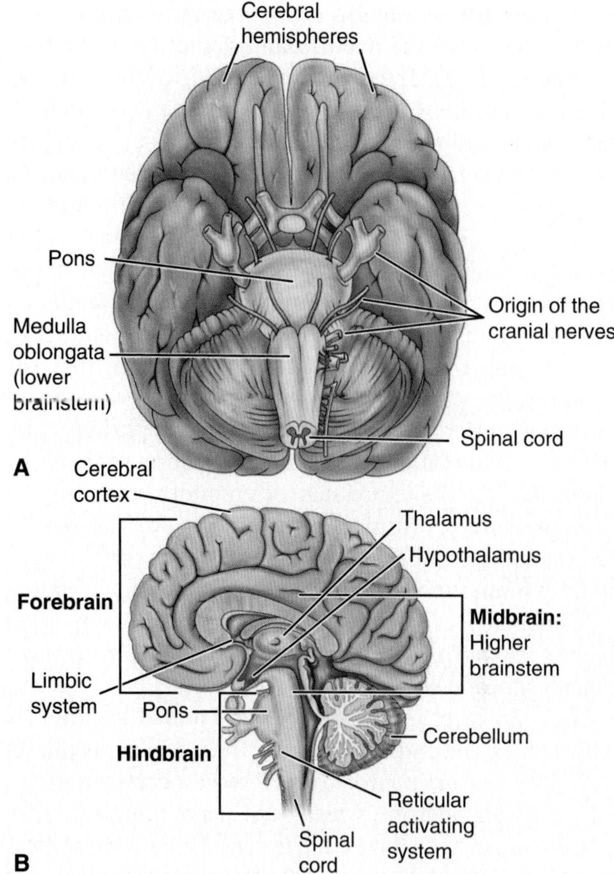

FIGURE 19.7 Anatomy of the brain. **A.** View of the underside of the brain. **B.** The medial or midsagittal view of the brain.

The **midbrain** sits above the hindbrain and is a small area. It contains cranial nerves related to the specific senses (sight, smell, hearing, balance, taste); some muscle activity of the head and neck (e.g., chewing, eye movement); and the reticular activating system (RAS), which transmits information via the thalamus, hypothalamus, and limbic system to the cerebral cortex. The RAS extends from the hindbrain to the midbrain and filters the billions of incoming messages, selecting only the most significant for response. Lesions or damage to the RAS leads to altered levels of consciousness that can range from mild confusion to coma.

 *Concept Mastery Alert*

Sleep–Wake Cycles

Sleep–wake cycles and wakefulness or alertness are modulated by several areas of the brain including the RAS, hypothalamus, thalamus, and cerebral cortex. The RAS and cortex are pivotal in modulating levels of consciousness. There are cells in the hypothalamus that regulate the circadian rhythms that are responsive to light and dark cycles. There are some nerves within the RAS that secrete serotonin, which can facilitate drowsiness and decreased alertness. The pineal gland, located in the midbrain, is also thought to secrete melatonin, a hormone that helps regulate sleep.

The **forebrain** contains the two cerebral hemispheres and the thalamus, the hypothalamus, and the limbic system (see Fig. 19.7). The thalamus sends direct information into the cerebrum to transfer sensations, such as cold, heat, pain, touch, and muscle sense. The hypothalamus, which is poorly protected by the blood–brain barrier, acts as a major sensor for activities in the body. Areas of the hypothalamus are responsible for temperature control, water balance, appetite, and fluid balance. In addition, the hypothalamus plays a central role in the endocrine system and in the autonomic nervous system.

The **limbic system** is an area of the brain that sits just above the thalamus and contains high levels of three neurotransmitters: epinephrine, norepinephrine, and serotonin. Stimulation of this area, which appears to be responsible for the expression of emotions, may lead to anger, pleasure, motivation, stress, and so on. This part of the brain seems to be largely responsible for the "human" aspect of brain function. Drug therapy aimed at alleviating emotional disorders such as depression and anxiety often involves attempting to alter the levels of epinephrine, norepinephrine, and serotonin.

The two cerebral hemispheres are joined together by an area called the corpus callosum. These two hemispheres contain the sensory neurons, which receive nerve impulses, and the motor neurons, which send nerve impulses. They also contain areas that coordinate speech and communication and seem to be the area where learning takes place (see Fig. 19.8). Different areas of the brain appear to be responsible for receiving and sending information to specific areas of the body. When the brain is viewed at autopsy, it looks homogeneous, but scientists have mapped the general areas that are responsible for sensory response, motor function, and other functions. In conjunction with the cerebellum, ganglia or groups of nerve cell bodies called the basal ganglia, located at the bottom of the brain, make up the extrapyramidal motor system. This system coordinates motor activity for unconscious activities such as posture and gait.

Anatomy of the Spinal Cord

The spinal cord is made up of 31 pairs of spinal nerves. Each spinal nerve has two components or roots, a sensory fiber (called the dorsal root) and a motor fiber (called the ventral root). The spinal sensory fibers bring information into the CNS from the periphery. The motor fibers carry information away from the brain and cause movement or reaction.

Functions of the Central Nervous System

The brain is responsible for coordinating reactions to the constantly changing external and internal environment. In all animals, the function of this organ is essentially the same. The human component involving emotions, learning, and conscious response takes the human nervous system beyond a simple reflex system and complicates the responses to any stimulus.

Sensory Functions

Millions of sensory impulses are constantly streaming into the CNS from peripheral receptors. Many of these impulses go directly to specific areas of the brain designated to deal with input from particular areas of the body or from the senses. The responses that occur as a result of these stimuli can be altered by efferent neurons that respond to emotions through the limbic system, to learned responses stored in the cerebral cortex, or to autonomic input mediated through the hypothalamus.

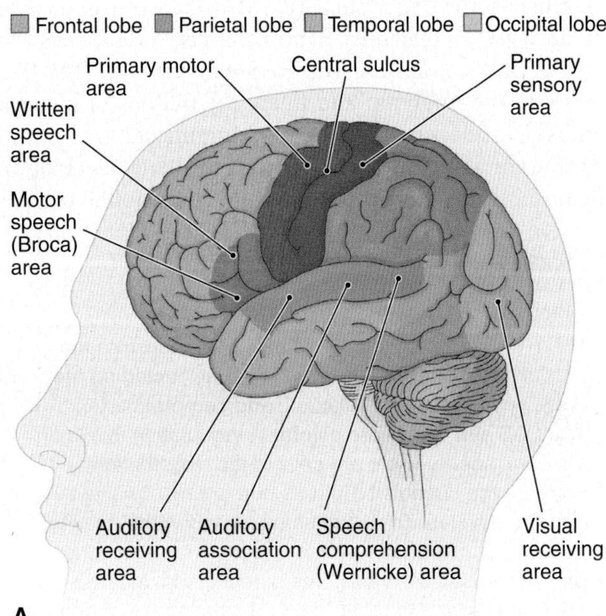

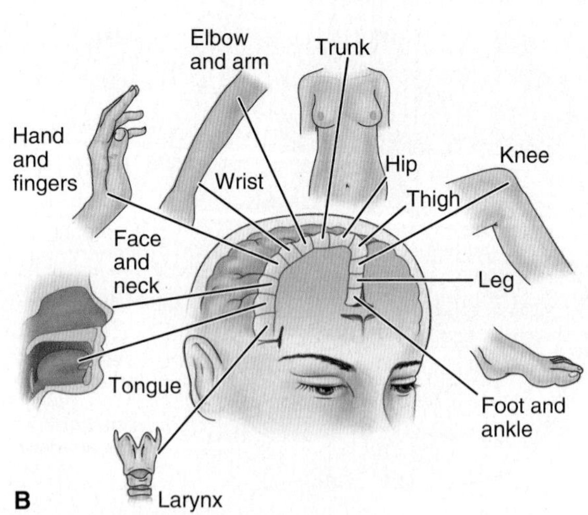

FIGURE 19.8 Functional areas of the brain. **A.** Topographical organization of functions of control and interpretation in the cerebral cortex. **B.** Areas of the brain that control specific areas of the body. Size indicates relative distribution of control.

The intricacies of the human brain can change the response to a sensation depending on the situation. People may react differently to the same stimulus. For example, if a person drops a can on their foot, the physiologic response is one of pain and a stimulation of the sympathetic branch of the autonomic nervous system. If the person is alone or in a very comfortable environment (e.g., fixing dinner at home), they may scream, swear, or jump around. However, if that person is in the company of other people (e.g., a cooking teacher working with a class), they may be much more composed and quieter, even though the physiologic effect on the body is the same.

Motor Functions

The sensory nerves that enter the brain react with related motor nerves to cause a reaction mediated by muscles or glands. The motor impulses that leave the cortex are further regulated or coordinated by the pyramidal system, which coordinates voluntary movement, and the extrapyramidal system, which coordinates unconscious motor activity that regulates control of position and posture. For example, some drugs may interfere with the extrapyramidal system and cause tremors, shuffling gait, and lack of posture and position stability. Motor fibers from the cortex cross to the other side of the spinal cord before emerging to interact with peripheral effectors. In this way, motor stimuli coming from the right side of the brain affect motor activity on the left side of the body. For example, an area of the left cortex may send an impulse down to the spinal cord that reacts with an interneuron, crosses to the other side of the spinal cord, and causes a finger on the right hand to twitch.

Intellectual and Emotional Functions

The way that the cerebral cortex uses sensory information is not clearly understood, but research has demonstrated that the two hemispheres of the brain process information in different ways. There is a theory that the right side of the brain is the more artistic side, concerned with forms and shapes; the left side is more analytical, concerned with names, numbers, and processes. Why the two hemispheres are different and how they develop differently is not known.

When learning takes place, distinct layers of the cerebral cortex are affected, and an actual membrane change occurs in a neuron to store information in the brain permanently. Learning begins as an electrical circuit called an **engram**, a reverberating circuit of action potentials that eventually becomes a long-term, permanent memory in the presence of the proper neurotransmitters and hormones. Scientists do not understand exactly how this happens, but it is known that the nerve requires oxygen, glucose, and sleep to process an engram into a permanent memory, and during that processing, structural changes occur to the cells involved in the engram. This reverberating circuit is responsible for short-term memory. When blood supply to a patient's brain decreases, short-term memory may be lost, and they are not able to remember new things. This happens because the engram requires a constant supply of oxygen and glucose to maintain that electrical circuit; if it cannot be maintained, it is lost. Because the patient is unable to remember new things, the brain falls back on long-term, permanent memory for daily functioning. For example, a patient may be introduced to a nurse and have no recollection of the nurse 2 hours later and yet be able to recall vividly the events of several years ago.

Several substances appear to affect learning. Antidiuretic hormone, which is released during reactions to stress, is one such substance. Although too much stress prevents learning, feeling slightly stressed may increase a person's ability to learn. A patient who is a little nervous about upcoming surgery, for example, seems to display better mastery of facts about the surgery and postoperative procedures than a patient who is very stressed and scared or one who appears to show no interest or concern. Oxytocin is another substance that seems to increase actual learning. Because childbirth is the only known time that oxytocin levels increase, the significance of this is not understood. Nurses who work with pregnant patients should know that patients in labor will very likely remember the smallest details about the whole experience; these nurses should use whatever opportunity is made available to do teaching.

The limbic system also appears to play an important role in how a person learns and reacts to stimuli. The emotions associated with a memory as well as with the present have an impact on stimulus response. The placebo effect is a documented effect of the mind on drug therapy. If a person perceives that a drug will be effective, it is much more likely to actually be effective. This effect, which uses the actions of the cerebrum and the limbic system, can have a tremendous impact on drug response.

Key Points

- The CNS consists of the brain and spinal cord, which are protected by bone and meninges. To ensure blood flow to the brain if a vessel should become damaged, the brain also has a protective blood supply moderated by the circle of Willis.
- The hindbrain, the most primitive area of the brain, contains the centers that control basic vital functions. The pons and the medulla are located in the hindbrain. The cerebellum, which helps to coordinate motor activity, is located at the back of the hindbrain.
- The midbrain consists of the cranial nerves and the RAS, which regulates arousal and awareness.
- The forebrain consists of the cerebral cortex composed of two hemispheres, which regulate the communication between sensory and motor neurons and are the sites of thinking and learning. The hypothalamus, thalamus, and the limbic system are also in the forebrain. The limbic system is responsible for the expression of emotion, and the thalamus and hypothalamus coordinate internal and external responses and direct information into the cerebral cortex.

Clinical Significance of Drugs That Act on the Nervous System

The features of the human nervous system, including the complexities of the human brain, sometimes make it difficult to predict the exact reaction of a particular patient to a given drug. When a drug is used to affect the nervous system, the occurrence of many systemic effects is always a possibility because the nervous system affects the entire body. The chapters in this part address the individual classes of drugs used to treat disorders of the nervous system, including their adverse effects. An understanding of the actions of specific drugs makes it easier to anticipate what therapeutic and adverse effects might occur. In addition, nurses should consider all of the learned, cultural, and emotional aspects of the patient's situation in an attempt to provide optimal therapeutic benefit and minimal adverse effects.

SUMMARY

- Although nerves do not reproduce, they can regenerate injured parts if the soma and axon hillock remain intact.
- Efferent fibers take information out of the CNS to effector cells; afferent fibers carry information into the CNS.
- When the transmission of action potentials reaches the axon terminal, it causes the release of chemicals called neurotransmitters, which cross the synaptic cleft to stimulate an effector cell, which can be another nerve, a muscle, or a gland.
- A neurotransmitter must be produced by a nerve (each nerve can produce only one kind), it must be released into the synapse when the nerve is stimulated, it must react with a very specific receptor site to cause a reaction, and it must be immediately broken down or removed from the synapse so that the cell can be ready to be stimulated again.
- Much of the drug therapy for the nervous system involves receptor sites and the release or reuptake and breakdown of neurotransmitters.
- The CNS consists of the brain and spinal cord, which are protected by bone and meninges. To ensure blood flow to the brain if a vessel should become damaged, the brain also has a protective blood supply moderated by the circle of Willis.
- The hindbrain, the most primitive area of the brain, contains the centers that control basic vital functions. The pons and the medulla are located in the hindbrain; the cerebellum, which helps to coordinate motor activity, is located at the back of the hindbrain.
- The midbrain consists of the RAS, which assists in the regulation of arousal and awareness, and the cranial nerves responsible for the special senses and control of head and neck muscles.
- The forebrain contains the hypothalamus, the thalamus, and the limbic system. The limbic system is responsible for the expression of emotion, and the thalamus and hypothalamus coordinate internal and external responses and direct information into the cerebral cortex.
- The cerebral cortex, also in the forebrain, consists of two hemispheres that regulate the communication between sensory and motor neurons and are the sites of thinking and learning.
- The mechanisms of learning and processing learned information are not understood. Emotion-related factors influence the human brain, which handles stimuli and responses in complex ways.
- Much remains to be learned about the human brain and how drugs influence it. The actions of many drugs that have known effects on human behavior are not understood.

CHECK YOUR UNDERSTANDING

Answers to the questions in this chapter can be found in Answers to Check Your Understanding Questions on thePoint®.

MULTIPLE CHOICE

Select the best answer.

1. The cerebellum
   a. initiates voluntary muscle movement.
   b. helps regulate the tone of skeletal muscles.
   c. if destroyed, would result in the loss of all voluntary skeletal activity.
   d. contains the centers responsible for the regulation of body temperature.

2. At those regions of the nerve membrane where myelin is present, there is
   a. low resistance to electrical current.
   b. high resistance to electrical current.
   c. high conductance of electrical current.
   d. energy loss for the cell.

3. The nerve synapse
   a. is not resistant to electrical current.
   b. cannot become exhausted.
   c. has a synaptic cleft.
   d. transfers information at the speed of electricity.

4. Which could result in the initiation of an action potential?
   a. Depolarizing the membrane
   b. Decreasing the extracellular potassium concentration
   c. Increasing the activity of the sodium–potassium active transport system
   d. Stimulating the nerve with a threshold electrical stimulus during the absolute refractory period of the membrane

5. Neurotransmitters are
   a. produced in the muscle to communicate with nerves.
   b. the chemicals used to stimulate or suppress effectors at the nerve synapse.
   c. usually found in the diet.
   d. nonspecific in their action on various nerves.

6. The limbic system is an area of the brain that is responsible for
   a. coordination of movement.
   b. the special senses.
   c. expression of emotions.
   d. control of sleep.

7. The most primitive area of the brain, the brainstem, contains areas responsible for
   a. vomiting, swallowing, respiration, arousal, and sleep.
   b. learning.
   c. motivation and memory.
   d. taste, sight, hearing, and balance.

8. A clinical indication of poor blood supply to the brain, particularly to the higher levels where learning takes place, would be loss of
   a. long-term memory.
   b. short-term memory.
   c. coordinated movement.
   d. ability to fall asleep.

MULTIPLE RESPONSE

Select all that apply.

1. In explaining the importance of a constant blood supply to the brain, the nurse would tell the student which?
   a. Energy is needed to maintain nerve membranes and cannot be produced without oxygen.
   b. Carbon dioxide must constantly be removed to maintain the proper pH.
   c. Little glucose is stored in nerve cells, so a constant supply is needed.
   d. The brain needs a constant supply of insulin and thyroid hormone.
   e. The brain swells easily and needs the blood supply to reduce swelling.
   f. Circulating aldosterone levels maintain the fluid balance in the brain.

2. The blood–brain barrier could be described in which ways?
   a. It is produced by the cells that make up the meninges.
   b. It is regulated by the microglia in the CNS.
   c. It is weaker in certain parts of the brain.
   d. It is uniform in its permeability throughout the CNS.
   e. It is an anatomical structure that can be punctured.
   f. It is more likely to block the entry of proteins into the CNS.

REFERENCES

Barrett, K. E., Barman, S. M., Brooks, H. L., & Yuan, J. (2019). *Ganong's review of medical physiology* (26th ed.). McGraw-Hill.

Brunton, L., Hilal-Dandan, R., & Knollman, B. (2018). *Goodman and Gilman's the pharmacological basis of therapeutics* (13th ed.). McGraw-Hill.

Guyton, A., & Hall, J. (2015). *Textbook of medical physiology* (13th ed.). W. B. Saunders.

Hendler, C. B. (Ed.) (2021). *Nursing 2021 drug handbook.* Wolters Kluwer.

Noback, C., Strominger, N. L., Demarest, R. J., et al. (2012). *The human nervous system: Structure and function* (7th ed.). Humana Press.

Norris, T. L. (2019). *Porth's pathophysiology concepts of altered health states.* Wolters Kluwer.

Parpura, V., & Hayden, P. (2009). *Astrocytes in the physiology of the nervous system.* Springer.

Thibodeau, G., & Patton, K. (2017). *Anthony's textbook of anatomy and physiology* (21st ed.). Mosby.

CHAPTER 20

Anxiolytic and Hypnotic Agents

Learning Objectives

Upon completion of this chapter, you will be able to:

1. Define the states that are affected by anxiolytic or hypnotic agents.
2. Discuss the use of anxiolytic or hypnotic agents across the lifespan.
3. Describe the therapeutic actions, indications, pharmacokinetics, contraindications, most common adverse reactions, and important drug–drug interactions associated with each class of anxiolytic or hypnotic agent.
4. Compare and contrast the prototype drugs for each class of anxiolytic or hypnotic drug with the other drugs in that class.
5. Outline the nursing considerations and teaching needs for patients receiving each class of anxiolytic or hypnotic agent.

Key Terms

anxiety: feeling of tension, fear, or nervousness in response to an environmental stimulus, whether actual or unknown

anxiolytic: drug used to depress the central nervous system (CNS); prevents or reduces the signs and symptoms of anxiety

barbiturates: CNS depressants that can cause sedation, hypnosis, and anesthesia

benzodiazepine: class of drug that acts in the limbic system and the reticular activating system (RAS) to make gamma-aminobutyric acid (GABA), an inhibitory neurotransmitter, more effective, causing interference with neuron firing; depresses CNS to block the signs and symptoms of anxiety; may cause sedation and hypnosis in higher doses

hypnosis: extreme sedation resulting in CNS depression and sleep

hypnotic: drug used to depress the CNS; causes sleep

sedation: loss of awareness of and reaction to environmental stimuli

sedative: drug that depresses the CNS; produces a loss of awareness of and reaction to the environment

Drug List

BENZODIAZEPINES USED AS ANXIOLYTIC–HYPNOTICS

alprazolam
chlordiazepoxide
clonazepam
clorazepate
(P) diazepam
estazolam
flurazepam
lorazepam
midazolam
oxazepam
quazepam
temazepam
triazolam

BARBITURATES USED AS ANXIOLYTIC–HYPNOTICS

pentobarbital
(P) phenobarbital
secobarbital

OTHER ANXIOLYTIC AND HYPNOTIC DRUGS

buspirone
dexmedetomidine
diphenhydramine
eszopiclone
meprobamate
promethazine
ramelteon
suvorexant
tasimelteon
zaleplon
zolpidem

The drugs discussed in this chapter are used to alter a person's responses to environmental stimuli. They have been called anxiolytics because they can reduce or prevent feelings of tension or fear, sedatives because they can calm patients and make them unaware of their environment, hypnotics because they can cause sleep, and minor tranquilizers because they can produce a state of tranquility in anxious patients. In the past, a given drug would simply be used at different doses to yield each of these effects. Further research into how the brain reacts to outside stimuli has resulted in the increased availability of specific agents that produce particular desired effects and avoid unwanted adverse effects. Use of these drugs also varies across the lifespan (Box 20.1).

States Affected by Anxiolytic and Hypnotic Drugs

Anxiety

Anxiety is a feeling of tension, nervousness, apprehension, or fear that usually involves unpleasant reactions to a stimulus, whether actual or unknown. Anxiety is often accompanied by signs and symptoms of the sympathetic stress reaction (see Chapter 29); this may include sweating, fast heart rate, rapid breathing, and elevated blood pressure. Mild anxiety may serve as a stimulus or motivator in some situations. A person who feels anxious about being alone in a poorly lit parking lot at night may be motivated to take extra safety precautions. When anxiety becomes overwhelming or severe, it can interfere with the activities of daily living and lead to medical problems related to chronic stimulation of the sympathetic nervous system. A severely anxious person may, for example, be afraid to leave the house or to interact with other people. In these cases, treatment is warranted. Anxiety disorders can be classified based on situations in which the person has symptoms and the characteristics of the stimuli. Generalized anxiety disorder, panic disorder, obsessive–compulsive disorder, social anxiety disorder, and posttraumatic stress disorder are some examples of how anxiety is diagnosed. **Anxiolytic** drugs are drugs that depress the central nervous system (CNS) and are used to lyse or break the feeling of anxiety. Medications that are used to treat anxiety but also have additional indications other than anxiety are discussed in other chapters. Antidepressants, especially the selective serotonin

Box 20.1 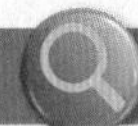 **Focus on Drug Therapy Across the Lifespan**

ANXIOLYTIC AND HYPNOTIC AGENTS

Children

Use of anxiolytic and hypnotic drugs with children is challenging. The response of the child to the drug may be unpredictable; inappropriate aggressiveness, crying, irritability, and tearfulness are common. Using good sleep hygiene measures is the preferred approach to insomnia in children.

Of the benzodiazepines, only chlordiazepoxide, clonazepam, clorazepate, midazolam, and diazepam have established pediatric dosages. Some of the others are used in pediatric settings; dosage may be calculated using age and weight.

The barbiturates, being older drugs, have established pediatric dosages. These drugs must be used with caution because of the often unexpected responses. Children must be monitored very closely for CNS depression and excitability.

The antihistamines diphenhydramine and promethazine are more popular for use in helping to calm children and to induce rest and sleep. Care must be taken to assess for possible dried secretions and effects on breathing. Dosage must be calculated carefully.

Adults

Adults using these drugs for the treatment of insomnia need to be cautioned that they are for short-term use only. The reason for the insomnia should be sought (e.g., medical, hormonal, or anxiety problems). Other methods for helping to induce sleep—established routine, quiet activities before bed, a back rub, or warm bath—should be encouraged before drugs are prescribed. Adults receiving anxiolytics also may need referrals for counseling and diagnosis of possible causes. Adults should be advised to avoid driving and making legal decisions when taking these drugs.

Liver function should be evaluated before and periodically during therapy.

These drugs are not recommended during pregnancy and lactation because of the potential for adverse effects on the fetus and possible sedation of the baby. The antihistamines, which have not been associated with congenital malformations, may be the safest to use, with caution, if an anxiolytic or hypnotic drug must be used.

Older Adults

Older patients may be more susceptible to the adverse effects of these drugs, from unanticipated CNS effects to increased sedation, dizziness, and even hallucinations. This is a major safety concern with this group. Dosages of all of these drugs should be reduced, and the patient should be monitored very closely for toxic effects and to provide safety measures if CNS effects do occur.

Baseline liver and renal function tests should be performed, and these values should be monitored periodically for any changes that would indicate a need to decrease dosage further or to stop the drug.

Nondrug measures to reduce anxiety and to help induce sleep are important with older patients. The patient should be screened for physical problems, neurological deterioration, or depression, which could contribute to the insomnia or anxiety.

reuptake inhibitors (SSRIs), have become the first-line treatment for chronic generalized anxiety (Chapter 21). Other medications that can be used for treatment of anxiety include anticonvulsants (Chapter 23), antipsychotics (Chapter 22), antihistamines (Chapter 54), and selective medications that act on the autonomic nervous system (Chapter 31).

Sedation

The loss of awareness of and reaction to environmental stimuli is termed **sedation.** This condition may be desirable in patients who are restless, nervous, irritable, or overreacting to stimuli. A **sedative** is a drug that depresses the CNS, thereby producing that loss of awareness of and reaction to the environment. Although sedation is anxiolytic, it may frequently lead to drowsiness. For example, sedative-induced drowsiness is a concern for outpatients who need to be alert and responsive in their normal lives. On the other hand, this tiredness may be desirable for patients who are about to undergo surgery or other procedures and who are receiving medical support. The choice of an anxiolytic drug depends on the situation in which it will be used, keeping the related adverse effects in mind. Anesthetic agents causing sedation are discussed in Chapter 27.

Hypnosis

Extreme sedation results in further CNS depression and sleep, or **hypnosis. Hypnotics** are used to help people fall asleep by causing sedation. Drugs that are effective hypnotics act on the reticular activating system (RAS) and block the brain's response to incoming stimuli. Hypnosis, therefore, is an extreme state of sedation in which the person no longer senses or reacts to incoming stimuli.

Alcohol and Alcohol Withdrawal

Alcohol is a commonly used CNS depressant. It enhances the inhibitory neurotransmitter gamma-aminobutyric acid (GABA) and inhibits the excitatory amino acid glutamate. When used regularly, people can become physically and psychologically dependent on alcohol. Withdrawal symptoms can range from nausea and vomiting to tonic–clonic seizures and delirium. Some people suffer from tremors and restlessness or irritability. Others may have variability in vital signs and cardiac arrhythmias. Benzodiazepines are often used first for acute treatment of alcohol withdrawal. Some antiseizure medications are also useful for treating alcohol withdrawal symptoms (Chapter 23). Naltrexone, discussed in Chapter 26, is an opioid antagonist that can be used to suppress alcohol cravings and opioid withdrawal. Two medications that can be used to enhance alcohol abstinence are discussed in Box 20.2.

Box 20.2 Focus on Safe Medication Administration

Some medications that support the withdrawal from alcohol are different than those that assist with maintaining alcohol abstinence. Disulfiram is a medication that blocks the metabolism of alcohol so that, if used concurrently with alcohol, highly unpleasant side effects occur. Disulfiram blocks the oxidation of alcohol, so acetaldehyde accumulates and causes unpleasant symptoms that can include nausea, vomiting, weakness, sweating, palpitations, hypotension, respiratory depression, and seizures. If enough alcohol is ingested with disulfiram, fatal reactions can occur. The drug is designed to be used as a behavioral deterrent, so that people do not ingest alcohol. It is best used in conjunction with supportive therapy.

Acamprosate is also a medication used to enhance alcohol abstinence, but its mechanism of action is different. It is hypothesized to act on the GABA neurotransmitter system influenced by alcohol and restore its natural function. It is helpful in decreasing the alcohol withdrawal symptoms of restlessness and anxiety. Dose reduction is required for people with moderate renal impairment, and the mediation is contraindicated if severe renal impairment is present.

Benzodiazepines Used as Anxiolytic–Hypnotics

Benzodiazepines, the most frequently used anxiolytic drugs, prevent anxiety without causing much associated sedation. In addition, they are able to relieve anxiety quickly. Table 20.1 lists the available benzodiazepines, including common indications and specific information about each drug. The benzodiazepines used as anxiolytics include alprazolam (*Xanax*), chlordiazepoxide (*Librium*), clonazepam (*Klonopin*), clorazepate (*Gen-Xene, Tranxene*), diazepam (*Valium*), estazolam (generic), flurazepam (generic), lorazepam (*Ativan*), midazolam (generic), oxazepam (generic), quazepam (*Doral*), temazepam (*Restoril*), and triazolam (*Halcion*). Box 20.3 provides an exercise in calculating dose for a pediatric patient receiving a sedative/hypnotic.

Therapeutic Actions and Indications

The benzodiazepines are indicated for the treatment of the following conditions: anxiety disorders, alcohol withdrawal, hyperexcitability and agitation, seizure disorders, insomnia, and preoperative relief of anxiety and tension to aid in balanced anesthesia. These drugs act in the limbic system and the RAS to make GABA more effective, causing interference with neuron firing (Fig. 20.1). GABA stabilizes the postsynaptic cell. This leads to an anxiolytic effect at doses lower than those required to induce sedation and hypnosis. The exact mechanism of action is not clearly understood. Benzodiazepines are classified as controlled substances and recommended only for short-term use due to potential for dependence.

Table 20.1 *Drugs in Focus:* Benzodiazepines Used as Anxiolytics[a]

Drug Name	Dosage/Route	Usual Indications
alprazolam (*Xanax*)	0.25–0.5 mg PO t.i.d. up to 1–10 mg/d PO have been used, reduced dosage in older adults	Anxiety, panic attacks *Onset:* 30 min *Duration:* 4–6 h
chlordiazepoxide (*Librium*)	*Adult:* 5–25 mg PO t.i.d. to q.i.d., may be repeated; reduce dosage with older patients *Pediatric (>6 y):* 5 mg PO b.i.d. to q.i.d.	Anxiety, alcohol withdrawal, preoperative anxiolytic *Onset:* 10–15 min *Duration:* 2–3 d
clonazepam (*Klonopin*)	*Adult:* 0.25 mg PO b.i.d., titrate as needed *Pediatric:* 0.01–0.03 mg/kg/d PO given in 2–3 doses, do not exceed 0.05 mg/kg/d	Panic disorders, restless leg syndrome, seizure disorders *Onset:* Slow *Duration:* 1–6 wk *Special considerations:* Monitor for suicidal ideation, liver function, and blood counts with long-term therapy.
clorazepate (*Gen-Xene, Tranxene*)	*Anxiety:* 30 mg/d PO in divided doses t.i.d. *Alcohol withdrawal:* dosing variable based on patient response	Anxiety, alcohol withdrawal
diazepam (*Valium*)	*Adult:* 2–10 mg PO b.i.d. to q.i.d. *or* 0.2 mg/kg PR, 2–2.5 mg PO b.i.d. for older adult patients; 2–10 mg IV/IM frequency will vary based on indication and patient response *Pediatric:* varies based on route, indication, and age. Weight-based dosing is common.	Anxiety, alcohol withdrawal, muscle relaxant, preoperative anxiolytic *Onset:* 5–60 min *Duration:* 3 h *Special considerations:* Taper after long-term therapy.
estazolam (generic)	1 mg PO at bedtime, start with 0.5 mg for older adult or debilitated patient	Hypnotic, insomnia *Onset:* 45–60 min *Duration:* 2 h *Special considerations:* Monitor liver and renal function, and CBC if used long term.
flurazepam (generic)	15–30 mg PO at bedtime, 15 mg PO at bedtime for older adults or debilitated patients	Hypnotic, insomnia *Onset:* Varies *Duration:* 30–60 min *Special considerations:* Monitor liver and renal function, and CBC if used long term.
lorazepam (*Ativan*)	2–6 mg/d PO in divided doses or 0.05 mg/kg IM and IV to max of 4 mg	Anxiety, preanesthetic anxiolytic, insomnia due to stress *Onset:* 1–30 min *Duration:* 12–24 h *Special considerations:* Monitor injection sites; reduce dosage of narcotics given with this drug.
midazolam (generic)	*Adult:* Sedation—5 mg IM; conscious sedation for short procedures—1–2.5 mg IV, maintenance dose 25% of initial dose; sedation in critical care—10–50 mcg/kg IV as a loading dose, repeat every 10–15 min until desired effect is seen, infusion of 20–100 mcg/kg/h maintenance *Pediatric:* Sedation—0.1–0.015 mg/kg IM or PO; conscious sedation for short procedures 50–100 mcg/kg IV; sedation in critical care—30–200 mcg/kg IV as a loading dose, maintenance infusion of 60–120 mcg/kg/h	Sedation, anxiety, conscious sedation for short procedures, continuous sedation of intubated or mechanically ventilated patients *Onset:* 3–15 min *Duration:* 2–6 h *Special considerations:* Do not administer intra-arterially; keep resuscitation equipment nearby; be prepared to breathe for the patient as needed.
oxazepam (generic)	10–15 mg PO t.i.d. to q.i.d.	Anxiety, alcohol withdrawal *Onset:* Slow *Duration:* 2–4 h *Special considerations:* Preferred for older adult patients

(continues on page 346)

Table 20.1 *Drugs in Focus:* Benzodiazepines Used as Anxiolytics[a] (*Continued*)

Drug Name	Dosage/Route	Usual Indications
quazepam (*Doral*)	15 mg PO at bedtime	Hypnotic, insomnia *Onset:* Varies *Duration:* 4–6 h *Special considerations:* Monitor liver and renal function, and CBC if used for long-term therapy; taper after long-term therapy.
temazepam (*Restoril*)	15–30 mg PO at bedtime for 7–10 d	Hypnotic, insomnia *Onset:* Varies *Duration:* 4–6 h *Special considerations:* Taper after long-term therapy.
triazolam (*Halcion*)	0.125–0.5 mg PO at bedtime, limit use to 7–10 d	Hypnotic, insomnia *Onset:* Varies *Duration:* 2–4 h *Special considerations:* Monitor liver and renal function, and CBC; taper after long-term therapy.

[a]Onset of action and duration are important in selecting the correct drug for a particular use.
CBC, complete blood count.

Pharmacokinetics

The benzodiazepines are well absorbed from the gastrointestinal (GI) tract, with peak level achieved in 30 minutes to 2 hours. They are lipid soluble and well distributed throughout the body, crossing the placenta and entering human milk. The benzodiazepines are metabolized extensively in the liver. Patients with liver disease must receive a smaller dose and be monitored closely. Excretion is primarily through the urine.

Box 20.3 Focus on Calculations

Your 3-year-old patient, weighing 10 kg, is prescribed phenobarbital as a hypnotic at bedtime. The order reads 6 mg/kg PO at bedtime. The drug comes in an elixir 4 mg/mL. How much of the elixir would you give at bedtime?

First, figure out what the correct dose would be

$$6\ \text{mg/kg} \times 10\ \text{kg} = 60\ \text{mg}$$

Set up the equation using available form = prescribed dose:

$$4\ \text{mg/mL} = 60\ \text{mg/dose}$$

Then, cross-multiply:

$$4\ \text{mg (dose)} = 60\ \text{mg (mL)}$$
$$\text{dose} = 60\ \text{mg (mL)}/4\ \text{mg}$$
$$\text{dose} = 15\ \text{mL}$$

Because the patient is a child, it is good practice to ask another nurse to calculate the correct dosage and then compare your work, so you can double-check the accuracy of your calculations.

Contraindications and Cautions

Contraindications to benzodiazepines include allergy to any benzodiazepine to prevent hypersensitivity reactions; psychosis, which could be exacerbated by sedation; and acute narrow-angle glaucoma, shock, coma, or acute alcoholic intoxication, all of which could be exacerbated by the depressant effects of these drugs.

In addition, these sedative–hypnotics are not recommended in pregnancy because a predictable syndrome of cleft lip or palate, inguinal hernia, cardiac defects, microcephaly, or pyloric stenosis occurs when they are taken in the first trimester. Neonatal withdrawal syndrome may also result. Breast or chestfeeding is also not recommended because of potential adverse effects on the neonate (e.g., sedation).

Use benzodiazepines with caution in older adults or debilitated patients because of the possibility of unpredictable reactions and in cases of renal or hepatic dysfunction, which may alter the metabolism and excretion of these drugs, resulting in direct toxicity. Dose adjustments usually are needed for such patients.

All of these drugs now have a boxed warning that concomitant use with opioids can result in profound sedation, respiratory depression, coma, or death. Because of this possibility, dosage should be limited, and patients should be monitored closely.

Adverse Effects

The adverse effects of benzodiazepines are associated with the impact of these drugs on the central and peripheral nervous systems. Nervous system effects include sedation, drowsiness, depression, lethargy, blurred vision, "sleep driving" and other complex behaviors, headaches, apathy, light-headedness, amnesia, and confusion. In addition, mild paradoxical excitatory reactions may occur during the first 2 weeks of therapy.

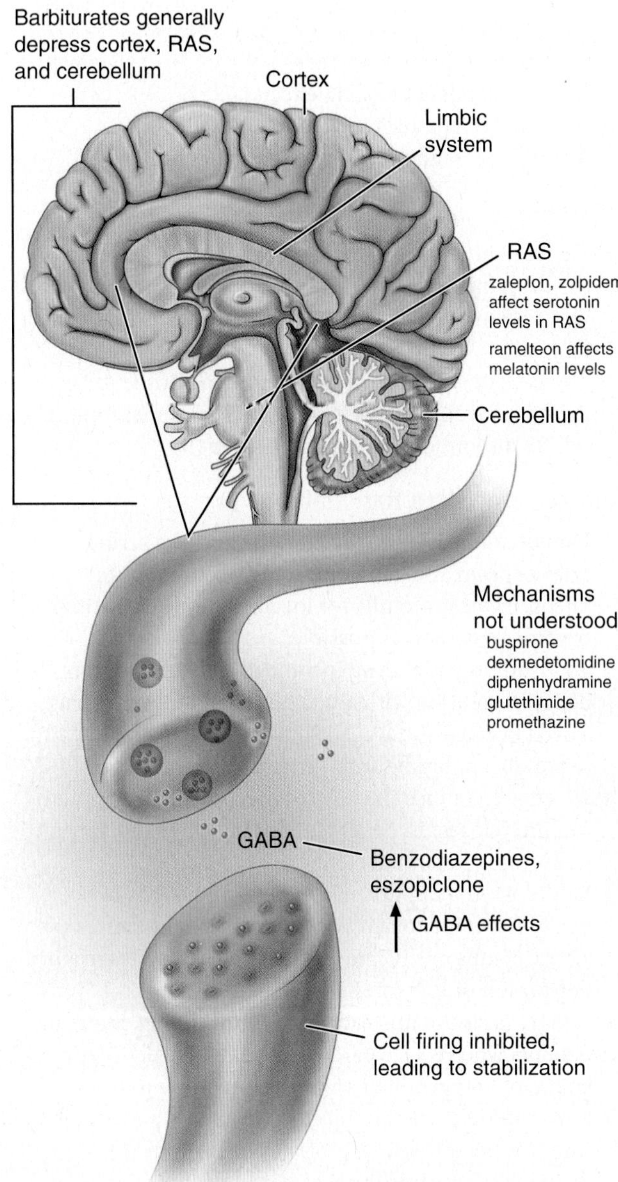

FIGURE 20.1 Sites of action of the benzodiazepines, barbiturates, and other anxiolytics. GABA, gamma-aminobutyric acid; RAS, reticular activating system.

Several other kinds of adverse effects may occur. GI conditions such as dry mouth, constipation, nausea, vomiting, and elevated liver enzymes may result. Cardiovascular problems may include hypotension, hypertension, arrhythmias, palpitations, and respiratory difficulties. Hematological conditions such as blood dyscrasias and anemia are possible. Genitourinary effects include urinary retention and hesitancy, loss of libido, and changes in sexual functioning. Because phlebitis, local reactions, and thrombosis may occur at local injection sites, such sites should be monitored. Abrupt cessation of these drugs may lead to a withdrawal syndrome characterized by nausea; headache; vertigo; malaise; nightmares; and, if severe, seizures. Patients taking these medications chronically should not stop taking them abruptly. They should be tapered slowly when possible (Fig. 20.2).

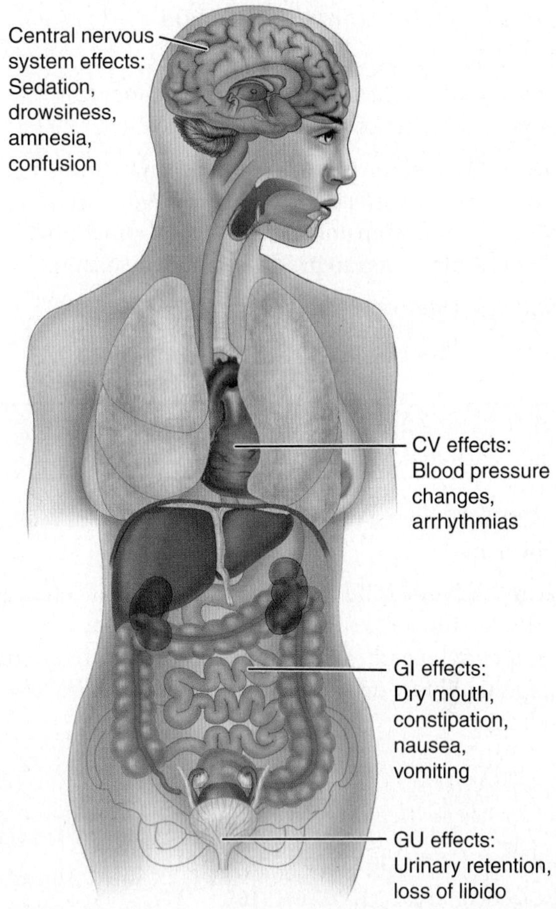

FIGURE 20.2 Variety of adverse effects and toxicities associated with anxiolytics and hypnotics.

Clinically Important Drug–Drug Interactions

The risk of CNS depression increases if benzodiazepines are taken with alcohol or other CNS depressants such as opioids, so such combinations should be avoided. In addition, the effects of benzodiazepines may increase if they are taken with cimetidine, oral contraceptives, or disulfiram. If one of these drugs is used with benzodiazepines, the patient should be monitored and the appropriate dose adjustments made. Finally, the impact of benzodiazepines may be decreased if they are given with theophyllines; therefore, dose adjustment may be necessary.

 *Concept Mastery Alert*

Benzodiazepine Toxicity Treatment

Flumazenil is used for benzodiazepine toxicity. It is a benzodiazepine receptor antagonist and can be used to reverse sedation and other adverse effects.

Prototype Summary: Diazepam

Indications: Management of anxiety disorders, acute alcohol withdrawal, muscle relaxation, and preoperative relief of anxiety and tension.

Actions: Acts in the limbic system and reticular formation to potentiate the effects of GABA, an inhibitory neurotransmitter; may act in spinal cord and supraspinal sites to produce muscle relaxation.

Pharmacokinetics:

Route	Onset	Peak	Duration (single dose)
Oral	30–60 min	1–2 h	3 h
Rectal	Rapid	1.5 h	3 h

$T_{1/2}$: 20 to 80 hours; metabolized in the liver; excreted in the urine.

Adverse Effects: Mild drowsiness, depression, lethargy, apathy, fatigue, restlessness, bradycardia, tachycardia, constipation, diarrhea, incontinence, urinary retention, changes in libido, drug dependence with withdrawal syndrome.

Nursing Considerations for Patients Receiving Benzodiazepines

Assessment: History and Examination

- Assess for contraindications or cautions: known allergies to benzodiazepines to prevent hypersensitivity reactions; impaired liver or kidney function, which could alter the metabolism and excretion of a particular drug; any condition that might be exacerbated by the depressant effects of the drugs (e.g., glaucoma, coma, psychoses, shock, acute alcohol intoxication); pregnancy and lactation; and use of other CNS depressing drugs such as opioids, which could lead to severe CNS depression.
- Assess for baseline status before beginning therapy to check for occurrence of any potential adverse effects. Assess for the following: temperature and weight; skin color and lesions; affect, orientation, reflexes, and vision; pulse, blood pressure, and perfusion; respiratory rate, adventitious sounds, and presence of chronic pulmonary disease; and bowel sounds on abdominal examination.
- Perform laboratory tests, including renal and liver function tests and complete blood count (CBC).

Refer to the "Critical Thinking Scenario" for a full discussion of nursing care for a patient dealing with anxiety.

Nursing Conclusions

Nursing conclusions related to drug therapy might include the following:

- Altered thought processes and disturbed sensory perception (visual, kinesthetic) related to CNS effects
- Injury risk related to CNS effects
- Altered sleep pattern related to CNS effects
- Knowledge deficit risk regarding drug therapy

Planning

- The patient will receive the best therapeutic effect from the drug therapy.
- The patient will have limited adverse effects to the drug therapy.
- The patient will have an understanding of the drug therapy, adverse effects to anticipate, and measures to relieve discomfort and improve safety.

Intervention With Rationale

- Do not administer intra-arterially because serious arteriospasm and gangrene could occur. Monitor injection sites carefully for local reactions to institute treatment as soon as possible.
- To avoid potential drug incompatibility, do not mix IV drugs in solution with any other drugs. Give IV drugs slowly because these agents have been associated with hypotension, bradycardia, and cardiac arrest.
- Arrange to reduce the dose of narcotic analgesics, and monitor closely in patients receiving a benzodiazepine to decrease potentiated effects and sedation.
- Be prepared to administer flumazenil if signs of benzodiazepine toxicity occur; this toxicity causes severe symptoms including life-threatening respiratory depression or extreme sedation.
- If there is risk of unsteadiness and/or falling, maintain patients who receive parenteral benzodiazepines in bed. Do not permit an ambulatory patient to operate a motor vehicle after an injection to ensure patient safety.
- Monitor hepatic and renal function, as well as CBC, during long-term therapy to detect dysfunction and to arrange to taper and discontinue the drug if dysfunction occurs.
- Taper dose gradually after long-term therapy, especially in epileptic patients. Acute withdrawal could precipitate seizures in these patients. It may also cause withdrawal syndrome.
- Provide comfort measures to help patients tolerate drug effects, such as having them void before dosing, giving food with the drug if GI upset is severe, providing environmental control (lighting, temperature, stimulation), taking safety precautions (use of side rails, assistance with ambulation), and aiding orientation.
- Provide thorough patient teaching, including drug name, prescribed dose, measures for avoidance of adverse effects, and warning signs that may indicate possible problems. Instruct patients about the need for periodic monitoring and evaluation to enhance patient knowledge about drug therapy and to promote adherence.

- Offer support and encouragement to help patients cope with the diagnosis and the drug regimen.

Evaluation

- Monitor patient response to the drug (alleviation of signs and symptoms of anxiety; sleep; sedation).
- Monitor for adverse effects (sedation, hypotension, cardiac arrhythmias, hepatic or renal dysfunction, blood dyscrasias, CNS depression, anterograde amnesia, paradoxical response).
- Evaluate the effectiveness of the teaching plan (patient can give the drug name, dosage, possible adverse effects to watch for, specific measures to help avoid adverse effects, and the importance of continued follow-up).
- Monitor the effectiveness of comfort measures and adherence to the regimen.

CRITICAL THINKING SCENARIO Benzodiazepines

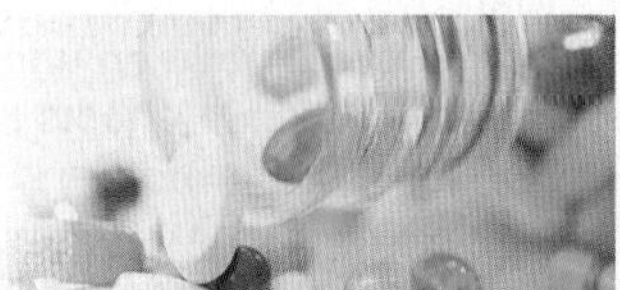

THE SITUATION

P.P., a 43-year-old parent of three teenagers, comes to the outpatient department for a routine physical examination. Results are unremarkable except for blood pressure of 145/90, pulse rate of 98, and apparent tension. P.P. is jittery, avoids eye contact, and sometimes appears teary-eyed. P.P. says they are having some problems dealing with "life in general." Their children present many stresses, and their spouse, who is busy with work, has little time to deal with issues at home; the spouse is very demanding when at home. In addition, P.P. is possibly beginning menopause and is having trouble coping with the idea of menopause as well as with some of the symptoms. Overall, P.P. feels lonely and has no outlet for anger, tension, or stress. A health care provider, who reassures P.P. that this problem is common at their age, prescribes the benzodiazepine diazepam (*Valium*) to help P.P. deal with anxiety.

CRITICAL THINKING

What sort of crisis intervention would be most appropriate for P.P.?

What nursing interventions are helpful at this point?

What nondrug interventions might be helpful?

What other support systems could be used to help P.P. deal with all that is going on in their life?

Think about the overwhelming problems that P.P. has to deal with on a daily basis and how the anxiolytic effects of diazepam might change their approach to these problems. Could the problems actually get worse?

Develop a care plan for the long-term care of P.P.

DISCUSSION

Anxiolytics are useful for controlling the acute unpleasant signs and symptoms of anxiety. The diazepam prescribed for P.P. may provide some immediate relief, enabling them to survive the "crisis" period and plan changes in their life in general. However, the associated drowsiness and sedation may make coping with the problems even more difficult. P.P. should be taught the adverse effects of diazepam, the warning signs of serious adverse effects, and the health problems to report. They should also have long-term therapy prescribed.

A follow-up evaluation should be scheduled. Additional meetings with the same health care provider are important for the long-term solution to P.P.'s anxiety. Their need for drug therapy should be reevaluated once P.P. can discover other support systems and develop other ways of coping. Although anxiolytic therapy may be beneficial initially, it will not solve the problems that are causing anxiety; in this case, the causes for the anxiety are specific. Anxiolytic therapy should be considered only as a short-term aid.

Unlike P.P., many patients in severe crisis do not consciously identify their causes of stress, or stressors. However, P.P. has identified a list of factors making life stressful. This facilitates the development of coping strategies. P.P. may find the following support measures helpful:

- Referral to a counselor and involvement of the entire family in identifying problems and ways to deal with them
- Support groups for people in various stages of life (e.g., entering menopause, parents of children who are entering the teen years). Just having the opportunity to discuss problems and explore ways of dealing with them helps many people.

NURSING CARE GUIDE FOR P.P.: DIAZEPAM

Assessment: History and Examination

Allergies to diazepam, psychoses, acute narrow-angle glaucoma, acute alcohol intoxication, impaired liver or kidney function, pregnancy, breast or chest-feeding, concurrent use of alcohol or opioids, or other medication interactions.

Cardiovascular: Blood pressure, pulse, perfusion
CNS: Orientation, affect, reflexes, vision
Skin: Color, lesions, texture
Respiratory: Respiration, adventitious sounds
GI: Abdominal examination, bowel sounds
Laboratory tests: Hepatic and renal function tests, CBC

(continues on page 350)

Nursing Conclusions

Altered thought processes and disturbed sensory perception (visual, kinesthetic) related to CNS effects
Injury risk related to CNS effects
Altered sleep patterns related to CNS effects
Knowledge deficit risk regarding drug therapy

Planning

The patient will receive the best therapeutic effect from the drug therapy.
The patient will have limited adverse effects to the drug therapy.
The patient will have an understanding of the drug therapy, adverse effects to anticipate, and measures to relieve discomfort and improve safety.

Intervention

Provide comfort and safety measures, small meals, drugs with food if GI upset occurs. Taper dosage after long-term use; reduce dosage if other medications include narcotics; lower dose with renal or hepatic impairment.
Provide support and reassurance to deal with drug effects.
Provide patient teaching regarding drug, dosage, adverse effects, safety precautions, and unusual symptoms to report.

Evaluation

Evaluate drug effects: Relief of signs and symptoms of anxiety.
Monitor for adverse effects, particularly sedation, dizziness, insomnia, blood dyscrasia, GI upset, hepatic or renal dysfunction, and cardiovascular effects.
Monitor for drug–drug interactions.
Evaluate effectiveness of patient teaching program.
Evaluate effectiveness of comfort and safety measures.

PATIENT TEACHING FOR P.P.

- The drug that has been prescribed for you is called diazepam, or *Valium*. It belongs to a class of drugs called benzodiazepines, which are used to relieve tension and nervousness. Exactly how the drug works is not completely understood, but it does relax muscle spasms, relieve insomnia, and promote calm. Common side effects of this drug include the following:
- Dizziness and drowsiness: Avoid driving or performing hazardous or delicate tasks that require concentration if these effects occur.
- Nausea, vomiting, and weight loss: Small, frequent meals may help to relieve nausea. If weight loss occurs, monitor the loss; if the loss is extensive, consult your health care provider. Do not take this drug with antacids.
- Constipation or diarrhea: These reactions usually pass with time. If they do not, consult with your health care provider for appropriate therapy.
- Vision changes, slurred speech, and unsteadiness: These effects also subside with time. Take extra care in your activities for the first few days. If these reactions do not go away after 3 or 4 days, consult your health care provider.
- Report to your health care provider any of the following conditions: rash, fever, sore throat, insomnia, depression, clumsiness, or nervousness.
- Tell any doctor, nurse, or other health care provider involved in your care that you are taking this drug.
- Keep this drug and all medications safely away from children or pets.
- Avoid the use of over-the-counter medications or herbal therapies while you are taking this drug. If you think that you need one of these products, consult with your health care provider about the best choice because many of these products can interfere with your medication.
- Avoid alcohol while you are taking this drug. Combining alcohol and a benzodiazepine can cause serious problems.
- If you have been taking this drug for a prolonged time, do not stop taking it suddenly. Your body will need time to adjust to stopping the drug, and the dosage will need to be reduced gradually to prevent serious problems. When discontinuing use of this drug, tell your health care provider if any of the following occur: trembling, muscle cramps, sweating, irritability, confusion, or seizures.

Key Points

- Anxiety is a feeling of tension, nervousness, apprehension, or fear. In the extreme, anxiety may produce physiologic manifestations and may interfere with activities of daily life. Anxiolytic drugs, such as the benzodiazepines, depress the CNS to diminish these feelings.
- CNS depressants may be used as sedatives or hypnotics, blocking the awareness of and reaction to environmental stimuli, or to induce drowsiness to facilitate sleep.
- Benzodiazepines are used for treatment of acute anxiety, alcohol withdrawal symptoms, and seizure disorders; for induction of anesthesia; and for similar indications. They work by enhancing the inhibitory effects of GABA.

Barbiturates Used as Anxiolytic–Hypnotics

Barbiturates were once the sedative–hypnotic drugs of choice. Not only is the likelihood of sedation and other adverse effects greater with these drugs than with newer sedative–hypnotic drugs, but the risk of addiction and dependence is also greater. For these reasons, newer anxiolytic drugs have replaced the barbiturates in most instances. The barbiturates used as anxiolytic–hypnotics include butabarbital (*Butisol*), pentobarbital (*Nembutal Sodium*), phenobarbital (generic), and secobarbital (*Seconal*). Table 20.2 lists the available barbiturates, including common indications and specific information about each drug.

Therapeutic Actions and Indications

Barbiturates are general CNS depressants that inhibit neuronal impulse conduction in the ascending RAS, depress the cerebral cortex, alter cerebellar function, and depress motor output (see Fig. 20.1). Thus, they can cause sedation, hypnosis, anesthesia, and in extreme cases coma. In general, barbiturates are indicated for the relief of the signs and symptoms of anxiety and for sedation, for insomnia, as a preanesthetic, and in the treatment of seizures (Table 20.2). Parenteral forms, which reach peak level faster and have a faster onset of action, may be used for the treatment of acute manic reactions and many forms of seizures (see Chapter 23).

Pharmacokinetics

Barbiturates are absorbed well, reaching peak level in 20 to 60 minutes. They are metabolized in the liver to varying degrees, depending on the drug, and excreted in the urine. The longer-acting barbiturates tend to be metabolized slower and excreted to a greater degree unchanged in the urine. They are known to induce liver enzyme systems, increasing the metabolism of the barbiturate broken down by that system, as well as that of any other drug that may be metabolized by the same system. Patients with hepatic or renal dysfunction require lower doses of the drug to avoid toxic effects and should be monitored closely. Barbiturates are lipid soluble; they readily cross the placenta and enter human milk.

Contraindications and Cautions

Contraindications to barbiturates include allergy to any barbiturate to avoid hypersensitivity reactions, and a previous history of addiction to sedative–hypnotic drugs or adverse effects, because the barbiturates are more likely to cause serious adverse effects than most other anxiolytics. Other contraindications are latent or manifest porphyria, which may be exacerbated; marked hepatic impairment or nephritis, which may alter the metabolism and excretion of these drugs; and respiratory distress or severe respiratory dysfunction, which could be exacerbated by the CNS depression caused by these drugs. Pregnancy is a contraindication because of potential adverse effects on the fetus; congenital anomalies have been reported with barbiturate use.

Use with caution in patients with acute or chronic pain because barbiturates can cause paradoxical excitement,

Table 20.2 *Drugs in Focus:* Barbiturates Used as Anxiolytic–Hypnotics[a]

Drug Name	Dosage/Route	Usual Indications
butabarbital (*Butisol*)	*Adult:* 15–30 mg PO t.i.d. to q.i.d., 50–100 mg PO at bedtime for sedation; reduce dosage in older adults *Pediatric:* 2–6 mg/kg PO based on age and weight with a maximum 100 mg/dose	Short-term sedative–hypnotic *Onset:* 45–60 min *Duration:* 6–8 h *Special considerations:* Taper gradually after long-term use; use caution in children, may produce aggressiveness, excitability.
pentobarbital (*Nembutal*)	*Adult:* 20 mg PO t.i.d. to q.i.d., 100 mg at bedtime for insomnia, 120–200 mg PR, 150–200 mg IM or 100 mg IV; reduce dosage in older adult patients *Pediatric:* 2–6 mg/kg/d, adjust dosage based on age and weight; 1–3 mg/kg IV	Sedative–hypnotic, preanesthetic *Onset:* 10–15 min *Duration:* 2–4 h *Special considerations:* Taper gradually after long-term use, give IV slowly, and monitor injection sites.
phenobarbital (generic)	*Adult:* 30–120 mg/d PO, IM, or IV; reduce dosage in older adult patients *Pediatric:* 1–3 mg/kg IV or IM	Sedative–hypnotic, control of seizures, preanesthetic *Onset:* 10–60 min *Duration:* 4–16 h *Special considerations:* Taper gradually after long-term use, give IV slowly, and monitor injection sites.
secobarbital (*Seconal*)	*Adult:* 100–300 mg PO; reduce dosage in older adult patients *Pediatric:* 2–6 mg/kg PO	Preanesthetic sedation, convulsive seizures of tetanus *Onset:* Rapid *Duration:* 1–4 h *Special considerations:* Taper gradually after long-term use.

[a]Onset of action and duration are important in selecting the correct drug for a particular use.

masking other symptoms; with seizure disorders because abrupt withdrawal of a barbiturate can precipitate status epilepticus; and with chronic hepatic, cardiac, or respiratory diseases, which could be exacerbated by the depressive effects of these drugs. Care should be taken with patients who are lactating because of the potential for adverse effects on the infant.

Adverse Effects

As previously stated, the adverse effects caused by barbiturates are more severe than those associated with other, newer sedative–hypnotics. For this reason, barbiturates are no longer considered the mainstay for the treatment of anxiety.

The most common adverse effects are related to general CNS depression. CNS effects may include drowsiness, somnolence, lethargy, ataxia, vertigo, a feeling of a "hangover," thinking abnormalities, paradoxical excitement, anxiety, and hallucinations. GI signs and symptoms such as nausea, vomiting, constipation, diarrhea, and epigastric pain may occur. Associated cardiovascular effects may include bradycardia, hypotension (particularly with IV administration), and syncope. Serious hypoventilation may occur, and respiratory depression and laryngospasm may also result, particularly with IV administration. Hypersensitivity reactions, including rash, serum sickness, and Stevens-Johnson syndrome, which is sometimes fatal, may also occur.

Clinically Important Drug–Drug Interactions

Increased CNS depression results if these agents are taken with other CNS depressants, including alcohol, antihistamines, and other tranquilizers. Dosing adjustments will probably be necessary if other CNS depressants are used simultaneously with barbiturate medications.

There often is an altered response to phenytoin if it is combined with barbiturates; evaluate the patient frequently if this combination cannot be avoided. If barbiturates are combined with monoamine oxidase (MAO) inhibitors, increased serum levels and effects occur. If the older sedative–hypnotics are combined with MAO inhibitors, monitor the patient closely and make necessary dose adjustments.

In addition, because of an enzyme induction effect of barbiturates in the liver, many medications may not be as effective. Some of the medications that can be altered include oral anticoagulants, digoxin, tricyclic antidepressants, corticosteroids, oral contraceptives, estrogens, acetaminophen, metronidazole, carbamazepine, beta-blockers, and doxycycline. Before administration of the barbiturate, it is recommended that the nurse check for any medication interactions. If these agents are given in combination with barbiturates, closely monitor the patient; frequent dose adjustments may be necessary to achieve the desired therapeutic effect.

P Prototype Summary: Phenobarbital

Indications: Sedation, short-term treatment of insomnia, long-term treatment of tonic–clonic seizures and cortical focal seizures, emergency control of certain acute convulsive episodes, preanesthetic.

Actions: Inhibits conduction in the ascending RAS; depresses the cerebral cortex; alters cerebellar function; depresses motor output; can produce excitation, sedation, hypnosis, anesthesia, and deep coma; and has anticonvulsant activity.

Pharmacokinetics:

Route	Onset	Peak	Duration
Oral	15 min	30–60 min	10–16 h
IM, subcutaneous	varies	10–30 min	4–6 h
IV	immediate	post administration	4–6 h

$T_{1/2}$: 79 hours; metabolized in the liver; excreted in the urine.

Adverse Effects: Somnolence, agitation, confusion, hyperkinesia, ataxia, vertigo, CNS depression, hallucinations, bradycardia, hypotension, syncope, nausea, vomiting, constipation, diarrhea, hypoventilation, apnea, withdrawal syndrome, rash, Stevens-Johnson syndrome.

Nursing Considerations for Patients Receiving Barbiturates

Assessment: History and Examination

- Assess for contraindications or cautions: known allergies to barbiturates to prevent hypersensitivity reactions or a history of addiction to sedative–hypnotic drugs to avert a similar problem with these drugs; impaired hepatic or renal function that could alter the metabolism and excretion of the drug; cardiac dysfunction or respiratory dysfunction; seizure disorders, which could be exacerbated by these drugs; acute or chronic pain disorders, which should be evaluated before using these drugs; and pregnancy or lactation, which would indicate a need for caution when using these drugs.
- Assess for baseline status before beginning therapy and for the occurrence of any potential adverse effects. Assess the following: temperature and weight; blood pressure and pulse, including perfusion; skin color and lesions; affect, orientation, and reflexes; respiratory rate and adventitious sounds; and bowel sounds.

Nursing Conclusions

Nursing conclusions related to drug therapy might include the following:

- Altered thought processes and altered sensory perception (visual, auditory, kinesthetic, tactile) related to CNS effects
- Injury risk related to CNS effects
- Altered gas exchange related to respiratory depression
- Knowledge deficit risk regarding drug therapy

Planning

- The patient will receive the best therapeutic effect from the drug therapy.
- The patient will have limited adverse effects to the drug therapy.
- The patient will have an understanding of the drug therapy, adverse effects to anticipate, and measures to relieve discomfort and improve safety.

Intervention With Rationale

- Do not administer these drugs intra-arterially because serious arteriospasm and gangrene could occur. Monitor injection sites carefully for local reactions.
- To avoid potential drug incompatibility, do not mix IV drugs in solution with any other drugs.
- Give parenteral forms only if oral forms are not feasible or available, and switch to oral forms as soon as possible to avoid serious reactions or adverse effects.
- Give IV medications slowly because rapid administration may cause cardiac problems.
- Provide standby life support facilities in case of severe respiratory depression or hypersensitivity reactions.
- Taper dose gradually after long-term therapy, especially in patients with epilepsy. Acute withdrawal may precipitate seizures or cause withdrawal syndrome in these patients.
- To help patients tolerate drug effects, provide comfort measures as needed, including small, frequent meals; access to bathroom facilities; bowel program as needed; consuming food with the drug if GI upset is severe; environmental control; safety precautions; orientation; and appropriate skin care.
- Provide thorough patient teaching, including drug name, prescribed dosage, measures for avoidance of adverse effects, and warning signs that may indicate possible problems. Instruct patients about the need for periodic monitoring and evaluation to enhance patient knowledge about drug therapy and to promote adherence.
- Offer support and encouragement to help the patient cope with the diagnosis and the drug regimen.

Evaluation

- Monitor patient response to the drug (alleviation of signs and symptoms of anxiety, sleep, sedation, reduction in seizure activity).
- Monitor for adverse effects (sedation, hypotension, cardiac arrhythmias, hepatic or renal dysfunction, skin reactions, dependence).
- Evaluate the effectiveness of the patient teaching plan (patient can give the drug name, dosage, possible adverse effects to watch for, specific measures to help avoid adverse effects, and the importance of continued follow-up).
- Monitor the effectiveness of comfort measures and adherence to the regimen.

Key Points

- Barbiturates are an older class of drugs used as anxiolytics, sedatives, and hypnotics.
- Because they are associated with potentially serious adverse effects and interact with many other drugs, barbiturates are less desirable than the benzodiazepines or other anxiolytics.

Other Anxiolytic and Hypnotic Drugs

Other drugs that do not fall into either the benzodiazepine or the barbiturate group are used to treat anxiety or to produce hypnosis. See Table 20.3 for a list of other anxiolytic–hypnotic drugs, including usual indications and special considerations. Such medications include the following:

- Antihistamines (promethazine [*Promethegan*], diphenhydramine [*Benadryl*]) can be very sedating in some people. They are used as preoperative medications and postoperatively to decrease the need for narcotics. These medications are discussed in Chapter 54.
- Buspirone (generic) has no sedative, anticonvulsant, or muscle relaxant properties. Its mechanism of action to decrease anxiety is unclear, but it does bind to both serotonin and dopamine receptors. It reduces the signs and symptoms of anxiety without many of the CNS effects and severe adverse effects associated with other anxiolytic drugs. However, it can take 1 to 4 weeks to take full effect. Adverse effects can include dizziness, nausea, constipation, headache, and agitation, but often these are self-limiting. Taking the medication with small meals can decrease the nausea. It is rapidly absorbed from the GI tract, metabolized in the liver, and excreted in the urine.
- Dexmedetomidine (*Precedex*) is an $alpha_2$-adrenergic agonist administered IV for sedation of ventilated patients in the intensive care unit or sedation of patient prior to and/or during surgical procedures.
- Eszopiclone (*Lunesta*) is indicated to treat insomnia. It is thought to react with GABA sites near benzodiazepine receptors, and it prolongs sleep and decreases awakenings. It is rapidly absorbed, metabolized in the liver, and excreted in the urine. It has been associated with "sleep driving" and other complex behaviors as well as next-day sedation, memory loss, and loss of coordination. Because of these concerns, patients should be instructed to take

Table 20.3 *Drugs in Focus:* Other Anxiolytic/Hypnotic Drugs

Drug Name	Dosage/Route	Usual Indications
buspirone (generic)	Initially 15 mg/d PO titrate to maximum dose of 60 mg/d	Treatment of anxiety *Special considerations*: May cause dry mouth, headache; use with caution in patients with hepatic or renal impairment and in older adult patients.
dexmedetomidine (*Precedex*)	1 mcg/kg IV over 10 min then 0.2–0.7 mcg/kg/h IV using controlled infusion device for up to 24 h	Sedation of intubated and mechanically ventilated patients during treatment in an intensive care setting or of patients prior to and/or during procedures *Special considerations*: Do not use longer than 24 h; monitor patient continually.
diphenhydramine (generic)	*Adult*: Oral, 25–50 mg PO q4–6 h; IV or IM, 10–50 mg; max 400 mg/d *Pediatric*: 12.5–25 mg PO t.i.d. to q.i.d. or 5 mg/kg/d PO or 5 mg/kg/d IV or deep IM injection	Sleep aid, motion sickness, allergic rhinitis; oral drug for short-term treatment of insomnia (up to 1 wk) *Special considerations*: Antihistamine, drying effects common; monitor patients for thickened respiratory secretions and breathing difficulties, a problem that can cause concern after anesthesia.
eszopiclone (*Lunesta*)	1 mg PO immediately before bed; max dose 3 mg	Insomnia *Special considerations*: Tablet must be swallowed whole; instruct the patient to take this drug just before bed and allow 8 h for sleep.
meprobamate (generic)	*Adult*: 1,200–1,600 mg/d PO in 3–4 divided doses *Pediatric*: 100–200 mg PO t.i.d. to q.i.d.	Short-term management of anxiety disorders *Special considerations*: Supervise dose in patients who are prone to substance use disorder; withdraw gradually over 2 wk if patient has been maintained on the drug for weeks or months.
promethazine (*Promethegan*)	*Adult*: 25–50 mg PO, PR, or IM *Pediatric*: 12.5–25 mg PO, PR, or IM	Decrease the need for postoperative pain relief and for preoperative sedation *Special considerations*: An antihistamine; monitor injection sites carefully; monitor patient for thickened respiratory secretions and breathing difficulties, a problem that can cause concern after anesthesia.
ramelteon (*Rozerem*)	8 mg PO 30 min before bed	Insomnia characterized by difficulty falling asleep *Special considerations*: Patient should take 30 min before bed and allow 8 h for sleep; monitor for depression and suicidal ideation.
suvorexant (*Belsomra*)	10 mg PO, max 20 mg/d	Insomnia with difficulty in sleep onset and/or sleep maintenance *Special considerations*: Take only once a night; should be in bed within 30 min of dose and plan to stay there for 7 h; safety issues during night of use and the next day as somnolence may persist.
tasimelteon (*Hetlioz*)	20 mg/d PO at bedtime	Treatment of non–24-hour sleep–wake disorder *Special considerations*: Take at bedtime, the same time each night; can impair mental alertness, safety precautions required; may cause fetal harm.
zaleplon (*Sonata*)	10 mg/d PO at bedtime	Short-term treatment of insomnia *Special considerations*: Patient should take before bed and devote 4–8 h to sleep; use with caution in patients with hepatic or renal impairment; older adult patients are especially sensitive to these drugs—administer a lower dose and monitor these patients carefully.
zolpidem (*Ambien, Intermezzo, Zolpimist*)	Initially 5 mg PO at bedtime, may increase to a max of 10 mg/d PO at bedtime or 6.25 mg PO (females) or 6.25–12.5 mg PO (males) using extended-release tablet or 2–3 sprays in mouth if using oral spray	Short-term treatment of insomnia *Special considerations*: Dispense the least amount possible to depressed and/or suicidal patients; withdraw gradually if used for prolonged period; patient should take before bed and devote 4–8 h to sleep; use with caution in patients with hepatic or renal impairment; older adult patients are especially sensitive to these drugs—administer a lower dose and monitor these patients carefully.

the medication in the evening and to allow for 8 hours of sleep, and they should be warned that the adverse effects can be enhanced if taking with other CNS depressants.

- Meprobamate (generic) is an older drug that is used to manage acute anxiety for up to 4 months. It works in the limbic system and thalamus and has some anticonvulsant properties and CNS muscle-relaxing effects. It is rapidly absorbed and is metabolized in the liver and excreted in the urine.
- Ramelteon (*Rozerem*) is a melatonin receptor agonist. This drug stimulates melatonin receptors, which are thought to be involved in the maintenance of circadian rhythm and the sleep–wake cycle. Ramelteon is used for the treatment of insomnia characterized by difficulty with sleep onset. It is rapidly absorbed, reaching peak level in 30 to 90 minutes. Absorption may be delayed if it is taken with a high fat meal. It is metabolized in the liver and excreted in the feces and urine. Side effects can include hormonal effects, due to increased levels of prolactin and decreased testosterone; worsening sleep apnea; abnormal thoughts and/or behaviors; depression; and impaired mental alertness.
- Suvorexant (*Belsomra*) was approved in 2014 and is one of a newer class of drugs called orexin receptor antagonists. It is used to treat insomnia. The orexin signaling system is thought to be a central promoter of wakefulness, and blocking these sites is thought to suppress the drive to wake up. It is absorbed quickly from the GI tract, reaching peak level in 30 minutes to 2 hours. It is metabolized in the liver and excreted in the feces, with a half-life of about 12 hours. It has been associated with "sleep driving" and other complex behaviors. To decrease safety risks of the CNS effects, the patient should be in bed within 30 minutes of taking the drug and plan to stay in bed for 7 hours.
- Tasimelteon (*Hetlioz*), another melatonin receptor agonist, was approved for the treatment of non–24-hour sleep–wake disorder, a common problem in patients with complete blindness who are not able to maintain circadian rhythm and the sleep–wake cycle because the retina does not experience light exposure. It is absorbed rapidly, reaching peak level in 30 to 180 minutes. It is metabolized in the tissues with a half-life of about 1.5 hours and is excreted in the urine.
- Zaleplon (*Sonata*) and zolpidem (*Ambien, Intermezzo, Zolpimist*), both of which cause sedation, are used for the short-term treatment of insomnia. They are thought to work by selectively binding to specific GABA receptors. They do not tend to bind as universally to GABA receptors compared to benzodiazepines or barbiturates. These drugs are metabolized in the liver and excreted in the urine. Zolpidem is available as a tablet, an orally disintegrating tablet, and a metered spray. These drugs are also associated with "sleep driving" and other complex behaviors and carry a warning about safety issues associated with these CNS effects.

SUMMARY

- Anxiolytics, once called minor tranquilizers, are drugs used to treat anxiety by depressing the CNS. When given at higher doses, these drugs may be sedatives or hypnotics.
- Sedatives block the awareness of and reaction to environmental stimuli, resulting in associated CNS depression that may cause drowsiness, lethargy, and other effects. This action can be beneficial when a patient is very excited or afraid.
- Hypnotics further depress the CNS, particularly the RAS, to inhibit neuronal arousal and induce sleep.
- Benzodiazepines are a group of drugs used as anxiolytics. They react with GABA inhibitory sites to depress the CNS. They can cause drowsiness, lethargy, and other CNS effects.
- Barbiturates are an older class of drugs used as anxiolytics, sedatives, and hypnotics. Because they are associated with potentially serious adverse effects and interact with many other drugs, they are less desirable than the benzodiazepines or other anxiolytics.
- Buspirone, another anxiolytic drug, does not cause sedation or muscle relaxation. Because of the absence of CNS effects, it is much preferred in certain circumstances (e.g., when a person must drive, go to work, or maintain alertness).
- Newer hypnotic agents act in the RAS to affect serotonin levels (zaleplon and zolpidem), affect melatonin levels in the brain (ramelteon, tasimelteon), or block orexin receptors (suvorexant).

CHECK YOUR UNDERSTANDING

Answers to the questions in this chapter can be found in Answers to Check Your Understanding Questions on thePoint®.

MULTIPLE CHOICE

Select the best answer.

1. Drugs that are best used to cause a patient to sleep are called
   a. hypnotics.
   b. sedatives.
   c. antiepileptics.
   d. anxiolytics.
2. The benzodiazepines are the most frequently used anxiolytic drugs because they
   a. are anxiolytic and act very rapidly to assist with sedation or hypnosis.
   b. can also be stimulating.
   c. are more likely to cause physical dependence than older anxiolytic drugs.
   d. do not affect any neurotransmitters.
3. Barbiturates cause liver enzyme induction, which could lead to
   a. rapid metabolism and loss of effectiveness of other drugs metabolized by those enzymes.
   b. increased bile production.
   c. CNS depression.
   d. the need to periodically lower the barbiturate dose to avoid toxicity.
4. A person who could benefit from an anxiolytic drug for short-term treatment of insomnia would not be prescribed
   a. zolpidem.
   b. zaleplon.
   c. buspirone.
   d. dexmedetomidine.
5. Anxiolytic drugs block awareness of and reaction to the environment. This effect would not be beneficial in
   a. relieving extreme fear.
   b. moderating anxiety related to unknown causes.
   c. treating a patient who must drive a vehicle for a living.
   d. treating a patient who is experiencing a stress reaction.
6. M.J. is the chief executive officer of a large company and has been experiencing acute anxiety attacks. Their physical examination was normal, and they were diagnosed with anxiety. Considering M.J.'s occupation and their need to be alert and present to large groups on a regular basis, which anxiolytic would be the drug of choice for them?
   a. Phenobarbital
   b. Diazepam
   c. Clorazepate
   d. Buspirone
7. The benzodiazepines react with
   a. GABA receptor sites in the RAS to cause inhibition of neural arousal.
   b. norepinephrine receptor sites in the sympathetic nervous system.
   c. acetylcholine receptor sites in the parasympathetic nervous system.
   d. monoamine oxidase to increase norepinephrine breakdown.
8. A pediatric patient is prescribed phenobarbital preoperatively to relieve anxiety and produce sedation. After giving the injection, you should assess the patient for
   a. acute Stevens-Johnson syndrome.
   b. bone marrow depression.
   c. paradoxical excitement.
   d. withdrawal syndrome.

MULTIPLE RESPONSE

Select all that apply.

1. In assessing a patient who is experiencing anxiety, the nurse would expect to find which conditions?
   a. Rapid breathing
   b. Rapid heart rate
   c. Fear and apprehension
   d. Constricted pupils
   e. Decreased abdominal sounds
   f. Hypotension
2. Your patient has a long history of anxiety and has always responded well to diazepam. They have just learned that they are pregnant; and the patient feels very anxious. They would like a prescription for diazepam to get through this early anxiety. What

rationale would the nurse use in explaining why this is not recommended?

a. This drug is known to cause a predictable syndrome of birth defects, including cleft lip and pyloric stenosis.
b. Babies born to birthing parents taking benzodiazepines may progress through a neonatal withdrawal syndrome.
c. Cardiac defects and small brain development may occur if this drug is taken in the first trimester.
d. This drug almost always causes loss of the pregnancy.
e. The hormones the body produces during pregnancy will make you unresponsive to diazepam.
f. This drug could have adverse effects on your baby; we should explore nondrug measures to help you deal with the anxiety.

REFERENCES

Bendz, L. M., & Scates, A. C. (2010). Melatonin treatment for insomnia in pediatric patients with attention-deficit/hyperactivity disorder. *Annals of Pharmacotherapy, 44*, 185–191. 10.1345/aph.1M365

Brunton, L., Hilal-Dandan, R., & Knollman, B. (2018). *Goodman and Gilman's the pharmacological basis of therapeutics* (13th ed.). McGraw-Hill.

Gotter, A. L., Garson, S. L., Stevens, J., Munden, R. L., Fox, S. V., Tannenbaum, P. L., Yao, L., Kuduk, S. D., McDonald, T., Uslaner, J. M., Tye, S. J., Coleman, P. J., Winrow, C. J., & Renger, J. J. (2014). Differential sleep-promoting effects of dual orexin antagonists and GABA A receptor modulators. *BMC Neuroscience, 15*, 109. https://bmcneurosci.biomedcentral.com/articles/10.1186/1471-2202-15-109

Hendler, C. B. (Ed.). (2021). *Nursing 2021 drug handbook.* Wolters Kluwer.

Norris, T. L. (2019). *Porth's pathophysiology concepts of altered health states.* Wolters Kluwer.

Roy-Byrne, P., Craske, M., Sullivan, G., Rose, R. D., Edlund, M. J., Lang, A. J., Bystritsky, A., Welch, S. S., Chavira, D. A., Golinelli, D., Campbell-Sills, L., Sherbourne, C. D., & Stein, M. B. (2010). Delivery of evidenced based treatment for multiple anxiety disorders in primary care. *Journal of the American Medical Association, 303*(19), 1921–1928. 10.1001/jama.2010.608

Sangal, R. B., Bluhm, J. L., Lankford, D. A., Grinnell, T. A., & Huang, H. (2014). Eszopiclone for insomnia associated with ADHD. *Pediatrics, 134*(4), 1095–1103. 10.1542/peds.2013-4221

Sobonsky, J. (2014). Overview and management of anxiety disorders. *US Pharmacist, 39*(11), 56–62. https://www.uspharmacist.com/article/overview-and-management-of-anxiety-disorders

Torpy, J., Burke, A., & Golub, R. (2011). Generalized anxiety disorders. *Journal of the American Medical Association, 305*(5), 522. 10.1001/jama.305.5.522

CHAPTER 21

Antidepressant Agents

Learning Objectives

Upon completion of this chapter, you will be able to:

1. Describe the biogenic theory of depression.
2. Discuss the use of antidepressants across the lifespan.
3. Describe the therapeutic actions, indications, pharmacokinetics, contraindications, most common adverse reactions, and important drug–drug interactions associated with each class of antidepressant.
4. Compare and contrast the prototype drugs for each class of antidepressant with the other drugs in that class and with drugs in the other classes of antidepressants.
5. Outline the nursing considerations and teaching needs for patients receiving each class of antidepressant.

Key Terms

affect: feeling that a person experiences when they respond emotionally to the environment

biogenic theory of depression: the idea that one of the amine neurotransmitters—norepinephrine, serotonin, or dopamine—is deficient in key areas of the brain, resulting in depression

depression: affective disorder in which a person experiences sadness that is much more severe and longer lasting than the event that seems to have precipitated it, with a more intense mood; the condition may not be traceable to a specific event or stressor

monoamine oxidase inhibitor (MAOI): drug that prevents the enzyme monoamine oxidase from breaking down norepinephrine (NE), serotonin (5HT), and dopamine (DA), leading to increased neurotransmitter levels in the synaptic cleft; relieves depression and also causes sympathomimetic effects

selective serotonin reuptake inhibitor (SSRI): drug that specifically blocks the reuptake of serotonin and increases its concentration in the synaptic cleft; relieves depression and is less associated with anticholinergic or sympathomimetic adverse effects

serotonin-norepinephrine reuptake inhibitors (SNRIs): drug that increases both serotonin and norepinephrine concentrations in synaptic cleft; relieves depression with varying serotonergic or noradrenergic activity

tricyclic antidepressants (TCAs): drug that blocks the reuptake of norepinephrine and serotonin; relieves depression and has anticholinergic and sedative effects

tyramine: an amine found in food that causes vasoconstriction and raises blood pressure; ingesting foods high in tyramine while taking an MAOI poses the risk of a severe hypertensive crisis

Drug List

TRICYCLIC ANTIDEPRESSANTS
- amitriptyline
- amoxapine
- clomipramine
- desipramine
- doxepin
- (P) imipramine
- maprotiline
- nortriptyline
- protriptyline
- trimipramine

MONOAMINE OXIDASE INHIBITORS
- isocarboxazid
- (P) phenelzine
- selegiline
- tranylcypromine

SELECTIVE SEROTONIN REUPTAKE INHIBITORS
- citalopram
- escitalopram
- (P) fluoxetine
- fluvoxamine
- paroxetine
- sertraline
- vilazodone
- vortioxetine

SEROTONIN-NOREPINEPHRINE REUPTAKE INHIBITORS
- desvenlafaxine
- (P) duloxetine
- levomilnacipran
- milnacipran
- venlafaxine

OTHER ANTIDEPRESSANTS
- bupropion
- esketamine
- mirtazapine
- nefazodone
- trazodone

When you ask people how they feel, they may say "pretty good" or "not so great." People's responses are usually appropriate to what is happening in their lives, and they describe themselves as being in a good mood or a bad mood. Some days are better than others.

Affect is a term that is used to refer to people's feelings in response to their environment, whether positive and pleasant or negative and unpleasant. All people experience different affective states at various times in their lives. These states of mind, which change in particular situations, usually do not last very long and do not often involve extremes of happiness or sadness. If a person's mood goes far beyond the usual normal "ups and downs," they are said to have an affective disorder.

Information regarding diagnosing psychiatric disorders is described in the *Diagnostic and Statistical Manual of Mental Disorders* (DSM-5). Psychiatric disorders include schizophrenia, mood disorders, anxiety disorders, obsessive–compulsive disorders (OCDs), and substance use disorders. This chapter includes the medications commonly used for treatment of the mood disorder of depression.

Depression and Antidepressants

Depression is a common affective disorder involving feelings of sadness that are much more severe and longer-lasting than the suspected precipitating event, and the mood of affected individuals is much more intense. The depression may not be traceable to a specific event or stressor (i.e., there are no external causes). Patients who are depressed may have little energy, sleep disturbances, altered appetite, altered libido, and reduced ability to perform activities of daily living. They may describe overwhelming feelings of sadness, despair, hopelessness, and disorganization. The DSM-5 describes multiple types of depressive disorders, including but not limited to major depressive disorder, persistent depressive disorder, premenstrual dysphoric disorder (PMDD), and disruptive mood dysregulation disorder. Each type of disorder has specific criteria for the diagnosis. For example, for the diagnosis of major depressive disorder, the individual must have symptoms that occur most of the day nearly every day for a period of at least 2 weeks, and the symptoms must interfere with daily life activities.

In many cases, depression is never diagnosed; the patient is instead treated for physical manifestations of the underlying disease, such as fatigue, malaise, obesity, eating disorder, or alcohol and drug dependence. Clinical depression is a disorder that can interfere with a person's personal life, work, and social participation. Left untreated, it can produce multiple physical problems that can lead to further depression and in extreme cases suicide.

Theories Connecting Neurophysiology With Depression

One of the theories regarding the cause of depression is the **biogenic theory of depression**. The hypothesis is that depression results from a deficiency of biogenic amines in key areas of the brain. These biogenic amines include norepinephrine (NE), dopamine, and serotonin (5HT). Both NE and 5HT are released throughout the brain by neurons that react with multiple receptors to regulate arousal, alertness, attention, moods, appetite, and sensory processing. Deficiencies of these neurotransmitters could be due to decreased release from the presynaptic neuron or decreased postsynaptic sensitivity. Many of the medications that are prescribed to treat clients who are experiencing depression work to increase the levels of these biogenic amines within the brain.

The amines are not the only chemicals that are thought to play a role in causing depression. Some researchers hypothesize that glutamate, which triggers nitric oxide release, may play a role in depression. Glutamate is released from the presynaptic nerve and facilitates a chemical to act with glutamate to stimulate the *N*-methyl-D-aspartate (NMDA) receptors on the postsynaptic nerve, which activate nitric oxide (NO). NO plays a crucial role in nerve health and plasticity, but in excess has been shown to be a factor in chronic inflammation and may decrease the synthesis of the biogenic amines. Many people with depression have been shown to have high inflammation markers in their blood plasma. There is also evidence that people who suffer from inflammatory disorders have a higher risk of developing mood disorders. Excessive NO could be the explanation of the link between inflammation and mood disorders.

Depression also may occur as a result of other, yet unknown factors. For example, early life stress that causes disturbance in the hypothalamic pituitary axis may result in higher levels of cortisol, which could increase feelings of depression. Vitamin D also has been shown to be low in some people suffering from depression. Research is ongoing to understand the etiology of mood disorders. Treatment is best for most people when both pharmacology and psychotherapy are combined.

Drug Therapy

The use of agents that alter the concentration of neurotransmitters in the brain is the most effective means of treating depression with drugs. Many antidepressant drugs used today counteract the effects of neurotransmitter deficiencies in three ways. First, they may inhibit the effects of monoamine oxidase (MAO), an enzyme that removes the neurotransmitters norepinephrine, serotonin, and dopamine from the neuron synaptic cleft. Inhibiting MAO can lead to more NE or 5HT in the synaptic cleft. Second, antidepressants may block reuptake of these neurotransmitters by the releasing nerve, leading to increased neurotransmitter levels in the synaptic cleft. Third, they may regulate receptor sites and the breakdown of neurotransmitters, leading to an accumulation of neurotransmitter in the synaptic cleft.

Antidepressants may be classified into four main groups: tricyclic antidepressants (TCAs), monoamine oxidase inhibitors (MAOIs), selective serotonin reuptake inhibitors (SSRIs), and serotonin-norepinephrine reuptake inhibitors (SNRIs). Other drugs that are used as antidepressants similarly increase the synaptic cleft concentrations of these neurotransmitters (Fig. 21.1). For information on how antidepressants affect people of all ages, see Box 21.1.

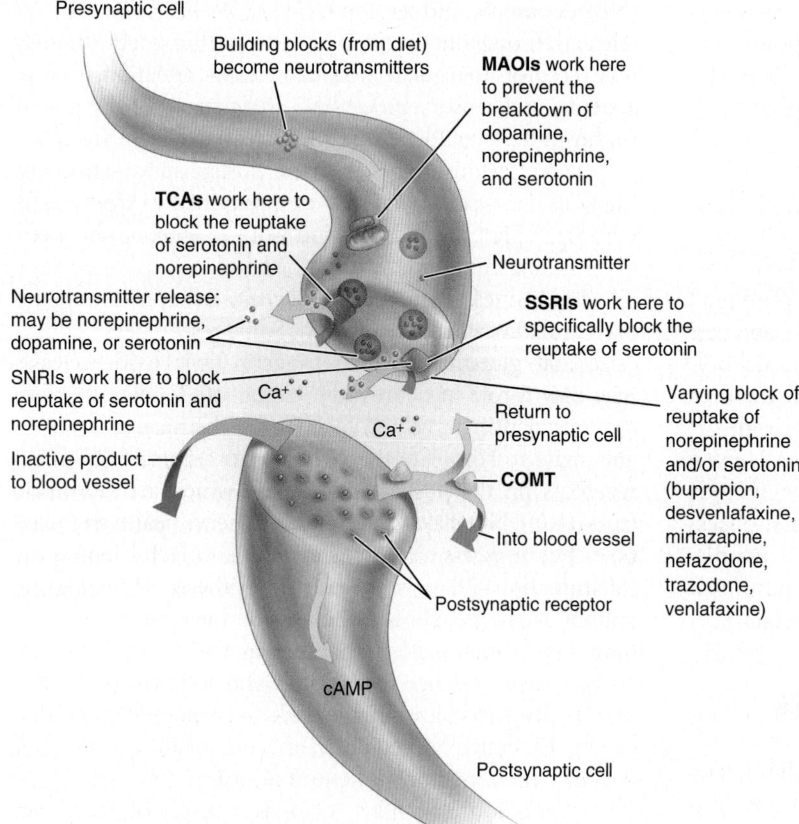

FIGURE 21.1 Sites of action for the antidepressants: monoamine oxidase inhibitors (MAOIs), tricyclic antidepressants (TCAs), selective serotonin reuptake inhibitors (SSRIs), and serotonin–norepinephrine reuptake inhibitors (SNRIs). cAMP, cyclic adenosine monophosphate; COMT, catecholamine-*O*-methyltransferase.

Box 21.1 Focus on Drug Therapy Across the Lifespan

ANTIDEPRESSANT AGENTS

Children

Use of antidepressant drugs with children poses a challenge. The response of the child to the drug may be unpredictable, and the long-term effects of many of these agents are not clearly understood. Studies have not shown efficacy in using these drugs to treat depression in children and also indicate that there may be an increase in suicidal ideation and suicidal behavior when antidepressants are used to treat depression in children.

Of the tricyclic drugs (TCAs), clomipramine, imipramine, nortriptyline, and trimipramine have established pediatric doses in children older than 6 years. Children should be monitored closely for adverse effects, and dose changes should be made as needed.

MAOIs should be avoided in children if at all possible because of the potential for drug–food interactions and the serious adverse effects.

The SSRIs and SNRIs can cause serious adverse effects in children; however, these medications are considered first line for pediatric patients. Fluvoxamine and sertraline have established pediatric dose guidelines for the treatment of OCDs. Fluoxetine is widely used to treat depression in adolescents, and a 2000 survey of off-label uses of drugs showed that it was being used in children as young as 6 months. Dosage regimens must be established according to the child's age and weight, and a child receiving an antidepressant should be monitored very carefully. Underlying medical reasons for the depression should be ruled out before antidepressant therapy is begun. Again, children should be monitored for any suicidal ideation.

Adults

Adults using these drugs should have medical causes for their depression ruled out before beginning antidepressant therapy. Thyroid disease, hormonal imbalance, and CV disorders can all lead to the signs and symptoms of depression. Screening for bipolar disease should also occur prior to medical treatment.

The patient needs to understand that the effects of drug therapy may not be seen for 4 weeks and that it is important to continue the therapy for at least that long.

It is encouraged that patients who are pregnant be enrolled in the pregnancy registry, which is evaluating effects of antidepressant medications on fetal outcomes. Untreated depression can be harmful for both parent and fetus, so thoughtful consideration of risks and benefits is required for patients who are pregnant.

Older Adults

Older patients may be more susceptible to the adverse effects of these drugs, from unanticipated CNS effects to increased sedation, dizziness, and even hallucinations. Doses of drugs may need to be reduced and the patient monitored very closely for toxic effects. Safety measures should be provided if CNS effects do occur.

Patients with hepatic or renal impairment should be monitored very closely while taking these drugs. Decreased doses may be needed. Because many older patients also have renal or hepatic impairment, they need to be screened carefully. TCAs may exacerbate benign prostate hypertrophy symptoms by decreasing bladder contractions.

Tricyclic Antidepressants

The **tricyclic antidepressants** (TCAs), including the amines, secondary amines, and tetracyclics, all reduce the reuptake of 5HT and NE into nerves. Because all TCAs are similarly effective, the choice of TCA depends on individual response to the drug and tolerance of adverse effects. A patient who does not respond to one TCA may respond to another drug from this class. Available TCAs include the amines amitriptyline (generic), amoxapine (generic), clomipramine (*Anafranil*), doxepin (generic), imipramine (*Tofranil*), and trimipramine (*Surmontil*); the secondary amines desipramine (*Norpramin*), nortriptyline (*Pamelor*), and protriptyline (*Vivactil*); and the tetracyclic drug maprotiline (generic).

Therapeutic Actions and Indications

The TCAs inhibit presynaptic reuptake of the neurotransmitters 5HT and NE, which leads to an accumulation of these neurotransmitters in the synaptic cleft and increased stimulation of the postsynaptic receptors. The exact mechanism of action in decreasing depression is not known but is thought to be related to the accumulation of NE and 5HT in certain areas of the brain.

TCAs are indicated for the relief of symptoms of depression. The sedative effects of these drugs may make them more effective in patients whose depression is characterized by anxiety and sleep disturbances. Some are effective for treating enuresis in children older than 6 years (see Box 21.1). Some of these drugs are used for the treatment of chronic, intractable pain, neuropathy, fibromyalgia, and anxiety disorders. In addition, the TCAs are anticholinergic. Clomipramine is now also approved for use in the treatment of obsessive–OCDs.

Pharmacokinetics

The TCAs are well absorbed from the gastrointestinal (GI) tract, reaching peak levels in 2 to 4 hours. They are highly bound to plasma proteins and are lipid soluble; this allows them to be distributed widely in the tissues, including the brain. TCAs are metabolized in the liver and excreted in the urine, with relatively long half-lives ranging from 8 to 46 hours. Clinically, they may take 10 to 14 days to have effect and maximum effect may not be seen for 4 to 8 weeks. The TCAs cross the placenta and enter human milk (see "Contraindications and Cautions").

Contraindications and Cautions

One contraindication to the use of TCAs is the presence of allergy to any of the drugs in this class because of the risk of hypersensitivity reactions. Other contraindications include recent myocardial infarction because of the potential occurrence of reinfarction or extension of the infarct with the cardiac effects of the drug, myelography within the previous 24 hours or in the next 48 hours because of a possible drug–drug interaction with the dyes used in these studies, and concurrent use of an MAOI because of the potential for serious adverse effects or toxic reactions. In addition, the risks of taking the medication during pregnancy and lactation are unknown so the medications should not be used unless the benefit to the parent clearly outweighs the potential risk to the neonate.

TCAs should be used with caution in patients with preexisting cardiovascular (CV) disorders because of the cardiac stimulatory effects of the drug and with any condition that would be exacerbated by the anticholinergic effects, such as angle-closure glaucoma, urinary retention, prostate hypertrophy, or gastrointestinal (GI) or genitourinary (GU) surgery. Care should also be taken with psychiatric patients, who may exhibit a worsening of psychoses or paranoia, and with manic–depressive patients, who may shift to a manic stage. There is a boxed warning on all of the TCAs bringing attention to a risk of suicidality, especially in children, adolescents, and young adults; caution should be used, and the amount of drug dispensed at any given time should be limited with potentially suicidal patients. In addition, caution is necessary in patients with a history of seizures because the seizure threshold may be decreased secondary to stimulation of the receptor

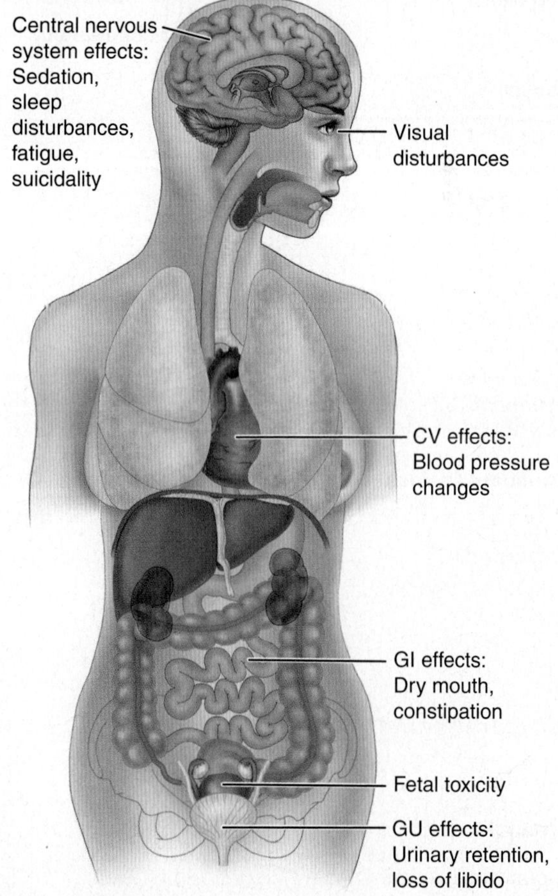

FIGURE 21.2 Variety of adverse effects and toxicities associated with antidepressants.

sites and in older adult patients. The presence of hepatic or renal disease, which could interfere with metabolism and excretion of these drugs and lead to toxic levels, also necessitates caution and the need for a lower dose of the drug.

Adverse Effects

The adverse effects of TCAs are associated with the effects of the drugs on the central nervous system (CNS) and on the peripheral nervous system (Fig. 21.2). Sedation, sleep disturbances, fatigue, hallucinations, disorientation, visual disturbances, difficulty in concentrating, weakness, ataxia, and tremors may occur.

Use of TCAs may lead to GI anticholinergic effects, such as dry mouth, constipation, nausea, vomiting, anorexia, and decreased salivation. Resultant GU effects may include urinary retention and hesitancy, loss of libido, and changes in sexual functioning. Anticholinergic effects can also cause ocular changes like blurred vision and/or photophobia. CV effects such as orthostatic hypotension, hypertension, tachycardia, other cardiac arrhythmias, myocardial infarction, angina, palpitations, and stroke may occur in some people. Miscellaneous reported effects include alopecia, weight gain or loss, flushing, chills, sweating, and nasal congestion.

These adverse effects may be intolerable to some patients, who then stop taking the particular TCA. Abrupt cessation of all TCAs causes a withdrawal syndrome characterized by nausea, headache, vertigo, malaise, and nightmares. Some of these side effects diminish over time. Table 21.1 shows the relative frequency of the occurrence of adverse effects by specific type of TCA.

Clinically Important Drug–Drug Interactions

If TCAs are given with cimetidine, fluoxetine, or ranitidine, an increase in TCA levels results with an increase in both therapeutic and adverse effects, especially anticholinergic conditions. Patients should be monitored closely, and appropriate dose reductions should be made.

Other drug combinations may also pose problems. The combination of TCAs and oral anticoagulants leads to higher serum levels of the anticoagulants and increased risk of bleeding. Blood tests should be done frequently, and appropriate dose adjustments in the oral anticoagulant should be made.

Table 21.1 *Drugs in Focus:* Tricyclic Antidepressants

Drug Name	Common Side Effects				Usual Dosage
	Sedation	Anticholinergic	Hypotension	Cardiovascular	
Amines					
amitriptyline (generic)	+ + + +	+ + + +	+ + + +	+ +	75–150 mg/d PO
amoxapine (generic)	+	+	+ +	+ +	50–100 mg PO b.i.d. to t.i.d.
clomipramine (*Anafranil*)	+ + +	+ + +	+ + +	+ + +	*Adult:* 25–50 mg PO q.i.d. *Pediatric:* 25 mg PO q.i.d. to a maximum of 3 mg/kg/d
doxepin (generic)	+ + +	+ + +	+ +	+ +	25–50 mg PO t.i.d.
imipramine (*Tofranil*)	+ +	+ +	+ + +	+ +	*Adult:* 50–200 mg/d PO *Pediatric:* 30–40 mg/d PO
trimipramine (*Surmontil*)	+ + +	+ +	+ +	+ +	*Adult:* 75–150 mg/d PO *Pediatric:* 50 mg/d PO *Older adults:* 50–100 mg/d PO
Secondary Amines					
desipramine (*Norpramin*)	+	+	+ +	+ +	100–200 mg/d PO
nortriptyline (*Aventyl, Pamelor*)	+	+	+	+	*Adult:* 25–50 mg PO t.i.d. to q.i.d. *Pediatric:* 30–50 mg/d PO in divided doses *Older adults:* 30–50 mg/d PO in divided doses
protriptyline (*Vivactil*)	+	+ + +	+	+	15–40 mg/d PO in three or four divided doses, 5 mg PO t.i.d. for older adult patients
Tetracyclic					
maprotiline (generic)	+ +	+	+ +	+ +	75–150 mg/d PO, reduce dose in older adult patients

+ + + +, marked effects; + + +, moderate effects; + +, mild effects; +, negligible effects.

If TCAs are combined with sympathomimetics or clonidine, the risk of arrhythmias and hypertension is increased. This combination should be avoided, especially in patients with underlying CV disease.

The combination of TCAs with MAOIs leads to a risk of severe serotonin syndrome or hyperpyretic symptoms with severe convulsions, hypertensive episodes, and death. This combination should be avoided. Although TCAs and MAOIs have been used together in selected patients who do not respond to a single agent, the risk of severe adverse effects is very high.

P Prototype Summary: Imipramine

Indications: Relief of symptoms of depression; enuresis in children older than 6 years; off-label consideration—control of chronic pain.

Actions: Inhibits presynaptic reuptake of norepinephrine and serotonin; anticholinergic at CNS and peripheral receptors; sedating.

Pharmacokinetics:

Route	Onset	Peak
Oral	Varies	2–4 h

$T_{1/2}$: 8 to 16 hours; metabolized in the liver; excreted in the urine.

Adverse Effects: Sedation, anticholinergic effects, confusion, anxiety, orthostatic hypotension, dry mouth, constipation, urinary retention, rash, bone marrow depression, suicidal ideation/behaviors.

Nursing Considerations for Patients Receiving Tricyclic Antidepressants

Assessment: History and Examination

- Assess for any known allergies to these drugs to avoid hypersensitivity reactions; impaired liver or kidney function, which could alter metabolism and excretion of the drug; glaucoma, benign prostatic hypertrophy, cardiac dysfunction, GI obstruction, surgery, or recent myocardial infarction, all of which could be exacerbated by the effects of the drug.
- Determine whether patients are pregnant or breast or chestfeeding because the effects of the medications during pregnancy or lactation are unknown.
- Assess whether the patient has a history of seizure disorders or a history of psychiatric problems or suicidal thoughts; myelography within the past 24 hours or in the next 48 hours; or is taking an MAOI, to avoid potentially serious adverse reactions.
- Assess temperature and weight; skin color and lesions; affect, orientation, and reflexes; vision; blood pressure, including orthostatic blood pressure; pulse and perfusion; respiratory rate and adventitious sounds; and bowel sounds on abdominal examination. This determines baseline status any potential adverse effects before beginning therapy. Also obtain an electrocardiogram as well as renal and liver function tests.

Nursing Conclusions

Nursing conclusions related to drug therapy might include the following:

- Impaired comfort related to anticholinergic effects, headache, and CNS effects
- Risk of activity intolerance related to CV effects
- Altered thought processes and altered sensory perception (visual, auditory, kinesthetic, tactile, or olfactory) related to CNS effects
- Injury risk related to CNS effects
- Knowledge deficiency regarding drug therapy

Planning

- The patient will receive the best therapeutic effect from the drug therapy, relief of depression.
- The patient will have limited adverse effects to the drug therapy.
- The patient will have an understanding of the drug therapy, adverse effects to anticipate, and measures to relieve discomfort and improve safety.

Intervention With Rationale

- Warn patient and family members about risk of worsening depression and even suicidal thoughts/behaviors, especially when initiating treatment in children and young adults.
- Maintain the initial dose for 4 to 8 weeks to evaluate the therapeutic effect.
- Administer parenteral forms of the drug only if oral forms are not feasible or available; switch to an oral form, which is less toxic and associated with fewer adverse effects, as soon as possible.
- Administer the dose at bedtime if drowsiness and anticholinergic effects are severe, to decrease the risk of patient injury. Warn patient to avoid hazardous activities, like driving, if daytime sleepiness, light-headedness, or dizziness occur.
- Reduce dose if minor adverse effects occur, and discontinue the drug if major or potentially life-threatening adverse effects occur, to ensure patient safety.
- Provide comfort measures to help the patient tolerate drug effects. These measures may include instituting a bowel program as needed for constipation, taking food with the drug if it assists with GI upset, chewing sugarless gum or sipping on water for dry mouth, wearing sunglasses if photophobia, and hydrating effectively to minimize orthostatic hypotension.
- Provide thorough patient teaching including drug name, prescribed dosage, measures for avoidance of adverse effects, and warning signs that may indicate

(continues on page 364)

possible problems. Instruct the patient about the need for periodic monitoring and evaluation to enhance patient knowledge about drug therapy and to promote compliance.

- Offer support and encouragement to help the patient cope with the diagnosis and the drug regimen.

Evaluation

- Monitor patient response to the drug (alleviation of signs and symptoms of depression).
- Monitor for adverse effects (sedation, anticholinergic effects, hypotension, cardiac arrhythmias, suicidal thoughts).
- Evaluate the effectiveness of the teaching plan (patient can give the drug name, dosage, possible adverse effects to watch for, specific measures to help avoid adverse effects, and importance of continued follow-up).
- Monitor the effectiveness of comfort measures and compliance with the regimen.

Table 21.2 *Drugs in Focus:* Monoamine Oxidase Inhibitors

Drug Name	Dosage/Route	Usual Indications
isocarboxazid (*Marplan*)	10 mg PO b.i.d., may reach a maximum of 40 mg/d	Treatment of depression not responsive to other agents
phenelzine (*Nardil*)	15 mg PO t.i.d., maintenance 15 mg/d PO	Treatment of depression not responsive to other agents
selegiline transdermal system (*Emsam*)	6 mg transdermal per 24 h initial and can be titrated to mass 12 mg transdermal per 24 h	Treatment of major depressive disorder
tranylcypromine (*Parnate*)	30 mg/d PO in divided doses, maximum 60 mg/d	Treatment of adult reactive depression

Key Points

- Affect is a term that refers to the feelings that people experience when they respond emotionally.
- Depression is an affective disorder characterized by inappropriate sadness, despair, and hopelessness.
- According to the biogenic theory, depression is caused by a brain deficiency of the biogenic amines. Antidepressant drugs are thought to raise the level of the biogenic amines.
- The tricyclic medications are often used to treat depression, but can also be used to treat chronic pain, anxiety disorders and insomnia.

Monoamine Oxidase Inhibitors

Monoamine oxidase inhibitors (MAOIs) (see Table 21.2) irreversibly inhibit MAO, which is an enzyme found in nerves and other tissues (including the liver) that breaks down the biogenic amines NE, dopamine, and 5HT. When the MAO is inhibited, there are higher levels of amines available, which correlates with lower levels of depression. At one time, MAOIs were used more often, but now they are used rarely because they require a specific dietary regimen to prevent toxicity from tyramine. This is due to the additional function of MAO to decrease tyramine levels in the body. Accumulation of tyramine can cause increased blood pressure and even hypertensive crisis. There are some patients, however, who only seem to respond to these particular drugs, so they remain available. Agents that can be taken orally include isocarboxazid (*Marplan*), phenelzine (*Nardil*), and tranylcypromine (*Parnate*). Selegiline (*Emsam*) can be administered transdermally for treatment of depression, and the oral form of selegiline (*Zelapar*) can be used as adjunctive treatment for patients with Parkinson's disease (Chapter 24). The choice of an MAOI depends on the prescriber's experience and individual response. A patient who does not respond to one MAOI may respond to another.

Therapeutic Actions and Indications

Blocking the breakdown of the biogenic amines NE, dopamine, and 5HT allows these amines to accumulate in the synaptic cleft and in neuronal storage vesicles, causing increased stimulation of the postsynaptic receptors. It is thought that this increased stimulation of the receptors causes relief of depression. The MAOIs are generally indicated for treatment of the signs and symptoms of depression in patients who cannot tolerate or do not respond to other safer antidepressants (see Table 21.2).

Pharmacokinetics

The MAOIs that are administered orally are well absorbed from the GI tract, reaching peak levels in 2 to 3 hours. However, clinical changes are slow to occur and it may take months to reach peak therapeutic effects. The MAOIs are metabolized in the liver primarily by acetylation and are excreted in the urine. Patients with liver or renal impairment and those known as "slow acetylators" may require lowered doses to avoid exaggerated effects of the drugs. The MAOIs cross the placenta and enter human milk (see "Contraindications and Cautions").

Contraindications and Cautions

Contraindications to the use of MAOIs include allergy to any of these antidepressants because of the risk of hypersensitivity reactions; pheochromocytoma because the sudden increases in NE levels could result in severe hypertension and CV emergencies; CV disease, including hypertension, coronary artery disease, angina, and congestive heart failure, which could be exacerbated by increased NE levels; and known abnormal CNS vessels or defects because the potential increase in blood pressure and vasoconstriction associated with higher NE levels could precipitate a stroke. A history of headaches may also be a contraindication.

Other contraindications include renal or hepatic impairment, which could alter the metabolism and excretion of these drugs and lead to toxic levels, and myelography within the past 24 hours or in the next 48 hours, because of the risk of severe reaction to the dye used in myelography.

In addition, caution should be used with patients who have been diagnosed with bipolar disorder, who could be overstimulated or experience mania as a result of the stimulation associated with MAOIs, and in patients with seizure disorders or hyperthyroidism, both of which could be exacerbated by the stimulation of these drugs. There is a boxed warning on all drugs of this class to bring awareness to a possible risk of suicidality in patients using these drugs, especially with children, adolescents, and young adults. Care should also be taken with patients who are soon to undergo elective surgery because of the potential for unexpected effects with NE accumulation during the stress reaction and with patients who are pregnant or breast or chestfeeding because of potential adverse effects on the fetus and neonate; these drugs should be used during pregnancy and lactation only if the benefit to the parent clearly outweighs the potential risk to the neonate since the effects are unknown.

Adverse Effects

The MAOIs are associated with some adverse effects, more of which are serious and/or fatal, than most other antidepressants. The effects relate to the accumulation of NE in the synaptic cleft. Dizziness, excitement, nervousness, mania, hyperreflexia, tremors, confusion, insomnia, agitation, and blurred vision may occur.

GI effects can include nausea, vomiting, diarrhea or constipation, anorexia, weight gain, dry mouth, and abdominal pain. Urinary retention, dysuria, incontinence, and changes in sexual function may also occur. CV effects can include orthostatic hypotension, arrhythmias, palpitations, angina, and the potentially fatal hypertensive crisis. This last condition is characterized by occipital headache, palpitations, neck stiffness, nausea, vomiting, sweating, dilated pupils, photophobia, tachycardia, and chest pain. It may progress to intracranial bleeding and fatal stroke.

Clinically Important Drug–Drug Interactions

Drug interactions of MAOIs with other antidepressants include increased risk of hypertensive crisis, coma, and severe convulsions with TCAs, and an increased risk of potentially life-threatening serotonin syndrome with serotonergic medications, including SSRIs. The exact timing will vary, but a period of 6 weeks after stopping an SSRI may be needed before beginning therapy with an MAOI.

If MAOIs are given with other sympathomimetic drugs (e.g., methyldopa), sympathomimetic effects increase. Combinations with insulin or oral antidiabetic agents may result in additive hypoglycemic effects. Patients who receive these combinations must be monitored closely, and appropriate dose adjustments should be made.

Clinically Important Drug–Food Interactions

Tyramine and other pressor amines that are found in food, which are normally broken down by MAO enzymes in the GI tract, may be absorbed in high concentrations in the presence of MAOIs, resulting in increased blood pressure. In addition, tyramine causes the release of stored NE from nerve terminals, which further contributes to high blood pressure and hypertensive crisis. Patients who take MAOIs should avoid the tyramine-containing foods listed in Table 21.3.

Table 21.3 Tyramine-Containing Foods

Foods High in Tyramine	Foods With Moderate Amounts of Tyramine	Foods With Low Amounts of Tyramine
Aged cheeses: cheddar cheese, blue cheese, Swiss cheese, Camembert Aged or fermented meats, fish, or poultry: chicken paté, beef liver paté, caviar Brewer's yeast Fava beans Red wines: Chianti, burgundy, sherry, vermouth Smoked or pickled meats, fish, or poultry: Herring, sausage, corned beef, salami, pepperoni Soy sauce	Meat extracts: Consommé, bouillon Pasteurized light and pale beer Avocados	Distilled liquors: vodka, gin, scotch, rye Cheeses: American, mozzarella, cottage cheese, cream cheese Chocolate Fruits: figs, raisins, grapes, pineapple, oranges Sour cream Yogurt

Prototype Summary: Phenelzine

Indications: Treatment of patients with depression who are unresponsive to other antidepressive therapy or who have an "atypical" presentation, often with a mixture of depression, anxiety, and/or phobic features.

Actions: Irreversibly inhibits MAO, allowing norepinephrine, 5HT, and dopamine to accumulate in the synaptic cleft; this accumulation is thought to be responsible for the clinical effects.

Pharmacokinetics:

Route	Onset	Duration
Oral	Slow	48–96 h

$T_{1/2}$: Approx. 11 hours; metabolized by monoamine oxidase; excreted in the urine.

Adverse Effects: Dizziness, vertigo, headache, overactivity, hyperreflexia, tremors, mania, weakness, drowsiness, fatigue, sweating, orthostatic hypotension, constipation, diarrhea, dry mouth, edema, anorexia, potential for hypertensive crisis.

Nursing Considerations for Patients Receiving Monoamine Oxidase Inhibitors

Assessment: History and Examination

- Assess for any known allergies to these drugs to avoid hypersensitivity reactions; cardiac dysfunction; GI or GU obstruction, which could be exacerbated by the drug; surgery, including elective surgery, because the effects of changes in norepinephrine levels are unpredictable following surgery; seizure disorders; psychiatric conditions or suicidality; and occurrence of myelography within the past 24 hours or in the next 48 hours to avoid the possibility of severe reactions.
- Determine whether patients are pregnant or breast or chestfeeding because the effects of drugs during pregnancy or lactation are unknown.
- Assess temperature and weight; skin color and lesions; affect, orientation, and reflexes; vision; blood pressure, including orthostatic blood pressure; pulse and perfusion; respiratory rate and adventitious sounds; and bowel sounds on abdominal examination to determine baseline status and for any potential adverse effects before beginning therapy. Also obtain an electrocardiogram and renal and liver function tests.

Nursing Conclusions

Nursing conclusions related to drug therapy might include the following:

- Impaired comfort related to sympathomimetic effects, headache, and CNS effects
- Risk of activity intolerance related to CV effects
- Altered thought processes and altered sensory perception (visual, kinesthetic) related to CNS effects
- Injury risk related to CNS effects
- Knowledge deficiency regarding drug therapy

Planning

- The patient will receive the best therapeutic effect from the drug therapy, relief of depression.
- The patient will have limited adverse effects to the drug therapy.
- The patient will have an understanding of the drug therapy, adverse effects to anticipate, and measures to relieve discomfort and improve safety.

Intervention With Rationale

- Limit drug access to a potentially suicidal patient to decrease the risk of self-harm.
- Monitor the patient for 2 to 12 weeks to ascertain the onset of the full therapeutic effect.
- Monitor blood pressure and orthostatic blood pressure carefully to arrange for a slower increase in dose as needed for patients who show a tendency toward altered blood pressures.
- Discontinue drug and monitor the patient carefully at any complaint of severe headache to decrease the risk of severe hypertension and cerebrovascular effects.
- Have phentolamine or another adrenergic blocker on standby as treatment in case of hypertensive crisis.
- Provide comfort measures to help the patient tolerate drug effects. These include instituting a bowel program as needed for constipation, taking food with the drug if GI upset is better with food, and ensuring proper hydration to decrease risk of orthostatic hypotension.
- Provide a list of potential drug–food interactions that can cause severe toxicity to decrease the risk of a serious drug–food interaction. Provide a diet that is low in tyramine-containing foods and a list of medications to avoid.
- Provide thorough patient teaching, including drug name, prescribed dosage, measures for avoidance of adverse effects, and warning signs that may indicate possible problems. Instruct the patient about the need for periodic monitoring and evaluation to enhance patient knowledge about drug therapy and to promote compliance.
- Offer support and encouragement to help the patient cope with the disease and the drug regimen.

Evaluation

- Monitor patient response to the drug (alleviation of signs and symptoms of depression).
- Monitor for adverse effects (sedation, sympathomimetic effects, hypotension, cardiac arrhythmias, GI disturbances, hypertensive crisis, suicidal ideation/behaviors).
- Evaluate the effectiveness of the teaching plan (patient can give the drug name, dosage, possible adverse effects to watch for, specific measures to help avoid adverse effects, importance of continued follow-up, and importance of avoiding foods high in tyramine).
- Monitor the effectiveness of comfort measures and compliance with the regimen.

Key Points

- The MAOIs prevent the breakdown of NE and 5HT by MAO, leading to an increased level of these biogenic amines in the synaptic cleft. This accumulation of the amines is thought to relieve the signs and symptoms of depression.
- Patients taking MAOIs need to avoid foods high in tyramine to prevent serious increases in blood pressure and hypertensive crises.

Selective Serotonin Reuptake Inhibitors

Selective serotonin reuptake inhibitors (SSRIs) (see Table 21.4) are a group of antidepressant drugs that specifically block the reuptake of 5HT with little to no known effect on NE. Because SSRIs do not have the many adverse effects associated with TCAs and MAOIs, they are a better choice for many patients. They are often prescribed first before the TCAs and MAOIs. SSRIs include fluoxetine (*Prozac*), the first SSRI; citalopram (*Celexa*); escitalopram (*Lexapro*); fluvoxamine (*Luvox*); paroxetine (*Paxil*); sertraline (*Zoloft*); vilazodone (*Viibryd*); and vortioxetine (*Brintellix*).

Therapeutic Actions and Indications

The action of SSRIs blocking the reuptake of 5HT increases the levels of 5HT in the synaptic cleft and may contribute to the antidepressant and other effects attributed to these drugs. Vilazodone is not only an inhibitor of 5HT uptake but is also a partial agonist at the 5HT receptors.

SSRIs are indicated for the treatment of depression, OCDs, panic attacks, bulimia, PMDD, posttraumatic stress disorders, social phobias, and social anxiety disorders. A period of up to 4 weeks is necessary for realization of the full therapeutic effect. Patients may respond well to one SSRI and yet show little or no response to another one. The choice of drug depends on the indications and individual response. The SSRIs are currently used as first-line therapy for both depression and anxiety disorders (see Table 21.4).

Table 21.4 *Drugs in Focus:* Selective Serotonin Reuptake Inhibitors

Drug Name	Dosage/Route	Usual Indications
citalopram (*Celexa*)	20 mg/d PO daily, up to 40 mg/d may be needed. Adults older than 60 should not be prescribed doses greater than 20 mg daily	Treatment of depression in adults has also been used to treat panic disorder, PMDD, OCDs, social phobias, trichotillomania, and posttraumatic stress disorders
escitalopram (*Lexapro*)	10 mg/d PO as a single dose, 10–20 mg/d PO maintenance	Treatment of major depressive disorder, maintenance of patients with major depressive disorder and generalized anxiety disorder
fluoxetine (*Prozac, Sarafem*)	20 mg/d PO in the a.m.; do not exceed 60 mg/d; reduce dose with hepatic impairment; also available in a 90-mg, once-a-week formulation	Treatment of depression, bulimia, OCDs, panic disorders, PMDD in adults; also under investigation for treatment of other psychiatric disorders, including obesity, alcohol use disorder, chronic pain, and various neuropathies
fluvoxamine (*Luvox*)	*Adult:* 50 mg PO at bedtime to a maximum of 300 mg/d; reduce dose with hepatic impairment *Pediatric (8–17 y):* 25 mg PO at bedtime; do not exceed 250 mg/d	Treatment of OCDs; also under investigation for treatment of depression, bulimia, panic disorder, and social phobia
paroxetine (*Paxil*)	10–20 mg/d PO, do not exceed 50 mg/d, *or* 62.5 mg/d controlled release tablets; reduce dose in hepatic or renal dysfunction and with older adults	Treatment of depression, OCDs, PMDD, posttraumatic stress reaction, social anxiety disorders, general anxiety disorders, and various panic disorders in adults; also under investigation for treatment of chronic headache, diabetic neuropathy, and hot flashes
sertraline (*Zoloft*)	*Adult:* 25–50 mg/d PO; reduce dose with hepatic dysfunction, OCD *Pediatric:* 25–50 mg/d PO based on age and severity of OCD	Treatment of depression, OCDs, social anxiety disorder, posttraumatic stress disorder, panic disorders, PMDD
vilazodone (*Viibryd*)	10 mg/d PO for 7 d, followed by 20 mg/d for 7 d, then the maintenance dose of 40 mg/d PO taken with food	Treatment of adult patients with major depressive disorder
vortioxetine (*Brintellix*)	10–20 mg/d PO as tolerated	Treatment of adult patients with major depressive disorder

PMDD, premenstrual dysphoric disorder; OCDs, obsessive–compulsive disorders.

Pharmacokinetics

The SSRIs are well absorbed from the GI tract, metabolized in the liver, and excreted in the urine and feces. The half-life varies widely with the drug being used.

Contraindications and Cautions

The SSRIs are contraindicated in the presence of allergy to any of these drugs because of the risk of hypersensitivity reactions. Caution should be used in patients with impaired renal or hepatic function that could alter the metabolism and excretion of the drug, leading to toxic effects, or with diabetes, which could be exacerbated by the stimulating effects of these drugs. Caution should also be used with severely depressed or suicidal patients, especially children, adolescents, and young adults because of a risk of increased suicidality. The SSRIs have been associated with congenital abnormalities in animal studies and should be used during pregnancy only if the benefits to the parent clearly outweigh the potential risks to the fetus. Recent reports have linked use of SSRIs during pregnancy with pulmonary and cardiac problems in the newborn; however, study results have been inconsistent and there are many confounding factors that inhibit clear cause-and-effect relationships between the medications and pregnancy outcomes. The SSRIs enter human milk and can cause adverse effects in the baby. However, the benefits generally outweigh the risks for many of the medications. All patients who are pregnant and those who plan to breast or chestfeed should discuss their medications with their health care provider.

Adverse Effects

The adverse effects associated with SSRIs, which are related to the effects of increased 5HT levels, include CNS effects such as headache, drowsiness, dizziness, insomnia, anxiety, activation of mania/hypomania, tremor, agitation, and seizures. GI effects such as nausea, vomiting, diarrhea, dry mouth, anorexia, constipation, and changes in taste often occur, as do GU effects, including painful menstruation, cystitis, sexual dysfunction, urgency, and impotence. Respiratory changes may include cough, dyspnea, upper respiratory infections, and pharyngitis. SSRIs may also cause serious intraocular pressure changes if used in patients with untreated narrow-angle glaucoma. Other reported effects are sweating, rash, fever, and pruritus. Recent studies have linked the incidence of suicidal ideation and suicide attempts to the use of these drugs in pediatric patients and adolescents (Box 21.2). Serotonin syndrome is a rare but potentially lethal adverse effect that is manifested by confusion, agitation, disorientation, hallucinations, delirium, seizures, tachycardia, labile blood pressure, diaphoresis, fever, hyperreflexia, tremors, nausea, vomiting, diarrhea, abdominal pain, and even coma.

Clinically Important Drug–Drug Interactions

Because of the risk of serotonin syndrome if SSRIs are used with MAOIs, this combination should be avoided. The exact timing will vary, but a period of 6 weeks after stopping an SSRI may be needed before beginning therapy with an MAOI.

In addition, the use of SSRIs with TCAs results in increased therapeutic and toxic effects. If these combinations are used, patients should be monitored closely, and appropriate dose adjustments should be made. Serotonin syndrome, a serious to potentially fatal reaction, can occur if these drugs are combined with any drug or herb

Box 21.2 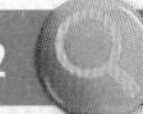 **Focus on The Evidence**

CHILDHOOD SUICIDE AND ANTIDEPRESSANTS

The Food and Drug Administration (FDA) issued a talk paper in late spring 2003 after reports from the British press cited an increase in suicidal behavior in children being treated with paroxetine (*Paxil*). The FDA compiled a review of reports for eight different antidepressant drugs—citalopram, fluoxetine, fluvoxamine, mirtazapine, nefazodone, paroxetine, sertraline, and venlafaxine—that were being studied for use in pediatric populations.

The data from these studies did not clearly establish a link between increased suicidal ideation and the use of these antidepressants, but the data also did not establish effectiveness in major depressive disorder in children for any of the drugs, except fluoxetine. A meta-analysis of randomized control trials was published in 2016 that found treatment with antidepressants caused a small increased risk of suicide in teenagers and young adults but was protective from suicide for older adults.

In 2006, a boxed warning was added to all antidepressant FDA labels bringing attention to the increase in suicidality, especially in children and adolescents, when these drugs were used. Currently the FDA recommends that people prescribed antidepressants who are younger than 30 years of age be closely monitored for worsening depression and/or suicidal thoughts or behaviors. A follow-up visit after about a week when starting a new antidepressant is recommended, especially since there is some evidence that the risk of suicide is greatest when first starting the medication. The increased risk of suicide could be related to undiagnosed bipolar disorder, so it is also recommended that patients be screened for bipolar prior to initiating medication.

Unfortunately, despite better side effect profiles, there is evidence that the newer antidepressants have the potential to increase risk of suicide. Therefore, all of these drugs should be used with caution, prescriptions should be written in the smallest quantity feasible, and parents should be educated about the warning signs of suicide. Continued research is being carried out to study the cause-and-effect relation.

Box 21.3 Focus on Herbal and Alternative Therapies

Patients being treated with SSRIs and SNRIs are at an increased risk of developing a severe reaction, including serotonin syndrome, as well as an increased sensitivity to light if they are also taking St. John's wort. Because this herbal therapy is often used to self-treat depression, it is important to forewarn any patient who is taking an SSRI not to combine it with taking St. John's wort.

Also caution patients that there is an increased risk of seizures if evening primrose is used with antidepressants, and patients should be cautioned against this combination. Interactions have also been reported when antidepressants are combined with ginkgo, ginseng, and valerian. Patients should be cautioned against using herbs without checking for potential interactions while taking antidepressants.

that increases 5HT levels—other SSRIs, serotonin–norepinephrine reuptake inhibitors (SNRIs), St. John's wort, and triptans. There is an increased risk of bleeding if these drugs are combined with aspirin, nonsteroidal anti-inflammatory drugs (NSAIDs), antiplatelet drugs, or drugs that affect coagulation. For more information, see Box 21.3.

Prototype Summary: Fluoxetine

Indications: Treatment of depression, OCDs, bulimia, premenstrual dysphoric disorder, panic disorders; off-label uses include chronic pain, alcohol dependency, neuropathies, obesity.

Actions: Inhibits CNS neuronal reuptake of 5HT with little effect on NE and little affinity for cholinergic, histaminic, or alpha-adrenergic sites.

Pharmacokinetics:

Route	Onset	Peak
Oral	Slow	6–8 h

$T_{1/2}$: Parent drug acute dosing 1 to 3 days; chronic dosing 4 to 6 days; active metabolite (norfluoxetine) 4 to 16 days; metabolized in the liver, so longer half-life with liver dysfunction; excreted in the urine and feces.

Adverse Effects: Headache, nervousness, insomnia, drowsiness, anxiety, tremor, dizziness, sweating, rash, nausea, vomiting, diarrhea, dry mouth, anorexia, sexual dysfunction, upper respiratory infections, weight loss, fever.

CRITICAL THINKING SCENARIO
Selective Serotonin Reuptake Inhibitors

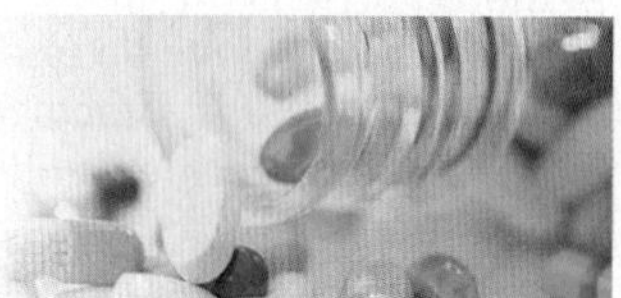

THE SITUATION

D.J., a 46-year-old patient, complains of weight gain, malaise, fatigue, sleeping during the day, loss of interest in daily activities, and bouts of crying for no apparent reason. On examination, they weigh 8 pounds more than the standard weight for their height; all other findings are within normal limits. In conversation with a nurse, D.J. says that in the past 10 months, several events have occurred. D.J. lost both of their parents, their only child graduated from high school and went away to college, their nephew died of renal failure, one of their siblings learned they had metastatic breast cancer, and D.J. lost their job as a day care provider when the client family moved out of town. In addition, the family cat of 17 years was diagnosed with terminal leukemia. D.J. is prescribed fluoxetine (*Prozac*) and is given an appointment with a counselor.

Critical Thinking

What nursing interventions are appropriate at this time?

What sort of crisis intervention would be most appropriate? Balance the benefits of pointing out all of the losses and points of grief that you detect in D.J.'s story with the risks of upsetting their strained coping mechanisms.

What can D.J. expect to experience as a result of the SSRI therapy?

How can you help D.J. cope during the lengthy period it takes to reach therapeutic effects?

What other future interventions should be planned with D.J.?

DISCUSSION

Many patients in severe crisis do not consciously identify the many things that are causing them stress. They have developed coping mechanisms to help them survive and cope with their day-to-day activities. However, D.J. seems to have reached their limit, and they exhibit many of the signs and symptoms of depression. However, it is important to make sure that they do not have some underlying medical condition that could be contributing to their complaints. Because of D.J.'s age, they may also be perimenopausal, which could account for some of their problems.

It is hoped that the fluoxetine, an SSRI, will enable D.J. to regain their ability to cope and their normal affect. The drug should give their brain a chance to reach a new biochemical balance. Before they begin taking the fluoxetine, they should receive a written sheet listing the pertinent drug information, adverse effects to watch for, warning signs to report, and a telephone number to call in case they have questions later or just need to talk. The written information is especially important because they may not remember drug-related discussions or instructions clearly.

Once the SSRI reaches therapeutic levels, which can take as long as 4 weeks, D.J. may start to feel like their "old self" and may be strong enough to begin processing their grief. They may recover from their need for the SSRI over time and use of the medication can then be discontinued.

(continues on page 370)

NURSING CARE GUIDE FOR D.J.: FLUOXETINE

Assessment: History and Examination

Allergies to fluoxetine or any other antidepressant SSRI, hepatic dysfunction, pregnancy or lactation, diabetes

Concurrent use of tricyclic antidepressants, cyproheptadine, lithium, MAOIs, benzodiazepines, alcohol, other SSRIs, NSAIDs and anticoagulants

CV: Blood pressure, pulse

CNS: Orientation, affect, reflexes, vision

Skin: Color, lesions, texture

Respiratory: Respiration, adventitious sounds

GI: Abdominal examination, bowel sounds

Laboratory tests: Hepatic function tests

Nursing Conclusions

Impaired comfort related to GI, GU, CNS effects

Altered thought processes related to CNS effects

Malnutrition risk related to GI effects

Knowledge deficiency regarding drug therapy

Planning

The patient will receive the best therapeutic effect from the drug therapy.

The patient will have limited adverse effects to the drug therapy.

The patient will have an understanding of the drug therapy, adverse effects to anticipate, and measures to relieve discomfort and improve safety.

Intervention

Administer drug in morning; divide doses if GI upset occurs.

Provide comfort, safety measures; small meals; void before dosing; side rails if dizziness occurs; limit dosage with patients who are potentially suicidal; consider lower dose with hepatic impairment.

Provide support and reassurance to help D.J. deal with drug effects (4-week delay in full effectiveness).

Provide patient teaching regarding drug dosage, adverse effect conditions to report, and the need to notify provider if they become pregnant.

Evaluation

Evaluate drug effects: relief of signs and symptoms of depression.

Monitor for adverse effects: sedation, dizziness, insomnia; respiratory dysfunction; GI upset; GU problems; rash; sexual dysfunction/decreased libido.

Monitor for drug–drug interactions.

Evaluate effectiveness of patient teaching program.

Evaluate effectiveness of comfort and safety measures.

PATIENT TEACHING FOR D.J.

- The drug that has been prescribed is called a selective serotonin reuptake inhibitor (SSRI). SSRIs change the concentration of serotonin (5HT) in specific areas of the brain. An increase in 5HT level is believed to relieve depression.
- The drug should be taken once a day in the morning. If your dosage has been increased or if you are having stomach upset, the dose may be divided.
- It may take as long as 4 weeks before you feel the full effects of this drug. Continue to take the drug every day during that time so that the concentration of the drug in your body eventually reaches effective levels.
- Common side effects of SSRIs include the following:
  - Dizziness, drowsiness, nervousness, and insomnia: If these effects occur, avoid driving or performing hazardous or delicate tasks that require concentration.
  - Nausea, vomiting, and weight loss: Small frequent meals may help. Monitor your weight loss; if it becomes excessive, consult your health care provider.
  - Sexual dysfunction and flulike symptoms: These effects may be temporary. Consult with your health care provider if these conditions become bothersome.
  - Report any of the following conditions to your health care provider: Rash mania, seizures, severe weight loss, increasing depression or thoughts of suicide.
- Tell your physicians, nurses, and other health care providers that you are taking this drug. Keep this drug and all medications out of the reach of children and pets. If you think that you are pregnant or would like to become pregnant, consult with your health care provider; there is a pregnancy registry into which patients who are pregnant patients can enroll.

Key Points

- The SSRIs prevent the reuptake of serotonin into the presynaptic nerve, leading to an accumulation of these biogenic amines in the synaptic cleft. This accumulation causes increased stimulation of the postsynaptic nerve and may be responsible for the antidepressant effects of these drugs.
- The SSRIs are not associated with many of the CNS, CV, and anticholinergic effects of other antidepressants.
- Combination of SSRIs with other SSRIs or with other drugs that are known to increase 5HT levels increases the risk of serotonin syndrome.
- SSRIs may take weeks for clinical effects to be apparent. Patients should be monitored for risk of increased depression and/or suicidal thoughts/behaviors.

Serotonin-Norepinephrine Reuptake Inhibitors (SNRIs)

The **serotonin-norepinephrine reuptake inhibitors (SNRIs)** work by decreasing the neuronal reuptake of both serotonin and norepinephrine and more weakly inhibit dopamine. This classification of medications may be more effective for treating depression than other antidepressants for some people. They should be used before MAOIs or TCAs due to fewer side effects. As with the other antidepressants, these drugs have a boxed warning to be alert for the possibility of increased suicidality, especially in children, adolescents, and young adults. The SNRIs are desvenlafaxine (*Pristiq*), duloxetine (*Cymbalta*), levomilnacipran (*Fetzima*), milnacipran (*Savella*), and venlafaxine (*Effexor, Effexor XR*). See Table 21.5 for usual indications.

Table 21.5 *Drugs in Focus:* Serotonin–Norepinephrine Reuptake Inhibitors

Drug Name	Dosage/Route	Usual Indications
desvenlafaxine (*Pristiq*)	50 mg/d PO with or without food, range 50–400 mg/d	Treatment of major depressive disorder in adults
duloxetine (*Cymbalta*)	20 mg/d PO b.i.d., up to 60 mg/d may be needed; may be given as a single daily dose	Treatment of major depressive disorder, neuropathic pain, fibromyalgia
levomilnacipran (*Fetzima*)	40 to 120 mg PO once daily without or without food	Treatment of major depressive disorder in adults
milnacipran (*Savella*)	12.5 mg/d PO, increase over a week to 50 mg PO b.i.d., up to 200 mg/d has been used	Management of fibromyalgia in adults
venlafaxine (*Effexor, Effexor XR*)	75 mg/d PO in divided doses to 375 mg/d; 75 mg/d PO sustained release formulation to a maximum 225 mg/d; reduce dose with hepatic and renal impairment	Treatment and prevention of depression in generalized anxiety disorder; social anxiety disorder; decreases addictive behavior

Therapeutic Actions and Indications

The SNRIs increase the levels of both serotonin and norepinephrine in the synaptic cleft. Some may weakly inhibit dopamine reuptake as well. They do not inhibit MAO. They are all indicated for treatment of major depressive disorder except for milnacipran. Milnacipran is approved for management of fibromyalgia in adult patients. The SNRIs often will not have therapeutic effect for 4 to 6 weeks.

Pharmacokinetics

The SNRIs are readily absorbed from the GI tract, metabolized in the liver, and excreted in the urine. The half-lives vary, so dosing can vary from once to twice a day.

Contraindications and Cautions

The SNRIs are contraindicated in the presence of allergy to any of the drugs. The drugs should not be used in conjunction with MAOIs due to risk of hypertensive crisis and serotonin syndrome. Caution should be used with patients who are severely depressed or suicidal, especially children, adolescents, and young adults, because of risk of increased suicidality. Patients should be screened for bipolar disease and risk of seizures before starting these medications. There is no clear evidence of whether the SNRIs will cause significant congenital abnormalities; however, there is some evidence of increased risk of pulmonary and cardiac problems in newborns exposed to SNRIs in third trimester. The medications should only be used if benefits to the parent clearly outweigh the potential risks to the fetus. The SNRIs are present in human milk, so a parent who is breast or chestfeeding may need to select a different method of feeding.

Adverse Effects

The adverse effects associated with the SNRIs are related to the effects on 5HT and NE levels. Some of the most common side effects are nausea, constipation, dizziness, headache, higher heart rates, hyperhidrosis, erectile dysfunction, decreased libido, tachycardia, vomiting, and palpitations. There is a risk of serotonin syndrome, hypertension, abnormal bleeding, angle closure glaucoma, and urinary retention.

Clinically Important Drug–Drug Interactions

Because of the increased risk of serotonin syndrome when SNRIs are used with MAOIs, the combination should be avoided. There is increased risk of side effects when coadministered with SSRIs or TCAs. Any substance that is serotonergic (including triptans, tricyclics, fentanyl, lithium, tramadol, tryptophan, buspirone, amphetamines, and St. John's wort) can increase the risk of serotonin syndrome. There is increased risk of bleeding if these medications are combined with aspirin, NSAIDs, antiplatelet drugs, or other drugs that affect coagulation.

Prototype Summary: Duloxetine

Indications: Treatment of depression, anxiety disorder, diabetic peripheral neuropathic pain, fibromyalgia, and chronic musculoskeletal pain.

Actions: Inhibits CNS neuronal reuptake of 5HT and norepinephrine with less potent inhibition of dopamine reuptake.

Pharmacokinetics:

Route	Onset	Peak
Oral	Slow	6–8 h

$T_{1/2}$: 8 to 17 hours; metabolized in the liver; excreted in the urine and feces.

Adverse Effects: Nausea, dry mouth, dizziness, blurred vision, somnolence, constipation, anorexia, hyperhidrosis, fatigue, vomiting, weight loss, rash, hepatotoxicity, orthostatic hypotension.

Key Points

- The SNRIs prevent the reuptake of primarily serotonin and norepinephrine to the presynaptic neuron, which increases the effect of the neurotransmitters.
- The side effects of this classification are related to potential serotonergic and noradrenergic activity.
- They have a boxed warning about increased risk of suicide thoughts and behaviors in children, adolescents, and young adults.

Nursing Considerations for Patients Receiving Selective Serotonin Reuptake Inhibitors (SSRIs) or Serotonin-Norepinephrine Reuptake Inhibitors (SNRIs)

Assessment: History and Examination

Assess for any known allergies to SSRIs or SNRIs to avoid hypersensitivity reactions; severe depression or suicidality, angle-closure glaucoma, and bipolar disorder, which could be exacerbated by these drugs; impaired liver function, which could alter metabolism of the drug; and diabetes mellitus. Find out whether patients are pregnant or breast or chestfeeding because there is a pregnancy registry that monitors pregnancy outcomes in patients who take antidepressants during pregnancy.

Assess temperature and weight; skin color and lesions; affect, orientation, and reflexes; vision; blood pressure and pulse; respiratory rate and adventitious sounds; and bowel sounds on abdominal examination for baseline status before beginning therapy and for any potential adverse effects. Also obtain renal and liver function tests.

Refer to "Critical Thinking Scenario" for a full discussion of nursing care for a patient who is dealing with depression.

Nursing Conclusions

Nursing conclusions related to drug therapy might include the following:

- Impaired comfort related to GI, GU, and CNS effects
- Altered thought processes and altered sensory perception (kinesthetic, tactile) related to CNS effects
- Malnutrition risk related to GI effects
- Knowledge deficiency regarding drug therapy

Planning

- The patient will receive the best therapeutic effect from the drug therapy, relief of depression.
- The patient will have limited adverse effects to the drug therapy.
- The patient will have an understanding of the drug therapy, adverse effects to anticipate, and measures to relieve discomfort and improve safety.

Intervention With Rationale

- Consider lower dose in older adult patients and in those with hepatic impairment because of the potential for severe adverse effects.
- Monitor the patient for up to 4 weeks to ascertain the onset of full therapeutic effect before adjusting dose.
- Establish suicide precautions for patients who are severely depressed, and limit the quantity of the drug dispensed to decrease the risk of overdose to cause harm.
- Administer the drug once a day in the morning to achieve optimal therapeutic effects unless the patient benefits from a sedative effect by taking at night. If dose is increased or if the patient is having severe GI effects, the dose can be divided. Serious name confusion has been reported with some of the SSRIs.
- Discuss potential for decreased sexual function and strategies for coping with any of those adverse effects.
- Provide comfort measures to help the patient tolerate drug effects. These may include taking food with the drug if GI upset is severe, dosing at night if sedating, or dosing in the morning if restlessness/insomnia occurs.
- Provide thorough patient teaching, including the drug name, prescribed dosage, measures for avoidance of adverse effects, and warning signs that may indicate possible problems. Instruct patients about the need for periodic monitoring and evaluation to enhance patient knowledge about drug therapy and to promote adherence.
- Offer support and encouragement to help the patient cope with the disease and the drug regimen.

Evaluation

- Monitor patient response to the drug (alleviation of signs and symptoms of depression, OCD, bulimia, panic disorder).
- Monitor for adverse effects of SSRIs (sedation, dizziness, GI upset, respiratory dysfunction, GU problems, skin rash, sexual dysfunction) or SNRIs (nausea, constipation, higher heart rates, hyperhidrosis, erectile dysfunction, tachycardia, vomiting, and palpitations). There is a risk of serotonin syndrome with both classifications of medications.
- Evaluate the effectiveness of the teaching plan (patient can give the drug name, dosage, possible adverse effects to watch for, specific measures to help avoid adverse effects, importance of continued follow-up, and importance of avoiding pregnancy).
- Monitor the effectiveness of comfort measures and adherence to the regimen.

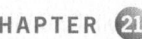

Table 21.6 *Drugs in Focus:* Other Antidepressants

Drug Name	Dosage/Route	Usual Indications
bupropion (*Wellbutrin, Wellbutrin SR, Wellbutrin XL, Zyban*)	300 mg/d PO given in three doses or 150 mg PO b.i.d. in sustained release form or 150–300 mg/d as a single dose of extended-release form	Treatment of depression in adults, smoking cessation
mirtazapine (*Remeron*)	15 mg/d PO, may be increased to a maximum of 45 mg/d; reduce dose in older adult patients and those with renal or hepatic dysfunction	Treatment of depression in adults
nefazodone (generic)	100 mg PO b.i.d., to a maximum of 600 mg/d; reduce dose in older adults	Treatment of depression in adults
trazodone (generic)	150 mg/d PO in divided doses; up to 600 mg/d, reduce dose with the older adults *Pediatric:* 1.5–2 mg/kg/d PO in divided doses; do not exceed 6 mg/kg/d	Treatment of depression in adults and children 6–18 y

Other Antidepressants

Some other effective antidepressants do not fit into any of the three groups that have been discussed in this chapter. These drugs have varying effects on NE, 5HT, and dopamine. Although it is not known how their actions are related to clinical efficacy, these agents may also be effective in treating depression in patients who do not respond to other antidepressants. As with the other antidepressants, these drugs have a boxed warning to be alert for the possibility of increased suicidality, especially in children, adolescents, and young adults. Other antidepressants include the following (see Table 21.6 for usual indications).

Bupropion (*Wellbutrin, Zyban*) weakly blocks the reuptake of NE and dopamine. At lower doses, this drug is effective in smoking cessation. It is well absorbed from the GI tract, metabolized in the liver, and excreted in the urine. There is a pregnancy registry to enroll pregnant patients that will gather data on effects of the medication on the pregnancy. No major adverse effects have been found on a developing fetus to date. The drug is available in a sustained release formulation as well as an extended-release formula, which some patients find to be more convenient.

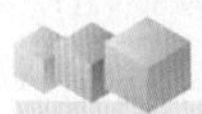

Concept Mastery Alert

Client Assessment

For clients taking bupropion who have denied a history of depression, it is important to know whether the client is in the process of quitting smoking. Bupropion (*Wellbutrin, Zyban*) weakly blocks the reuptake of norepinephrine and dopamine at lower doses. This drug is effective in clients undergoing smoking cessation.

Mirtazapine (*Remeron*) is indicated for treatment of major depression in adult patients. It is rapidly absorbed from the GI tract, extensively metabolized in the liver, and excreted in the urine. Mirtazapine has a half-life of 20 to 40 hours. Its mechanism of action is not completely understood but likely related to its ability to antagonize alpha2 receptors that increase both norepinephrine and serotonin in the CNS. It also antagonizes histamine receptors, which can cause somnolent effects. The adverse side effect of orthostatic hypotension may be due to its inhibitory effect on peripheral alpha1 receptors. There is a pregnancy registry to enroll pregnant patients that will gather data on effects of the medication on the pregnancy. No major adverse effects have been found on the developing fetus to date.

Nefazodone (generic) has a short half-life of 2 to 4 hours. It is well absorbed from the GI tract, metabolized in the liver, and excreted in the urine. It has been associated with severe liver toxicity in some patients; because of this, its use has become limited. Little is known about its effects during pregnancy and lactation, and it should be used during those times only if the benefit to the parent clearly outweighs the potential risk to the fetus or neonate.

Trazodone (generic), which blocks 5HT and some 5HT precursor reuptake, is effective in some forms of depression but has many adverse effects associated with its use (orthostatic hypotension, priapism, drowsiness, fatigue, syncope, and potential for cognitive and motor impairment). It is readily absorbed from the GI tract, extensively metabolized in the liver, and excreted in the urine and feces. There is a pregnancy registry to enroll pregnant patients that will gather data on effects of the medication on the pregnancy. No major adverse effects have been found on the developing fetus to date. A boxed warning has been added to this drug, cautioning about risk of and need for close monitoring of suicidal thoughts and behaviors in young adult patients; however, it is not approved for use in pediatric patients.

SUMMARY

- Depression is a very common affective disorder associated with many physical manifestations and is often misdiagnosed. It could be that depression is caused by a series of events that are not yet understood.

- Antidepressant drugs—TCAs, MAOIs, SSRIs, and SNRIs—increase the concentrations of the biogenic amines in the brain.
- Selection of an antidepressant depends on individual drug response and tolerance of associated adverse effects. The majority of patients will be treated with SSRIs or SNRIs. The adverse effects of TCAs are sedating and anticholinergic; those of MAOIs are CNS related and sympathomimetic. The adverse effects of SSRIs are fewer but may cause GI discomfort and sexual dysfunction. The SNRIs can have serotonergic and noradrenergic effects.
- Other antidepressants with unknown mechanisms of action are also effective in treating depression.
- All of these drugs have a boxed warning of the risk of suicidality, particularly in children, adolescents, and young adults.

CHECK YOUR UNDERSTANDING

Answers to the questions in this chapter can be found in Answers to Check Your Understanding Questions on thePoint®.

MULTIPLE CHOICE

Select the best answer.

1. The biogenic theory of depression states that depression is a result of
   a. an unpleasant childhood.
   b. gamma-aminobutyric acid (GABA) inhibition.
   c. deficiency of NE, dopamine, or 5HT in key areas of the brain.
   d. blockages within the limbic system, which controls emotions and affect.

2. When teaching a patient receiving TCAs, it is important to remember that TCAs are associated with many anticholinergic adverse effects. Teaching about these drugs should include anticipation of
   a. increased libido and increased appetite.
   b. polyuria and polydipsia.
   c. urinary retention, arrhythmias, and constipation.
   d. hearing changes, cataracts, and nightmares.

3. Adverse effects may limit the usefulness of TCAs with some patients. Nursing interventions that could alleviate some of the unpleasant aspects of these adverse effects include
   a. always administering the drug when the patient has an empty stomach.
   b. reminding the patient not to void before taking the drug.
   c. increasing the dose to override the adverse effects.
   d. taking the major portion of the dose at bedtime to avoid experiencing drowsiness and the unpleasant anticholinergic effects.

4. You might question an order for an MAOI as a first step in the treatment of depression remembering that these drugs are reserved for use in cases in which there has been no response to other agents because MAOIs
   a. can cause hair loss.
   b. are associated with potentially serious drug–food interactions.
   c. are mostly recommended for use in surgical patients.
   d. are more expensive than other agents.

5. Your patient is being treated for depression and is started on a regimen of fluoxetine (*Prozac*). They call you 10 days after the drug therapy has started to report that nothing has changed and they want to try a different drug. You should
   a. tell them to try sertraline (*Zoloft*) because some patients respond to one SSRI and not another.
   b. ask them to try a few days without the drug to see whether there is any difference.
   c. add an MAOI to their drug regimen to get an increased antidepressant effect.
   d. encourage them to keep taking the drug as prescribed because it usually takes up to 4 weeks to see the full antidepressant effect.

6. Which of the following medications is NOT indicated for obsessive–compulsive disorder, depression, and panic disorder?
   a. Citalopram (*Celexa*)
   b. Paroxetine (*Paxil*)
   c. Fluvoxamine (*Luvox*)
   d. Vortioxetine (*Brintellix*)

7. Venlafaxine (*Effexor*) is an antidepressant that might be very effective for use in patients who
   a. are being treated effectively with an SSRI.
   b. can tolerate multiple side effects.
   c. are reliable at taking multiple daily dosings.
   d. have not responded to other antidepressants and would benefit from once-a-day dosing.

8. Depression is an affective disorder that is
   a. always precipitated by a specific event.
   b. most common in patients with head injuries.
   c. characterized by overwhelming sadness, despair, and hopelessness.
   d. very evident and easy to diagnose in the clinical setting.

MULTIPLE RESPONSE

Select all that apply.

1. Depression is a common affective disorder that strikes many people. In assessing a client who might be suffering from depression, the nurse would expect to find which conditions?
   a. Lack of energy
   b. Hyperactivity
   c. Sleep disturbances
   d. Libido problems
   e. Confusion
   f. Decreased reflexes
2. A client reports that they think they are taking an antidepressant but are not sure. In reviewing their medication history, which drugs would be considered antidepressants?
   a. Tetracyclic drugs
   b. Cholinergics
   c. SSRIs
   d. MAOIs
   e. Angiotensin II receptor blockers
   f. Benzodiazepine

REFERENCES

American Psychiatric Association. (2010). *Practice guideline for the treatment of patients with major depressive disorder* (3rd ed.). American Psychiatric Association Publishing. https://psychiatryonline.org/pb/assets/raw/sitewide/practice_guidelines/guidelines/mdd.pdf

American Psychiatric Association. (2013). *Diagnostic and statistical manual of mental disorders* (5th ed.).

Brent, D. A. (2016). Antidepressants and suicidality. *Psychiatry Clinics of North America, 39*(3), 503–512. https://doi.org/10.1016/j.psc.2016.04.002

Brunton, L. L., Hilal-Dandan, R., & Knollman, B. C. (2018). *Goodman and Gilman's the pharmacological basis of therapeutics* (13th ed.). McGraw-Hill.

Courtet, P., & Lopez-Castroman, J. (2017). Antidepressants and suicide risk in depression. *World Psychiatry, 16*(3), 317–318. https://doi.org/10.1002/wps.20460

Häuser, W., Bernardy, K., Üçeyler, N., & Sommer, C. (2009). Treatment of fibromyalgia syndrome with antidepressants: A meta-analysis. *Journal of the American Medical Association, 301*(2), 198–209. https://doi.org/10.1001/jama.2008.944

Hendler, C. B. (Ed.) (2021). *Nursing 2021 drug handbook.* Wolters Kluwer.

Hengartner, M. P., & Plöderl, M. (2019). Newer-generation antidepressants and suicide risk in randomized controlled trials: A re-analysis of the FDA database. *Psychotherapy and Psychosomatics, 88*, 247–248. https://doi.org/10.1159/000501215

Nischal, A., Tripathi, A., Nischal, A., & Trivedi, J. K. (2012). Suicide and antidepressants: What current evidence indicates. *Mens Sana Monographs, 10*(1), 33–44. https://doi.org/10.4103/0973-1229.87287

Norris, M. M. (2013). Use of antidepressants during pregnancy and lactation. *Mental Health Clinician, 3*(2), 58–60. https://doi.org/10.9740/mhc.n163520

Norris, T. L. (2018). *Porth's pathophysiology: Concepts of altered health states* (10th ed.). Wolters Kluwer.

Rey, J. M., & Birmaher, B. (Eds.). (2009). *Treating child and adolescent depression.* Wolters Kluwer, Lippincott William & Wilkins.

Robinson, D. (2009). Antidepressant treatment and pregnancy: An update. *Primary Psychiatry, 16*(7), 19–22.

CHAPTER 22

Psychotherapeutic Agents

Learning Objectives

Upon completion of this chapter, you will be able to:

1. Define the term psychotherapeutic agent, and list conditions that the psychotherapeutic agents are used to treat.
2. Discuss the use of psychotherapeutic agents across the lifespan.
3. Describe the therapeutic actions, indications, pharmacokinetics, contraindications, most common adverse reactions, and important drug–drug interactions associated with each class of psychotherapeutic agent.
4. Compare and contrast the prototype drugs for each class of psychotherapeutic agent with other drugs in that class and with drugs in the other classes of psychotherapeutic agents.
5. Outline the nursing considerations and teaching needs for patients receiving each class of psychotherapeutic agents.

Key Terms

antipsychotic: drug used to treat disorders involving thought processes; dopamine receptor blocker that helps affected people to organize their thoughts and respond appropriately to stimuli

attention deficit hyperactivity disorder (ADHD): behavioral syndrome characterized by persistent behaviors demonstrating difficulty sustaining attention, hyperactivity, and impulsive behavior

bipolar disorder: behavioral disorder that involves extremes of depression alternating with hyperactivity, euphoria, and excitement

mania: state of hyperexcitability; one phase of bipolar disorder, which alternates between periods of severe depression and mania

narcolepsy: mental disorder characterized by daytime sleepiness and periods of sudden loss of wakefulness

neuroleptic: drug used to treat disorders that involve thought processes (e.g., schizophrenia); has many associated neurological adverse effects

schizophrenia: the most common type of psychosis; characteristics include hallucinations, paranoia, delusions, speech abnormalities, and affective problems

Drug List

ANTIPSYCHOTIC/NEUROLEPTIC DRUGS

Typical Antipsychotics

- chlorpromazine
- fluphenazine
- (P) haloperidol
- loxapine
- perphenazine
- pimozide
- prochlorperazine
- thioridazine
- thiothixene
- trifluoperazine

Atypical Antipsychotics

- aripiprazole
- asenapine
- brexpiprazole
- cariprazine
- (P) clozapine
- iloperidone
- lumateperone
- lurasidone
- olanzapine
- paliperidone
- quetiapine
- risperidone
- ziprasidone

DRUGS FOR BIPOLAR DISORDERS

- aripiprazole
- cariprazine
- (P) lithium
- lurasidone
- olanzapine
- quetiapine
- risperidone
- ziprasidone

DRUGS FOR ATTENTION DEFICIT HYPERACTIVITY DISORDER AND NARCOLEPSY

- armodafinil
- atomoxetine
- clonidine hydrochloride
- dexmethylphenidate
- dextroamphetamine
- guanfacine
- lisdexamfetamine
- (P) methylphenidate
- modafinil

The drugs discussed in this chapter are used to treat psychoses, perceptual and behavioral disorders. These psychotherapeutic agents are targeted at thought processes rather than affective states. Although they do not cure any psychotic disorders, psychotherapeutic agents do help both adult and pediatric patients function in a healthier manner, carry on activities of daily living, and increase their quality of life (Box 22.1).

Mental Disorders and Their Classifications

Mental disorders were once attributed to environmental influences and life experiences such as poor parenting or trauma. Mental disorders are now thought to be caused by some inherent dysfunction within the brain that leads to abnormal thought processes and responses. Most theories attribute these disorders to a chemical imbalance in specific areas within the brain. Diagnosis of a mental disorder is often based on distinguishing characteristics as described in the *Diagnostic and Statistical Manual of Mental Disorders*, 5th edition, text revision (DSM-IV-TR). Because no diagnostic laboratory tests are available, patient assessment and response must be carefully evaluated to determine the basis of a particular problem. Selected disorders are discussed here.

Schizophrenia, the most common type of psychosis, can be debilitating and prevent individuals from functioning in conventional society. Characteristics of schizophrenia can include positive or negative symptoms. Positive symptoms appear after the person has developed schizophrenia, and negative symptoms reflect more of what the person may lose after developing schizophrenia. Both positive and negative symptoms affect the person's thoughts and behaviors. The positive symptoms include hallucinations, paranoia, delusions, disorganized speech, and disorganized behavior. Negative symptoms reflect the absence of typical social behaviors; these symptoms can include avolition, apathy, lack of emotional expression, anhedonia, and mismatched affect. Schizophrenia, which seems to have a strong genetic association, may reflect a fundamental biochemical abnormality. It could be related to dysregulation of the dopamine and serotonin neurotransmitters.

Box 22.1 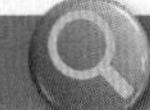 **Focus on Drug Therapy Across the Lifespan**

PSYCHOTHERAPEUTIC AGENTS

Children

Many of these agents are used in children, often in combination with other CNS drugs in an attempt to control symptoms and behavior. They can be indicated for treatment of symptoms of autism spectrum disorder, conduct disorder, attention deficit hyperactivity disorder (ADHD), and obsessive–compulsive disorders. Long-term effects of some of these agents are not known, and parents should be informed of this fact.

There are multiple antipsychotic medications that have specific dosing for children and adolescents. The child should be monitored carefully for adverse effects and developmental progress. Monitor for weight gain, impaired blood glucose control, hypercholesterolemia, orthostatic hypotension, tremor, agitation and/or sleep disturbance, neutropenia, effects of hyperprolactinemia, and anticholinergic effects.

Lithium does not have a recommended pediatric dose, and the drug should not ordinarily be used in children. If it is used, the dose should be carefully calculated from the child's age and weight and adjusted to maintain a level between 0.8 and 1.2 mEq/L. The child should be monitored closely for renal, CNS, CV, and endocrine function.

The CNS stimulants are often used in children to manage ADHD. Caution should be used with extended-release preparations because they differ markedly in timing and effectiveness. A baseline ECG should be done to rule out congenital heart problems. The child should be assessed carefully and challenged periodically for the necessity of continuing the drug. Treatment should be part of an interdisciplinary approach.

Adults

Adults using these drugs should be under regular care and should be monitored regularly for adverse effects. The QTc interval should be evaluated before thioridazine or ziprasidone is prescribed and periodically during use.

Patients receiving lithium should be encouraged to maintain hydration and salt intake. They need to understand the importance of periodic monitoring of their serum lithium level.

These drugs should be used cautiously during pregnancy and lactation because of the potential for adverse effects on the fetus or neonate. There is a pregnancy registry that monitors effects of the antipsychotic medications on pregnancy outcomes. Neonates exposed to antipsychotic medications during the third trimester are at risk for extrapyramidal and/or withdrawal symptoms after delivery. Patients who can become pregnant and who need to take lithium should be advised to use barrier contraceptives while taking the drug because of the potential for serious congenital abnormalities.

Older Adults

Older patients may be more susceptible to the adverse effects of these drugs. Patients need to be monitored closely for toxic effects and to provide safety measures if CNS effects do occur. They should not be used to control behavior with dementia.

Patients with renal impairment should be monitored closely while taking lithium. Decreased doses may be needed. Because many older patients may also have renal impairment, they need to be screened carefully. They should be urged to maintain hydration and salt intake, which can be a challenge with some older patients.

Prolongation of the QTc interval—associated with use of thioridazine or ziprasidone—may be a concern in older patients with coronary disease. Careful screening and monitoring should be done if these drugs are needed for such patients.

However, gamma-aminobutyric acid (GABA) may be deficient in the cortex of people diagnosed with schizophrenia. There are strong genetic links as well as environmental influences that are associated with increased risk of schizophrenia.

Bipolar disorder involves extremes of depression alternating with hyperactivity, euphoria, and excitement. There are four types of bipolar disorder. With bipolar I disorder, a person has one or more manic episodes alternating with major depression episodes. With bipolar II disorder, a person has a major depressive episode alternated with at least one hypomanic or less severe manic episode. Cyclothymia is similar to bipolar I, but with less severe symptoms. The rapid cycling type is characterized by a person having four or more manic episodes for at least 2 weeks in a year. This condition may reflect a biochemical imbalance followed by overcompensation on the part of neurons and their inability to reestablish stability. Causation is not completely understood, but there are genetic links.

Narcolepsy is characterized by daytime sleepiness and sudden periods of loss of wakefulness. This disorder may reflect problems with rapid eye movement (REM) sleep regulation, since REM sleep is noted to occur at sleep onset or within 10 to 15 minutes of sleep onset. A high rate of human leukocyte antigen (HLA) subtype DQB1-0602 has been shown in people who have narcolepsy. There is also some research that shows hypocretin 1 and 2 (neurotransmitters secreted by cells near the hypothalamus) may be deficient in people who suffer from narcolepsy with cataplexy (brief periods of muscle weakness often brought on by emotional situations). There may be an autoimmune process that causes the deficit in hypocretin neurons in people with the HLA DQB1-0602 allele.

Attention deficit hyperactivity disorder (ADHD) involves persistent behaviors demonstrating inattention, hyperactivity, and/or impulsivity that generally first emerge during childhood but can persist into adulthood. The exact pathophysiology is not known, but there is evidence of both genetic and environmental influences that cause alterations in the dopaminergic, serotonergic, and glutamatergic neurotransmitter systems. There may be an inflammatory component involved that precipitates alterations in the neurotransmitter systems and causes a reduction in cortical gray matter volume in specific areas of the brain.

Antipsychotic/Neuroleptic Drugs

The **antipsychotic** drugs, which are essentially dopamine receptor blockers, are used to treat disorders that involve thought processes. They help affected people to organize their thoughts and respond appropriately to stimuli. While the therapeutic effects may be due to blocking dopamine, these medications impact multiple other receptors, leading to many of their adverse effects. Because of their associated neurological adverse effects, these medications are also called **neuroleptic** agents. At one time, these drugs were known as major tranquilizers. However, that name is no longer used because the primary action of these drugs is not sedation but a change in neuron stimulation and response (Fig. 22.1).

Antipsychotics are classified as either typical or atypical. They are separated into these categories based on their mechanisms of action, which are described below. Typical antipsychotics include chlorpromazine (generic), fluphenazine (*Prolixin*), haloperidol (*Haldol*), loxapine (*Loxitane*), perphenazine (*Trilafon*), pimozide (*Orap*), prochlorperazine (generic), thiothixene (*Navane*), and trifluoperazine (generic). Atypical antipsychotics include aripiprazole (*Abilify*), asenapine (*Saphris*), brexpiprazole (*Rexulti*), cariprazine (*Vraylar*), clozapine (*Clozaril*), iloperidone (*Fanapt*), lumateperone (*Caplyta*), lurasidone (*Latuda*), olanzapine (*Zyprexa*, *Zyprexa Zydis*), paliperidone (*Invega*), quetiapine (*Seroquel*, *Seroquel XR*), risperidone (*Risperdal*, *Risperdal Consta*), and ziprasidone (*Geodon*). Table 22.1 lists both typical and atypical antipsychotic agents, including the specific type and the occurrence of sedation and other adverse effects.

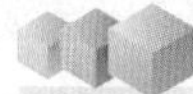
Concept Mastery Alert

Potency in Antipsychotic Medications

A highly potent antipsychotic agent can evoke a given effect with relatively low concentrations or doses. A medication with lower potency requires higher concentrations to evoke the same response.

Therapeutic Actions and Indications

The typical antipsychotic drugs block dopamine receptors, preventing the stimulation of the postsynaptic neurons by dopamine. They depress the reticular activating system (RAS), limiting the stimuli coming into the brain. They also have anticholinergic, antihistamine, and alpha-adrenergic blocking effects, all related to the blocking of the dopamine receptor sites. Newer atypical antipsychotics block both dopamine and serotonin receptors. This dual action may help alleviate some of the unpleasant neurological effects and depression associated with the typical antipsychotics (see Table 22.1).

The antipsychotics are indicated for schizophrenia and for manifestations of other psychotic disorders, including hyperactivity, combative behavior, and severe behavioral problems in children (short-term control); some of them are also approved for the treatment of bipolar disorder and/or major depressive disorder. Chlorpromazine, one of the older antipsychotics, is also used to decrease preoperative restlessness and apprehension; to treat intermittent porphyria; as an adjunct in the treatment of tetanus; and to control nausea, vomiting, and intractable hiccups. Haloperidol is frequently used to treat acute psychiatric

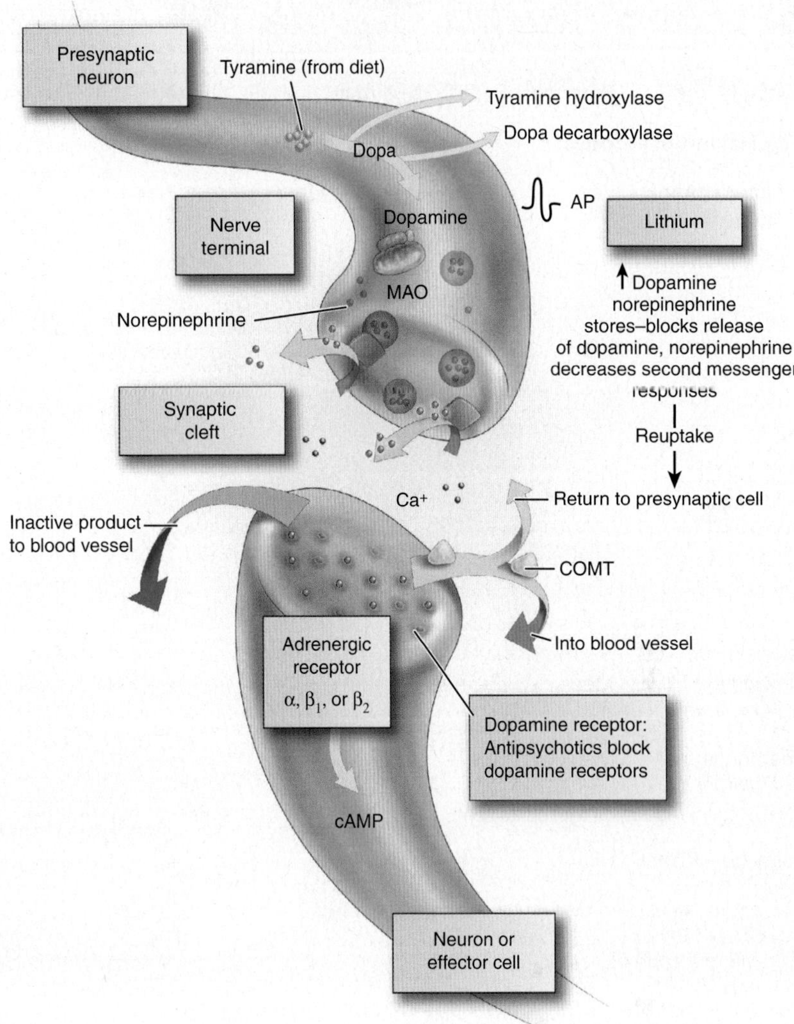

FIGURE 22.1 Sites of action of the drugs used to treat mental disorders: antipsychotics, central nervous system (CNS) stimulants, lithium. AP, action potential; COMT, catechol-*O*-methyltransferase; cAMP, cyclic adenosine monophosphate.

situations and is available for intravenous (IV) use when prolonged parenteral therapy is required because of swallowing difficulties or the acuity of the behavioral problems.

Prochlorperazine is also frequently used to control severe nausea and vomiting associated with surgery and chemotherapy. It has the advantage of being available in oral, rectal, and parenteral forms. Aripiprazole is indicated for treating schizophrenia, major depressive disorder, bipolar disorders, irritability associated with autism spectrum disorder, and Tourette's syndrome. It can be administered parenterally for the treatment of acute agitation associated with schizophrenia or bipolar mania. Lurasidone and lumateperone are indicated for treatment of schizophrenia in adults. Olanzapine and ziprasidone are also used for bipolar disorders and parenterally to treat acute agitation. Quetiapine is also approved for short-term treatment of acute manic episodes associated with bipolar disease. Risperidone is used frequently to treat irritability and aggression associated with autism spectrum disorder in children and adolescents, as well as for acute manic episodes of bipolar disorder. Paliperidone is now also approved for treatment of schizoaffective disorders. Brexpiprazole is indicated for treatment of schizophrenia and adjunctive therapy with antidepressants for major depressive disorder. Cariprazine is approved for treating schizophrenia in adults and acute treatment of bipolar I disorder. Any of these drugs may be effective in a particular patient; the selection of a specific drug depends on the desired potency and patient tolerance of the associated adverse effects. A patient who does not respond to one drug may react successfully to another agent. To determine the best therapeutic regimen for a particular patient, it may be necessary to try more than one drug.

Pharmacokinetics

The antipsychotics are erratically absorbed from the gastrointestinal (GI) tract, depending on the drug and the preparation of the drug. Intramuscular (IM) doses provide four to five times the active dose as oral doses, and caution is required when switching between routes. The antipsychotics are widely distributed in the tissues; they

Table 22.1 *Drugs in Focus:* Antipsychotic/Neuroleptic Drugs

		Common Side Effects				
Drug Name	**Potency**	**Sedation**	**Anticholinergic**	**Hypotension**	**Extrapyramidal**	**Usual Dosage**
Typical Antipsychotics						
chlorpromazine (generic)	Low	+ + + +	+ + +	+ + +	+ +	*Adult:* 25 mg IM for acute episode, may be repeated; switch to 25–50 mg PO t.i.d. *Pediatric:* 0.5–1 mg/kg q4–8h PO, IM, or PR
fluphenazine (*Prolixin*)	High	+	+	+	+ + + +	*Adult:* 0.5–10 mg/d PO in divided doses; 1.25–10 mg/d IM in divided doses *Geriatric:* 1–2.5 mg/d PO, adjust dose based on response
haloperidol (*Haldol*)	High	+	+/–	+	+ + + +	*Adult:* 0.5–2 mg PO t.i.d. *or* 2–5 mg IM, may be repeated in 1 h, 4–8 h more common *Geriatric:* Reduce dose *Pediatric (3–12 y):* 0.5 mg/d PO; 0.05–0.075 mg/kg/d PO for Tourette's syndrome and behavioral syndromes
loxapine (*Loxitane*)	Medium	+ + +	+ +	+ +	+ + +	*Adult:* 20–60 mg/d PO; 12.5–50 mg IM or IV for acute states
perphenazine (*Trilafon*)	Medium	+ +	+	+ +	+ + +	*Adult:* 4–8 mg PO t.i.d. *or* 5–10 mg IM q6h; switch to oral as soon as possible *Geriatric:* 1/2–1/3 of adult dose
pimozide (*Orap*)	High	+	+	+ +	+ + +	*Adult:* 1–2 mg/d PO in divided doses *Pediatric (> 12 y):* 0.05 mg/kg PO at bedtime; do not exceed 10 mg/d
prochlorperazine (generic)	Low	+	+ +	+	+ + +	*Adult:* 5–10 mg PO t.i.d. to q.i.d.; 10–20 mg IM for acute states *Geriatric:* Reduce dose *Pediatric:* 2.5 mg PO t.i.d.; 0.03 mg/kg IM for acute states; 20–25 mg/d PR
thioridazine (generic)	Low	+ + + +	+ + +	+ + +	+	*Adult:* 50–100 mg PO t.i.d., monitor QTc intervals *Pediatric:* up to 3 mg/kg/d PO
thiothixene (*Navane*)	High	+	+	+	+ + + +	*Adult:* 2 mg PO t.i.d.; up to a maximum 60 mg/d in severe cases
trifluoperazine (generic)	High	+	+	+	+ + + +	*Adult:* 2–5 mg PO b.i.d.; 1–2 mg IM q4–6h in severe cases *Geriatric:* Reduce dose *Pediatric (6–12 y):* 1 mg PO daily or b.i.d.: 1 mg IM daily or b.i.d. for severe cases
Atypical Antipsychotics						
aripiprazole (*Abilify*)	Medium	+	+	+ +	+	*Adult:* 10–15 mg/d PO *Pediatric (13–17 y):* 10–30 mg/d PO
brexpiprazole (*Rexulti*)	High	+		+/–	+	*Adult:* 0.5–1 mg/d PO initially; may titrate to a maximum of 3–4 mg/d PO; reduce dose with hepatic or renal impairment
cariprazine (*Vraylar*)	High	+	+	+	+ + +	*Adult:* 1.5 mg PO daily initial; may titrate up to 6 mg/d PO

Table 22.1 *Drugs in Focus:* Antipsychotic/Neuroleptic Drugs (*Continued*)

Drug Name	Potency	Common Side Effects: Sedation	Anticholinergic	Hypotension	Extrapyramidal	Usual Dosage
clozapine (*Clozaril*)	Low	+ + + +	+ +	+ + +	+/–	*Adult:* Initially 25 mg PO b.i.d. to t.i.d.; up to 500 mg/d; available only through the *Clozaril* Patient Management System, which monitors white blood cell count and adherence issues, only 1-wk supply given at a time
lumateperone (*Caplyta*)	Low	+ +	+ +	+/–	+	*Adult:* 42 mg/d PO w/food
luracidono (*Latuda*)	Low	I I	I I	I	I	*Adult:* 40 mg/d PO with food, titrotcd to a maximum 80 mg/d; do not exceed 40 mg/d with renal or hepatic dysfunction
olanzapine (*Zyprexa, Zyprexa Zydis*)	High	+ + + +	+ +	+ + +	+	*Adult:* 5–10 mg/d PO, up to 20 mg/d PO for bipolar mania; available in disintegrating tablets, which can be taken without swallowing
paliperidone (*Invega*)	Medium	+	+	+ +	+ +	*Adult:* 6 mg/d PO; maximum dose 12 mg/d *Renal impairment:* Maximum dose 6 mg/d with moderate impairment, maximum dose 3 mg/d with severe impairment
quetiapine (*Seroquel, Seroquel XR*)	Medium	+ + + +	+ +	+ +	+/–	*Adult:* Initially 25 mg PO b.i.d., up to 300–400 mg/d; 400–900 mg/d PO (XR) *Geriatric, hepatic impairment, or hypotensives:* Reduce dose and titrate very slowly
risperidone (*Risperdal, Risperdal Consta*)	High	+ + +	+	+ +	+ +	*Adult:* 1 mg PO b.i.d. up to 8 mg/d *or* 25 mg IM once every 2 wk *Pediatric 10–17 y:* 0.5–6 mg/d PO (bipolar disorders) *13–17 y:* 1–6 mg/d PO (schizophrenia) *Geriatric, renal impaired, or hypotensives:* 0.5 mg PO b.i.d. initially, titrate slowly
ziprasidone (*Geodon*)	Medium	+ + +	+ +	+	+	*Adult:* 20–80 mg PO b.i.d.; rapid control of as-stated behavior 10–20 mg IM (maximum dose 40 mg/d IM); monitor QTc intervals

Each plus sign indicates increased incidence of the given adverse effect.
XR, extended release.

are often stored there and are released for up to 6 months after the drug is stopped. They are metabolized in the liver and excreted through the bile and urine. Children tend to metabolize these drugs faster than do adults, and older adult patients tend to metabolize them more slowly, making it necessary to carefully monitor these patients and adjust doses as needed. Clinical effects may not be seen for several weeks, and patients should be encouraged to continue taking the drugs even if they see no immediate effects. The antipsychotics cross the placenta and enter human milk (see "Contraindications and Cautions").

Contraindications and Cautions

Antipsychotic drugs are contraindicated in the presence of underlying diseases that could be exacerbated by the dopamine-blocking effects of these drugs, such as Parkinson's disease. Most of the antipsychotic medications have been shown to prolong the QTc interval, leading to increased risk of serious cardiac arrhythmias, so QTc may need to be monitored in at-risk patients. Antipsychotics are contraindicated for use in older adult patients with dementia because this use is associated with an increased risk of cardiovascular (CV) events and death. Antipsychotics have a boxed warning on the prescribing information outlining this safety information and contraindication. Despite this warning, antipsychotics are still prescribed in this population.

Some of the antipsychotic medications have anticholinergic effects; caution should be used in the presence of medical conditions that could be exacerbated by the anticholinergic effects of the drugs, such as glaucoma, peptic ulcer, and urinary or intestinal obstruction. In addition, care should be taken in patients with seizure disorders because the threshold for seizures could be lowered by some antipsychotic medications. Caution should be taken with patients with active alcohol use disorder because of potentiation of the central nervous system (CNS) depression. There are fewer cautions and contraindications with the atypical medications compared to the typical antipsychotics. There is a pregnancy exposure registry that monitors pregnancy outcomes with use of atypical antipsychotic medications. There is evidence that neonates exposed to antipsychotic medications in the third trimester have risk of extrapyramidal effects and/or withdrawal symptoms. Because children are more apt to develop dystonia from the drugs, which could confuse the diagnosis of Reye's syndrome, caution should be used with children younger than 12 years of age who have a CNS infection or chickenpox. The use of antipsychotics may result in bone marrow suppression, leading to blood dyscrasias, so care should be taken with patients who are immunosuppressed and those who have cancer.

Adverse Effects

The adverse effects associated with the antipsychotic drugs are related to their dopamine-blocking, anticholinergic, antihistamine, and alpha-adrenergic activities. The most common CNS effects are sedation, weakness, tremor, drowsiness, and extrapyramidal side effects (pseudoparkinsonism, dystonia, akathisia, tardive dyskinesia). There are prescription medications designed to treat tardive dyskinesia symptoms (Box 22.2). Neuroleptic malignant syndrome is a rare but potentially fatal side effect that is manifested by hyperpyrexia, muscle rigidity, altered mental status, and autonomic instability. See Box 22.3 for more details regarding this adverse effect (see also Fig. 22.2). Anticholinergic effects include dry mouth, nasal congestion, flushing, constipation, urinary retention, impotence, glaucoma, blurred vision, and photophobia. Blocking of dopamine leads to an increase in prolactin levels and subsequent gynecomastia (breast development and occasionally milk production). Patients should be advised of that possibility. CV effects, which are probably related to the dopamine-blocking effects, include hypotension, orthostatic hypotension, cardiac arrhythmias, congestive heart failure, and pulmonary edema. Several of these agents (haloperidol, thioridazine, mesoridazine, ziprasidone) are associated with prolongation of the QTc interval, which could lead to serious or even fatal cardiac arrhythmias. Patients receiving these drugs should have a baseline and periodic electrocardiogram (ECG) during therapy. All of the atypical antipsychotics include warnings that there is a risk for the development of diabetes mellitus and weight gain when these drugs are used (Fig. 22.3). Ziprasidone has been associated with serious to fatal skin reactions and the systemic symptoms of DRESS (drug reaction with eosinophilia and systemic symptoms). Consequently, when patients are maintained on any of the atypical antipsychotics, they should be monitored regularly for the signs and symptoms of diabetes mellitus.

Respiratory effects such as laryngospasm, dyspnea, and bronchospasm may also occur. In addition, bone marrow suppression is a possibility with some antipsychotic agents. The phenothiazines (chlorpromazine, fluphenazine, prochlorperazine, promethazine, and thioridazine) often turn the urine pink to reddish brown as a result of their excretion. Although this effect may cause great patient concern, it has no clinical significance.

Box 22.2 Focus on Safe Medication Administration

MANAGING TARDIVE DYSKINESIA

There are two medications that are approved to treat one of the side effects of the antipsychotic medications, tardive dyskinesia. They are deutetrabenazine (*Austedo*) and valbenazine (*Ingrezza*) and are both vesicular monoamine transporter 2 inhibitors. These transporters are important for dopamine release, and modulating them has been shown to help with tardive dyskinesia symptoms. Deutetrabenazine is also indicated to treat chorea associated with Huntington's disease. There is a boxed warning with this medication cautioning about increased risk of depression and suicidal thoughts/behavior in patients with Huntington's disease.

Box 22.3 Focus on Safe Medication Administration

MANAGING NEUROLEPTIC MALIGNANT SYNDROME

Neuroleptic malignant syndrome is a rare but potentially life-threatening adverse effect of the antipsychotic medications. It is thought to be related to the blockade of dopamine receptors that triggers in some people excessive calcium release from the sarcoplasmic reticulum of the skeletal muscle cells. The signs/symptoms include sudden high-grade fever, blood pressure fluctuations, dysrhythmias including extreme tachycardia, muscle rigidity, sweating, and change in level of consciousness that can lead to coma and death. Males are at higher risk than females, and there is a genetic component. Nursing interventions include stopping the medication that triggered the syndrome, cooling the patient with ice packs and/or cool fluids, and administering antipyretic medication. The patient will require close monitoring of vital signs and mental status. Medication such as dantrolene can be administered to decrease muscle rigidity. The patient may also require medications to treat dysrhythmias.

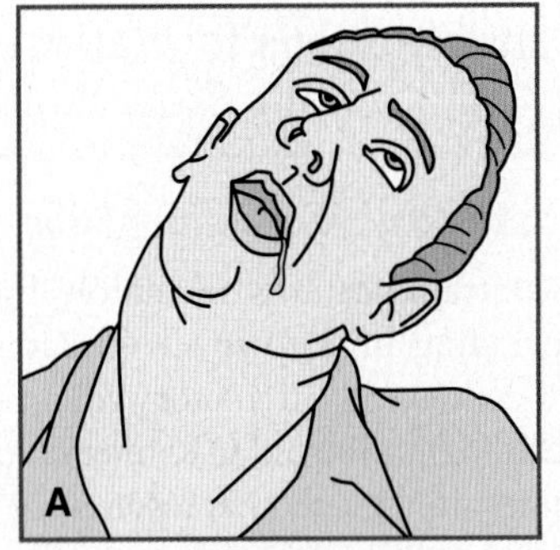

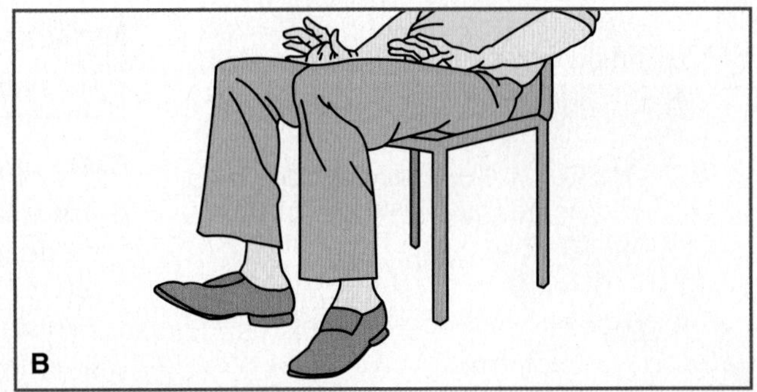

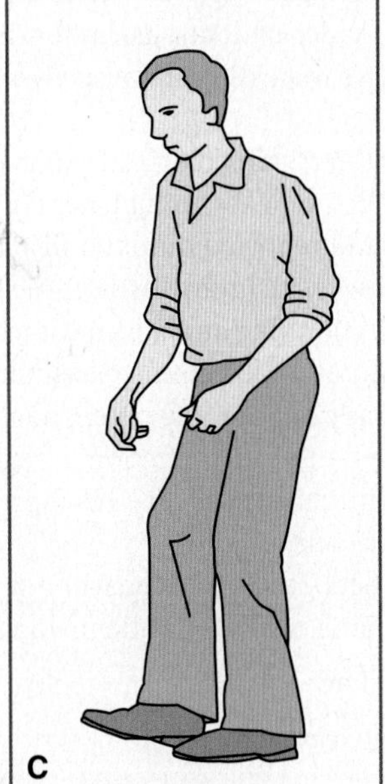

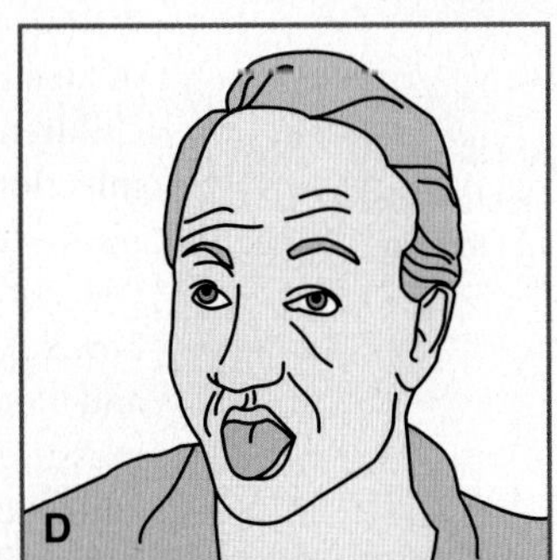

FIGURE 22.2 Neuroleptic malignant syndrome, a common neurological effect of antipsychotic drugs. **A.** Dystonia—spasms of the tongue, neck, back, and legs. Spasms may cause unnatural positioning of the neck, abnormal eye movements, excessive salivation. **B.** Akathisia—continuous restlessness, inability to sit still. Constant moving, foot tapping, hand movements may be seen. **C.** Pseudoparkinsonism—muscle tremors, cogwheel rigidity, drooling, shuffling gait, slow movements. **D.** Tardive dyskinesia—abnormal muscle movements such as lip smacking, tongue darting, chewing movements, slow and aimless arm and leg movements.

Clinically Important Drug–Drug Interactions

Antipsychotic–alcohol (or other CNS depressant) combinations result in an increased risk of CNS depression, and antipsychotic–anticholinergic combinations lead to increased anticholinergic effects, so dose adjustments may be necessary. Patients who take either of these combinations should be monitored closely for adverse effects, and supportive measures should be provided. Patients should be monitored closely if taking thioridazine or ziprasidone with any other drug that is associated with prolongation of the QTc interval.

Prototype Summary: Haloperidol

Indications: Treatment of patients with schizophrenia.

Actions: Blocks central type 2 dopamine receptors in the brain; some but minimal anticholinergic, antihistaminic, alpha$_1$-adrenergic blocking activity.

Pharmacokinetics:

Route	Onset	Peak	Duration
Oral	30–60 min	2–4 h	Varies
Intramuscular	10–15 min	15–20 min	About 4 wk
Intravenous	Immediate	After administration	4–6 h

$T_{1/2}$: 14 to 26 hours (IV), 21 hours (IM), 14 to 37 hours (oral); metabolized extensively in the liver; excreted in the urine and feces.

Adverse Effects: Drowsiness, insomnia, vertigo, extrapyramidal symptoms, orthostatic hypotension, photophobia, blurred vision, dry mouth, nausea, vomiting, anorexia, urinary retention, photosensitivity, prolonged QT interval, neuroleptic malignant syndrome.

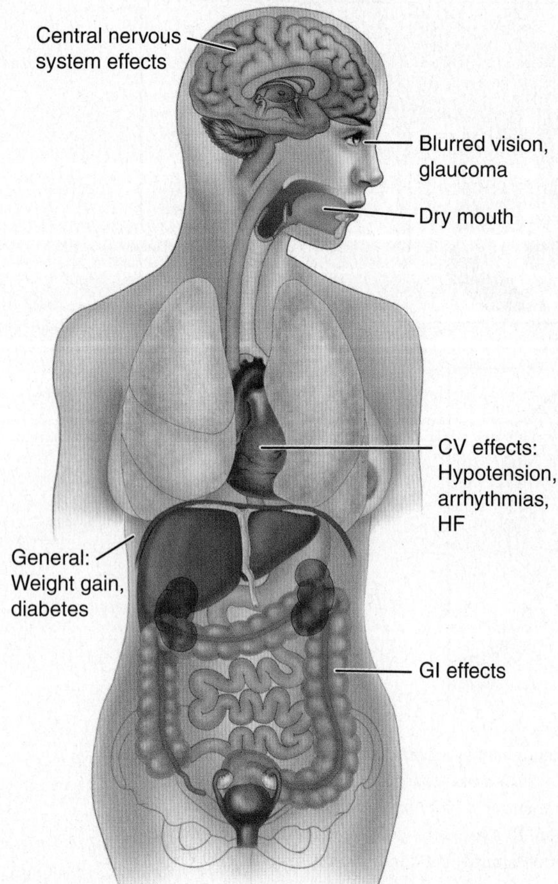

FIGURE 22.3 Adverse effects and toxicities associated with psychotherapeutic agents.

Prototype Summary: Clozapine

Indications: Management of severely ill patients with schizophrenia who are unresponsive to standard drugs; reduction of risk of recurrent suicidal behavior in patients with schizophrenia or schizoaffective disorder.

Actions: Blocks dopamine and serotonin receptors; depresses the RAS; anticholinergic, antihistaminic, alpha-adrenergic blocking.

Pharmacokinetics:

Route	Onset	Peak	Duration
Oral	Varies	1–6 h	Weeks

$T_{1/2}$: 4 to 12 hours; metabolized in the liver; excreted in the urine and feces.

Adverse Effects: Drowsiness, sedation, seizures, dizziness, syncope, headache, tachycardia, nausea, vomiting, fever, neuroleptic malignant syndrome, neutropenia, orthostatic hypotension, seizures, myocarditis, cardiomyopathy.

Nursing Considerations for Patients Receiving Antipsychotic/Neuroleptic Drugs

Assessment: History and Examination

- Assess for contraindications or cautions for the use of the drug including any known allergies to these drugs, severe CNS depression, circulatory collapse, cardiac disease including prolonged QTc interval or congenital, severe hypotension, glaucoma, respiratory depression, diabetes, urinary or intestinal obstruction, seizure disorder, bone marrow suppression, and pregnancy or lactation. In older patients, assess for dementia. In children younger than 12 years of age, screen for CNS infections.
- Assess temperature; skin color and lesions; CNS orientation, affect, reflexes, and bilateral grip strength; bowel sounds and reported output; pulse, auscultation, and blood pressure, including orthostatic blood pressure; respiration rate and adventitious sounds; and urinary output to determine baseline status before beginning therapy and for any potential adverse effects. Also obtain liver and renal function tests, blood glucose levels, thyroid function tests, ECG if appropriate, and complete blood count (CBC).

Refer to the "Critical Thinking Scenario" for a full discussion of nursing care for a patient who is prescribed antipsychotic drugs.

Nursing Conclusions

Nursing conclusions related to drug therapy might include the following:

- Impaired physical mobility related to extrapyramidal effects
- Fall risk related to orthostatic hypotensive effects
- Injury risk related to CNS effects and sedation
- Urinary retention and constipation risk related to anticholinergic effects
- Knowledge deficiency regarding drug therapy

Planning

- The patient will receive the best therapeutic effect from the drug therapy.
- The patient will have limited adverse effects to the drug therapy.
- The patient will have an understanding of the drug therapy, adverse effects to anticipate, and measures to relieve discomfort and improve safety.

Intervention With Rationale

- Do not allow the patient to crush or chew sustained-release capsules, which will speed up their absorption and may cause toxicity.
- If administering parenteral forms, keep the patient recumbent for 30 minutes to reduce the risk of orthostatic hypotension.

- Consider warning the patient or the patient's guardians about the risk of development of tardive dyskinesias and other extrapyramidal side effects with continued use so they are able to recognize and report any changes to the provider.
- To prevent undue stress, caution the patient/guardians about the risk of gynecomastia and sexual dysfunction when using these drugs.
- Teach comfort strategies for coping with the anticholinergic effects (dry mouth, photophobia) to enhance medication adherence.
- Monitor CBC to arrange to discontinue the drug at signs of bone marrow suppression.
- Monitor blood glucose levels with long-term use to detect the development of glucose intolerance.
- Arrange for gradual dose reduction after long-term use. Abrupt withdrawal has been associated with gastritis, nausea, vomiting, dizziness, arrhythmias, and insomnia.
- Provide positioning of legs and arms to decrease the discomfort of dyskinesias.
- Provide sugarless candy and ice chips to increase secretions, and provide frequent mouth care to prevent dry mouth from becoming a problem.
- If CNS effects or orthostatic hypotension occurs, provide safety measures such as side rails and assistance with ambulation to prevent patient injury.
- Provide for vision examinations to determine ocular changes and arrange appropriate dose change.
- Provide thorough patient teaching, including drug name, prescribed dosage, measures for avoidance of adverse effects, caution that it may take weeks to see the desired clinical effects, warning signs that may indicate possible problems, and the need for monitoring and evaluation to enhance patient knowledge about drug therapy and to promote adherence. (Refer to "Critical Thinking Scenario.") Warn the patient that their urine may have a pink to reddish-brown color.
- Offer support and encouragement to help the patient to cope with the drug regimen.

Evaluation

- Monitor patient response to the drug (decrease in signs and symptoms of psychotic disorder).
- Monitor for adverse effects (sedation, anticholinergic effects, orthostatic hypotension, extrapyramidal effects, bone marrow suppression).
- Evaluate the effectiveness of the teaching plan (the patient can give the drug name and dosage, possible adverse effects to watch for, specific measures to prevent adverse effects, and warning signs to report).
- Monitor the effectiveness of comfort measures and adherence to the regimen.

CRITICAL THINKING SCENARIO
Antipsychotic Drugs

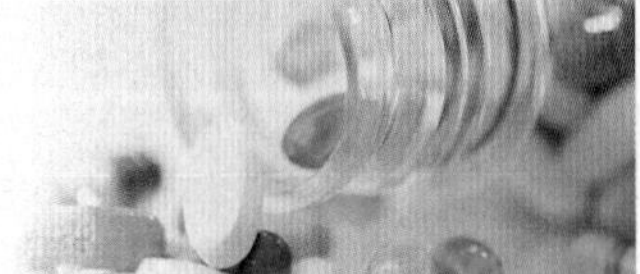

THE SITUATION

B.A., a 36-year-old single professional, was diagnosed with schizophrenia as a senior in high school. B.A.'s condition has been well controlled with chlorpromazine (generic), and they are able to maintain steady employment, live in their own home, and carry on a fairly active social life. At their last evaluation, B.A. appeared to be developing bone marrow suppression, and their physician decided to try to taper the drug dosage. As the dosage was being lowered, B.A. became withdrawn and listless, missed several days of work, and canceled most social engagements. Afraid of interacting with people, B.A. stayed in bed most of the time. B.A. reported having thoughts of death and paranoid ideation about their neighbors that B.A. was beginning to think might be true.

CRITICAL THINKING

What nursing interventions are appropriate at this time?
What supportive measures might be useful to help B.A. cope with this crisis and allow them to function normally again?
What happens to brain chemistry after long term therapy with phenothiazines?
What drug options should be tried?
Are there any other options that might be useful?

DISCUSSION

Schizophrenia is not a disorder that can be resolved simply with proper counseling. B.A., an educated person with a long history of taking phenothiazines, realizes the necessity of drug therapy to correct the chemical imbalance in their brain. They may need an antipsychotic to return to the level of functioning they had reached before experiencing this setback. B.A.'s knowledge of their individual responses can be used to help select an appropriate drug and dosage. Their experiences may also facilitate care planning and a new drug regimen.

B.A. will need support to cope with problems at work, to address their inability to go in to work, to cope with feelings about not meeting social obligations, and to find the motivation to get up and become active again. B.A. might do well with behavior modification techniques that give them some control over their activities and

(continues on page 386)

allow them to use their knowledge and experience with their own situation to their advantage in forming a new medical regimen. B.A. may need support in explaining the problem to their employer and social contacts in ways that will help B.A. avoid the prejudice associated with mental illness and will allow them every opportunity to return to a regular routine as soon as they can.

Because it may take several months to find the drug or drugs that will bring B.A. back to a point of stabilization, it is important to have a consistent, reliable health care team in place to support them through this stabilization period. B.A. should have a reliable contact person to call when they have questions and when they need support.

NURSING CARE GUIDE FOR B.A.: ANTIPSYCHOTIC/ NEUROLEPTIC DRUGS

Assessment: History and Examination

Allergies to any of these drugs, CNS depression, CV disease, pregnancy or lactation, myelography, glaucoma, hypotension, thyrotoxicosis, seizures

Concurrent use of anticholinergics, barbiturate anesthetics, alcohol, meperidine, beta-blockers, epinephrine, norepinephrine

CV: Blood pressure, pulse, orthostatic blood pressure

CNS: Orientation, affect, reflexes, vision

Skin: Color, lesions, texture

Respiratory: Respiration, adventitious sounds

GI: Abdominal examination, bowel sounds

Laboratory tests: Thyroid, liver, and renal function tests; CBC

Nursing Conclusions

Impaired activity related to extrapyramidal effects

Injury risk related to CNS effects

Altered tissue perfusion related to CV effects

Urinary retention and constipation related to anticholinergic effects

Knowledge deficiency regarding drug therapy

Planning

The patient will receive the best therapeutic effect from the drug therapy.

The patient will have limited adverse effects to the drug therapy.

The patient will have an understanding of the drug therapy, adverse effects to anticipate, and measures to relieve discomfort and improve safety.

Intervention

Instruct the patient to swallow sustained-release capsules whole without chewing or crushing.

Provide comfort and safety measures: Provide sugarless lozenges, mouth care; institute safety measures if CNS effects occur; position patient to relieve dyskinesia discomfort; taper dosage after long-term therapy.

Provide support and reassurance to help the patient cope with drug effects.

Teach the patient about drug, dosage, adverse effects, conditions to report, and precautions.

Evaluation

Evaluate drug effects: relief of signs and symptoms of psychotic disorders.

Monitor for adverse effects: sedation, dizziness, insomnia; anticholinergic effects; extrapyramidal effects; bone marrow suppression; skin rash; neuroleptic malignant syndrome.

Monitor for drug–drug interactions as listed.

Evaluate effectiveness of the patient teaching program.

Evaluate effectiveness of comfort and safety measures.

PATIENT TEACHING FOR B.A.

- The drugs that are useful for treating schizophrenia are called antipsychotic or neuroleptic drugs. These drugs affect the activities of certain chemicals in your brain and are used to treat certain mental disorders.
- Drugs in this group should be taken exactly as prescribed. Because these drugs affect many body systems, it is important that you have medical checkups regularly.
- Common effects of these drugs include the following:
  - Dizziness, drowsiness, and fainting: Avoid driving or performing hazardous tasks or delicate tasks that require concentration if these occur. Change position slowly. The dizziness usually passes after 1 to 2 weeks of drug use.
  - Pink or reddish urine (with phenothiazines): These drugs sometimes cause urine to change color. Do not be alarmed by this change; it does not mean that your urine contains blood.
  - Sensitivity to light: Bright light might hurt your eyes, and sunlight might burn your skin more easily. Wear sunglasses and protective clothing when you must be out in the sun.
  - Constipation: Consult with your health care provider if this becomes a problem.
- Report any of the following conditions to your health care provider: Sore throat, fever, rash, tremors, weakness, and vision changes.
- Tell any doctor, nurse, or other health care provider that you are taking this drug.
- Keep this drug and all medications out of the reach of children.
- Avoid the use of alcohol or other depressants while you are taking this drug. You also may want to limit your use of caffeine if you feel very tense or cannot sleep.
- Avoid the use of over-the-counter drugs while you are on this drug. Many of them contain ingredients that could interfere with the effectiveness of your drug. If you feel that you need one of these preparations, consult with your health care provider about the most appropriate choice.
- Take this drug exactly as prescribed. If you run out of medicine or find that you cannot take your drug for any reason, consult your health care provider. After this drug has been used for a period of time, additional adverse effects may occur if it is suddenly stopped. This drug dosage will need to be tapered over time.

Key Points

- Mental disorders are thought process disorders that may be caused by some inherent dysfunction within the brain. A psychosis is a thought disorder. Schizophrenia is the most common psychosis; delusions and hallucinations are hallmarks.
- Antipsychotic drugs are generally dopamine receptor blockers that are effective in helping people organize thought patterns and respond appropriately to stimuli.
- Antipsychotics can cause hypotension, anticholinergic effects, sedation, and extrapyramidal effects, including parkinsonism, dystonia, akathisia, and tardive dyskinesia.

Drugs for Bipolar Disorders

Mania, a state of hyperexcitability at the opposite pole from depression, occurs in people with bipolar disorder who experience a period of depression followed by a period of mania. The cause of mania is not completely understood, but it is thought to be an instability of certain neurons in the brain. The traditional treatment of mania has been lithium (*Lithobid*). Today, many other drugs are used successfully in treating bipolar disorder, including aripiprazole (*Abilify*), cariprazine (*Vraylar*), lurasidone (*Latuda*), olanzapine (*Zyprexa, Zyprexa Zydis*), quetiapine (*Seroquel*), risperidone (*Risperdal*), and ziprasidone (*Geodon*), which are atypical antipsychotics (see Table 22.2). There are also several antiepileptic agents that are indicated for treatment of bipolar disorder; these are discussed in greater detail in Chapter 23.

Lithium salts (*Lithobid*) are taken orally for the management of manic episodes and prevention of future episodes. These potentially toxic drugs can cause severe CNS, renal, and pulmonary problems that may lead to death. Despite the potential for serious adverse effects, lithium is used, albeit with caution, because it is consistently effective in the treatment of mania. The therapeutically effective serum level is 0.6 to 1.2 mEq/L.

Therapeutic Actions and Indications

Lithium functions in several ways. It alters sodium transport in nerve and muscle cells, inhibits the release of

Table 22.2 ***Drugs in Focus:*** **Drugs for Bipolar Disorders**

Drug Name	Typical Adult Dosage/Route	Usual Indications
aripiprazole (*Abilify*)	Initial 2–15 mg/d PO; may be titrated to maximum of 10–30 mg/d PO based on response and indication	Treatment of acute manic and mixed episodes of bipolar disorder in adults and pediatric patients; treatment of schizophrenia in adolescents and adults; treatment of major depressive disorder as adjunct to antidepressants in adults; irritability with autism spectrum disorder in pediatric patients, Tourette's syndrome
cariprazine (*Vraylar*)	Initial 1.5 mg/d PO; max dose for bipolar 3 mg/d PO	Treatment of schizophrenia, bipolar mania, and bipolar depression in adults
lithium salts (*Lithobid*)	600 mg PO t.i.d. for acute episodes; 300 mg PO t.i.d. to q.i.d. for maintenance; reduce dose with older patients	Treatment of manic episodes of manic-depressive or bipolar disorder; maintenance therapy to prevent or diminish the frequency and intensity of future manic episodes; currently being studied for improvement of neutrophil counts in patients with cancer chemotherapy-induced neutropenia and as prophylaxis of cluster headaches and migraine headaches; not recommended for children <12 y
lurasidone (*Latuda*)	Initial 20–40 mg/d PO; titrated to 40–160 mg/d PO; adjust doses for renal and hepatic impairment	Treatment of schizophrenia in adults and adolescents, bipolar I disorder in adult and pediatric patients
olanzapine (*Zyprexa, Zyprexa Zydis*)	10 mg/d PO; range 5–20 mg/d	Management of acute manic episodes associated with bipolar disorder, in combination with lithium or valproate, or as monotherapy
quetiapine (*Seroquel*)	50 mg PO b.i.d., titrate to a maximum 800 mg/d	Adjunct or monotherapy for the treatment of manic episodes associated with bipolar disorder
risperidone (*Risperdal*)	Initial 2 mg/d PO; dose adjustments needed with severe renal or hepatic dysfunction	Treatment of schizophrenia, acute manic or mixed episodes with bipolar I disorder as monotherapy or with lithium, irritability associated with autism spectrum disorder
ziprasidone (*Geodon*)	40 mg PO b.i.d. with food; maximum 80 mg b.i.d.	Treatment of acute manic and mixed episodes of bipolar disorder

norepinephrine and dopamine (but not serotonin) from stimulated neurons, increases the intraneuronal stores of norepinephrine and dopamine slightly, and decreases intraneuronal content of second messengers. This last mode of action may allow it to selectively modulate the responsiveness of hyperactive neurons that might contribute to the manic state. Although the biochemical actions of lithium are known, the exact mechanism of action in decreasing the manifestations of mania is not understood.

Pharmacokinetics

Lithium is readily absorbed from the GI tract and reaches peak level in 30 minutes to 3 hours. It follows the same distribution pattern in the body as water. It slowly crosses the blood–brain barrier, so toxic effects may be delayed. Lithium is excreted from the kidney, though about 80% is reabsorbed. During periods of sodium depletion or dehydration, the kidney reabsorbs more lithium into the serum, often leading to toxic levels. Therefore, patients must be encouraged to maintain consistent hydration while taking this drug. Lithium crosses the placenta, enters human milk, and has been associated with congenital abnormalities (see "Contraindications and Cautions").

Contraindications and Cautions

Lithium is contraindicated in the presence of hypersensitivity to lithium to prevent hypersensitivity reactions. In addition, it is contraindicated in the following conditions: Significant renal or cardiac disease that could be exacerbated by the toxic effects of the drug; a history of leukemia; metabolic disorders, including sodium depletion; dehydration; and diuretic use because lithium decreases sodium reabsorption and severe hyponatremia may occur. (Hyponatremia leads to lithium retention and toxicity.)

Pregnancy and lactation are also contraindications because of the potential for adverse effects on the fetus or neonate; breast or chestfeeding should be discontinued while using lithium, and patients who can become pregnant should be advised to use birth control while taking this drug. Caution should be used in any condition that could alter sodium levels, such as protracted diarrhea or excessive sweating; in suicidal or impulsive patients; and in patients who have infection with fever, which could be exacerbated by the toxic effects of the drug.

Adverse Effects

The adverse effects associated with lithium are often directly related to serum levels of the drug. There is risk of weight gain, renal toxicity, and goiter and hypothyroidism with long-term use.

- Serum levels of less than 1.5 mEq/L: CNS problems, including lethargy, slurred speech, muscle weakness, and fine tremor; polyuria, which relates to renal toxicity; and beginning of gastric toxicity, with nausea, vomiting, and diarrhea
- Serum levels of 1.5 to 2 mEq/L: Intensification of all of the foregoing reactions, with ECG changes demonstrating bradycardia and sometimes Brugada's syndrome
- Serum levels of 2 to 2.5 mEq/L: Possible progression of CNS effects to ataxia, clonic movements, hyperreflexia, and seizures; possible CV effects such as severe ECG changes and hypotension; large output of dilute urine secondary to renal toxicity; fatalities secondary to pulmonary toxicity
- Serum levels greater than 2.5 mEq/L: Complex multiorgan toxicity with a significant risk of death

Clinically Important Drug–Drug Interactions

There are many medication interactions that are clinically relevant. It is recommended that all medications that a patient is taking be evaluated for potential effects on serum lithium level. A lithium–haloperidol combination may result in an encephalopathic syndrome, consisting of weakness, lethargy, confusion, tremors, extrapyramidal symptoms, leukocytosis, and irreversible brain damage. Lithium may prolong effects of neuromuscular-blocking agents. Use of lithium with other serotonergic medications can trigger serotonin syndrome. See Box 22.4 for a serious lithium–herbal interaction.

If lithium is given with carbamazepine, increased CNS toxicity may occur, and a lithium–iodide salt combination results in increased risk of hypothyroidism. Patients who receive either of these combinations should be monitored carefully. In addition, a thiazide diuretic–lithium combination increases the risk of lithium toxicity because of the loss of sodium and increased retention of lithium. If this combination is used, the dose of lithium should be decreased, and the patient should be monitored closely.

In the following instances, the serum lithium level should be monitored closely and appropriate dose adjustments made. With the combination of lithium and some urine-alkalinizing drugs, including antacids and tromethamine, there is a possibility of decreased effectiveness of lithium. If lithium is combined with indomethacin or with some nonsteroidal antiinflammatory drugs, higher plasma levels of lithium occur.

Box 22.4 Focus on Herbal and Alternative Therapies

PSYLLIUM

Patients being treated with lithium should be encouraged not to use the herbal therapy psyllium, which is used to treat constipation and to lower cholesterol levels. If this agent is combined with lithium, the absorption of the lithium may be blocked, and the patient will not receive a therapeutic level. If the patient feels a need for a drug to relieve constipation or is concerned about their cholesterol level, they should be encouraged to discuss alternative measures with their health care provider.

Prototype Summary: Lithium

Indications: Treatment of manic episodes of bipolar disorder and maintenance treatment of bipolar disorder.

Actions: Alters sodium transport in nerve and muscle cells; inhibits the release of norepinephrine and dopamine (but not serotonin) from stimulated neurons; increases the intraneuronal stores of norepinephrine and dopamine slightly; and decreases the intraneuronal content of second messengers.

Pharmacokinetics:

Route	Onset	Peak	Duration
Oral	Unknown	0.5–3 h	8–12 h
Oral, extended release	Unknown	4–12 h	12–18 h

$T_{1/2}$: 24 hours; excreted in the urine.

Adverse Effects: CNS problems, including lethargy, slurred speech, muscle weakness, and fine tremor; polyuria, gastric toxicity, with nausea, vomiting, and diarrhea progressing; renal toxicity; CV collapse, com. Adverse effects are related to serum drug level.

Nursing Considerations for Patients Receiving Lithium

Assessment: History and Examination

- Assess for contraindications or cautions for the use of the drug, including any known allergies to lithium; renal or CV disease; dehydration; sodium depletion, use of diuretics, protracted sweating, or diarrhea; suicidal ideation or impulsiveness in patients with severe depression; pregnancy or lactation; and infection with fever.
- Assess temperature; skin color and lesions; CNS orientation, affect, and reflexes; bowel sounds and reported output; pulse, auscultation, and blood pressure, including orthostatic blood pressure; respiration rate and adventitious sounds; and urinary output for baseline status before beginning therapy and for any potential adverse effects. Also obtain liver and renal function tests, thyroid function tests, CBC, and baseline ECG, and obtain serum lithium levels. Often levels will need to be monitored with every dosage change, and there should be periodic monitoring even with stable dosing therapy.

Nursing Conclusions

Nursing conclusions related to drug therapy might include the following:

- Impaired comfort related to GI, CNS, and vision effects
- Injury risk related to CNS effects
- Impaired urinary elimination related to renal toxic effects
- Altered thought processes related to CNS effects
- Knowledge deficiency regarding drug therapy

Planning

- The patient will receive the best therapeutic effect from the drug therapy.
- The patient will have limited adverse effects to the drug therapy.
- The patient will have an understanding of the drug therapy, adverse effects to anticipate, and measures to relieve discomfort and improve safety.

Intervention With Rationale

- Administer drug cautiously, with frequent monitoring of serum lithium level, to patients with significant renal or CV disease, dehydration, or debilitation, as well as those taking diuretics to monitor for toxic levels and to arrange for appropriate dose adjustment.
- Administer drug with food or milk to alleviate GI irritation if GI upset is severe.
- Arrange to decrease dose after treatment of acute manic episodes. Lithium tolerance is greatest during acute episodes and decreases when the acute episode is over.
- Ensure that the patient maintains adequate intake of salt and fluid to decrease toxicity. Teach the patient about risk of dehydration in hot weather and in conjunction with exercise.
- Monitor the patient's clinical status closely, especially during the initial stages of therapy, to provide appropriate supportive management and dosage titrations as needed. Hemodialysis can be instituted if severe toxicity occurs.
- Arrange for small, frequent meals; sugarless lozenges to suck; and frequent mouth care to increase secretions and decrease discomfort as needed.
- If CNS effects occur, provide safety measures such as side rails and assistance with ambulation to prevent patient injury.
- Provide thorough patient teaching, including drug name, prescribed dosage, measures for avoidance of adverse effects, cautions that it may take time to see the desired therapeutic effects, warning signs that may indicate possible problems, and the need to avoid pregnancy while taking lithium to enhance patient knowledge about drug therapy and to promote adherence.
- Offer support and encouragement to help the patient to cope with the drug regimen.

Evaluation

- Monitor patient response to the drug (decreased manifestations and frequency of manic episodes).

(continues on page 390)

- Monitor for adverse effects (CV toxicity, renal toxicity, GI upset, respiratory complications, CNS changes).
- Evaluate effectiveness of the teaching plan (patient can give the drug name and dosage and describe the possible adverse effects to watch for, specific measures to help avoid adverse effects, warning signs to report, and the need to avoid pregnancy).
- Monitor effectiveness of comfort measures and adherence to the regimen.

Key Points

- Lithium, a membrane stabilizer, is the traditional antimanic drug. Because it can accumulate and cause severe toxicity, its serum level must be carefully monitored.
- Many other CNS drugs, including many of the atypical antipsychotics, are now approved for use in bipolar disorder. Many patients respond to a combination of these drugs to control their bipolar signs and symptoms.

Drugs for Attention Deficit Hyperactivity Disorder and Narcolepsy

CNS stimulants are commonly used to treat both ADHD and narcolepsy. Paradoxically, these drugs calm hyperkinetic children and help them focus on one activity for a longer period. They also redirect and excite the arousal stimuli from the RAS (Fig. 22.4; see also Fig. 22.1). The CNS stimulants that are used to treat ADHD and narcolepsy include methamphetamine hydrochloride (*Desoxyn*), several formulations of amphetamine (*Adderall XR, Adzenys ER, Dyanavel XR, Evekeo ODT, Mydayis*); methylphenidate (*Ritalin, Concerta,* and others); dexmethylphenidate (*Focalin*), an isomer of methylphenidate used in lower doses than methylphenidate; dextroamphetamine (*Dexedrine*); lisdexamfetamine (*Vyvanse*), an amphetamine; modafinil (*Provigil*), which is not associated with many of the systemic stimulatory effects of some of the other CNS stimulants; armodafinil (*Nuvigil*), which is thought to act through dopaminergic mechanisms but is not associated with the cardiac and systemic stimulatory effects seen with other CNS stimulants; and atomoxetine (*Strattera*), which is a selective norepinephrine reuptake inhibitor with anticholinergic effects but without the CV and stimulatory effects, making it preferable in patients who cannot tolerate the systemic stimulatory effects. There are also alpha$_2$-adrenergic agonists that are indicated for treatment of ADHD: guanfacine (*Intuniv*) and clonidine hydrochloride (*Kapvay*). Chapter 30 discusses the alpha$_2$-adrenergic agonists in more detail (Table 22.3).

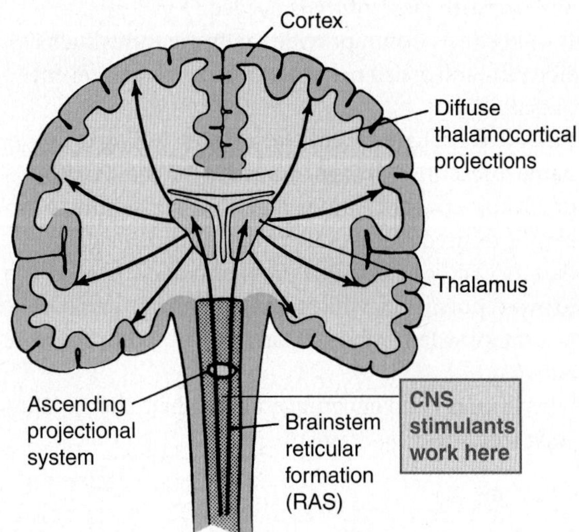

FIGURE 22.4 Site of action of the central nervous system (CNS) stimulants in the reticular activating system (RAS).

Therapeutic Actions and Indications

The CNS stimulants possibly act by increasing the release of catecholamines from presynaptic neurons, leading to an increase in stimulation of the postsynaptic neurons. The paradoxical effect of calming hyperexcitability through CNS stimulation seen in ADHD is not completely understood. The amphetamine stimulants block the reuptake of norepinephrine and dopamine in the presynaptic neuron and also increase more of their release.

The CNS stimulants are indicated, as part of a comprehensive treatment program, for the treatment of ADHD, as well as for narcolepsy and improvement of wakefulness in people with various sleep disorders. Most of these drugs are controlled substances, and it is important to include that point in the teaching plan; the drugs should be secured at home to prevent inappropriate use or distribution. In 2015, lisdexamfetamine was also approved for the treatment of binge-eating disorders in adults; it carries a warning that it is not approved as a weight loss agent and that there is high potential for misuse and dependence.

Pharmacokinetics

These drugs are rapidly absorbed from the GI tract, reaching peak level in 2 to 4 hours. They are metabolized in the liver and excreted in the urine, with half-lives ranging from 2 to 15 hours, depending on the drug. Premature delivery and low birth weight have been noted for infants born to people taking amphetamines. There is a pregnancy registry available to monitor fetal outcomes due to unknown risk of major congenital anomalies or miscarriage.

Contraindications and Cautions

The CNS stimulants are contraindicated in the presence of known allergy to the drug, which could lead to hypersensitivity reactions. Other contraindications include the

Table 22.3 *Drugs in Focus:* Drugs for Attention Deficit Hyperactivity Disorder and Narcolepsy

Drug Name	Dosage/Route	Usual Indications
amphetamine (*Adderall XR, Adzenys ER, Dyanavel XR, Evekeo ODT, Mydayis*)	Varies per formulation. Starts low with slow titrations; some will need dose modification for renal impairment	Treatment of ADHD
armodafinil (*Nuvigil*)	150–250 mg/d PO as a single dose in the morning *Shift work sleep disorder:* 150 mg/d PO at 1 h before the start of shift	Management of patients with obstructive sleep disorders (including sleep apnea), narcolepsy, and shift work sleep disorders to improve wakefulness
atomoxetine (*Strattera*)	*Adults and children >70 kg:* 40 mg/d PO, slowly increase to a target daily dose of 80 mg *Children ≤70 kg:* 0.5 mg/kg/d, increase to a target daily dose of 1.2 mg/kg/d *Hepatic impairment:* Decrease dose by 50%	Treatment of ADHD as part of a total treatment program
clonidine hydrochloride (*Kapvay*)	Start with 0.1 mg HS PO. Increase daily dosage in increments of 0.1 mg/d at weekly intervals to max of 0.4 mg/d. Take twice a day with either higher or equal dose at bedtime. Taper slowly when discontinuing	Treatment of ADHD
dexmethylphenidate (*Focalin*)	2.5–5 mg PO b.i.d.; do not exceed 10 mg PO b.i.d.	Treatment of ADHD in patients aged ≥6 y
dextroamphetamine (*Dexedrine*)	*Narcolepsy:* 5–60 mg/d PO in divided doses *Attention deficit disorders:* 2.5–5 mg/d PO taken in the morning *Obesity:* 5–30 mg/d PO (not recommended for children <12 y)	Treatment of narcolepsy, ADHD, behavioral syndromes, exogenous obesity
guanfacine (*Intuniv*)	*Children 6–17 y:* 1 mg/d PO, ER tablet, may be titrated to maximum 7 mg/d (0.05–0.12 mg/kg target weight-based dose range). Taper when discontinuing	Treatment of ADHD in ER tablet form
lisdexamfetamine (*Vyvanse*)	*Pediatric (6–12 y):* 30 mg/d PO; maximum dose 70 mg/d	Treatment of ADHD in children 6–12 y of age
methamphetamine (*Desoxyn*)	*Pediatric (>6 y):* 5–10 mg/d PO in one or two doses/d; may increase by 5 mg at weekly intervals as needed; usual effective dose 20–5 mg/d PO	Treatment of ADHD in children aged >6 y
methylphenidate (*Ritalin, Concerta*, and others)	*Adult:* 10–60 mg/d PO in divided doses, depending on preparation *Pediatric:* 5 mg PO b.i.d.; increase gradually, do not exceed 60 mg/d	Treatment of ADHD and other behavioral syndromes associated with hyperactivity, as well as narcolepsy; currently available in various forms allowing for dosing one, two, or three times a day
modafinil (*Provigil*)	200 mg/d PO as a single dose; reduce dose with hepatic impairment and in the older adults	Treatment of narcolepsy in adults, for improving wakefulness in various sleep disorders, and for improving wakefulness in people with obstructive sleep apnea/hypopnea syndrome

ER, extended release; ADHD, attention deficit/hyperactivity disorder.

following conditions: marked anxiety, agitation, tension, severe fatigue, or glaucoma, which could be exacerbated by the CNS stimulation caused by these drugs; and cardiac disease, which could be aggravated by the stimulatory effects of these drugs, making it important to rule out congenital heart problems.

Caution should be used in patients with a history of seizures, which could be potentiated by the CNS stimulation; in patients with a history of drug dependence, including alcohol use disorder, because these drugs may result in physical and psychological dependence; and in patients with hypertension, which could be exacerbated by the stimulatory effects of these drugs. Caution should be used with these medications during pregnancy, and it is not recommended that patients breast or chestfeed if taking the CNS stimulants.

Adverse Effects

The adverse effects associated with these drugs are related to the CNS stimulation they cause. CNS effects can include nervousness, insomnia, dizziness, headache, blurred vision, and difficulty with accommodation. GI effects such as anorexia, nausea, growth suppression, and weight loss may occur. CV effects can include hypertension, arrhythmias, and angina. Sudden cardiac death has been associated with the use of these drugs. Studies have shown that the majority of these deaths occurred in children with undocumented cardiac defects; because of this, a baseline ECG should be done before beginning therapy. Skin rashes are a common reaction to some of these drugs. Physical and psychological dependence may also develop. Because CNS stimulants have this effect, many of the drugs are controlled substances. Atomoxetine, which does not show dependence development, is not a controlled substance. The adverse effects associated with this drug are mainly anticholinergic (dry mouth, constipation, nausea, urinary hesitancy). Guanfacine and clonidine may cause sedation, dry mouth, constipation, hypotension, bradycardia, and impotence, but these drugs have not been associated with risk of dependence.

Clinically Important Drug–Drug Interactions

The combination of a CNS stimulant with a monoamine oxidase inhibitor leads to increased risk of adverse effects and increased toxicity and should be avoided if possible.

In addition, the combination of CNS stimulants with tricyclic antidepressants or phenytoin leads to a risk of increased drug levels. Patients who receive such a combination should be monitored for toxicity.

Caffeine and some over-the-counter cold medications also may increase the CNS stimulant effects.

Prototype Summary: Methylphenidate

Indications: Narcolepsy and ADHD.

Actions: Mild cortical stimulant with CNS actions similar to those of amphetamines.

Pharmacokinetics:

Route	Onset	Peak	Duration
Oral	Varies	1–3 h (short-acting) or 12 h (long-acting)	4–6 h (short-acting) or 24 h (long-acting)

$T_{1/2}$: 1 to 7 hours; metabolized in the liver; excreted in the urine.

Adverse Effects: Hypersensitivities, nervousness, insomnia, dry mouth, increased pulse rate and blood pressure, loss of appetite, nausea, growth impairment, priapism, and abdominal pain.

Nursing Considerations for Patients Receiving Central Nervous System Stimulants

Assessment: History and Examination

- Assess for contraindications or cautions for the use of the drug, including any known allergies to the drug; glaucoma, anxiety, psychosis, hyperthyroidism, or seizure disorder; cardiac disease and hypertension; pregnancy or lactation; a history of leukemia; and a history of drug dependency, including alcohol use disorder.
- Assess temperature; body weight, skin color, and lesions; CNS orientation, affect, and reflexes; ophthalmic examination; bowel sounds and reported output; pulse, auscultation, and blood pressure, including orthostatic blood pressure; respiration rate and adventitious sounds; and urinary output to determine baseline status before beginning therapy and for any potential adverse effects. Also obtain a CBC.

Nursing Conclusions

Nursing conclusions related to drug therapy might include the following:

- Altered thought processes related to CNS effects of the drug
- Altered vital signs related to CV effects of the drug
- Injury risk related to CNS and visual effects of the drug
- Knowledge deficiency regarding drug therapy

Planning

- The patient will receive the best therapeutic effect from the drug therapy.
- The patient will have limited adverse effects to the drug therapy.
- The patient will have an understanding of the drug therapy, adverse effects to anticipate, and measures to relieve discomfort and improve safety.

Intervention With Rationale

- Ensure proper diagnosis of behavioral syndromes and narcolepsy because these drugs should not be used until underlying medical causes of the problem are ruled out.
- Arrange for an overall treatment plan that includes family and cognitive–behavior therapy when possible.
- Arrange to interrupt the drug periodically in children who are receiving it for behavioral syndromes to determine whether symptoms recur and therapy should be continued.
- Arrange to dispense the least amount of drug possible to minimize the risk of overdose and misuse.
- Administer the drug regularly based on the prescription label instructions for best therapeutic effects.

- Monitor weight, CBC, and ECG to ensure early detection of adverse effects and proper interventions.
- Consult with the school nurse or counselor to ensure comprehensive care of school-aged children receiving CNS stimulants (see Box 22.5).
- Provide thorough patient/family teaching, including drug name, prescribed dosage, the need to secure the drug as a controlled substance, measures for avoidance of adverse effects, warning signs that may indicate possible problems, and the need for monitoring and evaluation to enhance patient knowledge about drug therapy and to promote adherence. Offer support and encouragement to help the patient cope with the drug regimen.

Evaluation

- Monitor patient response to the drug (decrease in manifestations of behavioral syndromes, decrease in daytime sleep and narcolepsy).
- Monitor for adverse effects (CNS stimulation, CV effects, rash, physical or psychological dependence, GI dysfunction).
- Evaluate effectiveness of the teaching plan (patient/family can give the drug name and dosage, name possible adverse effects to watch for and specific measures to help avoid adverse effects, and describe the need for follow-up and evaluation).
- Monitor effectiveness of comfort measures and adherence to the regimen.

Key Points

- ADHD is a behavioral syndrome characterized by hyperactivity, impulsivity, and a short attention span.
- Narcolepsy is a disorder characterized by daytime sleepiness and sudden loss of wakefulness.
- CNS stimulants, which stimulate more norepinephrine and dopamine in the CNS and periphery, are often used to treat ADHD and narcolepsy. These drugs improve concentration and the ability to filter and focus incoming stimuli.

Box 22.5 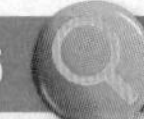 Focus on The Evidence

SCHOOL NURSING AND CNS STIMULANT ADMINISTRATION

As more has become known about ADHD, more children have been prescribed CNS stimulants. At first, the medications needed to be dosed multiple times per day, so school nurses were often required to administer the midday dose to the child. However, there are many longer-acting formulations available now. Both amphetamine and methylphenidate have multiple formulations that are dosed differently. The school nurse may not need to administer the medication, but they would need to be able to be a part of the comprehensive treatment plan for the student. For example, the school nurse is responsible for assessing response to the drug and for coordinating the teacher's and health care provider's input into each individual case, including the incidence of adverse effects and the appropriateness of the drug therapy.

The nurse should:

- Ensure that the proper diagnosis is made before supporting the use of the drug.
- Monitor for adverse effects including weight loss, growth suppression, restlessness, anxiety, tachycardia, and high blood pressure.
- Constantly evaluate and work with the primary health care provider, teacher, and parents to provide a comprehensive treatment plan for the child.

SUMMARY

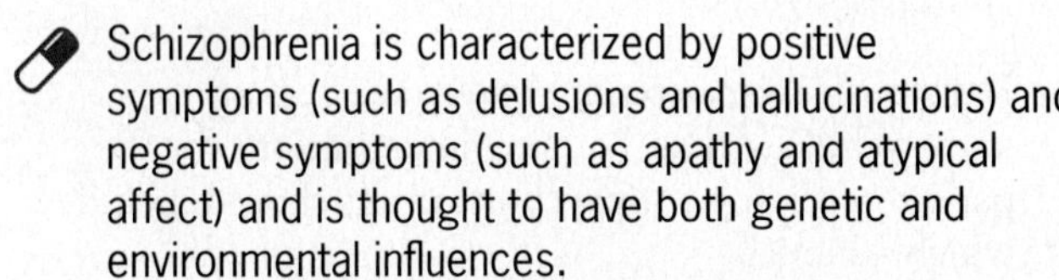

- Schizophrenia is characterized by positive symptoms (such as delusions and hallucinations) and negative symptoms (such as apathy and atypical affect) and is thought to have both genetic and environmental influences.
- Bipolar disorder is an affective disorder that involves extremes of depression alternating with hyperactivity and excitement.
- ADHD is a behavioral syndrome characterized by hyperactivity, impulsivity, and a short attention span.
- Narcolepsy is a disorder characterized by daytime sleepiness and sudden loss of wakefulness.
- Antipsychotic medications that inhibit dopamine can be used to treat schizophrenia, and some can be used to treat bipolar disorder.
- Lithium, a membrane stabilizer, is the traditional antimanic drug. Because it is potentially very toxic, serum level must be carefully monitored to prevent severe adverse effects. Many other CNS drugs are now approved for use in bipolar disorder.
- CNS stimulants, which stimulate more norepinephrine and dopamine in the CNS and periphery, are commonly used to treat ADHD and narcolepsy. These drugs improve concentration and the ability to filter and focus incoming stimuli.

CHECK YOUR UNDERSTANDING

Answers to the questions in this chapter can be found in Answers to Check Your Understanding Questions on thePoint®.

MULTIPLE CHOICE

Select the best answer.

1. Mental disorders are now thought to be caused by some inherent dysfunction within the brain that leads to abnormal thought processes and responses. They include
   a. depression.
   b. anxiety.
   c. seizures.
   d. schizophrenia.

2. Antipsychotic drugs are basically
   a. serotonin reuptake inhibitors.
   b. norepinephrine blockers.
   c. dopamine receptor blockers.
   d. acetylcholine stimulators.

3. Adverse effects associated with antipsychotic drugs are related to the drugs' effects on receptor sites and can include
   a. insomnia and hypertension.
   b. dry mouth, hypotension, and glaucoma.
   c. diarrhea and excessive urination.
   d. increased sexual drive and improved concentration.

4. Lithium toxicity can be dangerous. Patient assessment to evaluate for an appropriate lithium level would look for a serum lithium level
   a. >3 mEq/L.
   b. >4 mEq/L.
   c. <1.5 mEq/L.
   d. that is undetectable.

5. Your patient, a 6-year-old child, is starting a regimen of methylphenidate (*Ritalin*) to control ADHD. Family teaching should include which of the following?
   a. This drug can be shared with other family members who might seem to need it.
   b. This drug may cause insomnia, weight loss, and GI upset.
   c. Do not alert the school nurse to the fact that this drug is being taken because the child could have problems later.
   d. This drug should not be stopped for any reason for several years.

6. Antipsychotic drugs are also known as neuroleptic drugs because they
   a. cause numerous neurological effects.
   b. frequently cause epilepsy.
   c. are also minor tranquilizers.
   d. are the only drugs known to directly affect nerves.

7. Attention deficit hyperactivity disorder (the inability to concentrate or focus on an activity) and narcolepsy (sudden episodes of sleep) are both most effectively treated with the use of
   a. neuroinhibitors.
   b. dopamine receptor blockers.
   c. major tranquilizers.
   d. CNS stimulants.

8. Haloperidol (*Haldol*) is a potent antipsychotic that is associated with severe
   a. extrapyramidal effects.
   b. hyperactivity.
   c. hypotension.
   d. anticholinergic effects.

MULTIPLE RESPONSE

Select all that apply.

1. Before administering lithium to a patient, the nurse should check for the concomitant use of which drugs, which could cause serious adverse effects?
   a. Ibuprofen
   b. Haloperidol
   c. Thiazide diuretics
   d. Antacids
   e. Ketoconazole
   f. Theophylline

2. Dyskinesias are a common adverse effect of antipsychotic drugs. Nursing interventions for the patient receiving antipsychotic drugs should include which actions?
   a. Positioning to decrease discomfort of dyskinesias
   b. Implementing safety measures to prevent injury
   c. Encouraging the patient to chew tablets to prevent choking
   d. Careful teaching to alert the patient and family about this adverse effect
   e. Applying ice to the joints to prevent damage
   f. Pureeing all food to decrease the risk of aspiration

REFERENCES

American Psychiatric Association. (2013). *Diagnostic and statistical manual of mental disorders* (5th ed., text revision).

Brown, T. E. (2013). *A new understanding of ADHD in children and adults.* Routledge.

Brunton, L., Hilal-Dandan, R., & Knollman, B. (2018). *Goodman and Gilman's the pharmacological basis of therapeutics* (13th ed.). McGraw-Hill.

Dunn, G. A., Nigg, J. T., & Sullivan, E. L. (2019). Neuroinflammation as a risk factor for attention deficit hyperactivity disorder. *Pharmacology, Biochemistry and Behavior, 182*, 22–34. https://doi.org/10.1016/j.pbb.2019.05.005

Fahira, A., Li, Z., Liu, N., & Shi, Y. (2019). Prediction of causal genes and gene expression analysis of attention-deficit hyperactivity disorder in the different brain region, a comprehensive integrative analysis of ADHD. *Behavioral Brain Research, 364*, 183–192. https://doi.org/10.1016/j.bbr.2019.02.010

Hedges, D., Jeppson, K., & Whitehead, P. (2003). Antipsychotic medication and seizures: A review. *Drugs Today, 39*(7), 551–557. 10.1358/dot.2003.39.7.799445.

Hendler, C. B. (Ed.) (2021). *Nursing 2021 drug handbook.* Wolters Kluwer.

Kuehn, B. (2008). Antipsychotics risky for the elderly. *Journal of the American Medical Association*, 300(4), 379–380. 10.1001/jama.300.4.379

Madgulkar, A. R., Rao, M. R. P., & Warrier, D. (2014). Characterization of psyllium (*Plantago ovata*) polysaccharide and its uses. *Polysaccharides,* 1–17. 10.1007/978-3-319-03751-6_49-1

Mattingly, G. W., Wilson, J., Ugarte, L., & Glaser, P. (2020). *Individualization of attention-deficit/hyperactivity disorder treatment: Pharmacotherapy considerations by age and co-occurring conditions.* Cambridge University Press. https://www.cambridge.org/core/journals/cns-spectrums/article/individualization-of-attentiondeficithyperactivity-disorder-treatment-pharmacotherapy-considerations-by-age-and-cooccurring-conditions/D5ED66EFED3BEB1C830183101185D8D4

Norris, T. L. (2019). *Porth's pathophysiology concepts of altered health states* (10th ed.). Wolters Kluwer.

Oruch, R., Pryme, I. F., Engelsen, B. A., & Lund, A. (2017). Neuroleptic malignant syndrome: An easily overlooked neurologic emergency. *Neuropsychiatric Disease Treatment, 13*, 161–175. 10.2147/NDT.S118438

Sikich, L., Frazier, J., Mcclellan, J., Findling, R. L., Vitiello, B., Ritz, L., Ambler, D., Puglia, M., Maloney, A. E., Michael, E., De Jong, S., Slifka, K., Noyes, N., Hlastala, S., Pierson, L., McNamara, N. K., Delporto-Bedoya, D., Anderson, R., Hamer, R. M., & Lieberman, J. A. (2008). Children and antipsychotics. *American Journal of Psychiatry, 165*, 1420–1431. 10.1176/appi.ajp.2008.08050756

Tiihonen, J., Haukka, J., Taylor, M., Haddad, P. M., Patel, M. X., & Korhonen, P. (2011). A nationwide cohort study of oral and depot antipsychotics after first hospitalization or schizophrenia. *American Journal of Psychiatry, 168*(6), 603–609. 10.1176/appi.ajp.2011.10081224.

CHAPTER 23

Antiseizure Agents

Learning Objectives

Upon completion of this chapter, you will be able to:

1. Discuss the use of antiepileptic drugs across the lifespan.
2. Define the terms generalized seizure, tonic–clonic seizure, absence seizure, focal seizure, and status epilepticus.
3. Describe the therapeutic actions, indications, pharmacokinetics, contraindications, most common adverse reactions, and important drug–drug interactions associated with each class of antiseizure agents.
4. Compare and contrast the prototype drugs for each class of antiepileptic drug with the other drugs in that class and with drugs from the other classes.
5. Outline the nursing considerations and teaching needs for patients receiving each class of antiepileptic agents.

Key Terms

absence seizure: type of generalized seizure that is characterized by sudden, temporary loss of consciousness, sometimes with staring or blinking for 3 to 5 seconds; formerly known as a petit mal seizure

antiepileptic: drug used to treat the abnormal and excessive energy bursts in the brain that are characteristic of epilepsy

atonic seizure: generalized or focal seizure in which there is sudden loss of muscle tone that can cause the person to fall immediately to the ground; also called "drop attacks"

epilepsy: chronic disorder characterized by recurrent abnormal discharges from the neurons; recurrent seizure activity

focal seizures: seizures involving one area of the brain; they do not spread to both hemispheres of the brain; formerly known as partial seizures

generalized seizure: seizure that begins in both hemispheres of the brain and rapidly spreads throughout the brain

myoclonic seizures: generalized seizures that involve short, involuntary periods of muscle contractions that can be isolated or bilateral; initiated by cerebral stimuli

seizure: sudden abnormal discharge of excessive electrical energy from nerve cells in the brain that correspond to various associated signs and symptoms based on the area of the brain affected

status epilepticus: state in which seizures rapidly recur without cognitive recovery between seizures; most severe form of generalized seizure and a medical emergency

tonic–clonic seizure: type of motor generalized seizure that is characterized by both tonic (stiffening) and clonic (jerking) muscle contractions on both sides of the body; formerly known as a grand mal seizure

Drug List

DRUGS FOR TREATING GENERALIZED SEIZURES

Hydantoins
fosphenytoin
(P) phenytoin

Barbiturates and Barbituratelike Drugs
(P) phenobarbital
primidone

Benzodiazepines
clobazam
clonazepam
(P) diazepam

Succinimides
(P) ethosuximide
methsuximide

Drugs that Modulate the Inhibitory Neurotransmitter GABA
acetazolamide
divalproex sodium
(P) valproic acid
zonisamide

DRUGS WITH OTHER MECHANISMS OF ACTION
(P) carbamazepine
lamotrigine
levetiracetam
topiramate

DRUGS FOR TREATING FOCAL SEIZURES
clorazepate
(P) eslicarbazepine
ezogabine
felbamate
(P) gabapentin
lacosamide
oxcarbazepine
perampanel
pregabalin
rufinamide
tiagabine
vigabatrin

Epilepsy, the most prevalent of the neurological disorders, is not a single disease but a chronic disorder characterized by **seizures**. A seizure is the sudden abnormal discharge of excessive electrical energy from nerve cells in the brain that correspond to various associated signs and symptoms based on the area of the brain affected. In some cases, the release stimulates motor nerves, with tonic–clonic or myoclonic muscle contractions that have the potential to cause injury, tics, or spasms. Other discharges may stimulate autonomic or sensory nerves and cause different effects, such as a barely perceptible, temporary lapse in consciousness, or a sympathetic reaction. The effect of seizure activity will vary based on the location of the neurons that are firing abnormally and the spread of the abnormal electrical activity. The electrical activity of the brain can be studied with an electroencephalogram (EEG) that examines brain wave patterns. Because a seizure can result in a person losing control of their body, it can be frightening (Box 23.1).

The treatment of epilepsy varies widely depending on the exact problem and its manifestations. The drugs that are used to manage epilepsy are called **antiepileptics**, or antiseizure agents. They are sometimes referred to as anticonvulsants; however, because not all types of epilepsy involve convulsions, this term is not generally applicable. The drug of choice for any given situation depends on the type of epilepsy, patient age (Box 23.2), specific patient characteristics such as genetic variations (Box 23.3), and patient tolerance for associated adverse effects. Drugs can be used to treat more than one type of seizure. Table 23.1 lists drugs and the types of seizures that they can be used to treat.

Nature of Seizures

The form that a particular seizure takes depends on the location of the cells that initiate the electrical discharge and the neural pathways that are stimulated by the initial volley of electrical impulses. There are several theories regarding the etiology of seizure activity. There could be impairment of the cell membranes of certain neurons that changes membrane permeability or distribution of ions. There also may be structural differences in the cortical or thalamic nerves that result in decreased inhibition. Another theory involves having higher amounts of the neurotransmitter acetylcholine or a deficiency of gamma aminobutyric acid (GABA). There also could be genetic mutations that cause ion channel defects and lead to some epilepsy syndromes. For the most part, epilepsy seems to be caused by abnormal neurons that are very sensitive to stimulation or overrespond for some reason. Seizures caused by these abnormal cells are called primary seizures because no underlying cause can be identified. In many cases, however, outside factors—head injury, drug overdose, electrolyte alterations, environmental exposure, and so on—may precipitate seizures. Such seizures are often referred to as secondary seizures.

Classification of Seizures

Accurate diagnosis of seizure type is important for determining the correct medication to prevent future seizures while causing the fewest problems and adverse effects. Seizures are generally categorized as tonic–clonic (formerly

Box 23.1 Focus on Patient and Family Teaching

TEACHING AND COUNSELING PATIENTS WITH EPILEPSY

Epilepsy can be frightening to people due to its unpredictability, sudden onset, and frequent difficulty to control. Just having one seizure episode can be very frightening to the patient and their loved ones. (Keep in mind that many people who have a seizure do not necessarily have epilepsy.) What does having epilepsy mean? Epilepsy is a chronic disorder characterized by recurrent abnormal discharges from the neurons resulting in seizure activity. Many times chronic medication is needed to suppress the abnormal neuronal action potentials. In addition to medication, there are lifestyle changes that people with epilepsy must make.

People who are newly diagnosed with epilepsy must consider restrictions on their independence. For example, driving privileges will be restricted until medications are shown to have inhibited the seizure activity. The state restrictions on driving after a seizure vary from state to state; however, in all states, patients should be instructed to refrain from driving until cleared by a health care provider. The inability to drive and the seizure activity may adversely affect the person's quality of life in other ways as well. The person may not be able to work, go to school, or participate in hobbies or sports. It is best for the nurse to explain that, even if it might take time, medications are often able to help inhibit the seizure activity so that people are able to have very good quality of life and return to their previous activities.

Thorough patient teaching should include the following:

- Explanations of specific medication dosing and titration plans including risk of seizures if medication is stopped abruptly
- Ways in which people may react to the diagnosis and empathy for the person's feelings
- Actions to take if a seizure happens to promote safety
- Information about the availability of public transportation and/or a strategy for arranging rides to work or school
- Encouragement for patients with epilepsy to carry or wear MedicAlert identification to alert any emergency caregivers to their condition and to what drugs they are taking if they are not able to speak for themselves
- Contact information regarding other community support services

Many communities have epilepsy support groups that can supply information on valuable resources as well as updated facts about the laws in each area. While patients are first adjusting to epilepsy and its implications, it may help to put them in contact with such organizations. The local chapter of the Epilepsy Foundation of America may be able to offer support groups, lists of resources, and support. People with epilepsy should have several options for getting around without feeling that they are being a burden or an imposition.

Box 23.2 Focus on Drug Therapy Across the Lifespan

ANTISEIZURE AGENTS

Children

Antiepileptic drugs can have an impact on a child's learning and social development. Children's dosing of medications is often specific to age and weight. Children should be monitored closely and often require a switch to a different agent or dosage adjustments based on their response.

Newborns (1 to 10 days of age) respond best to intramuscular phenobarbital if an antiepileptic is needed.

After the age of 10 to 14 years, many of these drugs can be given in the standard adult dose.

Parents of children receiving these drugs should receive consistent support and education about the seizure disorder and the medications being used to treat it. Many communities have local support groups that can offer educational materials and support programs. It is a frightening experience to watch a child have a tonic–clonic seizure, and parents and other family members should be supported.

Adults

Adults using these drugs should be under regular care and should be monitored regularly for adverse effects. They should be encouraged to carry or wear MedicAlert identification to alert emergency personnel that the person is taking an antiepileptic drug. Adults also need education and support to deal with the old stigma of seizures as well as the lifestyle changes and drug effects with which they may need to cope.

There is an Antiepileptic Drug Pregnancy Registry that is monitoring pregnancy outcomes; pregnant patients can enroll in this registry. Some of the medications have documented fetal risks based on either human or animal data. For other medications, the evidence is less clear. Patients who can become pregnant should be educated regarding the specific risks of the medication they are taking and be encouraged to notify their providers if they plan to and/or do become pregnant. Several of the medications may decrease efficacy of oral contraceptives. If a pregnancy does occur, or if a patient taking one of these drugs desires to become pregnant, the importance of the drug to the patient should be weighed against the potential risk to the fetus. Stopping an antiepileptic can precipitate seizures that could cause anoxia and related problems for the patient and the baby. Patients who are breast or chestfeeding should be encouraged to find another way of feeding the baby to avoid the sedating and central nervous system (CNS) effects that these drugs can have on the infant.

Older Adults

Older patients may be more susceptible to the adverse effects of these drugs. Dosages of these drugs may need to be reduced, and the patient should be monitored closely for toxic effects and to provide safety measures if CNS effects do occur.

Patients with renal or hepatic impairment should be monitored closely. Baseline renal and liver function tests should be done and dosages adjusted as appropriate. Serum levels of the drug should be monitored closely in such cases to prevent serious adverse effects.

The older patient should also be encouraged to wear or carry MedicAlert identification in case there is an emergency and the patient is not able to communicate information about the drug or disorder.

grand mal) seizures or absence (formerly petit mal) seizures, but the International League Against Epilepsy has described a multilevel classification system of types of seizures based on their onset. First, the seizure is classified

Box 23.3 Focus on Cultural Considerations

ANTISEIZURE AGENTS AND GENETIC DIFFERENCES

There are genetic and ethnic risk factors that are associated with varying risk of medication hypersensitivities. For example, aspirin hypersensitivity is associated with a variety of genetic polymorphisms related to leukotriene overproduction, eosinophil infiltration, and histamine-related genes. A genetic risk factor associated with serious dermatologic reactions has been identified with some of the antiseizure agents. Having the inherited alle variant of the HLA-B gene, HLA-B*1502, has been shown to increase risk of developing toxic epidermal necrolysis and Steven Johnson syndrome in people taking carbamazepine. This alle has been demonstrated more strongly in people of Asian descent. Further evidence has shown that this same association with the HLA-B*1502 allele and severe dermatologic reactions can occur with phenytoin, lamotrigine, oxcarbazepine, and phenobarbital. The FDA recommends screening people of Asian descent for the HLA-B*1502 genotype prior to prescribing carbamazepine. There is also genetic research investigating adverse reactions of antiseizure medications for other ethnic groups.

Table 23.1 Antiepileptic Drug Therapy Grouped by Seizure Class

Focal Seizures	Generalized Seizures (Except Status Epilepticus)	Status Epilepticus
Carbamazepine	Carbamazepine	Diazepam
Clobazam	Clonazepam	Fosphenytoin
Clonazepam	Divalproex	Lorazepam
Clorazepate	Ethosuximide	Midazolam
Felbamate	Felbamate (Lennox-Gastaut syndrome)	Pentobarbital
Eslicarbazepine	Lamotrigine	Phenobarbital
Gabapentin	Levetiracetam	Phenytoin
Lacosamide	Methsuximide	
Lamotrigine	Phensuximide	
Levetiracetam	Phenytoin	
Oxcarbazepine	Topiramate	
Perampanel	Valproic acid	
Phenytoin	Zonisamide	
Pregabalin		
Rufinamide		
Tiagabine		
Topiramate		
Valproic acid		
Vigabatrin		
Zonisamide		

Adapted with permission from Aschenbrenner, D. S., & Venable, S. J. (2011). *Drug therapy in nursing* (4th ed.). Lippincott Williams & Wilkins.

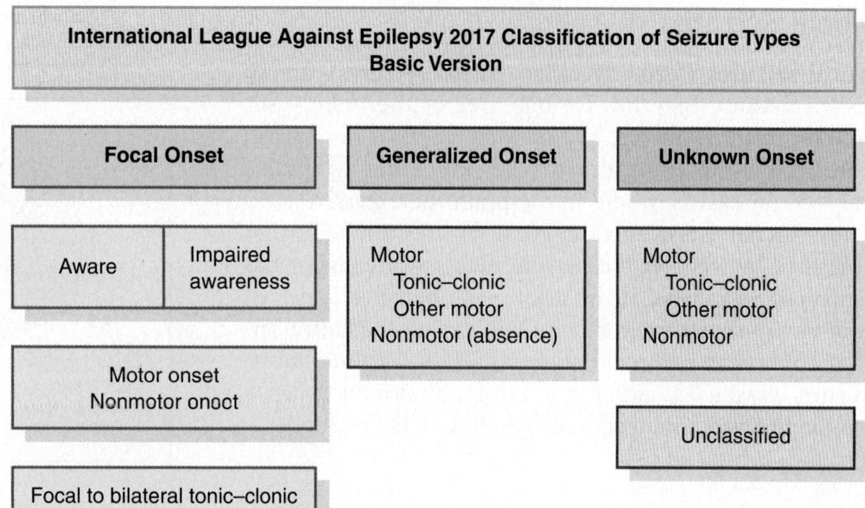

FIGURE 23.1 International League Against Epilepsy 2017 Classification of Seizure Types, Basic Version. (Reprinted with permission from Fisher, R. S., Cross, J. H., French, J. A., Higurashi, N., Hirsch, E., Janson, F. E., Lagae, L., Moshe, S. L., Peltola, J., Perez, E. R., Scheffer, I. E., & Zuberi, S. M. (2017). Operational classification of seizure types by the International League Against Epilepsy: Position paper of the ILAE commission for classification and terminology. *Epilepsia, 58*(4), 522–530. © 2017 International League Against Epilepsy. doi: 10.1111/epi.13670.)

as either focal onset, generalized onset, focal to bilateral, or unknown onset. After a focal onset seizure, it is important to note if there is impaired awareness or consciousness associated with the seizure. It is assumed that there will be some impaired awareness with all generalized onset seizures. The focal to bilateral seizure initiates in one area of the brain and then spreads to both hemispheres, so it is a secondary generalized seizure. The third part of the classification of seizure types is to diagnose whether there are motor symptoms. All seizure types can be categorized as either motor or nonmotor onset. There are times when the classification will stop at the seizure level. However, if there is the information available to diagnose epilepsy, the epilepsy type can be categorized as focal, generalized, combined, or unknown. Epilepsy is defined as recurrent seizure activity and is a complex neurologic disorder that may be diagnosed with comprehensive history and physical assessments. However, EEG is often used to diagnose epilepsy by demonstrating voltage fluctuations in brain wave tracings (Fig. 23.1).

Generalized Seizures

Generalized seizures begin in both hemispheres of the brain and rapidly spread throughout the brain. Patients who have a generalized seizure experience a loss of consciousness resulting from this massive electrical activity throughout the brain.

Generalized seizures are further classified into motor and nonmotor types. Some of the types are further defined as follows:

1. **Tonic–clonic seizures** are a motor type of seizure with both tonic (stiffening) and clonic (jerking) muscle contractions on both sides of the body. These types of seizures were formerly termed grand mal seizures. Often a person will have a vague sensation that warns them before the tonic contraction begins, which could be focal seizure activity. It can be common for incontinence of both the bladder and bowel to occur. After the tonic–clonic contractions, the person will have a recovery period characterized by unconsciousness and/or confusion and lethargy. This recovery period is termed the postictal phase.
2. **Absence seizures** are nonmotor generalized seizures that typically involve abrupt, brief (3- to 5-second) periods of loss of consciousness, sometimes with staring or blinking. Absence seizures occur commonly in children, starting at about 3 years of age, and frequently disappear by puberty. Typical absence seizures do not usually involve muscle contractions; the person will often demonstrate a blank stare and be motionless and unresponsive. Atypical absence seizures are difficult to diagnose without an EEG; however, people with these type of seizures will often have more prolonged symptoms with more muscle tone alteration.
3. **Myoclonic seizures** can be either motor or nonmotor (absence type) and involve short, sporadic periods of muscle contractions. The contractions can be isolated to the face, trunk, or one extremity or can be bilateral. Myoclonic seizures are initiated by cerebral stimuli. They are relatively rare and are often secondary seizures.
4. Febrile seizures are related to very high fevers and usually involve tonic–clonic seizures. Febrile seizures most frequently occur in children aged 3 months to 6 years. They are more likely to occur if there is a family history of febrile seizures. They do not generally require daily antiseizure medication. They are usually self-limiting and do not reappear once the temperature is reduced.
5. **Atonic seizures** can be either generalized or focal. They are characterized as a seizure that causes sudden loss of muscle tone. This will cause limp extremities and facial muscles. If the person is standing, they will fall immediately to the ground. Another term for these seizures is "drop attacks."
6. **Status epilepticus** is a state in which seizures rapidly recur without cognitive recovery in between. This is the most severe form of generalized seizure and is a medical emergency.

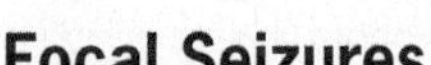

Focal Seizures

Focal seizures (formerly called partial seizures), are so called because they involve one area of the brain, usually originate from one site or focus and do not spread throughout the entire organ. The presenting symptoms depend on exactly where in the brain the excessive electrical discharge is occurring. Focal seizures can be further classified by whether the person retains awareness or has impaired awareness. If the person can perceive their self and environment even if immobile during the entire seizure, they have retained awareness. Focal seizures can be further classified as either motor or nonmotor onset based on the first prominent sign or symptom of the seizure.

> **Key Points**
>
> - Epilepsy is a chronic disorder characterized by seizures, or recurrent abnormal discharges from the neurons. There are two major categories of seizures: generalized and focal seizures.
> - Generalized seizures are further classified as either motor or nonmotor (absence) types.
> - Focal seizures may or may not cause impaired awareness and can be either motor onset or nonmotor onset.

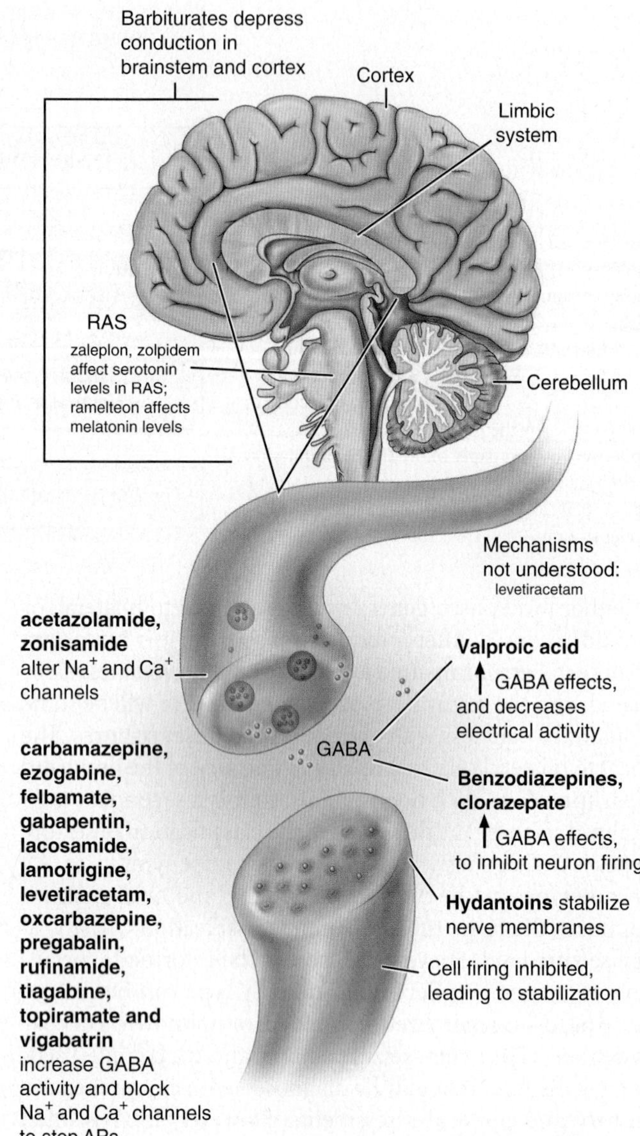

FIGURE 23.2 Sites of action of drugs used to treat various types of epilepsy. AP, action potential; GABA, gamma-aminobutyric acid; RAS, reticular activating system.

Drugs for Treating Generalized Seizures

Drugs typically used to treat generalized seizures stabilize the nerve membranes by blocking channels in the cell membrane or altering receptor sites. Because they work generally on the CNS, sedation and other CNS effects often result. Various drugs are used to treat generalized seizures, including hydantoins, barbiturates, barbituratelike drugs, benzodiazepines, and succinimides. These drugs affect the entire brain and reduce the chance of sudden electrical outburst. Associated adverse effects are often related to total brain stabilization (Fig. 23.2).

Absence seizures, another type of generalized seizure, may require drugs that are different than those used to treat or prevent other types of generalized seizures. The succinimides and drugs that modulate the inhibitory neurotransmitter GABA are most frequently used (Table 23.2).

Hydantoins

Hydantoins include fosphenytoin (*Cerebyx, Sesquient*) and phenytoin (*Dilantin*). The hydantoins are older medications and can be cost effective. They are less sedating and less dependency forming than the barbiturates or benzodiazepines.

Therapeutic Actions and Indications

The hydantoins stabilize nerve membranes throughout the CNS directly by influencing ionic channels in the cell membrane, thereby decreasing excitability and hyperexcitability to stimulation. By decreasing conduction through nerve pathways, they reduce the tonic–clonic, muscular, and emotional responses to stimulation. See Table 23.2 for usual indications.

Pharmacokinetics

Phenytoin is well absorbed from the gastrointestinal (GI) tract, metabolized in the liver, and excreted in the urine. Therapeutic serum phenytoin levels range from 10 to 20 mcg/mL. Fosphenytoin is given intramuscularly or intravenously. It is metabolized in the liver and excreted

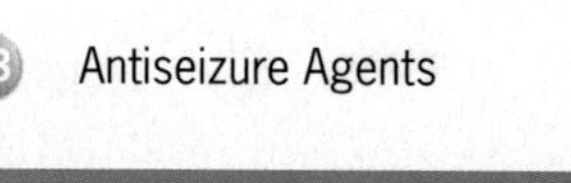

Table 23.2 *Drugs in Focus:* Drugs for Treating Generalized Seizures

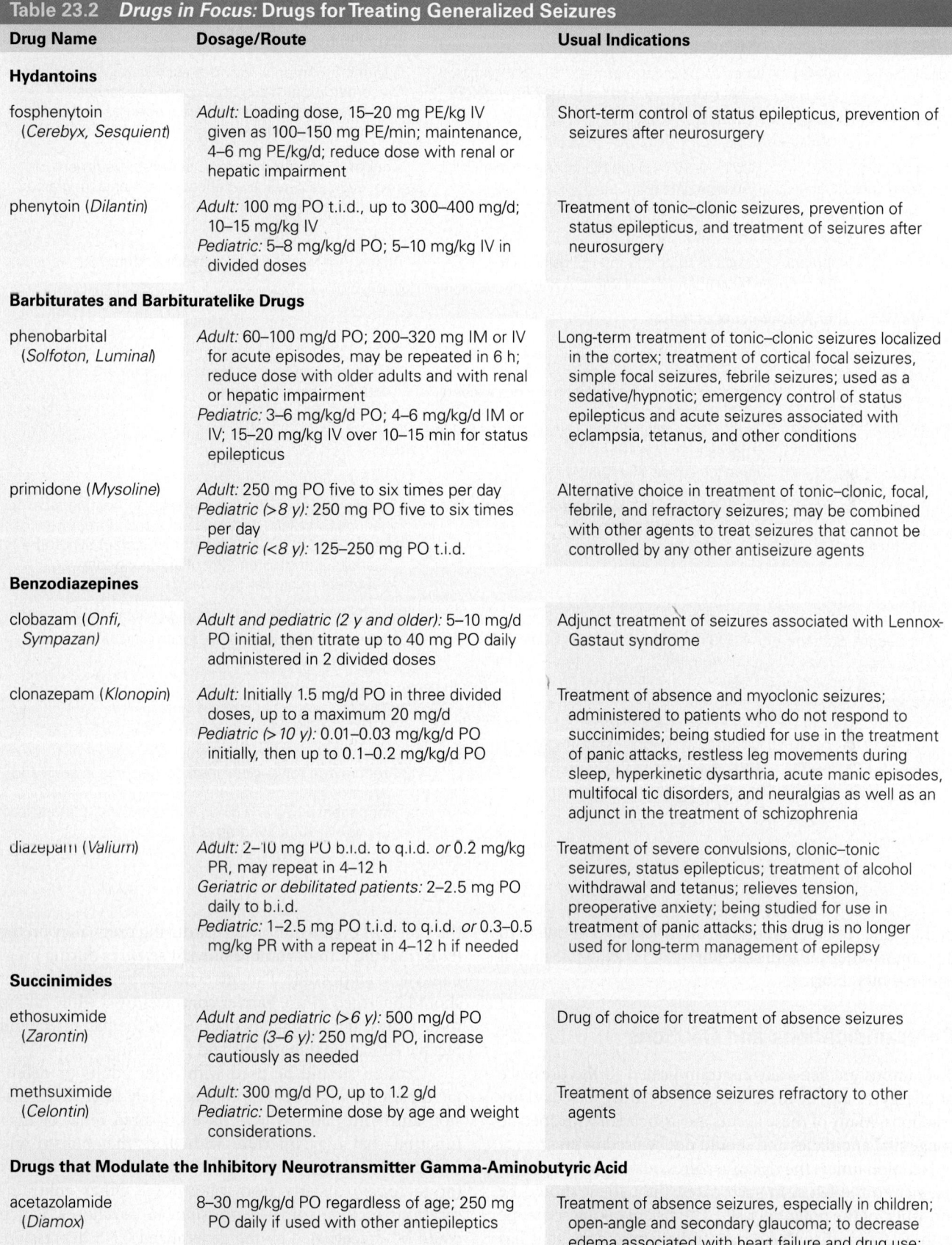

Drug Name	Dosage/Route	Usual Indications
Hydantoins		
fosphenytoin (*Cerebyx, Sesquient*)	*Adult:* Loading dose, 15–20 mg PE/kg IV given as 100–150 mg PE/min; maintenance, 4–6 mg PE/kg/d; reduce dose with renal or hepatic impairment	Short-term control of status epilepticus, prevention of seizures after neurosurgery
phenytoin (*Dilantin*)	*Adult:* 100 mg PO t.i.d., up to 300–400 mg/d; 10–15 mg/kg IV *Pediatric:* 5–8 mg/kg/d PO; 5–10 mg/kg IV in divided doses	Treatment of tonic–clonic seizures, prevention of status epilepticus, and treatment of seizures after neurosurgery
Barbiturates and Barbituratelike Drugs		
phenobarbital (*Solfoton, Luminal*)	*Adult:* 60–100 mg/d PO; 200–320 mg IM or IV for acute episodes, may be repeated in 6 h; reduce dose with older adults and with renal or hepatic impairment *Pediatric:* 3–6 mg/kg/d PO; 4–6 mg/kg/d IM or IV; 15–20 mg/kg IV over 10–15 min for status epilepticus	Long-term treatment of tonic–clonic seizures localized in the cortex; treatment of cortical focal seizures, simple focal seizures, febrile seizures; used as a sedative/hypnotic; emergency control of status epilepticus and acute seizures associated with eclampsia, tetanus, and other conditions
primidone (*Mysoline*)	*Adult:* 250 mg PO five to six times per day *Pediatric (>8 y):* 250 mg PO five to six times per day *Pediatric (<8 y):* 125–250 mg PO t.i.d.	Alternative choice in treatment of tonic–clonic, focal, febrile, and refractory seizures; may be combined with other agents to treat seizures that cannot be controlled by any other antiseizure agents
Benzodiazepines		
clobazam (*Onfi, Sympazan*)	*Adult and pediatric (2 y and older):* 5–10 mg/d PO initial, then titrate up to 40 mg PO daily administered in 2 divided doses	Adjunct treatment of seizures associated with Lennox-Gastaut syndrome
clonazepam (*Klonopin*)	*Adult:* Initially 1.5 mg/d PO in three divided doses, up to a maximum 20 mg/d *Pediatric (> 10 y):* 0.01–0.03 mg/kg/d PO initially, then up to 0.1–0.2 mg/kg/d PO	Treatment of absence and myoclonic seizures; administered to patients who do not respond to succinimides; being studied for use in the treatment of panic attacks, restless leg movements during sleep, hyperkinetic dysarthria, acute manic episodes, multifocal tic disorders, and neuralgias as well as an adjunct in the treatment of schizophrenia
diazepam (*Valium*)	*Adult:* 2–10 mg PO b.i.d. to q.i.d. *or* 0.2 mg/kg PR, may repeat in 4–12 h *Geriatric or debilitated patients:* 2–2.5 mg PO daily to b.i.d. *Pediatric:* 1–2.5 mg PO t.i.d. to q.i.d. *or* 0.3–0.5 mg/kg PR with a repeat in 4–12 h if needed	Treatment of severe convulsions, clonic–tonic seizures, status epilepticus; treatment of alcohol withdrawal and tetanus; relieves tension, preoperative anxiety; being studied for use in treatment of panic attacks; this drug is no longer used for long-term management of epilepsy
Succinimides		
ethosuximide (*Zarontin*)	*Adult and pediatric (>6 y):* 500 mg/d PO *Pediatric (3–6 y):* 250 mg/d PO, increase cautiously as needed	Drug of choice for treatment of absence seizures
methsuximide (*Celontin*)	*Adult:* 300 mg/d PO, up to 1.2 g/d *Pediatric:* Determine dose by age and weight considerations.	Treatment of absence seizures refractory to other agents
Drugs that Modulate the Inhibitory Neurotransmitter Gamma-Aminobutyric Acid		
acetazolamide (*Diamox*)	8–30 mg/kg/d PO regardless of age; 250 mg PO daily if used with other antiepileptics	Treatment of absence seizures, especially in children; open-angle and secondary glaucoma; to decrease edema associated with heart failure and drug use; and as a prophylaxis and for mountain sickness

(continues on page 402)

Table 23.2 *Drugs in Focus:* Drugs for Treating Generalized Seizures *(Continued)*

Drug Name	Dosage/Route	Usual Indications
divalproex *(Depakote)*	*Dose for seizure treatment:* 10–15 mg/kg/d that may be titrated up to max 60 mg/kg/d Dosing for other indications can vary	Treatment of manic episodes associated with bipolar disorder; prophylaxis of migraine headaches; treatment of focal and absence seizures and patients with multiple seizure types
valproic acid *(Depakene)*	*Adult:* 10–15 mg/kg/d PO up to a maximum 60 mg/kg/d *Pediatric:* Use extreme caution, determine dose by age and weight	Drug of choice for myoclonic seizures; treatment of absence seizures; also effective in mania, migraine headaches, and complex focal seizures
zonisamide *(Zonegran)*	*Adults (> 16 y):* 100 mg PO daily up to 600 mg/d	Adjunct for treatment of absence seizures
Drugs with other Mechanisms of Action		
carbamazepine *(Tegretol, Epitol)*	*Adult:* 800–1,200 mg/d PO in divided doses q6–8h *Pediatric (> 12 y):* Adult doses, do not exceed 1,000 mg/d *Pediatric (6–12 y):* 20–30 mg/kg/d PO in divided doses t.i.d. to q.i.d. *Pediatric (<6 y):* 35 mg/kg/d PO	Drug of choice for treatment of focal seizures and tonic–clonic seizures; treatment of trigeminal neuralgia, bipolar disorder
lamotrigine *(Lamictal)*	*Dosing based on concomitant medications, indication, and patient age*	Used as adjunct or for monotherapy in treating focal or generalized tonic–clonic seizures and in treatment of seizures associated with Lennox-Gastaut syndrome in adults and children ≥2 y of age; long-term treatment of bipolar disorder
levetiracetam *(Elepsia XR, Keppra, Spritam)*	*Adult:* 500 mg PO b.i.d. up to 3,000 mg/d; 1,000 mg PO daily up to 3,000 mg PO daily *(Elepsia XR)* *Pediatric:* Varies based on formulation, age, and weight Decrease dose if there is renal impairment	Treatment of focal seizures; adjunctive therapy for myoclonic and generalized tonic–clinic *(Keppra* and *Spritam)*
topiramate *(Qudexy XR, Topamax, Trokendi XR)*	*Dosing based on indication, age, and presence of renal impairment*	Used as adjunct or monotherapy in treating generalized tonic–clonic or focal seizures in adult and pediatric patients; prevention of migraine headaches for patients 12 y and older, and as adjunct therapy in Lennox-Gastaut syndrome

PE, phenytoin sodium equivalent.

in the urine. The therapeutic serum level peaks about 10 to 20 minutes after the infusion. Phenytoin is available in oral and parenteral forms.

Contraindications and Cautions

Hydantoins are generally contraindicated in the presence of allergy to any of these drugs to avoid hypersensitivity reactions. Many of these agents are associated with specific congenital anomalies and should not be used in pregnancy or lactation unless the risk of seizures outweighs the potential risk to the fetus. In such cases, the patient should be informed of the potential risks. The risk of taking someone with a seizure disorder off an antiepileptic drug that has stabilized their condition may be greater than the risk of the drug to the fetus. Discontinuing the drug could result in status epilepticus, which has a high risk of hypoxia for the patient and the fetus. Research has not been able to show the effects of even a minor seizure during pregnancy on the fetus, making it important to prevent seizures during pregnancy if at all possible. Patients who can become pregnant should be urged to use barrier contraceptives while taking these drugs. If a pregnancy does occur, the patient should receive educational materials and counseling.

Caution should be used with older adults or debilitated patients who may respond adversely to CNS depression and with patients who have impaired renal or liver function that may interfere with drug metabolism and excretion. Patients with hepatic impairment are at risk for increased toxicity from phenytoin. Other contraindications include coma, depression, or psychoses, which could be exacerbated by the generalized CNS depression. Patients receiving fosphenytoin intravenously require careful monitoring of their cardiovascular status during the infusion period. Some potentially serious name confusion has occurred with fosphenytoin (Box 23.4).

Box 23.4 Focus on Safe Medication Administration

Be aware that name confusion has been reported among fosphenytoin (*Cerebyx*), celecoxib (*Celebrex*; a nonsteroidal antiinflammatory agent), citalopram (*Celexa*, a selective serotonin reuptake inhibitor antidepressant), and alprazolam (*Xanax*, an antianxiety drug). Because these drugs have sound-alike, look-alike names, if your patient is prescribed any of these drugs, make sure you know what the drug is being used for and that the patient is getting the correct prescribed drug.

Adverse Effects

The most common adverse effects relate to CNS depression and its effects on body function: depression, confusion, drowsiness, lethargy, fatigue, constipation, dry mouth, anorexia, cardiac arrhythmias and changes in blood pressure, urinary retention, and loss of libido.

Specifically, the hydantoins may cause severe liver toxicity, bone marrow suppression, gingival hyperplasia, potentially serious dermatological reactions (e.g., hirsutism, Stevens-Johnson syndrome), and frank malignant lymphoma, all of which are directly related to cellular toxicity (Fig. 23.3).

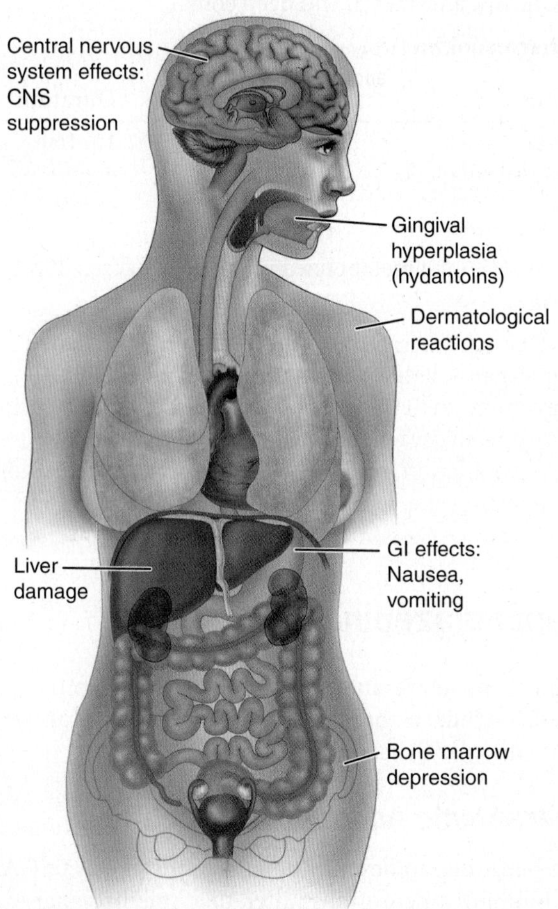

FIGURE 23.3 Common adverse effects associated with antiseizure agents. CNS, central nervous system; GI, gastrointestinal.

Box 23.5 Focus on Herbal and Alternative Therapies

Patients being treated for epilepsy should be advised not to use the herb evening primrose because it increases the risk of having seizures. Patients being treated with divalproex or phenytoin should be advised not to use ginkgo because it may lower the medication's effectiveness. Many medications used to treat epilepsy have significant drug and herbal interactions. Patients should be advised to check with a provider before starting or stopping any new medications.

Clinically Important Drug–Drug Interactions

Because the risk of CNS depression is increased with hydantoins taken with alcohol or other CNS depressants, patients should be advised to limit alcohol and other CNS depressants while they are taking these agents. Always consult a drug reference before any drug is added to or withdrawn from a therapeutic regimen that involves any of these agents. Box 23.5 describes hazardous drug–herbal therapy interactions associated with antiepileptic medications.

Prototype Summary: Phenytoin

Indications: Control of tonic–clonic and psychomotor seizures, prevention of seizures during neurosurgery, control of status epilepticus.

Actions: Stabilizes neuronal membranes and prevents hyperexcitability caused by excessive stimulation; limits the spread of seizure activity from an active focus; has cardiac antiarrhythmic effects similar to those of lidocaine.

Pharmacokinetics:

Route	Onset	Peak	Duration
Oral	Slow	2–12 h	6–12 h
IV	1–2 h	Rapid	12–24 h

$T_{1/2}$: 6 to 24 hours; metabolized in the liver; excreted in the urine.

Adverse Effects: Ataxia, dysarthria, slurred speech, mental confusion, dizziness, fatigue, tremor, headache, dermatitis, Stevens-Johnson syndrome, nausea, gingival hyperplasia, liver damage, hematopoietic complications, sometimes fatal. Nystagmus is possible at higher doses and with toxicity.

Barbiturates and Barbituratelike Drugs

Barbiturates and barbituratelike drugs include phenobarbital (*Solfoton*, *Luminal*), and primidone (*Mysoline*). These drugs are associated with significant CNS depression.

Therapeutic Actions and Indications

The barbiturates and barbiturate-type drugs inhibit impulse conduction in the ascending reticular activating system (RAS), depress the cerebral cortex, alter cerebellar function, and depress motor nerve output. They stabilize nerve membranes throughout the CNS directly by influencing ionic channels in the cell membrane, thereby decreasing excitability and hyperexcitability to stimulation. By decreasing conduction through nerve pathways, they reduce the tonic–clonic, muscular, and emotional responses to stimulation. Phenobarbital depresses conduction in the lower brainstem and the cerebral cortex and depresses motor conduction. See Table 23.2 for usual indications for each of these agents. Note that phenobarbital is not approved by the FDA but is marketed and distributed in the United States to be used in emergency situations.

Pharmacokinetics

Phenobarbital, which is available in oral and parenteral forms, is well absorbed from the GI tract, metabolized in the liver, and excreted in the urine. This drug has very low lipid solubility, giving it a slow onset and a very long duration of activity. The therapeutic serum level range is 10 to 40 mcg/mL. Adverse effects are more apparent with levels 30 mcg/mL and higher.

Primidone, available only as an oral agent, is well absorbed from the GI tract, metabolized in the liver to phenobarbital metabolites, and excreted in the urine. It tends to have a longer half-life than phenobarbital. The therapeutic serum levels are 5 to 12 mcg/mL.

Contraindications and Cautions

Contraindications and cautions for barbiturates are the same as those discussed for hydantoins.

Adverse Effects

The most common adverse effects associated with barbiturates relate to CNS depression and its effects on body function: depression, confusion, drowsiness, lethargy, fatigue, constipation, dry mouth, anorexia, cardiac arrhythmias and changes in blood pressure, urinary retention, and loss of libido. The degree of depression is dose related. Because barbiturates and barbituratelike drugs depress nerve function, they can produce sedation, hypnosis, anesthesia, respiratory depression, and deep coma. At doses below those needed to cause hypnosis, these drugs block seizure activity.

In addition, phenobarbital may be associated with physical dependence and withdrawal syndrome. The drug has also been linked to severe dermatological reactions and the development of drug tolerance related to changes in drug metabolism over time.

Clinically Important Drug–Drug Interactions

Because the risk of CNS depression is increased when barbiturates are taken with alcohol and other CNS depressants, patients should be advised to limit intake of other CNS depressants while they are taking these agents. There may be decreased synthesis of vitamin K and D and decreased effectiveness of warfarin. Always consult a drug reference before any drug is added to or withdrawn from a therapeutic regimen that involves any of these agents.

Prototype Summary: Phenobarbital

Indications: Long-term treatment of generalized tonic–clonic and cortical focal seizures, emergency control of certain acute convulsive episodes (status epilepticus, tetanus, eclampsia, meningitis), and anticonvulsant treatment of generalized tonic–clonic seizures and focal seizures (parenteral). Not approved by FDA but is marketed and available for use in the United States.

Actions: General CNS depressant; inhibits impulse conduction in the ascending RAS; depresses the cerebral cortex; alters cerebellar function; depresses motor output; and can produce excitation, sedation, hypnosis, anesthesia, and deep coma.

Pharmacokinetics:

Route	Onset	Duration
Oral	30–60 min	10–16 h
IM, subcutaneous	10–30 min	4–6 h
IV	5 min	4–6 h

$T_{1/2}$: 79 hours; metabolized in the liver, excreted in the urine.

Adverse Effects: Somnolence, insomnia, vertigo, nightmares, lethargy, nervousness, hallucinations, insomnia, anxiety, dizziness, bradycardia, hypotension, syncope, nausea, vomiting, constipation, diarrhea, hypoventilation, respiratory depression, tissue necrosis at injection site, withdrawal syndrome.

Benzodiazepines

Some benzodiazepines are used as antiepileptic agents. These include clobazam (*Onfi, Sympazan*), clonazepam (*Klonopin*), and diazepam (*Valium*).

Therapeutic Actions and Indications

The benzodiazepines may potentiate the effects of GABA, an inhibitory neurotransmitter that stabilizes nerve cell membranes. These drugs, which appear to act primarily in the limbic system and the RAS, also cause muscle relaxation and relieve anxiety without substantially affecting cortical functioning. The benzodiazepines stabilize nerve membranes throughout the CNS to decrease excitability and hyperexcitability to stimulation. By decreasing conduction through nerve pathways, they reduce the tonic–clonic, muscular, and emotional responses to stimulation. In general, these drugs have limited toxicity and are well tolerated by most people. (See Chapter 20 for the use of benzodiazepines as sedatives and anxiolytics.) See Table 23.2 for usual indications for each of these agents. Clonazepam may lose its effectiveness within 3 months (affected patients may respond to dose adjustment). Clobazam is indicated for adjunct treatment of seizures associated with Lennox-Gastaut syndrome in patients 2 years of age and older.

Pharmacokinetics

Diazepam is available in oral and rectal forms. Clonazepam is now available in an orally disintegrating tablet, making it a good choice for patients who have difficulty swallowing capsules or tablets. Clobazam is available in oral form only. These agents are well absorbed from the GI tract, metabolized in the liver, and excreted in the urine. They have a long half-life of 18 to 50 hours.

Contraindications and Cautions

Contraindications for benzodiazepines are the same as those discussed for hydantoins.

Adverse Effects

The most common adverse effects associated with benzodiazepines relate to CNS depression and its effects on body function: depression, confusion, drowsiness, lethargy, fatigue, constipation, dry mouth, anorexia, cardiac arrhythmias and changes in blood pressure, urinary retention, and loss of libido. Benzodiazepines may be associated with physical dependence and withdrawal syndrome, especially with rapid reduction in dose.

Clinically Important Drug–Drug Interactions

Because the risk of CNS depression is increased when benzodiazepines are taken with alcohol or other CNS depressants, patients should be advised not to drink alcohol or take other CNS depressants while they are taking these agents. There is a boxed warning on these drugs regarding risk of profound sedation, respiratory depression, coma, and death when benzodiazepines and opioids are taken together. Always consult a drug reference before any drug is added to or withdrawn from a therapeutic regimen that involves any of these agents.

Prototype Summary: Diazepam

Indications: Management of anxiety disorders, acute alcohol withdrawal, muscle relaxant, treatment of tetanus, adjunct in status epilepticus and severe recurrent convulsive seizures, preoperative relief of anxiety and tension, management of epilepsy in patients who require intermittent use to control bouts of increased seizure activity.

Actions: Acts in the limbic system and reticular formation, potentiates the effects of GABA, has little effect on cortical function.

Pharmacokinetics:

Route	Onset	Peak	Duration
Oral	30–60 min	1–2 h	3 h
IM	15–30 min	30–45 min	3 h
IV	1–5 min	30 min	15–60 min
Rectal	Rapid	1.5 h	3 h

$T_{1/2}$: 20 to 80 hours; metabolized in the liver; excreted in the urine.

Adverse Effects: Drowsiness, sedation, depression, lethargy, apathy, fatigue, disorientation, bradycardia, tachycardia, paradoxical excitatory reactions, constipation, diarrhea, incontinence, urinary retention, drug dependence with withdrawal syndrome.

Succinimides

The succinimides include ethosuximide (*Zarontin*) and methsuximide (*Celontin*). The succinimides are most frequently used to treat absence seizures, a form of generalized seizure.

Therapeutic Actions and Indications

Although the exact mechanism of action is not understood, the succinimides suppress the abnormal electrical activity in the brain that is associated with absence seizures. The action may be related to activity in inhibitory neural pathways in the brain (see Fig. 23.2).

Ethosuximide and methsuximide are indicated for the control of absence seizures (see Table 23.2). Ethosuximide should be tried first; methsuximide should be reserved for the treatment of seizures that are refractory to other agents because it is associated with more severe adverse effects.

Pharmacokinetics

Ethosuximide and methsuximide are available for oral use. These drugs cross the placenta and enter human milk (see "Contraindications and Cautions"). The succinimides are readily absorbed from the GI tract and reach peak level in 1 to 7 hours, depending on the drug. They are metabolized in the liver and excreted in the urine. The half-life of ethosuximide is 30 hours in children and 60 hours in adults; the half-life of methsuximide is 2.6 to 4 hours. The established therapeutic serum level for ethosuximide is 40 to 100 mcg/mL.

Contraindications and Cautions

The succinimides are contraindicated in the presence of allergy to any of these drugs to avoid hypersensitivity reactions. Caution should be used with succinimides in patients with intermittent porphyria, which could be exacerbated by the adverse effects of these drugs, and those with renal or hepatic disease, which could interfere with the metabolism and excretion of these drugs and lead to toxic levels. Use during pregnancy should be discussed with the patient because of the potential for adverse effects on the fetus. Another method of feeding the baby should be used if one of these drugs is needed during lactation because of the potential for adverse effects on the baby.

Adverse Effects

Ethosuximide has relatively few adverse effects compared with many other antiepileptic drugs. Many of the adverse effects associated with the succinimides are related to their depressant effects in the CNS. These may include depression, drowsiness, fatigue, ataxia, insomnia, headache, and blurred vision. Decreased GI activity with nausea, vomiting, anorexia, weight loss, GI pain, and constipation or diarrhea may also occur. Bone marrow suppression, including potentially fatal pancytopenia, and dermatological reactions such as pruritus, urticaria, alopecia, and Stevens-Johnson syndrome may occur as a result of direct chemical irritation of the skin and bone marrow. Antiepileptic medications, including the succinimides, are associated with increased risk of suicidal behavior and ideation.

Clinically Important Drug–Drug Interactions

Use of succinimides with primidone may cause a decrease in serum levels of primidone. Patients should be monitored and appropriate dose adjustments made if these two agents are used together.

Prototype Summary: Ethosuximide

Indications: Control of absence seizures.

Actions: May act in inhibitory neuronal systems, suppresses the electroencephalographic pattern associated with absence seizures, reduces frequency of attacks.

Pharmacokinetics:

Route	Peak
Oral	3–7 h

$T_{1/2}$: 30 hours (children), 60 hours (adults); metabolized in the liver; excreted in the urine and bile.

Adverse Effects: Drowsiness, ataxia, dizziness, irritability, nervousness, headache, blurred vision, pruritus, Stevens-Johnson syndrome, nausea, vomiting, epigastric pain, anorexia, diarrhea, and pancytopenia.

Drugs That Modulate the Inhibitory Neurotransmitter GABA

Other drugs that are used in the treatment of absence seizures work by modulating the inhibitor neurotransmitter GABA (see Table 23.2). These include acetazolamide (*Diamox*), divalproex (*Depakote*), valproic acid (generic), and zonisamide (*Zonegran*).

Prototype Summary: Valproic Acid

Indications: Drug of choice for myoclonic seizures; treatment of absence seizures; also effective in mania, migraine headaches, and complex focal seizures.

Actions: May act to increase GABA in brain.

Pharmacokinetics:

Route	Peak
Oral	3–8 h

T1/2: 9 to 16 hours; metabolized in liver.

Adverse effects: Hepatotoxicity, birth defects, pancreatitis, GI effects, headache, tinnitus, blurred vision, ataxia, hyperammonemia, thrombocytopenia, and infection.

Therapeutic Actions and Indications

Valproic acid reduces abnormal electrical activity in the brain and may also increase GABA activity at inhibitory receptors. It has been used for migraine prevention. Divalproex is indicated for treatment of manic episodes, treatment of absence and focal seizures, and prevention of migraine headaches. The therapeutic action is thought to be related to increased GABA levels in the brain. Acetazolamide—a sulfonamide—alters electrolyte movement, stabilizing nerve cell membranes, but it is rarely used for seizures. Another sulfonamide—zonisamide—is a newer agent that inhibits voltage-sensitive sodium and calcium channels, thus stabilizing nerve cell membranes and modulating calcium-dependent presynaptic release of excitatory neurotransmitters. See Table 23.2 for usual indications related to these drugs.

Pharmacokinetics

Valproic acid, available for oral use, is readily absorbed from the GI tract, reaching peak level in 1 to 4 hours. It is metabolized in the liver and excreted in the urine with a half-life of 6 to 16 hours. Acetazolamide, which can be given orally, IM, or IV, is readily absorbed from the GI tract and is excreted unchanged in the urine with a half-life of 2.5 to 6 hours. Divalproex is administered orally and is absorbed from the GI tract. It is almost entirely metabolized in the liver. The terminal half-life is 9 to 16 hours. Zonisamide, an oral drug, is well absorbed from the GI tract, reaching peak level in 2 to 6 hours. It is primarily excreted unchanged in the urine, with a half-life of 63 hours.

Contraindications and Cautions

These drugs are contraindicated with known allergy to any component of the drug. The sulfonamides are also contraindicated with known allergy to antibacterial sulfonamides and thiazide diuretics to avoid hypersensitivity reactions. When it is discontinued, zonisamide should be tapered over 2 weeks because of a risk of precipitating seizures. Patients who take this drug should be well hydrated due to risk of renal calculi development.

Caution should be used in patients with hepatic or renal impairment, which could alter metabolism and excretion of the drug. These drugs should not be used during pregnancy or lactation unless the benefit clearly outweighs the risk to the fetus or neonate because of the potential for serious adverse effects on the baby. There is teratogenic risk if valproic acid or divalproex are administered during pregnancy.

Adverse Effects

Valproic acid and divalproex are associated with liver toxicity, hyperammonemia, thrombocytopenia, and pancreatitis. They can also cause a rare hypersensitivity, Drug Reaction with Eosinophilia and Systemic Symptoms (DRESS). All of these drugs cause CNS effects related to CNS suppression—weakness, fatigue, drowsiness, dizziness, and paresthesias. Acetazolamide and zonisamide may cause rash and dermatological changes. Zonisamide is associated with bone marrow suppression, renal calculi development, and GI upset.

Clinically Important Drug–Drug Interactions

Acetazolamide increases the serum levels of quinidine, tricyclic antidepressants, and amphetamines and may increase salicylate toxicity when given with salicylates. Valproic acid and divalproex can increase serum levels and potential toxicity of phenobarbital, ethosuximide, diazepam, primidone, phenytoin, and zidovudine. If any of these drugs are used in combination, the patient should be monitored carefully and doses adjusted appropriately. Breakthrough seizures have been reported when valproic acid is combined with phenytoin, and extreme care should be taken if this combination must be used. Zonisamide levels and toxicity are increased if it is combined with carbamazepine, and the patient should be monitored and zonisamide dose reduced as needed.

Other Medications That Are Used to Treat Generalized Seizures

Some of the medications that are indicated for treatment of generalized seizures do not fit in the previous classifications. Carbamazepine (*Tegretol*, *Epitol*, and others), lamotrigine (*Lamictal*), levetiracetam (*Elepsia XR*, *Keppra*, *Spritam*), and topiramate (*Qudexy XR*, *Topamax*, *Trokendi XR*) are depicted in Table 23.2.

Therapeutic Actions and Indications

Carbamazepine is indicated for treatment of generalized and focal seizures in addition to trigeminal neuralgia. It is thought to inhibit polysynaptic responses and block sodium channels to prevent the formation of repetitive action potentials in the abnormal focus.

Lamotrigine may inhibit voltage-sensitive sodium and calcium channels, stabilize nerve cell membranes, and modulate calcium-dependent presynaptic release of excitatory neurotransmitters. Levetiracetam's mechanism of action is not completely understood; its antiepileptic action may be related to suppression of rapid action potentials without affecting normal neuronal excitability. See Box 23.6 for information about potentially serious name confusion that has occurred with levetiracetam.

Topiramate is a medication used to treat focal and generalized tonic–clonic seizures, including seizures associated with Lennox-Gastaut Syndrome. It is also indicated for prevention of migraines. The exact mechanisms of action are not known, but the theories include blocking sodium channels in neurons with sustained depolarization, increasing GABA activity, inhibiting a subtype of the glutamate receptor, and inhibiting the carbonic anhydrase enzyme.

Pharmacokinetics

Carbamazepine is absorbed from the GI tract and metabolized in the liver by the cytochrome P450 system. It is excreted in the urine with a half-life of 25 to 65 hours. Lamotrigine is rapidly absorbed from the GI tract, metabolized in the liver, and primarily excreted in the urine. The half-life of lamotrigine is approximately 25 hours. Levetiracetam is rapidly absorbed from the GI tract, reaching peak level in 1 hour. It goes through very little metabolism, with most of the drug being excreted unchanged in the urine with a half-life of 6 to 8 hours. Topiramate is absorbed via the GI tract. It is not metabolized and is excreted primarily unchanged in urine. The half-life is about 31 hours for *Trokendi XR*.

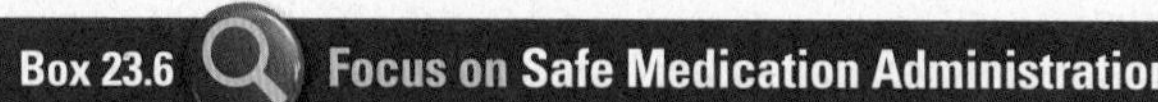
Box 23.6 Focus on Safe Medication Administration

Name confusion has been reported between levetiracetam (*Keppra*) and lopinavir/ritonavir (*Kaletra*), an HIV antiviral combination drug. Both drugs come in a liquid form, and confusion has been reported in the administration of the two drugs, causing serious adverse effects. Use extreme caution when administering these drugs.

Contraindications and Cautions

There is a boxed warning for carbamazepine regarding serious dermatologic reactions that are more frequent in people with the HLA-B*1502 Allele (see Box 23.3). There is also a caution to monitor for aplastic anemia and agranulocytosis. There is an association of congenital anomalies, specifically spina bifida, when administered during pregnancy.

Lamotrigine has a boxed warning regarding life-threatening rashes, including Stevens-Johnson syndrome and toxic epidermal necrolysis. The risk is greater in pediatric patients, when coadministered with valproate, when higher initial dose is used, and/or when dose escalation is exceeded.

There is a pregnancy registry that pregnant patients taking lamotrigine or levetiracetam can enroll in to monitor pregnancy outcomes. Pregnancy may decrease serum levels of levetiracetam. There is evidence that topiramate administered during pregnancy can cause fetal defects including cleft lip, cleft palate, and low birth weight.

Adverse Effects

Carbamazepine can cause CNS effects, including nystagmus, double vision, vertigo, staggering gait, and headache. Blood dyscrasias may also occur (leukopenia, anemia, and thrombocytopenia). Due to promotion of secretion of antidiuretic hormone, it may cause edema, HTN, and fluid overload, especially in patients with heart failure. Dermatitis, rash, photosensitivity, and Stevens-Johnson syndrome have been noted.

Lamotrigine can cause CNS effects similar to those of carbamazepine. There can be both mild and life-threatening rashes, as well. There is also a risk of developing aseptic meningitis.

Side effects associated with levetiracetam are dizziness, weakness, fatigue, agitation, anxiety, depression, and in rare cases suicidal ideation.

A reduced dose of topiramate is recommended for patients with renal impairment. The drug also has been associated with marked CNS depression. It can also cause metabolic acidosis, angle closure glaucoma, hyperthermia in the setting of decreased ability to sweat, visual field defects, suicidal thoughts and behavior, and serious rash reactions.

Clinically Important Drug–Drug Interactions

CNS depressants may increase CNS side effects of the medications. CYP3A4 inhibitors may increase carbamazepine levels, and CYP3A4 inducers may decrease carbamazepine levels. Carbamazepine may also influence plasma levels of other concomitant medications. Close monitoring is recommended when changing medication regimens. Concurrent use of topiramate and phenytoin or carbamazepine can decrease topiramate levels. Oral contraceptives may have decreased efficacy when taken with topiramate.

Prototype Summary: Carbamazepine

Indications: Treatment of generalized and focal seizures in addition to trigeminal neuralgia.

Actions: Inhibits polysynaptic responses and blocks posttetanic potentiation; mechanism of action is not completely understood.

Pharmacokinetics:

Route	Onset	Peak
Extended release	Slow	4–5 h
	Slow	3–12 h

$T_{1/2}$: 25 to 65 hours, then 12 to 17 hours; metabolized in the liver; excreted in the urine and feces. Initial half-life is longer due to process of "autoinduction." The medication induces liver enzymes to increase metabolism, which results in a shorter half-life over time. The half-life will stabilize with a fixed regimen in 3 to 5 weeks. Male children may have faster clearance and may require higher doses compared to female children.

Adverse Effects: Drowsiness, ataxia, dizziness, nausea, vomiting, cardiovascular (CV) complications, hepatitis, hematological disorders, Stevens-Johnson syndrome.

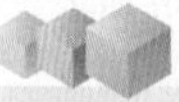
Concept Mastery Alert

Adverse Effects of Antiseizure Agents

For patients taking antiseizure agents, CNS depression is common, especially if the drug is administered with other CNS depressing agents. All such agents have a warning about the potential increased risk of suicidal thoughts and behavior. Furthermore, there is a pregnancy registry monitoring pregnancy outcomes for patients taking antiseizure medications, since many have been associated with increased risk of fetal abnormalities.

Nursing Considerations for Patients Receiving Drugs for Treating Generalized Seizures

The information that follows primarily relates to drug therapy with hydantoins, succinimides, medications that modulate GABA, and other medications that are used to treat generalized seizures. See Chapter 20 for nursing considerations for patients receiving barbiturates or benzodiazepines.

Assessment: History and Examination

- Assess for contraindications or cautions to the use of the medications, including known history of allergy to avoid hypersensitivity reactions, renal impairment that may indicate dosing adjustments, and current status related

to pregnancy and lactation to be able to advise regarding the pregnancy registry and to avoid fetal or infant harm.
- Obtain a description of seizures, including onset, aura, duration, and recovery, to determine type of seizure and establish a baseline.
- Perform a physical assessment to establish baseline data for determining the effectiveness of therapy and the occurrence of any potential adverse effects.
- Inspect the skin for color and lesions to determine evidence of possible skin effects; assess pulse and blood pressure and auscultate heart to evaluate for possible cardiac effects; assess level of orientation, affect, reflexes, and bilateral grip strength to evaluate any CNS effects; monitor bowel sounds and urine output to determine possible GI or genitourinary (GU) effects; and evaluate gums and mucous membranes to establish baseline and monitor changes associated with adverse effects.
- If appropriate, obtain a baseline electroencephalogram to evaluate brain function.
- Assess the patient's renal and liver function, including renal and liver function tests, to determine appropriateness of therapy and determine the need for possible dose adjustment.

Refer to the "Critical Thinking Scenario" for a full discussion of nursing care for a patient who is being prescribed antiepileptic drugs.

Nursing Conclusions

Nursing conclusions related to drug therapy might include the following:

- Impaired comfort related to GI, CNS, and GU effects
- Altered thought processes related to CNS effects
- Infection risk related to bone marrow suppression (succinimides, zonisamide)
- Injury risk related to CNS effects or toxic drug levels
- Altered skin integrity related to dermatological effects
- Knowledge deficit regarding drug therapy

Planning

- The patient will receive the best therapeutic effect from the drug therapy.
- The patient will have limited adverse effects to the drug therapy.
- The patient will have an understanding of the drug therapy, adverse effects to anticipate, and measures to relieve discomfort and improve safety.

Intervention With Rationale

- Discontinue the drug at any sign of hypersensitivity reaction, liver dysfunction, or severe skin rash to limit reaction and prevent potentially serious reactions.
- Administer the drug with food to alleviate GI irritation if GI upset is a problem.
- Monitor for adverse effects and provide appropriate supportive care as needed to help the patient cope with these effects.
- Monitor complete blood count (CBC) before and periodically during therapy if indicated for that medication to detect bone marrow suppression early and provide appropriate interventions.
- Discontinue the drug if skin rash, bone marrow suppression, or unusual depression or personality changes (including suicidal thoughts or behaviors) occur to prevent the development of more serious adverse effects.
- Discontinue the drug slowly, and refrain from withdrawing the drug quickly if possible, because rapid withdrawal may precipitate seizures.
- Monitor for drug–drug interactions to arrange to adjust doses appropriately if any drug is added to or withdrawn from the drug regimen.
- Arrange for counseling for patients who can become pregnant who are taking these drugs. Because these drugs have the potential to cause serious damage to the fetus, patients should understand these risks, use barrier contraceptives to avoid pregnancy, and be told about the pregnancy registry available for pregnant patients taking antiseizure medications.
- Offer support and encouragement to help the patient cope with the drug regimen and diagnosis.
- Provide thorough patient teaching to enhance patient knowledge about drug therapy and to promote adherence, including drug name and prescribed dosage, measures for avoidance of adverse effects, warning signs that may indicate possible problems, and the possible need for periodic blood tests to evaluate blood counts to reduce the risk for infection and for drug level tests to evaluate therapeutic effectiveness and minimize the risk for toxicity.
- Suggest the wearing or carrying of a MedicAlert ID to alert emergency workers and health care providers about the use of an antiepileptic drug.

Evaluation

- Monitor patient response to the drug (decrease in incidence or absence of seizures; serum drug levels within the therapeutic range); evaluate for therapeutic blood levels (40 to 100 mcg/mL) for ethosuximide to ensure the most appropriate dose of the drug.
- Monitor for adverse effects (CNS changes, GI depression, urinary retention, arrhythmias, blood pressure changes, liver toxicity, bone marrow suppression, severe dermatological reactions, suicidal thoughts or behaviors).
- Evaluate the effectiveness of the teaching plan (patient can give the drug name and dosage and name possible adverse effects to watch for and specific measures to prevent them; patient is aware of the risk of birth defects and the need to carry information about the diagnosis and use of this drug).
- Monitor the effectiveness of comfort measures and adherence to the regimen.

CRITICAL THINKING SCENARIO Antiepileptic Drugs

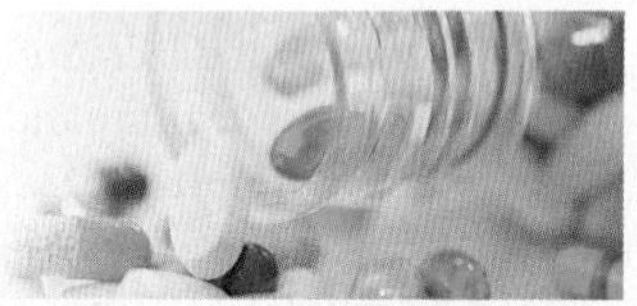

THE SITUATION

J.M., an athletic, 18-year-old high school senior, suffered their first seizure during math class. J.M. seemed attentive and alert and then suddenly slumped to the floor and suffered a full tonic–clonic seizure. The other students were frightened and did not know what to do. Fortunately, the teacher was familiar with seizures and quickly reacted to protect J.M. from hurting themself and to explain what was happening.

J.M. was diagnosed with idiopathic generalized epilepsy with tonic–clonic seizures. The topiramate that J.M. began taking made them quite drowsy during the day. J.M. was started on the medication due to it being the least expensive with their insurance plan. However, at the current dose, it was unable to control the seizures, and J.M. suffered three more seizures in the next month—one at school and two at home. J.M. is now undergoing reevaluation for possible dose and/or drug adjustment.

CRITICAL THINKING

What teaching implications should be considered when meeting with J.M.? Consider their age and the setting of their first seizure.

What problems might J.M. encounter in school and in athletics related to the diagnosis and the prescribed medication? Consider measures that may help J.M. avoid some of the unpleasant side effects related to the drug therapy. Driving a car may be a central social focus in the life of a high school senior.

What problems can be anticipated and confronted before they occur concerning laws that forbid people with newly diagnosed and/or poorly controlled epilepsy from driving?

Develop a teaching protocol for J.M. How will you involve the entire family in the teaching plan?

DISCUSSION

On their first meeting, it is important for the nurse to establish a trusting relationship with J.M. and their family. J.M., who is at a sensitive stage of development, requires a great deal of support and encouragement to cope with the diagnosis of epilepsy and the need for drug therapy. J.M. may need to ventilate their feelings and concerns and discuss how they can reenter school without worrying about having a seizure in class. The nurse should implement a thorough drug teaching program, including a description of warning signs to watch for that should be reported to a health care professional. J.M. should be encouraged to take the following preventive measures:

- Avoid operating dangerous machinery or performing tasks that require alertness while drowsy or confused.
- Pace activities as much as possible to help deal with any fatigue and malaise.
- Take the drugs with meals if GI upset is a problem.
- Report any eyesight changes, rashes or skin changes, high fever, depression, and/or thoughts of suicide immediately.

This information, along with the name of a health care professional and a telephone number to call with questions or comments, should be given to both J.M. and their family in written form for future reference. The importance of continuous medication to suppress the seizures should be stressed. The adverse effects of many of these drugs make it difficult for some patients to maintain adherence to their drug regimen.

After the discussion with J.M., the nurse should meet with their family members, who also need support and encouragement to deal with J.M.'s diagnosis and its implications. They need to know what seizures are, how the prescribed antiepileptic drug affects the seizures, what they can do when seizures occur, and complete information about the drugs J.M. must take and their anticipated effects. In addition, it is important to work with family members to determine whether any particular occurrence precipitated the seizures. In other words, was there any warning or aura? This may help with adjustment of drug dosages or avoidance of certain situations or stimuli that precipitate seizures. Family members should be encouraged to report and record any seizure activity that occurs.

Most states do not permit people with newly diagnosed epilepsy to drive, and states have varying regulations about the return of the driver's license after a seizure-free interval. If driving makes up a major part of J.M.'s social activities, this news may be even more unacceptable than the diagnosis. J.M. and their family should be counseled and helped to devise other ways of getting to places and coping with this restriction. J.M. may be interested in a referral to a support group for teens with similar problems, where they can share ideas, support, and frustrations.

J.M.'s condition is a chronic one that will require continual drug therapy and evaluation. They will need periodic reteaching and should have the opportunity to ask additional questions and to ventilate feelings. J.M. should be encouraged to wear or carry a MedicAlert ID so that emergency medical personnel are aware of their diagnosis and the medications they are taking.

NURSING CARE GUIDE FOR J.M.: ANTIEPILEPTIC AGENTS

Assessment: History and Examination

Assess for allergies to any of the drugs; depression, mood problems, and/or suicidal thoughts/behaviors; history of metabolic acidosis; weak or brittle bones; lung or breathing problems; eye problems (specifically glaucoma); growth problems; ketogenic diet; and hepatic or renal dysfunction. Assess whether the patient is pregnant and/or planning to become pregnant. Ask about any other medication (prescription or over-the-counter) or supplement use. Concurrent use of other antiseizure medications and any CNS depressants should be assessed.

Cardiovascular: Blood pressure, pulse, peripheral perfusion

CNS: Orientation, reflexes, affect, strength, electroencephalograph (EEG)

Skin: Color, lesions, texture, temperature
GI: Abdominal evaluation, bowel sounds
Respiratory: Respiration, adventitious sounds
Laboratory tests: CBC, liver and renal function tests

Nursing Conclusions

Impaired comfort related to GI, CNS, and GU effects
Injury risk related to CNS effects
Altered thought processes related to CNS effects
Knowledge deficit regarding drug therapy
Altered skin integrity related to dermatological effects

Planning

The patient will receive the best therapeutic effect from the drug therapy.
The patient will have limited adverse effects to the drug therapy.
The patient will have an understanding of the drug therapy, adverse effects to anticipate, and measures to relieve discomfort and improve safety.

Intervention

Discontinue drug at first sign of ocular impairment, skin rash, or suicidal ideation.
Provide comfort and safety measures: administer drugs with meals if GI discomfort occurs, and restrict activities and driving until the seizures are under control and J.M. has less fatigue.
Provide support and reassurance to cope with the diagnosis, restrictions, and drug effects.
Provide patient teaching regarding drug name, dosage, side effects, symptoms to report, the need to wear a MedicAlert ID, and other drugs to avoid.

Evaluation

Evaluate drug effects: decrease in incidence and frequency of seizures.
Monitor for adverse effects: CNS effects (multiple); rash or skin changes; GI effects such as anorexia or weight loss; eyesight changes; heat intolerance.
Monitor for drug–drug interactions: Increased depression with CNS depressants, alcohol, and any other antiseizure medication.
Evaluate effectiveness of patient teaching program.
Evaluate effectiveness of comfort/safety measures.

PATIENT TEACHING FOR J.M.

- The drug that has been prescribed is an antiepileptic agent. They are used to stabilize abnormal cells in the brain that have been firing excessively and causing seizures.
- The timing of these doses is important. To be effective, this drug must be taken at regular intervals and slowly titrated up to an effective dose.
- Do not stop taking this drug suddenly. If for any reason you are unable to continue taking the drug, notify your health care provider at once. This drug must be slowly withdrawn when its use is discontinued.
- Common effects of this drug include the following:
  - Fatigue, weakness, dizziness, and drowsiness: Try to space activities evenly throughout the day and allow rest periods to avoid these effects. Take safety precautions and avoid driving or operating dangerous machinery if these conditions occur.
  - Fever and decreased sweating: Monitor decreased sweating and body temperature; stay hydrated, especially in hot weather.
  - GI upset, loss of appetite, weight loss, and diarrhea: Taking the drug with food or eating small, frequent meals may help alleviate this problem.
- Report any of the following conditions to your health care provider: skin rash, severe nausea and vomiting, impaired coordination, eyesight changes, fever, personality changes, and depression and/or suicidal thoughts.
- It is advisable to wear or carry a MedicAlert ID so that any person who takes care of you in an emergency will know that you are taking this drug.
- Tell any doctor, nurse, or other health care provider involved in your care that you are taking this drug.
- Keep this drug and all medications out of the reach of children.
- Do not take any other drug, including over-the-counter medications and alcohol, without consulting with your health care provider. Many of these preparations interact with the drug and could cause adverse effects.
- Report and record any seizure activity that you have while you are taking this drug.
- Take this drug exactly as prescribed. Regular medical follow-up, which may include blood tests, may be necessary to evaluate the effects of this drug on your body.

Key Points

- There are several classifications of medications indicated to treat generalized tonic–clonic and absence seizures.
- All of these drugs stabilize nerve membranes throughout the CNS to decrease excitability and hyperexcitability to stimulation.
- Adverse effects associated with these drugs reflect CNS depression—lethargy, somnolence, fatigue, dry mouth, constipation, and dizziness. Serious liver, bone marrow, and dermatological problems can occur with specific drugs.
- All antiseizure medications can increase risk of suicidal thoughts and/or behaviors.

Drugs for Treating Focal Seizures

Focal seizures may be simple (involving only a single muscle or reaction) or complex (involving a series of reactions or emotional changes). Drugs used in the treatment of focal seizures include clorazepate (*Tranxene*, *Gen-Xene*, and others), eslicarbazepine (*Aptiom*), felbamate (*Felbatol*), gabapentin (*Neurontin*), lacosamide (*Vimpat*), oxcarbazepine (*Oxtellar XR*, *Trileptal*), pregabalin (*Lyrica*), perampanel (*Fycompa*), rufinamide (*Banzel*), tiagabine (*Gabitril*), and vigabatrin (*Sabril*) (Table 23.3). Some of the drugs used to treat generalized seizures have also been found useful in treating focal seizures (see Table 23.1).

Table 23.3 *Drugs in Focus:* Drugs for Treating Focal Seizures

Drug Name	Dosage/Route	Usual Indications
clorazepate (*Tranxene, Gen-Xene*)	*Adult:* 7.5 mg PO t.i.d., up to 90 mg/d *Pediatric (9–12 y):* 7.5 mg PO b.i.d., up to 60 mg/d	Used as adjunct for treatment of focal seizures; also used for anxiety disorders, acute symptoms of alcohol withdrawal
eslicarbazepine (*Aptiom*)	400 mg PO daily initially, up to 1,200 mg PO daily; half of dose if there is moderate or severe renal impairment	Used as adjunct for treatment of focal seizures
felbamate (*Felbatol*)	*Adult and pediatric > 14 y:* 2,600 mg/d PO *Pediatric (2–14 y):* 15 mg/kg/d PO in divided doses three to four times per day	Used as monotherapy or adjunctive therapy for treatment of focal seizures; adjunctive therapy for Lennox-Gastaut syndrome in children; however, drug is reserved for those cases that are unresponsive to other therapies due to its risks for severe adverse effects
gabapentin (*Gralise, Horizant, Neurontin*)	*Adult and pediatric:* Dosing varies based on formulation, indication, and age; decrease dose with renal impairment	Management of postherpetic neuralgia (all); treatment of restless legs syndrome (*Horizant*); used as adjunct in treating focal seizures (*Neurontin*)
lacosamide (*Vimpat*)	*Adult:* Initially 50 mg PO b.i.d., titrate to maintenance dose of 200–400 mg/d PO, IV dose is the same; decrease dose with renal or hepatic impairment	Adjunctive therapy for adults with focal seizures, reserve IV use for short term when oral is not possible
oxcarbazepine (*Oxtellar XR, Trileptal*)	*Adult:* 600 mg PO b.i.d. or daily for XR, increase up to 2,400 mg PO daily *Older adults:* Decrease initial dose *Pediatric:* Dosing based on body weight	Used for monotherapy or adjunctive therapy in treatment of focal seizures in adults and children
perampanel (*Fycompa*)	2 mg PO daily at bedtime initially; may be increased to max dose of 12 mg PO daily at bedtime; dose to be reduced if mild to moderate hepatic impairment; not recommended if severe renal or hepatic impairment	Used for adjunctive treatment of focal seizures for patients 12 y and older with or without secondarily generalized seizures
pregabalin (*Lyrica, Lyrica CR*)	300–600 mg/d PO in divided doses (*Lyrica*); 165 mg PO daily (*Lyrica CR*)	Used for adjunctive treatment of adult and pediatric patients with focal seizures (*Lyrica*); management of neuropathic pain associated with diabetic peripheral neuropathy and postherpetic neuralgia; fibromyalgia
rufinamide (*Banzel*)	*Adult:* Initially 400–800 mg/d PO, titrate to a target dose of 3,200 mg/d *Pediatric (4 and older):* 10 mg/kg/d PO in divided doses, titrate to a target dose of 45 mg/kg/d or 3,200 mg/d whichever is less	Adjunctive treatment of seizures associated with Lennox-Gastaut syndrome
tiagabine (*Gabitril*)	*Adult:* 4 mg PO daily up to 56 mg/d in two to four divided doses *Pediatric (12–18 y):* 4 mg PO daily up to a maximum 32 mg/d in two to four divided doses	Used as adjunct in treating focal seizures in adults and in children 12–18 y of age
vigabatrin (*Sabril*)	*Adult:* 500 mg PO b.i.d. to a maximum of 1.5 g PO b.i.d. with other antiepileptics *Pediatric (1 mo to 2 y):* 50 mg/kg PO b.i.d. of oral solution to a maximum 150 mg/kg PO b.i.d.	Monotherapy for children 1 mo to 2 y for infantile spasm; adjunctive therapy for adults with complex focal seizures not controlled by other therapy

ALS, amyotrophic lateral sclerosis.

Therapeutic Actions and Indications

The drugs used to control focal seizures stabilize nerve membranes in different ways—by altering sodium or calcium channels or by increasing the activity of GABA, an inhibitory neurotransmitter, and thereby decreasing excessive activity (see Fig. 23.2). Felbamate and oxcarbazepine can be used as monotherapy, and the remaining drugs are used as adjunctive therapy (see Table 23.3 for usual indications for each agent). Each of the drugs used for treating focal seizures has a slightly different mechanism of action.

Clorazepate and felbamate are thought to potentiate the effects of the inhibitory neurotransmitter GABA. Gabapentin's mechanism of action is unknown. It is found to be structurally related to GABA, and it binds to voltage-activated calcium channels, but it is unclear how this action causes the therapeutic effects. Gabapentin is also approved to be used in the treatment of postherpetic neuralgia and restless leg syndrome. It has many off-label uses and is often seen as a drug in the polypharmacy needed to achieve therapeutic results with psychiatric patients.

The drugs eslicarbazepine, lacosamide, and rufinamide inhibit voltage-sensitive sodium channels, which results in stabilization of nerve membranes and inhibition of neuronal firing.

Oxcarbazepine's exact mechanism of action is also unknown. It inhibits voltage-sensitive sodium channels, stabilizing hyperexcited nerve cell membranes. It also increases potassium conductance and modulates calcium-dependent presynaptic release of excitatory neurotransmitters. Any or all of these effects may be responsible for the antiseizure effects of the drug.

Perampanel acts as a noncompetitive glutamate receptor inhibitor. Glutamate is an excitatory neurotransmitter in the CNS. This medication has a boxed warning stating that there is a risk of serious or life-threatening psychiatric and behavioral adverse reactions that can include aggression, hostility, irritability, anger, and homicidal ideation and threats.

Pregabalin is indicated to treat postherpetic neuralgia, neuropathic pain associated with diabetic peripheral neuropathy or spinal cord injury, and fibromyalgia; it is also indicated for adjunctive therapy in treatment of focal seizures. It has a high binding affinity for voltage-gated calcium channels in the cerebrovascular system. It seems to modulate the calcium function in these neurons, leading to decreased release of neurotransmitters into the synaptic cleft and a decrease in cell activity.

Tiagabine binds to GABA reuptake receptors, causing an increase in GABA levels in the brain. Because GABA is an inhibitory neurotransmitter, the result is stabilization of nerve membranes and a decrease in excessive activity.

Vigabatrin blocks the enzyme GABAase, which increases GABA at the nerve synapse, leading to better stabilization of the nerve.

Pharmacokinetics

These drugs are all given orally. Lacosamide is also available for IV use.

Clorazepate is rapidly absorbed from the GI tract, reaching peak level in 1 to 2 hours. After metabolism in the liver, it is excreted in the urine with a half-life of 30 to 100 hours.

Eslicarbazepine reaches peak level in 1 to 4 hours. It is metabolized in the liver and excreted via the urine. The half-life is 13 to 20 hours.

Felbamate is absorbed well from the GI tract and is primarily excreted unchanged in the urine with a half-life of 20 to 23 hours.

Gabapentin is well absorbed from the GI tract and widely distributed in the body. It is excreted unchanged in the urine with a half-life of 5 to 7 hours.

Lacosamide is well absorbed from the GI tract, reaching peak level in 1 to 4 hours; if given IV, peak level is achieved at the end of the infusion. It is metabolized in the liver with a 13-hour half-life and is excreted in the urine.

Oxcarbazepine is completely absorbed from the GI tract and extensively metabolized in the liver. It is excreted in the urine with a half-life of 2 and then 9 hours.

Perampanel is readily absorbed orally, reaching peak level in 30 minutes to 2.5 hours. It is metabolized in the liver. It is excreted in urine and feces. The half-life is 105 hours.

Pregabalin is rapidly absorbed orally, reaching peak level in 1.5 hours. It is not metabolized but is eliminated unchanged in the urine with a half-life of 6.3 hours.

Rufinamide is well absorbed from the GI tract and reaches peak level in 4 to 6 hours. It is metabolized in the liver and excreted in the urine and has a half-life of 6 to 10 hours.

Tiagabine is rapidly absorbed from the GI tract, reaching peak level in 45 minutes. It is metabolized in the liver by the cytochrome P450 system. It is excreted in the urine with a half-life of 4 to 7 hours.

Vigabatrin is completely absorbed from the GI tract, does not undergo metabolism, and is excreted in the urine with a half-life of 7.5 hours.

Contraindications and Cautions

Contraindications to the drugs used to control focal seizures include the presence of any known allergy to the drug (due to possible hypersensitivity reactions) and severe hepatic dysfunction, which could be exacerbated and could interfere with the metabolism of the drugs.

There are pregnancy registries that monitor pregnancy outcomes in patients taking antiepileptic medications. Oxcarbazepine may be associated with increased risk of fetal congenital malformations, including ventricular septal defects and oral clefts. Patients who can become pregnant should be counseled regarding the risk of both seizure activity and medications on fetal development so that a safe plan can be made. These drugs enter human milk and can cause serious adverse effects in the baby. If any of these drugs is needed during lactation, another method of feeding the baby should be used.

Patients should be advised that in animal studies, males receiving pregabalin had decreased fertility and associated birth defects in offspring.

Caution should also be used with renal or hepatic dysfunction, which could alter the metabolism and excretion of the drugs, and with renal stones, which could be exacerbated by the effects of some of these agents.

Adverse Effects

The most frequently occurring adverse effects associated with the drugs used for focal seizures relate to the CNS depression that results. The following conditions may occur: drowsiness, fatigue, weakness, confusion, headache, and insomnia; GI depression with nausea, vomiting, and anorexia; and upper respiratory infections. Some antiepileptics can also be directly toxic to the liver and the bone marrow, causing dysfunction. The exact effects of each drug vary. All of these drugs carry warnings about the potential for increased suicidality. These drugs should also be tapered when discontinued because of the risk for precipitating seizures with sudden withdrawal. Felbamate has been associated with severe liver failure and aplastic anemia.

The adverse effects most commonly seen with pregabalin are related to CNS depression—tremor, dizziness, somnolence, and visual changes. It can also cause weight gain, edema, and, rarely, angioedema and hypersensitivity reactions. This drug has a controlled substance rating of category V. It can cause feelings of well-being and euphoria. Because of this, its use should be limited in patients who have a history of substance or alcohol use disorders.

Tiagabine has also been associated with serious skin rash. Vigabatrin is associated with a loss of vision, and the patient should be monitored before and during treatment. If vision changes begin to occur, the drug should be stopped.

Clinically Important Drug–Drug Interactions

If any of these drugs is taken with other CNS depressants or alcohol, a potential for increased CNS depression exists. Caution patients to take extreme precautions if such drug combinations cannot be avoided and to avoid alcohol while taking drugs for focal seizure.

Hormonal contraceptives may lose effectiveness if combined with oxcarbazepine and rufinamide. Patients needing a contraceptive when on rufinamide should consider a barrier contraceptive.

Prototype Summary: Gabapentin (*Neurontin*)

Indications: Treatment of focal onset seizures with and without secondary generalization, postherpetic neuralgia.

Actions: Exact mechanism of action is not understood; may bind to voltage-activated calcium channels; is structurally related to GABA, but does not affect GABA levels.

Pharmacokinetics:

Route	Onset	Peak
Oral	fast	1.7–4 h

$T_{1/2}$: 5 to 7 hours; not metabolized; excreted in the urine. Percentage of bioavailability decreases and time to peak increases with higher doses.

Adverse Effects: Drowsiness, ataxia, dizziness, edema, fatigue, nystagmus, nausea, vomiting, hypersensitivity and angioedema, drug reaction with eosinophilia and systemic symptoms.

Nursing Considerations for Patients Receiving Drugs to Treat Focal Seizures

Assessment: History and Examination

- Assess for contraindications and cautions: any known allergies to these drugs to avoid hypersensitivity reactions; history of renal or hepatic dysfunction that might interfere with drug metabolism and excretion; and current status of pregnancy or lactation, which require caution when using these drugs.
- Perform a physical assessment to establish baseline data for determining the effectiveness of therapy and the occurrence of any potential adverse effects.
- Inspect the skin for color and lesions to determine evidence of possible skin effects; assess pulse and blood pressure and auscultate heart to evaluate for possible cardiac effects; assess level of orientation, affect, reflexes, and bilateral grip strength to evaluate any CNS effects; monitor bowel sounds and urine output to determine possible GI or GU effects.
- If appropriate, obtain a baseline EEG to evaluate brain function.
- Assess the patient's renal and liver function, including renal and liver function tests, to determine the appropriateness of therapy and determine the need for possible dose adjustment.
- Monitor the results of laboratory tests such as urinalysis and CBC with differential to identify changes in bone marrow function.

Nursing Conclusions

Nursing conclusions related to drug therapy might include the following:

- Impaired comfort related to GI and CNS effects
- Altered thought processes related to CNS effects
- Injury risk and/or suicidal thoughts or behaviors related to CNS effects
- Knowledge deficit regarding drug therapy

Planning

- The patient will receive the best therapeutic effect from the drug therapy.
- The patient will have limited adverse effects to the drug therapy.
- The patient will have an understanding of the drug therapy, adverse effects to anticipate, and measures to relieve discomfort and improve safety.

Intervention With Rationale

- Administer the drug with food to alleviate GI irritation if GI upset is a problem.
- Monitor CBC before and periodically during therapy to detect and prevent serious bone marrow suppression for any medications for which this is a side effect.
- Protect the patient from exposure to infection if bone marrow suppression occurs.
- Discontinue the drug if skin rash, bone marrow suppression, unusual depression, or personality changes occur to prevent further serious adverse effects.
- Discontinue the drug slowly, and refrain from withdrawing the drug quickly when possible because rapid withdrawal may precipitate seizures.
- Arrange for counseling for patients who can become pregnant who are taking these drugs. Because some of these drugs have the potential to cause serious damage to the fetus, patients should understand the risk of congenital anomalies and use barrier contraceptives to avoid pregnancy or should be switched to a safer medication.
- Provide safety measures to protect the patient from injury or falls if CNS changes occur.
- Provide patient teaching, including drug name and prescribed dosage, measures for avoidance of adverse effects, warning signs that may indicate possible problems, the need for periodic laboratory testing, and monitoring and evaluation to enhance patient knowledge about drug therapy and to promote adherence.
- Suggest that the patient wear or carry a MedicAlert ID to alert emergency workers and health care providers about the use of an antiepileptic drug.
- Offer support and encouragement to help the patient cope with the drug regimen and diagnosis.

Evaluation

- Monitor patient response to the drug (decrease in incidence or absence of seizures).
- Monitor for adverse effects (CNS changes, GI depression, bone marrow suppression, severe dermatological reactions, liver toxicity, renal stones).
- Evaluate the effectiveness of the teaching plan (patient can give the drug name and dosage and name possible adverse effects to watch for and specific measures to prevent them; patient is aware of the risk of congenital anomalies and the need to carry information about the diagnosis and use of this drug).

Key Points

- Drugs used in the treatment of focal seizures include drugs that stabilize the nerve membrane by altering electrolyte movement or increasing GABA activity.
- Some of the drugs used to treat generalized seizures have also been found to be useful in treating focal seizures.
- Adverse effects associated with the use of drugs used in treating focal seizures include CNS depressive effects, dermatological disorders, and risk of suicidal thoughts and/or behaviors.

SUMMARY

- Epilepsy is a chronic disorder that includes seizure activity, a sudden discharge of excessive electrical energy from nerve cells located within the brain.
- Seizures can be divided into two groups: generalized and focal (formerly called partial).
- Generalized seizures can be further classified as motor and nonmotor (absence) types.
- Focal seizures can be further classified by whether or not awareness is impaired and whether there is motor or nonmotor onset.
- Drug treatment depends on the type of seizure that the patient has experienced and the toxicity associated with the available agents.
- Drug treatment is directed at stabilizing the overexcited nerve membranes and/or increasing the effectiveness of GABA, an inhibitory neurotransmitter.
- Adverse effects commonly associated with antiepileptics (e.g., insomnia, fatigue, confusion, GI depression, bradycardia) reflect the CNS depression caused by the drugs.
- Patients being treated with an antiepileptic should be advised to wear or carry a MedicAlert ID to alert emergency medical professionals to their epilepsy and their use of antiepileptic drugs.
- Patients being treated with an antiepileptic are often on long-term therapy, which requires adherence to their drug regimen and restrictions associated with their disorder and the drug effects.

CHECK YOUR UNDERSTANDING

Answers to the questions in this chapter can be found in Answers to Check Your Understanding Questions on thePoint®.

MULTIPLE CHOICE

Select the best answer.

1. When teaching a group of students about epilepsy, which characteristic should the nurse include?
   a. Always characterized by tonic–clonic seizures
   b. Only a genetic problem
   c. The most prevalent neurological disorder
   d. The name given to one brain disorder
2. Which type of seizure would the nurse be least likely to include as a type of generalized seizure?
   a. Absence seizures
   b. Febrile seizures
   c. Tonic–clonic seizures
   d. Complex seizures
3. Which would the nurse encourage a patient receiving an antiepileptic drug to do?
   a. Give up their driver's license.
   b. Wear or carry MedicAlert identification.
   c. Take antihistamines to help dry up secretions.
   d. Keep the diagnosis a secret to avoid prejudice.
4. Drugs that can be used to treat generalized seizures include
   a. barbiturates, benzodiazepines, and hydantoins.
   b. barbiturates, antihistamines, and local anesthetics.
   c. pregabalin, phenobarbital, and gabapentin.
   d. benzodiazepines, gabapentin, and pregabalin.
5. The drug of choice for the treatment of absence seizures is
   a. gabapentin.
   b. methsuximide.
   c. pregabalin.
   d. ethosuximide.
6. Focal seizures
   a. start at one point and spread quickly throughout the brain.
   b. are best treated with benzodiazepines.
   c. involve only part of the brain.
   d. are easily diagnosed and recognized.
7. One drug that is used alone in the treatment of focal seizures is
   a. carbamazepine.
   b. topiramate.
   c. lamotrigine.
   d. gabapentin.
8. Treatment of epilepsy is directed at
   a. blocking the transmission of nerve impulses into the brain.
   b. stabilizing overexcited nerve membranes.
   c. blocking peripheral nerve terminals.
   d. thickening the meninges to dampen brain electrical activity.

MULTIPLE RESPONSE

Select all that apply.

1. A patient has been stabilized on phenytoin (*Dilantin*) for several years and has not experienced a tonic–clonic seizure in more than 3 years. The patient decides to stop the drug because it no longer seems to be needed. In counseling, the nurse should include which points?
   a. The patient will always need this drug.
   b. This drug needs to be slowly tapered to avoid potentially serious adverse effects.
   c. The patient is probably correct, and the drug is not needed.
   d. The drug should not be stopped until appropriate blood tests are done.
   e. Stopping the drug suddenly could precipitate seizures because the nerves will be more sensitive.
   f. The patient's insurance company won't cover any problems that might occur if the drug is stopped without physician approval.
2. The most common adverse effects associated with antiepileptic therapy reflect the depression of the CNS. In assessing a patient on antiepileptic therapy, the nurse would monitor the patient for which conditions?
   a. Hypertension
   b. Insomnia
   c. Confusion
   d. GI depression
   e. Increased salivation
   f. Tachycardia

REFERENCES

Brunton, L., Hilal-Dandan, R., & Knollman, B. (2018). *Goodman and Gilman's the pharmacological basis of therapeutics* (13th ed.). McGraw-Hill.

Chang, G. B., Buchhalter, J., & Mullan, B. (2004). Mechanism of disease: Epilepsy. *New England Journal of Medicine, 349*, 1257–1266.

Delanty, N. (2010). *Seizures: Medical causes and management.* Humana Press.

Fisher, R. S., Cross, J. H., French, J. A., Higurashi, N., Hirsch, E., Janson, F. E., Lagae, L., Moshe, S. L., Peltola, J., Perez, E. R., Scheffer, I. E., & Zuberi, S. M. (2017). Operational classification of seizure types by the International League Against Epilepsy: Position paper of the ILAE commission for classification and terminology. *Epilepsia, 58*(4), 522–530. https://doi.org/10.1111/epi.13670

Kim, S., Ye, Y., Palikhe, N. S., Kim, J., & Park, H. (2010). Genetic and ethnic risk factors associated with drug hypersensitivity. *Current Opinion in Allergy and Clinical Immunology, 10*(4), 280–290. https://doi.org/10.1097/ACI.0b013e32833b1eb3

Kupiec, T., & Raj, V. (2005). Fatal seizures due to potential herb-drug interactions with Ginkgo Biloba. *Journal of Analytical Toxicology, 29*, 755–758. https://doi.org/10.1093/jat/29.7.755

Man, C. B. L., Kwan, P., Baum, L., Yu, E., Lau, K. M., Cheng, A. S. H., &, Ng, M. H. L. (2007). Association between HLA-B*1502 allele and antiepileptic drug-induced cutaneous reactions in Han Chinese. *Epilepsia, 48*(5), 1015–1018. https://doi.org/10.1111/j.1528-1167.2007.01022.x

Norris, T. L. (2019). *Porth's pathophysiology concepts of altered health states* (13th ed.). Wolters Kluwer.

Pandolfo, M. (2011). Genetics of epilepsy. *Seminars in Neurology, 31*(5), 506–518. https://doi.org/10.1055/s-0031-1299789

Scheffer, I. E., Berkovic, S., Capovilla, G., Connolly, M. B., French, J., Guilhoto, L., Hirsch, E., Jain, S., Mathern, G. W., Moshe, S. L., Nordli, D. R., Perucca, E., Tomson, T., Wiebe, S., Zhang, Y., & Zuberi, S. M. (2017). ILAE classification of the epilepsies: Position paper of the ILAE commission for the classification and terminology. *Epilepsia, 58*(4), 512–521. https://doi.org/10.1111/epi.13709

Sun, D., Yu, C. Y., He, X., Hu, J., Wu, G., Mao, B., Wu, S., & Xiang, H. (2014). Association of HLA-B*1502 and *1511 allele with antiepileptic drug-induced Stevens-Johnson syndrome in central China. *Journal of Huazhong University of Science and Technology, 34*, 146–150. https://link.springer.com/article/10.1007/s11596-014-1247-7

Wyllie, E., Cascino, G. D., Gidal, B. E., & Goodkin, H. P. (2010). *Treatment of epilepsy: Principles and practice.* Lippincott Williams & Wilkins.

CHAPTER 24

Antiparkinsonism Agents

Learning Objectives

Upon completion of this chapter, you will be able to:

1. Describe the current theory of the cause of Parkinson's disease and correlate this with the clinical presentation of the disease.
2. Discuss the use of antiparkinsonism agents across the lifespan.
3. Describe the therapeutic actions, indications, pharmacokinetics, contraindications, most common adverse reactions, and important drug–drug interactions associated with antiparkinsonism agents.
4. Compare and contrast the prototype drugs for each class of antiparkinsonism agents with the other drugs in that class and with drugs from the other classes used to treat the disease.
5. Outline the nursing considerations and teaching needs for patients receiving each class of antiparkinsonism agents.

Key Terms

anticholinergic: drug that opposes the effects of the neurotransmitter acetylcholine at acetylcholine receptor sites

basal ganglia: located in the brain just beneath the cerebral hemispheres, lateral to the thalamus; consist of the caudate nucleus, putamen, globus pallidus, substantia nigra, and subthalamic nucleus; function with the cerebral cortex as an accessory motor system

bradykinesia: difficulty in performing intentional movements and extreme slowness and sluggishness; characteristic of Parkinson's disease

dopaminergic: drug that increases the effects of dopamine at receptor sites

Parkinson's disease: debilitating disease characterized by progressive loss of coordination and function, which results from the degeneration of dopamine-producing cells in the substantia nigra

parkinsonism: clinical syndrome related to basal ganglia function due to medications blocking the effects of dopamine, damage caused by cerebral vascular disease, brain tumors, traumatic brain injury, or other causes

substantia nigra: a part of the basal ganglia rich in dopamine-secreting neurons; area of the brain where nerve cells atrophy in people diagnosed with Parkinson's disease

Drug List

DOPAMINERGIC AGENTS
- amantadine
- apomorphine
- bromocriptine
- (P) carbidopa–levodopa
- levodopa
- pramipexole
- rasagiline
- ropinirole
- rotigotine

ANTICHOLINERGIC AGENTS
- (P) benztropine
- diphenhydramine
- trihexyphenidyl

ADJUNCTIVE AGENTS
- entacapone
- safinamide
- selegiline
- tolcapone

In the 1990s, several prominent figures—former heavyweight boxing champion Muhammad Ali, former U.S. Attorney General Janet Reno, and actor Michael J. Fox—revealed that they had **Parkinson's disease**, a progressive, chronic neurological disorder. In general, Parkinson's disease may develop in people of any age, but it usually affects those who are past middle age and entering their 60s or even later years. Therefore, the occurrence of Parkinson's disease in these well-known individuals who were relatively young at the time of diagnosis is that much more interesting. The cause of the condition is not known; the etiology is suspected to be a combination of genetic predisposition and environmental factors.

At this time, there is no cure for Parkinson's disease. Therapy is aimed at management of signs and symptoms to provide optimal functioning for as long as possible.

Parkinson's Disease and Parkinsonism

Lack of coordination is characteristic of Parkinson's disease. Rhythmic tremors develop, insidiously at first. These tremors lead to rigidity in some muscle groups and to weakness in others. Affected patients may have trouble maintaining position or posture, and they may develop the condition known as **bradykinesia**, marked by difficulties in performing intentional movements and by extreme slowness or sluggishness.

As Parkinson's disease progresses, walking becomes a problem; a shuffling gait is a hallmark of the condition. In addition, patients may drool, and their speech may be slow and slurred. As the cranial nerves are affected, patients may develop a masklike expression. Difficulty swallowing, often leading to aspiration pneumonia, is a major issue as the disease progresses. It may be difficult to safely administer oral drugs to these patients. Parkinson's disease generally affects the higher levels of the cerebral cortex, so a person's alertness and cognition are maintained as they experience a progressively degenerating body. However, about 20% of people who suffer from Parkinson's disease will have severe cognitive dementia that causes deficits in visuospatial discrimination, memory retrieval, and frontal lobe executive functioning skills (planning, starting, and carrying out the steps of day-to-day tasks).

Parkinsonism is a term used to describe the Parkinson's disease–like extrapyramidal symptoms (tremor, rigidity, akinesia/bradykinesia, and postural changes) that are adverse effects associated with dopamine-blocking medications, brain tumors, severe carbon monoxide poisoning, cerebral vascular disease, or brain injuries.

Pathophysiology

Although the cause of Parkinson's disease is not known, it is known that the signs and symptoms of the disease relate to damaged neurons in the **basal ganglia** of the brain. The neurons of the basal ganglia are located just beneath the cerebral hemispheres, lateral to the thalamus, and consist of the caudate nucleus, putamen, globus pallidus, substantia nigra, and subthalamic nucleus. All of the sections of the basal ganglia work with the cerebral cortex and thalamus as an accessory motor control system. The basal ganglia help with both coordination of complex patterns of motor activity and cognitive control of motor activity. The dopamine neurotransmitter in this area of the brain acts as an inhibitory or stabilizing neurotransmitter. Another inhibitory neurotransmitter, gamma-aminobutyric acid, is secreted from the caudate nucleus and putamen and acts on the globus pallidus and substantia nigra. The excitatory neurotransmitter acetylcholine from the cortex acts on the caudate nucleus and putamen. There are also multiple glutamate pathways that are excitatory in this area of the brain, and the brain stem secretes several other neurotransmitters that can act on receptors in the basal ganglia. The neurotransmitters are designed to work together to balance excitation and inhibition to best facilitate coordination and smooth motor movements; for example, coordinating arm swinging with a graceful gait, putting the pattern of motor movements together required to throw a baseball, or hammering a nail require the motor pathways of the basal ganglia. See Figure 24.1 that demonstrates the motor circuit for learned patterns of movement and the neuronal pathways in the basal ganglia.

Theories about the cause of the degeneration of the basal ganglia range from viral infection, blows to the head,

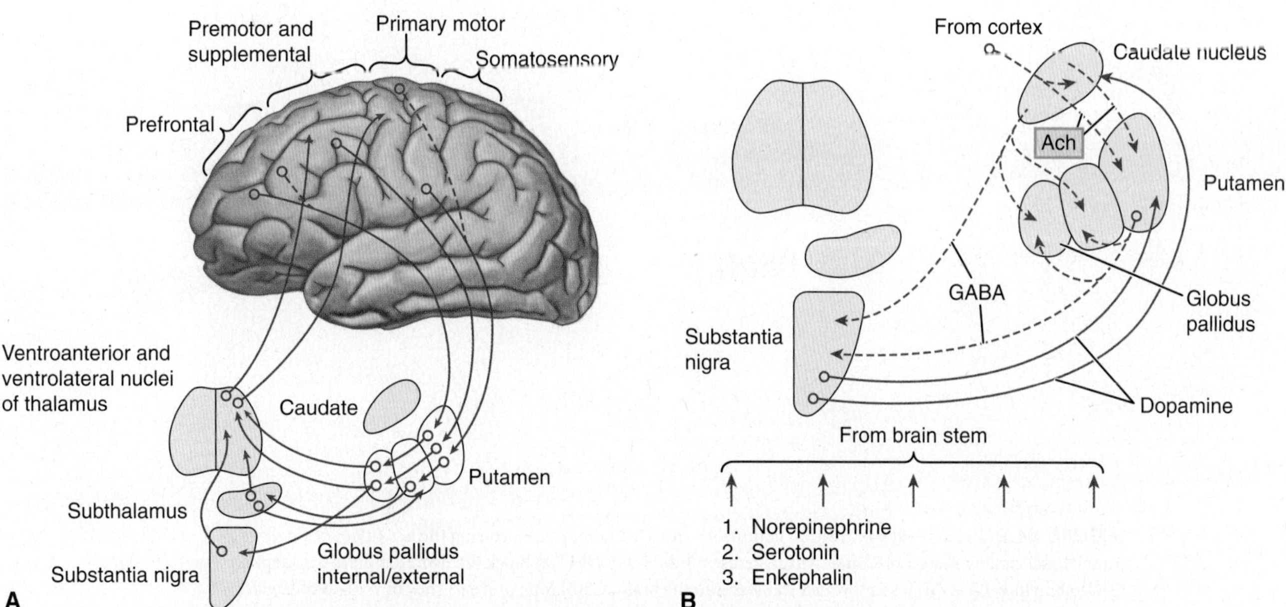

FIGURE 24.1 **A.** Putamen circuit through the basal ganglia for subconscious execution of learned patterns of movement. **B.** Close up of neuronal pathways that secrete different types of neurotransmitter substances in the basal ganglia. Ach, acetylcholine; GABA, gamma-aminobutyric acid. (Reprinted from *Guyton and Hall textbook of medical physiology*, 14th ed. Hall JE & Hall ME, Contributions of the Cerebellum and Basal Ganglia to Overall Motor Control, pp 711–726, Copyright 2021, with permission from Elsevier.)

brain infection, atherosclerosis, and exposure to certain drugs and environmental factors. There is most likely an interaction between genetic predisposition and environmental factors. Even though the actual cause is not known, the mechanism that causes the signs and symptoms of Parkinson's disease is understood. In a part of the basal ganglia called the **substantia nigra**, which has nerves that secrete dopamine, the nerve cell bodies progressively degenerate. This process results in a reduction of the amount of dopamine sent to the putamen and caudate nucleus. When dopamine decreases in the basal ganglia, a chemical imbalance occurs that allows the cholinergic or excitatory cells to dominate. This affects the functioning of the basal ganglia and of the cortical and cerebellar components of the extrapyramidal motor system. The extrapyramidal system is one that provides coordination for unconscious muscle movements, including those that control position, posture, and movement. The result of this imbalance in the motor system is apparent as the manifestations of Parkinson's disease.

Treatment

At this time, there is no treatment that arrests the neuron degeneration of Parkinson's disease and the eventual decline in patient function. Surgical procedures involving the basal ganglia have been tried, with varying levels of success at prolonging the degeneration caused by this disease. Drug therapy remains the primary treatment.

Therapy is aimed at restoring the balance between the declining levels of dopamine, which has an inhibitory effect on the neurons in the basal ganglia, and the now-dominant cholinergic neurons, which are excitatory.

This may help to reduce the signs and symptoms of parkinsonism and restore normal function for a time (Fig. 24.2).

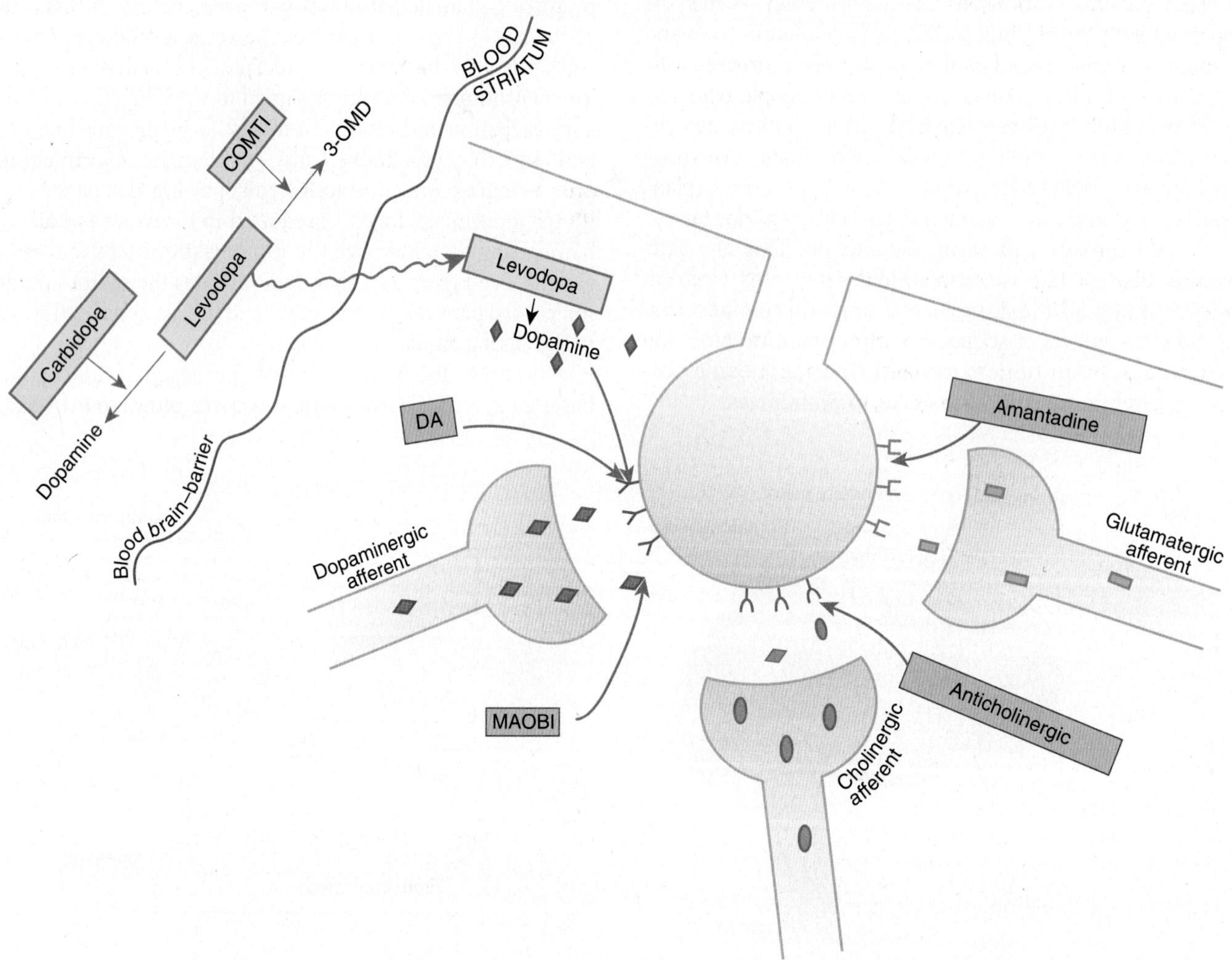

FIGURE 24.2 Drug therapy in treating Parkinson's disease is aimed at increasing the activity of dopamine in the basal ganglia. Catechol-*O*-methyltransferase inhibitors (COMTIs) block the degradation of levodopa to 3-*O*-methyldopa (3-OMD) so more can transfer into the brain. Carbidopa prevents the conversion of levodopa before it crosses the blood–brain barrier. Once levodopa is in the central nervous system, it can act on dopamine receptors. Dopamine agonists bind to and activate dopamine receptors. Monoamine oxidase type B inhibitors (MAOBIs) inhibit the breakdown of dopamine. Anticholinergic drugs bind and block the acetylcholine receptors. Amantadine binds and blocks *N-methyl*-D-aspartate (NMDA) glutamate receptors, which will enhance dopamine in this area of the brain. (Reprinted with permission from: Arcangelo, V. P., Peterson, A. M., Wilbur, V., & Kang, T. M. (2021). *Pharmacotherapeutics for advanced practice. A practical approach* (5th ed.). Wolters Kluwer.)

Box 24.1 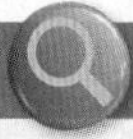 Focus on Drug Therapy Across the Lifespan

ANTIPARKINSONISM AGENTS

Children

The safety and effectiveness of most of these drugs has not been established in children. The incidence of Parkinson's disease in children is very small. Children do, however, experience parkinsonian symptoms as a result of drug effects.

If a child needs an antiparkinsonian drug, diphenhydramine is the drug of choice. If further relief is needed and another drug is tried, careful dosage calculations should be done based on age and weight, and the child should be monitored closely for adverse effects.

Adults

The eventual dependence and lack of control that accompany Parkinson's disease are devastating to all patients and their families but may be particularly overwhelming to individuals in their prime of life who value high degrees of autonomy, self-determination, and independence. Although these characteristics are not associated with any particular ethnic group, they are valued more highly among certain cultures than others. It is important for the nurse to assess all families with sensitivity to determine what convictions they hold and plan nursing care accordingly.

Adults diagnosed with Parkinson's disease require extensive teaching and support and help coping with the disease as well as with the effects of the drugs.

With the increasing interest in herbal and alternative therapies, it is important to stress the need to inform the health care provider about any other treatment being used. Vitamin B_6 or iron salts can pose a serious problem for patients who are taking some of these drugs.

Patients of childbearing age should be advised to use contraception when they are on these drugs. If a pregnancy does occur or is desired, the patient needs counseling about the potential for adverse effects. Patients who are nursing should be encouraged to find another method of feeding the baby because of the potential for adverse drug effects on the baby.

Older Adults

Although Parkinson's disease may affect individuals of any age, gender, or race or ethnicity, the frequency of the disease increases with age. This debilitating condition, which affects more males than females, may be one of many chronic problems associated with aging.

The drugs that are used to manage Parkinson's disease are associated with more adverse effects in older people with long-term problems. Both anticholinergic and dopaminergic drugs aggravate glaucoma, benign prostatic hypertrophy, constipation, cardiac problems, and chronic obstructive pulmonary diseases. Special precautions and frequent follow-up visits are necessary for older patients with Parkinson's disease, and their drug dosages may need to be adjusted frequently to avoid serious problems. In many cases, other agents are given to counteract the effects of these drugs, and patients then have complicated drug regimens with many associated adverse effects and problems. Consequently, it is essential for these patients to have extensive written drug-teaching protocols.

Total management of patient care in individuals with Parkinson's disease presents a challenge. Patients should be encouraged to be as active as possible, to perform exercises to prevent the development of skeletal deformities, and to attend to their own care as long as they can. Physical and occupational therapy can help slow the decline of motor function and teach the patient how to use adapted tools and strategies to maintain independence in their daily activities. When swallowing becomes an issue, a speech therapist may be helpful in teaching the patient to swallow safely, and thickening agents may be needed to help facilitate swallowing. Both the patient and family need instruction about following drug protocols and monitoring adverse effects, as well as encouragement and support for coping with the progressive nature of the disease (Box 24.1). Because of the degenerative effects of this disease, patients may experience episodes of depression or be emotionally upset. Psychological support, as well as physical support, is a crucial aspect of care.

Key Points

- Parkinson's disease is a progressive nervous system disease characterized by tremors, rigidity, bradykinesia, and changes in posture and gait.
- The loss of dopamine-secreting cells within the substantia nigra of the basal ganglia results in a loss of the inhibitory dopamine effect and is thought to be responsible for Parkinson's disease.

Dopaminergic Agents

Dopaminergic agents—drugs that increase the effects of dopamine at receptor sites—have been proven to be more effective than anticholinergics in the treatment of parkinsonism (Table 24.1). Dopaminergic agents include amantadine (*Gocovri, Osmolex ER*), apomorphine (*Apokyn*), bromocriptine (*Parlodel*), levodopa (*Inbrija*), carbidopa–levodopa (*Duopa, Rytary*), pramipexole (*Mirapex, Mirapex ER*), rasagiline (*Azilect*), ropinirole (*Requip, Requip ER*), and rotigotine (*Neupro*).

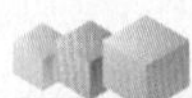 *Concept Mastery Alert*

Administration Route for Apomorphine

Apomorphine (used in the treatment of Parkinson's disease) is administered subcutaneously, not orally, and it is often given with trimethobenzamide. It is recommended that trimethobenzamide be started 3 days prior to the first dose of apomorphine and should only be continued as needed to control nausea and vomiting, generally no longer than 2 months.

Therapeutic Actions and Indications

Dopamine does not cross the blood–brain barrier. Therefore, other drugs that act like dopamine or increase dopamine concentrations indirectly must be used to increase dopamine levels in the basal ganglia or to directly stimulate

Table 24.1 *Drugs in Focus:* Dopaminergic Agents

Drug Name	Dosage/Route	Usual Indications
amantadine (*Gocovri, Osmolex ER*)	100 mg PO b.i.d. or 200 mg PO daily, up to 400 mg/d has been used; 129–322 mg PO daily (*Osmolex ER*); 137 mg PO daily for 1 week and then increase to 274 mg PO daily (*Gocovri*). Reduce dose with renal impairment.	Antiviral (generic), treatment of idiopathic and drug-induced parkinsonism in adults
apomorphine (*Apokyn, Kynmobi*)	2–6 mg subcutaneous PRN doses separated by at least 2 hours (*Apokyn*) 10–30 mg sublingual PRN; doses separated by at least 2 hours (*Kynmobi*)	Intermittent treatment of hypomobility "off" episodes of advanced Parkinson's disease
bromocriptine (*Parlodel*)	1.25 mg PO b.i.d., titrate up to 10–40 mg/d	Treatment of idiopathic Parkinson's disease may be beneficial in later stages when response to levodopa decreases; treatment of hyperprolactinemia, acromegaly
carbidopa–levodopa (*Duopa, Rytary*)	Initial dosing: 100 mg levodopa with 10–25 mg carbidopa PO t.i.d. (generic); 23.75/95 mg PO t.i.d. (*Rytary*) Max dose: 2000 mg enteral infusion over 16 hours (*Duopa*)	Treatment of idiopathic Parkinson's disease (both); treatment of postencephalitic parkinsonism, and parkinsonism that can follow intoxication with manganese or carbon monoxide (generic and *Rytary*)
levodopa (*Inbrija*)	84-mg capsules inhaled PRN, up to 5 times per day	Intermittent treatment of off episodes in patients with idiopathic Parkinson's disease treated with carbidopa/levodopa
pramipexole (*Mirapex, Mirapex ER*)	0.125 mg PO t.i.d., titrate up to 1.5 mg PO t.i.d. 0.375–4.5 mg PO daily (ER)	Treatment of idiopathic Parkinson's disease
rasagiline (*Azilect*)	1 mg/d PO, 0.5 mg/d PO if used with levodopa	Initial monotherapy and as adjunct to levodopa to treat idiopathic Parkinson's disease
ropinirole (*Requip, Requip XL*)	0.25 mg PO t.i.d., titrate up to maximum dose of 24 mg/d 2–24 mg PO daily (XL)	Treatment of idiopathic Parkinson's disease in early stages and in later stages when combined with levodopa; treatment of restless legs syndrome
rotigotine (*Neupro*)	2- to 8-mg/24-h transdermal patch, based on patient response and tolerance; 1- to 3-mg/24-h patch for restless leg syndrome	Treatment of all stages of Parkinson's disease; treatment of restless leg syndrome

the dopamine receptors in that area. This action helps restore the balance between the inhibitory and stimulating neurotransmitters. Dopaminergic agents are designed to promote dopamine synthesis, activate dopamine receptors, prevent dopamine breakdown, or decrease the degradation of levodopa. The agents do not stop the progression of Parkinson's disease but can offer relief from the symptoms (tremor, rigidity, and bradykinesia). See Table 24.1 for usual indications for each of these agents.

Levodopa is the mainstay of treatment for Parkinson's disease. This precursor of dopamine crosses the blood–brain barrier and is converted into dopamine. In this way, it acts like a replacement therapy. Levodopa is given in combination form with carbidopa as a fixed combination drug. When used with carbidopa, the enzyme dopa decarboxylase is inhibited in the periphery, diminishing the metabolism of levodopa in the gastrointestinal (GI) tract and in peripheral tissues, thereby leading to higher levels crossing the blood–brain barrier. Because the carbidopa increases the amount of levodopa that reaches the basal ganglia, the medication can have more therapeutic effect with less side effects.

In 2015, an extended-release combination of levodopa/carbidopa (*Rytary*) was approved for use in Parkinson's disease, postencephalitic parkinsonism, and post–carbon monoxide poisoning parkinsonism.

Amantadine is an antiviral drug that also seems to increase the release of dopamine. *Gocovri* is indicated for treatment of dyskinesia in patients with Parkinson's disease who are receiving levodopa-based therapy. *Osmolex ER* is indicated for treatment of Parkinson's disease and drug-induced extrapyramidal reactions in adults.

Apomorphine directly binds to postsynaptic dopamine receptors and is FDA approved for "off" episodes associated with advanced Parkinson's disease. Similar to apomorphine, bromocriptine, pramipexole, ropinirole, and rotigotine act as direct dopamine agonists on dopamine receptor sites in the basal ganglia. Because bromocriptine does not depend on cells in the area to biotransform it or to increase the release of already produced dopamine, it may be effective longer than levodopa or amantadine. Ropinirole can also be used to treat restless leg syndrome. Rotigotine is available in transdermal form, which is beneficial for patients having difficulty with swallowing. It is also indicated for treatment of restless leg syndrome.

Rasagiline is a dopamine agonist that increases dopamine in the nerve synapse, particularly in areas of the brain responsible for controlling movement and coordination. It inhibits monoamine oxidase (MAO) type B, which is found primarily in the central nervous system (CNS) and regulates the degradation of dopamine and other catecholamines. Because this drug works on an enzyme found mostly inside the CNS, it has fewer peripheral adverse effects. It can be used as initial monotherapy or as an adjunct therapy with levodopa for Parkinson's disease.

Pharmacokinetics

The dopaminergics are usually given orally and are generally well absorbed from the GI tract and widely distributed in the body. Apomorphine, however, must be given subcutaneously, and rotigotine is given transdermally. The dopaminergics are metabolized in the liver and peripheral cells and excreted in the urine. They cross the placenta and enter human milk.

Contraindications and Cautions

The dopaminergics are contraindicated in the presence of any known allergy to the drug or drug components to prevent hypersensitivity reactions and in angle-closure glaucoma, which could be exacerbated by these drugs. Dopaminergics enter human milk and should not be used during lactation because of the potential for adverse effects in the baby. In addition, levodopa (*Inbrija*) is contraindicated in patients who are taking or have recently taken (within 2 weeks) a nonselective MAO inhibitor. Extended-release forms of amantadine should not be administered if the patient has end-stage renal disease.

Administer dopaminergic agents cautiously with patients who have any condition that could be exacerbated by dopamine receptor stimulation, such as cardiovascular disease, including myocardial infarction, arrhythmias, and hypertension; bronchial asthma; history of peptic ulcers; urinary tract obstruction; and psychiatric disorders. Care also is necessary during pregnancy because these drugs cross the placenta and data with animals show potential for fetal harm and in patients with renal and hepatic disease, which could interfere with the metabolism and excretion of the drug. Closely monitor cardiac status in patients receiving apomorphine because of the associated risk for hypotension and prolonged QT interval.

Adverse Effects

The adverse effects associated with the dopaminergics usually result from stimulation of dopamine receptors. CNS effects may include anxiety, nervousness, headache, malaise, fatigue, confusion, mental changes including psychosis, blurred vision, muscle twitching, and ataxia. Peripheral effects may include anorexia, nausea, vomiting, dysphagia, and constipation or diarrhea; cardiac arrhythmias, orthostatic hypotension, and palpitations; bizarre breathing patterns; urinary retention; and flushing, increased sweating, and hot flashes. Bone marrow depression and hepatic dysfunction have also been reported (Fig. 24.3).

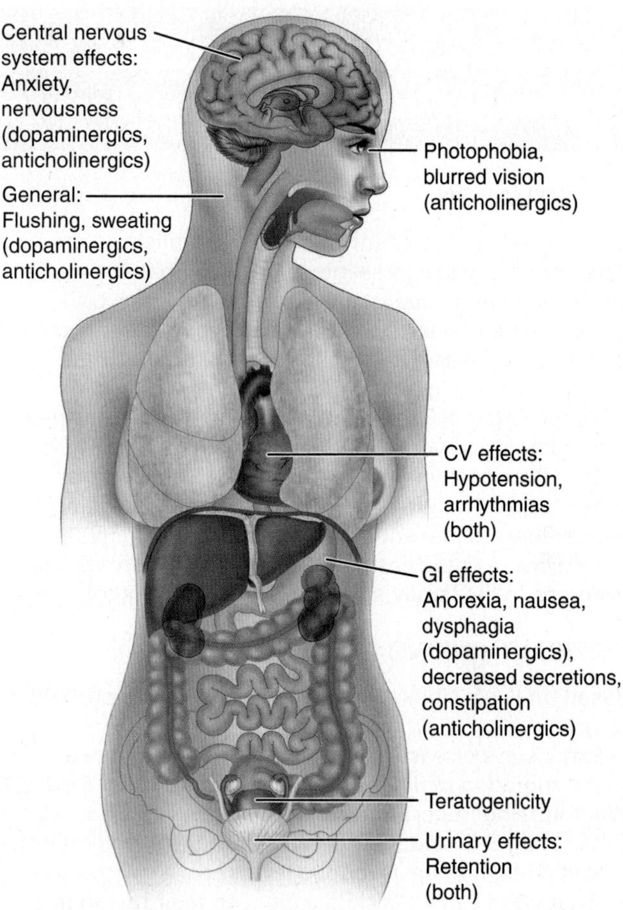

FIGURE 24.3 Common adverse effects and toxicities associated with antiparkinsonism agents.

Clinically Important Drug–Drug Interactions

If dopaminergics are combined with monoamine oxidase inhibitors (MAOIs), therapeutic effects increase and a risk of hypertensive crisis exists. The MAOI should be stopped 14 days before beginning therapy with a dopaminergic.

The combination of carbidopa–levodopa with iron salts or dopamine antagonists may lead to decreased efficacy of the medication (see "Critical Thinking Scenario"). In addition, patients who take dopaminergics should be cautioned to avoid over-the-counter vitamins; if such medications are used, the patient should be monitored closely because a decrease in dopaminergic effectiveness can result.

Patients using rasagiline should avoid tyramine-containing foods, as well as St. John's wort, meperidine, and acetaminophen, to avoid potentially serious reactions.

CRITICAL THINKING SCENARIO
Effects of Iron Salt Intake on Carbidopa–Levodopa Levels

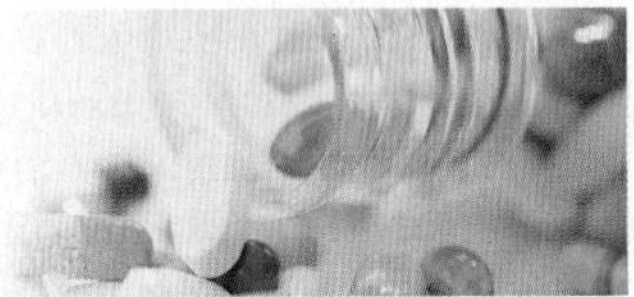

THE SITUATION

S.S., a 58-year-old patient with well-controlled Parkinson's disease, presents with severe nausea, anorexia, fainting spells, and heart palpitations. S.S. has been maintained on carbidopa–levodopa for the Parkinson's disease, and claims to have followed the drug regimen religiously.

According to S.S., the only change in lifestyle has been the addition of several health foods and vitamins. Their child, who recently returned from their freshman year in college, has begun a new health regimen, including natural foods and plenty of supplemental vitamins. They were so enthusiastic about their new approach that everyone in the family agreed to give this diet a try.

CRITICAL THINKING

Based on S.S.'s signs and symptoms, what has probably occurred?

In Parkinson's disease, is it possible to differentiate a deterioration of illness from a toxic reaction to a drug?

What nursing implications should be considered when teaching S.S. and their family about the effects of iron salt on carbidopa–levodopa levels?

In what ways can S.S's child cope with their role in this crisis?

Develop a new care plan for S.S. that involves all family members and includes drug teaching.

DISCUSSION

The presenting symptoms reflect an increase in Parkinson's symptoms as well as an increase in peripheral dopamine reactions (e.g., palpitations, fainting, anorexia, nausea). It is necessary to determine whether the problem involves a further degeneration in the neurons in the substantia nigra or the particular medication that S.S. has been taking. In many patients, responsiveness to levodopa is lost as neural degeneration continues.

The explanation of the new lifestyle—full of grains, natural foods, and vitamins—alerted the nurse to the possibility of excessive iron intake. In reviewing the vitamin bottles and some of the food packages supplied by S.S., it seemed that too much iron salt, which can bind with the medication and decrease effectiveness, might be the reason the patient's symptoms recurred.

The status of S.S.'s Parkinson's disease should be evaluated, and then, they can be restarted on carbidopa–levodopa. The smallest dose possible should be used initially, with gradual increases to achieve the maximum benefit with the fewest side effects. S.S. may also be prescribed an adjunctive medication to help with their symptoms.

In addition, S.S. should receive thorough drug teaching in written form for future reference. The need to avoid iron supplements should be emphasized. The entire family should be involved in an explanation of what happened and how this situation can be avoided in the future. Because the child may feel guilty about their role, they should have the opportunity to discuss their feelings and explore the positive impact of healthy food on nutrition and quality of life. This situation can serve as a good teaching example for staff as well as present them with an opportunity to review drug therapy in Parkinson's disease and the risks and benefits of certain diets.

NURSING CARE GUIDE FOR S.S.: LEVODOPA

Assessment: History and Examination

Allergies to carbidopa–levodopa; chronic obstructive pulmonary disease; dysrhythmias, hypotension, hepatic or renal dysfunction; psychoses; peptic ulcer; glaucoma

Concurrent use of MAOIs, phenytoin, pyridoxine, or tricyclic antidepressants

Focus physical examination on:

CV: Blood pressure, pulse rate, peripheral perfusion, electrocardiogram results

CNS: Orientation, affect, reflexes, grip strength

Renal: Output, bladder palpation

GI: Abdominal examination, bowel sounds

Respiratory: Respiration, adventitious sounds

Laboratory tests: Renal and liver function tests, complete blood count

Nursing Conclusions

Injury risk related to CNS effects

Altered thought processes related to CNS effects

Knowledge deficit regarding drug therapy

Constipation risk related to GI effects

Planning

The patient will receive the best therapeutic effect from the drug therapy.

The patient will have limited adverse effects to the drug therapy.

The patient will have an understanding of the drug therapy, adverse effects to anticipate, and measures to relieve discomfort and improve safety.

Intervention

Ensure safe and appropriate administration of drug.

Provide comfort and safety: Slow positioning changes; assess orientation, provide pain medication as needed; give drug with food; administer with carbidopa.

Provide support and reassurance for managing disease and drug effects.

Instruct the patient regarding drug dose, effects, and adverse symptoms to report.

Evaluation

Evaluate drug effects: relief of signs and symptoms of Parkinson's disease.

Monitor for adverse effects: CNS effects; renal changes, urinary retention; GI effects (constipation); increased sweating or flushing.

Monitor for drug–drug interactions: hypertensive crisis with MAOIs, decreased effects with iron salts or dopamine antagonists.

Evaluate the effectiveness of the patient teaching program.

Evaluate the effectiveness of comfort and safety measures.

PATIENT TEACHING FOR S.S.

- The drug that has been prescribed is called carbidopa–levodopa. It increases the levels of dopamine in the central areas of the brain and helps reduce the signs and symptoms of Parkinson's disease.
- People who take this drug must have their individual dose needs adjusted over time and sometimes adjunctive medication is prescribed. Common effects of this drug include the following:
  - Fatigue, weakness, and drowsiness: Try to space activities evenly through the day; allow rest periods to avoid these side effects. Take safety precautions and avoid driving or operating dangerous machinery if these conditions occur.
  - Dizziness, fainting: Change position slowly to avoid dizzy spells.
  - Increased sweating, darkened urine: This is a normal reaction. Avoid very hot environments.
  - Headaches, difficulty sleeping: These usually pass as the body adjusts to the drug. If they become too uncomfortable and persist, consult with your health care provider.
- Report any of the following to your health care provider: uncontrolled movements of any body part, chest pain or palpitations, depression or mood changes, difficulty in voiding, or severe or persistent nausea and vomiting.
- Be aware that iron salt interferes with the effects of carbidopa–levodopa. If you feel that you need a vitamin product, consult with your health care provider about using an agent that does not contain iron salts.
- Avoid eating large quantities of foods that contain iron, such as red meat.
- Tell any doctor, nurse, or other health care provider involved in your care that you are taking this drug.
- Keep this drug and all medications out of the reach of children.
- Do not overexert yourself when you begin to feel better. Pace yourself.
- Take this drug exactly as directed, and schedule regular medical checkups to evaluate its effects.

Prototype Summary: Carbidopa–Levodopa

Indications: Treatment of parkinsonism and Parkinson's disease.

Actions: Levodopa is a precursor of dopamine, which is deficient in parkinsonism; it crosses the blood–brain barrier, where it is converted to dopamine and acts as a replacement neurotransmitter. Carbidopa decreases the peripheral metabolism of levodopa so that more of the levodopa crosses the blood–brain barrier.

Pharmacokinetics:

Route	Onset	Peak	Duration
Oral	Varies	0.5–3 h	5 h

$T_{1/2}$: About 2 hours; metabolized in the liver; excreted in the urine.

Adverse Effects: Adventitious movements, ataxia, increased hand tremor, dizziness, numbness, weakness, agitation, anxiety, anorexia, nausea, vomiting, dry mouth, dysphagia, urinary retention, flushing, cardiac irregularities, psychosis.

Nursing Considerations for Patients Receiving Dopaminergic Agents

Assessment: History and Examination

- Assess for contraindications or cautions: Any known allergies to these drugs to avoid hypersensitivity reactions; GI depression or obstruction, urinary hesitancy or obstruction, benign prostatic hypertrophy, or glaucoma, which may be exacerbated by these drugs; cardiac arrhythmias, hypertension, or respiratory disease, which may be exacerbated by dopamine receptor stimulation; current status of pregnancy or lactation, which are cautions or contraindications to use of the drug; and renal or hepatic dysfunction, which could interfere with the drug's excretion or metabolism.
- Perform a physical assessment before beginning therapy to determine baseline status, to determine the effectiveness of drug therapy, and to monitor for any potential adverse effects.
- Inspect the skin for evidence of skin lesions or history of melanoma if the patient is to receive levodopa, which could cause or exacerbate melanoma.
- Assess level of orientation and neurological status, including affect, reflexes, bilateral grip strength, gait, tremors, and spasticity, to evaluate any CNS effects.

(continues on page 426)

- Auscultate lungs and assess respiratory status to evaluate for changes that could be exacerbated by the drug's effect.
- Monitor pulse, blood pressure, and cardiac output to evaluate for possible adverse effects.
- Auscultate bowel sounds to evaluate GI motility to assess for adverse effects.
- Assess urine output and palpate bladder to determine adequate bladder and renal function.
- Monitor the results of laboratory tests, such as liver and renal function studies, to determine need for possible dose adjustment, and complete blood count with differential to evaluate for possible bone marrow suppression.

Nursing Conclusions

Nursing conclusions related to drug therapy might include the following:

- Altered thought processes related to CNS effects
- Urinary retention related to dopaminergic effects
- Constipation risk related to dopaminergic effects
- Injury risk related to CNS effects and incidence of orthostatic hypertension
- Knowledge deficit regarding drug therapy

Planning

- The patient will receive the best therapeutic effect from the drug therapy.
- The patient will have limited adverse effects to the drug therapy.
- The patient will have an understanding of the drug therapy, adverse effects to anticipate, and measures to relieve discomfort and improve safety.

Intervention With Rationale

- Arrange to decrease the dose of the drug if therapy has been interrupted for any reason to prevent systemic dopaminergic effects.
- Evaluate disease progress and signs and symptoms periodically and record for reference of disease progress and drug response.
- Give the drug with meals to alleviate GI irritation if GI upset is a problem.
- Monitor bowel function and institute a bowel program if constipation is severe.
- Monitor urinary output, palpate bladder, and check for residual urine if urinary retention becomes a problem.
- Establish safety precautions if CNS or vision changes occur to prevent patient injury.
- Monitor hepatic, renal, and hematological tests periodically during therapy to detect early signs of dysfunction and consider reevaluation of drug therapy.
- Provide support services and comfort measures as needed to improve patient compliance.
- Provide thorough patient teaching about topics, such as the drug name and prescribed dose, measures to help avoid adverse effects, warning signs that may indicate problems, and the need for periodic monitoring and evaluation, to enhance patient knowledge about drug therapy and to promote adherence.
- Offer support and encouragement to help the patient cope with the disease and drug regimen.

Evaluation

- Monitor patient response to the drug (improvement in signs and symptoms of Parkinson's disease).
- Monitor for adverse effects (CNS changes, urinary retention, GI depression, tachycardia, increased sweating, flushing).
- Evaluate the effectiveness of the teaching plan (patient can give the drug name and dosage, name possible adverse effects to watch for and specific measures to prevent them, and discuss the importance of continued follow-up).
- Monitor the effectiveness of support measures and compliance with the regimen.

Key Points

- Dopaminergic drugs are used to increase the effects of dopamine at receptor sites, restoring the balance of neurotransmitters in the basal ganglia.
- The adverse effects most commonly associated with these drugs are related to the systemic effects of dopamine, increased heart rate, increased blood pressure, decreased GI activity, and urinary retention.
- Carbidopa–levodopa is the standard dopaminergic used to treat parkinsonism and Parkinson's disease. Several other dopaminergics are now used as monotherapy or adjuncts to carbidopa–levodopa to increase the dopamine effects as long as possible.

Anticholinergic Agents

Anticholinergic agents (Table 24.2) are drugs that oppose the effects of acetylcholine at receptor sites in the basal ganglia, thus helping to restore chemical balance in the area. Anticholinergics used to treat Parkinson's disease include benztropine (*Cogentin*), diphenhydramine (*Benadryl*), and trihexyphenidyl (generic).

Therapeutic Actions and Indications

The anticholinergics used to treat parkinsonism are synthetic drugs that have been developed to have a greater affinity for cholinergic receptor sites in the CNS than for those in the peripheral nervous system. However, to some extent, they still block the cholinergic receptors that are responsible for stimulation of the parasympathetic nervous system's postganglionic effectors. This blockage is

Table 24.2 ***Drugs in Focus:* Anticholinergic Agents**

Drug Name	Dosage/Route	Usual Indications
benztropine (*Cogentin*)	0.5–6 mg/d PO may be needed, 1–2 mg IM or IV; reduce dose in older patients	Adjunctive treatment of parkinsonism and drug-induced parkinsonism resulting from drug effects of phenothiazines
diphenhydramine (*Benadryl*)	*Adult:* 25–50 mg PO t.i.d. to q.i.d.; 10–50 mg IM or IV, maximum dose 400 mg/d *Pediatric:* 12.5–25 mg PO t.i.d. to q.i.d.; do not exceed 300 mg/d, 5 mg/kg/d IM or IV divided into four equal doses, maximum daily dose 300 mg	Adjunctive agent for treatment of Parkinson's disease; treatment of parkinsonism, including drug-induced disease particularly in the older adults and in patients at the early stages of disease; also used to treat allergy symptoms and motion sickness
trihexyphenidyl (generic)	1–2 mg PO daily initially, titrate up to 6–10 mg/d; up to 15 mg/d may be needed	Adjunct to levodopa in treatment of parkinsonism; can be used alone for the control of drug-induced extrapyramidal disorders

associated with adverse effects (see Chapter 33), including slowed GI motility and secretions with dry mouth and constipation, urinary retention, blurred vision, and dilated pupils.

Anticholinergic drugs are indicated for the treatment of parkinsonism, whether idiopathic, atherosclerotic, or postencephalitic, and for the relief of symptoms of extrapyramidal disorders associated with the use of some drugs, including phenothiazines. Although these drugs are not as effective as levodopa in the treatment of advancing cases of the disease, they may be useful as adjunctive therapy and for patients who no longer respond to levodopa. See Table 24.2 for usual indications.

Pharmacokinetics

The anticholinergic drugs are variably absorbed from the GI tract, reaching peak levels in 1 to 4 hours. They are metabolized in the liver and excreted by cellular pathways. All of them cross the placenta and enter human milk (see "Contraindications and Cautions"). Benztropine and diphenhydramine are available in oral and intramuscular/intravenous forms. Trihexyphenidyl is only available in an oral form.

Contraindications and Cautions

Anticholinergics are contraindicated in the presence of allergy to any of these agents to avoid hypersensitivity reactions. In addition, they are contraindicated in narrow-angle glaucoma, GI obstruction, genitourinary (GU) obstruction, and prostatic hypertrophy, all of which could be exacerbated by the peripheral anticholinergic effects of these drugs, and in myasthenia gravis, which could be exacerbated by the blocking of acetylcholine receptor sites at neuromuscular synapses. The safety and efficacy for use in children have not been established.

Administer these agents cautiously with tachycardia and other dysrhythmias and hypertension or hypotension because the blocking of the parasympathetic system may cause a dominance of sympathetic stimulatory activity and hepatic dysfunction, which could interfere with the metabolism of the drugs and lead to toxic levels. They should be used during pregnancy and lactation only if the benefit to the parent clearly outweighs the potential risk to the fetus or neonate. In addition, use caution in individuals who work in hot environments because reflex sweating may be blocked, placing the individuals at risk for heat prostration.

Adverse Effects

The use of anticholinergics for Parkinson's disease and parkinsonism is associated with CNS effects that relate to the blocking of central acetylcholine receptors, such as disorientation, confusion, and memory loss. Agitation, nervousness, delirium, dizziness, light-headedness, and weakness may also occur.

Anticipated peripheral anticholinergic effects include dry mouth, nausea, vomiting, paralytic ileus, and constipation related to decreased GI secretions and motility. In addition, other adverse effects may occur, including the tachycardia, palpitations, and hypotension related to the blocking of the suppressive cardiac effects of the parasympathetic nervous system; urinary retention and hesitancy related to a blocking of bladder muscle activity and sphincter relaxation; blurred vision and photophobia related to pupil dilation and blocking of lens accommodation; and flushing and reduced sweating related to a blocking of the cholinergic sites that stimulate sweating and blood vessel dilation in the skin.

Clinically Important Drug–Drug Interactions

When these anticholinergic drugs are used with other drugs that have anticholinergic properties, including the tricyclic antidepressants and the phenothiazines, there is a risk of potentially fatal paralytic ileus and an increased risk of toxic psychoses. If such combinations must be given, monitor patients closely and implement supportive measures. Dose adjustments often are necessary. In addition, when antipsychotic drugs are combined with anticholinergics, a risk for decreased antipsychotic therapeutic effectiveness may occur, possibly as a result of a central antagonism of the two agents.

Prototype Summary: Benztropine

Indications: Adjunctive therapy for Parkinson's disease, relief of symptoms of extrapyramidal disorders (parkinsonism) that accompany neuroleptic therapy.

Actions: Acts as an anticholinergic, principally in the CNS, returning balance to the basal ganglia and reducing the severity of rigidity, akinesia, and tremors; peripheral anticholinergic effects help to reduce drooling and other secondary effects of parkinsonism.

Pharmacokinetics:

Route	Onset	Peak	Duration
Oral	1 h	Unknown	6–10 h
IM, IV	15 min	Unknown	6–10 h

$T_{1/2}$: Unknown, metabolized in the liver.

Adverse Effects: Disorientation, confusion, memory loss, nervousness, light-headedness, dizziness, depression, blurred vision, mydriasis, dry mouth, constipation, urinary retention, urinary hesitation, flushing, decreased sweating.

Nursing Considerations for Patients Receiving Anticholinergic Agents

Assessment: History and Examination

- Assess for contraindications or cautions: Any known allergies to these drugs to avoid hypersensitivity reactions; GI depression or obstruction, urinary hesitancy or obstruction, benign prostatic hypertrophy, or glaucoma, which may be exacerbated by the peripheral anticholinergic effect of the drug; cardiac arrhythmias, hypertension, or hypotension, which may be increased due to the dominance of sympathetic stimulatory activity due to blockage of parasympathetic activity; myasthenia gravis, which may be exacerbated by blockage of acetylcholine receptors; and exposure to a hot environment, which may block the individual's reflex sweating.
- Perform a physical assessment to determine baseline data for determining the effectiveness of the drug and the occurrence of adverse effects associated with drug therapy.
- Assess level of orientation and neurological status, including affect, reflexes, bilateral grip strength, gait, tremors, and spasticity to evaluate any CNS effects.
- Monitor pulse, blood pressure, and cardiac output to evaluate for possible adverse effects related to blocking of suppressive action on the heart.
- Auscultate bowel sounds to evaluate GI motility and detect possible indications of paralytic ileus.
- Assess urine output and palpate bladder to determine adequate renal and bladder function.
- Monitor the results of laboratory tests such as renal and liver function tests to determine the need for possible dose adjustment and identify potential toxic effects.

Nursing Conclusions

Nursing conclusions related to drug therapy might include the following:

- Dry oral mucous membranes related to anticholinergic effects
- Risk for impaired thermoregulation related to anticholinergic effects
- Impaired urinary elimination related to genitourinary effects
- Constipation risk related to GI effects
- Altered thought processes related to CNS effects
- Injury risk related to CNS effects
- Knowledge deficit regarding drug therapy

Planning

- The patient will receive the best therapeutic effect from the drug therapy.
- The patient will have limited adverse effects to the drug therapy.
- The patient will have an understanding of the drug therapy, adverse effects to anticipate, and measures to relieve discomfort and improve safety.

Intervention With Rationale

- Arrange to decrease dose or discontinue the drug if dry mouth becomes so severe that swallowing becomes difficult. Provide sugarless lozenges to suck and frequent mouth care to help with this problem.
- Give drug with caution and arrange for a decrease in dose in hot weather or with exposure to hot environments because patients are at increased risk for heat prostration due to decreased ability to sweat.
- Give drug with meals if GI upset is a problem, before meals if dry mouth is a problem, and after meals if drooling occurs and the drug causes nausea, to facilitate adherence to drug therapy.
- Monitor bowel function and institute a bowel program if constipation is severe.
- Ensure that the patient voids before taking the drug; monitor urinary output and palpate for bladder distention and residual urine if urinary retention is a problem.
- To prevent patient injury, establish safety precautions if CNS or vision changes occur.
- Provide thorough patient teaching about topics, such as the drug name and prescribed dose, measures to help avoid adverse effects, warning signs that may indicate problems, and the need for periodic monitoring and evaluation, to enhance patient knowledge about drug therapy and promote adherence.
- Offer support and encouragement to help the patient cope with the progressive nature of the disease and long-term drug regimen.

Evaluation

- Monitor patient response to the drug (improvement in signs and symptoms of Parkinson's disease or parkinsonism).
- Monitor for adverse effects (CNS changes, urinary retention, GI slowing, tachycardia, decreased sweating, flushing).
- Evaluate the effectiveness of the teaching plan (patient can give the drug name and dosage, name possible adverse effects to watch for and specific measures to prevent them, and discuss the importance of continued follow-up).
- Monitor the effectiveness of support measures and compliance with the regimen.

Key Points

- Anticholinergic agents are used to suppress the stimulatory effects of acetylcholine in the basal ganglia, bringing balance into the control of movement.
- The adverse effects associated with the anticholinergic drugs are related to blocking of the acetylcholine in the parasympathetic nervous system—dry mouth, constipation, urinary retention, increased heart rate, and decreased sweating.

Adjunctive Agents

Adjunctive agents used to improve patient response to traditional therapy include entacapone (*Comtan*), safinamide (*Xadago*), selegiline (*Eldepryl*), and tolcapone (*Tasmar*). See Table 24.3 for additional information.

Entacapone is used with carbidopa–levodopa to increase the plasma concentration and duration of action of levodopa. It is also available in fixed combination tablets containing levodopa, carbidopa, and entacapone called *Stalevo*. It works by inhibiting catecholamine-*O*-methyltransferase (COMT), a naturally occurring enzyme that eliminates catecholamines, including dopamine. By inhibiting COMT, the plasma levels of levodopa are higher and there may be more constant dopamine receptor stimulation. It is given with the carbidopa–levodopa at a dose of 200 mg PO with a maximum of eight doses a day. It is readily absorbed from the GI tract, metabolized in the liver, and excreted in the urine and feces. Patients of childbearing age should be encouraged to use barrier contraceptives while taking this drug, which crosses the placenta and could have adverse effects on a fetus.

Tolcapone is also a COMT inhibitor and works with carbidopa levodopa to further increase plasma levels of levodopa. Because this drug has been associated with fulminant and potentially fatal liver damage, it is contraindicated in the presence of liver disease. Entacapone is always used preferentially to tolcapone. It undergoes hepatic metabolism after GI absorption and is excreted in the urine and feces. It is given in doses of 100 or 200 mg PO three times a day up to a maximum of 600 mg/d. Patients of childbearing age should be encouraged to use barrier contraceptives while taking this drug, which crosses the placenta and could have adverse effects on a fetus.

Safinamide is indicated to work with carbidopa–levodopa in patients with Parkinson's that are having "off" episodes. It is an MAO type B inhibitor, which in effect blocks the breakdown of dopamine levels. Recommended doses are 50 or 100 mg once a day, and these doses are tolerated without having to decrease tyramine intake. It is absorbed well via the GI tract with negligible first-pass effect, metabolized by the liver, and excreted via the kidneys. The half-life is 20 to 26 hours.

Selegiline is used with carbidopa–levodopa after patients have shown signs of deteriorating response to this treatment. It also irreversibly inhibits MAO, which has an important role in the breakdown of catecholamines, including dopamine. It is also approved in a dermal system for the treatment of depression. The maximum daily

Table 24.3 *Drugs in Focus:* Adjunctive Antiparkinsonism Drugs

Drug Name	Dosage/Route	Usual Indications
entacapone (*Comtan*)	200 mg PO taken with levodopa–carbidopa, maximum of eight doses per day	Adjunctive treatment of idiopathic Parkinson's disease with carbidopa–levodopa for patients who are experiencing "wearing off" of drug effects
tolcapone (*Tasmar*)	100 mg PO t.i.d., maximum daily dose 600 mg	Adjunctive treatment of idiopathic Parkinson's disease with carbidopa–levodopa
safinamide (*Xadago*)	Adult: 50 mg PO daily; may increase to 100 mg PO daily after 2 weeks Reduce dose with hepatic impairment	Adjunctive treatment with carbidopa–levodopa in patients with Parkinson's disease having "off" episodes
selegiline (*Emsam*, *Zelapar*)	5 mg PO b.i.d. (at breakfast and lunch); attempt to decrease carbidopa–levodopa dose after 2–3 days *Orally disintegrating tablet:* 1.25 mg/d PO with breakfast *Xadago:* 50–100 mg PO daily Reduce dose with hepatic impairment	Adjunctive treatment of idiopathic Parkinson's disease with carbidopa–levodopa in patients whose response to that therapy has decreased

dose of the drug is 10 mg, and the dose of levodopa needs to be reduced when this drug is started. It is well absorbed from the GI tract, extensively metabolized in the liver, and excreted in the urine. It is not known whether this drug crosses the placenta, but it should be used in pregnancy only if the benefits to the parent clearly outweigh any potential risks to the fetus. Because of the risk of MAOI-induced hypertensive effects, patients should be urged to immediately report severe headache and any other unusual symptoms that they have not experienced before.

Nursing Considerations for Patients Receiving Adjunctive Agents

Nursing considerations for patients receiving the drugs listed in this section are similar to those for patients receiving the dopaminergic drugs. Details related to each individual drug can be found in the specific drug monograph in your nursing drug guide or the prescribing label approved by the FDA.

Key Points

- Adjunctive drugs are only used in combination with carbidopa–levodopa and are usually reserved for use when the patient stops responding adequately to traditional therapy.
- The mechanism of action of the adjunctive medications varies. Some increase the plasma concentration and duration of action of carbidopa–levodopa by inhibiting COMT. Some inhibit the MAO enzyme that breaks down several neurotransmitters, including dopamine.

SUMMARY

- Parkinson's disease is a progressive, chronic neurological disorder for which there is currently no cure.
- Loss of dopamine-secreting neurons in the substantia nigra is characteristic of Parkinson's disease. Destruction of dopamine-secreting cells leads to an imbalance between excitatory cholinergic cells and inhibitory dopaminergic cells.
- Signs and symptoms of Parkinson's disease include tremor, changes in posture and gait, slow and deliberate movements (bradykinesia), and eventually drooling and changes in speech.
- Drug therapy for Parkinson's disease is aimed at restoring the neurotransmitter balance in the basal ganglia. The signs and symptoms of the disease can be managed until the degeneration of neurons is so extensive that a therapeutic response no longer occurs.
- Anticholinergic drugs are used to block the excitatory cholinergic receptors, and dopaminergic drugs are used to increase dopamine levels or to directly stimulate dopamine receptors.
- Many adverse effects are associated with the drugs used for treating Parkinson's disease, including CNS changes, anticholinergic effects when using the anticholinergics (atropinelike or parasympathetic blocking effects), and dopamine stimulation (sympathetic-type effects) in the peripheral nervous system when using the dopaminergics.

CHECK YOUR UNDERSTANDING

Answers to the questions in this chapter can be found in Answers to Check Your Understanding Questions on thePoint®.

MULTIPLE CHOICE

Select the best answer.

1. Parkinson's disease is a progressive, chronic neurological disorder that is caused by
   a. severe head injury.
   b. chronic diseases.
   c. old age.
   d. a combination of genetic and environmental factors.
2. Parkinson's disease reflects an imbalance between inhibitory and stimulating neurotransmitters in the
   a. reticular activating system.
   b. cerebellum.
   c. basal ganglia.
   d. limbic system.
3. The main underlying problem with Parkinson's disease seems to be a decrease in the neurotransmitter
   a. acetylcholine.
   b. norepinephrine.
   c. dopamine.
   d. serotonin.
4. Anticholinergic drugs are effective by acting to
   a. block stimulating effects of acetylcholine in the brain to facilitate balance of neurotransmitters in the basal ganglia.

b. block the signs and symptoms of the disease, making it more acceptable.
c. inhibit dopamine effects in the brain and increase neuron activity.
d. increase the effectiveness of the inhibitory neurotransmitter gamma-aminobutyric acid.

5. A patient receiving an anticholinergic drug for Parkinson's disease is planning a winter trip to Tahiti. The temperature in Tahiti is 70 degrees warmer than at home. What precautions should the patient be urged to take?
   a. Take the drug with plenty of water to stay hydrated.
   b. Reduce the dose, and take precautions to reduce the risk for heat stroke.
   c. Wear sunglasses and use sunscreen because of photophobia that will develop.
   d. Avoid drinking the water to prevent gastric distress.

6. Replacing dopamine in the brain would seem to be the best treatment for Parkinson's disease. This is difficult because dopamine
   a. is broken down in gastric acid.
   b. is not available in drug form.
   c. cannot cross the blood–brain barrier.
   d. is used peripherally before reaching the brain.

7. A patient taking levodopa and over-the-counter megavitamins might experience
   a. a cure from Parkinson's disease.
   b. the return of Parkinson's symptoms.
   c. improved health and well-being.
   d. a resistance to viral infections.

8. A patient who has been diagnosed with Parkinson's disease for many years and whose symptoms were controlled using *carbidopa–levodopa* has started to exhibit increasing signs of the disease. Possible treatment might include
   a. an increased exercise program.
   b. adding iron to the person's diet.
   c. adding an adjunctive agent like entacapone.
   d. changes in diet to eliminate vitamin B_6.

MULTIPLE RESPONSE

Select all that apply.

1. A patient asks the nurse to explain parkinsonism. Which possible causes of parkinsonism might be included in the explanation?
   a. Adverse effects of drug therapy
   b. Brain injury
   c. Viral infection
   d. Dementia
   e. Bacterial infection
   f. Birth defect

2. No therapy is available that will stop the loss of neurons and the eventual decline of function in clients with Parkinson's disease. As a result, nursing care should involve which interventions?
   a. Regular exercises to slow loss of function
   b. Supportive education as drugs fail and new therapy is needed
   c. Community and family support networking
   d. Discontinuation of drug therapy to test for a cure
   e. Special vitamin therapy to slow the loss of the neurons
   f. Explanations of the adjunctive drug therapy that may be used

REFERENCES

Arcangelo, V. P., Peterson, A. M., Wilbur, V., & Kang, T. M. (2022). *Pharmacotherapeutics for advanced practice. A practical approach* (5th ed.). Wolters Kluwer.

Bjorklund, A., & Cenci, M. A. (2010). *Recent advances in Parkinson's disease part I: Basic research*. Elsevier.

Bjorklund, A., & Cenci, M. A. (2010). *Recent advances in Parkinson's disease part II: Translational and clinical research*. Elsevier.

Bjorklund, A., & Kordower, J. H. (2013). Cell therapy for Parkinson's disease: What next? *Movement Disorders, 28*(1), 110–115. https://doi.org/10.1002/mds.25343

Brunton, L. L., Hilal-Dandan, R., & Knollman, B. C. (2018). *Goodman and Gilman's the pharmacological basis of therapeutics* (13th ed.). McGraw-Hill.

Hall, J. E., & Hall, M. E. (2021). *Guyton and Hall textbook of medical physiology* (14th ed.). Elsevier.

Hanin, I., Nitsch, R. M., Windisch, M., & Fisher, A. (Eds.). (2013). Alzheimer's and Parkinson's diseases: Mechanisms, clinical strategies, and promising treatments of neurodegenerative diseases. *Neurodegenerative Diseases, 11*(suppl. 1).

Leader, L., & Leader, G. (2009). *Parkinson's disease: Dopamine metabolism, applied biochemistry, and nutrition*. Denor Press.

Nitsch, R. M., Fisher, A., Windisch, M., & Hanin, I. (Eds.). (2011). Alzheimer's and Parkinson's disease: Advances, concepts and new challenges. *Neurodegenerative Diseases, 10*(1–4).

Norris, T. L. (2019). *Porth's pathophysiology: Concepts of altered health states* (13th ed.). Wolters Kluwer.

CHAPTER 25

Muscle Relaxants

Learning Objectives

Upon completion of this chapter, you will be able to:

1. Describe a spinal reflex and discuss the pathophysiology of muscle spasm and muscle spasticity.
2. Discuss the use of muscle relaxants across the lifespan.
3. Describe the therapeutic actions, indications, pharmacokinetics, contraindications, most common adverse reactions, and important drug–drug interactions associated with the centrally acting and the direct-acting skeletal muscle relaxants.
4. Compare and contrast the prototype drugs baclofen and dantrolene with other muscle relaxants in their classes.
5. Outline the nursing considerations, including important teaching points for patients receiving muscle relaxants as adjuncts to anesthesia.

Key Terms

basal ganglia: located in the brain just beneath the cerebral hemispheres, lateral to the thalamus; consist of the caudate nucleus, putamen, globus pallidus, substantia nigra, and subthalamic nucleus; functions with the cerebral cortex as an accessory motor system; active in coordination of smooth motor movements in conjunction with other motor areas of the central nervous system (CNS)

cerebellum: lower portion of the brain, associated with coordination of muscle movements, including voluntary motion as well as extrapyramidal control of unconscious muscle movements

extrapyramidal tract: portions of the CNS outside the pyramidal (corticospinal) tract that contribute to motor control; cells from the cortex and subcortical areas, including the basal ganglia and the cerebellum, which coordinate unconsciously controlled muscle activity; allows the body to make automatic adjustments in posture or position and balance

Golgi tendon organ: sensory receptor in skeletal muscle tendons that sense muscle tension; with excessive tension the Golgi tendon organ signals an inhibitor interneuron in the spinal cord that inhibits motor neuron activity, causing the muscle to relax; the organ responsible for the Golgi tendon reflex

hypertonia: state of excessive muscle contraction or tension and decreased ability to stretch

interneuron: neuron in the CNS that communicates with other neurons, not with muscles or glands

muscle spasm: sudden involuntary tightening or contraction of muscle, often due to damage or injury of the musculoskeletal system; repeated and/or severe spasms can cause significant pain

muscle spindles: intrafusal fibers within skeletal muscle tissue that help to modulate muscle tone by innervating alpha motor nerves after being stretched; fibers that are responsible for initiating the stretch reflex

pyramidal (corticospinal) tract: fibers from the motor cortex down through the brain stem, the majority of which cross to the opposite side before descending down the spinal cord; these nerve fibers within the CNS are the most important tracts for controlling precise, intentional movements

sliding filament mechanism: theory of the process of muscle contraction and relaxation

spasticity: sustained muscle contractions that prevent normal movement due to extreme resistance to any stretch or flexibility during the contractions; often caused by damage to areas of the brain and/or spinal cord responsible for controlling muscle and stretch reflexes

Drug List

CENTRALLY ACTING SKELETAL MUSCLE RELAXANTS
- baclofen
- carisoprodol
- chlorzoxazone
- cyclobenzaprine
- metaxalone
- methocarbamol
- orphenadrine
- tizanidine

DIRECT-ACTING SKELETAL MUSCLE RELAXANTS
- dantrolene
- incobotulinumtoxinA
- onabotulinumtoxinA
- rimabotulinumtoxinB

Many injuries and accidents result in local damage to muscles or the skeletal anchors of muscles. These injuries may lead to muscle spasm and pain, which may last for long periods of time and interfere with normal functioning. The perception of pain and response to pain is an individual response, as discussed further in Chapter 26. In a situation in which muscle spasm is causing pain, relaxing the muscle can often remove the physiological stimulus for pain. Damage to central nervous system (CNS) neurons may cause a permanent state of muscle **spasticity**—sustained muscle contractions—as a result of damage to nerves that help to maintain balance in controlling muscle activity.

Neuron damage, whether temporary or permanent, may be treated with skeletal muscle relaxants. Most skeletal muscle relaxants work in the brain and spinal cord, where they interfere with the cycle of muscle spasm and pain. However, botulinum toxins and dantrolene enter muscle fibers directly. See Box 25.1 for discussion of the use of these muscle relaxants in various age groups.

Nerves and Movement

Posture, balance, and movement are the result of a constantly fluctuating sequence of muscle contraction and

Box 25.1 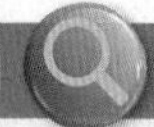 **Focus on Drug Therapy Across the Lifespan**

SKELETAL MUSCLE RELAXANTS

Children

The safety and effectiveness of some of these drugs have not been established in children. If a child older than 12 years requires a skeletal muscle relaxant after an injury, metaxalone has an established pediatric dosage. Other agents have been used with adjustments to the adult dosage based on the child's age and weight.

Baclofen is indicated for the use in children. It can be used to relieve the muscle spasticity associated with cerebral palsy. A caregiver needs intensive education in the use of the intrathecal infusion pump and how to monitor the child for therapeutic as well as adverse effects.

Methocarbamol is the drug of choice if a child needs to be treated for tetanus.

Dantrolene is used to treat upper motor neuron spasticity in children. The dosage is based on body weight and increases over time. The child should be screened regularly for CNS and GI (including hepatic) toxicity.

IncobotulinumtoxinA and onabotulinumtoxinaA are approved for use in children for treatment of muscle spasticity. The most common side effect in children was upper respiratory infection. RimabotulinumtoxinB is only approved for use in adults.

Adults

Adults being treated for acute musculoskeletal pain should be cautioned to avoid driving and to take safety precautions against injury because of the related CNS effects, including dizziness and drowsiness. Rest of the muscle, heat, massage, and physical therapy are key components to recovery from any muscular injury or pain.

Adults complaining of muscle spasm pain that may be related to anxiety often respond effectively to diazepam, which is a muscle relaxant and anxiolytic.

Patients who are able to become pregnant should be advised to use contraception when they are taking these drugs. If a pregnancy does occur or is desired, they need counseling about any known potential risks. Patients who are nursing should be encouraged to find another method of feeding the baby because of the potential for adverse drug effects on the baby.

Female patients and patients who are over 35 years of age have an increased risk for the hepatotoxicity associated with dantrolene and should be monitored closely for any change in hepatic function and given written information about the prodrome syndrome that often occurs with the hepatic toxicity.

Older Adults

Older adult patients are more likely to experience the adverse effects associated with these drugs—CNS, GI, and cardiovascular. Because older adult patients often also have renal or hepatic impairment, they are also more likely to have toxic levels of the drug related to changes in metabolism and excretion.

Carisoprodol is the centrally acting skeletal muscle relaxant of choice for older adult patients and for those with hepatic or renal impairment.

If dantrolene is required for an older adult patient, lower doses and more frequent monitoring are needed to assess for potential cardiac, respiratory, and liver toxicity.

Older female adults who are receiving hormone replacement therapy are at the same risk for development of hepatotoxicity as those who are premenopausal and should be monitored accordingly.

relaxation. A body at rest continues to engage in muscle contraction to maintain position in space; this is known as muscle tone, and it varies from person to person. The nerves that regulate these actions are the spinal motor neurons. These neurons are influenced by higher-level brain activity (motor and premotor cortex) in the lower areas of the brain, including the **cerebellum** and the **basal ganglia**. The cerebellum is associated with the coordination of muscle movements, including voluntary motion, as well as extrapyramidal control of unconscious muscle movements; the basal ganglia, which are located in the brain just beneath the cerebral hemispheres lateral to the thalamus, consist of the caudate nucleus, putamen, globus pallidus, substantia nigra, and subthalamic nucleus, function with the cerebral cortex as an accessory motor system, and are associated with the coordination of smooth motor movements in conjunction with other motor areas of the CNS. This brain activity provides coordination of muscle contraction. The cerebral cortex allows conscious thought to regulate intentional movement.

Spinal Reflexes

The spinal reflexes are the simplest nerve pathways that monitor movement and posture (Fig. 25.1). Spinal reflexes can be simple, involving an incoming sensory neuron and an outgoing motor neuron, or more complex, involving **interneurons** that communicate with other neurons in the related centers in the brain. Simple reflex arcs involve sensory receptors in the periphery and spinal motor nerves. Such reflex arcs make up what is known as the muscle stretch, or Golgi tendon reflex, which involves **muscle spindles**, or intrafusal fibers within skeletal muscle tissue that help to modulate muscle tone by innervating alpha motor nerves after being stretched. Muscle spindles are sensitive to the stretch of muscle tissue and when they are innervated they cause a muscle fiber contraction that relieves the stretch. In this system, nerves from stretch receptors form a synapse with gamma (motor) nerves in the spinal cord, which send an impulse to the stretched muscle fibers to stimulate their contraction. This process can assist in maintaining muscle tone and keeping the person in an upright position against the pull of gravity. Skeletal muscle tension in lower extremities can also be important in helping venous return when the contracting muscle fibers massage veins to help move the blood toward the heart. Other spinal reflexes may involve synapses with interneurons within the spinal cord, which adjust movement and response based on information from higher brain centers to coordinate movement and position. For example, when the **Golgi tendon organs**, sensory receptors in the skeletal muscle tendons that sense muscle tension, are excited by excessive muscle tension, they will excite an interneuron in the spinal cord that inhibits the motor neuron so the muscle will relax. The higher brain centers will also be signaled so that the individual will become aware of the muscle changes and react appropriately to whatever is triggering the excessive muscle tension.

Brain Control

Many areas within the brain influence the spinal motor nerves. Areas of the brainstem, the basal ganglia, and the cerebellum modulate spinal motor nerve activity and help coordinate activity among various muscle groups, thereby allowing coordinated movement and control of body

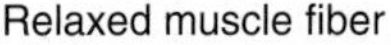

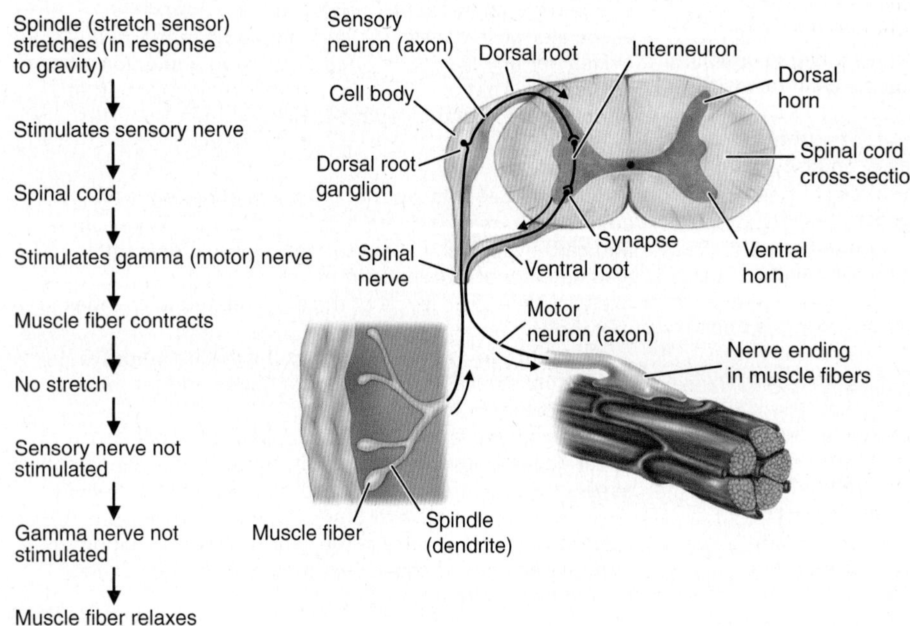

FIGURE 25.1 Reflex arc showing the pathway of impulses of the stretch reflex. The relaxing and contracting of muscle fibers causes muscle tone, facilitates the ability to stand upright, and promotes venous return.

muscle motions. Nerve areas within the cerebral cortex allow conscious, or intentional, movement. Nerves within the cerebral cortex send signals down the spinal cord, where they cross to the opposite side of the spinal cord before sending out nerve impulses to cause muscle contraction. In this way, each side of the cortex controls muscle movement on the opposite side of the body.

Different fibers control different types of movements. The fibers that initiate from the motor cortex and control precise, intentional movement make up the **pyramidal (corticospinal) tract** within the CNS. The **extrapyramidal tract** is composed of cells from the cerebral cortex, as well as those from several subcortical areas, including the basal ganglia and the cerebellum. This tract modulates or coordinates unconsciously controlled muscle activity, and it allows the body to make automatic adjustments in posture or position and balance. The extrapyramidal tract controls lower level, or crude, movements. Many health professionals no longer use the terms pyramidal and extrapyramidal tracts to describe movement since so many movements can't be clearly classified into one or the other tract.

The nerves are responsible for innervating the muscle via the neuromuscular junction. The nerve secretes the neurotransmitter acetylcholine, which binds to the muscle fiber membrane. Acetylcholine opens channels that allow sodium ions to diffuse and cause depolarization of the muscle tissue. This triggers the sarcoplasmic reticulum to release calcium ions, which binds to the muscle protein troponin. This allows the myosin cross bridges to attach to the actin. The myosin will contract and pull the actin, release the actin, and then attach again. This is called myosin–actin cycling. The muscle is contracted by shortening the sarcomere. When the nerve stimulation stops, calcium ions are transported back to the sarcoplasmic reticulum. Troponin is released by the calcium, the myosin are no longer able to attach to the actin, and the muscle fibers lengthen (relax). This process of muscle contraction is called the **sliding filament mechanism** (Fig. 25.2).

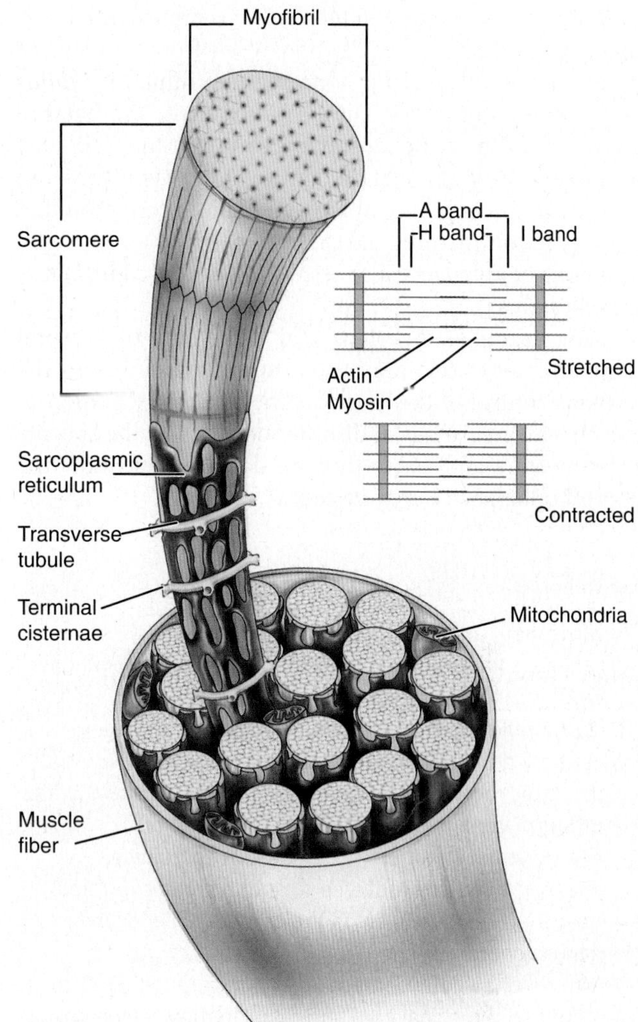

FIGURE 25.2 This process of muscle contraction is called the sliding filament mechanism. When muscles are stimulated, calcium ions are released and allow for actin and myosin to interact via cross bridges. This will contract (shorten) the muscle. When stimulation stops, calcium ions are actively transported back into the sarcoplasmic reticulum, resulting in decreased calcium ions in the sarcoplasm. The removal of calcium ions restores the inhibitory action of troponin–tropomyosin; cross bridge action is impossible in this state. The muscle will then relax (lengthen).

Neuromuscular Abnormalities

All of the areas mentioned work together to allow for a free flow of impulses into and out of the CNS to coordinate posture, balance, and movement. When injuries, diseases, and toxins affect the normal flow of information into and out of the CNS motor pathways, many clinical signs and symptoms may develop, ranging from simple muscle spasms to spasticity (sustained muscle spasm), and paralysis.

Muscle Spasm

Muscle spasms often result from injury to the musculoskeletal system—for example, overstretching a muscle, wrenching a joint, or tearing a tendon or ligament. These injuries can cause violent and painful involuntary muscle contractions. It is thought that these spasms are caused by the flood of sensory impulses coming to the spinal cord from the injured area. These impulses can be passed through interneurons to spinal motor nerves, which stimulate an intense muscle contraction. The contraction cuts off blood flow to the muscle fibers in the injured area, causing lactic acid to accumulate and resulting in pain. The new flood of sensory impulses caused by the pain may lead to further muscle contraction, and a vicious cycle may develop.

Muscle Spasticity

Muscle spasticity is the result of damage to neurons within the CNS rather than injury to peripheral structures. People with muscle spasticity will often report stiffness and/or heavy muscles and have difficulty with movement. Muscle spasticity can also be painful. Because the spasticity is caused by nerve damage in the CNS, it is more likely a permanent condition. Spasticity may result from an increase in excitatory influences or a decrease in inhibitory influences within the CNS. The interruption in the balance among all of these higher influences within the CNS may lead to excessive stimulation of muscles, or **hypertonia**, in opposing muscle groups at the same time, a condition that may cause contractures and permanent structural changes. This control imbalance also results in a loss of coordinated muscle activity.

For example, the signs and symptoms of cerebral palsy and paraplegia are related to the disruption in the nervous control of the muscles. The exact presentation of any chronic neurological disorder depends on the specific nerve centers and tracts that are damaged and how the control imbalance is manifested.

Key Points

- Movement and muscle control are regulated by spinal reflexes and the upper CNS, including the basal ganglia, cerebellum, and cerebral cortex.
- Spinal reflexes can be simple, involving an incoming sensory neuron and an outgoing motor neuron, or more complex, involving interneurons that communicate with other neurons in the related centers in the brain.
- The pyramidal tract in the cerebellum coordinates intentional muscle movement, and the extrapyramidal tract that includes fibers in the cerebellum and basal ganglia coordinates involuntary muscle activity.
- Muscle or skeletal damage may send a multitude of stimuli to the spinal cord and result in muscle spasms or extended contraction.
- Damaged motor neurons can cause muscle spasticity and impaired movement and coordination.

Centrally Acting Skeletal Muscle Relaxants

Centrally acting skeletal muscle relaxants (Table 25.1) include baclofen (*Lioresal*), carisoprodol (*Soma*), chlorzoxazone (generic), cyclobenzaprine (*Amrix*), metaxalone (*Skelaxin*), methocarbamol (*Robaxin*), orphenadrine (generic), and tizanidine (*Zanaflex*). Diazepam (*Valium*), a drug widely used as an anxiety agent (see Chapters 20 and 23), has also been shown to be an effective centrally acting skeletal muscle relaxant. It may be advantageous in situations in which anxiety may be precipitating the muscle spasm.

Other measures in addition to these drugs should be used to alleviate muscle spasm and pain. These include rest of the affected muscle, ice for acute injuries to decrease inflammation, and compression and elevation to decrease swelling. Heat applications have been shown to increase blood flow to the area and remove the pain-causing chemicals. Physical and occupational therapy are helpful to facilitate the return of the muscle to normal tone and activity so a person can regain independence in their daily life. Anti-inflammatory agents, including nonsteroidal anti-inflammatory drugs (NSAIDs), are also often used to decrease pain if the underlying problem is related to injury or inflammation.

Therapeutic Actions and Indications

The centrally acting skeletal muscle relaxants work in the CNS to interfere with the reflexes that are causing the muscle spasm. Because these drugs lyse or destroy spasm, they are often referred to as spasmolytics. Although the exact mechanism of action of some of these skeletal muscle relaxants is not known, most are thought to alter spinal or subcortical neurons to inhibit muscle innervation; it is perhaps accomplished by increasing the neurotransmitter gamma aminobutyric acid. Tizanidine is an alpha-adrenergic agonist and is thought to increase inhibition of presynaptic motor neurons in the CNS. The primary indication for the use of centrally acting skeletal muscle agents is the relief of discomfort associated with acute, painful musculoskeletal conditions as an adjunct to rest, physical and occupational therapy, and other measures. Because these drugs work in the upper levels of the CNS, possible depression must be anticipated with their use. See Table 25.1 for usual indications for each of these agents.

Pharmacokinetics

Baclofen is available in oral and intrathecal forms and can be administered via a delivery pump for the treatment of central spasticity. Cyclobenzaprine is available in a controlled release oral form for continual control of the discomfort without repeated dosings. Methocarbamol is available in both oral and parenteral forms. Most of these agents are rapidly absorbed and metabolized in the liver. Baclofen is not metabolized, but like the other skeletal muscle relaxants, it is excreted in the urine.

Contraindications and Cautions

Centrally acting skeletal muscle relaxants are contraindicated in the presence of any known allergy to any of these drugs to prevent hypersensitivity reactions, and with skeletal muscle spasms resulting from rheumatic disorders, which would not benefit from these drugs. In addition, baclofen should not be used to treat any spasticity that contributes to locomotion, upright position, or increased function. Blocking this spasticity results in loss of these functions. All centrally acting skeletal muscle relaxants should be used cautiously in the following circumstances: for those with a history of epilepsy, because the CNS depression and imbalance caused by these drugs may exacerbate the seizure disorder; with cardiac dysfunction, because muscle function may be depressed; with any

Table 25.1 *Drugs in Focus:* Centrally Acting Skeletal Muscle Relaxants

Drug Name	Dosage/Route	Usual Indications
baclofen (*Gablofen, Lioresal, Ozobax*)	*Adult:* 15–80 mg PO daily in divided doses, 12–1,500 mcg/d per intrathecal infusion pump *Pediatric:* Intrathecal infusion pump, 24–1,199 mcg/d—base dose on patient response	Treatment of muscle spasticity associated with neuromuscular diseases such as multiple sclerosis, muscle rigidity, and spinal cord injuries
carisoprodol (*Soma*)	250–350 mg PO t.i.d. to q.i.d.	Relief of discomfort of acute musculoskeletal conditions in adults
chlorzoxazone (generic)	250–500 mg PO t.i.d. to q.i.d.	Relief of discomfort of acute musculoskeletal conditions in adults
cyclobenzaprine (*Amrix*)	15 or 30 mg PO once daily (*Amrix*); 5–10 mg PO t.i.d.	Relief of discomfort of acute musculoskeletal conditions in adults; short term use (2–3 weeks)
metaxalone (*Skelaxin*)	*Adult and pediatric (>12 y):* 800 mg PO t.i.d. to q.i.d.; reduce dose with hepatic impairment	Relief of discomfort of acute musculoskeletal conditions, one of the few skeletal muscle relaxants with an established pediatric dose for children >12 y
methocarbamol (*Robaxin*)	*Adult:* 1.5 g PO q.i.d., up to 30–60 mg/d; 1–2 g IV or IM for tetanus *Pediatric:* 15 mg/kg IV for tetanus, 0.4 mg/kg/d PO initially, maintenance 0.2 mg/kg/d	Relief of discomfort of acute musculoskeletal conditions in adults, treatment of tetanus in children to alleviate signs and symptoms of tetanus
orphenadrine (generic)	100 mg PO, AM and at bedtime or 60 mg IV or IM q12h	Relief of discomfort of acute musculoskeletal conditions in adults, under investigation for relief of quinidine-induced leg cramps
tizanidine (*Zanaflex*)	2–4 mg PO; dose may be repeated q6–8h as needed up to 3 doses in 24 hours; total daily dose max 36 mg	Relief of discomfort of acute musculoskeletal conditions in adults, provides acute and intermittent management of increased muscle tone associated with spasticity

condition marked by muscle weakness, which the drugs could make much worse; and with hepatic or renal dysfunction (especially with metaxalone and tizanidine), which could interfere with the metabolism and excretion of the drugs, leading to toxic levels. There has not been adequate research examining the effects of these agents during pregnancy and lactation; therefore, use should be limited to those situations in which the benefit to the parent clearly outweighs any potential risk to the fetus or neonate.

Adverse Effects

The most frequently seen adverse effects associated with these drugs relate to the associated CNS depression: drowsiness, fatigue, weakness, confusion, headache, and insomnia. Gastrointestinal (GI) disturbances, including nausea, dry mouth, anorexia, and constipation, which may be linked to CNS depression of the parasympathetic reflexes, can occur with some of the medications. In addition, hypotension and arrhythmias may occur, again as a result of depression of normal reflex arcs. Urinary frequency, enuresis, and feelings of urinary urgency reportedly may occur. Chlorzoxazone may discolor the urine, becoming orange to purplish-red when metabolized and excreted. Patients should be warned about this effect to prevent any fears of blood in the urine. Tizanidine has been associated with liver toxicity and hypotension in some patients (Fig. 25.3).

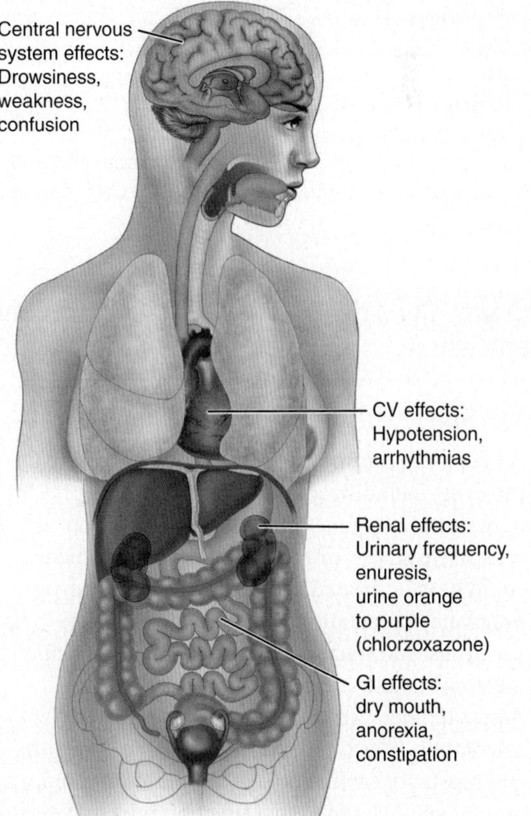

FIGURE 25.3 Common adverse effects and toxicities associated with muscle relaxants.

Clinically Important Drug–Drug Interactions

If any of the centrally acting skeletal muscle relaxants are taken with other CNS depressants or alcohol, CNS depression may increase. Patients should be cautioned to avoid alcohol while taking these muscle relaxants; if this combination cannot be avoided, they should take extreme precautions.

Prototype Summary: Baclofen

Indications: Alleviation of signs and symptoms of spasticity; may be of use in spinal cord injuries or spinal cord diseases.

Actions: Gamma-aminobutyric acid analogue, exact mechanism of action is not understood; inhibits monosynaptic and polysynaptic spinal reflexes; CNS depressant.

Pharmacokinetics:

Route	Onset	Peak	Duration
Oral	1 h	2 h	4–8 h
Intrathecal	30–60 min	4 h	4–8 h

$T_{1/2}$: 3 to 4 hours; not metabolized; excreted in the urine.

Adverse Effects: Transient drowsiness, dizziness, weakness, fatigue, constipation, headache, insomnia, hypotension, nausea, urinary retention.

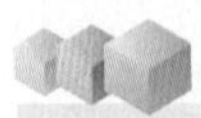

Concept Mastery Alert

Important Interaction

For a client receiving centrally acting skeletal muscle relaxants, taking other CNS depressants can increase adverse side effects and cause increased CNS depression.

Nursing Considerations for Patients Receiving Centrally Acting Skeletal Muscle Relaxants

Assessment: History and Examination

- Assess for contraindications or cautions for the use of the drug, including any known allergies, to prevent hypersensitivity reactions; cardiac depression, epilepsy, muscle weakness, or rheumatic disorder, which could be exacerbated by the effects of these drugs; pregnancy or lactation, which require caution to use the drugs; and renal or hepatic dysfunction, which alter metabolism and excretion of the drugs.
- Assess temperature; skin color and lesions; CNS orientation, affect, reflexes, bilateral grip strength, and spasticity evaluation; bowel sounds and reported output; and liver and renal function tests to determine baseline status before beginning therapy and for any potential adverse effects.

Nursing Conclusions

Nursing conclusions related to drug therapy might include the following:

- Impaired comfort related to GI and CNS effects
- Altered thought processes related to CNS effects
- Injury risk related to CNS effects
- Knowledge deficit regarding drug therapy

Planning

- The patient will receive the best therapeutic effect from the drug therapy, relaxation of muscle, and relief of discomfort.
- The patient will have limited adverse effects to the drug therapy.
- The patient will have an understanding of the drug therapy, adverse effects to anticipate, and measures to relieve discomfort and improve safety.

Intervention With Rationale

- Provide additional measures to relieve discomfort—heat, rest for the muscle, NSAIDs, and positioning—to augment the effects of the drug at relieving the musculoskeletal discomfort.
- Discontinue drug at any sign of hypersensitivity reaction or liver dysfunction to prevent severe health risks.
- If using baclofen, taper the drug slowly over 1 to 2 weeks to prevent the development of psychoses and hallucinations. Use baclofen cautiously in patients whose spasticity contributes to mobility, posture, or balance to prevent loss of this function.
- If patient is receiving baclofen through a delivery pump, the patient should understand the pump, the reason for frequent monitoring, and how to adjust the dose and program the unit to enhance patient knowledge and promote compliance.
- Monitor respiratory status to evaluate adverse effects and arrange for appropriate dose adjustment or discontinuation of the drug.
- Provide thorough patient teaching, including drug name, prescribed dosage, measures for avoidance of adverse effects, warning signs that may indicate possible problems, and the need for monitoring and evaluation to enhance patient knowledge about drug therapy and to promote compliance.
- Offer support and encouragement to help the patient cope with the drug regimen.

Evaluation

- Monitor patient response to the drug (improvement in muscle spasm and relief of pain; improvement in muscle spasticity).
- Monitor for adverse effects (CNS changes, GI depression, urinary retention).
- Evaluate the effectiveness of the teaching plan (patient can give the drug name and dosage, name possible adverse effects to watch for and specific measures to prevent them, and describe, if necessary, proper intrathecal administration).
- Monitor the effectiveness of comfort measures and compliance with the regimen.

Key Points

- The centrally acting skeletal muscle relaxants interfere with the nerves that are causing the muscle spasm.
- The centrally acting skeletal muscle relaxants can cause CNS depression, and the adverse effects associated with them are related to the CNS depression (insomnia, dizziness, confusion, anticholinergic effects).
- The centrally acting muscle relaxants are used for the relief of discomfort associated with acute, painful musculoskeletal conditions as an adjunct to rest, physical and occupational therapy, and other measures.

Direct-Acting Skeletal Muscle Relaxants

The direct-acting skeletal muscle relaxants enter the muscle to prevent muscle contraction directly. Direct-acting skeletal muscle relaxants (Table 25.2) include dantrolene (*Dantrium*), onabotulinumtoxinA (*Botox, Botox Cosmetic*), incobotulinumtoxinA (*Xeomin*), and rimabotulinumtoxinB (*Myobloc*).

Refer to the "Critical Thinking Scenario" for a full discussion of nursing care for a patient who is receiving *Botox* to treat migraines.

Table 25.2 ***Drugs in Focus:*** **Direct-Acting Skeletal Muscle Relaxants**

Drug Name	Dosage/Route	Usual Indications
dantrolene (*Dantrium*)	*Adult:* Initially 25 mg PO, increase based on spinal cord injuries, prevention and management of response to a maximum 400 mg/d for spasticity *Prevention of malignant hyperthermia:* 4–8 mg/kg/d PO for 1–2 d before surgery or 2.5 mg/kg IV over 1 h, given 1 h before surgery; postcrisis, 4–8 mg/kg/d PO for 1–3 d *Pediatric:* Initially 0.5 mg/kg/d PO b.i.d., titrate to a maximum 100 mg PO q.i.d. for spasticity; for malignant hyperthermia, follow adult dose	Management of upper motor neuron–associated muscle spasticity such as spinal cord injury, myasthenia gravis, cerebral palsy, multiple sclerosis, muscular dystrophy, polio, tetanus, quadriplegia, and amyotrophic lateral sclerosis; prevention or treatment of malignant hyperthermia—a state of intense muscle contraction and resulting hyperpyrexia; used orally as preoperative prophylaxis in susceptible patients who must undergo anesthesia and after acute episodes to prevent recurrence
incobotulinumtoxinA (*Xeomin*)	*Glabellar lines:* Five injections of four units each per session, may repeat in 3 mo *Limb spasticity, cervical dystonia, blepharospasm:* Based on age, severity and response to prior treatments *Chronic sialorrhea:* 30 units per parotid gland and 20 units per submandibular gland injected no sooner than every 16 weeks for adults; dosing for pediatrics based on body weight	Treatment of cervical dystonia; treatment of blepharospasm in adult previously treated with onabotulinumtoxin A; improvement in appearance of glabellar (frown) lines with corrugator or procerus muscle activity in adults; treatment of upper limb spasticity in adults and pediatric patients; treatment of chronic sialorrhea
onabotulinumtoxinA (*Botox, Botox Cosmetic*)	*Adult and pediatric:* Injection sites and doses will vary for treatment indication, severity and age of patient; max dose for adult in 3 mo interval 400 units, and for pediatric the lesser of 10 units/kg or 340 units	Treatment of spasticity; improvement of appearance in glabellar (frown) lines associated with corrugator or procerus muscle activity in adults; canthal lines, treatment of cervical dystonia, treatment of strabismus and blepharospasm associated with dystonia in patients ≥12 y of age; treatment of severe primary axillary hyperhidrosis (sweating) when injected into the axillary area; treatment of overactive bladder, detrusor overactivity associated with neurological conditions; treatment of chronic migraine
rimabotulinumtoxinB (*Myobloc*)	*Cervical dystonia:* 2,500–5,000 units IM injected locally into affected muscles *Chronic sialorrhea:* 1,500–3,500 units injected no more frequently than every 12 weeks	Reduction of severity of abnormal head position and neck pain associated with cervical dystonia; treatment of chronic sialorrhea in adults

CRITICAL THINKING SCENARIO
Direct-Acting Muscle Relaxant: IncobotulinumtoxinA

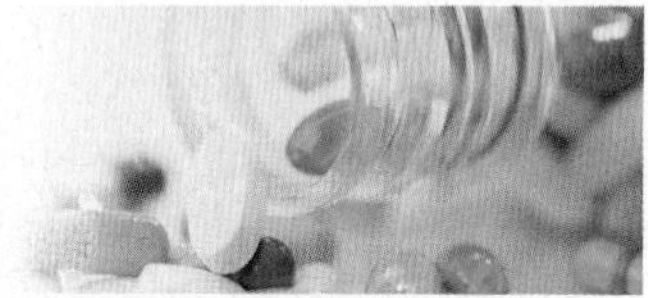

THE SITUATION

M.D. is a 38-year-old teacher with a long history of chronic migraines. They report that they have tried everything but still experience migraines 15 to 20 days a month. This continuous problem has caused them to take a leave of absence from their teaching job. M.D. saw an ad for *Botox* for chronic migraines and has come to the clinic to see if that is an option for them. They report that they know several people who go to *Botox* parties and was wondering if this is the same drug and if it can be given at one of these parties. M.D. has some concerns about *Botox* treatments that did not seem to have good results.

CRITICAL THINKING

What basic principles must be included in the nursing care plan for M.D.? Think about the action of this drug and the potential problems that could occur. Since M.D. associates the drug with Botox parties, what other information do they need to know?

What therapeutic goals might the nurse set for M.D.?

What additional drug-related information needs to be shared with M.D. to make them comfortable with any treatment choice that they might make?

DISCUSSION

Botox (incobotulinumtoxinA) has a strong reputation in the media for giving people instant "face lifts" and helping people look younger. There are places where these injections are given in homes or beauty spas, and consequently, the drug may not be seen as having any potential adverse effects. The drug is a neurotoxin and paralyzes muscles by blocking nerve transmission by inhibiting acetylcholine release. When used for improving the appearance of lines on the face, the drug is injected into the affected areas and can be repeated every 3 months. The muscles can no longer move, so any folds seem to disappear. People have reported visual changes, lopsided response, or no response. There is a boxed warning on the FDA label about the potential risk of the toxin effect to spread away from the area of injection. This adverse effect may occur even weeks after the injection and have the potential to cause swallowing and/or breathing difficulties that could be life threatening. When used to treat chronic migraines, the drug is injected into multiple sites bilaterally across seven head and neck muscles. This injection sequence can be repeated every 12 weeks. The studies done on this use of the drug found that some people began to feel better quickly, and overall, all patients had fewer headache days. However, as with all pain treatments, the actual response is individual.

The patient should be praised for taking the initiative to come in and explore this option for treatment. The nurse would need to review all of M.D.'s history and various methods that have been used to treat their migraines. Their neurologist should be brought into the discussion to weigh the pros and cons of this approach. When a patient has a chronic problem that traditional methods don't seem to be able to help, it is important to support their search for possible alternative treatments. Other nontraditional approaches might include acupuncture, massage, herbal therapies, or stimulus reduction. In M.D.'s case, after careful consideration of their status, it was decided to try the incobotulinumtoxinA injections to relieve their chronic migraines. The nurse needs to explain the series of injections that will need to be done in a medical facility and not at a *Botox* party. This will allow the health care professionals to ensure safe injections, decrease the risk of infection, and keep careful records of each site used for the repeat injections.

NURSING CARE GUIDE FOR M.D.: INCOBOTULINUMTOXINA

Assessment: History and Examination

Obtain a full history of migraine incidence, treatments, and response to treatment.

Assess for any active infection, known allergy to any ingredient in the drug, difficulty swallowing, and history of anaphylactic reactions.

Perform a physical assessment:

CV: Arrhythmias, hypertension

CNS: Orientation, affect

Skin: Color, lesions in head and neck area

Respiratory: Respiration, adventitious sounds

Nursing Conclusions

Acute pain related to injection effects

Breathing and/or swallowing impairment risk related to potential spread of effect

Knowledge deficit regarding drug therapy

Planning

The patient will receive the best therapeutic effect from the drug therapy.

The patient will have limited adverse effects to the drug therapy.

The patient will have an understanding of the drug therapy, adverse effects to anticipate, and measures to relieve discomfort and improve safety.

Intervention

Ensure ready access to epinephrine in case of anaphylactic reaction to injections.

Mark chart with sites of each injection given.

Ensure that there is no sign of infection or open areas near injection sites.

Provide comfort and safety measures, positioning, and pain medication as needed.

Provide support and reassurance to encourage M.D.

Teach M.D. about drug, drug effects, and symptoms of reportable serious adverse effects.

Evaluation

Evaluate drug effects: relief of migraine frequency, relief of migraine pain.

Monitor for adverse effects: headache, infection at injection sites, potential for spread of toxin (difficulty breathing and/or swallowing).

Evaluate effectiveness of patient teaching program.

PATIENT TEACHING FOR M.D.

- The drug prescribed for you is a direct-acting muscle relaxant called *Botox* (incobotulinumtoxinA). This drug stops muscles from moving. It is not really understood how the many injections into your head and neck actually help relieve migraines, but it is thought to be related to the muscle relaxation and changes in certain chemicals in the area.
- Common side effects of this drug include the following:
  - Pain at the injection sites: Report this to your provider.
  - Headache: An analgesic may be ordered to help.
- Report any of the following to your health care provider: fever, chills, appearance of any signs of infection at your injection sites; difficulty breathing or swallowing.
- You will need to return for another series of injections in 12 weeks; if your migraines become worse in that time, call your health care provider.

Therapeutic Actions and Indications

Dantrolene directly affects peripheral muscle contraction and has become important in the management of spasticity associated with neuromuscular diseases. Dantrolene is also used for treatment and prevention of malignant hyperthermia. Dantrolene acts within skeletal muscle fibers, interfering with the release of calcium from the muscle tubules (see Fig. 25.2). This action prevents the fibers from contracting. Dantrolene does not interfere with neuromuscular transmissions, and it does not affect the surface membrane of skeletal muscle. The botulinum toxins A and B bind directly to the receptor sites of motor nerve terminals and inhibit the release of acetylcholine, leading to local muscle paralysis. These drugs are injected locally and used to paralyze or prevent the contractions of specific muscle groups. RimabotulinumtoxinB is used to reduce the severity of abnormal head position and neck pain associated with cervical dystonia and can also be used to treat chronic sialorrhea. OnabotulinumtoxinA is used to improve the appearance of moderate to severe glabellar lines, canthal lines, and to treat cervical dystonia, muscle spasticity, severe primary axillary hyperhidrosis, strabismus and blepharospasm associated with dystonia, chronic migraines, overactive bladder, and detrusor overactivity associated with neurological disorders. IncobotulinumtoxinA is also used to decrease the severity of head position with cervical dystonia and to treat blepharospasm, upper limb spasticity, chronic sialorrhea, and improve glabellar lines in adults.

Long-term use of dantrolene commonly results in a decrease of the amount and intensity of required nursing care. Continued long-term use is justified as long as the drug reduces painful and disabling spasticity. This agent is not used for the treatment of muscle spasms associated with musculoskeletal injury or rheumatic disorders. Table 25.2 presents additional information about these agents, including usual indications.

Pharmacokinetics

Dantrolene is available in oral or parenteral forms. Dantrolene is slowly absorbed from the GI tract and metabolized in the liver with a half-life of 4 to 8 hours. Excretion is through the urine. Dantrolene crosses the placenta and was found to be embryotoxic in animal studies. Use should be reserved for those situations in which the benefit to the parent clearly outweighs the risk to the fetus, like with the treatment of malignant hyperthermia. Dantrolene enters human milk and is contraindicated for use during lactation. Safety for use in children younger than 5 years of age has not been established; because the long-term effects are not known, careful consideration should be given to use of the drug in children. The botulinum toxins are not generally absorbed systemically, and there is no pharmacokinetic information available.

Contraindications and Cautions

Dantrolene is contraindicated in the presence of any known allergy to the drug to prevent hypersensitivity reactions. It is also contraindicated in the following conditions: spasticity that contributes to locomotion, upright position, or increased function, which would be lost if that spasticity were blocked; active hepatic disease, which might interfere with metabolism of the drug and because of known liver toxicity; and lactation because the drug may cross into human milk and cause adverse effects in the infant. The botulinum toxins are contraindicated in the presence of allergy to any component of the drug to prevent hypersensitivity reactions or with active infection at the site of the injection because injecting the drug could aggravate the infection.

Caution should be used with dantrolene in female patients and in all patients older than 35 years because of increased risk of potentially fatal hepatocellular disease (Box 25.2); in patients with a history of liver disease or previous dysfunction, which could make the liver more

Box 25.2 Focus on Sex Differences

UNDERSTANDING THE RISKS OF LIVER DAMAGE WITH DANTROLENE

Dantrolene (*Dantrium*) is associated with potentially fatal hepatocellular injury. When liver damage begins to occur, patients often experience a prodrome, or warning syndrome, which includes anorexia, nausea, and fatigue. The incidence of such hepatic injury is greater in female patients and in patients older than 35 years of age.

In female patients, a combination of dantrolene and estrogen seems to affect the liver, thus posing a greater risk. Patients older than 35 years of age are at increased risk of liver injury because of the changing integrity of the liver cells that comes with age and exposure to toxins over time.

If a particular female patient needs dantrolene for relief of spasticity, they should not be taking any estrogens (e.g., birth control pills, hormone replacement therapy), and they should be monitored closely for any sign of liver dysfunction. For safer relief of spasticity in these patients, baclofen may be helpful.

susceptible to cellular toxicity; in patients with respiratory depression, which could be exacerbated by muscular weakness; in patients with cardiac disease because cardiac muscle depression may be a risk; and during pregnancy because of the potential for adverse effects on the fetus. Caution should be used with the botulinum toxins with any peripheral neuropathic disease; with neuromuscular disorders, which could be exacerbated by the effects of the drug; with pregnancy and lactation because the potential effects on the fetus or baby are not known; and with any known cardiovascular disease because of the potential changes in tissue perfusion and risk of systemic absorption.

Adverse Effects

The most frequently seen adverse effects associated with dantrolene relate to drug-caused CNS depression: drowsiness, fatigue, weakness, confusion, headache and insomnia, and visual disturbances. GI disturbances may be linked to direct irritation or to alterations in smooth muscle function caused by the drug-induced calcium effects. Such adverse GI effects may include GI irritation, diarrhea, constipation, and abdominal cramps. Dantrolene may also cause direct hepatocellular damage and hepatitis that can be fatal. Urinary frequency, enuresis, and feelings of urinary urgency reportedly occur, and crystalline urine with pain or burning on urination may result. In addition, several unusual adverse effects may occur, including acne, abnormal hair growth, rashes, photosensitivity, abnormal sweating, chills, and myalgia.

The botulinum toxins have been associated with anaphylactic reactions; with headache, dizziness, muscle pain, and paralysis; and with redness and edema at the injection site. Adverse effects associated with use of botulinum toxin A for cosmetic purposes include headache, respiratory infections, flulike syndrome, and droopy eyelids in severe cases. Pain, redness, and muscle weakness also have been reported. Children treated with these drugs have reportedly developed botulism. The reactions tended to be temporary, but there have been reports of reactions that lasted several months. The U.S. Food and Drug Administration strongly reminds providers that this is a prescription drug and should be used only under close medical supervision and not injected at trendy "Botox parties."

Clinically Important Drug–Drug Interactions

If dantrolene is combined with estrogens, the incidence of hepatocellular toxicity is apparently increased. If possible, this combination should be avoided. If the botulinum toxins are used with other drugs that interfere with neuromuscular transmission—neuromuscular junction blockers, lincosamides, quinidine, magnesium sulfate, anticholinesterases, succinylcholine, or polymyxin—or with aminoglycosides, there is a risk of additive effects. If any of these must be given in combination, extreme caution should be used.

Prototype Summary: Dantrolene

Indications: Control of clinical spasticity resulting from upper motor neuron disorders; preoperatively to prevent or attenuate the development of malignant hyperthermia in susceptible patients; IV for management of fulminant malignant hyperthermia.

Actions: Interferes with the release of calcium from the sarcoplasmic reticulum within skeletal muscles, preventing muscle contraction; does not interfere with neuromuscular transmission.

Pharmacokinetics:

Route	Onset	Peak	Duration
Oral	Slow	4–6 h	8–10 h
IV	Rapid	5 h	6–8 h

$T_{1/2}$: 9 hours (oral), 4 to 8 hours (IV); excreted in the urine.

Adverse Effects: Drowsiness, dizziness, weakness, fatigue, diarrhea, hepatitis, myalgia, tachycardia, transient blood pressure changes, rash, urinary frequency.

Nursing Considerations for Patients Receiving Direct-Acting Skeletal Muscle Relaxants

Assessment: History and Examination

- Assess for contraindications or cautions for the use of the drug including any known allergies to prevent hypersensitivity reactions; cardiac depression; epilepsy; muscle weakness; respiratory depression, which could be exacerbated by the effects of these drugs; pregnancy and lactation, which require cautious use; renal or hepatic dysfunction, which could alter the metabolism and excretion of the drug; and local infections (if using the botulinum toxins) to prevent exacerbation of the infections.
- Assess temperature; skin color and lesions; CNS orientation, affect, reflexes, bilateral grip strength, and spasticity; respiration and adventitious sounds; pulse, electrocardiogram, and cardiac output; bowel sounds and reported output; and liver and renal function tests to determine baseline status before beginning therapy and for any potential adverse effects.

Refer to the "Critical Thinking Scenario" for a full discussion of nursing care for a patient who is receiving a direct-acting skeletal muscle relaxant.

Nursing Conclusions

Nursing conclusions related to drug therapy might include the following:

- Impaired comfort related to GI and CNS effects
- Altered thought processes related to CNS effects
- Injury risk related to CNS effects
- Knowledge deficit regarding drug therapy

Planning

- The patient will receive the best therapeutic effect from the drug therapy.
- The patient will have limited adverse effects to the drug therapy.
- The patient will have an understanding of the drug therapy, adverse effects to anticipate, and measures to relieve discomfort and improve safety.

Intervention With Rationale

- Discontinue the drug at any sign of liver dysfunction. Early diagnosis of liver damage may prevent permanent dysfunction. Arrange for the drug to be discontinued if signs of liver damage appear. A prodrome, with nausea, anorexia, and fatigue, is present in 60% of patients with evidence of hepatic injury.
- Do not administer botulinum toxins into any area with an active infection because of the risk of exacerbation of the infection.
- Monitor intravenous access sites of dantrolene for potential extravasation because the drug is alkaline and irritating to tissues.
- Institute other supportive measures (e.g., ventilation, anticonvulsants as needed, cooling blankets) for the treatment of malignant hyperthermia to support the patient through the reaction.
- Periodically discontinue dantrolene for 2 to 4 days to monitor therapeutic effectiveness. A clinical impression of exacerbation of spasticity indicates a positive therapeutic effect and justifies continued use of the drug.
- Establish a therapeutic goal before beginning oral therapy with dantrolene (e.g., to gain or enhance the ability to engage in a therapeutic exercise program, to use braces, to accomplish transfer maneuvers) to promote patient compliance and a sense of success with therapy.
- Discontinue dantrolene if diarrhea becomes severe to prevent dehydration and electrolyte imbalance. The drug may be restarted at a lower dose.
- Provide thorough patient teaching, including drug name, prescribed dosage, measures for avoidance of adverse effects, warning signs that may indicate possible problems, and the need for monitoring and evaluation to enhance patient knowledge about drug therapy and to promote compliance.
- Offer support and encouragement to help the patient cope with the drug regimen.

Evaluation

- Monitor patient response to the drug (improvement in spasticity, improvement in movement and activities, improvement in continence, migraines, dystonia, facial lines, sweating with botulinum toxins).
- Monitor for adverse effects (CNS changes, diarrhea, liver toxicity, urinary urgency).
- Evaluate the effectiveness of the teaching plan (patient can give the drug name and dosage, possible adverse effects to watch for and specific measures to prevent adverse effects, and therapeutic goals).
- Monitor the effectiveness of comfort measures and compliance with the regimen.

Key Points

- Direct-acting skeletal muscle relaxants are used to relieve the effects of muscle spasm. Dantrolene, a direct-acting skeletal muscle relaxant, is used to control spasticity and prevent malignant hyperthermia.
- RimabotulinumtoxinB, onabotulinumtoxinA, and incobotulinumtoxinA are indicated to treat muscle spasticity in addition to a variety of other indications. They have a warning the effects could spread from injection site areas and cause swallowing and/or breathing difficulties.

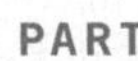

CRITICAL THINKING SCENARIO
Skeletal Muscle Relaxants for Cerebral Palsy

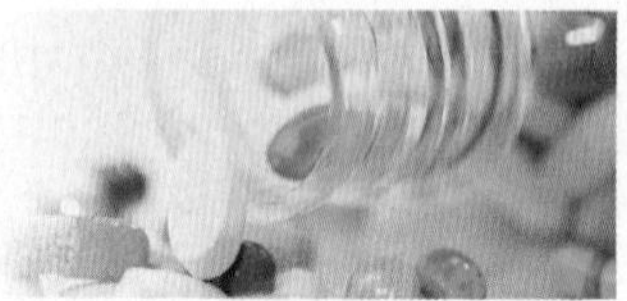

THE SITUATION

L.G. is 26 years old. They were diagnosed with cerebral palsy shortly after birth. L.G. lives in the community in a group home with six other people with cerebral palsy. Two adult caregivers provide supervision. In the past few months, L.G.'s spasticity has progressed severely, making it impossible for them to carry out daily activities without extensive assistance.

Following a clinical evaluation, their health care team suggests trying a course of dantrolene therapy. After learning about the risks of dantrolene-related hepatic dysfunction, L.G. decides that the benefits of dantrolene therapy are more important to them than the risks of hepatotoxicity. The health care team proceeds with a complete physical examination, including liver enzyme analysis. Therapy begins, and a clinic staff member schedules L.G. for a visit by a public health nurse in 4 days.

CRITICAL THINKING

What basic principles must be included in the nursing care plan for L.G. for the visiting nurses? Think about the importance of including the adult caregivers in any teaching or evaluation programs. Consider specific problems that could develop that L.G. would be unable to handle on their own.

What therapeutic goals might the nurse set with L.G. and their caregiver? How might these be evaluated?

What additional drug-related information should be posted in the group home and reviewed with L.G. and their caregivers?

DISCUSSION

In the first visit to the home, the nurse needs to establish a relationship with L.G. and their caregivers. They should all realize that drug therapy and other measures are needed to help L.G. attain their full potential and make use of their existing assets. Step-by-step therapeutic goals should be established and written down for future reference. Small reachable goals, such as partially dressing themselves, walking to the table for meals, and managing parts of their daily hygiene routine, are best at the beginning. Written goals provide a good basis for future evaluation when drug therapy is stopped briefly to determine its therapeutic effectiveness. It also helps L.G. see progress and improvement.

In addition, the nurse should perform a complete examination to obtain baseline data. The patient should be asked about any noticeable changes or problems since starting the drug. If improvement appears to have occurred, the dosage may be slowly increased until the optimal level of functioning has been achieved. The nurse is in a position to evaluate this and report it to the primary caregiver.

While in the home, the nurse can also evaluate resources and environmental limitations and suggest improvements in collaboration with rehabilitative therapists (e.g., use of leg braces). L.G. and their caregivers should receive a drug teaching card that includes a telephone number to call with questions or concerns, warning signs of liver disease, and a list of findings to report. The nurse should discuss anticipated appointments for liver function tests to ensure that L.G. can keep the appointments. The health care team should work closely with L.G. to maximize their involvement in their care and to minimize unnecessary problems and confusion. Because the treatment involves a long-term commitment, a good working relationship among all members of the health care team is important to ensure continuity of care and optimal results.

NURSING CARE GUIDE FOR L.G.: MUSCLE RELAXANTS

Assessment: History and Examination

Concentrate the health history on allergies to any skeletal muscle relaxants, respiratory depression, muscle weakness, hepatic or renal dysfunction, and concurrent use of verapamil or alcohol.

Focus the physical examination on the following:

CV: Blood pressure pulse rate, peripheral perfusion, electrocardiogram

CNS: Orientation, affect, reflexes, grip strength

Skin: Color, lesions, texture, temperature

GI: Abdominal examination, bowel sounds

Respiratory: Respiration, adventitious sounds

Laboratory tests: Renal and hepatic function

Nursing Conclusions

Impaired comfort related to GI, GU, and CNS effects

Injury risk related to CNS effects

Altered thought processes related to CNS effects

Knowledge deficit regarding drug therapy

Planning

The patient will receive the best therapeutic effect from the drug therapy.

The patient will have limited adverse effects to the drug therapy.

The patient will have an understanding of the drug therapy, adverse effects to anticipate, and measures to relieve discomfort and improve safety.

Intervention

Discontinue drug at first sign of liver dysfunction.

Provide comfort and safety measures: positioning, orientation, safety measures, pain medication as needed.

Provide support and reassurance to help L.G. deal with spasticity and drug effects.

Teach L.G. about drug, dosage, drug effects, and symptoms of reportable serious adverse effects.

Evaluation

Evaluate drug effects: relief of spasticity, improved daily function.

Monitor for adverse effects: multiple CNS effects, respiratory depression, rash, skin changes, GI problems (diarrhea, hepatotoxicity), urinary urgency, or weakness.

Monitor for drug–drug interactions: myocardial suppression with verapamil or alcohol.

Evaluate effectiveness of patient teaching program.

PATIENT TEACHING FOR L.G.

- The drug prescribed for you is a direct-acting skeletal muscle relaxant called dantrolene (*Dantrium*). This drug makes spastic muscles relax. Because this drug may cause liver damage, it is important that you have regular medical checkups.
- Common side effects of skeletal muscle relaxants, such as dantrolene, include the following:
  - Fatigue, weakness, and drowsiness: Try to pace activities evenly throughout the day and allow rest periods to avoid discouraging side effects. If they become too severe, consult your health care provider.
  - Dizziness and fainting: Change position slowly to avoid dizzy spells. If these effects should occur, avoid activities that require coordination and concentration.
  - Diarrhea: Be sure to be near bathroom facilities if this occurs. This effect usually subsides after a few weeks.
- Report any of the following to your health care provider: fever, chills, rash, itching, changes in the color of your urine or stool, or a yellowish tint to the eyes or skin.
- Keep this drug and all medications out of the reach of children.
- Do not overexert yourself when you begin to feel better. Pace yourself.
- Take this drug exactly as directed, and schedule regular medical checkups to evaluate the effects of this drug on your body.

SUMMARY

- Muscle contractions are controlled by multiple areas of the CNS: motor cortex, cerebellum, basal ganglia and spinal cord.
- Damage to a muscle or anchoring skeletal structure may result in the arrival of a flood of impulses to the spinal cord. Such overstimulation may lead to a muscle spasm or a state of increased contraction.
- Damage to motor neurons can cause muscle spasticity with a lack of coordination between muscle groups and loss of coordinated activity, including the ability to perform intentional tasks and maintain posture, position, and locomotion.
- Centrally acting skeletal muscle relaxants are used to relieve the effects of muscle spasm and/or spasticity and act on the nerves in the CNS.
- Dantrolene, a direct-acting skeletal muscle relaxant, is used to control spasticity and prevent or treat malignant hyperthermia.
- RimabotulinumtoxinB, onabotulinumtoxinA, and incobotulinumtoxinA are indicated to treat muscle spasticity in addition to a variety of other indications. They have a warning the effects could spread from injection site areas and cause swallowing and/or breathing difficulties.

CHECK YOUR UNDERSTANDING

Answers to the questions in this chapter can be found in Answers to Check Your Understanding Questions on thePoint®.

MULTIPLE CHOICE

Select the best answer.

1. A muscle spasm often results from
   a. damage to the basal ganglia.
   b. CNS damage.
   c. injury to the musculoskeletal system.
   d. chemical imbalance within the CNS.

2. Muscle spasticity is the result of
   a. direct damage to a muscle cell.
   b. overstretching of a muscle.
   c. tearing of a ligament.
   d. damage to neurons within the CNS.

3. Signs and symptoms of tetanus, which include severe muscle spasm, are best treated with
   a. baclofen.
   b. diazepam.
   c. carisoprodol.
   d. methocarbamol.

4. The drug of choice for a patient experiencing severe muscle spasms and pain precipitated by anxiety is
   a. methocarbamol.
   b. baclofen.
   c. diazepam.
   d. carisoprodol.

5. Dantrolene (*Dantrium*) differs from the other skeletal muscle relaxants because
   a. it acts in the highest levels of the CNS.
   b. it is used to treat muscle spasms as well as muscle spasticity.
   c. it cannot be used to treat neuromuscular disorders.
   d. it acts directly within the skeletal muscle fiber and not within the CNS.

6. The use of neuromuscular junction blockers may sometimes cause a condition known as malignant hyperthermia. The drug of choice for prevention or treatment of this condition is
   a. baclofen.
   b. diazepam.
   c. dantrolene.
   d. methocarbamol.

7. Patients treated with dantrolene should
   a. have repeated complete blood counts during therapy.
   b. have renal function tests done monthly.
   c. be monitored for signs of liver damage and have liver function tests done regularly.
   d. have a thorough eye examination before and periodically during therapy.

MULTIPLE RESPONSE

Select all that apply.

1. Spasmolytics, or centrally acting muscle relaxants, block the reflexes in the CNS that lead to spasm. While a patient is taking one of these drugs, which interventions should be implemented?
   a. Rest for the affected muscle
   b. Heat to the affected area
   c. Ice packs to the affected area
   d. Use of anti-inflammatory agents
   e. Body temperature check every 2 hours to watch for malignant hyperthermia
   f. Positioning to decrease pain and spasm

2. Muscle relaxants would be used in which circumstances?
   a. To treat spasticity related to spinal cord injury
   b. To treat spasticity that contributes to locomotion, upright position, or increase in function
   c. To treat spasticity that is related to toxins, such as tetanus
   d. To treat spasticity that is a result of neuromuscular degeneration
   e. To reduce the severity of head position associated with cervical dystonia
   f. To reduce the appearance of frown lines (glabellar lines)

REFERENCES

Albanese, A. (2011). Terminology for preparations of botulinum neurotoxins: What a difference a name makes. *Journal of the American Medical Association, 305*(1), 89–90. https://doi.org/10.1001/jama.2010.1937

Brunton, L. L., Hilal-Dandan, R., & Knollman, B. C. (2018). *Goodman and Gilman's the pharmacological basis of therapeutics* (13th ed.). McGraw-Hill.

Delgado, M. R., Hirtz, D., Aisen, M., Ashwal, S., Fehlings, D. L., McLaughlin, J., Morrison, L. A., Shrader, M. W., Tilton, A., & Vargus-Adams, J. (2010). Practice parameter: Pharmacologic treatment of spasticity in children and adolescents with cerebral palsy (an evidence-based review). *Neurology, 74*(4), 336–343. https://doi.org/10.1212/WNL.0b013e3181cbcd2f

Hall, J. E. (2016). *Guyton and Hall textbook of medical physiology* (13th ed.). Elsevier.

Kuehn, B. M. (2008). Studies, reports say botulinum toxins may have effects beyond injection site. *Journal of the American Medical Association, 299*(19), 2261–2263. https://doi.org/10.1001/jama.299.19.2261

Litman, R. S., & Rosenberg, H. (2005). Malignant hyperthermia: Update on susceptibility testing. *Journal of the American Medical Association, 293*(23), 2918–2924. https://doi.org/10.1001/jama.293.23.2918

Norris, T. L. (2019). *Porth's pathophysiology: Concepts of altered health states* (13th ed.). Wolters Kluwer.

Rössler, R., Donath, L., Verhagen, E., Junge, A., Schweizer, T., & Faude, O. (2014). Exercise-based injury prevention in child and adolescent sport: A systematic review and meta-analysis. *Sports Medicine, 44*(12), 1733–1748. https://doi.org/10.1007/s40279-014-0234-2

CHAPTER 26

Opioid Agonists, Opioid Antagonists, and Antimigraine Agents

Learning Objectives

Upon completion of this chapter, you will be able to:

1. Outline the gate theory of pain and explain therapeutic ways to block pain using the gate theory.
2. Discuss the use of the different classes of opioid agonists, opioid antagonists, and antimigraine agents across the lifespan.
3. Describe the therapeutic actions, indications, pharmacokinetics, contraindications, most common adverse reactions, and important drug–drug interactions associated with opioids and antimigraine agents.
4. Compare and contrast the prototype drugs with other drugs in their respective classes.
5. Outline the nursing considerations, including important teaching points, for patients receiving opioid agonists, opioid antagonists, or antimigraine drugs.

Key Terms

A fibers: medium and large-diameter nerve fibers that are typically myelinated and carry peripheral impulses associated with vibration, stretch, and pressure to the spinal cord; they are further divided into alpha, beta, gamma, and delta types

A-delta fibers: medium-diameter myelinated nerve fibers that carry peripheral impulses associated with pain to the spinal cord

C fibers: unmyelinated, small, slow-conducting fibers that carry peripheral impulses associated with pain to the spinal cord

ergot derivative: drug that causes a vascular constriction in the brain and the periphery; relieves or prevents migraine headaches but is associated with many adverse effects

gate control theory: theory that states the transmission of a nerve impulse can be modulated at various points along its path by the activation of larger sensory fibers transmitting tactile information to the brain, closing the "gate" and blocking transmission of pain information being communicated by the smaller A-delta and C fibers

migraine headache: headache characterized by severe, unilateral, pulsating head pain associated with systemic effects, including gastrointestinal (GI) upset and sensitization to light and sound; related to a hyperperfusion of the brain from arterial dilation

nociception: transmission of unpleasant stimuli from the point of initial injury to the brain via specialized nerve fibers

opioid agonists: drugs designed to react with specific opioid receptors throughout the body to stimulate the effects of the receptors

opioid agonists–antagonists: drugs that react at some opioid receptor sites to stimulate their activity and at other opioid receptor sites to block activity

opioid antagonists: drugs that block the opioid receptor sites; used to counteract the effects of opioids or to treat an overdose

opioid receptors: receptor sites on nerves that react with endorphins and enkephalins, which are receptive to opioid drugs

pain: a sensory and emotional experience associated with actual or potential tissue damage

spinothalamic tracts: nerve pathways from the spine to the thalamus along which pain impulses are carried to the brain

triptan: selective serotonin receptor blocker that causes a vascular constriction of cranial vessels; used to treat acute migraine attacks

Drug List

OPIOIDS

Opioid Agonists
alfentanil hydrochloride
codeine
fentanyl
hydrocodone
hydromorphone
levorphanol
meperidine
methadone
P morphine
opium
oxycodone
oxymorphone
remifentanil
sufentanil
tapentadol
tramadol

Opioid Agonists–Antagonists
P buprenorphine
butorphanol
nalbuphine

Opioid Antagonists
P naloxone
naltrexone

ANTIMIGRAINE AGENTS

Ergot Derivatives
dihydroergotamine
P ergotamine

Triptans
almotriptan
eletriptan
frovatriptan
naratriptan
rizatriptan
P sumatriptan
zolmitriptan

Calcitonin Gene–Related Peptide Inhibitors and Serotonin Agonist
eptinezumab
erenumab
fremanezumab
P galcanezumab
lasmiditan
rimegepant
ubrogepant

Pain, by definition, is a sensory and emotional experience associated with actual or potential tissue damage. The perception of pain is part of the clinical presentation in many disorders and is one of the hardest sensations for patients to cope with during the course of a disease or dysfunction. The drugs involved in the management of severe pain, whether acute or chronic, are discussed in this chapter. These agents all work in the central nervous system (CNS)—the brain and the spinal cord—to alter the way that pain impulses arriving from peripheral nerves are processed. These agents can change the perception and tolerance of pain. Two major types of drugs are considered here: the opium derivatives that are used to treat many types of pain and the antimigraine drugs, which are reserved for the treatment of migraine headache, a type of severe headache. Opioid antagonists, which are used to block the effects of the opioids in cases of overdose, also are discussed. Anti-inflammatory agents, which are often first-line treatment for pain, are discussed in Chapter 16. Some medications within the following classifications are commonly used as adjuvant medications for pain control: tricyclic antidepressants (TCAs) (Chapter 21) and antiseizure medications (Chapter 23).

Pain

Pain is described as an unpleasant sensation and an emotional experience. In many ways, it is a subjective experience. Pain occurs whenever tissues are damaged. The injury to cells releases many chemicals, including kinins and prostaglandins, which stimulate specific sensory nerves. The physiological processes that cause pain are perceived and reacted to in different ways because of learned experiences, cultural differences, and environmental stimuli.

Pain can be acute or chronic. Acute pain occurs in response to recent tissue damage or injury. This type of pain makes a person aware of an injury and should lead to measures to care for the injury and teaches the person to avoid similar situations that could cause this pain. Chronic pain can be constant or intermittent pain that keeps occurring past the time the injured area would be expected to heal. Chronic pain can cause a stress reaction, interrupt sleep, interfere with activities of daily living, and decrease quality of life. There are often circumstances in which people suffer from components of both chronic and acute pain.

Pain can also be classified by location. "Where does it hurt?" is a common question in assessing pain. Sometimes the location of the pain is a direct indicator of where the tissue damage has occurred. In some cases, referred pain occurs. A person experiencing pain from damage to the heart muscle may actually feel the pain in the neck or jaw. The sensation of pain is experienced in a different area of the body. Referred pain often follows predictable pathways, which helps health care providers figure out where the injury has occurred. Pain can be further classified by its originating source as nociceptive, neuropathic, or psychogenic. Nociceptive pain is caused by a direct stimulus to a pain receptor. Neuropathic pain is caused by nerve injury. Psychogenic pain is pain that is associated with emotional, psychological, or behavioral stimuli.

Pain Impulse Transmission and Perception

The transmission of unpleasant stimuli from the point of initial injury to the brain via specialized nerve fibers is labeled **nociception**. Two small-to-medium-diameter sensory nerves, called the A-delta and C fibers, respectively, respond to stimulation by generating nerve impulses that produce pain sensations. The **A-delta fibers** are medium, myelinated fibers that respond quickly to acute pain. The **C fibers** are small, unmyelinated, and slow conducting. Pain impulses from the skin, subcutaneous tissues, muscles, and deep visceral structures are conducted to the dorsal, or posterior, horn of the spinal cord on these fibers. In the spinal cord, these nerves form synapses with spinal cord nerves that then send impulses to the brain (Fig. 26.1).

In addition, large-diameter sensory nerves enter the dorsal horn of the spinal cord. These larger **A fibers** do

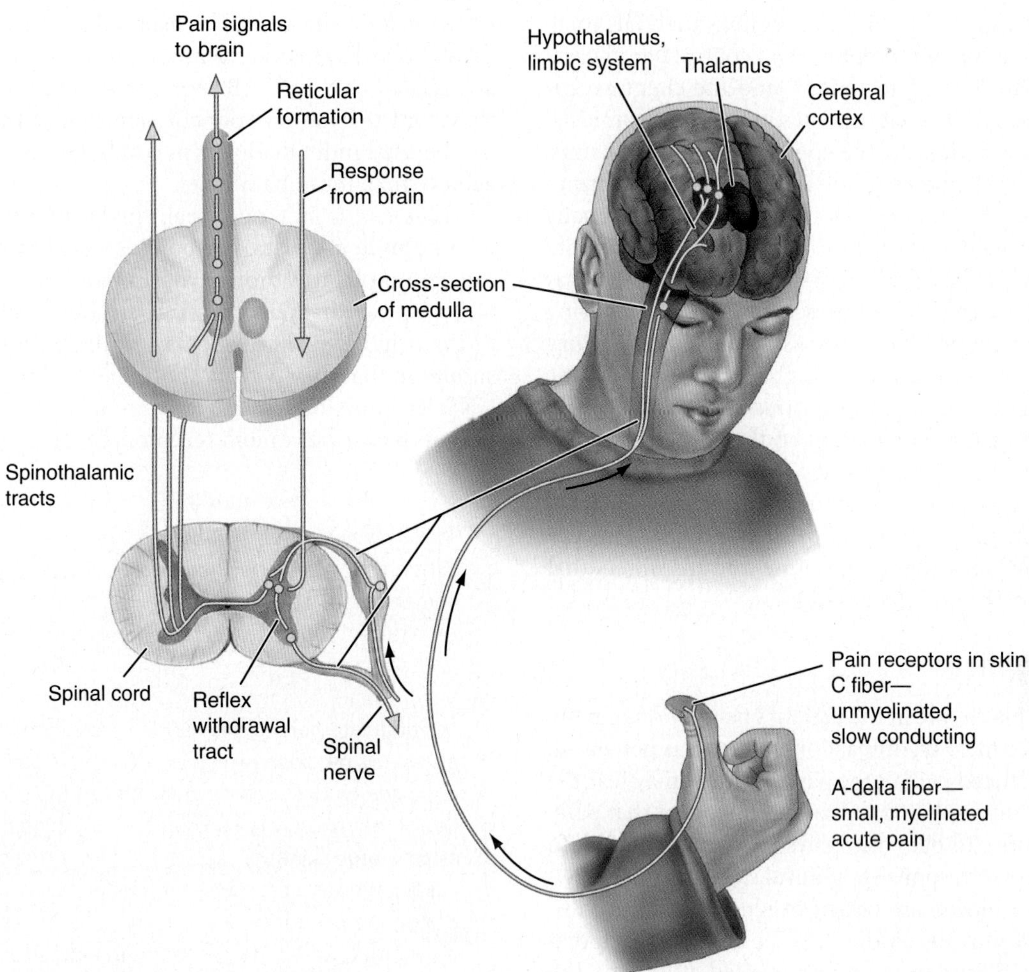

FIGURE 26.1 Neural pathways of pain.

not transmit pain impulses; instead, they transmit sensations associated with pressure, stretch, and vibration. A fibers, which are larger and conduct impulses more rapidly than the smaller fibers, can actually block the ability of the smaller fibers to transmit their signals to the secondary neurons in the spinal cord. The dorsal horn, therefore, can be both excitatory and inhibitory with regard to pain impulses that are transmitted from the periphery.

The impulses reaching the dorsal horn are transmitted upward toward the brain by a number of specific ascending nerve pathways. These pathways, known as **spinothalamic tracts**, run from the spinal cord into the thalamus, where they form synapses with various nerve cells that transmit the information to the cerebral cortex. According to the **gate control theory**, the transmission of these impulses can be modulated or adjusted all along these tracts. All along the spinal cord, the interneurons can act as "gates" by blocking the ascending transmission of pain impulses. It is thought that the gates can be closed by stimulation of the larger A fibers and by descending impulses coming down the spinal cord from higher levels in such areas as the cerebral cortex, the limbic system, and the reticular activating system.

The inhibitory influence of the higher brain centers on the transmission of pain impulses helps to explain much of the mystery associated with pain. Several factors, including learned experiences, cultural expectations, individual tolerance, and the placebo effect, can activate the descending inhibitory nerves coming from the upper CNS. Serotonin and norepinephrine are key substances secreted by the CNS that can modulate pain, and this may be why some of the antidepressant medications that increase these substances may be used as adjunctive pain treatment. All influencing factors need to be considered and incorporated into pain management strategies, which usually involve both pharmacologic and nonpharmacologic strategies. For example, relaxation, imagery, meditation, biofeedback, stress reduction, acupuncture, and back rubs (which stimulate the large A fibers) all can play important roles in the effective management of pain.

Pain Receptors

Opioid receptors are receptor sites that respond to naturally occurring peptides, the endorphins and the enkephalins. These receptor sites are found in the CNS, on nerves in the periphery, and on cells in the gastrointestinal (GI) tract. In the brainstem, opioid receptors help control blood pressure, pupil diameter, GI secretions, and the chemoreceptor trigger zone (CTZ) that regulates nausea and vomiting, cough, and respiration. In the spinal cord and thalamus, these receptors help integrate and relate incoming information about pain. The endorphins and enkephalins normally modulate the pain information coming into the brain. Endorphins are released during stress to block the sensation of pain. Professional athletes may be injured during an important game and have no sensation of pain or injury because their stress reaction is highly activated and the endorphins are blocking pain transmission into the brain. In the hypothalamus, stimulation of the opioid receptors may interrelate the endocrine and neural responses to pain. In the limbic system, the receptors incorporate emotional aspects of pain and response to pain. At peripheral nerve sites, they may block the release of neurotransmitters that are related to pain and inflammation.

Pain Perception

Many factors play a role in the patient's perception of pain. Past experience has a big impact on how pain is perceived. Having experienced pain in the past, a patient may fear the intensity it could reach and the overall impact of that pain. Learned response to pain also plays a large role. Children learn the accepted response to painful stimuli when growing up. Some children are taught to ignore pain and deal with it without showing emotion. Some children learn that reacting to pain can lead to much-wanted attention. The environmental setting in which the pain occurs also has an influence on perception and response to pain. A parent may not be willing to admit pain when the children are present, feeling that the role of the parent is to be strong. If you cut your finger when you are alone, you may perceive pain and react loudly. If you cut your finger when you are surrounded by young children, you may show no reaction and just go on with your activities. These varied influences on pain perception and response often make it very difficult to effectively evaluate and manage pain.

Pain Management

Accurately assessing pain can lead to effective pain management. Because so many factors play a role in pain perception and it is very subjective, assessment has to depend on the patient's report of pain. Health care providers often use a scale system to evaluate a patient's pain. Patients may be asked to rank their pain on a scale from 0 to 10, with 0 being no pain and 10 being the worst possible pain. Some pain scales use drawings of faces and ask the patient to pick the face that most reflects the pain they feel. Numerous methods, both nonpharmacological and pharmacological, may be used to manage pain. Nonpharmacological treatments can include warmth, massage, positioning, acupuncture, or meditation. Pharmacological methods often include the use of nonsteroidal anti-inflammatory drugs (NSAIDs) or acetaminophen (Chapter 16) for tissue-related pain or GABAergic or serotoninergic medications for the treatment of neurogenic pain. These methods can be used individually or in combination. The goal is to achieve maximum pain relief.

One major method of pain management involves the use of **opioid agonists.** The opioids were first derived from the opium plant. Although most opioids are now synthetically prepared, their chemical structure resembles that of the original plant alkaloids. All drugs in this class are similar in that they occupy specific opioid receptors in the CNS. Their actions in the body are related to the stimulation of the various opioid receptors that they occupy.

Key Points

- When tissue is injured, various chemicals are released, and pain can result.
- A-delta and C fibers carry pain impulses to the spinal cord.
- According to the gate control theory of pain, impulses travel from the spine to the cortex via tracts that can be modulated along the way at specific gates. These gates can be closed to block the transmission of pain impulses by descending nerves from the upper CNS (which often secrete serotonin or norepinephrine) and by large-diameter sensory A fibers, which are associated with pressure and vibration.
- Endogenous endorphins and enkephalins react with opioid receptors to regulate the transmission of pain.
- Opioids were originally derived from the opium plant; they bind to opioid receptors to relieve pain and promote feelings of well-being or euphoria.

Opioids

The opioid drugs used vary with the type of opioid receptors with which they react. This accounts for a change in pain relief as well as a variation in the side effects that can be anticipated. There are mu (m) and kappa (k) opioid receptors. The mu-receptors are primarily pain-blocking receptors. Besides analgesia, mu-receptors also account for respiratory depression, a feeling of euphoria, decreased GI activity, pupil constriction, and the development of physical dependence. The kappa-receptors are associated with some analgesia and with pupillary constriction, sedation, and dysphoria. The adverse effects of opioids can lead to death, and there is an opioid crisis in the United States. Some of the fatalities are caused by overdoses of opioids that are legally prescribed, but many are due to illicit opioid use. These substances are controlled substances due to the risk of abuse (Chapter 1), so the Drug Enforcement Agency closely regulates the prescription, distribution, and use of these substances. The administration of opioids requires specific considerations related to age (Box 26.1).

Box 26.1 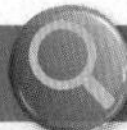 **Focus on Drug Therapy Across the Lifespan**

OPIOIDS

Children

The safety and effectiveness of many of these drugs have not been established in children. If an opioid is used, the dose should be calculated carefully, and the child should be monitored closely for the adverse effects associated with opioid use. The dosing for each formulation of opioid can vary, so careful review of the appropriate dosing is essential for all patients.

Methadone is not recommended as an analgesic in children. If a child older than 13 years of age requires an opioid agonist–antagonist, buprenorphine is the drug of choice. Naloxone is the drug of choice for reversal of opioid effects and opioid overdose in children.

Adults

Adults being treated for acute pain should be reassured regarding the positives of appropriate pain control. Opioids used for treatment of moderate and severe pain should be used in conjunction with other pharmacological and nonpharmacological pain reduction techniques. Patients should be encouraged to ask for pain medication before the pain is severe to get better coverage for their pain. Many institutions allow patients to self-regulate intravenous drips to control their pain postoperatively for a short time.

The opioids are used with caution during pregnancy because of the potential for adverse effects on the fetus. There are boxed warnings regarding potential for neonatal opioid withdrawal syndrome, which may be life threatening if not recognized and treated. These drugs enter human milk and can cause opioid effects in the baby, so caution should be used during lactation. Some of the opioids can be used for analgesia during labor. The birthing parent should be monitored closely for adverse reactions affecting them or the infant.

Older Adults

Older patients should be specifically asked whether they would like pain medication.

Older patients are more likely to experience the adverse effects associated with these drugs, including CNS, GI, and CV effects. Older adults who tolerated opioids well at a younger age may have a different response with age. These patients should be monitored when the drugs are started to evaluate response and toxicity.

Because older patients often have renal or hepatic impairment, they are also more likely to have toxic levels of the drug related to changes in metabolism and excretion. The older patient should have safety measures in effect—side rails, call light, and assistance to ambulate—when receiving one of these drugs in the hospital setting.

Opioid Agonists

The opioid agonists (Table 26.1) are drugs that react with the opioid receptors throughout the body to cause analgesia, sedation, or euphoria (Fig. 26.2). Anticipated effects other than analgesia are mediated by the types of opioid receptors affected by each drug. Because of the potential for the development of physical dependence while taking these drugs, the opioid agonists are classified as controlled substances. The degree of control is determined by the relative ability of each drug to cause physical dependence. With the rising problem of addiction and overuse of prescription drugs, measures are being taken to help better control these drugs. Hydrocodone and oxycodone have moved to C-II, providing more restrictions on their use and sale. In addition, manufacturers are working to develop tamper-resistant and abuse-resistant tablets. Some states have set up prescription registries for tracking the prescriptions of all controlled substances that allow providers and pharmacists to see all the controlled substances that have been prescribed to the patient. Opioid agonists include alfentanil hydrochloride (*Alfenta*), codeine, fentanyl (*Actiq, Duragesic, Lazanda, Subsys*), hydrocodone (*Hysingla ER, Zohydro ER*), hydromorphone (*Dilaudid*), levorphanol (generic), meperidine (*Demerol*), methadone (*Methadose*), morphine (*Infumorph, Kadian, Mitigo, MS Contin*), opium (*Paregoric*), oxycodone (*OxyContin, Roxicodone, Xtampza ER*), oxymorphone (generic), remifentanil (*Ultiva*), sufentanil (*Dsuvia, Sufenta*), tapentadol (*Nucynta, Nucynta ER*), and tramadol (*ConZip, Qdolo, Ultram*).

Therapeutic Actions and Indications

The opioid agonists act at specific opioid receptor sites in the CNS to produce analgesia, sedation, and a sense of well-being. They are also infrequently used as antitussives and as adjuncts to general anesthesia to produce rapid analgesia, sedation, and respiratory depression. Indications for opioid agonists include relief of severe acute or chronic pain, preoperative medication, analgesia during anesthesia, and specific individual indications, depending on their receptor affinity (see Table 26.1 for usual indications for each opioid agonist). Accurate calculation of a dose is crucial to prevent overdosing patients. Box 26.2 describes how to calculate the dose for one opioid agonist.

In deciding which opioid to use in any particular situation, it is important to consider all of these aspects of the patient's condition and to select the drug that will be most effective in each situation with the fewest adverse effects for the patient. Each patient is different, and their response to a drug is also different (Box 26.3). An extended-release formulation is probably best for patients that would like to minimize the sedative effects of the medications. However, short-acting formulations may be ordered for patients in the hospital or patients requiring fast relief. Fentanyl, which is available for injection, is also available as a lozenge for treating breakthrough pain, as a buccal tablet, transdermal patch, and sublingual tablet or nasal spray to be used as needed for treating breakthrough pain in cancer patients. See the "Critical Thinking Scenario" for information about using morphine to relieve pain.

Table 26.1 *Drugs in Focus*: Opioids

Drug Name	Dosage/Route	Usual Indications
Opioid Agonists		
alfentanil hydrochloride (*Alfenta*)	*Adult*: Induction and maintenance doses will vary based on the desired level of sedation and other coanesthetic agents *Pediatric*: Data for use in children 12 y are not available Reduce doses for older adults	As an analgesic adjunct given in incremental doses in the maintenance of anesthesia; as a primary anesthetic agent for the induction of anesthesia in patients undergoing general surgery in which endotracheal intubation and mechanical ventilation are required
codeine (generic)	*Adult*: 15–60 mg PO, IM, IV, or subcutaneous q4–6h; 10–20 mg PO q4–6h for cough *Pediatric*: 0.5 mg/kg PO, IM, or subcutaneous q4–6h; 2.5–10 mg PO q4–6h for cough. Not recommended for use due to unpredictable response	Relief of mild to moderate pain; relief of coughing induced by mechanical or chemical irritation of the respiratory tract
fentanyl (*Actiq, Duragesic, Lazanda, Subsys*)	*Adult*: 0.05–0.1 mg IM, 30–60 min before surgery; 0.002 mg/kg IV or IM during surgery; 0.05–0.1 mg postoperatively; 5 mcg/kg transmucosally; for transdermal patch, calculate the previous day's narcotics need and use table to convert to patch strength; sublingual tablet or nasal spray—initially a dose of 100 mcg to a maximum of 800 mcg sublingually or as a nasal spray in one nostril for treatment of breakthrough cancer pain *Pediatric (>2 y)*: 2–3 mcg/kg IM or IV; base transmucosal dose on weight and do not exceed 400 mcg	For analgesia before, during, and after surgery; transdermal patch for management of chronic pain; control of breakthrough pain
hydrocodone (*Hysingla ER, Zohydro ER*)	*Adult*: 10 mg PO q12h in combination products for pain; may increase in 10-mg increments as needed	Relief of pain requiring continuous analgesia for prolonged periods
hydromorphone (*Dilaudid*)	2–4 mg PO q4–6h *or* 3 mg PR q6–8h *or* 1–4 mg subcutaneous or IM q4–6h	Relief of moderate to severe pain in adults
levorphanol (generic)	1 mg IV by slow injection *or* 1–2 mg IM or subcutaneous q6–8h *or* 2 mg PO q6–8h	Management of moderate to severe pain in adults; postoperative pain in adults
meperidine (*Demerol*)	*Adult*: 50–150 mg PO, IM, or subcutaneous q3–4h; during labor, 100 mg IM or subcutaneous q1–3h *Pediatric*: 1–1.8 mg/kg IM, subcutaneous, or PO q3–4h	Relief of moderate to severe pain, preoperative analgesia and support of anesthesia, and obstetrical analgesia
methadone (*Methadose*)	2.5–10 mg IM, subcutaneous, or PO q3–4h for pain; 15–20 mg PO for withdrawal and then 20 mg PO q4–8h for maintenance treatment	Relief of severe pain; detoxification and temporary maintenance treatment of opioid use disorder in adults
morphine (*Infumorph, Kadian, Mitigo, MS Contin*)	*Adult*: 10- to 20-mg solution PO *or* 15- to 30-mg tablets PO q4h *or* 10 mg subcutaneous or IM q4h *or* 2–10 mg/70 kg IV over 4–5 min *or* 10–20 mg PR q4h *Pediatric*: 0.1–0.2 mg/kg IM or subcutaneous q4h	Relief of moderate to severe chronic and acute pain; preoperatively and postoperatively and during labor
opium (*Paregoric*)	*Adult*: 0.6 mL liquid PO q.i.d. or 5–10 mL camphorated tincture one to four times per day PO *Pediatric*: 0.005–0.02 mg/kg PO q3–4h or 0.25–0.5 mL/kg PO q1–4h of camphorated tincture	Treatment of diarrhea, relief of moderate pain
oxycodone (*OxyContin*, Roxicodone, *Xtampza ER*)	10 mg PO q12h as needed to start; immediate release 10 mg PO q4h as needed	Relief of moderate to severe pain in adults
oxymorphone (generic)	0.5 mg IV initially; 1–1.5 mg IM or subcutaneous q4–6h as needed; 0.5–1 mg IM for labor; 5 mg PR q4–6h	Relief of moderate to severe pain in adults; preoperative medication; obstetrical analgesia

Table 26.1 *Drugs in Focus*: Opioids (*continued*)

Drug Name	Dosage/Route	Usual Indications
remifentanil (*Ultiva*)	*Adult and pediatric* (>2 *y*): Dose determined by general anesthetic being used	Analgesic for use during general anesthesia *Special considerations*: Must be under the direct supervision of anesthesia practitioner
sufentanil (*Dsuvia, Sufenta*)	*Adult*: 1–2 mcg/kg IV with general anesthesia; *Dsuvia:* 30 mcg sublingual PRN with at least 1 hour between doses *Pediatric*: 10–25 mcg/kg IV	Analgesic for use during general anesthesia; used as an epidural agent in labor and delivery *Special considerations*: Must be under the direct supervision of anesthesia practitioner *Dsuvia*: Management of acute pain in supervised health care setting
tapentadol (*Nucynta, Nucynta ER*)	50–100 mg PO q4–6h; 50 mg PO q12h (ER)	Relief of moderate to severe pain or neuropathic pain associated with diabetic peripheral neuropathy in patients 18 y and older *Special considerations*: Risk of serious serotonin syndrome if combined with SSRIs, MAOIs, TCAs, and St. John's wort
tramadol (*ConZip, Qdolo, Ultram, Ultram XR*)	*Adults*: Rapid relief of pain, 50–100 mg PO q4–6h to a maximum of 400 mg/d; chronic pain, 25 mg/d PO titrated slowly to a maximum of 400 mg/d; *ConZip:* 100–300 mg PO/d	Relief of moderate to moderately severe pain *Special considerations*: Limit use in patients with a history of addictions
Opioid Agonists–Antagonists		
buprenorphine (*Belbuca, Buprenex, Butrans, Sublocade*)	*Adult and pediatric* (> *13 y*): 0.3 mg IM or slow IV q6h as needed; 5 mcg/h transdermal patch initially; *Belbuca:* 75–300 mcg buccal administration daily or twice a day; *Sublocade*: 2 monthly subcutaneous injections of 300 mg followed by 100 mg monthly maintenance doses	Treatment of chronic pain requiring an opioid; moderate to severe opioid use disorder (*Sublocade*)
butorphanol (generic)	*Adult*: 0.5–2 mg IV q3–4h *or* 1–4 mg IM q3–4h; 1 mg nasal spray, repeated in 60–90 min, and then in 3–4 h as needed *Older adults*: Use one-half of the adult dose at twice the usual interval *Pediatric*: Not recommended for children <18 y	Used as preoperative medication to relieve moderate to severe pain; treatment of migraine headaches, with fewer peripheral adverse effects than many of the traditional antimigraine drugs
nalbuphine (generic)	10 mg/70 kg IM, subcutaneous, or IV q3–6h as needed; do not exceed 160 mg/d	Relief of pain during labor and delivery; used as adjunct to general anesthesia; treatment of moderate to severe pain in adults
Opioid Antagonists		
naloxone (generic)	*Adult*: For overdose, 0.4–2 mg IV, may repeat at 2- to 3-min intervals; for reversal of opioid effects, 0.1–0.2 mg IV, may repeat at 2- to 3-min intervals *Pediatric*: For overdose, 0.01 mg/kg IV, repeat as needed; for reversal of opioid effects, 0.005–0.01 mg IV at 2- to 3-min intervals *Adult and pediatric*: 0.4 mg/0.4 mL using prefilled autoinjector IM or subcutaneously	Diagnosis of opioid overdose, reversal of opioid effects
naltrexone (*Vivitrol*)	*Adult*: 50 mg/d PO or 380 mg IM every 4 weeks	Adjunct treatment of alcohol or opioid dependence in adults

SSRI, selective serotonin reuptake inhibitor; MAOI, monoamine oxidase inhibitor; TCA, tricyclic antidepressant.

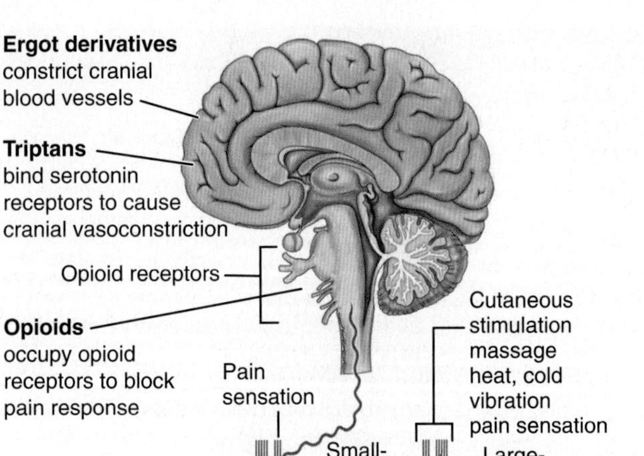

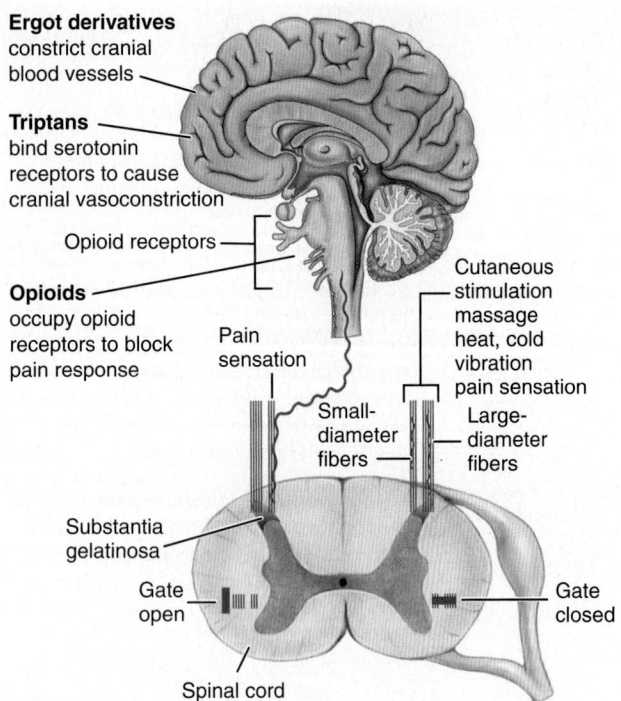

FIGURE 26.2 Sites of action. Opioids occupy opioid receptors to block pain response. Ergot derivatives constrict cranial blood vessels, and triptans bind serotonin receptors to cause cranial vasoconstriction.

Pharmacokinetics

Intravenous (IV) administration is the fastest way to achieve therapeutic levels of opioids. Intramuscular (IM) and subcutaneous administration offer varying rates of absorption, and absorption is usually slower in female patients than male patients because of the normal fat content of female muscles and tissue. These drugs undergo hepatic metabolism and are generally excreted in the urine and bile. Half-life periods vary widely, depending on the drug being used. These agents cross the placenta and are known to enter human milk.

Box 26.2 Focus on Calculations

You are taking care of a 4-year-old child after surgery. An order has been written for 0.15 mg/kg morphine IV q 2 to 4 hours as needed for pain control. The child is waking up and crying, so you decide to start the pain medication. The morphine is available as 5 mg/10 mL vial. You note that the child weighs 20 kg. How much morphine would you inject into the IV solution for each dose?

$$20\ \text{kg} \times 0.15\ \text{mg/kg} = 3\ \text{mg needed}$$
$$5\ \text{mg}/10\ \text{mL} = 3\ \text{mg}/X$$
$$5\ \text{mg}\ X = 30\ \text{mg mL}$$
$$X = 6\ \text{mL}$$

6 mL of the morphine would need to be injected into the IV solution for each dose.

Box 26.3 Focus on Cultural Considerations

DIFFERENCES IN RESPONSES TO OPIOID THERAPY

Because of physical and cultural differences among various ethnic groups, patients from certain groups respond differently to pain and analgesic medications. There is evidence regarding genetic differences that can predispose individuals to metabolize medications differently. For example, the genes that code the enzymes responsible for metabolism of opioids are highly polymorphic, which has the potential of causing significant variations in the pharmacokinetics of the medications. The polymorphisms of the genes may also be responsible for the variations in the severity of adverse effects potentiated by opioid agonists. Additional research is needed to facilitate the development of individualized dosing or treatment plans based on genetic variations. Based on these findings and variability in genetics, it is very important in the clinical setting to assess each individual's pain control and side effects and to refrain from assuming a certain dose of a medication "should" work effectively.

Contraindications and Cautions

The opioid agonists are contraindicated in the following conditions: presence of any known allergy to any opioid agonist, to avoid hypersensitivity reactions; diarrhea caused by toxins, because depression of GI activity could lead to increased absorption and toxicity; and some are contraindicated if GI obstruction is present, including paralytic ileus, because they may cause spasm of the sphincter of Oddi. Use extreme caution with opioid agonists in patients with biliary tract disease.

Caution should be used in patients with respiratory dysfunction, asthma, or emphysema, which could be exacerbated by the respiratory depression caused by these drugs; recent GI or genitourinary (GU) surgery and acute abdomen or inflammatory bowel disease, which could become worse with the GI depressive effects of the narcotics; head injuries, alcohol use disorder, delirium tremens, or cerebral vascular disease, which could be exacerbated by the CNS effects of the drugs; liver or renal dysfunction, which could alter the metabolism and excretion of the drugs; and during pregnancy, labor, or lactation because of potential adverse effects on the fetus or neonate, including respiratory depression. Prolonged use during pregnancy can result in neonatal opioid withdrawal syndrome, which may be life threatening if not recognized and treated.

Adverse Effects

The most frequently seen adverse effects associated with opioid agonists relate to their effects on various opioid receptors. Respiratory depression with apnea, cardiac arrest, and shock may result from narcotic-induced respiratory center depression. Orthostatic hypotension is commonly seen with some narcotics. GI effects such as nausea, vomiting, constipation, and biliary spasm may occur as a result of CTZ stimulation and negative effects on GI motility. Box 26.4 discusses drugs approved to treat opioid-induced constipation, a significant issue with long-term use in hospice situations and cancer care. Neurological effects such as light-headedness, dizziness, psychoses, anxiety, fear, hallucinations, pupil constriction, sedation, and impaired mental processes may occur as a result of the stimulation of CNS opioid receptors in the cerebrum, limbic system, and hypothalamus (Fig. 26.3). GU effects, including ureteral spasm, urinary retention, hesitancy, sweating, and loss of libido, may be related to direct receptor stimulation or to CNS activation of sympathetic pathways. Cough suppression is another side effect. This may be a wanted effect in people who need rest and are kept awake by their coughing; however, postsurgical patients often need to take deep breaths and perform coughing to decrease atelectasis postanesthesia. In addition, dependence (both physical and psychological) are possible, more so with some agents than with others. The medications have a boxed warning regarding the risk of addiction and misuse that can lead to overdose and death.

BOX 26.4

Combination Medications That Act on Opioid Receptors

There are several types of combination medications available that act on opioid receptors. The first combination type links an opioid agonist with either an NSAID or acetaminophen. *Percocet* (acetaminophen and oxycodone), *Norco* (acetaminophen and hydrocodone), and *Reprexain* (hydrocodone and ibuprofen) are examples of this type of combination medication. These medications are used to treat moderate to severe pain. They act through multiple mechanisms to alleviate pain, so patients will often have greater relief than if they were taking only one type of medication.

Another type of combination medication is indicated for treatment of opioid dependence. *Suboxone* and *Zubsolv* (naloxone and buprenorphine) are examples. These combine an opioid antagonist and opioid agonist–antagonist. People prescribed these medications should be monitored very carefully for signs of opioid withdrawal and should be enrolled in a complete treatment plan that includes counseling to assist with their opioid dependence.

Contrave (bupropion and naltrexone) is a combination medication with an opioid antagonist and antidepressant medication (see Chapter 21). It is indicated for weight management in people who are overweight with weight related comorbidity (hypertension, diabetes mellitus type 2, or dyslipidemia) or who are obese. This medication should be used in conjunction with a reduced-calorie diet and increased physical activity and is only indicated for adults.

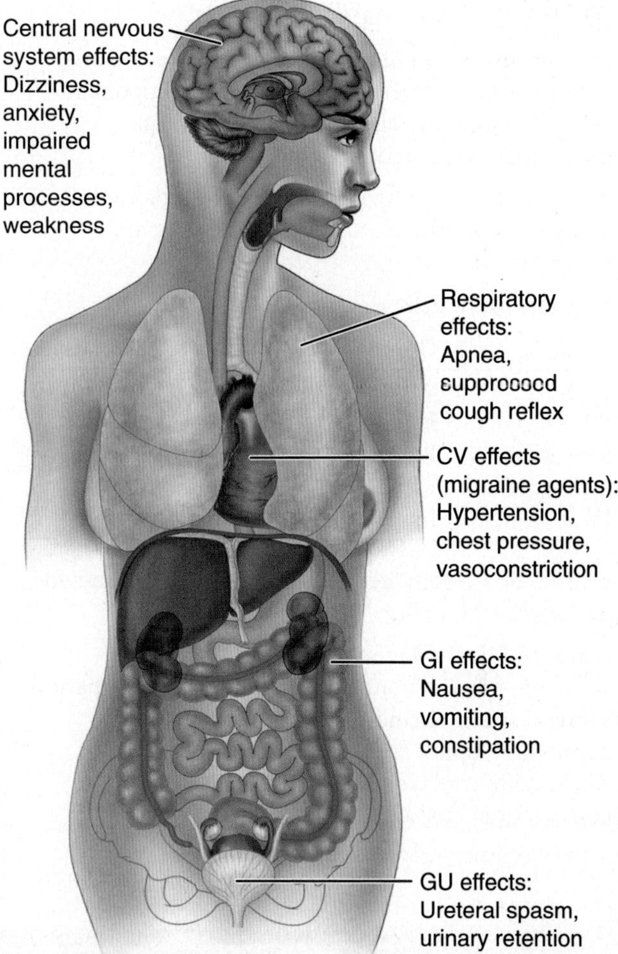

FIGURE 26.3 Common adverse effects and toxicities associated with narcotics, antimigraine agents.

Clinically Important Drug–Drug Interactions

When opioid agonists are given with barbiturate general anesthetics, other CNS depressants (including alcohol), or with some phenothiazines and monoamine oxidase inhibitors (MAOIs), the likelihood of respiratory depression, hypotension, and sedation or coma is increased. If these drug combinations cannot be avoided, patients should be monitored closely and appropriate supportive measures taken. Tapentadol also blocks norepinephrine reuptake in the CNS, and patients taking this drug should be cautioned if they are also taking selective serotonin reuptake inhibitors (SSRIs), MAOIs, TCAs, and St. John's wort because of the increased risk of potentially life-threatening serotonin syndrome. Use with anticholinergic agents may exacerbate GI and GU effects like constipation and urinary retention. Use with antihypertensive agents may increase the risk of systolic hypotension and orthostatic hypotension.

Prototype Summary: Morphine

Indications: Relief of moderate to severe acute or chronic pain; preoperative medication; component of combination therapy for severe chronic pain; intraspinal to reduce intractable pain.

Actions: Acts as an agonist at specific opioid receptors in the CNS to produce analgesia, euphoria, and sedation.

Pharmacokinetics:

Route	Onset	Peak	Duration
Oral	Varies	60 min	5–7 h
PR	Rapid	20–60 min	5–7 h
Subcutaneous	Rapid	50–90 min	5–7 h
IM	Rapid	30–60 min	5–6 h
IV	Immediate	20 min	5–6 h

$T_{1/2}$: 1.5 to 2 hours; metabolized in the liver; excreted in the urine and bile.

Adverse Effects: Light-headedness, dizziness, sedation, nausea, vomiting, dry mouth, constipation, ureteral spasm, urinary retention, respiratory depression, apnea, circulatory depression, respiratory arrest, shock, cardiac arrest, pupil constriction, coma.

Opioid Agonists–Antagonists

The **opioid agonists–antagonists** (see Table 26.1) stimulate certain opioid receptors but block other such receptors. These drugs also have boxed warnings regarding potential for abuse, although when closely monitored some can be used for treatment of opioid use disorder. Like morphine, they may cause sedation, respiratory depression, and constipation. They have also been associated with side effects including anxiety, fear, hallucinations, and impaired mental processes. They may induce a withdrawal syndrome in patients who have been taking opioids for a long period.

Available opioid agonists–antagonists include buprenorphine (*Buprenex*), butorphanol (generic), and nalbuphine (generic). Pentazocine has been discontinued as a single agent but is still manufactured as a combination medication with naloxone.

Therapeutic Actions and Indications

The opioid agonists–antagonists act as partial agonists at the mu-opioid receptors (and some at delta-opioid receptors) and antagonist at the kappa-opioid receptor in the CNS to produce analgesia, sedation, euphoria, and hallucinations. These drugs are used to treat moderate to severe pain that requires opioid medication, and some can be used to treat opioid use disorder. See Table 26.1 for usual indications for each opioid agonist–antagonist agent.

CRITICAL THINKING SCENARIO
Using Morphine to Relieve Pain

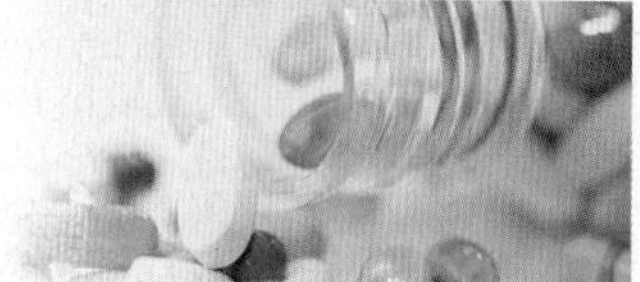

THE SITUATION

L.M., a 25-year-old businessperson, was in a car crash and suffered a fractured pelvis, a fractured left tibia, a fractured right humerus, and multiple contusions and abrasions. For the first 2 days after surgery, to reduce the fractures, L.M. was heavily sedated. As healing progressed, they were taught to use a patient-controlled analgesia (PCA) system using morphine. PCA provides a baseline, constant infusion of morphine and gives the patient control of the system to add bolus doses of morphine if they feel that pain is not being controlled. The system reduces the possibility of overdose by locking out extra doses until a specific period of time has elapsed. L.M. became agitated when they were not able to give themselves a bolus because the appropriate time between boluses had not elapsed. The nurse working with L.M. noted an increase in blood pressure, pulse, and respirations. L.M. had no fever. They did seem very anxious and rated their pain at 10. The nurse tried several nonpharmacological measures to alleviate the pain and spent time talking with L.M. and reassuring them. By day 5, L.M. was switched to oral morphine, and plans were made to wean them from opioid treatment.

CRITICAL THINKING

What basic principles must be included in the nursing care plan for this patient? Think about the difficult position the floor nurse is in when L.M. begins demanding pain relief before the prescribed time limit.

What implications will L.M.'s agitation have on the way that the staff responds to them and on other patients in the area?

What other nursing measures could be used to help relieve pain and make the medication more effective?

What plans could the health care team make with L.M. to give them more control over their situation and increase the chances that the pain relief will be effective?

DISCUSSION

In assessing L.M.'s response to drug therapy, you suspect that the morphine was not providing the desired therapeutic effect. It could be that the dose of morphine ordered for L.M. was not sufficient to relieve their pain. This patient has many causes of acute pain and will heal more quickly if the pain is managed better. They have requested more drugs because the dose may be too small or the intervals between doses may be too long to effectively relieve their pain. Other measures may be successful in helping the morphine relieve the pain. Back rubs, environmental controls to decrease excessive stimuli (e.g., noise, lighting, temperature, interruptions), and stress reduction may all be useful. It is often helpful to use adjunctive therapy with nonopioid medication to enhance analgesia. Discussing the possibility of enhancing the pain treatment plan with the provider would be appropriate.

L.M. may be anxious about their injuries, and the opportunity to vent their feelings and concerns may alleviate some of the tension associated with pain. They may fear that if they do not cover the pain before it gets too bad, it will be hard to get any pain relief. The nursing staff can work on this concern and figure out a way to reassure them.

The health care team should try to discuss the concerns with L.M., including the concern about physical dependency. L.M. is a businessperson and may respond positively to having some input into their care; they may even offer suggestions as to how they could cope better and adjust to their situation. Cortical impulses can close gates as effectively as descending inhibitory pathways, and stimulation of the cortical pathways through patient education and active involvement should be considered an important aspect of pain relief. Because L.M.'s injuries are extensive, a long-term approach should be taken to their care. The sooner L.M. can be involved, the better the situation will be for everyone.

NURSING CARE GUIDE FOR L.M.: OPIOIDS

Assessment: History and Examination

Assess history of allergies to any opioid drug, respiratory depression, GI or biliary surgery, hepatic or renal dysfunction, alcohol use disorder, or convulsive disorders.

Focus the physical examination on the following:

Cardiovascular (CV): Blood pressure, pulse rate, peripheral perfusion, electrocardiogram

CNS: Orientation, awareness, affect, reflexes, grip strength

Skin: Color, lesions, texture, temperature

GI: Abdominal examination, bowel sounds

Respiratory: Respiration rate and depth, adventitious sounds

Laboratory tests: Renal and liver function tests

Nursing Conclusions

Acute pain related to injuries

Impaired comfort from adverse effects of medication: GI, CNS, GU effects

Altered sensory perceptions (visual, auditory, kinesthetic) related to CNS effects

Altered gas exchange related to respiratory depression

Knowledge deficit regarding drug therapy

Anxiety related to injuries, drug regimen

Constipation risk due to inactivity, increased stress, and medication side effects

Planning

The patient will receive the best therapeutic effect from the drug therapy.

The patient will have limited adverse effects to the drug therapy.

The patient will have an understanding of the drug therapy, adverse effects to anticipate, and measures to relieve discomfort and improve safety.

Intervention

Ensure an opioid antagonist is available and facilities for assisted ventilation during intravenous administration.

Provide comfort and safety measures: orientation, accurate timing of doses, monitoring for extravasation, and additional measures for pain relief to increase effects.

Provide support and reassurance to deal with drug effects and addiction potential.

Provide patient teaching about the drug, dosage, drug effects, and symptoms of serious reactions to report.

Evaluation

Evaluate drug effects: relief of pain, sedation.

Monitor for adverse effects: CNS effects (multiple), respiratory depression, rash, skin changes, constipation, nausea, vomiting.

Monitor drug–drug interactions: increased respiratory depression, sedation, coma with barbiturate anesthetics, MAOIs, phenothiazines, SSRIs, TCAs, benzodiazepines, and other CNS depressants.

Evaluate the effectiveness of the patient teaching program.

Evaluate the effectiveness of comfort and safety measures.

PATIENT TEACHING FOR L.M.

- An opioid is used to relieve moderate to severe pain. Do not hesitate to take this drug if you feel uncomfortable. Remember that it is important to use the drug before the pain becomes severe and thus more difficult to treat.
- Common effects of these drugs include the following:
  - Constipation: Your health care provider will suggest appropriate measures to alleviate this common problem.
  - Dizziness, drowsiness, and visual changes: If any of these occur, avoid driving, operating complex machinery, or performing delicate tasks. If these effects occur in the hospital, the side rails on the bed may be raised for your protection.
  - Nausea, vomiting, and loss of appetite: Taking the drug with small sips of liquid or small meals may help. Lying quietly until these sensations pass may also help to alleviate this problem. If vomiting occurs, this may be treated with antiemetic medication.
- Report any of the following to your health care provider: severe nausea or vomiting, skin rash, or shortness of breath or difficulty breathing.
- Avoid the use of alcohol, antihistamines, and other over-the-counter drugs while taking this drug. Many of these drugs could interact with this medication.
- Tell any doctor, nurse, dentist, or other health care provider involved in your care that you are taking this drug.
- Keep this drug and all medications out of the reach of children.
- Do not take any leftover medication for other disorders, and do not let anyone else take your medication.
- Take this drug exactly as prescribed. Regular medical follow-up is necessary to evaluate the effects of this drug on your body.

Pharmacokinetics

Opioid agonists–antagonists are readily absorbed after IM administration and reach peak levels rapidly when given IV. They are metabolized in the liver and are excreted in the urine or feces. They are known to cross the placenta and enter human milk.

Buprenorphine is available for use in IM, IV, PO, transdermal, and transmucosal forms. Butorphanol is available for IM or IV administration and as a nasal spray. Nalbuphine is administered parenterally (subcutaneous, IM, or IV). Pentazocine was available in parenteral and oral forms, but now it is only available as an oral combination medication with naloxone.

Contraindications and Cautions

Opioid agonists–antagonists are contraindicated in the presence of any known allergy to any opioid agonist–antagonist to avoid hypersensitivity reactions.

Nalbuphine should not be given to patients who are allergic to sulfites to avoid a cross-hypersensitivity reaction.

Caution should be used in cases of physical dependence on opioids because a withdrawal syndrome may be precipitated; the opioid antagonistic properties can block the analgesic effect and intensify the pain. Opioid agonists–antagonists may be desirable for relieving chronic pain in patients who are susceptible to opioid dependence, but extreme care must be used if patients are switched directly from an opioid agonist to one of these drugs.

Caution should also be exercised in the following conditions: chronic obstructive pulmonary disease or other respiratory dysfunction, which could be exacerbated by respiratory depression; acute myocardial infarction (MI), documented coronary artery disease (CAD), or hypertension, which could be exacerbated by the cardiac stimulatory effects of these drugs; and renal or hepatic dysfunction, which could interfere with the metabolism and excretion of the drug.

With prolonged use during pregnancy, there is risk of neonatal opioid withdrawal syndrome that can be life threatening if not treated appropriately. These medications should be used during pregnancy only if the benefit to the parent clearly outweighs the risk to the fetus because of potential adverse effects on the neonate, including respiratory depression. Nalbuphine can be used to relieve pain during labor and delivery, which provides short-term exposure to the fetus. They are known to enter human milk and should be used with caution during lactation because of the potential for adverse effects on the baby.

Adverse Effects

The most frequently seen adverse effects associated with opioid agonists–antagonists relate to their effects on various opioid receptors. Respiratory depression with apnea and suppression of the cough reflex is associated with the respiratory center depression. Nausea, vomiting, constipation, and biliary spasm may occur as a result of CTZ stimulation and the negative effects on GI motility. Light-headedness, dizziness, headache, psychoses, anxiety, fear, hallucinations, and impaired mental processes may occur as a result of the activation of CNS opioid receptors in the cerebrum, limbic system, and hypothalamus. GU effects, including ureteral spasm, urinary retention, hesitancy, and loss of libido, may be related to direct receptor stimulation or to CNS activation of sympathetic pathways. Although sweating and both physical and psychological dependence are possible, their occurrence is considered less likely than with opioid agonists.

Clinically Important Drug–Drug Interactions

When opioid agonists–antagonists are given with barbiturate general anesthetics and other CNS depressant substances, the likelihood of respiratory depression, hypotension, and sedation or coma increases. If this combination cannot be avoided, patients should be monitored closely, and appropriate supportive measures taken.

Use of opioid agonists–antagonists in patients who are physically dependent on opioid agonists can put the patient at risk for abstinence syndrome that includes withdrawal symptoms like abdominal pain/cramping, hypertension, anxiety, vomiting, and fever. Patients should be monitored carefully in this situation and will require supportive care if symptoms are severe.

Prototype Summary: Buprenorphine

Indications: Relief of moderate to severe pain; treatment of moderate to severe opioid use disorder.

Actions: A partial agonist at specific opioid receptors in the CNS and antagonist at the kappa-opioid receptors, producing analgesia and sedation.

Pharmacokinetics:

Route	Onset	Peak	Duration
Buccal, IM, IV	15–30 min	1–3 h	3 h
Subcutaneous implant	Not quantified	~12 h	~20 weeks

$T_{1/2}$: About 30 hours to 60 days; metabolized in the liver; excreted in the urine and feces.

Adverse Effects: Light-headedness, dizziness, sedation, euphoria, nausea, vomiting, constipation, tachycardia, palpitations, sweating, ureteral spasm, physical dependence.

Nursing Considerations for Patients Receiving Opioid Agonists and Opioid Agonists–Antagonists

Assessment: History and Examination

- Assess for contraindications or cautions: known allergies to these drugs or to sulfites if using nalbuphine, to avoid hypersensitivity reactions; respiratory dysfunction, which may be exacerbated by the respiratory depression caused by these drugs; MI or CAD, which could be exacerbated by the effects of these drugs; renal or hepatic dysfunction, which might interfere with drug metabolism or excretion; current status of pregnancy and lactation, which require cautious use of the drugs; diarrhea caused by toxins because depression of GI activity could lead to increased absorption and toxicity; and after biliary surgery or surgical anastomoses because of the adverse effects associated with slowed GI activity due to narcotics.
- Perform a pain assessment with the patient to establish baseline and evaluate the effectiveness of drug therapy.
- Perform a physical assessment before beginning therapy to establish baseline status, determine drug effectiveness, and evaluate for any potential adverse effects.
- Assess orientation, affect, reflexes, and pupil size to evaluate any central CNS effects; monitor respiratory rate and auscultate lungs for adventitious sounds to evaluate respiratory effects.
- Monitor pulse, blood pressure, and cardiac output to evaluate for cardiac effects.
- Palpate abdomen for distension and auscultate bowel sounds to monitor for GI effects; assess urine output and palpate for bladder distension to evaluate for GU effects.
- Monitor the results of laboratory tests such as liver and renal function tests to determine the need for possible dose adjustment and identify toxic drug effects.

Nursing Conclusions

Nursing conclusions related to drug therapy might include the following:

- Altered sensory perception (visual, auditory, kinesthetic) related to CNS effects
- Constipation, nausea, vomiting related to GI effects
- Altered gas exchange related to respiratory depression
- Injury risk related to CNS effects of the drug

Planning

- The patient will receive the best therapeutic effect from the drug therapy.
- The patient will have limited adverse effects to the drug therapy.
- The patient will have an understanding of the drug therapy, adverse effects to anticipate, and measures to relieve discomfort and improve safety.

Intervention With Rationale

- Perform baseline and periodic pain assessments with the patient to monitor drug effectiveness and provide appropriate changes in pain management protocol as needed.
- Have an opioid antagonist and equipment for assisted ventilation readily available when administering the drug to provide patient support in case of severe reaction or overdose.
- Monitor injection sites for irritation and extravasation to provide appropriate supportive care if needed.
- Monitor timing of analgesic doses. Prompt administration may provide a more acceptable level of analgesia and lead to quicker resolution of the pain.
- Use extreme caution when injecting these drugs into any body area that is chilled or has poor perfusion or shock because absorption may be delayed, and after repeated doses, an excessive amount is absorbed all at once.
- Use additional measures to relieve pain (e.g., back rubs, stress reduction, hot packs, ice packs) to increase the effectiveness of the opioid being given and reduce pain.
- Monitor respiratory status before beginning therapy and periodically during therapy to monitor for potential respiratory depression.
- Institute comfort and safety measures, such as side rails and assistance with ambulation, to ensure patient safety; bowel program as needed to treat constipation; environmental controls to decrease stimulation; and small, frequent meals to relieve GI distress if GI upset is severe.
- Offer support and encouragement to help the patient cope with the drug regimen.
- Provide thorough patient teaching, including drug name, prescribed dose, and schedule of administration; measures for avoidance of adverse effects; warning signs that may indicate possible problems; safety measures such as avoiding driving, getting assistance with ambulation, avoiding making important decisions, or signing important papers; and the need for monitoring and evaluation to enhance patient knowledge about drug therapy and to promote compliance.

Evaluation

- Monitor patient response to the drug (relief of pain, sedation).
- Monitor for adverse effects (CNS changes, GI depression, respiratory depression, arrhythmias, hypotension).
- Evaluate the effectiveness of the teaching plan (the patient can state the drug name and dosage and describe possible adverse effects to watch for, specific measures to prevent them, and warning signs to report).
- Monitor the effectiveness of comfort measures and compliance with the regimen.

Opioid Antagonists

The **opioid antagonists** (see Table 26.1) are drugs that bind strongly to opioid receptors but do not activate them. They block the effects of the opioid receptors and are often used to block the effects of too many opioids in the system. The opioid antagonists in use include naloxone (generic) and naltrexone (*Vivitrol*). There are opioid antagonists that are indicated to treat opioid-related constipation that are discussed in Chapter 58.

Therapeutic Actions and Indications

The opioid antagonists block opioid receptors and reverse the effects of opioids, including respiratory depression, sedation, psychotomimetic effects, and hypotension.

These agents are indicated for reversal of the adverse effects of opioid use, including respiratory depression and sedation, and for treatment of opioid overdose (see Table 26.1 for usual indications for each opioid antagonist agent). The opioid antagonists do not have an appreciable effect in most people, but individuals who are dependent on opioid agonists experience the signs and symptoms of withdrawal when receiving these drugs rapidly. In 2014, naloxone was released in an autoinjector for use by first responders, family members of known opioid users who could be at risk for overdose, and emergency care workers. Rapid response to overdose can save many lives.

Pharmacokinetics

Opioid antagonists may be administered parenterally or orally. If administered orally, naloxone is not absorbed. When formulated with an opioid receptor agonist, it serves as an abuse deterrent. Naltrexone is well absorbed orally. These drugs are widely distributed in the body. They undergo hepatic metabolism and are excreted primarily in the urine. They often have shorter half-lives than opioids so may need to be dosed more frequently to have therapeutic effect.

Contraindications and Cautions

Opioid antagonists are contraindicated in the presence of any known allergy to any opioid antagonist to avoid hypersensitivity reactions. Caution should be used during pregnancy and lactation because of potential of the fetus having withdrawal symptoms and/or respiratory depression. However, treating with opioid antagonists that may prevent opioid overdose and/or severe withdrawal symptoms in the person who is pregnant is often thought to be safer than withholding the opioid antagonist.

Adverse Effects

The most frequently seen adverse effects associated with these drugs relate to the blocking effects of the opioid receptors. The most common effect is an acute opioid abstinence syndrome that is characterized by nausea, vomiting, sweating, tachycardia, hypertension, tremulousness, and feelings of anxiety.

CNS excitement and reversal of analgesia are especially common after surgery. CV effects related to the reversal of the opioid depression can include tachycardia, blood pressure changes, dysrhythmias, and pulmonary edema.

Clinically Important Drug–Drug Interactions

To reverse the effects of buprenorphine, butorphanol, nalbuphine, or pentazocine, larger doses of opioid antagonists may be needed.

Prototype Summary: Naloxone

Indications: Complete or partial reversal of effects of opioids; diagnosis of suspected opioid overdose.

Actions: Pure opioid antagonist; reverses the effects of the opioids, including respiratory depression, sedation, and hypotension.

Pharmacokinetics:

Route	Peak	Onset	Duration
IV	Unknown	2 min	2 h
IM, subcutaneous	Unknown	3–5 min	2 h

$T_{1/2}$: 30 to 81 minutes; metabolized in the liver; excreted in the urine.

Adverse Effects: Acute opioid abstinence syndrome (nausea, vomiting, sweating, tachycardia, fall in blood pressure), hypotension, hypertension, pulmonary edema.

Nursing Considerations for Patients Receiving Opioid Antagonists

Assessment: History and Examination

- Assess for contraindications or cautions: any known allergies to these drugs to avoid hypersensitivity reactions; history of opioid dependence (unless being used in an overdose), which may lead to opioid abstinence syndrome; history of MI or CAD, which may be exacerbated by the reversal of opioid depression; and current status of pregnancy and lactation, which require cautious use of these drugs.
- Perform a physical assessment before beginning therapy to establish baseline status and any potential adverse effects.
- Assess the patient's neurological status, including level of orientation, affect, reflexes, and pupil size to evaluate CNS effects; monitor respiratory rate and auscultate

lungs for adventitious sounds to evaluate respiratory status.
- Monitor vital signs, including pulse and blood pressure, to identify changes and risks to the CV system.
- Obtain an electrocardiogram as appropriate to evaluate for cardiac effects.

Nursing Conclusions

Nursing conclusions related to drug therapy might include the following:

- Acute pain related to withdrawal and CV effects
- Altered cardiac output related to CV effects
- Injury risk related to CNS effects
- Knowledge deficit regarding drug therapy

Planning

- The patient will receive the best therapeutic effect from the drug therapy.
- The patient will have limited adverse effects to the drug therapy.
- The patient will have an understanding of the drug therapy, adverse effects to anticipate, and measures to relieve discomfort and improve safety.

Intervention With Rationale

- Maintain open airway and provide artificial ventilation and cardiac massage as needed to support the patient. Administer vasopressors as needed to manage opioid overdose.
- Provide continuous monitoring of the patient, adjusting the dose as needed, during treatment of acute overdose.
- Provide comfort and safety measures to help the patient cope with withdrawal syndrome.
- Ensure that patients receiving naltrexone have been opioid-free for 7 to 10 days to prevent severe withdrawal syndrome. Check urine opioid levels if there is any question.
- If the patient is receiving naltrexone as part of a comprehensive opioid or alcohol withdrawal program, advise the patient to wear or carry a MedicAlert warning so that medical personnel know how to treat the patient in an emergency.
- Institute comfort and safety measures, such as side rails and assistance with ambulation, to ensure patient safety; institute bowel program as needed for treatment of constipation; use environmental controls to decrease stimulation; and provide small frequent meals to relieve GI irritation if GI upset is severe.
- Offer support and encouragement to help the patient cope with the effects of the drug regimen.
- Provide thorough patient teaching, including drug name and prescribed dosage; measures to avoid adverse effects; warning signs to report immediately that may indicate possible problems; safety measures such as avoiding driving, avoiding making important decisions, and having a responsible person available for assistance; and the importance of continued monitoring and evaluation to enhance patient knowledge about drug therapy and to promote adherence.

Evaluation

- Monitor patient response to the drug (reversal of opioid effects, treatment of alcohol dependence).
- Monitor for adverse effects (CV changes, arrhythmias, hypertension).
- Evaluate the effectiveness of the teaching plan (patient can give the drug name and dosage and describe possible adverse effects to watch for, specific measures to prevent them, and warning signs to report).
- Monitor the effectiveness of comfort measures and compliance with the regimen.

Key Points

- Opioid agonists react with opioid receptor sites to stimulate their activity.
- Opioid agonists–antagonists react with some opioid receptor sites to stimulate activity and block other opioid receptor sites.
- Opioid antagonists are used to treat opioid overdose or to reverse unacceptable adverse effects.

Migraine Headaches

There are several types of headaches. Tension headaches are the most common and often are not so severe that they drastically interfere with daily activities. Cluster headaches are uncommon and the etiology is not completely known, though they do occur more in males. They seem to have a neurovascular component that activates the trigeminovascular system and the cranial autonomic parasympathetic reflexes to cause acute and severe pain that is often unilateral and behind the eye, radiating to the temple, cheek, and gums. Associating symptoms include sweating, flushing, tearing, and nasal congestion.

Migraine headaches are also due to the activation of the trigeminal nerve that causes inflammation within the meningeal blood vessels. One of the chemicals secreted during this process is the calcitonin gene–related peptide (CGRP). There is a component of vasodilation of blood vessels during this process, which can further activate the nocioreceptors to cause pain. Often migraines cause severe, throbbing headaches on one side of the head. This pain can be so severe that it can cause widespread disturbances, affecting GI (nausea and vomiting) and CNS function, including mood and personality changes, with photo and/or phonophobia. Females suffer more from migraine headaches, and hormonal variations in estrogen levels can affect the timing of migraine headaches (Box 26.5).

Box 26.5 Focus on Sex Differences

HEADACHE DISTRIBUTION

Headaches are distributed in the general population in a definite sex-related pattern. For example:

- Migraine headaches are three times more likely to occur in females than in males.
- Cluster headaches are more likely to occur in males than in females.
- Tension headaches are more likely to occur in females than in males.

There is some speculation that the predisposition of females to experiencing migraine headaches may be related to the vascular sensitivity to hormones, especially estrogen. Some people assigned female can directly plot migraine occurrence to periods of fluctuations in their menstrual cycle.

Migraines generally are classified as common or classic. Common migraines, which occur without an aura, cause severe, unilateral, pulsating pain that is frequently accompanied by nausea, vomiting, and sensitivity to light and sound. Such migraine headaches are often aggravated by physical activity. Classic migraines are usually preceded by an aura—a sensation involving sensory or motor disturbances—that usually occurs about 30 minutes before the pain begins. The pain and adverse effects are the same as those of the common migraine.

Antimigraine Agents

Many people will appropriately first use over-the-counter pain medications to treat headaches. Often an NSAID, caffeine, acetaminophen, or combination of over-the-counter analgesics will be able to alleviate pain caused by a tension headache or mild migraine. However, for more severe headaches, prescription medications are available. For many years, the standard treatment for migraine headaches was acute analgesia, often involving a narcotic, together with control of lighting and sound and the use of ergot derivatives. In the late 1990s, a new class of drugs, the triptans, was found to be extremely effective in treating migraine headaches without the adverse effects associated with ergot derivative use. Because these agents are associated with many systemic adverse effects, their usefulness is limited in some patients (Box 26.6). In recent years, the calcitonin gene–related peptide (CGRP) inhibitors and a serotonin receptor agonist have been approved for prevention and/or treatment of migraine headaches. Other classes of drugs have been used with some success in the prevention of migraines, including the beta-adrenergic blockers, the TCA amitriptyline, several anticonvulsants, and the calcium channel blocker verapamil. Table 26.2 includes additional information about each class of antimigraine agents used to abort headaches.

Ergot Derivatives

The **ergot derivatives** cause constriction of cranial blood vessels and decrease the pulsation of cranial arteries. As a result, they reduce the hyperperfusion of the basilar artery vascular bed. Available ergot derivatives include dihydroergotamine (*Migranal, D.H.E. 45*) and ergotamine (*Ergomar*).

Box 26.6 Focus on Drug Therapy Across the Lifespan

ANTIMIGRAINE AGENTS

Children

There are not many medications to treat migraines that are recommended for use in children. The ergot derivatives can have many adverse effects in children. Almotriptan may be used for adolescents, and rizatriptan can be prescribed to children 6 years and older. As with adults, children with headaches should be first treated with over-the-counter analgesics. If headaches are frequent and/or severe, children need to be evaluated for secondary causes of headache before they are prescribed medication to alleviate the pain.

Adults

Adults requesting treatment for migraine headaches should be carefully evaluated before one of the antimigraine drugs is used. This ensures that the headache being treated is of the type that can benefit from these drugs and rules out secondary type headaches that can be caused by a variety of disease processes including tumors, infections, and structural abnormalities.

The ergots and the triptans are contraindicated during pregnancy because of the potential for adverse effects in the parent and fetus. People who can become pregnant should be advised to use contraception while they are taking these drugs. People who are breast or chestfeeding should be encouraged to find another method of feeding the baby because of the potential for adverse drug effects on the baby. Caution should be taken with the CGRP inhibitors and lasmiditan during pregnancy due to lack of data in humans.

Older Adults

Older adults are more likely to have chronic diseases such as CV disease or renal or hepatic impairment that would be exacerbated by the ergot and triptan antimigraine drugs. They should be used with extreme caution in older adults. The older adult should be encouraged to take the least amount of the drug possible and should be monitored closely for any sign of chest pain, MI, or acute vascular changes. Safety measures are extremely important with the older adult.

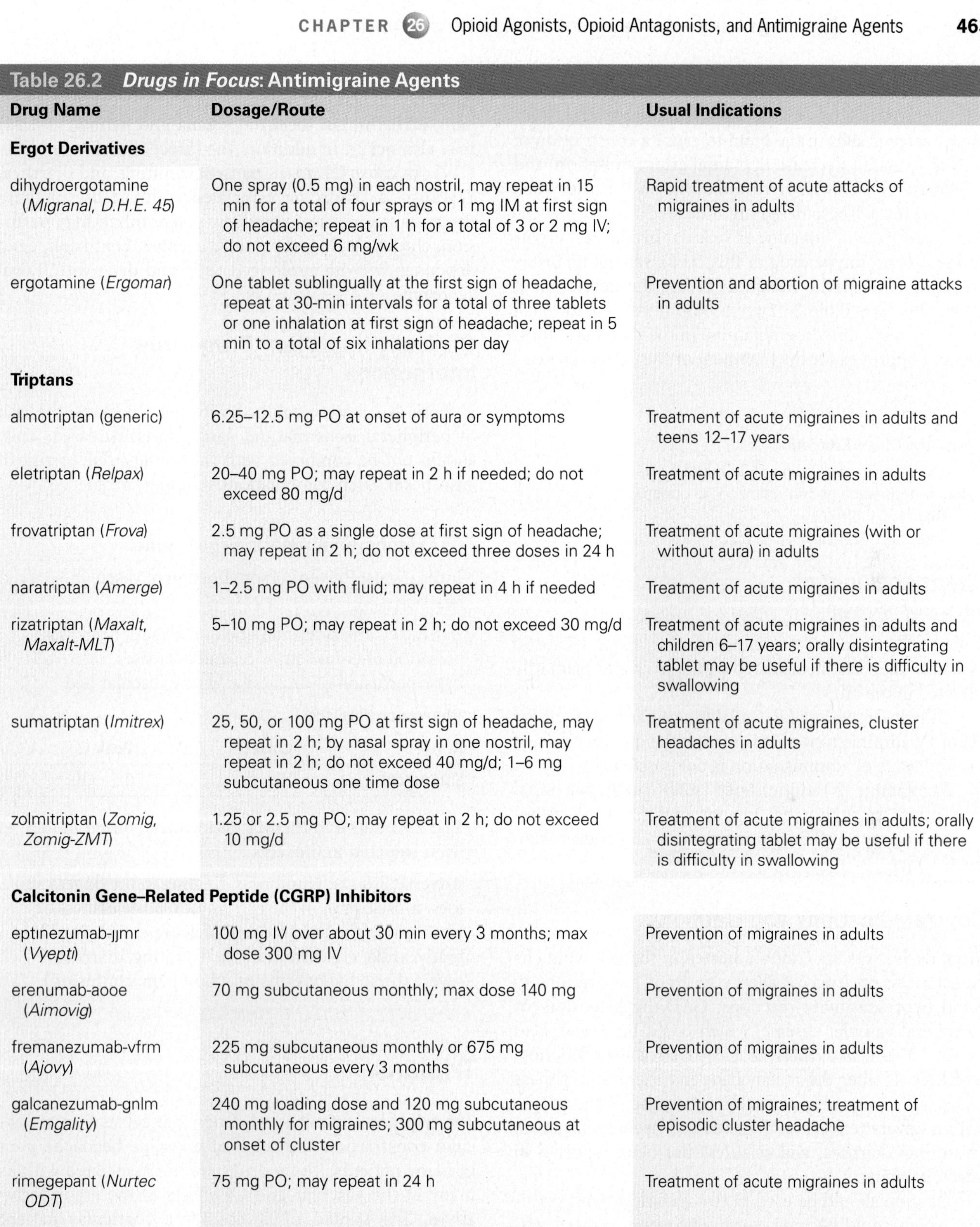

Table 26.2 *Drugs in Focus*: Antimigraine Agents

Drug Name	Dosage/Route	Usual Indications
Ergot Derivatives		
dihydroergotamine (*Migranal, D.H.E. 45*)	One spray (0.5 mg) in each nostril, may repeat in 15 min for a total of four sprays or 1 mg IM at first sign of headache; repeat in 1 h for a total of 3 or 2 mg IV; do not exceed 6 mg/wk	Rapid treatment of acute attacks of migraines in adults
ergotamine (*Ergomar*)	One tablet sublingually at the first sign of headache, repeat at 30-min intervals for a total of three tablets or one inhalation at first sign of headache; repeat in 5 min to a total of six inhalations per day	Prevention and abortion of migraine attacks in adults
Triptans		
almotriptan (generic)	6.25–12.5 mg PO at onset of aura or symptoms	Treatment of acute migraines in adults and teens 12–17 years
eletriptan (*Relpax*)	20–40 mg PO; may repeat in 2 h if needed; do not exceed 80 mg/d	Treatment of acute migraines in adults
frovatriptan (*Frova*)	2.5 mg PO as a single dose at first sign of headache; may repeat in 2 h; do not exceed three doses in 24 h	Treatment of acute migraines (with or without aura) in adults
naratriptan (*Amerge*)	1–2.5 mg PO with fluid; may repeat in 4 h if needed	Treatment of acute migraines in adults
rizatriptan (*Maxalt, Maxalt-MLT*)	5–10 mg PO; may repeat in 2 h; do not exceed 30 mg/d	Treatment of acute migraines in adults and children 6–17 years; orally disintegrating tablet may be useful if there is difficulty in swallowing
sumatriptan (*Imitrex*)	25, 50, or 100 mg PO at first sign of headache, may repeat in 2 h; by nasal spray in one nostril, may repeat in 2 h; do not exceed 40 mg/d; 1–6 mg subcutaneous one time dose	Treatment of acute migraines, cluster headaches in adults
zolmitriptan (*Zomig, Zomig-ZMT*)	1.25 or 2.5 mg PO; may repeat in 2 h; do not exceed 10 mg/d	Treatment of acute migraines in adults; orally disintegrating tablet may be useful if there is difficulty in swallowing
Calcitonin Gene–Related Peptide (CGRP) Inhibitors		
eptinezumab-jjmr (*Vyepti*)	100 mg IV over about 30 min every 3 months; max dose 300 mg IV	Prevention of migraines in adults
erenumab-aooe (*Aimovig*)	70 mg subcutaneous monthly; max dose 140 mg	Prevention of migraines in adults
fremanezumab-vfrm (*Ajovy*)	225 mg subcutaneous monthly or 675 mg subcutaneous every 3 months	Prevention of migraines in adults
galcanezumab-gnlm (*Emgality*)	240 mg loading dose and 120 mg subcutaneous monthly for migraines; 300 mg subcutaneous at onset of cluster	Prevention of migraines; treatment of episodic cluster headache
rimegepant (*Nurtec ODT*)	75 mg PO; may repeat in 24 h	Treatment of acute migraines in adults
ubrogepant (*Ubrelvy*)	50 or 100 mg PO at first sign of headache, may repeat in 2 h; do not exceed 200 mg/d	Treatment of acute migraines
Serotonin Agonist		
lasmiditan (*Reyvow*)	50–200 mg PO dosed PRN	Treatment of acute migraines in adults

Therapeutic Actions and Indications

The ergot derivatives block alpha-adrenergic and serotonin receptor sites in the brain to cause a constriction of cranial vessels, a decrease in cranial artery pulsation, and a decrease in the hyperperfusion of the basilar artery bed (see Fig. 26.2). These drugs are indicated for the prevention or abortion of migraine or vascular headaches. Ergotamine, the prototype drug in this class, was the mainstay of migraine headache treatment before the development of triptans (see Table 26.2 for usual indications for each drug). In 2003, dihydroergotamine in the parenteral form was also approved for the treatment of cluster headaches.

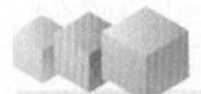 Concept Mastery Alert

Migraine Client Education

Vasodilation occurs during most migraine headaches; medications such as triptans work to constrict blood vessels.

Pharmacokinetics

The ergot derivatives are rapidly absorbed from many routes with an onset of action ranging from 15 to 30 minutes. They are metabolized in the liver and primarily excreted in the bile.

Dihydroergotamine is available as a nasal spray or for IM or IV administration. This agent is the drug of choice if the oral route of administration is not possible.

Ergotamine is administered sublingually for rapid absorption. *Cafergot*, the popular oral form, combines ergotamine with caffeine to increase its absorption from the GI tract.

Contraindications and Cautions

Ergot derivatives are contraindicated in the following circumstances: presence of allergy to ergot preparations to avoid hypersensitivity reactions; CAD, hypertension, or peripheral vascular disease, which could be exacerbated by the CV effects of these drugs; impaired liver function, which could alter the metabolism and excretion of these drugs; and pregnancy or lactation because of the potential for adverse effects on the fetus and neonate. Ergotism (vomiting, diarrhea, and seizures) has been reported in affected infants.

Caution should be used in two instances: with pruritus, which could become worse with drug-induced vascular constriction, and with malnutrition, because ergot derivatives stimulate the CTZ and can cause severe GI reactions, possibly worsening malnutrition.

Adverse Effects

The adverse effects of ergot derivatives can be related to the drug-induced vascular constriction. CNS effects include numbness, tingling of extremities, and muscle pain; CV effects such as pulselessness, weakness, chest pain, arrhythmias, localized edema and itching, and MI may also occur. In addition, the direct stimulation of the CTZ can cause GI upset, nausea, vomiting, and diarrhea. Ergotism, a syndrome associated with the use of these drugs, causes nausea, vomiting, severe thirst, hypoperfusion, chest pain, blood pressure changes, confusion, drug dependency (with prolonged use), and drug withdrawal syndrome.

Clinically Important Drug–Drug Interactions

If these drugs are combined with beta-blockers, the risk of peripheral ischemia and gangrene is increased. They should not be combined with the triptans due to risk of vasospasm. Such combinations should be avoided.

Prototype Summary: Ergotamine

Indications: Prevention or abortion of vascular headaches.

Actions: Constricts cranial blood vessels, decreases pulsation of cranial arteries, and decreases hyperperfusion of the basilar artery vascular bed.

Pharmacokinetics:

Route	Onset	Peak
Sublingual	Rapid	0.5–3 h

$T_{1/2}$: 2.7 hours and then 21 hours; metabolized in the liver; excreted in the feces.

Adverse Effects: Numbness, tingling in the fingers and toes, muscle pain in the extremities, pulselessness or weakness in the legs, precordial distress, tachycardia, bradycardia, ergotism (nausea, vomiting, diarrhea, severe thirst, hypoperfusion, chest pain, confusion).

Triptans

The **triptans** are a class of drugs that cause cranial vascular constriction and relief of migraine headache pain in many patients. These drugs are not associated with as many of the vascular and GI effects of the ergot derivatives. The triptan of choice for a particular patient depends on personal experience, kinetic factors, and preexisting medical conditions. A patient may have a poor response to one triptan and respond well to another (see Box 26.5).

Available triptans include almotriptan (generic), eletriptan (*Relpax*), frovatriptan (*Frova*), naratriptan (*Amerge*), rizatriptan (*Maxalt*, *Maxalt-MLT*), sumatriptan (*Imitrex*), and zolmitriptan (*Zomig*, *Zomig-ZMT*).

Therapeutic Actions and Indications

The triptans bind to selective serotonin receptor sites to cause vasoconstriction of cranial vessels, relieving the signs and symptoms of migraine headache (see Fig. 26.2). They are indicated for the treatment of acute migraine and are not used for prevention of migraines (see Table 26.2 for usual indications for each of the triptans).

Sumatriptan, the first drug of this class, is used for the treatment of acute migraine attacks and for the treatment of cluster headaches in adults. It can be given orally, subcutaneously, or by nasal spray.

Naratriptan, rizatriptan, zolmitriptan, and eletriptan are used orally only for the treatment of acute migraines. Rizatriptan and zolmitriptan are also available as fast-dissolving tablets.

CRITICAL THINKING SCENARIO
Relieving Migraine Pain

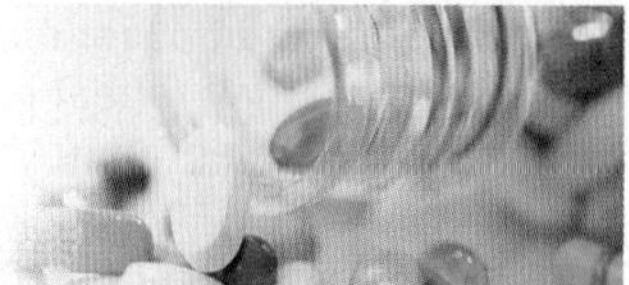

THE SITUATION

B.F., a 32-year-old financial planner, was experiencing severe headaches that they attributed to long hours at the computer and eye fatigue related to screen use. When standard NSAID therapy and rest periods did not seem to help, B.F. began keeping a log of what they experienced, how they felt, and what was going on in their environment. After watching a TV documentary, B.F. became concerned that they may have a brain tumor and made an appointment to see their health care provider. Their provider reviewed B.F.'s logs and did a complete physical exam, including a brief neurological exam. The provider came to the conclusion that B.F. was actually having migraine headaches. The pain was on one side of the head; they were often nauseous, had visual disturbances, and on several occasions had to stay in bed and call in sick to work because they could not function. The headaches occurred about every 3 weeks and did not seem to be related to their menstrual cycle. B.F. requested a CAT (computed tomography) scan to make sure they did not have a brain tumor. It was explained that their physical findings were otherwise normal, and B.F. agreed to try zolmitriptan the next time they felt a headache coming on to see what happened.

CRITICAL THINKING

What basic principles must be included in the nursing care plan for this patient? Think about the patient's fears, the impact of the media on health care decisions, and the impact of the loss of work and function on a young adult.

What other nursing measures could be used to help relieve pain and ease the patient's anxiety? What measures can be used to relax the patient and relieve their anxiety?

What teaching points need to be covered to help facilitate a safe and therapeutic response to the drug therapy prescribed? Think about timing of doses, adverse effects that could occur, and other nondrug measures to help alleviate pain and discomfort.

DISCUSSION

The patient suffered from headaches for quite some time before seeking medical assistance. This may reflect a lack of confidence in the health care system or a fear of what was really going on in their head. The impact of the TV documentary was impressive and caused a great deal of concern and anxiety for the patient. These responses are known to activate the sympathetic nervous system, which could further add to discomfort and headache pain. The nurse working with this patient needs to listen to their fears, try to explain what the patient saw on TV, and work to provide support and assurance and develop trust with the patient.

Although the physical exam was negative, it is still important to discuss with the patient what that means. B.F. should be praised for keeping a detailed log surrounding their headaches and encouraged to continue to log them when they occur. It will be important to explain what a migraine headache is, what happens in the brain, and the reasons for the various responses that they experienced. B.F. will need thorough teaching about the timing of zolmitriptan administration, the use of the disintegrating tablet, as well as the adverse effects that they might experience. Numbness and tingling may cause added concerns, so warning them that this may occur is important. Environmental controls should also be discussed, as controlling them can make the drug therapy more effective, and the patient will be more comfortable, leading to decreased anxiety, which will further help relieve the situation.

NURSING CARE GUIDE FOR B.F.: TRIPTANS

Assessment: History and Examination

Assess history of allergies to zolmitriptan, active CAD or angina, pregnancy, or breast or chestfeeding.

Focus the physical examination on the following:

CV: Blood pressure, pulse rate, peripheral perfusion, and reflexes

CNS: Orientation, affect

Skin: Color, lesions, texture, temperature

Laboratory tests: Renal tests

Nursing Conclusions

Altered sensory perceptions (visual, auditory, kinesthetic) related to CNS effects

Knowledge deficit regarding drug therapy

Anxiety related to diagnosis, drug regimen

(continues on page 466)

Planning

The patient will receive the best therapeutic effect from the drug therapy.
The patient will have limited adverse effects to the drug therapy.
The patient will have an understanding of the drug therapy, adverse effects to anticipate, and measures to relieve discomfort and improve safety.

Intervention

Administer drug at onset of headache, not for prevention; may repeat in 2 hours if pain persists.
Place orally disintegrating tablet on tongue, let it dissolve, and then have patient swallow.
Monitor blood pressure if any risk of CAD or angina.
Provide comfort and safety measures: monitor lighting, sound, room temperature, and positioning.
Provide safety measures if dizziness, vertigo, or visual changes occur.
Provide patient teaching about the drug, dosage, drug effects, and symptoms of serious reactions to report.

Evaluation

Evaluate drug effects: relief of pain.
Monitor for adverse effects: CNS effects, numbness or tingling, blood pressure changes.
Monitor drug–drug interactions: risk of MAOI toxicity with MAOIs, increased vasoactive reactions with ergots, cimetidine, hormonal contraceptives; serotonin syndrome with sibutramine; prolonged QT interval with other QT-prolonging drugs.
Evaluate the effectiveness of the patient teaching program.
Evaluate the effectiveness of comfort and safety measures.

PATIENT TEACHING FOR B.F.

- The drug prescribed for your migraine headaches is called a triptan. This drug works to constrict the blood vessels in your brain to prevent the vasodilation that occurs and causes migraines.
- Take this drug exactly as prescribed, at the onset of your headache. Place the disintegrating tablet on your tongue and let it dissolve and then swallow. You should lower the lights, turn off noise, regulate the room temperature, and try to relax while the drug works. If the headache persists after 2 hours, you can take another tablet. Do not take more than two per day. If the headache still persists, call your health care provider.
- Common effects of these drugs include the following:
  - Dizziness, drowsiness, and visual changes: If any of these occur, avoid driving, operating complex machinery, or performing delicate tasks.
  - Numbness, tingling, feelings of pressure or heaviness: The drug causes blood vessels to constrict so you may feel like your arms or legs have "gone to sleep"; this will pass when the drug wears off.
- Report any of the following to your health care provider: feelings of heat, flushing, nausea, chest pain or pressure, swelling of the lips or eyelids.
- Tell any doctor, nurse, dentist, or other health care provider involved in your care that you are taking this drug.
- Keep this drug and all medications out of the reach of children.
- Do not use this drug if you think you are pregnant or want to become pregnant; consult with your health care provider.

Pharmacokinetics

The triptans are rapidly absorbed from many sites; they are metabolized in the liver (sumatriptan by monoamine oxidase) and are primarily excreted in the urine. They cross the placenta and have been shown to be toxic to the fetus in animal studies. They also enter human milk. In most, the safety and efficacy of use in children have not been established, but almotriptan can be prescribed to adolescents and rizatriptan can be prescribed to children 6 and older.

Contraindications and Cautions

Triptans are contraindicated with any of the following conditions: allergy to any triptan to avoid hypersensitivity reactions; pregnancy because of the possibility of severe adverse effects on the fetus; and active CAD, which could be exacerbated by the vessel-constricting effects of these drugs. These drugs should be used with caution in older adult patients because of the possibility of underlying vascular disease; in patients with risk factors for CAD; in patients who are lactating because of the possibility of adverse effects on the infant; and in patients with renal or hepatic dysfunction, which could alter the metabolism and excretion of the drug. Rizatriptan seems to have more angina-related effects, and it is not recommended for patients with a history of CAD, which could be exacerbated by its cardiac effects.

Adverse Effects

The adverse effects associated with the triptans are related to the vasoconstrictive effects of the drugs. CNS effects may include numbness, tingling, burning sensation, feelings of coldness or strangeness, dizziness, weakness, myalgia, and vertigo. GI effects such as dysphagia and abdominal discomfort may occur. CV effects can be severe and include blood pressure alterations and tightness or pressure in the chest. Almotriptan is reported to have fewer side effects than the other triptans, and it is also thought that the longer half-life of this drug will prevent the rebound headaches that may be seen with other triptans.

Clinically Important Drug–Drug Interactions

Combining triptans with ergot-containing drugs results in a risk of prolonged vasoactive reactions.

There is a risk of severe adverse effects if these drugs are used within 2 weeks after discontinuation of an MAOI. If triptans are to be given, it is imperative that the patient has not received an MAOI in more than 2 weeks.

There is risk of serotonin syndrome if combined with selective SSRIs and other serotonergic medications.

Prototype Summary: Sumatriptan

Indications: Treatment of acute migraine; treatment of cluster headaches (subcutaneous route).

Actions: Binds to serotonin receptors to cause vasoconstrictive effects on cranial blood vessels.

Pharmacokinetics:

Route	Onset	Peak	Duration
Nasal spray	Varies, rapid	5–20 min	Unknown
Oral	30–60 min	2–4 h	Up to 24 h
Subcutaneous	Rapid	1–5 h	Up to 24 h

$T_{1/2}$: 115 minutes; metabolized in the liver; excreted in the urine.

Adverse Effects: Dizziness, vertigo, weakness, myalgia, blood pressure alterations, tightness or pressure in the chest, injection site discomfort, tingling, burning sensations.

Calcitonin Gene–Related Peptide (CGRP) Inhibitors and Serotonin Agonist

The CGRP inhibitors are a class of drugs that help to block CGRP receptors or target the peptide directly. They are indicated for the prevention and/or treatment of headaches.

Available CGRP inhibitors are eptinezumab-jjmr (*Vyepti*), erenumab-aooe (*Aimovig*), fremanezumab-vfrm (*Ajovy*), galcanezumab-gnlm (*Emgality*), rimegepant (*Nurtec ODT*), and ubrogepant (*Ubrelvy*). Lasmiditan (*Reyvow*) is a serotonin agonist that is more selective than the triptans so it is less likely to cause vasoconstriction adverse side effects. See Table 26.2 for indications and dosing.

Therapeutic Actions and Indications

The CGRP is a potent vasodilator chemical released during migraine headache attacks. There are two main types of CGRP inhibitors. The first is a small molecule called "gepants" that block the CGRP receptor. Rimegepant and ubrogepant are medications of this type and are indicated for treatment of acute migraine headache. The second type of CGRP inhibitor includes the monoclonal antibodies that can target either the receptor or the CGRP directly. They are indicated for the prevention of migraine headaches; galcanezumab has the added indication for treatment of cluster headaches.

Lasmiditan is a very selective serotonin agonist that is indicated for treatment of acute migraine with or without aura in adults. Due to its more selective action on a specific serotonin receptor, it has less of the vasoconstriction actions compared to the triptans that target more of the serotonin receptors.

Pharmacokinetics

The gepants CGRP inhibitors and lasmiditan are administered orally or sublingually and absorbed via the GI tract. The monoclonal antibodies that are CGRP inhibitors are injected subcutaneously or intravenously.

Lasmiditan is absorbed quickly (about 2 hours), metabolized in and outside the liver, eliminated renally, and the half-life is about 6 hours. The gepant CGRP inhibitors reach maximum concentrations in about 1.5 hours; portions are metabolized and then mostly eliminated through bile and feces, with some through urine. The monoclonal antibody CGRP inhibitors have long half-lives (27 to 31 days) so they do not have be administered frequently.

There are no human data of the effects on pregnancy outcomes for any of these medications. Animal studies have shown potential of fetal harm with lasmiditan and the gepant CGRP inhibitors, but not with the monoclonal antibody CGRP inhibitors.

Contraindications and Cautions

These medications are contraindicated with signs of allergy to the medication to avoid hypersensitivity reactions and should be used cautiously during pregnancy because of lack of data on fetal outcomes in humans.

Adverse Effects

The adverse effects associated with lasmiditan include dizziness, fatigue, paresthesia, and sedation. It is a Scheduled V medication.

The CGRP inhibitors have risk of causing hypersensitivity reactions. The gepant substances may also cause nausea. The monoclonal antibodies have risk of injection site reactions.

Clinically Important Drug–Drug Interactions

Lasmiditan should be used with caution with CNS depressants, heart rate lowering medications, and other serotonergic medications, due to risk of increased adverse effects.

Lasmiditan and the gepant CGRP inhibitors may inhibit Pgp or BCRP, so these substrates should be avoided. The gepant CGRP inhibitors have interactions with CYP3A4 inducers and inhibitors as well.

Prototype Summary: Galcanezumab

Indications: Preventative treatment of migraines; treatment of episodic cluster headache.

Actions: Binds to the CGRP ligand and prevents it from attaching to the receptor.

Pharmacokinetics:

Route	Onset	Peak	Duration
Subcutaneous	Unknown	5 days	Long acting

$T_{1/2}$: 27 days; metabolized in the liver; excreted in the urine.

Adverse Effects: Hypersensitivity and injection site reactions.

Nursing Considerations for Patients Receiving Antimigraine Agents

Assessment: History and Examination

- Assess for contraindications or cautions: known allergies to any component of the drugs to avoid hypersensitivity reactions; history of MI, CAD, or hypertension, which may be exacerbated by the drug (ergots or triptans); hepatic or renal dysfunction, which could alter the metabolism and excretion of the drug; pruritus or malnutrition, which could be exacerbated by ergot derivatives; and current status of pregnancy and lactation, which would be cautions to the use of these drugs.
- Perform a physical assessment to establish baseline status before beginning therapy, determine drug effectiveness, and evaluate for any potential adverse effects.
- Assess the patient's neurological status, including level of orientation, affect, and reflexes to evaluate CNS effects of the drugs.
- Monitor for complaints of extremity numbness and tingling to identify effects on vascular constriction.
- Inspect the skin for localized edema, itching, or breakdown with ergot derivatives to evaluate potential dermatological effects.
- Assess vital signs, including pulse rate and blood pressure; obtain an electrocardiogram as appropriate to evaluate cardiac status for changes.
- Monitor the results of laboratory tests, including liver and renal function tests, to determine the need for dose adjustment and identify possible toxic effects.

Nursing Conclusions

Nursing conclusions related to drug therapy might include the following:

- Impaired comfort related to CV and vasoconstrictive effects
- Altered cardiac output related to CV effects
- Altered sensory perception (visual, auditory, kinesthetic, and tactile) related to CNS effects
- Injury risk related to changes in peripheral sensation, CNS effects
- Knowledge deficit regarding drug therapy

Planning

- The patient will receive the best therapeutic effect from the drug therapy.
- The patient will have limited adverse effects to the drug therapy.
- The patient will have an understanding of the drug therapy, adverse effects to anticipate, and measures to relieve discomfort and improve safety.

Intervention With Rationale

- Administer the drug to prevent or relieve acute migraines based on their specific indication.
- For abortion of headache, administer at the first sign of a headache and do not wait until it is severe, to improve therapeutic effectiveness.
- Arrange for safety precautions if CNS or visual changes occur to prevent patient injury.
- Provide comfort and safety measures such as environmental controls and stress reduction for the relief of headache. Provide additional pain relief as needed.
- Monitor the blood pressure of any patient with a history of CAD, and discontinue the drug if any sign of angina or prolonged hypertension occurs to prevent severe vascular effects.
- Offer support and encouragement to help the patient cope with the disorder and associated drug regimen.
- Provide thorough patient teaching, including drug name, prescribed dose, and schedule for administration; measures to avoid adverse effects; warning signs that may indicate possible problems; signs of ergotism if taking ergot derivatives; safety measures such as avoiding driving and avoiding overdose; and importance of follow-up monitoring and evaluation to enhance patient knowledge about drug therapy and to promote compliance.

Evaluation

- Monitor patient response to the drug (relief of acute or prevention of migraine headaches).
- Monitor for adverse effects (CV changes, arrhythmias, hypertension, CNS changes).
- Evaluate the effectiveness of the teaching plan (patient can give the drug name and dosage and describe possible adverse effects to watch for, specific measures to prevent them, and warning signs to report).
- Monitor the effectiveness of comfort measures and compliance with the regimen.

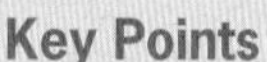

Key Points

- Migraine headaches are severe, throbbing headaches on one side of the head that may be associated with an aura or warning syndrome. These headaches are thought to be caused by activation of the trigeminovascular system causing release of chemicals that can trigger vasodilation and pain.
- Treatment of acute migraines may involve ergot derivatives, triptans, lasmiditan, or CGRP receptor antagonists.
- There are monoclonal antibody CGRP receptor antagonists that are indicated for prevention of migraine headaches.

SUMMARY

- Pain can occur any time tissue is injured and various chemicals are released. The pain impulses are carried to the spinal cord by small and medium-diameter A-delta and C fibers, which form synapses with interneurons in the dorsal horn of the spinal cord.
- Opioid receptors found throughout various tissues in the body react with endogenous endorphins and enkephalins to modulate the transmission of pain impulses.
- The effectiveness and adverse effects associated with specific opioids are associated with their particular affinity for various types of opioid receptors.
- Opioid agonists react with opioid receptors to relieve pain. In addition, they can cause constipation, respiratory depression, sedation, and suppression of the cough reflex; they also stimulate feelings of well-being or euphoria.
- Because opioid agonists and agonist–antagonists are associated with the development of physical dependency, they are controlled substances.
- Opioid agonists–antagonists react with some opioid receptor sites to stimulate activity and block other opioid receptor sites. These drugs have less of a risk of causing physical dependency compared to opioid agonists.
- Opioid antagonists, which work to reverse the effects of opioids, are used to treat opioid overdose or to reverse unacceptable adverse effects.
- Migraine headaches are severe, throbbing headaches on one side of the head that may be associated with an aura or warning syndrome.
- Acute treatment of migraines may involve either ergot derivatives or triptans.
- The CGRP inhibitors can be used for both prevention and treatment of migraine headaches.

Unfolding Patient Stories: Yoa Li • Part 1

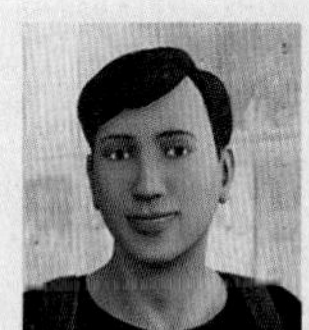

Yoa Li is a 26-year-old male admitted to the hospital for surgical repair of a strangulated groin hernia. He is experiencing symptoms of allergic rhinitis. Recognizing he is NPO pending surgery, what are medication options to relieve nasal congestion and drainage that the nurse can recommend when informing the provider of his symptoms? (Yoa Li's story continues in Chapter 54.)

Care for Yoa and other patients in a realistic virtual environment: ***vSim** for Nursing* (thepoint.lww.com/vSimPharm). Practice documenting these patients' care in DocuCare (thepoint.lww.com/DocuCareEHR).

CHECK YOUR UNDERSTANDING

Answers to the questions in this chapter can be found in Answers to Check Your Understanding Questions on thePoint®.

MULTIPLE CHOICE

Select the best answer.

1. Which of the following is correct about pain according to the gate control theory?
   a. It is caused by gates in the CNS.
   b. It can be blocked or intensified by gates in the CNS.
   c. It is caused by gates in peripheral nerve sensors.
   d. It cannot be affected by learned experiences.

2. Opioid receptors are found throughout the body
   a. only in people who have become addicted to opiates.
   b. in increasing numbers with chronic pain conditions.
   c. to incorporate pain perception and blocking.
   d. to initiate the release of endorphins.

3. Opioid agonists are controlled substances because they
   a. are very expensive.
   b. can cause respiratory depression.
   c. can cause physical dependency and addiction.
   d. can be used only in a hospital setting.

4. Injecting an opioid into an area of the body that is chilled can be dangerous because
   a. an abscess will form.
   b. the injection will be very painful.
   c. an excessive amount may be absorbed all at once.
   d. narcotics are inactivated in cold temperatures.

5. Proper administration of an ordered opioid
   a. will frequently lead to addiction.
   b. should be done promptly to prevent increased pain and the need for larger doses.
   c. would include holding the drug as long as possible until the patient really needs it.
   d. should rely on the patient's request for medication.

6. Migraine headaches
   a. occur during sleep and involve sweating and eye pain.
   b. occur with stress and feel like a dull band around the entire head.
   c. often occur when drinking coffee.
   d. are throbbing headaches on one side of the head.

7. The triptans are a class of drugs that bind to serotonin receptor sites and cause
   a. cranial vascular dilation.
   b. cranial vascular constriction.
   c. clinical depression.
   d. nausea and vomiting.

8. The only triptan that has been approved for use in treating cluster headaches as well as migraines is
   a. naratriptan.
   b. rizatriptan.
   c. sumatriptan.
   d. zolmitriptan.

MULTIPLE RESPONSE

Select all that apply.

1. Opioid agonists are drugs that react with opioid receptors throughout the body. Which conditions would the nurse expect to find when assessing a patient who was taking an opioid agonist?
   a. Hypnosis
   b. Sedation
   c. Analgesia
   d. Euphoria
   e. Orthostatic hypotension
   f. Increased salivation

2. The nurse would expect to administer an opioid agonist as the analgesic of choice for which patients?
   a. A patient with severe postoperative pain
   b. A patient with severe chronic obstructive pulmonary disease and difficulty in breathing
   c. A patient with severe, chronic pain
   d. A patient with ulcerative colitis
   e. A patient with recent biliary surgery
   f. A patient with cancer and severe bone pain

REFERENCES

Arcangelo, V. P., Peterson, A. M., Wilbur, V., & Kang, T. M. (2022). *Pharmacotherapeutics for advanced practice. A practical approach* (5th ed.). Wolters Kluwer.

Beaulieu, P., Lussier, D., Porreca, F., & Dickenson, A. H. (2010). *Pharmacology of pain.* IASP Press.

Brunton, L. L., Hilal-Dandan, R., & Knollman, B. C. (2018). *Goodman and Gilman's the pharmacological basis of therapeutics* (13th ed.). McGraw-Hill.

deVries, T., Villalón, C. M., & MaassenVanDenBrink, A. (2020). Pharmacological treatment of migraine: CGRP and 5-HT beyond the triptans. *Pharmacology and Therapeutics, 211*, 107528. https://doi.org/10.1016/j.pharmthera.2020.107528

Hall, J. E., & Hall, M. E. (2021). *Guyton and Hall textbook of medical physiology* (14th ed.). Elsevier.

Hendler, C. B. (Ed.) (2021). *Nursing 2021 drug handbook.* Wolters Kluwer.

Lipton, R. B., Bigal, M. E., Steiner, T. J., & Olesen, J. (2004). Classification of primary headaches. *Neurology, 63*(3), 427–435. https://doi.org/10.1212/01.wnl.0000133301.66364.9b

Miaskowski, C. (2005). Patient-controlled modalities for acute postoperative pain management. *Journal of Perianesthesia Nursing, 20*(4), 255–267. https://doi.org/10.1016/j.jopan.2005.05.005

Norris, T. L. (2019). *Porth's pathophysiology: Concepts of altered health states* (13th ed.). Wolters Kluwer.

Obeng, A. O., Hamadeh, I., & Smith, M. (2017). Review of opioid pharmacogenetics and considerations for pain management. *Pharmacotherapy, 37*(9), 1105–1121. https://doi.org/10.1002/phar.1986

Rivera-Mancilla, E., Villalón, C. M., & MaassenVanDenBrink, A. (2020). CGRP inhibitors for migraine prophylaxis: A safety review. *Expert Opinion on Drug Safety, 19*(10), 1237–1250. https://doi.org/10.1080/14740338.2020.1811229

Stannard, C., Kalso, E., & Ballantyne, J. (Eds.) (2010). *Evidence-based chronic pain management.* Wiley-Blackwell.

Vadivelu, N., Urman, R. D., & Hines, R. L. (Eds.) (2011). *Essentials of pain management.* Springer.

CHAPTER 27

General and Local Anesthetic Agents

Learning Objectives

Upon completion of this chapter, you will be able to:

1. Describe the concept of balanced anesthesia.
2. Describe the actions and uses of local anesthesia.
3. Describe the therapeutic actions, indications, pharmacokinetics, contraindications, most common adverse reactions, and important drug–drug interactions associated with general and local anesthetics.
4. Outline the preoperative and postoperative needs of a patient receiving general or local anesthesia.
5. Compare and contrast the prototype drugs methohexital, midazolam, nitrous oxide, desflurane, and lidocaine with other drugs in their respective classes.
6. Outline the nursing considerations, including important teaching points, for patients receiving general and local anesthetics.

Key Terms

amnesia: loss of memory of an event or procedure

analgesia: loss of pain sensation

anesthetic: drug used to cause complete or partial loss of sensation

balanced anesthesia: use of several different types of drugs to achieve the quickest, most effective anesthesia with the fewest adverse effects

general anesthesia: use of drugs to induce a loss of consciousness, amnesia, analgesia, and loss of reflexes to allow performance of painful surgical procedures

induction: time from the beginning of anesthesia until achievement of surgical anesthesia

local anesthesia: loss of sensation in limited areas of the body

maintenance: the period from stage 3 until the surgical procedure is complete

plasma esterase: enzyme found in plasma that immediately breaks down ester-type local anesthetics

recovery: the period from discontinuation of the anesthetic until the patient has regained consciousness, movement, and the ability to communicate

unconsciousness: loss of awareness of one's surroundings

volatile liquid: liquid that is unstable at room temperature and releases gases; used as an inhaled general anesthetic, usually in the form of a halogenated hydrocarbon

Drug List

GENERAL ANESTHETIC AGENTS

Barbiturate Anesthetics
- (P) methohexital

Nonbarbiturate General Anesthetics
- etomidate
- ketamine
- (P) midazolam
- propofol

Anesthetic Gases
- (P) nitrous oxide

Volatile Liquids
- (P) desflurane
- isoflurane
- sevoflurane

LOCAL ANESTHETIC AGENTS

Esters
- benzocaine
- chloroprocaine
- cocaine
- tetracaine

Amides
- bupivacaine
- dibucaine
- (P) lidocaine
- mepivacaine
- prilocaine
- ropivacaine

Others
- pramoxine

Anesthetics are drugs that are used to cause complete or partial loss of sensation. The anesthetics can be subdivided into general and local anesthetics, depending on their site of action. General anesthetics are central nervous system (CNS) depressants used to produce loss of pain sensation and consciousness. Local anesthetics are drugs used to cause loss of pain sensation and feeling in a designated area of the body without the systemic effects associated with severe CNS depression. This chapter discusses various general and local anesthetics. Box 27.1 highlights information about using anesthetics with various age groups.

General Anesthesia

General anesthesia involves the administration of a combination of several different general anesthetic agents to achieve the following goals: **analgesia**, or loss of pain sensation; **unconsciousness**, or loss of awareness of one's surroundings; and **amnesia**, or the loss of memory of an event or procedure. Ideally, the drugs are combined to achieve the best effects with the fewest adverse effects. General anesthesia also blocks the body's reflexes. Blockage of autonomic reflexes prevents involuntary reflex response to bodily injury that might compromise a patient's cardiac, respiratory, gastrointestinal (GI), and immune status. Blockage of muscle reflexes prevents jerking movements that might interfere with the success of the surgical procedure.

Risk Factors Associated With General Anesthesia

Widespread CNS depression, which is not without risks, occurs with general anesthesia. In addition, all other body systems are affected. Because of the wide systemic effects, patients must be evaluated for factors that may increase their risk. These factors include the following:

- CNS factors: Underlying neurological disease (e.g., epilepsy, stroke, myasthenia gravis) that presents a risk for abnormal reaction to the CNS-depressing and muscle-relaxing effects of these drugs.
- Cardiovascular (CV) factors: Underlying vascular disease, coronary artery disease, or hypotension, which put patients at risk for severe reactions to anesthesia, such as hypotension and shock, dysrhythmias, and ischemia.
- Respiratory factors: Obstructive pulmonary disease (e.g., asthma, chronic obstructive pulmonary disease, bronchitis), which can complicate the delivery of gas anesthetics, as well as the intubation and mechanical ventilation that must be used in most applications of general anesthesia.

Box 27.1 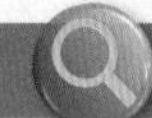 **Focus on Drug Therapy Across the Lifespan**

ANESTHETIC AGENTS

Children

Children are at greater risk for complications after anesthesia, including laryngospasm, bronchospasm, aspiration, and even death. They require careful monitoring and support, and the anesthetist needs to be skilled at calculating dosage and balance during the procedure. Propofol is widely used for diagnostic tests and short procedures in children older than 3 years of age because of its rapid onset and metabolism and generally smooth recovery. Sevoflurane has a minimal impact on intracranial pressure and allows rapid induction and recovery with minimal sympathetic reaction. It is still quite expensive, however, which may limit its use.

Nursing care until full recovery after general anesthesia should include support and reassurance, assessment of the child for any skin breakdown related to immobility, and safety precautions.

The very young have higher risk of developing methemoglobinemia associated with some local anesthetic use. The FDA wrote a warning against using formulations of benzocaine for teething pain on children 2 and younger.

Bupivacaine and tetracaine do not have established doses for children younger than 12 years of age.

Tight diapers can act like occlusive dressings and increase systemic absorption. Children need to be cautioned not to bite themselves when receiving dental anesthesia.

Adults

Adults require a considerable amount of teaching and support when receiving anesthetics, including what will happen, what they will feel, how it will feel when they recover, and the approximate time to recovery.

Adults should be monitored closely until fully recovered from general anesthetics and should be cautioned to prevent injury when receiving local anesthetics. It is important to remember to reassure and talk to adults who may be aware of their surroundings yet unable to speak.

Most of the general anesthetics are not recommended for use during pregnancy because of the potential risk to the fetus. Short-onset and local anesthetics are frequently used at delivery. Use of a regional or other local anesthetic is usually preferred if surgery is needed during pregnancy. During lactation, it is recommended that the patient wait 4 to 6 hours to feed the baby after the anesthetic is used.

Older Adults

Older patients are more likely to experience the adverse effects associated with these drugs, including CNS, CV, and dermatological effects. Thinner skin and the possibility of decreased perfusion to the skin make them especially susceptible to skin breakdown during immobility. Because older patients often also have renal or hepatic impairment, they are also more likely to have toxic levels of drugs related to changes in metabolism and excretion. The older patient should have in effect safety measures, such as side rails, a call light, and assistance to ambulate; special efforts to provide skin care to prevent skin breakdown are especially important with older skin. The older patient may require longer monitoring and regular orienting and reassuring. After general anesthesia, it is important to promote vigorous pulmonary hygiene to decrease the risk of pneumonia.

- Renal and hepatic function: Conditions that interfere with the metabolism and excretion of anesthetics (e.g., acute renal failure, hepatitis) and could result in prolonged anesthesia and the need for continued support during recovery. Toxic reactions to the accumulation of abnormally high levels of anesthetic agents may even occur.

Balanced Anesthesia

With the wide variety of drugs available, the therapeutic effects required need to be balanced with the potential for adverse effects. This is accomplished by **balanced anesthesia**. Rather than using one drug, balanced anesthesia combines several drugs, each with a specific effect, to achieve analgesia, muscle relaxation, unconsciousness, and amnesia quickly and effectively with the fewest adverse effects. Balanced anesthesia commonly involves the following agents:

- *Preoperative medications*, which may include the use of anticholinergics that decrease secretions to facilitate intubation and prevent bradycardia associated with neural depression
- *Sedative–hypnotics* to relax the patient, facilitate amnesia, and decrease sympathetic stimulation
- *Antiemetics* to decrease the nausea and vomiting associated with the slowing of GI activity
- *Antihistamines* to decrease the chance of allergic reaction and help to dry secretions
- *Opioids* to aid analgesia and sedation (see Chapter 26)

Many of these drugs are given before the general anesthetic is administered to facilitate the process. Some are continued during surgery to aid the general anesthetic, allowing therapeutic effects at lower doses. For example, a patient may receive a neuromuscular junction (NMJ) blocker (see Chapter 28) to stop muscle activity and a rapid-acting intravenous (IV) general anesthetic to induce anesthesia, and then a gas general anesthetic to balance the anesthetic effect during the procedure and allow for easier recovery. Careful selection of appropriate general anesthetic agents, along with monitoring and support of the patient, helps alleviate many of the potential risks of anesthesia.

Administration of General Anesthesia

General anesthesia is delivered by a physician or nurse anesthetist trained in the delivery of these potent drugs along with intubation, mechanical ventilation, and full life support. During the delivery of anesthesia, the patient can go through predictable stages (Fig. 27.1), referred to as the depth of anesthesia:

Stage 1, the analgesia stage, refers to the loss of pain sensation with the patient still conscious and able to communicate.

Stage 2, the excitement stage, is a period of excitement and often combative behavior with many signs of sympathetic stimulation (e.g., tachycardia, increased respirations, blood pressure changes).

Stage 3, surgical anesthesia, involves relaxation of skeletal muscles, return of regular respirations, and progressive loss of eye reflexes and pupil dilation. Surgery can be safely performed in stage 3.

Stage 4, medullary paralysis, is very deep CNS depression with loss of respiratory and vasomotor center stimuli in which death can occur rapidly. If a patient reaches this level, the anesthesia has become too intense, and the situation is critical.

General anesthesia administration is also divided into three phases: induction, maintenance, and recovery.

Induction

Induction is the period from the beginning of anesthesia until stage 3, or surgical anesthesia, is reached. The danger period for many patients during induction is stage 2 because of the systemic stimulation that occurs. Often, a rapid-acting anesthetic is used to move quickly through this phase and into stage 3. NMJ blockers may be used during induction to facilitate intubation, which is necessary to support the patient with mechanical ventilation during anesthesia (see Chapter 28).

Maintenance

Maintenance is the period from stage 3 until the surgical procedure is complete. A more predictable anesthetic,

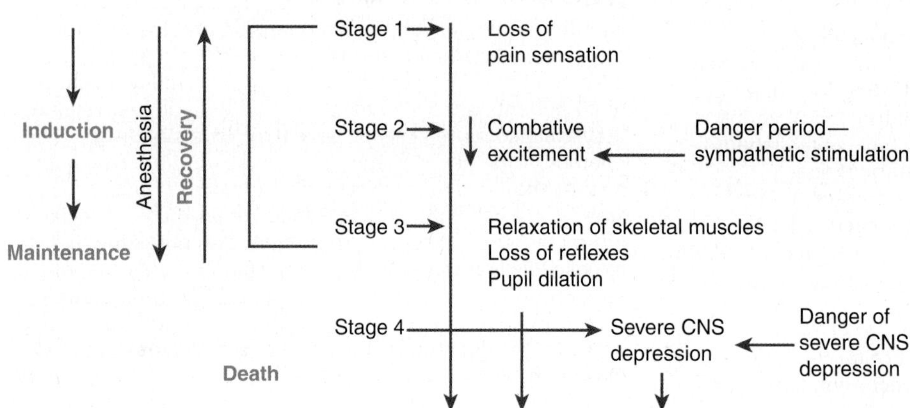

FIGURE 27.1 Stages of general anesthesia.

such as a gas anesthetic, may be used to maintain the anesthesia once the patient is in stage 3.

Recovery

Recovery is the period from discontinuation of the anesthetic until the patient has regained consciousness, movement, and the ability to communicate. During recovery, the patient requires continuous monitoring for any adverse effects of the drugs used while ensuring support of the patient's vital functions as necessary.

Key Points

- General anesthesia produces analgesia, amnesia, and unconsciousness.
- General anesthesia places the patient at risk for problems because of its extensive CNS depression and widespread effects on other body systems.
- Balanced anesthesia involves the administration of several drugs rather than a single drug to achieve analgesia, muscle relaxation, unconsciousness, and amnesia.
- Induction of anesthesia is the period ranging from administration of the anesthetic to the point of surgical anesthesia.

General Anesthetic Agents

Several different types of drugs are used as general anesthetics. These include barbiturate and nonbarbiturate anesthetics, gas anesthetics, and volatile liquids. See Table 27.1 for a listing of general anesthetic agents.

Barbiturate Anesthetics

Barbiturate anesthetics (see Table 27.1) are IV drugs used to induce rapid anesthesia; they are then maintained with an inhaled drug. Methohexital (*Brevital*) is a barbiturate that is used primarily as an anesthetic. Other barbiturates that can be used for sedative purposes are discussed in more detail in Chapter 20.

Table 27.1 *Drugs in Focus*: General Anesthetic Agents

Drug Name	Onset	Recovery
methohexital (*Brevital*)	10–30 s	3–4 min
etomidate (*Amidate*)	1 min	3–5 min
ketamine (*Ketalar*)	30 s	45 min
midazolam (generic)	15 min	30 min
propofol (*Diprivan*)	30–60 s	25–100 min
nitrous oxide (*Blue*)	1–2 min	Rapid
desflurane (*Suprane*)	1–2 min	15–20 min
isoflurane (*Forane*)	1–2 min	15–20 min
sevoflurane (*Sojourn, Ultane*)	30 s	10 min

Therapeutic Actions and Indications

Methohexital is an ultrashort-acting barbiturate anesthetic. It is indicated to be used as an adjunct medication with other agents for general anesthesia, an agent to induce a hypnotic state, or as solitary anesthesia agent for procedures that have minimal pain stimuli. The medication lacks analgesic properties, and the patient may require postoperative analgesics.

Pharmacokinetics

Methohexital has a rapid onset of action and a recovery period that is usually 3 to 4 minutes. This drug is lipophilic. It is dissolved and rapidly absorbed through the lipid blood–brain barrier and diffuses into the brain rapidly.

Contraindications and Cautions

Methohexital should only be used in a clinical setting that can provide continuous monitoring of respiratory and cardiac function. The setting should have resuscitative drugs and equipment for ventilation including intubation because of the rapid onset and because these drugs can cause respiratory depression and apnea. The medication is contraindicated in patients who cannot undergo general anesthesia, have known hypersensitivity to barbiturates, or who have latent or manifest porphyria. This drug should not be used during pregnancy or lactation unless the benefit clearly outweighs the potential risk to the fetus or neonate because of the CNS-depressive effects of these drugs. This medication should only be used in rectal or IM forms in pediatric patients and should not be used in children less than 1 month old. IV administration is approved for adults only.

Adverse Effects

The adverse effects associated with these drugs are related to the suppression of the CNS with decreased pulse, hypotension, suppressed respirations, and decreased GI activity. Nausea and vomiting after recovery are common.

Clinically Important Drug–Drug Interactions

Caution must be used when these drugs are used with any other CNS suppressants. Barbiturates can cause decreased effectiveness of theophylline, oral anticoagulants, beta-blockers, corticosteroids, hormonal contraceptives, phenylbutazones, metronidazole, quinidine, and carbamazepine. Combinations of barbiturate anesthetics with opioids or alcohol may produce apnea more commonly than occurs with other analgesics.

Prototype Summary: Methohexital

Indications: Induction of anesthesia, maintenance of anesthesia; induction of a hypnotic state.

Actions: Depresses the CNS to produce hypnosis and anesthesia without analgesia.

Pharmacokinetics:

Route	Onset	Duration
IV	30 s	3–4 min
IM	2–10 min	20–30 min
Rectal	5–15 min	20–30 min

$T_{1/2}$: 3 to 8 hours; metabolized in the liver; excreted in the urine.

Adverse Effects: Emergence delirium, headache, restlessness, anxiety, CV depression, respiratory depression, apnea, salivation, hiccups, skin rashes.

Nonbarbiturate Anesthetics

The other parenteral drugs used for IV administration in anesthesia are nonbarbiturates with a wide variety of effects. Such anesthetics include etomidate (*Amidate*), ketamine (*Ketalar*), midazolam (well known as *Versed*, but IV is only available in a generic form as that brand name has been retired; *Seizalam*—IM; *Nayzilam*—nasal spray), and propofol (*Diprivan*) (see Table 27.1).

Therapeutic Action and Indications

Midazolam is the prototype nonbarbiturate anesthetic. It is a potent amnesiac and in the benzodiazepine classification (see Chapter 20). These drugs are thought to act in the reticular activating system and limbic system to potentiate the effects of gamma-aminobutyric acid. Midazolam's amnesiac effects occur at doses below those needed to cause sedation. It is widely used to produce amnesia or sedation for many diagnostic, therapeutic, and endoscopic procedures. Midazolam can also be used to induce anesthesia and to provide continuous sedation for intubated and mechanically ventilated patients. Etomidate is used as a general anesthetic and is sometimes used to sedate patients receiving mechanical ventilation. Ketamine has been associated with a state of unconsciousness in which the patient appears to be awake but is unconscious and cannot feel pain. This drug, which causes sympathetic stimulation with increases in blood pressure and heart rate, may be helpful in situations when cardiac depression is dangerous. Propofol is often used for short procedures because it has a very rapid clearance, produces much less of a hangover effect, and allows for quick recovery. It is also used to maintain patients on mechanical ventilation.

Pharmacokinetics

Midazolam has a rapid onset but does not reach peak effectiveness for 30 to 60 minutes. Etomidate has an onset within 1 minute and a rapid recovery period within 3 to 5 minutes. Ketamine has an onset of action within 30 seconds and a slow recovery period (45 minutes). Propofol is a short-acting anesthetic with a rapid onset of action of 30 to 60 seconds.

Contraindications and Cautions

Midazolam has been associated with respiratory depression and respiratory arrest, and so life support equipment should be readily available whenever it is used. There are no data to support the use of etomidate in children less than 10 years of age.

Adverse Effects

Patients receiving any general anesthetic are at risk for skin breakdown because they will not be able to move. Care must be taken to prevent decubitus ulcer formation. Patients receiving midazolam should be monitored for respiratory depression and CNS suppression (Fig. 27.2). During the recovery period with etomidate, many patients experience myoclonic and tonic movements, as well as nausea and vomiting. Ketamine crosses the blood–brain barrier and can cause hallucinations, dreams, and

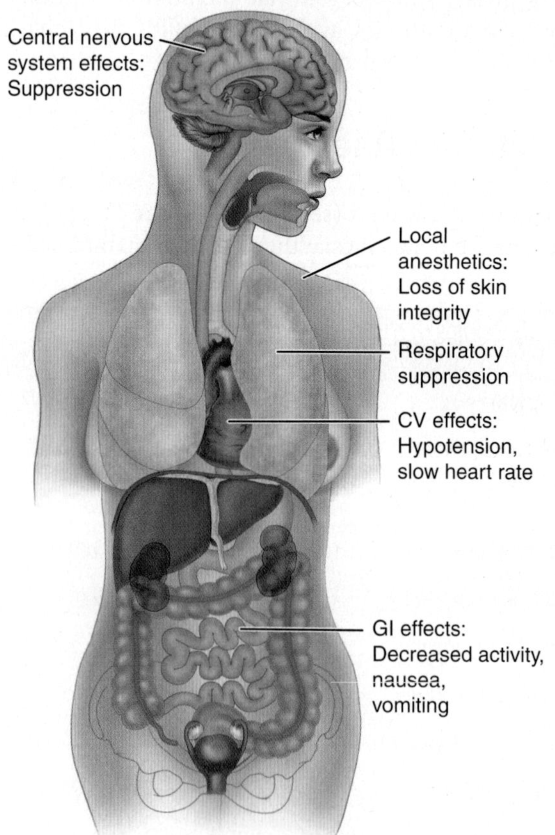

FIGURE 27.2 Common adverse effects associated with anesthetic agents.

psychotic episodes. Propofol often causes local burning on injection and should be administered into a large vein. It can cause bradycardia, hypotension, and, in extreme cases, pulmonary edema.

Clinically Important Drug–Drug Interactions

Ketamine may also potentiate the muscular blocking of NMJ blockers, and the patient may require prolonged periods of respiratory support. Midazolam is associated with increased toxicity and length of recovery when used in combination with inhaled anesthetics, other CNS depressants, opioids, alcohol, or propofol. If any of these agents are used in combination, careful balancing of drug doses is necessary.

Prototype Summary: Midazolam

Indications: Sedation, anxiolysis, and amnesia before diagnostic, therapeutic, or endoscopic procedures; induction of anesthesia; continuous sedation of intubated patients; acute treatment of seizure activity.

Actions: Acts mainly at the limbic system and reticular activating system; potentiates the effects of gamma-aminobutyric acid; has little effect on cortical function; exact mechanism of action is not understood.

Pharmacokinetics:

Route	Onset	Peak	Duration
Nasal spray	10 min	30 min–2 h	4 h
Oral	30–60 min	12 h	2–6 h
IM	15 min	30 min	2–6 h
IV	3–5 min	<30 min	2–6 h

$T_{1/2}$: 1.8 to 6.8 hours; metabolized in the liver; excreted in the urine.

Adverse Effects: Transient drowsiness, sedation, drowsiness, lethargy, apathy, fatigue, disorientation, restlessness, constipation, diarrhea, incontinence, urinary retention, bradycardia, tachycardia, phlebitis at IV injection site.

Anesthetic Gases

Like all inhaled drugs, anesthetic gas enters the bronchi and alveoli, rapidly passes into the capillary system (because gases flow from areas of higher concentration to areas of lower concentration), and is transported to the heart to be pumped throughout the body. This type of gas has a high affinity for fatty tissue and is lipophilic, including the lipid membrane of the nerves in the CNS. The gas passes quickly into the brain and causes severe CNS depression. Once the patient is in stage 3 of anesthesia, the anesthetist regulates the amount of gas that is delivered to ensure that it is sufficient to keep the patient unconscious but not enough to cause severe CNS depression. This is done by decreasing the concentration of the gas that is flowing into the bronchi, creating a concentration gradient that results in the movement of gas in the opposite direction—out of the tissues and back to expired air. The anesthetic gases were once the best way to achieve anesthesia, but they are highly flammable and associated with toxic adverse effects. Newer agents that are safer and less toxic have replaced these drugs in most cases.

One anesthetic gas, nitrous oxide (blue cylinder), is still used (see Table 27.1).

Therapeutic Actions and Indications

Nitrous oxide is a very potent analgesic. It moves so quickly in and out of the body that it can actually accumulate and cause pressure in closed body compartments such as the sinuses. Because nitrous oxide is such a potent analgesic, it is used frequently for dental surgery. It does not cause muscle relaxation. Nitrous oxide is usually combined with other agents for anesthetic use.

Pharmacokinetics

Nitrous oxide has a rapid onset of action, usually within 1 to 2 minutes, and a rapid recovery period. Timing of recovery depends on the other drugs being used.

Contraindications and Cautions

Nitrous oxide can block the reuptake of oxygen after surgery and cause hypoxia. Because of this reaction, it is always given in combination with oxygen. Susceptible patients should be monitored for signs of hypoxia, chest pain, and stroke. This drug should not be used during pregnancy unless the benefit clearly outweighs the potential risk to the fetus. Patients who are breast or chestfeeding should wait 4 hours before feeding a baby when they have been administered nitrous oxide.

Adverse Effects

As with other general anesthetics, patients need to be monitored for skin integrity when they are not able to move for periods of time. Nitrous oxide can cause acute sinus and middle-ear pain, bowel obstruction, and pneumothorax because it so rapidly moves into and accumulates in closed spaces. Because nitrous oxide inactivates vitamin B_{12}, patients should also be monitored for signs of low vitamin B_{12} levels, including neurological, immune, and hematological complications.

Clinically Important Drug–Drug Interactions

Caution should be used if these drugs are combined with any other drug that causes CNS depression. If these agents must be used together, the patient should be monitored closely.

Prototype Summary: Nitrous Oxide

Indications: Induction and maintenance of anesthesia.

Actions: Depresses the CNS to produce anesthesia and analgesia.

Pharmacokinetics:

Route	Onset	Duration
Inhalation	1–2 min	20 min

$T_{1/2}$: Minutes; not metabolized; excreted in the lungs.

Adverse Effects: CV depression, respiratory depression, apnea, earache, sinus pain, vomiting, malignant hyperthermia.

Volatile Liquids

Inhaled anesthetics also can be **volatile liquids**—liquids that are unstable at room temperature and release gases. These gases are then inhaled by the patient. Volatile liquids act like gas anesthetics.

Most of the volatile liquids in use are halogenated hydrocarbons such as desflurane (*Suprane*), isoflurane (*Forane*), and sevoflurane (*Ultane*) (see Table 27.1).

Therapeutic Actions and Indications

Desflurane is widely used in outpatient surgery because of its rapid onset and quick recovery time. Isoflurane is widely used to maintain anesthesia after inductions. It can cause muscle relaxation. Sevoflurane is used in outpatient surgery as an induction agent and is rapidly cleared for quick recovery.

Pharmacokinetics

Desflurane and isoflurane have a rapid onset—within 1 to 2 minutes—and rapid recovery—usually within 15 to 20 minutes. Sevoflurane, the newest of the volatile liquids, has a very rapid onset of action—within 30 seconds—and a rapid clearance, lasting only about 10 minutes. These drugs are all cleared through the lungs.

Contraindications and Cautions

Desflurane use should be avoided in patients with respiratory problems and in those with increased sensitivity because of its irritation to the airways and tendency to cause respiratory depression. In addition, it is not recommended for induction in pediatric patients because of its irritation of the airways. Isoflurane and sevoflurane should be used with caution in patients with respiratory depression to avoid severe respiratory depression. All of these drugs have the potential to trigger malignant hyperthermia and should be used with caution in any patient at high risk for developing it. Dantrolene, the preferred treatment for malignant hyperthermia, should be readily available whenever any of these drugs is used. These drugs should be avoided in pregnancy and lactation unless the benefit clearly outweighs the risk to the fetus or baby because of the CNS-depressive effects of the drugs.

Adverse Effects

Desflurane is associated with a collection of respiratory reactions, including cough, increased secretions, and laryngospasm. Isoflurane is associated with hypotension, hypercapnia, muscle soreness, and a bad taste in the mouth, but it does not cause cardiac arrhythmias or respiratory irritation as do some other volatile liquids. Adverse effects of sevoflurane are thought to be minimal.

Clinically Important Drug–Drug Interactions

Caution should be used when any of these drugs are combined with other CNS suppressants.

Prototype Summary: Desflurane

Indications: Induction and maintenance of general anesthesia.

Actions: Depresses the CNS, causing anesthesia; relaxes muscles; sensitizes the myocardium to the effects of norepinephrine and epinephrine.

Pharmacokinetics:

Route	Onset	Peak	Duration
Inhaled	Rapid	Rapid	End of inhalation

$T_{1/2}$: Unknown; metabolized in the liver; excreted in the urine.

Adverse Effects: Transient drowsiness, sedation, lethargy, apathy, fatigue, disorientation, restlessness, bradycardia, tachycardia, hypoxia, acidosis, apnea, cough, laryngospasm.

Nursing Considerations for Patients Receiving General Anesthetic Agents

Assessment: History and Examination

- Assess for contraindications or cautions: any known allergies to general anesthetics to avoid hypersensitivity reactions; myasthenia gravis or cardiac or respiratory disease, which may be exacerbated by the depressive effects of the drug; or personal or family history of malignant hyperthermia, which may be triggered by the use of general anesthetics.
- Perform a physical assessment, including weighing the patient, before beginning therapy to determine the

appropriate dosing of the drug, establish a baseline status, and evaluate for any potential adverse effects.

- Assess the patient's neurological status, including level of consciousness, affect, reflexes, and pupil size and reaction, and evaluate muscle tone and response to monitor CNS depression, and provide appropriate support, including ventilation and/or intubation as needed.
- Monitor vital signs, including temperature, pulse, and blood pressure, for changes, and auscultate lung and heart sounds to monitor for adverse effects of the drugs.
- Obtain an electrocardiogram (ECG) to evaluate for underlying cardiac problems that may be exacerbated by the drug.
- Assess skin color and lesions to monitor for potential skin breakdown resulting from patient paralysis and immobility while under anesthesia.
- Auscultate the abdomen for bowel sounds to evaluate GI motility.

Nursing Conclusions

Nursing conclusions related to drug therapy might include the following:

- Impaired gas exchange related to respiratory depression
- Altered skin integrity related to immobility secondary to effects of positioning during anesthesia and immobility
- Injury risk related to CNS-depressive effects of the drug
- Altered thought processes and sensory perception related to CNS depression
- Knowledge deficit regarding drug therapy

Planning

- The patient will receive the best therapeutic effect from the drug therapy.
- The patient will have limited adverse effects to the drug therapy.
- The patient will have an understanding of the drug therapy, adverse effects to anticipate, and measures to relieve discomfort and improve safety.

Intervention With Rationale

- Keep in mind that the drug must be administered by trained personnel (usually an anesthesiologist) because of the potential risks associated with its use.
- Have emergency equipment to maintain airway readily available and provide mechanical ventilation when the patient is not able to maintain respiration because of CNS depression.
- Monitor temperature for prompt detection and treatment of malignant hyperthermia. Maintain dantrolene on standby.
- Monitor pulse, respiration, blood pressure, ECG, and cardiac output continually during administration to assess systemic response to CNS depression and provide appropriate support as needed.
- Monitor temperature and reflexes to maximize overall benefit with the least toxicity and because dose adjustment may be needed to alleviate potential problems.
- To ensure patient safety, institute safety precautions, such as side rails, and monitor the patient until the recovery phase is complete and the patient is conscious and able to move and communicate.
- Provide comfort measures to help the patient tolerate drug effects. Provide pain relief as appropriate, along with reassurance and support, to deal with the effects of anesthesia and loss of control; skin care and turning to prevent skin breakdown; and supportive care for conditions such as hypotension and bronchospasm.
- Offer support and encouragement to help the patient cope with the procedure and the drugs being used.
- Provide preoperative patient teaching, realizing that most patients who receive the drug will be unconscious or will be receiving teaching about a particular procedure. Teaching should include the following:
  - Information about the anesthetic (e.g., what to expect, rate of onset, time to recovery)
  - Medications that may be used preoperatively
  - Effects of the medication on the patient preoperatively
  - Measures to maintain the patient's safety preoperatively and during recovery
  - How the patient will feel during the recovery phase
  - Signs and symptoms to report during recovery and afterward
- Provide postprocedure information to the patient and another responsible adult (caregiver or significant other) who is with the patient because after the procedure the patient may not be able to remember the information. This information should include the following:
  - Patient should not drive or operate machinery the day of the procedure.
  - Patient should not sign any legal documents and/or make any significant decisions for 24 hours after the anesthetic procedure.
  - Patient and caregiver should be informed it is normal for the patient to be drowsy for 12 to 24 hours postprocedure but should *always* be arousable. If the patient is not arousable, a provider should be called.

Evaluation

- Monitor patient response to the drug (analgesia, loss of consciousness).
- Monitor for adverse effects (respiratory depression, hypotension, bronchospasm, slowed GI activity, skin breakdown, malignant hyperthermia).
- Evaluate the effectiveness of the teaching plan (patient can relate anticipated effects of the drug and the recovery process).
- Monitor the effectiveness of comfort and safety measures.

Key Points

- General anesthetics must be administered by physicians or nurse anesthetists trained in their administration and prepared to provide constant monitoring and life support measures to assist the patient when the CNS is depressed.
- General anesthetics include barbiturates and nonbarbiturate drugs, which are administered parenterally, and anesthetic gases and volatile liquids, which are administered through inhalation.
- Patients receiving general anesthetics must be constantly monitored because the CNS depression can cause respiratory arrest, CV reactions including hypotension, and alterations in GI activity that can lead to nausea and vomiting.

Local Anesthesia

Local anesthesia refers to a loss of sensation in limited areas of the body. Local anesthesia can be achieved by several different methods: topical administration, infiltration, field block, nerve block, and IV regional anesthesia.

Topical Administration

Topical local anesthesia involves the application of a cream, lotion, ointment, or drop of a local anesthetic to traumatized skin to relieve pain. It can also involve applying these forms to the mucous membranes in the eye, nose, throat, mouth, urethra, anus, or rectum to relieve pain or to anesthetize the area to facilitate a medical procedure. Although systemic absorption is rare with topical application, it can occur if there is damage or breakdown of the tissues in the area, if large portions of the body are covered in topical anesthetic, or if an occlusive barrier is placed over the topical anesthetic.

Infiltration

Infiltration local anesthesia involves injecting the anesthetic directly into the tissues to be treated (e.g., sutured, drilled, cut). This injection brings the anesthetic into contact with the nerve endings in the area and prevents them from transmitting nerve impulses to the brain.

Field Block

Field block local anesthesia involves injecting the anesthetic all around the area that will be affected by the procedure or surgery. This is more intense than infiltration anesthesia because the anesthetic agent comes in contact with all of the nerve endings surrounding the area. This type of block is often used for tooth extractions.

Nerve Block

Nerve block local anesthesia involves injecting the anesthetic at some point along the nerve or nerves that run to and from the region in which the loss of pain sensation or muscle paralysis is desired. These blocks are performed not in the surgical field but at some distance from the field. They involve a greater area with potential for more adverse effects. Several types of nerve blocks are possible:

- Peripheral nerve block: Blockage of the sensory and motor aspects of a particular nerve for relief of pain or for diagnostic purposes
- Central nerve block: Injection of anesthetic into the roots of the nerves in the spinal cord
- Epidural anesthesia: Injection of the drug into the epidural space where the nerves emerge from the spinal cord
- Caudal block: Injection of anesthetic into the sacral canal, below the epidural area
- Spinal anesthesia: Injection of anesthetic into the spinal subarachnoid space

Intravenous Regional Local Anesthesia

IV regional local anesthesia, or "Bier block," involves carefully exsanguinating blood from the patient's arm or leg by compression tourniquets. The anesthetic is injected into the vein of the limb that requires the anesthesia, and tourniquets are used to prevent the anesthetic from entering the general circulation. This technique is used for specific surgical procedures on limbs, more commonly in procedures on the upper extremities.

Local Anesthetic Agents

Local anesthetic agents (Table 27.2) are used primarily to prevent the patient from feeling pain for varying periods of time after the agents have been administered in the peripheral nervous system. In increasing concentrations, local anesthetics can also cause loss of the following sensations (in this sequence): temperature, touch, proprioception (position sense), and skeletal muscle tone. If these other aspects of nerve function are progressively lost, recovery occurs in the reverse order of the loss.

The local anesthetics are very powerful nerve blockers, and it is important that their effects be limited to a particular area of the body. At very high doses, systemic absorption could produce toxic effects on the nervous system and the heart (e.g., severe CNS depression, cardiac arrhythmias).

Local anesthetics are classified as esters or amides. The agent of choice depends on the method of administration, the length of time for which the area is to be anesthetized, and consideration of potential adverse effects. Esters include benzocaine (*Dermoplast, Lanacane, Unguentine*), chloroprocaine (*Clorotekal, Nesacaine*), cocaine

Table 27.2 *Drugs in Focus*: Local Anesthetic Agents

Drug Name	Onset	Duration	Administration	Special Considerations
Esters				
benzocaine (*Dermoplast, Lanacane, Unguentine*)	1 min	30–60 min	Skin, mucous membranes	Avoid tight bandages with skin preparation. Not indicated for children aged ≤2 years due to risk of methemoglobinemia.
chloroprocaine (*Clorotekal, Nesacaine*)	6–15 min	15–75 min	Peripheral nerve block, subarachnoid (spinal anesthesia)	Different formulations may have different indications and dosing.
cocaine hydrochloride (*Goprelto, Numbrino*)	15–30 min	5–8 h	Nasal solution indicated for the induction of local anesthesia of the mucous membranes of the nasal cavities for adults	Has high potential for abuse and dependence; may lower seizure threshold; may increase heart rate and blood pressure.
tetracaine (generic)	10–20 s	10–20 min	Ophthalmic	Rapid, short-acting topical ophthalmic anesthetic.
Amides				
bupivacaine (*Exparel, Marcaine, Sensorcaine, Xaracoll*)	5–20 min	2–7 h	Local, epidural, dental, caudal, subarachnoid, sympathetic, retrobulbar, interscalene brachial plexus (*Exparel*), implant post inguinal hernia repair (*Xaracoll*)	*Sensorcaine* (0.75% concentration) not recommended for obstetrical anesthesia due to reports of cardiac arrest post epidural anesthesia in obstetrical patients.
dibucaine (*Nupercainal*)	<15 min	3–4 h	Skin, mucous membranes	Monitor for local reactions.
lidocaine (*Akten, Dilocaine, Glydo, Solarcaine, Xylocaine, Lidoderm, Zingo, Ztlido*)	5–15 min	30–90 min	Ophthalmic, caudal, epidural, spinal, cervical, dental, skin, mucous membrane, topical patch	Different formulations may have very specific indications and dosing.
mepivacaine (*Carbocaine, Polocaine, Scandonest Plain*)	3–15 min	45–90 min	Nerve block, obstetric, cervical, epidural, dental, local infiltration	Caution with renal impairment.
prilocaine (generic)	1–15 min	0.5–3 h	Nerve block, dental	Advise patients not to bite themselves.
ropivacaine (*Naropin*)	1–5 min	2–6 h	Nerve block, epidural, caudal	Avoid rapid infusion; offers good pain management post-op and obstetrics.
Others				
pramoxine (*Tronothane, PrameGel, Itch-X, Prax*)	3–5 min	<60 min	Skin, mucous membranes	Do not cover with tight bandages; used for treatment of pruritus.

hydrochloride (*Goprelto, Numbrino*), and tetracaine (generic). Amides include bupivacaine (*Exparel, Marcaine, Sensorcaine, Xaracoll*), dibucaine (*Nupercainal*), lidocaine (*Akten, Dilocaine, Glydo, Solarcaine, Xylocaine, Lidoderm, Zingo, Ztlido*), mepivacaine (*Carbocaine, Polocaine, Scandonest Plain*), prilocaine (generic), and ropivacaine (*Naropin*). Pramoxine (*Tronothane, PrameGel, Itch-X, Prax*) is a topical-only local anesthetic agent that does not fit into either of these classes.

Therapeutic Actions and Indications

Local anesthetics work by causing a temporary interruption in the production and conduction of nerve impulses. They affect the permeability of nerve membranes to sodium ions, which normally infuse into the cell in response to stimulation. By preventing the sodium ions from entering the nerve, they stop the nerve from depolarizing. A particular section of the nerve cannot be stimulated, and nerve impulses directed toward that section are lost when they reach that area.

The way in which a local anesthetic is administered helps to increase its effectiveness by delivering it directly to the area that is causing or will cause the pain, thereby decreasing systemic absorption and related toxic effects (Fig. 27.3). Local anesthetics are indicated for infiltration anesthesia, peripheral nerve block, spinal anesthesia, and the relief of local pain. Some of the local anesthetic products are in combination forms (see Box 27.2).

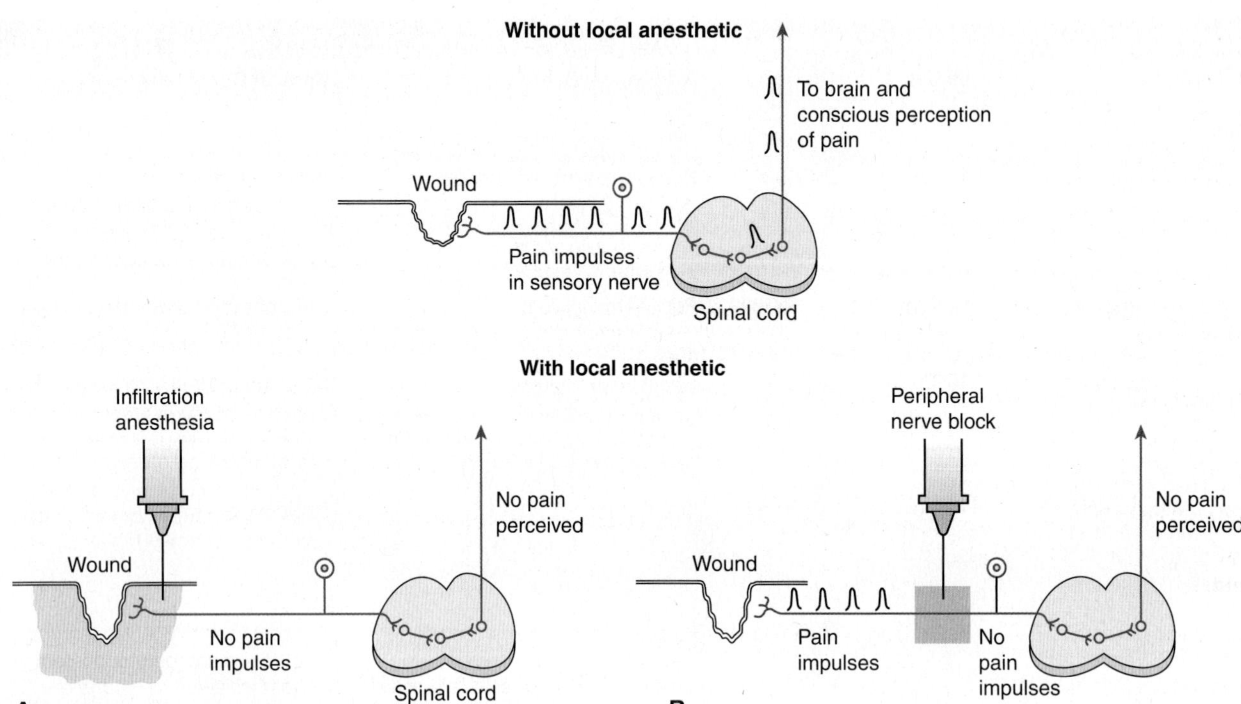

FIGURE 27.3 Mechanism of action of local anesthetics. **Top.** An injury produces pain impulses (action potentials) that are conducted and transmitted in an area of the brain in which pain is perceived. **A.** Conduction of the pain impulse has been blocked by infiltration anesthetics at the site of the injury. **B.** A nerve block at some distance from the injury. Local anesthetics block the movement of sodium into the nerve and prevent nerve depolarization, stopping the transmission of the pain impulse.

Pharmacokinetics

The ester local anesthetics are broken down immediately in the plasma by enzymes called **plasma esterases.** The amide local anesthetics are metabolized more slowly in the liver, and serum levels of these drugs can increase and lead to toxicity.

Contraindications and Cautions

The local anesthetics are contraindicated with any of the following conditions: history of allergy to any one of these agents or to parabens to avoid hypersensitivity reactions; heart block, which could be greatly exacerbated with systemic absorption at very high levels; shock, which could alter the local delivery and absorption of these drugs; and decreased plasma esterases, which could result in toxic levels of the ester-type local anesthetics.

They should be used during pregnancy and lactation only if the benefit outweighs any potential risk to the fetus or neonate. Several local anesthetics are indicated for treating pain during labor and delivery; fetal monitoring

Box 27.2 Focus on Safe Medication Administration

EXAMPLES OF COMBINATION LOCAL ANESTHETICS

EMLA cream is a mixture of lidocaine and prilocaine that is administered for dermal analgesia for clinical procedures (e.g., IV catheter placement or skin graft harvesting). It should be applied to skin at least 1 hour prior to the procedure but may need earlier administration if the procedure requires deeper puncture. The amount of medication systemically absorbed is related to duration of application and the area to which it is applied.

There are several local anesthetic combinations that are used for dental procedures. *Octocaine* is a combination of lidocaine and epinephrine, *Citanest Forte Dental* is a combination of prilocaine and epinephrine, and *Kovanaze* is a combination of tetracaine HCl and oxymetazoline HCl. The epinephrine and oxymetazoline HCl act as vasoconstrictors and decrease the spread of the anesthetic from the local area.

Synera, a local anesthetic product that is a combination of lidocaine and tetracaine and is available in a dermal patch, is approved for use on intact skin to provide local dermal anesthesia when doing venipunctures or inserting IV cannulae or for superficial dermatological procedures that could cause discomfort to the patient. When using it for venipunctures or inserting an IV, one patch is applied 20 to 30 minutes before the procedure. If a superficial dermatological procedure is being performed, one patch is applied to the area 30 minutes before the procedure. The patch must be removed if the patient is undergoing a magnetic resonance imaging scan to prevent burning related to the dermal patch. The site should be monitored for any local irritation.

Pliaglis is a cream combining lidocaine and tetracaine. It is indicated for topical analgesia during superficial dermatological procedures such as dermal filler injections, pulsed dye laser therapy, and laser-assisted tattoo removal. The cream should be applied to intact skin 20 to 60 minutes prior to the procedure.

should be used due to potential for fetal bradycardia. Patients with glucose-6-phosphate dehydrogenase deficiency, infants younger than 6 months of age, and patients with compromised cardiac or pulmonary function have increased risk of methemoglobinemia. Signs include cyanotic skin discoloration and abnormal coloration of the blood. Medication should be discontinued immediately with these occurrences.

Adverse Effects

The adverse effects of these drugs may be related to their local blocking of sensation (e.g., skin breakdown, self-injury, biting oneself if used in the oral cavity). Loss of skin integrity is always a problem if the patient is unable to move, and care must be taken to prevent skin breakdown. Other problematic effects are associated with the route of administration and the amount of drug that is absorbed systemically. There are risks of CNS effects such as headache (especially with epidural and spinal anesthesia), restlessness, anxiety, dizziness, tremors, blurred vision, and backache; GI effects such as nausea and vomiting; CV effects such as peripheral vasodilation, myocardial depression, arrhythmias, and blood pressure changes, all of which may lead to fatal cardiac arrest; and respiratory arrest.

Clinically Important Drug–Drug Interactions

When local anesthetics and succinylcholine are given together, increased and prolonged neuromuscular blockade occurs. When used in combination with epinephrine, there is risk of vasoconstriction causing gangrene.

Prototype Summary: Lidocaine

Indications: Infiltration anesthesia; peripheral and sympathetic nerve blocks; central nerve blocks; spinal and caudal anesthesia; topical anesthetic for skin or mucous membrane disorders.

Actions: Blocks the generation and conduction of action potentials in sensory nerves by reducing sodium permeability, reducing the height and rate of rise of the action potential, increasing the excitation threshold, and slowing the conduction velocity.

Pharmacokinetics:

Route	Onset	Peak	Duration
IM	5–10 min	5–15 min	2 h
Topical	Not generally absorbed systemically		

$T_{1/2}$: 10 minutes, then 1.5 to 3 hours; metabolized in the liver; excreted in the urine.

Adverse Effects: Headache, backache, hypotension, urinary retention, urinary incontinence, pruritus, seizures; when locally applied, burning, stinging, swelling, tenderness.

Nursing Considerations for Patients Receiving Local Anesthetic Agents

Assessment: History and Examination

- Assess for contraindications and cautions: any known allergies to these drugs or to parabens to avoid hypersensitivity reactions; impaired liver function, which could alter metabolism and clearance of the drug; low plasma esterases in people who have history or family history of prolonged apnea with anesthesia, which may cause prolonged effects of the muscle relaxant; heart block, which could be exacerbated by the drug effects; shock, to prevent altered local delivery and absorption; and current status of pregnancy or lactation, which are cautions to the use of the drug.
- Perform a physical assessment before beginning therapy to establish a baseline status and any potential adverse effects.
- Inspect the site for local anesthetic application to ensure integrity of the skin and to prevent inadvertent systemic absorption of the drug.
- Assess the patient's neurological status, including level of orientation, reflexes, pupil size and reaction, muscle tone and response, and sensation to evaluate the effectiveness of the drug and monitor for potential toxic neurological effects.
- Monitor vital signs, including temperature, pulse, and blood pressure, and assess respiratory rate and auscultate lungs *for* adventitious sounds to identify changes and possible systemic absorption.
- Monitor laboratory test results, such as liver function tests and plasma esterases (if appropriate), to determine possible need for dose adjustment.

Refer to the "Critical Thinking Scenario" for a full discussion of nursing care for a patient who is receiving local anesthesia.

Nursing Conclusions

Nursing conclusions related to drug therapy might include the following:

- Altered sensory perception (kinesthetic, tactile) related to local anesthetic effect
- Altered skin integrity related to immobility caused by actions of the drug
- Injury risk related to loss of sensation and mobility
- Knowledge deficit regarding drug therapy

Planning

- The patient will receive the best therapeutic effect from the drug therapy.
- The patient will have limited adverse effects to the drug therapy.

(continues on page 484)

- The patient will have an understanding of the drug therapy, adverse effects to anticipate, and measures to relieve discomfort and improve safety.

Intervention With Rationale

- For systemic administration, have emergency equipment readily available to maintain airway and provide mechanical ventilation if needed.
- For systemic administration, ensure that drugs for managing hypotension, cardiac arrest, and CNS alterations are readily available in case of severe reaction and toxicity.
- Ensure that patients receiving spinal anesthesia or epidural anesthesia are well hydrated and remain lying down for up to 12 hours after the anesthesia to minimize headache.
- Establish safety precautions to prevent injury during the time that the patient has a loss of sensation and/or mobility.
- Provide meticulous skin care to the site of administration to reduce the risk of breakdown.
- Provide comfort measures to help the patient tolerate drug effects. Provide pain relief, as well as skin care and turning to prevent skin breakdown.
- Offer support and encouragement to help the patient cope with the procedure and drugs being used.
- Provide thorough patient teaching, including anesthetic to be given, method for administration, activities involved with administering and monitoring the drug, and safety precautions.

Evaluation

- Monitor patient response to the drug (loss of feeling in designated area).
- Monitor for adverse effects (respiratory depression, blood pressure changes, arrhythmias, GI upset, skin breakdown, injury, CNS alterations, fetal heart rate changes).
- Evaluate the effectiveness of the teaching plan (the patient can relate the anticipated effects of the drug and the recovery process).

CRITICAL THINKING SCENARIO
Local Anesthesia

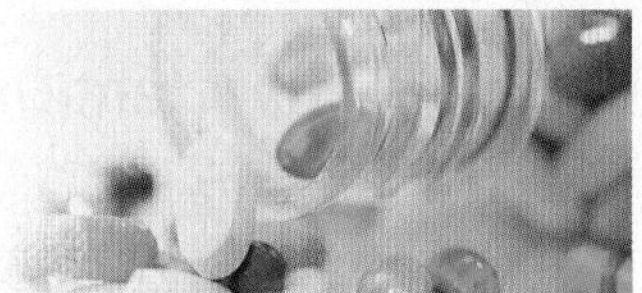

THE SITUATION

A.M., a 32-year-old athlete with a history of asthma (which could indicate pulmonary dysfunction), was admitted to the hospital for an inguinal hernia repair. At the patient's request, the surgeon elected to use a local anesthetic employing spinal anesthesia. Because the extent of the repair was unknown (A.M. had undergone two previous repairs), bupivacaine, a long-acting anesthetic, was selected. A.M. remained alert (blood pressure 120/64 mm Hg, pulse 62 beats/min, respiration rate 10/min) and stable throughout the procedure. Two hours after the conclusion of the procedure, A.M. appeared agitated (blood pressure 154/68 mm Hg, pulse 88 beats/min, respiration rate 12/min). Although A.M. did not complain of discomfort, they did state that they still had no feeling and had only limited movement of their legs.

CRITICAL THINKING

What safety precautions need to be taken?

What nursing interventions should be done at this point?

How could the patient be reassured? Think about the anxiety level of the patient—an athlete who elected to have local anesthesia may have an urge to control the outcome and may feel somewhat invincible. Consider the anxiety that loss of mobility and sensation in the legs may cause in a person who makes their living as an athlete.

In addition, consider the expected duration of action of bupivacaine and the rate of return of function.

DISCUSSION

Bupivacaine is a long-acting anesthetic with effects that may persist for several hours. The timing of the drug's effects should be explained to A.M., and they should be monitored for a period of time to determine whether their agitated state and slightly elevated vital signs are a result of anxiety or an unanticipated reaction to the surgery or the drug. Life support equipment should be on standby in case A.M.'s condition is a toxic drug reaction or some unanticipated problem occurring after surgery.

The nurse is in the best position to perform the following interventions: explaining the effects of the drug and the anticipated recovery schedule, keeping the patient as flat as possible to decrease the headache usually associated with spinal anesthesia, encouraging the patient to turn from side to side periodically to allow skin care to be performed and to alleviate the risk of pressure sore development, and staying with the patient as much as possible to reassure them, to answer their questions, and to encourage them to talk about their feelings and reaction.

If the agitated state is caused by a stress reaction, the patient should return to normal; comfort measures, teaching, and reassurance should be provided. An elevated systolic pressure with a normal diastolic pressure often is an indication of a sympathetic stress response. An athlete is more likely than most people to suffer great anxiety and fear if their legs become numb and they are unable to move them. Teaching and comfort measures may be all that are needed to relieve the anxiety and ensure a good recovery.

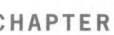

NURSING CARE GUIDE FOR A.M.: LOCAL ANESTHESIA

Assessment: History and Examination

Assess for allergies to local anesthetics or to parabens, cardiac disorders, vascular problems, hepatic dysfunction; also assess for concurrent use of succinylcholine.
Focus physical examination on the following:
CV: Blood pressure, pulse, peripheral perfusion, ECG
CNS: Orientation, affect, reflexes, vision
Skin: Color, lesions, texture, sweating
Respiratory: Respiration, adventitious sounds
Laboratory tests: Liver function tests

Nursing Conclusions

Altered sensory perception (kinesthetic, tactile) related to anesthesia
Anxiety related to drug effects or procedure
Altered skin integrity related to immobility
Injury risk related to loss of sensation and mobility
Knowledge deficit regarding drug therapy

Planning

The patient will receive the best therapeutic effect from the drug therapy.
The patient will have limited adverse effects to the drug therapy.
The patient will have an understanding of the drug therapy, adverse effects to anticipate, and measures to relieve discomfort and improve safety.

Intervention

Provide comfort and safety measures: positioning, skin care, side rails, pain medication as needed, maintaining airway, antidotes on standby.
Provide support and reassurance to deal with loss of sensation and mobility.
Provide patient teaching about the procedure being performed and what to expect.
Provide life support as needed.

Evaluation

Evaluate drug effects: loss of sensation, loss of movement.
Monitor for adverse effects: CV effects (blood pressure changes, arrhythmias), respiratory depression, GI upset, CNS alterations, skin breakdown, anxiety, and fear.
Monitor for drug–drug interactions as indicated for each drug.
Evaluate the effectiveness of the patient teaching program and comfort and safety measures.
Constantly monitor vital signs and muscular function and sensation as it returns.

PATIENT TEACHING FOR A.M.

Teaching about local anesthetics is usually incorporated into the overall teaching plan about the procedure that the patient will undergo. Things to highlight with the patient include the following:

- Discussion of the overall procedure:
  - What it will feel like (possible numbness, tingling, inability to move, pressure, pain, choking).
  - Any anticipated discomfort.
  - How long it will last.
  - Concerns during the procedure: Report any discomfort and ask any questions as they arise.
- Discussion of the recovery:
  - How long it will take.
  - Feelings to expect: tingling, numbness, pressure, itching.
  - Pain that will be felt as the anesthesia wears off.
  - Measures to reduce pain in the area.
  - Signs and symptoms to report (e.g., pain along a nerve route, palpitations, feeling faint, disorientation).

Key Points

- Local anesthetics block the depolarization of nerve membranes, preventing the transmission of pain sensations and motor stimuli.
- Local anesthetics are administered to deliver the drug directly to the desired area and to prevent systemic absorption, which could lead to serious interruption of nerve impulses and response.
- Ester-type local anesthetics are immediately metabolized by plasma esterases. Amide local anesthetics are biotransformed in the liver and have a greater risk of accumulation and systemic toxicity.

SUMMARY

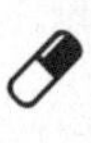
General anesthetics result in analgesia, amnesia, and unconsciousness; they also block muscle reflexes that could interfere with a surgical procedure or put the patient at risk for harm.

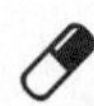
The use of general anesthetics involves widespread CNS depression that could be harmful, especially in patients with underlying CNS, CV, or respiratory diseases.

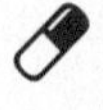
Anesthesia proceeds through four predictable stages from loss of sensation to total CNS depression, in which death can rapidly occur.

- Induction of anesthesia is the period of time from the beginning of anesthesia administration until the patient reaches surgical anesthesia.
- Balanced anesthesia involves giving a variety of drugs, including anticholinergics, rapid intravenous anesthetics, inhaled anesthetics, NMJ blockers, and opioids.
- Patients receiving general anesthetics should be monitored for any adverse effects; they need reassurance and safety measures until the recovery of sensation, mobility, and ability to communicate.
- Local anesthetics block the depolarization of nerve membranes, preventing the transmission of pain sensations and motor stimuli.
- Local anesthetics are administered to deliver the drug directly to the desired area and to prevent systemic absorption, which could lead to serious interruption of nerve impulses and response.
- Ester-type local anesthetics are immediately destroyed by plasma esterases. Amide local anesthetics are destroyed in the liver and have a greater risk of accumulation and systemic toxicity.
- Nursing care of patients receiving general or local anesthetics should include safety precautions to prevent injury and skin breakdown; support and reassurance to deal with the loss of sensation and mobility; and patient teaching regarding what to expect, to decrease stress and anxiety.

CHECK YOUR UNDERSTANDING

Answers to the questions in this chapter can be found in Answers to Check Your Understanding Questions on thePoint®.

MULTIPLE CHOICE

Select the best answer.

1. The highest risk period for many patients undergoing general anesthesia is during which stage?
   a. Stage 1, when communication becomes difficult
   b. Stage 2, when systemic stimulation occurs
   c. Stage 3, when skeletal muscles relax
   d. There is no real danger during general anesthesia

2. Recovery after a general anesthetic refers to the period of time
   a. from the beginning of anesthesia until the patient is ready for surgery.
   b. during the surgery when anesthesia is maintained at a certain level.
   c. from discontinuation of the anesthetic until the patient has regained consciousness, movement, and the ability to communicate.
   d. when the patient is in the most danger of CNS depression.

3. While a patient is receiving a general anesthetic, they must be continually monitored because the patient
   a. has no pain sensation.
   b. experiences generalized CNS depression that affects all body functions.
   c. cannot move.
   d. cannot communicate.

4. The nursing instructor determines that teaching about general anesthetics was successful when the students identify which person as being most qualified to administer general anesthetics?
   a. Nursing supervisor
   b. Graduate nurse
   c. Trained physician
   d. Surgeon

5. Local anesthetics are used to block feeling in specific body areas. If given in increasing concentrations, local anesthetics can cause loss in which order?
   a. Temperature sensation, touch sensation, proprioception, and skeletal muscle tone
   b. Touch sensation, skeletal muscle tone, temperature sensation, and proprioception
   c. Proprioception, skeletal muscle tone, touch sensation, and temperature sensation
   d. Skeletal muscle tone, touch sensation, temperature sensation, and proprioception

MULTIPLE RESPONSE

Select all that apply.

1. Which comfort measures are important for a patient receiving a local anesthetic?
   a. Skin care and turning
   b. Reassurance over loss of control and sensation
   c. Use of antihypertensive agents
   d. Use of analgesics as needed
   e. Ice applied to the area involved
   f. Safety precautions to prevent injury
2. A nurse would anticipate the use of general anesthetics for which reasons?
   a. Produce analgesia
   b. Produce amnesia
   c. Activate the reticular activating system
   d. Block muscle reflexes
   e. Cause unconsciousness
   f. Prevent nausea
3. Balanced anesthesia combines different classes of drugs to achieve the best effects with the fewest adverse effects. Balanced anesthesia usually involves the use of which types of drugs?
   a. Anticholinergics
   b. Narcotics
   c. Sedative/hypnotics
   d. Adrenergic beta-blockers
   e. Dantrolene
   f. Neuromuscular blocking agents

REFERENCES

Barash, P. G., Cullen, B. F., Stoelting, R. K., et al. (2015). *Clinical anesthesia fundamentals.* Wolters Kluwer.

Brunton, L., Hilal-Dandan, R., & Knollman, B. (2018). *Goodman and Gilman's the pharmacological basis of therapeutics* (13th ed.). McGraw-Hill.

Candido, K. D., Tharian, A. R., & Winnie, A. P. (2021). *Intravenous regional block for upper and lower extremity surgery.* https://www.nysora.com/techniques/intravenous-regional-anesthesia/intravenous-regional-block-upper-lower-extremity-surgery/

Clifford, T. (2011). Peripheral nerve blocks. *Journal of Perianesthesia Nursing, 26*(2), 120–121. 10.1016/j.jopan.2011.01.004

Fleisher, L., & Roizen, M. (2011). *Essence of anesthesia practice: Expert consultant.* Saunders.

Hall, J. E., & Hall, M. E. (2021). *Guyton and Hall's textbook of medical physiology* (14th ed.). Elsevier.

Hendler, C. B. (Ed.) (2021). *Nursing 2021 drug handbook.* Wolters Kluwer.

Meier, G., & Buettner, J. (2009). *Peripheral regional anesthetics.* Thieme.

Norris, T. L. (2019). *Porth's pathophysiology concepts of altered health states* (13th ed.). Wolters Kluwer.

Pine, M., Holt, K. D., & Lou, Y. (2003). Surgical mortality and type of anesthesia provider. *American Association of Nurse Anesthetists Journal, 71,* 109–116.

CHAPTER 28

Neuromuscular Junction Blocking Agents

Learning Objectives

Upon completion of this chapter, you will be able to:

1. Describe the structure and function of the neuromuscular junction.
2. Discuss the use of neuromuscular junction blockers across the lifespan.
3. Describe the therapeutic actions, indications, pharmacokinetics, contraindications, most common adverse reactions, and important drug–drug interactions associated with the depolarizing and nondepolarizing neuromuscular junction blockers.
4. Compare and contrast the prototype drugs pancuronium and succinylcholine with other neuromuscular junction blockers.
5. Outline the nursing considerations, including important teaching points, for patients receiving a neuromuscular junction blocker.

Key Terms

acetylcholine receptor site: muscarinic or nicotinic receptor that can be activated by acetylcholine; the area on the muscle cell membrane where acetylcholine (ACh) reacts is a type of nicotinic receptor, and stimulation of the receptor will cause contraction of the muscle

depolarizing neuromuscular junction (NMJ) blocker: chemical that can stimulate a muscle cell, causing it to contract with no allowance for repolarization and restimulation of the muscle; will cause paralysis once the muscle is contracted

malignant hyperthermia: reaction to some NMJ blocking drugs in susceptible people; characterized by extreme muscle rigidity, severe hyperpyrexia, acidosis, and in some cases death

neuromuscular junction (NMJ): the synapse between a nerve and a muscle cell

nondepolarizing neuromuscular junction (NMJ) blocker: chemical that will inhibit depolarization of the muscle cell; prevents depolarization and stimulation by blocking the effects of acetylcholine

paralysis: loss of muscle function

sarcomere: functional unit of a muscle cell, composed of actin and myosin molecules arranged in layers to give the unit a striped or striated appearance

sliding filament theory: theory explaining muscle contraction as a reaction of actin and myosin molecules when they are freed to react by the inactivation of troponin after calcium enters the cell during depolarization

Drug List

NEUROMUSCULAR JUNCTION BLOCKING AGENTS

Nondepolarizing NMJ Blockers

atracurium
cisatracurium
(P) pancuronium
rocuronium
vecuronium

Depolarizing NMJ Blocker

(P) succinylcholine

Nerves communicate with muscles at a synapse called the neuromuscular junction (NMJ). At this point, a nerve stimulates a muscle to contract. If the nerve is not able to communicate with the muscle cell, the muscle will not be able to contract, and paralysis will result. Preventing a patient from moving their muscles is required in certain clinical situations, including surgery, diagnostic procedures, and mechanical ventilation. Anesthetics (discussed in Chapter 27) can prevent muscle movement by suppressing function through the central nervous system (CNS). The NMJ blocking drugs are used to prevent the nerve stimulation at the muscle cell and cause paralysis of the muscle directly without total CNS depression and its many systemic effects. They are often used in conjunction with general anesthetic medication as part of balanced anesthesia for surgeries.

The Neuromuscular Junction

The **neuromuscular junction** is the point at which a motor neuron communicates with a skeletal muscle fiber to cause muscular contraction. NMJ blocking agents affect the normal functioning of muscles by interfering with the normal processes that occur at the junction of nerve and muscle cell.

The functional unit of a muscle, called a **sarcomere**, is made up of light and dark filaments formed by actin and myosin molecules. These molecules are arranged in orderly stacks that give the sarcomere a striated or striped appearance. Normal muscle function involves the arrival of a nerve impulse at the motor nerve terminal, followed by the release of the neurotransmitter acetylcholine (ACh) into the synaptic cleft. At the **acetylcholine receptor site** on the effector side of the synapse, the ACh interacts with the nicotinic cholinergic receptors, causing depolarization of the muscle membrane. ACh is then broken down by the enzyme acetylcholinesterase, freeing the receptor for further stimulation. With stimulation, this depolarization allows the release of calcium ions, stored in tubules, into the cell. The calcium binds to troponin, a chemical found throughout the sarcomere. This binding of troponin releases the actin- and myosin-binding sites, allowing them to react with each other. The actin and myosin molecules react with each other again and again, sliding along the filament and making it shorter. This is a contraction of the muscle fiber according to the **sliding filament theory** (Fig. 28.1). As the calcium is removed from the cell during repolarization of the muscle membrane, the troponin is freed and once again prevents the actin and myosin from reacting with each other. The muscle filament then relaxes or slides back to the resting position.

A dynamic balance of excitatory and inhibitory impulses to the muscle results in muscle tone. However, if ACh cannot react with the cholinergic muscle receptor or if the muscle cells cannot repolarize to allow new stimulation and muscle contraction, **paralysis**, or loss of muscle function, occurs.

> **Key Points**
> - The nerves and muscles communicate at the NMJ.
> - ACh acts as the neurotransmitter at the NMJ.
> - NMJ blockers interfere with muscle function.

Neuromuscular Junction Blocking Agents

Drugs that affect the NMJ can be divided into two groups. One group, the **nondepolarizing neuromuscular junction blockers**, includes those agents that act as antagonists to ACh at the NMJ and prevent depolarization of muscle cells. The other group, the **depolarizing neuromuscular junction**

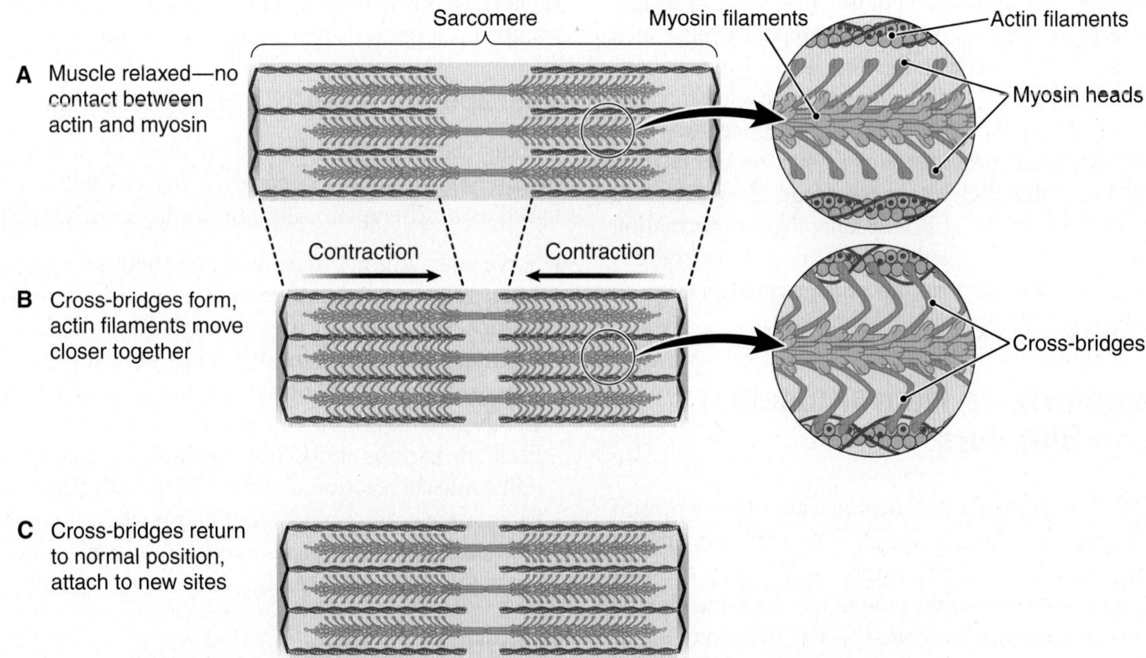

FIGURE 28.1 Sliding filament mechanism of skeletal muscle contraction. **A.** Muscle is relaxed, and there is no contact between the actin and myosin filaments. **B.** Cross bridges form, and the actin filaments are moved closer together as the muscle fiber contracts. **C.** The cross bridges return to their original position and attach to new sites to prepare for another pull on the actin filaments and further contraction.

TABLE 28.1 *Drugs in Focus*: Neuromuscular Junction (NMJ) Blockers

Drug Name	Preferred Uses	Special Considerations
Nondepolarizing NMJ Blockers		
atracurium (generic)	Mechanical ventilation; long duration of action; surgical procedures	Has no effect on pain perception or consciousness; do not use before induction of anesthesia; bradycardia is more common with this drug; reduce dose in renal failure
cisatracurium (*Nimbex*)	Intermediate action; used for surgical procedures and to facilitate intubation	No known effect on pain perception or consciousness; contains benzyl alcohol, avoid use in children <1 month old; not recommended for rapid sequence intubation due to time of onset
pancuronium (generic)	Surgical procedures; mechanical ventilation	Long-term use for mechanical ventilation; monitor for prolonged adverse effects
rocuronium (generic)	Rapid onset; indicated for rapid intubation and routine tracheal intubation; also for muscle relaxation during surgery or mechanical ventilation	No known effect on pain perception or consciousness; may be associated with pulmonary hypertension
vecuronium (generic)	Short surgical procedures; intubation; mechanical ventilation	May contain benzyl alcohol; avoid use in neonates, can cause fatalities in premature infants; monitor long-term use during ventilation; may be associated with permanent muscle damage; if response does not occur with the first twitch test, discontinue
Depolarizing NMJ Blocker		
succinylcholine (*Anectine, Quelicin*)	Surgical procedures; intubation; mechanical ventilation	Should only be used in emergent situations for pediatric patients due to risk of cardiac arrest from hyperkalemic rhabdomyolysis; may cause myalgia secondary to muscle contraction; associated with increased intraocular pressure; associated with increased intragastric pressure, which may cause vomiting; more likely to cause malignant hyperthermia

blocker (of which there is one drug), acts as an ACh agonist at the junction, causing stimulation of the muscle cell and staying on the receptor site, preventing it from repolarizing, which results in muscle paralysis with the muscle in a constant contracted state. Both of these types of drugs are used to cause paralysis for the performance of surgical procedures and endoscopic diagnostic procedures or facilitation of mechanical ventilation. Table 28.1 lists these drugs, their preferred uses, and potential problems. Box 28.1 highlights information about using NMJ blockers with various age groups (see also the "Critical Thinking Scenario" for nursing care related to an older adult patient receiving an NMJ blocker).

Nondepolarizing Neuromuscular Junction Blockers

The first NMJ blocker to be discovered was curare, a poison used on the tips of arrows or spears by hunters to paralyze their game. Animals died when their respiratory muscles became paralyzed. Because the poison was destroyed by the cooking process or by gastric acid if the meat were eaten raw, it was safe for humans. Curare was first purified for clinical use as the NMJ blocker tubocurarine, which has since been replaced with more refined drugs with which onset and duration of effect can be controlled.

Nondepolarizing NMJ blockers include atracurium (generic), cisatracurium (*Nimbex*), pancuronium (generic), rocuronium (generic), and vecuronium (generic).

Therapeutic Actions and Indications

Nondepolarizing NMJ blockers are used when clinical situations require or desire muscle paralysis (see Table 28.1 for preferred uses). Therapeutically, nondepolarizing NMJ blockers

- Serve as an adjunct to general anesthetics during surgery when reflex muscle movement could interfere with the surgical procedure or the delivery of anesthesia.
- Facilitate mechanical intubation by preventing resistance to passing of the endotracheal tube and in situations in which patients "fight" or resist the ventilator.
- Facilitate various endoscopic diagnostic procedures when reflex muscle reaction could interfere with the procedure.
- Facilitate electroconvulsive therapy when intense skeletal muscle contractions as a result of electric shock could cause the patient broken bones or other injuries.

Pharmacokinetics

All nondepolarizing NMJ blockers are similar in structure to ACh and compete with ACh for the muscle ACh receptor site (Fig. 28.2). As a result, they occupy the muscular

Box 28.1 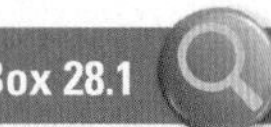 **Focus on Drug Therapy Across the Lifespan**

NMJ BLOCKING AGENTS

Children

Children require careful monitoring and support after the use of NMJ blockers. These agents are used by anesthetists skilled in their use and with full support services available.

The nondepolarizing NMJ blockers are preferable because of the lack of muscle contraction with its resultant discomfort on recovery. Succinylcholine is only indicated for emergent intubation due to risk of cardiac arrest from hyperkalemic rhabdomyolysis in some pediatric patients.

Adults

Adults need to be monitored closely for full return of muscle function. If succinylcholine is used, they need to be told that they may experience muscle pain and discomfort when the procedure is over.

The NMJ blockers are used during pregnancy and lactation only if the benefit to the patient outweighs the potential risk to the fetus or neonate.

Older Adults

Because older patients often also have renal or hepatic impairment, they are more likely to have toxic levels of the drug related to changes in metabolism and excretion. The older patient should receive special efforts to provide skin care to prevent skin breakdown, which is more likely with older skin. The older patient may require longer monitoring and regular orienting and reassuring.

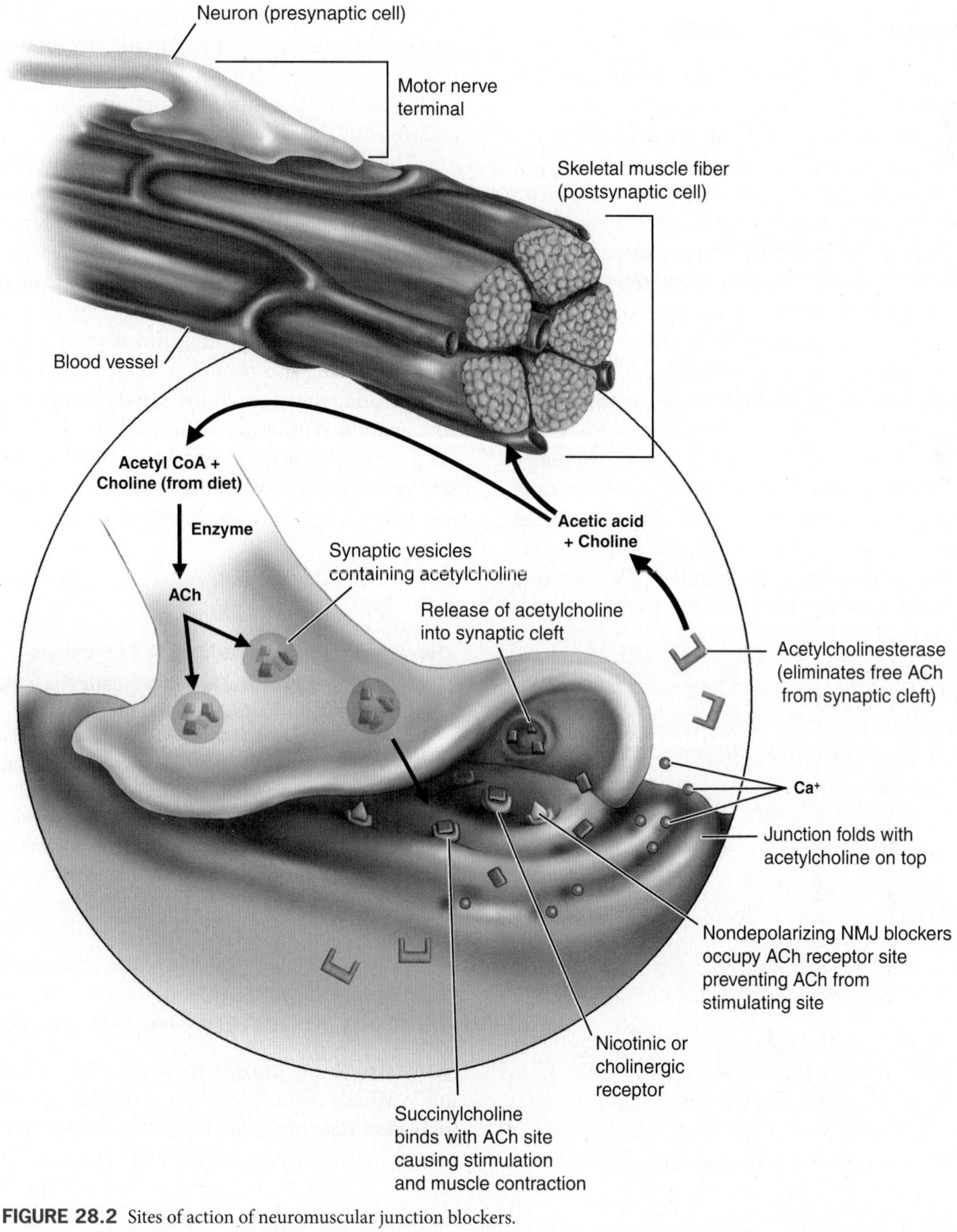

Neuron (presynaptic cell)
Motor nerve terminal
Skeletal muscle fiber (postsynaptic cell)
Blood vessel
Acetyl CoA + Choline (from diet)
Enzyme
ACh
Acetic acid + Choline
Synaptic vesicles containing acetylcholine
Release of acetylcholine into synaptic cleft
Acetylcholinesterase (eliminates free ACh from synaptic cleft)
Ca^{+}
Junction folds with acetylcholine on top
Nondepolarizing NMJ blockers occupy ACh receptor site preventing ACh from stimulating site
Nicotinic or cholinergic receptor
Succinylcholine binds with ACh site causing stimulation and muscle contraction

FIGURE 28.2 Sites of action of neuromuscular junction blockers.

cholinergic receptor site and do not allow stimulation to occur. These agents do not cause the activation of muscle cells; consequently, muscle contraction does not occur. Because they are not broken down by acetylcholinesterase, their effect is longer lasting than that of ACh. The nondepolarizing NMJ blockers are hydrophilic instead of lipophilic, so they do not readily cross the blood–brain barrier and have little effect on the ACh receptors in the brain.

Nondepolarizing NMJ blockers are metabolized in the serum, although metabolism is dependent on the liver to produce the needed plasma cholinesterases. Most of the metabolites are excreted in the urine.

Each nondepolarizing NMJ blocker differs in terms of time of onset and duration (Fig. 28.3). The drug of choice in any given situation is determined by the procedure being performed, including the estimated time involved.

Contraindications and Cautions

Nondepolarizing NMJ blockers are contraindicated when there is a known allergy, to prevent hypersensitivity reactions. Caution should be used with myasthenia gravis because blocking of the ACh cholinergic receptors aggravates the neuromuscular disease (which results from destruction of the ACh receptor sites) and increases its effects (see Chapter 32); renal or hepatic disease, which could interfere with the metabolism or excretion of these drugs, leading to toxic effects; and pregnancy due to lack of well-controlled studies informing of the risks.

Caution should be used in patients with any family or personal history of **malignant hyperthermia**, a serious adverse effect associated with these drugs that is characterized by extreme muscle rigidity, severe hyperpyrexia (fever), acidosis, and death in some cases, because malignant hyperthermia can occur with the use of these drugs. Caution should also be used in the following circumstances: pulmonary or cardiovascular (CV) dysfunction, which could be exacerbated by the paralysis of the respiratory muscles and resulting changes in perfusion and respiratory function; altered fluid and electrolyte imbalance, which could affect membrane stability and subsequent muscular function; some respiratory conditions that could be made worse by the histamine release associated with some of these agents; and lactation because of the potential for adverse effects on the baby.

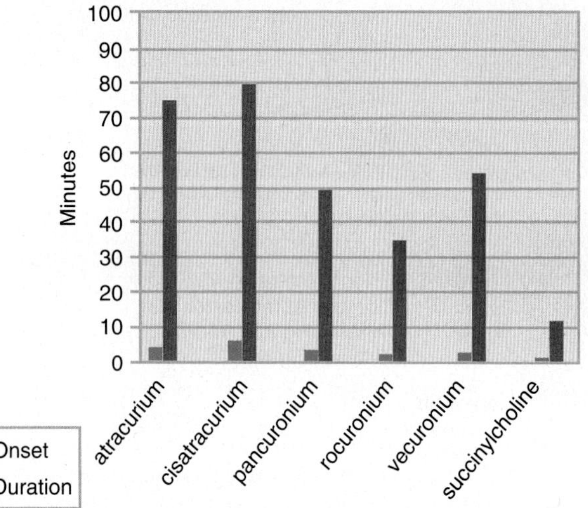

FIGURE 28.3 Onset and duration of neuromuscular junction blockers.

Adverse Effects

The adverse effects related to the use of nondepolarizing NMJ blockers are associated with the paralysis of muscles. Profound and prolonged muscle paralysis is always possible, and patients must be supported until they are able to resume voluntary and involuntary muscle movement. When the respiratory muscles are paralyzed, depressed respiration, bronchospasm, and apnea are anticipated adverse effects. These agents are never used without an anesthesiologist or nurse anesthetist present who can provide assisted ventilatory measures and deliver oxygen under positive pressure. Intubation is an anticipated procedure with these drugs.

The histamine release associated with many of the nondepolarizing NMJ blockers can cause respiratory obstruction with wheezing and bronchospasm. Hypotension and cardiac arrhythmias may occur in patients who do not adapt to the drugs effectively, use the drugs for prolonged periods, have certain underlying conditions, or take certain drugs (e.g., vecuronium) that are known to affect CV receptors. Prolonged drug use may also result in gastrointestinal (GI) dysfunction related to paralysis of the muscles in the GI tract; constipation, vomiting, regurgitation, and aspiration may occur. Pressure ulcers may develop because the patient loses reflex muscle movement that protects the body. Hyperkalemia may occur as a result of muscle membrane alterations.

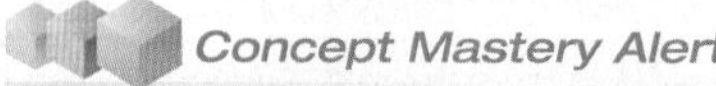

Reversal of Nondepolarizing NMJ Blockers

Neostigmine (*Bloxiverz*) is a cholinesterase inhibitor that can be used to help reverse the effects of nondepolarizing NMJ blockers after surgery. It acts by inhibiting the enzyme cholinesterase, which breaks down acetylcholine. This allows for more acetylcholine to be in the NMJ; therefore, more is able to compete with the nondepolarizing NMJ blocker for muscle receptor sites. This can help to decrease the effect of the medication and allow the person to move.

Clinically Important Drug–Drug Interactions

Many drugs are known to react with the nondepolarizing NMJ blockers. Some drug combinations result in an increased neuromuscular effect. General anesthetics that are commonly used with the NMJ blockers during surgery

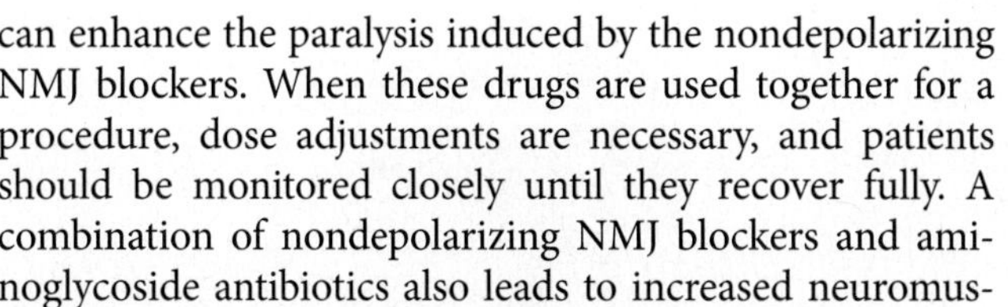

can enhance the paralysis induced by the nondepolarizing NMJ blockers. When these drugs are used together for a procedure, dose adjustments are necessary, and patients should be monitored closely until they recover fully. A combination of nondepolarizing NMJ blockers and aminoglycoside antibiotics also leads to increased neuromuscular blockage. Patients who receive this drug combination require a lower dose of the nondepolarizing NMJ blockers and prolonged support and monitoring after the procedure.

Calcium channel blockers may also increase the paralysis caused by nondepolarizing NMJ blockers because of their effects on the calcium channels in the muscle. If this combination cannot be avoided, the dose of the nondepolarizing NMJ blocker should be lowered, and the patient should be monitored closely until complete recovery occurs.

If nondepolarizing NMJ blockers are combined with cholinesterase inhibitors, the effectiveness of the nondepolarizing NMJ blockers is decreased because of an increase in ACh in the synaptic cleft.

Combination with xanthines (e.g., theophylline, aminophylline) could result in reversal of the neuromuscular blockage. Patients receiving this combination of drugs should be monitored closely during the procedure for the potential of early arousal and return of muscle function.

Do not mix the drug with any alkaline solutions such as barbiturates because a precipitate may form, making it inappropriate for use.

Clinically Important Drug–Herb Interactions

Concurrent use of valerian, melatonin, and kava may cause increased sedation and slower recovery. Assess patients before any procedure for the use of these herbs, and monitor closely during and after the use of the NMJ blocker for any potential recovery issues if the patient reports the use of these herbs.

Prototype Summary: Pancuronium

Indications: As an adjunct to general anesthesia; to induce skeletal muscle relaxation; to reduce the intensity of muscle contractions in electroconvulsive therapy; to facilitate the care of patients undergoing mechanical ventilation.

Actions: Occupies the muscular cholinergic receptor site, preventing ACh from reacting with the receptor; does not cause activation of muscle cells; causes flaccid paralysis.

Pharmacokinetics:

Route	Onset	Duration
IV	4–6 min	120–180 min

$T_{1/2}$: 89 to 161 minutes; metabolized in the tissues; excreted unchanged in the urine.

Adverse Effects: Respiratory depression, apnea, bronchospasm, cardiac arrhythmias.

Depolarizing Neuromuscular Junction Blocker

There is only one agent classified as a depolarizing NMJ blocker: succinylcholine (*Anectine, Quelicin*).

Therapeutic Actions and Indications

Succinylcholine, a depolarizing NMJ blocker, attaches to the ACh receptor site on the muscle cell, causing a prolonged depolarization of the muscle. This depolarization causes stimulation of the muscle and muscle contraction (seen as twitching) and then flaccid paralysis. Both effects cause muscles to stop responding to stimuli, and paralysis occurs.

Succinylcholine has a rapid onset and a short duration of action because it is broken down by cholinesterase in the plasma. Unlike endogenous ACh, however, succinylcholine is not broken down instantly. The result is a prolonged contraction of the muscle, which cannot be restimulated. Eventually, a gradual repolarization occurs as continually stimulated channels in the cell membrane close. Some patients have a genetic predisposition for a prolongation of paralysis (Box 28.2).

Pharmacokinetics

Succinylcholine, like the nondepolarizing NMJ blockers, is metabolized in the serum, although metabolism is dependent on the liver to produce the needed plasma cholinesterases. Patients with hepatic impairment may experience prolonged effects of this drug. Onset of action is usually within 1 minute, and duration of effect is 10 to 12 minutes.

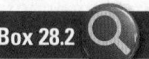

Box 28.2 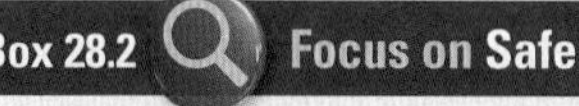 **Focus on Safe Medication Administration**

SUCCINYLCHOLINE AND PARALYSIS

Succinylcholine is broken down in the body by cholinesterase, an enzyme found in the plasma. Some groups of people have a genetic predisposition to low plasma cholinesterase levels. Patients should be asked whether they have or any family member has a history of either low plasma cholinesterase levels or prolonged recovery from anesthetics. Several conditions may also cause the body to produce less of this enzyme, including cirrhosis, metabolic disorders, carcinoma, burns, dehydration, malnutrition, hyperpyrexia, thyrotoxicosis, collagen diseases, and exposure to neurotoxic insecticides. If plasma cholinesterase levels are low, the serum level of succinylcholine will remain elevated, and the paralysis can last much longer than anticipated. These patients need support and ventilation for long periods after surgery.

People who are homozygous for atypical plasma cholinesterase gene are extremely sensitive to the medication effect; they should only be administered succinylcholine in low levels via very slow infusion. Longer times to muscle activity recovery should also be expected, and special care must be taken to monitor their response and to ensure their breathing for an extended postoperative period.

Most of the metabolites are excreted in the urine. Patients with renal impairment may be at risk for increased toxicity from the drugs. Succinylcholine crosses the placenta. Effects on lactation are not known.

Contraindications and Cautions

Some of the contraindications and cautions for succinylcholine are the same as for nondepolarizing NMJ blockers. However, there is a boxed warning regarding use of succinylcholine with pediatric patients. There have been cases of acute rhabdomyolysis with hyperkalemia causing ventricular dysrhythmias, cardiac arrest, and death in some pediatric patients who were found to have undiagnosed skeletal muscle myopathy. Due to this rare but fatal risk, succinylcholine should only be used for pediatrics when emergency intubation is necessary.

Succinylcholine is contraindicated in patients with personal or family history of malignant hyperthermia, skeletal muscle myopathies, or known hypersensitivity to the medication.

In addition, succinylcholine should be used with caution in patients with fractures because the muscle contractions it causes might lead to additional trauma; in patients with narrow-angle glaucoma or penetrating eye injuries because intraocular pressure increases; and in patients with paraplegia or spinal cord injuries, which could cause loss of potassium from the overstimulated cells and hyperkalemia. Extreme caution is necessary in the presence of genetic or disease-related conditions causing low plasma cholinesterase levels, such as cirrhosis, metabolic disorders, carcinoma, burns, dehydration, malnutrition, hyperpyrexia, thyrotoxicosis, collagen diseases, and exposure to neurotoxic insecticides. Low plasma cholinesterase levels may result in prolonged paralysis because succinylcholine is not broken down in the plasma and continues to stimulate the receptor site, leading to a need for prolonged support after use of the drug is discontinued.

Adverse Effects

The adverse effects of succinylcholine are the same as those for nondepolarizing NMJ blockers. In addition, succinylcholine is associated with muscle pain related to the initial muscle contraction reaction. A nondepolarizing NMJ blocker may be given first to prevent some of these contractions and the associated discomfort. Aspirin also alleviates much of this pain after the procedure. Malignant hyperthermia, which may occur in susceptible patients, is a serious condition characterized by massive muscle contraction, sharply elevated body temperature, severe acidosis, and—if uncontrolled—death (Fig. 28.4). This reaction is most likely with succinylcholine, and treatment involves dantrolene (see Chapter 25) to inhibit the muscle effects of the NMJ blocker.

Clinically Important Drug–Drug Interactions

Potential drug–drug interactions for succinylcholine are the same as for the nondepolarizing NMJ blockers.

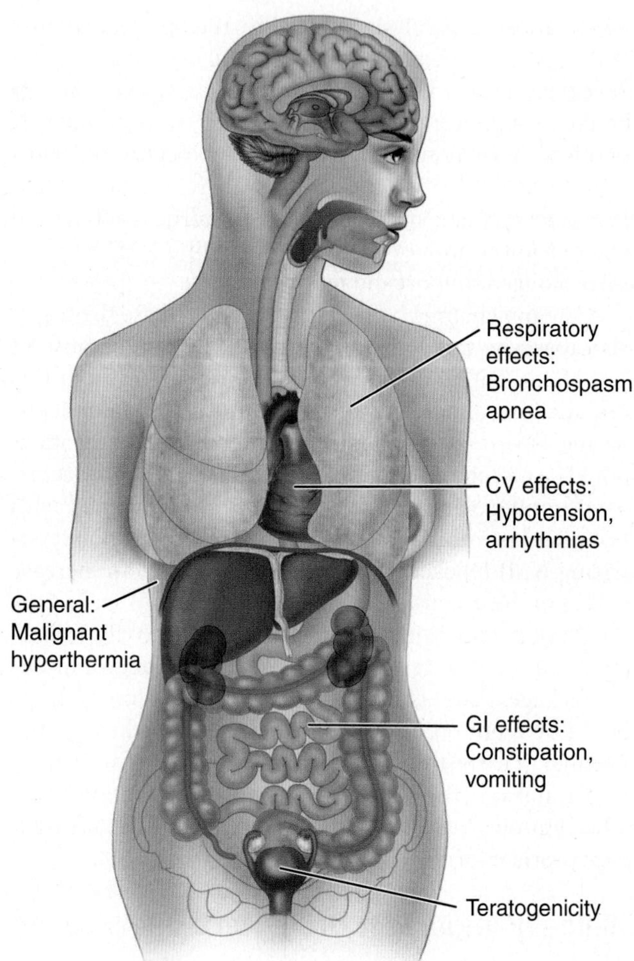

FIGURE 28.4 Common adverse effects associated with neuromuscular junction blockers.

Prototype Summary: Succinylcholine

Indications: As an adjunct to general anesthesia; to facilitate endotracheal intubation; to induce skeletal muscle relaxation during surgery or mechanical ventilation.

Actions: Combines with ACh receptors at the motor endplate to produce depolarization; this inhibits neuromuscular transmission, causing flaccid paralysis.

Pharmacokinetics:

Route	Onset	Duration
IV	30–60 s	4–6 min

$T_{1/2}$: 2 to 3 minutes; metabolized in the tissues; excreted unchanged in the urine.

Adverse Effects: Muscle pain related to the contraction of the muscles as a first reaction; respiratory depression, apnea, hyperkalemia, malignant hyperthermia.

Nursing Considerations for Patients Receiving Neuromuscular Junction Blocking Agents

Assessment: History and Examination

- Assess for contraindications or cautions: any known allergies to these drugs to avoid hypersensitivity reactions; impaired liver or kidney function, which might interfere with metabolism or excretion of the drug; myasthenia gravis, which may be exacerbated by the use of this drug; impaired cardiac or respiratory function, which may be worsened due to the drug's effect on respiratory muscles and changes in perfusion; personal or family history of malignant hyperthermia, which may increase the patient's risk for this condition; fractures, which might lead to additional trauma with administration of succinylcholine; narrow-angle glaucoma because an increase in intraocular pressure can occur with succinylcholine; paraplegia, which might lead to potassium imbalance with administration of succinylcholine; and current status of pregnancy or lactation.
- Perform a physical assessment before beginning therapy to establish baseline status and any potential adverse effects.
- Assess the patient's neurological status, including level of orientation, affect, reflexes, pupil size and reactivity, and muscle tone and response, to monitor drug effects and recovery.
- Monitor respiratory rate and auscultate lung sounds for evidence of adventitious sounds to evaluate effects on respiratory muscles and monitor for adverse reactions.
- Monitor vital signs, including temperature, pulse rate, and blood pressure, to identify changes.
- Auscultate the abdomen for evidence of bowel sounds to monitor effects on GI muscles and recovery.
- Inspect the skin for color and evidence of pressure areas or breakdown, which could result when movement ceases.
- Monitor the results of laboratory tests, including liver function tests, to determine the need for possible dose adjustment, and serum electrolyte levels to determine potential cautions to the use of the drugs.

Refer to the "Critical Thinking Scenario" for a full discussion of nursing care for an older patient who is receiving succinylcholine.

Nursing Conclusions

Nursing conclusions related to drug therapy may include the following:

- Impaired gas exchange related to depressed muscle function for respiration
- Impaired skin integrity related to immobility from prolonged drug effects
- Impaired verbal communication related to effects on muscle activity
- Fear related to paralysis
- Injury risk related to loss of muscle control
- Acute muscle pain related to prolonged muscle contraction with succinylcholine use
- Knowledge deficit regarding drug therapy

Planning

- The patient will receive the best therapeutic effect from the drug therapy.
- The patient will have limited adverse effects to the drug therapy.
- The patient will have an understanding of the drug therapy, adverse effects to anticipate, and measures to relieve discomfort and improve safety.

Intervention With Rationale

- Be aware that administration of the drug should be performed by trained personnel (usually an anesthesiologist) because of the potential for serious adverse effects and the need for immediate ventilatory support.
- Ensure that emergency supplies and equipment are readily available to maintain airway and provide mechanical ventilation.
- Do not mix the drug with any alkaline solutions such as barbiturates because a precipitate may form, making it inappropriate for use.
- If the drug is being given over a long period, test patient response and recovery periodically to maintain mechanical ventilation. Discontinue the drug if response does not occur or is greatly delayed.
- Monitor patient temperature for prompt detection and treatment of malignant hyperthermia; have dantrolene readily available for treatment of malignant hyperthermia if it should occur.
- Arrange for a small dose of a nondepolarizing NMJ blocker before the use of succinylcholine to reduce the adverse effects associated with muscle contraction.
- Ensure that a cholinesterase inhibitor is readily available to overcome excessive neuromuscular blockade caused by nondepolarizing NMJ blockers.
- Have a peripheral nerve stimulator on standby to assess the degree of neuromuscular blockade, if appropriate.
- Provide comfort measures to help the patient tolerate drug effects, such as pain relief as appropriate; reassurance, support, and orientation for conscious patients unable to move or communicate; skin care and turning to prevent skin breakdown; and supportive care for emergencies such as hypotension and bronchospasm.
- Monitor patient response closely (blood pressure, temperature, pulse, respiration, reflexes) to determine

(continues on page 496)

effectiveness; expect dose adjustment to ensure the greatest therapeutic effect with minimal risk of toxicity.
- Provide thorough patient preoperative teaching about this drug because most patients who receive the drug will be receiving teaching about a particular procedure and will be unconscious when the drug is given. Teaching includes drug to be given, method for administration, effects of the drug (i.e., what to expect), and safety precautions.
- Offer support and encouragement to help the patient cope with drug effects.

Evaluation

- Monitor patient response to the drug (adequate muscle paralysis).
- Monitor for adverse effects (respiratory depression, hypotension, bronchospasm, GI slowdown, skin breakdown, fear related to helplessness and inability to communicate).
- Evaluate effectiveness of the teaching plan (the patient can relate anticipated effects of the drug and the recovery process).
- Monitor the effectiveness of comfort measures and adherence to the regimen.

Key Points

- Nondepolarizing NMJ blockers prevent ACh from exciting the muscle, and paralysis ensues because the muscle cannot respond.
- The depolarizing NMJ blocker, succinylcholine, causes muscle paralysis by acting like ACh. It excites (depolarizes) the muscle and prevents repolarization and further stimulation.

CRITICAL THINKING SCENARIO
Using Succinylcholine in an Older Adult Patient

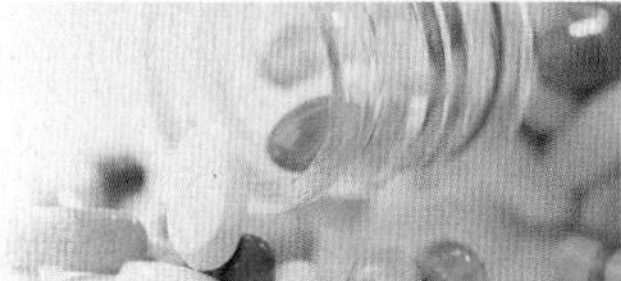

THE SITUATION

S.N., an 82-year-old patient in good health, has been admitted to the hospital for an exploratory laparotomy to evaluate a probable abdominal mass. On admission, health care practitioners learned that S.N. had a history of mild hypertension that was well regulated by diuretic therapy. They received a baseline physical examination and preoperative instruction. On the morning of the surgery, it was noted that the anesthesiologist planned to give S.N. a general anesthetic and succinylcholine to ensure muscle paralysis.

CRITICAL THINKING

What areas must be considered for S.N.? Consider the patient's age and associated chronic problems that often occur with aging. Also consider the support that S.N. has available and potential physical and emotional support that they might need before and after this procedure. Use of an NMJ blocker in older adult patients brings some nursing challenges that may not be seen with younger patients.

What particular nursing care activities should be considered with S.N.? Because S.N. has been maintained on long-term diuretic therapy, they are at special risk for electrolyte imbalance.

What, if any, complications could arise if S.N. has electrolyte disturbances before surgery?

DISCUSSION

Before surgery, the preoperative teaching protocol should be reviewed with the patient. S.N. should be advised that they may experience back and neck pain secondary to the muscle contractions caused by succinylcholine and throat pain after the procedure. Reassure S.N. that this is normal and that a medication will be made available to alleviate the discomfort. Review deep breathing and coughing; S.N. may need encouragement to clear secretions from their lungs and ensure full inflation. This is usually easier to do if it is a familiar activity. S.N.'s serum electrolytes should be evaluated before surgery because potassium imbalance can cause unexpected effects with succinylcholine. Renal and hepatic function tests should also be performed to ensure that the dose of the NMJ blocker is not excessive.

During the procedure, S.N.'s cardiac and respiratory status should be monitored carefully for any potential problems; such effects are more common in people with underlying physical problems. Because of S.N.'s age and potential circulatory problems, they should receive meticulous skin care and turning as soon as the procedure allows this kind of movement. S.N. should be turned frequently during the recovery period, and their skin should be checked for any breakdown. Nursing personnel must remain close by the patient until they have regained muscle control and the ability to communicate. S.N. should be evaluated for the need of pain medication and position adjustments.

S.N. will require additional teaching about their diagnosis and potential treatment. This should wait until S.N. has regained full ability to communicate and is able to respond and participate in any discussion that may be held. At that time, S.N. may require emotional support and encouragement. It may be necessary to contact available family or social service agencies regarding S.N.'s physical and medical needs.

NURSING CARE GUIDE FOR S.N.: SUCCINYLCHOLINE

Assessment: History and Examination

Assess allergies to the drug, and assess for history of respiratory or cardiac disorders, myasthenia gravis, hepatic or renal dysfunction, fractures, and glaucoma

Concurrent use of aminoglycosides or calcium channel blockers

Focus the physical examination on the following:

CV: Blood pressure, pulse rate, peripheral perfusion, and electrocardiogram

CNS: Orientation, affect, reflexes, and vision

Skin: Color, lesions, texture, and sweating

Genitourinary: Urinary output and bladder tone

GI: Abdominal examination

Respiratory: Respirations and adventitious sounds

Nursing Conclusions

Impaired gas exchange related to depressed respirations

Risk for impaired skin integrity related to immobility

Pain related to prolonged muscle contractions with succinylcholine use

Knowledge deficit regarding drug therapy

Impaired verbal communication due to paralysis and inability to communicate

Planning

The patient will receive the best therapeutic effect from the drug therapy.

The patient will have limited adverse effects to the drug therapy.

The patient will have an understanding of the drug therapy, adverse effects to anticipate, and measures to relieve discomfort and improve safety.

Intervention

Provide comfort and safety measures: positioning, skin care, temperature control, pain medication as needed, maintenance of airway, ventilating patient, antidotes on standby.

Provide support and reassurance to deal with paralysis and inability to communicate.

Provide patient teaching about the procedure being performed and what to expect.

Assist with life support as needed.

Evaluation

Evaluate drug effects: muscle paralysis.

Monitor for adverse effects: CV effects (tachycardia, hypotension, respiratory distress, increased respiratory secretions), GI effects (constipation, nausea), skin breakdown, anxiety, and fear.

Monitor for drug–drug interactions as indicated.

Evaluate the effectiveness of the patient teaching program and comfort and safety measures.

Constantly monitor vital signs and watch for return of normal muscular function.

PATIENT TEACHING FOR S.N.

- Before the surgery is performed, you will be given a drug to paralyze your muscles. This drug is called a neuromuscular blocking agent. It is important that your muscles do not move at this time because it could interfere with the procedure.
- Common effects of these drugs include complete paralysis:
  - You will not be able to move or to speak while you are receiving this drug.
  - You will not be able to breathe on your own, and you will receive mechanical assistance in breathing.
- This drug may not affect your level of consciousness, and it can be frightening to be unable to communicate with anyone around you. Someone will be with you, will try to anticipate your needs, and will explain what is going on at all times.
- This drug may have no effect on your pain perception. Every effort will be made to make sure that you do not experience pain.
- You will be receiving succinylcholine; with this drug, you may experience back and throat pain related to muscle contractions that occur. You will be able to take medication to relieve this discomfort, and a warm compress may also help.
- Recovery of your muscle function may take 2 to 3 hours, and someone will be nearby at all times until you have recovered from the paralysis.

SUMMARY

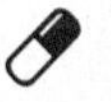
The nerves communicate with muscles at a point called the NMJ, using ACh as the neurotransmitter.

NMJ blockers interfere with muscle function. The two groups of NMJ blockers are nondepolarizing agents and a single depolarizing agent.

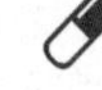
The nondepolarizing NMJ blockers include those agents that act as antagonists to ACh at the NMJ and prevent depolarization of muscle cells. The depolarizing NMJ blocker acts as an ACh agonist at the junction, causing stimulation of the muscle cell, and then prevents it from repolarizing.

- NMJ blockers are primarily used as adjuncts to general anesthesia to facilitate endotracheal intubation, to facilitate mechanical ventilation, and to prevent injury during electroconvulsive therapy.
- Adverse effects of NMJ blockers, such as prolonged paralysis, inability to breathe, weakness, muscle pain and soreness, and effects of immobility, are related to muscle function blocking.

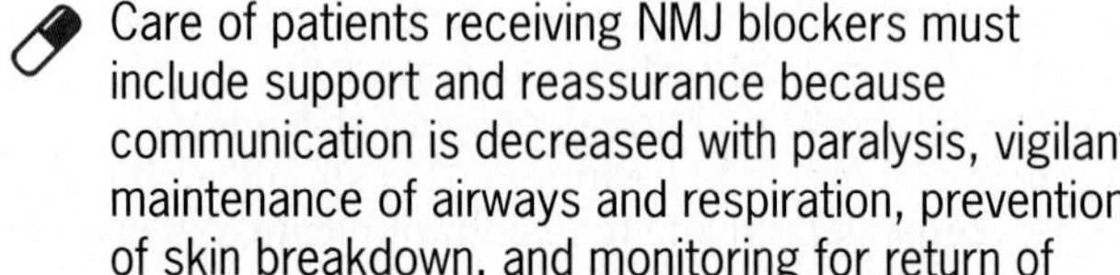

- Care of patients receiving NMJ blockers must include support and reassurance because communication is decreased with paralysis, vigilant maintenance of airways and respiration, prevention of skin breakdown, and monitoring for return of function.

CHECK YOUR UNDERSTANDING

***Answers to the questions in this chapter can be found in Answers to Check Your Understanding Questions on** thePoint®.*

MULTIPLE CHOICE

Select the best answer.

1. Nondepolarizing NMJ blockers
   a. antagonize ACh to prevent depolarization of muscle cells.
   b. act as agonists of ACh, leading to depolarization of muscle cells.
   c. prevent the repolarization of muscle cells.
   d. are associated with painful muscle contractions on administration.

2. Which of the following is correct about the NMJ blockers?
   a. Can routinely be administered to pediatric patients
   b. Decrease pain by blocking ACh
   c. Have very short half-lives
   d. Can cause respiratory arrest

3. Succinylcholine has a more rapid onset of action and a shorter duration of activity than the nondepolarizing NMJ blockers because it
   a. does not bind well to receptor sites.
   b. rapidly crosses the blood–brain barrier and is lost.
   c. is broken down by acetylcholinesterase that is found in the plasma.
   d. is very unstable.

4. When planning the care of a patient who is to receive an NMJ blocker, the nurse would expect which about the patient?
   a. Transfer to an intensive care unit will be essential.
   b. Intubation will be necessary to maintain respirations.
   c. The patient will have no memory of any events.
   d. No adverse effects will occur after the drug is stopped.

5. Malignant hyperthermia can occur with any NMJ blocker, but it most often occurs with succinylcholine. The nurse would expect to see which drug ordered?
   a. Phenobarbital
   b. Pancuronium
   c. Dantrolene
   d. Diazepam

6. Patient recovery from an NMJ blocker
   a. is predictable based on the drug given.
   b. can be affected by genetic enzyme deficiency.
   c. is always ensured because of the drug half-life.
   d. can be shortened by administration of oxygen.

7. When preparing NMJ blockers for administration, it is important that they are not
   a. mixed in with any alkaline solutions.
   b. exposed to light.
   c. mixed with any other drug.
   d. combined with heparin.

MULTIPLE RESPONSE

Select all that apply.

1. The nurse would expect administration of an NMJ blocker as the drug of choice to accomplish which actions?
   a. Facilitate endotracheal intubation.
   b. Facilitate mechanical ventilation.
   c. Prevent injury during electroconvulsive therapy.
   d. Relieve pain during labor and delivery.
   e. Treat myasthenia gravis.
   f. Treat a patient with a history of malignant hyperthermia.

REFERENCES

Brunton, L., Hilal-Dandan, R., & Knollman, B. (2018). *Goodman and Gilman's the pharmacological basis of therapeutics* (13th ed.). McGraw-Hill.

Gibbs, N. M. (2012). Risks of anesthesia and surgery in elderly patients. *Journal of Anesthesia and Intensive Care, 40*(1), 14–16. https://doi.org/10.1177/0310057X1204000103

Hall, J. E. (2018). *Guyton and Hall textbook of medical physiology* (13th ed.). Elsevier.

Hendler, C. B. (Ed.). (2021). *Nursing 2021 drug handbook.* Wolters Kluwer.

Kaye, A. D., Mahakian, T., Kaye, A. J., Pham, A. A., Hart, B. M., Gennuso, S., Cornett, E. M., Gabriel, R. A., & Urman, R. D. (2016). Pharmacogenomics, precision medicine, and implications for anesthesia care. *Best Practice and Research Clinical Anaesthesiol, 32*, 61–81. https://doi.org/10.1016/j.bpa.2018.07.001

Miller, R. D., & Pardo, M. (2011). *Basics of anesthesia* (6th ed.). Saunders.

Nagelhout, J. J., & Plaus, K. (2013). *Nurse anesthesia* (5th ed.). Saunders.

Norris, T. L. (2019). *Porth's pathophysiology concepts of altered health states* (13th ed.). Wolters Kluwer.

Rosenberg, H., Davis, M., James, D., Pollock, N., & Stowell, K. (2007). Malignant hyperthermia. *Orphanet Journal of Rare Diseases, 2*(21), 21. https://doi.org/10.1186/1750-1172-2-21

Wadlund, D. L. (2006). Prevention, recognition and management of nursing complications in the intraoperative and postoperative surgical patient. *Nursing Clinics of North America, 41*, 219–229. 10.1016/j.cnur.2006.01.005

PART 5

Drugs Acting on the Autonomic Nervous System

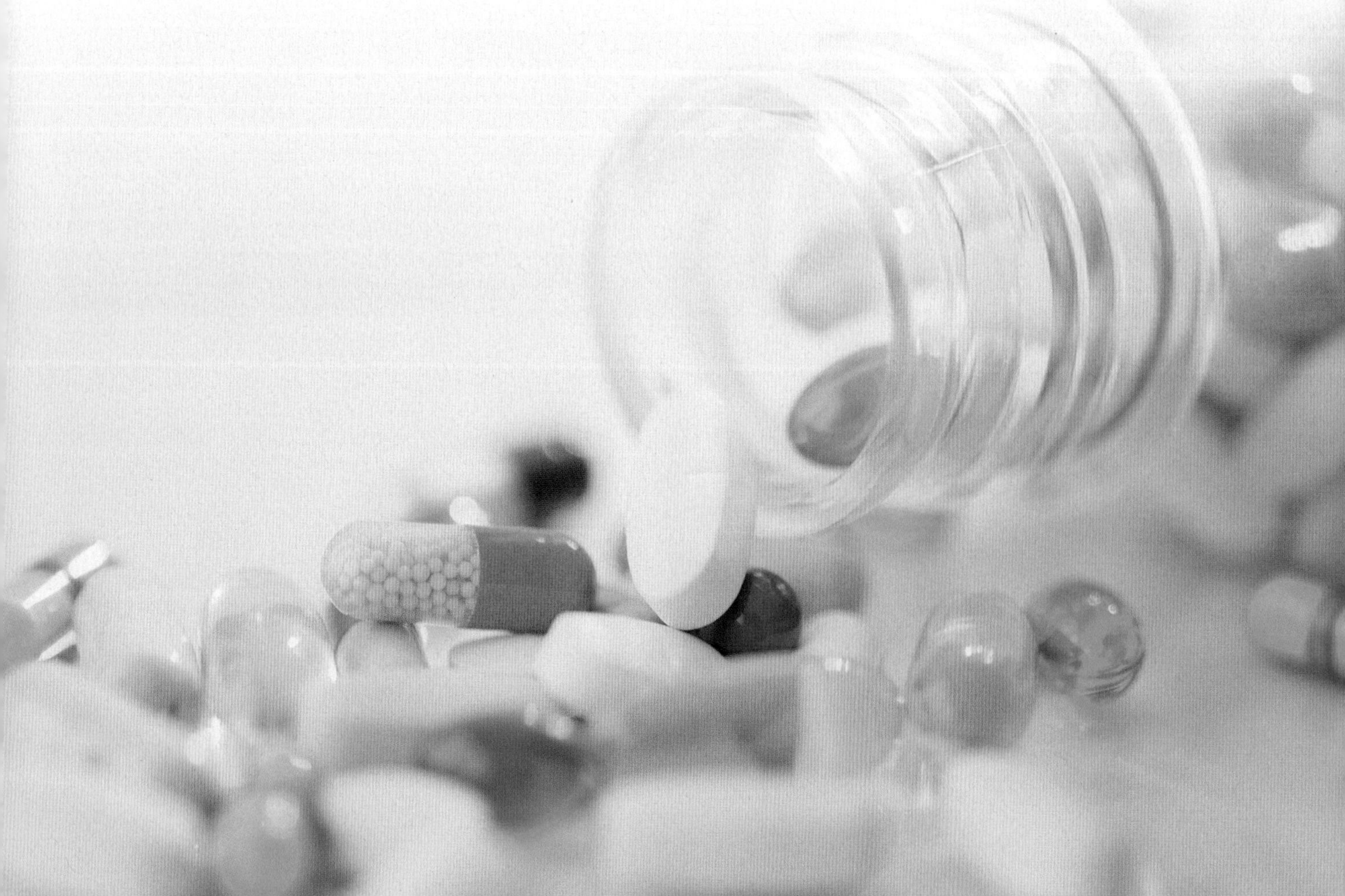

CHAPTER 29

Introduction to the Autonomic Nervous System

Learning Objectives

Upon completion of this chapter, you will be able to:

1. Describe how the autonomic nervous system differs anatomically from the rest of the nervous system.
2. Outline a sympathetic response and the clinical manifestation of this response.
3. Describe the alpha- and beta-receptors found within the sympathetic nervous system by sites and actions that follow the stimulation of each kind of receptor.
4. Outline the events that occur with stimulation of the parasympathetic nervous system.
5. Define the terms muscarinic receptor and nicotinic receptor, giving an example of each.

Key Terms

acetylcholinesterase: enzyme responsible for the immediate breakdown of acetylcholine when released from the nerve ending; prevents overstimulation of cholinergic receptor sites

adrenergic receptors: receptor sites on effectors that respond to norepinephrine/epinephrine

alpha-receptors: adrenergic receptors that are found in smooth muscles of blood vessels, the eyes, and a variety of other organs

autonomic nervous system (ANS): portion of the central and peripheral nervous systems that, with the endocrine system, functions to maintain internal homeostasis

beta-receptors: adrenergic receptors that are found in the heart, lungs, bladder, uterus, and vascular smooth muscle

cholinergic receptors: receptor sites on effectors that respond to acetylcholine

ganglia: groups of closely packed nerve cell bodies

monoamine oxidase: enzyme that breaks down norepinephrine, dopamine, and serotonin to make them inactive

muscarinic receptors: cholinergic receptors that are stimulated by postganglionic nerves; located in visceral effector organs such as the GI tract, bladder, and heart; in sweat glands; and in some vascular smooth muscle

nicotinic receptors: cholinergic receptors that respond to stimulation by nicotine; located between pre- and postganglionic nerves and also at the neuromuscular junctions

parasympathetic nervous system (PNS): contains central nervous system (CNS) cells from the cranium or sacral area of the spinal cord, long preganglionic axons, ganglia near or within the effector tissue, and short postganglionic axons that react with cholinergic receptors; responsible for most unconscious actions; sometimes called the "rest-and-digest" or "feed-and-breed" system

sympathetic nervous system (SNS): composed of CNS cells from the thoracic or lumbar areas, short preganglionic axons, ganglia near the spinal cord, and long postganglionic axons that react primarily with adrenergic receptors; functions as the antagonist of the parasympathetic system; and prepares the body to respond to stress; sometimes called the "fight-or-flight" system.

The **autonomic nervous system** (ANS) is sometimes called the involuntary or visceral nervous system because it mostly functions with the person having little conscious awareness of its activity. Working closely with the endocrine system, the ANS helps regulate and integrate the body's internal functions within a relatively narrow average range on a minute-to-minute basis. The ANS integrates parts of the central nervous system (CNS) and peripheral nervous system to automatically react to changes in the internal and external environments (Fig. 29.1).

Structure and Function of the Autonomic Nervous System

The main nerve centers for the ANS are located in the hypothalamus, the medulla, and the spinal cord. Nerve impulses that arise in peripheral structures are carried to these centers by afferent nerve fibers. These integrating centers in the CNS respond by sending out efferent impulses along the autonomic nerve pathways. These impulses adjust the functioning of various internal organs in ways that keep the body's internal environment constant or homeostatic.

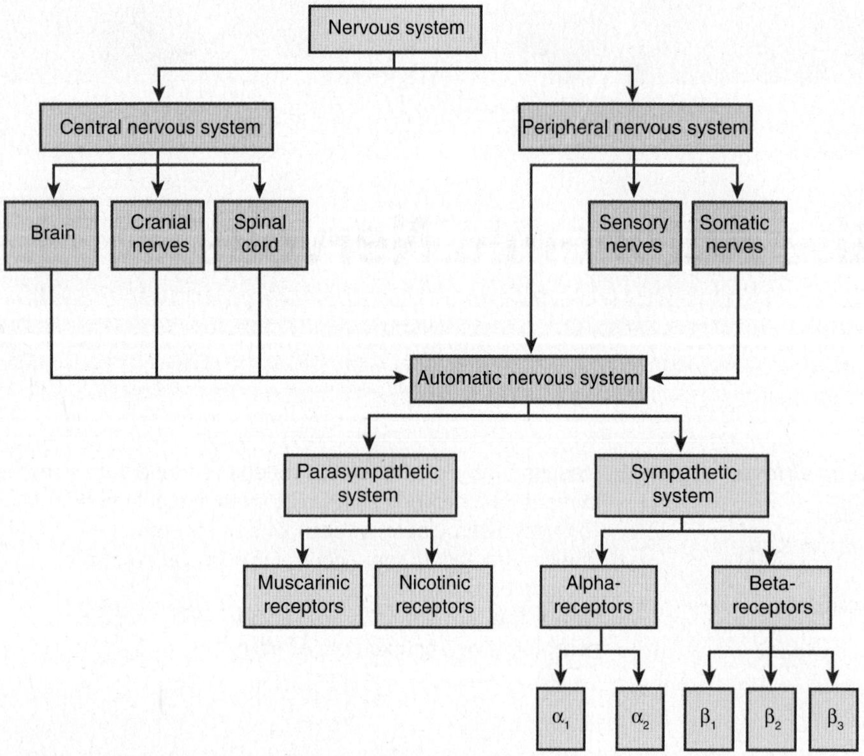

Nervous system
Central nervous system
Peripheral nervous system
Brain
Cranial nerves
Spinal cord
Sensory nerves
Somatic nerves
Automatic nervous system
Parasympathetic system
Sympathetic system
Muscarinic receptors
Nicotinic receptors
Alpha-receptors
Beta-receptors
α_1 α_2 β_1 β_2 β_3

FIGURE 29.1 Organization of the nervous system.

Nerve Impulse Transmission

Throughout the ANS, nerve impulses are carried from the CNS to the outlying organs by way of a two-neuron system. In most peripheral nervous system activities, the CNS nerve body sends an impulse directly to an effector organ or muscle. The ANS does not send impulses directly to the periphery. Instead, axons from CNS neurons end in **ganglia**, or groups of nerve cell bodies that are packed together, located outside of the CNS. These ganglia receive information from the preganglionic neuron that started in the CNS and relay that information along postganglionic neurons. The postganglionic neurons transmit impulses to the neuroeffector cells—muscles, glands, and organs.

Functions

The ANS works to regulate blood pressure, heart rate, respiration, body temperature, water balance, urinary excretion, and digestive functions, among other things. This system exerts minute-to-minute control of body responses, which is balanced by the two divisions of the ANS.

Divisions

The ANS is divided into two branches: the **sympathetic nervous system** (SNS) and the **parasympathetic nervous system** (PNS). These two branches differ in three basic ways: (a) the location of the originating cells in the CNS, (b) the location of the nerve ganglia, and (c) the preganglionic and postganglionic neurons (Table 29.1 and Fig. 29.2).

Table 29.1 Comparison of the Sympathetic and Parasympathetic Nervous Systems

Characteristic	Sympathetic	Parasympathetic
CNS nerve origin	Thoracic, lumbar spinal cord	Cranium, sacral spinal cord
Preganglionic neuron	Short axon	Long axon
Preganglionic neurotransmitter	ACh	ACh
Ganglia location	Next to spinal cord	Within or near effector organs
Postganglionic neuron	Long axon	Short axon
Postganglionic neurotransmitter	Norepinephrine, epinephrine	ACh
Neurotransmitter terminator	MAO, COMT	Acetylcholinesterase
General response	Fight-or-flight	Rest-and-digest

CNS, central nervous system; ACh, acetylcholine; MAO, monoamine oxidase; COMT, catechol-*O*-methyltransferase.

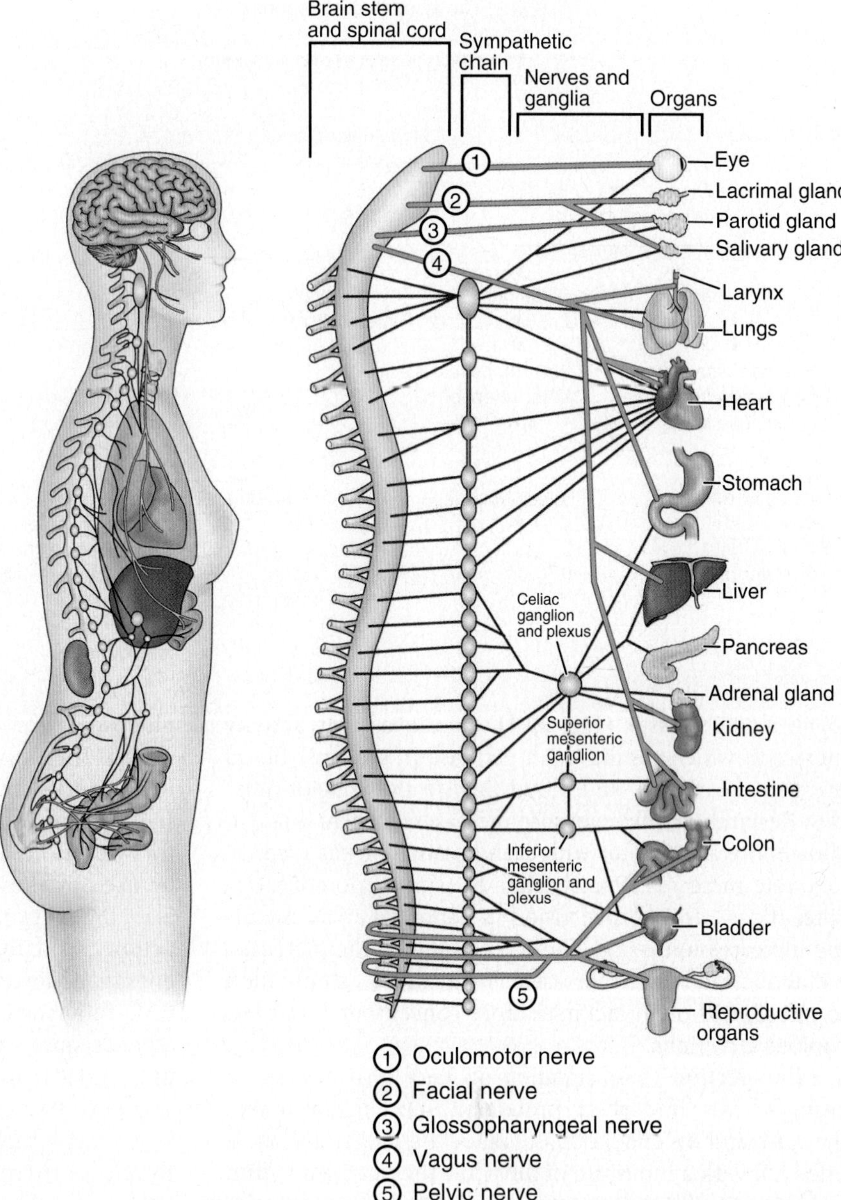

FIGURE 29.2 The autonomic nervous system. The sympathetic, or thoracolumbar, division sends relatively short preganglionic fibers to the chains of paravertebral ganglia and to certain outlying ganglia. The second cell, or postganglionic cell, sends relatively long postganglionic fibers to the organs it innervates. The parasympathetic, or craniosacral, division sends long preganglionic fibers that synapse with a second nerve cell in ganglia located close to or within the organs that are then innervated by short postganglionic fibers.

Sympathetic Nervous System

The SNS is sometimes referred to as the "fight-or-flight" system or the system responsible for preparing the body to respond to stress. Stress can be either internal, such as cell injury or death, or external, such as a perceived or learned reaction to various external situations or stimuli. For the most part, the SNS acts much like an accelerator, speeding things up for action.

Structure and Function

The SNS is also called the thoracolumbar system because the CNS cells that originate impulses for this system are located in the thoracic and lumbar sections of the spinal cord. These cells send out short preganglionic fibers that synapse or communicate with nerve ganglia located in chains running alongside the spinal cord. Acetylcholine (ACh) is the neurotransmitter released by these preganglionic nerves. The nerve ganglia, in turn, send out long postganglionic fibers that synapse with neuroeffectors, using primarily norepinephrine or epinephrine as the neurotransmitter. The exceptions are that the postganglionic sympathetic nerve fibers that innervate the sweat glands, and a few blood vessels, secrete ACh. One of the sympathetic ganglia, on either side of the spinal cord, does not develop postganglionic axons but produces norepinephrine and epinephrine, which are secreted directly into the bloodstream. These ganglia have evolved into the adrenal medullae. When the SNS is stimulated, the chromaffin cells of the adrenal medullae secrete epinephrine and norepinephrine directly into the bloodstream.

When stimulated, the SNS works in conjunction with the endocrine system to prepare the body respond

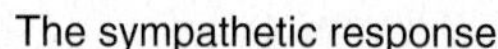

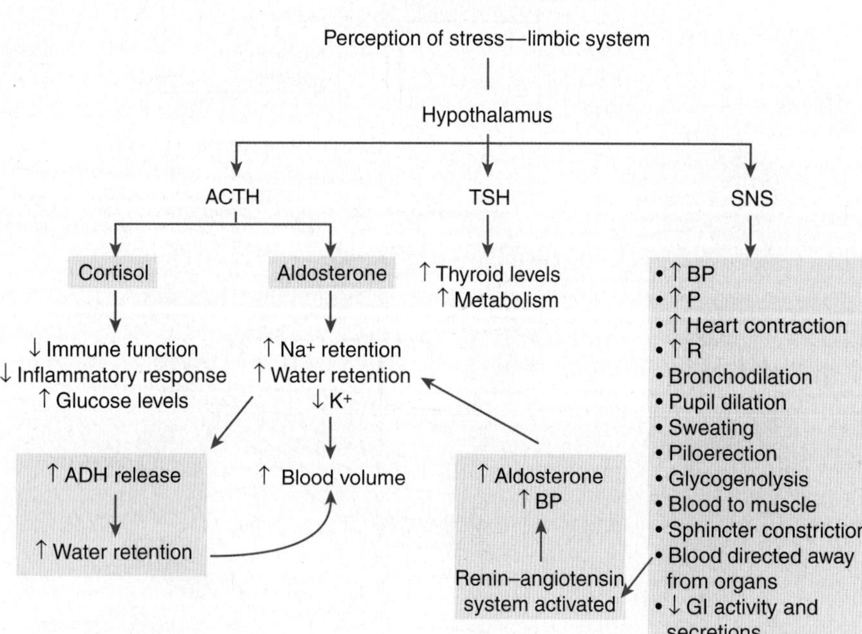

FIGURE 29.3 The acute stress or "fight-or-flight" response. The sympathetic stress reaction. ACTH, adrenocorticotropic hormone; ADH, antidiuretic hormone; BP, blood pressure; GI, gastrointestinal; P, pulse; R, respiratory rate; SNS, sympathetic nervous system; TSH, thyroid-stimulating hormone.

to an acute stressor (Fig. 29.3). Cardiovascular activity increases, which results in an increase in systemic blood pressure, heart rate, and blood flow to the skeletal muscles. Respiratory efficiency also increases; bronchi dilate to allow more air to enter with each breath, and the respiratory rate increases. Pupils dilate to permit more light to enter the eye to improve vision in darkened areas. Sweating increases to dissipate heat generated by the increased metabolic activity. Increased sympathetic stimulation to glands will often facilitate more concentrated and less copious secretions.

Piloerection (hair standing on end) also occurs. In animals, this important protection mechanism makes the fur stand on end so that an attacking larger animal is often left with a mouthful of fur while the intended victim scurries away. The actual benefit to humans is not known, except that this activity helps generate heat when the core body temperature is too low.

Stimulation of the SNS causes blood to be diverted away from the gastrointestinal (GI) tract because there is no real need to digest food when responding to an acute stressor. Subsequently, bowel sounds decrease and digestion slows dramatically; sphincters are constricted, and bowel evacuation is less likely to occur. Blood is also diverted away from other internal organs, including the kidneys, resulting in activation of the renin-angiotensin-aldosterone system (Chapter 42) and a further increase in blood pressure and blood volume as water is retained by the kidneys. Sphincters in the urinary bladder are also constricted, precluding urination.

Several other metabolic activities occur that prepare the body to respond to an acute stressor. For example, glucose is formed by glycogenolysis to increase blood glucose levels and provide energy. The hypothalamus causes the secretion of adrenocorticotropic hormone, leading to a release of the adrenal hormones, including cortisol, which suppress the immune and inflammatory reactions to preserve energy that otherwise might be used by these activities. The corticosteroid hormones also block protein production, another energy-saving activity, and increase the release of glucose to provide energy. Aldosterone, also released with adrenal stimulation, retains sodium and water and causes the excretion of potassium in the urine. This will increase blood volume and also usually increases blood pressure. The hypothalamus also causes the release of thyrotropin-releasing hormone, which stimulates the anterior pituitary gland to release thyroid-stimulating hormone. Thyroid-stimulating hormone facilitates the thyroid gland to produce and release thyroid hormone, which increases metabolism and the efficient use of energy. Together, all of these activities prepare the body to respond to an acute stressor more effectively. When overstimulated or when responding to chronic stress, however, they can lead to system overload and a variety of disorders.

Concept Mastery Alert

Acute Stress Response

Norepinephrine and epinephrine are the primary neurotransmitters that illicit the acute stress response. Aldosterone is secreted during the acute stress response and retains sodium and water; it causes the excretion of potassium in the urine. Cortisol, a corticosteroid hormone, is responsible for suppressing the immune system's inflammatory response.

Adrenergic Response

Sympathetic postganglionic nerves that synthesize, store, and release norepinephrine are referred to as adrenergic nerves. Adrenergic nerves are also found within the CNS. The chromaffin cells of the adrenal medulla also are adrenergic because they synthesize, store, and release norepinephrine as well as epinephrine.

Norepinephrine Synthesis and Storage

Norepinephrine belongs to a group of structurally related chemicals called catecholamines that also includes dopamine, serotonin, and epinephrine. Norepinephrine is made by the nerve cells using tyrosine, which is obtained in the diet. Dihydroxyphenylalanine (DOPA) is produced by a nerve, using tyrosine from the diet and other chemicals. With the help of the enzyme DOPA decarboxylase, the DOPA is converted to dopamine, which in turn is converted to norepinephrine in adrenergic cells. The norepinephrine then is stored in granules or storage vesicles within the cell. These vesicles move down the nerve axon to the terminals of the axon, where they line up along the cell membrane. To be an adrenergic nerve, the nerve must contain all of the enzymes and building blocks necessary to produce norepinephrine (Fig. 29.4). In the adrenal medulla, about 80% of the norepinephrine is converted to epinephrine to be released in the bloodstream.

Norepinephrine Release

When the nerve is stimulated, the action potential travels down the nerve axon and arrives at the axon terminal (see Chapter 19). The action potential depolarizes the axon membrane. This action allows calcium into the nerve, causing the membrane to contract and the storage vesicles to fuse with the cell membrane, releasing their load of norepinephrine into the synaptic gap or cleft. The norepinephrine travels across the very short gap to specific adrenergic receptor sites on the effector cell on the other side of the synaptic gap.

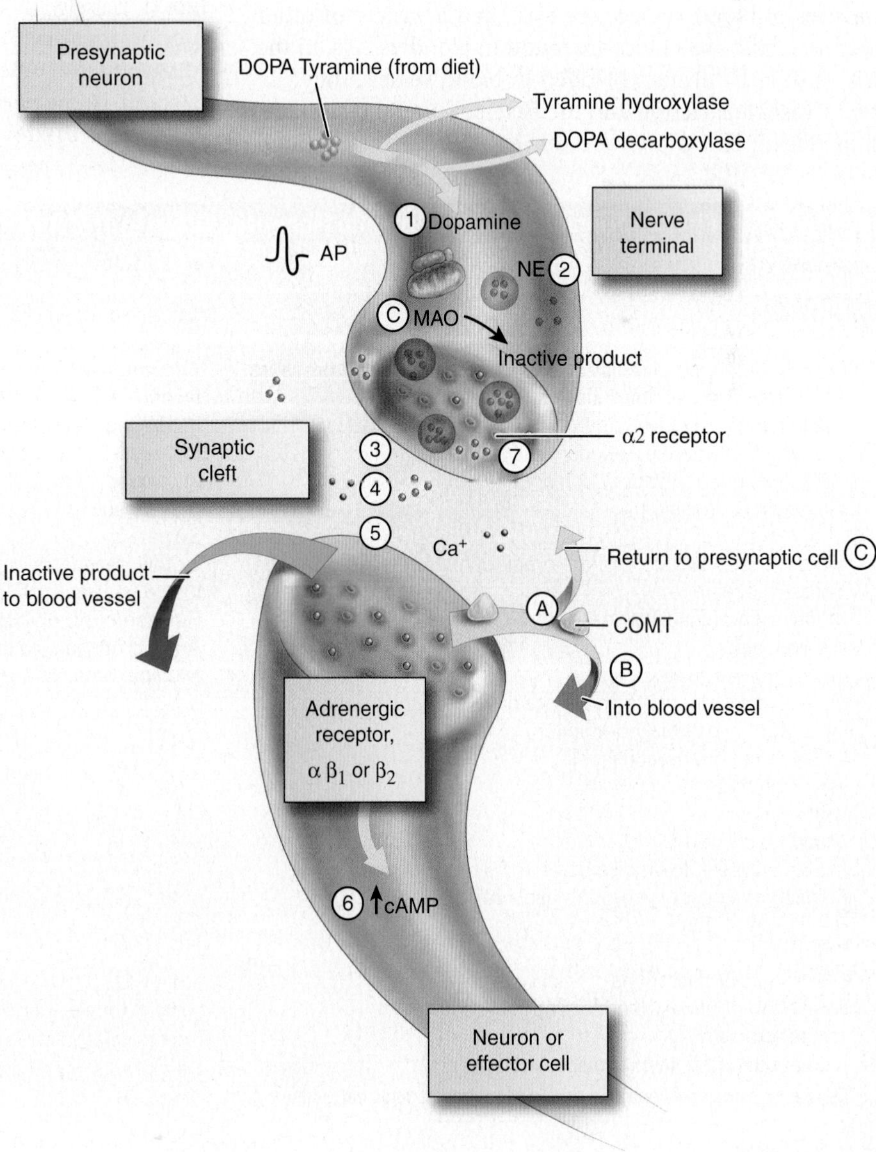

FIGURE 29.4 Sequence of events at an adrenergic synapse. (*1*) Dopamine, a precursor of norepinephrine (*NE*), is synthesized from tyrosine in several steps. (*2*) Dopamine is taken into the storage vesicle and converted to NE. (*3*) Release of neurotransmitter by an action potential (*AP*) in the presynaptic nerve. (*4*) Diffusion of neurotransmitter across synaptic cleft. (*5*) Combination of neurotransmitter with receptor. The events resulting from NE's occupation of receptor sites depend on the nature of the postsynaptic cell. (*6*) Interaction of NE with many beta-receptors leads to increased synthesis of cyclic adenosine monophosphate (*cAMP*). (*7*) Feedback control at alpha$_2$-receptor leads to decreased NE relapse from presynaptic neuron. Deactivation of NE occurs by breakdown of NE by the enzyme catechol-*O*-methyltransferase (*COMT*) (*A*) or more importantly by reuptake into the presynaptic neuron (*C*) where it may be reused or inactivated by another enzyme, monoamine oxidase (*MAO*). Some of the neurotransmitter may also diffuse away from the synaptic cleft (*B*).

Adrenergic Receptors

Adrenergic receptors have receptor sites on effectors that respond to norepinephrine and epinephrine. These receptor sites can be stimulated by the neurotransmitter released from the axon in the immediate vicinity, and they can be further stimulated by circulating norepinephrine and epinephrine secreted directly into the bloodstream by the adrenal medulla. The receptor sites that react with neurotransmitters at adrenergic sites have been classified as alpha-receptors and beta-receptors. These receptors are further classified as $alpha_1$-, $alpha_2$-, $beta_1$-, $beta_2$-, and $beta_3$-receptors (Table 29.2). It is thought that receptors may respond to different concentrations of norepinephrine or different ratios of norepinephrine and epinephrine. Different drugs that are known to affect the SNS may affect parts of the sympathetic response but not all of it, because they are designed to stimulate specific adrenergic receptors.

Alpha-Receptors

Alpha-receptors are adrenergic receptors found in smooth muscles of blood vessels, the eyes, and a variety of other organs. $Alpha_1$-receptors are found in blood vessels, in the iris, and in the urinary bladder. In blood vessels, they can cause vasoconstriction and increase peripheral resistance, thus raising blood pressure. In the iris, they cause pupil dilation. In the urinary bladder, they cause the increased closure of the internal sphincter.

$Alpha_2$-receptors are located on presynaptic nerve membranes and act as modulators of norepinephrine release. When norepinephrine is released from a nerve ending, it crosses the synaptic cleft to react with its specific receptor site. Some of it also flows back to react with the alpha-receptor on the nerve membrane. This causes a reflex decrease in norepinephrine release. In this way, the $alpha_2$-receptor helps prevent overstimulation of effector sites. These receptors are also found on the beta cells in the pancreas, where they help moderate the insulin release stimulated by SNS activation.

Beta-Receptors

Beta-receptors are adrenergic receptors that are found in the heart, lungs, bladder, uterus, and vascular smooth muscle. $Beta_1$-receptors are found in cardiac tissue, where they can stimulate increased myocardial activity and increased heart rate. They are also responsible for increased lipolysis or breakdown of fat for energy in peripheral tissues.

$Beta_2$-receptors are found in the smooth muscle in blood vessels, in the bronchi, in the periphery, and in uterine muscle. In blood vessels, $beta_2$ stimulation leads to vasodilation. $Beta_2$-receptors also cause dilation in the bronchi. In the periphery, they can cause increased muscle and liver breakdown of glycogen and increased release of

Table 29.2 Physiological Effects of Specific Receptor Sites in the Autonomic Nervous System

Sympathetic System	Parasympathetic System
$Alpha_1$-receptors	Muscarinic receptors
Vasoconstriction	Pupil constriction
Increased peripheral resistance with increased blood pressure	Accommodation of the lens
Contracted piloerection muscles	Decreased heart rate
Pupil dilation	Increased GI motility
Thickened salivary secretions	Increased GI secretions
Closure of urinary bladder sphincter	Increased urinary bladder contraction
Male sexual emission	Male erection
$Alpha_2$-receptors	Sweating
Negative feedback control of norepinephrine release from presynaptic neuron	Nicotinic receptors
Moderation of insulin release from the pancreas	Muscle contractions
$Beta_1$-receptors	Release of norepinephrine from the adrenal medulla
Increased heart rate	Autonomic ganglia stimulation
Increased conduction through the atrioventricular node	Multiple areas in the brain
Increased myocardial contraction	
Lipolysis in peripheral tissues	
$Beta_2$-receptors	
Vasodilation	
Bronchial dilation	
Increased breakdown of muscle and liver glycogen	
Release of glucagon from the pancreas	
Relaxation of uterine smooth muscle	
Decreased GI muscle tone and activity	
Decreased GI secretions	
Relaxation of urinary bladder detrusor muscle	
$Beta_3$-receptors	
Increased metabolism and lipolysis	
Detrusor muscle relaxation and increased bladder capacity	

GI, gastrointestinal.

glucagon from the alpha cells of the pancreas. Stimulation of beta$_2$-receptors in the uterus results in relaxed uterine smooth muscle.

Beta$_3$-receptors are found in adipose tissue, the GI tract, the bladder, and the heart. When stimulated, metabolism and lipolysis are increased. These receptors are often resistant to blockade from antagonists. Stimulation with agonists may help treat overactive bladder (see Chapter 52).

Termination of Response

Once norepinephrine has been released into the synaptic cleft, stimulation of the receptor site is terminated and disposal of any extra norepinephrine, as well as the neurotransmitter that has reacted with the receptor site, must occur. Most of the free norepinephrine molecules are taken up by the nerve terminal that released them in a process called reuptake. This neurotransmitter is then repackaged into vesicles to be released later with nerve stimulation. This is an effective recycling effort by the nerve. Some of the norepinephrine can diffuse into the bloodstream. Enzymes are also in the area, as well as in the liver, to metabolize or biotransform any remaining norepinephrine or any norepinephrine that is absorbed into circulation. These enzymes are **monoamine oxidase** (MAO) and catechol-*O*-methyltransferase (COMT). MAO and COMT are enzymes that facilitate metabolism of neurotransmitters (epinephrine, norepinephrine, dopamine, and serotonin) to make them inactive.

Key Points

- The ANS, which is divided into two branches—the SNS and the PNS—works with the endocrine system to regulate internal functioning and maintain homeostasis.
- The SNS is responsible for the acute stress response.
- The SNS is composed of CNS cells arising in the thoracic or lumbar area of the spinal cord and long postganglionic axons that react with effector cells. The neurotransmitter used by the preganglionic cells is ACh; the primary neurotransmitter used by the postganglionic cells is norepinephrine.
- SNS adrenergic receptors are classified as alpha$_1$-, alpha$_2$-, beta$_1$-, beta$_2$-, or beta$_3$-receptors.

Parasympathetic Nervous System

The PNS contains CNS cells from the cranium or sacral area of the spinal cord, long preganglionic axons, ganglia near or within the effector tissue, and short postganglionic axons that react with cholinergic receptors. In many areas, the PNS works in opposition to the SNS. This allows the autonomic system to maintain a fine control over internal homeostasis. For example, the SNS increases heart rate, while the PNS decreases it. Thus, the ANS can influence heart rate by increasing or decreasing sympathetic activity or by increasing or decreasing parasympathetic activity. This is like controlling the speed of a car by moving between the accelerator and the brake or combining the two. While the SNS is associated with the stress reaction and expenditure of energy, the PNS is responsible for most unconscious actions. It increases the digestion, absorption, and metabolism of nutrients and slows metabolism and function to save energy—sometimes called a "rest-and-digest" or "feed-and-breed" response (Table 29.3).

Structure and Function

The PNS is sometimes called the craniosacral system because the CNS neurons that originate parasympathetic impulses are found in the cranium (one of the most important being the vagus, or 10th cranial nerve) and in the sacral area of the spinal cord (see Fig. 29.2). The terms "cholinergic," "muscarinic," and "vagal" are often used interchangeably when discussing the PNS. It has long preganglionic axons that meet in ganglia located close to or within the organ to be affected. The postganglionic axon is very short, going directly to the effector cell. The neurotransmitter used by both the preganglionic and postganglionic neurons is ACh.

PNS stimulation results in the following actions:

- Increased motility and secretions in the GI tract to promote digestion and absorption of nutrients
- Decreased heart rate and contractility to conserve energy and provide rest for the heart
- Constriction of the bronchi, with increased secretions
- Relaxation of the GI and urinary bladder sphincters, allowing evacuation of waste products
- Pupillary constriction, which decreases the light entering the eye and decreases stimulation of the retina

These activities are aimed at increasing digestion, absorption of nutrients, and building of essential proteins, as well as a general conservation of energy.

Cholinergic Response

Neurons that use ACh as their neurotransmitter are called cholinergic neurons. There are four basic kinds of cholinergic nerves:

1. All preganglionic nerves in the ANS, both sympathetic and parasympathetic
2. Postganglionic nerves of the parasympathetic system and a few SNS nerves, such as those that reenter the spinal cord and cause general body reactions such as sweating
3. Motor nerves on skeletal muscles
4. Cholinergic nerves within the CNS

Acetylcholine Synthesis and Storage

ACh is an ester of acetic acid and an organic alcohol called choline. Cholinergic nerves use choline, obtained in the

Table 29.3 Comparing the Effects of Autonomic Stimulation

Effector Site	Sympathetic Reaction	Parasympathetic Reaction
Eye Structures		
Iris radial muscle	Contraction (pupil dilates)	—
Iris sphincter muscle	—	Contraction (pupil constricts)
Ciliary muscle	Slight relaxation (better for far vision)	Contraction (lens accommodates for near vision)
Lacrimal glands	—	↑ Secretions
Heart	↑ Rate, contractility ↑ Atrioventricular conduction	↓ Rate ↓ Atrioventricular conduction
Blood Vessels		
Skin, mucous membranes	Constriction	—
Skeletal muscle	Dilation	—
Bronchial muscle	Relaxation (dilation)	Constriction
GI System		
Muscle motility and tone	↓ Activity	↑ Activity
Sphincters	Contraction	Relaxation
Secretions	↓ Secretions	↑ Activity
Salivary glands	Thick secretions	Copious, watery secretions
Gallbladder	Relaxation	Contraction
Liver	Gluconeogenesis	Slight glycogen synthesis
Kidneys and Urinary Bladder		
Kidneys	Decreased urine output and increased renin secretion	—
Detrusor muscle	Relaxation	Contraction
Trigone muscle and sphincter	Contraction	Relaxation
Sex Organs		
Male	Emission	Erection (vascular dilation)
Female	Uterine relaxation	—
Skin Structures		
Sweat glands	↑ Sweating	Sweat on palms of hands
Piloerector muscles	Contracted (goose bumps)	—

—, no reaction or response; GI, gastrointestinal.

diet, to produce ACh. The last step in the production of the neurotransmitter involves choline acetyltransferase, an enzyme that is also produced within cholinergic nerves. Just like norepinephrine, ACh is produced in the nerve and travels to the end of the axons, where it is packaged into vesicles. To be a cholinergic nerve, the nerve must contain all of the enzymes and building blocks necessary to produce ACh.

Acetylcholine Release

The vesicles full of ACh move to the nerve membrane; when an action potential reaches the nerve terminal, calcium entering the cell causes the membrane to contract and secrete the neurotransmitter into the synaptic cleft. The ACh travels across the synaptic cleft and reacts with specific cholinergic receptor sites on the effector cell (Fig. 29.5).

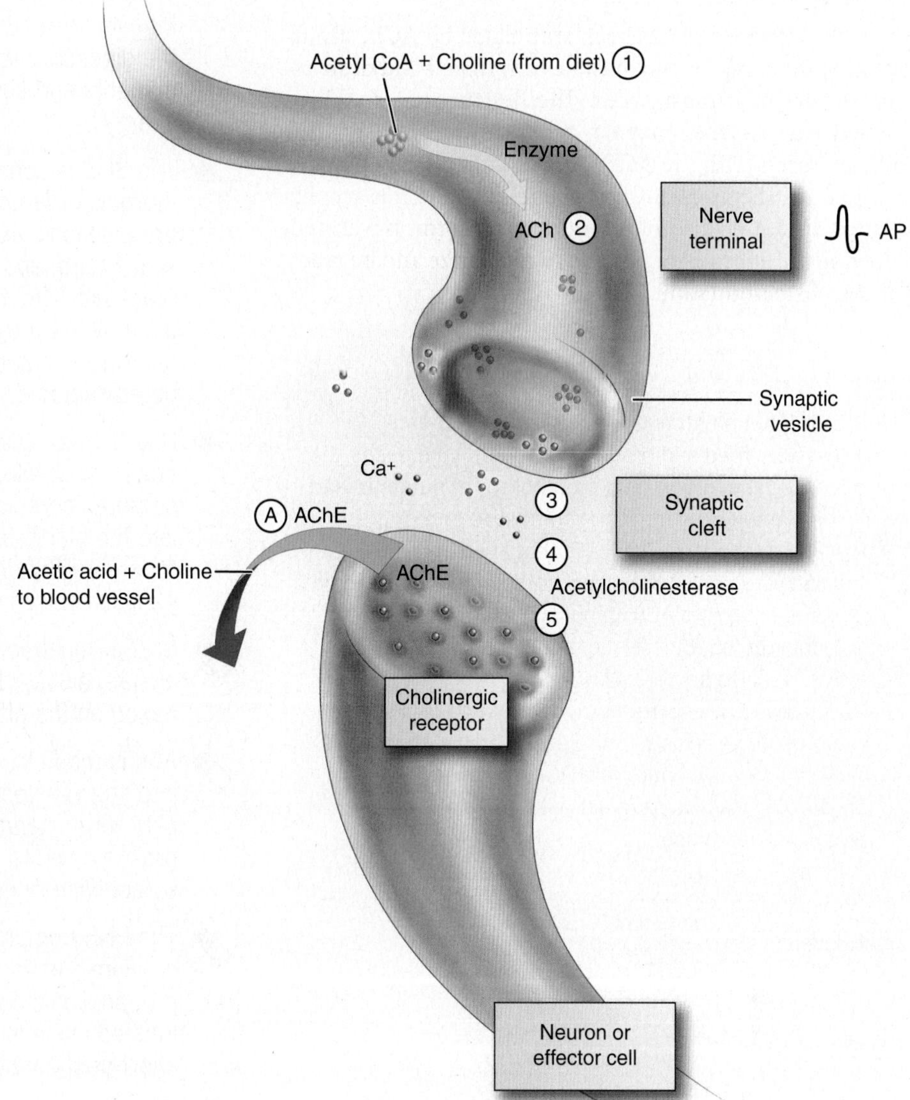

FIGURE 29.5 Sequence of events at a cholinergic synapse. (*1*) Synthesis of acetylcholine (*ACh*) from choline (a substance in the diet) and a cofactor (the enzyme is choline acetyltransferase, *CoA*). (*2*) Uptake of neurotransmitter into storage (synaptic) vesicle. (*3*) Release of neurotransmitter by an action potential (*AP*) in the presynaptic nerve. (*4*) Diffusion of neurotransmitter across the synaptic cleft. (*5*) Combination of neurotransmitter with receptor. The events resulting from ACh's occupation of receptor sites depend on the nature of the postsynaptic cell. ACh excites some cells and inhibits others. An enzyme, acetylcholinesterase (*AChE*), found in the tissues and on the postsynaptic cell inactivates ACh (*A*). Some of the products diffuse into the circulation, but most of the choline formed is taken up and reused by the cholinergic neuron.

Cholinergic Receptors

Cholinergic receptors or ACh receptors are found on organs and muscles—effectors that respond to ACh. They have been classified as muscarinic receptors and nicotinic receptors. This classification is based on early research of the ANS that used muscarine (a plant alkaloid from mushrooms) and nicotine (a plant alkaloid found in tobacco plants) to study the actions of the parasympathetic system.

Muscarinic Receptors

Muscarinic receptors are cholinergic receptors that are stimulated by postganglionic nerves. They are found in visceral effector organs, such as the GI tract, bladder, and heart; in sweat glands; and in some vascular smooth muscle. Stimulation of muscarinic receptors causes pupil constriction, increased GI motility and secretions (including saliva), increased urinary bladder contraction, and a slowing of the heart rate.

Nicotinic Receptors

Nicotinic receptors are located in the CNS, the adrenal medulla, the autonomic ganglia, and the neuromuscular junction. These cholinergic receptors respond to stimulation by nicotine located between pre- and postganglionic nerves and also at the neuromuscular junctions. Stimulation of nicotinic receptors causes skeletal muscle contractions, autonomic responses such as signs and symptoms of a stress reaction, and release of norepinephrine and epinephrine from the adrenal medulla. When nicotinic receptors are stimulated in the brain, there are a variety of different neurotransmitters released. However, dopamine seems to be a prominent one released in the mesolimbic area that can cause strong feelings of reward and addiction.

Termination of Response

Once the effector cell has been stimulated by ACh, stimulation of the receptor site must be terminated and destruction of any ACh must occur. The destruction of ACh is carried out by the enzyme **acetylcholinesterase**. This enzyme reacts with the ACh to form a chemically inactive compound. The breakdown of the released ACh is accomplished in 1/1,000 second, and the receptor is vacated, allowing the effector membrane to repolarize and be ready for the next stimulation.

Key Points

- The PNS, when stimulated, acts as a "rest-and-digest" or "feed-and-breed" response. It increases the digestion, absorption, and metabolism of nutrients and slows metabolism and function to save energy.
- The PNS comprises CNS cells that arise in the cranium and sacral region of the spinal cord, long preganglionic axons that secrete ACh, ganglia located very close to or within the effector tissue, and short postganglionic axons that also secrete ACh.
- ACh is made by choline from the diet and packaged into storage vesicles to be released by the cholinergic nerve into the synaptic cleft. ACh is broken down to an inactive form almost immediately by acetylcholinesterase.
- PNS receptors are classified as muscarinic or nicotinic, depending on what response they have to these plant alkaloids.

SUMMARY

- The ANS works with the endocrine system to regulate internal functioning and maintain homeostasis.
- The two branches of the ANS, the SNS and the PNS, work in opposition to maintain minute-to-minute regulation of the internal environment and to allow rapid response to stress situations.
- The SNS, when stimulated, is responsible for the acute stress response. It prepares the body for immediate reaction to stressors by increasing metabolism, diverting blood to big muscles, and increasing cardiac and respiratory function.
- The PNS, when stimulated, acts as a "rest-and-digest" or "feed-and-breed" response. It increases the digestion, absorption, and metabolism of nutrients and slows metabolism and function to save energy.
- The SNS is composed of CNS cells arising in the thoracic or lumbar area of the spinal cord, short preganglionic axons, ganglia located near the spinal cord, and long postganglionic axons that react with effector cells. The neurotransmitter used by the preganglionic cells is ACh; the primary neurotransmitter used by the postganglionic cells is norepinephrine.
- One SNS ganglion on either side of the spinal cord does not develop postganglionic axons but instead secretes norepinephrine and epinephrine directly into the bloodstream to travel throughout the body to react with adrenergic receptor sites. These ganglia evolve into the adrenal medulla.
- SNS adrenergic receptors are classified as being $alpha_1$-, $alpha_2$-, $beta_1$-, $beta_2$-, or $beta_3$-receptors based on the effectors that they stimulate.
- ACh is made by choline from the diet and packaged into storage vesicles to be released by the cholinergic nerve into the synaptic cleft. ACh is broken down to an inactive form almost immediately by acetylcholinesterase.
- The PNS comprises CNS cells that arise in the cranium and sacral region of the spinal cord, long preganglionic axons that secrete ACh, ganglia located close to or within the effector tissue, and short postganglionic axons that also secrete ACh.
- Norepinephrine is made by adrenergic nerves using tyrosine from the diet. It is packaged in storage vesicles that align on the axon membrane and is secreted into the synaptic cleft when the nerve is stimulated. It reacts with specific receptor sites and is then is recycled to the presynaptic nerve, diffuses into the bloodstream, or broken down by MAO or COMT to relax the receptor site and recycle the building blocks of norepinephrine.
- Parasympathetic system receptors are classified as muscarinic or nicotinic, depending on what response they have to these plant alkaloids.

CHECK YOUR UNDERSTANDING

Answers to the questions in this chapter can be found in Answers to Check Your Understanding Questions on thePoint®.

MULTIPLE CHOICE

Select the best answer.

1. When describing the functions of the ANS, which would the instructor include?
   a. Maintenance of balance and posture
   b. Maintenance of the special senses
   c. Regulation of integrated internal body functions
   d. Coordination of peripheral and central nerve pathways

2. The ANS differs from other systems in the CNS in that it
   a. uses only peripheral pathways.
   b. affects organs and muscles via a two-neuron system.
   c. uses a unique one-neuron system.
   d. bypasses the CNS in all of its actions.

3. If you suspect that a person is very stressed and is experiencing a sympathetic stress reaction, you would expect to find
   a. increased bowel sounds and urinary output.
   b. constricted pupils and warm, flushed skin.
   c. slow heart rate and decreased systolic blood pressure.
   d. dilated pupils and elevated systolic blood pressure.

4. The nurse determines that the beta$_2$-receptors in the SNS have been stimulated by which finding?
   a. Increased heart rate
   b. Increased myocardial contraction
   c. Bronchial dilation
   d. Uterine contraction

5. Once a postganglionic receptor site has been stimulated, the neurotransmitter must be broken down immediately. The sympathetic system breaks down postganglionic neurotransmitters by using
   a. liver enzymes and acetylcholinesterase.
   b. acetylcholinesterase and MAO.
   c. COMT and liver enzymes.
   d. MAO and COMT.

6. The parasympathetic nervous system, in most situations, opposes the actions of the SNS, allowing the ANS to
   a. generally have no effect.
   b. maintain a fine control over internal homeostasis.
   c. promote digestion.
   d. respond to stress most effectively.

7. Cholinergic neurons, those using ACh as their neurotransmitter, would be least likely to be found in
   a. motor nerves on skeletal muscles.
   b. preganglionic nerves in the sympathetic and parasympathetic systems.
   c. postganglionic nerves in the parasympathetic system.
   d. the adrenal medulla.

8. Stimulation of the parasympathetic nervous system would cause
   a. slower heart rate and increased GI secretions.
   b. faster heart rate and urinary retention.
   c. vasoconstriction and bronchial dilation.
   d. pupil dilation and muscle paralysis.

MULTIPLE RESPONSE

Select all that apply.

1. The SNS
   a. is called the thoracolumbar system.
   b. is called the fight-or-flight system.
   c. is called the craniosacral system.
   d. uses ACh as its sole neurotransmitter.
   e. uses epinephrine as its sole neurotransmitter.
   f. is active during a stress reaction.

2. The sympathetic system uses catecholamines at the postganglionic receptors. Which are considered catecholamines?
   a. Dopamine
   b. Norepinephrine
   c. ACh
   d. Epinephrine
   e. MAO
   f. Serotonin

REFERENCES

Barrett, K. E., Barman, S. M., Boitano, S., & Brooks, H. L. (2012). *Ganong's review of medical physiology* (24th ed.). McGraw-Hill.

Brunton, L. L., Hilal-Dandan, R., & Knollmann, B. C. (2018). *Goodman and Gilman's the pharmacological basis of therapeutics* (13th ed.). McGraw-Hill.

Edwards, D., & Burnard, P. (2003). A systemic review of stress and stress management for mental health nurses. *Journal of Advanced Nursing, 42*(2), 169–200. https://doi.org/10.1046/j.1365-2648.2003.02600.x

Hall, J. E. (2016). *Guyton and Hall textbook of medical physiology* (13th ed.). Elsevier.

Jänig, W. (2008). *Integrative action of the autonomic nervous system: Neurobiology of homeostasis*. Cambridge University Press.

Motzer, S. A., & Hertig, V. (2004). Stress, stress response, and health. *Nursing Clinics of North America, 39*(1), 1–17. https://doi.org/10.1016/j.cnur.2003.11.001

Norris, T. L. (2019). *Porth's pathophysiology: Concepts of altered health states* (10th ed.). Wolters Kluwer.

Rider, S. H. (2004). Psychological distress: Concept analysis. *Journal of Advanced Nursing, 45*(5), 536–545. https://doi.org/10.1046/j.1365-2648.2003.02938.x

CHAPTER 30

Adrenergic Agonists

Learning Objectives

Upon completion of this chapter, you will be able to:

1. Describe two ways that sympathomimetic drugs act to produce effects at adrenergic receptors.
2. Discuss the use of adrenergic agents across the lifespan.
3. Describe the therapeutic actions, indications, pharmacokinetics, contraindications, most common adverse reactions, and important drug–drug interactions associated with adrenergic agonists.
4. Compare and contrast the prototype drugs dopamine, phenylephrine, and isoproterenol with other adrenergic agonists.
5. Outline the nursing considerations, including important teaching points, for patients receiving an adrenergic agent.

Key Terms

adrenergic agonist: drug that stimulates the adrenergic receptors of the sympathetic nervous system, either directly (by reacting with receptor sites) or indirectly (by increasing norepinephrine levels)

alpha-agonist: drug that specifically stimulates the alpha-receptors within the sympathetic nervous system, causing body responses seen when the alpha-receptors are stimulated

beta-agonist: drug that specifically stimulates the beta-receptors within the sympathetic nervous system, causing body responses seen when the beta-receptors are stimulated

glycogenolysis: breakdown of stored glucose so that the glucose can be used as energy

sympathomimetic: drug that mimics the sympathetic nervous system (SNS) with the signs and symptoms seen when the SNS is stimulated

Drug List

ALPHA- AND BETA-ADRENERGIC AGONISTS
dobutamine
(P) dopamine
ephedrine
epinephrine
norepinephrine
pseudoephedrine

ALPHA-SELECTIVE ADRENERGIC AGONISTS
clonidine (alpha$_2$-selective)
dexmedetomidine (alpha$_2$-selective)
guanfacine (alpha$_2$-selective)
midodrine
(P) phenylephrine

BETA-SELECTIVE ADRENERGIC AGONISTS (Also See Beta-Adrenergic Agonists in Chapter 55)
albuterol
arformoterol
formoterol
(P) isoproterenol
levalbuterol
metaproterenol
olodaterol
salmeterol
terbutaline

An **adrenergic agonist** is also called a **sympathomimetic** drug because it mimics the effects of the sympathetic nervous system (SNS). The therapeutic and adverse effects associated with these drugs are related to their stimulation of adrenergic receptor sites. That stimulation can be either direct, by occupation of the adrenergic receptor, or indirect, by modulation of the release of neurotransmitters from the axon. Some drugs act in both ways. Adrenergic agonists also can affect both the alpha- and beta-receptors, or they can act at specific receptor sites.

The use of adrenergic agonists varies from ophthalmic preparations for dilating pupils to systemic preparations used

Box 30.1 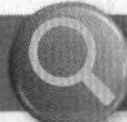 **Focus on Drug Therapy Across the Lifespan**

ADRENERGIC AGONISTS

Children

Children are at risk for complications associated with the use of adrenergic agonists, including tachycardia, hypertension, tachypnea, and GI complications. The dosage for an adrenergic agonist administered intravenously often needs to be calculated using the child's body weight. It is good practice to have a second person check the dosage calculation before administering the drug to avoid potential toxic effects. Children should be carefully monitored and supported during the use of these drugs.

Phenylephrine is often found in OTC allergy and cold preparations, and parents need to be instructed to be careful with the use of these drugs; they should check the labels for ingredients, monitor the recommended dose, and avoid combining drugs that contain similar ingredients.

Adults

Adults being treated with adrenergic agonists for cardiogenic shock or hypotensive states require constant monitoring and dosage adjustments based on their response. Patients who may be at increased risk for cardiac or vascular complications may need to be started on lower doses. Adults using these agents for glaucoma or for seasonal rhinitis need to be cautioned about the use of OTC drugs and alternative therapies that might increase the drug effects and cause serious adverse effects.

Many of these drugs are used in emergency situations and may be used during pregnancy and lactation. In general, there are no adequate studies about their effects during pregnancy and lactation; in those situations, they should be used only if the benefit to the patient is greater than the risk to the fetus or neonate.

Older Adults

Older patients commonly experience the adverse CNS, CV, GI, and respiratory effects associated with these drugs. Because older patients often have renal or hepatic impairment, they are also more likely to have a toxic level of the drug related to changes in metabolism and excretion. Older patients may need to be started on lower doses of the drugs and should be monitored closely for potentially serious arrhythmias or blood pressure changes.

They also should be cautioned about the use of OTC drugs and complementary therapies that could increase drug effects and cause serious adverse reactions.

to support patients experiencing acute hypotension. They are used for patients of all ages (see Boxes 30.1 and 30.2).

Alpha- and Beta-Adrenergic Agonists

Drugs that are generally sympathomimetic (Fig. 30.1) are called **alpha-agonists** (stimulate alpha-receptors) and **beta-agonists** (stimulate beta-receptors). General adrenergic agonists stimulate all of the adrenergic receptors; that is, they affect both alpha- and beta-receptors (Table 30.1). Agents that affect both alpha- and beta-receptor sites include dobutamine (generic), dopamine (generic), ephedrine (*Akovaz, Corphedra, Emerphed*), epinephrine (*Adrenalin, Adrenaclick, Auvi-Q, Epipen, Primatene Mist, Symjepi*), and norepinephrine (*Levophed*). Some of these drugs are naturally occurring catecholamines.

Therapeutic Actions and Indications

The effects of the sympathomimetic drugs are mediated by the adrenergic receptors in target organs: Heart rate increases with increased myocardial contractility; bronchi dilate and respirations increase in rate and depth; blood vessels constrict, causing an increase in blood pressure; intraocular pressure decreases; **glycogenolysis** (breakdown of glucose stores so that the glucose can be used as energy) occurs throughout the body; pupils dilate; and sweating can increase (see Fig. 30.1). These drugs generally are indicated for the treatment of hypotensive states or shock, bronchospasm, and some types of asthma. Table 30.1 discusses usual indications for each of these agents.

Dopamine, a naturally occurring catecholamine, is the sympathomimetic drug of choice for the treatment of shock. It

BOX 30.2

Rapid Response for Anaphylaxis

Epinephrine is available in a number of different autoinjectors for use in the emergency treatment of acute allergic reactions including anaphylaxis. Dosing varies between adults and children, and it is important to make sure the correct injector is used. The traditional *EpiPen* (0.3 mg/0.3 mL) and *EpiPen Jr.* (0.15 mg/0.15 mL) are well known to people. *Adrenaclick* comes in the same volumes and concentrations but provides color-coded use for immediate injection into the upper thigh. In 2014, an updated *Auvi-Q* injector was introduced; it has a protective carrying case, is easy to inject subcutaneously or IM through clothing, and has a voice instruction system to assure proper use and actual injection. Any patient at risk for anaphylaxis should be carefully instructed in the carrying and use of these autoinjectors. They are for emergency use only, and the patient should seek immediate medical care following use. Proper disposal of the autoinjector varies with the injector and should be part of the instructional session. Patients should know that they may experience sweating, tremors, anxiety, fast heart rate, weakness, dizziness, or GI upset following the use of this drug.

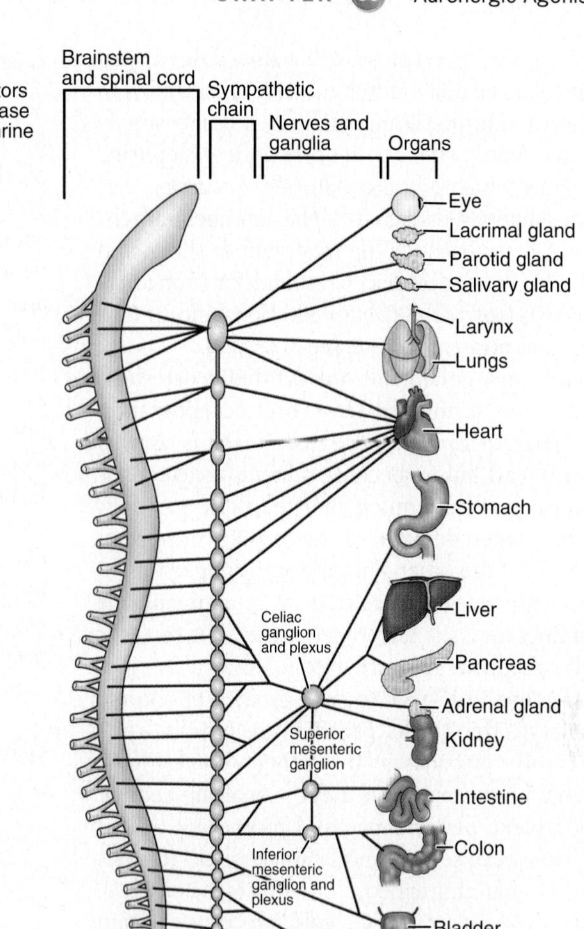

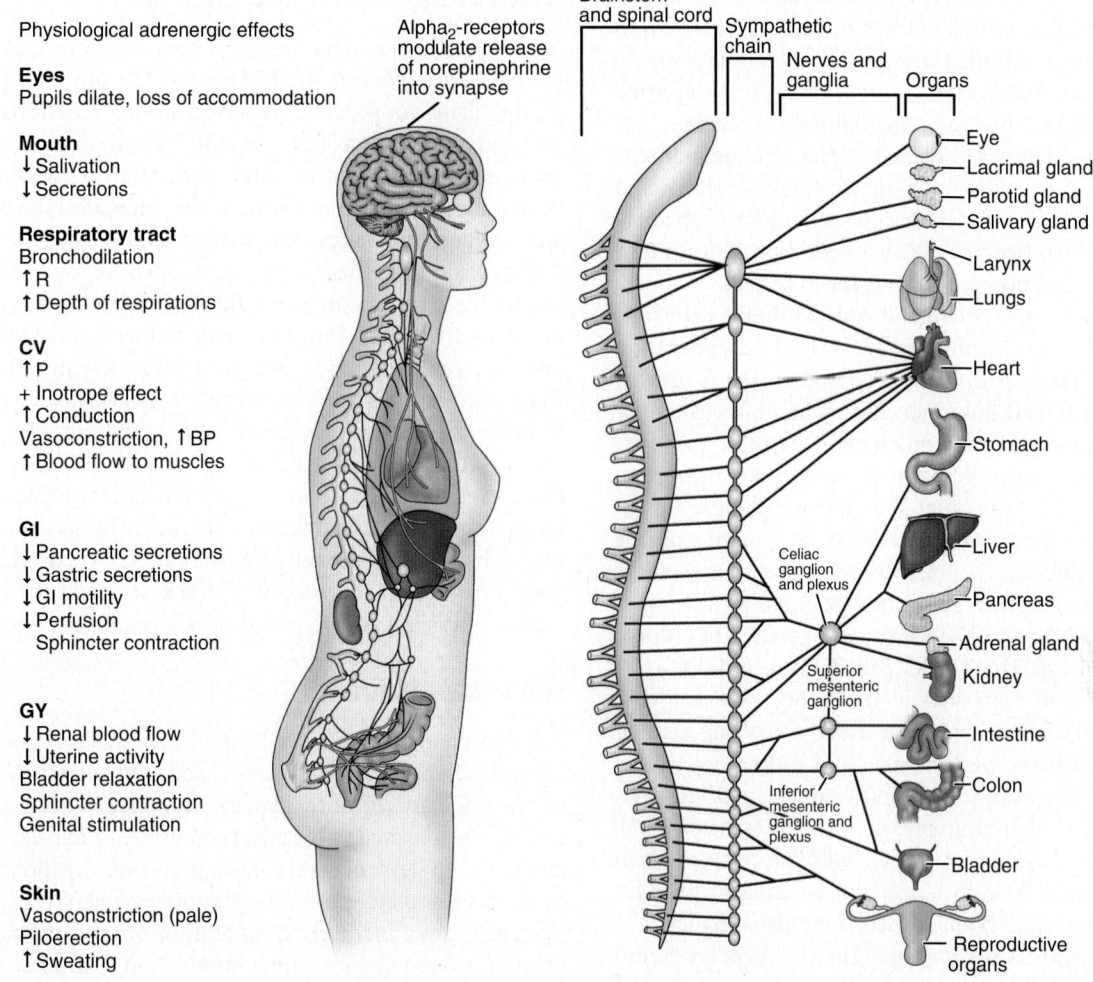

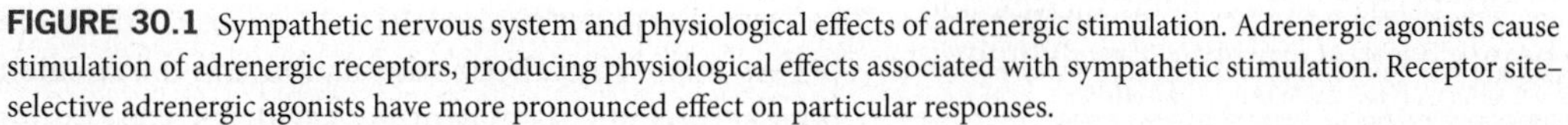
FIGURE 30.1 Sympathetic nervous system and physiological effects of adrenergic stimulation. Adrenergic agonists cause stimulation of adrenergic receptors, producing physiological effects associated with sympathetic stimulation. Receptor site–selective adrenergic agonists have more pronounced effect on particular responses.

Table 30.1 ***Drugs in Focus*: Alpha- and Beta-Adrenergic Agonists**

Drug Name	Dosage/Route	Usual Indications
dobutamine (generic)	2.5–10 mcg/kg/min IV with dose adjusted based on patient response	Treatment of heart failure
dopamine (generic)	Initially 5–10 mcg/kg/min IV with incremental increases up to 20–50 mcg/kg/min based on patient response	Treatment of shock
ephedrine (*Akovaz, Corphedra, Emerphed*)	5–10 mg IV bolus	Treatment of hypotensive episodes in the setting of anesthesia
epinephrine (*Adrenalin, Adrenaclick, Auvi-Q, Epipen, Primatene Mist, Symjepi*)	Specific formulations may have unique dosing *Adult*: 0.05–2 mcg/kg/min IV for acute treatment; 0.3–0.5 mg subcutaneous or IM for respiratory distress; may be used in a nebulizer or as topical nasal drops; dilute 1 mL with 100–1,000 mL of ophthalmic irrigation fluid for ophthalmic irrigation or intracameral injection *Pediatric*: 0.01–0.3 mg IM or subcutaneous (30 kg or less); 0.3–0.5 mg IM or subcutaneous (>30 kg) *Adult and pediatric (12 years and older)*: 1–2 inhalations every 4 hours as needed; no more than 8 inhalations in 24 hours (*Primatene Mist*)	Treatment of hypotension associated with shock; to prolong effects of regional anesthetic; primary treatment for bronchospasm; to produce a local vasoconstriction that prolongs the effects of local anesthetics; emergency treatment of allergic reactions; maintenance of mydriasis during intraocular surgery
norepinephrine (*Levophed*)	8–12 mcg base/min IV; with rate and dose adjusted based on patient response	Treatment of acute hypotensive states

stimulates the heart and blood pressure but also causes a renal and splanchnic arteriole dilation that increases blood flow to the kidneys, preventing the diminished renal blood supply and possible renal shutdown that can occur with epinephrine or norepinephrine, which are also naturally occurring catecholamines that interact with both alpha- and beta-adrenergic receptors and are used for the treatment of shock and to stimulate the body after cardiac arrest and for immediate relief of anaphylaxis (see Table 30.1; for additional indications for epinephrine and norepinephrine, see Box 30.2).

Dobutamine and ephedrine are synthetic catecholamines. Dobutamine, although it acts at both receptor sites, has a slight preference for beta$_1$-receptor sites. It is used in the treatment of heart failure because it can increase myocardial contractility without much change in rate and does not increase the oxygen demand of the cardiac muscle, an advantage over all of the other sympathomimetic drugs.

Ephedrine stimulates the release of norepinephrine from nerve endings and acts directly on adrenergic receptor sites. Although ephedrine was once used for situations ranging from the treatment of shock to management of chronic asthma and allergic rhinitis, its primary use now is treatment of hypotensive episodes in the setting of anesthesia. The herb ephedra has been used as a nutritional supplement for enhancing athletic performance and promoting weight loss, but there have been serious and fatal reactions. This has resulted in the FDA banning ephedra as a drug (see Box 30.3).

Many over-the-counter (OTC) cold products contain pseudoephedrine. These products can be used to produce methamphetamine, an often-abused street drug. By law, the sale of these products is restricted. The products are found behind the counter at pharmacies, not on open shelves, and the amount that can be purchased at any given time is limited.

Pharmacokinetics

These drugs are generally absorbed rapidly after injection or passage through mucous membranes. They are metabolized in the liver and excreted in the urine. When used in emergency situations, they are given intravenously (IV) to achieve rapid onset of action.

BOX 30.3 Focus on Herbal and Alternative Therapies

Ephedra, an herb that acts like ephedrine, was formerly used as a treatment for asthma and nasal congestion. It was also used to promote weight loss and athletic performance. However, due to its sympathomimetic side effects, there are serious cardiovascular risks that can result in sudden death. The U.S. Food and Drug Administration (FDA) has banned ephedra as a drug and prohibited ephedrine alkaloids from being used in supplements. There are many nutritional supplements that are advertised as increasing energy and/or weight loss. These formulations may include herbs that act similarly to ephedra (e.g., guarana, caffeine, and others). Educate patients to read nutritional labels carefully to fully understand the risks and benefits of supplements.

Contraindications and Cautions

The alpha- and beta-agonists are contraindicated in patients with known hypersensitivity to any component of the drug to prevent hypersensitivity reactions; with pheochromocytoma because the systemic overload of catecholamines could be fatal; with tachyarrhythmias or ventricular fibrillation because the increased heart rate and oxygen consumption usually caused by these drugs could exacerbate these conditions; with hypovolemia, for which fluid replacement would be the treatment for the associated hypotension; and with halogenated hydrocarbon general anesthetics, which sensitize the myocardium to catecholamines and could cause serious cardiac effects. Caution should be exercised with any kind of peripheral vascular disease (e.g., atherosclerosis, Raynaud's disease, diabetic endarteritis), which could be exacerbated by systemic vasoconstriction. Because the sympathomimetic drugs stimulate the SNS, they should be used during pregnancy and lactation only if the benefits to the patient clearly outweigh any potential risks to the fetus or neonate.

Adverse Effects

The adverse effects associated with the use of alpha- and beta-adrenergic agonists may be associated with the drugs' effects on the SNS: arrhythmias, hypertension, palpitations, angina, and dyspnea related to the effects on the heart and cardiovascular (CV) system; nausea, vomiting, and constipation related to the depressant effects on the gastrointestinal (GI) tract; and headache, sweating, feelings of tension or anxiety, and piloerection related to sympathetic stimulation (Fig. 30.2). Hypokalemia can occur as a result of the release of aldosterone that occurs with sympathetic stimulation and the resultant loss of potassium. Patients may present with muscle cramps related to the shift in potassium. Because all of these drugs cause vasoconstriction, care must be taken to avoid extravasation of any infused drug. The vasoconstriction in the area of extravasation can lead to necrosis and cell death in that area.

Clinically Important Drug–Drug Interactions

Increased effects of tricyclic antidepressants (TCAs) and monoamine oxidase inhibitors (MAOIs) can occur because of the increased norepinephrine levels or increased receptor stimulation that occurs with both drugs. There is an increased risk of hypertension if alpha- and beta-adrenergic agonists are given with any other drugs that cause hypertension, including herbal therapies and OTC preparations. Any adrenergic agonist will lose effectiveness if combined with any adrenergic antagonist. This may be beneficial if there is extravasation, since an alpha adrenergic blocking agent (phentolamine) can be used to block the vasoconstrictive actions. Halogenated hydrocarbon general anesthetics can cause the heart tissue to be more sensitive to catecholamines and cause dysrhythmias. Monitor the patient's drug regimen for appropriate use of the drugs.

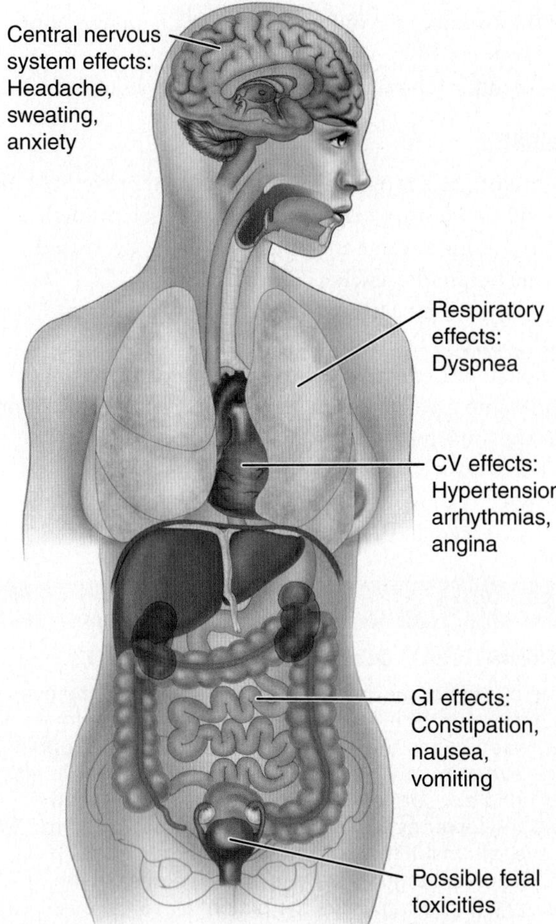

FIGURE 30.2 Common adverse effects associated with adrenergic agonists.

Prototype Summary: Dopamine

Indications: Correction of hemodynamic imbalances present in shock.

Actions: Acts directly and by the release of norepinephrine from sympathetic nerve terminals; mediates dilation of vessels in the renal and splanchnic beds to maintain renal perfusion while stimulating the sympathetic response.

Pharmacokinetics:

Route	Onset	Peak	Duration
IV	1–2 min	10 min	Length of infusion

$T_{1/2}$: 2 minutes; metabolized in the liver; excreted in the urine.

Adverse Effects: Tachycardia, ectopic beats, anginal pain, dyspnea, nausea, vomiting, headache.

Nursing Considerations for Patients Receiving Alpha- and Beta-Adrenergic Agonists

Assessment: History and Examination

Assess for contraindications or cautions: any known allergies to these drugs to avoid hypersensitivity reactions; pheochromocytoma, which could lead to fatal reactions due to systemic overload of catecholamines; tachyarrhythmias or ventricular fibrillation, which could be exacerbated by these drugs; hypovolemia, which would require fluid replacement as treatment for the associated hypotension; general anesthesia with halogenated hydrocarbon anesthetics, which could lead to serious cardiac effects; the presence of vascular disease, which could be exacerbated with the use of these drugs; and current status of pregnancy and lactation.

- Perform a physical assessment to establish baseline status before beginning therapy and during therapy to evaluate for any potential adverse effects and to determine the effectiveness of therapy.
- Assess vital signs, especially pulse and blood pressure, to monitor for possible excess stimulation of the cardiac system; obtain an electrocardiogram (ECG) to evaluate for possible arrhythmias.
- Note respiratory rate and auscultate lungs for adventitious sounds to evaluate effects on bronchi and respirations.
- Monitor urine output to evaluate perfusion of the kidneys and therapeutic effects.
- Monitor the results of laboratory tests, such as renal and liver function tests, to determine the need for possible dose adjustment, and serum electrolyte levels to evaluate fluid loss and appropriateness of therapy.

Refer to the "Critical Thinking Scenario" for a full discussion of nursing care for a patient who is being treated with an adrenergic agonist.

Nursing Conclusions

Nursing conclusions related to drug therapy may include the following:

- Decreased cardiac output related to CV effects
- Altered tissue perfusion related to CV effects or possible extravasation
- Knowledge deficit regarding drug therapy

Planning

- The patient will receive the best therapeutic effect from the drug therapy.
- The patient will have limited adverse effects from the drug therapy.

(continues on page 520)

- The patient will have an understanding of the drug therapy, adverse effects to anticipate, and measures to relieve discomfort and improve safety.

Intervention With Rationale

- Use extreme caution in calculating and preparing doses of these drugs because even small errors could have serious effects. Always dilute a parenteral drug before use if it is not prediluted to prevent tissue irritation on infection.
- Use proper technique when administering ophthalmic or nasal agents to assure the therapeutic effectiveness of the drug. (See Box 30.4.)
- Monitor patients receiving the drug ophthalmically or nasally for all of the systemic effects associated with parenteral administration to prevent potentially serious adverse effects if the drug is absorbed systemically.
- Monitor patient response closely (blood pressure, ECG, urine output, cardiac output) and adjust dose accordingly to ensure the most benefit with the least amount of toxicity.
- Maintain phentolamine on standby in case extravasation occurs; infiltration of the site with 10 mL of saline containing 5 to 10 mg of phentolamine is usually effective in saving the area.
- Offer support and encouragement for managing the drug regimen.
- Provide comfort measures to help the patient cope with sympathomimetic effects of the drug and relaxation measures to deal with feelings of tension and anxiety.
- Monitor light exposure to prevent sensitivity to light caused by pupil dilation.
- Encourage voiding before giving the drug to alleviate urinary retention caused by sphincter contraction and monitor bowel function and provide assistance as needed to deal with GI suppression.
- Provide appropriate patient teaching to patients using these drugs orally or ophthalmically. Most of these drugs are given in emergency situations, and teaching will be based on the patient's condition and awareness. Teaching includes the following:
  - Drug name, prescribed dosage, and schedule for administration
  - Rationale for the drug
  - Proper technique for administration
  - Measures to prevent or avoid adverse effects
  - Need to check with prescriber before taking any OTC medication
  - Warning signs that might indicate a problem
  - Importance of avoiding intake of caffeine-containing products
  - Need for follow-up monitoring and evaluation

Evaluation

- Monitor patient response to the drug (improvement in blood pressure, ocular pressure, bronchial airflow).
- Monitor for adverse effects (CV changes, decreased urine output, headache, GI upset).
- Monitor the effectiveness of comfort measures and adherence to the regimen.
- Evaluate the effectiveness of the teaching plan (patient can name the drug, dosage, adverse effects to watch for, and specific measures to avoid them).

Box 30.4 Focus on Safe Medication Administration

ADMINISTERING OPHTHALMIC MEDICATIONS

Some of the adrenergic agonists are applied in the eye; it is important to review the administration technique. First, wash hands thoroughly. Do not touch the dropper to the eye or to any other surfaces. Have the patient tilt their head back or lie down and stare upward. Gently grasp the lower eyelid and pull the eyelid away from the eyeball. Instill the prescribed number of drops into the lower conjunctival sac and then release the lid slowly (Fig. 30.3). Have the patient close the eye and look downward. The patient may slowly blink or keep their eyes closed for a short time. Do not rub the eyeball, and do not rinse the dropper. If more than one type of eyedrop is being used, wait 5 minutes before administering the next one.

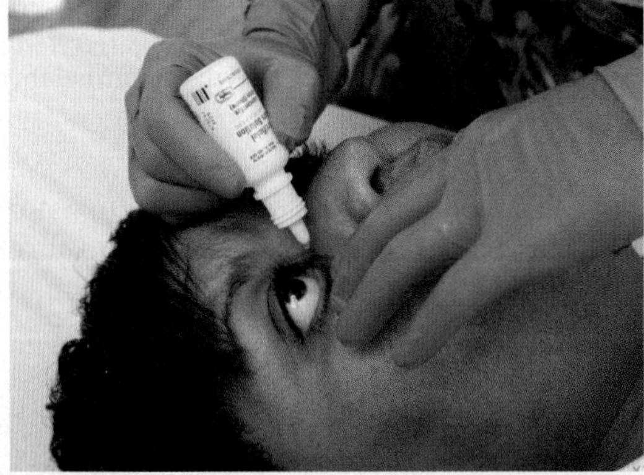

FIGURE 30.3 After gently exposing the lower conjunctival sac, the nurse administers an eyedrop. (Reprinted with permission from Lynn, P. (2018). *Taylor's clinical nursing skills: A nursing process approach* (5th ed., p. 244). Wolters Kluwer, Figure 4.)

CRITICAL THINKING SCENARIO
Treatment With Adrenergic Agonist

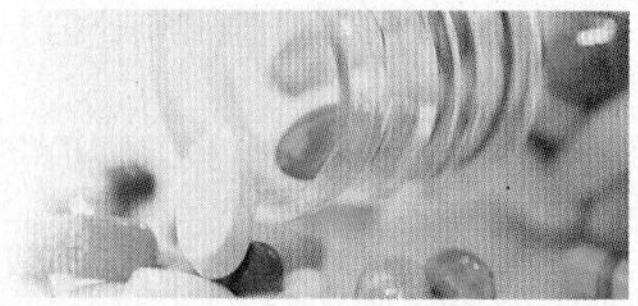

THE SITUATION

M.C., who is 26 years old, has recently moved to the northeastern United States from New Mexico with their spouse. The two have been enjoying the early fall weather by going on many hikes in the nearby parks and wooded areas. For 2 days, M.C. had been complaining of fatigue and said they did not feel like going on the walks. This morning M.C.'s spouse had a difficult time rousing M.C., and M.C. was barely responsive. They called 911, and M.C. was transferred to the emergency room. M.C. was found to be in complete heart block with a ventricular rate of 25 beats per minute and a blood pressure reading of 69/40. They were administered a dose of atropine and also started on a continuous infusion of norepinephrine while waiting for the team to place a temporary pacemaker. During the physical assessment, the nurse noticed a rash that resembled a "bull's eye" shape on M.C.'s right lower leg. The nurse talked to the provider about this, and Lyme titers were sent to be evaluated for possible Lyme carditis.

CRITICAL THINKING

What are the important nursing implications for M.C.? Think about the problems that confront a patient in a new area seeking health care for the first time.

What could be causing the problems with which M.C. presents? There is the possible diagnosis of Lyme's disease, but could there be other causes of heart block that should be considered?

Keeping in mind that this diagnosis means that M.C. could have an understimulated sympathetic stress reaction, what other physical problems can be anticipated? Lyme carditis is caused by an infection in the heart after being bit by a tick. If this is causing the heart block, then antibiotics will be needed to treat the infection. However, if there is not a reversable cause of the heart block, M.C. may need a permanent pacemaker.

Given these facts, how may the nurse best deal with explaining the problem to the patient and their spouse?

What treatment should be planned, and what teaching points should be covered for M.C.?

DISCUSSION

The first step in caring for M.C. is establishing a trusting relationship to help alleviate some of the anxiety they and their spouse are probably feeling. Being in a new state and seeking health care in a new setting can be stressful for patients under normal circumstances and especially in emergency situations.

A careful review of any medications including OTC drugs and supplements should be performed. The patient should be asked about any allergies or intolerances to medications. This will be especially important if M.C. will need to be started on any antibiotics. There will also need to be a discussion with MC and their spouse about the need for careful monitoring due to M.C.'s heart arrhythmia and the continuous infusion of norepinephrine. Once a temporary pacemaker is placed, M.C. may become more stable and may not need the norepinephrine, but their heart rate and blood pressure will be monitored closely.

A careful patient history will help determine whether there are any underlying medical problems that could be exacerbated by drug effects. This questioning will also reassure M.C. that they are an important member of the health team and that the information they have to offer is valued.

To ensure that the underlying cause of the problem was Lyme's disease, titers are sent for analysis, but it may take 2 to 3 days to receive results. During this time, it is common for a temporary pacemaker to be used to keep the patient stable. The treatment plan should be communicated to M.C. and their spouse to help to decrease anxiety.

NURSING CARE GUIDE FOR M.C.: TREATMENT WITH ADRENERGIC AGONIST

Assessment: History and Examination

Assess the patient's history of drug allergies, CV dysfunction, pheochromocytoma, narrow-angle glaucoma, prostatic hypertrophy, thyroid disease, or diabetes, as well as concurrent use of MAOIs, TCAs, reserpine, ephedrine, or urinary alkalinizers.

Focus the physical examination on the following:

CV: Blood pressure, pulse rate, peripheral perfusion, and ECG

Central nervous system (CNS): Orientation, affect, reflexes, peripheral sensation, and vision

Skin: Color and temperature

GI: Abdominal examination

Genitourinary (GU): Urine output

Respiratory: Respiratory rate and adventitious sounds

Nursing Conclusions

Decreased cardiac output related to CV effects

Activity intolerance related to CV and systemic effects

Altered tissue perfusion related to CV effects

Knowledge deficit regarding drug therapy

Altered skin integrity related to requirement to be sedentary

Planning

The patient will receive the best therapeutic effect from the drug therapy.

(continues on page 522)

The patient will have limited adverse effects from the drug therapy.
The patient will have an understanding of the drug therapy, adverse effects to anticipate, and measures to relieve discomfort and improve safety.

Intervention

Ensure safe and appropriate administration of the drug.
Provide comfort and safety measures: temperature and lighting control (patient may have pupil dilation secondary to sympathetic effects), mouth care, and skin care.
Monitor blood pressure, pulse rate, and respiratory status throughout drug therapy.
Provide support and reassurance to deal with drug therapy and drug effects.
Provide patient teaching about drug name, dosage, side effects, precautions, and warning signs to report.

Evaluation

Evaluate drug effects: increased heart rate and blood pressure.
Monitor for adverse effects: tachycardia, ventricular arrythmia, dizziness, confusion, headache, rash, difficulty voiding, sweating, flushing, and pupillary dilation.
Monitor for drug–drug interactions as indicated.
Evaluate the effectiveness of the patient teaching program and comfort and safety measures.

PATIENT TEACHING FOR M.C.

- The drug that is being administered is norepinephrine. It is an adrenergic agonist (or a sympathomimetic drug). It acts by mimicking the effects of the SNS, which is the part of your nervous system that is responsible for your response to fear or danger (this is called the "fight or flight" response). It is being used to increase your heart rate and blood pressure since your own heart is beating too slowly. This is used only temporarily until a pacemaker can be placed or your heart rate otherwise increases back to a normal rate. Because this drug triggers many effects in the body, you may experience some undesired adverse effects. It is crucial to discuss the effects of the drug with your health care provider so we can try to make the effects as tolerable as possible.
- You will need to stay in bed until your heart rate and blood pressure are more stable.
- If the heart block was caused by a Lyme infection, antibiotics can be used to treat it.
- Some of the following adverse effects may occur:
  - *Restlessness, shaking, or jitteriness*: If these occur, please tell you nurse.
  - *Flushing or sweating*: Nurses will be able to help to cool you down; cool wash cloths and/or fans may help.
  - *Heart palpitations*: If you feel that your heart is beating too fast or skipping beats, alert the nurse. Your heart rhythm is being monitored. If your heart rate is going faster, the dosage of the drug may need to be decreased, or medication may need to be stopped.
  - *Sensitivity to light*: Avoid glaring lights, or wear sunglasses if you are in bright light.
  - Report any of the following to your health care provider: difficulty voiding, chest pain, difficulty breathing, dizziness, headache, or changes in vision.
- The medication is only a temporary treatment while your heart rate and blood pressure are low. It will be titrated down and stopped as your vital signs become more stable.
- All of your medications will be administered by the nurse while you are in the hospital. Do not take any medications you typically take at home.

Key Points

- Adrenergic agonists (sympathomimetics) stimulate the adrenergic receptors in the SNS.
- Alpha- and beta-adrenergic agonists stimulate all of the adrenergic receptors in the SNS. They induce a fight or flight response and are frequently used to treat shock.

Alpha-Selective Adrenergic Agonists

Alpha-selective adrenergic agonists (Table 30.2), or alpha-agonists, are drugs that bind primarily to alpha-receptors rather than to beta-receptors. Three drugs are primarily alpha$_2$ agonists: clonidine (*Catapres, Kapvay*), dexmedetomidine (*Precedex*), and guanfacine (*Intuniv*). Midodrine (*Orvaten*) and phenylephrine (*Biorphen, Vazculep*) target more of the alpha$_1$ receptors.

Therapeutic Actions and Indications

Therapeutic effects of the alpha-selective adrenergic agonists result from the stimulation of alpha-receptors within the SNS (see Fig. 30.1). The uses are varied, depending on the specific drug and the route of administration (see Table 30.2).

Phenylephrine, a potent vasoconstrictor and alpha$_1$-agonist with little or no effect on the heart or bronchi, is used in many combination cold and allergy products. Parenterally, it is used to treat shock or shocklike states, to overcome paroxysmal supraventricular tachycardia, to prolong local anesthesia, and to maintain blood pressure during spinal anesthesia. Topically, it is used to treat allergic rhinitis and to relieve the symptoms of otitis media. Ophthalmically, it is used to dilate the pupils for eye examination, before surgery, or to relieve elevated eye pressure associated with glaucoma. Phenylephrine is found in many cold and allergy products because it is so effective in constricting topical vessels and decreasing the swelling, signs,

Table 30.2 ***Drugs in Focus*: Alpha-Selective Adrenergic Agonists**

Drug Name	Dosage/Route	Usual Indications
clonidine hydrochloride (*Catapres*)	0.1 mg PO b.i.d. initially up to a maximum 2.4 mg/d if needed; transdermal system may increase from 0.1 to 0.3 mg/d	Treatment of essential hypertension; chronic pain; to ease opiate withdrawal; used only for adults
clonidine hydrochloride (*Kapvay*)	Start with 0.1 mg HS PO. Increase daily dosage in increments of 0.1 mg/d at weekly intervals to max of 0.4 mg/d. Take twice a day with either higher or equal dosage at bedtime	Treatment of ADHD; taper slowly when discontinuing
dexmedetomidine (*Precedex*)	1 mcg/kg IV over 10 min then 0.2–0.7 mcg/kg/h IV using controlled infusion device for up to 24 h *Special considerations:* Do not use longer than 24 h; monitor patient continually	Sedation of intubated and mechanically ventilated patients during treatment in an intensive care setting or of patients prior to and/or during procedures
guanfacine (*Intuniv*)	Initial dose 1 mg PO daily; adjust by increments of no more than 1 mg/wk	Treatment of ADHD
midodrine (*Orvaten*)	10 mg PO t.i.d. during daytime hours when patient is upright	Treatment of orthostatic hypotension
phenylephrine (*Biorphen, Vazculep*)	1–10 mg PO subcutaneous or IV *or* 40–250 mcg IV bolus, 0.5–1.4 mcg/kg/min IV continuous infusion; 0.5 mg IV by rapid injection to convert tachycardias; 1–2 gtt in affected eye(s) for glaucoma or dilation of pupil	Cold and allergies; perioperative hypotension; vasodilatory shock; supraventricular tachycardias; glaucoma; allergic rhinitis; otitis media

and symptoms of rhinitis. See Box 30.5 for information regarding brimonidine, a topical alpha-agonist that can be used to treat rosacea and high intraocular pressure.

Midodrine is an oral drug that is used to treat orthostatic hypotension in patients who do not respond to traditional therapy. It activates $alpha_1$-adrenergic receptors, leading to peripheral vasoconstriction and an increase in vascular tone and blood pressure. This effect can cause serious supine hypertension. Patients need to be monitored in the standing, sitting, and supine positions to determine whether this will be a problem. See Box 30.6 regarding droxidopa, a drug for treating orthostatic hypotension. Droxidopa is discussed in more detail in Chapter 43.

Clonidine specifically stimulates CNS $alpha_2$-receptors. This leads to decreased sympathetic outflow from the CNS because the $alpha_2$-receptors moderate the release of norepinephrine from the nerve axon. Clonidine is available in oral and transdermal forms to control hypertension and as an injection for epidural infusion to control pain in cancer patients. One of the oral formulations has been approved for the treatment of attention deficit hyperactivity disorder (ADHD). Because of its centrally acting effects, clonidine is associated with many more CNS effects (bad dreams, sedation, drowsiness, fatigue, headache) than other sympathomimetics. It can also cause extreme hypotension, heart failure, and bradycardia due to decreased effects of the sympathetic outflow from the CNS.

Guanfacine has also been approved to treat ADHD. Its mechanism of action is as a central $alpha_2$-receptor agonist. It acts to decrease sympathetic nerve action potentials from the CNS to the heart and blood vessels, so there will often be a decrease in blood pressure and heart rate. The

BOX 30.5

Alpha-Agonist for Treatment of Rosacea and High Intraocular Pressure

Brimonidine (*Mirvaso*) is an alpha adrenergic receptor agonist. When used topically, brimonidine is indicated to treat rosacea. Rosacea is a persistent facial erythema or redness that might be related to a vascular sensitivity in certain patients. In the past, topical steroids were often used to help patients with this disorder, but the use of corticosteroids often made the condition worse. Brimonidine is an alpha-agonist and causes a local vasoconstriction at the site of application, decreasing the redness associated with vasodilation and improving the appearance of the skin. It is applied in pea-size amounts each day to the head, chin, nose, and each cheek. The eyes and lips are avoided. It is not for oral, ophthalmic, or intravaginal use. Patients are advised to wash their hands immediately after applying the gel and to avoid application to any area that is eroded or has open skin. In some cases, vascular insufficiency can occur, so the area should be monitored closely. Since the drug is not generally absorbed systemically, there are few systemic effects.

Another brand name of brimonidine, *Alphagan P*, is indicated to treat elevated intraocular pressure in people with open-angle glaucoma or ocular hypertension. Patients are to place one drop in the affected eye(s) three times a day. As with other alpha adrenergic receptor agonists, there is risk of vasoconstriction causing vascular insufficiency. Most common side effects are allergic conjunctivitis, burning sensation in the eye, eye pruritus, ocular allergic reactions, and visual disturbances.

BOX 30.6

Droxidopa for Orthostatic Hypotension

Droxidopa (*Northera*) is approved for the treatment of orthostatic hypotension, dizziness, and light-headedness in adults with symptomatic neurogenic orthostatic hypotension caused by primary autonomic failure, dopamine beta-hydroxylase deficiency, and nondiabetic autonomic neuropathy. Droxidopa is a synthetic amino acid precursor of norepinephrine. It is metabolized to norepinephrine in the tissues throughout the body. It is not completely understood how that affects orthostatic hypotension, but the conversion to norepinephrine in the tissues is thought to cause vasoconstriction leading to a higher blood pressure. The efficacy of the drug beyond 2 weeks of use has not been reported. *Northera* has a boxed warning that there is a risk of supine hypertension and CV risk. Supine blood pressure should be monitored prior to and during treatment. If the patient has high supine blood pressure that is not relieved by elevation of the bed, the medication dose should be lowered or the medication should be stopped.

exact way it helps people with ADHD is not completely understood.

Dexmedetomidine is also a selective alpha$_2$-adrenergic agonist, but its indications are very different from clonidine and guanfacine. It is indicated for sedation of patients who are undergoing surgical procedures and/or are mechanically intubated and ventilated in an intensive care setting. Sedation with dexmedetomidine should not exceed 24 hours due to risk of tolerance and ineffectiveness.

Pharmacokinetics

These drugs are generally well absorbed from all routes of administration. IV and immediate-release oral products are rapid acting and reach peak levels in a short period. They are widely distributed in the body, metabolized in the liver, and primarily excreted in the urine. The transdermal form of clonidine is slow-release and has a 7-day duration of effects, so it only needs to be replaced once a week. Phenylephrine can be given intramuscularly (IM), subcutaneously, IV, orally, and as a nasal or an ophthalmic solution.

Contraindications and Cautions

The alpha-selective adrenergic agonists are contraindicated in the presence of allergy to the specific drug to avoid hypersensitivity reactions; severe hypertension because of possible vasoconstriction; and narrow-angle glaucoma, which could be exacerbated by arterial constriction. Alpha$_2$-selective medications should not be used in the presence of hypotension or bradycardia due to the effect on modulation of norepinephrine. There is limited data regarding use during pregnancy and lactation, so use should be reserved for situations in which the benefit to the patient outweighs any potential risk to the fetus or neonate.

They should be used with caution in the presence of CV disease or vasomotor spasm because these conditions could be aggravated by the vascular effects of the drug; thyrotoxicosis or diabetes because of the thyroid-stimulating and glucose-elevating effects of sympathetic stimulation; or renal or hepatic impairment, which could interfere with metabolism and excretion of the drug.

Adverse Effects

Patients receiving these drugs often experience adverse effects that are extensions of the therapeutic effects or other sympathetic stimulatory reactions. CNS effects include feelings of anxiety, restlessness, depression, fatigue, strange dreams, and personality changes. Blurred vision and sensitivity to light may occur because of the pupil dilation that occurs when the sympathetic system is stimulated. CV effects can include arrhythmias, ECG changes, blood pressure changes, and peripheral vascular problems. Nausea, vomiting, and anorexia can occur related to the depressant effects of the SNS on the GI tract. GU effects can include decreased urinary output, difficulty urinating, dysuria, and changes in sexual function related to the sympathetic stimulation of these systems. These drugs should not be stopped suddenly; adrenergic receptors will be sensitive to catecholamines, and sudden withdrawal can lead to tachycardia, hypertension, arrhythmias, flushing, and even death. Avoid these effects by tapering the drug over 2 to 4 days when it is being discontinued when possible. As with other sympathomimetic drugs, if phenylephrine is given IV, care should be taken to avoid extravasation. The vasoconstricting effects of the drug can lead to necrosis and cell death in the area of extravasation.

Clinically Important Drug–Drug Interactions

Phenylephrine combined with MAOIs can cause severe hypertension, headache, and hyperpyrexia; this combination should be avoided. Increased sympathomimetic effects occur when phenylephrine is combined with TCAs; if this combination must be used, the patient should be monitored closely.

Clonidine and guanfacine have potential for decreased antihypertensive effect if taken with TCAs, and paradoxical hypertension occurs if it is combined with propranolol. They can cause increased CNS effects if taken with other CNS depressants, and exaggerated hypotension if taken with other antihypertensive medications. If these combinations are used, the patient response should be monitored closely and dose adjustment made as needed.

When midodrine is administered with cardiac glycosides (like digoxin), there can be increased risk of bradycardia, heart block, and arrhythmia. Alpha-adrenergic blocking agents (like prazosin, terazosin, and doxazosin) can antagonize the effects of midodrine. Midodrine should not be administered with MAO inhibitors due to increased risk of hypertension.

When combined with anesthetics, sedatives, hypnotics, or opioids, dexmedetomidine may have increased effect; dosage reduction may be indicated.

Any adrenergic agonist will lose effectiveness if combined with another adrenergic antagonist. Monitor the patient's drug regimen for appropriate use of the drugs.

Prototype Summary: Phenylephrine

Indications: Treatment of vascular failure in shock or drug-induced hypotension to overcome paroxysmal supraventricular tachycardia and to prolong spinal anesthesia; as a vasoconstrictor in regional anesthesia to maintain blood pressure during anesthesia; topically for symptomatic relief of nasal congestion and as adjunctive therapy in middle-ear infections; ophthalmically to dilate pupils; and as a decongestant to provide temporary relief of eye irritation.

Actions: Powerful postsynaptic alpha-adrenergic receptor stimulant causing vasoconstriction and raising systolic and diastolic blood pressure with little effect on the beta-receptors in the heart.

Pharmacokinetics:

Route	Onset	Duration
IV	Immediate	15–20 min
Topically	Very little systemic absorption occurs	

$T_{1/2}$: Approximately 2.5 hours; metabolized in the tissues and liver; excreted in the urine and bile.

Adverse Effects: Fear, anxiety, restlessness, headache, nausea, decreased urine formation, pallor, hypertension.

Nursing Considerations for Patients Receiving Alpha-Selective Adrenergic Agonists

Assessment: History and Examination

- Assess for contraindications or cautions: any known allergies to the drug to avoid hypersensitivity reactions; presence of any CV diseases, which could be exacerbated by the vascular effects of these drugs; thyrotoxicosis or diabetes, which would lead to an increase in thyroid stimulation or glucose elevation; chronic renal failure, which could be exacerbated by drug use; renal or hepatic impairment, which could interfere with drug excretion or metabolism; and current status of pregnancy or lactation.
- Perform a physical assessment to establish baseline status before beginning therapy to determine effectiveness and during therapy to evaluate for any potential adverse effects.
- Assess level of orientation, affect, reflexes, and vision to monitor for CNS changes related to drug therapy.
- Monitor blood pressure and pulse, assess peripheral perfusion, and obtain an ECG, if indicated, to determine drug effectiveness and evaluate for adverse CV effects.
- Assess urinary output to evaluate renal function and monitor for adverse effects of the drug.
- Evaluate the patient for nausea and constipation to assess adverse effects of the drug and establish appropriate interventions.
- Monitor laboratory test results, such as renal and liver function tests, to determine drug effects on renal and hepatic systems.

Nursing Conclusions

Nursing conclusions related to drug therapy might include the following:

- Altered sensory perception (visual, kinesthetic, tactile) related to CNS effects
- Altered comfort levels related to GI and GU effects of the drug and pupil dilation causing sensitivity to light
- Injury risk related to CNS or CV effects of the drug and potential for extravasation
- Altered tissue perfusion related to blood pressure changes, arrhythmias, or vasoconstriction
- Knowledge deficit regarding drug therapy

Planning

- The patient will receive the best therapeutic effect from the drug therapy.
- The patient will have limited adverse effects from the drug therapy.
- The patient will have an understanding of the drug therapy, adverse effects to anticipate, and measures to relieve discomfort and improve safety.

Intervention With Rationale

- Do not discontinue the drug abruptly because sudden withdrawal can result in rebound hypertension, arrhythmias, flushing, and even hypertensive encephalopathy and death; taper the drug over 2 to 4 days when possible.
- Mark the patient's chart and monitor blood pressure carefully during surgery. Sympathetic stimulation may alter the normal response to anesthesia as well as recovery from anesthesia.

(continues on page 526)

- Monitor blood pressure, orthostatic blood pressure, pulse, rhythm, and cardiac output regularly, even with ophthalmic preparations, to adjust dose or discontinue the drug if CV effects are severe.
- When giving phenylephrine intravenously, ensure that an alpha-blocking agent is readily available to counteract the effects in case severe reaction occurs; infiltrate any area of extravasation with phentolamine within 12 hours after extravasation to preserve tissue.
- Arrange for supportive care and comfort measures, including rest and environmental control to decrease CNS irritation; analgesics for headache to relieve discomfort; safety measures, such as use of side rails and assistance with ambulation, if CNS effects occur to protect the patient from injury; and protective measures if CNS effects are severe.
- Provide thorough patient teaching about drug name, dose, and schedule for administration; technique for administration if appropriate; measures to prevent potential adverse effects such as voiding before taking the drug and use of bowel-training activities if constipation is a problem; safety measures such as avoiding driving and operating dangerous machinery if CNS effects occur and getting up and down slowly if orthostatic hypotension is an issue; warning signs of problems; and importance of monitoring and follow-up to improve adherence and ensure safe and effective use of the drug.

Evaluation

- Monitor patient response to the drug (improvement in condition being treated).
- Monitor for adverse effects (GI upset, CNS, and CV changes).
- Monitor the effectiveness of comfort measures and adherence to the regimen.
- Evaluate the effectiveness of the teaching plan (patient can name the drug, dosage, adverse effects to watch for, and specific measures to avoid them).

Key Points

- Alpha-selective adrenergic agonists stimulate only the alpha receptors within the SNS. Some are more selective for only alpha$_1$ or only alpha$_2$ receptors.
- Care must be taken to prevent extravasation when used IV; the vasoconstrictive properties of the drug can cause necrosis and cell death in the area of extravasation.
- These drugs should be tapered when discontinued when possible because the adrenergic receptors will be sensitive, and rebound hypertension, tachycardia, arrhythmias, and even death can occur.

Beta-Selective Adrenergic Agonists

Most of the drugs that belong to the class of beta-selective adrenergic agonists (Table 30.3), or beta-agonists, are beta$_2$-selective agonists and are used to manage and treat bronchial spasm, asthma, and other obstructive pulmonary conditions. These drugs, including albuterol (*AccuNeb, Proair Respiclick, Proair HFA, Proventil HFA, Ventolin HFA, Vospire ER*), arformoterol (*Brovana*), formoterol (*Foradil, Perforomist*), levalbuterol (*Xopenex*), metaproterenol (generic), olodaterol (*Striverdi Respimat*), salmeterol (*Serevent Diskus*), and terbutaline (generic), are discussed at length in Chapter 55, which deals with drugs used to treat obstructive pulmonary diseases. Beta$_3$-agonists act to relax the bladder and are used to help treat overactive bladder as discussed in Chapter 52. This chapter specifically addresses isoproterenol (*Isuprel*), which is used as a sympathomimetic drug for its overall stimulatory properties.

Therapeutic Actions and Indications

Therapeutic effects of isoproterenol are related to its stimulation of all beta-adrenergic receptors. Desired effects of the drug include increased heart rate, conductivity, and contractility; bronchodilation; increased blood flow to skeletal muscles and splanchnic beds; and relaxation of the uterus. Its use has decreased over the years as more specific drugs with less toxicity have been developed to treat the cardiac problems isoproterenol was developed to treat. Some research has shown that isoproterenol exerts a "coronary steal" effect, diverting blood away from injured or hypoxic areas of the heart muscle, an effect that can increase the size and extent of an evolving myocardial infarction, further decreasing the drug's usefulness in the clinical setting. There are some emergency situations, however, that respond well to isoproterenol. See Table 30.3 for usual indications.

Pharmacokinetics

Isoproterenol is rapidly distributed after injection; it is metabolized in the liver and excreted in the urine. The half-life is relatively short—less than 1 hour.

Contraindications and Cautions

Isoproterenol is contraindicated in the presence of allergy to the drug or any components of the drug to avert hypersensitivity reactions; with pulmonary hypertension, which could be exacerbated by the effects of the drug; in patients with tachyarrhythmias, heart block caused by digitalis intoxication, or during angina pectoris due to potential for worsening clinical status; during anesthesia with halogenated hydrocarbons, which sensitize the myocardium to catecholamines and could cause a severe reaction; with eclampsia, uterine hemorrhage, and intrauterine

Table 30.3 *Drugs in Focus*: Beta-Selective Adrenergic Agonists

Drug Name	Dosage/Route	Usual Indications
albuterol (*AccuNeb, Proair Respiclick, Proair HFA, Proventil HFA, Ventolin HFA, Vospire ER*)	*Adult*: 2–4 mg t.i.d.–q.i.d. PO or 1–2 inhalations q4–6h *Pediatric*: 2 mg t.i.d.–q.i.d. PO *or* 1.25–2.5 mg b.i.d. by inhalation	Treatment and prevention of bronchospasm; treatment of acute bronchospasm and exercise-induced bronchospasm when used by inhalation
arformoterol (*Brovana*)	*Adult*: 15 mcg b.i.d. by nebulization, do not exceed 30 mcg/d	Long-term maintenance treatment of bronchospasm in adult patients with chronic obstructive pulmonary disease
formoterol (*Foradil, Perforomist*)	*Adult*: Oral inhalation of 12 mcg every 12 h *or* 20 mcg/2 mL by oral inhalation using a jet nebulizer twice daily *Pediatric (12 y and older for exercise-induced bronchospasm)*: Oral inhalation of 12 mcg 15 min before exercise *Pediatric (5 y and older for maintenance treatment of asthma)*: Oral inhalation of 12 mcg every 12 h	Long-term maintenance treatment of asthma in adults and children 5 y and older; prevention of exercise-induced bronchospasm
isoproterenol (*Isuprel*)	*Adult*: IV injection bolus, 0.02–0.06 mg; IV infusion, 5 mcg/min; 0.2 mg IM or subcutaneous *Pediatric*: 0.1–1.0 mcg/kg/min IV has been used	Treatment of shock with low cardiac output, cardiac arrest, and certain ventricular arrhythmias; treatment of heart block; prevention of bronchospasm during anesthesia, treatment of acute hyperkalemia in the hospital setting
levalbuterol (*Xopenex*)	*Adult and pediatric (12 y and older)*: 0.63 mg t.i.d. by nebulization *Pediatric (6–11 y)*: 0.31 mg t.i.d. by nebulization *Pediatric (4 y and older)*: Two inhalations q4–6h	Treatment and prevention of bronchial asthma and reversible bronchospasm in patients 4 y and older
metaproterenol (generic)	*Adult and pediatric (12 y and older)*: 2–3 inhalations every 3–4 h; 2.5 mL by nebulization; 20 mg PO t.i.d.–q.i.d. *Pediatric (6–9 y)*: 10 mg PO t.i.d.–q.i.d.; 0.1–0.2 mL in saline by nebulization	Treatment of bronchial asthma and reversible bronchospasm; by inhalation, treatment of acute asthma attacks in children 6 y and older
olodaterol (*Striverdi Respimat*)	*Adult*: Two oral inhalations once daily at the same time each day: 2.5 mcg/inhalation	Long-term maintenance treatment of bronchospasm in adult patients with chronic obstructive pulmonary disease
salmeterol (*Serevent Diskus*)	*Adult and pediatric (12 y and older)*: One inhalation b.i.d.; 30 min before exercise with exercise-induced bronchospasm	Treatment and prevention of bronchial asthma and reversible bronchospasm, including exercise-induced bronchospasm (patients 4 y and older); maintenance treatment of bronchospasm associated with chronic obstructive pulmonary disease
terbutaline (generic)	*Adult and pediatric (15 y and older)*: 5 mg PO t.i.d.; 0.25 mg subcutaneous, may be repeated in 15 min to a maximum of 0.5 mg/4 h *Pediatric (12–15 y)*: 2.5 mg PO t.i.d.	Treatment and prevention of bronchial asthma and reversible bronchospasm

death, which could be complicated by uterine relaxation or increased blood pressure; and during pregnancy and lactation because of potential effects on the fetus or neonate. Caution should be exercised with diabetes, thyroid disease, vasomotor problems, degenerative heart disease, or history of stroke, all of which could be exacerbated by the sympathomimetic effects of the drug, and with severe renal impairment, which could alter excretion of the drug.

Adverse Effects

Patients receiving isoproterenol often experience adverse effects related to the stimulation of sympathetic adrenergic receptors. CNS effects include restlessness, anxiety, fear, tremor, fatigue, and headache. CV effects can include tachycardia, angina, myocardial infarction, and palpitations. Pulmonary effects can be severe, ranging from difficulty breathing, coughing, and bronchospasm to severe pulmonary edema. GI upset, nausea, vomiting, and anorexia can occur as a result of the slowing of the GI tract with SNS stimulation. Hypokalemia can occur as a result of the release of aldosterone that occurs with sympathetic stimulation and the resultant loss of potassium. Other anticipated effects can include sweating, pupil dilation, rash, and muscle cramps that occur as a result of the potassium shift.

Clinically Important Drug–Drug Interactions

Increased sympathomimetic effects can be expected if this drug is taken with other sympathomimetic drugs. Decreased therapeutic effects can occur if this drug is combined with beta-adrenergic blockers.

P Prototype Summary: Isoproterenol

Indications: Treatment of shock when there is low cardiac output, cardiac arrest, and certain ventricular arrhythmias; treatment of heart block; prevention of bronchospasm during anesthesia, treatment of acute hyperkalemia in the hospital setting.

Actions: Acts on beta-adrenergic receptors to produce increased heart rate, positive inotropic effect, bronchodilation, and vasodilation.

Pharmacokinetics:

Route	Onset	Duration
IV	Immediate	1–2 min

$T_{1/2}$: Unknown; metabolized in the tissues.

Adverse Effects: Restlessness, apprehension, anxiety, fear, cardiac arrhythmias, tachycardia, nausea, vomiting, heartburn, respiratory difficulties, coughing, pulmonary edema, sweating, pallor.

Nursing Considerations for Patients Receiving Beta-Selective Adrenergic Agonists

Assessment: History and Examination

- Assess for contraindications or cautions: any known allergies to any drug or any components of the drug to avoid possible hypersensitivity reactions; pulmonary hypertension, which could be exacerbated by the effects of the drug; anesthesia with halogenated hydrocarbons, which sensitize the myocardium to catecholamines and could cause severe reaction; eclampsia, uterine hemorrhage, and intrauterine death, which could be complicated by uterine relaxation or increased blood pressure; diabetes, thyroid disease, vasomotor problems, degenerative heart disease, or history of stroke, all of which could be exacerbated by the sympathomimetic effects of the drugs; severe renal impairment, which could interfere with the excretion of the drug; and current status of pregnancy or lactation.
- Perform a physical assessment to establish a baseline before beginning therapy and during therapy to determine the drug's effectiveness and identify any potential adverse effects.
- Assess CV status, including pulse rate and blood pressure, to evaluate for any CV effects associated with SNS stimulation; obtain an ECG to evaluate for changes indicating excessive SNS stimulation.
- Assess respiratory status and listen for adventitious sounds to monitor drug effects and assess for any adverse effects.
- Monitor urine output to evaluate renal function and kidney perfusion.
- Monitor laboratory test results, including thyroid function tests, blood glucose levels, and renal function, to monitor drug effects and potential adverse effects.

Nursing Conclusions

Nursing conclusions related to drug therapy might include the following:

- Altered tissue perfusion related to CV effects
- Altered breathing pattern due to effects on bronchial tissue
- Knowledge deficit risk regarding drug therapy

Planning

- The patient will receive the best therapeutic effect from the drug therapy.
- The patient will have limited adverse effects from the drug therapy.
- The patient will have an understanding of the drug therapy, adverse effects to anticipate, and measures to relieve discomfort and improve safety.

Intervention With Rationale

- Monitor pulse and blood pressure carefully during administration to arrange to discontinue the drug at any sign of toxicity.
- Ensure that a beta-adrenergic blocker is readily available when giving parenteral isoproterenol in case severe reaction occurs.
- Use minimal doses of isoproterenol needed to achieve desired effects to prevent adverse effects and maintain patient safety.
- Arrange for supportive care and comfort measures, including rest and environmental control, to relieve CNS effects; provide analgesics for headache and safety measures if CNS effects occur to provide comfort and

prevent injury; and avoid overhydration to prevent pulmonary edema.
- Provide thorough patient teaching, including drug name, dosage, and frequency of administration; rationale for administration; monitoring required; anticipated adverse effects, including measures to reduce these; and warning signs of problems to report immediately to improve adherence and ensure safe and effective use of the drug.

Evaluation

- Monitor patient response to the drug (improvement in condition being treated, stabilization of blood pressure, prevention of preterm labor, cardiac stimulation).
- Monitor for adverse effects (GI upset, CNS changes, respiratory problems, cardiac arrhythmias).
- Evaluate the effectiveness of the teaching plan (patient can name drug, dosage, adverse effects to watch for, and specific measures to reduce them).
- Monitor the effectiveness of comfort measures and adherence to the regimen.

Concept Mastery Alert

Nursing Care for Patients Taking Adrenergic Agonists

When caring for a patient taking an adrenergic agonist, be sure to review the indication, route, and dosing of the medication. Keep in mind that these medications can have opposite effects from each other depending on which receptors are targeted. For patients on any of these medications, be sure to assess CNS status, heart rate, blood pressure, GI function, and urinary output since all adrenergic agonists can affect these major functions.

Key Points

- Most of the $beta_2$-selective adrenergic agonists are used to manage and treat asthma, bronchospasm, and other obstructive pulmonary diseases.
- Isoproterenol, a nonselective beta-specific adrenergic agent, is used for its sympathomimetic effects to treat heart block and shock due to low cardiac output.
- Because of its many adverse effects, isoproterenol is reserved for use in emergency situations that do not respond to other safer therapies.

SUMMARY

- Adrenergic agonists, also called sympathomimetics, are drugs that mimic the effects of the SNS and are used to stimulate the adrenergic receptors within the SNS. The adverse effects associated with these drugs are usually a result of sympathetic stimulation.
- Adrenergic agonists include alpha- and beta-adrenergic agonists, which stimulate both types of adrenergic receptors in the SNS, and alpha-selective and beta-selective adrenergic agonists, which stimulate only alpha-receptors or only beta-receptors, respectively.
- $Alpha_1$-selective adrenergic agonists can increase blood pressure by causing vasoconstriction. $Alpha_2$-selective adrenergic agonists can lower blood pressure by modulating the norepinephrine release.
- Many of the $beta_2$-selective adrenergic agonists are used to manage and treat asthma, bronchospasm, and other obstructive pulmonary diseases.
- Isoproterenol, a nonselective beta-specific adrenergic agent, is used for its sympathomimetic effects to treat heart block and shock that is due to low cardiac output.

CHECK YOUR UNDERSTANDING

Answers to the questions in this chapter can be found in Answers to Check Your Understanding Questions on thePoint®.

MULTIPLE CHOICE

Select the best answer.

1. The instructor determines that teaching about adrenergic drugs has been successful when the class identifies the drugs are also called
   a. sympatholytic agents.
   b. cholinergic agents.
   c. sympathomimetic agents.
   d. anticholinergic agents.
2. The adrenergic agent of choice for treating the signs and symptoms of allergic rhinitis is
   a. norepinephrine.
   b. phenylephrine.
   c. dobutamine.
   d. dopamine.

3. An adrenergic agent being used to treat shock infiltrates into the tissue with IV administration. Which action by the nurse would be most appropriate?
   a. Watch the area for any signs of necrosis, and report it to the provider.
   b. Notify the provider, and decrease the rate of infusion.
   c. Remove the IV, and prepare phentolamine for administration to the area.
   d. Apply ice, and elevate the arm.
4. Phenylephrine, an alpha-selective agonist, is found in many cold and allergy preparations. The nurse instructs the patient to be alert for which adverse effects?
   a. Urinary retention and pupil constriction
   b. Hypotension and slow heart rate
   c. Personality changes and increased appetite
   d. Cardiac arrhythmias and difficulty urinating
5. Adverse effects associated with adrenergic agonists are related to the generalized stimulation of the SNS and could include
   a. slowed heart rate.
   b. constriction of the pupils.
   c. hypertension.
   d. increased GI secretions.
6. A patient has elected to take an OTC cold preparation that contains phenylephrine. The nurse would advise the patient not to take that drug if the patient has
   a. thyroid or CV disease.
   b. a cough and runny nose.
   c. chronic obstructive pulmonary disease.
   d. hypotension.

MULTIPLE RESPONSE

Select all that apply.

1. Isoproterenol is a nonselective beta-agonist. The nurse might expect to administer this drug for which condition?
   a. Preterm labor
   b. Bronchospasm
   c. Cardiac standstill
   d. Shock
   e. Heart block in transplanted hearts
   f. Heart failure
2. A nurse would question the order for an adrenergic agonist for a patient who is also receiving which of the following?
   a. Anticholinergic drugs
   b. Halogenated hydrocarbon anesthetics
   c. Beta-blockers
   d. Benzodiazepines
   e. MAOIs
   f. TCAs

REFERENCES

American Association of Critical Care Nurses. (2009). *Core curriculum for progressive nursing care.* Saunders/Elsevier.

Brunton, L., Hilal-Dandan, R., & Knollman, B. (2018). *Goodman and Gilman's the pharmacological basis of therapeutics.* (13th ed.). McGraw-Hill.

Gheorghiade, M., Filippatos, G. S., & Felker, G. M. (2011). Diagnosis and management of acute failure syndromes. In R. O. Bonow, D. L. Mann, D. P. Zipes, & P. Libby (Eds.), *Braunwald's heart disease: A textbook of cardiovascular medicine* (9th ed.). Saunders; chap. 27.

Hasdai, D., Berger, P. B., Battler, A., & Holmes, D. R., Jr. (Eds.). (2010). *Cardiogenic shock.* Humana Press.

Hendler, C. B. (Ed.) (2021). *Nursing 2021 drug handbook.* Wolters Kluwer.

Norris, T. L. (2019). *Porth's pathophysiology concepts of altered health states* (10th ed.). Wolters Kluwer.

CHAPTER 31

Adrenergic Antagonists

Learning Objectives

Upon completion of this chapter, you will be able to:

1. Describe the effects of adrenergic blocking agents on adrenergic receptors, correlating these effects with their clinical effects.
2. Discuss the use of adrenergic blocking agents across the lifespan.
3. Describe the therapeutic actions, indications, pharmacokinetics, contraindications and cautions, most common adverse reactions, and important drug–drug interactions associated with adrenergic blocking agents.
4. Compare and contrast the prototype drugs labetalol, phentolamine, doxazosin, propranolol, and atenolol with other adrenergic blocking agents.
5. Outline the nursing considerations, including important teaching points, for patients receiving an adrenergic blocking agent.

Key Terms

adrenergic receptor–site specificity: a drug's affinity for only adrenergic receptor sites; certain drugs may have specific affinity for only alpha- or only beta-adrenergic receptor sites

alpha$_1$-selective adrenergic blocking agents: drugs that block the postsynaptic alpha$_1$-receptor sites, causing a decrease in vascular tone and vasodilation that leads to a fall in blood pressure; these drugs do not block the presynaptic alpha$_2$-receptor sites, and therefore, the reflex tachycardia that accompanies a fall in blood pressure is less likely to occur

beta-adrenergic blocking agents: drugs that, at therapeutic levels, block the beta-receptors of the sympathetic nervous system

beta$_1$-selective adrenergic blocking agents: drugs that, at therapeutic levels, specifically block the beta$_1$-receptors in the sympathetic nervous system while not blocking the beta$_2$-receptors with resultant effects on the respiratory system

bronchodilation: relaxation of the smooth muscles in the bronchi, resulting in a widening of the bronchi; an effect of sympathetic stimulation

pheochromocytoma: tumor of the chromaffin cells of the adrenal medulla that periodically releases large amounts of norepinephrine and epinephrine into the system with resultant severe hypertension and tachycardia

sympatholytic: drug that lyses, or blocks, the effects of the sympathetic nervous system

Drug List

NONSELECTIVE ADRENERGIC BLOCKING AGENTS
- amiodarone
- carvedilol
- (P) labetalol

NONSELECTIVE ALPHA-ADRENERGIC BLOCKING AGENTS
- (P) phentolamine

ALPHA$_1$-SELECTIVE ADRENERGIC BLOCKING AGENTS
- alfuzosin
- (P) doxazosin
- prazosin
- silodosin
- tamsulosin
- terazosin

NONSELECTIVE BETA-ADRENERGIC BLOCKING AGENTS
- carteolol
- levobunolol
- nadolol
- nebivolol
- (P) propranolol
- sotalol
- timolol

BETA$_1$-SELECTIVE ADRENERGIC BLOCKING AGENTS
- acebutolol
- (P) atenolol
- betaxolol
- bisoprolol
- esmolol
- metoprolol

Adrenergic antagonists or adrenergic blocking agents are also called **sympatholytic** drugs because they lyse, or block, the effects of the sympathetic nervous system (SNS). The therapeutic and adverse effects associated with these drugs are related to their **adrenergic receptor–site specificity**, that is, the ability to react with specific adrenergic receptor sites without activating them, thus preventing the typical manifestations of SNS activation. By occupying the adrenergic receptor site, they prevent norepinephrine released from the nerve terminal or from the adrenal medulla from activating the receptor, thus blocking the SNS effects.

The adrenergic blockers have varying degrees of specificity for the adrenergic receptor sites. For example, some can interact with both alpha- and beta-receptors. Some are specific to alpha-receptors, with some being even more specific to just alpha$_1$-receptors. Other adrenergic blockers interact with both beta$_1$- and beta$_2$-receptors, whereas others interact with either beta$_1$- or beta$_2$-receptors only. This specificity allows the provider to select a drug that will have the desired therapeutic effects without the undesired effects that occur when the entire SNS is blocked. In general, however, the specificity of adrenergic blocking agents depends on the concentration of drug in the body. Most specificity is lost with higher serum drug levels (Fig. 31.1).

The effects of the adrenergic blocking agents vary with the age of the patient (Box 31.1). Various alternative and herbal remedies can also affect these drugs (see Chapter 60).

Nonselective Adrenergic Blocking Agents

Drugs that block both alpha- and beta-adrenergic receptors are primarily used to treat cardiac-related conditions. These drugs include amiodarone (*Nexterone, Pacerone*), carvedilol (*Coreg, Coreg CR*), and labetalol (*Trandate*) (Table 31.1).

Therapeutic Actions and Indications

Adrenergic blocking agents competitively block the effects of norepinephrine at alpha- and beta-receptors throughout the SNS. This results in lower blood pressure, slower pulse rate, and increased renal perfusion with decreased renin levels.

Labetalol is used intravenously (IV) and orally to treat hypertension. It has been used to treat hypertension associated with **pheochromocytoma** (tumor of the chromaffin cells of the adrenal medulla that periodically releases large amounts of norepinephrine and epinephrine into the system with resultant severe hypertension and tachycardia) and clonidine withdrawal. Amiodarone, which is available in oral and IV forms, is indicated to treat life threatening ventricular arrhythmias and is used as an antiarrhythmic (see Chapter 45). It is generally thought of as a class III antiarrhythmic. However, it blocks sodium channels (like class I), is an antisympathetic (like class II), and has negative chronotropic effects (like class IV). Carvedilol is only available orally and is used to treat hypertension as well as heart failure (HF) and left ventricular dysfunction after myocardial infarction (MI). Table 31.1 shows usual indications for each of these agents.

Pharmacokinetics

These drugs are well absorbed when given orally and are distributed throughout the body when given IV or orally. They are metabolized in the liver and excreted in feces and urine. The half-life varies with the particular drug and preparation.

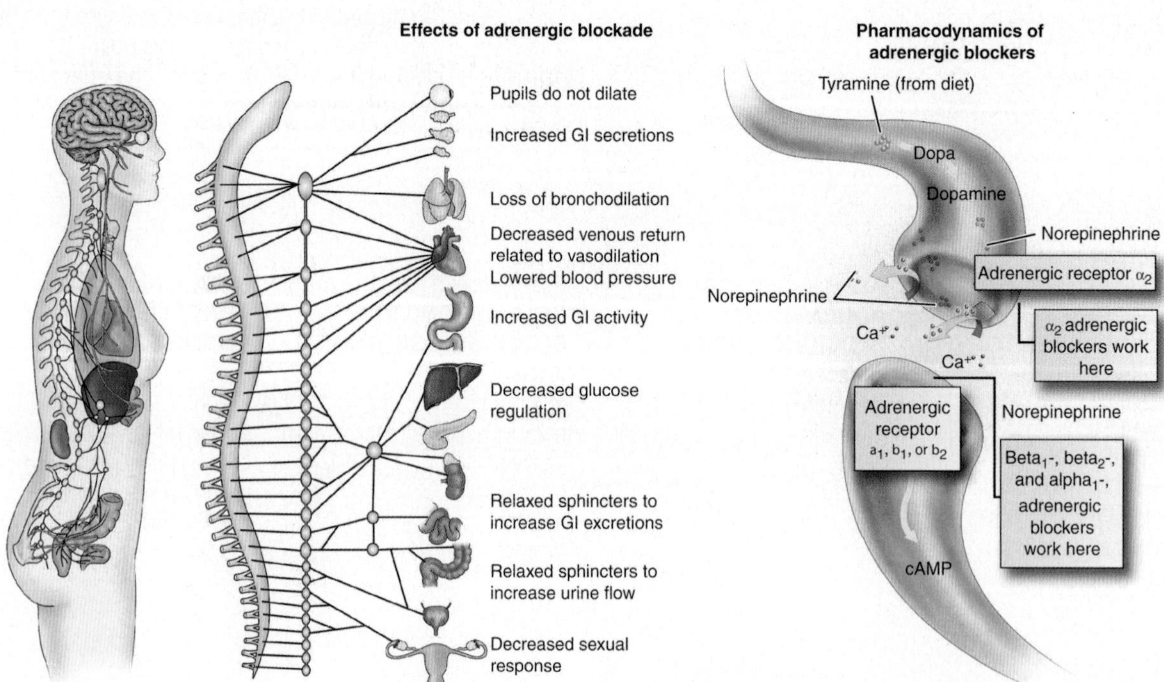

FIGURE 31.1 Site of action of adrenergic receptors and resultant physiological responses. These responses are blocked by adrenergic blockers.

Box 31.1 Focus on Drug Therapy Across the Lifespan

ADRENERGIC BLOCKING AGENTS

Children

The safety and efficacy for many of these drugs have not been established for children younger than 18 years of age. If one of these drugs is used, the dose needs to be calculated from the child's body weight and age. It is good practice to have a second person check the dose calculation before administering the drug to avoid potential toxic effects. Prazosin is used to treat hypertension, and phentolamine is used during surgery for pheochromocytoma. Children should be carefully monitored and supported when adrenergic blocking agents are given. Propranolol as an oral solution form is used for the treatment of proliferating infantile hemangioma in children 5 weeks to 5 months of age.

Adults

Adults being treated with adrenergic blocking agents should be cautioned about the many adverse effects associated with the drugs. Patients with diabetes need to be reeducated about ways to monitor themselves for hyperglycemia and hypoglycemia because the sympathetic reaction (sweating, feeling tense, increased heart rate, rapid breathing) usually alerts patients that there is a problem with their glucose levels. Patients with severe thyroid disease are also at high risk for serious adverse effects when taking these drugs; if one of them is needed, the patient should be monitored closely. Propranolol and metoprolol are associated with more CNS adverse effects than are other adrenergic blockers, and patients who have CNS complications already or who develop CNS problems while taking an adrenergic blocker might do better with a different agent.

In general, there is little data about the effects of adrenergic blockers during pregnancy and lactation, and they should be used only in those situations in which the benefit to the patient is greater than the risk to the fetus or neonate. Adrenergic blockers can affect labor, and babies born to people taking these drugs may exhibit adverse CV, respiratory, and CNS effects. Many of these drugs were teratogenic in animal studies. Because of a similar risk of adverse reactions to the baby, patients who are breast or chestfeeding should find another way to feed the baby if an adrenergic blocking drug is needed.

Older Adults

Older patients are more likely to experience the adverse CNS, CV, GI, and respiratory effects associated with these drugs. Because older patients often also have renal or hepatic impairment, they are more likely to have toxic levels of these drugs related to changes in metabolism and excretion. The older patient should be started on a lower dose of the drug and should be monitored closely for potentially serious arrhythmias or blood pressure changes.

Contraindications and Cautions

The nonselective adrenergic blocking agents are contraindicated in patients with known hypersensitivity to any component of the drug to avoid potentially serious hypersensitivity reactions; with bradycardia or heart blocks, which could be worsened by the slowed heart rate and conduction; with shock or HF requiring inotropic support, which could become worse with the loss of the sympathetic reaction; and who are lactating because of the potential adverse effects on neonates (amiodarone especially).

These drugs should be used with caution in patients with diabetes because the disorder could be aggravated by the blocked sympathetic response and because the usual signs and symptoms of hypoglycemia and hyperglycemia can be masked with the SNS blockade. Caution also should be exercised in patients with bronchospasm and/or asthma, which could progress to respiratory distress due to the loss of norepinephrine's bronchodilating actions, and in pregnancy because there is little data to evaluate the potential risk to the fetus (labetalol and carvedilol). Amiodarone is known to cross the placenta and cause neonatal bradycardia, hypothyroidism, fetal growth retardation, premature birth, and other

Table 31.1 *Drugs in Focus*: Nonselective Adrenergic Blocking Agents

Drug Name	Dosage/Route	Usual Indications
amiodarone (*Nexterone*, *Pacerone*)	Loading dose PO, 800–1,600 mg/d PO, reduce to 100–400 mg/d for maintenance; *or* loading dose IV 150 mg over 10 min followed by 360 mg over 6 h at 1 mg/min and then 540 mg over 18 h at 0.5 mg/min; switch to PO as soon as possible	Treatment of life-threatening ventricular arrhythmias (ventricular fibrillation or ventricular tachycardia), atrial fibrillation
carvedilol (*Coreg*, *Coreg CR*)	6.25–25 mg PO b.i.d. for hypertension; 3.125–25 mg PO b.i.d. for HF/LV dysfunction *CR:* 2–80 mg PO daily for hypertension; 10–80 mg PO daily for HF/LV dysfunction	Treatment of hypertension, left ventricular dysfunction after myocardial infarction (MI), and HF in adults, alone or as part of combination therapy
labetalol (*Trandate*)	100 mg PO b.i.d. initially, maintenance at 200–400 mg PO b.i.d.; 20 mg IV, slowly with additional doses given at 10-min intervals to a maximum dose of 300 mg for severe hypertension	Treatment of hypertension, hypertension associated with pheochromocytoma, and clonidine withdrawal

HF, heart failure.

adverse effects. The drugs should only be used if the benefit to the patient clearly outweighs the potential risk to the fetus.

Adverse Effects

The adverse effects associated with the use of nonselective adrenergic blocking agents are usually associated with the drug's effects on the SNS. These effects can include dizziness, paresthesia, insomnia, depression, fatigue, and vertigo, which are related to the blocking of norepinephrine's effect in the central nervous system (CNS). Nausea, vomiting, diarrhea, anorexia, and flatulence are associated with the loss of the balancing sympathetic effect on the gastrointestinal (GI) tract and increased parasympathetic dominance. Cardiac arrhythmias, hypotension, HF, pulmonary edema, and cerebrovascular accident, or stroke, are related to the lack of stimulatory effects and loss of vascular tone in the cardiovascular (CV) system. Bronchospasm, cough, rhinitis, and bronchial obstruction are related to loss of **bronchodilation**—the relaxation of the smooth muscles in the bronchi, resulting in a widening of the bronchi—of the respiratory tract and vasodilation of mucous membrane vessels (Fig. 31.2). Other effects reported include decreased exercise tolerance, hypoglycemia, and rash related to the sympathetic blocking effects. Abruptly stopping these drugs after long-term therapy can result in MI, stroke, and arrhythmias related to an increased hypersensitivity to catecholamines that develops when the receptor sites have been blocked. Carvedilol and labetalol have been associated with hepatic failure related to its effects on the liver. Amiodarone has been associated with hepatic injury, pulmonary fibrosis, loss of vision, and thyroid abnormalities.

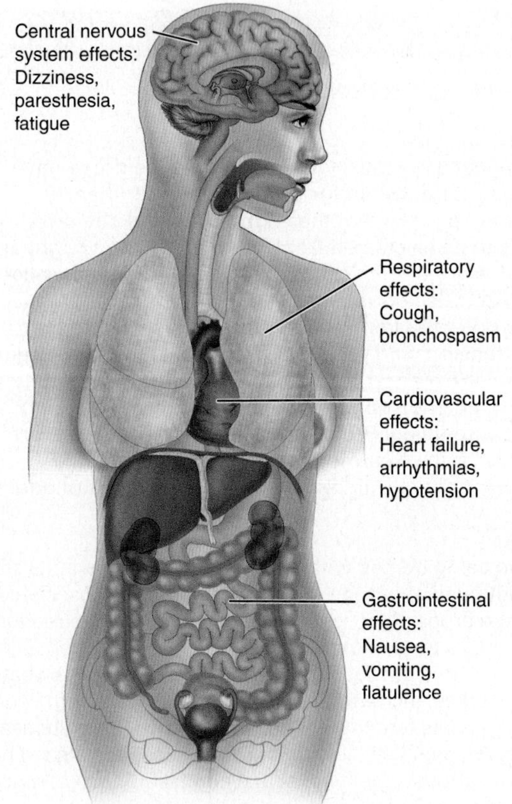

FIGURE 31.2 Variety of adverse effects and toxicities associated with adrenergic blocking antagonists.

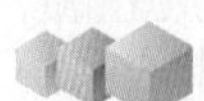 *Concept Mastery Alert*

Nursing Intervention for Adrenergic Blocking Medication

For patients who were on long-term nonselective adrenergic blocking medications and who report ceasing all medications because they began feeling nauseated and started vomiting, a primary step in assessing the severity of adverse effects (such as cardiovascular incidents) is to perform a bedside electrocardiogram to assess for any arrhythmias. Abruptly stopping these drugs after long-term therapy can result in myocardial infarction, stroke, and arrhythmias related to the increased hypersensitivity to catecholamines that develops when the receptor sites have been blocked.

Clinically Important Drug–Drug Interactions

There is increased risk of excessive hypotension if any of these drugs is combined with volatile liquid general anesthetics such as enflurane, halothane, or isoflurane. The effectiveness of some diabetic agents is increased, leading to hypoglycemia when such agents are used with these drugs; patients should be monitored closely and dose adjustments made as needed. In addition, carvedilol has been associated with potentially dangerous conduction system disturbances when combined with verapamil or diltiazem; use of amiodarone with carvedilol may increase levels of carvedilol. Coadministration of amiodarone and other antiarrhythmics that can prolong the QT interval may increase risk of torsade de pointes.

Prototype Summary: Labetalol

Indications: Hypertension, alone or in combination with other drugs; off-label uses, including control of blood pressure in pheochromocytoma and clonidine withdrawal hypertension.

Actions: Competitively blocks $alpha_1$- and beta-receptor sites in the SNS, leading to lower blood pressure without reflex tachycardia and decreased renin levels.

Pharmacokinetics:

Route	Onset	Peak	Duration
Oral	Varies	1–2 h	8–12 h
IV	Immediate	5 min	5.5 h

$T_{1/2}$: 6 to 8 hours (oral); metabolized in the liver; excreted in the urine and feces.

Adverse Effects: Dizziness, vertigo, fatigue, gastric pain, flatulence, impotence, bronchospasm, dyspnea, cough, decreased exercise tolerance, hypotension, hepatic injury.

Nursing Considerations for Patients Receiving Nonselective Adrenergic Blocking Agents

Assessment: History and Examination

- Assess for contraindications or cautions: any known allergies to these drugs to avoid hypersensitivity reactions; presence of bradycardia or heart blocks, which could be worsened by the slowing of heart rate and conduction; asthma or bronchospasm, which could be exacerbated by the loss of the bronchodilation effect of norepinephrine; shock or HF requiring inotropic support, which could worsen with the loss of the sympathetic reaction; diabetes, which could be aggravated by the blocking of the sympathetic response and the masking of the usual signs and symptoms of hypoglycemia and hyperglycemia; and pregnancy or lactation status because of the potential adverse effects on the fetus or neonate.
- Perform a physical assessment to establish baseline data for determining the effectiveness of the drug and the occurrence of any adverse effects associated with drug therapy; assess the level of orientation and for any complaints of dizziness, paresthesia, or vertigo.
- Monitor vital signs and assess CV status, including pulse, blood pressure, and cardiac output, to evaluate for possible cardiac effects; obtain an electrocardiogram (ECG) as ordered to assess for possible irregularities in rate or rhythm; assess respiratory rate and auscultate lungs to determine the presence of any adventitious sounds; observe for ease of breathing, and report any signs and symptoms of bronchospasm or respiratory distress; and monitor GI activity to determine the need for interventions to deal with increased activity.
- Monitor the results of laboratory tests such as renal and liver function studies and electrolyte levels to determine the need for possible dose adjustment; monitor blood glucose levels to evaluate for hyperglycemia or hypoglycemia.

Nursing Conclusions

Nursing conclusions related to drug therapy might include the following:

- Altered cardiac output related to CV effects
- Altered breathing pattern related to lack of bronchodilating effects
- Injury risk related to CNS effects
- Diarrhea related to increased parasympathetic activity
- Knowledge deficit regarding drug therapy

Planning

- The patient will receive the best therapeutic effect from the drug therapy.
- The patient will have limited adverse effects from the drug therapy.
- The patient will have an understanding of the drug therapy, adverse effects to anticipate, and measures to relieve discomfort and improve safety.

Intervention With Rationale

- Do not discontinue abruptly after chronic therapy but taper drug slowly when possible because long-term use of medication can sensitize the receptors to catecholamines, and the patient may have very high heart rates and blood pressures. Monitor heart rate and blood pressure as the drug is tapered.
- Encourage the patient to adopt lifestyle changes, including diet, exercise, smoking cessation, and stress reduction, to aid in lowering blood pressure.
- Assess heart rate for changes that might suggest arrhythmias. Obtain blood pressure in various positions to assess for orthostatic hypotension.
- Institute safety precautions especially if the patient complains of dizziness, fatigue, or vertigo, or if orthostatic hypotension occurs, to prevent injury to the patient.
- Monitor GI function and need for increased access to bathroom facilities and for increased fluid intake related to diarrhea.
- Monitor for any sign of liver failure to arrange to discontinue the drug if this occurs.
- Offer support and encouragement to help the patient deal with the drug regimen.
- Provide thorough patient teaching, including drug name, dosage, and schedule for administration; measures to prevent adverse effects and warning signs of problems; the need to avoid herbal or alternative therapies unless allowed by the prescriber; safety measures, such as changing position slowly and avoiding driving or operating hazardous machinery; and the need for monitoring and evaluation to enhance patient knowledge about drug therapy and to promote adherence.

Evaluation

- Monitor patient response to the drug (improvement in blood pressure and HF).
- Monitor for adverse effects (CV changes, headache, GI upset, bronchospasm, liver failure).
- Evaluate the effectiveness of the teaching plan (patient can name drug, dosage, adverse effects to watch for, specific measures to avoid adverse effects).
- Monitor the effectiveness of comfort measures and adherence to the regimen.

Key Points

- Adrenergic blocking agents block the effects of the SNS.
- The nonselective adrenergic blocking agents block all adrenergic receptors, that is, both alpha- and beta-receptors. Selective adrenergic blocking agents have specific affinity for alpha- or beta-receptors or for specific $alpha_1$-, $beta_1$-, or $beta_2$-receptor sites.
- Blocking all of the receptor sites within the SNS results in a lowering of blood pressure.

Nonselective Alpha-Adrenergic Blocking Agents

Some adrenergic blocking agents have a specific affinity for alpha-receptor sites. Their use is limited because of the development of even more specific and safer drugs. Only one of these drugs, phentolamine (*Oraverse, Regitine*), is still used (Table 31.2).

Therapeutic Actions and Indications

Phentolamine blocks the postsynaptic $alpha_1$-adrenergic receptors, decreasing sympathetic tone in the vasculature and causing vasodilation, which leads to a lowering of blood pressure. It also blocks presynaptic $alpha_2$-receptors, preventing the feedback control of norepinephrine release. The result is an increase in reflex tachycardia that occurs when blood pressure is lowered. Phentolamine is most frequently used to prevent cell death and tissue sloughing after extravasation of intravenous norepinephrine or dopamine, causing local vasodilation and a return of blood flow to the area. Table 31.2 shows the usual indications for this agent.

Pharmacokinetics

Phentolamine is rapidly absorbed after IV or intramuscular (IM) injection and is excreted in the urine. There is little data on its metabolism and distribution.

Contraindications and Cautions

Phentolamine is contraindicated in the presence of allergy to this or similar drugs and in the presence of coronary artery disease or MI because of the potential exacerbation of these conditions; it should be used cautiously in pregnancy or lactation because of the potential adverse effects on the fetus or neonate.

Adverse Effects

Patients receiving phentolamine often experience extensions of the therapeutic effects, including hypotension, orthostatic hypotension, angina, MI, cerebrovascular accident, flushing, tachycardia, and arrhythmia—all of which are related to vasodilation and decreased blood pressure. Headache, weakness, and dizziness often occur in response to hypotension. Nausea, vomiting, and diarrhea may also occur.

Clinically Important Drug–Drug Interactions

Ephedrine and epinephrine may have decreased hypertensive and vasoconstrictive effects if they are taken concomitantly with phentolamine because these agents work in opposing ways in the body. Increased hypotension may occur if this drug is combined with alcohol, which is also a vasodilator.

Prototype Summary: Phentolamine

Indications: Prevention or control of hypertensive episodes associated with pheochromocytoma; test for diagnosis of pheochromocytoma; prevention and treatment of dermal necrosis and sloughing associated with IV extravasation of norepinephrine or dopamine.

Actions: Competitively blocks postsynaptic $alpha_1$- and presynaptic $alpha_2$-receptors, causing vasodilation and lowering of blood pressure, accompanied by increased reflex tachycardia.

Pharmacokinetics:

Route	Onset	Peak	Duration
Intramuscular	Rapid	20 min	30–45 min
IV	Immediate	2 min	15–30 min

$T_{1/2}$: Metabolism and excretion are unknown.

Adverse Effects: Acute and prolonged hypotensive episodes, MI, tachycardia, arrhythmias, nausea, flushing.

Table 31.2 *Drugs in Focus*: Nonselective Alpha-Adrenergic Blocking Agent

Drug Name	Dosage/Route	Usual Indications
phentolamine (*Oraverse, Regitine*)	*Adult*: 5 mg IV or IM 1–2 h before surgery; 5–10 mg in 10 mL of saline injected into the area of extravasation within 12 h after extravasation *Pediatric*: 1 mg IM or IV 1–2 h before surgery; treat extravasation as in the adult *Oraverse:* dosing based on amount of local anesthesia administered	Prevention of cell death and tissue sloughing after extravasation of IV norepinephrine or dopamine, and of severe hypertension reactions caused by manipulation of the pheochromocytoma before and during surgery; diagnosis of pheochromocytoma; reversal of soft tissue anesthesia (*Oraverse*)

Nursing Considerations for Patients Receiving the Nonselective Alpha-Adrenergic Blocking Agent

Assessment: History and Examination

- Assess for contraindications or cautions: any known allergies to the drug to avoid hypersensitivity reactions; presence of any CV diseases, which may be exacerbated by the use of this drug; and current status of pregnancy or lactation because of the potential for adverse effects to the fetus or neonate.
- Perform a physical assessment to establish baseline data for determining the effectiveness of the drug and occurrence of any adverse effects.
- Assess orientation, affect, and reflexes to monitor for CNS changes related to drug therapy; monitor CV status, including pulse, blood pressure, peripheral perfusion, and cardiac output, to determine changes in function, and urine output, which will reflect perfusion of the kidney as another assessment of cardiac function.

Nursing Conclusions

Nursing conclusions related to drug therapy might include the following:

- Injury risk related to CNS and CV effects of the drug
- Altered cardiac output related to blood pressure changes, arrhythmias, and vasodilation
- Knowledge deficit regarding drug therapy

Planning

- The patient will receive the best therapeutic effect from the drug therapy.
- The patient will have limited adverse effects from the drug therapy.
- The patient will have an understanding of the drug therapy, adverse effects to anticipate, and measures to relieve discomfort and improve safety.

Intervention With Rationale

- Monitor heart rate and blood pressure closely and frequently for changes to anticipate the need to discontinue the drug if adverse reactions are severe; provide supportive management if needed.
- Inject phentolamine directly into the area of extravasation of epinephrine or dopamine to prevent local cell death.
- Arrange for supportive care and comfort measures such as rest, environmental control, and other measures to decrease CNS irritation; provide headache medication to alleviate patient discomfort.
- Institute safety measures to prevent injury if the patient experiences weakness, dizziness, or orthostatic hypotension.
- Provide thorough patient teaching, including drug name, dosage, and schedule for administration; potential adverse effects and measures to prevent them; and warning signs of problems to enhance patient knowledge about drug therapy and to promote adherence.
- Offer support and encouragement to help the patient deal with the need for the drug.

Evaluation

- Monitor patient response to the drug (improvement in signs and symptoms of pheochromocytoma, improvement in tissue condition after extravasation).
- Monitor for adverse effects (orthostatic hypotension, arrhythmias, CNS effects such as headache or dizziness).
- Evaluate the effectiveness of the teaching plan (patient can name drug, dosage, adverse effects to watch for, and specific measures to avoid them).
- Monitor the effectiveness of support measures.

Key Points

- A nonselective alpha-adrenergic blocking agent is used to treat pheochromocytoma, a tumor of the adrenal medulla. A reflex tachycardia commonly occurs when the blood pressure falls.
- Phentolamine is a nonselective alpha-adrenergic blocker used most commonly for the prevention and treatment of dermal necrosis and sloughing associated with IV extravasation of norepinephrine or dopamine.

Alpha$_1$-Selective Adrenergic Blocking Agents

Alpha1-selective adrenergic blocking agents are drugs that have a specific affinity for alpha$_1$-receptors. These drugs include alfuzosin (*Uroxatral*), doxazosin (*Cardura*), prazosin (*Minipress*), silodosin (*Rapaflo*), tamsulosin (*Flomax*), and terazosin (generic) (Table 31.3).

Therapeutic Actions and Indications

The therapeutic effects of the alpha$_1$-selective adrenergic blocking agents come from their ability to block the postsynaptic alpha$_1$-receptor sites. This causes a decrease in vascular tone and vasodilation, which leads to a fall in blood pressure. Because these drugs do not block the presynaptic alpha$_2$-receptor sites, the reflex tachycardia that accompanies a fall in blood pressure does not occur. They also block smooth muscle receptors in the prostate, prostatic capsule, prostatic urethra, and urinary bladder neck, which leads to relaxation of the bladder and prostate and improved flow of urine in male patients with benign prostatic hyperplasia

Table 31.3 *Drugs in Focus*: Alpha$_1$-Selective Adrenergic Blocking Agents

Drug Name	Dosage/Route	Usual Indications
alfuzosin (*Uroxatral*)	10 mg/d PO	Treatment of BPH
doxazosin (*Cardura*)	1 mg/d PO up to 16 mg/d PO for hypertension; 1–8 mg/d PO for BPH	Treatment of hypertension and BPH
prazosin (*Minipress*)	*Adult*: 1 mg PO b.i.d. to t.i.d. with maintenance at 6–15 mg/d PO in divided doses *Pediatric*: 0.5–7 mg PO t.i.d.	Treatment of hypertension, alone or in combination with other drugs
silodosin (*Rapaflo*)	*Adult*: 8 mg/d PO with meal; dose adjustment with renal impairment	Treatment of signs/symptoms of BPH
tamsulosin (*Flomax*)	0.4–0.8 mg/d PO 30 min after the same meal each day	Treatment of BPH
terazosin (generic)	1–5 mg/d PO, preferably at bedtime for hypertension; 10 mg/d PO for BPH	Treatment of hypertension and BPH

BPH, benign prostatic hyperplasia.

(BPH). These drugs are available in oral form and can be used to treat BPH (see Chapter 52 for further discussion on BPH) and hypertension. Alfuzosin, silodosin, and tamsulosin are only indicated for treatment of BPH and not for hypertension due to their actions on a subtype of alpha receptor found predominately in the prostate. The drugs may be used alone or as part of a combination therapy. Table 31.3 shows usual indications for each of these agents.

Pharmacokinetics

The alpha$_1$-selective adrenergic blocking agents are well absorbed after oral administration and undergo extensive hepatic metabolism. They are excreted in the urine.

Contraindications and Cautions

The alpha$_1$-selective adrenergic blocking agents are contraindicated in the presence of allergy to any of these drugs to avoid hypersensitivity reactions and also with lactation because the drugs cross into human milk and could have adverse effects on the neonate. They should be used cautiously in the presence of HF or renal failure because their blood pressure–lowering effects could exacerbate these conditions and with hepatic impairment, which could alter the metabolism of these drugs. Caution also should be exercised during pregnancy because of the potential for adverse effects on the fetus.

Adverse Effects

The adverse effects associated with the use of these drugs are usually related to their effects of SNS blockage. CNS effects include headache, dizziness, weakness, fatigue, drowsiness, and depression. Nausea, vomiting, abdominal pain, and diarrhea may occur as a result of direct effects on the GI tract and sympathetic blocking. Anticipated CV effects include arrhythmias, hypotension, edema, HF, and angina. The vasodilation caused by these drugs can also cause flushing, rhinitis, reddened eyes, nasal congestion, retrograde ejaculation, and priapism.

Clinically Important Drug–Drug Interactions

Increased hypotensive effects may occur if these drugs are combined with any other vasodilating or antihypertensive drugs, such as nitrates, calcium channel blockers, drugs used for erectile dysfunction, and angiotensin-converting enzyme inhibitors.

Prototype Summary: Doxazosin

Indications: Treatment of mild to moderate hypertension as monotherapy or in combination with other antihypertensives; treatment of BPH.

Actions: Reduces total peripheral resistance through alpha blockade; does not affect heart rate or cardiac output; increases high-density lipoproteins while lowering total cholesterol levels.

Pharmacokinetics:

Route	Onset	Peak	Duration
Oral	Varies	2–3 h	Not known

$T_{1/2}$: 22 hours; metabolized in the liver; excreted in the bile, feces, and urine.

Adverse Effects: Hypotension, headache, fatigue, dizziness, postural dizziness, vertigo, tachycardia, edema, nausea, dyspepsia, diarrhea, retrograde ejaculation.

Nursing Considerations for Patients Receiving Alpha$_1$-Selective Adrenergic Blocking Agents

Assessment: History and Examination

- Assess for contraindications or cautions: any known allergies to these drugs to avoid hypersensitivity reactions; heart failure or renal failure, which could be exacerbated by drug use; hepatic dysfunction, which could alter the drug's metabolism; and current status of pregnancy or lactation because of unknown or adverse effects to the fetus or neonate.
- Perform a physical assessment to establish baseline data for determining the effectiveness of drug therapy and the occurrence of any adverse effects.
- Monitor the level of orientation, affect, and reflexes to monitor for CNS changes related to drug therapy.
- Monitor vital signs and assess CV status, including pulse, blood pressure, peripheral perfusion, and cardiac output, to evaluate for possible cardiac effects; obtain an electrocardiogram as ordered to assess for possible irregularities in rate or rhythm.
- Assess renal function, including urinary output, to evaluate effects on the renal system and assess BPH and its effects on urinary output.
- Monitor renal and hepatic function tests to evaluate potential need for dose adjustment.

Nursing Conclusions

Nursing conclusions related to drug therapy might include the following:

- Impaired comfort related to headache, GI upset, flushing, nasal congestion
- Injury risk related to CNS or CV effects of the drug
- Altered cardiac output related to blood pressure changes, arrhythmias, vasodilation
- Knowledge deficit regarding drug therapy

Planning

- The patient will receive the best therapeutic effect from the drug therapy.
- The patient will have limited adverse effects from the drug therapy.
- The patient will have an understanding of the drug therapy, adverse effects to anticipate, and measures to relieve discomfort and improve safety.

Intervention With Rationale

- Monitor blood pressure, pulse, rhythm, and cardiac output regularly to evaluate for changes that may indicate a need to adjust dose or discontinue the drug if CV effects are severe.
- Establish safety precautions if CNS effects or orthostatic hypotension occurs to prevent patient injury.
- Arrange for small, frequent meals if GI upset is severe to relieve discomfort and maintain nutrition.
- Arrange for supportive care and comfort measures (rest, environmental control, other measures) to decrease CNS effects; provide headache medication to alleviate patient discomfort; and arrange safety measures if CNS effects occur to prevent patient injury.
- Offer support and encouragement to help the patient deal with the drug regimen.
- Provide thorough patient teaching, including drug name, dosage, and administration; measures to prevent adverse effects and warning signs to report to prescriber; safety measures such as changing positions slowly and avoiding driving or operating hazardous machinery; and the need to report the use of other drugs, including drugs for erectile dysfunction and dietary measures in conjunction with drug therapy to promote blood pressure control or alleviate GI upset to enhance patient knowledge about drug therapy and to promote adherence.
- Offer support and encouragement to help the patient deal with the drug regimen.

Evaluation

- Monitor patient response to the drug (lowering of blood pressure, improved urine flow with BPH).
- Monitor for adverse effects (GI upset, CNS or CV changes).
- Evaluate effectiveness of the teaching plan (patient can name drug, dosage, adverse effects to watch for, and specific measures to avoid them).
- Monitor the effectiveness of comfort measures and adherence to the regimen.

Key Points

- Alpha$_1$-selective adrenergic blocking agents decrease blood pressure by blocking the postsynaptic alpha$_1$-receptor sites, decreasing vascular tone, and promoting vasodilation.
- Alpha$_1$-selective adrenergic blocking agents are used to treat hypertension and are often used to treat BPH because of their relaxing effects on the bladder and prostate.

Nonselective Beta-Adrenergic Blocking Agents

The **beta-adrenergic blocking agents** (Table 31.4) are used to treat migraine headaches and CV problems (hypertension, angina) and to prevent reinfarction after MI. These drugs are widely used and include carteolol (generic), levobunolol (*Akbeta*, *Betagan*), nadolol (*Corgard*), nebivolol (*Bystolic*), propranolol (*Hemangeol*, *Inderal*, *Innopran XL*), sotalol (*Betapace*, *Betapace AF*, *Sorine*, *Sotylize*), and timolol

(*Betimol, Istalol, Timolol Maleate, Timoptic*). The prototype drug propranolol has a variety of uses that range from prophylaxis of migraine headaches to treatment of arrhythmias.

Therapeutic Actions and Indications

The therapeutic effects of these drugs are related to their competitive blocking of the beta-adrenergic receptors in the SNS. The blockade of the beta-receptors in the heart and in the juxtaglomerular apparatus of the nephron accounts for the majority of the therapeutic benefit. Decreased heart rate, contractility, and excitability, as well as a membrane-stabilizing effect, lead to decreases in arrhythmias, cardiac workload, and oxygen consumption. The juxtaglomerular cells are not stimulated to release renin, which further decreases blood pressure. These effects are useful in treating hypertension and chronic angina and can help to prevent reinfarction after an MI by decreasing cardiac workload and oxygen consumption. Sotalol is used for treating life-threatening ventricular arrhythmias and to maintain sinus rhythm in patients with atrial flutter or atrial fibrillation (see Chapter 45). It is both a beta-blocker (class II antiarrhythmic) and a class III antiarrhythmic.

Propranolol is effective in blocking all of the beta-receptors in the SNS and was one of the first drugs of the class (see Table 31.4 for usual indications). Since the introduction of propranolol, newer and more selective drugs have become available that are not associated with some of the adverse effects seen with total blockade of the SNS beta-receptors. In 2014, propranolol (*Hemangeol*) was approved in an oral solution form for the treatment of proliferating infantile hemangioma in children 5 weeks to 5 months of age. Nebivolol is indicated for treatment of hypertension alone or in combination with other medications. Timolol has several recommended uses, which are listed in Table 31.4; timolol, carteolol, and levobunolol are available in an ophthalmic form for reduction of intraocular pressure in patients with open-angle glaucoma. When these drugs are used topically, eye muscle relaxation occurs. Because they are applied topically, if used properly they have limited systemic absorption.

Pharmacokinetics

The drugs that are indicated for oral use are absorbed from the GI tract and undergo hepatic metabolism. Food has been found to increase the bioavailability of propranolol, though this effect was not found with other beta-adrenergic blocking agents. Absorption of sotalol is decreased by the presence of food. Propranolol also crosses the blood–brain barrier, but nadolol and sotalol do not, making them

Table 31.4 *Drugs in Focus*: Nonselective Beta-Adrenergic Blocking Agents

Drug Name	Dosage/Route	Usual Indications
carteolol (generic)	One drop in affected eye(s) b.i.d.	Treatment of chronic open-angle glaucoma
levobunolol (*Akbeta, Betagan*, generic)	1–2 drops in affected eye(s) q.d. or b.i.d.	Treatment of chronic open-angle glaucoma, ocular hypertension
nadolol (*Corgard*)	*Hypertension*: 40–80 mg/d PO, up to 320 mg/d may be needed; reduce dose in renal impairment *Angina*: 40–80 mg/d PO	Treatment of hypertension, management of chronic angina in adults
nebivolol (*Bystolic*)	Initially 5 mg/d PO, increase at 2-wk intervals based on patient response; maximum dose of 40 mg/d	Treatment of hypertension, alone or as part of combination therapy in adults
propranolol (*Inderal, Hemangeol, Innopran XL*)	Dose varies widely based on indication; check drug guide for specific information	Treatment of hypertension, angina, idiopathic hypertrophic subaortic stenosis–induced palpitations, angina and syncope, certain cardiac arrhythmias induced by catecholamines or digoxin, and pheochromocytoma; prevention of reinfarction after MI; prophylaxis for migraine headache (which may be caused by vasodilation and is relieved by vasoconstriction, although the exact action is not clearly understood); prevention of stage fright (which is a sympathetic stress reaction to a particular situation); treatment of essential tremors; treatment of proliferating infantile hemangioma
sotalol (*Betapace, Betapace AF, Sorine, Sotylize*)	80 mg PO b.i.d., up to 320 mg PO b.i.d. may be needed; dose adjustment based on QT interval, renal function, and patient response	Treatment of potentially life-threatening ventricular arrhythmias; maintenance of normal sinus rhythm in patients with symptomatic atrial fibrillation/flutter
timolol (*Betimol, Istalol, Timolol Maleate, Timoptic*)	10 mg PO b.i.d., increase based on patient response; 1–2 drops (gtt) in affected eye(s) for glaucoma	Treatment of hypertension; prevention of reinfarction after MI; prophylaxis for migraine; in ophthalmic form, reduction of intraocular pressure in open-angle glaucoma

MI, myocardial infarction.

a better choice if CNS effects occur with propranolol. These drugs are all excreted in the urine. Carteolol and levobunolol are only available in an ophthalmic form.

Contraindications and Cautions

Nonselective beta-adrenergic blocking agents are contraindicated in the presence of allergy to any of these drugs or any components of the drug being used, to avoid hypersensitivity reactions; with bradycardia or heart blocks, shock, or HF, which could be exacerbated by the cardiac-suppressing effects of these drugs; with bronchospasm or acute asthma, which could worsen due to the blocking of sympathetic bronchodilation; with pregnancy because teratogenic effects have occurred in animal studies with all of these drugs except sotalol, and because neonatal apnea, bradycardia, and hypoglycemia could occur; and with lactation because of the potential effects on the neonate, which could include slowed heart rate, hypotension, and hypoglycemia. The safety and efficacy for use of these drugs in children have not been established.

These drugs should be used cautiously in patients with diabetes and hypoglycemia because of the blocking of the normal signs and symptoms of hypoglycemia and hyperglycemia; in patients with chronic obstructive pulmonary disease (COPD) and asthma, which could worsen due to the blocking of sympathetic bronchodilation; or with renal or hepatic dysfunction, which could interfere with the excretion and metabolism of these drugs.

Adverse Effects

Patients receiving these drugs often experience adverse effects related to blockage of beta-receptors in the SNS. CNS effects include headache, fatigue, dizziness, depression, paresthesia, sleep disturbances, memory loss, and disorientation. CV effects can include bradycardia, heart block, HF, hypotension, and peripheral vascular insufficiency. Pulmonary effects can range from difficulty breathing, coughing, and bronchospasm to severe pulmonary edema and bronchial obstruction. GI upset, nausea, vomiting, diarrhea, gastric pain, and even colitis can occur as a result of unchecked parasympathetic activity and the blocking of the sympathetic receptors. Genitourinary (GU) effects can include decreased libido, impotence, dysuria, and Peyronie's disease. Other effects that can occur include decreased exercise tolerance (patients often report that their "get up and go" is gone), hypoglycemia or hyperglycemia, and liver changes. If these drugs are stopped abruptly after long-term use, there is risk of angina, MI, hypertension, and stroke because the receptor sites become hypersensitive to catecholamines after being blocked by the drugs.

Clinically Important Drug–Drug Interactions

When beta-adrenergic blocking agents are used with calcium channel blockers (verapamil and diltiazem), increased negative inotropic effects may occur. Increased antihypertensive effect may be seen with use of other antihypertensives with beta-adrenergic blocker medications.

There may be an enhanced parasympathetic response when beta-blockers are administered with clonidine. If they are to be discontinued, there is risk of severe hypertension response. If the medications need to be stopped, it is recommended to first discontinue the beta-blocker for several days and to then taper the clonidine.

A decreased antihypertensive effect may occur when beta-blockers are given with nonsteroidal anti-inflammatory drugs (NSAIDs); if this combination is used, the patient should be monitored closely, and dose adjustment should be made to achieve the desired control of blood pressure.

An initial hypertensive episode followed by bradycardia may occur if these drugs are given with epinephrine. Peripheral ischemia may occur if beta-blockers are taken in combination with ergot alkaloids.

When these drugs are given with insulin or other antidiabetic agents, there is a potential for change in blood glucose levels. The patient may not display the usual signs and symptoms of hypoglycemia or hyperglycemia, which are caused by activation of the SNS. Because these effects are blocked, the patient will need new indications to alert them to potential problems. If this combination is used, the patient should monitor blood glucose levels frequently throughout the day and should be alert to new manifestations indicating glucose imbalance.

Prototype Summary: Propranolol

Indications: Treatment of hypertension, angina pectoris, idiopathic hypertrophic subaortic stenosis, supraventricular tachycardia, and tremor; prevention of reinfarction after MI; adjunctive therapy in pheochromocytoma; prophylaxis of migraine headache; management of situational anxiety, treatment of proliferating infantile hemangioma.

Actions: Competitively blocks beta-adrenergic receptors in the heart and juxtaglomerular apparatus; reduces vascular tone in the CNS.

Pharmacokinetics:

Route	Onset	Peak	Duration
Oral	20–30 min	60–90 min	6–12 h
IV	Immediate	1 min	4–6 h

$T_{1/2}$: 3 to 5 hours; metabolized in the liver; excreted in the urine.

Adverse Effects: Allergic reaction, bradycardia, heart failure, cardiac arrhythmias, cerebrovascular accident, pulmonary edema, gastric pain, flatulence, impotence, decreased exercise tolerance, bronchospasm, hypotension, fatigue.

Nursing Considerations for Patients Receiving Nonselective Beta-Adrenergic Blocking Agents

Assessment: History and Examination

- Assess for contraindications or cautions: known allergy to any drug or to any components of the drug to avoid hypersensitivity reactions; bradycardia or heart blocks, shock, or heart failure, which could be exacerbated by the cardiac-suppressing effects of these drugs; bronchospasm, COPD, or acute asthma, which could worsen with blocking of sympathetic bronchodilation; diabetes or hypoglycemia, which could lead to altered blood glucose levels; renal or hepatic dysfunction, which could interfere with the excretion or metabolism of these drugs; and status of pregnancy and lactation because of the potential effects on the fetus or neonate.
- Perform a physical assessment to establish baseline data for determining the effectiveness of the drug and the occurrence of any adverse effects.
- Assess level of orientation and sensory function to evaluate for possible CNS effects.
- Monitor cardiopulmonary status, including pulse, blood pressure, and respiratory rate; auscultate lungs for adventitious breath sounds; obtain an ECG as ordered to evaluate for changes in heart rate or rhythm; and check color, sensation, and capillary refill of extremities to evaluate for possible peripheral vascular insufficiency.
- Assess the abdomen, including auscultating bowel sounds, to monitor for GI effects.
- Monitor the results of laboratory tests, such as electrolyte levels, to observe for risks for arrhythmias, and adrenal and hepatic function studies to determine the need for possible dose adjustment.

Refer to the "Critical Thinking Scenario" for a full discussion of nursing care for a patient who is receiving beta-adrenergic blocking agents.

Nursing Conclusions

Nursing conclusions related to drug therapy might include the following:

- Impaired comfort related to CNS, GI, and systemic effects
- Decreased cardiac output related to CV effects
- Altered tissue perfusion related to CV effects
- Injury risk related to CNS effects
- Activity intolerance related to suppression of the sympathetic system
- Knowledge deficit regarding drug therapy

Planning

- The patient will receive the best therapeutic effect from the drug therapy.
- The patient will have limited adverse effects from the drug therapy.
- The patient will have an understanding of the drug therapy, adverse effects to anticipate, and measures to relieve discomfort and improve safety.

Intervention With Rationale

- Do not stop these drugs abruptly after chronic therapy; instead, taper gradually if possible because long-term use of these drugs can sensitize the myocardium to catecholamines and severe reactions could occur.
- Continuously monitor any patient receiving an intravenous form of these drugs to avert serious complications caused by rapid sympathetic blockade.
- Monitor blood pressure, pulse, rhythm, and cardiac output regularly to evaluate drug effectiveness and to monitor for changes that may indicate a need to adjust dose or discontinue the drug if CV effects are severe.
- Arrange for supportive care and comfort measures (rest, environmental control, other measures) to relieve CNS effects; institute safety measures if CNS effects *occur to prevent patient injury*; provide small, frequent meals and mouth care to help relieve the discomfort of GI effects; establish a daily activity program, spacing activities to help the patient deal with activity intolerance.
- Offer support and encouragement to help the patient deal with the drug regimen.
- Provide thorough patient teaching, including drug name, dose, and schedule of administration; use of drug with food or meals, if appropriate; possible adverse effects and measures to prevent them; warning signs to report; safety measures, such as changing position slowly, avoiding driving or using hazardous machinery, and pacing activities; and the need for follow-up evaluation and possible changes in dose to achieve therapeutic effectiveness to enhance patient knowledge about drug therapy and to promote adherence.

Evaluation

- Monitor patient response to the drug (lowering of blood pressure, decrease in anginal episodes, improvement in condition being treated).
- Monitor for adverse effects (GI upset, CNS changes, respiratory problems, CV effects, loss of libido, and impotence).
- Evaluate the effectiveness of the teaching plan (patient can name drug, dosage, adverse effects to watch for, and specific measures to avoid them).
- Monitor the effectiveness of comfort measures and adherence to the regimen.

CRITICAL THINKING SCENARIO
Nonselective Beta-Blockers (Propranolol)

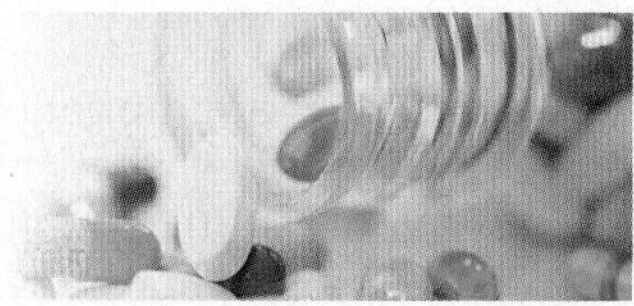

THE SITUATION

M.R., who is 69 years old, has been seen several times complaining of tremor in their hands that eventually made it difficult for them to work as a computer programmer. A diagnosis of essential tremor was made, and M.R. was prescribed propranolol (*Inderal*) 20 mg twice daily. M.R. had good effects with the drug and had no further problems until they ran out of prescriptions for the inhalers that treated their COPD. After several days without the inhalers, M.R. reported significant increase in difficulty breathing. They had gone a few days without an inhaler before so did not understand why the COPD symptoms were so bad this time. M.R. was planning on calling their primary care provider on Monday, but on Sunday evening, they developed acute respiratory distress, and their spouse called for an ambulance. M.R. was admitted to the hospital and placed in the respiratory intensive care unit.

CRITICAL THINKING

Why did M.R. have such a severe reaction? What appropriate measures should be taken to ensure that M.R. recovers fully and does not reexperience this event?

What sort of support will M.R. and their family need after going through such a frightening experience? Think about the support M.R.'s spouse may need and the fear that may now be associated with M.R.'s condition. M.R. has been taking propranolol for several months and needs to decide whether they feel comfortable continuing the medication with the effects it can have on their COPD.

What kind of teaching program will need to be developed to help M.R. deal with this drug and its potential adverse effects?

DISCUSSION

Propranolol, a nonselective beta-blocker, was prescribed to decrease the tremor M.R. was experiencing. The exact action of this drug to decrease the tremor is thought to be related to its membrane-stabilizing properties. The desired therapeutic effect is the reduction of the tremor, but all of the beta-blocking effects will occur and need to be monitored. M.R. did well on the drug until running out of COPD medication. That is because propranolol, a nonselective beta-blocker, prevented the compensatory bronchodilation that is beneficial to keep airways patent. People who have COPD are often prescribed bronchodilation medication. When M.R. ran out of this medication, their airways narrowed, causing difficulty breathing and subsequent respiratory distress requiring hospitalization. Before M.R. began taking propranolol, they probably had been effectively compensating when they ran out of medication for a few days, but this time the propranolol blocked the compensating response. There are few other drugs for treating essential tremor. M.R. and their health care providers will need to decide whether the benefit that the drug has brought is worth the potential for adverse effects, or if there is a safer medication to try. The providers might be able to suggest ways to keep M.R. from running out of COPD medication to make the use of propranolol safer for this patient.

M.R. may want to discuss this frightening incident with their health care provider. They may also want to include their family in this discussion. M.R. and their family should receive support and be encouraged to talk about what happened and how they reacted to it. It is normal to feel frightened and unsure when a loved one is in distress. The family should be involved in the discussion of what medical regimen would be most appropriate for M.R. at this point.

NURSING CARE GUIDE FOR M.R.: PROPRANOLOL

Assessment: History and Examination

Review the patient's history for allergy to propranolol, HF, shock, bradycardia, heart block, hypotension, COPD, thyroid disease, diabetes, respiratory impairment, and concurrent use of barbiturates, NSAIDs, piroxicam, sulindac, lidocaine, cimetidine, phenothiazines, clonidine, theophylline, and rifampin.

Focus the physical examination on the following:

CV: Blood pressure, pulse, peripheral perfusion, ECG
CNS: Orientation, affect, reflexes, vision
Skin: Color, lesions, texture
GU: Urinary output, sexual function
GI: Abdominal, liver evaluation
Respiratory: Respirations, adventitious sounds

Nursing Conclusions

Decreased cardiac output related to CV effects
Impaired comfort related to CNS, GI, systematic effects
Altered tissue perfusion related to CV effects
Knowledge deficit regarding drug therapy

Planning

The patient will receive the best therapeutic effect from the drug therapy.

The patient will have limited adverse effects from the drug therapy.

The patient will have an understanding of the drug therapy, adverse effects to anticipate, and measures to relieve discomfort and improve safety.

(continues on page 544)

Intervention

Ensure safe and appropriate administration of the drug.
Provide comfort and safety measures: assistance/side rails; temperature control; rest periods; mouth care; small, frequent meals.
Monitor blood pressure, pulse, and respiratory status throughout drug therapy.
Taper the drug gradually if it is to be discontinued to decrease the risk of severe hypertension, MI, or stroke related to abrupt withdrawal.
Provide support and reassurance to deal with drug effects and discomfort, sexual dysfunction, and fatigue.
Provide patient teaching regarding drug name, dosage, side effects, precautions, and warning signs to report.

Evaluation

Evaluate drug effects: blood pressure within normal limits, decrease in essential tremors, and stabilized cardiac rhythm.
Monitor for adverse effects: CV effects, HF and block, dizziness and confusion, sexual dysfunction, GI effects, hypoglycemia, and respiratory problems.
Monitor for drug–drug interactions as indicated.
Evaluate the effectiveness of the patient teaching program.
Evaluate the effectiveness of comfort and safety measures.

PATIENT TEACHING FOR M.R.

- The drug that has been prescribed for you, propranolol, is a nonselective beta-adrenergic blocking agent. A beta-adrenergic blocking agent works to prevent certain stimulating activities that normally occur in the body in response to such factors as stress, injury, or excitement. It stabilizes certain nerve membranes, which helps to decrease your tremor.
- You should learn to take your pulse and monitor it daily, writing the pulse rate on the calendar. Your current pulse rate is 82 beats/min.
- Do not discontinue this medication suddenly unless instructed by a medical care professional. If you find that your prescription is running low, notify your health care provider at once. This drug needs to be tapered over time to prevent severe reactions when its use is discontinued. Some of the following adverse effects may occur:
  - *Fatigue, weakness*: Try to stagger your activities throughout the day to allow rest periods.
  - *Dizziness, drowsiness*: If these should occur, take care to avoid driving, operating dangerous machinery, or doing delicate tasks. Change position slowly to avoid dizzy spells.
  - *Change in sexual function*: Be assured that this is a drug effect and discuss it with your health care provider.
  - *Nausea, diarrhea*: These GI discomforts often diminish with time. If they become too uncomfortable or do not improve, talk to your health care provider.
  - *Dreams, confusion*: These are drug effects. If they become too uncomfortable, discuss them with your health care provider.
- Report any of the following to your health care provider: very slow pulse, need to sleep on more pillows at night, difficulty breathing, swelling in the ankles or fingers, sudden weight gain, mental confusion or personality change, fever, or rash.
- Avoid over-the-counter medications, including cold and allergy remedies and diet pills. Many of these preparations contain drugs that could interfere with this medication. If you feel that you need one of these, check with your health care provider first.
- Tell any doctor, nurse, or other health care provider that you are taking these drugs, keep all medications out of the reach of children, and do not share these drugs with other people.

Key Points

- Beta-blockers are drugs used to block the beta-receptors within the SNS. These drugs are used for a wide range of conditions, including hypertension, stage fright, migraines, angina, and essential tremors.
- Nonselective blockade of all beta-receptors results in a loss of the reflex bronchodilation that occurs with sympathetic stimulation. This limits the use of these drugs in patients who smoke or have allergic or seasonal rhinitis, asthma, or COPD.

Beta$_1$-Selective Adrenergic Blocking Agents

Beta1-selective adrenergic blocking agents (Table 31.5) have an advantage over the nonselective beta-blockers in some cases. Because at lower doses they do not usually block beta$_2$-receptor sites, they do not block the sympathetic bronchodilation that is important for patients with lung diseases or allergic rhinitis. Consequently, these drugs are preferred for patients who smoke or who have asthma, any other obstructive pulmonary disease, or seasonal or allergic rhinitis. These selective beta-blockers are also used for treating hypertension, angina, and some cardiac arrhythmias. Beta$_1$-selective adrenergic blocking agents include acebutolol (generic), atenolol (*Tenormin*), betaxolol (*Betoptic*), bisoprolol (generic), esmolol (*Brevibloc*), and metoprolol (*Lopressor*, *Toprol XL*).

Therapeutic Actions and Indications

The therapeutic effects of these drugs are related to their ability to selectively block beta$_1$-receptors in the SNS at therapeutic doses. As a result, these drugs do not block

Table 31.5 *Drugs in Focus*: Beta$_1$-Selective Adrenergic Blocking Agents

Drug Name	Dosage/Route	Usual Indications
acebutolol (generic)	400 mg/d PO, up to 1,200 mg/d may be used; decrease dose in older adult patients and with renal and hepatic impairment	Treatment of hypertension and premature ventricular contractions in adults
atenolol (*Tenormin*)	Initially 50 mg/d PO, may be increased to 100 mg/d; reduce dose with renal impairment	Treatment of MI, chronic angina, and hypertension in adults (atenolol is more widely used than the other drugs of this class for hypertension)
betaxolol (*Betoptic*)	10–20 mg/d PO; reduce to 5 mg/d PO in older adult patients; 1–2 drops (gtt) in affected eye(s) for glaucoma	Treatment of hypertension in adults; available as ophthalmic agent for treatment of ocular hypertension, open-angle glaucoma
bisoprolol (*Zebeta*)	Initially 5 mg/d PO, up to 20 mg/d PO may be needed; reduce dose with renal or hepatic impairment	Treatment of hypertension in adults, alone or as part of combination therapy
esmolol (*Brevibloc*)	Loading dose 500 mcg/kg IV over 1 min; then 50–200 mcg/kg/min IV, with dose based on patient response	Treatment of supraventricular tachycardias (e.g., atrial flutter, atrial fibrillation) in adults and noncompensatory tachycardia when the heart rate must be slowed (IV use only)
metoprolol (*Lopressor, Toprol XL*)	100–400 mg/d PO, based on patient response; XL preparation for treatment of angina: 50–200 mg/d PO based on patient response; acute MI: three IV bolus doses of 5 mg each at 2-min intervals; if tolerated, start PO therapy 15 min after last IV dose	Treatment of hypertension; prevention of reinfarction after MI; early acute MI treatment; treatment of stable and symptomatic HF (extended-release preparation only)

MI, myocardial infarction; HF, heart failure.

the beta$_2$-receptors and, therefore, do not prevent sympathetic bronchodilation. However, the selectivity is lost with higher doses.

The blockade of the beta$_1$-receptors in the heart and in the juxtaglomerular apparatus accounts for most of the therapeutic benefits. Decreased heart rate, contractility, and excitability, as well as a membrane-stabilizing effect, lead to decreases in arrhythmias, cardiac workload, and oxygen consumption. The juxtaglomerular cells are not stimulated to release renin, which further decreases blood pressure. These drugs are useful in treating cardiac arrhythmias, hypertension, and chronic angina and can help prevent reinfarction after an MI by decreasing cardiac workload and oxygen consumption.

Beta$_1$-selective adrenergic blocking agents in ophthalmic form are used to decrease intraocular pressure and to treat open-angle glaucoma. See Table 31.5 for usual indications for each drug.

Pharmacokinetics

The beta$_1$-selective adrenergic blockers are absorbed from the GI tract after oral administration, reach peak levels directly with IV infusion, and are not usually absorbed when given in ophthalmic form. The bioavailability of metoprolol is increased if it is taken in the presence of food. These drugs are metabolized in the liver and excreted in the urine. Metoprolol readily crosses the blood–brain barrier and may cause more CNS effects than acebutolol and atenolol, which do not cross the barrier.

Contraindications and Cautions

The beta$_1$-selective adrenergic blockers are contraindicated in the presence of allergy to the drug or any components of the drug, to avoid hypersensitivity reactions; with sinus bradycardia, heart block, cardiogenic shock, HF requiring inotropic support, or hypotension, all of which could be exacerbated by the cardiac-depressing and blood pressure–lowering effects of these drugs; and with lactation because of the potential adverse effects on the neonate. They should be used with caution in patients with diabetes, thyroid disease, or COPD because of the potential for adverse effects on these diseases with sympathetic blockade and in pregnancy because of the potential for adverse effects on the fetus. The safety and efficacy of the use of these drugs in children have not been established.

Adverse Effects

Patients receiving these drugs often experience adverse effects related to the blocking of beta$_1$-receptors in the SNS. CNS effects include headache, fatigue, dizziness, depression, paresthesia, sleep disturbances, memory loss, and disorientation. CV effects can include bradycardia, heart block, HF, hypotension, and peripheral vascular insufficiency. Pulmonary effects ranging from rhinitis to bronchospasm and dyspnea can occur; these effects are not as likely to occur with these drugs as with the nonselective beta-blockers. GI upset, nausea, vomiting, diarrhea, gastric pain, and even colitis can occur as a result of unchecked parasympathetic activity and the blocking of the sympathetic receptors. GU effects can include decreased libido, impotence, dysuria, and Peyronie's disease. Other effects that can occur include decreased exercise tolerance (patients often report that their "get up and go" is gone), hypoglycemia or hyperglycemia, and liver changes that are reflected in increased concentrations of liver enzymes. If these drugs are stopped abruptly after long-term use, there is a risk of severe hypertension, angina, MI, and stroke because the receptor sites become hypersensitive to catecholamines after being blocked by the drug.

Clinically Important Drug–Drug Interactions

A decreased antihypertensive effect may occur if these drugs are given with NSAIDs, rifampin, or barbiturates. If such a combination is used, the patient should be monitored closely and dose adjustment made. An increased antihypertensive effect may occur if the medications are given with clonidine, and patients should be monitored closely with this combination and when titrating or discontinuing the medications.

There is an initial hypertensive episode followed by bradycardia if these drugs are given with epinephrine. Increased serum levels and increased toxicity of intravenous lidocaine will occur if it is given with these drugs.

Increased risk for orthostatic hypotension occurs if these drugs are taken with prazosin. If this combination is used, the patient must be monitored closely and safety precautions taken.

The selective $beta_1$-blockers have increased effects if they are taken with verapamil, cimetidine, methimazole, or propylthiouracil. The patient should be monitored closely and appropriate dose adjustment made.

Prototype Summary: Atenolol

Indications: Treatment of angina pectoris, hypertension, and MI; off-label uses are prevention of migraine headaches, alcohol withdrawal syndrome, and supraventricular tachycardia.

Actions: Blocks $beta_1$-adrenergic receptors, decreasing the excitability of the heart, cardiac output, and oxygen consumption; decreases renin release, which lowers blood pressure.

Pharmacokinetics:

Route	Onset	Peak	Duration
Oral	Varies	2–4 h	24 h
IV	Immediate	5 min	24 h

$T_{1/2}$: 6 to 7 hours; excreted in the bile, feces, and urine.

Adverse Effects: Allergic reaction, dizziness, bradycardia, heart block, hypotension, heart failure, arrhythmias, gastric pain, flatulence, impotence, bronchospasm, decreased exercise tolerance.

Nursing Considerations for Patients Receiving $Beta_1$-Selective Adrenergic Blocking Agents

Assessment: History and Examination

- Assess for contraindications or cautions: known allergies to any drug or any components of the drug to avoid hypersensitivity reactions; bradycardia or heart blocks, shock, or heart failure requiring inotropic support, which could be exacerbated by the cardiac-suppressing effects of these drugs; diabetes, thyroid disease, or COPD to reduce risk of adverse effects on these conditions due to sympathetic blockade; and current status of pregnancy or lactation because of the potential effects on the fetus or neonate.
- Perform a physical assessment before beginning therapy to establish baseline status to determine the effectiveness of therapy and evaluate for any potential adverse effects.
- Assess neurological status, including level of orientation and sensation, to evaluate for CNS effects.
- Monitor cardiac status, including pulse, blood pressure, and heart rate, to identify changes, and obtain an ECG as ordered to evaluate for changes in heart rate or rhythm.
- Assess pulmonary status, including respirations, and auscultate lungs for adventitious sounds to monitor respiratory status.
- Examine the abdomen and auscultate bowel sounds to evaluate GI effects.
- Monitor urine output to monitor the effectiveness of cardiac output and any changes in renal perfusion.
- Monitor the results of laboratory tests, including electrolyte levels, to observe for risk of arrhythmias, and renal and hepatic function studies to determine the need for possible dose adjustment.

Nursing Conclusions

Nursing conclusions related to drug therapy might include the following:

- Impaired comfort related to CNS, GI, and systemic effects
- Altered cardiac output related to CV effects
- Altered tissue perfusion related to CV effects
- Injury risk related to CNS effects
- Activity intolerance related to sympathetic blocking
- Knowledge deficit regarding drug therapy

Planning

- The patient will receive the best therapeutic effect from the drug therapy.
- The patient will have limited adverse effects from the drug therapy.

- The patient will have an understanding of the drug therapy, adverse effects to anticipate, and measures to relieve discomfort and improve safety.

Intervention With Rationale

- Do not stop these drugs abruptly after chronic therapy; instead, taper gradually if possible to prevent the possibility of hypertensive crisis, tachycardia, angina, MI, and stroke. Long-term use of these drugs can sensitize the myocardium to catecholamines, and severe reactions could occur.
- Consult with the physician about discontinuing these drugs before surgery because withdrawal of the drug before surgery when the patient has been maintained on the drug is controversial.
- Give oral forms of metoprolol with food to facilitate absorption.
- Continuously monitor any patient receiving an IV form of these drugs to detect severe reactions to sympathetic blockade and to ensure rapid response if these reactions occur.
- Arrange for supportive care and comfort measures, including rest, environmental control, and other measures, to relieve CNS effects; safety measures if CNS effects occur to protect the patient from injury; small, frequent meals and mouth care to relieve the discomfort of GI effects; and an activity program and daily energy management ideas to help to deal with activity intolerance.
- Offer support and encouragement to help the patient deal with the drug regimen.
- Provide thorough patient teaching, including drug name, dosage, and schedule for administration; use of drug with food or meals if appropriate; technique for ophthalmic administration if indicated; potential adverse effects, measures to avoid drug-related problems, and warning signs of problems; safety measures such as changing position slowly and avoiding driving or operating hazardous machinery; and energy conservation measures as appropriate to provide drug education and improve adherence to the drug regimen.

Evaluation

- Monitor patient response to the drug (lowered blood pressure, fewer anginal episodes, lowered intraocular pressure).
- Monitor for adverse effects (GI upset, CNS changes, CV effects, loss of libido and impotence, potential respiratory effects).
- Evaluate the effectiveness of the teaching plan (patient can name drug, dosage, adverse effects to watch for, and specific measures to avoid them).
- Monitor the effectiveness of comfort measures and adherence to the regimen.

Key Points

- At low doses, $beta_1$-selective adrenergic blocking agents do not block the $beta_2$-receptors that are responsible for bronchodilation and, therefore, are preferred in patients with respiratory problems.
- $Beta_1$-selective adrenergic blocking agents are used to treat hypertension, tachycardia, and angina. Some are indicated to treat heart failure.
- All of the adrenergic blocking drugs should be tapered when they are discontinued after long-term use. The blocking of the receptor sites makes them hypersensitive to catecholamines and extreme hypertension, angina, MI, or stroke could occur.

SUMMARY

- Adrenergic blocking agents, or sympatholytic drugs, lyse, or block, the effects of the SNS.
- Both the therapeutic and the adverse effects associated with these drugs are related to their blocking of the normal responses of the SNS.
- The alpha- and beta-adrenergic blocking agents block all of the receptor sites within the SNS, which results in lower blood pressure, slower pulse, and increased renal perfusion with decreased renin levels. These drugs are indicated for the treatment of essential hypertension. They are associated with many adverse effects, including the blocking of reflex bronchodilation, cardiac suppression, and diabetic reactions.
- Selective adrenergic blocking agents have been developed that at therapeutic levels have specific affinity for alpha- or beta-receptors or for specific $alpha_1$-, $beta_1$-, or $beta_2$-receptor sites. This specificity is lost at levels higher than the therapeutic range.
- Alpha-adrenergic drugs specifically block the alpha-receptors of the SNS. At therapeutic levels, they do not block beta-receptors.
- Nonspecific alpha-adrenergic blocking agents are used to treat pheochromocytoma, a tumor of the adrenal medulla.

- Alpha$_1$-selective adrenergic blocking agents block the postsynaptic alpha$_1$-receptor sites, causing a decrease in vascular tone and vasodilation that leads to a fall in blood pressure without the reflex tachycardia that occurs when the presynaptic alpha$_2$-receptor sites are also blocked.
- Beta-blockers are drugs used to block the beta-receptors within the SNS. These drugs are used for a wide range of conditions, including hypertension, stage fright, migraines, angina, and essential tremors.
- Blockade of all beta-receptors results in a loss of the reflex bronchodilation that occurs with sympathetic stimulation. This limits the use of these drugs in patients who smoke or have allergic or seasonal rhinitis, asthma, or COPD.
- At low doses, beta$_1$-selective adrenergic blocking agents do not block the beta$_1$-receptors that are responsible for bronchodilation and, therefore, are preferred in patients with respiratory problems.

CHECK YOUR UNDERSTANDING

Answers to the questions in this chapter can be found in Answers to Check Your Understanding Questions on thePoint®.

MULTIPLE CHOICE

Select the best answer.

1. Adrenergic blocking drugs, because of their clinical effects, are also known as
   a. anticholinergics.
   b. sympathomimetics.
   c. parasympatholytics.
   d. sympatholytics.

2. The nurse would anticipate administering drugs that generally block all adrenergic receptor sites to treat
   a. allergic rhinitis.
   b. COPD.
   c. cardiac-related conditions.
   d. premature labor.

3. Phentolamine (*Regitine*), an alpha-adrenergic blocker, is most frequently used to
   a. prevent cell death after extravasation of intravenous dopamine or norepinephrine.
   b. treat COPD in patients with hypertension or arrhythmias.
   c. treat hypertension and BPH in male patients.
   d. block bronchoconstriction during acute asthma attacks.

4. A patient with which conditions would most likely be prescribed an alpha$_1$-selective adrenergic blocking agent?
   a. COPD and hypotension
   b. Hypertension and BPH
   c. Erectile dysfunction and hypotension
   d. Shock states and bronchospasm

5. The beta-blocker of choice for a patient who has chronic open-angle glaucoma is
   a. sotalol.
   b. propranolol.
   c. timolol.
   d. carteolol.

6. A nurse would question an order for beta$_1$-selective adrenergic blocker for a patient with
   a. cardiac arrhythmias.
   b. hypertension.
   c. cardiogenic shock.
   d. open-angle glaucoma.

7. A smoker who is being treated for hypertension with a beta-blocker is most likely receiving
   a. a nonspecific beta-blocker.
   b. an alpha$_1$-specific beta-blocker.
   c. beta- and alpha-blockers.
   d. a beta$_1$-specific blocker.

8. You would caution a patient who is taking an adrenergic blocker to avoid
   a. exposure to infection.
   b. the drug if they experience flulike symptoms.
   c. stopping the drug abruptly because it can be dangerous.
   d. exposure to the sun.

MULTIPLE RESPONSE

Select all that apply.

1. A nurse would question an order for a beta-adrenergic blocker if the patient was also receiving what other drugs?
   a. Clonidine
   b. Ergot alkaloids
   c. Aspirin
   d. NSAIDs
   e. Triptans
   f. Epinephrine

2. The beta-adrenergic blocker propranolol is approved for a wide variety of uses. Which of the following are approved indications?
   a. Migraine headaches
   b. Stage fright
   c. Bronchospasm
   d. Reinfarction after an MI
   e. Erectile dysfunction
   f. Hypertension

REFERENCES

Andrews, M., & Boyle, J. (2011). *Transcultural concepts in nursing care* (6th ed.). Lippincott Williams & Wilkins.

Brunton, L., Hilal-Dandan, R., & Knollman, B. (2018). *Goodman and Gilman's the pharmacological basis of therapeutics* (13th ed.). McGraw-Hill.

Cleland, J. G. (2003). Beta blockers for heart failure: Why, which, when and where. *The Medical Clinics of North America, 87*, 339–371. 10.1016/s0025-7125(02)00173-6

Dakin, C. (2008). New approaches to heart failure in the ED. *American Journal of Nursing, 108*(3), 68–71. 10.1097/01.NAJ.0000312259.79367.75

Greenberg, B., Barnard, D., Narayan, S., et al. (2010). *Management of heart failure.* Wiley-Blackwell.

Norris, T. L. (2019). *Porth's pathophysiology concepts of altered health states* (10th ed.). Wolters Kluwer.

Wiysonge, C. S., Bradley, H. A., Volmink, J., Mayosi, B. M., Opie, L. H., & Cochrane Hypertension Group. (2017). Beta-blockers for hypertension. *Cochrane Database System Review (1).* 10.1002/14651858.CD002003.pub5

CHAPTER 32

Cholinergic Agonists

Learning Objectives

Upon completion of this chapter, you will be able to:

1. Describe the effects of cholinergic receptors, correlating these effects with the clinical effects of cholinergic agonists.
2. Discuss the use of cholinergic agonists across the lifespan.
3. Describe the therapeutic actions, indications, pharmacokinetics, contraindications and cautions, most common adverse effects, and important drug–drug interactions associated with the direct- and indirect-acting cholinergic agonists.
4. Compare and contrast the prototype drugs bethanechol, varenicline, donepezil, and pyridostigmine with other cholinergic agonists.
5. Outline the nursing considerations, including important teaching points, for patients receiving a cholinergic agonist.

Key Terms

acetylcholinesterase: enzyme responsible for the immediate breakdown of acetylcholine when released from the nerve ending; prevents overstimulation of cholinergic receptor sites

Alzheimer's disease: degenerative disease of the cortex with loss of acetylcholine-producing cells and cholinergic receptors; characterized by progressive dementia

cholinergic agonist: substance that mimics actions of acetylcholine; refers to receptor sites stimulated by acetylcholine as well as neurons that release acetylcholine

miosis: constriction of the pupil; relieves intraocular pressure in some types of glaucoma

myasthenia gravis: autoimmune disease characterized by antibodies to cholinergic receptor sites leading to destruction of the receptor sites and decreased response at the neuromuscular junction; it is progressive and debilitating, leading to paralysis

nerve gas: irreversible acetylcholinesterase inhibitor used in warfare to cause paralysis and death by prolonged muscle contraction and parasympathetic crisis

parasympathomimetic: mimicking the effects of the parasympathetic nervous system leading to bradycardia, hypotension, pupil constriction, increased gastrointestinal secretions and activity, increased bladder tone, relaxation of sphincters, and bronchoconstriction

Drug List

DIRECT-ACTING CHOLINERGIC AGONISTS (MUSCARINIC)
- acetylcholine chloride
- (P) bethanechol
- carbachol
- cevimeline
- pilocarpine

DIRECT-ACTING CHOLINERGIC AGONISTS (NICOTINIC) AND AGENTS FOR NICOTINE WITHDRAWAL/ABSTINENCE
- bupropion
- nicotine
- (P) varenicline

INDIRECT-ACTING CHOLINERGIC AGONISTS
- echothiophate iodide
- neostigmine
- (P) pyridostigmine

Agents for Alzheimer's Disease
- (P) donepezil
- galantamine
- rivastigmine

Cholinergic agonists act at the same site as the neurotransmitter acetylcholine (ACh) and increase the activity of the ACh receptor sites throughout the body. Because these sites are found extensively throughout the parasympathetic nervous system, their stimulation produces a response similar to what is seen when the parasympathetic system is activated. As a result, these drugs are often called **parasympathomimetic** because their action mimics the action of the parasympathetic nervous system. Because the action of these drugs cannot be limited to a specific site, their effects can be widespread throughout the body, and they are usually associated with many undesirable systemic effects.

Cholinergic agonists work either directly or indirectly. Direct-acting cholinergic agonists occupy receptor sites for ACh on the membranes of the effector cells of the postganglionic cholinergic nerves, causing increased stimulation of the cholinergic receptor. In contrast, indirect-acting cholinergic agonists cause increased stimulation of the ACh receptor sites by reacting with **acetylcholinesterase**, the enzyme responsible for the immediate breakdown of ACh when released from a nerve ending. This enzyme prevents overstimulation of cholinergic receptor sites. Indirect-acting cholinergic agonists prevent acetylcholinesterase from breaking down the ACh released from the nerve. These drugs produce their effects indirectly by producing an increase in the level of ACh in the synaptic cleft, leading to increased stimulation of the cholinergic receptor site (Fig. 32.1). See Box 32.1 for use of these drugs across the lifespan.

Direct-Acting Cholinergic Agonists (Muscarinic)

The direct-acting cholinergic agonists are similar to ACh and react directly with receptor sites to cause the same reaction as if ACh had stimulated the receptor sites. These drugs usually stimulate muscarinic receptors within the parasympathetic system. They are used as systemic agents to increase bladder tone, urinary excretion, and gastrointestinal (GI) secretions and as ophthalmic agents to induce **miosis** (constriction of the pupil) to relieve the increased intraocular pressure of glaucoma (see Table 32.1). Systemic absorption usually does not occur when these drugs are used ophthalmically.

Direct-acting cholinergic agonists include acetylcholine chloride (*Miochol-E*), bethanechol (*Duvoid*), carbachol (*Miostat*), cevimeline (*Evoxac*), and pilocarpine (*Isopto Carpine*, *Salagen*). These agents are used infrequently today because of their widespread parasympathetic activity. More specific and less toxic drugs are now available and preferred.

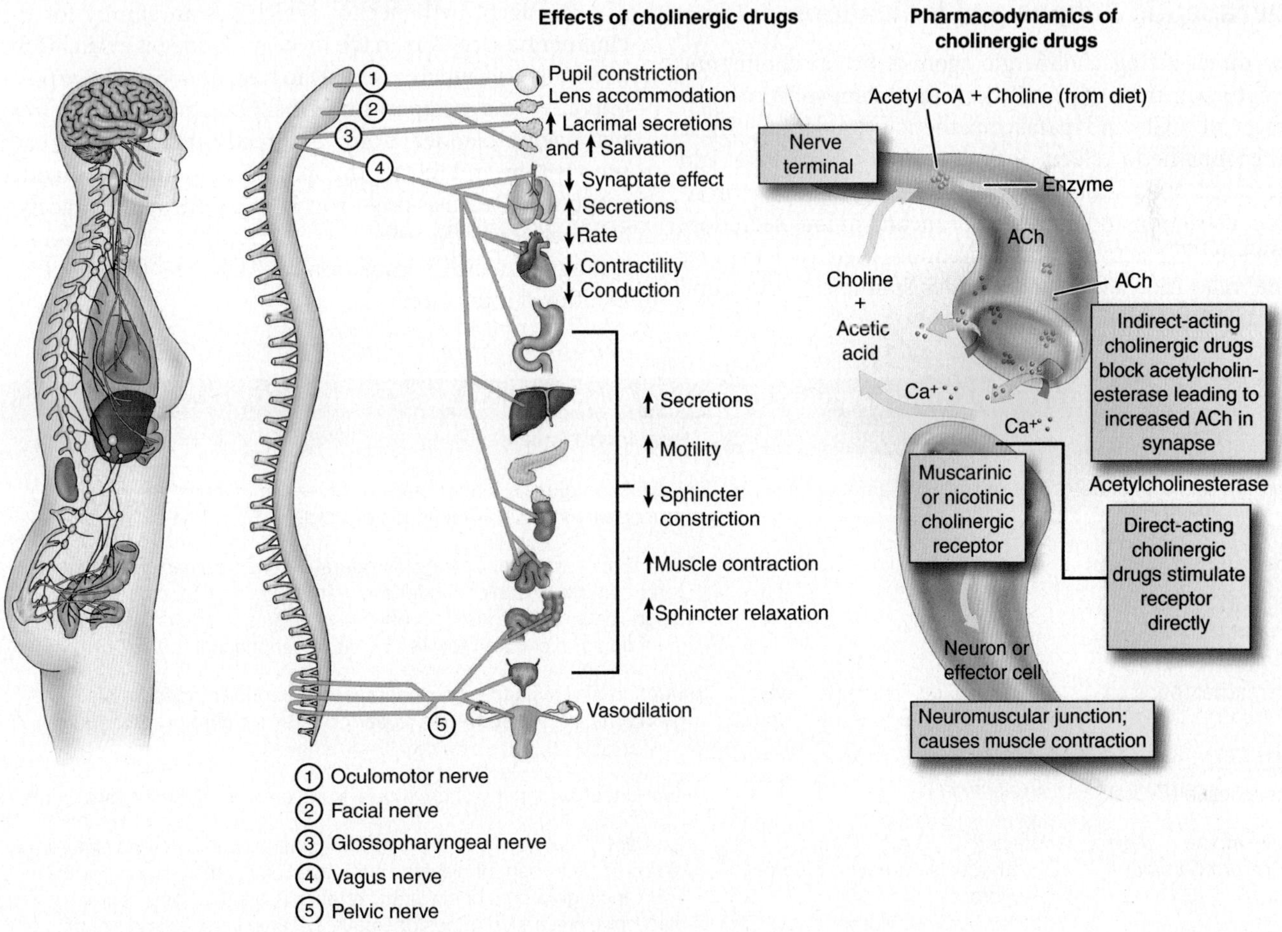

FIGURE 32.1 Pharmacodynamics of cholinergic drugs and associated physiological responses.

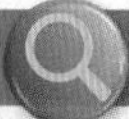

Box 32.1 Focus on Drug Therapy Across the Lifespan

CHOLINERGIC AGONISTS

Children

Children may be more susceptible to the adverse effects associated with the cholinergic agonists, including GI upset, diarrhea, increased salivation that could lead to choking, and loss of bowel and bladder control, a problem that could cause stress in children. Children should be monitored closely if these agents are used and should receive appropriate supportive care.

Bethanechol is approved for the treatment of neurogenic bladder in children older than 8 years of age. Neostigmine and pyridostigmine are used in the control of myasthenia gravis and for reversal of neuromuscular junction blocker effects in children. Care should be taken in determining the appropriate dose based on weight. Edrophonium is used for diagnosis of myasthenia gravis only.

Adults

Adults should be cautioned about the many adverse effects that can be anticipated when using a cholinergic agonist. Flushing, increased sweating, increased salivation and GI upset, and urinary urgency often occur. The patient also needs to be aware that dizziness, drowsiness, and blurred vision may occur and that driving and operating dangerous machinery should be avoided.

In general, there are no adequate studies about the effects of these drugs during pregnancy and lactation. Therefore, the cholinergic agonist should be used only in those situations in which the benefit to the patient is greater than the risk to the fetus or neonate. Patients who are breast or chestfeeding and who require one of these drugs should find another way to feed the baby.

Older Adults

Older patients are more likely to experience the adverse CNS, cardiovascular, GI, respiratory, and urinary effects associated with these drugs. Because older patients often have renal or hepatic impairment, they are also more likely to have toxic levels of the drug related to changes in metabolism and excretion.

The older patient should be started on lower doses of the drugs and should be monitored very closely for potentially serious arrhythmias or hypotension. Safety precautions should be established if the drug causes dizziness or drowsiness. Special efforts may also be needed to help the patient maintain fluid intake and nutrition if the GI effects become uncomfortable. Taking the drug with food and eating several small meals throughout the day may alleviate some of these problems.

Therapeutic Actions and Indications

The direct-acting cholinergic agonists act at cholinergic receptors in the peripheral nervous system to mimic the effects of ACh and parasympathetic stimulation. These parasympathetic effects include slowed heart rate and decreased myocardial contractility, vasodilation, bronchoconstriction and increased bronchial mucus secretion, increased GI activity and secretions, increased bladder tone, relaxation of GI and bladder sphincters, and pupil constriction (see Fig. 32.1).

The agent bethanechol, which has an affinity for the cholinergic receptors in the urinary bladder, is available for use orally and subcutaneously to treat nonobstructive postoperative and postpartum urinary retention and to treat neurogenic bladder atony. It directly increases detrusor muscle tone and relaxes the sphincters to improve bladder emptying. Because this drug is not destroyed by acetylcholinesterase, the effects on the receptor site are longer lasting than with stimulation by ACh. See Table 32.1 for additional indications.

Table 32.1 *Drugs in Focus:* Direct-Acting Cholinergic Agonists

Drug Name	Dosage/Route	Usual Indications
acetylcholine chloride (*Miochol-E*)	Instilled into the anterior chamber of the eye	Introduction of miosis after delivery of lens in cataract surgery; other procedures in which rapid miosis is required
bethanechol (*Duvoid*)	10–50 mg PO b.i.d. to q.i.d.	Treatment of nonobstructive postoperative and postpartum urinary retention, neurogenic bladder atony in adults and children >8 y; diagnosis and treatment of reflux esophagitis in adults; used orally in infants and children for treatment of esophageal reflux
carbachol (*Miostat*)	1–2 drops (gtt) in affected eye(s) as needed, up to three times a day	Induction of miosis to relieve increased intraocular pressure of glaucoma; allows surgeons to perform certain surgical procedures
cevimeline (*Evoxac*)	30 mg PO t.i.d.	Treatment of symptoms of dry mouth in patients with Sjögren's syndrome
pilocarpine (*Salagen, Isopto Carpine*)	*Salagen*: 5–10 mg PO t.i.d. with meals if treating Sjögren syndrome *Isopto Carpine*: 1 drop (gtt) in eye(s) up to four times daily	Treatment of symptoms of dry mouth in patients with Sjögren's syndrome (*Salagen*); treatment of elevated intraocular pressure in patients with open-angle glaucoma or ocular hypertension, acute angle-closure glaucoma; prevention of postoperative elevated intraocular pressure associated with laser surgery; induction of miosis (*Isopto Carpine*)

Acetylcholine chloride (*Miochol-E*) is instilled into the eye during eye procedures that require rapid miosis. Carbachol and pilocarpine are also available as ophthalmic agents. They are used to induce miosis, or pupil constriction; to relieve the increased intraocular pressure of glaucoma; and to allow surgeons to perform certain surgical procedures.

Cevimeline and pilocarpine, which bind to muscarinic receptors throughout the system, are used to increase secretions in the mouth and GI tract and relieve the symptoms of dry mouth that are seen in Sjögren's syndrome. They are approved for use in adults and are given three times a day, often with meals.

Pharmacokinetics

The direct-acting cholinergic agonists are generally well absorbed after oral administration and have relatively short half-lives, ranging from 1 to 6 hours. The metabolism and excretion of these drugs are not known but are believed to occur at the synaptic level using normal processes similar to the way that ACh is handled. Drugs used topically are not generally absorbed systemically.

Contraindications and Cautions

These drugs are used sparingly because of the potential undesirable systemic effects of parasympathetic stimulation. They are contraindicated with hypersensitivity to any component of the drug to avoid hypersensitivity reaction and in the presence of any condition that would be exacerbated by parasympathetic effects, such as bradycardia, hypotension, vasomotor instability, and coronary artery disease, which could be made worse by the cardiac- and cardiovascular-suppressing effects of the parasympathetic system. Peptic ulcer, intestinal obstruction, or recent GI surgery could be negatively affected by the GI-stimulating effects of the parasympathetic nervous system. Asthma could be exacerbated by the increased parasympathetic effect, overriding the protective sympathetic bronchodilation. Bladder obstruction or impaired healing of sites from recent bladder surgery could be aggravated by the stimulatory effects on the bladder. Epilepsy and parkinsonism could be affected by the stimulation of ACh receptors in the brain. Caution should be used during pregnancy and lactation because it is unknown if there could be adverse effects on the fetus or neonate.

Adverse Effects

Patients should be cautioned about the potential adverse effects of these drugs. Even if the drug is being given as a topical ophthalmic agent, there is always a possibility that it can be absorbed systemically. The adverse effects associated with these drugs are related to parasympathetic

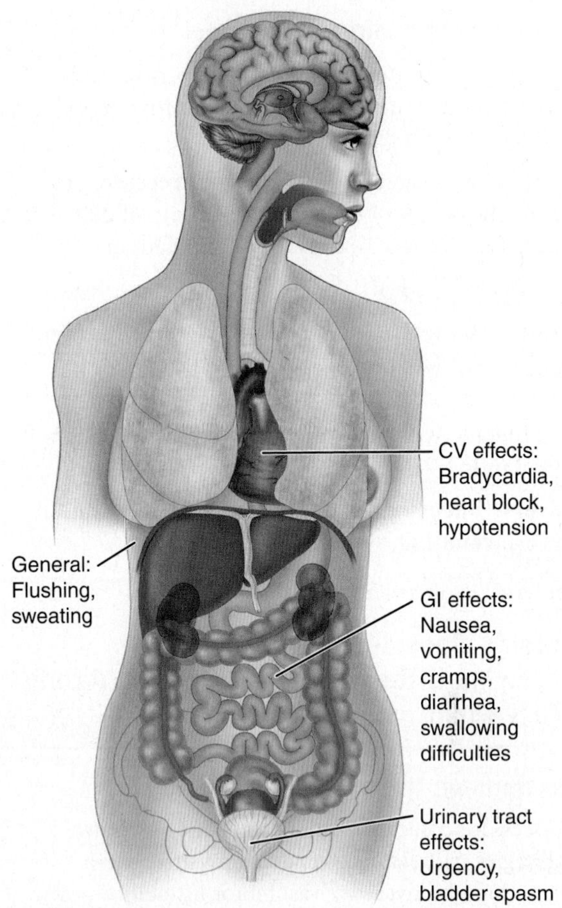

FIGURE 32.2 Variety of adverse effects and toxicities associated with cholinergic agonists.

nervous system stimulation. Cardiovascular effects can include bradycardia, heart block, hypotension, and even cardiac arrest related to the cardiac-suppressing effects of the parasympathetic nervous system. GI effects can include nausea, vomiting, cramps, diarrhea, increased salivation, and involuntary defecation related to the increase in GI secretions and activity (Fig. 32.2). Swallowing difficulties leading to aspiration may occur with cevimeline or oral pilocarpine due to the increase in salivary secretions. Dehydration is possible due to the increase in GI motility and resultant diarrhea. Urinary tract effects can include a sense of urgency related to the stimulation of the bladder muscles and sphincter relaxation. Other effects may include flushing and increased sweating secondary to stimulation of the cholinergic receptors in the sympathetic nervous system.

Clinically Important Drug–Drug Interactions

There is an increased risk of cholinergic effects if these drugs are combined or given with acetylcholinesterase inhibitors, such as neostigmine. The patient should be monitored and appropriate dose adjustments made.

Prototype Summary: Bethanechol

Indications: Acute postoperative or postpartum nonobstructive urinary retention, neurogenic atony of the bladder with retention.

Actions: Acts directly on cholinergic receptors to mimic the effects of ACh, increases tone of detrusor muscles, and causes emptying of the bladder.

Pharmacokinetics:

Route	Onset	Peak	Duration
Oral	30–90 min	60–90 min	1–6 h

$T_{1/2}$: Metabolism and excretion unknown, thought to be synaptic.

Adverse Effects: Abdominal discomfort, salivation, nausea, vomiting, sweating, flushing.

Nursing Considerations for Patients Receiving Direct-Acting Cholinergic Agonists (Muscarinic)

Assessment: History and Examination

- Assess for contraindications or cautions: known allergies to these drugs to avoid hypersensitivity reactions; bradycardia, vasomotor instability, peptic ulcer, and obstructive urinary or GI diseases; recent GI or genitourinary (GU) surgery; asthma; parkinsonism or epilepsy, which could be exacerbated or complicated by parasympathetic stimulation; and current status of pregnancy and lactation because of the potential for adverse effects on the fetus or neonate.
- Perform a physical assessment before beginning therapy to establish a baseline status, determine the effectiveness of therapy, and evaluate for any potential adverse effects.
- Assess vital signs, including pulse and blood pressure, and cardiopulmonary status, including heart and lung sounds, to evaluate for changes related to cardiovascular effects of parasympathetic activity; obtain an electrocardiogram (ECG) as indicated to evaluate heart rate and rhythm.
- Assess abdomen, auscultating for bowel sounds; palpate bladder for distention.
- Monitor intake and output, noting any complaints of urinary urgency to monitor for drug effects on the urinary system.

Nursing Conclusions

Nursing conclusions related to drug therapy might include the following:

- Impaired comfort related to GI effects
- Altered cardiac output related to cardiovascular effects
- Impaired urinary elimination related to effects on the bladder
- Injury risk related to blurred vision and changes in visual acuity
- Diarrhea related to GI stimulatory effects
- Knowledge deficit regarding drug therapy

Planning

- The patient will receive the best therapeutic effect from the drug therapy.
- The patient will have limited adverse effects from the drug therapy.
- The patient will have an understanding of the drug therapy, adverse effects to anticipate, and measures to relieve discomfort and improve safety.

Intervention With Rationale

- Ensure proper administration of ophthalmic preparations to increase the effectiveness of drug therapy and minimize the risk of systemic absorption.
- Administer oral drug on an empty stomach to decrease nausea and vomiting.
- Monitor patient response closely, including blood pressure, ECG, urine output, and cardiac output, and arrange to adjust dose accordingly to ensure the most benefit with the least amount of toxicity. Maintain on standby a cholinergic-blocking drug such as atropine to use as an antidote for excessive doses of cholinergic drugs (see more in Box 3.5, "Focus on Safe Medication Administration: Myasthenic Crisis Versus Cholinergic Crisis") to reverse overdose or counteract severe reactions (see Chapter 33 for further discussion of atropine).
- Provide safety precautions if the patient reports poor visual acuity in dim light to prevent injury.
- Monitor urinary output to evaluate effects on the bladder; ensure ready access to bathroom facilities as needed with GI stimulation.
- Provide thorough patient teaching, including drug name, dosage, and schedule of administration; administration of oral forms before meals or without food; proper administration for ophthalmic preparations as indicated; measures to prevent or minimize adverse effects; need for readily available access to toileting facilities; warning signs of problems; and importance of follow-up and evaluation to increase patient knowledge and improve adherence to the drug regimen.

Evaluation

- Monitor patient response to the drug (improvement in bladder function, increased salivation, miosis).
- Monitor for adverse effects (cardiovascular changes, GI stimulation, urinary urgency, respiratory distress).
- Evaluate the effectiveness of the teaching plan (patient can name drug, dosage, adverse effects to watch for and specific measures to avoid them, proper administration of ophthalmic drugs).
- Monitor the effectiveness of comfort and safety measures and adherence to the regimen.

Key Points

- Cholinergic agonists stimulate the parasympathetic nerves, some nerves in the brain, and the neuromuscular junction at the same sites that ACh does.
- Cholinergic agonists are used topically in the eye to produce miosis (pupillary constriction) and treat glaucoma.
- Systemically, these agents are used to increase bladder tone (e.g., postoperative or postpartum) and to increase secretions to relieve dry mouth associated with Sjögren's syndrome.

Direct-Acting Cholinergic Agonists (Nicotinic) and Medications for Nicotine Withdrawal/Abstinence

Nicotine is a substance that binds to nicotinic cholinergic receptors in the peripheral and central nervous systems. Nicotine increases neuronal activity in the prefrontal cortex, thalamus, and visual system. Dopamine is the predominant neurotransmitter released; it acts in the mesolimbic area, corpus striatum, and frontal cortex. This release of dopamine is responsible for the drug-induced reward feeling that facilitates dependence on nicotine. Nicotine is used for mood control and may be associated with both improved concentration and performance levels on certain tasks. Nicotine withdrawal and the subsequent decrease in dopamine decreases the brain reward and is a key barrier to abstinence. Other neurotransmitters that are released with nicotine use are norepinephrine, acetylcholine, serotonin, GABA, glutamate, and endorphins. Nicotine withdrawal is associated with negative emotional states including anxiety and increased stress. People can become irritable, depressed, or restless; may have difficulty concentrating and/or sleeping; and may experience strain in their relationships with others. Nicotine addiction is reinforced by environmental cues and habits developed over time. For example, if a person repeatedly smokes a cigarette after dinner, the timing and environmental cues can potentiate strong urges for the person to use nicotine at that specific time of day. Medications have been developed to facilitate smoking and chewing tobacco cessation (Box 32.2).

BOX 32.2

Smoking Cessation

The effects of smoking on morbidity and mortality are well known. Multimedia campaigns that illustrate the detrimental effects of smoking have an impact on smokers and health care providers. The Agency for Health Care Policy and Research (AHCPR) published guidelines for health care providers to promote smoking cessation as a regular and vital part of any health care visit. Nicotine is very addictive, and those who try to quit smoking usually struggle to succeed. The AHCPR developed multiple programs and offers free access to consumers to help in the process. A real desire to quit is essential for success, so patient interactions should include counseling, offering insights, and sharing statistics about the detrimental effects of smoking.

Nicotine patches and nicotine gum are available by prescription to help the patient ease off the addicting effects of nicotine. Buproprion (*Zyban*), an antidepressant, is approved to help with smoking cessation as well as alleviate some of the depression that may occur as nicotine is removed from the body. Varenicline (*Chantix*) is a nicotine receptor agonist that binds to the nicotine receptors in the CNS and prevents nicotine from binding to and stimulating the receptors. The patient should pick a date to stop smoking, begin the drug 1 week before that date, and quit smoking between days 8 and 35 of the treatment plan. The drug therapy should be part of a complete support and education program. If the patient has not been able to stop smoking in 12 weeks, the drug should be stopped. The treatment regimen can be restarted after factors that prevented success are addressed. This drug has a boxed warning for potentially serious mental health events, including behavioral changes, depression, hostility, aggression, and suicidality. It is also associated with potentially dangerous CV events. Weighing the health risks of smoking versus the adverse effects of the drug is an important part of deciding to try this approach. Patients who opt to use varenicline should be monitored closely for mental health effects. Log on to therealcost.betobaccofree.hhs.gov/costs/health-costs/index.html to access the smoking cessation information available for health care providers and consumers.

Therapeutic Actions and Indications

Nicotine replacement therapy is available in a variety of routes (patch, gum, lozenge, nasal spray, and inhaler). The replacement therapy is safer than smoking cigarettes due to the absence of toxic combustion products; however, long-term nicotine exposure via any route may have risks. The direct-acting cholinergic agonists and medications used for nicotine withdrawal/abstinence are listed in Table 32.2.

Bupropion hydrochloride is a prescription medication that has a formulation used as an antidepressant (see Chapter 21) and a different formulation to aid in smoking cessation. It may act by weakly inhibiting the neuronal reuptake of norepinephrine and dopamine; however, the exact mechanism of how it helps with smoking cessation is not entirely known. Varenicline (*Chantix*) is an oral medication indicated as aid for smoking cessation; it acts as nicotinic receptor partial agonist. It stimulates the nicotinic ACh receptors, but at a lower level than nicotine. It can also block nicotine from activating the receptors.

Table 32.2 *Drugs in Focus:* Direct-Acting Cholinergic Agonists (Nicotinic) and Medications for Nicotine Withdrawal/Abstinence		
Drug Name	**Dosage/Route**	**Usual Indications**
bupropion (generic)	Begin 1 wk before date to stop smoking; start 150 mg PO daily for 3 d, then increase to 150 mg PO twice a day; reduce dose recommended with hepatic or renal impairment	Aid in smoking cessation treatment
nicotine (*Habitrol, Nicoderm CQ, Nicorette, Nicotrol*)	*Transdermal patch*: Initial 14–21 mg patch/d, titrate down gradually *Gum or lozenge*: Initial 2–4 mg every 1–2 h, titrate to every 2–4 h, and then every 4–8 h *Nasal spray*: Dosing individualized based on level of nicotine dependence; initial recommendation is 1–2 sprays in each nostril (1–2 mg) per hour; max 5 doses/h, max 40 doses/d *Inhaler*: Dosing individualized based on level of nicotine dependence; initial recommendation 6–16 cartridges/d for first 12 wk then gradual reduction	Nicotine replacement therapy to aid smoking or chewing tobacco cessation
varenicline (*Chantix*)	Begin 1 wk before date to stop smoking; start 0.5 mg PO daily, slowly titrate up per insert instructions to 1 mg PO twice day for a total of 12–24 wk; reduce dosage with severe renal impairment	Treatment for smoking cessation

Pharmacokinetics

Nicotine replacement therapy allows for slower absorption of nicotine than cigarette smoking. The rates of absorption, distribution, and half-life vary by the delivery system. The principle action of the slower rate of nicotine delivery is to decrease withdrawal symptoms. Positive reinforcement feelings are more likely to occur with rapid delivery systems (e.g., a nasal spray versus a transdermal patch). Nicotine is metabolized into more than 20 different metabolites by the liver (primary), kidneys, and lungs. The half-life is 1 to 2 hours, and it is mostly eliminated in the urine.

Bupropion has low bioavailability after oral administration (5% to 20%), and peak concentrations occur in about 3 hours. Administration of food does not alter absorption. It is almost entirely metabolized into active metabolites via enzymes in the liver, the half-life is about 20 hours, and it is primarily eliminated (87%) via the renal system.

Varenicline is absorbed within 3 to 4 hours after oral administration. Bioavailability is high (90%) and is not affected by food or time of dosing. The half-life is about 24 hours. Most of the drug is eliminated unchanged via the renal system.

Contraindications and Cautions

Nicotine withdrawal medications are contraindicated with hypersensitivity to any component of the drug to avoid hypersensitivity reaction. Bupropion is contraindicated for patients with seizure disorder due to lower seizure threshold, especially with higher doses. There are cautions regarding use during pregnancy and lactation due to possible harm to the fetus or neonate; however, tobacco smoke is known to be harmful, so benefits and risks should be weighed. It is preferred that the pregnant patient attempt to cease smoking with educational and behavioral interventions before pharmacological approaches.

Adverse Effects

Adverse effects of nicotine replacement may include tachycardia and hypertension; however, those risks must be weighed against health benefits of smoking cessation. Caution is necessary with nicotine replacement for patients in an acute setting with myocardial infarction, angina, or arrhythmia. Nicotine is an irritant to the airways, so the inhaled forms of nicotine replacement may need to be avoided in people with severe bronchospastic airway disease.

Bupropion and varenicline have been associated with increased risk of seizures and neuropsychiatric adverse events including depression, mania, agitation, anxiety, paranoia, hallucinations, and delusions. Other adverse effects to monitor for include nausea, dry mouth, dizziness, skin rash, strange dreams, and hypertension.

Clinically Important Drug–Drug Interactions

There are several clinically important interactions with bupropion and other medications. Bupropion should not be used with monoamine oxidase inhibitors due to increased risk of hypertensive crisis. The doses of medications metabolized by CYP2D6 enzymes should be reduced when taken with bupropion due to bupropion inhibiting CYP2D6. Examples of these medications include venlafaxine, nortriptyline, fluoxetine, sertraline, haloperidol, and metoprolol. Check for interactions before administering this medication.

Smoking cessation with or without nicotine replacement may affect other medication concentrations. Some medications may need a decreased dose (e.g., insulin, propranolol, acetaminophen, and caffeine). Adrenergic agonists may need to be dosed higher. Patients need to be monitored carefully while undergoing smoking cessation.

There may be increased effects of alcohol when used with varenicline.

Prototype Summary: Varenicline

Indications: Aid to smoking cessation treatment.

Actions: Binds to a specific type of neuronal nicotinic acetylcholine receptor and acts as an agonist while preventing nicotine from binding to those receptors.

Pharmacokinetics:

Route	Onset	Peak	Duration
Oral	Varies based on dose titration	3–4 hours	About 24 hours

$T_{1/2}$: 24-hour half-life; metabolism is minimal and 92% of the drug is excreted unchanged in urine.

Adverse Effects: Nausea; vivid, unusual, or strange dreams; constipation; flatulence; vomiting; seizures; neuropsychiatric adverse events, including depression, mania, psychosis, hallucinations, paranoia, delusions, aggression, homicidal ideation, panic, and suicidal ideation; skin reactions; angioedema; and hypersensitivity reactions.

Nursing Considerations for Patients Receiving Direct-Acting Cholinergic Agonists (Nicotinic) and Medications for Nicotine Withdrawal/Abstinence

Assessment: History and Examination

- Assess for contraindications or cautions: known allergies to these drugs to avoid hypersensitivity reactions; tachycardia, hypertension, seizure activity, or neuropsychiatric events, which could be exacerbated or complicated by these medications; and current status of pregnancy and lactation because of the potential for adverse effects on the fetus or neonate.
- Perform a physical assessment to establish a baseline status before beginning therapy, determine the effectiveness of therapy, and evaluate for any potential adverse effects.
- Assess amount of current tobacco use, to assist with appropriate dosing and duration of medications.
- Assess vital signs, including pulse and blood pressure, and cardiopulmonary status, including heart and lung sounds, to evaluate for changes related to cardiovascular effects of increased sympathetic activity; obtain an electrocardiogram (ECG) as indicated to evaluate heart rate and rhythm.
- Assess mood, sleep, suicidal thoughts and behaviors, and level of agitation to evaluate for worsening conditions based on the smoking cessation process or adverse effects of the medication.

Nursing Conclusions

Nursing conclusions related to drug therapy might include the following:

- Impaired comfort related to GI effects
- Altered cardiac output related to cardiovascular effects
- Injury risk related to seizures or neuropsychiatric side effects
- Knowledge deficit regarding drug therapy

Planning

- The patient will receive the best therapeutic effect from the drug therapy.
- The patient will have limited adverse effects from the drug therapy.
- The patient will have an understanding of the drug therapy, adverse effects to anticipate, and measures to relieve discomfort and improve safety.

Intervention With Rationale

- Ensure proper administration of nicotine replacement preparations to increase the effectiveness of drug therapy and minimize the risk of adverse side effect.
- Check for medication interactions to best ensure safety and proper dosing of all medications. Note that oral drugs may be taken with or without food.
- Monitor patient response closely, including blood pressure, heart rate, moods, urge to smoke cigarettes, and sleep quality; arrange to adjust dose accordingly to ensure the most benefit with the least amount of toxicity.
- Provide safety precautions if the patient reports neuropsychiatric events or seizure activity to prevent injury.
- Provide thorough patient teaching, including drug name, dosage, and schedule of administration; proper administration of nicotine replacement preparations as indicated; measures to prevent or minimize adverse effects; warning signs of problems; and importance of follow-up and evaluation to increase patient knowledge and improve adherence to the drug regimen.

Evaluation

- Monitor patient response to the drug (improvement in smoking cessation and stability of moods/behaviors).
- Monitor for adverse effects (cardiovascular changes, GI discomfort, seizures, neuropsychiatric effects).
- Evaluate the effectiveness of the teaching plan (patient can name drug, dosage, adverse effects to watch for and specific measures to avoid them, proper administration of drugs).
- Monitor the effectiveness of comfort and safety measures and adherence to the regimen.

Key Points

- Direct-acting cholinergic agonists (nicotinic) and medications for nicotine withdrawal/abstinence act as a nicotine replacement, act as a partial nicotinic receptor agonist, and/or assist in decreasing nicotine cravings or symptoms of withdrawal.
- There are many preparations of nicotine replacement, including transdermal, gum, lozenges, nasal spray, and inhaler.
- With oral preparations, check medication interactions prior to administration and closely monitor potential side effects.

Indirect-Acting Cholinergic Agonists

The indirect-acting cholinergic agonists (Table 32.3) do not react directly with ACh receptor sites; instead, they react chemically with acetylcholinesterase (the enzyme responsible for the breakdown of ACh) in the synaptic cleft to prevent it from breaking down ACh. As a result, the ACh that is released from the presynaptic nerve remains in the area and accumulates, stimulating the ACh receptors for a longer period of time than normally expected. These drugs work at all ACh receptors, in the parasympathetic nervous system, in the central nervous system, and at the neuromuscular junction. Most of these drugs bind reversibly to acetylcholinesterase, so their effects pass with time when the acetylcholinesterase is released and allowed to break down ACh. However, there are certain indirect-acting cholinergic agonists that irreversibly bind to acetylcholinesterase and have effects for a longer period of time. Echothiophate iodide (*Phospholine Iodide*) is a long-acting cholinesterase inhibitor for topical use in the eye (see Table 32.3). Systemic irreversible cholinesterase inhibitors are not used therapeutically; rather, they are toxic and can be used as weapons in the form of **nerve gas** (Box 32.3). Because these drugs might be encountered in a war situation, it is important to have an antidote readily available to military personnel and any civilians who might be affected. Pralidoxime is the antidote developed for the irreversible indirect-acting cholinergic agonists; it is also used to reverse poisoning associated with organophosphate pesticides (Box 32.4).

The reversible (shorter-acting) indirect-acting cholinergic agonists include neostigmine (*Bloxiverz*), pyridostigmine (*Mestinon, Reginol*), donepezil (*Aricept*), galantamine (*Razadyne*), and rivastigmine (*Exelon*) (see Table 32.3). Some are used for reversal of neuromuscular junction-blocking agents (Chapter 28). Pyridostigmine can be used for management of myasthenia gravis, and others are indicated for management of Alzheimer dementia or dementia related to Parkinson's disease.

Table 32.3 *Drugs in Focus:* Indirect-Acting Cholinergic Agonists

Drug Name	Dosage/Route	Usual Indications
echothiophate iodide (*Phospholine Iodide*)	0.03% ophthalmic solution instilled in eye(s) twice a day	Treatment of chronic open-angle glaucoma; subacute or chronic angle-closure glaucoma after iridectomy or when surgery is not able to be performed; glaucoma following cataract surgery
neostigmine (*Bloxiverz*)	*Antidote:* 0.03 mg/kg IV for reversal of neuromuscular junction blockers with short half-lives or 0.07 mg/kg IV for reversal of nondepolarizing neuromuscular junction blockers with long half-lives (max up to total of 5 mg); administered with anticholinergic agent	Reversal of toxicity from nondepolarizing neuromuscular junction–blocking drugs, which are used to paralyze muscles during surgery (see Chapter 28)
pyridostigmine (*Mestinon, Reginol*)	*Adult:* Average, 180–540 mg daily PO for myasthenia gravis; 0.1–0.25 mg/kg IV for antidote; 30 mg q8h starting several hours before exposure to nerve gas *Pediatric:* 7 mg/d PO in five or six divided doses for myasthenia gravis	Management of myasthenia gravis; antidote to neuromuscular junction blockers; increases survival after exposure to nerve gas
Agents for Alzheimer's Disease		
donepezil (*Aricept*)	5–23 mg PO daily at bedtime; available as an oral disintegrating tablet	Management of Alzheimer dementia, including severe dementia
galantamine (*Razadyne*)	4–12 mg PO b.i.d.; reduce dose to 16 mg/d maximum with renal or hepatic impairment; available as an oral solution 4 mg/mL; range 16–32 mg/d; extended-release tablets, range 16–24 mg/d taken as a single dose	Management of mild to moderate Alzheimer dementia; delays progression of disease
rivastigmine (*Exelon*)	1.5–6 mg PO b.i.d., based on patient response and tolerance; transdermal system, one 4.6 mg/24 h patch placed once a day, maximum 9.5 mg/24 h	Management of mild to moderate Alzheimer dementia; treatment of dementia related to Parkinson's disease

BOX 32.3

Nerve Gas: An Irreversible Indirect-Acting Cholinergic Agonist

Worldwide events and conflicts have made the potential use of nerve gas a major news story. Developed as a weapon, nerve gas is an irreversible acetylcholinesterase inhibitor. The drug is inhaled and quickly spreads throughout the body, where it permanently binds with acetylcholinesterase. This causes an accumulation of ACh at nerve endings and a massive cholinergic response. The heart rate slows and becomes ineffective, pupils and bronchi constrict, the GI tract increases activity and secretions, and muscles contract and remain that way. The muscle contraction soon immobilizes the diaphragm, causing breathing to stop. The bodies of people who are killed by nerve gas have a characteristic rigor of muscle contraction.

If an attack using nerve gas is expected, people who may be exposed are given intramuscular injections of atropine (to temporarily block cholinergic activity and to activate ACh sites in the CNS) and pralidoxime (to free up the acetylcholinesterase to start breaking down acetylcholine). An autoinjector is provided to military personnel who may be at risk. The injector is used to give atropine and then pralidoxime. The injections are repeated in 15 minutes. If symptoms of nerve gas exposure exist after an additional 15 minutes, the injections are repeated. If symptoms still persist after a third set of injections, medical help should be sought.

BOX 32.4

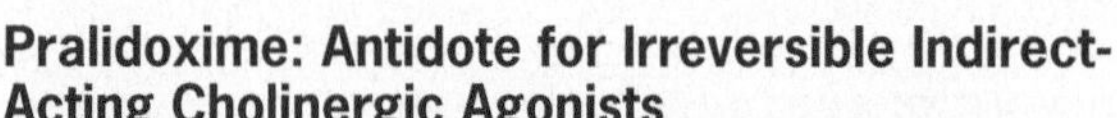

Pralidoxime: Antidote for Irreversible Indirect-Acting Cholinergic Agonists

Pralidoxime (*Protopam Chloride*), the antidote for irreversible acetylcholinesterase-inhibiting drugs, or nerve gas, is given IM or IV to reactivate the acetylcholinesterase that has been blocked by these drugs. Freeing up the acetylcholinesterase allows it to break down accumulated acetylcholine that has overstimulated ACh receptor sites, causing paralysis.

Pralidoxime does not readily cross the blood–brain barrier, and it is most useful for treating peripheral drug effects. It reacts within minutes after injection and should be available for any patient receiving indirect-acting cholinergic agonists to treat myasthenia gravis. The patient and a family member should understand when to use the drug and how to administer it.

Pralidoxime is also used with atropine (which does cross the blood–brain barrier and will block the effects of accumulated acetylcholine at CNS sites) to treat organophosphate pesticide poisoning and nerve gas exposure (see Box 32.2), both of which cause inactivation of acetylcholinesterase.

Adverse effects associated with the use of pralidoxime include dizziness, blurred vision, diplopia, headache, drowsiness, hyperventilation, and nausea. These effects are also seen with exposure to nerve gas and organophosphate pesticides, so it can be difficult to differentiate drug effects from the effects of the poisoning.

Myasthenia Gravis

Myasthenia gravis is a chronic disorder of the neuromuscular junction. It is thought to be an autoimmune disease in which patients make antibodies to their nicotinic ACh receptors. These antibodies cause gradual destruction of the ACh receptors, resulting in fewer receptor sites being available for stimulation and in widened synaptic space. These both impair transmission of action potentials from the nerve to the muscle. ACh is the neurotransmitter that is used at the nerve–muscle synapse. If the ACh receptors are blocked and cannot be stimulated, muscle activity is decreased. The disease is marked by progressive weakness and lack of muscle control, with periodic acute episodes. Some patients have a mild clinical presentation, such as drooping eyelids, and go into remission with no further signs and symptoms for several years. Other patients have a more severe course of the disease, with progressive skeletal muscle weakness that may require the use of a wheelchair. The disease can further progress to paralysis of the diaphragm, which interferes with breathing and is fatal without intervention. Often, during the course of the disease, the patient will experience an intense phase of the disease, called a myasthenic crisis. Management of this crisis can be challenging (Box 32.5).

Alzheimer's Disease

Alzheimer's disease is a progressive disorder involving neural degeneration in the cortex that leads to a marked loss of memory, difficulty with language, and changes in behavior. It progresses to a point at which the person is unable to carry on activities of daily living. Because of this, Alzheimer's disease can have very negative effects on the patient and their family (Box 32.6).

The cause of the disease is not yet known, but it is known that there is a progressive loss of ACh-producing neurons and their target neurons in the cortex of the brain. These neurons seem to be related to memory and associations among memories that allow for connections between thoughts and stimuli (e.g., seeing a face, being able to know that it is a face, and being able to name the person the face belongs to). Within the brain of a person with Alzheimer's disease, there are amyloid beta plaques that accumulate, cause neurofibrillary tangles, and further disrupt signaling in the cholinergic and glutamatergic systems in the cortex. This causes poor functioning in the hippocampus, amygdala, frontal cortex, and parietal nerves. There is not a cure for this disease, but cholinesterase inhibitors slow progression by increasing the availability of Ach.

There are three reversible indirect-acting cholinergic agonists available to slow the progression of Alzheimer's disease. These include galantamine (*Razadyne*), rivastigmine (*Exelon*), and donepezil (*Aricept*) (see Table 32.3). The other type of medication that is used to help manage Alzheimer's disease is an *N*-methyl-D-aspartate (NMDA) receptor antagonist, memantine (*Namenda*). This drug works in a unique way to block NMDA receptor sites in the brain that are activated by glutamate. It has been theorized that the excitatory amino acid glutamate can contribute to

Box 32.5 Focus on Safe Medication Administration

MYASTHENIC CRISIS VERSUS CHOLINERGIC CRISIS

Myasthenia gravis is an autoimmune disease that runs an unpredictable course throughout the patient's life. Often, the disease goes through an intense phase called a myasthenic crisis, marked by extreme muscle weakness and respiratory difficulty.

Because of the variability of the disease and the tendency to have crises and periods of remission, management of the drug dose for a patient with myasthenia gravis is a nursing challenge. If a patient goes into remission, a smaller dose is needed. If a patient has a crisis, an increased dose is needed. To further complicate the clinical picture, the presentation of a cholinergic overdose or cholinergic crisis is similar to the presentation of a myasthenic crisis. The patient with a cholinergic crisis presents with progressive muscle weakness and respiratory difficulty as the accumulation of ACh at the cholinergic receptor site leads to reduced impulse transmission and muscle weakness. This is a crisis when the respiratory muscles are involved.

For a myasthenic crisis, the correct treatment is increasing the cholinergic drug. Treatment of a cholinergic crisis requires withdrawal of the drug. The patient's respiratory difficulty usually necessitates acute medical attention. At this point, the drug edrophonium can be used as a diagnostic agent to distinguish the two conditions. If the patient improves immediately after the edrophonium injection, the problem is a myasthenic crisis, which is improved by administration of the cholinergic drug. If the patient gets worse, the problem is probably a cholinergic crisis, and withdrawal of the patient's cholinergic drug along with intense medical support is indicated. Atropine helps alleviate some of the parasympathetic reactions to the cholinergic drug. However, because atropine is not effective at the neuromuscular junction, only time will reverse the drug toxicity.

The patient and a family member will need support, teaching, and encouragement to deal with the tricky regulation of the cholinergic medication throughout the course of the disease. Nurses in the acute care setting need to be mindful of the difficulty in distinguishing drug toxicity from the need for more drugs and be prepared to respond appropriately.

The drugs used to help patients with this progressive disease are several indirect-acting cholinergic agonists that do not cross the blood–brain barrier and do not affect ACh transmission in the brain (Table 32.3). These drugs include neostigmine (*Bloxiverz*) and pyridostigmine (*Mestinon*).

some of the symptoms of Alzheimer's disease. There is no evidence that memantine prevents or slows neurodegeneration (Box 32.7). In 2015, an extended-release capsule containing a combination of memantine and donepezil (*Namzaric*) was approved for treatment of Alzheimer's disease, targeting two different sites of action.

Therapeutic Actions and Indications

Echothiophate iodide (*Phospholine Iodide*) is a long-acting cholinesterase inhibitor for topical use in the eye to treat glaucoma and accommodative esotropia. It acts by increasing the effect of ACh in the iris, ciliary muscle, and other structures in the eye to cause miosis, increase aqueous humor outflow, and lower intraocular pressure.

Box 32.6 Focus on Cultural Considerations

ALZHEIMER'S DISEASE

Alzheimer's disease is a chronic, progressive disease of the brain's cortex. Eventually it results in memory loss so severe that the patient may not remember how to perform basic activities of daily living and may not recognize close family members. Although Alzheimer's disease primarily strikes older adults, it has a tremendous impact on family members of all ages. For example, Alzheimer patients' adult children, many of whom are busy raising children of their own, may find themselves in the caregiver role—in essence, becoming parents of their parent. This new role can put tremendous stress on people who are trying to balance work, family, and issues related to their parent's care.

When caring for an Alzheimer's patient and their family, the nurse must remember that the patient's cultural background can affect how the family copes. For instance, those who have a solid extended family or who are part of a community offering strong social support and interdependence may be better equipped to deal with caring for the patient as the disease progresses. In contrast, families whose lifestyles may include more autonomy and independence may find themselves overwhelmed by the patient's needs and may require more support and referrals to community resources.

The nurse is in the best position to evaluate the family situation. By approaching each situation as unique and striving to incorporate cultural and social considerations into care, the nurse can help ease the family's burden while also maintaining the dignity of the patient and the family through this difficult experience.

BOX 32.7

Another Treatment for Alzheimer's Disease

In late 2003, the U.S. Food and Drug Administration approved a new drug for treating Alzheimer's disease. The drug, memantine hydrochloride (*Namenda*), had been used in Europe for several years and had been reported to slow memory loss in patients with moderate to severe dementia associated with Alzheimer's disease. Memantine has a low to moderate affinity for NMDA receptors with no effects on dopamine, gamma-aminobutyric acid, histamine, glycine, or adrenergic receptor sites. It is thought that persistent activation of the CNS NMDA receptors contributes to the symptoms of Alzheimer's disease. By blocking these sites, it is thought that the symptoms are reduced or delayed.

The drug is available in a tablet form and an oral solution and is started at 5 mg/d PO, increasing by 5 mg/d at weekly intervals. The target dose is 20 mg/d given as 10 mg twice daily. Dose reduction should be considered in patients with renal impairment. Headache, dizziness, fatigue, confusion, and constipation are common adverse effects. The drug should not be taken with anything that alkalinizes the urine. Patients and family members need to understand that this drug is not a cure but may offer some extended time with mild symptoms.

The indirect-acting cholinergic agonists work by reversibly blocking acetylcholinesterase at the synaptic cleft. This blocking allows the accumulation of ACh released from the nerve endings and leads to increased and prolonged stimulation of ACh receptor sites at all of the postsynaptic cholinergic sites. Indirect-acting cholinergic agonists work to relieve the signs and symptoms of myasthenia gravis or toxicity from nondepolarizing neuromuscular junction blockers and increase muscle strength by allowing ACh to accumulate in the synaptic cleft at neuromuscular junctions. Treatment of Alzheimer's disease makes use of indirect-acting cholinergic agonists that more readily cross the blood–brain barrier and seems to affect mostly the cells in the cortex to increase ACh concentration in the area of the brain where ACh-producing cells are dying, affecting memory and the ability to access and link different memories. In addition to usual indications, pyridostigmine has also been approved for military personnel to increase survival after exposure to particular nerve gases and to reverse the effects of nondepolarizing neuromuscular junction blockers used to cause paralysis in surgery. See Table 32.3 for usual indications for each drug.

Pharmacokinetics

Many of the anticholinesterase inhibitors are well absorbed after oral administration and are distributed throughout the body. Some are metabolized by liver enzymes; others remain primarily unchanged. The major elimination pathway is via the kidneys.

Echothiophate iodide is an ophthalmic solution for topical use only. It has been found to lower plasma and erythrocyte cholinesterase levels in patients for weeks after administration.

Neostigmine is a synthetic drug that has a strong influence at the neuromuscular junction. Neostigmine has duration of action of 2 to 4 hours and, therefore, must be given every few hours based on patient response to maintain a therapeutic level.

Pyridostigmine has a longer duration of action than neostigmine (3 to 6 hours) and is preferred in some cases for the management of myasthenia gravis because it does not need to be taken as frequently. Pyridostigmine is available in oral and parenteral forms; the latter can be used if the patient is having trouble swallowing.

The drugs used to treat Alzheimer's disease are well absorbed and distributed throughout the body. They are metabolized in the liver by the cytochrome P450 system, so caution must be used for patients with hepatic impairment and for cases in which many interacting drugs are used. The drugs used to treat Alzheimer's disease are excreted in the urine.

Galantamine is available in tablet and oral solution forms. It has a half-life of 7 hours and is taken twice a day. An extended-release form, recently available, can be taken just once a day. Rivastigmine is available in capsule and solution forms to help with patients who have swallowing difficulties, as well as a transdermal patch that is applied once a day. The duration of effects for rivastigmine is 12 hours. Donepezil, which has a 70-hour half-life, is available in oral forms as tablets and as a rapidly dissolving tablet. It can be given in once-a-day dosing, which is advantageous with a disease that affects memory and the patient's ability to remember to take pills throughout the day. None of these drugs reverse the effects of Alzheimer's disease. However, studies show that they may somewhat delay the losses seen with the disease.

Contraindications and Cautions

Anticholinesterase inhibitors are contraindicated in the presence of allergy to any of these drugs to avoid hypersensitivity reactions and with bradycardia or intestinal or urinary tract obstruction, which could be exacerbated by the stimulation of cholinergic receptors.

Caution should be used with any condition that could be exacerbated by cholinergic stimulation. Although the effects of these drugs are generally more localized to the cortex and the neuromuscular junction, the possibility of parasympathetic effects must be considered carefully in patients with asthma, coronary disease, peptic ulcer, arrhythmias, epilepsy, or parkinsonism, which could be exacerbated by the effects of parasympathetic stimulation. Drugs used to treat Alzheimer's disease are metabolized in the liver and excreted in the urine, so caution should be used in the presence of hepatic or renal dysfunction, which could interfere with the metabolism and excretion of the drugs. Caution should be taken if administering to a patient who is pregnant or lactating due to lack of studies in humans and some animal data that indicates potential of harm to the fetus or infant.

Adverse Effects

The adverse effects associated with agents for treating myasthenia gravis or Alzheimer's disease are related to stimulation of the parasympathetic nervous system. GI effects can include nausea, vomiting, cramps, diarrhea, increased salivation, and involuntary defecation related to the increase in GI secretions and activity due to parasympathetic nervous system stimulation. Cardiovascular effects can include bradycardia, heart block, hypotension, and even cardiac arrest related to the cardiac-suppressing effects of the parasympathetic nervous system. Urinary tract effects can include a sense of urgency related to stimulation of the bladder muscles and sphincter relaxation. Miosis and blurred vision, headaches, dizziness, and drowsiness can occur related to CNS cholinergic effects. Other effects may include flushing and increased sweating secondary to stimulation of the cholinergic receptors in the sympathetic nervous system. Cholinergic crisis can occur with overdose of medications causing excessive muscarinic and nicotinic stimulation that causes extreme symptoms including abdominal cramps, increased salivation, lacrimation, muscular weakness, paralysis, muscular fasciculation, diarrhea, blurry vision, and respiratory depression.

Clinically Important Drug–Drug Interactions

There may be an increased risk of GI bleeding if these drugs are used with nonsteroidal anti-inflammatory drugs (NSAIDs) because of the combination of increased GI secretions and the GI mucosal erosion associated with the use of NSAIDs. If this combination is used, the patient should be monitored closely for any sign of GI bleeding. The effect of anticholinesterase drugs is decreased if they are taken in combination with any cholinergic drugs because these work in opposition to each other. Cholinesterase inhibitors increase the neuromuscular blockage of depolarizing neuromuscular blockers (succinylcholine).

Prototype Summary: Pyridostigmine

Indications: Treatment of myasthenia gravis; antidote for nondepolarizing neuromuscular junction blockers; increased survival after exposure to nerve gas.

Actions: Reversible cholinesterase inhibitor that increases the levels of ACh, facilitating transmission at the neuromuscular junction.

Pharmacokinetics:

Route	Onset	Duration
Oral	35–45 min	3–6 h
IM	15 min	3–6 h
IV	5 min	3–6 h

$T_{1/2}$: 1.9 to 3.7 hours; metabolized in the liver and tissue; excreted in the urine.

Adverse Effects: Bradycardia, cardiac arrest, tearing, miosis, salivation, dysphagia, nausea, vomiting, increased bronchial secretions, urinary frequency, and incontinence.

Prototype Summary: Donepezil

Indications: Treatment of mild to moderate Alzheimer's disease.

Actions: Reversible cholinesterase inhibitor that causes elevated ACh levels in the cortex, which slows the neuronal degradation of Alzheimer's disease.

Pharmacokinetics:

Route	Onset	Peak
Oral	Varies	2–4 h

$T_{1/2}$: 70 hours; metabolized in the liver; excreted in the urine.

Adverse Effects: Insomnia, fatigue, rash, nausea, vomiting, diarrhea, dyspepsia, abdominal pain, muscle cramps.

Nursing Considerations for Patients Receiving Indirect-Acting Cholinergic Agonists

Assessment: History and Examination

- Assess for contraindications or cautions: known allergies to any of these drugs to avoid hypersensitivity reactions; arrhythmias, coronary artery disease, hypotension, urogenital or GI obstruction, or peptic ulcer, which could be exacerbated by cholinergic stimulation; recent GI or GU surgery, which could limit use of the drugs because of the stimulatory effects of the parasympathetic system, which could aggravate healing; regular use of NSAIDs, cholinergic drugs, or theophylline, which could cause a drug–drug interaction; and current status of pregnancy and lactation because of potential effects on the fetus or neonate.
- Perform a physical assessment before beginning therapy to establish baseline status and any potential adverse effects; assess orientation, affect, reflexes, ability to carry on activities of daily living (Alzheimer's drugs), and vision to monitor for CNS changes related to drug therapy.
- Assess blood pressure, pulse, ECG, peripheral perfusion, and cardiac output to monitor the parasympathetic effects on the vascular system; perform urinary output and renal and liver function tests to monitor drug effects on the renal system and liver, which could change the metabolism and excretion of the drugs.

Refer to the "Critical Thinking Scenario" for a full discussion of nursing care for a patient who is receiving indirect-acting cholinergic agonists.

Nursing Conclusions

Nursing conclusions related to drug therapy might include the following:

- Altered thought processes related to CNS effects
- Impaired comfort related to GI effects
- Decreased cardiac output related to blood pressure changes, arrhythmias, and vasodilation
- Knowledge deficit regarding drug therapy
- Injury risk related to CNS effects
- Diarrhea related to GI stimulatory effects

Planning

- The patient will receive the best therapeutic effect from the drug therapy.
- The patient will have limited adverse effects from the drug therapy.
- The patient will have an understanding of the drug therapy, adverse effects to anticipate, and measures to relieve discomfort and improve safety.

Intervention With Rationale

- If the drug is given intravenously, administer it slowly to avoid severe cholinergic effects.
- Maintain on standby atropine sulfate as an antidote in case of overdose or severe cholinergic reaction.
- Discontinue the drug if diarrhea, emesis, excessive salivation, or frequent urination becomes a problem, to decrease the risk of severe adverse reactions.
- Administer the oral drug with meals to decrease GI upset if it is a problem.
- Mark the patient's chart and notify the surgeon if the patient is to undergo surgery because prolonged muscle relaxation may occur if succinylcholine-type

anesthetics are used. The patient will require prolonged support and monitoring.

- Monitor the patient being treated for Alzheimer's disease for any progress because the drug is not a cure and only slows progression; refer their family to supportive services.
- The patient who is being treated for myasthenia gravis and a significant other should receive instruction in drug administration, warning signs of drug overdose, and signs and symptoms to report immediately to enhance patient knowledge about drug therapy and to promote adherence.
- Arrange for supportive care and comfort measures, including rest, environmental control, and other measures, to decrease CNS irritation; headache medication to relieve pain; safety measures if CNS effects occur to prevent injury; protective measures if CNS effects are severe to prevent patient injury; and small, frequent meals if GI upset is severe to decrease discomfort and maintain nutrition.
- Provide thorough patient teaching, including dosage, adverse effects to anticipate and measures to avoid them, and warning signs of problems, as well as proper administration for each route used, to enhance patient knowledge about drug therapy and to promote adherence.
- Offer support and encouragement to help the patient manage the diagnosis and drug regimen.

Evaluation

- Monitor patient response to the drug (improvement in condition being treated).
- Monitor for adverse effects (GI upset, CNS changes, cardiovascular changes, GU changes).
- Evaluate the effectiveness of the teaching plan (patient can name drug, dosage, adverse effects to watch for and specific measures to avoid them, and proper administration).
- Monitor the effectiveness of comfort measures and adherence to the regimen.

CRITICAL THINKING SCENARIO
Indirect-Acting Cholinergic Agonists

THE SITUATION

A.J., who is 75 years old and has an unremarkable medical history, is seen in the clinic for evaluation of memory loss and confusion. Three years ago, A.J.'s spouse began to notice A.J. exhibiting memory gaps and confusion when driving around town. A.J. would get lost only a few blocks from home. The problem has gotten steadily worse. A.J. is diagnosed with Alzheimer's disease after neurological tests and medical evaluation ruled out other causes for the problem. A.J. did not want to take any drugs, but when they hear the diagnosis, they become quite frightened and agree to try medication. A.J.'s spouse voices concern about giving A.J. medication because they sometimes have trouble swallowing and choke on their food. A.J.'s spouse excitedly tells them that with the medication, A.J.'s memory will return, and things will be normal again. A.J. is placed on rivastigmine.

CRITICAL THINKING

What could be responsible for A.J.'s symptoms?

What modifications can be made to the prescription to ensure patient safety if A.J. is having trouble swallowing?

What important information about the disease and the effectiveness of drug therapy needs to be discussed with A.J. and their spouse? Will things return to normal?

What potential adverse effects can be anticipated with rivastigmine, and how might these effects complicate the situation for this patient and their spouse?

DISCUSSION

Alzheimer's disease is a chronic, progressive disease that involves the loss of neurons in the cortex of the brain, which are responsible for making connections between different memories. A.J. has had the problem for at least 3 years, and their loss of memory and confusion have gotten worse over that period of time. Unfortunately, there is nothing available at this time that can stop the loss of neurons or restore the function that has already been lost.

One of the problems that occurs with Alzheimer's disease is difficulty swallowing. Swallowing is a complex CNS reflex that requires coordination of impulses; with this disease, the ability to swallow in a coordinated manner is often lost. This can lead to aspiration and pneumonia, which are often the underlying causes of death with Alzheimer's disease. Since A.J. already has some difficulty swallowing, it would be important to look into the forms in which rivastigmine is provided. The drug is available in capsule form and as an oral solution. The oral solution might be suggested because it could be much easier to swallow. The drug is also available as a transdermal system, which would eliminate the need to swallow the drug as the disease progresses. The status of A.J.'s swallowing should be evaluated before starting therapy and periodically as time goes on to determine how safe the dosage form of the drug is for their particular situation.

A.J. and their spouse should receive information on Alzheimer's disease and its progression. The drugs available at this time do not reverse the memory loss, and they do not cure the disease. A.J.'s spouse may be encouraged to monitor A.J.'s behavior, ability to perform activities of daily living, and other significant markers of importance to them. The drug should slow the progression

(continues on page 564)

of the disease, and it might be helpful to monitor progress to see if the drug is effective. A.J.'s spouse might also want to become involved in an Alzheimer's support group or organization, which could provide valuable support, educational materials, and access to community resources. This is an overwhelming diagnosis, and it might be necessary to approach A.J. and their spouse over several visits to give them both time to adjust. It is important to always include a family member and provide information in writing for later reference when providing teaching to a patient with Alzheimer's disease.

Many of the adverse effects associated with the indirect-acting cholinergic agonists are a result of the parasympathetic stimulation caused by these drugs. This may complicate A.J.'s care as the disease progresses. GI effects can include increased salivation, which may further add to A.J.'s difficulty swallowing; nausea and vomiting, which could make it difficult to maintain nutrition; and cramps, diarrhea, and involuntary defecation related to the increase in GI secretions and activity, which could make toileting difficult and add to A.J.'s spouse's home care burden. Cardiovascular effects can include bradycardia, heart block, and hypotension, which could lead to dizziness and weakness and further complicate safety issues. Urinary tract effects can include a sense of urgency related to stimulation of the bladder muscles and sphincter relaxation, which could lead to incontinence as the patient becomes less responsive to normal reflexes. Miosis and blurred vision, headaches, dizziness, and drowsiness can occur, further complicating safety issues. The benefits of slowing the progression of the disease often need to be weighed against all of the potential adverse effects that can complicate care and safety.

NURSING CARE GUIDE FOR A.J.: INDIRECT-ACTING CHOLINERGIC AGONISTS

Assessment: History and Examination

Assess for contraindications or cautions: known allergies to any of components of this drug, arrhythmias, coronary artery disease, hypotension, urogenital or GI obstruction, peptic ulcer, recent GI or GU surgery, and regular use of NSAIDs, cholinergic drugs, or theophylline.

Focus the physical exam on the following:

CNS: Orientation, affect, reflexes, memory response, ability to carry out simple commands, vision

CV: Blood pressure, pulse, peripheral perfusion, electrocardiography

GI: Abdominal exam

GU: Urinary output, bladder tone

Respiratory: Respirations, adventitious sounds

Skin: Color, temperature, texture

Nursing Conclusions

Altered cardiac output related to CV effects
Injury risk related to CNS effects
Risk for diarrhea
Knowledge deficit regarding drug therapy

Planning

The patient will receive the best therapeutic effect from the drug therapy.

The patient will have limited adverse effects from the drug therapy.

The patient will have an understanding of the drug therapy, adverse effects to anticipate, and measures to relieve discomfort and improve safety.

Intervention

Ensure safe and appropriate administration of the drug; monitor ability to swallow and the appropriateness of dosage form.

Provide comfort and safety measures (e.g., physical assistance, raising side rails on the bed); temperature control; pain relief; small, frequent meals.

Monitor cardiac status and urine output throughout drug therapy.

Provide support and reassurance to deal with side effects, discomfort, and GI effects.

Provide patient and family teaching regarding drug name, dosage, side effects, precautions, and warning signs of serious adverse effects to report.

Evaluation

Evaluate drug effects: slowing of progression of dementia.

Monitor for adverse effects: CV effects—bradycardia, heart block, hypotension; urinary problems; GI effects; respiratory problems.

Monitor for drug–drug interactions.

Evaluate the effectiveness of patient and teaching program and comfort and safety measures.

Patient/Family Teaching for A.J.

- The drug that was ordered for you is called rivastigmine. It is called a cholinergic agonist or a parasympathetic drug because it mimics the effects of the parasympathetic nervous system. Cholinergic drugs get this name because they act at certain nerve–nerve and nerve–muscle junctions in the body that are called cholinergic sites. They use a chemical called acetylcholine to carry out their functions. The nerves in your brain that are affected by Alzheimer's disease use acetylcholine to help you to remember things and make connections between memories. This drug will not reverse the losses of memory but may slow the loss.
- Some of the following adverse effects may occur:
  - *Nausea, vomiting, diarrhea*: It is wise to be near bathroom facilities after taking your drug. If these symptoms become too severe, consult with your health care provider.
  - *Flushing, sweating*: Staying in a cool environment and wearing lightweight clothing may help.
  - *Increased salivation*: This may increase your difficulty in swallowing.
  - *Urgency to void*: Maintaining access to a bathroom may relieve some of this discomfort.
  - *Headache*: Aspirin or another headache medication (if not contraindicated in your particular case) will help to alleviate this pain.
  - *Changes in vision, dizziness*: These might lead to falls or more confusion.
- Report any of the following to your health care provider: very slow pulse, light-headedness, fainting, excessive salivation, abdominal cramping or pain, weakness or confusion, blurring of vision, further signs of dementia.
- Tell any doctor, nurse, or other health care provider involved in your care that you are taking this drug.

Key Points

- Myasthenia gravis is an autoimmune disease characterized by antibodies to ACh receptors. This results in a loss of ACh receptors and eventual loss of response at the neuromuscular junction.
- Acetylcholinesterase inhibitors are used to treat myasthenia gravis because they allow the accumulation of ACh in the synaptic cleft, prolonging stimulation of any ACh sites that remain.
- Alzheimer's disease is a progressive dementia characterized by a loss of ACh-producing neurons and ACh receptor sites in the neurocortex.
- Acetylcholinesterase inhibitors that cross the blood–brain barrier are used to manage Alzheimer's disease by increasing ACh levels in the brain and slowing the progression of the disease.

SUMMARY

- Cholinergic drugs are chemicals that act at the same site as the neurotransmitter ACh, stimulating the parasympathetic nerves, some nerves in the brain, and the neuromuscular junction.
- Direct-acting cholinergic drugs react with the ACh receptor sites to cause cholinergic stimulation.
- Use of direct-acting cholinergic drugs is limited by the systemic effects of the drug. One drug is used to induce miosis and to treat glaucoma, another agent is available to treat neurogenic bladder and bladder atony postoperatively or postpartum, and another agent is available to increase GI secretions and relieve the dry mouth of Sjögren's syndrome.
- All indirect-acting cholinergic drugs are acetylcholinesterase inhibitors. They block acetylcholinesterase to prevent it from breaking down ACh in the synaptic cleft.
- Cholinergic stimulation by acetylcholinesterase inhibitors is due to accumulation of the ACh released from the nerve ending.
- Myasthenia gravis is an autoimmune disease characterized by antibodies to the ACh receptors. This results in a loss of ACh receptors and eventual loss of response at the neuromuscular junction.
- Acetylcholinesterase inhibitors are used to treat myasthenia gravis because they allow the accumulation of ACh in the synaptic cleft, prolonging stimulation of any ACh sites that remain.
- Alzheimer's disease is a progressive dementia characterized by a loss of ACh-producing neurons and ACh receptor sites in the neurocortex.
- Acetylcholinesterase inhibitors that cross the blood–brain barrier are used to manage Alzheimer's disease by increasing ACh levels in the brain and slowing the progression of the disease.
- Side effects associated with the use of these drugs (bradycardia, hypotension, increased GI secretions and activity, increased bladder tone, relaxation of GI and GU sphincters, bronchoconstriction, pupil constriction) are related to stimulation of the parasympathetic nervous system and may limit the usefulness of some of the drugs.

CHECK YOUR UNDERSTANDING

Answers to the questions in this chapter can be found in Answers to Check Your Understanding Questions on thePoint®.

MULTIPLE CHOICE

Select the best answer.

1. Indirect-acting cholinergic agents
   a. react with acetylcholine receptor sites on the membranes of effector cells.
   b. react chemically with acetylcholinesterase to increase acetylcholine concentrations.
   c. are used to increase bladder tone and urinary excretion.
   d. should be given with food to slow absorption.
2. A patient is to receive pilocarpine. The nurse understands that this drug would be most likely used to treat which of the following?
   a. Myasthenia gravis
   b. Neurogenic bladder
   c. Sjögren's disease dry mouth
   d. Alzheimer's disease

3. Myasthenia gravis is treated with indirect-acting cholinergic agents that
   a. lead to accumulation of acetylcholine in the synaptic cleft.
   b. block the GI effects of the disease, allowing for absorption.
   c. directly stimulate the remaining acetylcholine receptors.
   d. can be given only by injection because of problems associated with swallowing.

4. A patient with myasthenia gravis is no longer able to swallow. Which of the following would the nurse expect the physician to order?
   a. Rivastigmine
   b. Memantine
   c. Pyridostigmine
   d. Edrophonium

5. Alzheimer's disease is marked by a progressive loss of memory and is associated with
   a. degeneration of dopamine-producing cells in the basal ganglia.
   b. loss of acetylcholine-producing neurons and their target neurons in the CNS.
   c. loss of acetylcholine receptor sites in the parasympathetic nervous system.
   d. increased levels of acetylcholinesterase in the CNS.

6. The nurse would expect to administer donepezil to a patient with Alzheimer's disease who
   a. cannot remember family members' names.
   b. is mildly inhibited and can still follow medical dosing regimens.
   c. is able to carry on normal activities of daily living.
   d. has memory problems and would benefit from once-a-day dosing.

7. Adverse effects associated with the use of cholinergic drugs include
   a. constipation and insomnia.
   b. diarrhea and urinary urgency.
   c. tachycardia and hypertension.
   d. dry mouth and tachycardia.

8. Nerve gas is an irreversible acetylcholinesterase inhibitor that can cause muscle paralysis and death. An antidote to such an agent is
   a. atropine.
   b. propranolol.
   c. pralidoxime.
   d. neostigmine.

MULTIPLE RESPONSE

Select all that apply.

1. A nurse is explaining myasthenia gravis to a family. Which of the following points would be included in the explanation?
   a. It is thought to be an autoimmune disease.
   b. It is associated with destruction of acetylcholine receptor sites.
   c. It is best treated with potent antibiotics.
   d. It is a chronic and progressive muscular disease.
   e. It is caused by demyelination of the nerve fiber.
   f. Once diagnosed, it has a 5-year survival rate.

2. A nurse would question an order for a cholinergic drug if the patient was also taking which drugs?
   a. Theophylline
   b. NSAIDs
   c. Cephalosporin
   d. Atropine
   e. Propranolol
   f. Memantine

REFERENCES

Andrews, M., & Boyle, J. (2011). *Transcultural concepts in nursing care* (6th ed.). Lippincott Williams & Wilkins.

Benowitz, N. L. (2010). Pharmacology of nicotine: Addiction, smoking-induced disease, and therapeutics. *Annual Review of Pharmacology Toxicology*, *49*, 57–71. 10.1146/annurev.pharmtox.48.113006.094742

Bird, S. J., & Levine, J. M. (2021). Myasthenic crisis. *UptoDate*. https://www.uptodate.com/contents/myasthenic-crisis/print?search=myasthenia%20gravis%20crisis&source=search_result&selectedTitle=1~81&usage_type=default&display_rank=1

Brunton, L., Hilal-Dandan, R., & Knollman, B. (2018). *Goodman and Gilman's the pharmacological basis of therapeutics* (13th ed.). McGraw-Hill.

Iqbal, K., & Grundke-Iqbal, I. (2004). Inhibition of neurofibrillary degeneration: A promising approach to Alzheimer disease and other tauopathies. *Current Drug Targets*, 5(6), 495–501.

Kaminski, H. (2011). *Myasthenia gravis and related disorders*. Springer Publishing.

Naylor, M. D., Stephen, C., Bowles, K. H., & Bixby, M. B. (2005). Cognitively impaired older adults: From hospital to home. *American Journal of Nursing*, *105*, 52–61.

Norris, T. L. (2019). *Porth's pathophysiology concepts of altered health states* (10th ed.). Wolters Kluwer.

Reisberg, B., Doody, R., Stöffler, A., Schmitt, F., Ferris, S., Möbius, H. J., & Memantine Study Group. (2003). Memantine in moderate-to-severe Alzheimer disease. *New England Journal of Medicine*, *348*, 1333–1341.

CHAPTER 33

Anticholinergic Agents

Learning Objectives

Upon completion of this chapter, you will be able to:

1. Define anticholinergic agents.
2. Discuss the use of anticholinergic agents across the lifespan.
3. Describe the therapeutic actions, indications, pharmacokinetics, contraindications and cautions, most common adverse effects, and important drug–drug interactions of anticholinergic agents.
4. Compare and contrast the prototype drug atropine with other anticholinergic agents.
5. Outline the nursing considerations, including important teaching points, for patients receiving anticholinergic agents.

Key Terms

anticholinergic: opposes the effects of acetylcholine at acetylcholine receptor sites

belladonna: plant that contains atropine as an alkaloid; used to dilate the pupils as a fashion statement in the past; used in herbal medicine much as atropine is used today

cycloplegia: inability of the lens in the eye to accommodate to near vision, causing blurring and inability to see near objects

mydriasis: relaxation of the muscles around the pupil, leading to pupil dilation

parasympatholytic: lysing or preventing parasympathetic effects

Drug List

ANTICHOLINERGIC AGENTS/ PARASYMPATHOLYTICS
aclidinium
(P) atropine
darifenacin
dicyclomine
fesoterodine
flavoxate
glycopyrrolate
hyoscyamine
ipratropium
methscopolamine
oxybutynin chloride
propantheline
revefenacin
scopolamine
solifenacin
tiotropium
tolterodine
trospium
umeclidinium

Drugs that are used to block the effects of acetylcholine are called **anticholinergic** agents. Because this action lyses, or blocks, the effects of the parasympathetic nervous system, they are also called **parasympatholytic** agents. This class of drugs was once widely used to decrease gastrointestinal (GI) activity and secretions in the treatment of ulcers and to decrease other parasympathetic activities to allow the sympathetic system to become more dominant. Today, more specific and less systemically toxic drugs are available for many of the conditions that would benefit from these effects. Therefore, this class of drugs is less commonly used for treating GI ailments, but there are a few still on the market. Other uses of these medications are for bronchodilation and treatment of overactive bladder. Atropine is a widely used anticholinergic drug used to treat symptomatic bradycardia, as an antidote for cholinergic medication, to cause pupil dilation, and to decrease secretions. Box 33.1 discusses the use of anticholinergics across the lifespan.

Anticholinergics/Parasympatholytics

Anticholinergic agents include aclidinium (*Tudorza Pressair*), atropine (*Atropen*), darifenacin (*Enablex*), dicyclomine

Box 33.1 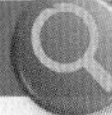 Focus on Drug Therapy Across the Lifespan

ANTICHOLINERGIC AGENTS/PARASYMPATHOLYTICS

Children

The anticholinergic agents are often used in children. Children may suffer from the adverse effects of the drugs, including constipation, urinary retention, heat intolerance, and confusion. If a child is given one of these drugs, they should be closely watched and monitored for adverse effects, and appropriate supportive measures should be instituted. Dicyclomine is not recommended for use in children.

Adults

Adults need to be made aware of the potential for adverse effects associated with the use of these drugs. They should be encouraged to void before taking the medication if urinary retention or hesitancy is a problem. They should be encouraged to drink plenty of fluids and to avoid hot temperatures because heat intolerance can occur, and it will be important to maintain hydration should this happen. Safety precautions may be needed if blurred vision and dizziness occur. The patient should be urged not to drive or perform tasks that require concentration and coordination.

There should be caution with use of these drugs during pregnancy because they cross the placenta and could cause adverse effects on the fetus. Sometimes there are emergent situations that require their use, with the benefit to the patient clearly outweighing the potential risk to the fetus. Patients who are breast or chestfeeding should find another method of feeding the baby if an anticholinergic drug is needed because of the potential for serious adverse effects on the baby.

Older Adults

Older adults may be more likely to experience the adverse effects associated with these drugs. Older adults may not eliminate the medications as quickly as younger adults due to changes in renal function. The dose may need to be reduced, and the patient should be monitored very closely. Because older patients are more susceptible to heat intolerance owing to decreased body fluid and decreased sweating, extreme caution should be used when an anticholinergic drug is given. The patient should be urged to drink plenty of fluids and to avoid extremes of temperature on exertion in warm temperatures. The older adult is more likely to experience confusion, hallucinations, and psychotic syndromes when taking an anticholinergic drug. Safety precautions may be needed if CNS effects are severe.

(*Bentyl*), fesoterodine (*Toviaz*), flavoxate (generic), glycopyrrolate (*Cuvposa, Glyx-PF, Lonhala Magnair*), hyoscyamine (*Symax* and others), ipratropium (*Atrovent HFA*), methscopolamine (generic), oxybutynin chloride (*Ditropan XL, Gelnique, Oxytrol*), propantheline (generic), revefenacin (*Yupelri*), scopolamine (*Transderm Scop*), solifenacin (*VESIcare*), tiotropium (*Spiriva*), tolterodine (*Detrol*), trospium (generic), and umeclidinium (*Incruse Ellipta*) (see Table 33.1).

Therapeutic Actions and Indications

The anticholinergic drugs competitively block the acetylcholine receptors at the muscarinic cholinergic receptor sites that are responsible for mediating the effects of parasympathetic postganglionic impulses (Fig. 33.1). Some are more specific to particular receptors in the respiratory, genitourinary (GU), or GI tracts, making them preferred for treating specific conditions, and others more generally

Table 33.1 *Drugs in Focus:* Anticholinergic Agents/Parasympatholytics

Drug Name	Dosage/Route	Usual Indications
aclidinium (*Tudorza Pressair*)	400 mcg b.i.d. by oral inhalation	Long-term maintenance treatment of bronchospasm associated with COPD
atropine (*Atropen*)	*Adult*: Dosing varies per indication and titrated based on HR and BP response; 0.4–3 mg IM, subcutaneous, or IV *Pediatric*: 0.1–0.4 mg/kg, IM, or subcutaneous	Decrease secretions; bradycardia; pylorospasm; ureteral colic; relaxing of bladder; emotional lability with head injuries; antidote for cholinergic drugs; pupil dilation
darifenacin (*Enablex*)	7.5–15 mg/d PO	Treatment of overactive bladder with symptoms of urge urinary incontinence, urgency, and urinary frequency
dicyclomine (*Bentyl*)	80–160 mg/d PO in four divided doses; 40–80 mg/d IM in four divided doses—do not give IV	Treatment of irritable or hyperactive bowel in adults
fesoterodine (*Toviaz*)	4–8 mg/d PO	Treatment of overactive bladder with symptoms of urge urinary incontinence, urgency, and urinary frequency
flavoxate (generic)	100–200 mg PO t.i.d. to q.i.d.	Symptomatic relief of dysuria, urgency, nocturia, suprapubic pain, frequency and incontinence associated with cystitis, prostatitis, urethritis, urethrocystitis, or urethrotrigonitis

Table 33.1 ***Drugs in Focus:*** **Anticholinergic Agents/Parasympatholytics *(Continued)***

Drug Name	Dosage/Route	Usual Indications
glycopyrrolate (*Cuvposa, Glyrx-PF, Lonhala Magnair*)	*Adult and pediatric*: Dosing varies based on indication and route of administration	Decrease secretions before anesthesia or intubation; treatment of ulcers (although not drug of choice); reduction of severe drooling; protects the patient from the peripheral effects of cholinergic drugs; reverses neuromuscular blockade; inhalation for maintenance treatment of COPD
hyoscyamine (*Symax*, others)	0.125–0.25 mg t.i.d. to q.i.d. PO or sublingually; 0.25–0.5 mg b.i.d. to q.i.d. IM, IV, or subcutaneous	Adjunctive therapy for peptic ulcer; overactive GI disorders; neurogenic bladder or cystitis; parkinsonism; biliary or renal colic; decrease secretions preoperatively; treatment of partial heart block associated with vagal activity; treatment of rhinitis or anticholinesterase poisoning
ipratropium (*Atrovent HFA*)	2 inhalations or nasal sprays t.i.d. or q.i.d. (do not exceed 12 inhalations/d)	Maintenance treatment of bronchospasm associated with COPD; nasal spray for symptomatic relief of perennial and seasonal rhinitis
methscopolamine (*Pamine*)	2.5 mg PO 30 min before meals and 2.5–5 mg PO at bedtime	Adjunctive therapy for the treatment of peptic ulcer
oxybutynin chloride (*Ditropan XL, Gelnique, Oxytrol*)	*Adult*: 5 mg PO b.i.d. or t.i.d.; ER tablets 5 mg PO daily; transdermal patch, 1 patch every 3–4 days (twice a week) will administer 3.9 mg/d; topical gel 1 mL applied every 24 h *Pediatric*: ER tablets 5 mg PO daily (over 6 y); 5 mg PO b.i.d. or t.i.d. (over 5 y)	Relief of bladder instability; treatment of overactive bladder
propantheline (generic)	*Adult*: 15 mg PO 30 min before meals and at bedtime *Pediatric*: As antisecretory agent, 1.5 mg/kg/d PO in divided doses t.i.d. to q.i.d. as antispasmodic, 2–3 mg/kg/d PO in divided doses q4–6 h and at bedtime	Decrease GI secretions and stop GI spasms in conditions that would benefit from these actions; adjunctive therapy in treatment of peptic ulcer
revefenacin (*Yupelri*)	*Adult*: one 175 mcg vial inhaled daily	Maintenance treatment of patients with COPD
scopolamine (*Transderm Scop*)	*Adult*: 0.32–0.65 mg subcutaneous or IM; 1–2 drops (gtt) in eye(s) for refraction; 1.5 mg transdermal every 3 d for motion sickness; use caution with older patients *Pediatric*: Do not use PO or transdermal system with children; 0.006 mg/kg subcutaneous, IM, or IV	Decrease nausea and vomiting associated with motion sickness; decrease GI secretions; induce obstetric amnesia and relax the pregnant patient; relieve urinary problems; adjunctive therapy for ulcers; dilate pupils to aid examination of the eye and preoperatively and postoperatively with eye surgery
solifenacin (*VESIcare*)	5–10 mg/d PO	Treatment of overactive bladder with symptoms of urge urinary incontinence, urgency, and urinary frequency
tiotropium (*Spiriva*)	Two inhalations of the contents of one capsule (18 mcg) each day using an inhalation device	Maintenance treatment of bronchospasm associated with COPD, for long-term use
tolterodine (*Detrol, Detrol LA*)	2 mg PO b.i.d. or 4 mg/d PO extended release; reduce dose if severe renal or hepatic impairment	Treatment of overactive bladder with symptoms of urge urinary incontinence, urgency, and urinary frequency
trospium (generic)	20 mg PO b.i.d. or 60-mg extended release tablet PO once a day	Treatment of urinary incontinence, urgency, and frequency associated with overactive bladder
umeclidinium (*Incruse Ellipta*)	One inhalation/d (62.5 mcg)	Long-term, once-daily maintenance treatment of COPD

COPD, chronic obstructive pulmonary disease; GI, gastrointestinal.

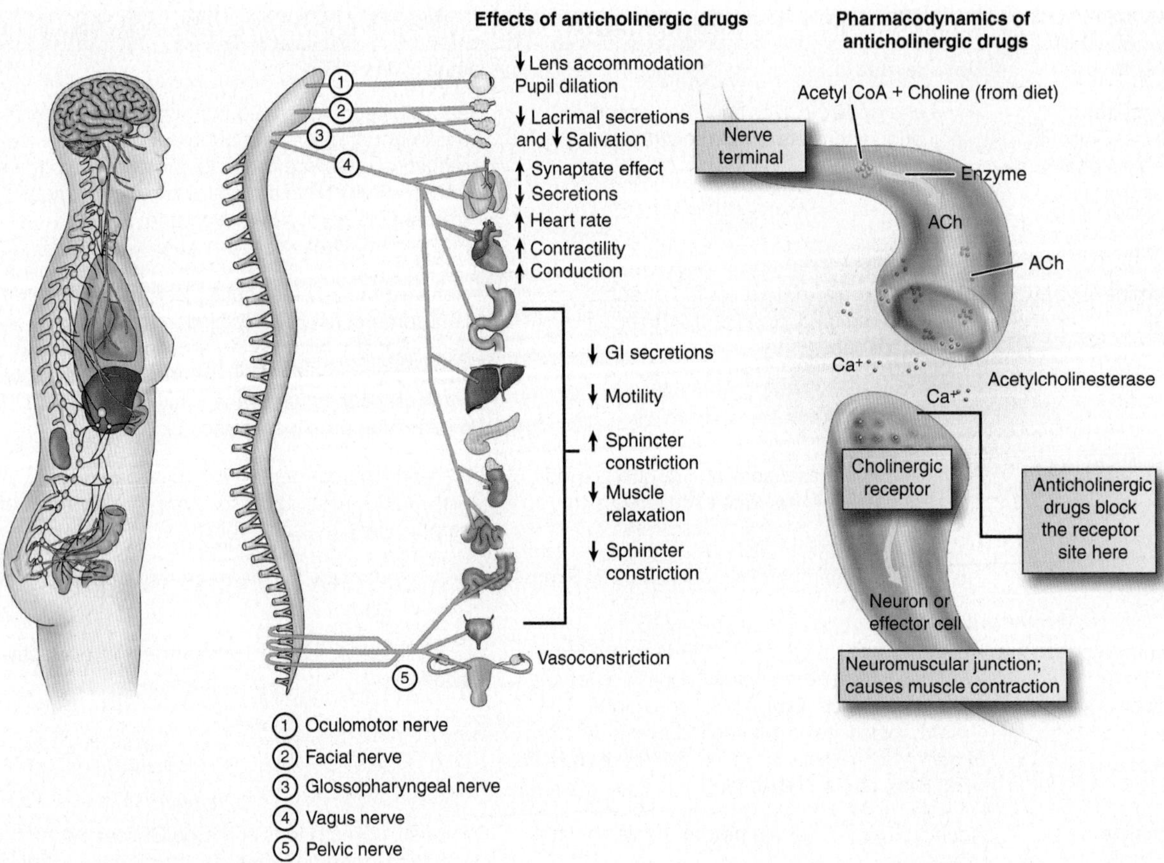

FIGURE 33.1 Pharmacodynamics of anticholinergic drugs and associated physiological responses.

depress the parasympathetic system. When the parasympathetic system is blocked, the effects of the sympathetic system are more prominently seen. These drugs can be used to decrease secretions before anesthesia, to treat parkinsonism (by blocking the stimulating effects of acetylcholine), to restore cardiac rate and blood pressure after vagal stimulation during surgery, to relieve bradycardia caused by a hyperactive carotid sinus reflex, to relieve pylorospasm and hyperactive bowel, to prevent the signs and symptoms of motion sickness and vomiting, to relax biliary and ureteral colic, to relax bladder detrusor muscles and tighten sphincters, to help to control crying or laughing episodes in patients with brain injuries, to relax uterine hypertonicity, to help in the management of peptic ulcer, to control rhinorrhea associated with hay fever, as an antidote for cholinergic drugs and poisoning by certain mushrooms, as maintenance treatment of bronchospasm associated with chronic obstructive pulmonary disease (COPD), and as an ophthalmic agent to cause mydriasis or cycloplegia in acute inflammatory conditions (see Table 33.1). Anticholinergic drugs also are thought to block the effects of acetylcholine in the central nervous system (CNS), which may account for their effectiveness in treating motion sickness and preventing nausea and vomiting.

Atropine, the prototype drug, has been used for many years and is derived from the plant **belladonna**. Belladonna was once used by fashionable ladies of the European courts to dilate their pupils in an effort to make them more innocent looking and alluring. It is still used in herbal medicine today, much as atropine is. Atropine is used to depress salivation and bronchial secretions and to dilate the bronchi, but it can thicken respiratory secretions (causing obstruction of airways). Atropine is also used to inhibit vagal responses in the heart, which will increase heart rate and blood pressure; to relax the GI and GU tracts; to inhibit GI secretions; to cause **mydriasis** or relaxation of the pupil of the eye (also called a mydriatic effect; see Box 33.2); and to cause **cycloplegia**, or inhibition of the ability of the lens in the eye to accommodate to near vision (also called a cycloplegic effect).

Box 33.2 Focus on **Cultural Considerations**

THE MYDRIATIC EFFECT

Nurses working in eye clinics or administering preoperative medications for eye surgery should be aware that mydriatics (including atropine) may take longer to have effectiveness and require higher doses in people with dark-pigmented eyes. There may be better effect of dilation when combination medications are used. Also keep in mind that younger patients may have a better response to the medication than older patients.

Both atropine and scopolamine work by blocking only the muscarinic effectors in the parasympathetic nervous system and the few cholinergic receptors in the sympathetic nervous system (SNS), such as those that control sweating. They act by competing with acetylcholine for the muscarinic acetylcholine receptor sites. They do not block the nicotinic receptors and therefore have little or no effect at the neuromuscular junction.

Darifenacin, fesoterodine, flavoxate, oxybutynin chloride, solifenacin, tolterodine, and trospium are used to treat overactive bladder with symptoms of urinary incontinence, urgency, and urinary frequency. These medications act to inhibit muscarinic receptors of the detrusor muscle of the bladder to help relax the bladder and decrease spasms. Some of the medications act more specifically on receptors than others. See Chapter 52 for further discussion of these drugs. Aclidinium, glycopyrrolate, ipratropium, revefenacin, tiotropium, and umeclidinium act more specifically to decrease respiratory secretions and cause bronchodilation and are used as bronchodilators for long-term maintenance of COPD. These agents are discussed in more detail in Chapter 55. Dicyclomine, hyoscyamine, propantheline, scopolamine, and methscopolamine act on the receptors in the GI tract and are used as adjuncts in the treatment of peptic ulcers, irritable bowel syndrome, and GI disorders. These agents are discussed in more detail in Chapters 57 to 59.

Pharmacokinetics

The anticholinergics are administered via a variety of routes. Some are well absorbed after oral administration. Some are administered by IV, IM, and subcutaneous injections. Some are inhaled. Scopolamine and oxybutynin chloride can be administered via transdermal systems (see Box 33.3). Onset, peak, and half-lives vary by drug. Because many are metabolized in the liver and excreted in the urine, there are often dosage reductions recommended with severe hepatic and/or renal impairment.

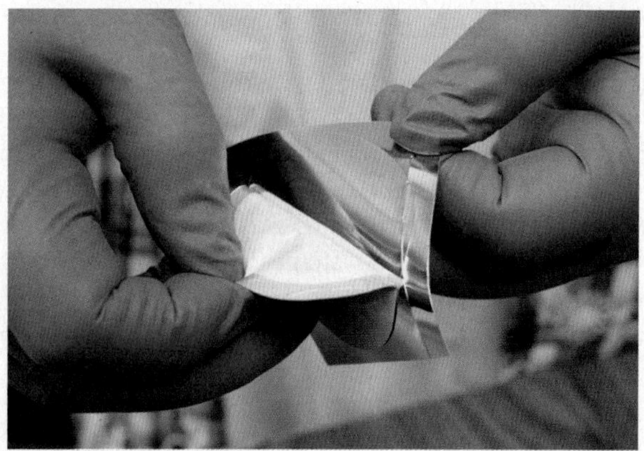

FIGURE 33.2 Carefully remove the backing from the patch without touching the adhesive.

Box 33.3 Focus on Safe Medication Administration

APPLYING DERMAL PATCH DELIVERY SYSTEMS

If a drug has been ordered to be given via a transdermal patch, review the proper technique for applying a transdermal patch. The patch should be applied to a clean, dry, intact, and hairless area of the body. Do not shave an area of application; doing so could abrade the skin and lead to increased absorption. Hair may be clipped if necessary. Peel off the backing without touching the adhesive side of the patch (Fig. 33.2). Place the patch at a new site each time to avoid skin irritation or degradation. Be sure to remove the old patch and clean the area when putting on a new transdermal patch. It is important to remember that many transdermal systems contain an aluminized barrier that could cause an electrical charge with arcing, smoke, and severe transdermal burns if a defibrillator is discharged over it or if the patient has magnetic resonance imaging (MRI). Remove any transdermal patches in the area if a defibrillator is to be used or before the patient has an MRI.

Contraindications and Cautions

Anticholinergics are contraindicated in the presence of known allergy to any of these drugs to avoid hypersensitivity reactions. They are also contraindicated with any condition that could be exacerbated by blockade of the parasympathetic nervous system. These conditions include glaucoma because of the possibility of increased intraocular pressure with pupil dilation; stenosing peptic ulcer, intestinal atony, paralytic ileus, GI obstruction, severe ulcerative colitis, and toxic megacolon, all of which could be exacerbated with a further slowing of GI activity; prostatic hypertrophy and bladder obstruction, which could be further compounded by a blocking of bladder muscle activity and a blocking of sphincter relaxation in the bladder; and myasthenia gravis, which could worsen with further blocking of the cholinergic receptors. (Low doses of atropine are sometimes used in myasthenia gravis to block unwanted GI and cardiovascular effects of the cholinergic drugs used to treat that condition.)

Caution should be used in patients with cardiac arrhythmias, tachycardia, and myocardial ischemia, which could be exacerbated by the increased sympathetic influence, including tachycardia and increased contractility that occurs when the parasympathetic nervous system is blocked; with impaired liver or kidney function, which could alter the metabolism and excretion of the drug; in patients who are breast or chestfeeding because of possible suppression of lactation; in patients who are pregnant because of the potential for adverse effects to the fetus; in patients with hypertension because of the possibility of additive hypertensive effects from the sympathetic system's dominance with parasympathetic nervous system blocking; and with spasticity or brain damage, which could be exacerbated by cholinergic blockade within the CNS.

Adverse Effects

The adverse effects associated with the use of anticholinergic drugs are caused by the systemic blockade of cholinergic receptors. What are adverse effects in some cases may be the desired therapeutic effects in others (Table 33.2). The intensity of adverse effects is related to drug dose; the more of the drug in the system, the greater the systemic effects. These adverse effects could include ocular effects such as blurred vision, pupil dilation, and resultant photophobia; cycloplegia; and increased intraocular pressure, all of which are related to the blocking of the parasympathetic effects in the eye.

Weakness, dizziness, insomnia, mental confusion, and psychosis are effects related to cholinergic receptor blockade within the CNS (Fig. 33.3). Dry mouth results from the blocking of GI secretions. Altered taste perception, nausea, heartburn, constipation, bloated feelings, and paralytic ileus are related to a slowing of GI activity. Tachycardia and palpitations are possible effects related to blocking of the parasympathetic effects on the heart. Urinary hesitancy and retention are related to the blocking of bladder muscle activity and sphincter relaxation. Decreased sweating and an increased predisposition to heat prostration are related to the inability to cool the body by sweating, a result of blocking of the sympathetic cholinergic receptors responsible for sweating. Suppression of

Table 33.2 Effects of Parasympathetic Blockade and Associated Therapeutic Uses

Physiological Effect	Therapeutic Uses
Gastrointestinal	
Smooth muscle: Blocks spasm, blocks peristalsis *Secretory glands*: Decreases acid and digestive enzyme production	Decreases motility and secretory activity in peptic ulcer, gastritis, cardiospasm, pylorospasm, enteritis, diarrhea, hypertonic constipation
Urinary Tract	
Decreases tone and motility in the ureters and fundus of the bladder; increases tone in the bladder sphincter	Increases bladder capacity in children with enuresis and in people with spastic paraplegia; decreases urinary urgency and frequency in cystitis; antispasmodic in renal colic and to counteract bladder spasm caused by morphine
Biliary Tract	
Relaxes smooth muscle, antispasmodic	Relief of biliary colic; counteracts spasms caused by narcotics
Bronchial Muscle	
Weakly relaxes smooth muscle	Aerosol form may be used in asthma; may counteract bronchoconstriction caused by drugs
Cardiovascular System	
Increases heart rate (may decrease heart rate at very low doses); causes local vasodilation and flushing	Counteracts bradycardia caused by vagal stimulation, carotid sinus syndrome, surgical procedures; used to overcome heart blocks following MI; used to counteract hypotension caused by cholinergic drugs
Ocular Effects	
Pupil dilation, cycloplegia	Allows ophthalmological examination of the retina, optic disk; relaxes ocular muscles and decreases irritation in iridocyclitis, choroiditis
Secretions	
Reduces sweating, salivation, respiratory tract secretions	Preoperatively before inhalation of anesthesia; reduces nasal secretions in rhinitis, hay fever; may be used to reduce excessive sweating in hyperhidrosis
Central Nervous System	
Decreases extrapyramidal motor activity; atropine may cause excessive stimulation, psychosis, delirium, disorientation; scopolamine causes depression, drowsiness	Decreases tremor in parkinsonism; helps prevent motion sickness; scopolamine may be in OTC sleep aids

MI, myocardial infarction; OTC, over the counter.

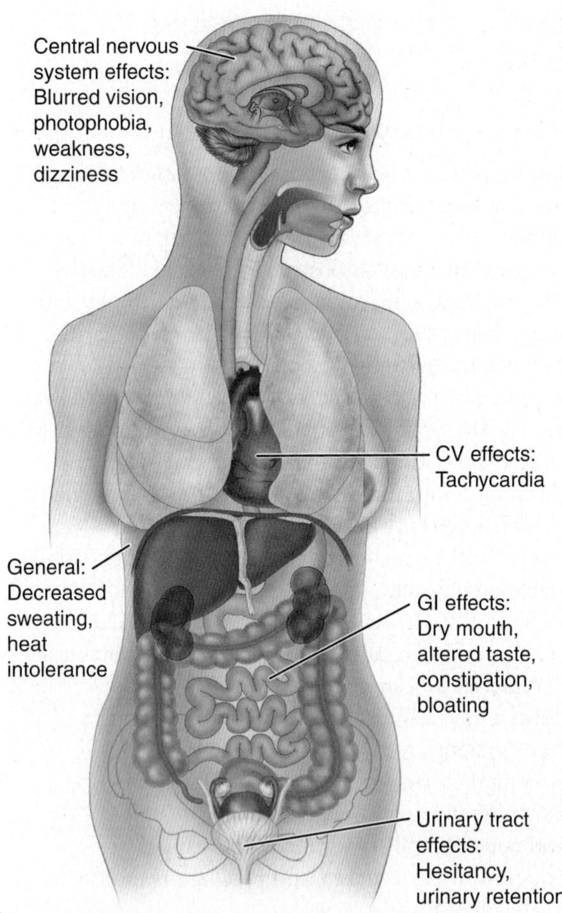

FIGURE 33.3 Variety of adverse effects and toxicities associated with anticholinergic agents.

lactation is related to anticholinergic effects in the breasts and in the CNS. The severity of the adverse effects is related to the dose of the drug, and additive effects can occur if more than one anticholinergic substance is administered (Box 33.4).

Box 33.4 Focus on Safe Medication Administration

ANTICHOLINERGIC TOXICITY

Anticholinergic medications are used in a large variety of clinical settings (see Table 33.1 for usual indications). These drugs can cause severe toxicity. Because many compounds including plants, over-the-counter medications, and prescription medications have anticholinergic properties, toxicity can occur inadvertently. Anticholinergic toxicity should be considered whenever a patient receiving an anticholinergic drug presents with a sudden onset of atypical mental and neurological symptoms. There are additive effects from simultaneous use of more than one anticholinergic medication.

Toxicity due to anticholinergic medication is usually a clinical diagnosis. Serum medication levels are often not helpful or available in the clinical setting. Tachycardia is the first and most reliable symptom. Decreased or absent bowel sounds are often common. The other classic clinical signs are as follows:

"Red as a beet"—The skin flushes due to vasodilation of the capillaries near the skin that assist with dissipating heat by shunting blood to the skin. This is to compensate for the loss of sweat production.

"Dry as a bone" (anhidrosis)—Sweat glands are innervated by muscarinic receptors. Since anticholinergic medications will decrease their effect, the person often will have dry skin.

"Hot as a hare" (anhidrotic hyperthermia)—Interference with normal heat dissipation mechanisms (e.g., sweating) frequently leads to hyperthermia.

"Blind as a bat" (nonreactive mydriasis)—Muscarinic input contributes to both pupillary constriction and effective accommodation. Anticholinergic medications generally produce pupillary dilation and ineffective accommodation; this frequently manifests as blurry vision.

"Mad as a hatter" (delirium; hallucinations)—Blockade of muscarinic receptors in the CNS accounts for these findings. Manifestations may include anxiety, agitation, dysarthria, confusion, disorientation, visual hallucinations, bizarre behavior, delirium, psychosis (usually paranoia), coma, and seizures.

"Full as a flask"—The detrusor muscle of the bladder and the urethral sphincter are both under muscarinic control. Anticholinergic substances reduce detrusor contraction (thereby reducing or eliminating the desire to urinate) and prevent normal opening of the urethral sphincter (contributing to urinary retention).

Treatment may vary based on the severity of symptoms and timing of the administration of the medication. As with any acute situation, the priority is to first stabilize the patient's airway, breathing, and circulation. Cooling may be needed if the patient is hyperthermic. Administration of sodium bicarbonate can be beneficial for treating anticholinergic poisoning in the presence of prolonged QRS intervals or arrhythmias, so an EKG is helpful with guiding management. Benzodiazepines may be administered to treat severe agitation and/or seizure activity. Many patients will recover from anticholinergic toxicity with supportive care. However, there are instances when physostigmine can be administered to act as an acetylcholinesterase inhibitor that can decrease the anticholinergic blockade. The use of physostigmine is controversial due to lack of randomized control trials. It is not used frequently; therefore, it is recommended that clinicians consult with a medical toxicologist and/or pharmacist when considering it as treatment for anticholinergic toxicity.

Clinically Important Drug–Drug Interactions

The incidence of anticholinergic effects increases if these drugs are combined with any other drugs with anticholinergic activity, including antihistamines, antiparkinsonism drugs, monoamine oxidase inhibitors, and tricyclic antidepressants. If such combinations must be used, the patient should be monitored closely and dose adjustments made. Patients should be advised to avoid over-the-counter products that contain these drugs. The effectiveness of phenothiazines decreases if they are combined with anticholinergic drugs, and the risk of paralytic ileus increases. This combination should be avoided. Anticholinergics may also interact with certain herbal therapies (Box 33.5).

Box 33.5 **Focus on Herbal and Alternative Therapies**

The risk of anticholinergic effects can be exacerbated if anticholinergic medications are combined with plants or herbs that also have anticholinergic properties. Some examples of plants that can increase anticholinergic effects are belladonna, mandrake, moonflower, and several types of muscarinic mushroom species. Advise patients who are taking anticholinergic medications to ask about interactions before starting any new herbal therapy.

Key Points

- At cholinergic receptor sites, anticholinergic drugs block the effects of acetylcholine. Because they block the effects of the parasympathetic nervous system, they are also known as parasympatholytic drugs.
- When the parasympathetic system is blocked, the pupils dilate, the heart rate rises, and GI activity and urinary bladder tone and function decrease.

Prototype Summary: Atropine

Indications: To decrease secretions before surgery; treatment of parkinsonism; restoration of cardiac rate and arterial pressure following vagal stimulation; relief of bradycardia and syncope due to hyperactive carotid sinus reflex; relief of pylorospasm; relaxation of the spasm of biliary and ureteral colic and bronchospasm; control of crying and laughing episodes associated with brain lesions; relaxation of uterine hypertonicity; management of peptic ulcer; control of rhinorrhea associated with hay fever; antidote for cholinergic overdose; and poisoning from various mushrooms.

Actions: Competitively blocks acetylcholine muscarinic receptor sites, blocking the effects of the parasympathetic nervous system.

Pharmacokinetics:

Route	Onset	Peak	Duration
IM	10–15 min	30 min	4 h
IV	Immediate	2–4 min	4 h
Subcutaneous	Varies	1–2 h	4 h
Ophthalmic	Unknown	30–40 min	7–14 d

$T_{1/2}$: 2.5 hours; metabolized in the liver; excreted in the urine.

Adverse Effects: Blurred vision, mydriasis, cycloplegia, photophobia, palpitations, tachycardia, dry mouth, altered taste perception, urinary hesitancy and retention, decreased sweating, and predisposition to heat prostration (see Box 33.4).

Nursing Considerations for Patients Receiving Anticholinergic Agents

Assessment: History and Examination

- Assess for contraindications or cautions: any known allergies to these drugs to avoid hypersensitivity reactions; glaucoma; stenosing peptic ulcer, intestinal atony, paralytic ileus, GI obstruction, severe ulcerative colitis, and toxic megacolon; prostatic hypertrophy and bladder obstruction; cardiac arrhythmias, tachycardia, and myocardial ischemia, all of which could be exacerbated by parasympathetic blockade; impaired liver or kidney function, which could alter the metabolism and excretion of the drug; myasthenia gravis, which could worsen with further blocking of the cholinergic receptors; pregnancy because of the potential for adverse effects on the fetus; lactation because of possible suppression of lactation; hypertension because of the possible additive hypertensive effects; and muscle spasticity and brain damage, which could be exacerbated by cholinergic blockade.
- Perform a physical assessment, including a review of all body systems, to establish baseline status before beginning therapy, determine drug effectiveness, and evaluate for any potential adverse effects.
- Assess neurological status, including level of orientation, affect, reflexes, and papillary response, to evaluate any CNS effects.
- Monitor vital signs and cardiopulmonary status, including pulse, blood pressure, heart rate, and heart sounds; auscultate lung sounds. Obtain an electrocardiogram if ordered to identify changes in heart rate or rhythm.
- Assess abdomen; auscultate bowel sounds; evaluate bowel and bladder patterns; monitor urinary output; palpate bladder for possible distention to evaluate for GI and GU adverse effects.
- Monitor the results of laboratory tests, including renal function studies, to determine need for possible dose adjustment and to identify potential toxicity.

See the "Critical Thinking Scenario" to learn more about nursing care for the patient who has heart disease and is taking anticholinergic drugs.

Nursing Conclusions

Nursing conclusions related to drug therapy might include the following:

- Impaired comfort related to GI, CNS, GU, and cardiovascular effects
- Altered cardiac output related to cardiovascular effects
- Constipation related to GI effects
- Urinary retention related to bladder relaxation effects
- Injury risk related to CNS effects
- Thermal injury risk related to decrease in ability to sweat

- Nonadherence related to adverse drug effects
- Knowledge deficiency regarding drug therapy

Planning

- The patient will receive the best therapeutic effect from the drug therapy.
- The patient will have limited adverse effects from the drug therapy.
- The patient will have an understanding of the drug therapy, adverse effects to anticipate, and measures to relieve discomfort and improve safety.

Intervention With Rationale

- Ensure proper administration of the drug to ensure effective use and decrease the risk of adverse effects.
- Provide comfort measures to help the patient tolerate drug effects; sugarless lozenges to suck and frequent mouth care to alleviate problems associated with dry mouth; lighting control to alleviate photophobia; small and frequent meals to alleviate GI discomfort; a bowel program, including a high-fiber diet, to alleviate constipation; safety precautions, such as side rails if appropriate, assistance with ambulation, and advice to avoid driving or operating hazardous machinery to prevent injury if CNS effects are severe; analgesics to relieve pain if headaches occur; advice to void before taking medication if urinary retention is a problem (commonly occurs with benign prostatic hyperplasia); and encouragement to increase fluid intake and monitor heat exposure because the ability to sweat will be reduced.
- Monitor patient response closely, including blood pressure, electrocardiogram, urine output, and cardiac output, for changes that may indicate a need to adjust dose to ensure benefit with the least amount of toxicity.
- Offer support and encouragement to help the patient manage the drug regimen.
- Provide thorough patient teaching about drug name, dosage, and schedule for administration; proper technique for application, measures to minimize or prevent adverse effects; safety measures such as avoiding driving, operating hazardous machinery, staying hydrated, and monitoring exposure to heat; dietary recommendations if appropriate; avoidance of over-the-counter medications, unless recommended by the provider; warning signs of problems and the need to report these; and importance of follow-up monitoring and evaluation to improve patient knowledge and help increase adherence to the drug regimen.

Evaluation

- Monitor patient response to the drug (improvement in disorder being treated).
- Monitor for adverse effects (cardiovascular changes, GI problems, CNS effects, urinary hesitancy and retention, pupil dilation and photophobia, decrease in sweating, and heat intolerance).
- Evaluate the effectiveness of the teaching plan (patient can name drug, dosage, adverse effects to watch for and specific measures to avoid them, proper administration of drugs).
- Monitor the effectiveness of comfort measures and adherence to the regimen.

CRITICAL THINKING SCENARIO
Anticholinergic Drugs and Heart Disease

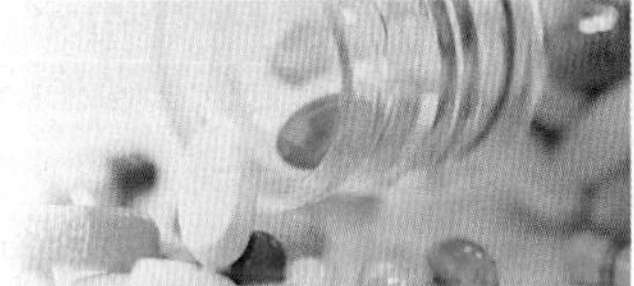

THE SITUATION

E.K., a 74-year-old patient with a long history of coronary artery disease that has been medically managed, presents to the emergency room due to shortness of breath, fatigue, and lightheadedness. E.K. also feels nauseous. E.K. says when they had their heart attacks, they also felt short of breath, so they are concerned they may be having another heart attack. Once E.K. is put on telemetry, bradycardia is noted, and an electrocardiogram demonstrates third-degree heart block with a ventricular rate of 35 beats per minute. The provider orders atropine 1 mg IV and pages the cardiology team to request a temporary pacemaker. E.K.'s heart rate increases to 45 beats per minute, and their blood pressure is measured at 78/40. After 3 minutes, the provider asks the nurse to administer another 1 mg of atropine IV. After this second dose, E.K.'s heart rate increases to greater than 120 beats per minute. E.K. reports they are now experiencing chest pain and palpitations.

CRITICAL THINKING

E.K. presents many nursing care problems. What are the implications of giving an anticholinergic drug to a person with a long history of heart disease?

Could the age of the patient have influenced the effects of the medication?

Given the emergent circumstances of how E.K. presented to the emergency room, were the risks of administering the medication worth the benefits?

What nursing actions can monitor for adverse effects of the medication?

What information is important to communicate to E.K.?

DISCUSSION

It is not known what caused E.K. to go into heart block. In the emergent situation, it is often necessary to administer medications that are designed to stabilize a patient to give time to figure out the cause of the

(continues on page 576)

problem. However, there are times when administering the medication can cause dangerous side effects. The anticholinergic medication that E.K. was administered helped to increase their heart rate. Due to E.K.'s age, they may be eliminating the atropine at a slower rate than expected for a younger patient. The tachycardia that was induced increased the heart muscle's need for oxygen. Due to E.K.'s coronary artery disease, the oxygen need may be greater than what can be provided. This could be causing the new feeling of chest pain.

The cardiology team will not only be able to place a temporary pacemaker, but they also can evaluate potential causes of the heart block. E.K. may need a permanent pacemaker, but they also may need another evaluation to see if their coronary artery disease has become worse.

The nurse can educate E.K. and their family regarding the short-term indication of atropine. Assure E.K. that this medication will not be needed long-term and that they will be closely monitored while it is in their system. An explanation of the side effects of atropine as well as of the management plan may help E.K. and their family understand more of what occurred and have less anxiety.

NURSING CARE GUIDE FOR E.K.: HEART DISEASE

Assessment: History and Examination

Assess for a history of allergy to anticholinergic drugs, COPD, narrow-angle glaucoma, myasthenia gravis, bowel or urinary obstruction, tachycardia, and recent GI or urinary surgery.

Focus the physical examination on the following:

CV: Blood pressure, pulse rate, peripheral perfusion, electrocardiogram (ECG)

CNS: Orientation, affect, reflexes, vision

Skin: Color, lesions, texture, sweating

GU: Urinary output, bladder tone

GI: Abdominal examination

Respiratory: Respiratory rate, adventitious sounds

Nursing Conclusions

Altered cardiac output related to cardiovascular effects

Constipation risk related to GI effects

Impaired urinary elimination related to bladder relaxation effects

Injury risk related to CNS effects

Risk for hyperthermia related to decreased ability to sweat

Knowledge deficit regarding drug therapy

Planning

The patient will receive the best therapeutic effect from the drug therapy.

The patient will have limited adverse effects from the drug therapy.

The patient will have an understanding of the drug therapy, adverse effects to anticipate, and measures to relieve discomfort and improve safety.

Intervention

Ensure safe and appropriate administration of the drug.

Provide comfort and safety measures, including bed rest during the acute situation, temperature control, dark glasses if there is photophobia, artificial saliva if needed for dry mouth, sugarless lozenges, and mouth care; bowel program.

Provide support and reassurance to deal with drug effects, discomfort, and GI effects.

Provide patient teaching regarding drug name, dosage, adverse effects, precautions, and warnings to report.

Monitor blood pressure and pulse rate, and adjust or hold dose as needed.

Evaluation

Evaluate drug effects: pupil dilation, decrease in signs and symptoms being treated.

Monitor for adverse effects: CV effects (tachycardia, heart failure), CNS effects (confusion, dreams), urinary retention, GI effects (constipation), visual blurring, and photophobia.

Monitor for drug–drug interactions as indicated for each drug.

Evaluate effectiveness of the patient teaching program and comfort and safety measures.

PATIENT TEACHING FOR E.K.

- Anticholinergics are drugs that block or decrease the actions of a group of nerves that are part of the parasympathetic nervous system. These drugs may decrease the activity of your GI tract, dilate your pupils, or speed up your heart.
- Some of the following adverse effects may occur:
  - *Dry mouth, difficulty swallowing*: Frequent mouth care will help to remove dried secretions and keep the mouth fresh. Sucking on sugarless candies will help to keep the mouth moist.
  - *Blurred vision, sensitivity to light*: If your vision is blurred, this is only temporary. Dark glasses and/or dimming the lights can help decrease irritation to your eyes while your pupils are dilated.
  - *Retention of urine*: The medication may decrease your ability to void. Because the medication will only be used in this emergent situation, this will not be a long-term problem.
  - *Constipation*: The medication may cause temporary constipation. Once the acute situation is over and you are able to resume normal meals and fluids, the constipation will resolve. Laxatives can be prescribed if needed.
  - *Flushing, intolerance to heat, decreased sweating*: This drug blocks sweating, which is your body's way of cooling off. This places you at increased risk for heat stroke. Your temperature will be monitored and the environment adjusted to avoid this complication.
  - Report any of the following to your health care provider: eye pain, skin rash, fever, rapid heartbeat, chest pain, difficulty breathing, agitation, or mood changes. A dose adjustment may help to alleviate these problems.
- Some medications may interact with this medication and increase risk of severe adverse reactions. Please report all medication (including over-the-counter medications) and any herbal supplements that you normally use.
- Tell any doctor, nurse, or other health care provider involved in your care that you are taking these drugs.

CHECK YOUR UNDERSTANDING

Answers to the questions in this chapter can be found in Answers to Check Your Understanding Questions on thePoint®.

MULTIPLE CHOICE

Select the best answer.

1. Anticholinergic drugs are used to
   a. enhance the sympathetic system.
   b. block the sympathetic system.
   c. treat ulcers as the common drug of choice.
   d. stimulate GI activity.

2. Atropine and scopolamine work by blocking
   a. nicotinic receptors only.
   b. muscarinic and nicotinic receptors.
   c. muscarinic receptors only.
   d. adrenergic receptors only.

3. Which of the following suggestions would the nurse make to help a patient who is receiving an anticholinergic agent reduce the risks associated with decreased sweating?
   a. Covering the head and using sunscreen
   b. Ensuring hydration and temperature control
   c. Changing position slowly and protecting from the sun
   d. Monitoring for difficulty swallowing and breathing

4. Which of the following would the nurse be least likely to include when developing a teaching plan for a patient who is receiving an anticholinergic agent?
   a. Encouraging the patient to void before dosing
   b. Setting up a bowel program to deal with constipation
   c. Encouraging the patient to use sugarless lozenges to combat dry mouth
   d. Performing exercises to increase the heart rate

MULTIPLE RESPONSES

Select all that apply.

1. A nurse would expect atropine to be used to do which of the following?
   a. Depress salivation.
   b. Dry up bronchial secretions.
   c. Increase the heart rate.
   d. Promote uterine contractions.
   e. Treat myasthenia gravis.
   f. Treat Alzheimer's disease.

2. Remembering that anticholinergics block the effects of the parasympathetic nervous system, the nurse would question an order for an anticholinergic drug for patients with which conditions?
   a. Ulcerative colitis
   b. Asthma
   c. Bradycardia
   d. Inner ear imbalance
   e. Glaucoma
   f. Prostatic hyperplasia

Key Points

- Atropine is a commonly used anticholinergic drug. It is indicated for a wide variety of conditions and is available in oral, parenteral, and topical forms.
- Patients receiving anticholinergic drugs must be monitored for dry mouth, difficulty swallowing, constipation, urinary retention, tachycardia, pupil dilation and photophobia, cycloplegia and blurring of vision, and heat intolerance caused by a decrease in sweating.

SUMMARY

- Anticholinergic drugs, also called parasympatholytic drugs, block the effects of acetylcholine at cholinergic receptor sites, thus blocking the effects of the parasympathetic nervous system.
- Parasympathetic nervous system blockade causes an increase in heart rate, decrease in GI activity, decrease in urinary bladder tone and function, and pupil dilation and cycloplegia.
- These drugs also block cholinergic receptors in the CNS and sympathetic postganglionic cholinergic receptors, including those that cause sweating.
- Many systemic adverse effects associated with the use of anticholinergic drugs are due to the systemic cholinergic blocking effects that also produce the desired therapeutic effect.
- Atropine is a commonly used anticholinergic drug. It is indicated for a wide variety of conditions and is available in oral, parenteral, and topical forms.
- Patients receiving anticholinergic drugs must be monitored for dry mouth, difficulty swallowing, constipation, urinary retention, tachycardia, pupil dilation and photophobia, cycloplegia and blurring of vision, and heat intolerance caused by a decrease in sweating.

REFERENCES

Anderson, H. A., Bertrand, K. C., Manny, R. E., Hu, Y., & Fern, K. D. (2010). A comparison of two drug combinations for dilating dark irides. *Otometry and Vision Science, 87*(2), 120–124. 10.1097/OPX.0b013e318cc8da3

Andrews, M., & Boyle, J. (2011). *Transcultural concepts in nursing care* (6th ed.). Lippincott Williams & Wilkins.

Brunton, L., Hilal-Dandan, R., & Knollman, B. (2018). *Goodman and Gilman's the pharmacological basis of therapeutics* (13th ed.). McGraw-Hill.

Norris, T. L. (2019). *Porth's pathophysiology concepts of altered health states* (10th ed.). Wolters Kluwer.

Su, M., & Goldman, M. (2020). Anticholinergic poisoning. *UpToDate*. https://www.uptodate.com/contents/anticholinergic-poisoning?search=atropine%20toxicity&source=search_result&selectedTitle=2~145&usage_type=default&display_rank=1

PART 6

Drugs Acting on the Endocrine System

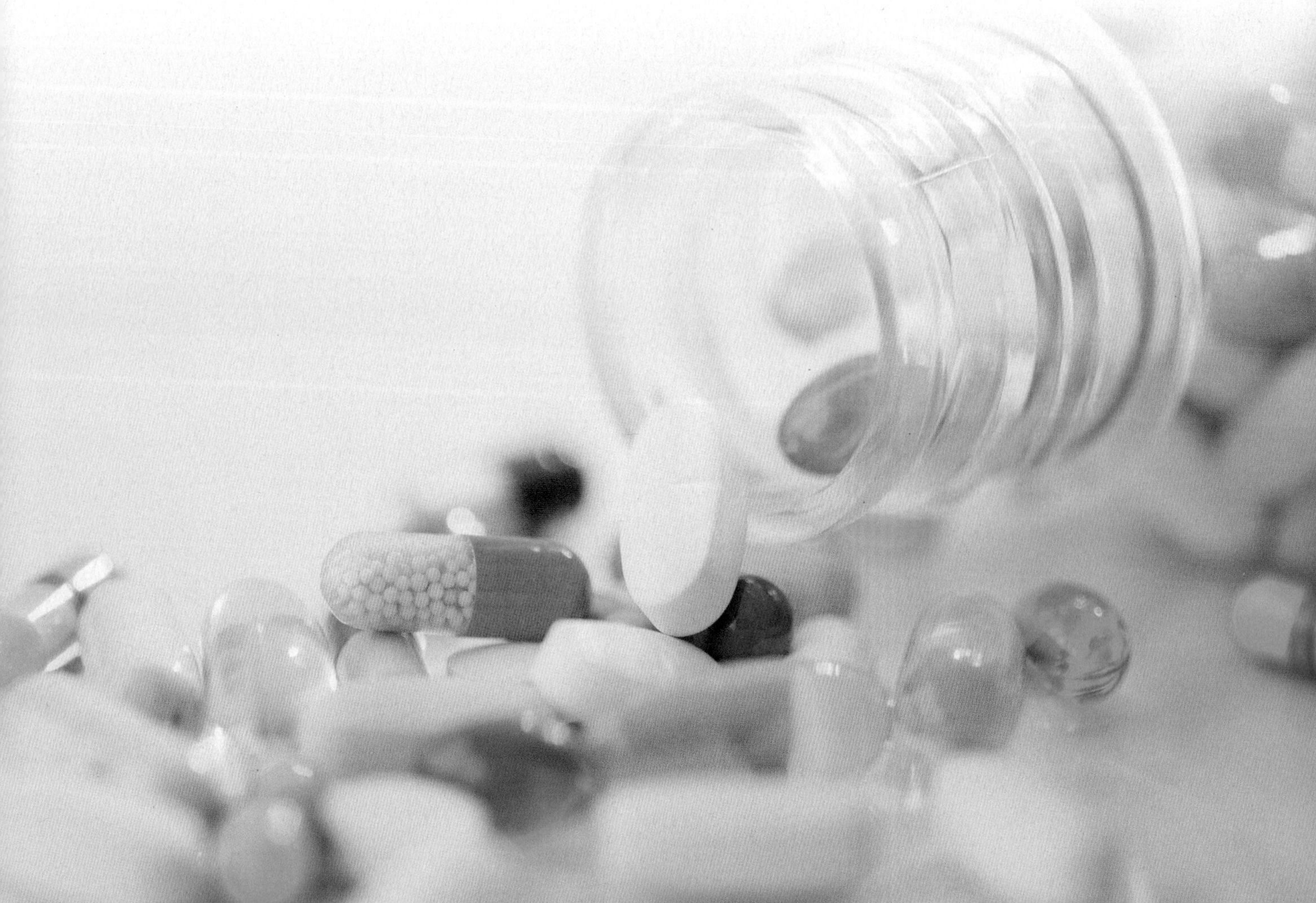

CHAPTER 34

Introduction to the Endocrine System

Learning Objectives

Upon completion of this chapter, you will be able to:

1. List the glands of the traditional endocrine system and the hormones produced by each.
2. Describe two theories of hormone action.
3. Discuss the role of the hypothalamus as the master gland of the endocrine system, including influences on the actions of the hypothalamus.
4. Outline a negative feedback system within the endocrine system and explain the ways that this system controls hormone levels in the body.
5. Describe the hypothalamic–pituitary axis (HPA) and what would happen if a hormone level was altered within the HPA.

Key Terms

anterior pituitary: lobe of the pituitary gland that produces stimulating hormones as well as growth hormone, prolactin, and melanocyte-stimulating hormone

diurnal rhythm: response of the hypothalamus and then the pituitary and adrenals to wakefulness, sleeping, and light exposure

glands: organized groups of specialized cells that secrete hormones directly into the bloodstream to communicate within the body

hormones: chemical messengers working within the endocrine system to communicate within the body

hypothalamic–pituitary axis: interconnection of the hypothalamus and pituitary gland to regulate levels of certain endocrine hormones through a complex series of negative feedback systems

hypothalamus: "master gland" of the neuroendocrine system; regulates both nervous and endocrine responses to internal and external stimuli

negative feedback system: control system in which increasing levels of a hormone lead to decreased levels of releasing and stimulating hormones, leading to decreased hormone levels, which stimulates the release of releasing and stimulating hormones; allows tight control of the endocrine system

neuroendocrine system: the combination of the nervous and endocrine systems, which work closely together to maintain regulatory control and homeostasis in the body

pituitary gland: gland found in the sella turcica of the brain; produces hormones, endorphins, and enkephalins and stores two hypothalamic hormones

posterior pituitary: lobe of the pituitary that receives antidiuretic hormone and oxytocin via nerve axons from the hypothalamus and stores them to be released when stimulated by the hypothalamus

releasing hormones or factors: chemicals released by the hypothalamus into the anterior pituitary to stimulate the release of anterior pituitary hormones

The endocrine system, in conjunction with the nervous system, works to maintain internal homeostasis and to integrate the body's response to the external environment. The activities and functions of the endocrine and nervous systems are so closely related that it is probably more correct to refer to them as the **neuroendocrine system**. However, this section deals with drugs affecting the "traditional" endocrine system, which includes **glands**—organized groups of specialized cells that produce and secrete **hormones**, or chemical messengers, directly into the bloodstream to communicate within the body.

Some organs function like endocrine glands, but they are not considered part of the traditional endocrine system. In addition, certain hormones that influence body functioning are not secreted by endocrine glands. For example, prostaglandins are tissue hormones produced in various tissues; they do not enter the bloodstream but exert their effects right in the area where they are released. Moreover, neurotransmitters, such as norepinephrine and dopamine, can be classified as hormones because they are secreted directly into the bloodstream for dispersion throughout the body. There are also many gastrointestinal (GI) hormones that are

Table 34.1 Endocrine Glands With Associated Hormones and Clinical Effects

Gland	Hormones Produced	Principal Effects
Adrenal cortex	Cortisol Aldosterone	Metabolism of nutrients, assists regulation of blood glucose levels, anti-inflammatory Sodium retention, potassium and hydrogen ion excretion
Intestine	Secretin Cholecystokinin	Stimulates pancreas to release bicarbonate and water Stimulates bile release from gallbladder and pancreatic enzyme secretion
Kidney	Erythropoietin Renin 1,25-Dihydroxycholecalciferol	Increases red blood cell production Stimulates increase in blood pressure and vascular volume via converting angiotensinogen to angiotensin I Increase calcium absorption and bone mineralization
Ovaries	Estrogen Progesterone	Promotes growth and development of female reproductive system; female secondary sex characteristics Stimulates growth of uterine wall; promotes secretory apparatus of breast tissue
Pancreas	Insulin, glucagon, somatostatin	Regulation of glucose, fat metabolism (islets of Langerhans)
Parathyroid glands	Parathyroid hormone	Increases serum calcium levels
Pineal gland	Melatonin	Affects secretion of hypothalamic hormones, particularly gonadotropin-releasing hormone
Placenta	Human chorionic gonadotropin Estrogen and progesterone	Promotes growth of corpus luteum and enhances secretion of estrogen and progesterone Same actions as when secreted from ovaries
Stomach	Gastrin	Stimulates stomach acid production
Testes	Testosterone	Development of male reproductive system and stimulates secondary male sex characteristics
Thyroid	Thyroid hormones (T_3 and T_4) Calcitonin	Stimulates basal metabolic rate (how the body uses energy) by increase rate of reactions in most cell Decreases serum calcium levels

produced in GI cells and act locally. All of these hormones are addressed in the chapters most related to their effects.[1]

Structure and Function of the Endocrine System

The endocrine system provides communication within the body and helps regulate growth and development, reproduction, energy use, and electrolyte balance. The endocrine system is closely interconnected with the nervous system, and the two systems work to maintain homeostasis within the body to ensure maximum function and adequate response to various internal and external stressors.

[1]GI hormones are discussed in Part 11: Drugs Acting on the Gastrointestinal System. Neurotransmitters acting like hormones are discussed in Chapter 29: Introduction to the Autonomic Nervous System. The reproductive hormones are discussed in Chapter 39: Introduction to the Reproductive System. Hormones active in the inflammatory and immune response are discussed in Part 3: Drugs Acting on the Immune System. Specific traditional endocrine glands and hormones are discussed in Chapter 35: Hypothalamic and Pituitary Hormones, Chapter 36: Adrenocortical Hormones, Chapter 37: Thyroid and Parathyroid Hormones, and Chapter 38: Agents to Control Blood Glucose Levels.

Glands

The endocrine glands are collections of specialized cells that produce hormones that cause an effect at hormone receptor sites. These glands do not have ducts, so they secrete their hormones directly into the bloodstream. There are many endocrine glands in the body. Table 34.1 lists the endocrine glands, the hormones they produce, and the clinical effects the hormones cause.

Hormones

Hormones are chemicals that are transported in bodily fluids and act on specific target cells. Most hormones

- Are produced in small amounts
- Are secreted directly into the bloodstream
- Travel through the blood to specific receptor sites throughout the body
- Act to increase or decrease the normal metabolic cellular processes when they react with their specific receptor sites
- Are present in the body at all times, but their amount may fluctuate

Hormones may be classified by their chemical structure. The protein and polypeptide hormones, which are made of groups of amino acids, are the most prominent type of hormones. Hormones secreted by the anterior pituitary, posterior pituitary, pancreas, and parathyroid are in this category. Another class of hormones is the steroid hormones secreted by the adrenal cortex, ovaries, testes, and placenta. They are usually made from cholesterol and are lipid soluble. A third type of hormones is the amine hormones that are derived from tyrosine. The thyroid hormones and secretions from the adrenal medulla (epinephrine and norepinephrine) are examples of this type.

Hormones may link to receptors on the cell surface or inside of the cell. The peptide, protein, and catecholamine hormones primarily attach to receptors on the cell membrane. They tend to be both water soluble and polarized (electrically charged), so they do not easily cross the cell membrane. Hormones attached to cell membrane receptors may cause intracellular actions via activation of specialized guanosine triphosphate (GTP)-binding proteins or G proteins. These proteins may be activated to change the cell membrane or even stimulate a second messenger system within the cytoplasm of the cell. For example, thyroid-stimulating hormone will attach to a receptor on a thyroid cell and trigger the adenylyl cyclase–cyclic adenosine monophosphate (cAMP) second messenger system to facilitate formation of the thyroid hormones. Other hormones that attach to cell membrane receptors may cause changes in the cell via an enzyme second messenger system.

Other hormones that are lipid soluble and nonpolar actually enter the cell and react with a receptor site inside the cytoplasm or cell nucleus. When the appropriate gene regulatory proteins are present, the hormone-receptor complex can bind to a regulatory sequence of DNA. This will either activate or repress transcription of genes to form messenger RNA. This messenger RNA can enter the cell nucleus to affect cellular DNA and thereby alter the cell's function and the proteins the cell is able to make. These intracellular hormones may take hours, months, or years to produce an effect. For example, the full effects of estrogen may not be seen for months to years, as evidenced by the changes that occur at puberty. Because the neuroendocrine system tightly regulates the body's processes within a narrow range of normal limits, overproduction or underproduction of any hormone can affect the body's activities and other hormones within the system.

Key Points

- The endocrine system and the nervous system regulate body functions and maintain homeostasis largely with the help of hormones, which are chemicals produced within the body. Hormones increase or decrease cellular activity.
- The endocrine system regulates growth and development, reproduction, energy use in the body, and electrolyte balance.
- Some hormones can react with cell surface receptors to cause effect via G-proteins or enzyme systems. Other hormones are able to bind to receptors in the cytoplasm or cell nucleus.

The Hypothalamus

The **hypothalamus** is the coordinating center for the nervous and endocrine responses to internal and external stimuli. The hypothalamus constantly monitors the body's homeostasis by analyzing input from the periphery and the central nervous system (CNS) and coordinating responses through the autonomic, endocrine, and nervous systems. In effect, it is the "master gland" of the neuroendocrine system. This title was once given to the pituitary gland because of its many functions and well-protected location.

The hypothalamus has various regions or clusters of neurons that are sensitive to certain stimuli. It is responsible for regulating a number of body functions, including body temperature, thirst, hunger, water retention, blood pressure, respiration, reproduction, and emotional reactions. Situated at the base of the forebrain, the hypothalamus receives input from virtually all other areas of the brain, including the limbic system, cerebral cortex, and the special senses that are controlled by the cranial nerves—smell, sight, touch, taste, and hearing. Because of its positioning, the hypothalamus is able to influence and be influenced by emotions and thoughts. The hypothalamus is also located in an area of the brain that is poorly protected by the blood–brain barrier, so it is able to act as a sensor to various electrolytes, chemicals, and hormones that are in circulation and do not affect other areas of the brain.

The hypothalamus maintains internal homeostasis by sensing blood chemistries and by stimulating or suppressing endocrine, autonomic, and CNS activity. In essence, it can modulate the autonomic nervous system (ANS). The hypothalamus also produces and secretes a number of **releasing hormones or factors**, chemicals that stimulate the anterior pituitary, which in turn stimulates or inhibits various endocrine glands throughout the body (Fig. 34.1). These releasing hormones include growth hormone (GH)-releasing hormone, thyrotropin-releasing hormone (TRH), gonadotropin-releasing hormone (GnRH), corticotropin-releasing hormone (CRH), and prolactin (PRL)-releasing hormone. The hypothalamus also produces two inhibiting factors that act as regulators to shut off the production of hormones when levels become too high: GH release–inhibiting factor (somatostatin) and prolactin-inhibiting factor (PIF), which is the same chemical structure as the catecholamine dopamine. Patients who are taking dopamine-blocking drugs often develop galactorrhea (milky discharge from nipple/s unrelated to breast or chestfeeding) and breast enlargement, theoretically because PIF is also blocked and PRL levels continue to rise, stimulating breast tissue and milk production. Research is ongoing about the chemical structure of several of the releasing factors.

The hypothalamus is connected to the pituitary gland by two networks: a vascular capillary network carries the hypothalamic-releasing factors directly into the anterior pituitary, and a neurological network delivers two other hypothalamic hormones—antidiuretic hormone (ADH) and oxytocin—to the posterior pituitary to be stored. These hormones are released as needed by the body when stimulated by the hypothalamus.

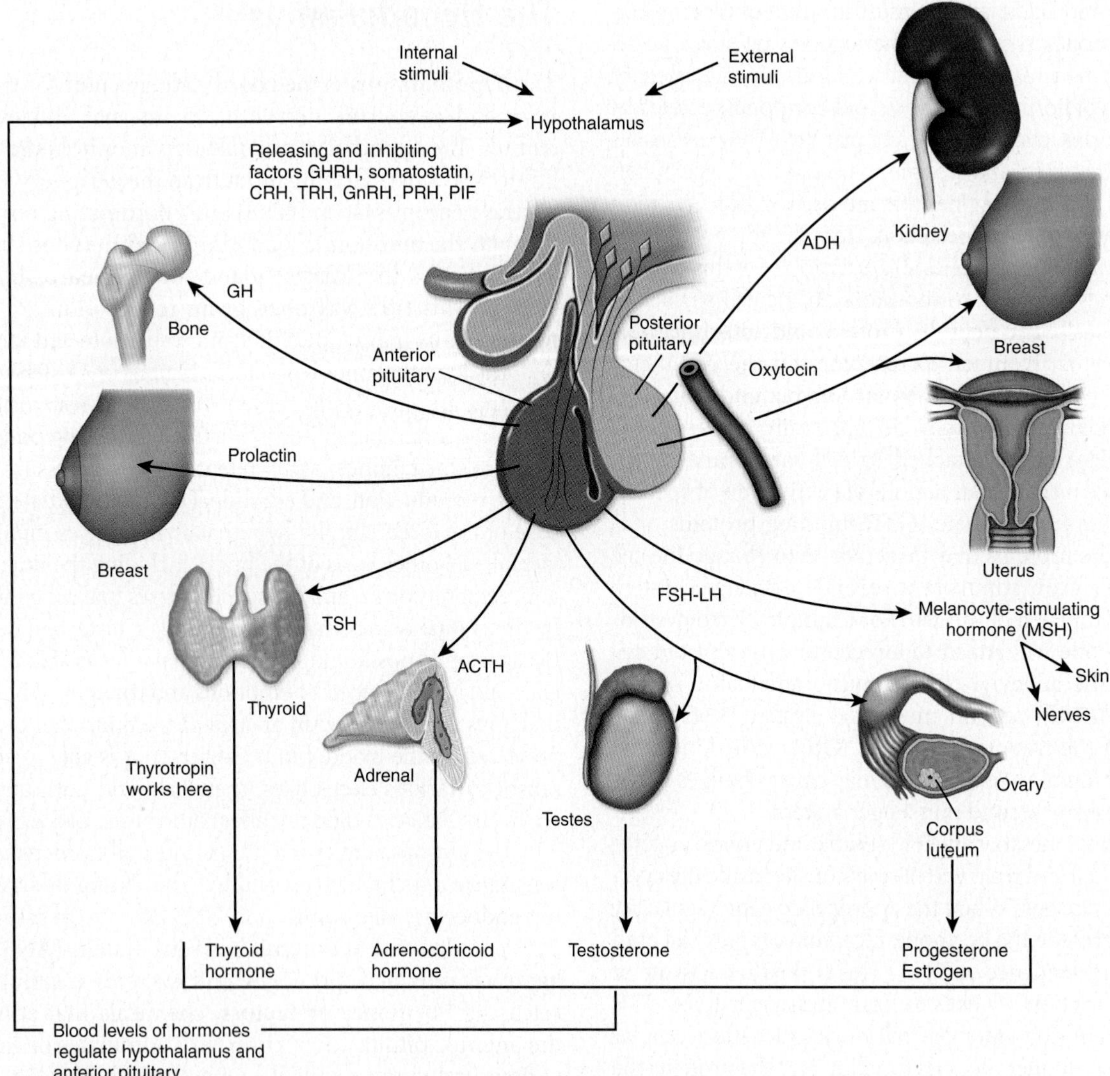

FIGURE 34.1 The traditional endocrine system. The hypothalamus secretes releasing factors to stimulate the pituitary gland to produce stimulating factors that enter the circulation and react with specific target glands, which produce endocrine hormones.

Key Points

- As the "master gland" of the neuroendocrine system, the hypothalamus helps regulate the central and autonomic nervous systems and the endocrine system to maintain homeostasis.
- The hypothalamus produces stimulating and inhibiting factors that travel through a capillary system to the anterior pituitary to stimulate the release of pituitary hormones or block the production of certain pituitary hormones when levels of target hormones get too high.
- The hypothalamus is connected to the posterior pituitary by a nerve network that delivers the hypothalamic hormones ADH and oxytocin to be stored in the posterior pituitary until the hypothalamus stimulates their release.

The Pituitary Gland

The **pituitary gland** is located in the skull in the bony sella turcica under a layer of dura mater. It is divided into three lobes: an anterior lobe, a posterior lobe, and an intermediate lobe. It produces hormones, endorphins, and enkephalins and stores two hypothalamic hormones. Traditionally, the anterior pituitary was known as the body's master gland because it has so many important functions and through feedback mechanisms regulates the function of many other endocrine glands. In addition, its unique and protected position in the brain led early scientists to believe that it must be the chief control gland. However, as knowledge of the endocrine system has grown, scientists now designate the hypothalamus as the master gland because it has even greater direct regulatory effects over the neuroendocrine system, including stimulation of the pituitary gland to produce its hormones.

The Anterior Pituitary

The **anterior pituitary** produces six major hormones: GH, adrenocorticotropic hormone (ACTH), follicle-stimulating hormone (FSH), luteinizing hormone (LH), PRL, and thyroid-stimulating hormone (TSH, also called thyrotropin) (Table 34.2; see also Fig. 34.1). These hormones are essential for the regulation of growth, reproduction, and some metabolic processes. Deficiency or overproduction of these hormones disrupts this regulation.

The anterior pituitary hormones are released in a rhythmic manner into the bloodstream. Their secretion varies with wakefulness, sleeping, and light exposure (often referred to as **diurnal rhythm**) or with physiological conditions such as exercise. Their release is affected by activity in the CNS, by hypothalamic hormones, by hormones of the peripheral endocrine glands, by certain diseases that can alter endocrine functioning, and by a variety of drugs, which can directly or indirectly upset the homeostasis in the body and cause an endocrine response. Normally, diurnal rhythm occurs when the hypothalamus begins secretion of corticotropin-releasing factor (CRF) in the evening, peaking at about midnight; adrenocortical peak response is between 6 and 9 AM; levels fall during the day until evening, when the low level is picked up by the hypothalamus and CRF secretion begins again.

The anterior pituitary also produces melanocyte-stimulating hormone (MSH) and various lipotropins. MSH plays an important role in animals that use skin color changes as an adaptive mechanism. It might also be important for nerve growth and development in humans. Lipotropins stimulate fat mobilization but have not been clearly isolated in humans.

The Posterior Pituitary

The **posterior pituitary** is the lobe of the pituitary gland that stores two hormones, ADH and oxytocin, that are produced by the hypothalamus and deposited in the posterior lobe via the nerve axons where they are produced. These two hormones are ADH, also referred to as vasopressin, and oxytocin. ADH is directly released in response to increased plasma osmolarity or decreased blood volume (which often results in increased osmolarity). The osmoreceptors in the hypothalamus stimulate the release of ADH. ADH acts in the kidneys to increase retention of water in order to decrease the osmolarity of the blood volume. Oxytocin stimulates uterine smooth muscle contraction in late phases of pregnancy and also causes milk release or "let-down" reflex in people who are lactating. Its release is stimulated by various hormones and neurological stimuli associated with labor and with lactation.

Table 34.2 Hypothalamic Hormones, Associated Anterior Pituitary Hormones, and Target Organ Response

Hypothalamus Hormones	Anterior Pituitary Hormones	Target Organ Response
Stimulating Hormones		
CRH	ACTH	Stimulates production of adrenal cortex hormones including glucocorticoids and androgens
TRH	TSH	Stimulates production of thyroid hormones and maintains size of follicular cells
GHRH	GH	Cell growth, secretion of insulinlike growth factor-1, stimulates lipolysis, inhibits actions of insulin on carbohydrate and lipid metabolism
GnRH	LH and FSH	Estrogen and progesterone (females), testosterone (males)
PRH	PRL	Milk production and secretion
	MSH	Melanin stimulation (color change in animals, nerve growth in humans)
Inhibiting Hormones		
Somatostatin (growth hormone–inhibiting factor)		Inhibits release of GH
PIF (prolactin-inhibiting factors)		Inhibits synthesis and release of PRL

CRH, corticotropin-releasing hormone; ACTH, adrenocorticotropic hormone; TRH, thyroid-releasing hormone; TSH, thyroid-stimulating hormone; GHRH, growth hormone–releasing hormone; GH, growth hormone; GnRH, gonadotropin-releasing hormone; LH, luteinizing hormone; FSH, follicle-stimulating hormone; PRH, prolactin-releasing hormone; PRL, prolactin; MSH, melanocyte-stimulating hormone.

The Intermediate Lobe

The intermediate lobe of the pituitary produces endorphins and enkephalins, which are released in response to severe pain or stress and occupy specific endorphin receptor sites in the brainstem to block the perception of pain. These hormones are also produced in peripheral tissues and in other areas of the brain. They are released in response to overactivity of pain nerves, sympathetic stimulation, transcutaneous stimulation, guided imagery, and vigorous exercise. The intermediate lobe secretes MSH, which is also produced in the anterior pituitary.

> **Key Points**
>
> The pituitary gland has three lobes:
>
> - The anterior lobe produces stimulating hormones in response to hypothalamic stimulation.
> - The posterior lobe of the pituitary stores ADH and oxytocin, which are two hormones produced by the hypothalamus.
> - The intermediate lobe of the pituitary produces endorphins and enkephalins to modulate pain perception.

Endocrine Regulation

The production and release of hormones need to be tightly regulated within the body. Hormones are released in small amounts to accomplish what needs to be done to maintain homeostasis within the body. The fine tuning and regulation of hormone release through the hypothalamus are often regulated by a series of negative feedback systems. Other hormones are not controlled in this fashion but respond to other direct stimuli.

Hypothalamic–Pituitary Axis

Because of its position in the brain, the hypothalamus is stimulated by many things, such as light, emotion, cerebral cortex activity, and a variety of chemical and hormonal stimuli. Together, along what is called the **hypothalamic–pituitary axis** (HPA), the hypothalamus and the pituitary function closely using a series of negative feedback systems to maintain endocrine activity and regulate levels of certain endocrine hormones.

A **negative feedback system** works much like the law of supply and demand in business. In business, when there is an adequate supply of a product, production of that product slows down because there is an adequate supply and no current demand for it. When the supply is used up, demand increases, and so production picks up. Production continues until the supply is adequate and demand is reduced. In a negative feedback system, when the hypothalamus senses a need for a particular hormone—for example, thyroid hormone—it secretes the releasing hormone or factor TRH directly into the anterior pituitary. In response to the TRH, the anterior pituitary secretes TSH, which in turn stimulates the thyroid gland to produce thyroid hormone. When the hypothalamus senses the rising levels of thyroid hormone, it stops secreting TRH, resulting in decreased TSH production and subsequently reduced thyroid hormone levels. The hypothalamus, sensing the falling thyroid hormone levels, secretes TRH again. The negative feedback system continues in this fashion, maintaining the levels of thyroid hormone within a relatively narrow range of normal (Fig. 34.2).

It is thought that this feedback system is more complex than once believed. The hypothalamus probably also senses TRH and TSH levels and regulates TRH secretion within a narrow range, even if thyroid hormone is not produced. The anterior pituitary may also be sensitive to TSH levels and thyroid hormone, regulating its own production of TSH. This complex system provides backup controls and regulation if any part of the HPA fails. This system also can create complications, especially when there is a need to override or interact with the total system, as is the case with hormone replacement therapy or the treatment of endocrine disorders. Supplying an exogenous hormone, for example, may increase the hormone levels in the body but then may affect the HPA to stop production of releasing and stimulating hormones, leading to a decrease in the body's normal production of the hormone.

Two of the anterior pituitary hormones (i.e., GH and PRL) do not have a target organ to produce hormones and so cannot be regulated by the same type of feedback mechanism. The hypothalamus in this case responds directly to rising levels of GH and PRL. When levels rise, the hypothalamus directly releases the inhibiting factors somatostatin and PIF to inhibit the pituitary's release of GH and PRL, respectively. The HPA functions through negative feedback loops or the direct use of inhibiting factors to constantly keep these hormones regulated.

Other Forms of Regulation

Hormones other than stimulating hormones also are released in response to stimuli. For example, the pancreas produces and releases insulin, glucagon, and somatostatin from different cells in response to varying blood glucose levels and to stimulatory factors released by the GI tract. The parathyroid glands release parathyroid hormone, or parathormone, in response to local calcium levels. The juxtaglomerular cells in the kidney release erythropoietin and renin in response

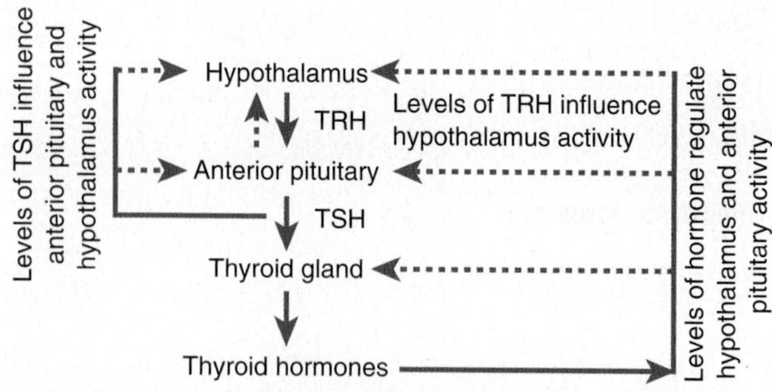

FIGURE 34.2 Negative feedback system. Thyroid hormone levels are regulated by a series of negative feedback systems influencing thyrotropin-releasing hormone (TRH), thyroid-stimulating hormone (TSH), and thyroid hormone levels.

to decreased pressure or decreased oxygenation of the blood flowing into the glomerulus. GI hormones are released in response to local stimuli in areas of the GI tract, such as acid, proteins, or calcium. The thyroid gland produces and secretes another hormone, called calcitonin, in direct response to serum calcium levels. Many different prostaglandins are released throughout the body in response to local stimuli in the tissues that produce them. Activation of the sympathetic nervous system directly causes release of ACTH and the adrenocorticoid hormones to prepare the body for the acute stress response. Aldosterone, an adrenocorticoid hormone, is released in response to ACTH but also is released directly in response to high potassium levels.

As more is learned about the interactions of the nervous and endocrine systems, new ideas are being formed about how the body controls its intricate homeostasis. When administering any drug that affects the endocrine or nervous systems, it is important for the nurse to remember how closely related all of these activities are. Expected or unexpected adverse effects involving areas of the endocrine and nervous systems often occur.

Key Points

- The hypothalamus and pituitary operate by a series of negative feedback mechanisms called the HPA. The hypothalamus secretes releasing factors to cause the anterior pituitary to release stimulating hormones, which act with specific endocrine glands to cause the release of hormones.
- GH and PRL are released by the anterior pituitary and directly influence cell activity. These hormones are regulated by the release of the hypothalamic-inhibiting factors somatostatin and PIF in response to the levels of the pituitary hormones GH and PRL.
- Some hormones are not influenced by the HPA and are released in response to direct local stimulation.

SUMMARY

- The endocrine system is a regulatory system that communicates through the use of hormones.
- Because the endocrine and nervous systems are tightly intertwined in the regulation of body homeostasis, they are often referred to as the neuroendocrine system.
- A hormone is a chemical that is produced within the body, is needed in only small amounts, travels to specific receptor sites to cause an increase or decrease in cellular activity, and is broken down immediately.
- As the "master gland" of the neuroendocrine system, the hypothalamus helps regulate the central and autonomic nervous systems and the endocrine system to maintain homeostasis.
- The pituitary is made up of three lobes: anterior, posterior, and intermediate. The anterior lobe produces stimulating hormones in response to hypothalamic stimulation. The posterior lobe stores two hormones produced by the hypothalamus—ADH and oxytocin. The intermediate lobe produces endorphins and enkephalins to modulate pain perception.
- The hypothalamus and pituitary operate by a series of negative feedback mechanisms called the HPA. The hypothalamus secretes releasing factors to cause the anterior pituitary to release stimulating hormones, which act with specific endocrine glands to cause the release of hormones or, in the case of GH and PRL, to stimulate cells directly. This stimulation shuts down the production of releasing factors, which leads to decreased stimulating factors and subsequently decreased hormone release.
- GH and PRL are released by the anterior pituitary and directly influence cell activity. These hormones are regulated by the release of hypothalamic-inhibiting factors in response to hormone levels or a cellular mediator.
- Some hormones are not influenced by the HPA and are released in response to direct local stimulation.
- When any drug that affects either the endocrine or the nervous system is given, adverse effects may occur throughout both systems because they are closely interrelated.

CHECK YOUR UNDERSTANDING

Answers to the questions in this chapter can be found in Answers to Check Your Understanding Questions on thePoint®.

MULTIPLE CHOICE

Select the best answer.

1. Which of the following best describes aldosterone?
   a. It causes the loss of sodium and water from the renal tubules.
   b. It is under direct hormonal control from the hypothalamus.
   c. It is released into the bloodstream in response to angiotensin I.
   d. It is released into the bloodstream in response to high potassium levels.

2. When explaining the role of ADH to a group of students, which fact would the instructor include?
   a. It is produced by the anterior pituitary.
   b. It causes the retention of water by the kidneys.
   c. It is released by the hypothalamus.
   d. It causes the retention of sodium by the kidneys.
3. The endocrine glands
   a. form part of the communication system of the body.
   b. cannot be stimulated by hormones circulating in the blood.
   c. cannot be viewed as integrating centers of reflex arcs.
   d. are only controlled by the hypothalamus.
4. The hypothalamus maintains internal homeostasis and could be considered the master endocrine gland because
   a. it releases stimulating hormones that cause endocrine glands to produce their hormones.
   b. no hormone-releasing gland responds unless stimulated by the hypothalamus.
   c. it secretes releasing hormones that are an important part of the HPA.
   d. it regulates temperature control and arousal as well as hormone release.
5. The posterior lobe of the pituitary gland
   a. secretes a number of stimulating hormones.
   b. produces endorphins to modulate pain perception.
   c. has no function that has yet been identified.
   d. stores ADH and oxytocin, which are produced in the hypothalamus.
6. After teaching a group of students about the negative feedback system, identification of which of the following as an example would indicate that the students have understood the teaching?
   a. Growth hormone control
   b. Prolactin control
   c. Melanocyte-stimulating hormone control
   d. Thyroid hormone control
7. Internal body homeostasis and communication are regulated by
   a. the cardiovascular and respiratory systems.
   b. the nervous and cardiovascular systems.
   c. the endocrine and nervous systems.
   d. the endocrine and cardiovascular systems.

MULTIPLE RESPONSE

Select all that apply.

1. Hormones exert their influence on human cells by influencing which of the following?
   a. Enzyme-controlled reactions
   b. Messenger RNA
   c. Lysosome activity
   d. Transcription RNA
   e. Cellular DNA
   f. Cyclic AMP activity
2. The specific criteria that define a hormone would include which of the following?
   a. It is produced in small amounts.
   b. It is secreted directly into the bloodstream.
   c. It is slowly metabolized in the liver and lungs.
   d. It reacts with a specific receptor set on a target cell.
   e. A mechanism is always available to immediately destroy it.
   f. It can change a cell's basic function.
3. Some endocrine glands do not respond to the HPA. These glands include the
   a. thyroid gland.
   b. ovaries.
   c. parathyroid glands.
   d. adrenal cortex.
   e. endocrine pancreas.
   f. GI gastrin-secreting cells.

REFERENCES

Brunton, L. L., Hilal-Dandan, R., & Knollmann, B. C. (2018). *Goodman and Gilman's the pharmacological basis of therapeutics* (13th ed.). McGraw-Hill.

Hall, J. E., & Hall, M. E. (2021). *Guyton and Hall textbook of medical physiology* (14th ed.). Elsevier.

Norris, T. L. (2019). *Porth's pathophysiology: Concepts of altered health states* (10th ed.). Wolters Kluwer.

CHAPTER 35

Hypothalamic and Pituitary Agents

Learning Objectives

Upon completion of this chapter, you will be able to:

1. Describe the anatomical and physiological relationship between the hypothalamus and the pituitary gland, and list the hormones produced by each.
2. Discuss the use of hypothalamic and pituitary agents across the lifespan.
3. Describe the therapeutic actions, indications, pharmacokinetics, contraindications, most common adverse reactions, and important drug–drug interactions associated with the hypothalamic and pituitary agents.
4. Compare and contrast the prototype drugs leuprolide, somatropin, bromocriptine mesylate, and desmopressin with other hypothalamic and pituitary agents.
5. Outline the nursing considerations and nursing care, including important teaching points, for patients receiving a hypothalamic or pituitary agent.

Key Terms

acromegaly: excessive GH secretion that occurs after puberty and epiphyseal plate closure, causing thickening of bones and enlargement of tissues

diabetes insipidus: condition resulting from a lack of antidiuretic hormone, which results in the production of copious amounts of glucose-free urine

dwarfism: small stature, resulting from lack of growth hormone in children

gigantism: response to excess levels of growth hormone before the epiphyseal plates fuse; can result in heights of 7 to 8 ft

hypopituitarism: lack of adequate function of the pituitary; reflected in many endocrine disorders

Drug List

DRUGS AFFECTING HYPOTHALAMIC HORMONES

Agonists
goserelin
histrelin
(P) leuprolide
nafarelin
tesamorelin

Antagonists
cetrorelix
degarelix
ganirelix

DRUGS AFFECTING ANTERIOR PITUITARY HORMONES

Growth Hormone Agonists
somapacitan-beco
(P) somatropin

Growth Hormone Antagonists
(P) bromocriptine mesylate
lanreotide
octreotide acetate
pegvisomant

DRUGS AFFECTING OTHER ANTERIOR PITUITARY HORMONES
chorionic gonadotropin
chorionic gonadotropin alpha
cosyntropin
pasireotide
thyrotropin alpha

DRUGS AFFECTING POSTERIOR PITUITARY HORMONES
conivaptan
(P) desmopressin
tolvaptan
vasopressin

The endocrine system's main function is to maintain homeostasis. This is achieved through a complex balance of glandular activities that either stimulate or suppress hormone release. Too much or too little glandular activity disrupts the body's homeostasis, leading to various disorders and interfering with the normal functioning of other endocrine glands. The drugs presented in this chapter are those used to either replace or interact with the hormones or factors produced by the hypothalamus and pituitary. See Figure 35.1 for sites of action of hypothalamic and pituitary agents. Box 35.1 discusses the use of these drugs in various age groups.

Drugs Affecting Hypothalamic Hormones

The hypothalamus uses a number of hormones or factors to either stimulate or inhibit the release of hormones from the anterior pituitary. Factors that stimulate the release of hormones are growth hormone–releasing hormone (GHRH), thyrotropin-releasing hormone (TRH), gonadotropin-releasing hormone (GnRH), corticotropin-releasing hormone (CRH), and prolactin-releasing hormone (PRH). Factors that inhibit the release of hormones are somatostatin (growth hormone–inhibiting factor) and

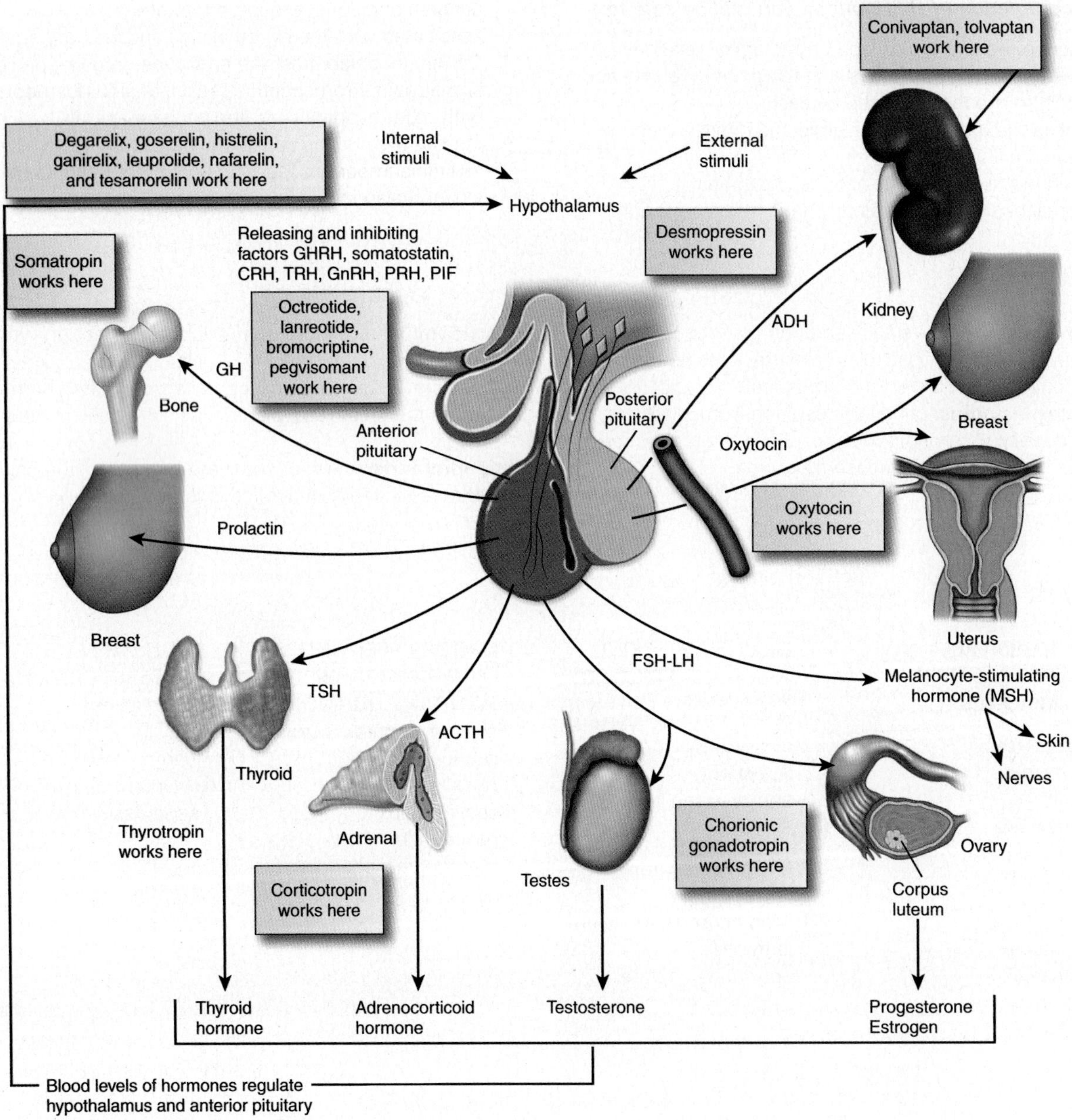

Conivaptan, tolvaptan work here
Degarelix, goserelin, histrelin, ganirelix, leuprolide, nafarelin, and tesamorelin work here
Internal stimuli
External stimuli
Hypothalamus
Desmopressin works here
Somatropin works here
Releasing and inhibiting factors GHRH, somatostatin, CRH, TRH, GnRH, PRH, PIF
Octreotide, lanreotide, bromocriptine, pegvisomant work here
Kidney
ADH
GH
Bone
Posterior pituitary
Anterior pituitary
Oxytocin
Breast
Oxytocin works here
Prolactin
Breast
Uterus
FSH-LH
Melanocyte-stimulating hormone (MSH)
TSH
ACTH
Skin
Nerves
Thyroid
Thyrotropin works here
Adrenal
Chorionic gonadotropin works here
Ovary
Testes
Corticotropin works here
Corpus luteum
Thyroid hormone
Adrenocorticoid hormone
Testosterone
Progesterone Estrogen
Blood levels of hormones regulate hypothalamus and anterior pituitary

CRH, corticotropin-releasing hormone; ACTH, adrenocorticotropic hormone; TRH, thyroid-releasing hormone; TSH, thyroid-stimulating hormone; GHRH, growth hormone-releasing hormone; GH, growth hormone; GnRH, gonadotropin-releasing hormone; FSH, follicle-stimulating hormone; LH, luteinizing hormone; PRH, prolactin-releasing hormone; MSH, melanocyte-stimulating hormone; ADH, antidiuretic hormone.

FIGURE 35.1 Sites of action of hypothalamic/pituitary agents.

Box 35.1 Focus on Drug Therapy Across the Lifespan

HYPOTHALAMIC AND PITUITARY AGENTS

Children

Children who receive any of the hypothalamic or pituitary agents need to be monitored closely for adverse effects associated with changes in overall endocrine function, particularly growth and development and metabolism. Periodic radiograph of the long bones, as well as monitoring of blood sugar levels and electrolytes, should be a standard part of the treatment plan. Children receiving growth hormone (GH) pose many challenges. Before the drug is prescribed, the child must undergo screening procedures and specific testing (including radiographs and blood tests) and must display a willingness to have regular injections. The child taking this drug will need to have pretherapy and periodic tests of thyroid function, blood glucose levels, glucose tolerance tests, and tests for GH antibodies (a risk that increases with the length of therapy). In addition, radiographs of the long bones will need to be taken to monitor for closure of the epiphyses, a sign that the drug must be stopped. Because the child who is taking GH may experience sudden growth, they will need to be monitored for nutritional needs, as well as psychological trauma that may occur with the sudden change in body image. Insulin therapy and replacement thyroid therapy may be needed, depending on the child's response to the drug. Children who are using desmopressin for diabetes insipidus need to have the administration technique monitored and should have an adult responsible for the overall treatment protocol.

Adults

Adults also need frequent monitoring of electrolytes and blood sugar levels when receiving any of these agents. Adults using nasal forms of drugs to control diabetes insipidus should review periodically the proper administration of the drug with the primary care provider; inappropriate administration can lead to complications and lack of therapeutic effect. Adults receiving regular injections of these drugs should learn the proper storage, preparation, and administration of the drug, including rotation of injection sites.

These drugs should not be used during pregnancy or lactation unless the benefit to the patient clearly outweighs any risk to the fetus or neonate, because most have not been adequately studied for this population.

Older Adults

Older adults may be more susceptible to the imbalances associated with alterations in the endocrine system. They should be evaluated periodically during treatment for hydration and nutrition, as well as for electrolyte balance. Proper administration technique should be reviewed, and nasal mucous membranes should be evaluated regularly because older adult patients are more apt to develop dehydrated membranes and possibly ulcerations, leading to improper dosing of drugs delivered nasally. Some of the medications require dosing adjustments with renal or hepatic impairment, and older adults have higher potential for these impairments.

prolactin-inhibiting factor (PIF). Not all of these hormones are available for pharmacological use.

Available hypothalamic-releasing hormones include goserelin (*Zoladex*; synthetic GnRH), histrelin (*Supprelin LA*, *Vantas*), leuprolide (*Eligard Kit*, *Fensolvi Kit*, *Lupron Depot*) and nafarelin (*Synarel*; GnRH agonists that will block gonadotropin secretion with continuous use), and tesamorelin (*Egrifta*; a GRH analogue used to stimulate the release of GH from the pituitary). Available antagonists that block the effects of hypothalamic-releasing hormones include cetrorelix (*Cetrotide*), ganirelix acetate (generic; GnRH antagonists and fertility drugs), and degarelix (*Firmagon*; blocks GnRH and is used as an antineoplastic agent). See Table 35.1 for a complete list of these drugs with their indications and usual dosing.

Therapeutic Actions and Indications

The hypothalamic hormones are found in such minute quantities that the actual chemical structures of all of these hormones have not been clearly identified. Not all of the hypothalamic hormones are used as pharmacological agents. The hypothalamic-releasing hormones described here can be used as antineoplastic agents, treatment for precocious puberty, and fertility medications. It is important to note that several of the agonists will actually inhibit pituitary gonadotropin secretion. For example, goserelin, histrelin, leuprolide, and nafarelin are analogues of GnRH. Following an initial burst of follicle-stimulating hormone (FSH) and/or luteinizing hormone (LH) release, they inhibit pituitary gonadotropin secretion, with a resultant drop in the production of sex hormones. Tesamorelin is used to stimulate GH and its lipolytic effects, helping to decrease the excess abdominal fat in HIV-infected patients with lipodystrophy. Tesamorelin is an analogue of human GH–releasing factor that stimulates the release of GH from the pituitary. Cetrorelix, degarelix, and ganirelix acetate are antagonists of GnRH.

Pharmacokinetics

The pharmacokinetics of the medications will vary based on the formulation of the medication and how each medication is administered. The medications that are designed to be administered as depot injections are absorbed slowly. They tend to have long half-lives of days to weeks. Cetrorelix and ganirelix are administered subcutaneously, are indicated as fertility medications, and have shorter absorption times and half-lives. Nafarelin is administered via a nasal spray, and it has fast absorption and a shorter half-life.

Table 35.1 *Drugs in Focus:* Drugs Affecting Hypothalamic Hormones

Drug Name	Dosage/Route	Usual Indications
Agonists		
goserelin (*Zoladex*)	3.6 mg subcutaneous implant every 28 d or 6 mo for management of endometriosis	Used as an antineoplastic agent for treatment of specific hormone-stimulated prostate or breast cancers; management of endometriosis
histrelin (*Supprelin LA, Vantas*)	One implant (50 mg) implanted subcutaneously every 12 mo	Palliative treatment of advanced prostate cancer; treatment of children with central precocious puberty
leuprolide (*Lupron*)	*Prostate cancer*: 1 mg/d subcutaneously or various depot preparations *Endometriosis*: 3.75 mg IM once a month *Precocious puberty*: 45 mg subcutaneously every 6 mo or various depot preparations	Used as antineoplastic agent for treatment of specific cancers; treatment of endometriosis and precocious puberty that results from hypothalamic activity
nafarelin (*Synarel*)	400 mcg/d divided as one spray in left nostril a.m. or p.m.; one spray in right nostril a.m. or p.m. *Precocious puberty*: 1,600–1,800 mcg/d intranasally	Treatment of endometriosis and precocious puberty
tesamorelin (*Egrifta*)	2 mg subcutaneously once a day	Reduction of excessive abdominal fat in patients with HIV with lipodystrophy
Antagonists		
cetrorelix (*Cetrotide*)	3 mg subcutaneously during early follicular phase or 0.25 mg subcutaneously on day 5 or 6 and then every day until HCG is administered	Inhibition of premature LH surges in patients undergoing controlled ovarian stimulation
degarelix (*Firmagon*)	Initially 240 mg by subcutaneous injection of two 120-mg injections at separate sites; maintenance 80 mg subcutaneously every 28 d	Treatment of advanced prostate cancer
ganirelix acetate (generic)	250 mcg subcutaneously initiated on day 2 or 3 of the menstrual cycle and continued daily until day of human chorionic gonadotropin (hCG) administration	Inhibition of premature luteinizing hormone surge in patients undergoing controlled ovarian hyperstimulation

Metabolism has not been studied for all of these medications. Some are known to be broken down into peptides and others are found to be unchanged when excreted. Most hypothalamic hormones are excreted in urine, but some are partially excreted in feces. Because they are hormones or similar to hormones, they cross the placenta and cross into human milk.

Contraindications and Cautions

These drugs are contraindicated with known hypersensitivity to any component of the drug because of the risk of hypersensitivity reactions, and during pregnancy and lactation, because of the potential adverse effects to the fetus or baby. Caution should be used with patients at risk for cardiovascular disorders, due to cases of myocardial infarction in males taking GnRH analogs, and with rhinitis or sneezing immediately after administration when using nafarelin, which could alter the absorption of the nasal spray.

Adverse Effects

Adverse effects associated with these drugs are related to the stimulation or blocking of regular hormone control. The GnRH agonists lead to initial increased release of sex hormones, but then with continuous use lead to a decrease in the sex hormones. The GnRH antagonist will also decrease testosterone levels. Common side effects are hot flashes, decreased libido, erectile dysfunction, changes in menstrual flow, fluid and electrolyte changes, irritability, decreased muscle/bone mass, and gynecomastia. The agonists may trigger an initial disease flare due to a transient increase in hormone levels. Injection site reactions can occur with medications that are administered subcutaneously. Emotional lability and increased risk of seizure activity have been noted with some of the GnRH agonists. GnRH agonists may also increase the blood glucose, and androgen lowering medication can prolong the QT interval. See Figure 35.2 for a variety of adverse effects from hypothalamic and pituitary agents.

Prototype Summary: Leuprolide

Indications: Treatment of advanced prostatic cancer, endometriosis, central precocious puberty, uterine leiomyomata.

Actions: GnRH agonist that occupies pituitary GnRH receptors and desensitizes them; causes an initial increase and then profound decrease in LH and FSH levels.

Pharmacokinetics:

Route	Peak post initial dose	Time at steady state	Duration
Subcutaneous depot	2–4 h	Variable	1–6 months

$T_{1/2}$: 3 hours; metabolized into peptides; excretion via urine.

Adverse Effects: Dizziness, headache, pain, peripheral edema, myocardial infarction, nausea, vomiting, anorexia, constipation, urinary frequency, hematuria, hot flashes, increased sweating, malaise, fatigue, emotional lability, injection site pain, convulsions, testicular atrophy, decreased bone density, hyperglycemia.

Nursing Considerations for Patients Receiving Drugs Affecting Hypothalamic Hormones

The specific nursing care of the patient who is receiving a hypothalamic-releasing factor is related to the hormone (or hormones) that the drug is affecting and the indication that the medication is being used for. For example, a male prescribed a GnRH agonist for palliative treatment for prostate cancer will have very unique nursing assessment, conclusions, planning requirements, intervention strategies, and evaluation needs compared to a female being administered a GnRH antagonist as part of fertility treatment. However, for all hypothalamic agonists and antagonists that are injected, be sure to monitor for injection site reactions. Since several of the medications have varied dosing amounts and frequencies, educate patients and families about timing for follow-up and next scheduled doses. In addition to advising patients on the common side effects, warn patients receiving GnRH agonists that there may be an initial worsening of their disease process due to a rise in the LH and FSH; however, reassure them that over time those levels will decrease, and symptoms will lessen. Bone density, blood glucose, and QT intervals may need to be monitored with some patients.

Key Points

- The hypothalamus releases hormones that act as releasing factors, stimulating the anterior pituitary to release specific stimulating factors, and inhibiting factors that act to decrease the production of specific anterior pituitary hormones.
- Not all of the hypothalamic hormones are available for pharmacological use; those that are available are indicated for treatment of prostate and breast cancers, endometriosis, precocious puberty, reduction in lipodystrophy, and as fertility medications.

Drugs Affecting Anterior Pituitary Hormones

Agents that affect pituitary function are used mainly to mimic or antagonize the effects of specific pituitary hormones. They may be used either as replacement therapy for conditions resulting from a hypoactive pituitary or for diagnostic purposes. Antagonists are also available that may be used to block the effects of the anterior pituitary hormones (Table 35.2).

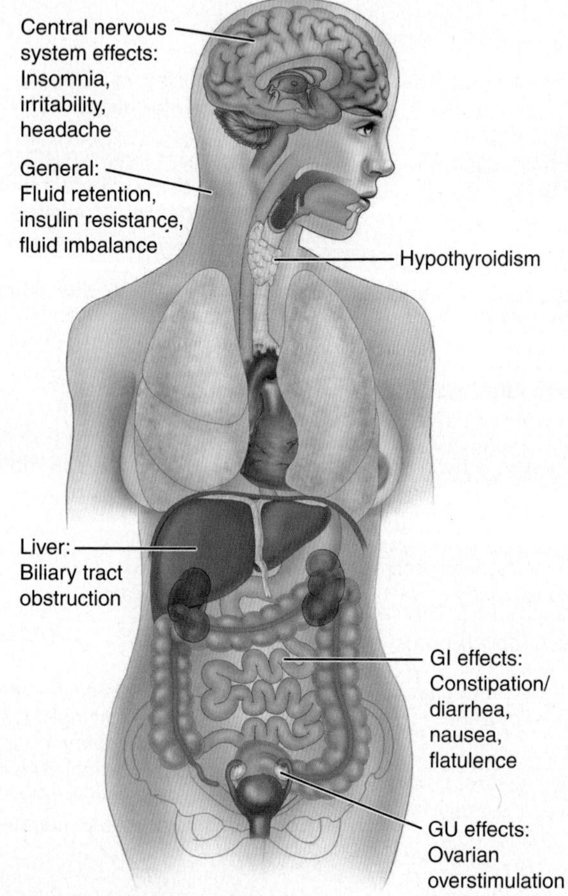

FIGURE 35.2 Variety of adverse effects and toxicities associated with hypothalamic and pituitary agents.

Table 35.2 *Drugs in Focus:* Drugs Affecting Anterior Pituitary Hormones

Drug Name	Dosage/Route	Usual Indications
Growth Hormone Agonists		
somapacitan-beco (*Sogroya*)	Initial 1.5 mg subcutaneously weekly; titrated based on clinical response and serum insulinlike growth factor; max dose 8 mg subcutaneously weekly	Replacement of endogenous growth hormone in adults with growth hormone deficiency
somatropin (*Genotropin, Norditropin Flexpro, Nutropin, Nutropin AQ Nuspin, Omnitrope, Serostim, Zomacton, Saizen, Humatrope, Zorbtive*)	Dose varies based on indication and product, check manufacturer's instructions; must be given subcutaneously or IM daily	Treatment of children with growth failure due to lack of GH or to chronic renal failure; replacement of GH in patients with GH deficiency; long-term treatment of growth failure in children born small for gestational age who do not achieve catch-up growth by 2 y of age; treatment of short stature associated with Turner's syndrome or Prader-Willi syndrome; also approved to increase protein production and growth in various AIDS-related states. Replacement of endogenous GH in adults with GH deficiency. Treatment of adults with short bowel syndrome who are receiving specialized nutritional support (*Zorbtive* only)
Growth Hormone Antagonists		
bromocriptine mesylate (*Parlodel*)	1.25–2.5 mg/d PO initially and may titrate up to usual adult dose of 20–30 mg/d; max dose 100 mg/d	Treatment of acromegaly, hyperprolactinemia-associated dysfunctions, adjunctive treatment for Parkinson's disease
lanreotide (*Somatuline Depot*)	Initially 90–120 mg depending on indication subcutaneously every 4 wk for 3 mo; then adjust dose based on patient response	Long-term treatment of acromegaly in patients with inadequate response to or who cannot be treated with surgery or radiation; treatment of adults with advanced or metastatic gastroenteropancreatic neuroendocrine tumors; treatment of adults with carcinoid syndrome
octreotide (*Bynfezia Pen, Mycapssa, Sandostatin, Sandostatin LAR Depot*)	Subcutaneous dosing varies based on formulation and indication	Treatment of acromegaly in adults who are not candidates for or cannot tolerate other therapy; treatment of severe diarrhea/flushing associated with metastatic carcinoid tumors and vasoactive intestinal peptide secreting tumors
	Initial 20 mg PO twice a day; titrate based on insulinlike growth factor-1 levels and clinical response to max dose 80 mg/d (*Mycapssa*)	Maintenance treatment of patients with acromegaly who have tolerated treatment with octreotide or lanreotide (*Mycapssa*)
pegvisomant (*Somavert*)	40 mg subcutaneously as a loading dose, then 10–30 mg/d subcutaneously titrated on serum insulinlike growth factor-1 levels	Treatment of acromegaly in adults who are not candidates for or who cannot tolerate other therapy
Drugs Affecting Other Anterior Pituitary Hormones		
chorionic gonadotropin (*Pregnyl*, others)	Dose varies with indication; 4,000–10,000 IU IM 1 to 3 times per wk is common	Treatment of male hypogonadism, to induce ovulation in assigned females with functioning ovaries, for treatment of prepubertal cryptorchidism when there is no anatomical obstruction to testicular movement
chorionic gonadotropin alpha (*Ovidrel*)	250 mcg subcutaneously given 1 d after last dose of a FSH stimulator	Induction of ovulation in infertile females who have been pretreated with FSH
cosyntropin (*Cortrosyn*)	0.25–0.75 mg IV or IM	Diagnosis of adrenal function
pasireotide (*Signifor, Signifor LAR*)	*Signifor* 0.6 or 0.9 mg SQ b.i.d. initially and titrate for response (Cushing's disease) *Signifor LAR*: 40 mg IM every 4 wk (acromegaly); 10 mg IM initially every 4 wk and titrate for response (Cushing's disease) Reduce dose with moderate hepatic impairment	Treatment of Cushing's disease when pituitary surgery is not an option Treatment of acromegaly if inadequate response to or if surgery is not an option (*Signifor LAR*)
thyrotropin alpha (*Thyrogen*)	0.9 mg IM, followed by 0.9 mg IM in 24 h	Adjunctive treatment for postradioiodine ablation of thyroid tissue in patients with near-total thyroidectomy and well-differentiated thyroid cancer without metastasis; adjunctive diagnostic tool for thyroid cancer

GH, growth hormone; FSH, follicle-stimulating hormone.

Growth Hormone Agonists

The anterior pituitary hormone that is most commonly used pharmacologically is GH. GH is responsible for linear skeletal growth, the growth of internal organs, protein synthesis, and the stimulation of many other processes that are required for normal growth. **Hypopituitarism**, or a lack of adequate functioning of the pituitary, is often seen as GH deficiency before any other signs and symptoms occur. Hypopituitarism may occur as a result of developmental differences or congenital anomalies of the pituitary, circulatory disturbances (e.g., hemorrhage, infarction), acute or chronic inflammation of the pituitary, and pituitary tumors. GH deficiency in children results in short stature (**dwarfism**). Adults with somatotropin deficiency syndrome (SDS) may have hypopituitarism as a result of pituitary tumors or trauma, or they may have been treated for GH deficiency as children, resulting in a shutdown of the pituitary production of somatotropin.

GH deficiency was once treated with GH injections extracted from the pituitary glands of cadavers. The supply of GH was, therefore, rather limited and costly. Synthetic human GH is now available from recombinant DNA (rDNA) sources, using genetic engineering. Somatropin (*Humatrope, Nutropin, Saizen, Genotropin, Serostim, Zorbtive*, and others) and somapacitan-beco (*Sogroya*; a GH analog) are available for GH replacement today. Box 35.2 discusses an alternate treatment for growth failure in pediatric patients.

Therapeutic Actions and Indications

GH agonists stimulate overall growth and production of protein. They bind to GH receptors on target tissues. Some of their effects are mediated by insulinlike growth factor that can stimulate skeletal growth and protein building. Lypolysis (break down of fats) is another direct effect of GH agonists. Somatropin is indicated to treat GH deficiencies in both adults and children, but somapacitan-beco is only approved for treatment of adults (Table 35.2).

BOX 35.2

Treatment for Growth Failure in Children

In late 2005, the U.S. Food and Drug Administration approved two drugs that contain human insulinlike growth factor-1 (IGF-1) and human insulinlike growth factor–binding protein-3. These factors promote linear growth in children and also have anabolic effects, sensitize cells to insulin, and have insulinlike effects on metabolism. They do not directly alter GH levels. The drugs mecasermin (*Increlex*) and mecasermin rinfabate (*Iplex*) were approved for the long-term treatment of growth failure in children with severe primary IGF-1 deficiency or with GH gene depletion who have developed neutralizing antibodies to GH. Mecasermin rinfabate has since been withdrawn from the market. *Increlex* is given by subcutaneous injection, initially 0.04–0.08 mg/kg (40–80 mcg/kg) b.i.d., and then increased by 0.04 mg/kg per dose to a maximum dose of 0.12 mg/kg b.i.d. When using this drug, hypoglycemia is common, and patients must be monitored to ensure that they eat after administration. Tonsillar hypertrophy, local and systemic hypersensitivity are also common, and the child should be monitored appropriately.

Pharmacokinetics

Somatropin is injected and reaches peak level within 7 hours. Somapacitan-beco is also injected, takes 4 to 24 hours to reach max concentration, and 1 to 2 weeks for steady state to be achieved. These two drugs are widely distributed in the body and localize in highly perfused tissues, particularly the liver and kidney. Excretion occurs through the urine and feces. Patients with liver or renal dysfunction may experience reduced clearance and increased concentrations of the drugs.

Contraindications and Cautions

Somatropin is contraindicated with any known allergy to the drug or ingredients in the drug, to avoid hypersensitivity reactions. It is also contraindicated in the presence of closed epiphyses when indication for use is linear growth, and if active malignancy is present, due to potential for enhanced tumor growth. Caution should be taken with patients who have underlying cranial lesions because of the risk of increased intracranial pressure; with acute critical illness (including immediately postabdominal or heart surgery; acute respiratory distress; trauma), because of increased mortality rates; and with people with glucose intolerance due to worsening of glycemic control. There is little data regarding these medications and human pregnancy or lactation outcomes; however, animal studies do not demonstrate high risk.

Adverse Effects

The adverse effects that most often occur when using GH replacement include injection site reactions, edema, myalgia, and arthralgia. It is possible for the client to develop antibodies which inactivate the hormone replacement. Insulin resistance and hyperglycemia should be monitored, and antihyperglycemic agent doses may need to be increased. GH analogs may also cause hypoadrenalism, hypothyroidism, and pancreatitis.

Clinically Important Drug–Drug Interactions

Concurrent use with glucocorticoids may counteract the growth-promoting effects. However, glucocorticoid treatment may be indicated if GH replacement induces hypoadrenalism. Caution should be used when these agents are combined with any drugs using the cytochrome P450 liver enzyme system because of a risk for change in metabolism of the combined drugs.

Prototype Summary: Somatropin

Indications: Treatment of children with growth failure due to lack of GH or to chronic renal failure; replacement of GH in patients with GH deficiency; long-term treatment of growth failure in children born small for gestational age who do not achieve catch-up growth by 2 years of age; treatment of short stature associated with Turner's syndrome or Prader-Willi syndrome; also approved to increase protein production and growth in various AIDS-related states. Replacement of endogenous GH in adults with GH deficiency. Treatment of adults with short bowel syndrome who are receiving specialized nutritional support (*Zorbtive* only).

Actions: Replaces human GH; stimulates skeletal growth, growth of internal organs, and protein synthesis.

Pharmacokinetics:

Route	Onset	Peak
IM, subcutaneous	Varies	5–7.5 h

$T_{1/2}$: 15 to 50 minutes; metabolized in the liver and excreted in the urine and feces.

Adverse Effects: Development of antibodies to growth hormone, insulin resistance, swelling, joint/muscle pain, headache, injection-site pain.

Nursing Considerations for Patients Receiving Growth Hormone Agonists

Assessment: History and Examination

- Assess history of allergy to any ingredient in the medication, presence of closed epiphyses, acute illness including active malignancy, glucose intolerance, and pregnancy or lactation status due to potential contraindications or cautions to the use of the drug.
- Assess height, weight, thyroid function tests, glucose tolerance tests, and GH levels to determine baseline status before beginning therapy and for any potential adverse effects.

Nursing Conclusions

Nursing conclusions related to drug therapy might include the following:

- Altered nutrition: less than body requirements related to metabolic changes
- Acute pain related to need for injections
- Knowledge deficit regarding drug therapy

Planning

- The patient will receive the best therapeutic effect from the drug therapy.
- The patient will have limited adverse effects to the drug therapy.
- The patient will have an understanding of the drug therapy, adverse effects to anticipate, and measures to relieve discomfort and improve safety.

Intervention With Rationale

- Reconstitute the drug following manufacturer's directions because individual products vary; administer IM or subcutaneously for appropriate delivery of drug.
- Monitor response carefully when beginning therapy to allow appropriate dose adjustments as needed.
- Monitor thyroid function, glucose tolerance, and GH levels periodically to monitor endocrine changes and to institute treatment as needed.
- Provide thorough patient teaching, including measures to take to avoid adverse effects, warning signs of problems, and the need for regular evaluation (including blood tests) to enhance patient knowledge about drug therapy and promote compliance. Instruct a family member or caregiver in the following points:
  - Storage of the drug (refrigeration is required)
  - Preparation of the drug (the reconstitution procedure varies depending on the brand name product used)
  - Administration techniques (sterile technique, need to rotate injection sites, and need to monitor injection sites for atrophy or extravasation)
  - Report any lack of growth as well as signs of glucose intolerance (thirst, hunger, voiding pattern changes) or thyroid dysfunction (fatigue, thinning hair, slow pulse, puffy skin, intolerance to the cold)

Evaluation

- Monitor patient response to the drug (return of GH levels to normal, growth and development).
- Monitor for adverse effects (hypothyroidism, glucose intolerance, nutritional imbalance).
- Evaluate the effectiveness of the teaching plan (patient can name drug, dosage, adverse effects to watch for, and specific measures to avoid them; family member can demonstrate proper technique for preparation and administration of the drug).
- Monitor the effectiveness of comfort measures and compliance with the regimen.

Growth Hormone Antagonists

GH hypersecretion is usually caused by pituitary tumors and can occur at any time of life. This is often referred to as hyperpituitarism. If hyperpituitarism occurs before the epiphyseal plates of the long bones fuse, it causes an acceleration in linear skeletal growth, producing heights of 7 to 8 ft with fairly normal body proportions (**gigantism**). In adults, after epiphyseal closure, linear growth is impossible. Instead, hypersecretion of GH causes enlargement in the peripheral parts of the body, such as the hands and feet, and the internal organs, especially the heart. **Acromegaly** is the term used to describe the onset of excessive GH secretion that occurs after puberty and epiphyseal plate closure causing thickening of bones and enlargement of tissues.

Most conditions of GH hypersecretion are treated by radiation therapy or surgery. Drug therapy for GH excess can be used for those patients who are not candidates for surgery or radiation therapy. The drugs include a dopamine agonist (bromocriptine [*Parlodel*]), two somatostatin analogues (octreotide acetate [*Sandostatin* and others] and lanreotide [*Somatuline Depot*]), and a GH analogue (pegvisomant [*Somavert*]).

Therapeutic Actions and Indications

Somatostatin is an inhibitory factor released from the hypothalamus. It is not used to decrease GH levels, though it does do that effectively. Because it has multiple effects on many secretory systems (e.g., it inhibits release of gastrin, glucagon, and insulin) and a short duration of action, it is not desirable as a therapeutic agent. Analogues of somatostatin, octreotide acetate, and lanreotide are considerably more potent in inhibiting GH release with less of an inhibitory effect on insulin release. Consequently, they are used instead of somatostatin.

Bromocriptine, a semisynthetic ergot alkaloid, is a dopamine agonist that can be used to treat acromegaly and hyperprolactinemia-associated dysfunctions, and as an adjunctive treatment for Parkinson disease. It may be used alone or as an adjunct to irradiation. Bromocriptine is a postsynaptic dopamine receptor agonist that modulates secretion of prolactin from the anterior pituitary by acting in the corpus striatum. It may inhibit GH by increasing the dopamine that facilitates more somatostatin release from the hypothalamus.

Lanreotide, which acts like somatostatin, is given as a monthly depot subcutaneous injection. It also affects insulin growth factor levels and is used long-term for patients with acromegaly who have had no response to or cannot be treated with surgery or radiation. It is also indicated in treatment of adults with advanced or metastatic gastroenteropancreatic neuroendocrine tumors or adults with carcinoid syndrome.

Pegvisomant is a GH analogue that was approved for the treatment of acromegaly in patients who do not respond to other therapies. It binds to GH receptors on cells, inhibiting GH effects. It must be given by daily subcutaneous injections. Table 35.2 shows usual indications for each of these agents.

Pharmacokinetics

Octreotide and lanreotide are primarily administered subcutaneously. Octreotide is rapidly absorbed and widely distributed throughout the body, and it is metabolized in the tissues with about 30% excreted unchanged in the urine. Lanreotide forms a depot in the subcutaneous tissue and is slowly released into circulation with a half-life of 23 to 30 days. It is metabolized in the tissues and excretion is not known. There is an oral formulation of octreotide (*Mycapssa*). The peak absorption concentration is about 2 hours and the half-life is about 2.5 hours; about 32% is excreted unchanged in urine.

Bromocriptine is administered orally and effectively absorbed from the gastrointestinal (GI) tract. The drug undergoes extensive first-pass metabolism in the liver and is primarily excreted in the bile.

Pegvisomant is given by subcutaneous injection and is slowly absorbed, reaching peak effects in 33 to 77 hours. It also clears from the body at a slow rate, with a half-life of 6 days. The drug is excreted in the urine.

Contraindications and Cautions

Bromocriptine should be used during pregnancy with extreme caution due to increased risk of inducing hypertension. It should not be used during lactation because of effects on the fetus and because it blocks lactation. There are no adequate human studies of effects of octreotide, lanreotide, and pegvisomant in pregnancy and during lactation, but animal studies have not shown harm with most doses. GH antagonists are contraindicated in the presence of any known allergy to the drug to prevent hypersensitivity reactions. They should be used cautiously in the presence of any other endocrine disorder (e.g., diabetes, thyroid dysfunction) that could be exacerbated by the blocking of GH.

Adverse Effects

Patients with renal dysfunction may accumulate higher levels of octreotide. GI complaints (e.g., constipation or diarrhea, flatulence, and nausea) are not uncommon because of the drug's effects on the GI tract. Octreotide and lanreotide have also been associated with the development of acute cholecystitis, cholestatic jaundice, biliary tract obstruction, and pancreatitis. Patients must be assessed for the possible development of any of these problems. Other less common adverse effects include headache, sinus bradycardia or other cardiac arrhythmias, and decreased glucose tolerance. The medications that are administered subcutaneously can be associated with discomfort and/or inflammation at injection sites.

Lanreotide is associated with changes in blood glucose levels, and glucose should be followed carefully while on the drug.

Bromocriptine is also associated with GI disturbances. Because of its dopamine-blocking effects, it may cause drowsiness and postural hypotension. It blocks lactation and should not be used by nursing parents.

Pegvisomant may cause pain and inflammation at the injection site (common). Increased incidence of infection, nausea, and diarrhea and changes in liver function may also occur.

Clinically Important Drug–Drug Interactions

Increased serum bromocriptine levels were noted with concurrent use of macrolide antibiotics, like erythromycin, lanreotide, and octreotide. There are several medications that may decrease effectiveness of bromocriptine, so medication interactions should be checked for each patient. Use of lanreotide or octreotide with cyclosporin can decrease the absorption of cyclosporine. These medications may enhance bradycardic effect if used concurrently with other medications that can lower heart rate, so dosage adjustments may be needed. Glycemic medication doses also may need to be altered based on changes of serum glucose levels.

Patients receiving pegvisomant may require higher doses to receive adequate GH suppression if they are also taking opioids.

Prototype Summary: Bromocriptine Mesylate

Indications: Treatment of acromegaly and hyperprolactinemia-associated dysfunctions; adjunctive treatment for Parkinson's disease.

Actions: Acts directly on postsynaptic dopamine receptors in the brain and as a dopamine agonist.

Pharmacokinetics:

Route	Onset	Peak	Duration
PO	Varies	1–3 h	14 h

$T_{1/2}$: 5 hours, extensively metabolized in the liver and excreted primarily via feces.

Adverse Effects: Dizziness, fatigue, light-headedness, nasal congestion, drowsiness, nausea, vomiting, abdominal cramps, constipation, diarrhea, headache.

Nursing Considerations for Patients Receiving Growth Hormone Antagonists

Assessment: History and Examination

- Assess for history of allergies to any GH antagonist or binder to prevent hypersensitivity reactions; other endocrine disturbances, which could be exacerbated when blocking GH; and pregnancy and lactation if client is prescribed bromocriptine, because of the potential for inducing hypertension and the blocking of lactation.
- Assess orientation, affect, and reflexes; blood pressure, pulse, and orthostatic blood pressure; abdominal examination; glucose tolerance tests; and GH levels, to determine baseline status before beginning therapy and for any potential adverse effects.

Nursing Conclusions

Nursing conclusions related to drug therapy might include the following:

- Altered nutrition: more than body requirements related to metabolic changes
- Acute pain related to need for injections (octreotide, lanreotide, pegvisomant)
- Knowledge deficit regarding drug therapy

Planning

- The patient will receive the best therapeutic effect from the drug therapy.
- The patient will have limited adverse effects to the drug therapy.
- The patient will have an understanding of the drug therapy, adverse effects to anticipate, and measures to relieve discomfort and improve safety.

Intervention With Rationale

- Reconstitute octreotide and pegvisomant following manufacturer's directions; administer these drugs subcutaneously and rotate injection sites regularly to prevent skin breakdown and to ensure proper delivery of the drug.
- Inject lanreotide deep into the subcutaneous fat in the superior quadrant of the buttocks; alternate injection sites from right to left to ensure proper delivery of the drug and prevent local reactions.
- Monitor thyroid function, glucose tolerance, and GH levels periodically to detect problems and to institute treatment as needed.
- Arrange for baseline and periodic ultrasound evaluation of the gallbladder if using octreotide or lanreotide to detect any gallstone development and to arrange for appropriate treatment.
- Provide thorough patient teaching, including measures to avoid adverse effects, warning signs of problems, and need for regular evaluation (including blood tests), to enhance patient knowledge about drug therapy and promote compliance. Instruct a family member in proper preparation and administration techniques to ensure that there is another responsible person to administer the drug if needed.

Evaluation

- Monitor patient response to the drug (return of GH levels to normal, growth and development).
- Monitor for adverse effects (hypothyroidism, glucose intolerance, nutritional imbalance, GI disturbances, headache, dizziness, cholecystitis).
- Evaluate the effectiveness of the teaching plan (patient can name drug, dosage, adverse effects to watch for, and specific measures to avoid them; family member can demonstrate proper technique for preparation and administration of drug).
- Monitor the effectiveness of comfort measures and compliance with the regimen.

Drugs Affecting Other Anterior Pituitary Hormones

Drugs that affect GH are the most prevalent drugs affecting anterior pituitary hormones. There are several other anterior pituitary hormones that can now be affected by drugs. The other anterior pituitary hormones that are available for pharmacological use include chorionic gonadotropin (*Pregnyl* and others), chorionic gonadotropin alpha (*Ovidrel*), cosyntropin (*Cortrosyn*), pasireotide (*Signifor, Signifor LAR*), and thyrotropin alpha (*Thyrogen*). Usual indications and doses are presented in Table 35.2.

Chorionic gonadotropin acts like LH and stimulates the production of testosterone and progesterone. Chorionic gonadotropin alpha is used as a fertility drug to induce ovulation in females treated with FSH. Due to their indications, these drugs are better discussed in Chapter 40 (Drugs Affecting the Female Reproductive System).

Cosyntropin is used for diagnostic purposes to test adrenal function and responsiveness. It acts as natural adrenocorticotropic hormone (ACTH). Clients with primary adrenal insufficiency (Addison's disease) will not respond to the cosyntropin. However, clients with adrenal insufficiency due to a secondary process will have increased levels of cortisol after cosyntropin injections. Cosyntropin has a rapid onset and short duration of activity and, therefore, is not used for therapeutic purposes.

Pasireotide is a somatostatin analog that is indicated for treatment of Cushing disease when surgery is not an option (see Chapter 36, Box 36.2 for more info). It ultimately acts to decrease secretion of ACTH due to attaching on somatostatin receptors in the adrenal gland that tend to be overactive with Cushing disease. *Signifor LAR* also is indicated for treatment of acromegaly due to its ability to suppress GH.

Thyrotropin alpha is recombinant human thyroid stimulating hormone. It can be used as adjunctive treatment for radioiodine ablation of thyroid tissue remnants in patients who have undergone a near-total to total thyroidectomy for well-differentiated thyroid cancer and who do not have evidence of metastatic thyroid cancer. It can also be used as an adjunctive diagnostic tool for thyroid cancer.

Key Points

- Hypothalamic-releasing factors stimulate the anterior pituitary to release hormones, which in turn stimulate endocrine glands or cell metabolism.
- The anterior pituitary hormones may be used for diagnostic testing, for treating some cancers, or in fertility programs.
- GH may be replaced by synthetic replacement to treat children with growth failure or adults with short bowel syndrome.
- Growth hormone antagonists may be used for treatment of acromegaly.

Drugs Affecting Posterior Pituitary Hormones

The posterior pituitary stores two hormones produced in the hypothalamus: antidiuretic hormone (ADH, also known as vasopressin) and oxytocin. Oxytocin stimulates milk ejection or "let down" during lactation. In pharmacological doses, it can be used to initiate or improve uterine contractions in labor. Oxytocin is discussed in Chapter 40.

ADH possesses antidiuretic, hemostatic, and vasopressor properties. Posterior pituitary disorders can occur secondary to head trauma or surgery, metastatic cancer, lymphoma, disseminated intravascular coagulation, or septicemia. Posterior pituitary disorders that are seen clinically involve ADH release and include **diabetes insipidus**, which results from insufficient secretion of ADH, and syndrome of inappropriate antidiuretic hormone (SIADH), which occurs with excessive secretion of ADH. Both conditions can now be treated pharmacologically. (See the "Critical Thinking Scenario" related to diabetes insipidus and posterior pituitary hormones.)

Diabetes insipidus is caused by either a deficiency in the amount of posterior pituitary ADH or a decrease in the ability of the kidneys to respond to ADH. It may result from pituitary disease or injury (e.g., head trauma, surgery, tumor) and can also be due to genetic or acquired renal deficiencies that impair the urine concentrating ability. The condition can be acute and short in duration, or chronic and lifelong. It is characterized by the production of a large amount of dilute urine. If the person has a normal thirst mechanism and is able to intake enough fluids to balance out the loss of fluid, the person may stay hemodynamically stable. However, with the excessive fluid loss, it is easy for the person to become dehydrated. Blood becomes concentrated if the person does not hydrate enough to keep up with the fluid loss. The patient typically presents with polyuria (increased urine production), polydipsia (increased thirst), and various level of dehydration.

SIADH presents with fluid retention, dilution of the blood and all of the blood elements, and serious issues with water balance and fluid volume. This disorder is now treated with drugs that block the ADH or vasopressin receptors so water is no longer retained and urine is produced, helping to restore water balance. Keeping the fluid balance in check can be tricky, and patients receiving these drugs need to be closely monitored in the hospital.

ADH itself is never used as therapy for diabetes insipidus. Instead, synthetic preparations of ADH, which are purer and have fewer adverse effects, are used. Desmopressin (*DDAVP, Nocdurna*) is a synthetic analogue of the natural posterior pituitary hormone ADH. It is indicated to treat diabetes insipidus, von Willebrand disease, and hemophilia. There is also a sublingual form that is indicated for the treatment of nocturia due to nocturnal polyuria in adults. Vasopressin (*Vasostrict*) is synthetic also synthetic ADH, but it is indicated for increasing blood pressure in adults with vasodilatory shock or in clients who remain hypotensive despite fluids and catecholamines (Table 35.3).

Table 35.3 *Drugs in Focus:* Drugs Affecting Posterior Pituitary Hormones

Drug Name	Dosage/Route	Usual Indications
conivaptan (*Vaprisol*)	20 mg IV loading dose over 30 min, then 20–40 mg by continuous IV infusion over 24 h Decrease dose if moderate or severe hepatic impairment	Treatment of hypervolemic or euvolemic hyponatremia in hospitalized patients
desmopressin (*DDAVP, Nocdurna*)	*Adult*: dosing can vary per indication and formulation; 0.1–0.4 mL/d IV, subcutaneously, 0.05–0.8 mg daily PO may be divided in two doses, intranasal for diabetes insipidus; 0.3 mcg/kg IV over 15–30 min for von Willebrand disease; 20 mcg intranasal at bedtime for nocturnal enuresis; 27.7 mcg sublingual (female) or 55.3 mcg sublingual (male) 1 h before bedtime (*Nocdurna*) *Pediatric*: Dosing can vary per indication; 0.05–0.3 mL/d intranasal for diabetes insipidus; 0.3 mcg/kg IV over 15–30 min for von Willebrand disease	Treatment of neurogenic diabetes insipidus, von Willebrand disease, hemophilia; treatment of nocturia due to nocturnal polyuria in adults (*Nocdurna*)
tolvaptan (*Jynarque, Samsca*)	Initial dosage 60 mg PO daily split in 2 doses separated by 8 h (45 and 15 mg); titration dose 90 mg PO daily split in 2 doses separated by 8 h (60 and 30 mg); target dose 120 mg PO daily split in 2 doses separated by 8 h (90 and 30 mg) (*Jynarque*) Initially 15 mg PO; titrate to a maximum of 60 mg/d PO based on patient response (*Samsca*)	Slows kidney function decline in adults at risk for rapidly progressing autosomal-dominant polycystic kidney disease (*Jynarque*) Treatment of hypervolemic and euvolemic hyponatremia that is resistant to correction with fluid restriction including patients with heart failure or SIADH (*Samsca*)
vasopressin (*Vasostrict*)	0.01–0.1 units/min IV titrated to maintain blood pressure	Increase blood pressure in adults with vasodilatory shock or who remain hypotensive despite fluids and catecholamines

SIADH, syndrome of inappropriate antidiuretic hormone.

There are currently two drugs available that selectively block vasopressin or ADH receptors: conivaptan (*Vaprisol*) and tolvaptan (*Jynarque, Samsca*). These drugs are used to treat clinically significant hypervolemic or euvolemic hyponatremia, including patients with SIADH. By blocking the vasopressin receptors, they cause an increased excretion of water, which results in an increase in serum sodium concentrations and a return to fluid balance.

Therapeutic Actions and Indications

ADH is released from the posterior pituitary in response to increases in plasma osmolarity or decreases in blood volume. It produces its antidiuretic activity in the kidneys, causing the cortical and medullary parts of the collecting duct to become permeable to water, thereby increasing water reabsorption and decreasing urine formation. These activities reduce plasma osmolarity and increase blood volume.

The vasopressin blockers cause a loss of water through the urine and, therefore, increase in serum sodium levels as the water level decreases. They must be given under close supervision in the hospital to monitor fluid volume carefully. See Table 35.3 for usual indications for these drugs.

Pharmacokinetics

Desmopressin is rapidly absorbed and metabolized; it is excreted in the liver and kidneys. Desmopressin is available for oral, IV, subcutaneous, and nasal administration (Box 35.3). Vasopressin is administered IV, it is predominately metabolized by the liver and kidney and has a half-life of about 10 minutes. Tolvaptan is given orally, is readily absorbed, and has a half-life of 12 hours. Conivaptan is given by continuous IV infusion, has a half-life of 5 hours, and is excreted in the urine and feces.

Contraindications and Cautions

Drugs affecting the anterior pituitary hormones are contraindicated with any known allergy to the drug or its components to avoid potential hypersensitivity reactions or with severe renal dysfunction, which could alter the effects of the drug. Caution should be used with any known vascular disease because of its effects on vascular smooth muscle, asthma, and hyponatremia, which could be exacerbated by the effects of the drug. Studies have not been conducted to evaluate the safety of these medications when used during pregnancy or lactation.

Box 35.3 Focus on Safe Medication Administration

ADMINISTERING A NASAL SPRAY

Instruct the patient to sit upright and press a finger over one nostril to close it. Then, with the spray bottle held upright, have the patient place the tip of the bottle about 1.5 cm (1/2 in.) into the open nostril. A firm squeeze should deliver the drug to the desired mucosal area for absorption. Caution the patient not to use excessive force and not to tip the head back because these actions could result in ineffective administration.

Adverse Effects

The adverse effects associated with the use of desmopressin and vasopressin include water intoxication (drowsiness, light-headedness, headache, coma, convulsions) related to the shift to water retention and resulting electrolyte imbalance; tremor, sweating, vertigo, and headache related to water retention (a "hangover" effect); abdominal cramps, flatulence, nausea, and vomiting related to stimulation of GI motility; and local nasal irritation related to nasal administration (desmopressin). Local reaction at injection sites is fairly common (desmopressin). Hypersensitivity reactions have also been reported, ranging from rash to bronchial constriction. There is risk of myocardial ischemia due to vasoconstriction when administering vasopressin. The adverse effects associated with conivaptan and tolvaptan are associated with rapid volume shifts (polyuria, blood pressure changes, hyperglycemia, arrhythmias). Constipation, dry mouth, and thirst have also been reported. Patients need to be monitored for liver injury when administered tolvaptan.

Clinically Important Drug–Drug Interactions

There is an increased risk of antidiuretic effects if desmopressin is combined with carbamazepine or tricyclic antidepressants. Use of alcohol or other diuretic medications can decrease antidiuretic effects. The vasopressor effects are enhanced if vasopressin is administered with catecholamines. Tolvaptan and conivaptan are metabolized via CYP 3A enzymes, so interactions with CYP 3A inducers and inhibiters can be expected. Potential medication interactions should be checked when administering these medications.

Prototype Summary: Desmopressin

Indications: Treatment of neurogenic diabetes insipidus, von Willebrand disease, hemophilia; treatment of nocturia due to nocturnal polyuria in adults.

Actions: Has pressor and antidiuretic effects; increases levels of clotting factor VIII.

Pharmacokinetics:

Route	Onset	Peak	Duration
Oral	1 h	60–90 min	7 h
IV, subcutaneous	30 min	90–120 min	Varies
Nasal	15–60 min	1–5 h	5–21 h

$T_{1/2}$: 7.8 minutes, then 75.5 minutes (IV); 1.5 to 2.5 hours (oral); 3.3 to 3.5 hours (nasal); metabolized in the tissues; excretion is mainly via urine.

Adverse Effects: Headache, dry mouth, facial flushing, nausea, fluid retention, slight increase in blood pressure, local reaction at injection site, water intoxication at high doses.

Nursing Considerations for Patients Receiving Drugs Affecting Posterior Pituitary Hormones

Assessment: History and Examination

- Assess for history of allergy to any antidiuretic hormone preparation or components, to avoid hypersensitivity reactions; assess for vascular diseases, renal dysfunction, pregnancy, and lactation, which could be cautions or contraindications to use of the drug.
- Assess skin for lesions; orientation, affect, and reflexes; blood pressure and pulse; respiration and adventitious sounds; abdominal examination; renal function tests; and serum electrolytes, to determine baseline status before beginning therapy and for any potential adverse effects.

Nursing Conclusions

Nursing conclusions related to drug therapy might include the following:

- Altered urinary elimination
- Altered fluid volume related to water retention or excretion
- Knowledge deficit regarding drug therapy

Planning

- The patient will receive the best therapeutic effect from the drug therapy.
- The patient will have limited adverse effects to the drug therapy.
- The patient will have an understanding of the drug therapy, adverse effects to anticipate, and measures to relieve discomfort and improve safety.

Intervention With Rationale

- Monitor patient fluid volume to watch for signs of water intoxication and fluid excess or excessive fluid loss; arrange to decrease dose as needed.
- Monitor patients with vascular disease for any sign of exacerbation to provide for immediate treatment.
- Monitor condition of nasal passages if given intranasally to observe for nasal ulceration, which can occur and could affect absorption of the drug.
- Monitor for injection site reactions if administered IV, subcutaneous, or IM to observe for any ulceration or trauma.
- Provide thorough patient teaching, including measures to avoid adverse effects, warning signs of problems, and the need for regular evaluation, including blood tests, to enhance patient knowledge about drug therapy and promote compliance.

(continues on page 602)

Evaluation

- Monitor patient response to the drug (maintenance of fluid balance).
- Monitor for adverse effects (GI problems, cardiac or peripheral vascular changes, water intoxication, fluid loss, headache, skin rash).
- Evaluate the effectiveness of the teaching plan (patient can name drug, dosage, adverse effects to watch for, and specific measures to avoid them; patient can demonstrate proper administration of nasal preparations).
- Monitor the effectiveness of comfort measures and compliance with the regimen.

CRITICAL THINKING SCENARIO
Diabetes Insipidus and Posterior Pituitary Hormones (Desmopressin)

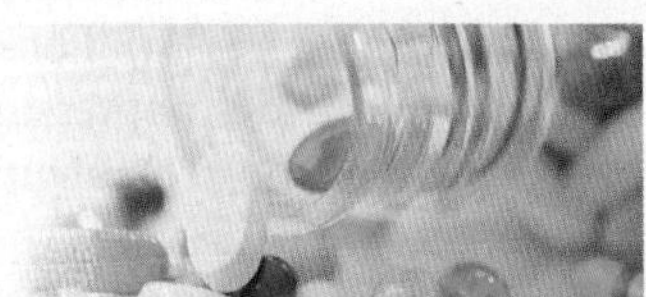

THE SITUATION

B.T. is a 56-year-old teacher with diabetes insipidus. Their condition was eventually regulated on desmopressin nasal spray, one or two sprays per nostril four times a day. B.T. seemed highly interested in their disease and therapy and learned to control their dose by symptom control. For several years, their symptoms were well controlled. Then, at B.T.'s last clinical visit, it was noted that they had postnasal ulcerations and nasal rhinitis. They also complained of several GI symptoms, including upset stomach, abdominal cramps, and diarrhea.

CRITICAL THINKING

Think about the pathophysiology of diabetes insipidus. What are the effects of desmopressin on the body, and what adverse effects might occur if the drug was being absorbed inappropriately?

Because B.T. has used the drug for so many years, they may have forgotten some of the teaching points about their disease and drug administration. Outline a care plan for B.T. that includes necessary teaching points and takes into consideration their long experience with their disease and drug therapy. Think about specific warning signs that should be highlighted for B.T. and ways to involve them in the teaching program that might make it more pertinent to them and their needs.

DISCUSSION

An essential aspect of the ongoing nursing process is continual evaluation of the effectiveness of the drug therapy. An evaluation of this situation shows that B.T.'s postnasal mucosa was ulcerated, possibly as a result of overexposure to the vasoconstrictive properties of the drug. B.T.'s GI tract also seemed to show evidence of increased ADH effects. These factors suggest that perhaps the drug was being administered incorrectly, resulting in excessive exposure of the nasal mucosa to the drug, increased absorption, and increased levels of the drug reaching the systemic circulation.

The nurse should watch B.T. administer a dose of the drug to themselves and then discuss the signs and symptoms of problems that B.T. should watch for. In this case, B.T. remembered most of the details of their drug teaching. But when administering the drug, B.T. tilted their head back, tipped the bottle upside down, and then squirted the drug into each nostril. When the nurse questioned B.T. about the technique, they explained that they had seen an advertisement on TV about nasal sprays and realized that they had been doing it wrong all these years. The nurse explained the difference in the types of nasal sprays and reviewed the entire teaching plan with B.T. The drug was discontinued and B.T. was placed on subcutaneous ADH until the nasal ulcerations healed. As a patient becomes more familiar with drug therapy, the details about the drug may be forgotten.

It is important to remember that patient teaching needs regular updating and evaluation. This point is often forgotten when dealing with patients who have been taking a drug for years. However, remembering to assess the patient's knowledge about the drug can prevent problems such as B.T.'s from developing. Because B.T. is a teacher, they might be interested in developing a teaching protocol that will meet their needs and serve as an appropriate reminder about the disease and drug therapy. If B.T. is actively involved in preparing such a plan, it will be more effective and might be remembered much longer.

NURSING CARE GUIDE FOR B.T.: DIABETES INSIPIDUS AND POSTERIOR PITUITARY HORMONES

Assessment: History and Examination

Also assess for a history of coronary artery disease, decreased peripheral circulation, moderate to severe renal impairment or hyponatremia.

Focus the physical assessment on the following:

Cardiovascular (CV): Blood pressure, pulse rate, peripheral perfusion, electrocardiogram
CNS: Orientation, affect, reflexes, vision
Skin: Color, lesions, texture, sweating
Genitourinary (GU): Urinary output, bladder tone
GI: Abdominal examination
Respiratory: Respiratory rate, adventitious sounds

Nursing Conclusions

Altered cardiac output related to CV effects
Impaired comfort related to GI, GU, CNS, CV effects
Knowledge deficit regarding drug therapy

Planning

The patient will receive the best therapeutic effect from the drug therapy.

The patient will have limited adverse effects to the drug therapy.

The patient will have an understanding of the drug therapy, adverse effects to anticipate, and measures to relieve discomfort and improve safety.

Intervention

Ensure safe and appropriate administration of the drug.

Provide comfort and safety measures, such as physical assistance or raised side rails if B.T. is hospitalized and showing any signs of unsteadiness or confusion.

Provide support and reassurance to deal with drug effects, and probable need to restrict fluid intake.

Teach patient about drug therapy, including drug name, dosage, adverse effects, precautions, and warning signs of serious adverse effects to report.

Monitor blood pressure and pulse rate, and adjust dosage as needed.

Evaluation

Evaluate drug effects, including decrease in signs and symptoms being treated.

Monitor for adverse effects: CV effects—tachycardia, heart failure, weight gain, elevated blood pressure; CNS—confusion, drowsiness, headache, visual blurring, photophobia; GU—urinary retention; GI effects—constipation.

Monitor for drug–drug interactions as indicated for each drug.

Evaluate the effectiveness of patient teaching program and comfort and safety measures.

PATIENT TEACHING FOR B.T.

- The anterior pituitary hormone desmopressin or ADH acts to promote the reabsorption of water in your kidneys, replacing the ADH that you are missing in your body. This lack of ADH is the cause of your diabetes insipidus. This drug will replace the missing hormone. This drug also causes your blood vessels to contract and may increase the activity of your GI tract. Some of the following adverse effects may occur:
  - Sleepiness, headache, confusion: If these occur, you should avoid driving a car, operating dangerous machinery, or performing any other tasks that require alertness. You should alert your health care provider as well, because a dose change may be indicated.
  - Weight gain due to fluid overload: If you have weight gain and urinary retention, please alert your health care provider, because a dose change may be indicated.
  - GI cramping, passing of gas: Eating small, frequent meals may help.
  - Nasal irritation, development of lesions: Proper administration of the drug will decrease this effect.
- Use caution to administer the nasal solution correctly. Sit upright and press a finger over one nostril to close it. Hold the spray bottle upright and place the tip of the bottle about 1.5 cm into the open nostril. A firm squeeze on the bottle will deliver the drug. Do not use excessive force when squeezing the bottle. Do not tip your head back during administration.
- Tell any doctor, nurse, or other health care provider involved in your care that you are taking this drug.
- Watch for any signs of water intoxication (drowsiness, light-headedness, headache, seizures, coma) and report this to your health care provider immediately.
- Report any nasal pain or runny nose, which might indicate that you are not administering the drug correctly.
- Keep this drug, and all medications, out of the reach of children. Do not share this drug with other people.

Key Points

- Posterior pituitary hormones are produced in the hypothalamus and stored in the posterior pituitary. They include oxytocin and ADH.
- Lack of ADH produces diabetes insipidus, which is characterized by large amounts of dilute urine and excessive thirst.
- ADH replacement uses an analogue of ADH, desmopressin, and can be administered parenterally or intranasally.
- Vasopressin is administered IV for increasing blood pressure in adults with vasodilatory shock or who remain hypotensive despite fluids and catecholamines.
- Vasopressin blockers are used to restore sodium balance in patients with severe hyponatremia.
- Fluid balance needs to be monitored when patients are taking drugs that affect ADH.

SUMMARY

Hypothalamic-releasing factors stimulate the anterior pituitary to release hormones.

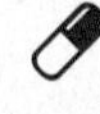
The anterior pituitary hormones may be used for diagnostic testing, for treating some cancers, or in fertility programs.

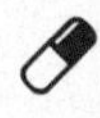
GH may be replaced by synthetic replacement to treat children with growth failure or adults with short bowel syndrome.

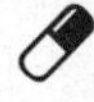
Growth hormone antagonists may be used for treatment of acromegaly. Posterior pituitary hormones are produced in the hypothalamus and stored in the posterior pituitary. They include oxytocin and ADH.

- Lack of ADH produces diabetes insipidus, which is characterized by large amounts of dilute urine and excessive thirst.
- ADH replacement uses desmopressin, an analogue of ADH, which can be administered enterally, parenterally, or intranasally.
- Vasopressin is administered IV for increasing blood pressure in adults with vasodilatory shock or who remain hypotensive despite fluids and catecholamines.
- Vasopressin blockers are used to restore sodium balance in patients with severe hyponatremia by preventing ADH from working and greater amounts of urine being produced leading to a concentration of serum.
- Fluid balance needs to be monitored when patients are taking drugs that affect ADH.

CHECK YOUR UNDERSTANDING

Answers to the questions in this chapter can be found in Answers to Check Your Understanding Questions on thePoint®.

MULTIPLE CHOICE

Select the best answer.

1. Hypothalamic hormones are normally present in small amounts. Which of the following is a common indication for an analogue of GnRH?
   a. Treatment of hormone stimulated cancers
   b. Treatment of multiple endocrine disorders
   c. Treatment of CNS-related abnormalities
   d. Treatment of autoimmune-related problems
2. Somatropin (*Nutropin* and others) is a genetically engineered GH that is used
   a. to diagnose hypothalamic failure.
   b. to treat precocious puberty.
   c. in the treatment of children with growth failure.
   d. to stimulate pituitary response.
3. GH deficiencies
   a. occur only in children.
   b. always result in dwarfism.
   c. are treated only in children because GH is usually produced only until puberty.
   d. can occur in adults as well as children.
4. Patients who are receiving GH replacement therapy must be monitored closely. Routine follow-up examinations would include
   a. a bowel program to deal with constipation.
   b. tests of thyroid function and glucose tolerance.
   c. a calorie check to control weight gain.
   d. tests of ADH levels.
5. Acromegaly and gigantism are both conditions related to excessive secretion of
   a. thyroid hormone.
   b. melanin-stimulating hormone.
   c. growth hormone.
   d. oxytocin.
6. Diabetes insipidus is a relatively rare disease characterized by
   a. excessive secretion of ADH.
   b. renal damage.
   c. the production of large amounts of dilute urine containing no glucose.
   d. insufficient pancreatic activity.
7. Treatment with ADH preparations is associated with adverse effects, including
   a. constipation and paralytic ileus.
   b. cholecystitis and bile obstruction.
   c. nocturia and bedwetting.
   d. "hangover" symptoms, including headache, sweating, and tremors.
8. A patient who is receiving an ADH preparation for diabetes insipidus may need instruction in administering the drug
   a. PO or IM.
   b. PO or intranasally.
   c. PR or PO.
   d. intranasally or by dermal patch.

MULTIPLE RESPONSE

Select all that apply.

1. Octreotide (*Sandostatin*) would be the drug of choice in the treatment of acromegaly in a client with which factors?
   a. Diabetes
   b. Gallbladder disease
   c. Adrenal insufficiency
   d. Hypothalamic lesions
   e. Intolerance to other therapies
   f. Age older than 18 years

2. A parent brought their 15-year-old child to the endocrine clinic because the child was only 5 ft tall. The parent wanted their child to receive GH therapy because the parent believed short stature would be a detriment to their child's success as an adult. The child would be considered for this therapy under which of the following circumstances?
   a. If they were against the use of cadaver parts
   b. If their epiphyses were closed
   c. If their GH levels were very low
   d. If they were also diabetic
   e. If they had chronic renal failure
   f. If they had hypothyroidism

REFERENCES

Andrews, M. M., & Boyle, J. S. (2012). *Transcultural concepts in nursing care* (6th ed.). Lippincott Williams & Wilkins.

Brunton, L. L., Hilal-Dandan, R., & Knollmann, B. C. (2018). *Goodman and Gilman's the pharmacological basis of therapeutics* (13th ed.). McGraw-Hill.

Hall, J. E. & Hall, M. E. (2021). *Guyton and Hall's textbook of medical physiology* (14th ed.). Elsevier.

John, C. A., & Day, M. W. (2012). Central neurogenic diabetes insipidus, syndrome of inappropriate secretion of antidiuretic hormone, and cerebral salt-wasting syndrome in traumatic brain injury. *Critical Care Nurse, 32*(2), e1–e7. https://doi.org/10.4037/ccn2012904

Lavin, N. (2009). *Manual of endocrinology and metabolism.* Lippincott Williams & Wilkins.

Melmed, S., Polonsky, K. S., Larsen, P. R., & Kronenberg, H. M. (2011). *Williams textbook of endocrinology* (12th ed.). Saunders.

Norris, T. L. (2019). *Porth's pathophysiology: Concepts of altered health states* (13th ed.). Wolters Kluwer.

Reichlin, S. (Ed.). (2012). *The neurohypophysis: Physiological and clinical aspects.* Springer.

CHAPTER 36

Adrenocortical Agents

Learning Objectives

Upon completion of this chapter, you will be able to:

1. Explain the control of synthesis and secretion and physiological effects of the adrenocortical agents.
2. Discuss the use of adrenocortical agents across the lifespan.
3. Describe the therapeutic actions, indications, pharmacokinetics, contraindications, most common adverse effects, and important drug–drug interactions associated with the adrenocortical agents.
4. Compare and contrast the prototype drugs prednisone and fludrocortisone with other adrenocortical agents.
5. Outline the nursing considerations, including important teaching points, for patients receiving an adrenocortical agent.

Key Terms

adrenal cortex: outer layer of the adrenal gland; produces glucocorticoids and mineralocorticoids in response to adrenocorticotropic hormone (ACTH) stimulation; also responds to sympathetic stimulation

adrenal medulla: inner layer of the adrenal gland; a sympathetic ganglion, it releases norepinephrine and epinephrine into circulation in response to sympathetic stimulation

corticosteroids: steroid hormones produced by the adrenal cortex; they include androgens, glucocorticoids, and mineralocorticoids

diurnal rhythm: response of the hypothalamus and then the pituitary and adrenals to wakefulness and sleeping; normally, the hypothalamus begins secretion of corticotropin-releasing factor (CRF) in the evening, peaking at about midnight; adrenocortical peak response is between 6 and 9 a.m.; levels fall during the day until evening, when the low level is picked up by the hypothalamus and CRF secretion begins again

glucocorticoids: steroid hormones released from the adrenal cortex; they increase blood glucose levels, fat deposits, and protein breakdown for energy

mineralocorticoids: steroid hormones released by the adrenal cortex; they cause sodium and water retention and potassium excretion

Drug List

ADRENOCORTICAL AGENTS

Glucocorticoids
beclomethasone
betamethasone
budesonide
cortisone
deflazacort
dexamethasone
flunisolide
hydrocortisone
methylprednisolone
prednisolone
(P) prednisone
triamcinolone

Mineralocorticoids
cortisone
(P) fludrocortisone
hydrocortisone
prednisone
prednisolone

Adrenocortical agents are widely used to suppress inflammation and the immune system and help people feel better. These drugs do not, however, cure inflammatory disorders. They may also be used to as replacement therapy for people with adrenal insufficiency. Due to significant side effects, they are not used as long-term therapy if there are safer alternatives.

The Adrenal Glands

The two adrenal glands are flattened bodies that sit on top of each kidney. Each gland is made up of an inner core called the adrenal medulla and an outer shell called the **adrenal cortex**.

The **adrenal medulla** is actually part of the sympathetic nervous system (SNS). It is a ganglion of neurons that releases the neurotransmitters norepinephrine and epinephrine into circulation when the SNS is stimulated. The secretion of these neurotransmitters directly into the bloodstream allows them to act as hormones, traveling from the adrenal medulla to react with specific receptor sites throughout the body. This is thought to be a backup system for the sympathetic system, adding an extra stimulus to the fight or flight response.

The adrenal cortex surrounds the medulla and consists of three layers of cells, each of which synthesizes chemically different types of steroid hormones that exert physiological effects throughout the body. The adrenal cortex produces hormones called **corticosteroids**. There are three types of corticosteroids: androgens, glucocorticoids, and mineralocorticoids. Androgens are a form of the male sex hormone testosterone; both males and females produce these hormones. They affect electrolytes, stimulate protein production, and decrease protein breakdown. They are used pharmacologically to treat hypogonadism or to increase protein growth and red blood cell production. These hormones are discussed in Chapter 41.

Controls

The adrenal cortex responds to adrenocorticotropic hormone (ACTH) released from the anterior pituitary. ACTH in turn responds to corticotropin-releasing hormone (CRH) released from the hypothalamus. This happens regularly during a normal day in what is called **diurnal rhythm** (Box 36.1). A person who has a regular cycle of sleep and wakefulness will produce high levels of CRH during sleep, usually around midnight. A resulting peak response of increased ACTH and adrenocortical hormones occurs sometime early in the morning, around 6 to 9 a.m. This high level of hormones then suppresses any further CRH or ACTH release. The corticosteroids are metabolized and excreted slowly throughout the day and fall to low levels by evening. At this point, the hypothalamus and pituitary sense low levels of the hormones and begin the production and release of CRH and ACTH again. This peaks around midnight, and the cycle starts again. It is thought that this diurnal rhythm is partly in response to exposure to light. People who work night shifts and have a different exposure to light cycling do not have the same diurnal schedule as do people who are awake in daylight and sleep at night.

Activation of the stress reaction through the SNS bypasses the usual diurnal rhythm and causes release of ACTH and secretion of the adrenocortical hormones—an important aspect of the stress ("fight or flight") response. The stress response is activated with cellular injury or when a person perceives fear or feels anx-

Box 36.1 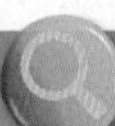 **Focus on The Evidence**

DIURNAL RHYTHM

Research over the years has shown that the adrenocortical hormones are released in a pattern called the diurnal rhythm. The secretion of CRH, ACTH, and cortisol are high in the morning in day-oriented people (those who have a regular cycle of wakefulness during the day and sleep during the night). In such people, the peak level of cortisol usually comes between 6 and 8 a.m. The level then falls off slowly (with periodic spurts) and reaches a low in the late evening, with the lowest level around midnight. Clinically you can see this action. In the morning, most patients will not have a fever because the high level of corticosteroid blocks inflammation and immunity, the reactions that cause an increase in body temperature. As the day progresses and the evening shift comes on, the fever rises. This is because the dropping corticosteroids allow the inflammatory and immune systems to get back into action, and fevers occur. It is thought that this cycle is related to the effects of sleeping on the hypothalamus and to the hypothalamus regulating its stimulation of the anterior pituitary in relation to sleep and activity. The cycle may also be connected to the hypothalamic response to light. This is important to keep in mind when treating patients with corticosteroids. In order to mimic the normal diurnal pattern, corticosteroids should be taken immediately upon waking in the morning.

Complications to this pattern arise, however, when patients work shifts or change their sleeping patterns (e.g., college students). In response, the hypothalamus shifts its release of CRH to correspond to the new cycle. For instance, if a person works all night and goes to bed at 8 a.m., rising at 3 p.m. to carry on the day's activities before going to work at 11 p.m., the hypothalamus will release CRH at about 3 p.m. in accordance with the new sleep–wake cycle. It usually takes 2 or 3 days for the hypothalamus to readjust. A patient on this schedule who is taking replacement corticosteroids would then need to take them at 3 p.m. or upon waking. A patient who works several different shifts in a single week may not have time to reregulate their hypothalamus, and the corticosteroid cycle may be thrown off. Patients who have to change their sleep patterns repeatedly often complain about feeling weak, getting sick more easily, or having trouble concentrating. College students frequently develop a pattern of sleeping all day and then staying up all night—a cycle that becomes hard to break as their bodies and endocrine systems try to readjust.

In nursing practice, it is a challenge to help patients understand how the body works and to offer ways to decrease the stress of changing sleep patterns—especially if the nurse is also working several different shifts. Many employers are willing to have employees work several days of the same shift before switching back, mainly because they have noticed an increase in productivity and a decrease in absences when employees have enough time to allow their bodies to adjust to the new shift.

ious. These hormones have many actions, including the following:

- Increasing the blood volume (aldosterone effect)
- Causing the release of glucose for energy
- Slowing the rate of protein production in most cells and increasing protein breakdown
- Mobilizing fatty acids into plasma
- Decreasing the activities of the inflammatory and immune systems (which preserves energy)

These actions are important during an acute stress situation, but they can cause adverse effects in periods of extreme or prolonged stress. For instance, a postoperative patient who is fearful and stressed may not heal well because protein building is blocked; infections may be hard to treat in such a patient because the inflammatory and immune systems are not functioning adequately.

ACTH stimulation is necessary for aldosterone release from the adrenal cortex. However, other factors influence the rate of release. High potassium ions in the blood and increased angiotensin II in the extracellular fluid both greatly increase the rate of aldosterone release. High plasma sodium and atrial natriuretic peptide slightly decrease the rate of aldosterone secretion. Aldosterone causes the kidneys to reabsorb sodium with a resultant excretion of potassium to restore homeostasis.

Adrenal Excess

Excessive adrenocortical excretion results in a disorder called Cushing's syndrome. This could be the result of an adrenal hyperplasia or tumor, an ACTH-secreting tumor, or an early sign of excessive administration of exogenous steroids. Cushing's disease is a type of Cushing's syndrome; this refers to when there is excess ACTH secreted due to a tumor in the pituitary gland. A person with Cushing's syndrome may have the following signs/symptoms: moonlike face, central obesity, dorsocervical adiposity, hypertension, protein breakdown, poor wound healing, muscle wasting, abdominal striae, and osteoporosis. Females also develop hirsutism (Table 36.1). A medication to treat Cushing's disease in patients for whom pituitary surgery is not an option is described in Box 36.2.

BOX 36.2

Cushing's Disease Alternative Therapy

Pasireotide (*Signifor*) is approved for the treatment of adults with Cushing's disease for whom pituitary surgery is not an option or for whom pituitary surgery was not curative. Pasireotide (*Signifor LAR*) is additionally approved for patients with acromegaly who have not had adequate response to surgery, or if surgery is not an option. These drugs are somatostatin analogs. Somatostatin is also known as a growth hormone inhibitor. The drugs bind to somatostatin receptors, causing corticotroph tumor cells from Cushing's disease patients to secrete less ACTH. This lowers release of cortisol from the adrenal gland. *Signifor LAR* has the additional action of binding to somatostatin receptors that inhibit growth hormone secretion in patients with acromegaly. Both medications are injected, and dosing may need to be adjusted for patients with hepatic impairment. There is a risk of hypocortisolism, hyperglycemia and diabetes, bradycardia, and prolonged QT intervals. Liver function impairment and gallstones have also been reported.

Adrenal Insufficiency

Some patients experience a shortage of adrenocortical hormones and develop signs of adrenal insufficiency (see Table 36.1). This can occur when a patient does not produce enough ACTH, when the adrenal glands are not able to respond to ACTH, when an adrenal gland is damaged and cannot produce enough hormones (as in Addison's disease), or secondary to surgical removal of the glands. There is a medication to assist with diagnosis with adrenocortical insufficiency if the diagnosis is unclear (Box 36.3).

Table 36.1 Signs and Symptoms of Adrenal Dysfunction

Clinical Effects	Hypoadrenal Function (Addison's Syndrome)	Hyperadrenal Function (Cushing's Disease)
CNS	Confusion, disorientation	Emotional disturbances
CV system	Hypotension, arrhythmias, CV collapse, loss of extracellular fluid	Cardiac hypertrophy, hypertension
Skin, hair, nails	Hyperpigmentation, sparse axillary and pubic hair, bluish-black oral mucosa	Thin, wrinkled skin; purpura; purple abdominal striae; hirsutism
Metabolic rate	Hyponatremia, hyperkalemia, hypoglycemia, lethargy, fatigue, weakness	Hyperglycemia, hypokalemia, hypernatremia, osteoporosis, renal calculi, amenorrhea
General	Dehydration, fatigue, poor response to stress, limited ability to respond to infection	Moon face, buffalo hump, obesity, immune and inflammatory suppression, risk of gastric ulcers and bleeding

CNS, central nervous system; CV, cardiovascular.

BOX 36.3

Diagnostic Medication for Patients With Presumed Adrenocortical Insufficiency

Cosyntropin is an injected medication that can be used as a diagnostic drug in screening patients who may have adrenocortical insufficiency. It acts as ACTH in the body to stimulate the adrenal cortex. Within an hour after injection of cosyntropin, the plasma cortisol level is tested. A level lower than 18 to 20 mcg/dL suggests that the adrenal cortex was not able to be stimulated and the patient has adrenocortical insufficiency.

A fairly common cause of adrenal insufficiency is prolonged use of corticosteroid hormones. When exogenous corticosteroids are used, they act to negate the regular feedback systems (Fig. 36.1). The adrenal glands begin to atrophy because ACTH release is suppressed by the exogenous hormones, so the glands are no longer stimulated to produce or secrete hormones. It takes several weeks to recover from the atrophy caused by this lack of stimulation. To prevent this from happening, patients who are receiving steroid therapy for more than 10 to 14 days should be weaned slowly from the hormones so that the adrenals have time to recover and start producing hormones again.

Adrenal Crisis

Patients who have an adrenal insufficiency may do quite well until they experience a period of extreme stress, such as a motor vehicle accident, a surgical procedure, or a massive infection. Because they are not able to supplement the energy-consuming effects of the sympathetic reaction, they enter an adrenal crisis, which can include physiological exhaustion, hypotension, fluid shift, shock, and even death. Patients in adrenal crisis are treated with massive infusion of replacement steroids, constant monitoring, and life support procedures.

Key Points

- There are two adrenal glands, one on top of each kidney.
- Each adrenal gland is composed of the adrenal medulla and the adrenal cortex.
- Corticosteroids help the body conserve energy for the fight or flight response and help maintain fluid balance.
- Prolonged use of corticosteroids suppresses the normal hypothalamic–pituitary axis and may lead to adrenal atrophy from lack of stimulation.

Adrenocortical Agents

There are three types of corticosteroids: androgens (discussed in Chapter 41), glucocorticoids, and mineralocorticoids. Not all adrenocortical agents are classified as only glucocorticoids or mineralocorticoids. Hydrocortisone, cortisone, prednisolone, and prednisone have glucocorticoid and some mineralocorticoid activity and affect potassium, sodium, and water levels in the body when present in high levels (Table 36.2). Box 36.4 discusses use of corticosteroids in different age groups. Figure 36.2 displays the sites of action of the glucocorticoids and the mineralocorticoids.

Glucocorticoids

Glucocorticoids (Table 36.3) are so named because they stimulate an increase in glucose levels for energy. They also increase the rate of protein breakdown and decrease the rate of protein formation in most cells. Glucocorticoids

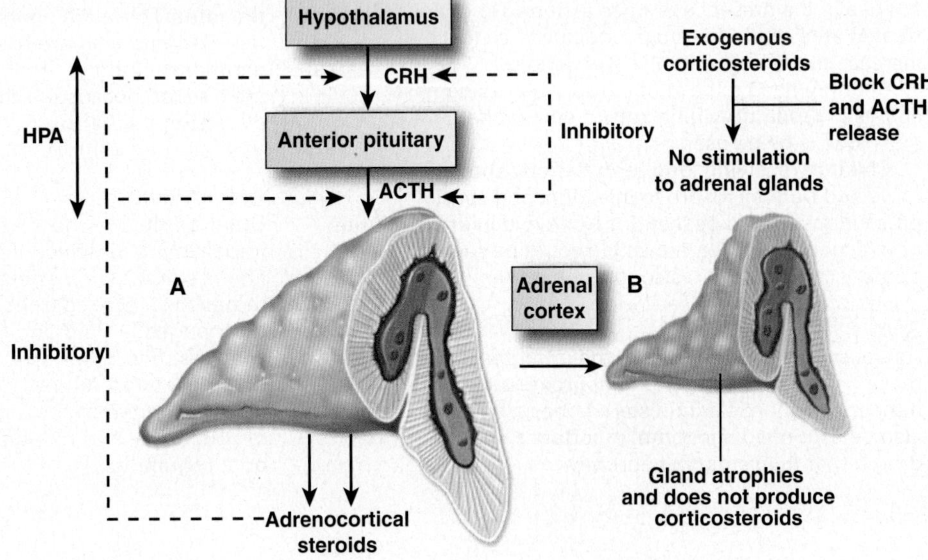

FIGURE 36.1 **A.** Normal controls of the adrenal gland. The hypothalamus releases corticotropin-releasing hormone (CRH), which causes release of corticotropin (ACTH) from the anterior pituitary. ACTH stimulates the adrenal cortex to produce and release corticosteroids. Increasing levels of corticosteroids inhibit the release of CRH and ACTH. **B.** Exogenous corticosteroids act to inhibit CRH and ACTH release; the adrenal cortex is no longer stimulated and atrophies. Sudden stopping of steroids results in a crisis of adrenal hypofunction until hypothalamic–pituitary axis controls stimulate the adrenal gland again.

Table 36.2 Selected Corticosteroids: Equivalent Strength, Glucocorticoid and Mineralocorticoid Effects, and Duration of Effects

Drug	Equivalent Dose (mg)	Duration of Effects (h)
Short-Acting Corticosteroids		
Cortisone	25	8–12
Hydrocortisone	20	8–12
Intermediate-Acting Corticosteroids		
Prednisone	5	18–36
Prednisolone	5	18–36
Triamcinolone	4	18–36
Methylprednisolone	4	18–36
Long-Acting Corticosteroids		
Dexamethasone	0.75	36–54
Betamethasone	0.75	35–54

also cause increased mobilization of fatty acids to be used as energy. With high levels, they are able to suppress the inflammatory response and immune response.

Several glucocorticoids are available for pharmacological use. They differ mainly by route of administration and duration of action. Glucocorticoids include beclomethasone (*Beconase AQ, QNASL, QVAR Redihaler*), betamethasone (*Celestone Soluspan* and others), budesonide (*Rhinocort, Entocort EC, Pulmicort Flexhaler, Pulmicort Respules, Ortikos, Uceris*), cortisone (generic), deflazacort (*Emflaza*), dexamethasone (*Hemady, Maxidex, Ozurdex, Tobradex, Decadron,* and others), flunisolide (generic), hydrocortisone (*Alkindi Sprinkle, Ala-cort, Cortinema, Cortef, Solu-cortef,* and others), methylprednisolone (*Depo-Medrol, Medrol, Solu-Medrol*), prednisolone (*Omnipred, Orapred ODT, Pediapred, Pred Forte, Pred Mild,* and others), prednisone (*Prednisone Intensol, Rayos*), and triamcinolone (*Aristospan, Kenalog, Nasacort Allergy, Triderm, Triesence, Zilretta*).

Therapeutic Actions and Indications

Glucocorticoids enter target cells and bind to cytoplasmic receptors, initiating many complex reactions that are

Box 36.4 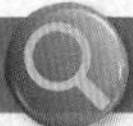 **Focus on Drug Therapy Across the Lifespan**

CORTICOSTEROIDS

Children

Corticosteroids are used in children for the same indications as in adults. The dose for children is determined by the severity of the condition being treated and the response to the drug—not on a weight or age formula.

Children need to be monitored closely for any effects on growth and development, and dose adjustments should be made or the drug discontinued if growth is severely diminished.

Topical use of corticosteroids should be limited in children; because their body surface area is comparatively large, the amount of the drug absorbed in relation to weight is greater than in an adult. Apply sparingly and do not use in the presence of open lesions. Do not occlude treated areas with dressings or diapers, as this may increase the risk of systemic absorption.

Children need to be supervised when using nasal sprays or respiratory inhalants to ensure that proper technique is being used.

Children receiving long-term therapy should be protected from exposure to infection, and special precautions should be instituted to avoid injury. If injuries or infections do occur, the child should be seen by a primary care provider as soon as possible.

Adults

Adults should be reminded of the importance of taking these drugs in the morning to approximate diurnal rhythm if the medication is administered once a day. They should also be cautioned about the importance of tapering the drug rather than stopping abruptly.

Several over-the-counter topical preparations contain corticosteroids, and adults should be cautioned to avoid combining these preparations with prescription topical corticosteroids. They also should be cautioned to apply any of these sparingly and to avoid applying them to open lesions or excoriated areas.

With long-term therapy, the importance of avoiding exposure to infection—crowded areas, people with colds or the flu, activities associated with injury—should be stressed. If an injury or infection should occur, the patient should be encouraged to seek medical care. Monitoring blood glucose levels should be done regularly.

There is caution with using these drugs during pregnancy because some have not been studied in humans, and others have shown potential for harm to the fetus. There are times that the benefit outweighs the risk. Patients who are breast or chestfeeding should find another method of feeding the baby if corticosteroids are needed because of the potential for serious adverse effects on the baby.

Older Adults

Older adults are more likely to have hepatic and/or renal impairment, which could lead to accumulation of drug and resultant toxic effects. They are also more likely to have medical conditions that could be imbalanced by changes in fluid and electrolytes, metabolism changes, and other drug effects. Such conditions include diabetes, heart failure, osteoporosis, coronary artery disease, and immune suppression. Careful monitoring of drug dose and response to the drug should be done on a regular basis.

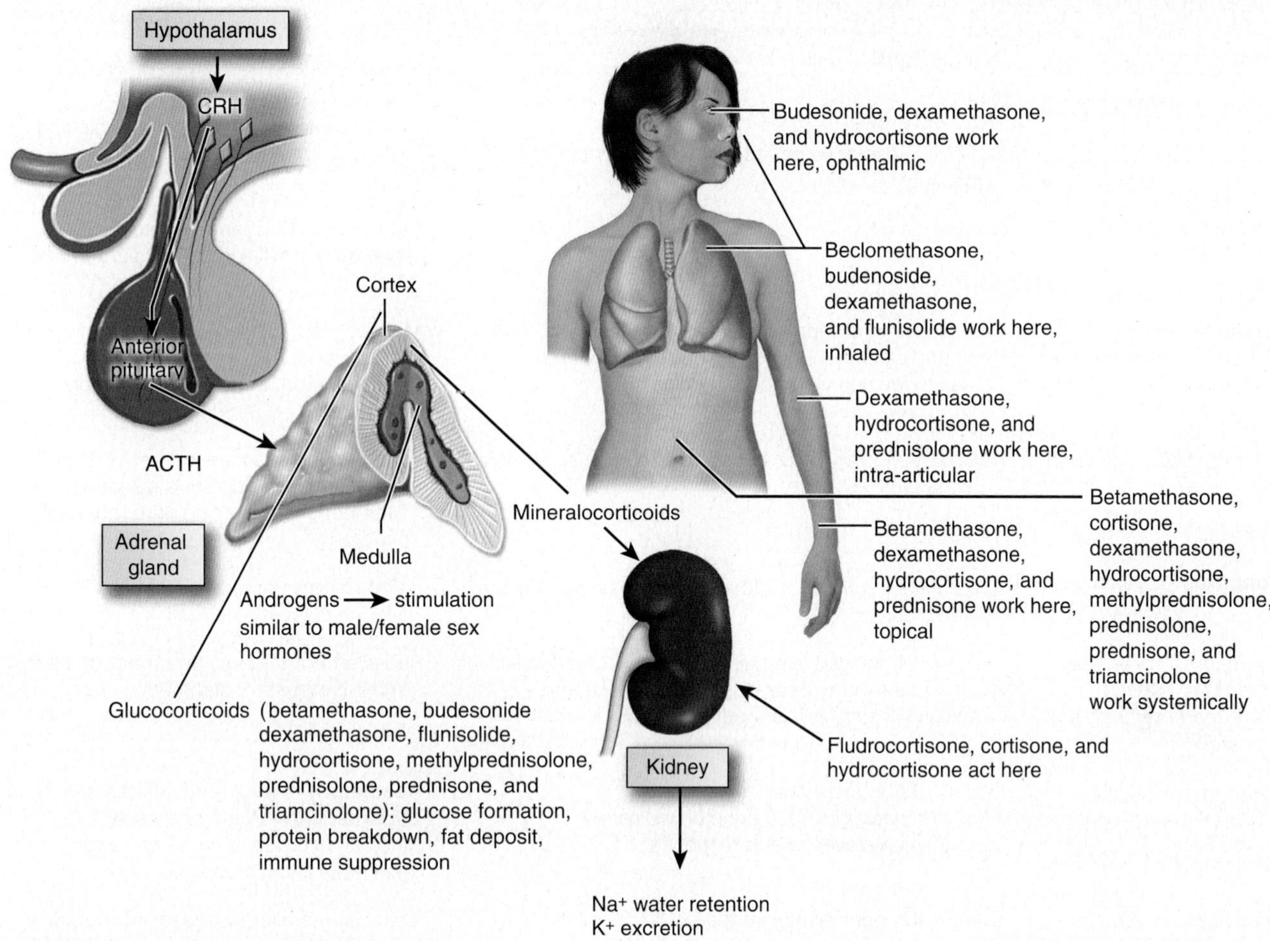

FIGURE 36.2 Sites of action of the adrenocortical agents.

Table 36.3 *Drugs in Focus:* Adrenocortical Agents

Drug Name	Dosage/Route	Usual Indications
Glucocorticoids and Mineralocorticoids		
beclomethasone (*Beconase AQ, QNASL QVAR Redihaler*)	*Beconase AQ and QNASL*: 1–2 intranasal administrations b.i.d. *QVAR Redihaler Adult and pediatric 12 y and older*: 40–320 mcg inhaled b.i.d. (each inhalation 40 or 80 mcg per actuation) *Pediatric 4–11 y*: 40 or 80 mcg inhaled b.i.d.	*Beconase AQ and QNASL*: Seasonal allergic and nonallergic rhinitis, prevention of recurrence of nasal polyps postsurgical removal *QVAR Redihaler*: Maintenance treatment of asthma
betamethasone (*Celestone Soluspan*, and multiple topical formulations)	Oral, IM, IV, intra-articular, topical *Adult and pediatric*: Base dose on indication, severity, response, and formulation	Management of allergic intra-articular, topical, and inflammatory disorders
budesonide (*Rhinocort, Entocort EC, Pulmicort Flexhaler, Pulmicort Respules, Ortikos, Uceris*)	Intranasal, inhalation, rectal *Adult and pediatric*: Base dose on indication, severity, response, and formulation Oral Mild to moderate active Crohn's disease *Adult*: 9 mg once daily for up to 8 wk; repeat 8-wk treatment courses recurring episodes of active disease. *Pediatric 8–17 y, weight >25 kg*: 9 mg once daily for up to 8 wk, followed by 6 mg once daily in the morning for 2 wk Maintenance of clinical remission of mild to moderate Crohn's disease *Adult*: 6 mg once daily for up to 3 mo; taper to complete cessation after 3 mo	Relief of symptoms of seasonal and allergic rhinitis with few side effects, maintenance treatment of asthma, as an oral or rectal agent for the treatment of mild to moderate active Crohn's disease

(continues on page 612)

Table 36.3 *Drugs in Focus*: Adrenocortical Agents (*Continued*)

Drug Name	Dosage/Route	Usual Indications
cortisone (generic)	Oral *Adult*: 25–300 mg/d PO *Pediatric*: Base dose on response; monitor patient closely	Replacement therapy in adrenal insufficiency, treatment of allergic and inflammatory disorders
deflazacort (*Emflaza*)	0.9 mg/kg/d PO	Treatment of Duchenne muscular dystrophy (DMD) in patients 2 y of age and older
dexamethasone (*Hemady, Maxidex, Ozurdex, Tobradex*, and others)	Oral, IV, IM, inhalation, intranasal, ophthalmic, topical *Adult and pediatric*: Base dose on response and severity; dosing will vary per indication	Management of allergic and topical inflammatory disorders, adrenal hypofunction, treatment of multiple myeloma
fludrocortisone (generic)	*Adult*: 0.1–0.2 mg/d PO; base dose on disease severity and patient response	Primary and secondary adrenocortical insufficiency in Addison's disease, treatment of salt-losing adrenogenital syndrome
flunisolide (generic)	*Adult and pediatric*: 50–300 mcg intranasal per day in divided doses	Relief of symptoms of seasonal and allergic rhinitis
hydrocortisone (*Alkindi Sprinkle, Ala-cort, Cortinema, Cortef*, and others)	Oral, IV, IM, topical, ophthalmic, rectal, intra-articular *Adult and pediatric*: Base dose on response and severity; dosing will vary per indication	Replacement therapy, treatment of allergic and inflammatory disorders
methylprednisolone (*Depo-Medrol, Medrol, Solu-Medrol*)	Oral, IV, IM, intra-articular *Adult and pediatric*: Base dose on indication, formulation, severity, and response	Treatment of allergic and inflammatory disorders, treatment of adrenal insufficiency, palliative treatment of leukemia and lymphoma
prednisolone (*Omnipred, Orapred ODT, Pediapred, Pred Forte, Pred Mild*, and others)	Oral, IV, IM, ophthalmic, intra-articular *Adult and pediatric*: Base dose on indication, formulation, severity, and response	Treatment of allergic and inflammatory disorders, treatment of certain endocrine conditions, palliation of certain neoplastic conditions
prednisone (*Prednisone Intensol, Rayos*)	Oral *Adult*: 5 mg/PO daily typical initial dosage and may be tapered for response *Pediatric*: Base dose on severity and response	Replacement therapy for adrenal insufficiency, treatment of allergic and inflammatory disorders, palliation of certain neoplastic conditions
triamcinolone (*Aristospan, Kenalog, Nasacort Allergy, Triderm, Triesence, Zilretta*)	Oral, IM, inhalant, intra-articular, topical *Adult and pediatric*: Base dose on indication, formulation, severity and response	Treatment of allergic and inflammatory disorders, management of asthma; treatment of adrenal insufficiency when combined with a mineralocorticoid; treatment of sympathetic ophthalmia, temporal arteritis, uveitis; visualization during vitrectomy (*Triesence*)

responsible for anti-inflammatory and immunosuppressive effects. Hydrocortisone, cortisone, and prednisone also have some mineralocorticoid activity and affect potassium, sodium, and water levels in the body. They may be used as replacement therapy for adrenal insufficiency.

Glucocorticoids are indicated for the treatment of many inflammatory disorders and to relieve discomfort. They block the actions of arachidonic acid, which leads to a decrease in the formation of prostaglandins and leukotrienes. Without these chemicals, the normal inflammatory reaction is blocked. Due to suppression of eosinophil production, these medications can be helpful with managing allergic reactions. They also impair the ability of phagocytes to leave the bloodstream and move to injured tissues, and they inhibit the ability of lymphocytes to act within the immune system, including a blocking of the production of antibodies. The effect of glucocorticoids on neutrophils is somewhat complex. The white blood cell count often will increase in people treated with glucocorticoids. This could be due to increased mobilization of neutrophils from the bone marrow, and a decrease in the rate that the cells die. However, the increased count does not indicate a greater response to infections or cancer. Due to their suppression of inflammation and the immune response, the glucocorticoid medications can be used in conjunction with other immunosuppressant medications to inhibit transplant rejection. They can be used to treat local inflammation as topical agents, intranasal or inhaled agents, intra-articular injections, and ophthalmic agents. Systemic use is indicated for the treatment of some cancers, hypercalcemia associated with cancer, hematological disorders, and some neurological infections. When combined with mineralocorticoids, some of these drugs can be used in replacement therapy for adrenal insufficiency. See Table 36.3 for information on each type of glucocorticoid agent.

Pharmacokinetics

These drugs are absorbed well from many sites. They are metabolized by natural systems, mostly within the liver, and are excreted in the urine. The glucocorticoids are known to cross the placenta and to enter human milk; they should be used during pregnancy and lactation only if the benefits to the patient clearly outweigh the potential risks to the fetus or neonate.

Beclomethasone is available in the form of a respiratory inhalant and nasal spray. Betamethasone is a long-acting steroid available for systemic, parenteral use in acute situations, as well as orally and as a topical application. Budesonide is available for intranasal, oral, and rectal use. Cortisone is used as oral preparation. Dexamethasone, hydrocortisone, and triamcinolone are available in multiple forms for dermatological, ophthalmological, intra-articular, parenteral, and inhalational uses. Flunisolide is available for intranasal dosing. Methylprednisolone is available in multiple forms, including oral, parenteral, intra-articular, and retention enema preparations. Prednisolone is an intermediate-acting corticosteroid with effects lasting only a day or so. It is used for intraocular and intra-articular injection and is also available in oral and topical forms. Prednisone is available only as an oral agent.

Contraindications and Cautions

These drugs are contraindicated in the presence of any known allergy to any steroid preparation to avoid hypersensitivity reactions.

Caution should be used in the presence of an acute infection not controlled with antibiotics, which could become serious or even fatal if the immune and inflammatory responses are blocked; in patients with diabetes because the glucose-elevating effects disrupt glucose control; with acute peptic ulcers because steroid use is associated with the development of ulcers and perforation; with lactation because the anti-inflammatory and immunosuppressive actions could be passed to the baby; and in pregnancy (especially first trimester) because of the potential for adverse effects on the fetus.

Adverse Effects

Children are at risk for diminished growth associated with suppression of the hypothalamic–pituitary system. Systemic adverse effects include hyperglycemia and retention of sodium and water, causing edema and weight gain, osteoporosis or decreased bone density, peptic ulcer, and infections. Administering glucocorticoids will interrupt the hypothalamic–pituitary axis and may cause adrenal insufficiency, so medications will need to be slowly tapered if they are administered for more than 10 to 14 days. Glucocorticoids have been known to precipitate behavioral and mood disturbances that could include euphoria, insomnia, mood swings, personality changes, severe depression, and psychosis. Additional adverse effects associated with the glucocorticoids are related to the route of administration that is used. Local use is associated with local inflammation and infection, as well as burning and stinging sensations (Box 36.5).

Box 36.5 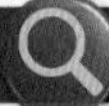 **Focus on Safe Medication Administration**

ADVERSE EFFECTS OF CORTICOSTEROID USE ASSOCIATED WITH VARIOUS ROUTES OF ADMINISTRATION

Systemic: Systemic effects are most likely to occur when the corticosteroid is given by the oral, IV, IM, or subcutaneous route. Systemic absorption is possible, however, if other routes of administration are not used correctly or if tissue breakdown or injury allows direct absorption.

Central nervous system (CNS): Vertigo, headache, paresthesia, insomnia, convulsions, psychosis

Gastrointestinal: Peptic or esophageal ulcers, pancreatitis, abdominal distention, nausea, vomiting, increased appetite, weight gain

Cardiovascular: Hypotension, shock, heart failure secondary to fluid retention, thromboembolism, thrombophlebitis, fat embolism, arrhythmias secondary to electrolyte disturbances

Hematological: Sodium and fluid retention, hypokalemia, hypocalcemia, increased blood sugar, increased serum cholesterol, decreased thyroid hormone levels, increased white blood cell counts

Musculoskeletal: Muscle weakness, steroid myopathy, loss of muscle mass, osteoporosis, spontaneous fractures

Eyes, ears, nose, and throat: Cataracts, glaucoma

Dermatological: Frail skin, petechiae, ecchymoses, purpura, striae, subcutaneous fat atrophy

Endocrine: Amenorrhea, irregular menses, diminished growth, decreased carbohydrate tolerance, diabetes, Cushing's syndrome

Other: Immunosuppression, aggravation or masking of infections, impaired wound healing, suppression of hypothalamic–pituitary axis

Intramuscular repository injections: Atrophy at the injection site

Retention enema: Local pain, burning; rectal bleeding

Intra-articular injection: Osteonecrosis, tendon rupture, infection

Intraspinal: Meningitis, adhesive arachnoiditis, conus medullaris syndrome

Intrathecal administration: Arachnoiditis

Topical: Local burning, irritation, acneiform lesions, striae, skin atrophy

Respiratory inhalant: Oral, laryngeal, and pharyngeal irritation; fungal infections

Intranasal: Headache, nausea, nasal irritation, fungal infections, epistaxis, rebound congestion, perforation of the nasal septum, anosmia, urticaria

Ophthalmic: Infections, glaucoma, cataracts

Intralesional: Blindness when used on the face and head (rare)

Prototype Summary: Prednisone

Indications: Replacement therapy in adrenal cortical insufficiency, management of various inflammatory and allergic disorders, hypercalcemia associated with cancer, hematological disorders, ulcerative colitis, acute exacerbations of multiple sclerosis, palliation in some leukemias, trichinosis with systemic involvement, COPD exacerbations.

Actions: Enters target cells and binds to intracellular corticosteroid receptors, initiating many complex reactions responsible for its anti-inflammatory and immunosuppressive effects.

Pharmacokinetics:

Route	Onset	Peak	Duration
PO	Varies	1–2 h	1–1.5 d

$T_{1/2}$: 3.5 hours; metabolized in the liver and excreted in the urine.

Adverse Effects: Vertigo, headache, hypotension, shock, sodium and fluid retention, amenorrhea, increased appetite, weight gain, immunosuppression, aggravation or masking of infections, impaired wound healing, mood disturbances, delirium.

Clinically Important Drug–Drug Interactions

There are many potential drug–drug interactions to monitor. Concurrent use with NSAIDs or alcohol may increase the risk of GI distress or bleeding. Concurrent use with potassium depleting agents (loop and thiazide diuretics) can cause hypokalemia. Use with vaccines may decrease antibody response. Use with an anticoagulant may change the anticoagulant's effectiveness. Due to multiple potential interactions, it is recommended that interactions be monitored for all patients taking glucocorticoid medications.

Nursing Considerations for Patients Receiving Glucocorticoids

Assessment: History and Examination

- Assess for history of allergy to any steroid preparations, acute infections, peptic ulcer disease or GI bleed, pregnancy, lactation, endocrine disturbances, and renal dysfunction, which could be cautions or contraindications to use of the drug.
- Assess weight; temperature; orientation and affect; grip strength; eye examination; blood pressure, pulse, peripheral perfusion, and vessel evaluation; respiration and adventitious breath sounds; and glucose tolerance, renal function, serum electrolytes, and endocrine function tests as appropriate before beginning therapy to determine baseline status and any potential adverse effects.

Refer to the "Critical Thinking Scenario" for a full discussion of nursing care for a patient who is receiving glucocorticoids.

Nursing Conclusions

Nursing conclusions related to drug therapy might include the following:

- Hypertension risk related to fluid retention
- Fluid overload risk related to water retention
- Altered skin and tissue integrity risk related to decreased protein synthesis
- Infection risk related to immunosuppression
- Ineffective coping related to body changes caused by the drug
- Self-harm risk related to possible mood and cognitive disturbances
- Knowledge deficit regarding drug therapy
- Hyperglycemia risk related to metabolic changes

Planning

- The patient will receive the best therapeutic effect from the drug therapy.
- The patient will have limited adverse effects from the drug therapy.
- The patient will have an understanding of the drug therapy, adverse effects to anticipate, and measures to relieve discomfort and improve safety.

Intervention With Rationale

- If using once-a-day dosing, administer the drug in the morning to mimic normal peak diurnal concentration levels and thereby minimize suppression of the hypothalamic–pituitary axis.
- Space multiple doses evenly throughout the day to try to achieve homeostasis.
- Use the minimal dose for the minimal amount of time to minimize adverse effects.
- Taper doses when discontinuing from high doses or from long-term therapy to give the adrenal glands a chance to recover and produce adrenocorticoids.
- If the patient is taking the drug for an extended period of time, arrange for an increased dose when the patient is under stress to supply the increased demand for corticosteroids associated with the stress reaction.
- Do not give live virus vaccines when the patient is immunosuppressed because there is an increased risk of infection.
- Protect the patient from unnecessary exposure to infection and invasive procedures because the steroids suppress the immune system and the patient is at increased risk for infection.
- Assess the patient carefully for any potential drug–drug interactions to avoid adverse effects.
- Provide thorough patient teaching, including measures to avoid adverse effects, warning signs of problems, and the need for regular evaluation, including blood tests, to enhance patient knowledge of drug therapy and

promote adherence. Explain the need to protect the patient from exposure to infections to prevent serious adverse effects.

Evaluation

- Monitor patient response to the drug (relief of signs and symptoms of inflammation, return of adrenal function to within normal limits).
- Monitor for adverse effects (increased susceptibility to infections, skin changes, endocrine dysfunctions, fatigue, fluid retention, peptic ulcer, psychological changes).
- Evaluate the effectiveness of the teaching plan (patient can name drug, dosage, adverse effects to watch for, and specific measures to avoid them).

CRITICAL THINKING SCENARIO
Adrenocortical Agents

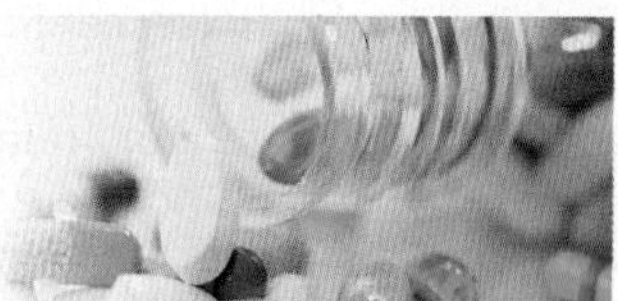

THE SITUATION

M.W., who is 48 years old, was diagnosed with severe rheumatoid arthritis 7 years ago. M.W. has been retired on disability from a job as an art teacher at the local high school. M.W.'s pain was no longer controlled by aspirin or NSAIDs, and their physician ordered 5-mg prednisone three times a day. Over the next 4 weeks, M.W.'s symptoms were markedly relieved; they were able to start painting again, and they became much more mobile. M.W. also noted that for the first time in years they felt "really good." M.W.'s appetite increased, they were no longer fatigued, and their outlook on life was markedly improved. At their follow-up visit, M.W. had gained 9 lb; they had slight edema in both ankles, and their blood pressure was 150/92 mmHg. An inflamed, oozing lesion was found on M.W.'s right hand, which they stated became infected after cutting their hand while peeling potatoes a few weeks ago. M.W.'s range of motion and joints were markedly improved. The physician decided that M.W. was past the crisis and that the prednisone should be tapered to 5 mg/d over a 4-week period.

CRITICAL THINKING

Think about the pathophysiology of rheumatoid arthritis.

What effects did the prednisone have on the process at work in M.W.'s joints?

What effects does the adrenocorticoid steroid have on the rest of M.W.'s body?

What can be expected to occur when a patient is on prednisone for a month?

What precautions should be taken?

What nursing interventions are appropriate for M.W. at this visit?

DISCUSSION

The most urgent problem for M.W. at this time is the infected lesion on their hand. Because steroids interfere with the normal inflammatory and immune response to infection, the lesion could progress to a serious problem. The lesion should be cultured, cleansed, and dressed. M.W. should be instructed in how to care for their hand and how to protect it from water or further injury. An antibiotic might be prescribed and then evaluated for its appropriateness when the culture report comes back.

The real nursing challenge with M.W. will be helping them cope with and understand the need to taper the prednisone. The drug teaching information for prednisone should be thoroughly reviewed with M.W., pointing out the side effects of drug therapy that they are already experiencing (weight gain, hypertension, edema, decreased ability to fight off infection) and explaining again the effect that prednisone has on their body. M.W. may be more eager to start the taper once they are reminded about the effects of weight gain and swelling that they have been experiencing on the medication. A calendar should be prepared for M.W. to help them schedule the tapering of the drug. It usually progresses from 5 mg twice daily for 2 weeks to 5 mg/d. M.W. will need a great deal of encouragement and support to cope with the decrease in therapeutic benefit caused by the need to reduce the prednisone dose. M.W. has felt so good and done so much better while receiving the drug that they may have a real dread of losing those benefits. M.W. should be encouraged to discuss their feelings and to call for support if needed. It is also important to discuss with M.W. nonpharmaceutical pain control strategies (gentle massage, alternating heat and cold, range-of-motion activities) that may help as they are weaning off the prednisone. M.W. should also be encouraged to call their provider if the pain increases and they would like to request pharmaceutical pain control options. M.W. should be given an appointment for a return visit in 2 weeks to evaluate the lesion on their hand and to check the progress of the tapering of the drug. M.W. should be urged to call if the lesion looks worse to them or if they have any difficulties with the drug therapy.

M.W.'s case is a common example of the clinical problems that are encountered when a patient with a chronic inflammatory condition begins steroid therapy. These patients require strong nursing support and continual teaching.

(continues on page 616)

NURSING CARE GUIDE FOR M.W.: ADRENOCORTICAL AGENTS

Assessment: History and Examination

Assess for any potential medication interactions and allergies to any steroids and for heart failure, pregnancy, hypertension, acute infection, peptic ulcer, vaccination with a live virus, or endocrine disorders (including diabetes mellitus).

Focus the physical examination on the following:

Neurological: Orientation, reflexes, affect

General: Temperature, weight, site of hand infection

Cardiovascular: Pulse, cardiac auscultation, blood pressure, edema

Respiratory: Respiratory rate, adventitious sounds

Laboratory tests: Urinalysis, blood glucose level, stool guaiac test, renal function tests, culture and sensitivity of wound specimen

Nursing Conclusions

Hypertension risk related to fluid retention

Fluid overload risk related to water retention

Altered skin and tissue integrity risk related to decreased protein synthesis

Infection risk related to immunosuppression

Ineffective coping related to body changes caused by the drug

Knowledge deficit regarding drug therapy

Hyperglycemia risk related to metabolic changes

Planning

The patient will receive the best therapeutic effect from the drug therapy.

The patient will have limited adverse effects from the drug therapy.

The patient will have an understanding of the drug therapy, adverse effects to anticipate, and measures to relieve discomfort and improve safety.

Intervention

Use the minimal dose for the minimal period of time that the dose is needed.

Arrange for increased doses during times of stress.

Taper gradually to allow adrenal glands to recover and produce their own steroids.

Protect the patient from unnecessary exposure to infection.

Provide support and reassurance to deal with drug therapy.

Provide patient teaching regarding drug name, dosage, adverse effects, precautions, and warning signs to report.

Evaluation

Evaluate drug effects: relief of signs and symptoms of inflammation.

Monitor for adverse effects: infection, peptic ulcer, fluid retention, hypertension, electrolyte imbalance, or endocrine changes.

Monitor for drug–drug interactions as listed.

Evaluate the effectiveness of the patient teaching program.

Evaluate the effectiveness of comfort and safety measures and support offered.

PATIENT TEACHING FOR M.W.

- The drug that has been prescribed for you is called prednisone. Prednisone is from a class of drugs called corticosteroids, which are similar to steroids produced naturally in your body. They affect a number of bodily functions, including increasing your body's glucose levels, blocking your body's inflammatory and immune responses, and slowing the healing process.
- It is best to slowly decrease this medication so that your body can adjust and begin to make its own steroids. You can take 5 mg twice a day for the next couple of weeks. Your provider will check in with you to see how you are doing with the decrease in the medication.
- Some of the following adverse effects may continue and/or occur:
  - *Increased appetite*: This may be a welcome change, but if you notice a continual weight gain, you may want to watch your calories.
  - *Restlessness, trouble sleeping*: Some people experience elation and a feeling of new energy; take frequent rest periods.
  - *Increased susceptibility to infection and decreased wound healing*: Your body's normal defenses will be decreased. If you notice any signs of illness or worsening infection, notify your health care provider at once.
  - Report any of the following to your health care provider: sudden weight gain; fever or sore throat; black, tarry stools; swelling of the hands or feet; any signs of infection; or easy bruising.
- If you are taking this drug for a prolonged period, limit your intake of salt and salted products and add proteins to your diet.
- Avoid the use of any over-the-counter medication without first checking with your health care provider. Several of these medications can interfere with the effectiveness of this drug.
- Tell any doctor, nurse, or other health care provider involved in your care that you are taking this drug.
- Because this drug affects your body's natural defenses, you will need special care during any stressful situations. You may want to wear or carry medical identification showing that you are taking this medication. This identification alerts any medical personnel taking care of you in an emergency to the fact that you are taking this drug.
- It is important to have regular medical follow-up. If your drug dose is being tapered, notify your health care provider if any of the following occurs: fatigue, nausea, vomiting, diarrhea, weight loss, weakness, or dizziness.
- Keep this drug out of the reach of children. Do not give this medication to anyone else or take any similar medication that has not been prescribed for you.

Key Points

- The glucocorticoids increase glucose production, stimulate fat acid mobilization and protein breakdown, and inhibit protein formation. They are used clinically to block inflammation and the immune response and in conjunction with mineralocorticoids to treat adrenal insufficiency.
- Patients receiving glucocorticoids need to be protected from exposure to infection, have their blood sugar monitored regularly and dietary changes made as needed, and will not heal as quickly due to decreased cellular protein synthesis.

Mineralocorticoids

Mineralocorticoids (see Table 36.3) affect electrolyte levels and homeostasis. These steroid hormones directly affect the levels of electrolytes in the system. The mineralocorticoid secreted by the adrenal gland is aldosterone. Aldosterone causes the retention of sodium—and with it, water—in the body and causes the excretion of potassium by acting on the renal tubule. Aldosterone is no longer available for pharmacological use. Mineralocorticoids that are available include cortisone (generic), fludrocortisone (generic), hydrocortisone (*Alkindi Sprinkle*, *Ala-cort*, *Cortinema*, *Cortef*, and others), prednisolone (*Omnipred*, *Pred Forte*, and others), and prednisone (*Rayos*). These medications have glucocorticoid properties as well.

Therapeutic Actions and Indications

The mineralocorticoids increase sodium reabsorption in renal tubules, leading to sodium and water retention, and increase potassium excretion (see Fig. 36.2). Fludrocortisone is a potent mineralocorticoid and is preferred for replacement therapy over cortisone and hydrocortisone; it is used in combination with a glucocorticoid. Hydrocortisone and cortisone also exert mineralocorticoid effects at high doses; however, this effect usually is not enough to maintain electrolyte balance in adrenal insufficiency. These drugs are indicated (in combination with a glucocorticoid) for replacement therapy in primary and secondary adrenal insufficiency. They are also indicated for the treatment of salt-wasting adrenogenital syndrome when taken with appropriate glucocorticoids. See Table 36.3 for usual indications for each mineralocorticoid.

Pharmacokinetics

These drugs are absorbed slowly and distributed throughout the body. They undergo hepatic metabolism to inactive forms. They are known to cross the placenta and to enter human milk. They should be avoided during pregnancy and lactation because of the potential for adverse effects in the fetus or baby.

Contraindications and Cautions

These drugs are contraindicated in the presence of any known allergy to the drug to avoid hypersensitivity reactions. Caution is necessary in administering to people with severe hypertension, heart failure, or cardiac disease because of the resultant increased blood pressure. Caution should be used in pregnancy and during lactation due to potential adverse effects on the fetus or baby. Caution should be taken with high sodium intake because severe hypernatremia could occur. With the mineralocorticoid medications that also have glucocorticoid properties, caution should be taken in the presence of any systemic infection, which can be exacerbated due to suppression of the inflammation and immune responses.

Adverse Effects

Adverse effects commonly associated with the use of mineralocorticoids are related to the increased fluid volume seen with sodium and water retention (e.g., headache, edema, hypertension, heart failure, arrhythmias, weakness) and possible hypokalemia (Fig. 36.3). Allergic reactions, ranging from skin rash to anaphylaxis, have also been reported.

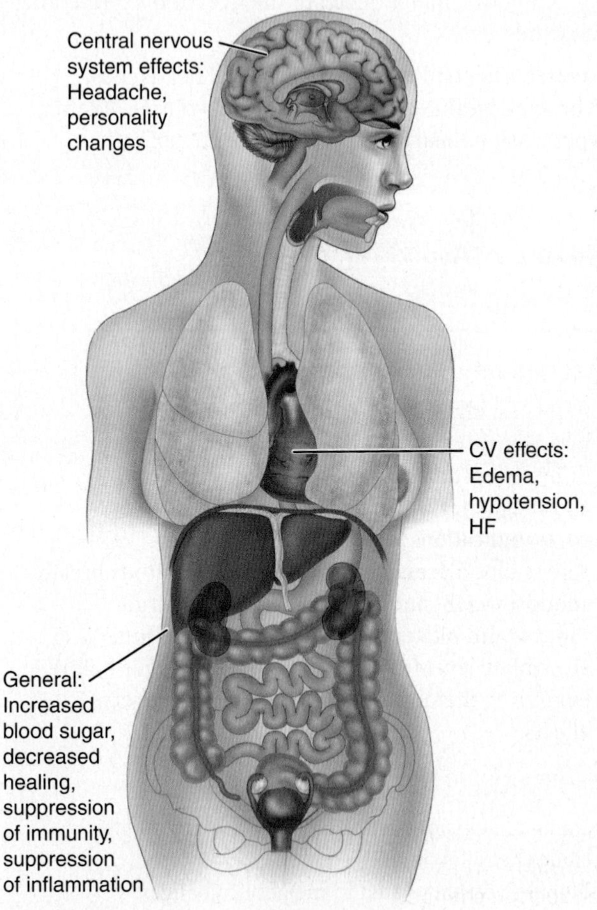

FIGURE 36.3 Variety of adverse effects and toxicities associated with adrenocortical agents.

Clinically Important Drug–Drug Interactions

When mineralocorticoids are combined with barbiturates, phenytoin, or rifampin, effectiveness may be decreased due to faster metabolic clearance. Decreased effectiveness of antidiabetic medications has been reported when these drugs are combined with mineralocorticoids. Multiple other interactions may occur. Patients should be monitored closely when being treated with mineralocorticoids, and dose titrations should be based on individual responses.

Prototype Summary: Fludrocortisone

Indications: Partial replacement therapy in cortical insufficiency conditions, treatment of salt-losing adrenogenital syndrome; off-label use: treatment of hypotension.

Actions: Increases sodium reabsorption in the renal tubules and increases potassium and hydrogen excretion, leading to water and sodium retention.

Pharmacokinetics:

Route	Onset	Peak	Duration
PO	Gradual	1.7 h	18–36 h

$T_{1/2}$: 3.5 hours; metabolized in the liver and excreted in the urine.

Adverse Effects: Frontal and occipital headaches, arthralgia, weakness, increased blood volume, edema, hypertension, heart failure, rash, anaphylaxis.

Nursing Considerations for Patients Receiving Mineralocorticoids

Assessment: History and Examination

- Assess for allergy to these drugs to avoid hypersensitivity reactions; history of heart failure or hypertension, high sodium intake, lactation, and pregnancy, which could be cautions or contraindications to use of the drug.
- Assess blood pressure, pulse, and adventitious breath sounds; weight and temperature; tissue turgor; reflexes and bilateral grip strength; and serum electrolyte levels to determine baseline status before beginning therapy and for any potential adverse effects.

Nursing Conclusions

Nursing conclusions related to drug therapy might include the following:

- Hyperglycemia related to metabolic changes
- Fluid overload risk related to sodium retention
- Urinary retention risk related to sodium retention
- Knowledge deficit regarding drug therapy

Planning

- The patient will receive the best therapeutic effect from the drug therapy.
- The patient will have limited adverse effects from the drug therapy.
- The patient will have an understanding of the drug therapy, adverse effects to anticipate, and measures to relieve discomfort and improve safety.

Intervention With Rationale

- Increase dose in times of stress to prevent adrenal insufficiency and to meet increased demands for corticosteroids under stress.
- Monitor for hypokalemia (weakness, serum electrolytes) to detect the loss early and treat appropriately.
- Discontinue if signs of overdose (excessive weight gain, edema, hypertension, cardiomegaly) occur to prevent the development of more severe toxicity.
- Provide thorough patient teaching, including drug name, dosage, and administration; measures to avoid adverse effects; warning signs of problems; and the need for regular evaluation, including blood tests, to enhance patient knowledge about drug therapy and promote adherence.

Evaluation

- Monitor patient response to the drug (maintenance of electrolyte balance).
- Monitor for adverse effects (fluid retention, edema, hypokalemia, headache).
- Evaluate the effectiveness of the teaching plan (patient can name drug, dosage, adverse effects to watch for, and specific measures to avoid them).
- Monitor effectiveness of comfort measures and adherence to the regimen.

Key Points

- The mineralocorticoids stimulate retention of sodium and water and excretion of potassium. They are used therapeutically in conjunction with glucocorticoids to treat adrenal insufficiency.
- Patients receiving mineralocorticoids need to be evaluated for possible hypokalemia and its associated cardiac effects and for fluid retention that could exacerbate heart failure and cause electrolyte abnormalities.

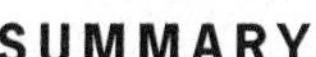

SUMMARY

- The adrenal medulla acts similarly to a sympathetic nerve ganglion; it releases norepinephrine and epinephrine into the bloodstream in response to sympathetic stimulation.
- The adrenal cortex produces three types of corticosteroids: androgens (similar to male sex hormones), glucocorticoids, and mineralocorticoids.
- The corticosteroids are released normally in a diurnal rhythm, with the hypothalamus producing a peak level of CRH around midnight; peak adrenal response occurs around 9 a.m. The steroid levels drop slowly during the day to reach low levels in the evening when the hypothalamus begins CRH secretion with a peak level again occurring around midnight. Corticosteroids are also released as part of the sympathetic stress reaction to help the body conserve energy for the fight or flight response.
- Prolonged use of corticosteroids suppresses the normal hypothalamic–pituitary axis and leads to adrenal atrophy from lack of stimulation. Corticosteroids need to be tapered slowly after prolonged use to allow the adrenals to resume steroid production.
- The glucocorticoids increase glucose production, stimulate fat deposition and protein breakdown, and inhibit protein formation. They are used clinically to block inflammation and the immune response and in conjunction with mineralocorticoids to treat adrenal insufficiency.
- The mineralocorticoids stimulate retention of sodium and water and excretion of potassium. They are used therapeutically in conjunction with glucocorticoids to treat adrenal insufficiency.
- Adverse effects of corticosteroids are related to exaggeration of the physiological effects; they include immunosuppression, peptic ulcer formation, fluid retention, and edema.
- Corticosteroids are used topically and locally to achieve the desired anti-inflammatory effects at a particular site without the systemic adverse effects that limit the usefulness of these drugs.

CHECK YOUR UNDERSTANDING

Answers to the questions in this chapter can be found in Answers to Check Your Understanding Questions on thePoint®.

MULTIPLE CHOICE

Select the best answer.

1. Adrenocortical agents are widely used
   a. to cure chronic inflammatory disorders.
   b. for treatment to relieve moderate to severe inflammation.
   c. for long-term treatment of chronic infections.
   d. to relieve minor aches and pains and to make people feel better.

2. If a nurse is asked to explain the adrenal medulla to a patient, it would be appropriate for them to tell that patient that it
   a. is the outer core of the adrenal gland.
   b. is the site of production of aldosterone and corticosteroids.
   c. secretes substances that enhance the stress response.
   d. consists of three layers of cells that produce different hormones.

3. Glucocorticoids are hormones that
   a. are released in response to high glucose levels.
   b. help regulate electrolyte levels.
   c. help regulate water balance in the body.
   d. promote the preservation of energy through increased glucose levels, protein breakdown, and fatty acid mobilization.

4. Diurnal rhythm in a person with a regular sleep cycle would show
   a. high levels of ACTH during the night while sleeping.
   b. rising levels of corticosteroids throughout the day.
   c. peak levels of ACTH and corticosteroids early in the morning.
   d. hypothalamic stimulation to release CRH around noon.

5. Patients who have been receiving corticosteroid therapy for a prolonged period and suddenly stop the drug may experience an adrenal crisis because their adrenal glands will not be producing any adrenal hormones. Your assessment of a patient for the possibility of adrenal crisis may include
   a. physiological exhaustion, shock, and fluid shift.
   b. acne development and hypertension.
   c. water retention and increased speed of healing.
   d. hyperglycemia and water retention.

6. A patient is started on a regimen of prednisone because of a crisis in their ulcerative colitis. Nursing care of this patient would need to include
   a. immunizations to prevent infections.
   b. increased calories to deal with metabolic changes.
   c. fluid restriction to decrease water retention.
   d. teaching regarding the common side effects of weight gain and hyperglycemia.

7. A patient who is taking corticosteroids is at increased risk for infection and should
   a. be protected from exposure to infections and invasive procedures.
   b. take anti-inflammatory agents regularly throughout the day.
   c. receive live virus vaccines to protect them from infection.
   d. be at no risk if elective surgery is needed.

8. Mineralocorticoids are used to maintain electrolyte balance in situations of adrenal insufficiency, and they are
   a. usually given alone.
   b. given only IV.
   c. always given in conjunction with appropriate glucocorticoids.
   d. separate in their function from the glucocorticoids.

MULTIPLE RESPONSE

Select all that apply.

1. Patients who are taking corticosteroids would be expected to report which findings?
   a. Weight gain
   b. Round or "moon face" appearance
   c. Feeling of well-being
   d. Weight loss
   e. Excessive hair growth
   f. Fragile skin

2. Corticosteroid hormones are released during a sympathetic stress reaction. They would cause which actions?
   a. Increased blood volume
   b. Release of glucose for energy
   c. Increased rate of protein production
   d. Blocked effects of the inflammatory and immune systems
   e. Storage of glucose to preserve energy
   f. Blocked protein production to save energy

REFERENCES

Andrews, M., & Boyle, J. (2012). *Transcultural concepts in nursing care* (6th ed.). Lippincott Williams & Wilkins.

Brunton, L., Hilal-Dandan, R., & Knollman, B. (2018). *Goodman and Gilman's the pharmacological basis of therapeutics* (13th ed.). McGraw-Hill.

Chung, S., Son, G. H., & Kim, K. (2011). Circadian rhythm of adrenal glucocorticoid: Its regulation and clinical implications. *Biochimica et Biophysica Acta, 1812*, 581–591. 10.1016/j.bbadis.2011.02.003

Goulding, N., & Flower, R. (Eds.). (2013). *Glucocorticoids, milestones in drug therapy*. Birkhauser.

Hall, J. E., & Hall, M. E. (2021). *Guyton and Hall's textbook of medical physiology* (14th ed.). Saunders.

Kasiske, L. B., Snyder, J. J., Gilbertson, D., & Matas, A. J. (2003). Diabetes mellitus after kidney transplantation in the United States. *American Journal of Transplantation, 3*(2), 178–185. 10.1034/j.1600-6143.2003.00010.x

Lavin, N. (2009). *Manual of endocrinology and metabolism*. Lippincott Williams & Wilkins.

Linos, D. A., & van Heerden, J. A. (2011). *Adrenal glands, diagnostic aspects and surgical therapy*. Springer.

Melmed, S., Polonsky, K., Larson, P. R., & Kronenberg, H. (2011). *Williams textbook of endocrinology* (12th ed.). Saunders.

Norris, T. L. (2019). *Porth's pathophysiology concepts of altered health states* (13th ed.). Wolters Kluwer.

Ronchetti, S., Ricci, E., Migliorati, G., Gentili, M., & Riccardi, C. (2018). How glucocorticoids affect the neutrophil life. *International Journal of Molecular Sciences, 19*(1), 4090. 10.3390/ijms19124090

CHAPTER 37

Thyroid and Parathyroid Agents

Learning Objectives

Upon completion of this chapter, you will be able to:

1. Explain the control of synthesis and secretion of thyroid hormones and parathyroid hormones.
2. Discuss the use of thyroid and parathyroid drugs across the lifespan.
3. Describe the therapeutic actions, indications, pharmacokinetics, contraindications, most common adverse effects, and important drug–drug interactions associated with thyroid and parathyroid agents.
4. Compare and contrast thyroid and parathyroid prototype drugs with agents in their classes.
5. Outline nursing considerations, including important teaching points, for patients receiving drugs used to affect thyroid or parathyroid functions.

Key Terms

bisphosphonates: drugs used to block bone resorption and lower serum calcium levels in several conditions

calcitonin: hormone produced by the parafollicular cells of the thyroid; counteracts the effects of parathyroid hormone to maintain calcium levels

follicle: structural unit of the thyroid gland; cells arranged in a circle

hypercalcemia: excessive calcium levels in the blood

hyperparathyroidism: excessive parathormone

hyperthyroidism: excessive thyroid hormone

hypocalcemia: calcium deficiency

hypoparathyroidism: rare condition of absence of parathormone; may be seen after thyroidectomy

hypothyroidism: lack of sufficient thyroid hormone to maintain normal metabolism

iodine: important dietary element used by the thyroid gland to produce thyroid hormone

metabolism: rate at which the cells burn energy

myxedema: severe lack of thyroid hormone in adults causing hypometabolic rate and accumulation of nonpitting edema in connective tissues throughout the body

Paget's disease: genetically linked disorder of overactive osteoclasts that are eventually replaced by enlarged and softened bony structures

parathormone: hormone produced by the parathyroid glands; responsible for maintaining calcium levels in conjunction with calcitonin

postmenopausal osteoporosis: condition in which dropping levels of estrogen allow calcium to be pulled out of the bone, resulting in a weakened and honeycombed bone structure

thioamides: drugs used to prevent the formation of thyroid hormone in the thyroid cells, lowering thyroid hormone levels

thyroxine: thyroid hormone that is converted to triiodothyronine in the tissues; it has a half-life of 1 week

Drug List

THYROID AGENTS

Thyroid Hormones

- (P) levothyroxine
- liothyronine
- liotrix
- thyroid desiccated

ANTITHYROID AGENTS

Thioamides

- (P) methimazole
- propylthiouracil

Iodine Solutions

- sodium iodide I^{131}
- (P) strong iodine solution
- potassium iodide

PARATHYROID AGENTS

Antihypocalcemic Agents

- abaloparatide
- (P) calcitriol
- parathyroid hormone
- teriparatide

Antihypercalcemic Agents

Bisphosphonates

- (P) alendronate
- etidronate
- ibandronate
- pamidronate
- risedronate
- zoledronic acid

Calcitonins

- (P) calcitonin salmon

This chapter reviews drugs that are used to affect the function of the thyroid and parathyroid glands. These two glands are closely situated in the middle of the neck and share a common goal of calcium homeostasis. Serum calcium levels need to be maintained within a narrow range to promote effective blood coagulation, as well as nerve and muscle function. In most respects, however, these glands are different in structure and function.

The Thyroid Gland

The thyroid gland is located in the middle of the neck, where it surrounds the trachea like a shield (Fig. 37.1). Its name comes from the Greek words *thyros* (shield) and *eidos* (gland). It produces thyroid hormones (triiodothyronine—T_3 and thyroxine—T_4) and calcitonin.

Structure and Function

The thyroid is a vascular gland with two lobes—one on each side of the trachea—and a small isthmus connecting the lobes. The gland is made up of cells arranged in circular **follicles**. The center of each follicle is composed of colloid tissue in which the thyroid hormones produced by the gland are stored. Cells found around the follicle of the thyroid gland are called parafollicular cells (see Fig. 37.1). These cells produce another hormone, **calcitonin**, which affects calcium levels and acts to balance the effects of the parathyroid hormone (PTH), **parathormone**. Calcitonin will be discussed later in connection with the parathyroid glands.

Using iodine that is found in the diet, the thyroid gland produces two slightly different thyroid hormones: **thyroxine**, or tetraiodothyronine (T_4), so named because it contains four iodine atoms, which is given therapeutically in the synthetic form levothyroxine, and triiodothyronine (T_3), so named because it contains three iodine atoms, which is given in the synthetic form liothyronine. The thyroid cells remove iodine from the blood, concentrate it, and prepare it for attachment to tyrosine, an amino acid. A person must obtain sufficient amounts of dietary iodine to produce thyroid hormones. Thyroid hormone regulates the rate of **metabolism**—that is, the rate at which energy is burned—in almost all the cells of the body. The thyroid hormones affect heat production and body temperature; oxygen consumption and cardiac output; blood volume; enzyme system activity; and metabolism of carbohydrates, fats, and proteins. Thyroid hormone is also an important regulator of growth and development, especially within the reproductive and nervous systems. Because the thyroid has such widespread effects throughout the body, any dysfunction of the thyroid gland will have numerous systemic effects.

When thyroid hormone is needed in the body, the stored thyroid hormone molecule is absorbed into the thyroid cells, where the T_3 and T_4 are released into circulation. These hormones are carried on plasma proteins, which can

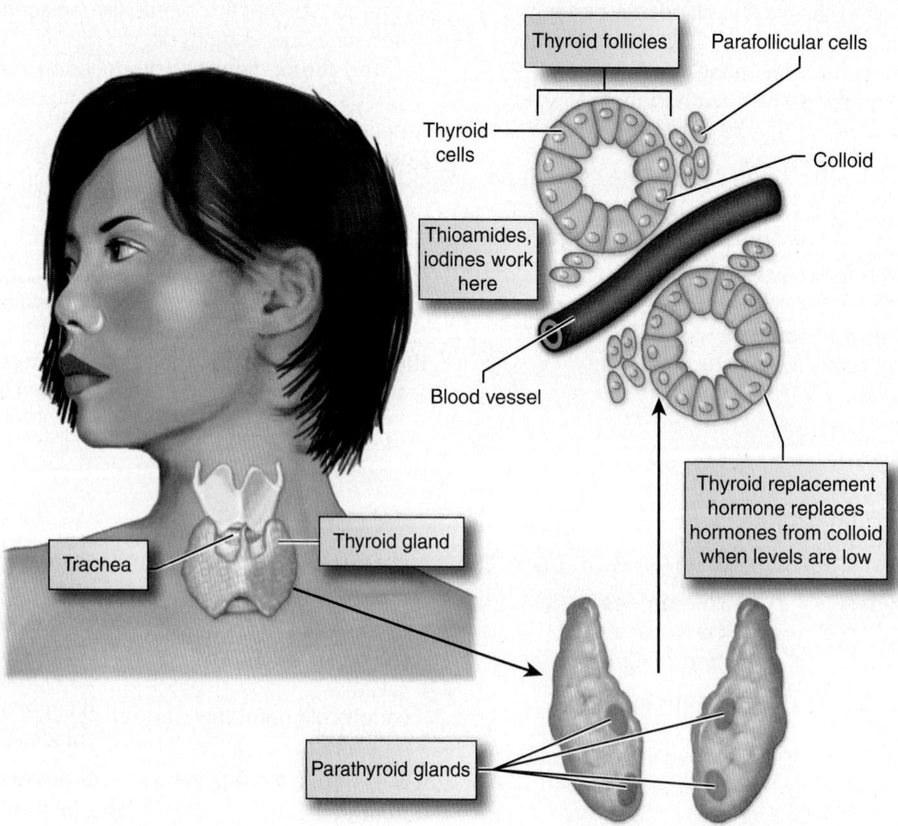

FIGURE 37.1 The thyroid and parathyroid glands. The basic unit of the thyroid gland is the follicle.

be measured as protein-bound iodine levels. The thyroid gland produces more T_4 than T_3. More T_4 is released into circulation, but T_3 is approximately four times more active than T_4. However, T_4 has a longer half-life in the blood and can be converted to T_3 when needed.

Control

Thyroid hormone production and release are regulated by the anterior pituitary hormone called thyroid-stimulating hormone (TSH). The secretion of TSH is regulated by thyrotropin-releasing hormone (TRH), a hypothalamic regulating factor. A delicate balance exists among the thyroid, the pituitary, and the hypothalamus in regulating the level of thyroid hormone. See Chapter 34 for a review of the negative feedback system and the hypothalamic–pituitary axis. The thyroid gland produces increased thyroid hormones in response to increased levels of TSH. The increased levels of thyroid hormones send a negative feedback message to the pituitary to decrease TSH release and, at the same time, to the hypothalamus to decrease TRH release. A drop in TRH levels subsequently results in a drop in TSH levels, which in turn leads to a drop in thyroid hormone levels. In response to low blood serum levels of thyroid hormone, the hypothalamus sends TRH to the anterior pituitary, which responds by releasing TSH, which in turn stimulates the thyroid gland to again produce and release thyroid hormone. The rising level of thyroid hormone is sensed by the hypothalamus, and the cycle begins again. This intricate series of negative feedback mechanisms keeps the level of thyroid hormone within a narrow range of normal (Fig. 37.2).

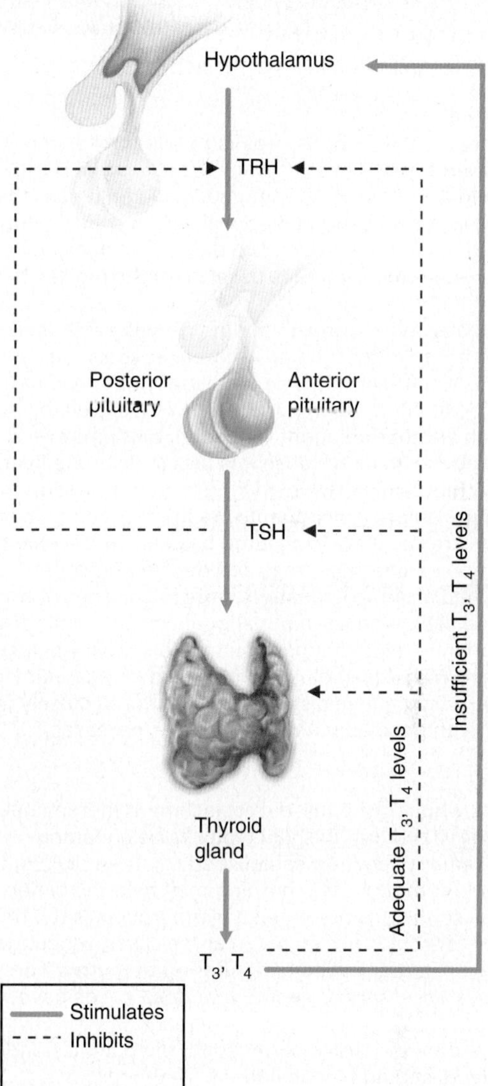

FIGURE 37.2 In response to low blood serum levels of thyroid hormone, the hypothalamus sends thyrotropin-releasing hormone (TRH) to the anterior pituitary, which responds by releasing thyroid-stimulating hormone (TSH) to the thyroid gland; it, in turn, responds by releasing thyroid hormone (T_3 and T_4) into the bloodstream. The anterior pituitary is also sensitive to the increase in blood serum levels of the thyroid hormone and responds by decreasing production and release of TSH. As thyroid hormone production and release subside, the hypothalamus senses the lower serum levels, and the process is repeated by the release of TRH again. This intricate series of negative feedback mechanisms keeps the level of thyroid hormone within normal limits.

Thyroid Dysfunction

Thyroid dysfunction involves either underactivity (hypothyroidism) or overactivity (hyperthyroidism). This dysfunction can affect any age group. Box 37.1 explains the use of thyroid agents across the lifespan.

Hypothyroidism

Hypothyroidism is a lack of sufficient levels of thyroid hormones to maintain normal metabolism. This condition occurs in a number of pathophysiological states:

- Absence of the thyroid gland
- Lack of sufficient iodine in the diet to produce the needed level of thyroid hormone
- Lack of sufficient functioning thyroid tissue due to tumor or autoimmune disorder
- Lack of TSH due to pituitary disease
- Lack of TRH related to a tumor or disorder of the hypothalamus

Hypothyroidism is the most common type of thyroid dysfunction. It is estimated that approximately 5% to 10% of females older than 50 years of age have hypothyroidism. Hypothyroidism is also a common finding in older adult males. The symptoms of hypothyroidism can be varied and vague, such as obesity and fatigue, and are frequently overlooked or mistaken for signs of normal aging (Table 37.1).

Children who are born without a thyroid gland or who have a nonfunctioning gland develop a condition called congenital hypothyroidism. If untreated, these children will experience poor growth and development and cognitive impairment because of the lack of thyroid hormone stimulation.

Box 37.1 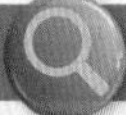 **Focus on Drug Therapy Across the Lifespan**

THYROID AND PARATHYROID AGENTS

Children

Thyroid replacement therapy is required when a child has hypothyroidism. Levothyroxine is the drug of choice in children. The dose is determined based on serum thyroid hormone levels and the response of the child, including growth and development. The dose for children tends to be higher than that for adults because of the higher metabolic rate of the growing child.

Regular monitoring, including growth records, is necessary to determine an accurate dose as the child grows. Maintenance levels are usually obtained at the adult dose after puberty and when active growing stops.

If an antithyroid agent is needed, methimazole is the drug of choice because it is less toxic to the liver. Propylthiouracil (PTU) is no longer recommended for children. Unless other agents are ineffective, radioactive agents are not used in children because of the effects of radiation on chromosomes and developing cells.

Hypercalcemia is relatively rare in children, although it may be seen with certain malignancies. If a child develops malignancy-related hypercalcemia, bisphosphonates may be used with dose adjustments based on age and weight. Serum calcium levels should be monitored closely in the child, with dose adjustments made as necessary.

Adults

Adults who require thyroid replacement therapy need to understand that this will typically be a lifelong replacement need. An established routine of taking the tablet first thing in the morning may help the patient adhere to the drug regimen. Levothyroxine is the drug of choice for replacement, but in some cases, other agents may be needed. Periodic monitoring of thyroid hormone levels is necessary to ensure that dose needs have not changed.

If antithyroid drugs are needed, the patient's underlying problems should be considered. Methimazole is associated with bone marrow suppression and more GI and CNS effects than is PTU, but PTU is associated with more liver toxicity. Sodium iodide I^{131} should not be used in adults in their reproductive years unless they are aware of the possibility of adverse effects on fertility.

Bisphosphonates are commonly used drugs for osteoporosis and calcium lowering if plasma levels are too high. Serum calcium levels need to be monitored carefully with any of the drugs that affect calcium levels. Patients should be encouraged to take calcium and vitamin D in their diet or as supplements in cases of hypocalcemia and also for the prevention and treatment of osteoporosis.

Thyroid replacement therapy is necessary during pregnancy for patients who have been maintained on this regimen. It is not uncommon for hypothyroidism to develop during pregnancy. Levothyroxine is again the drug of choice.

If an antithyroid drug is essential during pregnancy, PTU is the drug of choice because it is less likely to cross the placenta and cause problems for the fetus. Radioactive agents should not be used. Bisphosphonates should be used during pregnancy only if the benefit to the patient clearly outweighs the potential risk to the fetus. Breast or chestfeeding patients who need thyroid replacement therapy should continue with their prescribed regimen and report any adverse effects in the baby. Bisphosphonates and antithyroid drugs should not be used during lactation because of the potential for adverse effects on the baby; another method of feeding the baby should be used.

Older Adults

Because the signs and symptoms of thyroid disease mimic many other problems that are common in older adults—hair loss, slurred speech, fluid retention, heart failure, and so on—it is important to screen older adults for thyroid disease carefully before beginning any therapy. The dose should be started at a very low level and increased based on patient response. Levothyroxine is the drug of choice for hypothyroidism. Periodic monitoring of thyroid hormone levels, as well as cardiac and other responses, is essential with this age group.

If antithyroid agents are needed, sodium iodide I^{131} may be the drug of choice because it has fewer adverse effects than the other agents and surgery. The patient should be monitored closely for the development of hypothyroidism, which usually occurs within a year after initiation of antithyroid therapy.

Older adults may have dietary deficiencies related to calcium and vitamin D. They should be encouraged to eat dairy products and foods high in calcium and to supplement their diet if necessary. Postmenopausal females, who are prone to developing osteoporosis, may want to consider hormone replacement therapy and calcium supplements to prevent osteoporosis, though this decision has to be made with full consideration of the risks of using hormone replacement therapy. Many postmenopausal patients and some older males respond well to the effect of bisphosphonates in moving calcium back into the bone. They need specific instructions on the proper way to take these drugs and may not be able to adhere to the restrictions about staying upright and swallowing the tablet with a full glass of water.

Older adults have a greater incidence of renal impairment, and kidney function should be evaluated before starting any of these drugs. Bisphosphonates should be used in lower doses in patients with moderate renal impairment and are not recommended for those who have severe renal impairment. With any of these drugs, regular monitoring of calcium levels is important to ensure that therapeutic effects are achieved with a minimum of adverse effects.

Severe adult hypothyroidism is called **myxedema**, which results in hypometabolic rate and accumulation of nonpitting edema in connective tissues throughout the body. Myxedema usually develops gradually as the thyroid slowly stops functioning. It can develop as a result of autoimmune thyroid disease (Hashimoto's disease), viral infection, overtreatment with antithyroid drugs, or surgical removal or irradiation of the thyroid gland. Patients

Table 37.1 Signs and Symptoms of Thyroid Dysfunction

Clinical Effects	Hypothyroidism	Hyperthyroidism
CNS	*Depressed*: Hypoactive reflexes, lethargy, sleepiness, slow speech, emotional dullness	*Stimulated*: Hyperactive reflexes, anxiety, nervousness, insomnia, tremors, restlessness, increased basal temperature
CV system	*Depressed*: Bradycardia, hypotension, anemia, oliguria, decreased sensitivity to catecholamines	*Stimulated*: Tachycardia, palpitations, increased pulse pressure, systolic hypertension, increased sensitivity to catecholamines
Skin, hair, and nails	Skin is pale, coarse, dry, thickened; puffy eyes and eyelids; hair is coarse and thin; hair loss; nails are thick and hard	Skin is flushed, warm, thin, moist, and sweating; hair is fine and soft; nails are soft and thin
Metabolic rate	*Decreased*: Lower body temperature, intolerance to cold, decreased appetite, higher levels of fat and cholesterol, weight gain, hypercholesterolemia	*Increased, overactive cellular metabolism*: Low-grade fever, intolerance to heat, increased appetite with weight loss, muscle wasting and weakness, thyroid myopathy
Generalized myxedema	Accumulation of mucopolysaccharides in the heart, tongue, and vocal cords; periorbital edema; cardiomyopathy; hoarseness and thickened speech	Localized with accumulation of mucopolysaccharides in eyeballs, ocular muscles; periorbital edema, lid lag, exophthalmos; pretibial edema
Ovaries	*Decreased function*: Menorrhagia, habitual abortion, sterility, decreased sexual function	*Altered*: Tendency toward oligomenorrhea, amenorrhea
Goiter	Rare; simple nontoxic type may occur	Frequent; diffuse, highly vascular

CNS, central nervous system; CV, cardiovascular.

with myxedema exhibit many signs and symptoms of hypothyroidism (Table 37.1). Hypothyroidism is treated with replacement thyroid hormone therapy.

Hyperthyroidism

Hyperthyroidism occurs when excessive amounts of thyroid hormones are produced and released into circulation. Graves' disease is the most common cause of hyperthyroidism. With Graves' disease, there is an autoimmune process in which antibodies abnormally stimulate the thyroid gland to release excessive amounts of thyroid hormone. Goiter (enlargement of the thyroid gland) can occur when a person is hypo-, hyper-, or euthyroid. However, it is often an effect of hyperthyroidism, which occurs when the thyroid is overstimulated by TSH. This can happen if the thyroid gland does not make sufficient thyroid hormones to suppress the hypothalamus and anterior pituitary; in the body's attempt to produce the needed amount of thyroid hormone, the thyroid is continually stimulated by increasing levels of TSH. Additional signs and symptoms of hyperthyroidism can be found in Table 37.1.

Hyperthyroidism may be treated by surgical removal of the gland or portions of the gland, treatment with radiation to destroy parts or all of the gland, or drug treatment to block the production of thyroxine in the thyroid gland or to destroy parts or all of the gland. The metabolism of these patients then must be regulated with replacement thyroid hormone therapy.

Key Points

- The thyroid gland uses iodine to produce the thyroid hormones that regulate body metabolism.
- Control of the thyroid gland involves an intricate balance among TRH, TSH, and circulating levels of thyroid hormone.
- Hypothyroidism is treated with replacement thyroid hormone; hyperthyroidism is treated with thioamides or iodines.

Thyroid Agents

When thyroid function is low, thyroid hormone needs to be replaced to ensure adequate metabolism and homeostasis in the body. When thyroid function is too high, the resultant systemic effects can be serious, and the thyroid will need to be removed or destroyed pharmacologically, and then the hormone normally produced by the gland will need to be replaced with thyroid hormone. Thyroid agents include thyroid hormones and antithyroid drugs, which are further classified as thioamides and iodine solutions. Table 37.2 includes a complete list of each type of thyroid agent.

Thyroid Hormones

Several replacement hormone products are available for treating hypothyroidism. These hormones replace the low

Table 37.2 *Drugs in Focus:* Thyroid Agents

Drug Name	Dosage/Route	Usual Indications
Thyroid Hormones		
levothyroxine (*Synthroid, Levoxyl, Levothroid,* others)	*Adult*: 12.5–200 mcg/d PO; 300–500 mcg IV loading dose followed by 50–100 mcg/d IV maintenance dose for myxedema coma *Pediatric*: Varies based on age and weight	Replacement therapy in hypothyroidism; suppression of TSH release; treatment of myxedema coma and thyrotoxicosis; synthetic hormone used in patients allergic to desiccated thyroid
liothyronine (*Cytomel, Triostat*)	*Adult*: 25–100 mcg/d PO; reduced dosing for older adults *Pediatric*: 5–50 mcg/d PO; 65–100 mcg/d IV	Replacement therapy in hypothyroidism; suppression of TSH release; thyroid suppression test; treatment of myxedema coma and thyrotoxicosis; synthetic hormone used in patients allergic to desiccated thyroid
thyroid desiccated (*Armour Thyroid*)	*Adult*: 60–120 mg/d PO *Pediatric*: 15–90 mg/d PO	Thyroid hormone supplement
Antithyroid Agents		
Thioamides		
methimazole (*Tapazole*)	*Adult*: 15 mg/d PO initially, up to 30–60 mg/d may be needed; maintenance, 5–15 mg/d PO *Pediatric*: 0.4 mg/kg/d PO initially; maintenance, 15–20 mg/m²/d PO in three divided doses	Treatment of hyperthyroidism
propylthiouracil (PTU)	*Adult*: 300–900 mg/d PO initially; maintenance, 100–150 mg/d PO	Treatment of hyperthyroidism
Iodine Solutions		
sodium iodide I^{131} or I^{123} (*Hicon*, generic, radioactive iodine)	*Adult*: Dose varies based on formulation and indication	Treatment of hyperthyroidism; thyroid blocking in radiation emergencies; destruction of thyroid tissue in patients who are not candidates for surgical removal of the gland
strong iodine solution, potassium iodide (*Thyrosafe, Thyroshield*)	*Adult and pediatric*: One to two tablets, or 2–6 drops (gtt) PO daily to t.i.d.	Treatment of hyperthyroidism, thyroid blocking in radiation emergencies; presurgical suppression of the thyroid gland; treatment of acute thyrotoxicosis until thioamide levels can take effect

TSH, thyroid-stimulating hormone.

or absent levels of natural thyroid hormone and suppress the overproduction of TSH by the pituitary. These products can contain both natural and synthetic thyroid hormone. Levothyroxine (*Synthroid, Levoxyl, Levothroid, Unithroid, Tirosint*), a synthetic salt of T_4, is the most frequently used replacement hormone because of its predictable bioavailability and reliability. Desiccated thyroid (*Armour Thyroid* and others) is prepared from dried animal thyroid glands and contains both T_3 and T_4. Although the ratio of the hormones is unpredictable and the required dose and effects vary widely, this drug is inexpensive, making it attractive to some. An additional thyroid hormone is liothyronine (*Cytomel, Triostat*), which is a synthetic salt of T_3.

Therapeutic Actions and Indications

The thyroid replacement hormones increase the metabolic rate of body tissues, increasing oxygen consumption, respiration, heart rate, growth and maturation, and the metabolism of fats, carbohydrates, and proteins. They are indicated for replacement therapy in hypothyroid states, treatment of myxedema coma, suppression of TSH in the treatment and prevention of goiters, and management of thyroid cancer. In conjunction with antithyroid drugs, they are also indicated to treat thyroid toxicity, prevent goiter formation during thyroid overstimulation, and treat thyroid overstimulation during pregnancy. These drugs are not approved for weight loss and carry a warning that they are not to be used for weight loss (see Box 37.2). See Table 37.2 for usual indications for each drug.

Pharmacokinetics

These drugs are well absorbed from the gastrointestinal (GI) tract. They are best absorbed when taken on an empty stomach. They are distributed bound to serum

Box 37.2 Focus on The Evidence

THYROID HORMONES ARE NOT INDICATED AS TREATMENT FOR OBESITY

Treatment trends for obesity have changed over the years. Not long ago, one of the suggested treatments was the use of thyroid hormone. The thinking was that people with obesity had slower metabolisms and, therefore, would benefit from a boost in metabolism from extra thyroid hormone.

If patient with obesity truly has hypothyroidism, this might be a good idea. Unfortunately, many patients who received thyroid hormone for weight loss were not tested for thyroid activity and ended up with excessive thyroid hormone in their systems. This situation triggered a cascade of events. The exogenous thyroid hormone disrupted the hypothalamic–pituitary–thyroid control system, resulting in decreased production of TRH and TSH as the hypothalamus and pituitary sensed the rising level of thyroid hormone. Because the thyroid was no longer stimulated to produce and secrete thyroid hormone, the thyroid level would actually fall. Lacking stimulation by TSH, the thyroid gland would start to atrophy. If exogenous thyroid hormone were stopped, the atrophied thyroid would not be able to immediately respond to the TSH stimulation and produce thyroid hormone. Ultimately, these patients experienced an endocrine imbalance. They also did not lose weight; in the long run, they may have actually gained weight as the body's compensatory mechanisms tried to deal with the imbalances.

Today, thyroid hormone is no longer considered a good choice for treating obesity. Other drugs have come and gone, and new drugs are released each year to attack other aspects of the problem. Many patients, especially middle-aged people who may recall that thyroid hormone was once used for weight loss, ask for it as an answer to weight management. Patients have even been known to "borrow" thyroid replacement hormones from others for a quick weight loss solution or to order the drug over the internet without supervision or monitoring.

Patients with obesity need reassurance, understanding, and education about the risks of borrowed thyroid hormone. Insistent patients should undergo thyroid function tests. If the results are normal, patients should receive teaching about the controls and actions of thyroid hormone in the body and an explanation of why taking these hormones can cause problems. Obesity is a chronic and frustrating problem that poses continual challenges for health care providers.

proteins. Because it contains only T_3, liothyronine has a rapid onset and a long duration of action. Deiodination of the drugs occurs at several sites, including the liver, kidney, and other body tissues. Elimination is primarily by the kidney, but some is eliminated in feces. Thyroid hormone does not cross the placenta and seems to have no effect on the fetus. Thyroid replacement therapy should not be discontinued during pregnancy, and the need for thyroid replacement often becomes apparent or increases during pregnancy. Thyroid hormone does enter human milk in small amounts. Caution should be used during lactation.

Contraindications and Cautions

These drugs should not be used with any known allergy to the drugs or their binders to prevent hypersensitivity reactions, during acute thyrotoxicosis (unless used in conjunction with antithyroid drugs), or during acute myocardial infarction (unless complicated by hypothyroidism), because the thyroid hormones could exacerbate these conditions. Caution should be used during lactation because the drug enters human milk and could suppress the infant's thyroid production and with hypoadrenal conditions such as Addison's disease because the body will not be able to deal with the drug effects. Caution should be used when dosing for older adults because they often will require lower doses to become euthyroid.

Adverse Effects

When the correct dose of the replacement therapy is being used, few, if any, adverse effects are associated with these drugs. Thyroid function tests should be checked annually in long-term therapy to ensure that the correct levels are being maintained. Skin reactions and loss of hair are sometimes seen, especially during the first few months of treatment in children. Symptoms of hyperthyroidism (anxiety, tremors, weight loss, palpitations, tachycardia, chest pain, sweating) may occur if the dose is too high. Some of the less predictable effects are associated with cardiac stimulation (arrhythmias, hypertension), central nervous system (CNS) effects (anxiety, sleeplessness, headache), and difficulty swallowing and esophageal atresia (taking the drug with a full glass of water is strongly recommended to alleviate this effect) (Fig. 37.3).

Clinically Important Drug–Drug Interactions

Oral formulations should be taken on an empty stomach 30 to 60 minutes before eating breakfast and without any other medications. There are several medications that will bind to the thyroid hormone and decrease absorption. There may be increased responsiveness to catecholamines with thyroid hormone, which could increase the risk of arrhythmias. Increased insulin and digoxin could be required with concurrent use of thyroid hormone replacement.

The effectiveness of oral anticoagulants is increased if they are combined with thyroid hormone. Because this may lead to increased bleeding, the dose of the oral anticoagulant should be reduced and the bleeding time checked periodically.

There are many medications that can affect the pharmacokinetics of thyroid hormone replacement. All concurrent medications should be checked for potential interactions.

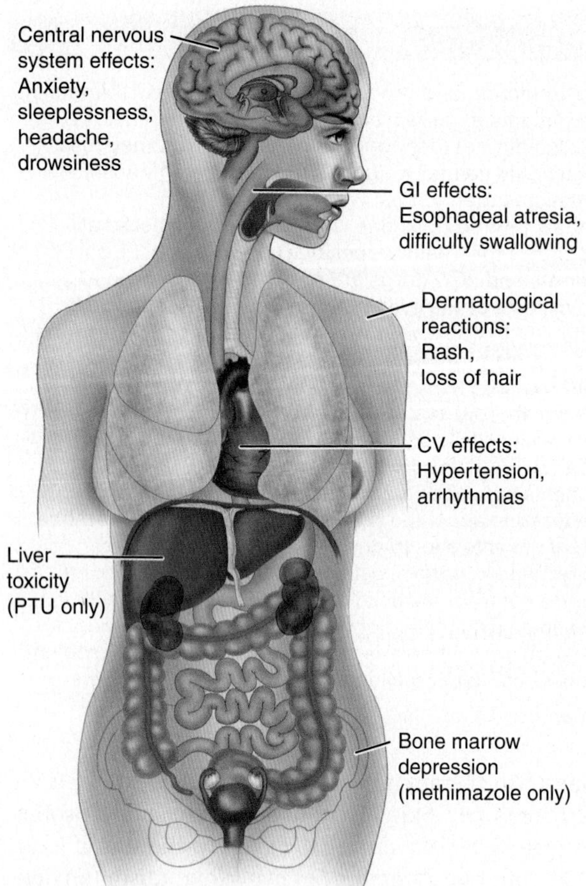

FIGURE 37.3 Variety of adverse effects and toxicities associated with thyroid and parathyroid drugs.

Prototype Summary: Levothyroxine

Indications: Replacement therapy in hypothyroidism; pituitary TSH suppression in the treatment of euthyroid goiters and in the management of thyroid cancer; thyrotoxicosis in conjunction with other therapy; myxedema coma.

Actions: Increases metabolic rate of body tissues, oxygen consumption, respiration, and heart rate; the rate of fat, protein, and carbohydrate metabolism; and growth and maturation.

Pharmacokinetics:

Route	Onset	Peak	Duration
PO	Slow	1–3 wk	1–3 wk
IV	6–8 h	24–48 h	Unknown

$T_{1/2}$: 6 to 7 days; metabolized in the liver and excreted in the bile.

Adverse Effects: Tremors, headache, nervousness, palpitations, tachycardia, allergic skin reactions, loss of hair in the first few months of therapy in children, diarrhea, nausea, vomiting.

Nursing Considerations for Patients Receiving Thyroid Hormones

Assessment: History and Examination

- Assess for history of allergy to any thyroid hormone or binder, lactation, Addison's disease, acute myocardial infarction not complicated by hypothyroidism, and thyrotoxicosis, which could be contraindications or cautions to use of the drug.
- Assess for the presence of any skin lesions; orientation and affect; baseline pulse and blood pressure; respiration and adventitious sounds; and thyroid function tests to determine baseline status and any potential adverse effects before beginning therapy.

Refer to the "Critical Thinking Scenario" for a full discussion of nursing care for a patient who is receiving a thyroid hormone.

Nursing Conclusions

Nursing conclusions related to drug therapy might include the following:

- Altered cardiac output related to cardiac effects
- Malnutrition risk: less than body requirements related to changes in metabolism
- Altered tissue perfusion related to thyroid activity
- Knowledge deficit regarding drug therapy

Planning

- The patient will receive the best therapeutic effect from the drug therapy.
- The patient will have limited adverse effects from the drug therapy.
- The patient will have an understanding of the drug therapy, adverse effects to anticipate, and measures to relieve discomfort and improve safety.

Intervention With Rationale

- Administer a single daily dose before breakfast each day to ensure consistent therapeutic levels.
- Monitor response carefully when beginning therapy to adjust dose according to patient response.
- Monitor cardiac response to detect cardiac adverse effects.
- Assess patient carefully to detect any potential drug–drug interactions if giving thyroid hormone in combination with other drugs.
- Arrange for periodic blood tests of thyroid function to monitor the effectiveness of the therapy.
- Provide thorough patient teaching, including drug name, dosage and administration, measures to avoid adverse effects, warning signs of problems, and the need for regular evaluation if used for longer than

recommended to enhance patient knowledge of drug therapy and promote adherence.

Evaluation

- Monitor patient response to the drug (return of metabolism to normal, resolution of any symptoms of hypothyroidism, prevention of goiter).
- Monitor for adverse effects (tachycardia, hypertension, anxiety, tremor, weight loss, heat intolerance, skin rash).
- Evaluate the effectiveness of the teaching plan (patient can name drug, dosage, adverse effects to watch for, and specific measures to avoid them).

CRITICAL THINKING SCENARIO Hypothyroidism

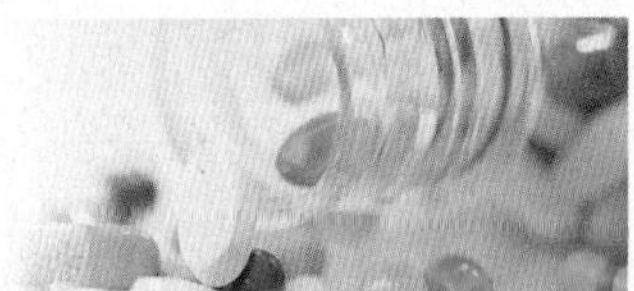

THE SITUATION

H.R., a 38-year-old patient, complains of "exhaustion, lethargy, and sleepiness." Their reported history is inconsistent, their speech seems slurred, and their attention span is limited. H.R.'s spouse reports feeling frustrated with H.R., stating that they have become increasingly lethargic, disorganized, and uninvolved at home. The spouse also notes that H.R. has gained weight and lost interest in their appearance. Physical examination reveals the following remarkable findings: pulse rate, 52/min; blood pressure, 90/62 mm Hg; temperature, 96.8°F (oral); pale, dry, and thick skin; periorbital edema; thick and asymmetric tongue; height, 5 ft 5 in.; and weight, 165 lb. The immediate impression is that of hypothyroidism. Laboratory tests confirm this, revealing elevated TSH and very low levels of triiodothyronine and thyroxine. *Synthroid*, 125 mcg daily PO, is prescribed.

CRITICAL THINKING

What teaching plans should be developed for this patient?

What interventions would be appropriate in helping the couple accept the diagnosis and the pathophysiological basis for H.R.'s complaints and problems?

What body image changes will H.R. experience as their body adjusts to the thyroid therapy?

How can H.R. be helped to adjust to these changes and reestablish body image and self-concept?

DISCUSSION

Hypothyroidism develops slowly. With it come fatigue, lethargy, and lack of emotional affect—conditions that result in the patient losing interest in appearance, activities, and responsibilities. In this case, the patient's spouse, not knowing that there was a physical reason for the problem, became increasingly frustrated and even angry. H.R.'s spouse should be involved in the teaching program so that their feelings can be taken into consideration. Any teaching content should be written down for later reference. (When H.R. starts to return to normal, their attention span and interest should return; anything that was missed or forgotten can be referred to in the written teaching program.)

H.R. may be encouraged to bring a picture of themselves from a year or so ago to help them understand and appreciate the changes that have occurred. Many patients are totally unaware of changes in their appearance and activity level because the disease progresses so slowly and brings on lethargy and lack of emotional affect.

The teaching plan should include information about the function of the thyroid gland and the anticipated changes that will be occurring for H.R. over the next week and beyond. The importance of taking the medication daily should be emphasized. The need to return for follow-up to evaluate the effectiveness of the medication and the effects on H.R.'s body should also be stressed. Both H.R. and their spouse will need support and encouragement to deal with past frustrations and the return to normal. Lifelong therapy will probably be needed, so further teaching will be important once things have stabilized.

NURSING CARE GUIDE FOR H.R.: THYROID HORMONE

Assessment: History and Examination

Review the patient's history for allergies to any of these drugs, Addison's disease, acute myocardial infarction not complicated by hypothyroidism, lactation, and thyrotoxicosis.

Focus the physical examination on the following:

Neurological: Orientation and affect

Skin: Color and lesions

Cardiovascular (CV): Pulse, cardiac auscultation, blood pressure, and electrocardiogram findings

Respiratory: Respirations, adventitious sounds

Hematological: Thyroid function tests

Nursing Conclusions

Altered cardiac output related to cardiac effects

Malnutrition risk: less than body requirements related to effects on metabolism

(continues on page 630)

Altered tissue perfusion related to thyroid effects
Knowledge deficit regarding drug therapy

Planning

The patient will receive the best therapeutic effect from the drug therapy.
The patient will have limited adverse effects from the drug therapy.
The patient will have an understanding of the drug therapy, adverse effects to anticipate, and measures to relieve discomfort and improve safety.

Intervention

Administer the drug once a day 30 to 60 minutes before breakfast. Avoid taking other medications or vitamins at the same time you are taking your thyroid medication.
Provide comfort and safety measures (e.g., temperature control, rest as needed, safety precautions).
Provide support and reassurance to deal with drug effects and lifetime need.
Provide patient teaching regarding drug name, dosage, adverse effects, precautions, and warning signs to report. Advise the patient to not use a drug past its expiration date.

Evaluation

Evaluate drug effects: return of metabolism to normal, resolution of symptoms of hypothyroidism, prevention of goiter.
Monitor for adverse effects: anxiety, tachycardia, hypertension, tremor, or skin reaction.
Monitor for drug–drug interactions as indicated for each drug.
Evaluate the effectiveness of the patient teaching program and comfort and safety measures.

PATIENT TEACHING FOR H.R.

- This hormone is designed to replace the thyroid hormone that your body is not able to produce. The thyroid hormone is responsible for regulating your body's metabolism, or the speed with which your body's cells burn energy. Thyroid hormone actions affect many body systems, so it is important that you take this medication only as prescribed.
- Never stop taking this drug without consulting with your health care provider. The drug is used to replace an important hormone and will probably have to be taken for life. Stopping the medication can lead to serious problems.
- Take this drug before breakfast each day with water and without any other medications or supplements.
- Make sure that you do not use the drug after its expiration date; this drug is known to lose effectiveness over time.
- Thyroid hormone usually causes no adverse effects. You may notice a slight skin rash or hair loss in the first few months of therapy. You should notice the signs and symptoms of your thyroid deficiency subsiding, and you will feel "back to normal."
- Report any of the following to your health care provider: chest pain, difficulty breathing, sore throat, fever, chills, weight gain, sleeplessness, nervousness, unusual sweating, or intolerance to heat.
- Avoid taking any over-the-counter medication without first checking with your health care provider because several of these medications can interfere with the effectiveness of this drug.
- Tell any doctor, nurse, or other health care provider involved in your care that you are taking this drug. You may also want to wear or carry medical identification showing that you are taking this medication. This would alert any health care personnel taking care of you in an emergency to the fact that you are taking this drug.
- While you are taking this drug, you will need regular medical follow-up, including blood tests to check the activity of your thyroid gland, to evaluate your response to the drug, and to monitor for any possible underlying problems.
- Keep this drug and all medications out of the reach of children. Do not give this medication to anyone else or take any similar medication that has not been prescribed for you.

Antithyroid Agents

Drugs used to block the production of thyroid hormone and to treat hyperthyroidism include the thioamides and iodide solutions (see Table 37.2). Although these groups of drugs are not chemically related, they both block the formation of thyroid hormones within the thyroid gland.

Therapeutic Actions and Indications

Thioamides

Thioamides lower thyroid hormone levels by preventing the formation of thyroid hormone in the thyroid cells, which lowers the serum levels of thyroid hormone. They also partially inhibit the conversion of T_4 to T_3 at the cellular level. These drugs are indicated for the treatment of hyperthyroidism. Thioamides include propylthiouracil (PTU) and methimazole (*Tapazole*).

Iodine Solutions

Low doses of **iodine** are needed in the body for the formation of thyroid hormone. High doses, however, block thyroid function. Therefore, iodine preparations are sometimes used to treat hyperthyroidism but are not used as often as they once were in the clinical setting. The iodine solutions cause the thyroid cells to become oversaturated with iodine and stop producing thyroid hormone. In some cases, the thyroid cells are actually destroyed. Radioactive iodine (sodium iodide I^{131} and I^{123}) is taken up into the thyroid cells, which are then destroyed by the beta-radiation given off by the radioactive iodine. At low doses, radioactive iodine may be used for diagnostic purposes to evaluate thyroid function. At high doses, radioactive iodine can be used for people who have not responded to other treatments or if other treatments are contraindicated. Iodine solutions include strong iodine solution, potassium iodide (*Thyrosafe, Thyroshield*), and sodium iodide I^{131} and I^{123} (*Hicon*, generic). See Table 37.2 for usual indications for each drug.

Pharmacokinetics

Thioamides

These drugs are well absorbed from the GI tract and are then concentrated in the thyroid gland. The onset and duration of PTU varies with each patient. Methimazole has an onset of action of 30 to 40 minutes and peaks in about 60 minutes. Some excretion can be detected in the urine. Methimazole crosses the placenta and is found in a high ratio in human milk. PTU has a low potential for crossing the placenta and for entering human milk.

Iodine Solutions

These drugs are rapidly absorbed from the GI tract and widely distributed throughout the body fluids. Excretion occurs through the urine. Strong iodine products, potassium iodide, and sodium iodide are taken orally and have a rapid onset of action, with effects seen within 24 hours and peak effects seen in 10 to 15 days. The effects are short-lived and may even precipitate further thyroid enlargement and dysfunction. For this reason, and because of the availability of the more predictable thioamides, iodides are not used as often as they once were in the clinical setting. They are used in cases of radiation emergencies or for diagnostic purposes.

The strong iodine products cross the placenta and are known to enter human milk. Use during pregnancy and when breast or chestfeeding can be detrimental to the fetus or infant and can cause hypothyroidism.

Contraindications and Cautions

Antithyroid agents are contraindicated in the presence of any known allergy to antithyroid drugs to prevent hypersensitivity reactions and during pregnancy because of the risk of adverse effects on the fetus and the development of hypothyroidism. (If an antithyroid drug is absolutely essential and the pregnant patient has been informed about the risk of hypothyroidism in the infant, PTU is the drug of choice, but caution should still be used.) Another method of feeding the baby should be chosen if an antithyroid drug is needed during lactation because of the risk of antithyroid activity in the infant, including the development of signs and symptoms of hypothyroidism. PTU has been associated with severe liver toxicity and is not recommended for use in children except in rare circumstances where other therapy is not appropriate.

Adverse Effects

Thioamides

The adverse effects most commonly seen with thioamides are the effects of thyroid suppression or hypothyroidism. PTU is associated with nausea, vomiting, GI complaints, and severe liver toxicity. GI effects and liver toxicity are less pronounced with methimazole; it is the drug of choice for nonpregnant patients. Methimazole is also associated with bone marrow suppression, so the patient using this drug must have frequent blood tests to monitor for this effect.

Iodine Solutions

The most common adverse effect of iodine solutions is hypothyroidism; the patient will need to be started on replacement thyroid hormone to maintain homeostasis. Other adverse effects include iodism (metallic taste and burning in the mouth, sore teeth and gums, diarrhea, cold symptoms, and stomach upset), staining of teeth, skin rash, and the development of goiter.

Clinically Important Drug–Drug Interactions

Thioamides

An increased risk for bleeding exists when PTU is administered with oral anticoagulants. Changes in serum levels of theophylline, metoprolol, propranolol, and digitalis may lead to changes in the effects of PTU as the patient moves from the hyperthyroid to the euthyroid state.

Iodine Solutions

Because the use of drugs to destroy thyroid function moves the patient from hyperthyroidism to hypothyroidism, patients who are taking drugs that are metabolized differently in hypothyroid and hyperthyroid states or drugs that have a small margin of safety that could be altered by the change in thyroid function should be monitored closely. These drugs include anticoagulants, theophylline, digoxin, metoprolol, and propranolol. Eating foods high in iodine will increase risk of toxicity. Concurrent use of other antithyroid medication reduces uptake of radioactive iodine.

Prototype Summary: Methimazole

Indications: Treatment of hyperthyroidism.

Actions: Inhibits the synthesis of thyroid hormones.

Pharmacokinetics:

Route	Onset	Duration
PO	30–60 min	2–4 h

$T_{1/2}$: 6 to 13 hours; excreted in the urine.

Adverse Effects: Paresthesia, neuritis, vertigo, drowsiness, skin rash, urticaria, skin pigmentation, nausea, vomiting, epigastric distress, nephritis, bone marrow suppression, arthralgia, myalgia, edema.

Prototype Summary: Strong Iodine Solutions

Indications: Adjunct therapy for hyperthyroidism; thyroid blocking in a radiation emergency.

Actions: Inhibit the synthesis of thyroid hormones and inhibit the release of these hormones into the circulation.

Pharmacokinetics:

Route	Onset	Peak	Duration
PO	24 h	10–15 d	6 wk

$T_{1/2}$: Unknown; metabolized in the liver and excreted in the urine.

Adverse Effects: Rash, hypothyroidism, goiter, swelling of the salivary glands, iodism (metallic taste, burning mouth and throat, sore teeth and gums, head cold symptoms, stomach upset, diarrhea), allergic reactions.

Nursing Considerations for Patients Receiving Antithyroid Agents

Assessment: History and Examination

- Assess for history of allergy to any antithyroid drug; pregnancy and lactation status, liver dysfunction; and pulmonary edema or pulmonary tuberculosis if using strong iodine solutions, which could be cautions or contraindications to use of the drug.
- Assess for skin lesions; orientation and affect; baseline pulse, blood pressure, and electrocardiogram; respiration and adventitious sounds; and thyroid function tests to determine baseline status and any potential adverse effects before beginning therapy.

Nursing Conclusions

Nursing conclusions related to drug therapy might include the following:

- Altered cardiac output related to cardiac effects
- Malnutrition risk: more than body requirements related to changes in metabolism
- Infection and bleeding risk related to bone marrow suppression
- Knowledge deficit regarding drug therapy

Planning

- The patient will receive the best therapeutic effect from the drug therapy.
- The patient will have limited adverse effects from the drug therapy.
- The patient will have an understanding of the drug therapy, adverse effects to anticipate, and measures to relieve discomfort and improve safety.

Intervention With Rationale

- Administer methimazole and propylthiouracil three times a day in about 8-hour intervals to ensure consistent therapeutic levels.
- Give iodine solution through a straw to decrease staining of teeth; tablets can be crushed.
- Monitor response carefully, and arrange for periodic blood tests to assess patient response and to monitor for adverse effects.
- Monitor patients receiving iodine solution for any sign of iodism so the drug can be stopped immediately if such signs appear.
- Provide thorough patient teaching, including measures to avoid adverse effects, warning signs of problems, and the need for regular evaluation if used for longer than recommended to enhance patient knowledge of drug therapy and promote adherence.

Evaluation

- Monitor patient response to the drug (lowering of thyroid hormone levels).
- Monitor for adverse effects (bradycardia, drowsiness, cold intolerance, changes in blood counts, liver injury, blood dyscrasias, skin rash).
- Evaluate the effectiveness of the teaching plan (patient can name drug, dosage, adverse effects to watch for, and specific measures to avoid them).
- Monitor the effectiveness of comfort measures and adherence to the regimen.

Key Points

- Hypothyroidism, or lower-than-normal levels of thyroid hormone, is treated with replacement thyroid hormone.
- Hyperthyroidism, or higher-than-normal levels of thyroid hormone, is treated with thioamides, which block the thyroid from producing thyroid hormone, or with iodines, which prevent thyroid hormone production or destroy parts of the gland.

The Parathyroid Glands

The parathyroid glands are four very small groups of glandular tissue located on the back of the thyroid gland. The parathyroid glands produce PTH, an important regulator of serum calcium levels (Fig. 37.4).

Structure and Function

As mentioned earlier, the parafollicular cells of the thyroid gland produce the hormone calcitonin. Calcitonin responds to high calcium levels to cause lower serum calcium levels and acts to balance the effects of the PTH, which works to elevate calcium levels. PTH is the most

Increases calcium resorption
Parathyroid glands
Teriparatide works here
Parathormone
Increases calcium resorption
Parathyroid hormone works here
Increases serum calcium
Calcitonin
Inhibits calcium resorption
Parafollicular cells
Bisphosphonates work here to increase calcium deposition in bones and decrease serum calcium
Calcitonin salmon works here to decrease serum calcium and inhibit bone resorption
Reduces serum calcium

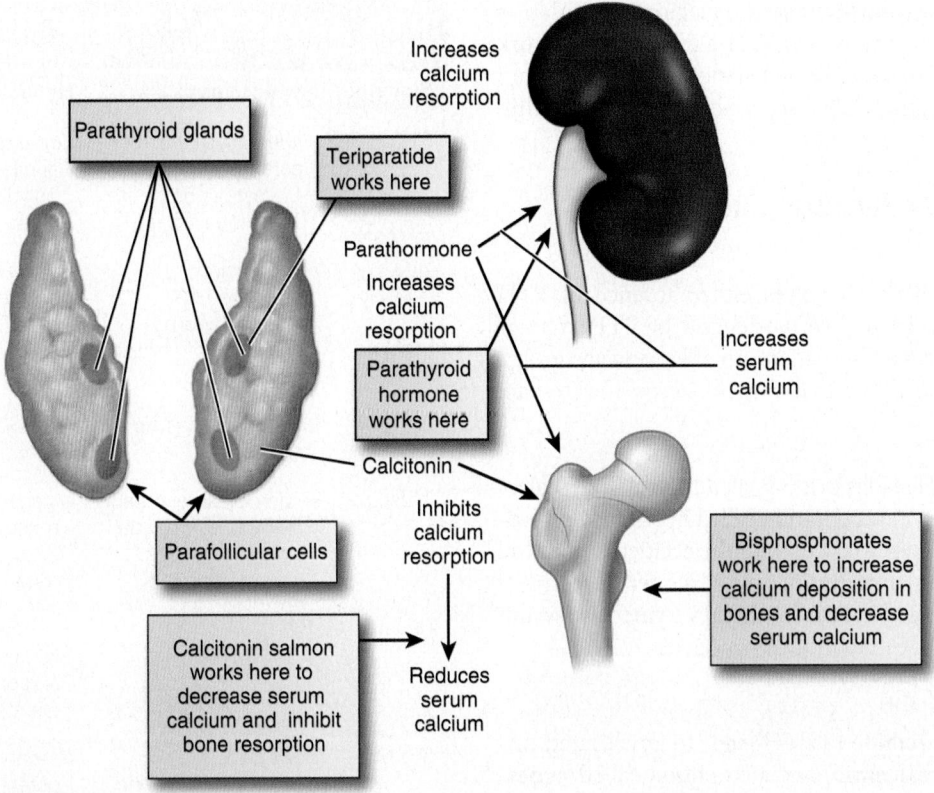

FIGURE 37.4 Calcium control. Parathormone and calcitonin work to maintain calcium homeostasis in the body.

important regulator of serum calcium levels in the body. PTH has many actions, including the following:

- Stimulation of osteoclasts or bone cells to release calcium from the bone
- Increased intestinal absorption of calcium
- Increased calcium reabsorption from the kidneys
- Stimulation of cells in the kidney to produce calcitriol, the active form of vitamin D, which stimulates intestinal transport of calcium into the blood

Control

Calcium is an electrolyte that is used in many of the body's metabolic processes. These processes include membrane transport systems, conduction of nerve impulses, muscle contraction, and blood clotting. To achieve all of these effects, the serum levels of calcium must be maintained within the normal range. This is achieved through regulation of serum calcium by PTH and calcitonin (Fig. 37.5).

The release of calcitonin is not controlled by the hypothalamic–pituitary axis but is regulated locally at the cellular level. Calcitonin is released when serum calcium levels rise. Calcitonin works to reduce calcium levels by blocking bone resorption and enhancing bone formation. This action pulls calcium out of the serum for deposit into the bone. When serum calcium levels are low, PTH release is stimulated. When serum calcium levels are high, PTH release is blocked.

Another electrolyte—magnesium—also affects PTH secretion by mobilizing calcium and inhibiting the release of PTH when concentrations rise above or fall below normal. An increased serum phosphate level indirectly stimulates parathyroid activity. Renal tubular phosphate reabsorption is balanced by calcium secretion into the

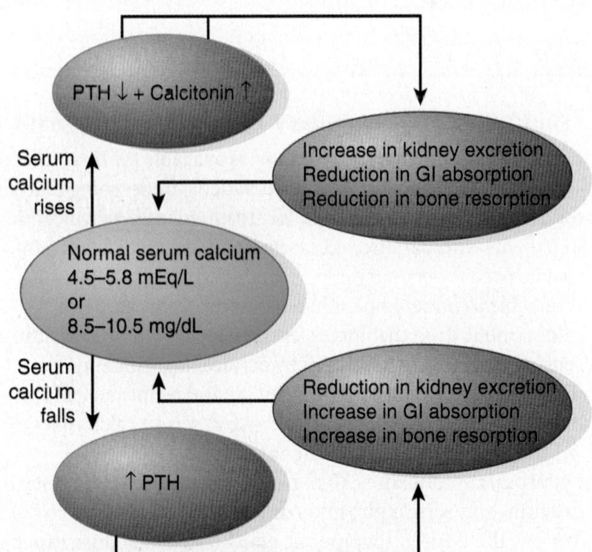

FIGURE 37.5 Regulation of serum calcium. Parathyroid hormone (PTH) and calcitonin regulate normal serum calcium. As serum calcium rises, PTH is inhibited by calcitonin. The kidney then excretes more calcium, the gastrointestinal (GI) system absorbs less, and a reduction in bone resorption occurs. As serum calcium falls, PTH is secreted and raises the calcium level by decreasing the amount of calcium lost in the kidney, increasing the amount absorbed in the GI tract and increasing bone resorption.

urine, which causes a drop in serum calcium, stimulating PTH secretion. The hormones PTH and calcitonin work together to maintain the delicate balance of serum calcium levels in the body and to keep serum calcium levels within the normal range.

Parathyroid Dysfunction and Related Disorders

Parathyroid dysfunction involves either absence of PTH (hypoparathyroidism) or overproduction of PTH (hyperparathyroidism). This dysfunction can affect any age group. See Box 37.1 for use of parathyroid agents across the lifespan.

Hypoparathyroidism

The absence of PTH results in a low calcium level (**hypocalcemia**) and a relatively rare condition called **hypoparathyroidism**. This is most likely to occur with the accidental removal of the parathyroid glands during thyroid surgery. Treatment consists of calcium and vitamin D therapy to increase serum calcium levels (see "Antihypocalcemic Agents").

Hyperparathyroidism

The excessive production of PTH leads to an elevated calcium level (**hypercalcemia**) and a condition called **hyperparathyroidism**. This can occur as a result of parathyroid tumor or certain genetic disorders. The patient presents with signs of high calcium levels (Table 37.3). Primary hyperparathyroidism occurs more often in females between 60 and 70 years of age. Secondary hyperparathyroidism occurs most frequently in patients with chronic renal failure (see Box 37.3 for more information). When the plasma concentrations of calcium are elevated secondary to high PTH levels, inorganic phosphate levels are usually decreased. Pseudorickets (renal fibrocystic osteosis or renal rickets) may occur as a result of this phosphorus retention (hyperphosphatemia), which results from increased stimulation of the parathyroid glands and increased PTH secretion.

Table 37.3 Signs and Symptoms of Calcium Imbalance

System	Hypocalcemia	Hypercalcemia
CNS	Hyperactive reflexes, paresthesia, positive Chvostek and Trousseau signs	Lethargy, personality and behavior changes, polydipsia, stupor, coma
CV	Hypotension, prolonged QT interval, edema, and signs of cardiac insufficiency	Hypertension, shortening of the QT interval, atrioventricular block
GI	Abdominal spasms and cramps	Anorexia, nausea, vomiting, constipation
Muscular	Tetany, skeletal muscle cramps, carpopedal spasm, laryngeal spasm, tetany	Muscle weakness, muscle atrophy, ataxia, loss of muscle tone
Renal		Polyuria, flank pain, kidney stones, acute and/or chronic renal insufficiency
Skeletal	Bone pain, osteomalacia, bone deformities, fractures	Osteopenia, osteoporosis

CNS, central nervous system; CV, cardiovascular; GI, gastrointestinal.

BOX 37.3

Treatments for Secondary Hyperparathyroidism

Cinacalcet hydrochloride (*Sensipar*) is available for treatment of secondary hyperparathyroidism in patients undergoing dialysis for chronic kidney disease and for treatment of hypercalcemia in patients with parathyroid carcinoma. This medication can also be used for primary hyperparathyroidism if the person is not able to undergo parathyroidectomy. Cinacalcet is a calcimimetic drug that increases the sensitivity of the calcium-sensing receptors to activation by extracellular calcium. In increasing the receptors' sensitivity, cinacalcet lowers PTH levels, causing a concomitant decrease in serum calcium levels.

The usual initial adult dose for secondary hyperparathyroidism is 30 mg/d PO, after which PTH, serum calcium, and serum phosphorus levels are monitored to achieve the desired therapeutic effect. The usual dose range is 60 to 180 mg/d. The drug must be used in combination with vitamin D and/or phosphate binders.

For parathyroid carcinoma, the initial dose is 30 mg PO twice a day titrated every 2 to 4 weeks to maintain serum calcium levels within a normal range; 30 to 90 mg twice a day up to 90 mg three to four times daily may be needed.

Side effects that the patient may experience include nausea, vomiting, diarrhea, and dizziness.

Another treatment available for secondary hyperparathyroidism related to renal failure is paricalcitol (*Zemplar*). Paricalcitol is an analogue of vitamin D. Vitamin D levels are decreased in renal disease, leading to an increase in PTH levels and signs and symptoms of hyperparathyroidism. *Zemplar* is taken orally or can be injected during hemodialysis. The body recognizes the vitamin D and subsequently decreases the synthesis and storage of PTH, allowing control over calcium levels.

The usual dose is 1 to 4 mcg PO from once a day to three times a week based on the patient's calcium levels, or 0.04 to 0.1 mcg/kg injected during hemodialysis. The drug is rapidly absorbed and reaches peak level within 3 hours. The drug has a half-life of 12 to 20 hours. Patients will need regular serum calcium checks, and the dose will be adjusted based on individual response. Adverse effects are usually mild as long as calcium levels are monitored. Diarrhea, headache, and mild hypertension have been reported.

Box 37.4 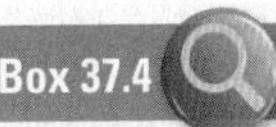 Focus on Sex Differences

OSTEOPOROSIS

Osteoporosis is the most common bone disease found in adults. It results from a lack of bone-building cell (osteoclast) activity and a decrease in bone matrix and mass with less calcium and phosphorus being deposited in the bone. This can occur with advancing age, when the endocrine system is slowing down and the stimulation to build bone is absent; with menopause, when the calcium-depositing effects of estrogen are lost; with malnutrition states, when vitamin C and proteins essential for bone production are absent from the diet; and with a lack of physical stress on the bones from lack of activity, which promotes calcium removal and does not stimulate osteoclast activity. The inactive, older, postmenopausal person with a poor diet is a prime candidate for osteoporosis. Fractured hips and wrists, shrinking size, and curvature of the spine are all evidence of osteoporosis in this age group. Besides the use of bisphosphonates to encourage calcium deposition in the bone, several other interventions can help prevent severe osteoporosis in this group or in any other people with similar risk factors.

- *Aerobic exercise*: Walking, even for just 10 minutes a day, has been shown to help increase osteoclast activity. Encourage people to walk around the block or to park their cars far from the door and walk. Exercise does not have to involve vigorous gym activity to be beneficial.
- *Proper diet*: Calcium and proteins are essential for bone growth. For example, the person who eats only pasta and avoids milk products could benefit from calcium supplements and encouragement to eat protein at least two or three times a week. Weight loss can also help improve activity and decrease pressure on bones at rest.
- *Hormone replacement therapy (HRT)*: For females, HRT has been successful in decreasing the progression of osteoporosis. However, research showed an increase in CV events and dementia with long-term HRT, making it a less desirable treatment. The use of HRT has often been linked to increased risk of breast cancer. The use of bisphosphonates might be a better choice of drug therapy for many patients.

The risk of osteoporosis should be taken into consideration as part of the health care regimen for all people as they age. Prevention can save a great deal of pain and debilitation in the long run.

The genetically linked disorder **Paget's disease** is a condition of overactive osteoclasts that are eventually replaced by enlarged and softened bony structures. Patients with this disease complain of deep bone pain, headaches, and hearing loss and usually have cardiac failure and bone malformation.

Postmenopausal osteoporosis can occur when dropping levels of estrogen allow calcium to be pulled out of the bone, resulting in a weakened and honeycombed bone structure. Estrogen normally causes calcium deposits in the bone; osteoporosis is one of the many complications that accompany the loss of estrogen at menopause (Box 37.4).

Key Points

- Parathyroid glands produce PTH, which, together with calcitonin, maintains the body's calcium balance.
- A low calcium level (hypocalcemia) is treated with vitamin D and calcium replacement therapy.
- Hypercalcemia and hypercalcemic states are associated with postmenopausal osteoporosis, Paget's disease, and malignancies.

Parathyroid Agents

The drugs used to treat disorders associated with parathyroid function are drugs that affect serum calcium levels. There are two parathyroid replacement hormones available and one form of calcitonin; other drugs affect calcium levels in different ways.

Antihypocalcemic Agents

Deficient levels of PTH result in hypocalcemia (calcium deficiency). Vitamin D stimulates calcium absorption from the intestine and restores the serum calcium to a normal level. Hypoparathyroidism is treated primarily with vitamin D and, if necessary, dietary supplements of calcium. However, there are several medications available for therapeutic use. Teriparatide (*Bonsity, Forteo*) and parathyroid hormone (*Natpara*) are recombinant human PTH analogs. Teriparatide is approved to increase bone mass in postmenopausal patients with primary or hypogonadal osteoporosis who are at high risk for fracture. Parathyroid hormone (*Natpara*) is approved to help control calcium levels in patients with hypoparathyroidism. Calcitriol (*Rocaltrol*) is a synthetic vitamin D analog that can be used to manage hypocalcemia. Other vitamin D analogs are discussed in Chapter 60. Abaloparatide (*Tymlos*) is a parathyroid hormone–related peptide that is indicated for treatment of patients with high risk of fracture due to osteoporosis (Table 37.4).

Therapeutic Actions and Indications

Vitamin D compounds regulate the absorption of calcium and phosphate from the small intestine, mineral resorption in bone, and reabsorption of phosphate from the renal tubules. Working along with PTH and calcitonin to regulate calcium homeostasis, vitamin D functions as a hormone. With once-daily administration, teriparatide stimulates new bone formation, leading to an increase in

Table 37.4 *Drugs in Focus:* Parathyroid Agents

Drug Name	Usual Dosage	Usual Indications
Antihypocalcemic Agents		
abaloparatide (*Tymlos*)	80 mcg/d subcutaneously in periumbilical region of abdomen	Treatment of postmenopausal patients with osteoporosis at high risk for fracture
calcitriol (*Rocaltrol*)	0.5–2 mcg/d PO in the morning	Management of hypocalcemia and reduction of parathormone levels; management of hypocalcemia and metabolic bone disease in patients with renal impairment
parathyroid hormone (*Natpara*)	50 mcg/d subcutaneously, adjust dose to maintain serum calcium levels in the lower range of normal	Maintenance of serum calcium levels in adults with hypoparathyroidism
teriparatide (*Bonsity, Forteo*)	20 mg subcutaneously daily	Management of osteoporosis in postmenopausal females and males with primary hypogonadal osteoporosis who do not respond to standard therapy; treatment of patients on sustained systemic glucocorticoid therapy at high risk for fractures
Antihypercalcemic Agents		
Bisphosphonates		
alendronate (*Bonosto, Fosamax*)	Dosing varies based on indication and formulation	Treatment of Paget's disease; postmenopausal osteoporosis treatment and prevention; treatment of glucocorticoid-induced osteoporosis; osteoporosis in males
ibandronate (*Boniva*)	2.5 mg/d PO or 150 mg PO once per month on the same day each month; 3 mg IV given over 15–30 s once every 3 mo	Treatment and prevention of osteoporosis in postmenopausal patients
pamidronate (*Aredia*)	30–90 mg IV as an infusion	Treatment of Paget's disease, postmenopausal osteoporosis, hypercalcemia of malignancy, osteolytic bone lesions in cancer patients
risedronate (*Actonel, Atelvia*)	30 mg/d PO for 2 mo; reduce dose in renal dysfunction; 5 mg/d PO for osteoporosis *or* 35 mg PO once per week *or* 150 mg PO once per month; 35 mg PO once per week for males to increase bone mass; 35 mg PO once a week (*Atelvia*)	Treatment of symptomatic Paget's disease in patients who are at risk for complications; treatment and prevention of osteoporosis (postmenopausal, glucocorticoid related and in males); treatment of postmenopausal osteoporosis (*Atelvia*)
zoledronic acid (*Zometa, Reclast*)	IV infusions; dosing and frequency varies based on indication and formulation	Treatment of Paget's disease, postmenopausal osteoporosis, hypercalcemia of malignancy, osteolytic bone lesions in certain cancer patients; prevention of new fractures in patients with low-trauma hip fractures
Calcitonins		
calcitonin salmon (*Miacalcin*)	*Paget's disease*: 50–100 IU/d subcutaneous or IM *Postmenopausal osteoporosis*: 100 IU/d subcutaneous or IM with calcium and vitamin D *Hypercalcemia*: 4–8 IU/kg subcutaneous or IM q12h	Treatment of Paget's disease, postmenopausal osteoporosis in conjunction with vitamin D and calcium supplements; emergency treatment of hypercalcemia
calcitonin salmon (generic)	200 IU/d intranasally; alternate nostrils daily	Treatment of postmenopausal osteoporosis in conjunction with calcium supplements and vitamin D

skeletal mass. It increases serum calcium and decreases serum phosphorus. Parathyroid hormone acts as a replacement for missing PTH. Abaloparatide acts to increase bone mineral content to strengthen bone.

Use of these agents is indicated for the management of hypocalcemia in patients undergoing chronic renal dialysis and for the treatment of hypoparathyroidism; teriparatide is also used for the treatment of postmenopausal or hypogonadal osteoporosis and osteoporosis associated with sustained systemic glucocorticoid therapy, which could lead to fractures (see Table 37.4). Parathyroid hormone is only approved for maintenance of calcium levels in patients with hypoparathyroidism.

Pharmacokinetics

Calcitriol is well absorbed from the GI tract and widely distributed throughout the body. It is stored in the liver, fat, muscle, skin, and bones. Calcitriol has a half-life of approximately 5 to 8 hours and a duration of action of 3 to 5 days. There are multiple pathways for metabolism. It is primarily excreted in the feces, with some found in the urine.

Teriparatide is given by subcutaneous injection every day. It is rapidly absorbed from the subcutaneous tissues, reaching peak concentration within 3 hours. The half-life of teriparatide is about 1 hour. Serum calcium levels will begin to decline after about 6 hours and return to baseline 16 to 24 hours after dosing. This drug is believed to be metabolized in the liver and excreted through the kidneys.

Parathyroid hormone is given as a daily subcutaneous injection. It reaches peak level in 5 to 30 minutes and has a half-life of 3 hours. It is thought to be metabolized in the liver and excreted through the kidneys. Abaloparatide is given as a daily subcutaneous injection. It reaches peak level in about 30 minutes and has a half-life of about 1.7 hours. It is primarily excreted by the kidneys.

Contraindications and Cautions

These drugs should not be used in the presence of any known allergy to any component of the drug to avoid hypersensitivity reactions, or hypercalcemia or vitamin D toxicity, which would be exacerbated by these drugs. At therapeutic levels, these drugs should be used during pregnancy only if the benefit to the patient clearly outweighs the potential for adverse effects on the fetus. Calcitriol has been associated with hypercalcemia (excessive calcium levels in the blood) in the baby when used by breast or chestfeeding patients; therefore, another method of feeding the baby should be used if these drugs are needed during lactation. Caution should be used with a history of renal stones or during lactation, when high calcium levels could cause problems.

Abaloparatide, teriparatide, and parathyroid hormone are associated with osteosarcoma—a bone cancer—in animal studies, so use caution with patients at higher risk for osteosarcoma. These agents are recommended for patients who cannot be managed with calcium supplements and active forms of vitamin D alone. Patients should be informed of the risk of osteosarcoma. These patients should also take supplemental calcium and vitamin D, increase weight-bearing exercise, and decrease risk factors such as smoking and alcohol consumption. Parathyroid hormone is only available through a limited access program.

Adverse Effects

The adverse effects most commonly seen with these drugs are related to GI effects: metallic taste, nausea, vomiting, dry mouth, constipation, and anorexia. CNS effects such as weakness, headache, somnolence, and irritability may also occur. These are possibly related to the changes in electrolytes that occur with these drugs. Patients with liver or renal dysfunction may experience increased levels of the drugs and/or toxic effects. Severe hypocalcemia can occur with interruption of treatment, and hypercalcemia can occur when starting or increasing the dose of parathyroid hormone.

Clinically Important Drug–Drug Interactions

The risk of hypermagnesemia increases if these drugs are taken with magnesium-containing antacids. This combination should be avoided.

Reduced absorption of calcitriol may occur if they are taken with cholestyramine or mineral oil because they are fat-soluble vitamins.

Digoxin toxicity can occur with hypercalcemia. If combining these drugs with digoxin, digoxin serum levels and serum calcium levels should be monitored closely.

Prototype Summary: Calcitriol

Indications: Management of hypocalcemia in patients on chronic renal dialysis, management of hypocalcemia associated with hypoparathyroidism.

Actions: A vitamin D compound that regulates the absorption of calcium and phosphate from the small intestine, mineral resorption in bone, and reabsorption of phosphate from the renal tubules, increasing the serum calcium level.

Pharmacokinetics:

Route	Onset	Peak	Duration
PO	Slow	4 h	3–5 d

$T_{1/2}$: 5 to 8 hours; metabolized in the kidneys and other body tissues; excreted in the bile and feces.

Adverse Effects: Weakness, headache, nausea, vomiting, dry mouth, constipation, muscle pain, bone pain, metallic taste.

Nursing Considerations for Patients Receiving Antihypocalcemic Agents

Assessment: History and Examination

- Assess for history of allergy to any component of the drugs, hypercalcemia, vitamin toxicity, renal stone, risk of osteosarcoma, and pregnancy or lactation, which could be cautions or contraindications to use of the drug.
- Assess for the presence of any skin lesions; orientation and affect; serum calcium, magnesium, and alkaline phosphate levels; and radiographs of bones as appropriate, to determine baseline status and any potential adverse effects before beginning therapy.

Nursing Conclusions

Nursing conclusions related to drug therapy might include the following:

- Impaired comfort related to GI or CNS effects
- Malnutrition risk: less than body requirements related to GI effects
- Knowledge deficit regarding drug therapy

Planning

- The patient will receive the best therapeutic effect from the drug therapy.
- The patient will have limited adverse effects from the drug therapy.
- The patient will have an understanding of the drug therapy, adverse effects to anticipate, and measures to relieve discomfort and improve safety.

Intervention With Rationale

- Monitor serum calcium concentration before and periodically during treatment to allow for adjustment of dose to maintain calcium levels within normal limits.
- Provide supportive measures to help the patient manage GI and CNS effects of the drug (analgesics, small and frequent meals, help with activities of daily living).
- Arrange for a nutritional consultation if GI effects are severe to ensure nutritional balance.
- Provide thorough patient teaching, including measures to avoid adverse effects, warning signs of problems, and the need for regular evaluation to enhance the patient's knowledge about drug therapy and promote adherence.

Evaluation

- Monitor patient response to the drug (return of serum calcium levels to normal).
- Monitor for adverse effects (weakness, headache, GI effects).
- Evaluate the effectiveness of the teaching plan (patient can name drug, dosage, adverse effects to watch for, and specific measures to avoid them).
- Monitor the effectiveness of comfort measures and adherence to the regimen.

Antihypercalcemic Agents

Drugs used to treat PTH excess or hypercalcemia include the bisphosphonates and calcitonin salmon. These drugs act on the serum levels of calcium and do not suppress the parathyroid gland or PTH (see Table 37.4).

Therapeutic Actions and Indications

Bisphosphonates

The **bisphosphonates** act to slow or block bone resorption; by doing this, they help to lower serum calcium levels, but they do not inhibit normal bone formation and mineralization. Bisphosphonates include ibandronate (*Boniva*), pamidronate (*Aredia*), risedronate (*Actonel, Atelvia*), alendronate (*Binosto, Fosamax*), and zoledronic acid (*Reclast, Zometa*). These drugs are used in the treatment of Paget's disease and of postmenopausal osteoporosis in females, and alendronate is also used to treat osteoporosis in males. Zoledronic acid is also used to prevent new fractures in patients with low-trauma hip fractures and to treat patients with multiple myeloma or documented bone metastases from solid tumors. See Table 37.4 for usual indications for each drug.

Calcitonins

The calcitonins are hormones secreted by the thyroid gland to balance the effects of PTH. Currently, the only calcitonin readily available is calcitonin salmon (generic, *Miacalcin*). This hormone inhibits bone resorption; lowers serum calcium levels in children and in patients with Paget's disease; and increases the excretion of phosphate, calcium, and sodium from the kidney. See Table 37.4 for usual indications of this drug.

Pharmacokinetics

Bisphosphonates

These drugs are well absorbed from the small intestine and do not undergo metabolism. They are excreted relatively unchanged in the urine. The onset of action is slow, and the duration of action is days to weeks. Pamidronate and zoledronic acid are administered via IV and eliminated renally. Patients with renal dysfunction may experience toxic levels of the drug and should be evaluated for a dose reduction.

Calcitonins

These medications have good bioavailability after injection. These drugs are metabolized in the body tissues to inactive fragments, which are excreted by the kidney. Calcitonins cross the placenta and have been associated with lower fetal birth weights in animals when administered in high doses, but no adequate studies in humans have been performed. These drugs inhibit lactation in animals; it is not known whether they are excreted in human milk. Calcitonin salmon can be given by injection or by nasal spray. By either route, the peak effect is seen within 40 minutes, and the duration of effect is 8 to 24 hours.

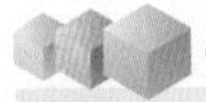 Concept Mastery Alert

Administering Calcitonin

The primary route of administration for calcitonin used to treat Paget's disease and postmenopausal osteoporosis is via subcutaneous injection. The intranasal route is only for patients with osteoporosis.

Contraindications and Cautions

Bisphosphonates

These drugs should not be used in the presence of hypocalcemia, which could be made worse by lowering calcium levels, or with a history of any allergy to bisphosphonates, to avoid hypersensitivity reactions. Fetal abnormalities have been associated with these drugs in animal trials, and they should not be used during pregnancy unless the benefit to the patient clearly outweighs the potential risk to the fetus or neonate. Extreme caution should be used when nursing because of the potential for adverse effects on the baby. Alendronate should not be used by breast or chestfeeding patients because of potential risk for adverse effects on the baby. Caution should be used in patients with renal dysfunction, which could interfere with excretion of the drug, or with upper GI disease, which could be aggravated by the drug.

Alendronate, ibandronate, and risedronate need to be taken on arising in the morning, with water and 30 to 60 minutes before any other food or beverage, and the patient must then remain upright for at least 30 minutes. These drugs should not be given to anyone who is unable to remain upright for 30 minutes after taking the drug because serious esophageal erosion can occur.

Zoledronic acid should be used cautiously in patients with asthma who are aspirin sensitive. It may be given as an intravenous (IV) infusion once every 2 years for osteoporosis. Alendronate and risedronate are available in a once-a-week formulation to decrease the number of times the patient must take the drug, which should increase adherence to the drug regimen. Ibandronate is available in a once-a-month formulation and in an IV preparation for use when oral drugs cannot be taken.

Calcitonins

This drug should be used in pregnancy only if the benefit to the patient clearly outweighs the potential risk to the fetus. It should not be used during lactation because the calcium-lowering effects could cause problems for the baby. Calcitonin salmon should not be used with a known allergy to salmon or fish products. This drug should be used with caution in patients with renal dysfunction or pernicious anemia, which could be exacerbated by these drugs. Prolonged use should be evaluated due to evidence of increased risk of malignancies with prolonged use.

Adverse Effects

Bisphosphonates

The most common adverse effects seen with bisphosphonates are abdominal pain, constipation, musculoskeletal pain, nausea, and diarrhea. There is also an increase in bone pain in patients with Paget's disease, but this effect usually passes after a few days to a few weeks. Esophageal ulceration has been associated with oral formulations. This risk can be decreased if the patient takes the medication with water and remains upright for at least 30 minutes after taking the dose. Long-term use of bisphosphonates, over 5 years, has been associated with increased risk of femoral shaft fractures. Osteonecrosis of the jaw has also been reported with use of bisphosphonates. Risk/benefit analysis of prolonged use should be evaluated for each patient. There is risk of renal toxicity with IV formulations.

Calcitonins

The most common adverse effects seen with this drug are flushing of the face and hands, skin rash, nausea and vomiting, urinary frequency, and local inflammation at the site of injection. Nasal dryness and irritation may be noted with intranasal route. Many of these side effects lessen with time, the length of time varying with each individual patient.

Clinically Important Drug–Drug Interactions

Bisphosphonates

Oral absorption of bisphosphonates is decreased if they are taken concurrently with antacids, calcium products, iron, or multiple vitamins. Bisphosphonates should be separated from all medications by at least 30 minutes.

Risk of GI ulceration may increase if bisphosphonates are combined with aspirin; this combination should be avoided if possible.

Calcitonins

Concomitant use of the IV formulation of calcitonin salmon and lithium may lead to a reduction in plasma lithium concentration due to increased urinary clearance of lithium, so the dose of lithium may require adjustment.

Prototype Summary: Alendronate

Indications: Treatment and prevention of osteoporosis in postmenopausal females and in males; treatment of glucocorticoid-induced osteoporosis; treatment of Paget's disease in certain patients.

Actions: Slows normal and abnormal bone resorption without inhibiting bone formation and mineralization.

Pharmacokinetics:

Route	Onset	Duration
PO	Slow	Days

$T_{1/2}$: Greater than 10 days; not metabolized but excreted in the urine.

Adverse Effects: Abdominal pain, constipation, nausea, diarrhea, increased or recurrent bone pain, esophageal erosion.

Prototype Summary: Calcitonin Salmon

Indications: Paget's disease, postmenopausal osteoporosis, emergency treatment of hypercalcemia.

Actions: Inhibits bone resorption; lowers elevated serum calcium in children and patients with Paget's disease; increases the excretion of filtered phosphate, calcium, and sodium by the kidney.

Pharmacokinetics:

Route	Onset	Peak	Duration
IM, subcutaneous	15 min	3–4 h	8–24 h
Nasal	Rapid	31–39 min	8–24 h

$T_{1/2}$: About 1 hour; metabolized in the kidneys and excreted in the urine.

Adverse Effects: Flushing of face and hands, nausea, vomiting, local inflammatory reactions at injection site, nasal irritation if nasal form is used.

Nursing Considerations for Patients Receiving Antihypercalcemic Agents

Assessment: History and Examination

- Assess for history of allergy to any of these products or to fish products with calcitonin salmon to avoid hypersensitivity reaction; pregnancy or lactation; hypocalcemia; and renal dysfunction, which could be cautions or contraindications to use of the drug.
- Assess for the presence of any skin lesions; orientation and affect; abdominal examination; serum electrolytes; and renal function tests to determine baseline status and any potential adverse effects before beginning therapy.

Nursing Conclusions

Nursing conclusions related to drug therapy might include

- Impaired comfort related to GI, musculoskeletal, or skin effects
- Malnutrition risk: less than body requirements related to GI effects
- Knowledge deficit regarding drug therapy

Planning

- The patient will receive the best therapeutic effect from the drug therapy.
- The patient will have limited adverse effects from the drug therapy.
- The patient will have an understanding of the drug therapy, adverse effects to anticipate, and measures to relieve discomfort and improve safety.

Intervention With Rationale

- Ensure adequate hydration with any of these agents to reduce the risk of renal complications.
- Arrange for concomitant vitamin D, calcium supplements, and hormone replacement therapy if used to treat postmenopausal osteoporosis.
- Rotate injection sites and monitor for inflammation if using calcitonins to prevent tissue breakdown and irritation.
- Monitor serum calcium regularly to allow for dose adjustment as needed.
- Assess the patient carefully for any potential drug–drug interactions if giving in combination with other drugs to prevent serious effects.
- Arrange for periodic blood tests of renal function if using gallium to monitor for renal dysfunction.
- Provide comfort measures and analgesics to relieve bone pain if it returns as treatment begins.
- Provide thorough patient teaching, including measures to avoid adverse effects, warning signs of problems, the need for regular evaluation if used for longer than recommended, and proper administration of nasal spray, to enhance patient knowledge about drug therapy and promote adherence.

Evaluation

- Monitor patient response to the drug (return of calcium levels to normal; prevention of complications of osteoporosis; control of Paget's disease).
- Monitor for adverse effects (skin rash; abdominal pain, nausea and vomiting; hypocalcemia; renal dysfunction).
- Monitor length of biphosphate use; limit duration of use based on risk/benefit analysis.
- Evaluate the effectiveness of the teaching plan (patient can name drug, dosage, adverse effects to watch for, and specific measures to avoid them).
- Monitor the effectiveness of comfort measures and adherence to the regimen.

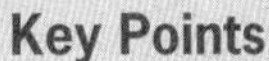

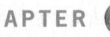

Key Points

- The parathyroid glands are located behind the thyroid gland and produce PTH, which works with calcitonin, produced by thyroid cells, to maintain the calcium balance in the body.
- Hypocalcemia, or low levels of calcium, is usually first treated with vitamin D products and calcium replacement therapy.
- Hypercalcemia can occur in postmenopausal osteoporosis and Paget's disease; hypercalcemia can also be related to malignancy.
- Hypercalcemia is treated with bisphosphonates, which slow or block bone resorption to lower serum calcium levels, or calcitonin, which inhibits bone resorption; lowers serum calcium levels in children and patients with Paget's disease; and increases the excretion of phosphate, calcium, and sodium from the kidney.

SUMMARY

- The thyroid gland uses iodine to produce thyroid hormones. Thyroid hormones control the rate at which most body cells use energy (metabolism).
- Control of the thyroid gland is an intricate process between TRH, released by the hypothalamus; TSH, released by the anterior pituitary; and circulating levels of thyroid hormone.
- Hypothyroidism, or lower-than-normal levels of thyroid hormone, is treated with replacement thyroid hormone.
- Hyperthyroidism, or higher-than-normal levels of thyroid hormone, is treated with thioamides, which block the thyroid from producing thyroid hormone, or with iodines, which prevent thyroid hormone production or destroy parts of the gland.
- The parathyroid glands are located behind the thyroid gland and produce PTH, which works with calcitonin, produced by thyroid cells, to maintain the calcium balance in the body.
- Hypocalcemia, or low levels of calcium, is usually first treated with vitamin D products and calcium replacement therapy.
- Hypercalcemia and hypercalcemic states include postmenopausal osteoporosis and Paget's disease, as well as hypercalcemia related to malignancy.
- Hypercalcemia is treated with bisphosphonates or calcitonin. Bisphosphonates slow or block bone resorption, which lowers serum calcium levels. Calcitonin inhibits bone resorption; lowers serum calcium levels in children and patients with Paget's disease; and increases the excretion of phosphate, calcium, and sodium from the kidney.

Unfolding Patient Stories: Suzanne Morris • Part 1

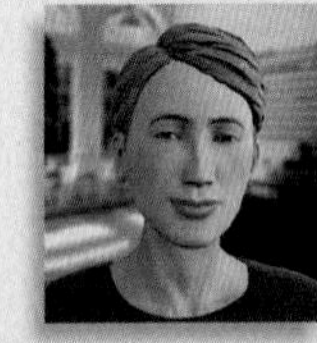

Suzanne Morris, age 43, is diagnosed with peptic ulcer disease. She is prescribed triple combination therapy with amoxicillin, clarithromycin, and pantoprazole for *H. pylori*. What patient education would the nurse provide for each medication? (Suzanne Morris's story continues in Chap. 57.)

Care for Suzanne and other patients in a realistic virtual environment: ***vSim** for Nursing* (thepoint.lww.com/vSimPharm). Practice documenting these patients' care in DocuCare (thepoint.lww.com/DocuCareEHR).

CHECK YOUR UNDERSTANDING

Answers to the questions in this chapter can be found in Answers to Check Your Understanding Questions on thePoint®.

MULTIPLE CHOICE

Select the best answer.

1. The thyroid gland produces the thyroid hormones triiodothyronine (T_3) and tetraiodothyronine (T_4), which are dependent on the availability of
   a. iodine produced in the liver.
   b. iodine found in the diet.
   c. iron absorbed from the GI tract.
   d. PTH to promote iodine binding.
2. The thyroid gland is dependent on the hypothalamic–pituitary axis for regulation.

Increasing the level of thyroid hormone (by taking replacement thyroid hormone) would

a. increase hypothalamic release of TRH.
b. increase pituitary release of TSH.
c. suppress hypothalamic release of TRH.
d. stimulate the thyroid gland to produce more T_3 and T_4.

3. Goiter, or enlargement of the thyroid gland, is usually associated with
   a. hypothyroidism.
   b. iodine deficiency.
   c. hyperthyroidism.
   d. underactive thyroid tissue.

4. Thyroid replacement therapy is indicated for the treatment of
   a. obesity.
   b. myxedema.
   c. Graves' disease.
   d. Cushing's disease.

5. Assessing a patient's knowledge of their thyroid replacement therapy would show good understanding if the patient stated,
   a. "My spouse may use some of my drug since they want to lose weight."
   b. "I should only need this drug for about 3 months."
   c. "I can stop taking this drug as soon as I feel like my old self."
   d. "I should call if I experience unusual sweating, weight gain, or chills and fever."

6. Administration of propylthiouracil would include giving the drug
   a. once a day in the morning.
   b. at regular intervals to assure therapeutic levels.
   c. once a day at bedtime to decrease adverse effects.
   d. if the patient is experiencing slow heart rate, skin rash, or excessive bleeding.

7. The parathyroid glands produce PTH, which is important in the body as
   a. a modulator of thyroid hormone.
   b. a regulator of potassium.
   c. a regulator of calcium.
   d. an activator of vitamin D.

8. Which should NOT be used for the treatment of postmenopausal osteoporosis?
   a. Risedronate
   b. Alendronate
   c. Zoledronic acid
   d. Parathyroid hormone

MULTIPLE RESPONSE

Select all that apply.

1. A patient who is receiving a bisphosphonate for the treatment of postmenopausal osteoporosis should be taught to do which of the following?
   a. Also take vitamin D, calcium, and hormone replacement
   b. Restrict fluids as much as possible
   c. Take the drug before any food for the day with a full glass of water
   d. Stay upright for at least 30 minutes after taking the drug
   e. Take the drug with meals to avoid GI upset
   f. Avoid exercise to prevent bone fractures

2. Hypothyroidism is a common and often missed disorder. Signs and symptoms of hypothyroidism include which of the following?
   a. Increased body temperature
   b. Thickening of the tongue
   c. Bradycardia
   d. Loss of hair
   e. Excessive weight loss
   f. Oily skin

REFERENCES

Brunton, L., Hilal-Dandan, R., & Knollman, B. (2018). *Goodman and Gilman's the pharmacological basis of therapeutics* (13th ed.). McGraw-Hill.

Cooper, D. S. (2005). Drug therapy: Antithyroid drugs. *New England Journal of Medicine*, *352*, 905–917. 10.1056/NEJMra042972

Hall, J. E., & Hall, M. E. (2021). *Guyton and Hall's textbook of medical physiology* (14th ed.). Saunders.

Khan, A., & Clark, O. (2011). *Parathyroid and calcium disorders.* Humana Press.

Licata, A., & Lerma, E. (Eds.). (2012). *Diseases of the parathyroid glands.* Springer.

Norris, T. L. (2019). *Porth's pathophysiology concepts of altered health states* (13th ed.). Wolters Kluwer.

Park-Willie, L., Mamdani, M., Juulink, D. N., Hawker, G. A., Gunraj, N., Austin, P. C., Whelan, D. B., Weiler, P. J., & Laupacis, A. (2011). Bisphosphonate use and the risk of subtrochanteric or femoral shaft fractures in older women. *Journal of the American Medical Association*, *305*(8), 783–789. 10.1001/jama.2011.190

Pearce, E. N. (2012). Thyroid hormone and obesity. *Current Opinion in Endocrinology and Diabetes and Obesity*, *19*(5), 408–413. 10.1097/MED.0b013e328355cd6c

CHAPTER 38

Agents to Control Blood Glucose Levels

Learning Objectives

Upon completion of this chapter, you will be able to:

1. Explain how the glands, hormones, and other factors work together to regulate the body's glucose levels.
2. Describe the pathophysiology of diabetes mellitus, including alterations in metabolic pathways and changes to basement membranes.
3. Discuss the use of antidiabetic and glucose-elevating agents across the lifespan.
4. Describe the therapeutic actions, indications, pharmacokinetics, contraindications, most common adverse effects, and important drug–drug interactions associated with insulin and other antidiabetic and glucose-elevating agents.
5. Compare and contrast the prototype drugs insulin, glyburide, metformin, liraglutide, sitagliptin, and canagliflozin with other antidiabetic agents in their classes.
6. Outline the nursing considerations, including important teaching points, for patients receiving an antidiabetic or glucose-elevating agent.

Key Terms

adiponectin: hormone produced by adipocytes that acts to increase insulin sensitivity, decrease the release of glucose from liver, and protect the blood vessels from inflammatory changes

diabetes mellitus: a metabolic disorder characterized by high blood glucose levels and altered metabolism of proteins and fats; associated with thickening of the basement membrane, leading to numerous complications

dipeptidyl peptidase-4 (DPP-4): enzyme that quickly metabolizes glucagonlike polypeptide-1

endocannabinoid receptors: receptors found in the adipose tissue, muscles, liver, satiety center, and gastrointestinal (GI) tract that are part of a signaling system within the body to keep the body in a state of energy gain

glucagonlike polypeptide-1 (GLP-1): a peptide produced in the GI tract in response to carbohydrates that increases insulin release, decreases glucagon release, slows GI emptying, and stimulates the satiety center in the brain

glycogen: storage form of glucose; can be broken down for rapid increase of glucose level during times of stress

glycosuria: presence of glucose in the urine

glycosylated hemoglobin: a blood glucose marker that provides a 3-month average of blood glucose levels

hyperglycemia: elevated blood glucose levels leading to multiple signs and symptoms and abnormal metabolic pathways

hypoglycemia: lower-than-normal blood sugar; often results from imbalance between insulin or oral agents and patient's eating, activity, and stress; symptoms of hypoglycemia may be seen if blood sugar is 70 mg/dL or lower

incretins: peptides produced in the GI tract in response to food that help modulate insulin and glucagon activity

insulin: hormone produced by the beta cells in the pancreas; stimulates insulin receptor sites to move glucose into the cells; promotes storage of fat and glucose in the body

ketosis: breakdown of fats for energy, resulting in an increase in ketones to be excreted from the body

polydipsia: increased thirst; seen in diabetes when loss of fluid and increased tonicity of the blood lead the hypothalamic thirst center to make the patient feel thirsty

polyphagia: increased hunger; sign of diabetes when cells cannot use glucose for energy and sense that they are starving, causing hunger

polyuria: increased urination; high glucose in blood is filtered by the kidneys without all of the glucose being reabsorbed into the blood, and the resulting higher filtrate osmolality causes more water to be lost in the urine

Drug List

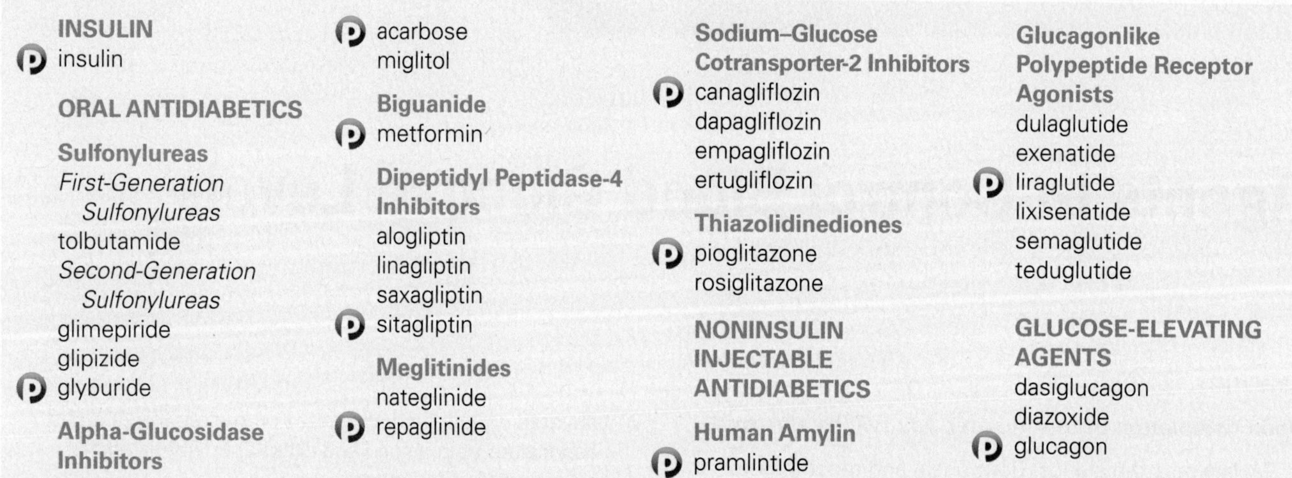

INSULIN
insulin

ORAL ANTIDIABETICS

Sulfonylureas
First-Generation Sulfonylureas
tolbutamide
Second-Generation Sulfonylureas
glimepiride
glipizide
glyburide

Alpha-Glucosidase Inhibitors
acarbose
miglitol

Biguanide
metformin

Dipeptidyl Peptidase-4 Inhibitors
alogliptin
linagliptin
saxagliptin
sitagliptin

Meglitinides
nateglinide
repaglinide

Sodium–Glucose Cotransporter-2 Inhibitors
canagliflozin
dapagliflozin
empagliflozin
ertugliflozin

Thiazolidinediones
pioglitazone
rosiglitazone

NONINSULIN INJECTABLE ANTIDIABETICS

Human Amylin
pramlintide

Glucagonlike Polypeptide Receptor Agonists
dulaglutide
exenatide
liraglutide
lixisenatide
semaglutide
teduglutide

GLUCOSE-ELEVATING AGENTS
dasiglucagon
diazoxide
glucagon

Antidiabetic agents, as the name implies, are used to treat diabetes mellitus, the most common metabolic disorder. It is estimated that 34 million people in the United States have diabetes. Diabetes is a complicated disorder that alters the metabolism of glucose, fats, and proteins, affecting many end organs and causing numerous clinical complications. It is part of metabolic syndrome, a collection of conditions that predispose people to cardiovascular (CV) disease (Chapter 47). Treatment of diabetes is aimed at regulating the blood glucose level through the use of insulin or other glucose-lowering drugs. Maintaining the level of serum glucose within a certain range is very important to the nervous system. The nerves in the central nervous system (CNS) receive glucose by diffusion; they do not have insulin receptor sites like all other cells. The presence of too much glucose, which is a large molecule, takes water into the CNS and can cause swelling and nerve instability. The presence of too little glucose results in less energy for the nerves to use to function and loss of cell membrane integrity. Maintaining an appropriate glucose level is a complicated process that involves diet, exercise, and drug therapy. At times, the blood glucose level is lowered too much, producing a state of hypoglycemia. When this occurs, glucose-elevating agents or carbohydrates need to be used to quickly return the serum glucose levels to a normal level.

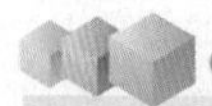

Concept Mastery Alert

Blood Glucose Assessment

An elevated blood glucose level is the diagnostic criteria for diabetes mellitus. Blood glucose level can be assessed by the fasting blood glucose, 2-hour plasma glucose, blood glucose after a glucose tolerance test, or HbA1c assessment.

Glucose Regulation

Glucose is the main energy source for the human body. Glucose is stored in the body for rapid release in times of stress. Typically, the blood glucose level can be readily maintained so that the neurons always receive a constant supply of glucose to function. The body's control of glucose is intricately related to fat and protein metabolism, balancing energy conservation with energy consumption to maintain homeostasis in a variety of situations. Many factors impact this balance and the body's ability to adapt and to maintain metabolism.

The Pancreas

The pancreas is both an endocrine gland, producing hormones, and an exocrine gland, releasing sodium bicarbonate and pancreatic enzymes directly into the common bile duct to be released into the small intestine, where they neutralize the acid chyme from the stomach and aid digestion. The endocrine part of the pancreas produces hormones in collections of tissue called the islets of Langerhans. These islets contain endocrine cells that produce specific hormones. The alpha cells release glucagon in direct response to low blood glucose levels. The beta cells release insulin in direct response to high blood glucose levels and when stimulated by incretins. Delta cells produce somatostatin (growth hormone–inhibiting factor) in response to low blood glucose levels; somatostatin blocks the secretion of both insulin and glucagon and slows absorption of food by decreasing gastrointestinal (GI) mobility. These hormones work together to maintain the blood glucose level within normal limits.

Insulin

Insulin is the hormone produced by the pancreatic beta cells of the islets of Langerhans. The hormone is released into circulation when the level of glucose around these cells rises. If there is an increase in free fatty acids (FFAs) or amino acids in the blood, the release of insulin is increased. It is also released in response to **incretins**, peptides that are produced in the GI tract in response to food. Incretins help modulate insulin and glucagon activity. One of these incretins, **glucagonlike polypeptide-1** (GLP-1), increases insulin release and decreases glucagon release in preparation for the nutrients that will soon be absorbed. GLP-1 also slows GI emptying to allow more absorption of nutrients and stimulates the satiety center in the brain to decrease the desire to eat because food is already in the GI tract. GLP-1 has a short half-life and is metabolized by the enzyme **dipeptidyl peptidase-4** (DPP-4).

Insulin circulates through the body and reacts with specific insulin receptor sites to stimulate the transport of glucose into the cells to be used for energy. The cell membrane also becomes more permeable to amino acids, and protein synthesis is increased. Insulin stimulates the liver to be able to uptake, store, and use glucose. The liver is responsible for slowly releasing glucose between meals so that blood glucose does not get too low.

Insulin is released after a meal in response to incretin release and when the blood glucose level rises. It circulates and affects metabolism, allowing the body to either store or use the nutrients from the meal effectively. As a result of the insulin release, the blood glucose level falls, and insulin release drops off. Sometimes, an insufficient amount of insulin is released. This may occur because the pancreas cannot produce enough insulin, the insulin receptor sites have lost their sensitivity to insulin and they require more insulin to lower glucose effectively, or the person does not have enough receptor sites to support their body size, as with obesity.

Glucagon

Glucagon is released from the alpha cells in the islets of Langerhans in response to a low blood glucose level. Glucagon causes an immediate mobilization of **glycogen**, the form of glucose stored in the liver. Glycogen can be broken down for rapid increase of glucose level during times of stress. This mobilization raises blood glucose levels. Glucagon also stimulates the liver to convert protein into glucose; this is called gluconeogenesis.

Other Factors Affecting Glucose Regulation

Other factors in the body have been found to impact glucose, fat, and protein metabolism. These factors play a role in the overall energy balance in the body.

Adipocytes, or fat cells, were once thought to just store fat for energy. However, they have been found to have a major impact on glucose and fat metabolism throughout the body through the secretion of **adiponectin**. This hormone acts to increase insulin sensitivity, decrease the release of glucose from the liver, and protect the blood vessels from inflammatory changes. When the adiponectin level is high, it exerts a protective effect on the body. When the level is low, as in cases of intra-abdominal fat accumulation, the glucose level rises and blood vessel injury increases.

Endocannabinoid receptors have been identified in adipose tissue, muscles, liver, the satiety center, and the GI tract. These receptors seem to be part of a signaling system within the body to keep the body in a state of energy gain to prepare for stressful situations. When stimulated, these receptors promote food intake, decrease adiponectin release, increase fat breakdown, decrease insulin sensitivity, increase fat storage, and alter gastric emptying to promote greater nutrient absorption. Patients who have obesity have been shown to have increased stimulation of these receptors.

The sympathetic nervous system (SNS), through norepinephrine and epinephrine effects, directly causes a decrease in insulin release, an increase in the release of stored glucose, and an increase in fat breakdown. A person under stress will have an increased glucose level and increased FFA level, which will provide the energy needed for the immediate "fight or flight" associated with a stress reaction. Prolonged stress can alter the control of metabolism that regulates the body's energy balance.

Corticosteroids, which are released diurnally but also during a stress reaction, decrease insulin sensitivity, increase glucose release, and decrease protein building. All of these actions conserve energy and provide immediate glucose for any stressful situation.

Growth hormone causes decreased insulin sensitivity, increase of FFAs, and increase in protein building. Fluctuating levels of growth hormone can upset metabolic homeostasis. Box 38.1 summarizes the effects of various factors on blood glucose levels.

Loss of Blood Glucose Control

When an insufficient amount of insulin is released or insulin receptors are less responsive, several metabolic changes occur, beginning with hyperglycemia, or increased blood sugar. Hyperglycemia results in **glycosuria**; sugar is spilled into the urine because the concentration of glucose in the blood is too high for complete reabsorption. Because this sugar-rich urine is an ideal environment for bacteria, cystitis is a common finding. Glucose in the urine filtrate has high osmotic pull, so more water is kept in the nephron and lost in the urine. This increased water in the nephron results in increased urination, or **polyuria**. The patient experiences fatigue because the body's cells cannot use the glucose that is there; they need insulin to facilitate transport of the glucose into the cells. **Polyphagia** (increased

BOX 38.1

Glucose Control Mechanisms

Insulin	Decreases blood glucose; glycogen storage; adipose tissue deposit; synthesis of proteins to form amino acids
Glucagon	Increases blood glucose
Somatostatin	Decreases insulin release; decreases glucagon release; slows GI emptying
Growth hormone	Decreases insulin sensitivity; increases protein building; increases FFA formation
Incretins	Increase insulin release; decrease glucagon release; stimulate satiety center; slow GI emptying
Adiponectin	Increases insulin sensitivity; decreases glucose output from liver; protects vessels from inflammatory reactions
Catecholamines	Decrease insulin release; increase glucose output from liver and muscles; increase breakdown of fat to FFAs
Corticosteroids	Increase glucose output; decrease insulin sensitivity
Endocannabinoid system	Increases food intake by blocking satiety signals; decreases adiponectin release; decreases insulin sensitivity; increases fat synthesis; alters gastric motility

hunger) occurs because the hypothalamic centers cannot take in glucose; thus, the cells sense that they are starving. **Polydipsia** (increased thirst) occurs because the tonicity of the blood is increased owing to the increased glucose and waste products in the blood and the loss of fluid with glucose in the urine. The hypothalamic cells that are sensitive to fluid levels sense a need to increase fluid in the system, which in turn causes the patient to feel thirsty.

Lipolysis, or fat breakdown, occurs as the body breaks down stored fat into FFAs for energy because glucose is not usable. The patient experiences **ketosis** as metabolism shifts to the use of fat for energy. Ketones are produced; they cannot be removed effectively. Acidosis also occurs because the liver cannot remove all of the waste products (acid being a primary waste product) that result from the breakdown of glucose, fat, and proteins. Muscles break down because proteins are being broken down for their essential amino acids. The breakdown of proteins results in an increase in nitrogen wastes, which is manifested by an elevated blood urea nitrogen concentration and sometimes by protein in the urine. Patients with hyperglycemia do not heal quickly because of this protein breakdown and the lack of a stimulus to initiate protein building. All of these actions eventually contribute to development of the complications associated with chronic hyperglycemia or diabetes.

Diabetes Mellitus

Diabetes mellitus (literally, "honey urine") is characterized by complex disturbances in metabolism. Diabetes affects carbohydrate, protein, and fat metabolism. The most frequently recognized clinical signs of diabetes are hyperglycemia (a fasting blood sugar level greater than 126 mg/dL) and glycosuria (the presence of sugar in the urine). The alteration in the body's ability to effectively deal with carbohydrate, fat, and protein metabolism over the long term results in vascular damage. The vascular damage is probably due to increased production of reactive oxygen species that decrease production of the vascular endothelial relaxing factor nitric oxide, which is important for endothelial cell health. The exact mechanisms of how chronic hyperglycemia affects the body tissues are not completely understood. However, chronic uncontrolled blood sugar can result in an increased incidence of a number of disorders, including the following:

- *Atherosclerosis*: Heart attacks, peripheral vascular disease, and strokes related to the development of atherosclerotic plaques in the vessel lining
- *Retinopathy*: Resultant loss of vision as tiny vessels in the eye are narrowed and closed
- *Neuropathies*: Motor and sensory changes in the feet and legs and progressive changes in other nerves as the oxygen supply to these nerves is slowly cut off
- *Nephropathy*: Renal dysfunction related to changes in the basement membrane of the glomerulus
- *Infections*: Increases in frequency and severity due to decreased blood flow and altered neutrophil function
- *Foot ulcers*: Decreased wound healing due to vascular insufficiency; unnoticed wounds and infections due to neuropathy decreasing perception of pain

The overall metabolic disturbances associated with diabetes were once thought to be caused by a lack of insulin. It is now thought that they are caused by a mosaic of problems, including low insulin secretion from the pancreas, cellular insulin resistance, and increased glucose production by the liver. There are also cases in which there is hypersecretion of insulin from the pancreas but severe insulin resistance. Insulin resistance, in which the receptor signaling is diminished, is often progressive over time. There is an overall change in energy metabolism due to the cell's decreased ability to utilize glucose; fats and proteins are metabolized at higher rates. People with type 2 diabetes are also at risk for metabolic syndrome, which includes obesity, high plasma triglycerides, low high-density lipoproteins, hypertension, systemic inflammation, and abnormal fibrinolysis. There is a genetic component

BOX 38.2

Focus on Diagnosis of Diabetes Mellitus

The American Diabetes Association (ADA) has published the criteria for the diagnosis of diabetes. The diagnosis requires two abnormal test results unless there is unequivocal hyperglycemia. Diagnosis requires meeting one of the following criteria:

- Fasting (no caloric intake for at least 8 h) plasma glucose ≥126 mg/dL
- 2-hour plasma glucose ≥200 mg/dL during oral glucose tolerance test
- HbA1c ≥ 6.5%
- In a patient with classic symptoms of hyperglycemia or hyperglycemic crisis, a random plasma glucose ≥200 mg/dL

to the development of diabetes. There is also a link to obesity (especially abdominal obesity) and the development of diabetes.

The American Diabetes Association (ADA) has defined criteria for the diagnosis of diabetes mellitus. Diagnostic tests include fasting blood glucose, a glucose tolerance test, HbA1c evaluation, or a random plasma glucose test in a patient with classic symptoms of hyperglycemia. See Box 38.2 for specific tests and criteria.

Glycosylated hemoglobin levels, or an HbA1c test, provide a 3-month average of glucose levels. Red blood cells are freely permeable to glucose, and this test gives an average range of glucose exposure over the life of the red blood cell, about 120 days. This test does not require fasting before blood is drawn or the oral intake of glucose before testing. Elevations at or above 6.5% may be an early indicator of diabetes before changes are noted in the fasting blood sugar level. Once a baseline is established, the goal of therapy for most patients with diabetes is an HbA1c level less than 7%. Researchers believe that early intervention—diet, exercise, and lifestyle changes—may delay the onset of diabetes and the complications, including coronary artery disease, that come with it.

Diabetes mellitus can be classified in four general categories:

1. *Type 1* was once called insulin-dependent diabetes mellitus. It is generally caused by autoimmune destruction of the beta cells of the pancreas. Due to lack of insulin release, patients need insulin replacement. This category also includes latent autoimmune diabetes of adulthood.
2. *Type 2* was once called noninsulin-dependent diabetes mellitus or adult-onset diabetes. There is a progressive loss of beta cell release of insulin, but there is also decreased insulin sensitivity in the peripheral cells. This decreased insulin sensitivity is called insulin resistance.
3. *Diabetes due to other causes* refers to development of hyperglycemia due to secondary causes, for example, medication-induced diabetes or diabetes caused by diseases of the exocrine pancreas (cystic fibrosis or pancreatitis).
4. Gestational diabetes is diagnosed in the second or third trimester of pregnancy.

There is good evidence that lifestyle habits can prevent and/or lessen severity of development of type 2 diabetes. The ADA recommends lifestyle habits that help prevent development of diabetes in people who have prediabetes. This term refers to a person having blood glucose levels that are higher than normal but not high enough to meet the criteria for diabetes. It was found that achieving and maintaining a minimum of a 7% weight loss reduced risk of diabetes. A reduced-calorie diet and at least 150 minutes per week of moderately intense physical activity were shown to assist with weight loss programs. The eating plans that worked for people attempting to lower their risk included Mediterranean-style, low-carbohydrate, vegetarian plans, and Dietary Approaches to Stop Hypertension (DASH). The moderately intense physical exercise was shown to improve insulin sensitivity and decrease abdominal obesity. Exercise was also shown to decrease risk of gestational diabetes mellitus.

When diet and exercise are not sufficient to control high glucose levels, it is beneficial to the individual to use medications. Control of blood glucose levels can decrease long-term adverse effects of hyperglycemia. For people with type 2 diabetes, oral or noninsulin injectable agents can often be effective. However, there are times when people with type 2 diabetes benefit from insulin treatment. Type 2 diabetes is a progressive disease, so people may slowly require increased doses and/or a variety of medications to control their blood sugar. People with type 1 diabetes always need insulin replacement. During acute stress, blood glucose levels are higher, so treatment of diabetes is often modified during stressful situations. See Box 38.3 for more information about managing glucose levels during stress.

Hyperglycemia

Hyperglycemia, or high blood sugar, results when there is an increase in glucose in the blood. Clinical signs and symptoms include fatigue, lethargy, irritation, glycosuria, polyphagia, polydipsia, frequent infections, and poor wound healing. Acute complications of high blood sugar include diabetic ketoacidosis (DKA) and hyperosmolar hyperglycemic state (HHS). DKA is more common in people with type 1 diabetes. The lack of insulin causes an increase in fat metabolism and ketone production, which results in metabolic acidosis. The hyperglycemia leads to osmotic dehydration. If hyperglycemia goes unchecked, the patient will experience ketoacidosis and CNS changes that can progress to coma. Signs of impending dangerous complications of hyperglycemia include the following:

- Fruity breath as the ketones build up in the system and are excreted through the lungs

Box 38.3 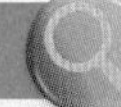 Focus on The Evidence

MANAGING GLUCOSE LEVELS DURING STRESS

The body has many compensatory mechanisms for ensuring that a person's blood glucose level stays within a safe range. The sympathetic stress reaction elevates the blood glucose level to provide ready energy for the fight or flight response (see Chapter 29). The stress reaction causes the breakdown of glycogen to release glucose and the breakdown of fat and proteins to release other energy.

Stress Reactions

The stress reaction elevates blood glucose concentration above the normal range. In severe stress situations—such as an acute myocardial infarction or an automobile accident—the blood glucose level can be high (200 to 300 mg/dL). The body uses that energy to fight the insult or flee from the stressor.

Nurses in acute care situations need to be aware of this reflex elevation in glucose when caring for patients in acute stress, especially patients in emergency situations whose medical history is unknown. The usual medical response to a blood glucose concentration of 400 mg/dL is the administration of insulin. In many situations, that is exactly what is done, especially if the patient's history is not known and the effects of such a high glucose level could cause severe systemic reactions. Insulin administration causes a drop in the blood glucose level as glucose enters cells to be either used for energy or converted to glycogen for storage.

However, a problem may arise in the acute care setting, particularly in a nondiabetic patient. Relieving the stress reaction can also drop glucose levels as the stimulus to increase these levels is lost and the glucose that was there is used for energy. A patient in this situation who has been treated with insulin is at risk for development of potentially severe hypoglycemia. The body's response to a low glucose level is a sympathetic stress reaction, which again elevates the blood glucose concentration. If treated, the patient can potentially enter a cycle of high and low glucose levels.

Best Nursing Practice

Nurses are often the ones in closest contact with the highly stressed patient—in the emergency room, the intensive care unit, and the postanesthesia room—and should be constantly aware of the normal and reflex changes in blood glucose that accompany stress. Careful monitoring with awareness of stress and the relief of stress can prevent a prolonged treatment program to maintain the blood glucose level within the range of normal, a situation that is not "normal" during a stress reaction.

Patients with diabetes who are in severe stress situations require changes in their insulin doses. They should be allowed some elevation of blood glucose, even though their inability to produce sufficient insulin will make it difficult for their cells to make effective use of the increased glucose level. It is a clinical challenge to balance glucose levels with the needs of the patient because so many factors can affect the glucose level.

- Dehydration as fluid and important electrolytes are lost through the kidneys
- Slow, deep respirations (Kussmaul respirations) as the body tries to rid itself of high acid levels
- Loss of orientation and coma

HHS, while it does not involve ketoacidosis, is also an acute situation. This is more common in people with type 2 diabetes. Both of these acute situations need emergent attention and treatment with insulin.

Hypoglycemia

Hypoglycemia, or lower-than-normal blood glucose concentration (70 mg/dL or lower), occurs in a number of clinical situations, including starvation, or if treatment of hyperglycemia with insulin or oral agents lowers the blood glucose level too far. The body immediately reacts to lowered blood glucose because the cells require glucose to survive, the neurons being among the cells most sensitive to the lack of glucose. The initial reaction to a falling blood glucose level is parasympathetic stimulation—increased GI activity to increase digestion and absorption. Rather rapidly, the SNS responds with a fight or flight reaction that increases the blood glucose level by initiating the breakdown of fat and glycogen to release glucose for rapid energy. The pancreas releases glucagon, a hormone that counters the effects of insulin and works to increase the glucose level and somatostatin, which helps the body conserve energy. In many cases, the response to the hypoglycemic state causes a hyperglycemic state. Balancing the body's responses to glucose is sometimes difficult when one is trying to treat and control diabetes. Table 38.1 offers a comparison of the signs and symptoms of hyperglycemia and hypoglycemia. Signs and symptoms of hypoglycemia can be divided in two main categories: altered nerve function and activation of the autonomic nervous system. People may report headache, difficulty focusing, anxiety, or sweating. Since symptoms of hypoglycemia vary from person to person, it is recommended to assess blood glucose whenever there is an acute mental status change.

Insulin

Insulin is the only parenteral antidiabetic agent available for exogenous replacement of low levels of insulin (Table 38.2). It is used to treat type 1 diabetes and to treat type 2 diabetes in adults who have no response to diet, exercise, and other

Table 38.1 Signs and Symptoms of Hypoglycemia and Hyperglycemia

Clinical Effects	Hypoglycemia	Hyperglycemia
CNS	Headache, blurred vision, diplopia; drowsiness progressing to coma; ataxia; hyperactive reflexes	Decreased level of consciousness, sluggishness progressing to coma; hypoactive reflexes
Neuromuscular	Paresthesia; weakness; muscle spasms; twitching progressing to seizures	Weakness, lethargy
CV	Tachycardia; palpitations; normal to high blood pressure	Tachycardia; hypotension
Respiratory	Rapid, shallow respirations	Rapid, deep respirations (Kussmaul); acetonelike or fruity breath
GI	Hunger, nausea	Nausea; vomiting; thirst
Other	Diaphoresis; cool and clammy skin; normal eyeballs	Dry, warm, flushed skin; soft eyeballs
Laboratory tests	Urine glucose negative; blood glucose low	Urine glucose strongly positive; urine ketone levels positive; blood glucose high
Onset	Sudden; patient appears anxious, drunk; associated with overdose of insulin, missing a meal, increased stress	Gradual; patient is slow and sluggish; associated with lack of insulin, increased stress

CNS, central nervous system; CV, cardiovascular; GI, gastrointestinal.

agents. Insulin is often substituted for other antidiabetic agents for patients during acute situations such as infection, trauma, undergoing a surgical procedure, or treatment for DKA or HHS. People with hyperglycemia in conjunction with severe liver and/or renal disease may need treatment with insulin. See Box 38.4 for considerations related to the use of insulin based on age.

The types of insulin are often categorized as rapid, short, intermediate, or long acting. The rapid-acting type includes lispro (*Humalog* and others), aspart (*NovoLog* and others), and glulisine (*Apidra* and others). Regular insulin (*Novolin R* and others) is short acting. NPH insulin (*Novolin N*) and insulin detemir (*Levemir* and others) are intermediate acting. At higher doses they can be long acting. Insulin glargine (*Lantus*, *Toujeo*, and others) and degludec (*Tresiba*) are long-acting insulins.

Originally, insulin was prepared from pig and cow pancreas. Today, virtually all insulin is prepared by recombinant DNA technology and is human insulin produced by genetically altered bacteria. This purer form of insulin is not associated with the sensitivity problems that many patients developed with the animal products. Box 38.5 describes the various forms of insulin delivery that are available or under study for future use.

Therapeutic Actions and Indications

Insulin is a hormone that promotes the storage of the body's fuels, facilitates the transport of various metabolites and ions across cell membranes, and stimulates the synthesis of glycogen from glucose, of fats from lipids, and of proteins from amino acids. Insulin does these things by

Table 38.2 *Drugs in Focus:* Insulin

Drug Name	Dosage/Route	Usual Indications
Insulin (various types)	Varies based on patient response, diet, and activity level ***Insulin*** *Aspart and Lispro*: Given within 20 min of start of a meal *Regular insulin*: Given within 30 min of a meal *Glulisine*: Given 15 min before or within 20 min of the start of a meal *Detemir and Glargine*: Given once daily at bedtime, or twice daily 12 h apart *Degludec*: Given once daily at same time of day	Treatment of type 1 diabetes mellitus; treatment of type 2 diabetes mellitus in patients whose diabetes cannot be controlled by diet or other agents; treatment of severe ketoacidosis or diabetic coma; treatment of hyperkalemia (in conjunction with a glucose infusion to produce a shift of potassium into the cells [polarizing solution]); also used for short courses of therapy during periods of stress (e.g., surgery, disease) in patients with type 2 diabetes, for newly diagnosed patients being stabilized, for patients with poor control of glucose levels, and for patients with gestational diabetes

Box 38.4 **Focus on Drug Therapy Across the Lifespan**

ANTIDIABETIC AGENTS

Children

Treatment of diabetes in children is a difficult challenge of balancing diet, activity, growth, stressors, and insulin requirements. Children need to be carefully monitored for any sign of hypoglycemia or hyperglycemia and treated quickly because their fast metabolism and lack of body reserves can push them into a severe state quickly.

Insulin dose, especially in infants, may be so small that it is difficult to calibrate. Insulin often needs to be diluted to a volume that can be detected on the syringe. A second person should always check the calculations and dose of insulin being given to small children.

Teenagers often present a challenge for diabetes management. The social pressure on adolescents to "fit in" can sometimes lead to resistance to dietary restrictions and insulin injections. The metabolism of the teenager is also in flux, leading to complications in regulating insulin dose. A team approach, including the child, family members, teachers, coaches, and even friends, may be the best way to help the child deal with the disease and the required therapy. New delivery methods for insulin may help this age group cope with the drug therapy in the future.

Metformin is the only oral antidiabetic drug approved for children. It has established dosing for children 10 years of age and older.

Adults

Adults need extensive education about the disease and about the drug therapy. Warning signs and symptoms should be stressed repeatedly as the adult learns to juggle insulin needs with exercise, stressors, other drug effects, and diet. Adults maintained on oral agents need to be monitored for changes in response to the drugs. Often, additional drugs are added or doses are changed as the disease progresses over time.

Exercise and diet should always be emphasized as the mainstay of dealing with diabetes. Adults need to be cautioned about the use of over-the-counter and herbal or alternative therapies. Many of these products contain agents that alter blood glucose levels and will change insulin or oral agent requirements. Adults should always be asked specifically whether they use any of these agents, and adjustments should be made accordingly.

Insulin therapy is the best choice for people with diabetes during pregnancy and lactation, which are times of high stress and metabolic demands. Needs may change on a daily basis, and the patient should have ready support and extensive teaching about what to do if hypoglycemia or hyperglycemia occurs. The period of labor and delivery is often a critical time in diabetes management because of the stress and sudden changes in body fluid volume and hormone levels. The obstetrician and the endocrinologist or primary care provider should consult frequently about the best way to support the patient through this period.

Older Adults

Older adults can have many underlying problems that complicate diabetic therapy. Poor vision and/or coordination may make it difficult to prepare injections.

Dietary deficiencies related to changes in taste, absorption, or attitude may lead to wide fluctuations in blood sugar levels, making it difficult to control diabetes. Many areas have nutritional assistance programs for older adults (e.g., Meals on Wheels) or have resources that can refer patients to appropriate agencies that might be able to offer assistance.

Older adults have a greater incidence of renal or hepatic impairment, and kidney and liver function should be evaluated before starting many of the noninsulin antidiabetic medications. Combinations of oral agents may not be feasible with severe dysfunction, and the patient may need to use insulin to control blood glucose levels.

Older adults should receive periodic educational reminders about diet, the need for exercise, skin and foot care, and warning signs to report to the health care provider.

The older patient is also more likely to experience end organ damage related to diabetes—loss of vision, kidney problems, coronary artery disease, and infections—and the drug regimen for these patients can become quite complex. Careful screening for drug interactions is an important aspect of the assessment of these patients.

reacting with specific receptor sites on the cell. Figure 38.1 shows the sites of action of replacement insulin and other drugs used to treat diabetic conditions. See Table 38.2 for usual indications.

Pharmacokinetics

Various preparations of insulin are available to provide short- and long-term coverage. These preparations are processed within the body like endogenous insulin. However, the peak, onset, and duration of each vary because of the placement or addition of glycine and/or arginine chains. Maintenance doses are given by subcutaneous or inhaled routes. Injection sites need to be rotated regularly to avoid damage to muscles and to prevent subcutaneous atrophy. Regular insulin is given intramuscularly (IM) or IV in emergency situations.

Insulin is available in various preparations with a wide range of peaks and durations of action. A patient may receive a long-acting formulation daily or twice a day to cover the basal insulin need and may receive a short-acting insulin for the increased glucose levels from meals. Some

BOX 38.5

Insulin Delivery: Past, Present, and Future

Past

Subcutaneous Insulin Injection: The delivery of insulin by subcutaneous injection was introduced in the 1920s and changed clinical management of patients with diabetes, giving them a chance for a normal lifestyle.

Present

Subcutaneous Insulin Injection: This remains the primary delivery system.

Insulin Jet Injector: This cylindrical device shoots a fine spray of insulin through the skin under high pressure. Although it is appealing for people who do not like needles or have problems disposing of needles properly, it can be expensive.

Insulin Pen: This syringelike device looks like a pen. It has a small needle at the tip and a barrel that holds insulin. The patient "dials" the amount of insulin to be given and injects the insulin subcutaneously by pressing on the top of the pen. This is advantageous for people who need insulin two or three times during the day but cannot easily transport syringes and needles. It is a subtle way to give insulin and is popular with students and business people on the go. It is important to rotate the syringe 15 to 20 times before injecting the insulin to disperse it. Patients often forget this point after using the pens for a while, and as a result may inject far too much or too little insulin when it is needed. Periodic reinforcement of the administration instructions is important.

External Insulin Pump: This pump device can be worn on a belt or hidden in a pocket and is attached to a small tube inserted into the subcutaneous tissue of the abdomen. The device slowly leaks a base rate of insulin into the abdomen all day; the patient can pump or inject booster doses throughout the day to correspond with meals and activity. The device does have several disadvantages. For example, it is awkward, the tubing poses an increased risk of infection and requires frequent changing, and the patient has to frequently check blood glucose levels throughout the day to monitor response.

IV Insulin: In emergency situations or when rapid and continuous control of blood glucose is needed, insulin can be given IV. Insulin is considered a high-risk drug when administered this way. There is potential for rapid changes in blood glucose and resultant risk to the CNS and heart. IV insulin should be given using a controlled delivery pump, the patient should be constantly monitored, and blood glucose levels should be checked frequently to adjust the dosage appropriately.

Inhaled Insulin: The lung tissue is one of the best sites for insulin absorption. An aerosol delivery system delivers a powdered insulin formulation directly into the lung tissue. *Afrezza* is a rapid-acting inhaled insulin that is indicated for adult patients with diabetes mellitus who are also prescribed long-acting insulin. There are warnings that acute bronchospasm could occur with people who have asthma, chronic obstructive pulmonary disease (COPD), or lung cancer, and a baseline and periodic spirometry is suggested. This rapid-acting insulin is inhaled at the beginning of a meal. If used in type 1 diabetes, it must be combined with a long-acting insulin. The most common adverse effects are cough, throat irritation, and hypoglycemia. Because of adverse effects seen in clinical studies, it is suggested that patients using this form of insulin may experience more ketoacidosis, hypokalemia, and life-threatening hypoglycemia than patients receiving insulin by injection. Careful monitoring and patient teaching is important.

Future

Implantable Insulin Pump: This pump is surgically implanted into the abdomen and delivers base insulin as well as insulin boluses as needed directly into the abdomen to be absorbed by the liver, just as pancreatic insulin is. The disadvantages are risk of infection, mechanical problems with the pump, and lack of long-term data on its effectiveness. This method is not yet available for general use.

Insulin Patch: The patch is placed on the skin and delivers a constant low dose of insulin. When the patient eats a meal, tabs are pulled on the patch to release more insulin. The problem with this delivery method is that insulin does not readily pass through the skin, so there is tremendous variability in its effects. This route is not yet commercially available.

The National Institute of Diabetes and Digestive and Kidney Diseases reports up-to-date research on insulin delivery.

patients with type 2 diabetes may take oral or noninsulin injectable antidiabetic medications in addition to insulin therapy.

Contraindications and Cautions

Because insulin is used as a replacement hormone, there are no contraindications other than episodes of hypoglycemia, which could be exacerbated. Care should be taken during pregnancy and lactation to monitor glucose levels closely and adjust the insulin dose accordingly. Insulin does not cross the placenta; therefore, it is the drug of choice for managing diabetes during pregnancy. Insulin does enter human milk, but it is destroyed in the GI tract and does not affect the nursing infant. However, insulin-dependent people may have inhibited milk production because of insulin's effects on fat and protein metabolism. The effectiveness of nursing the infant should be evaluated periodically. Patients using inhaled insulin are at risk for impairment of respiratory function; this route is contraindicated in people with asthma or COPD and in people with lung cancer or a history of lung cancer.

Adverse Effects

The most common adverse effect related to insulin use is hypoglycemia, which can be controlled with proper dose

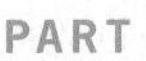
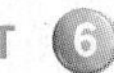

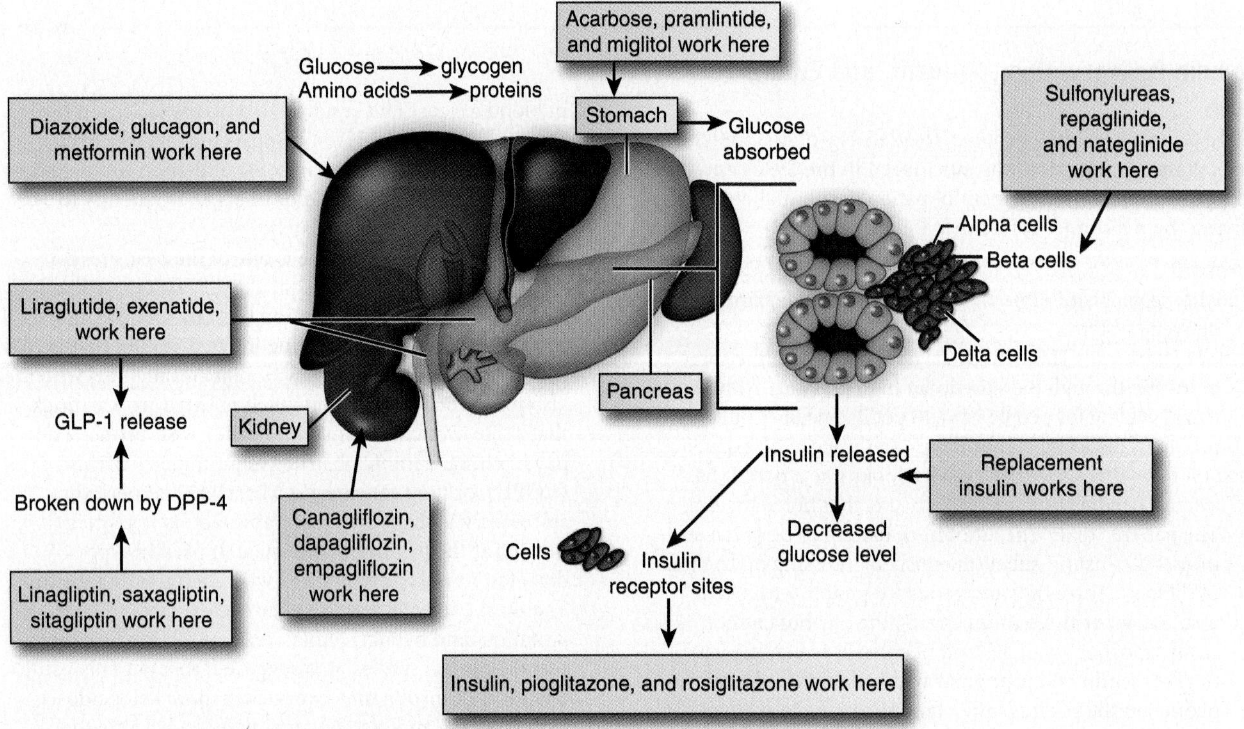

FIGURE 38.1 Sites of action of drugs used to treat diabetic conditions.

Box 38.6 Focus on Safe Medication Administration

Many of the antidiabetic agents need to be administered with specific timing around food intake. If a patient is not able to eat, adjustments need to be made. Use care in teaching patients about timing and eating and in administering insulin in institutions, where timing of food delivery may vary or patients may be NPO for tests or procedures. Often when patients are admitted to the hospital, the form of antidiabetic treatment may change from their home treatment. Careful assessment of blood glucose must be done to keep the patient from becoming hypo- or hyperglycemic. Insulin is considered a high-risk drug. The patient is in a precarious situation, and rapid swings in blood sugar can occur. Frequent assessment of blood glucose is required when administering IV insulin.

Box 38.7 Focus on Safe Medication Administration

Insulin is usually given by subcutaneous injection. Using an insulin syringe or insulin pen, inject the insulin into the loose connective tissue underneath the skin. The areas of the body that are best able to be pinched up to access this tissue are the abdomen, the upper thigh, and the upper arm. Insert the needle at a 45-degree angle (Fig. 38.2). Inject the insulin. Remove the needle and syringe and apply gentle pressure at the injection site. Rotate sites regularly to prevent tissue damage.

adjustments (Box 38.6). Local reactions at injection sites, including lipodystrophy, can also occur. This effect is lessened by rotation of injection sites and by proper injection administration (see Box 38.7 and Fig. 38.2). Insulin can also decrease blood potassium levels. People taking large doses of insulin should be monitored for hypokalemia, and potassium replacement should be given to treat if hypokalemia occurs. With inhaled insulin, the most common adverse effects also include cough and throat pain or irritation. Figure 38.3 shows adverse effects and toxicities associated with antidiabetic agents.

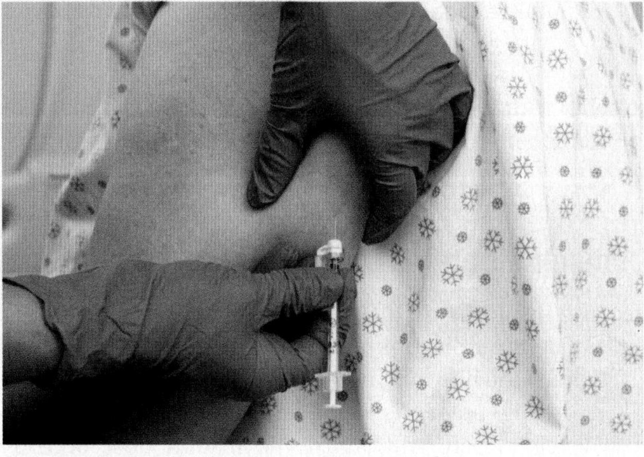

FIGURE 38.2 Insert the needle at a 45-degree angle.

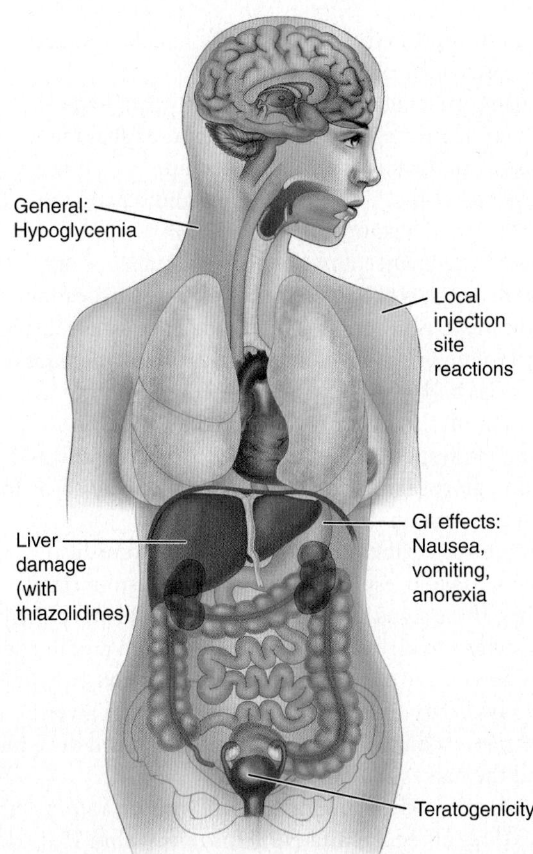

FIGURE 38.3 Variety of adverse effects and toxicities associated with antidiabetic agents.

Clinically Important Drug–Drug Interactions

Caution should be used when giving a patient stabilized on insulin any drug that decreases glucose levels (e.g., oral antidiabetic agents, beta-blockers, salicylates, alcohol). Dose adjustments may be needed when any of these drugs is added or removed. Care should also be taken when combining insulin with any beta-blocker. The blocking of the SNS also blocks many of the signs and symptoms of hypoglycemia, hindering the patient's ability to recognize problems. Patients may need higher doses of insulin if they are also using thiazide diuretics or glucocorticoids. Patients should also be warned about possible interactions with various herbal therapies (Box 38.8). Insulin is a medication that often requires frequent titrations and monitoring due to multiple drug–drug interactions.

Box 38.8 Focus on Herbal and Alternative Therapies

Patients being treated with antidiabetic therapies are at increased risk of developing hypoglycemia if they use aloe vera, cinnamon, juniper berries, ginseng, garlic, fenugreek, coriander, dandelion root, celery, and other alternative or herbal medicines. If a patient uses supplements or herbs to decrease blood glucose, levels should be monitored closely and appropriate dose adjustment made for the prescribed drug.

Prototype Summary: Insulin

Indications: Treatment of type 1 diabetes; treatment of type 2 diabetes when other agents are not able to better control blood glucose; short-term treatment of type 2 diabetes during periods of stress; management of diabetic ketoacidosis, hyperkalemia, and marked insulin resistance.

Actions: Replaces endogenous insulin.

Pharmacokinetics:

Route	Onset	Peak	Duration
Regular (*Humulin R, Novolin R*)	30–60 min	2–4 h	6–12 h
NPH (*Novolin N*)	1–1.5 h	4–12 h	24 h
Inhaled insulin (*Afrezza*)	12–15 min	60 min	2.5–3 h
lispro (*Humalog*)	<15 min	30–90 min	2–5 h
aspart (*NovoLog*)	10–20 min	1–3 h	3–5 h
glargine (*Lantus, Toujeo*)	60–70 min	None	24 h
glulisine (*Apidra*)	2–5 min	30–90 min	2 h
detemir (*Levemir*)	1–2 h	3–6 h	5.7–23.3 h
Combination Insulins			
Humalog 50/50, *Humalog* 75/25, *NovoLog* 70/30, *Humulin* 70/30, *Novolin* 70/30	varies	varies	varies

$T_{1/2}$: Varies with each preparation; metabolized at the cellular level.

Adverse Effects: Hypersensitivity reaction, local reactions at injection site, hypoglycemia, hypokalemia.

Nursing Considerations for Patients Taking Insulin

Assessment: History and Examination

- Assess for contraindications or cautions including any known allergy to any insulin and current status of pregnancy or lactation so that appropriate monitoring and dose adjustments can be completed. Assess for history of asthma or COPD if using inhaled insulin to prevent exacerbation of these conditions and decline in respiratory function.
- Perform a physical assessment to establish a baseline before beginning therapy and during therapy to evaluate the effectiveness of therapy and any potential adverse effects.
- Assess for indications of presence of any skin lesions; orientation and reflexes; baseline pulse and blood

(continues on page 654)

pressure; respiration or adventitious breath sounds; and spirometry if using inhaled form. These could indicate response to high or low glucose levels and potential risk factors in giving insulin.
- Assess body systems for changes suggesting possible complications associated with poor blood glucose control.
- Investigate nutritional intake, noting any problems with intake and adherence to prescribed diet that could alter the anticipated response to insulin therapy.
- Assess activity level, including amount and degree of exercise, which could alter anticipated response to insulin therapy.
- Inspect skin areas that will be used for injection of insulin; note any areas that are bruised, thickened, or scarred, which could interfere with insulin absorption and alter anticipated response to insulin therapy.
- Obtain blood glucose levels as ordered to monitor response to insulin and need to adjust dose.
- Monitor the results of laboratory tests, including urinalysis, for evidence of glycosuria, and HbA1c, for evidence or hyperglycemia in past 3 months.

Refer to the "Critical Thinking Scenario" for a full discussion of nursing care for a patient with type 1 diabetes mellitus.

Nursing Conclusions

Nursing conclusions related to drug therapy might include the following:
- Glucose and electrolyte imbalance risk related to the use of insulin and underlying disease processes
- Malnutrition risk related to changes in glucose transport
- Altered sensory perception (kinesthetic, visual, auditory, and tactile) related to glucose levels
- Infection risk related to injections and disease processes
- Injury risk related to potential hyperglycemia or hypoglycemia and injection technique
- Coping impairment related to diagnosis and the need for injection therapy
- Knowledge deficit risk regarding drug therapy

Planning

- The patient will receive the best therapeutic effect from the drug therapy.
- The patient will have limited adverse effects from the drug therapy.
- The patient will have an understanding of the drug therapy, adverse effects to anticipate, and measures to relieve discomfort and improve safety.

Intervention With Rationale

- Ensure that the patient is following a dietary and exercise regimen and is using good hygiene practices to improve the effectiveness of the insulin and decrease adverse effects of the disease.
- If using an insulin suspension, gently rotate the vial containing the agent and avoid vigorous shaking to ensure uniform suspension of insulin.
- Select a site that is free of bruising and scarring to ensure good absorption of the insulin.
- Give maintenance doses by the subcutaneous or inhaled routes only (see "Focus on Safe Medication Administration" under "Pharmacokinetics" for insulin), and rotate injection sites regularly to avoid damage to muscles and to prevent subcutaneous atrophy. Give regular insulin IM or IV in emergency situations.
- Monitor response carefully to avoid adverse effects; blood glucose monitoring is the most effective way to evaluate insulin dose.
- Monitor the patient for signs and symptoms of hypoglycemia, especially during peak insulin times, when these signs and symptoms would be most likely to appear, to assess the response to insulin and the need for dose adjustment or medical intervention.
- Always verify the name of the insulin being given because each insulin has a different peak and duration, and the names can be confused.
- Use caution when mixing types of insulin; administer mixtures of regular and NPH insulins within 15 minutes after combining them to ensure appropriate suspension and therapeutic effect.
- Read instructions for storage details and check expiration dates to ensure effectiveness.
- Monitor the patient during times of trauma or severe stress for potential dose adjustment needs.
- Monitor the patient's food intake; ensure that the patient eats when using insulin to ensure therapeutic effect and avoid hypoglycemia.
- Monitor the patient's exercise and activities; ensure that the patient considers the effects of exercise in relationship to eating and insulin dose to ensure therapeutic effect and avoid hypoglycemia.
- Protect the patient from infection, including ensuring good skin care and foot care, to prevent the development of serious infections and changes in therapeutic insulin doses.
- Monitor the patient's sensory losses to incorporate their needs into safety measures and to identify potential problems in drawing up and administering insulin.
- Help the patient manage necessary lifestyle changes, including diet and exercise needs, sensory loss, and the impact of a drug regimen that includes giving injections, to help encourage adherence to the treatment regimen.
- Instruct patients who are also receiving beta-blockers on ways to monitor glucose levels and signs and symptoms of glucose abnormalities to prevent hypoglycemic and hyperglycemic episodes when SNS and warning signs are blocked.

- Provide thorough patient teaching, including diet and exercise needs; measures to avoid adverse effects, including proper food care and screening for injuries; warning signs of problems, including signs and symptoms of hypoglycemia and hyperglycemia; the importance of increased screening when ill or unable to eat properly; proper administration techniques and proper disposal of needles and syringes in the provided sharps bucket and to return this when full to a community take-back center or pharmacy; to never reuse needles or lancets or share needles with other people; and the need to monitor disease status, to enhance patient knowledge about drug therapy and promote adherence.

Evaluation

- Monitor patient response to the drug (stabilization of blood glucose levels).
- Monitor for adverse effects (hypoglycemia, hypokalemia, lung function decline with inhaled insulin, and injection site irritation).
- Evaluate the effectiveness of the teaching plan (patient can name drug, dosage, adverse effects to watch for, specific measures to avoid them, and proper administration technique).
- Monitor the effectiveness of comfort measures and adherence to the regimen.

CRITICAL THINKING SCENARIO
Type 1 Diabetes Mellitus

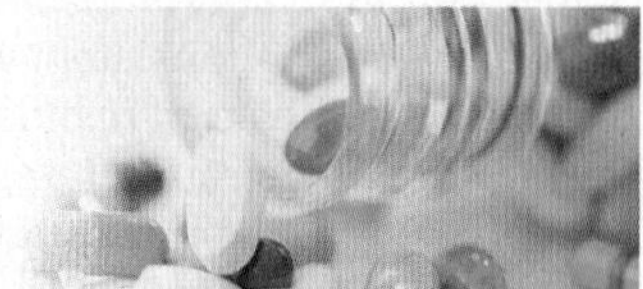

THE SITUATION

M.J. is 22 years old and has newly diagnosed type 1 diabetes mellitus. M.J. was stabilized on insulin while hospitalized for diagnosis and management. One week after discharge, M.J. experienced nausea and anorexia. They were unable to eat but took insulin as usual in the morning. That afternoon, M.J. experienced profuse sweating and was tremulous and apprehensive, so they went to the hospital emergency room. The initial diagnosis was hypoglycemia from taking insulin and not eating, combined with the stress of having GI upset. M.J. was treated at the emergency room with intravenous glucose. After they had rested and their glucose levels had returned to normal, M.J. was discharged to home.

CRITICAL THINKING

What instructions should M.J. receive before leaving? Think about the ways that stress can alter blood glucose levels. Then consider the stress that a patient with newly diagnosed type 1 diabetes undergoes while trying to cope with the diagnosis and learn self-injection. Think about complications of the disease that may arise in the future.

What teaching approaches could help M.J. decrease stress and effectively plan a medical regimen?

What sort of support would be useful for M.J. as they adjust to a new life?

DISCUSSION

The diagnosis of type 1 diabetes is a life-changing event. M.J. has to learn about the disease and how to test their blood and give themself injections, manage a new diet and exercise program, and cope with the knowledge that the long-term complications of diabetes can be devastating. Many patients who are regulated on insulin in the hospital experience a change in insulin demand after discharge. The SNS is active in the hospital, and one of the effects of SNS activity is increased glucose level—preparing the body for fight or flight. For some patients, returning home eases the stress that activated the SNS, and glucose levels fall. If the patient continues to use the same insulin dose, hypoglycemia can occur. Other patients may feel protected in the hospital and experience stress when they are sent home. They may feel anxious about taking care of themselves while coping with everyday problems and tensions. In addition, it may be overwhelming to learn the proper preparation and administration of a subcutaneous injection. Learning how to properly dispose of needles and syringes may be one more stressor. These patients need an increased insulin dose because their stress reaction intensifies when they get home, driving their blood glucose level up.

Patients are taught how to measure their blood glucose levels before they leave the hospital. After they get used to doing this and regulating their insulin based on glucose concentrations, they usually manage well. The first few days to weeks are often the hardest. The nurse should review with M.J. how to test their glucose, administer insulin, and regulate the dose. The nurse should also give M.J. written information that they can refer to later.

In addition, the nurse should give M.J. a chance to talk and to vent feelings about the diagnosis and their future. To help decrease M.J.'s stress and to avoid problems during this adjustment period, the nurse can give M.J. a telephone number to call if they have problems or questions. M.J. should return in a few days to review their progress and have any questions answered. In the meantime, the nurse should encourage M.J. to write down any questions or problems that arise so that they can be addressed during a follow-up visit.

(continues on page 656)

Support and encouragement will be crucial to helping M.J. adjust to the disease and the drug therapy. M.J. can also be referred to the American Diabetic Association, which in many communities offers support services to help diabetic patients.

NURSING CARE GUIDE FOR M.J.: TYPE 1 DIABETES MELLITUS

Assessment: History and Examination

Review the patient's history for allergies to drug products, pregnancy, breast or chestfeeding, and other drugs in current use. M.J. denies allergies, pregnancy, and lactation. They are taking no other medications.

Focus the physical examination on the following:

Neurological: Orientation, reflexes; M.J. appears shaky, and their pupils are dilated.

Skin: Coloration and/or lesions; M.J.'s appearance (pale and sweaty) is consistent with diaphoresis.

CV: Pulse, 110 beats/min; blood pressure, 155/92 mm Hg.

Respiratory: Respiratory rate, 24/min; lungs clear on auscultation; rapid respiratory rate is indicative of acidosis.

Laboratory tests: Urinalysis—negative for glucose, positive for ketones; blood glucose level, 72 mg/dL.

Nursing Conclusions

Malnutrition risk less than body requirements related to metabolic effects

Altered sensory perception (kinesthetic, visual, auditory, and tactile) related to effects on glucose levels

Infection risk related to injections and disease process

Coping impairment related to diagnosis and injections

Knowledge deficit regarding drug therapy

Planning

The patient will receive the best therapeutic effect from the drug therapy.

The patient will have limited adverse effects from the drug therapy.

The patient will have an understanding of the drug therapy, adverse effects to anticipate, and measures to relieve discomfort and improve safety.

Intervention

Provide patient teaching regarding drug name, dosage, adverse effects, precautions, warning signs to report, and proper administration technique.

Assist M.J. with restoring blood glucose to normal levels by using insulin and constantly monitoring blood glucose levels during normal times and during times of stress and trauma so that insulin dose can be adjusted as necessary.

Review proper subcutaneous injection technique and site rotation.

Provide support and reassurance to help M.J. deal with drug injections, this hypoglycemic episode, and their lifetime need for insulin.

Teach M.J. how to store insulin and to check expiration dates.

Review with M.J. the name and type of insulin, dosage, adverse effects, precautions, warning signs of adverse effects to report, proper administration technique, and proper disposal of needles and syringes.

Evaluation

Evaluate drug effects: return of glucose levels to normal.

Monitor for adverse effects: hypoglycemia and/or injection site reaction.

Monitor for drug–drug interactions as indicated for insulin.

Evaluate the effectiveness of patient teaching program and comfort and safety measures.

PATIENT TEACHING FOR M.J.

- Diet modifications and exercise are important aspects of your diabetes management. You should also practice good skin care and hygiene measures. Check for injuries or signs of infection regularly.
- Insulin is a hormone that is normally produced by your pancreas. It helps regulate your energy balance by affecting the way the body uses sugar, proteins, and fats. The lack of insulin produces a disease called diabetes mellitus. By injecting insulin each day, you can help your body effectively use the nutrients in your food.
- Check the expiration date on your insulin. Store the insulin based on the manufacturer's directions and avoid extremes of heat and light.
- Rotate your injection sites on a regular basis to prevent tissue damage and to ensure that the proper amount of insulin is absorbed.
- Depending on the type of insulin and state laws, a prescription may be required to get the supplies you will need to administer your insulin. Keep supplies sealed until ready to use, and dispose of them appropriately in the sharps bucket provided; when it is full, return it to a community drug take-back center or a pharmacy. Never reuse needles or lancets, and never share needles with other people.
- You should be aware of the signs and symptoms of hypoglycemia (too much insulin). If any of these occur, eat or drink something high in sugar, such as candy, orange juice, honey, or sugar. The signs and symptoms to watch for include nervousness, anxiety, sweating, pale and cool skin, headache, nausea, hunger, and shakiness. These may happen if you skip a meal, exercise too much, or experience extreme stress. If these symptoms happen often, notify your health care provider. If you cannot eat because of illness or other problems, do not take your usual insulin dose. Contact your health care provider for assistance.
- Avoid the use of any over-the-counter medications or herbal therapies without first checking with your health care provider. Several of these medications and many commonly used herbs can interfere

with the effectiveness of insulin. Avoid the use of alcohol because it increases the chances of having hypoglycemic attacks.

- Tell any doctor, nurse, or other health care provider involved in your care that you are taking this drug. You may want to wear or carry a MedicAlert tag showing that you are on this medication. This would alert any medical personnel taking care of you in an emergency to the fact that you are taking this drug.
- Report any of the following to your health care provider: loss of appetite, blurred vision, fruity odor to your breath, increased urination, increased thirst, nausea, or vomiting.
- While you are taking this drug, it is important to have regular medical follow-ups, including blood tests to monitor your blood glucose levels, to evaluate you for any adverse effects of your diabetes.
- Keep this drug and supplies out of the reach of children. Use proper disposal techniques for your needles and insulin supplies. Do not give this medication to anyone else or take any similar medication that has not been prescribed for you.

Key Points

- Insulin replaces the endogenous hormone when the body does not produce enough insulin or when there are not enough insulin receptor sites to provide adequate glucose control.
- Blood glucose levels vary with food intake, exercise, and stress levels, possibly necessitating a change in insulin dose.
- Patients need to learn to recognize the signs of hypoglycemia and hyperglycemia to effectively manage their drug therapy.

Oral Antidiabetics

There are oral medications that are designed to help with management of blood glucose levels. These agents include the sulfonylureas, alpha-glucosidase inhibitors, biguanide, dipeptidyl peptidase-4 inhibitors, meglitinides, sodium-glucose cotransporter-2 inhibitors, and thiazolidinediones (Table 38.3). The sulfonylureas were the first oral agents introduced to treat type 2 diabetes. They stimulate the pancreas to release insulin. Other oral agents discussed in this section have been introduced more recently for use in patients with type 2 diabetes.

Table 38.3 ***Drugs in Focus:*** **Oral Antidiabetic Agents and Noninsulin Injectable Antidiabetic Agents**

Drug Name	Dosage/Route	Usual Indications
Sulfonylureas		
First-Generation Sulfonylureas		
tolbutamide (generic)	0.25–3 g/d PO	Adjunct to diet for the management of type 2 diabetes; adjunct to insulin for management in certain type 2 diabetics, reducing the insulin dose and decreasing the risk of hypoglycemia
Second-Generation Sulfonylureas		
glimepiride (*Amaryl*)	1–8 mg/d PO; careful titration with older adults and people with renal impairment	Adjunct to diet for the management of type 2 diabetes; adjunct to insulin for management in certain patients with type 2 diabetes, reducing the insulin dose and decreasing the risks of hypoglycemia
glipizide (*Glucotrol, Glucotrol XL*)	5 mg PO daily, may divide into two doses per day; do not exceed 40 mg/d; use lower doses with older adults and hepatic-impaired patients; extended release: 5 mg/d, adjust to a maximum of 20 mg/d	Adjunct to diet for the management of type 2 diabetes; adjunct to insulin for management in certain type 2 diabetics, reducing the insulin dose and decreasing the risk of hypoglycemia
glyburide (*DiaBeta, Glynase*)	1.25–20 mg/d PO (*DiaBeta*), 0.75–12 mg/d PO (*Glynase*); reduce dose with older patients and those with renal and hepatic impairment	Adjunct to diet for the management of type 2 diabetes; adjunct to insulin for management in certain type 2 diabetics, reducing the insulin dose and decreasing the risk of hypoglycemia
Alpha-Glucosidase Inhibitors		
acarbose (generic)	25–100 mg PO t.i.d. at the start of each meal	Adjunct to diet to lower blood glucose in type 2 diabetics; may be used in combination with other antidiabetic agents
miglitol (*Glyset*)	25–100 mg PO t.i.d. at the start of each meal; not recommended with severe renal impairment	Adjunct to diet to lower blood glucose in type 2 diabetics; may be used in combination with other antidiabetic agents

(*continues on page 658*)

Table 38.3 *Drugs in Focus:* Oral Antidiabetic Agents and Noninsulin Injectable Antidiabetic Agents *(Continued)*

Drug Name	Dosage/Route	Usual Indications
Biguanide		
metformin (*Fortamet, Glumetza, Riomet*)	*Adult*: 500–2,550 mg/d PO in divided doses or single dose for extended-release form; reduce dose in geriatric and renal-impaired patients; maximum dose: 2,550 mg/d *Pediatric (10–16 y)*: 500 mg/d PO with a maximum dose of 2,000 mg/d; do not use extended-release form	Adjunct to diet and exercise to lower blood glucose in type 2 diabetics
DPP-4 Inhibitors		
alogliptin (*Nesina*)	25 mg/d PO; reduce dose with renal impairment	Adjunct to diet and exercise to improve glucose control in patients with type 2 diabetes
linagliptin (*Tradjenta*)	5 mg/d PO	Adjunct to diet and exercise to improve glucose control in patients with type 2 diabetes
saxagliptin (*Onglyza*)	2.5–5 mg/d PO; reduce dose with renal impairment	Adjunct to diet and exercise to improve glucose control in patients with type 2 diabetes
sitagliptin (*Januvia*)	100 mg/d PO; reduce dose with renal impairment	Adjunct to diet and exercise to improve glucose control in patients with type 2 diabetes
Meglitinides		
nateglinide (generic)	120 mg PO t.i.d. with each meal	Adjunct to diet to lower blood glucose in people with type 2 diabetes
repaglinide (generic)	0.5–4 mg PO before meals; do not exceed 16 mg/d; reduce dose with renal impairment	Adjunct to diet to lower blood glucose in patients with type 2 diabetes
SGLT-2 Inhibitors		
canagliflozin (*Invokana*)	100 mg/d PO with the first meal of the day; maximum 300 mg/d; reduce dose with moderate renal impairment; contraindicated with severe renal impairment	Adjunct to diet and exercise to improve glycemic control in people with type 2 diabetes; reducing risk of cardiovascular events in adults with type 2 diabetes and cardiovascular disease; reducing risk of end-stage kidney disease, doubling of serum creatinine, cardiovascular death, and hospitalization for heart failure in adults with type 2 diabetes and diabetic nephropathy with albuminuria
dapagliflozin (*Farxiga*)	5–10 mg/d PO in the morning; contraindicated with severe renal impairment	Adjunct to diet and exercise to improve glycemic control in people with type 2 diabetes; reducing risk of hospitalization for heart failure in adults with type 2 diabetes and established cardiovascular disease or multiple cardiovascular risk factors; reducing risk of cardiovascular death and hospitalization for heart failure in adults with heart failure with reduced ejection fraction (NYHA class II–IV)
empagliflozin (*Jardiance*)	10 mg/d PO in the morning; maximum 25 mg/d; contraindicated with severe renal impairment	Adjunct to diet and exercise to improve glycemic control in adults with type 2 diabetes; reducing risk of cardiovascular death in adult patients with type 2 diabetes and established cardiovascular disease
ertugliflozin (*Steglatro*)	5–15 mg/d PO in a.m. with or without food; contraindicated with severe renal impairment	Adjunct to diet and exercise to improve glycemic control in adults with type 2 diabetes
Thiazolidinediones		
pioglitazone (*Actos*)	15–45 mg/d PO as a single dose; use caution with hepatic impairment and heart failure	Adjunct to diet and exercise to lower blood glucose in patients with type 2 diabetes
rosiglitazone (*Avandia*)	4–8 mg/d PO as a single dose; use caution with hepatic impairment and heart failure	Adjunct to diet and exercise to lower blood glucose in patients with type 2 diabetes

Table 38.3 *Drugs in Focus:* Oral Antidiabetic Agents and Noninsulin Injectable Antidiabetic Agents *(Continued)*

Drug Name	Dosage/Route	Usual Indications
Human Amylin		
pramlintide (*Symlin*)	*Type 2 diabetes*: 60 mcg subcutaneous injection before major meals; may be increased to 120 mcg *Type 1 diabetes*: Initially 15 mcg subcutaneous injection before major meals; maintenance 30–60 mcg/dose	Treatment for patients with type 1 or type 2 diabetes who use mealtime insulin and have failed to achieve desired glycemic control despite optimal insulin therapy
GLP-1 Agonists		
dulaglutide (*Trulicity*)	0.75–4.5 mg by subcutaneous injection once a week	Adjunct to diet and exercise to improve glucose control in patients with type 2 diabetes; reducing risk of major adverse cardiovascular events in adults with type 2 diabetes who have established cardiovascular disease or multiple cardiovascular risk factors; consider risk of thyroid tumor and limit use to patients in whom the benefit outweighs the risk
exenatide (*Bydureon, Byetta*)	5–10 mcg by subcutaneous injection within 60 min before morning and evening meals; extended release 2 mg by subcutaneous injection every 7 d	Adjunct to diet and exercise to improve glycemic control in patients with type 2 diabetes
liraglutide (*Victoza, Saxenda*)	*Victoza*: 0.6 mg by subcutaneous injection once a day for 1 wk; increase dose based on patient response after 1 wk to a maximum of 1.8 mg/d *Saxenda*: Initiate 0.6 mg subcutaneous injection per day for 1 wk; in weekly intervals, increase dose until a dose of 3 mg is reached	*Victoza*: Adjunct to diet and exercise to improve glucose control in patients with type 2 diabetes; reducing risk of major adverse cardiovascular events in adults with type 2 diabetes and established cardiovascular disease; consider risk of thyroid tumor and limit use to patients in whom the benefit outweighs the risk *Saxenda*: Adjunct to a reduced-calorie diet and increased physical activity for chronic weight management
lixisenatide (*Adlyxin*)	10 mcg by subcutaneous injection daily for 14 d; then increase to 20 mcg subcutaneous injection daily; inject 1 h before first meal of day	Adjunct to diet and exercise to improve glycemic control in adults with type 2 diabetes; not for patients with pancreatitis or gastroparesis
semaglutide (*Ozempic, Rybelsus*)	*Ozempic*: 0.25 mg injected subcutaneously once a week; may increase after 4 wk; max dose 1 mg/wk *Rybelsus*: Initial 3 mg PO daily; may increase every 30 days to 7 mg and then max dose of 14 mg/d; swallow tablets whole at least 30 min before any other food, drink, or medications with only 4 oz of water	Adjunct to diet and exercise to improve glycemic control in adults with type 2 diabetes; reducing risk of major adverse cardiovascular events in adults with type 2 diabetes and established cardiovascular disease; not for patients with personal or family history of medullary thyroid carcinoma or multiple endocrine neoplasia syndrome type 2

DPP-4, dipeptidyl peptidase-4; GLP-1, glucagonlike peptide-1; SGLT-2, sodium–glucose cotransporter-2.

Sulfonylureas

The sulfonylureas stimulate the functioning beta cells in the pancreatic islets to release insulin. They may improve the binding of insulin to insulin receptors and increase the number of insulin receptors. They are also known to increase the effect of antidiuretic hormone on renal cells. They are effective only in patients who have functioning beta cells. They are not effective for all patients and may lose their effectiveness over time. Sulfonylureas are further classified as first-generation or second-generation sulfonylureas. All of the sulfonylureas can cause hypoglycemia.

First- and Second-Generation Sulfonylureas

The only first-generation sulfonylurea still on the U.S. market is tolbutamide (generic). The use of first-generation sulfonylureas has declined as safer drugs have become available.

The second-generation drugs include glimepiride (*Amaryl*), glipizide (*Glucotrol*), and glyburide (*DiaBeta* and others). See Table 38.3 for usual indications for each drug. Second-generation sulfonylureas have several advantages over the first-generation drugs, including the following:

- They do not interact with as many protein-bound drugs as the first-generation drugs do.
- They have a longer duration of action, making it possible to take them only once or twice a day, thus increasing adherence.

Prescribers may try different agents before finding the one that is most effective for a given patient.

Therapeutic Actions and Indications

The sulfonylureas stimulate insulin release from the beta cells in the pancreas (see Fig. 38.1). They improve the binding of insulin to insulin receptors and may actually increase the number of insulin receptors. They are indicated as an adjunct to diet and exercise to lower blood glucose levels in type 2 diabetes mellitus. They have the off-label use of being an adjunct to insulin and metformin to improve glucose control in type 2 diabetics (Box 38.9).

Pharmacokinetics

These drugs are rapidly absorbed from the GI tract and undergo hepatic metabolism. They are excreted in the urine. Glyburide is also excreted via bile. The peak effects and duration of effects differ because of the activity of various metabolites of the different drugs.

Contraindications and Cautions

Sulfonylureas are contraindicated in the presence of known allergy to any sulfonylureas to avoid hypersensitivity reactions and in diabetes complicated by fever, severe infection, severe trauma, major surgery, ketoacidosis, severe renal or hepatic disease, pregnancy, or lactation, which require tighter control of glucose levels using insulin. These drugs are also contraindicated for use in people diagnosed with type 1 diabetes because they do not have functioning beta cells and would have no benefit from the drug.

These drugs are not for use during pregnancy. Insulin should be used if an antidiabetic agent is needed during pregnancy. Some of these drugs cross into human milk, and adequate studies are not available on others. Because of the risk of hypoglycemic effects in the baby, these drugs should not be used during lactation. Another method of feeding the baby should be used. The safety and efficacy of these drugs for use in children have not been established.

Box 38.9 Focus on Safe Medication Administration

The sulfonylurea medications can cause hypoglycemia. Ensure that your patient and their family know how to monitor for signs and symptoms and how to treat hypoglycemia orally.

Adverse Effects

The most common adverse effects related to the sulfonylureas are hypoglycemia (caused by an imbalance in levels of glucose and insulin) and GI distress, including nausea, vomiting, epigastric discomfort, heartburn, and anorexia. Anorexia should be monitored because affected patients may not eat after taking the sulfonylurea, which could lead to hypoglycemia. Allergic skin reactions have been reported with some of these drugs. There is a small amount of evidence that treatment with the sulfonylureas may increase risk of CV events; however, the research was done with first-generation agents.

Clinically Important Drug–Drug Interactions

There are multiple medications that may have an additive hypoglycemic effect. Care should be taken to monitor blood glucose levels closely when adding or changing doses of medications. Caution should also be used with beta-blockers, which may mask the signs of hypoglycemia, and with alcohol, which can lead to altered glucose levels when combined with sulfonylureas. Caution must also be used with many herbal therapies that could alter blood glucose levels.

Prototype Summary: Glyburide

Indications: Adjunct to diet and exercise in the management of type 2 diabetes; used with metformin or insulin for stabilization of diabetic patients.

Actions: Stimulates insulin release from functioning beta cells in the pancreas; may improve binding of insulin to insulin receptor sites or increase the number of insulin receptor sites.

Pharmacokinetics:

Route	Onset	Duration
Oral	1 h	24 h

$T_{1/2}$: 10 hours; metabolized in the liver and excreted in the bile and urine.

Adverse Effects: GI discomfort, anorexia, nausea, vomiting, heartburn, diarrhea, allergic skin reactions, hypoglycemia.

Alpha-Glucosidase Inhibitors

The alpha-glucosidase inhibitors include acarbose (generic) and miglitol (*Glyset*) (see Table 38.3).

Therapeutic Actions and Indications

Acarbose and miglitol are inhibitors of alpha-glucosidase (an enzyme that breaks down glucose for absorption); they delay the absorption of glucose. They have been shown to assist in lowering HbA1c levels. They do not enhance insulin secretion, so their effects are additive to those of other agents in controlling blood glucose. These drugs are used in combination with other agents for patients whose glucose levels cannot be controlled with a single agent or diet and exercise alone. They are taken three times a day at the start of each meal.

Pharmacokinetics

The alpha-glucosidase inhibitors are absorbed orally at variable amounts; however, due to mechanism of action in GI tract, amount of absorption is not therapeutically pertinent. Acarbose is metabolized in the GI tract, and miglitol is excreted without being metabolized. Both are excreted by the kidneys, so renal impairment can increase plasma levels.

Contraindications and Cautions

Both alpha-glucosidase inhibitors are contraindicated for patients with known hypersensitivity or in patients diagnosed with DKA. They are also contraindicated in patients with GI disorders like inflammatory bowel disease, intestinal obstruction, or colonic ulceration due to their mechanism of action. Acarbose is contraindicated in patients with cirrhosis due to some evidence of hepatotoxicity. Caution should be used with both medications in patients with renal impairment.

Adverse Effects

The most common side effects are related to the GI system: abdominal distension, cramping, hyperactive bowel sounds, diarrhea, and excessive flatulence. There is risk of anemia due to decreased iron absorption.

Clinically Important Drug–Drug Interactions

Use of medications with other glucose-lowering agents increases risk of hypoglycemia. There may be decreased glucose control if alpha-glucosidase inhibitors are administered with medications that increase blood glucose.

P Prototype Summary: Acarbose

Indications: Adjunct to diet and exercise in the management of type 2 diabetes; used with other antidiabetic agents for stabilization of blood glucose in patients with type 2 diabetes.

Actions: Inhibits enzymes to delay glucose absorption and lower postprandial hyperglycemia.

Pharmacokinetics:

Route	Onset	Duration
Oral	1 h	Unknown

$T_{1/2}$: 2 hours; metabolized in the gastrointestinal tract and excreted in the urine.

Adverse Effects: GI discomfort, anorexia, nausea, vomiting, heartburn, diarrhea, allergic skin reactions, hypoglycemia.

Biguanide

Metformin (*Fortamet, Glumetza, Riomet*) is the medication in the biguanide classification (see Table 38.3). It is the first-line medication choice for people with type 2 diabetes.

Therapeutic Actions and Indications

Metformin decreases the production and increases the uptake of glucose. It is effective in lowering both basal and postprandial blood glucose levels. It decreases hepatic glucose production, decreases intestinal absorption of glucose, and improves insulin sensitivity of peripheral cells. The medication may allow for less or unchanged insulin secretion from the pancreas.

It is currently the first-line standard of care for people with type 2 diabetes. It is also being used off-label in the treatment of patients with polycystic ovary syndrome (Box 38.10).

Pharmacokinetics

Metformin is absorbed orally. It is not metabolized and is excreted primarily in urine. Absorption and elimination times vary based on the type of formulation of metformin. There are some that are available in extended-release forms.

Contraindications and Cautions

Metformin is contraindicated in patients with known hypersensitivity reactions. It is also contraindicated in patients with metabolic acidosis, including DKA, due to risk of acidotic state that can cause coma and death. It is also contraindicated in patients with severe renal impairment due to increased risks of side effects, including lactic acidosis. Caution should be used in administering

BOX 38.10

Polycystic Ovary Syndrome and Antidiabetic Drugs

Polycystic ovary syndrome is an ovarian function disorder associated with obesity, infrequent or absent menses, and infertility. People who have this disorder have elevated insulin levels with normal fasting blood glucose levels, elevated luteinizing hormone (LH) levels, and normal estrogen and follicle-stimulating hormone levels. Because of the alterations in hormone activity, follicles develop on the ovaries, but ovulation does not occur, and the developed follicles turn into cysts. High LH levels tend to cause an increase in androgen production, which is associated with insulin resistance.

Treatment is aimed at altering the metabolic changes to allow ovulation (if pregnancy is desired) or stop the follicle development (if pregnancy is not desired). Weight loss is important and may correct the alterations in metabolism and allow ovulation to occur without medical treatment. Metformin and pioglitazone have proven effective in increasing insulin sensitivity and decreasing androgen and LH levels to break the cycle and allow ovulation to occur if pregnancy is desired. A fertility drug is often used with the antidiabetic agent. If pregnancy is not desired, hormonal contraceptives are used to halt the development of the follicles and stop the cyst production.

metformin to people with hepatic impairment, who have excessive alcohol intake, who are not eating/drinking due to surgical procedures, who are undergoing radiologic studies with contrast, who are age 65 or older, and who are in hypoxic states due to increased risk of lactic acidosis. Metformin may lower vitamin B_{12}, so levels should be monitored.

Adverse Effects

There is a boxed warning regarding metformin-associated lactic acidosis; this is uncommon but can be fatal. Symptoms include malaise, myalgias, respiratory hyperventilation, somnolence, and severe abdominal pain. Common GI side effects include diarrhea, nausea, vomiting, abdominal discomfort and distention, constipation, dyspepsia, and flatulence. Some people also report dizziness, headache, upper respiratory infection, and taste disturbance.

Clinically Important Drug–Drug Interactions

Alcohol use and carbonic anhydrase inhibitors administered with metformin can increase the risk of lactic acidosis. Concurrent use of iodine-containing contrast media can result in acute kidney failure. Some medications can reduce metformin clearance, so drug interactions should be checked prior to administering metformin.

P Prototype Summary: Metformin

Indications: Adjunct to diet and exercise for the treatment of type 2 diabetics in patients older than 10 years of age, with an extended-release form used in adult patients; adjunct treatment for polycystic ovary syndrome.

Actions: May increase the peripheral use of glucose, increase production of insulin, decrease hepatic glucose production, and alter intestinal absorption of glucose.

Pharmacokinetics:

Route	Onset	Peak	Duration
Oral	Slow	2–2.5 h	10–16 h

$T_{1/2}$: 6.2 to 17 hours; excreted in the urine.

Adverse Effects: Hypoglycemia, lactic acidosis, GI upset, nausea, anorexia, diarrhea, heartburn, allergic skin reaction.

Dipeptidyl Peptidase-4 Inhibitors (DPP-4 inhibitors)

The DPP-4 inhibitors are alogliptin (*Nesina*), linagliptin (*Tradjenta*), saxagliptin (*Onglyza*), and sitagliptin (*Januvia*) (Table 38.3).

Therapeutic Actions and Indications

The DPP-4 inhibitors slow the inactivation of incretin hormones, such as glucagonlike peptide-1 (GLP-1). GLP-1 and other incretin hormones are released in the intestine, and they increase insulin release and lower glucagon secretion from the pancreas. The incretins are deactivated by DPP-4 enzyme. Therefore, the DPP-4 inhibitors can increase the actions of the hormones and help with blood glucose control. There are currently four drugs available in this class: alogliptin, linagliptin, saxagliptin, and sitagliptin. They are indicated to be used as an adjunct to diet and exercise to lower blood glucose levels in patients with type 2 diabetes.

Pharmacokinetics

The DPP-4 inhibitors are oral medications that are administered daily and can be taken with or without food. They are rapidly absorbed, with peak effects varying from 1 to 5 hours. The half-life and metabolism can vary. For example, sitagliptin is not extensively metabolized, while saxagliptin is primarily metabolized by cytochrome P450 enzymes. Excretion of the drugs is primarily via the kidneys.

Contraindications and Cautions

The DPP-4 inhibitors are contraindicated for treatment of DKA or type 1 diabetes. They are not to be used in patients with history of severe hypersensitivity reactions (angioedema, exfoliative skin conditions, or anaphylaxis) to these medications. Caution should be used when administering to patients with renal impairment; the dose may need to be reduced.

Adverse Effects

The DPP-4 inhibitors are generally well tolerated, and most people do not report adverse effects. There are rare instances of people developing pancreatitis, heart failure, severe arthralgia, hypersensitivity reactions, and exfoliative skin conditions that can require hospitalization.

Clinically Important Drug–Drug Interactions

Concurrent use with other medications that can lower blood glucose increases risk of hypoglycemia. Depending on the individual medication's metabolism, there may be other drug interactions, but there are none that are common to all DPP-4 inhibitors.

Prototype Summary: Sitagliptin

Indications: Adjunct to diet and exercise for the treatment of type 2 diabetes.

Actions: DPP-4 inhibitor; slows the breakdown of GLP-1, which leads to increased insulin release, decreased glucagon release, and slowed GI absorption.

Pharmacokinetics:

Route	Onset	Peak	Duration
Oral	Rapid	1–4 h	10–16 h

$T_{1/2}$: 12.4 hours; a small amount is metabolized in the liver, most excreted in the urine.

Adverse Effects: Hypoglycemia, headache, upper respiratory infection, acute pancreatitis, hypersensitivity reactions.

Meglitinides

The meglitinides include repaglinide (generic) and nateglinide (generic) (see Table 38.3).

Therapeutic Actions and Indications

The meglitinides act similarly to the sulfonylureas by stimulating insulin release from the beta cells in the pancreas. They are indicated as an adjunct to diet and exercise in treatment of type 2 diabetes. They are administered before each meal to stimulate insulin release during the postprandial period.

Pharmacokinetics

The meglitinides are rapidly absorbed, extensively metabolized by the cytochrome P-450 enzyme system in the liver, and quickly eliminated by the kidneys. These are rapidly acting drugs with a very short half-life.

Contraindications and Cautions

The meglitinides are contraindicated for use with patients with type 1 diabetes or DKA. They are also contraindicated if there is any known hypersensitivity to the medication or its inactive ingredients. There have not been studies regarding risks and benefits of taking these medications when pregnant. It is recommended for patients not to breast or chestfeed while taking the meglitinides due to risk of hypoglycemia in the infant.

Adverse Effects

Commonly reported adverse effects when taking the meglitinides are upper respiratory infection, headache, arthralgia, nausea, diarrhea, and hypoglycemia.

Clinically Important Drug–Drug Interactions

There are multiple drug–drug interactions that can occur with the meglitinides. It is recommended that a nurse check for potential interactions prior to administering the medication. Gemfibrozil should not be administered with repaglinide due to the inhibition of repaglinide metabolism and risk of hypoglycemia.

Prototype Summary: Repaglinide

Indications: Adjunct to diet and exercise for the treatment of type 2 diabetes.

Actions: Stimulates the beta cells in the pancreas to release more insulin.

Pharmacokinetics:

Route	Onset	Peak	Duration
Oral	Rapid	1 h	3–4 h

$T_{1/2}$: 1 hour; metabolized in the liver; most excreted in the urine.

Adverse Effects: Hypoglycemia, headache, upper respiratory infection, arthralgia, nausea and diarrhea.

Sodium-Glucose Cotransporter-2 Inhibitors (SGLT-2 Inhibitors)

The SGLT-2 inhibitors include canagliflozin (*Invokana*), dapagliflozin (*Farxiga*), empagliflozin (*Jardiance*), and ertugliflozin (*Steglatro*) (see Table 38.3).

Therapeutic Actions and Indications

The SGLT-2 inhibitors work in a unique way to promote the loss of glucose through the urine. Glucose is filtered at the glomerulus but is such a big molecule it needs to actively be reabsorbed using the sodium–glucose cotransporter. If all of the cotransporter sites are inhibited, glucose is concentrated in the urine, usually indicating a serum glucose over 200. These drugs block the cotransporter system, and glucose is not reabsorbed but lost in the urine. The serum glucose levels fall since glucose is not reabsorbed.

All of the SGLT-2 inhibitors are indicated for adjunctive treatment with diet and exercise of blood glucose control in patients with type 2 diabetes. Some also have been found to decrease risk of CV death and hospitalization due to heart failure in adults with and without type 2 diabetes and/or heart failure and to slow the progression of renal disease in patients with chronic kidney disease. Due to their mechanism of action, they would work to lower blood glucose levels in patients with type 1 diabetes mellitus; however, the FDA does not currently recommend them to be used in this population. There is ongoing research on their risk/benefit ratio for patients with type 1 DM, since there may be some increased risk of DKA.

Pharmacokinetics

These drugs are absorbed from the GI tract and may be taken with or without food. Peak levels are reached in about 1.5 hours. They are primarily metabolized in the liver and excreted via the kidneys and feces. The half-lives are 12 to 17 hours.

Contraindications and Cautions

The SGLT-2 inhibitors are contraindicated for use in patients with DKA or type 1 diabetes mellitus. They are also contraindicated in patients with severe renal impairment. There are data from animal research that show there could be adverse renal effects if these medications are taken during the second or third trimester. It is also not recommended that people breast or chestfeed if taking these medications.

Adverse Effects

The patient is at risk for dehydration and hypotension, as well as for urinary tract infections (UTIs) and genital fungal infections because of the large amount of glucose in the urine. Patients taking these drugs are at increased risk for DKA and need to be monitored accordingly. Canagliflozin has been linked to loss of bone density and bone fractures; patients receiving this drug need to be screened for risk of bone loss, and bone density should be monitored. There is also increased risk of lower limb amputation, so perfusion to extremities and any sores or cuts should be monitored regularly.

Clinically Important Drug–Drug Interactions

Medications that enhance metabolism of the SGLT-2 inhibitors may decrease their exposure and effectiveness. Rifampin has been shown to decrease effectiveness of canagliflozin. Before administering these medications, check for potential interactions.

Prototype Summary: Canagliflozin

Indications: Adjunct to diet and exercise for the treatment of type 2 diabetes; reduce risk of cardiovascular events in adults with and without type 2 diabetes and cardiovascular disease; reduce risk of end-stage kidney disease, cardiovascular death and hospitalization for adults with heart failure, diabetic nephropathy with albuminuria, and diabetes type 2.

Actions: Sodium–glucose cotransporter-2 inhibitor; increases the excretion of glucose from the kidney leading to lowered serum glucose levels.

Pharmacokinetics:

Route	Onset	Peak	Duration
Oral	Rapid	1–2 h	10–16 h

$T_{1/2}$: 10 to 13 hours; metabolized in the liver; excreted in the urine.

Adverse Effects: Dehydration due to increased urination, hypotension, urinary tract infection, genital fungal infections, hypoglycemia.

Thiazolidinediones

The thiazolidinediones include pioglitazone (*Actos*) and rosiglitazone (*Avandia*) (Table 38.3).

Therapeutic Actions and Indications

The thiazolidinediones decrease insulin resistance and are indicated as adjuncts to diet and exercise to lower blood glucose in patients with type 2 diabetes. They act by decreasing insulin resistance in peripheral cells and the liver. They increase responsiveness to insulin but do not lower blood glucose without the presence of insulin. These drugs are also being studied for use in increasing ovulation frequency in patients who have polycystic ovary syndrome (see Box 38.10).

Pharmacokinetics

The thiazolidinediones are absorbed orally, and peak concentrations are reached in 1 to 2 hours. Most if not all of the thiazolidinediones are metabolized by the liver and excreted via the kidneys and feces. The half-lives are 3 to 7 hours. There are limited data regarding the risk of medication use during pregnancy or lactation.

Contraindications and Cautions

Thiazolidinediones can increase the risk of heart failure exacerbation, so they are contraindicated in patients with moderate or severe heart failure. They should be discontinued if any signs or symptoms of heart failure occur. Pioglitazone has been strongly linked to an increased risk of bladder cancer if it is used for over 1 year. Patients should be monitored for any change in liver function while they are taking these drugs due to some evidence of increased risk of hepatic injury.

Adverse Effects

Commonly reported adverse effects with the thiazolidinediones include upper respiratory infections, headache, and muscle pains. Total cholesterol levels may increase when people take these medications, so cholesterol levels need to be monitored. Hepatic injury is a rare but dangerous risk. Fluid retention may cause rapid weight gain and edema in some people.

Clinically Important Drug–Drug Interactions

Concurrent use with insulin may increase risk of hypoglycemia and fluid retention. Use of the thiazolidinediones with CYP2C8 inhibitors my increase the medications' concentrations. Conversely, CYP2C8 inducers may decrease concentrations. Drug–drug interactions need to be assessed prior to administration.

Prototype Summary: Pioglitazone

Indications: Adjunct to diet and exercise for the treatment of type 2 diabetes.

Actions: Decreases insulin resistance in peripheral cells and the liver.

Pharmacokinetics:

Route	Onset	Peak	Duration
Oral	Rapid	1–2 h	16-24 h

$T_{1/2}$: 3 to 7 hours; metabolized in the liver; excreted in the urine and feces.

Adverse Effects: Upper respiratory infection, myalgia, headache, edema, weight gain, liver impairment, congestive heart failure, bladder cancer, elevated cholesterol level.

BOX 38.11

Available Fixed-Combination Oral Agents

Several fixed-combination oral antidiabetic agents have become available. These combination products are intended to decrease the number of tablets the patient needs to take each day and thereby increase adherence to the drug regimen. Some of the medications have a synergistic effect with each other, which may facilitate better blood glucose control. It is safest if the patient is stabilized on the individual product first and then switched to the combination product after the correct dose combination for that patient has been established; however, this is not always done in clinical practice. When combination products are used, it is imperative that the patient and nurse are aware of the side effects and cautions for all of the individual components in the combination formulation. The patient should be reminded that diet and exercise are still the key parts of the antidiabetic treatment regimen. The following are examples of combination antidiabetic agents:

- glyburide and metformin (generic)
- glipizide and metformin (generic)
- glimepiride and pioglitazone (generic)
- *Duetact* (pioglitazone and glimepiride)
- *Actoplus Met* (pioglitazone and metformin)
- *Janumet* and *Janumet XR* (sitagliptin and metformin)
- *Kombiglyze XR* (saxagliptin and extended-release metformin)
- *Kazano* (alogliptin and metformin)
- *Oseni* (alogliptin and pioglitazone)
- *Invokamet or Invokamet XR* (canagliflozin and metformin)
- *Glyxambi* (empagliflozin and linagliptin)
- *Jentadueto and Jentadueto XR* (linagliptin and metformin)
- *Synjardy and Synjardy XR* (empagliflozin and metformin)
- *Segluromet* (ertugliflozin and metformin)
- *Steglujan* (ertugliflozin and sitagliptin)
- *Trijardy XR* (empagliflozin, linagliptin, and metformin)
- *Xigduo XR* (dapagliflozin and metformin)

Box 38.11 describes some of the new fixed-combination oral agents, which provide two or more agents in one tablet to make it easier for the patient to adhere to the drug regimen.

In 2009, an old drug, bromocriptine, was approved for use to improve glycemic control in type 2 diabetics. This is a unique CNS approach to treating type 2 diabetes. The use of bromocriptine is explained in Box 38.12.

Noninsulin Injectable Antidiabetics

There are two classifications of medications that are indicated to treat patients with diabetes mellitus that are injected like insulin but have different mechanism of

BOX 38.12

Alternative Approach to Treating Type 2 Diabetes

In 2009, the FDA granted approval for a new use of an old drug, bromocriptine (*Cycloset*). Bromocriptine is a dopamine agonist that is used to treat Parkinson's disease (Chapter 24), and it is indicated as an adjunct to diet and exercise to improve glycemic control in adults with type 2 diabetes. *Cycloset* is taken orally in the morning, within 2 hours of waking, and with food. In patients with type 2 diabetes, timed morning administration of *Cycloset* is associated with increased insulin sensitivity, lower plasma glucose, and reduced fasting and postprandial hyperglycemia throughout the day without raising plasma insulin levels. It should not be used to treat type 1 diabetes or diabetic ketoacidosis. Safety has not been established for pediatric patients.

action. The classifications are human amylin and glucagonlike polypeptide receptor agonists.

Human Amylin

Pramlintide (*Symlin*) is a human amylin that can be used as an adjunctive treatment for people with type 1 or type 2 diabetes (see Table 38.3).

Therapeutic Actions and Indications

Pramlintide works to modulate gastric emptying after a meal, causes a feeling of fullness or satiety, and prevents the postmeal rise in glucagon that usually elevates glucose levels. It is a synthetic form of human amylin, a hormone produced by the beta cells in the pancreas that is important in regulating glucose levels after meals. Human amylin can slow gastric emptying, suppress glucagon secretion from the liver, and regulate food intake by modulating appetite. The synthetic form is injected subcutaneously immediately before a major meal. It is indicated for use in patients with both type 1 and type 2 diabetes who are also treated with insulin.

Pharmacokinetics

Pramlintide has a rapid onset of action and peaks in about 20 minutes, and the half-life is about 48 minutes. It should be injected before each major meal of the day, at least 2 in. away from any insulin injection site. It cannot be combined in the syringe with insulin.

Contraindications and Cautions

Pramlintide is contraindicated in patients who have had a serious hypersensitivity reaction to it or its ingredients, in patients who have gastroparesis due to the slowing of gastric emptying, and who are at risk of becoming hypoglycemic. There is a boxed warning regarding the risk of severe hypoglycemia, and it is recommended that when starting this medication, insulin dosing should be decreased.

Adverse Effects

The most commonly reported side effects are nausea, vomiting, anorexia, headache, and injection site reactions. Severe hypoglycemia is a risk, especially in those who do not decrease their insulin dose and/or are not closely monitored.

Clinically Important Drug–Drug Interactions

There is increased risk of hypoglycemia with concurrent administration of pramlintide and insulin or other antidiabetic medications. Due to the slowing of gastric emptying, absorption of oral medications may be inhibited. The slowing of gastric emptying can be worsened with concurrent administration with other gastric-slowing medications (opioids).

Prototype Summary: Pramlintide

Indications: Treatment of patients with type 1 or 2 diabetes who use meal-time insulin and have not achieved desired glycemic control despite optimal insulin therapy.

Actions: Modulates gastric emptying after a meal, causes a feeling of fullness or satiety, and prevents the post-meal rise in glucagon that usually elevates glucose levels.

Pharmacokinetics:

Route	Onset	Peak	Duration
Subcutaneous	Varies	30 min	30–50 min

$T_{1/2}$: 30 to 50 minutes; metabolized into an active metabolite.

Adverse Effects: Nausea, vomiting, anorexia, headache, hypoglycemia, and injection site reactions.

Glucagonlike Polypeptide Receptor Agonists (GLP-1 Agonists)

The GLP-1 receptor agonists include dulaglutide (*Trulicity*), exenatide (*Bydureon, Byetta*), liraglutide (*Victoza, Saxenda*), lixisenatide (*Adlyxin*), and semaglutide (*Ozempic, Rybelsus*) (Table 38.3).

Therapeutic Actions and Indications

The GLP-1 receptor agonists increase insulin release and decrease glucagon release in preparation for the nutrients that will soon be absorbed. GLP-1 agonists also slow GI emptying to allow more absorption of nutrients and stimulate the satiety center in the brain to decrease the desire to eat because food is already in the GI tract. GLP-1 agonists have a very short half-life and are metabolized by the enzyme DPP-4. These drugs are indicated as adjuncts to diet and exercise for people with type 2 diabetes. Some have additional indications to reduce risk of major CV events in adults with type 2 diabetes and CV disease.

Pharmacokinetics

Most of the GLP-1 receptor agonists are administered via subcutaneous injections. Semaglutide (*Rybelsus*) is an oral formulation. The frequency of dosing varies between twice a day and every 7 days. The metabolism and excretion of these medications vary.

Contraindications and Cautions

Liraglutide and semaglutide have boxed warnings for risk of thyroid C-cell tumors in animals, and patients need to be made aware of the risk and taught to monitor for the signs and symptoms of thyroid tumors. The drugs should not be used in patients with a history or family history of thyroid cancer or multiple endocrine neoplasia syndrome. These medications are not indicated for patients with type 1 diabetes or DKA. Based on animal studies, there may be risk of harm to the fetus or infant if taken during pregnancy or when breast or chestfeeding.

Adverse Effects

There is a risk of pancreatitis with these drugs, so they need to be held if the patient reports severe epigastric pain. Common side effects are primarily GI related and include nausea, vomiting, decreased appetite, constipation, and diarrhea.

Clinically Important Drug–Drug Interactions

The effects of oral medication administered concurrently may be delayed due to slowed gastric emptying. There is a risk of hypoglycemia when taken with other antidiabetic agents.

Prototype Summary: Liraglutide

Indications: Adjunct to diet and exercise for the treatment of adults with type 2 diabetes.

Actions: Acts on beta cells to increase insulin release and decrease glucagon release; slows GI absorption and stimulates the satiety center to decrease appetite.

Pharmacokinetics:

Route	Onset	Peak	Duration
Subcutaneous	Slow	8–12 h	24 h

$T_{1/2}$: 13 hours; metabolized in the tissues.

Adverse Effects: Hypoglycemia, headache, nausea, anorexia, diarrhea, allergic skin reaction, pancreatitis, renal impairment, thyroid C-cell tumors.

Nursing Considerations for Patients Taking Noninsulin Antidiabetic Agents

Assessment: History and Examination

- Assess for contraindications or cautions: history of allergy to any of these agents to avoid hypersensitivity reactions; severe renal or hepatic dysfunction, which could interfere with metabolism and excretion of some of the drugs; and status of pregnancy or lactation, which are contraindications to the use of some of these agents.
- Perform a complete physical assessment to establish baseline status before beginning therapy and to evaluate effectiveness and any potential adverse effects during therapy.
- Assess for the presence of any skin lesions for indication of possible infection and to establish appropriate sites for subcutaneous administration as appropriate; orientation and reflexes; baseline pulse and blood pressure; adventitious breath sounds; and abdominal sounds and function to monitor effects of altered glucose levels.
- Assess body systems for changes suggesting possible complications associated with poor blood glucose control.
- Investigate nutritional intake, noting any problems with intake and adherence to prescribed diet, to help prevent adverse reactions to drug therapy.
- Assess activity level, including amount and degree of exercise, which can alter serum glucose levels and dosage needs for these drugs.
- Monitor blood glucose levels as ordered to evaluate effectiveness of the drug and glycemic control.
- Monitor results of laboratory tests, including urinalysis, for evidence of glucosuria, and renal function tests, especially with the sodium–glucose cotransporter-2 inhibitors, and liver function tests, especially with use of the thiazolidinediones, which can cause liver failure, to determine the need for possible dose adjustment and evaluate for signs of toxicity.

Nursing Conclusions

Nursing conclusions related to drug therapy might include the following:

- Hyperglycemia risk related to diabetes mellitus disease process
- Hypoglycemia risk related to dosing of antidiabetic agents
- Coping impairment related to diagnosis and therapy
- Knowledge deficit regarding drug therapy

Planning

- The patient will receive the best therapeutic effect from the drug therapy.

(continues on page 668)

- The patient will have limited adverse effects from the drug therapy.
- The patient will have an understanding of the drug therapy, adverse effects to anticipate, and measures to relieve discomfort and improve safety.

Intervention With Rationale

- Administer the drug as prescribed in an appropriate relationship with meals to ensure therapeutic effectiveness.
- Ensure that the patient is following diet and exercise modifications to improve effectiveness of the drug and decrease adverse effects of diabetes mellitus.
- Monitor nutritional status to provide nutritional consultation as needed.
- Monitor response carefully; blood glucose monitoring is the most effective way to evaluate dose. Obtain blood glucose levels as ordered to monitor drug effectiveness.
- Monitor liver enzymes of patients receiving pioglitazone or rosiglitazone carefully to avoid liver toxicity; arrange to discontinue the drug to avert serious liver damage if liver toxicity develops.
- Monitor patients during times of trauma, pregnancy, or severe stress, and arrange to switch to insulin coverage if needed.
- Provide thorough patient teaching, including drug name, dosage, and schedule for administration; administration technique if appropriate; proper disposal of needles and syringes in a sharps bucket with return to a community take-back site or pharmacy; never to reuse needles or share needles with other people; need for food intake within specified time periods; signs and symptoms of hypoglycemia and hyperglycemia; skin assessment, including daily inspection of feet; signs and symptoms to report immediately; measures to use when ill or unable to eat; a proper diet and exercise program; hygiene measures; recommended schedule for follow-up and disease monitoring; and the need for follow-up lab testing to enhance patient knowledge of drug therapy and to promote adherence.

Evaluation

- Monitor patient response to the drug (stabilization of blood glucose levels).
- Monitor for adverse effects (hypoglycemia, UTI, pancreatitis, and GI distress).
- Evaluate the effectiveness of the teaching plan (patient can name drug, dosage, adverse effects to watch for, and specific measures to avoid them).
- Monitor the effectiveness of comfort measures and adherence to the regimen.

Key Points

- Oral antidiabetic agents have varied mechanisms of action, but all are indicated as adjuncts to diet and exercise to treat type 2 diabetes.
- There are also noninsulin injectable antidiabetic medications that can be used to help control blood glucose levels.
- In times of severe stress, patients regulated on other antidiabetic agents may need to be switched to insulin to control blood glucose levels.

Glucose-Elevating Agents

Glucose-elevating agents, as the name implies, raise the blood level of glucose when hypoglycemia occurs (lower than 70 mg/dL). Some adverse conditions are associated with increased risk of hypoglycemia, including pancreatic disorders, kidney disease, certain cancers, disorders of the anterior pituitary, and unbalanced treatment of diabetes mellitus, which can occur if the patient takes the wrong dose of insulin or antidiabetic agent or if something interferes with food intake or changes stress or exercise levels. Agents used to elevate glucose in these conditions include dasiglucagon (*Zegalogue*), diazoxide (*Proglycem*), and glucagon (*GlucaGen* and others). Pure glucose can also be given orally or IV to increase the blood glucose level. Oral glucose tablets or gels (*Glutose*, *Insta-Glucose*, and *BD Glucose*) are available over the counter for patients to keep on hand for management of moderate hypoglycemic episodes (Table 38.4).

Therapeutic Actions and Indications

These agents increase the blood glucose level by decreasing insulin release and accelerating the breakdown of glycogen in the liver to release glucose. They are indicated for the treatment of hypoglycemic reactions related to insulin or oral antidiabetic agents, for the treatment of hypoglycemia related to pancreatic or other cancers, and for short-term treatment of acute hypoglycemia related to anterior pituitary dysfunction (see Table 38.4).

Pharmacokinetics

Diazoxide is administered orally. Dasiglucagon is administered subcutaneously and is indicated for severe hypoglycemia. Glucagon dosing varies based on formulation. These drugs are rapidly absorbed and widely distributed throughout the body. They are excreted in the urine.

Contraindications and Cautions

Diazoxide is contraindicated with known allergies to sulfonamides or thiazides. Diazoxide has been associated with adverse effects on the fetus, including pulmonary hypertension, and

Table 38.4 *Drugs in Focus:* Glucose-Elevating Agents

Drug Name	Dosage/Route	Usual Indications
dasiglucagon (*Zegalogue*)	0.6 mg subcutaneous injection; additional dose may be administered after 15 min if no response	Treatment of severe hypoglycemia in pediatric (age ≥6 y) and adult patients with diabetes
diazoxide (*Proglycem*)	*Adult and pediatric*: 3–8 mg/kg/d PO in two to three divided doses q8–12h	Oral management of hypoglycemia
glucagon (*Baqsimi, GlucaGen, Gvoke*)	Dosing varies by formulation and patient age *Baqsimi*: Intranasal *GlucaGen*: Subcutaneous, IM, or IV *Gyoke*: Subcutaneous	To counteract severe hypoglycemic reactions

should not be used during pregnancy. There are no adequate studies on glucagon and pregnancy, so use should be reserved for those situations in which the benefits to the patient outweigh any potential risks to the fetus. Caution should be used during lactation because the drugs may cause hyperglycemic effects in the baby. Caution should be used in patients with renal or hepatic dysfunction or CV disease.

Adverse Effects

Glucagon and dasiglucagon are associated with GI upset, nausea, and vomiting. Diazoxide has been associated with vascular effects, including hypotension, headache, cerebral ischemia, weakness, heart failure, and arrhythmias; these reactions are associated with diazoxide's ability to relax arteriolar smooth muscle.

Clinically Important Drug–Drug Interactions

Taking diazoxide in combination with thiazide diuretics causes increased risk of toxicity because diazoxide is structurally similar to these diuretics.

Increased anticoagulation effects have been noted when glucagon and dasiglucagon are combined with oral anticoagulants. If this combination is needed, the dose should be adjusted.

Prototype Summary: Glucagon

Indications: Counteracts severe hypoglycemic reactions in diabetic patients treated with insulin.

Actions: Accelerates the breakdown of glycogen to glucose in the liver, causing an increase in the blood glucose level.

Pharmacokinetics:

Route	Onset	Peak	Duration
IV	1 min	15 min	9–20 min

$T_{1/2}$: 3 to 10 minutes; metabolized in the liver and excreted in the urine and bile.

Adverse Effects: Hypotension, hypertension, nausea, vomiting, respiratory distress with hypersensitivity reactions, hypokalemia with overdose.

Nursing Considerations for Patients Taking Glucose-Elevating Agents

Assessment: History and Examination

- Assess for contraindications and cautions including history of allergy to thiazides if using diazoxide, to avoid hypersensitivity reactions; severe renal or hepatic dysfunction, which could alter metabolism and excretion of the drug; CV disease, which could be exacerbated by the effects of the drug; and current status of pregnancy or lactation, which could require caution.
- Perform a complete physical assessment to establish a baseline before beginning therapy, monitor effectiveness of therapy, and evaluate for any potential adverse effects during therapy.
- Assess orientation and reflexes and baseline pulse, blood pressure, and adventitious sounds to monitor the effects of altered glucose levels, and abdominal sounds and function, which could be altered by these drugs.
- Monitor blood glucose levels as ordered to assess the effectiveness of the drug and patient response to treatment.
- Monitor the results of laboratory tests, including urinalysis, to evaluate for glucosuria, serum glucose levels to evaluate response to therapy, and renal and liver function tests to determine the need for possible dose adjustment or identify possible toxic effects.

Nursing Conclusions

Nursing conclusions related to drug therapy might include the following:

- Risk for unstable blood glucose related to ineffective dosing of the drug
- Malnutrition risk more than body requirements related to metabolic effects, and less than body requirements related to GI upset
- Altered sensory perception (kinesthetic, visual, auditory, and tactile) related to glucose levels
- Knowledge deficit regarding drug therapy

Planning

- The patient will receive the best therapeutic effect from the drug therapy.

(continues on page 670)

- The patient will have limited adverse effects from the drug therapy.
- The patient will have an understanding of the drug therapy, adverse effects to anticipate, and measures to relieve discomfort and improve safety.

Intervention With Rationale

- Monitor blood glucose levels to evaluate the effectiveness of the drug.
- Have insulin on standby during emergency use to treat severe hyperglycemia if it occurs as a result of overdose.
- Monitor nutritional status to provide nutritional consultation as needed.
- Monitor patients receiving diazoxide for potential CV effects, including blood pressure, heart rhythm and output, and weight changes, to avert serious adverse reactions.
- Provide thorough patient teaching, including drug name, dosage, and schedule for administration; signs and symptoms of hyperglycemia; administration technique if indicated; signs and symptoms of adverse effects; need for follow-up monitoring and laboratory testing if indicated; nutritional measures; and blood glucose monitoring, to improve patient knowledge and increase adherence to drug regimen.

Evaluation

- Monitor patient response to the drug (stabilization of blood glucose levels).
- Monitor for adverse effects (hyperglycemia and GI distress).
- Evaluate the effectiveness of the teaching plan (patient can name drug, dosage, adverse effects to watch for, and specific measures to avoid them).
- Monitor the effectiveness of comfort measures and adherence to the regimen.

Key Points

- Glucose-elevating agents are used to increase glucose when the level becomes dangerously low. Imbalance in glucose levels while taking insulin or oral agents is a common cause of hypoglycemia.
- Patients need to be carefully monitored to determine the effectiveness of therapy with these drugs and to prevent inadvertent overdose, which could lead to hyperglycemia.

SUMMARY

- Diabetes mellitus is the most common metabolic disorder. It is characterized by high blood glucose levels and alterations in the metabolism of nutrients.
- Glucose control is a complicated process affected by various hormones, enzymes, and receptor sites.
- Diabetes mellitus is complicated by many end organ problems if blood glucose levels are not controlled.
- Treatment of diabetes involves control of blood glucose levels using diet and exercise, a combination of other agents to stimulate insulin release or alter glucose absorption, and/or the injection of replacement insulin.
- The amount and type of insulin given must be regulated based on the patient's response and blood glucose levels. Patients taking insulin must learn to inject the drug, properly dispose of needles and syringes, test their blood glucose level, and recognize the signs of hypoglycemia and hyperglycemia.
- Insulin is used for type 1 diabetes and for type 2 diabetes in times of stress or when other therapies have failed.
- There are multiple other oral and noninsulin injectable medications that are indicated as adjuncts to diet and exercise for treatment of type 2 diabetes.
- Glucose-elevating agents are used to increase glucose when the level becomes dangerously low. Imbalance in glucose levels while taking insulin or oral agents is a common cause of hypoglycemia.

Unfolding Patient Stories: Juan Carlos • Part 2

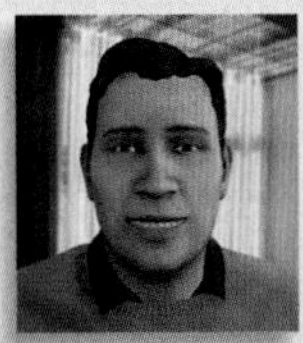

Recall Juan Carlos, a 52-year-old with diabetes type 2, hypertension, and hyperlipidemia, whom you first met in Chapter 18. He is hospitalized for antibiotic treatment and surgical debridement of a wound to his right great toe. He dropped a rock on his toe and sustained an open wound, which required surgical debridement. He is to receive his maintenance insulin detemir 5 units SC and a sliding-scale insulin aspart 4 units SC for a fingerstick glucose of 225. What factors may be causing an increase in Juan's insulin requirement? How would the nurse explain the characteristics of each insulin? What patient education would the nurse provide when Juan asks the nurse to combine the insulins for one injection and why he needs frequent fingersticks?

Care for Juan and other patients in a realistic virtual environment: ***vSim** for Nursing* (thepoint.lww.com/vSimPharm). Practice documenting these patients' care in DocuCare (thepoint.lww.com/DocuCareEHR).

CHECK YOUR UNDERSTANDING

Answers to the questions in this chapter can be found in Answers to Check Your Understanding Questions on thePoint®.

MULTIPLE CHOICE

Select the best answer.

1. The medical management of diabetes mellitus is aimed at
   a. controlling caloric intake.
   b. increasing exercise levels.
   c. regulating blood glucose levels.
   d. decreasing fluid loss.

2. The HbA1c blood test is a good measure of overall glucose control because
   a. it reflects the level of glucose after a meal.
   b. fasting for 8 hours before the test ensures accuracy.
   c. it reflects a 3-month average glucose level in the body.
   d. the test can be affected by the glucose challenge.

3. A patient with hyperglycemia will often present with
   a. polyuria, polydipsia, and polyphagia.
   b. polycythemia, polyuria, and polyphagia.
   c. polyadenitis, polyuria, and polydipsia.
   d. polydipsia, polycythemia, and polyarteritis.

4. The long-term alterations in nutrient metabolism associated with diabetes mellitus result in
   a. obesity.
   b. vascular changes that can increase risk of heart attack and/or stroke.
   c. chronic obstructive pulmonary disease.
   d. lactose intolerance.

5. Insulin is available in several forms or suspensions which differ in several ways. However, they do NOT differ in their
   a. effect on the pancreas.
   b. onset and duration of action.
   c. means of administration.
   d. tendency to cause adverse effects.

6. Which would be the first choice for a newly diagnosed patient with diabetes mellitus type II who does not have any other health problems?
   a. Canagliflozin
   b. Liraglutide
   c. Pioglitazone
   d. Metformin

7. Miglitol differs from the sulfonylureas in that it
   a. greatly stimulates pancreatic insulin release.
   b. greatly increases the sensitivity of insulin receptor sites.
   c. delays the absorption of glucose, leading to lower glucose levels.
   d. cannot be used in combination with other antidiabetic agents.

8. Teaching subjects for the patient with diabetes should include
   a. diet and exercise changes that are needed.
   b. the importance of avoiding exercise and eating one meal a day.
   c. protection from exposure to any infection and avoiding tiring activities.
   d. avoiding pregnancy and taking hygiene measures.

MULTIPLE RESPONSE

Select all that apply.

1. Treatment of diabetes may include which of the following?
   a. Replacement therapy with insulin
   b. Control of glucose absorption through the GI tract
   c. Drugs that stimulate insulin release or increase sensitivity of insulin receptor sites
   d. Surgical clearing of the capillary basement membranes
   e. Slowing of gastric emptying
   f. Diet and exercise programs

2. A patient is recently diagnosed with diabetes. In reviewing their past history, which would be early indicators of the problem?
   a. Lethargy
   b. Fruity-smelling breath
   c. Boundless energy
   d. Weight loss
   e. Increased sweating
   f. Getting up often at night to go to the bathroom

REFERENCES

American Diabetes Association (ADA). (2021). Classification and diagnosis of diabetes: Standards of medical care—2021. *Diabetes Care, 44(*Suppl. 1), S15–S33. https://doi.org/10.2337/dc21-S002

American Diabetes Association (ADA). (2018). Standards of medical care for patients with diabetes mellitus: 2018. *Diabetes Care,* 41(Suppl. 1), S1–S172. http://care.diabetesjournals.org/content/diacare/suppl/2017/12/08/41.Supplement_1.DC1/DC_41_S1_Combined.pdf

Anabtawi, A., Hurst, M., Titi, M., Patel, S., Palacio, C., & Rajamani, K. (2010). Incidence of hypoglycemia with tight glycemic control protocols: A comparative study. *Diabetes Technology & Therapeutics, 12*(8), 635–639. 10.1089/dia.2010.0009

Brunton, L., Hilal-Dandan, R., & Knollman, B. (2018). *Goodman and Gilman's the pharmacological basis of therapeutics* (13th ed.). McGraw-Hill.

Hall, J. E., & Hall, M. E. (2021). *Guyton and Hall's textbook of medical physiology* (14th ed.). Elsevier.

Norris, T. L. (2019). *Porth's pathophysiology concepts of altered health states* (13th ed.). Wolters Kluwer.

Patoulias, D., Imprialos, K., Stavropoulos, K., Athyros, V., & Doumas, M. (2018). SGLT-2 inhibitors in type 1 diabetes mellitus: A comprehensive review of the literature. *Current Clinical Pharmacology, 13*(4), 261–272. https://doi.org/10.2174/1574884713666180807150509

Trikudanathan, S. (2015). Polycystic ovarian syndrome. *Medical Clinics of North America, 99*(1), 221–235. 10.1016/j.mcna.2014.09.003

U.S. Department of Health and Human Services Centers for Disease Control and Prevention. (2020). *National diabetes statistics report 2020.* https://www.cdc.gov/diabetes/pdfs/data/statistics/national-diabetes-statistics-report.pdf

Wang, M. (2011). *Metabolic syndrome: Underlying mechanisms and drug therapy*. John Wiley & Sons.

Wilson, Y. (2013). Type 2 diabetes: An epidemic in children. *Nursing Children and Young People, 25*(2), 14–17. 10.7748/ncyp2013.03.25.2.14.e136

PART 7

Drugs Acting on the Reproductive System

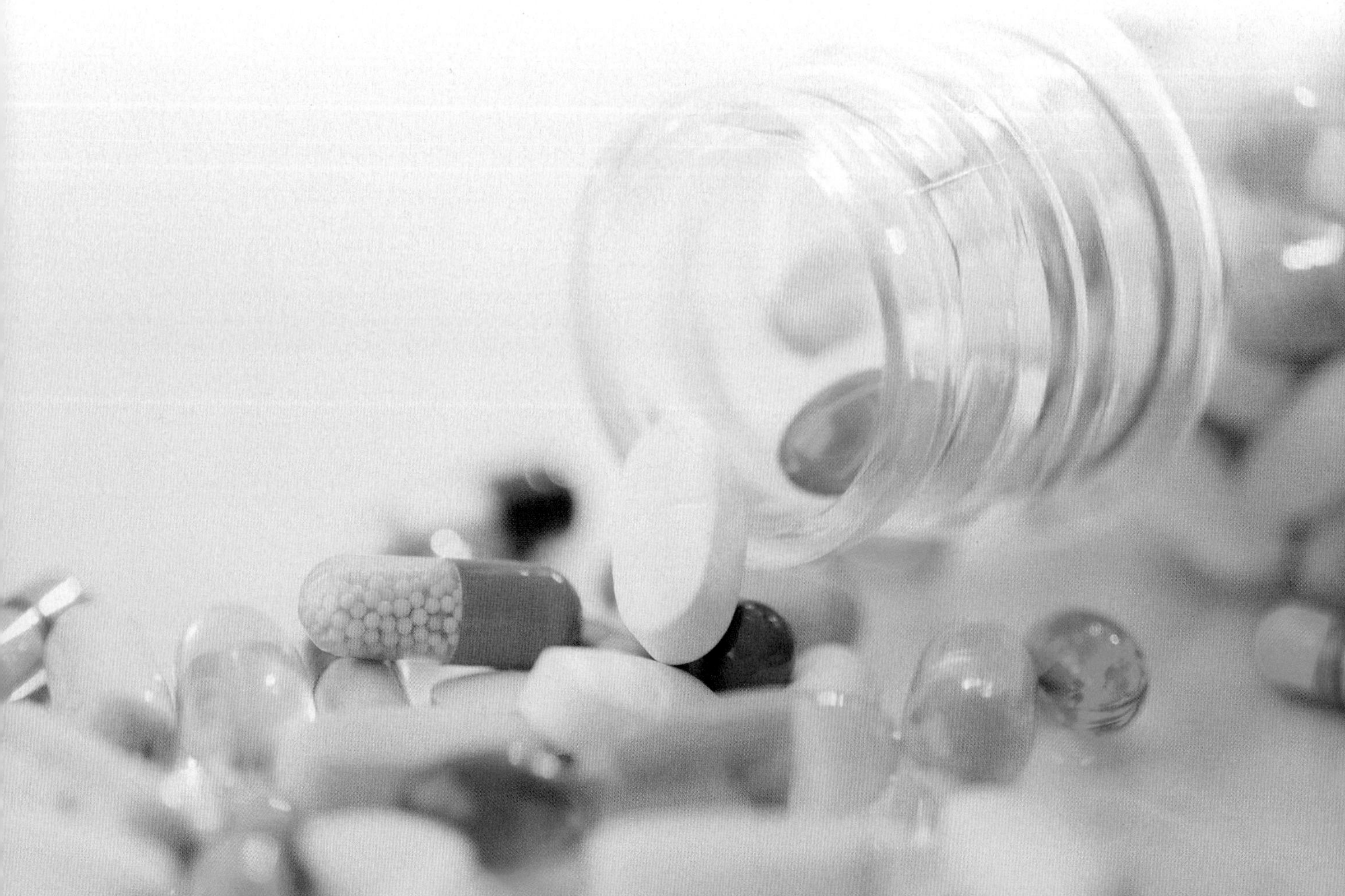

CHAPTER 39

Introduction to the Reproductive System

Learning Objectives

Upon completion of this chapter, you will be able to:

1. Label a diagram depicting the structures of the female and male reproductive systems and explain the function of each structure.
2. Outline the control mechanisms involved with the male and female reproductive systems, using this outline to explain the negative feedback systems involved with each system.
3. List five effects for each of the sex hormones: estrogen, progesterone, and testosterone.
4. Describe the changes that occur in the body during pregnancy.
5. Describe the progression of the human sexual response.

Key Terms

andropause: decrease in gonadal function in males associated with advancing age analogous to female menopause

corpus luteum: remains of a follicle that releases mature ovum at ovulation; becomes an endocrine gland producing estrogen and progesterone

estrogen: hormone produced by the ovary placenta, and adrenal gland; stimulates development of female characteristics and prepares the body for pregnancy

follicle: storage site of each ovum in the ovary; allows the ovum to grow and develop; produces estrogen and progesterone

inhibin: estrogenlike substance produced by seminiferous tubules during sperm production; acts as a negative feedback stimulus to decrease release of follicle-stimulating hormone (FSH)

interstitial or Leydig cells: part of the testes that produce testosterone in response to stimulation by luteinizing hormone (LH)

menarche: the onset of the menstrual cycle

menopause: depletion of the female ova; results in lack of estrogen and progesterone

menstrual cycle: cycling of female sex hormones in interaction with the hypothalamus and anterior pituitary feedback systems

menstruation: expulsion of the uterine lining occurring approximately every 28 to 32 days

ova: eggs the female gamete, contain half of the information needed in a human nucleus

ovaries: female sexual glands that store ova and produce estrogen and progesterone

ovulation: release of the ovum from the follicle into the abdomen

progesterone: hormone produced by the ovary placenta, and adrenal gland; promotes maintenance of pregnancy

puberty: point at which the hypothalamus starts releasing gonadotropin-releasing factor (GnRF) to stimulate the release of FSH and LH and begin sexual development

seminiferous tubules: part of the testes that produce sperm in response to stimulation by FSH

sperm: male gamete; contains half of the information needed for a human cell nucleus

testes: male sexual glands that produce sperm and testosterone

testosterone: male sex hormone; produced by the interstitial or Leydig cells of the testes

uterus: the womb; site of growth and development of the embryo and fetus

The reproductive systems in males and females are composed of the structures that support conception and development of a fetus and the endocrine glands that produce the hormones that facilitate reproduction and are necessary for the regulation and maintenance of these structures. Though anatomically the two systems appear to be very different, they have many underlying similarities. The same fetal cells in males and females give rise to the glands that produce sexual hormones. In the female, those cells remain in the abdomen and develop into the ovaries, the female sexual glands. In the male, the cells migrate out of the abdomen to form the testes (the male sexual glands), which are suspended from the body in the scrotum. Both male and female glands respond to follicle-stimulating hormone (FSH) and luteinizing hormone (LH), which are released from the anterior pituitary in response to stimulation from gonadotropin-releasing hormone (GnRH) released from the hypothalamus.

Female Reproductive System

The female reproductive system consists of two ovaries, two fallopian tubes, the uterus, and accessory structures, including the vagina, clitoris, labia, and breast tissue. The hormones that stimulate and maintain these structures are estrogen and progesterone. See Figure 39.1.

Structures

The **ovaries** are almond-shaped organs located on each side of the pelvic cavity. The ovaries store the **ova** or eggs. Eggs contain half of the genetic material needed to produce a whole cell. Ova develop in the fetus, and at birth, a female's ovaries contain all of their ova. No new ova will ever be produced by the ovaries. The ova are released into the abdomen throughout the person's life or slowly degenerate over time. Each ovum is contained in a storage site called a **follicle**; the follicles act as endocrine glands producing the hormones estrogen and progesterone. The primary function of these hormones is to prepare the body for pregnancy and to maintain the pregnancy until delivery. Near each ovary is a fallopian tube. The fallopian tube is a muscular tube with a ciliated lining that is constantly moving. This movement propels the ovum released into the abdomen down the fallopian tube and into the **uterus**, or womb, the site for the developing embryo and fetus. The uterus is a muscular organ that can develop a blood-filled inner lining, the endometrium, which allows for implantation of the fertilized egg and supports the development of the placenta, which provides nourishment for the developing fetus and acts as an endocrine gland producing the hormones needed to maintain the active metabolic state of pregnancy. The muscular walls of the uterus are important for expelling the developed fetus through the vagina at delivery. The external genitalia—the clitoris, labia, and vagina—are sites of erogenous stimulation; they are also the entryway for sperm to reach the uterus to allow conception and the exit path for the developed fetus at birth. Development of the breast tissue, considered a secondary sex characteristic—a quality that appears during puberty that is not directly involved in reproduction—is controlled by the female sex hormones. Breast tissue is necessary for producing milk for the nourishment of the baby when it has been expelled from the uterus and is no longer able to depend on the parent's blood supply for nourishment.

Hormones

The hormones produced in the ovaries are estrogen and progesterone. These two hormones influence many other body systems while preparing the body for pregnancy or maintenance of pregnancy.

Estrogen

The **estrogens** produced by the ovaries include estradiol, estrone, and estriol. The estrogens enter cells and bind

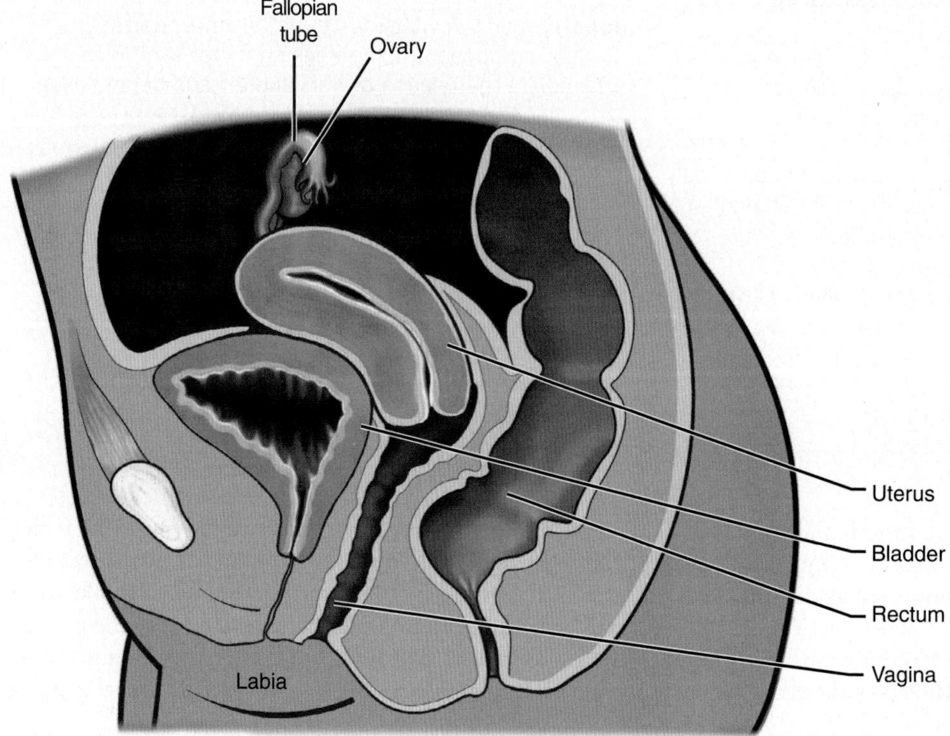

FIGURE 39.1 The female reproductive system.

to receptors within the cytoplasm to promote messenger ribonucleic acid (mRNA) activity, which results in specific proteins for cell activity or structure. Many of these effects are first noticed at **menarche** (the onset of the menstrual cycle), when the hormones begin cycling for the first time. Female characteristics are associated with the effects of estrogen on many of the body's systems—wider hips, soft skin, breast growth, and others. Box 39.1 summarizes the effects of estrogen on the body.

BOX 39.1

Effects of Estrogen

Growth of genitalia (in preparation for childbirth)
Growth of breast tissue (in preparation for pregnancy and lactation)
Characteristic female pubic hair distribution (a triangle)
Stimulation of protein building (important for the developing fetus)
Increased total blood cholesterol (for energy for the pregnant person as well as the developing fetus) with an increase in high-density lipoprotein levels ("good" cholesterol, which serves to protect the blood vessels against atherosclerosis)
Retention of sodium and water (to provide cooling for the heat generated by the developing fetus and to increase diffusion of sodium and water to the fetus through the placenta)
Inhibition of calcium resorption from the bones (helps deposit calcium in the fetal bone structure; when this property is lost at menopause, osteoporosis, or loss of calcium from the bone, is common)
Alteration of pelvic bone structure to a wider and flaring pelvis (to promote easier delivery)
Closure of the epiphyses (to conserve energy for the fetus by halting growth of the pregnant person)
Increased thyroid hormone globulin (metabolism needs to be increased greatly during pregnancy, and the increase in thyroid hormone facilitates this)
Increased elastic tissue in the skin (to allow for the tremendous stretch of the abdominal skin during pregnancy)
Increased vascularity of the skin (to allow for radiation loss of heat generated by the developing fetus)
Increased uterine motility (estrogen is high when the ovum first leaves the ovary, and increased uterine motility helps move the ovum toward the uterus and propel the sperm toward the ovum)
Thin, clear cervical mucus (allows easy penetration of the sperm into the uterus as ovulation occurs; used in fertility programs as an indication that ovulation will soon occur)
Proliferative endometrium (to prepare the lining of the uterus for implantation with the fertilized egg)
Anti-insulin effect with increased glucose levels (to allow increased diffusion of glucose to the developing fetus)
T-cell inhibition (to protect the nonself cells of the embryo from the immune surveillance of the pregnant person)

Progesterone

Progesterone is released into circulation after ovulation. Progesterone has many effects that support the early development of the fetus. Progesterone's effects on body temperature are monitored in the rhythm method of birth control as a sign that ovulation has just occurred. Box 39.2 summarizes the effects of progesterone on the body.

Control Mechanisms

The developing hypothalamus is sensitive to the androgens released by the adrenal glands and does not release GnRH during childhood. As the hypothalamus matures, it loses its sensitivity to the androgens and starts to release GnRH. This occurs at **puberty**, the beginning of sexual development. The onset of puberty leads to a number of hormonal changes. See Figure 39.2.

GnRH stimulates the anterior pituitary to release FSH and LH. FSH and LH stimulate growth and development of the follicles on the outer surface of the ovaries. These follicles, called graafian follicles, produce progesterone, which is retained in the follicle, and estrogen, which is released into circulation. When the circulating estrogen level rises high enough, it stimulates a massive release of LH from the anterior pituitary. This is called the LH surge. This burst of LH causes one of the developing follicles to burst and release the ovum with its stored hormones into the system. LH also causes the rest of the developing follicles to shrink in on themselves, or involute, and eventually disappear.

BOX 39.2

Effects of Progesterone

Decreased uterine motility (to provide increased chance that implantation can occur)
Development of a secretory endometrium (to provide glucose and a rich blood supply for the developing placenta and embryo)
Thickened cervical mucus (to protect the developing embryo and keep out bacteria and other pathogens; this is lost at the beginning of labor as the mucous plug)
Breast growth (to prepare for lactation)
Increased body temperature (a direct hypothalamic response to progesterone, which stimulates metabolism and promotes activities for the developing embryo; this increase in temperature is monitored in the rhythm method of birth control as a sign that ovulation has occurred)
Increased appetite (this is a direct effect on the satiety centers of the hypothalamus and results in increased delivery of nutrients to the developing embryo)
Depressed T-cell function (this protects the nonself cells of the developing embryo from the immune system)
Anti-insulin effect (to generate a higher blood glucose concentration to allow rapid diffusion of glucose to the developing embryo)

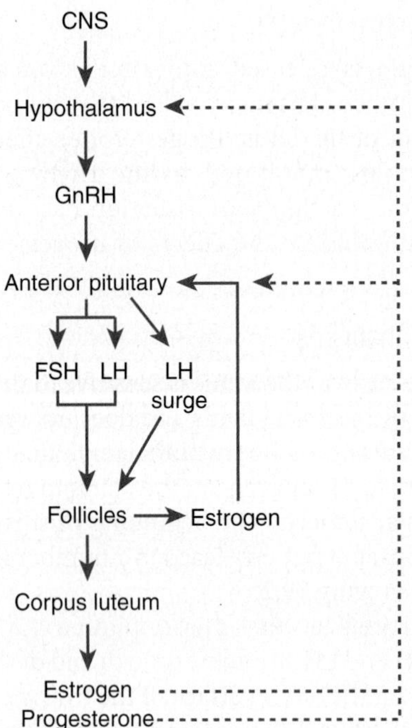

FIGURE 39.2 Interaction of the hypothalamic, pituitary, and ovarian hormones underlying the menstrual cycle. *Dotted lines* indicate negative feedback surge. CNS, central nervous system; FSH, follicle-stimulating hormone; GnRH, gonadotropin-releasing hormone; LH, luteinizing hormone.

The release of an ovum from the follicle is called **ovulation**.

The ovum is released into the abdomen near the end of one of the fallopian tubes, and the constant movement of cilia within the tube propels the ovum into the fallopian tube and then into the uterus. The ruptured follicle becomes a functioning endocrine gland called the **corpus luteum**. It will continue to produce estrogen and progesterone for 10 to 14 days unless pregnancy occurs.

Fertilization of the ovum and implantation in the uterine wall result in the production of human chorionic gonadotropin. This hormone stimulates the corpus luteum to continue to produce estrogen and progesterone until the placenta develops and becomes functional, producing these hormones at a level high enough to sustain the pregnancy.

If pregnancy does not occur, the corpus luteum involutes and becomes a white scar on the ovary. This scar is called the corpus albicans. Initially, the rising levels of estrogen and progesterone produced by the corpus luteum act as a negative feedback system to the hypothalamus and the pituitary, stopping the production and secretion of GnRH, FSH, and LH. Later in the cycle, the corpus luteum atrophies, the falling levels of estrogen and progesterone stimulate the hypothalamus to once again release GnRH, and the cycle begins again.

Factors Influencing Control Mechanisms

Because of its position in the brain, the hypothalamus is influenced by many internal and external factors. For example, high levels of stress can interrupt the reproductive cycle. Tremendous amounts of energy are expended in reproduction, and if the body needs energy for fight or flight, the hypothalamus shuts down the reproductive activities, stopping the release of GnRH, which results in no FSH or LH release and no stimulation of the follicles. This saves a tremendous amount of energy in the body that can be used for fight or flight. In addition to stress, starvation, extreme exercise, and emotional problems are all associated with a decrease in reproductive capacity related to the controls of the hypothalamus.

Light has also been found to have an influence on the functioning of the hypothalamus. Increased light levels boost the release of FSH and LH and increase the release of estrogen and progesterone. This is thought to contribute to the earlier sexual maturation of females who live near the equator. Longer and earlier exposure to light leads to earlier GnRH release by the hypothalamus and earlier sexual development. Females living in areas with prolonged periods of darkness (e.g., above the Arctic Circle) tend to go through puberty and sexual development at a much later age.

The Menstrual Cycle

The cyclical nature of the female sex hormones on the body produces the **menstrual cycle**. The onset of the menstrual cycle at puberty is called menarche. Each cycle starts with release of FSH and LH and stimulation of the ovarian follicles. For about the next 14 days, the developing follicles release estrogen into the body. Thus, a person who menstruates may notice the many effects of estrogen, such as breast tenderness and water retention. In addition, estrogen thins cervical mucosa and increases susceptibility to infections.

By about day 14, the higher estrogen level has caused the LH surge, and ovulation occurs. The menstruator experiences increased body temperature, increased appetite, breast tenderness, bloating and abdominal fullness, constipation, and other symptoms—the effects associated with progesterone, which is released into the system when the follicle ruptures. The uterus becomes thicker and more vascular as the cycle progresses, and it develops a proliferative endometrium. After ovulation, the lining of the uterus begins to produce glucose and other nutrients that would nurture a growing embryo; this is called a secretory endometrium. If pregnancy does not occur, after about 14 days, the corpus luteum involutes, and the levels of estrogen and progesterone drop off (Fig. 39.3).

The dropping levels of estrogen and progesterone trigger the release of GnRH and then FSH and LH again, along with the start of another menstrual cycle. Lowered hormone levels also cause the inner lining of the uterus to slough off because it is no longer stimulated by the hormones. High levels of plasminogen in the uterus prevent clotting of the lining as the vessels shear off. Prostaglandins in the uterus stimulate uterine contraction to clamp off vessels as the lining sheds. This causes menstrual cramps. This loss of the uterine lining, called **menstruation**, repeats approximately every 28 to 32 days. Figure 39.3 depicts the various phases of the menstrual cycle.

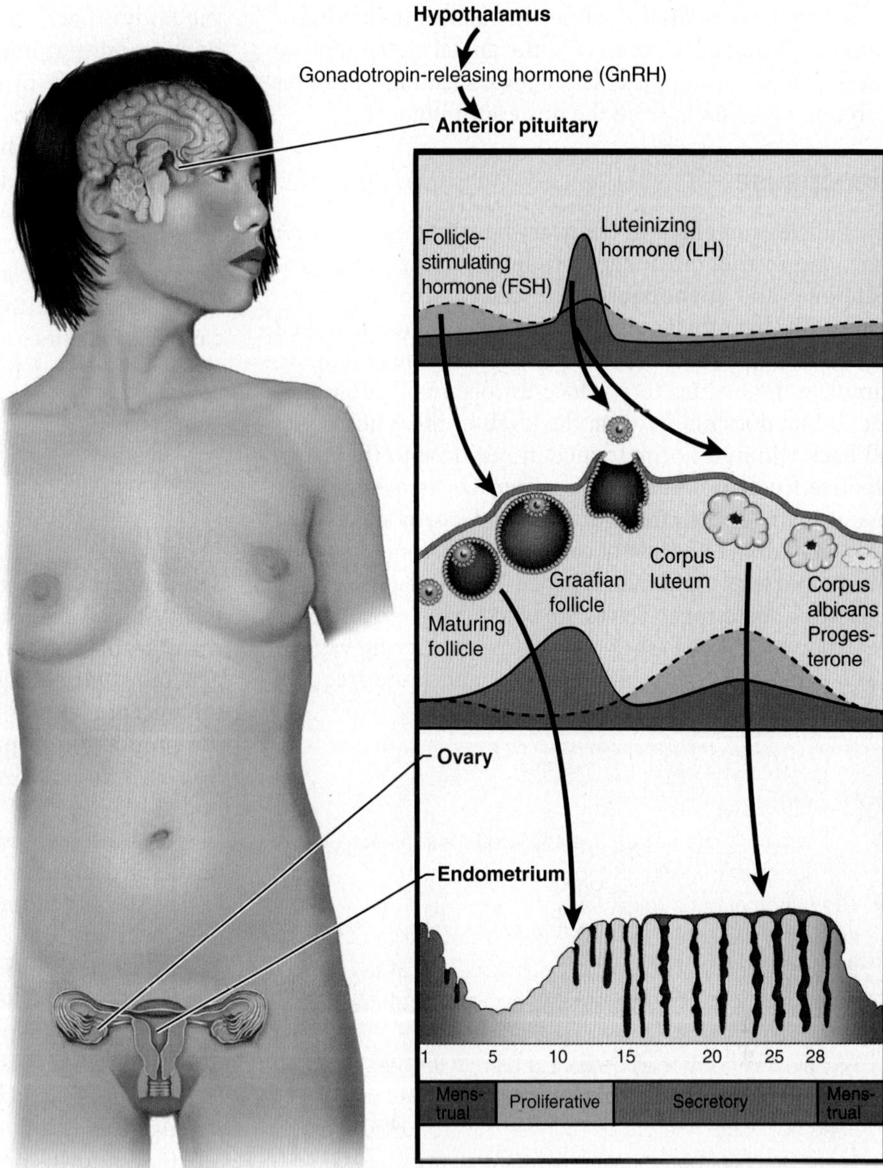

FIGURE 39.3 Relation of pituitary and ovarian hormone levels to the menstrual cycle and to ovarian and endometrial function.

Pregnancy

When the ovum is fertilized by a sperm, this produces a new cell that rapidly divides to produce the embryo. The embryo implants in the wall of the uterus, and the interface between the fetal cells and the uterus produces the placenta, a large vascular organ that serves as a massive endocrine gland and a transfer point for nutrients from the pregnant person to the fetus. The placenta maintains high levels of estrogens and progesterone to support the uterus and the developing fetus. It also secretes chorionic gonadotropin that can act on the corpus luteum to prolong its production of estrogen and progesterone for up to 4 months of pregnancy. When the placenta ages, the level of progesterone decreases in relation to the estrogen level. The increased uterine contractility at the end of pregnancy may be partially due to the higher level of estrogen compared to progesterone.

The stimulation of labor and strong uterine contractions is multifactorial. The stretch of uterine musculature and the cervix can stimulate uterine contractions. The fetus's hormonal secretion of higher levels of cortisol and prostaglandins also increase intensity of contractions. Increased release of oxytocin from the posterior pituitary also increases uterine contractility. Together, the mechanical and hormonal changes facilitate labor.

Once the fetus and the placenta have been expelled from the uterus, the estrogen and progesterone levels plummet toward the nonpregnant state. It often takes 6 to 8 weeks for stabilization of the hormonal cycle after labor and delivery. This postpartum period is a time of tremendous adjustment for the body as it works toward homeostasis. Prolactin is secreted from the anterior pituitary; its role is to promote milk secretion. The level of prolactin increases throughout the pregnancy, but estrogen and progesterone inhibit milk promotion until after delivery of the fetus. Oxytocin is the hormone that allows milk to flow from the alveoli of the breasts to the ductal system and be ejected from the nipples. The baby's suckling promotes secretion of oxytocin from the posterior pituitary.

Menopause

The follicles contained in the ovary become depleted over time, the ovaries no longer produce estrogen and progesterone, and **menopause**—the cessation of menses—occurs. The hypothalamus and pituitary produce increased levels of GnRH, FSH, and LH for a while in an attempt to stimulate the ovaries to produce estrogen and progesterone. If that does not happen, the levels of these hormones fall back within a normal range in response to their own negative feedback systems. Menopause is associated with loss of many of the effects of these two hormones on the body, including retention of calcium in the bones, lowered serum lipid levels, and maintenance of secondary sex characteristics. As estrogen leaves the blood vessels, many people experience "hot flashes" or vasospasm. Drying vaginal tissue can lead to painful intercourse and more frequent urinary tract infections (UTIs).

Key Points

- The female ovary stores ova and produces the sex hormones estrogen and progesterone.
- The hypothalamus releases GnRH at puberty to stimulate the anterior pituitary release of FSH and LH, thus stimulating the production and release of the sex hormones. Levels are controlled by a series of negative feedback systems.
- Female sex hormones prepare the body for pregnancy and the maintenance of the pregnancy. If pregnancy does not occur, the prepared inner lining of the uterus sloughs off as menstruation in the menstrual cycle.
- Menopause occurs when the supply of ova is depleted and the person's ovaries no longer produce the hormones estrogen and progesterone.

Male Reproductive System

The male reproductive system consists of two testes, the vas deferens, the prostate gland, the penis, and the urethra. The hormone that stimulates and maintains these structures is testosterone.

Structures

The male reproductive system originates from the same fetal cells as in the female. The major male reproductive system structure is the **testes**—the two endocrine glands that continually produce **sperm**—and the hormone testosterone. During fetal development, the two testes migrate down the abdomen and descend into the scrotum outside the body. There, they are protected from the heat of the body to prevent injury to the sperm-producing cells. The testes are made of two distinct parts, the **seminiferous tubules**, which produce the sperm, and the **interstitial or Leydig cells**, which produce the hormone testosterone. Other components include the vas deferens, which stores produced sperm and carries sperm from the testes to be ejaculated from the body; the prostate gland, which produces enzymes to stimulate sperm maturation, as well as lubricating fluid; the penis, which includes two corpora cavernosa and a corpus spongiosum, structures that allow greatly increased blood flow and erection; the urethra, through which urine and the sperm and seminal fluid are delivered; and other glands and ducts that promote sperm and seminal fluid development (Fig. 39.4).

Hormones

The primary hormone associated with the male reproductive system is **testosterone**. Testosterone is responsible for many sexual and metabolic effects in the male. Like estrogen, testosterone enters the cell and reacts with a cytoplasmic receptor site to influence mRNA activity, resulting in the production of proteins for cell structure or function. Box 39.3 summarizes the effects of testosterone on the body.

Castration, or removal of the testes, before puberty results in lack of development of male characteristics, as well as sterility. If the testes are lost before puberty occurs, there will be no development of the secondary male sex characteristics or the other effects seen when testosterone is released. The person would require testosterone replacement therapy to develop these characteristics. Once puberty and the physical changes brought about by testosterone have occurred, the androgens released by the adrenal glands are sufficient to sustain the male characteristics. Androgens are similar in structure to testosterone and are able to influence cells to maintain the changes caused by testosterone. This is important information for adult patients undergoing testicular surgery or chemical castration.

Control Mechanisms

The activity of the male sex glands is not thought to be cyclical like that of the female. The hypothalamus in the male child is also sensitive to circulating levels of adrenal androgens and suppresses GnRH release. After the hypothalamus matures, this sensitivity is lost, and the hypothalamus releases GnRH. This in turn stimulates the anterior pituitary to release FSH and LH, or what is sometimes called interstitial cell–stimulating hormone (ICSH) in males. FSH directly stimulates the seminiferous tubules to produce sperm, a process called spermatogenesis. FSH also stimulates the Sertoli cells in the seminiferous tubules to produce estrogens, which provide negative feedback to the pituitary and hypothalamus to cause a decrease in the release of GnRH, FSH, and LH.

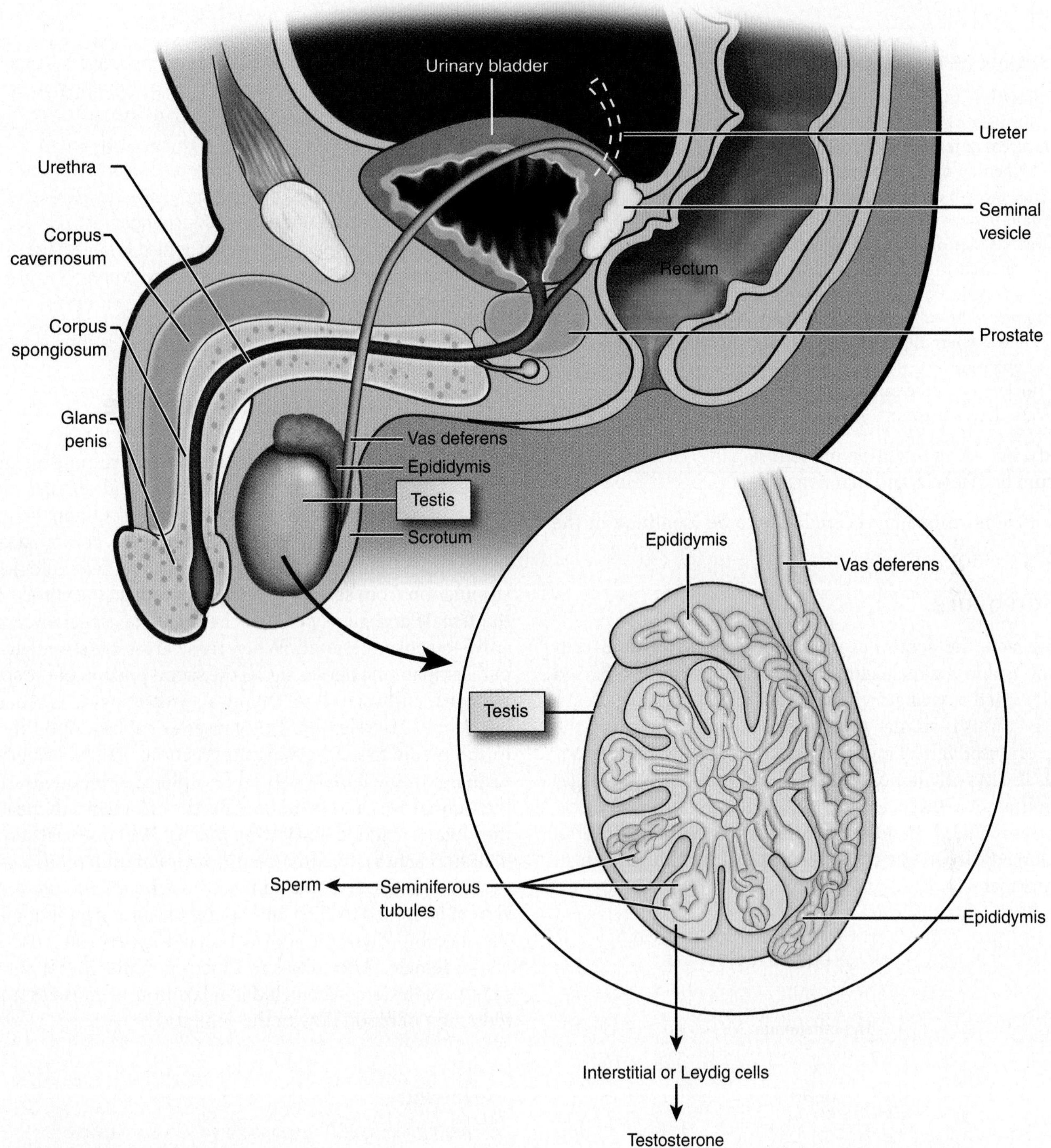

FIGURE 39.4 The male reproductive system.

The Sertoli cells also produce a substance called **inhibin**, an estrogenlike molecule. When the hypothalamus and anterior pituitary sense inhibin, a negative feedback response occurs, decreasing the circulating level of FSH. When the FSH level falls low enough, the hypothalamus is stimulated to again release GnRH to stimulate FSH release. This feedback system prevents overproduction of sperm in the testes (Fig. 39.5).

The LH or ICSH stimulates the interstitial (Leydig) cells to produce testosterone. The concentration of testosterone acts in a similar negative feedback system with the hypothalamus. When the concentration is high enough, the hypothalamus decreases GnRH release, leading to a subsequent decrease in FSH and LH release. The levels of testosterone are thought to remain within a fairly well-defined range of normal. It has been documented, however, that light affects the male sexual hormones in a similar fashion to its effect on female hormones. Increased exposure to sunlight increases testosterone levels in men. Other factors that may also have an influence

BOX 39.3

Effects of Testosterone

Growth of male and sexual accessory organs (penis, prostate gland, seminal vesicles, vas deferens)
Growth of testes and scrotal sac
Thickening of vocal cords, producing a deeper voice
Hair growth on the face, body, arms, legs, and trunk
Male-pattern baldness
Increased protein anabolism and decreased protein catabolism (this causes development of larger and stronger muscles)
Increased bone growth in length and width, which ends when the testosterone stimulates closure of the epiphyses
Thickening of the cartilage and skin
Vascular thickening
Increased hematocrit

on male hormone levels are likely to be identified in the future.

Andropause

With age, the seminiferous tubules and interstitial cells atrophy and the male climacteric or **andropause**, a period of lessened sexual activity and loss of testosterone effects, occurs. This is similar to female menopause; however, the age of onset varies, and the process is usually more gradual. The hypothalamus and anterior pituitary release larger amounts of GnRH, FSH, and LH in an attempt to stimulate the gland. If no increase in testosterone or inhibin occurs, the levels of GnRH, FSH, and LH eventually return to normal.

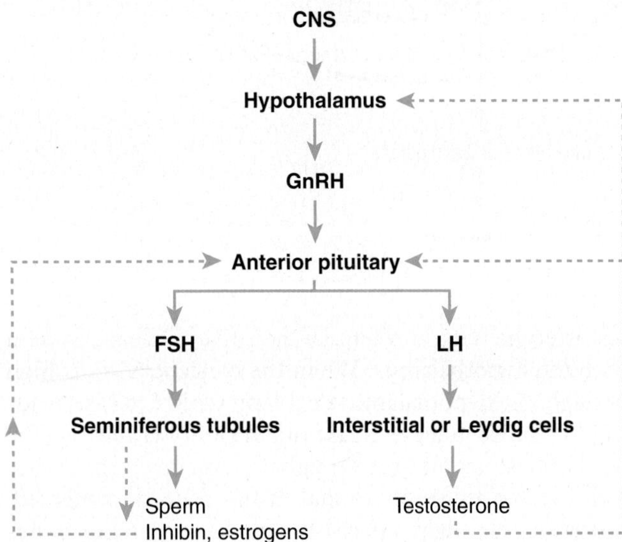

FIGURE 39.5 Interaction of the hypothalamic, pituitary, and testicular hormones underlying the male sexual hormone system. CNS, central nervous system; FSH, follicle-stimulating hormone; GnRH, gonadotropin-releasing hormone; LH, luteinizing hormone.

Key Points

- The testes produce sperm in the seminiferous tubules in response to FSH stimulation and testosterone in the interstitial cells in response to LH stimulation.
- Testosterone is responsible for the development of male sex characteristics. These characteristics can be maintained by the androgens from the adrenal gland once the body has undergone the changes of puberty.
- Andropause, or male climacteric, which is analogous to female menopause, occurs with age when the production of testosterone declines, with the subsequent loss of testosterone effects.

The Human Sexual Response

Sexual stimulation and activity are normal responses, and despite the physical differences of males and females, the stages of sexual activity are quite similar. Often, sexual excitement for both males and females is a combination of physical stimulation of sexual organs and psychological stimulation from sexually exciting thoughts. The clitoris of the female and glans penis of the male are especially sensitive to sensory stimuli. When these areas are stimulated, parasympathetic nerves signal the sacral portion of the spinal cord, and vasoactive chemicals (nitric oxide and acetylcholine) are released. This causes enhanced blood flow to the penile tissue, causing an erection. The same nerve response in the female also causes enhanced blood flow to the vaginal area and stimulates Bartholin's glands (beneath the labia) to secrete lubricating mucus. When sexual stimulation reaches a maximal point, a person undergoes a climax or orgasm. For this climax, the sympathetic nervous system is needed to elicit an impulse to cause ejaculation in the male and rhythmic contraction of the perineal muscles in the female. After orgasm, a person undergoes a stage called resolution that includes relaxation of muscles and reduction of blood flow to the genitals.

Key Points

- The human sexual response involves activation of the parasympathetic nervous system at first and the sympathetic nervous system for climax.
- Both males and females undergo similar stages during the sexual response despite different anatomic characteristics.

SUMMARY

- Male and female reproductive systems arise from the same fetal cells. The female ovaries store ova and produce the sex hormones estrogen and progesterone; the male testes produce sperm and the sex hormone testosterone.

- The hypothalamus releases GnRH at puberty to stimulate the anterior pituitary release of FSH and LH, thus stimulating the production and release of the sex hormones. Levels are controlled by a series of negative feedback systems.
- Female sex hormones are released in a cyclical fashion. Release of an ovum for possible fertilization is termed ovulation. The female hormones prepare the body for pregnancy, including maintenance of the pregnancy if fertilization occurs.
- If pregnancy does not occur, the prepared inner lining of the uterus is sloughed off as menstruation in the menstrual cycle so that the lining can be prepared again when ovulation reoccurs.
- Menopause and the male climacteric occur when the body no longer produces sex hormones; the hypothalamus and anterior pituitary respond by releasing increased levels of GnRH, FSH, and LH in an attempt to achieve higher levels of sex hormones.
- The testes produce sperm in the seminiferous tubules in response to FSH stimulation and testosterone in the interstitial cells in response to LH stimulation.
- Testosterone is responsible for the development of male sex characteristics. These characteristics can be maintained by the androgens from the adrenal gland once the body has undergone the changes of puberty.
- Both males and females undergo similar stages during the sexual response despite different anatomic characteristics.

CHECK YOUR UNDERSTANDING

Answers to the questions in this chapter can be found in Answers to Check Your Understanding Questions on thePoint®.

MULTIPLE CHOICE

Select the best answer.

1. In a nonpregnant female, the levels of the sex hormones fluctuate in a cyclical fashion until the
   a. ova are all depleted.
   b. FSH and LH are depleted.
   c. hypothalamus no longer senses FSH and LH.
   d. hypothalamus becomes more sensitive to androgens.

2. A female develops ova, or eggs,
   a. continually until menopause.
   b. during fetal life.
   c. until menopause.
   d. starting with puberty.

3. Control of the female sex hormones starts with the release of GnRH from the hypothalamus. Because of this, the cycling of these hormones may be influenced by
   a. body temperature.
   b. stress or emotional problems.
   c. age.
   d. androgen release.

4. The rhythm method of birth control depends on the effects of progesterone to
   a. increase uterine motility.
   b. decrease and thicken cervical secretions.
   c. elevate body temperature.
   d. depress appetite.

5. The menstrual cycle
   a. always repeats itself every 28 days.
   b. is associated with changing hormone levels.
   c. is necessary for a human sexual response.
   d. cannot occur if ovulation does not occur.

6. In the male reproductive system, the
   a. seminiferous tubules produce sperm and testosterone.
   b. interstitial cells produce sperm.
   c. seminiferous tubules produce sperm and the interstitial cells produce testosterone.
   d. interstitial cells produce sperm and testosterone.

7. Spring fever occurs as a result of increased light. In males, this increase in light causes an increase in the production of
   a. inhibin.
   b. adrenal androgens.
   c. estrogen.
   d. testosterone.

8. The human sexual climax depends on stimulation of the
   a. sympathetic nervous system.
   b. parasympathetic nervous system.
   c. hypothalamic sex drive center.
   d. adrenal androgens.

MULTIPLE RESPONSE

Select all that apply.

1. After teaching a group of students about the effects of the various sex hormones, the instructor determines that the teaching was successful when the group identifies which as related to estrogen?
   a. Increased levels of high-density lipoproteins
   b. Increased calcium density in the bone
   c. Closing of the epiphyses
   d. Development of a thick cervical plug
   e. Increased body temperature
   f. Triangle-shaped body hair distribution

2. A group of students are reviewing material in preparation for an examination on the sex hormones. If identified by the students as effects of testosterone, which demonstrate understanding of the information?
   a. Thickening of skin and vocal cords
   b. Development of a wide and flat pelvis
   c. Development of facial hair
   d. Closure of the epiphyses
   e. Increased hematocrit
   f. Increased aggression

REFERENCES

Basson, R. (2007). Women's sexual function and dysfunction. *Journal of the American Medical Association, 297*, 895–897. 10.1038/ijir.2008.23

Camacho, P. M., Gharib, H., & Sizemore, G. W. (Eds.). (2012). *Evidence-based endocrinology* (3rd ed.). Lippincott Williams & Wilkins.

Girard, J. (1992). *Endocrinology of puberty*. Karger Classic.

Greenspan, F. S., & Gardner, D. G. (Eds.). (2011). *Basic and clinical endocrinology* (9th ed.). Lange Medical Books.

Hall, J. E., & Hall, M. E. (2021). *Guyton and Hall's textbook of medical physiology* (14th ed.). Elsevier.

Jones, R. (2013). *Human reproductive biology* (4th ed.). Academic Press.

Kronenberg, H. M., Melmed, S., Polonsky, K. S., & Larsen, P. R. (Eds.). (2011). *Williams textbook of endocrinology* (12th ed.). W. B. Saunders.

Norris, T. L. (2019). *Porth's pathophysiology concepts of altered health states* (13th ed.). Wolters Kluwer.

CHAPTER 40

Drugs Affecting the Female Reproductive System

Learning Objectives

Upon completion of this chapter, you will be able to:

1. Discuss the use of drugs that affect the female reproductive system across the lifespan.
2. Integrate knowledge of the effects of sex hormones on the female body to explain the therapeutic and adverse effects of these agents when used clinically.
3. Describe the therapeutic actions, indications, pharmacokinetics, contraindications, most common adverse reactions, and important drug–drug interactions associated with drugs that affect the female reproductive system.
4. Compare and contrast the prototype drugs estradiol, raloxifene, norethindrone, clomiphene, oxytocin, and hydroxyprogesterone caproate with other agents in their class.
5. Outline the nursing considerations, including important teaching points to stress, for patients receiving drugs that affect the female reproductive system.

Key Terms

abortifacients: drugs used to stimulate uterine contractions and promote evacuation of the uterus to cause abortion or to empty the uterus after fetal death

fertility drugs: drugs used to stimulate ovulation and pregnancy in people with functioning ovaries who are having trouble conceiving

oxytocics: drugs that act like the hypothalamic hormone oxytocin; they stimulate uterine contraction and contraction of the lacteal glands, promoting milk ejection

progestins: the endogenous female hormone progesterone and its various derivatives; important in maintaining a pregnancy; supports many secondary sex characteristics

Drug List

SEX HORMONES AND ESTROGEN RECEPTOR MODULATORS

Sex Hormones

Estrogens

(P) estradiol
estrogens, conjugated
estrogens, esterified
estropipate

Progestins

desogestrel
drospirenone
etonogestrel
levonorgestrel
medroxyprogesterone
(P) norethindrone acetate
norgestrel
progesterone
ulipristal

Estrogen Receptor Modulator

(P) raloxifene

FERTILITY DRUGS

cetrorelix
chorionic gonadotropin
chorionic gonadotropin alpha
(P) clomiphene
follitropin alfa
follitropin beta
ganirelix
menotropins
urofollitropin

UTERINE MOTILITY DRUGS

Oxytocics and Abortifacients

carboprost
methylergonovine
mifepristone
(P) oxytocin

Tocolytic

(P) hydroxyprogesterone caproate

The female reproductive system functions in a cyclic fashion that typically completes a full cycle every 28 to 30 days. Altering any component of this cycle or the system can have a wide variety of effects on the entire body. Drugs that affect the female reproductive system typically include hormones and hormonal-like agents. Figure 40.1 reviews the female reproductive system and sites of action of the drugs used to affect the system. Box 40.1 highlights considerations related to the use of drugs discussed in this chapter as they affect the female reproductive system throughout the lifespan.

Sex Hormones and Estrogen Receptor Modulators

The female sex hormones can be used to replace hormones that are missing or to act on the control mechanisms of the endocrine system to decrease the release of endogenous hormones. Drugs that act like estrogen, particularly at specific estrogen receptors, are also used to stimulate the effects of estrogen in the body with fewer of the adverse effects. See Table 40.1 for information on these agents.

Sex Hormones

Female sex hormones include estrogens and **progestins** (the endogenous female hormone progesterone and its various derivatives). Estrogens that are available for use include estradiol (*Estrace*, *Climara*, and others), conjugated estrogens (*Premarin*), esterified estrogen (*Menest*), and estropipate (*Ogen*).

Progestins include etonogestrel (*Nexplanon*), levonorgestrel (*Mirena*, *Plan B One-Step*, and others), medroxyprogesterone (*Depo-Provera*), norethindrone (*Camila*, *Errin*, *Heather*, and others), progesterone (generic), and ulipristal (*Ella*, *Logilia*) used as a postcoital contraceptive.

Estrogens and progestins are most commonly used in combination medications.

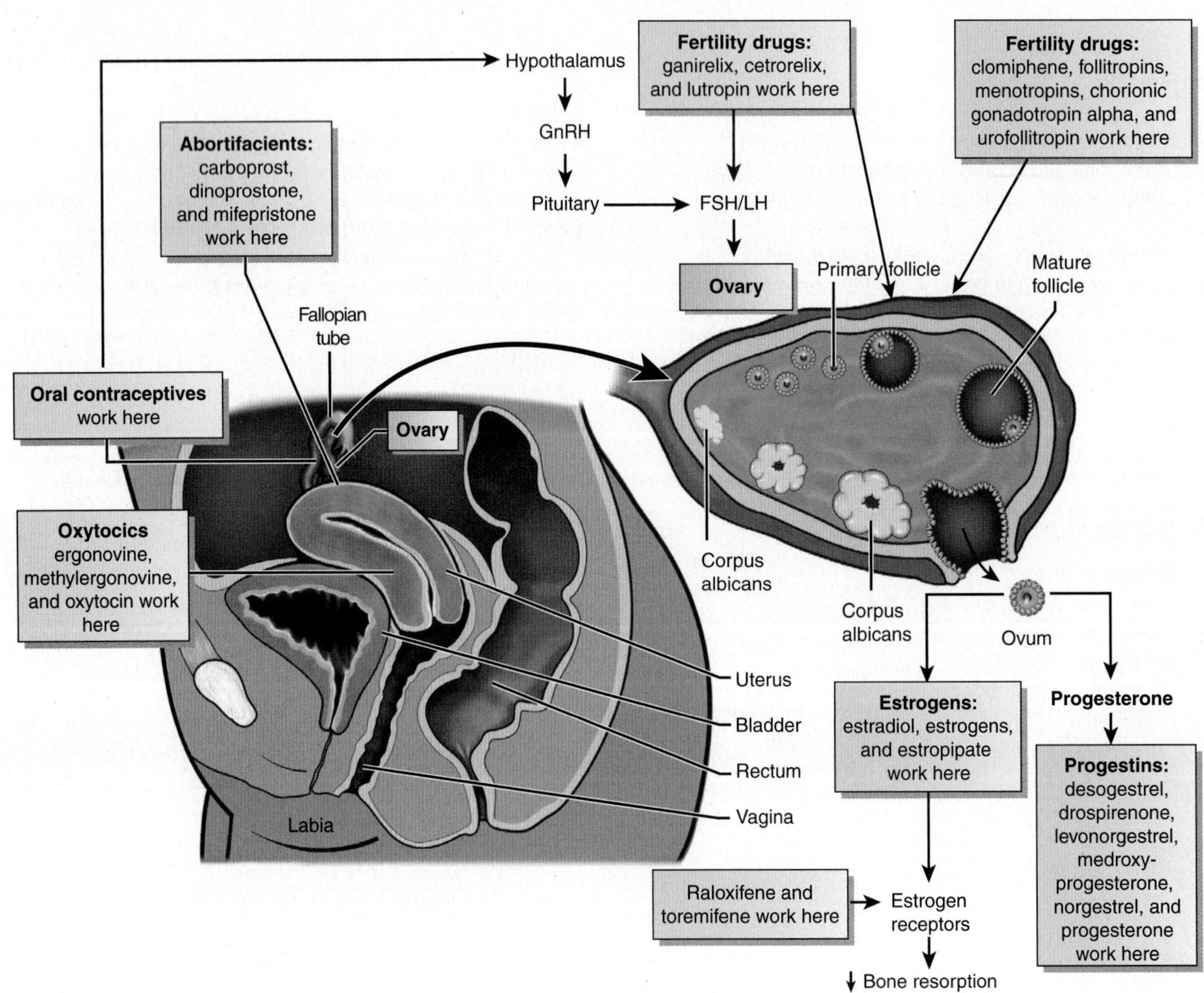

FIGURE 40.1 Sites of action of drugs affecting the female reproductive system.

Box 40.1 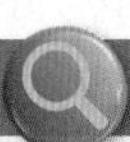 Focus on Drug Therapy Across the Lifespan

DRUGS AFFECTING THE FEMALE REPRODUCTIVE SYSTEM

Children

The estrogens and progestins have undergone little testing in children. Because of their effects on closure of the epiphyses, they should be used only with great caution in growing children.

If oral contraceptives are prescribed for teenage patients, the smallest dose possible should be used and the child should be monitored carefully for metabolic and other effects.

Adults

Patients who are receiving any of these drugs should receive an annual medical examination, including breast/chest examination and Pap smear to monitor for adverse effects and underlying medical conditions. The potential for adverse effects should be discussed and comfort measures provided. Patients taking estrogen should be advised not to smoke because of the increased risk of thrombotic events.

If one of these drugs is used in males for the treatment of specific cancers, the patient should be advised about the possibility of estrogenic effects, and appropriate support should be offered.

When combinations of these hormones are used as part of a fertility program, patients need a great deal of psychological support and comfort measures to cope with the many adverse effects associated with these drugs. The risk of multiple births should be explained, as should the need for frequent monitoring.

When abortifacients are used, patients need a great deal of psychological support. Written lists of signs and symptoms to report and what to expect are more effective than just verbal lists in this time of potential stress.

These agents are not for use during pregnancy or lactation because of the potential for adverse effects on the fetus or neonate.

Older Adults

Hormone replacement therapy (HRT) is no longer commonly used for long-term treatment by postmenopausal patients. Medication may be used short term for palliation of signs and symptoms of menopause. However, it is advisable to stop therapy as soon as possible due to increased risk of breast cancer, cardiovascular events, and even dementia (in patients 65 years or older). Topical therapy is safer and may relieve some of the symptoms of menopause without the risks associated with systemic therapy.

Table 40.1 *Drugs in Focus:* Sex Hormones and Estrogen Receptor Modulators

Name	Usual Dosage	Usual Indications
Sex Hormones		
Estrogens		
estradiol (*Climara, Estrace,* generic)	Dosing varies based on formulation; available in oral, transdermal, intravaginal, and IM formulations	Palliation of signs and symptoms of menopause, prostate cancer, inoperable breast cancer; treatment of female hypogonadism, postpartum breast engorgement; prevention of postmenopausal osteoporosis (transdermal)
estrogens, conjugated (*C.E.S., Premarin*)	0.3–1.25 mg/d PO	Palliation of signs and symptoms of menopause, prostate cancer, inoperable breast cancer; treatment of female hypogonadism, postpartum breast engorgement; to retard the progress of osteoporosis
estrogens, esterified (*Menest*)	0.3–1.25 mg/d PO	Palliation of signs and symptoms of menopause, prostate cancer, inoperable breast cancer; treatment of female hypogonadism
estropipate (*Ogen*)	0.625–5 mg/d PO	Palliation of signs and symptoms of menopause; treatment of female hypogonadism
Progestins		
etonogestrel (*Nexplanon*)	68 mg implanted subdermally for up to 3 y, may be replaced at that time	Contraceptive for female patients
levonorgestrel (*Kyleena, Liletta, Mirena, Plan B One-step, Skyla,* and multiple other over-the-counter forms)	*Intrauterine:* device inserted for up to 3–6 y *Plan B One-Step:* 1.5 mg PO taken within 72 h of sexual intercourse	Intrauterine contraceptive and treatment of heavy menstrual bleeding; also used as "morning-after" pill; component in many combination contraceptives
medroxyprogesterone (*Depo-Provera*)	5–10 mg/d PO for 5–10 d for amenorrhea; 400–1,000 mg/wk IM for cancer therapy	Treatment of amenorrhea (orally); palliation of certain cancers (injection)

(*Continued on page 688*)

Table 40.1 *Drugs in Focus:* Sex Hormones and Estrogen Receptor Modulators (*continued*)

Name	Usual Dosage	Usual Indications
norethindrone (*Camila, Errin, Heather, Incassia, Jencycla, Nor-QD*)	PO dosing varies based on formulation and indication	Used in combination contraceptives; used alone for treatment of amenorrhea, endometriosis, and bleeding disorders and for contraception
progesterone (generic)	5–10 mg/d IM for 6–8 d; 90 mg/d intravaginally	Used as contraceptive and in fertility programs; treatment of amenorrhea and abnormal uterine bleeding due to hormonal imbalance in the absence of organic pathology, such as submucous fibroids or uterine cancer
ulipristal (*Ella, Logilia*)	30 mg PO within 120 h (5 d) of unprotected intercourse	Postcoital contraception
Estrogen Receptor Modulators		
raloxifene (*Evista*)	60 mg/d PO	Treatment and prevention of osteoporosis in postmenopausal patients; reducing risk of invasive breast cancer in postmenopausal patients with osteoporosis; reducing risk of invasive breast cancer in postmenopausal patients at high risk

PMDD, premenstrual dysphoric disorder.

Therapeutic Actions and Indications

Estrogens

Estrogens are used in many clinical situations; for example, in small doses, they are used for HRT when ovarian activity is blocked or absent. (Box 40.2 lists combination products used as HRT.) Estrogens are also used as palliation for discomforts in the first few years of menopause, when many of the beneficial effects of estrogen are lost; to treat female hypogonadism and ovarian failure; to prevent postpartum breast engorgement; as part of combination contraceptives (Box 40.3 lists forms and dosing of contraceptives); to slow bone loss in osteoporosis; and for palliation in certain cancers that have known receptor sensitivity (see Chapter 14). See Table 40.1 for usual indications for each type of estrogen.

Estrogens are important for the development of the female reproductive system and secondary sex characteristics. They affect the release of pituitary follicle-stimulating hormone (FSH) and luteinizing hormone (LH); cause capillary dilation, fluid retention, and protein anabolism and thin the cervical mucus; conserve calcium and phosphorus and encourage bone formation; inhibit ovulation; and prevent postpartum breast discomfort. Estrogens also are responsible for the proliferation of the endometrial lining (see Fig. 40.1). An absence or decrease in estrogen produces the signs and symptoms of menopause in the uterus, vagina, breasts, and cervix. Estrogens are known to compete with androgens for receptor sites; this trait makes them beneficial in certain androgen-dependent prostate cancers. Estrogens produce a wide variety of systemic effects, including protecting the heart from atherosclerosis, retaining calcium in the bones, and maintaining the secondary female sex characteristics (see Box 39.1 for a complete list of estrogen

BOX 40.2

Combination Drugs Used for Menopause

Many fixed-combination drugs containing estrogen and a progestin are available specifically for relieving the signs and symptoms associated with menopause in patients who have an intact uterus. The benefits include reduction in the risk of osteoporosis. However, there is risk of endometrial cancer, stroke, DVT, and dementia associated with use of these drugs. They are not indicated for use to decrease coronary artery disease. The oral drugs are taken as one tablet once a day. There are also transdermal formulations available. Patients should receive regular medical follow-up and monitoring while taking these drugs.

Estrogen/bazedoxifene (*Duavee*)
Estradiol/norethindrone (*Activella, Amabelz, Aurovela, Blisovi, Chabelina Fe*)
Estradiol/progesterone (*Bijuva*)
Estradiol/norgestimate (*Ortho-Prefest*)
Estradiol/drospirenone (*Yaz*)
Ethinyl estradiol/norethindrone acetate (*Femhrt, Fyavolv, Gemmily, Gildess, Hailey, Junel, Larin, Leribane, Lo Loestrin Fe, Merzee, Mibelas 24 Fe, Taytulla*)
Estrogen/medroxyprogesterone (*Premphase*)
Estrogen/medroxyprogesterone/conjugated estrogens (*Prempro*)
Estradiol/drospirenone (*Angeliq*)
Estrogen/norethindrone (*CombiPatch*)
Estradiol/levonorgestrel (*Climara Pro*)

BOX 40.3

Contraceptives: Forms and Dosing

Oral contraceptives are available as monophasic, biphasic, triphasic, and quadriphasic preparations. With monophasic dosing, patients take one tablet orally for 21 days, beginning on day 5 of menstrual bleeding (day 1 of the cycle is the first day of menstrual bleeding). Inert tablets or no tablets are taken for the next 7 days, and then a new course of 21 days is started. Dosing instructions vary per specific formulation for the biphasic, triphasic, and quadriphasic preparations.

Missed doses: If one tablet is missed, the patient should take it as soon as possible; generally, backup contraceptive method is not necessary. If two consecutive tablets are missed, the patient should take the missed tablet as soon as possible and resume the prescribed schedule; generally, backup contraceptive method is not necessary. If three consecutive tablets are missed, the patient should follow the package insert directions and use additional contraceptive method until the start of their next menstrual period.

Postcoital or Emergency Contraception ("Morning After" Regimen)

levonorgestrel (*Plan B*)	Take one tablet within 72 h after intercourse and a second tablet 12 h later
levonorgestrel (*Plan B One-Step, Her Style, Next Choice One Dose, My Way, Opcicon One-Step, Fallback Solo*)	Take one tablet within 72 h after unprotected intercourse, available over the counter for patients 17 y and older
ulipristal (*Ella*)	Take one tablet within 5 d of unprotected intercourse

Monophasic Oral Contraceptive Agents

Afirmelle, Aviane, Balcoltra, Cerinta, Falmina, Lessina Lutera, Sronyx, Tyblume, Vienva	20-mcg estradiol, 0.10-mg levonorgestrel
Altavera, Ayuna, Iclevia, Introvale, Jolessa, Kurvelo, Levora 0.15/30, Marlissa, Portia, Quasense	30-mcg ethinyl estradiol, 0.15-mg levonorgestrel
Alyacen 1/35, Cyclafem 1/35, Dasetta 1/35, Necon 1/35, Norinyl 1 + 35, Nortrel 1/35, Nylia 1/35, Pirmella 1/35	35-mcg ethinyl estradiol, 1-mg norethindrone
Ashlyna, Daysee, Quasense, Seasonale, Seasonique, Setlakin, Sylevia	0.15-mg levonorgestrel, 30-mcg ethinyl estradiol; taken as 84 d active tablets, 7 d inactive
Aurovela 1/20, Blisovi Fe 1/20, Blisovi 24 Fe, Gemmily, Gildess 1/20, Gildess Fe 1/20, Gildess 24 Fe, Hailey FE 1/20, Junel Fe 1/20, Junel 21 Day 1/20, Larin 1/20, Larin FE 1/20, Loestrin 21 1/20, Loestrin Fe 21 1/20, Loestrin 24 Fe, Lomedia 24 FE, Merzee, Mibelas 24 Fe, Microgestin Fe 1/20, Minastrin 24 FE, Taytulla	20-mcg ethinyl estradiol, 1-mg norethindrone
Aurovela 1.5/30, Blisovi Fe 1.5/30, Gildess 1.5/20, Hailey 1.5/30, Hailey FE 1.5/30, Junel Fe 1.5/30, Junel 21 Day 1.5/30, FE 15/30, Larin Fe 1.5/30, Loestrin 21 1.5/30, Loestrin Fe 1.5/30, Microgestin Fe 1.5/30	30-mcg ethinyl estradiol, 1.5-mg norethindrone acetate
Balziva-28, Briellyn, Gildagia, Nexesta FE, Philith, Vyfemla, Wymzya FE, Zenchent	35-mcg ethinyl estradiol, 0.4-mg norethindrone
Beyaz	3-mg drospirenone, 0.2-mg ethinyl estradiol, 0.45-mg levomefolate
Cryselle, Elinest, Low-Ogestrel	30-mcg ethinyl estradiol, 0.3-mg norgestrel
Cyonanz, Modicon, Necon 0.5/35, Nortrel 0.5/35, Wera	35-mcg ethinyl estradiol, 0.5-mg norethindrone
Dolishale	20-mcg ethinyl estradiol, 0.09-mg levonorgestrel
Enskyce, Isibloom, Kalliga, Solia	30-mcg ethinyl estradiol, 0.15-mg desogestrel
Estarylla, Mono-Linyah, Mili, MonoNessa, Ortho-Cyclen, Previfem, Sprintec	35-mcg ethinyl estradiol, 0.25-mg norgestimate
Generess FE, Kaitlib FE	25-mg ethinyl estradiol, 0.8-mg norethindrone
Gianvi, Loryna, Melamisa, Nikki, Vestura, Yaz	20-mcg ethinyl estradiol, 3-mg drospirenone
Kelnor 1/35, Lo Malmorede, Norinyl 1/35, Zovia 1/35E	35-mcg ethinyl estradiol, 1-mg ethynodiol diacetate
Kemeya, Kyra, Lo Zumandimine, Ocella, Safryal, Syeda, Yaela, Yasmin 28, Zumandimine	30-mcg ethinyl estradiol, 3-mg drospirenone
Lo/Ovral FE	30-mcg ethinyl estradiol, 0.3-mg norgestrel, 75-mg ferrous fumarate
Malmorede, Zovia 1/50E	50-mcg ethinyl estradiol, 1-mg ethynodiol diacetate
Necon 1/50, Norinyl 1 + 50	50-mcg mestranol, 1-mg norethindrone
Norminest FE	35-mcg ethinyl estradiol, 0.5-mg norethindrone, 75-mg ferrous fumarate
Safyral, Tydemy	3-mg drospirenone, 30-mcg ethinyl estradiol, 45-mcg levomefolate

Biphasic Oral Contraceptive Agents

Camrese, Daysee, Jaimiess, Seasonique	Phase 1, 84 tablets: 0.15-mg levonorgestrel, 30-mcg ethinyl estradiol Phase 2, 7 tablets: 10-mcg ethinyl estradiol
Amethia Lo, Lo Simpesse	Phase 1, 84 tablets: 0.1-mg levonorgestrel, 20-mcg ethinyl estradiol Phase 2, 7 tablets: 10-mcg ethinyl estradiol

(*Continued on page 690*)

BOX 40.3

Contraceptives: Forms and Dosing (*Continued*)

Azurette, Bekyree, Kariva, Kimidess, Pimtrea, Simliya, Viorele, Volnea	Phase 1, 21 tablets: 0.15-mg desogestrel, 20-mcg ethinyl estradiol Phase 2, 5 tablets: 10-mcg ethinyl estradiol
Camrese Lo, LoSeasonique	Phase 1, 84 tablets: 0.15-mg levonorgestrel, 20-mcg ethinyl estradiol Phase 2, 7 tablets: 10-mcg ethinyl estradiol
Lo Loestrin Fe, Lo Minastrin Fe	Phase 1, 24 tablets: 1-mg norethindrone, 10-mcg ethinyl estradiol Phase 2, 2 tablets: 10-mcg ethinyl estradiol
Necon 10/11	Phase 1, 10 tablets: 0.5-mg norethindrone, 35-mcg ethinyl estradiol Phase 2, 11 tablets: 1-mg norethindrone, 35-mcg ethinyl estradiol
Simpesse	Phase 1, 84 tablets: 0.01-mg levonorgestrel, 30-mcg ethinyl estradiol Phase 2, 7 tablets: 15-mcg ethinyl estradiol

Triphasic Oral Contraceptive Agents

Aranelle, Leena, Tri-Norinyl	Phase 1, 7 tablets: 0.5-mg norethindrone, 35-mcg ethinyl estradiol Phase 2, 9 tablets: 1-mg norethindrone, 35-mcg ethinyl estradiol Phase 3, 5 tablets: 0.5-mg norethindrone, 35-mcg ethinyl estradiol
Alyacen 7/7/7, Cyclafem 7/7/7, Dasetta 7/7/7, Necon 7/7/7, Nortrel 7/7/7, Nylia 7/7/7, Pirmella 7/7/7	Phase 1, 7 tablets: 0.5-mg norethindrone (progestin), 35-mcg ethinyl estradiol (estrogen) Phase 2, 7 tablets: 0.75-mg norethindrone (progestin), 35-mcg ethinyl estradiol (estrogen) Phase 3, 7 tablets: 1-mg norethindrone (progestin), 35-mcg ethinyl estradiol (estrogen)
Caziant, Cyclessa, Velivet	Phase 1, 7 tablets: 0.1-mg desogestrel, 25-mcg ethinyl estradiol Phase 2, 7 tablets: 0.125-mg desogestrel, 25-mcg ethinyl estradiol Phase 3, 7 tablets: 0.15-mg desogestrel, 25-mcg ethinyl estradiol
Chabelina FE, Tri-Legest	Phase 1, 5 tablets: 1-mg norethindrone, 20-mcg ethinyl estradiol Phase 2, 7 tablets: 1-mg norethindrone, 30-mcg ethinyl estradiol Phase 3, 9 tablets: 1-mg norethindrone, 35-mcg ethinyl estradiol
Enpresse, Levonest, Myzilra, Trivora	Phase 1, 6 tablets: 0.5-mg levonorgestrel (progestin), 30-mcg ethinyl estradiol (estrogen) Phase 2, 5 tablets: 0.075-mg levonorgestrel (progestin), 40-mcg ethinyl estradiol (estrogen) Phase 3, 10 tablets: 0.125-mg levonorgestrel (progestin), 30-mcg ethinyl estradiol (estrogen)
Estrostep Fe, Tilia Fe, Tri-Legest Fe	Phase 1, 5 tablets: 1-mg norethindrone, 20-mcg ethinyl estradiol, 75-mg ferrous fumarate Phase 2, 7 tablets: 1-mg norethindrone, 30-mcg ethinyl estradiol, 75-mg ferrous fumarate Phase 3, 9 tablets: 1-mg norethindrone, 35-mcg ethinyl estradiol, 75-mg ferrous fumarate
Ortho Tri-Cyclen, Tri-Estarylla, Tri-Linyah, Tri-Mili, TriNessa, Tri-Sprintec	Phase 1, 7 tablets: 0.18-mg norgestimate, 35-mcg ethinyl estradiol Phase 2, 7 tablets: 0.215-mg norgestimate, 35-mcg ethinyl estradiol Phase 3, 7 tablets: 0.25-mg norgestimate, 35-mcg ethinyl estradiol
Tri Lo Estarylla, Tri Lo Mili, Tri Lo Sprintec	Phase 1, 7 tablets: 0.18-mg norgestimate, 25-mcg ethinyl estradiol Phase 2, 7 tablets: 0.025-mg norgestimate, 25-mcg ethinyl estradiol Phase 3, 7 tablets: 0.25-mg norgestimate, 25-mcg ethinyl estradiol

Quadriphasic Oral Contraceptive Agents

Natazia	Phase 1, 2 tablets: 3-mg estradiol valerate Phase 2, 5 tablets: 2-mg estradiol valerate, 2-mg dienogest Phase 3, 17 tablets: 2-mg estradiol valerate, 3-mg dienogest Phase 4, 2 tablets: 1-mg estradiol valerate
Leribane, Quartette	Phase 1, 42 tablets: 0.15-mg levonorgestrel, 0.02-mg ethinyl estradiol Phase 2, 21 tablets: 0.15-mg levonorgestrel, 0.025-mg ethinyl estradiol

BOX 40.3 (*Continued*)

Contraceptives: Forms and Dosing (*Continued*)

Drug	Forms and Dosing
	Phase 3, 21 tablets: 0.15-mg levonorgestrel, 0.03-mg ethinyl estradiol Phase 4, 7 tablets: 0.01-mg ethinyl estradiol
Progestin-only contraceptives Camila, Errin, Heather, Jencycla, Nor-QD, Ortho Micronor	0.35-mg norethindrone
Injectables	
Depo-Provera, Depo-SubQ Provera 104	*Depo Provera:* 150-mg medroxyprogesterone, given 1 mL by deep IM injection q3mo; *Depo-SubQ Provera 104:* 104-mg medroxyprogesterone, give 0.65 mL subcutaneously *Boxed Warning:* Risk of significant bone loss
Intrauterine System	
Liletta	52-mg levonorgestrel inserted into uterus for up to 6 y
Mirena	52-mg levonorgestrel, inserted into the uterus, releases low-dose levonorgestrel over a 5-y period
Skyla	13.5-mg levonorgestrel inserted into uterus for up to 3 y
Transdermal System	
Twirla	120-mcg levonorgestrel, 30-mcg ethinyl estradiol in transdermal system. Patch applied on same day of week for 3 consecutive wks, followed by 1 wk patch-free *Boxed Warning:* Contraindicated in patients w/BMI ≥ 30 kg/m² and in patients >35 y who smoke (increased risk of CV events)
Xulane	6-mg norelgestromin, 0.75-mg ethinyl estradiol; three patches per cycle, each worn for 1 wk followed by 1 wk patch-free *Boxed Warning:* Higher risk of thromboembolic events/death if combined w/smoking
Vaginal Ring	
Annovera	0.15-mg segesterone acetate, 0.013-mg ethinyl estradiol ring inserted vaginally and kept in place for 21 d, followed by 7-d ring-free interval. One ring provides contraception for 13 28-d cycles (1 y). *Boxed Warning:* Higher risk of thromboembolic events/death if combined w/smoking, especially in patients >35 y
EluRyng, NuvaRing	0.12-mg etonogestrel, 0.015-mg ethinyl estradiol ring inserted vaginally once a month and kept in place for 3 wk; after 1-wk rest, a new ring is inserted *Boxed Warning:* Higher risk of thromboembolic events/death if combined w/smoking, especially in patients >35 y
Subdermal Implant	
Implanon, Nexplanon	68-mg etonogestrel implanted subdermally, effective up to 3 y, may be replaced at that time if desired

effects). However, the results of a study by the Women's Health Initiative showed some serious negative reactions to exogenous estrogen in postmenopausal patients when used in HRT over a period of time (Box 40.4). Box 40.5 describes information about treating dyspareunia during menopause.

Progestins

Progestins are used as contraceptives, most effectively in combination with estrogens (see Box 40.3 for available contraceptives). They are used to treat primary and secondary amenorrhea and functional uterine bleeding and as part of fertility programs. Some are indicated for postcoital emergency contraception. Like estrogens, some progestins are useful in treating specific cancers with specific receptor site sensitivity (see Chapter 14). See Table 40.1 for usual indications for each type of progestin.

Progestins transform the proliferative endometrium into a secretory endometrium, inhibit the secretion of FSH and LH, prevent follicle maturation and ovulation, inhibit uterine contractions, and may have some anabolic and estrogenic effects. When they are used as contraceptives, the exact mechanism of action is not known, but it is thought that circulating progestins and estrogens "trick" the hypothalamus and pituitary and prevent the release of gonadotropin-releasing hormone (GnRH), FSH, and LH, thus preventing follicle development and ovulation. The low levels of these hormones do not produce a thick and vascular endometrium that is receptive to implantation; if ovulation and fertilization were to occur, the chances of implantation would be remote.

Box 40.4 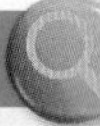 Focus on The Evidence

MENOPAUSE AND HORMONE REPLACEMENT THERAPY—THE WOMEN'S HEALTH INITIATIVE STUDY

Females experience menarche (onset of the menstrual cycle) in adolescence and menopause (cessation of the menstrual cycle) in midlife. The age at which a person experiences menopause varies. The family history of onset of menopause is a good guide for when the effects can be expected. Just as the physical changes associated with puberty can take a few years to be accomplished, so too can the changes associated with menopause. The signs and symptoms of menopause (vaginal dryness, hot flashes, moodiness, loss of bone density, increased risk of CV disease, somnolence) are related to the loss of estrogen and progesterone effects on the body.

HORMONE REPLACEMENT THERAPY OR NOT?

For centuries, people have proceeded through this time in their lives without pharmacologic intervention, though many herbal and alternative therapies may help to ease the transition through menopause (see Box 40.7). Patients who rely on these therapies need to be cautioned about potential drug–drug interactions and advised to always report the use of these agents to their health care providers. Today, with more research and safer drugs available to counteract some of the effects of menopause, many patients choose to use HRT if the adverse effects of menopause become too uncomfortable or difficult to tolerate. The use of HRT can decrease the discomforts associated with menopause, though various forms of HRT have been associated with increased risks for breast and cervical cancer, heart disease, and stroke. Many patients are reluctant to consider HRT because of these effects. The newer drugs used in HRT have been shown to be associated with only a possible increase in risk of breast and cervical cancer, but with long-term use, they are associated with increased risk of CV events. Patients with many risk factors for developing breast and cervical cancers are at a greater risk than patients with no risk factors. Other drugs—the estrogen receptor modulators—have antiestrogen effects on the breast and may remove the cancer risk. However, these drugs may be less reliable in their management of the signs and symptoms of menopause.

EARLY RESEARCH

The Women's Health Initiative was a long-term, multisite study of the effects of hormones during menopause. When the initial reports were published, after the 3rd and 4th years of the study, it seemed that the use of HRT was protective in many ways. It seemed that people using HRT had decreased coronary artery disease and CV events, decreased osteoporosis and bone fractures, decreased breast and colon cancer, and improved memory. HRT was then being prescribed to prevent a number of these chronic conditions.

LATER RESEARCH

In 2002, however, the study was stopped when it was found that participants using HRT for 5 or more years had an increased incidence of CV disease and stroke, as well as blood clots, gallstones, and ovarian cancer. The news headlines were confusing at best; many people simply stopped HRT, and those new to menopause would not even consider it.

APPLYING THE EVIDENCE

A person who is entering menopause should have all of the information available before deciding whether HRT is for them. This can be a difficult decision for many people because the risks involved may outweigh the benefits or vice versa. The nurse is often in the best position to provide information, listen to concerns, and help the patient to decide what is best for them.

A complete family and personal history of cancer and coronary artery disease risk factors should be completed to help the patient balance the benefits versus the risks of this therapy. If the patient decides to use HRT, they may need support in dealing with the effects of the drugs and may have to try several different preparations before the one best suited to them is found. This can be a frustrating time, so the patient will need a consistent, reliable person to turn to with questions and for support. As researchers continue to study health issues related to the female body, better therapies may be developed to help patients through this transition in life. Keeping up with the research as it is reported can be a difficult task, but for anyone who works with female patients in clinical practice, it is a necessity.

The current recommendation of the U.S. Preventative Services Task Force is that patients should feel comfortable taking HRT to reduce the symptoms of menopause for short-term therapy (fewer than 5 years). The task force summarized all of the studies and noted that long-term use of HRT provides a decreased risk of osteoporosis and related fractures, possibly a reduced risk of dementia, and a reduction in risk of colon cancer. The negative aspects of this therapy include a definite but small increased risk for heart disease, stroke, and breast cancer. The harms of long-term use outweigh the benefits for most patients. The benefits of short-term use, however, must be considered if a patient is having a difficult time getting through menopause, and HRT should not be used for primary prevention for chronic disease (USPSTF, 2017).

Critics of the study also point out that the participants in the study were much older than most early postmenopausal groups who could benefit from HRT; they concluded that more research is needed on this. Follow-up research using this study has found no correlation between the use of HRT and the prevention of Alzheimer's disease and no drop in bone fractures in patients using HRT.

Pharmacokinetics

Estrogens

Oral estrogens are well absorbed through the gastrointestinal (GI) tract and undergo extensive hepatic metabolism. They are excreted in the urine. Estrogens cross the placenta and enter human milk. Estrogen is available in multiple forms: tablets, solutions for injection, creams/gels, transdermal patches, and intravaginal rings.

Progestins

Progestins are well absorbed, undergo hepatic metabolism, and are excreted in the urine. They are known to cross

BOX 40.5

Treating Dyspareunia During Menopause

The FDA has approved a drug for the treatment of moderate to severe dyspareunia during menopause and for treatment of moderate to severe vaginal dryness. Dysparenunia is a condition of painful intercourse associated with the vaginal dryness and changes that occur with menopause. The drug, ospemifene (*Osphena*), is an estrogen agonist/antagonist. It is taken orally once a day. *Osphena* has a boxed warning that its use increases the risk of endometrial cancer and of CV events including stroke, myocardial infarction, and deep-vein thrombosis. Patients should be screened for appropriate use. The drug is contraindicated with any undiagnosed genital bleeding, known or suspected estrogen-dependent cancers, active thromboembolic disease, or known or suspected pregnancy. It is advised that a progestin be added to the drug regimen in people with an intact uterus to decrease the risk of endometrial cancer. When taking the drug, patients may experience hot flashes, vaginal discharge, muscle spasms, and increased sweating. Because of the potential risk associated with the use of the drug, it is recommended that every 3 to 6 months, the use of the drug be reevaluated.

the placenta and to enter human milk. Like estrogens, progestins are available in several forms: tablets, solutions for injection, cream/gel, transdermal patch, and implanted uterine devices.

Contraindications and Cautions

Estrogens

Estrogens are contraindicated or used with extreme caution in patients with undiagnosed atypical vaginal bleeding, breast cancer, or any estrogen-dependent cancer, all of which could be exacerbated by the drug; with a history of thromboembolic disorders, including cerebrovascular accident; with patients who are heavy smokers, because of the increased risk of thrombus and embolus development; or with hepatic dysfunction, because of the effects of estrogen on liver function.

Estrogens are contraindicated during pregnancy due to the risk of serious fetal defects. They should be avoided during breast or chestfeeding because of decreased quantity and quality of milk production. Estrogens should be used cautiously in patients with metabolic bone disease because of the bone-conserving effect of estrogen, which could exacerbate the disease; with renal insufficiency, which could interfere with the renal excretion of the drug and increase the risk for potential adverse effects on fluid and electrolyte balance; and with hepatic impairment, which could alter the metabolism of the drug and increase the risk for adverse effects, including those on the liver and GI tract.

Progestins

Contraindications and cautions for progestins are similar to those for estrogens. Progestins are also contraindicated in the presence of endometriosis or pelvic surgery because of the effects of progestins on the vasculature of the uterus. Drospirenone is contraindicated in patients who are at risk for hyperkalemia due to renal disorders, liver disease, adrenal dysfunction, or the use of other drugs that can affect potassium levels, because of its antimineralocorticoid effects and the risk of hyperkalemia.

Progestins should be used with caution in patients with epilepsy, migraine headaches, asthma, or cardiac or renal dysfunction because of potential exacerbation of these conditions. See Box 40.6 for more information about risks of estrogen and progesterone products.

Box 40.6 Focus on Safe Medication Administration

Estrogen, estrogenlike, and progesterone products have a boxed warning of potential risks. Estrogen-only products are associated with risk of endometrial cancer in people with an intact uterus and no concurrent progesterone therapy. Estrogen alone should not be used to prevent cardiovascular disease or dementia. There is increased risk for stroke and thrombotic disorders and possible increased risk for dementia in postmenopausal patients who are 65 years of age or older. When estrogen and progesterone products are used together, there is increased risk of stroke, deep-vein thrombosis, pulmonary embolism, and myocardial infarction; of invasive breast cancer; and of dementia in postmenopausal people. These products are also not approved for prevention of CV disease or dementia. Patients who take any of these products should be alerted to the possible risks, have annual pelvic and breast examinations and breast cancer screenings, be monitored for any signs of thrombotic disorders, and be alerted to what signs they need to report. Smoking increases the risk of thrombotic events; all patients taking these products should be advised not to smoke.

Adverse Effects

Estrogens

Many of the more common adverse effects associated with estrogens involve the genitourinary (GU) tract. They include breakthrough bleeding, menstrual irregularities, dysmenorrhea, amenorrhea, and changes in libido. Other effects can result from the systemic effects of estrogens; these include fluid retention, electrolyte disturbances, headache, dizziness, mental changes, weight changes, and edema. GI effects are also fairly common and include nausea, vomiting, abdominal cramps and bloating, and colitis. Potentially serious GI effects, including acute pancreatitis, cholestatic jaundice, and hepatic adenoma, have been reported with the use of estrogens (Fig. 40.2).

Progestins

Adverse effects associated with progestins vary with the administration route used. Systemic effects are similar to the adverse effects of estrogen. Dermal patch contraceptives are associated with the same systemic effects and

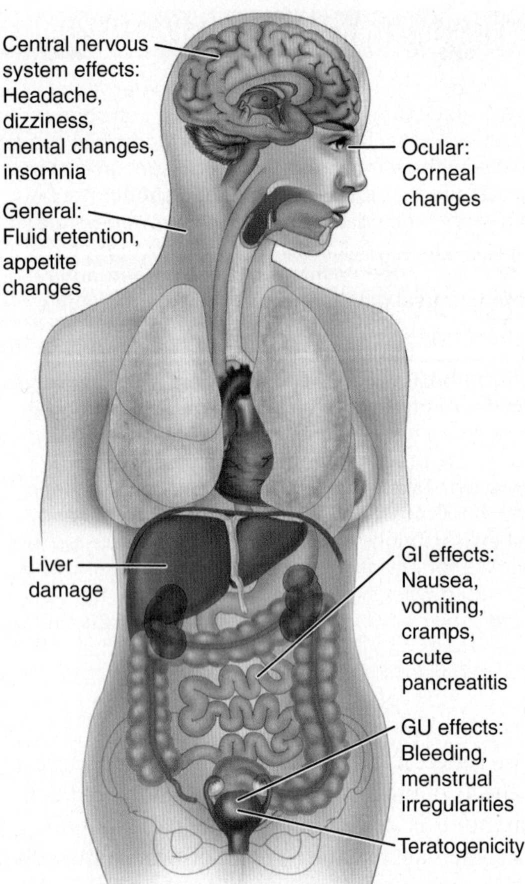

FIGURE 40.2 Variety of adverse effects and toxicities associated with drugs affecting the female reproductive system.

with local skin irritation. Vaginal gel use is associated with headache, nervousness, constipation, breast enlargement, and perineal pain. Intrauterine devices are associated with abdominal pain, intensified endometriosis symptoms, abortion, PID, and expulsion of the intrauterine device. Vaginal use is associated with local irritation and swelling. Drospirenone, used in combination contraceptives, has antimineralocorticoid activity and can block aldosterone, leading to increased potassium levels.

Clinically Important Drug–Drug Interactions

Estrogens

Estrogens are metabolized partially by cytochrome P450 3A4 (CYP3A4). Therefore, inducers or inhibitors of CYP3A4 may affect estrogen drug metabolism.

If estrogens are given in combination with drugs that enhance hepatic metabolism (e.g., barbiturates, rifampin, tetracyclines, phenytoin), serum estrogen levels may decrease.

Estrogens have been associated with increased therapeutic and toxic effects of corticosteroids, so patients taking both drugs should be monitored closely. Concurrent use with warfarin, other anticoagulants, some thyroid medications, and oral medications for diabetes may decrease effectiveness of the medications, so dosage adjustments may be necessary.

Smoking while taking estrogens should be strongly discouraged because the combination with nicotine increases the risk for development of thrombi and emboli.

Grapefruit juice can inhibit the metabolism of estradiols, leading to increased serum levels. Patients should be discouraged from drinking large quantities of grapefruit juice if they are taking estrogens. St. John's wort can affect the metabolism of estrogens and can make estrogen-containing contraceptives less effective. This combination should be discouraged. Other herbal and alternative therapies used for menopausal symptoms may also interact with estrogens (Box 40.7).

Progestins

Interaction with barbiturates, carbamazepine, phenytoin, griseofulvin, penicillins, tetracyclines, or rifampin may reduce the effectiveness of progestins. Patients using any of these

Box 40.7 Focus on Herbal and Alternative Therapies

There are herbal and alternative therapies that may help to alleviate hot flashes and/or other menopausal symptoms. Patients should be aware of the cautions associated with these therapies.

Black cohosh: No clear evidence of benefit, but some people have reported reduced symptoms; some evidence of use causing liver problems

Borage: May help relieve menopausal symptoms and act as anti-inflammatory; not for long-term use; use caution with seizure disorders or liver impairment

Chaste tree: May decrease anxiety and other menopausal symptoms; may cause increased blood pressure, avoid use with antihypertensives or beta-blockers; may cause rash and itching

Clary sage: Used as topical oil; may decrease hot flashes and have antidepressant-like effects; may slow development of osteoporosis; may cause sedation, avoid use with alcohol; not for internal use

Devil's claw: May help to alleviate joint pain; increases stomach acid and may interfere with many prescription drugs; use with caution

Dong quai: Has been used in traditional Chinese medicine for years; causes photosensitivity, avoid exposure to the sun; do not use with warfarin, increased bleeding can occur

False unicorn root: Do not use with estrogen or progestins, may alter uterine effects and cause uterine contractions

Ginseng: May help mood, enhance sleep, and increase overall sense of well-being; does not relieve hot flashes

Red clover: No clear evidence of benefit, but some people report reduced symptoms; do not combine with HRT because of risk for increased estrogenic effects

Soy: Do not use with calcium, iron, or zinc products; may decrease effects of estrogen, raloxifene, and tamoxifen—alert the health care provider if combining these drugs

Wild yam: Contains progesterone, do not use with HRT; may cause increased blood glucose and other toxic effects; do not combine with disulfiram or metronidazole, severe reaction may occur

drugs should use another method of contraception if birth control is needed. St. John's wort can affect the metabolism of progestins and can make progestin-containing contraceptives less effective. This combination should be discouraged.

Prototype Summary Estradiol

Indications: Palliation of moderate to severe vasomotor symptoms associated with menopause; prevention of postmenopausal osteoporosis; treatment of female hypogonadism, female castration, ovarian failure; palliation of inoperable and progressing breast cancer and inoperable prostatic cancer.

Actions: The most potent endogenous female sex hormone, responsible for estrogen effects on the body.

Pharmacokinetics:

Route	Onset	Peak	Duration
PO	Slow	Days	Unknown

Topical preparations are not generally absorbed systemically.

$T_{1/2}$: Not known; metabolized in the liver and excreted in the urine.

Adverse Effects: Corneal changes, photosensitivity, peripheral edema, chloasma, hepatic adenoma, nausea, vomiting, abdominal cramps, bloating, breakthrough bleeding, change in menstrual flow, dysmenorrhea, premenstrual-like syndrome, cardiovascular events (stroke or other thromboembolic disorders), breast cancer.

Prototype Summary Norethindrone Acetate

Indications: Treatment of amenorrhea, abnormal uterine bleeding due to hormonal imbalance; treatment of endometriosis symptoms; component of some hormonal contraceptives.

Actions: Progesterone derivative that transforms the proliferative endometrium into a secretory endometrium; inhibits the secretion of pituitary FSH and LH, which prevents ovulation; inhibits uterine contractions.

Pharmacokinetics:

Route	Onset	Peak	Duration
PO	Varies	Unknown	Unknown

$T_{1/2}$: Unknown; metabolized in the liver and excreted in the feces and urine.

Adverse Effects: Venous thromboembolism, loss of vision, diplopia, migraine headache, rash, acne, chloasma, alopecia, breakthrough bleeding, spotting, amenorrhea, fluid retention, edema, increase in weight.

Estrogen Receptor Modulators

There are several medications that are classified as selective estrogen receptor modulators or estrogen agonist/antagonists. Some are indicated for treating breast cancer; these are discussed in Chapter 14 with the other antineoplastic agents. Raloxifene (*Evista*) is indicated for treatment and prevention of osteoporosis in postmenopausal people and for reduction of risk of breast cancer but is not indicated for treatment of breast cancer.

Therapeutic Actions and Indications

Estrogen receptor modulators are not hormones but affect specific estrogen receptor sites, stimulating some and blocking others. They were developed to produce some of the positive effects of estrogen replacement while limiting the adverse effects. See Table 40.1 for usual indications for raloxifene. Raloxifene acts as an estrogen agonist in the bone, which decreases bone resorption, increases bone mineral density, and decreases bone fractures. Raloxifene acts as an estrogen antagonist in the uterine and breast tissues.

Pharmacokinetics

Administered orally, raloxifene is well absorbed from the GI tract and is metabolized in the liver. Excretion occurs through the feces. It is known to cross the placenta and to enter into human milk.

Contraindications and Cautions

Raloxifene is contraindicated in the presence of any known allergy to raloxifene to avoid hypersensitivity reactions and during pregnancy and lactation because of potential effects on the fetus or neonate. Caution should be used in patients with a history of venous thrombosis or smoking because of increased risk of blood clot formation if smoking and estrogen are combined. It is not indicated for use in premenopausal patients.

Adverse Effects

Raloxifene has been associated with GI upset, nausea, and vomiting. Changes in fluid balance may also cause headache, dizziness, visual changes, and mental changes. Hot flashes, skin rash, edema, and vaginal bleeding may occur secondary to specific estrogen receptor stimulation. Venous thromboembolism and pulmonary emboli have occurred with use of raloxifene. There was a trial that showed increased risk of death due to stroke in postmenopausal people with coronary heart disease or with risk factors for coronary events.

Clinically Important Drug–Drug Interactions

Cholestyramine reduces the absorption of raloxifene. Highly protein-bound drugs, such as diazepam (*Valium*), ibuprofen (*Motrin*), indomethacin (*Indocin*), and naproxen (*Naprosyn*), may interfere with binding sites. Warfarin taken with raloxifene may decrease the prothrombin time; patients using this combination must be monitored closely. It is not recommended to be taken concurrently with other systemic estrogens.

Prototype Summary Raloxifene

Indications: Prevention and treatment of osteoporosis in postmenopausal patients; reduction of risk of breast cancer in postmenopausal patients.

Actions: Increases bone mineral density without stimulating the endometrium; modulates effects of endogenous estrogen at specific receptor sites.

Pharmacokinetics:

Route	Onset	Peak	Duration
PO	Varies	4–7 h	24 h

$T_{1/2}$: 27.7 hours; metabolized in the liver and excreted primarily in the feces.

Adverse Effects: Venous thromboembolism, hot flashes, skin rash, nausea, vomiting, vaginal bleeding, depression, light-headedness, stroke, pulmonary embolism, high triglycerides, hepatic impairment.

Nursing Considerations for Patients Receiving Sex Hormones or Estrogen Receptor Modulators

Assessment: History and Examination

- Assess for contraindications or cautions: history of allergy to any sex hormone or component of the drug product to avoid hypersensitivity reactions; current status related to pregnancy and lactation due to adverse effects on the fetus and neonate; hepatic dysfunction, which might interfere with drug metabolism; CV disease, breast or genital cancer, renal disease, or metabolic bone disease, which could be exacerbated by estrogen use; history of thromboembolism or smoking, which may increase the patient's risk for embolic conditions; idiopathic vaginal bleeding or pelvic disease, which could represent an underlying problem that could be exacerbated with the use of these drugs; and history of asthma or epilepsy, which could be exacerbated by progestin use.
- Perform a physical assessment to establish baseline status before beginning therapy and during therapy to determine the effectiveness of therapy and evaluate for any potential adverse effects.
- Assess skin color, lesions, and texture; affect, orientation, mental status, and reflexes; and blood pressure, pulse, cardiac auscultation, edema, and perfusion, which will reflect circulatory status and show any changes associated with thromboembolism.
- Complete or assist with pelvic and breast/chest examinations. Ensure specimen collection for Pap smear; obtain a history of the patient's menstrual cycle to provide baseline data and to monitor for any adverse effects that could occur.
- Arrange for ophthalmic examination (particularly if the patient wears contact lenses) because hormonal changes can alter the fluid in the eye and curvature of the cornea, which can change the fit of contact lenses and alter visual acuity.
- Monitor the results of laboratory tests, including urinalysis and renal and/or hepatic function tests, to determine the need for possible dose adjustment and identify early indications of dysfunction.

See the "Critical Thinking Scenario" for additional information related to a patient who is taking contraceptives.

Nursing Conclusions

Nursing conclusions related to drug therapy might include the following:

- Fluid overload risk related to fluid retention
- Impaired comfort related to systemic side effects of GI pain and headache
- Altered tissue perfusion (cerebral, cardiopulmonary, peripheral) related to changes in the blood vessels concerning drug therapy and risk of thromboemboli
- Malnutrition risk related to GI distress associated with drug therapy
- Knowledge deficit regarding drug therapy

Planning

- The patient will receive the best therapeutic effect from the drug therapy.
- The patient will have limited adverse effects from the drug therapy.
- The patient will have an understanding of the drug therapy, adverse effects to anticipate, and measures to relieve discomfort and improve safety.

Intervention With Rationale

- Administer drug as prescribed to prevent adverse effects; administer with food if GI upset is severe to relieve GI distress.
- Provide analgesics for relief of headache as appropriate.

- Strongly urge the patient to stop smoking to reduce the risk of thromboemboli.
- Encourage small, frequent meals to assist with nausea and vomiting.
- Monitor for swelling and changes in vision or fit of contact lenses to monitor for fluid retention and fluid changes.
- Arrange for at least an annual physical examination, including pelvic examination, Pap smear, and breast/chest examination, to reduce the risk of adverse effects and to monitor drug effects.
- Assess the patient periodically for changes in perfusion or signs of vessel occlusion because of the risk of thromboemboli.
- Monitor liver function periodically for the patient on long-term therapy to evaluate liver function and ensure discontinuation of the drug at any sign of hepatic dysfunction.
- Offer support and reassurance to help the patient manage the drug and its effects.
- Provide thorough patient teaching, including steps to take if a dose is missed or lost, measures to avoid adverse effects, signs and symptoms that may indicate a problem, and the need for regular evaluation to enhance patient knowledge about drug therapy and to promote adherence.

Evaluation

- Monitor patient response to the drug (palliation of signs and symptoms of menopause, prevention of pregnancy, palliation of certain cancers).
- Monitor for adverse effects (liver changes, GI upset, edema, changes in secondary sex characteristics, headaches, thromboembolic episodes, breakthrough bleeding).
- Monitor for potential drug–drug interactions as indicated.
- Evaluate the effectiveness of the teaching plan (the patient can name the drug, dosage, adverse effects to watch for, specific measures to avoid them, and warning signs and symptoms).
- Monitor the effectiveness of comfort measures and adherence to the regimen.

CRITICAL THINKING SCENARIO
Birth Control

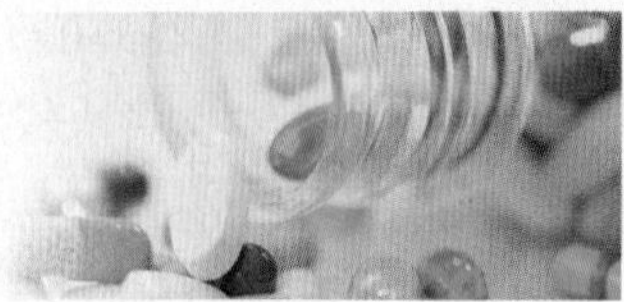

THE SITUATION

J.M. is a 25-year-old patient who is being seen in their gynecologist's office for a routine annual physical examination and Pap test. J.M. reports that they have just become sexually active and would like to start using contraceptives. J.M. has some concerns about stories they have heard about "the pill" and would like to know the safest and most effective birth control to use. J.M. is interested in what other methods are available and what the advantages and disadvantages of each form might be.

CRITICAL THINKING

What teaching and counseling issues will be important for J.M. at this time?

What important issues should be discussed when explaining the benefits and drawbacks of various contraceptive measures?

What teaching information needs to be stressed with J.M. if they elect to use oral contraceptives?

DISCUSSION

This appointment presents a good opportunity for the health care provider to allow J.M. to discuss this new aspect of their life. J.M. may have questions about the experience and about things they should be doing or questioning. The risk of sexually transmitted infections, as well as pregnancy, can be discussed. J.M. needs full information about the various forms of birth control that are available for use. Nonpharmacological measures such as condoms and the rhythm method and their reliability can be discussed.

The use of hormones for birth control should then be explained, including the 96% to 98% reliability of these methods when used correctly. The numerous delivery methods for these hormones should be outlined. A variety of possibilities exist, ranging from the transdermal patch, to injection, to the vaginal ring, to the traditional tablet, and to the use of the subdermal implant and intrauterine devices. J.M. elects to go with an oral contraceptive (OC). They state that they have a good memory, and taking them every day won't be a problem. J.M. swims regularly and thinks that the patch might be an issue if it came off and states they are not comfortable with anything being injected or inserted into their body. J.M. will need teaching about drug and herbal interactions with the OC and will need to have written instructions on what to do if a dose is missed. The action that should be taken if a dose is missed can be complicated and involves knowing on which day in J.M.'s cycle the dose was missed.

It is also important to stress that the OC will not protect J.M. from sexually transmitted infections and that barrier contraception should be used to avoid exposure to these infections. J.M. should also be advised not to smoke because smoking combined with

(Continued on page 698)

OC use increases the risk for emboli. The adverse effects that J.M. might experience should be reviewed, and the importance of an annual pelvic examination and Pap test should be stressed. A trusting nurse–patient relationship is important at this time so J.M. can feel free to call with questions or problems in the future.

NURSING CARE GUIDE FOR J.M.: ORAL CONTRACEPTIVES

Assessment: History and Examination

Assess the patient's health history for allergies to any estrogens; pregnancy or lactation status; breast or genital cancer; hepatic dysfunction; coronary artery disease; thromboembolic disease; renal disease; idiopathic vaginal bleeding; metabolic bone disease; diabetes; and smoking history.

Focus the physical examination on the following:

Neurological: Orientation, reflexes, affect, mental status

Skin: Color, lesions

CV: Pulse, cardiac auscultation, blood pressure, edema, perfusion

GI: Abdominal examination, liver examination

GU: Pelvic examination, Pap smear, urinalysis

Eye: Ophthalmological examination

Nursing Conclusions

Fluid overload risk related to fluid retention

Impaired comfort related to systemic side effects of GI pain or headache

Altered tissue perfusion (cerebral, cardiopulmonary, peripheral) related to changes in the blood vessels in connection with drug therapy, and risk of thromboemboli if also smoking

Knowledge deficit regarding drug therapy

Planning

The patient will receive the best therapeutic effect from the drug therapy.

The patient will have limited adverse effects from the drug therapy.

The patient will have an understanding of the drug therapy, adverse effects to anticipate, and measures to relieve discomfort and improve safety.

Intervention

Administer medication as prescribed.

Administer with meals if upset stomach is a problem.

Provide analgesics for headache if appropriate.

Advise the patient that if they wear contact lenses, the shape of the cornea may change and they may need a new prescription or may no longer be able to wear them.

Provide at least an annual physical examination, including Pap smear and breast/chest examination.

Monitor perfusion and complaints of pain, tingling, or numbness.

Provide support and reassurance to deal with drug therapy.

Provide patient teaching regarding drug name, dosage, what to do if a dose is missed, adverse effects, precautions, warnings to report, and safe administration.

Evaluation

Evaluate drug effects: prevention of pregnancy.

Monitor for adverse effects: signs of liver dysfunction, GI upset, edema, changes in secondary sex characteristics, headaches, thromboembolic episodes, breakthrough bleeding.

Evaluate the effectiveness of the patient teaching program and comfort and safety measures.

PATIENT TEACHING FOR J.M.

- An OC, or birth control pill, contains specific amounts of female sex hormones that work to make the body unreceptive to pregnancy and to prevent ovulation (the release of the egg from the ovary). Because these hormones affect many systems in your body, it is important to have regular physical checkups while you are taking this drug.
- Many drugs affect the way that OCs work. To be safe, avoid the use of over-the-counter (OTC) drugs, herbal therapies, and other drugs unless you first check with your health care provider.
- It is important to know that this drug does not protect you against sexually transmitted infections, and appropriate precautions should be taken.
- Some of the following adverse effects may occur:
  - *Headache, nervousness:* Check with your health care provider about the use of an analgesic; this effect usually passes after a few months on the drug.
  - *Nausea, loss of appetite:* This usually passes with time; consult your health care provider if it is a problem.
  - *Swelling, weight gain:* Water retention is a normal effect of these hormones. Limiting salt intake may help. You may have trouble with contact lenses if you wear them because the body often retains fluid, which may change the shape of your eye. This usually adjusts over time.
  - *Blood clots:* Cigarette smoking can aggravate serious side effects of OCs, such as the formation of blood clots. When taking OCs, it is advisable to cut down or preferably to stop cigarette smoking.
- Tell any doctor, nurse, or other health care provider that you are taking this drug.
- Report any of the following to your health care provider: pain in the calves or groin; chest pain or difficulty breathing; lump in the breast; severe headache, dizziness, visual changes; severe abdominal pain; yellowing of the skin; pregnancy.
- Bleeding (a false menstrual period) should occur during the time that the drug is withdrawn. Report bleeding at *any* other time to your health care provider.
- It is important to have regular medical checkups, including Pap tests, while you are taking this drug. If you decide to stop the drug to become pregnant, consult with your health care provider.
- A patient package insert is included with the drug. Read this information and feel free to ask any questions that you might have.
- Keep this drug and all medications out of the reach of children.

Key Points

- Estrogens are hormones associated with the development of the female reproductive system and secondary sex characteristics. Estrogens are used to prevent conception, to stimulate ovulation in patients with hypogonadism, and to a lesser extent to replace hormones after menopause.
- Progestins maintain pregnancy and are also involved with development of secondary sex characteristics. Progestins are used as part of combination contraceptives, to treat amenorrhea and functional uterine bleeding, and as part of fertility programs.
- Estrogen receptor modulators are used to stimulate specific estrogen receptors to achieve therapeutic effects of increased bone mass without stimulating the endometrium and causing other, less desirable estrogen effects.

Fertility Drugs

Fertility drugs stimulate the female reproductive system. The following fertility drugs are in use: cetrorelix (*Cetrotide*), chorionic gonadotropin (*Pregnyl*), chorionic gonadotropin alpha (*Ovidrel*), clomiphene (generic), follitropin alfa (*Gonal-F*), follitropin alpha/beta (*Follistim AQ, Gonal-F RFF, Gonal-F RFF Redi-ject*), ganirelix acetate (generic), menotropins (*Menopur*), and urofollitropin (*Bravelle*). Table 40.2 gives more information on these agents.

Therapeutic Actions and Indications

Patients without primary ovarian failure who cannot get pregnant after 1 year of trying may be candidates for the use of fertility drugs. Fertility drugs work either directly to stimulate follicles and ovulation or stimulate the hypothalamus to increase FSH and LH levels, leading to ovarian follicular development and maturation of ova. Given in sequence with human chorionic gonadotropin (HCG) to maintain the follicle and hormone production, these drugs are used to treat infertility in people with functioning ovaries whose partners are fertile. Fertility drugs may also be used to stimulate multiple follicle development for the harvesting of ova for in vitro fertilization. Follitropin alfa and follitropin alpha/beta are also indicated for induction of spermatogenesis in patients with primary and secondary hypogonadotropic hypogonadism not due to primary testicular failure.

Cetrorelix inhibits premature LH surges in patients undergoing controlled ovarian stimulation by acting as a GnRH antagonist. Chorionic gonadotropin is used to stimulate ovulation by acting like GnRH and affecting FSH and LH release. Follitropin alfa and follitropin alpha/beta are FSH molecules; they are injected to stimulate follicular development in the treatment of infertility and for harvesting of ova for in vitro fertilization. Menotropins, a purified gonadotropin (similar to FSH and LH), are also used to stimulate ovulation. Urofollitropin is indicated for induction of ovulation or stimulation of multiple follicles in ovulatory patients. See Table 40.2 for usual indications for each fertility drug.

Pharmacokinetics

These drugs are well absorbed and are treated like endogenous hormones within the body, undergoing hepatic metabolism and renal excretion. Drugs that are available in injectable form include cetrorelix, chorionic gonadotropin, chorionic gonadotropin alpha, follitropin alfa, follitropin alpha/beta, menotropins, ganirelix, and urofollitropin. Clomiphene is available as an oral agent.

Contraindications and Cautions

These drugs are contraindicated in the presence of primary ovarian failure (they only work to stimulate functioning ovaries); ovarian cysts, which could be stimulated and become larger due to the effects of the drugs; pregnancy, due to the potential for serious fetal effects; idiopathic uterine bleeding, which could represent an underlying problem that could be exacerbated by the stimulatory effects of these drugs; and known allergy to any fertility drug to avoid hypersensitivity reactions.

Caution should be used in patients who are breast or chestfeeding because of the risk of adverse effects on the baby and in those with thromboembolic diseases because of the risk of increased thrombus formation, as well as in patients with respiratory diseases because of alterations in fluid volume and blood flow that could overtax the respiratory system.

Adverse Effects

Adverse effects associated with fertility drugs include a greatly increased risk of multiple births and congenital anomalies; ovarian overstimulation (abdominal pain, distention, ascites, pleural effusion); and headache, fluid retention, nausea, bloating, uterine bleeding, ovarian enlargement, gynecomastia, and febrile reactions (possibly due to stimulation of progesterone release).

Table 40.2 *Drugs in Focus:* Fertility Drugs

Drug Name	Dosage/Route	Usual Indications
cetrorelix (*Cetrotide*)	3 mg subcutaneously during early follicular phase or 0.25 mg subcutaneously on day 5 or 6 of stimulation and then every day until HCG is administered	Inhibition of premature LH surges in patients undergoing controlled ovarian stimulation
chorionic gonadotropin (*Pregnyl*)	500–10,000 IU subcutaneously depending on timing and indication	Stimulation of ovulation, hypogonadism, prepubertal cryptorchidism
chorionic gonadotropin alpha (*Ovidrel*)	250 mcg subcutaneously, timing depending on indication	Induction of final follicular maturation and ovulation induction in infertile female patients
clomiphene (generic)	50–100 mg/d PO, with the length of therapy and timing dependent on the particular situation	Treatment of infertility; also found to be effective in the treatment of male infertility
follitropin alfa (*Gonal-F*)	75–150 IU/d subcutaneously, dose increases based on response; do not exceed 300 IU/d	Stimulation of follicular development in the treatment of infertility and for harvesting of ova for in vitro fertilization; induction of spermatogenesis in males with primary and secondary hypogonadotropic hypogonadism not due to primary testicular failure
follitropin alpha/beta (*Follistim AQ, Gonal-F RFF, Gonal-F RFF Redi-ject*)	75–225 IU/d subcutaneously, dose increases based on response; do not exceed 450 IU/d	Stimulation of follicular development in the treatment of infertility and for harvesting of ova for in vitro fertilization; induction of spermatogenesis in males with primary and secondary hypogonadotropic hypogonadism not due to primary testicular failure (*Follistim AQ*)
ganirelix acetate (generic)	250 mcg/d subcutaneously during early follicular phase	Inhibition of premature LH surges in patients undergoing controlled ovarian hyperstimulation as part of a fertility program
menotropins (*Menopur*)	Starting dose 225 IU/d subcutaneously; max dose 450 IU/d; may be administered with urofollitropin	Development of multiple follicles and pregnancy in ovulatory patients as part of Assisted Reproductive Technology treatment
urofollitropin (*Bravelle*)	150 IU/d subcutaneously or IM, maximum daily dose of 450 IU	Induction of ovulation in patients who have previously received pituitary suppression; stimulation of multiple follicles in ovulatory patients

HCG, human chorionic gonadotropin; LH, luteinizing hormone; FSH, follicle-stimulating hormone.

Prototype Summary Clomiphene

Indications: Treatment of ovarian failure in patients with normal liver function and normal endogenous estrogens; off-label use for treatment of male sterility.

Actions: Binds to estrogen receptors, decreasing the number of available estrogen receptors, which gives the hypothalamus the false signal to increase FSH and LH secretion, leading to ovarian stimulation.

Pharmacokinetics:

Route	Onset	Peak	Duration
PO	5–8 d	Unknown	6 wk

$T_{1/2}$: 5 days; metabolized in the liver and excreted in the urine.

Adverse Effects: Vasomotor flushing; visual changes; abdominal discomfort, distention, and bloating; nausea; vomiting; ovarian enlargement; breast tenderness; ovarian overstimulation; multiple births.

Nursing Considerations for Patients Receiving Fertility Drugs

Assessment: History and Examination

- Assess for contraindications or cautions: history of allergy to any fertility drug to avoid hypersensitivity reactions; current status of pregnancy and lactation, which are contraindications or cautions to the use of the drug; primary ovarian failure, which would not respond to these agents; thyroid or adrenal dysfunction due to effects on the hypothalamic–pituitary axis; ovarian cysts, which could be stimulated and become larger as a result of the drug's stimulatory effects; idiopathic uterine bleeding, which could reflect an underlying medical problem that could be exacerbated by the stimulatory effects of the drug; thromboembolic diseases, which could increase the patient's risk for thrombus formation; and respiratory diseases, which would be exacerbated by the effects of the drug.

- Perform a complete physical assessment to establish baseline status before beginning therapy and during therapy to monitor for any potential adverse effects.
- Perform a psychological assessment to determine teaching and support needs, as these patients are often stressed or anxious and can experience bouts of depression, which the nurse will need to be ready to address.
- Assess skin and lesions; orientation, affect, and reflexes; and blood pressure, pulse, respiration, and adventitious sounds to determine cardiac function and perfusion and to detect changes in blood flow or thromboemboli.
- Complete or assist with pelvic and breast/chest examinations and ensure collection of specimen for Pap smear to establish a baseline of GU health and detect early changes as a result of drug therapy.
- Monitor the results of laboratory tests, such as renal and hepatic function studies, to evaluate for possible dysfunction that might interfere with metabolism and excretion of the drug; and check hormonal levels as indicated to determine the effectiveness of therapy and reduce the risk of ovarian hyperstimulation.

Nursing Conclusions

Nursing conclusions related to drug therapy might include the following:

- Altered body image related to drug treatment and diagnosis
- Impaired comfort related to headache, fluid retention, or GI upset
- Sexual dysfunction related to alterations in normal hormone control
- Knowledge deficit regarding drug therapy
- Altered tissue perfusion risk (cardiopulmonary, peripheral) related to increased risk for thrombus formation
- Situational low self-esteem related to the need for fertility drugs

Planning

- The patient will receive the best therapeutic effect from the drug therapy.
- The patient will have limited adverse effects from the drug therapy.
- The patient will have an understanding of the drug therapy, adverse effects to anticipate, and measures to relieve discomfort and improve safety.

Intervention With Rationale

- Assess the cause of dysfunction before beginning therapy to ensure appropriate use of the drug.
- Complete a pelvic examination before each use of the drug to rule out ovarian enlargement, pregnancy, or uterine problems.
- Check urine estrogen and estradiol levels before beginning therapy to verify ovarian function.
- Administer with an appropriate dose of HCG as indicated to ensure beneficial effects.
- Discontinue the drug at any sign of ovarian overstimulation and arrange for hospitalization to monitor and support the patient if this occurs.
- Provide a calendar of treatment days, explanations of adverse effects to anticipate, and instructions on when intercourse should occur to increase the therapeutic effectiveness of the drug.
- Provide warnings about the risk and hazards of multiple births so the patient can make informed decisions about drug therapy.
- Offer support and encouragement for managing with low self-esteem, stress, anxiety, and possible depression issues associated with infertility.
- Provide patient teaching about proper administration technique, appropriate disposal of needles and syringes, measures to avoid adverse effects, warning signs of problems, and the need for regular evaluation to enhance patient knowledge about drug therapy and to promote adherence.

Evaluation

- Monitor patient response to the drug (ovulation).
- Monitor for adverse effects (abdominal bloating, weight gain, ovarian overstimulation, multiple births).
- Evaluate the effectiveness of the teaching plan (the patient can name the drug, dosage, adverse effects to watch for, and specific measures to avoid them).
- Monitor effectiveness of comfort measures and adherence to the regimen.

Key Points

- In patients with functioning ovaries, fertility drugs increase follicle development by stimulating FSH and LH to increase the chances for pregnancy.
- Patients receiving fertility drugs need to be monitored for ovarian overstimulation, need to be aware of the possibility of multiple births, and need support and encouragement to deal with the self-esteem issues associated with infertility.

Uterine Motility Drugs

Uterine motility drugs stimulate uterine contractions to assist labor (**oxytocics**) or induce abortion (**abortifacients**). Tocolytics are drugs used to slow uterine activity. Oxytocics, abortifacients, and tocolytics are discussed in detail in this section and in Table 40.3.

Oxytocics and Abortifacients

Oxytocics and abortifacients stimulate contraction of the uterus; they can be used to induce labor or terminate pregnancy depending on the specific medication and clinical situation. Some are used to control uterine bleeding. These drugs include carboprost (*Hemabate*), dinoprostone (*Cervidil, Prepidil Gel, Prostin E2*), methylergonovine (*Methergine*), mifepristone (*Mifeprex*), and oxytocin (*Pitocin*). Misoprostol (*Cytotec*) is indicated for reducing risk of gastric ulcers, but it can also have an abortifacient effect on pregnant patients. This medication is discussed in Chapter 57 due to its primary action on the GI tract.

Therapeutic Actions and Indications

The oxytocics directly affect neuroreceptor sites to stimulate contraction of the uterus. They are especially effective in the gravid uterus. Oxytocin, a synthetic form of the hypothalamic hormone, also stimulates the lacteal glands in the breast to contract, promoting milk ejection in lactating patients. Oxytocics are indicated for the prevention and treatment of uterine atony after delivery. This is important to prevent postpartum hemorrhage. See Table 40.3 for usual indications for each of these drugs.

Abortifacients stimulate uterine activity, dislodging any implanted trophoblasts and preventing implantation of any fertilized egg. These drugs are approved for use to terminate pregnancy at 12 to 20 weeks from the date of the last menstrual period. See Table 40.3 for usual indications for each of these agents.

Pharmacokinetics

The oxytocics and abortifacients are rapidly absorbed after parenteral or oral administration, metabolized in the liver, and excreted in the urine and feces. They cross the placenta and enter human milk.

Methylergonovine is administered IM or IV and then continued in the oral form to promote uterine involution. Oxytocin can be administered IV and IM but is also used in a nasal form to stimulate milk "letdown" in lactating patients. Mifepristone is administered orally and takes 5 to 7 days to produce the desired effect. Carboprost is available as an IM injection with onset of effects in 15 minutes and a duration of 2 hours. Dinoprostone is given by intravaginal suppository with onset of effects in 10 minutes and a duration of 2 hours.

Contraindications and Cautions

Oxytocics and abortifacients are contraindicated in the presence of any known allergy to avoid hypersensitivity reactions and with cephalopelvic disproportion, unfavorable fetal position, and complete uterine atony, which could

Table 40.3 ***Drugs in Focus:*** **Uterine Motility Drugs**

Drug Name	Dosage/Route	Usual Indications
Oxytocics/Abortifacients		
carboprost (*Hemabate*)	250 mcg IM at intervals of 1.5–3.5 h, not to exceed 12-mg total dose; 250 mcg IM to control postpartum bleeding, not to exceed 2-mg total dose	Stimulates uterine muscle contraction (similar to labor contractions) for termination of early pregnancy (within 13–20 wk of gestation); evacuation of missed abortion; control of postpartum hemorrhage and uterine atony that does not respond to other therapy
dinoprostone (*Cervidil, Prepidil Gel, Prostin E2*)	20-mg vaginal suppository, may repeat q3–5h as needed for termination of pregnancy; 0.5-mg gel via cervical catheter, repeated in 6 h if needed for cervical ripening, then wait 6–12 h before using oxytocin	A prostaglandin used for induction of labor; stimulation of cervical ripening before labor; termination of pregnancy (12th–20th gestational week); evacuation of missed abortion or intrauterine fetal death up to 28th gestational week (*Prostin E2*)
methylergonovine (*Methergine*)	0.2 mg IM or IV, may repeat q2–4h; 0.2 mg PO t.i.d. during the puerperium up to 1 wk	Promotion of postpartum uterine involution; control of uterine hemorrhage
mifepristone (*Mifeprex*)	200 mg PO *Mifeprex* on day 1, followed 24–48 h after *Mifeprex* dosing by 800 mcg buccal misoprostol	A progestin antagonist indicated, in a regimen with misoprostol, for the medical termination of intrauterine pregnancy through 70 days of gestation
oxytocin (*Pitocin*)	1–2 mU/min IV through an infusion pump, increase as needed, do not exceed 20 mU/min; 10 units IM after delivery of the placenta; one spray in each nostril 2–3 min before breast or chestfeeding	Induction of labor; delivery of placenta; promotion of uterine contractions postpartum; used nasally to stimulate milk letdown in lactating patients; also being evaluated as a diagnostic agent to test abnormal fetal heart rates (oxytocin challenge) and to treat breast engorgement
Tocolytic		
Hydroxyprogesterone caproate (*Makena*)	275 mg subcutaneous or IM injection once weekly	Reduction of risk of preterm birth in patients with a single-fetus pregnancy who have a history of singleton spontaneous preterm birth

be compromised by uterine stimulation. Oxytocin is used during lactation because of its effects on milk ejection, but the baby should be evaluated for any adverse effects associated with the hormone. Caution should be used in patients with coronary disease and hypertension due to the effect of causing arterial contraction, which could raise blood pressure or compromise coronary blood flow, or in patients who have had previous cesarean births because of the effects on uterine contraction, which could compromise scars from previous procedures. Caution should be used in hepatic or renal impairment, which could alter the metabolism or excretion of the drug.

Adverse Effects

The adverse effects most often associated with the oxytocics and abortifacients are related to excessive effects (e.g., uterine hypertonicity and spasm, uterine rupture, postpartum hemorrhage, decreased fetal heart rate). GI upset, nausea, headache, and dizziness also are common. Methylergonovine can produce ergotism, manifested by nausea, blood pressure changes, weak pulse, dyspnea, chest pain, numbness and coldness in extremities, confusion, excitement, delirium, convulsions, and even coma. Oxytocin has caused severe water intoxication with coma and even maternal death when used for a prolonged period. This is thought to occur because of related effects of antidiuretic hormone, which is also stored in the posterior pituitary and may be released in response to oxytocin activity, causing water retention by the kidneys.

Prototype Summary Oxytocin

Indications: To initiate or improve uterine contractions for early vaginal delivery; to stimulate or reinforce labor in selected cases of uterine inertia; to manage inevitable or incomplete abortion; for second-trimester abortion; to control postpartum bleeding or hemorrhage; to treat lactation deficiency.

Actions: Synthetic form stimulates the uterus, especially the gravid uterus; causes myoepithelium of the lacteal glands to contract, resulting in milk ejection in lactating patients.

Pharmacokinetics:

Route	Onset	Peak	Duration
IV	Immediate	Unknown	60 min
IM	3–5 min	Unknown	2–3 h

$T_{1/2}$: 1 to 6 minutes; metabolized in the tissue and excreted in the urine.

Adverse Effects: Cardiac arrhythmias, hypertension, fetal bradycardia, nausea, vomiting, uterine rupture, pelvic hematoma, uterine hypertonicity, severe water intoxication, anaphylactic reaction.

Nursing Considerations for Patients Receiving Oxytocics or Abortifacients

Assessment: History and Examination

- Assess for contraindications or cautions: history of allergy to avoid hypersensitivity reactions; early status of pregnancy (unless termination of pregnancy is the indication), which might lead to early onset of labor; current status of lactation; uterine atony, undesirable fetal position, and cephalopelvic disproportion, which could be compromised by the stimulatory effects of the drug; hypertension, which could be exacerbated due to the drug's effect on arteries; and history of cesarean birth, which could lead to uterine rupture or damage to previous surgical sites due to the drug's stimulatory effect on uterine contraction.
- Perform a complete physical assessment to establish a baseline before beginning therapy and during therapy to evaluate drug effectiveness and to determine potential adverse effects.
  - Assess the patient's neurological status, including level of orientation, affect, reflexes, and papillary response.
  - Monitor vital signs, including pulse and blood pressure; auscultate lungs for evidence of adventitious sounds.
  - Assess labor pattern, including uterine contractions, cervical dilation and effacement, and fetal status, including fetal heart rate, rhythm, and position. Institute electronic fetal monitoring as appropriate.
  - Evaluate uterine tone, noting any indications of atony; assess fundal height and uterine involution, and amount and characteristics of vaginal bleeding.
- Monitor the results of laboratory tests, including coagulation studies and complete blood count *to evaluate hematological status.*

Nursing Conclusions

Nursing conclusions related to drug therapy might include the following:

- Acute pain related to increased frequency and intensity of uterine contractions or headache
- Excess fluid volume related to ergotism or water intoxication
- Knowledge deficit regarding drug therapy

Planning

- The patient will receive the best therapeutic effect from the drug therapy.
- The patient will have limited adverse effects from the drug therapy.
- The patient will have an understanding of the drug therapy, adverse effects to anticipate, and measures to relieve discomfort and improve safety.

(Continued on page 704)

Intervention With Rationale

- Ensure fetal position (if appropriate) and cephalopelvic proportions to prevent serious complications of delivery.
- Regulate oxytocin delivery using an infusion pump between contractions if it is being given to stimulate labor to regulate dose appropriately.
- Monitor blood pressure and fetal heart rate frequently during and after administration to monitor for adverse effects. Discontinue the drug if blood pressure rises dramatically.
- Monitor uterine tone and involution and amount of bleeding to ensure safe and therapeutic drug use.
- Discontinue the drug at any sign of uterine hypertonicity to avoid potentially life-threatening effects; provide life support as needed.
- Monitor fetal heart rate and rhythm if given during labor to ensure safety of the fetus.
- Provide nasal oxytocin at bedside with the bottle sitting upright. Have the patient invert the squeeze bottle and exert gentle pressure to deliver the drug just before nursing to achieve greatest therapeutic effect to stimulate milk letdown.
- Provide patient teaching about administration technique for nasal oxytocin if indicated, required monitoring and assessments, danger signs and symptoms to report immediately, possible adverse effects, measures to be instituted to reduce the risk of adverse effects, safety and comfort measures, measures to promote effective breast or chestfeeding as appropriate (for nasal administration of oxytocin), and ongoing need for continued monitoring and evaluation to enhance patient knowledge of drug therapy and to promote adherence.

Evaluation

- Monitor patient response to the drug (uterine contraction, prevention of hemorrhage, milk letdown).
- Monitor for adverse effects (blood pressure changes, uterine hypertonicity, water intoxication, ergotism).
- Evaluate the effectiveness of the teaching plan (the patient can name the drug, dosage, adverse effects to watch for, and specific measures to avoid them).
- Monitor the effectiveness of comfort measures and adherence to the regimen.

Tocolytics

Tocolytics are used to calm or slow uterine contractions or prevent preterm labor. Nifedipine is a calcium channel blocker that can be used off-label to slow or suppress preterm labor. Indomethacin blocks prostaglandins and can slow labor progression. Terbutaline, a beta$_2$-selective adrenergic agonist, was widely used off-label as a tocolytic agent to relax the gravid uterus to prolong pregnancy. However, it is only to be used short term and for emergency situations due to risk of serious heart arrhythmias and maternal death; the FDA has stressed that terbutaline is not approved for obstetric indications. Hydroxyprogesterone caproate (*Makena*) is approved for reduction of the risk of preterm birth in patients with a single-fetus pregnancy who have a history of singleton spontaneous preterm birth (Table 40.3).

Therapeutic Actions and Indications

Hydroxyprogesterone caproate (*Makena*) was approved to reduce the risk of preterm birth in patients with a single-fetus pregnancy and a history of singleton spontaneous preterm birth. It is not approved for use in multiple-fetus pregnancies. It is a synthetic progestin and has the same effects and adverse effects as the progestins.

Pharmacokinetics

Hydroxyprogesterone caproate is given by IM or subcutaneous injection once a week. It is metabolized by the liver and excreted in both urine and feces.

Contraindications and Cautions

Hydroxyprogesterone caproate is contraindicated in patients with current or history of thrombosis or thromboembolic disorders; known or suspected breast cancer, other hormone-sensitive cancer, or history of these conditions; undiagnosed abnormal vaginal bleeding unrelated to pregnancy; cholestatic jaundice of pregnancy; benign or malignant liver tumors or active liver disease; or uncontrolled hypertension due to the medication potentially worsening these conditions.

Adverse Effects

Adverse effects associated with hydroxyprogesterone caproate include depression, fluid retention that can worsen hypertension, glucose intolerance, and thromboembolic events. Injection site reactions and allergic reactions are also a risk.

Prototype Summary Hydroxyprogesterone caproate

Indications: Reduction of the risk of preterm birth in patients with a single-fetus pregnancy who have a history of singleton spontaneous preterm birth; not intended for use in patients with a multiple-fetus pregnancy or other risk factors for preterm birth.

Actions: It acts as a synthetic progestin. The exact mechanism by which hydroxyprogesterone caproate reduces the risk of recurrent preterm birth is not known.

Pharmacokinetics:

Route	Onset	Peak	Duration
Subcutaneous or IM	Slow	Days	Unknown

$T_{1/2}$: 16 to 19 days; metabolized in the liver and excreted in the urine and feces.

Adverse Effects: Injection-site reactions, glucose intolerance, fluid retention, depression, hypertension, thrombosis, breast cancer, liver disease.

Nursing Considerations for Patients Receiving Tocolytics

Assessment: History and Examination

- Assess for contraindications or cautions: history of allergy to any preparation to avoid hypersensitivity reactions; active liver disease, which could be exacerbated by the medication; hypertension, which can be worsened by fluid retention; and history of thromboembolic events or breast cancer, which could cause increased risk to the patient.
- Perform a psychological assessment to determine teaching and support needs as these patients are often stressed or anxious and can experience bouts of depression, which the nurse will need to be ready to address.
- Perform a complete physical assessment before beginning therapy to establish baseline status and during therapy to determine drug effectiveness and evaluate for any potential adverse effects.
- Confirm date of last menstrual period and estimated duration of pregnancy to ensure appropriate use of the drug.
- Assess skin and lesions; orientation and affect; and vital signs including blood pressure, pulse, and respiration; and auscultate lung sounds to monitor for vascular effects, including bleeding and hypersensitivity reactions.
- Assist with or complete a pelvic examination, observe for vaginal discharge, and evaluate uterine tone to monitor effectiveness of the drug and the occurrence of adverse effects.
- Monitor the results of laboratory tests, including blood glucose levels, due to increased risk of glucose intolerance.

Nursing Conclusions

Nursing conclusions related to drug therapy might include the following:

- Ineffective coping related to pregnancy and potential for preterm labor
- Risk for fluid volume overload, edema, and hypertension
- Knowledge deficit risk regarding drug therapy

Planning

- The patient will receive the best therapeutic effect from the drug therapy.
- The patient will have limited adverse effects from the drug therapy.
- The patient will have an understanding of the drug therapy, adverse effects to anticipate, and measures to relieve discomfort and improve safety.

Intervention With Rationale

- Administer via route indicated and follow the manufacturer's directions for storage and preparation to ensure safe and therapeutic use of the drug.
- Confirm the duration of the pregnancy before administering the drug to ensure appropriate use of the drug.
- Monitor blood pressure frequently during and after administration to assess for adverse effects; discontinue the drug if blood pressure rises dramatically.
- Monitor fetal heart rate and uterine contractions to evaluate the safety of the fetus and the effectiveness of the medication.
- Provide patient teaching, including how patient will be monitored during drug administration, comfort measures, signs and symptoms of adverse effects, measures to minimize or prevent adverse effects, danger signs and symptoms to report immediately, need for follow-up monitoring and evaluation, and sources for support and referrals to enhance patient knowledge about drug therapy and to promote adherence.

Evaluation

- Monitor patient response to the drug (progression to full-term pregnancy; prevention of preterm labor).
- Monitor for adverse effects (GI upset, nausea, blood pressure changes, hypertension, injection site reactions, fluid accumulation).
- Evaluate the effectiveness of the teaching plan (the patient can name the drug, dosage, adverse effects to watch for, and specific measures to avoid them).
- Monitor the effectiveness of comfort measures and adherence to the regimen.

Key Points

- Oxytocic drugs act like the hypothalamic hormone oxytocin to stimulate uterine contractions and induce or speed up labor and to control bleeding and promote postpartum involution of the uterus.
- Abortifacients are drugs that stimulate uterine activity to cause uterine evacuation. These drugs can be used to induce abortion in early pregnancy or to promote uterine evacuation after intrauterine fetal death.
- Tocolytics are drugs that relax the uterine smooth muscle; they are used to stop premature labor in patients after 20 weeks of gestation.

SUMMARY

- Estrogens are primarily used pharmacologically to replace hormones lost at menopause to reduce the signs and symptoms associated with menopause, to stimulate ovulation in people with hypogonadism, and in combination with progestins for oral contraceptives.
- Progestins, which include progesterone and all of its derivatives, are female sex hormones that are responsible for the maintenance of a pregnancy and for the development of some secondary sex characteristics.
- Progestins are used in combination with estrogens for contraception, to treat uterine bleeding, and for palliation in certain cancers with sensitive receptor sites.
- Fertility drugs stimulate FSH and LH in patients with functioning ovaries to increase follicle development and improve the chances for pregnancy.
- Major adverse effects of fertility drugs are multiple births and congenital anomalies.
- Oxytocic drugs act like the hypothalamic hormone oxytocin to stimulate uterine contractions and induce or speed up labor and to control bleeding and promote postpartum involution of the uterus.
- Abortifacients are drugs that stimulate uterine activity to cause uterine evacuation. These drugs can be used to induce abortion in early pregnancy or to promote uterine evacuation after intrauterine fetal death.
- Tocolytics are drugs that relax the uterine smooth muscle; they are used to stop premature labor in patients after 20 weeks of gestation. Hydroxyprogesterone caproate is the only drug approved for this purpose in the United States.

Unfolding Patient Stories: Rachel Heidebrink • Part 1

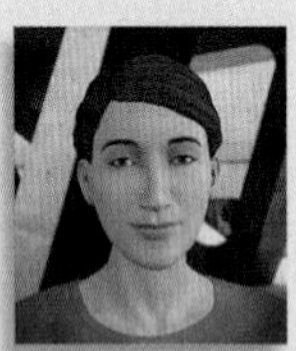

Rachel Heidebrink, a 22-year-old who sustained a fracture to the right greater trochanter in a motorcycle accident and had right hip hemiarthroplasty, developed a pulmonary embolism on postoperative day 1. The patient is on an oral estrogen–progestin combination for contraception. What actions should the nurse take when considering the diagnosis and adverse effects of the medication? (Rachel Heidebrink's story continues in Chapter 48.)

Care for Rachel and other patients in a realistic virtual environment: ***vSim** for Nursing* (thepoint.lww.com/vSimPharm). Practice documenting these patients' care in DocuCare (thepoint.lww.com/DocuCareEHR).

CHECK YOUR UNDERSTANDING

Answers to the questions in this chapter can be found in Answers to Check Your Understanding Questions on thePoint®.

MULTIPLE CHOICE

Select the best answer.

1. A postmenopausal patient is to receive short-term hormone replacement therapy to control menopausal symptoms. Which adverse effect would the nurse include in the patient teaching about this therapy?
   a. Constipation
   b. Breakthrough bleeding
   c. Weight loss
   d. Persistently elevated body temperature
2. An estrogen receptor modulator might be the drug of choice in the treatment of postmenopausal osteoporosis in a patient with a family history of breast or uterine cancer. The nurse would instruct the patient that they might experience which side effects?
   a. Constipation and dry, itchy skin
   b. Flushing and dry vaginal mucosa
   c. Hot flashes and vaginal bleeding
   d. Diarrhea and weight loss

3. Combination estrogens and progestins are commonly used as OCs. It is thought that this combination has its effect by
   a. acting to block the release of FSH and LH, preventing follicle development.
   b. directly suppressing the ovaries and preventing ovulation.
   c. keeping the endometrium constantly thick and blood filled.
   d. preventing menstruation, which prevents pregnancy.

4. Any patient who is taking estrogens, progestins, or combination products should be cautioned to avoid smoking because nicotine
   a. increases the metabolism of the hormones, making them less effective.
   b. increases the risk for potentially dangerous thromboembolic episodes.
   c. amplifies the adverse effects of the hormones.
   d. blocks hormone receptor sites, and they may no longer be effective.

5. Oxytocin, a synthetic form of the hypothalamic hormone, is used to
   a. induce abortion via uterine expulsion.
   b. stimulate milk letdown in the lactating person.
   c. increase fertility and the chance of conception.
   d. relax the gravid uterus to prevent preterm labor.

6. The use of an abortifacient drug is contraindicated in a patient who
   a. is 15 weeks pregnant.
   b. is older than 50 years of age.
   c. has a history of four previous cesarean births.
   d. is 10 weeks pregnant.

7. A young patient chooses oral contraceptive medication because they feel that it is not the right time to get pregnant. You would evaluate patient teaching about the drug to have been effective if they make which statement?
   a. "I shouldn't smoke for the first month to make sure I don't react severely to the pills."
   b. "If I forget to take a pill, I'll just start over the next day with a new series of pills."
   c. "I may not be able to wear my contact lenses while taking these pills, or I might have to be fitted for a new pair."
   d. "If I have to take an antibiotic while I am using these pills, I should take double pills on those days that I am using the antibiotic."

MULTIPLE RESPONSE

Select all that apply.

1. Estrogens produce a wide variety of systemic effects. Effects attributed to estrogen include
   a. protecting the heart from atherosclerosis.
   b. retaining calcium in the bones.
   c. maintaining the secondary female sex characteristics.
   d. relaxing the gravid uterus to prolong pregnancy.
   e. stimulating the uterus to increase the chances of conception.
   f. relaxing blood vessels.

2. A patient is taking clomiphene after 6 years of inability to conceive a child. The patient will need to be informed about which?
   a. Necessity of a complete physical and pelvic examination before each course of drug therapy
   b. Risks and hazards of multiple births
   c. Importance of scheduling treatments and intercourse to increase the chance of conception
   d. Necessity of using oral contraceptives during drug therapy
   e. Needing to report blurred vision
   f. Common adverse effects include light-headedness, dizziness, and drowsiness

3. A patient is receiving an oxytocic drug to stimulate labor. The nursing care of this patient would include which?
   a. Monitoring fetal heart rate during labor
   b. Regulation of drug delivery between contractions
   c. Administration of blood pressure–lowering drugs to balance hypertensive effects
   d. Monitoring maternal blood pressure periodically during and after administration
   e. Close monitoring of maternal blood loss following delivery
   f. Isolation of the patient and newborn to prevent infection

REFERENCES

Bernstein, P., & Pohost, G. (2010). Progesterone, progestins and the heart. *Reviews in Cardiovascular Medicine, 11*(4), 228–236.

Brunton, L., Hilal-Dandan, R., & Knollman, B. (2018). *Goodman and Gilman's the pharmacological basis of therapeutics* (13th ed.). McGraw-Hill.

FDA's decision regarding Plan B. U.S. Food and Drug Administration. http://www.fda.gov/Drugs/DrugSafety/PostmarketDrugSafetyInformationforPatientsandProviders/ucm109795.htm

Foster, D. G., Biggs, M. A., Phillips, K. A., Grindlay, K., & Grossman, D. (2015). Potential public sector cost-savings from OTC access to oral contraceptives. *Contraception, 91*(5), 373–379. 10.1016/j.contraception.2015.01.010

Heiss, G., Wallace, R., Anderson, G. L., Aragaki, A., Beresford, S. A. A., Brzyski, R., Chlebowski, R. T., Gass, M., LaCroix, A., Manson, J. E., Prentice, R. L., Rossouw, J., Stefanick, M. L., & WHI Investigators. (2008). Health risks and benefits 3 years after stopping randomized treatment with estrogen and progestin. *Journal of the American Medical Association, 299*, 1036–1045. 10.1001/jama.299.9.1036

Langer, R. D. (2010). The need to clarify and disseminate contemporary knowledge of hormone therapy initiated near menopause. *Climacteric, 13*(4), 303–306. 10.3109/13697137.2010.496316

Langer, R. D. (2017). The evidence base for HRT: What can we believe? *Climacteric, 20*(2), 91–96. 10.1080/13697137.2017.1280251

Moynihan, R. (2014). Evening the score on sex drugs: Feminist movement or marketing masquerade? *British Medical Journal, 349*, 8246. 10.1136/bmj.g6246

Naseri, R., Farnia, V., Yazdchi, K., Alikhani, M., Basanj, B., & Salemi, S. (2019). Comparison of *Vitex agnus-castus* extracts with placebo with reducing menopausal symptoms: A randomized double-blind study. *Korean Journal Family Medicine, 40*(6), 362–367. 10.4082/kjfm.18.0067

Panay, N., Hamoda, H., Arya, R., & Savvas, M. (2013). The 2013 British Menopause Society and Women's Health Concern recommendations on hormone replacement therapy. *Post Reproductive Health, 19*(2), 59–68. https://doi.org/10.1177/2053369116680501

Potera, C. (2011). Unneeded pelvic exams in women seeking birth control. *American Journal of Nursing, 111*(3), 17–20. 10.1097/10.1097/01.NAJ.0000395226.64552.63

Raymond, E. G., Halpern, V., & Lopez, L. M. (2011). Pericoital oral contraception with levonorgestrel: A systematic review. *Obstetrician Gynecology, 117*(3), 673–681. 10.1097/AOG.0b013e318209dc25

Taylor, H. S., & Manson, J. E. (2011). Update on hormone therapy use in menopause. *Journal of Clinical Endocrinology and Metabolism, 96*(2), 255–264. https://doi.org/10.1210/jc.2010-0536

The North American Menopause Society. (2021). *Natural remedies for hot flashes.* https://www.menopause.org/for-women/menopauseflashes/menopause-symptoms-and-treatments/natural-remedies-for-hot-flashes

Toh, S. D., Hernández-Díaz, S., Logan, R., Rossouw, J. E., & Hernán, M. A. (2010). Coronary heart disease in postmenopausal recipients of estrogen and progestin therapy: Does the risk ever disappear? *Annals of Internal Medicine, 152*, 211–217. https://www.ncbi.nlm.nih.gov/pmc/articles/PMC2936769

USPSTF. (2017). *Hormone replacement therapy for the prevention of chronic conditions in postmenopausal women.* U.S. Preventative Services Task Force. https://www.uspreventiveservicestaskforce.org/Page/Document/UpdateSummaryFinal/menopausal-hormone-therapy-preventive-medication

CHAPTER 41

Drugs Affecting the Male Reproductive System

Learning Objectives

Upon completion of this chapter, you will be able to:

1. Discuss the use of drugs that affect the male reproductive system across the lifespan.
2. Discuss the effects of testosterone and androgens on the male body and use this information to explain the therapeutic and adverse effects of these agents when used clinically.
3. Describe the therapeutic actions, indications, pharmacokinetics, contraindications, most common adverse effects, and important drug–drug interactions associated with drugs affecting the male reproductive system.
4. Compare and contrast the prototype drugs testosterone, oxandrolone, and sildenafil with other agents in their class.
5. Outline the nursing considerations, including important teaching points, for patients receiving drugs used to affect the male reproductive system.

Key Terms

anabolic steroids: androgens developed with more anabolic or protein-building effects than androgenic effects

androgenic effects: effects associated with development of male sexual characteristics and secondary characteristics (e.g., deepening of voice, hair distribution, genital development, acne)

androgens: male sex hormones, primarily testosterone; produced in the testes and adrenal glands

hirsutism: hair distribution associated with male secondary sex characteristics (e.g., increased hair on trunk, arms, legs, face)

hypogonadism: underdevelopment of the gonads (testes in the male)

penile erectile dysfunction: condition in which the corpus cavernosum does not fill with blood to allow for penile erection; can be related to aging or to neurological or vascular conditions

phosphodiesterase type 5 receptor inhibitors: drugs used in the treatment of erectile dysfunction; cause smooth muscle relaxation, allowing the flow of blood into the corpus cavernosum

priapism: a painful and continual erection of the penis

Drug List

ANDROGENS/ ANABOLIC STEROIDS
danazol
methyltestosterone
oxandrolone
oxymetholone
(P) testosterone

DRUGS FOR TREATING PENILE ERECTILE DYSFUNCTION
alprostadil
avanafil
(P) sildenafil
tadalafil
vardenafil

Drugs that are used to affect the male reproductive system include androgens (anabolic steroid hormones) and drugs that act to improve penile dysfunction. The male hormones are produced in the testes and affect the entire male reproductive system (Fig. 41.1). Box 41.1 describes the effect of these drugs across the lifespan. Drugs used to treat prostatic hypertrophy are discussed in Chapter 52.

Androgens

Androgens are male sex hormones and include testosterone, which is produced in the testes, and androgens, which are produced in the adrenal glands. Testosterone (*Androderm*, *Androgel*, and others), the primary natural androgen, is the classic androgen in use today. It is

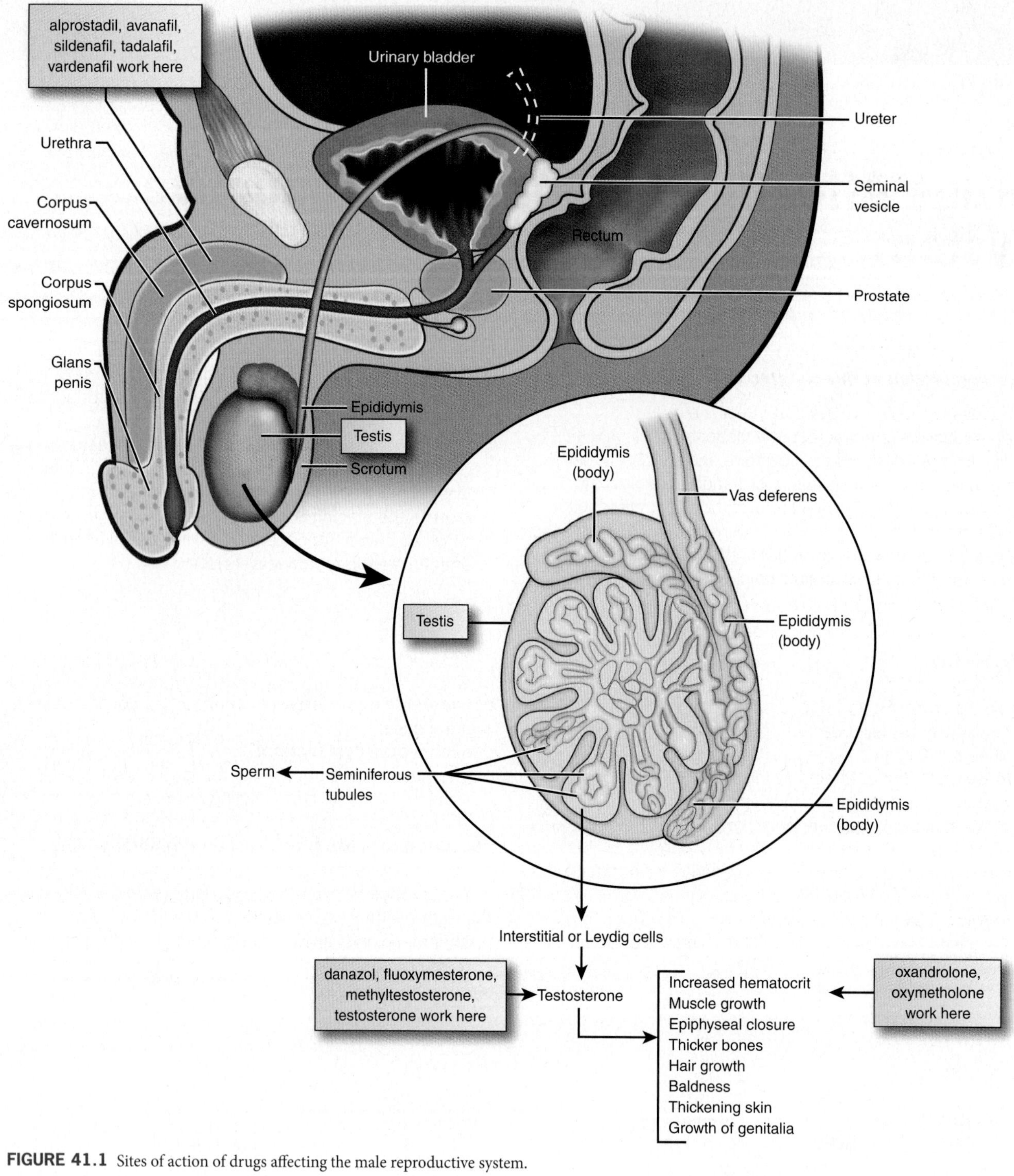

FIGURE 41.1 Sites of action of drugs affecting the male reproductive system.

used for replacement therapy in cases of **hypogonadism** (underdeveloped testes) and to treat certain breast cancers. Testosterones are class III controlled substances. Other androgens include danazol (generic) and methyltestosterone (*Android 25*). The **anabolic steroids** are analogues of testosterone that have been developed to produce the tissue-building effects of testosterone with less androgenic effect. Anabolic steroids include oxandrolone (generic) and oxymetholone (*Anadrol-50*). See Table 41.1 for more information about these agents.

Therapeutic Actions and Indications

Because androgens are forms of testosterone, they are responsible for the growth and development of male sex organs and the maintenance of secondary male sex characteristics. They act to increase the retention of nitrogen, sodium, potassium, and phosphorus and to decrease the urinary excretion of calcium. Testosterones increase protein anabolism and decrease protein catabolism (breakdown). They also increase the production

Box 41.1 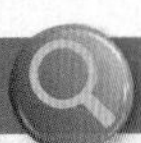 Focus on Drug Therapy Across the Lifespan

DRUGS AFFECTING THE MALE REPRODUCTIVE SYSTEM

Children

Anabolic steroids or androgens may be used in children as replacement therapy and to increase red blood cell production in renal failure. Because of the effects of these hormones on epiphyseal closure, children should be closely monitored with hand and wrist radiographs pretreatment and every 6 months. If precocious puberty occurs, the drug should be stopped.

Adolescents who are prescribed androgens should be alerted to the potential for increased acne and other effects.

Adolescent athletes need constant education about the risks associated with the use of anabolic steroids to improve athletic prowess and the lack of scientific evidence of beneficial effects.

Adults

Adults also need reinforcement of the information about anabolic steroid use and athletics.

Females who are prescribed these drugs may experience masculinizing effects and may need support in coping with these body changes if they are undesired by the patient. Patients who are receiving these drugs for replacement therapy may need to learn self-injection techniques and may benefit from information on depot forms or dermal systems. Periodic liver function tests are important in monitoring the effects of these drugs on the liver.

These drugs are not indicated for use in pregnancy or lactation because of the potential for serious effects on the fetus or neonate.

Older Adults

Older adults may have problems with androgen therapy because of underlying conditions that are aggravated by the drug effects. Hypertension, heart failure, and coronary artery disease may be aggravated by the fluid retention associated with these drugs. Benign prostatic hypertrophy, a common problem in older males, may be aggravated by androgenic effects that may enlarge the prostate further, leading to urinary difficulties and increased risk of prostate cancer.

Many older adults have hepatic dysfunction, and these drugs can be hepatotoxic. Older patients should be monitored carefully and dose should be reduced. If signs of liver failure or hepatitis occur, the drug should be stopped immediately.

of red blood cells. Danazol is used to treat symptoms of endometriosis and fibrocystic breast disease in females and to treat hereditary angioedema. Because it is an androgen, it is able to inhibit the hypothalamic–pituitary–adrenal axis and gonadotropin-releasing hormone, leading to a decrease in follicle-stimulating hormone and luteinizing hormone when used in females.

Anabolic steroids promote the processes of body tissue building, reverse catabolic or tissue-destroying processes, and increase hemoglobin and red blood cell mass. Indications for particular anabolic steroids vary with the drug. They can be used to treat anemias, certain cancers, and angioedema and to promote weight gain and tissue repair in debilitated patients and protein anabolism in patients who are receiving long-term corticosteroid therapy.

Table 41.1 *Drugs in Focus:* Androgens

Drug Name	Usual Dosage	Usual Indications
danazol (generic)	100–1,600 mg/d PO, depending on use and response	Treatment of endometriosis amenable to hormonal management; decreasing pain in patients with fibrocystic breast disease that is not treated with other measures; prevention of angioedema attacks
oxandrolone (generic)	*Adult*: 2.5 mg PO 2–4 times daily, maximum dose 20 mg/d *Pediatric*: <0.1 mg/kg/d PO, monitor closely, may be repeated intermittently	Promotion of weight gain in debilitated patients; treatment of certain cancers; relief of bone pain of osteoporosis; promotion of catabolism with prolonged corticosteroid use
oxymetholone (*Anadrol-50*)	1–5 mg/kg/d PO	Treatment of anemias cause by deficit in RBC production
testosterone (*Androderm, Depo-testosterone, Androgel, Fortesta, Natesto, Aveed*, and others)	Dosing varies based on formulation and indication; IM, transdermal, implantable pellets, and buccal tablets forms available	Replacement therapy in hypogonadism; treatment of delayed puberty in male patients and certain breast cancers in postmenopausal patients; prevention of postpartum breast engorgement
methyltestosterone (*Android 25*)	*Males*: 10–50 mg/d PO *Females*: 50–200 mg/d PO	Replacement therapy in hypogonadism; treatment of delayed puberty in male patients; treatment of certain breast cancers in postmenopausal patients

Anabolic steroids are also used illegally for the enhancement of athletic performance by promoting increased muscle mass, increased hematocrit, and (theoretically) an increase in strength and endurance. They are class III controlled substances. The adverse effects of these drugs can be significant when they are used in the amounts needed for enhanced athletic performance (see "Adverse Effects").

Pharmacokinetics

Testosterone is long acting and is available in several forms, including depot (deep, slow-release) injections, buccal systems, topical gels, topical sprays, implantable pellets, and a dermal patch. Danazol, a synthetic androgen, is also long acting but is available only in oral form. Methyltestosterone and fluoxymesterone have long half-lives and are available in the oral form. The androgens are well absorbed and widely distributed throughout the body. They are metabolized in the liver and excreted in the urine. It is not known whether androgens enter human milk (see "Contraindications and Cautions").

Oxandrolone and oxymetholone are available orally. Like androgens, anabolic steroids are well absorbed and widely distributed throughout the body. They are metabolized in the liver and excreted in the urine. Anabolic steroids are contraindicated for use in pregnancy because of the potential for adverse effects on the fetus. It is not known whether anabolic steroids enter human milk, but because of the potential for adverse effects, another method of feeding the baby should be used if these drugs are needed during lactation.

Contraindications and Cautions

These drugs are contraindicated with any known allergy to the drug or ingredients in the drug to prevent hypersensitivity reactions; during pregnancy and lactation because of potential adverse effects on the neonate (another method of feeding the baby should be used if these drugs are needed during lactation); and in the presence of prostate or breast cancer in males, which could be aggravated by the testosterone effects of the drugs. They should be used cautiously in the presence of any liver dysfunction or cardiovascular disease because these disorders could be exacerbated by the effects of the hormones. The topical forms of testosterone have a boxed warning alerting the user to the risk of virilization in children who come in contact with the drug from touching the clothes and skin of the patient using the drug. The patient is advised to cover all application areas if coming in contact with children and to wash all clothing that has touched the area before children come in contact with it. Danazol has a boxed warning regarding the risk for thromboembolic events, fetal abnormalities, hepatitis, and intracranial hypertension. Health care providers are advised that the drug is not for long-term use and to take appropriate precautions with all patients.

Adverse Effects

Androgenic effects include acne, edema, **hirsutism** (hair distribution associated with male secondary sex characteristics), deepening of the voice, oily skin and hair, weight gain, decrease in breast size, penile enlargement, and testicular atrophy. In prepubescent males, adverse effects include virilization (e.g., phallic enlargement, hirsutism, increased skin pigmentation). Postpubescent males may experience inhibition of testicular function, gynecomastia, testicular atrophy, **priapism** (a painful and continual erection of the penis), baldness, and change in libido (increased or decreased). There is an increased risk of prostate problems, especially in geriatric patients. Antiestrogen effects—flushing, sweating, vaginitis, nervousness, menstrual irregularity or cessation of menses, hirsutism, growth of the clitoris, and emotional lability—can be anticipated when these drugs are used in females. Other common effects include headache (possibly related to fluid and electrolyte changes), dizziness, sleep disorders and fatigue, rash, and altered serum electrolytes (Fig. 41.2). A potentially life-threatening effect that has been documented is hepatocellular cancer or hepatitis. This may occur because of the effect of testosterone on hepatic cells. Patients on long-term therapy should have hepatic func-

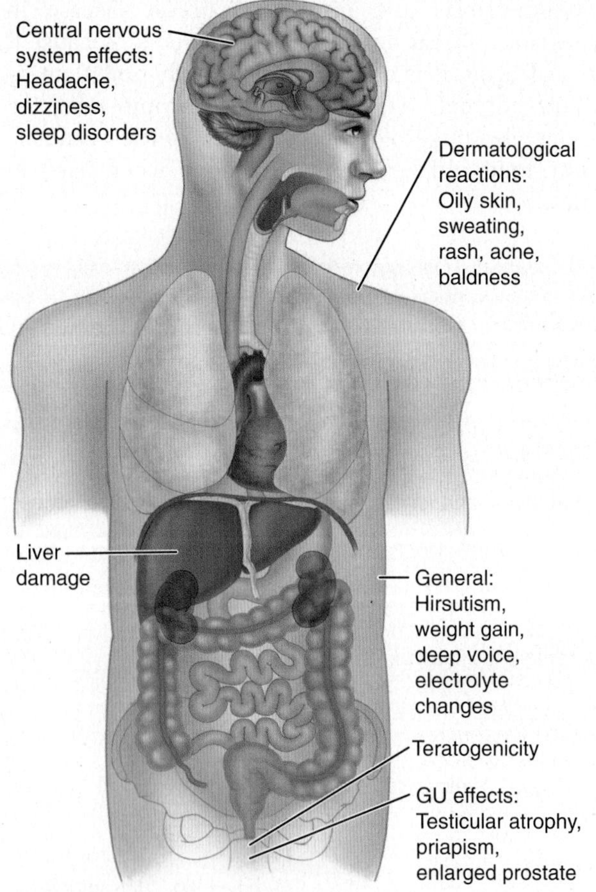

FIGURE 41.2 Variety of adverse effects and toxicities associated with the use of drugs that affect the male reproductive system.

BOX 41.2

Low-Testosterone Syndrome

In the past decade, there have been media ads promoting the use of testosterone for treating "low-T syndrome." The signs and symptoms that males were told to look for as they aged included fatigue, loss of hair, depression, muscle weakness, decreased sexual performance, and decreased energy. Many people could experience those signs and symptoms without a problem with testosterone. Low testosterone levels can be associated with many chronic diseases, such as chronic obstructive pulmonary disease (COPD), obesity in males, anemia, renal failure, or diabetes mellitus. Testosterone levels can be measured, and often testosterone replacement therapy can raise levels and relieve symptoms. When therapy is used appropriately, the treatment does not seem to increase risk of prostate cancer or cardiovascular events.

tion tests monitored regularly before beginning therapy and every 6 months during therapy. Fluid retention and/or hypercholesterolemia may also increase cardiovascular risk for patients taking these medications. Inappropriate use of testosterone has led to cardiovascular events including myocardial infarction (MI) and stroke and venous embolic events, including deep-vein thrombosis (DVT) and pulmonary embolism (PE). The U.S. Food and Drug Administration (FDA) has issued warnings for all testosterone products after follow-up studies showed the risks associated with using these products for unapproved indications. The media pushing treatment for "low-T syndrome" (Box 41.2) led to these warnings, and further studies are being conducted. All testosterone products now carry a general warning about the risks of cardiovascular events and the need to evaluate the patient carefully for appropriate use of the drugs. Premature closure of epiphysis that can reduce mature height can occur if male children are administered androgens, so serial X-rays may be indicated if a male child is being treated with one of these medications.

See the "Critical Thinking Scenario" for additional information about the risks and adverse effects of anabolic steroids.

Cardiomyopathy, hepatic carcinoma, personality changes, and sexual dysfunction are all associated with the excessive and off-label use of anabolic steroids. These drugs are class III controlled substances, which mean they are monitored by the Drug Enforcement Agency. There is an increased effort to encourage the use of herbal products to improve athletic performance. These products are advertised as "safe" alternatives (Box 41.3).

Clinically Significant Drug–Drug Interactions

While a patient is taking androgens, there may be decreased thyroid function as well as increased creatinine and creatinine clearance, results that are not associated with disease states. These effects can last up to 2 weeks after discontinuation of therapy. Androgens can alter effects of oral anticoagulants, insulin, and oral antidiabetic medications. The steroids may increase sensitivity to anticoagulants (particularly warfarin), so lower dosages may be needed.

Box 41.3 Focus on Herbal and Alternative Therapies

With increased awareness of the risks associated with anabolic steroid use and increased pressures to make it difficult to get these drugs even illegally, there is an increased push in advertising of alternative or "natural" products that are reported to enhance athletic performance.

Bee pollen: Reported to contain amino acids and other minerals and enzymes and to improve athletic stamina. There is no clear evidence regarding its effectiveness. Serious allergic reactions have been reported with the use of this product. Random studies have found a wide variety of ingredients in each product, depending on the season, growing conditions, and geographical area.

Creatine: Contains a substance that is found in muscle and naturally occurs in red meats and other dietary sources. There is mixed evidence regarding whether it can enhance performance. The strongest evidence is that it could help increase strength for resistance training. Short-term use is probably safe, but safety is not clear with long-term use. It can interact with many other drugs, including nonsteroidal anti-inflammatory drugs, cimetidine, probenecid, and trimethoprim, and can cause serious effects on kidney functioning. Users should be advised to drink plenty of fluids while taking this drug and to monitor for swelling, muscle cramps, and dizziness.

Damiana: Used to increase muscle strength, as an aphrodisiac, and to boost mental health. It can cause liver toxicity. It interferes with antidiabetic agents and causes elevated blood sugar concentrations. Users should report muscle spasms or hallucinations.

Spirulina: Used to increase energy and boost metabolism. It may contain toxic metals and can cause serious reactions in children and pets. It interferes with vitamin B_{12} absorption. No scientific studies validate the claims of its effectiveness.

Wild yam: Found to have many estrogenlike effects, this herb is used to increase athletic performance because it may contain a constituent of dehydroepiandrosterone used to slow the aging process and to improve energy and stamina. Preparations interact with disulfiram and metronidazole because they contain alcohol. It is known to be toxic to the liver. Users may experience estrogenlike effects, including breast pain. Users should be monitored closely and urged to report any adverse effects.

Patients who are taking a prescribed androgen or anabolic steroid for a medical condition should be advised to avoid taking any of these herbal remedies because of the risk of adverse effects.

CRITICAL THINKING SCENARIO
Adverse Effects of Anabolic Steroids

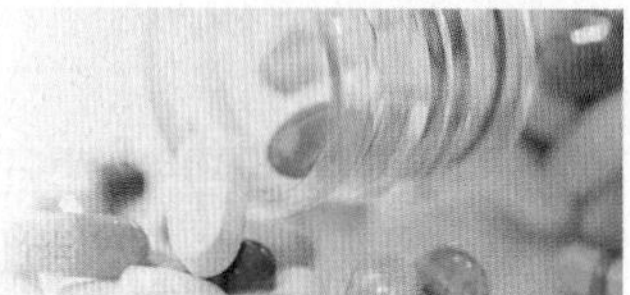

THE SITUATION

Senior nursing student K.S. recently became engaged. Their partner is a college senior who is training as a javelin thrower in hopes of competing in the Olympics. K.S. noticed that their partner had been suffering from gastrointestinal (GI) upset for the last 3 weeks and more recently had developed tremors and muscle cramps. K.S. first suspected their partner was suffering from a viral infection, but when the symptoms did not resolve, K.S. became concerned. K.S. tried to get their partner to see a doctor, but the partner refused. Eventually, they admitted that they had begun using anabolic steroids to develop muscles and improve their athletic prowess. They said that the friend who provided the drugs said that stomach upset was normal. K.S.'s partner refuses to see a physician because the use of these drugs is illegal and they don't want to get into any trouble. They believe that using the anabolic steroids for a while will help them achieve their goal. K.S. accepts the explanation but is upset about the use of anabolic steroids. K.S. consults with their clinical instructor about the effects of these drugs.

CRITICAL THINKING

What does K.S. need to know? Think about the systemic effects of anabolic steroids and the possible long-term effects from their abuse.

What implications do these effects have for the athlete? Consider the concern that K.S. must be experiencing. Suggest ways for K.S. to share the information about the actual effects of anabolic steroids with their partner and still cope with their own feelings and concerns.

What are the ethical and legal issues involved when a health care provider knows about illegal drug use and abuse? Outline a plan for helping K.S. and their partner cope with this issue and its implications for their futures.

DISCUSSION

Use of anabolic steroids is illegal in almost all organized athletic contests. Random drug testing is done to rule out use of these and other drugs. Not surprisingly, K.S. feels insecure about their partner's decision. K.S. needs to know that this discussion will be confidential and that they will receive support for their concerns and fears. K.S. needs to review the effects of anabolic steroids. Although anabolic steroids do promote muscle development, there has never been any evidence that they actually improve athletic performance. The potential adverse effects of these drugs can be deadly, especially if K.S.'s partner is receiving the drugs from a friend and has no medical evaluation or dosage guidance to reduce the risk. Personality changes, cardiomyopathy, liver cancer, and impotence are just a few of the possible adverse effects.

K.S. is in a precarious position. They do not want to interfere with their partner's dreams or cause problems in the relationship. K.S. should be encouraged to explain the adverse effects of the drugs to their partner, pointing out that their partner is already experiencing some of them. Adverse effects associated with the drugs can ultimately interfere with, not enhance, athletic performance. K.S. might be encouraged to practice what they will tell their partner and to seek other support as needed.

The sale or distribution of anabolic steroids without a prescription is illegal, and this fact further complicates the situation for K.S. Because they are planning to become a health care provider, K.S. may be obligated by state law to report this information to the authorities. K.S. should research these issues and discuss them further with the clinical instructor and other resource people.

NURSING CARE GUIDE: ANDROGENS, ANABOLIC STEROIDS

A patient receiving an androgen or anabolic steroid for a medical condition would have the following care plan.

Assessment: History and Examination

Assess the patient's health history for allergies to any steroids, breast or prostate cancer, hepatic dysfunction, coronary artery disease, pregnancy or breast or chestfeeding, or concurrent use of insulin or oral anticoagulants.

Focus the physical examination on the following:

Neurological: Orientation, reflexes, affect

Skin: Color, lesions, hair

CV: Pulse, cardiac auscultation, blood pressure, edema

Genitourinary (GI): Abdominal examination, liver examination

Laboratory tests: Serum electrolytes, hepatic function tests, long-bone x-ray studies

Nursing Conclusions

Altered body image perception related to drug effects

Altered sexual function

Knowledge deficit regarding drug therapy

Planning

The patient will receive the best therapeutic effect from the drug therapy.

The patient will have limited adverse effects from the drug therapy.

The patient will have an understanding of the drug therapy, adverse effects to anticipate, and measures to relieve discomfort and improve safety.

Intervention

Administer as prescribed.
Monitor liver function before and periodically during therapy.
Monitor patient response and adjust dose as appropriate.
Provide support and reassurance to deal with drug therapy.
Provide patient teaching regarding drug name, dosage, adverse effects, precautions, warnings to report, and safe administration.

Evaluation

Evaluate drug effects: maintenance of male sex characteristics, suppression of lactation.
Monitor for adverse effects: androgenic effects, hypoestrogenic effects, hepatic dysfunction, electrolyte imbalance, endocrine changes.
Monitor for drug–drug interactions: decreased need for insulin, increased bleeding with oral anticoagulants.
Evaluate the effectiveness of the patient teaching program and comfort and safety measures.

PATIENT TEACHING

If the patient is taking these drugs to increase body mass following severe weight loss due to trauma, you would teach about the following (sharing this information with people considering the unprescribed use of the drugs might also be helpful):

- Androgens or anabolic steroids have properties similar to those of the male sex hormones. Because the formulations have widespread effects, there are often many adverse effects associated with their use.
- These drugs are controlled substances because the tendency for people (athletes in particular) to abuse them can cause serious medical problems. When the drug is used as prescribed, it is safe, but you will need to be monitored.
- Some of the following adverse effects may occur:
  - *GI upset, nausea, vomiting*: Taking the drug with food usually helps to relieve these effects.
  - *Acne*: This is a hormonal effect; washing your face regularly and avoiding oily foods may help.
  - *Increased facial hair, decreased head hair*: These are hormonal effects; if they become bothersome, consult your health care provider.
  - *Menstrual irregularities (females)*: This is a normal effect of the androgens; if you suspect that you might be pregnant, consult with your health care provider immediately.
  - *Weight gain, increased muscle development*: These are common hormonal effects.
  - *Change in sex drive*: This can be distressing and difficult to deal with; consult with your health care provider if this is a serious concern.
- Report any of the following to your health care provider: swelling in fingers or legs; continual erection; uncontrollable sex drive; yellowing skin; fever, chills, or rash; chest pain or difficulty breathing; hoarseness; loss of hair or growth of facial hair (females).
  - Tell any doctor, nurse, or other health care provider involved in your care that you are taking this drug.
  - Take this medicine only as directed. In addition, schedule regular medical follow-ups, including blood tests, to monitor your response to this drug.
  - Keep this drug and all medications out of the reach of children. Do not give this medication to anyone else or take any similar medication that has not been prescribed for you.

When a patient is taking anabolic steroids, oral antidiabetic medications may not be metabolized as quickly. Dosing changes may be required. Concurrent use with other hepatotoxic medication can increase the risk for hepatotoxicity. The medications may alter lipid metabolism and reduce the effectiveness of lipid-lowering agents. Patients should be monitored closely, and appropriate dose adjustments should be made.

Nursing Considerations for Patients Receiving Androgens/Anabolic Steroids

Assessment: History and Examination

- Assess for contraindications or cautions to the use of the drug, including history of allergy to any testosterone or androgen to avoid hypersensitivity reactions; pregnancy or lactation to avoid potential adverse effects on the fetus or baby; hepatic dysfunction to avoid the risk of hepatocellular disorders; and cardiovascular disease and breast or prostate cancer, which could be aggravated by the drug.
- Perform a physical assessment before beginning therapy to determine baseline status and any potential adverse effects.
- Assess skin color, lesions, texture, and hair distribution to monitor for drug effects on the body and potential adverse effects.
- Monitor affect, orientation, and peripheral sensation to assess CNS effects related to drug use.
- Perform abdominal examination and serum electrolytes, serum cholesterol, and liver function tests to monitor for potential effects on liver function.
- Arrange for radiographs of the long bones in children to assess for testosterone effects on growth.

(continues on page 716)

Nursing Conclusions

Nursing conclusions related to drug therapy might include the following:

- Altered body image perception related to androgenic effects
- Impaired comfort related to need for injections
- Altered sexual function related to androgenic effects
- Knowledge deficit regarding drug therapy

Planning

- The patient will receive the best therapeutic effect from the drug therapy.
- The patient will have limited adverse effects from the drug therapy.
- The patient will have an understanding of the drug therapy, adverse effects to anticipate, and measures to relieve discomfort and improve safety.

Intervention With Rationale

- Reconstitute the drug according to the manufacturer's directions to ensure proper reconstitution and to administer as prescribed.
- Remove an old dermal system before applying a new system to clean, dry, intact skin to ensure accurate administration and decrease risk of toxic levels.
- When using any of the topical testosterones or nasal testosterone, follow the manufacturer's guidelines regarding placement, frequency, and protection of the area being used for application, to ensure therapeutic effectiveness and decrease the incidence of adverse effects. Instruct the patient to wash their hands after using topical formulations to decrease risk of transfer to others.
- Monitor response carefully when beginning therapy so that the dose can be adjusted accordingly.
- Monitor liver function periodically with long-term therapy and arrange to discontinue the drug at any sign of hepatic dysfunction.
- Monitor growth of prepubescent males getting therapy due to risk of epiphyseal closure.
- Provide thorough patient teaching including measures to avoid adverse effects, warning signs of problems, and the need for regular evaluation including blood tests. Instruct a family member or caregiver in proper preparation and administration techniques as appropriate to enhance patient knowledge about drug therapy and to promote adherence to the drug regimen.

Evaluation

- Monitor patient response to the drug (onset of puberty, maintenance of male sexual characteristics, palliation of breast cancer, blockage of ovulation, prevention of postpartum breast engorgement, relief of angioedema).
- Monitor for adverse effects (androgenic effects, hypoestrogenic effects, serum electrolyte imbalance, headache, sleep disturbances, rash, hepatocellular carcinoma).
- Evaluate the effectiveness of the teaching plan (patient can name drug, dosage, adverse effects to watch for, and specific measures to avoid them; family member or caregiver can demonstrate proper technique for preparation and administration of the drug as appropriate).
- Monitor the effectiveness of comfort measures and adherence to the regimen.

Prototype Summary Testosterone

Indications: Replacement therapy in hypogonadism; treatment of delayed puberty in male patients and certain breast cancers in postmenopausal patients; prevention of postpartum breast engorgement.

Actions: Primary natural androgen, responsible for growth and development of male sex organs and maintenance of secondary sex characteristics; increases the retention of nitrogen, sodium, potassium, and phosphorus; decreases urinary excretion of calcium; increases protein anabolism; stimulates red blood cell production.

Pharmacokinetics:

Route	Onset	Peak
Buccal	Slow	10–12 h
IM	Slow	1–3 d
IM cypionate	Slow	2–4 wk
IM enanthate	Slow	2–4 wk
Dermal	Rapid	24 h
Nasal	Rapid	40 min

$T_{1/2}$: 10 to 100 minutes; metabolized in the liver and excreted in the urine and feces.

Adverse Effects: Dizziness, headache, sleep disorders, fatigue, rash, androgenic effects (acne, deepening voice, oily skin), hypoestrogenic effects (flushing, sweating, vaginitis), polycythemia, nausea, hepatocellular carcinoma, hepatitis, fluid accumulation, electrolyte changes.

Key Points

- Androgens are the male sex hormones that are responsible for the development and maintenance of male sex characteristics and secondary sex characteristics or androgenic effects.
- Androgens are used for replacement therapy for males or to decrease the gonadotropin-releasing hormone in

females suffering from endometriosis or some types of breast cancer.
- There are significant side effects for both males and females taking these medications including the potential for androgenic effects, antiestrogen effects, hepatocellular cancer, and cardiovascular events.
- Anabolic steroids are testosterone analogues with more anabolic or protein-building effects than androgenic effects.
- Anabolic steroids may be prescribed for promotion of weight gain, treatment of anemia, and relief of bone pain of osteoporosis.
- There are the rare but life-threatening risks of cardiomyopathy and hepatic carcinoma from the abuse of anabolic steroids by athletes trying to build muscle mass and improve performance.

Drugs for Treating Penile Erectile Dysfunction

Penile erectile dysfunction is a condition in which the corpus cavernosum does not fill with blood to allow for penile erection. This can result from the aging process and in vascular and neurological conditions. Two very different types of drugs are approved for the treatment of this condition. These include the prostaglandin alprostadil (*Caverject*, *Muse*, and others) and the **phosphodiesterase type 5 (PDE5) receptor inhibitors** avanafil (*Stendra*), sildenafil (*Viagra*, also available as *Revatio* for the treatment of pulmonary hypertension), tadalafil (*Cialis*, also available as *Adcirca* and *Alyq* for treatment of pulmonary hypertension), and vardenafil (*Levitra*, *Staxyn*).

Therapeutic Actions and Indications

When injected directly into the cavernosum, alprostadil acts locally to relax the vascular smooth muscle and allow filling of the corpus cavernosum, causing penile erection. Alprostadil (*Muse*) is a urethral suppository. The PDE5 inhibitors avanafil, sildenafil, tadalafil, and vardenafil are selective inhibitors of cyclic guanosine monophosphate (cGMP). The PDE5 inhibitors are taken orally and act to increase nitrous oxide levels in the corpus cavernosum. Nitrous oxide activates the enzyme cGMP, which causes smooth muscle relaxation, allowing the flow of blood into the corpus cavernosum. They prevent the breakdown of cGMP by phosphodiesterase, leading to increased cGMP levels and prolonged smooth muscle relaxation, thus promoting the flow of blood into the corpus cavernosum, resulting in penile erection.

The prostaglandin alprostadil and the PDE5 inhibitors are indicated for the treatment of penile erectile dysfunction. The PDE5 inhibitors have the advantage of being oral drugs that can be timed in coordination with sexual activity based on the drug's onset. Sildenafil (*Revatio*) and tadalafil (*Alyq*, *Adcirca*) are also approved for the treatment of pulmonary arterial hypertension. These drugs are used for both male and female patients with the disease. By relaxing smooth muscle, the pulmonary artery relaxes and there is less resistance and pressure in the pulmonary bed. For this use, the drug is available in an oral tablet or suspension and in an IV form. Vardenafil is available in an orally disintegrating tablet, offering an advantage to patients who might have trouble swallowing tablets. See Table 41.2 for usual indications for all of these drugs.

Table 41.2 *Drugs in Focus:* Drugs Used to Treat Penile Erectile Dysfunction

Drug Name	Dosage/Route	Usual Indications
alprostadil (*Caverject*, *Edex*, *Muse*)	1.25 or 2.5 mcg injected intracavernously as initial dose; titrate the dose to one that will allow a satisfactory erection that is maintained no longer than 1 h; 125–1,000 mcg urethral suppository (*Muse*)	Treatment of penile erectile dysfunction
avanafil (*Stendra*)	50–200 mg PO 15–30 min before sexual stimulation	Treatment of penile erectile dysfunction
sildenafil (*Viagra*, *Revatio*)	*Viagra*: 25–100 mg PO taken 1 h before sexual stimulation *Revatio*: 5 or 20 mg PO t.i.d., at least 4–6 h apart, or 2.5 or 10 mg IV t.i.d.	Treatment of penile erectile dysfunction (*Viagra*); treatment of pulmonary arterial hypertension (*Revatio*)
tadalafil (*Cialis*, *Adcirca*, *Alyq*)	*Cialis*: 5–20 mg PO PRN taken before sexual activity or 2.5–5 mg PO daily for BPH or erectile dysfunction *Adcirca*, *Alyq*: 40 mg/d PO	Treatment of penile erectile dysfunction (*Cialis*); treatment of signs and symptoms of benign prostatic hyperplasia (BPH) (*Cialis*); treatment of pulmonary artery hypertension (*Adcirca*, *Alyq*)
vardenafil (*Levitra*, *Staxyn*)	5–20 mg PO taken 1 h before sexual stimulation, limit use to once a day; 10 mg/d PO orally disintegrating tablets	Treatment of penile erectile dysfunction

Pharmacokinetics

After injection, alprostadil is metabolized to inactive compounds in the lungs and excreted in the urine. The PDE5 inhibitors are well absorbed from the GI tract, undergo metabolism in the liver, and are excreted in the feces. The differences among the three PDE5 inhibitors lie in their onsets and durations of action. Sildenafil has a median onset of 27 minutes and a duration of 4 hours. Patients are encouraged to take the drug 1 hour before anticipated sexual stimulation. Vardenafil has a mean onset of action of 26 minutes and a duration of 4 hours; it is also intended to be taken 1 hour before sexual stimulation. Tadalafil has an onset of action of 45 minutes and a duration of 36 hours. Avanafil, the newest drug in this class, has a rapid onset with peak effects in 30 to 40 minutes and a duration of 2 to 3 hours. It can be taken 15 to 30 minutes before sexual stimulation.

Originally, these drugs were not indicated for use in female patients, so little was known about use during pregnancy and lactation. The drugs are now used to treat pulmonary hypertension in both female and male patients. It is suggested that they be used during pregnancy or lactation only if clearly indicated and if the benefits outweigh potential risks. Because the effects on pregnancy are not known, a patient taking alprostadil should use a condom during intercourse with a pregnant person.

Contraindications and Cautions

These drugs are contraindicated in the presence of any anatomic obstruction or condition that might predispose the patient to priapism because the risk could be exacerbated by these drugs.

They cannot be used with penile implants, and they are not indicated for use to improve sexual performance in female patients. However, sildenafil and tadalafil are used in females for the treatment of pulmonary arterial hypertension.

Caution should be used in patients with bleeding disorders. The PDE5 inhibitors should also be used cautiously in patients with coronary artery disease, active peptic ulcer, retinitis pigmentosa, optic neuropathy, hypotension or severe hypertension, congenital prolonged QT interval, or severe hepatic or renal disorders because of the risk of exacerbating these diseases. There may be interactions with certain foods and other medications with these drugs (Box 41.4).

Adverse Effects

Adverse effects associated with alprostadil are local effects such as pain at the injection site, infection, priapism, fibrosis, and rash. PDE5 inhibitors are associated with more systemic effects, including headache, flushing (related to relaxation of vascular smooth muscle), priapism, dyspepsia, urinary tract infection, diarrhea, dizziness, optic neuropathy, eighth cranial nerve toxicity and loss of hearing, increased risk of melanoma, and rash.

Box 41.4 Focus on Safe Medication Administration

Patients who are using PDE5 inhibitors need to be advised to avoid drinking grapefruit juice while using the drug. Grapefruit juice can cause a decrease in the metabolism of the PDE5 inhibitor, leading to increased serum levels and a risk of toxicity. They need to know that it takes 48 hours for grapefruit juice to be processed by the body and will, therefore, need to avoid it for several days around taking the drug. They should also be advised to avoid taking the drug with or just after a high-fat meal. The presence of fat in the GI tract will delay the absorption and onset of action of the drug, which could cause problems for patients who are timing onset of action with their sexual activity. Administration of the drug should balance these dietary factors.

Clinically Important Drug–Drug Interactions

The PDE5 inhibitors cannot be taken in combination with any organic nitrates (nitroglycerin or isosorbide dinitrate) or alpha-adrenergic blockers, drugs that cause a drop in blood pressure; serious cardiovascular effects including death due to severe hypotension have occurred. There is also a possibility of increased levels and effects of PDE5 inhibitors if taken with moderate or potent CYP3A4 inhibitors such as ketoconazole, itraconazole, or erythromycin; monitor the patient and reduce the dose as needed.

Vardenafil and tadalafil serum levels can increase if these drugs are combined with indinavir or ritonavir. If these drugs are being used, limit the dose of the PDE5 inhibitor.

Prototype Summary Sildenafil

Indications: Treatment of erectile dysfunction in the presence of sexual stimulation, treatment of pulmonary arterial hypertension.

Actions: Inhibits PDE5 receptors, leading to a release of nitrous oxide, which activates cyclic guanosine monophosphate to cause a prolonged smooth muscle relaxation, allowing the flow of blood into the corpus cavernosum and facilitating erection.

Pharmacokinetics:

Route	Onset	Peak	Duration
PO	15–30 min	30–120 min	4 h

$T_{1/2}$: 4 hours; metabolized in the liver and excreted in the urine and feces.

Adverse Effects: Headache, abnormal vision, flushing, dyspepsia, urinary tract infection, rash, hypotension, priapism, hearing loss.

Nursing Considerations for Patients Receiving Drugs to Treat Penile Erectile Dysfunction

Assessment: History and Examination

- Assess for the following conditions, which could be cautions or contraindications to the use of the drug: history of allergy to any of the preparations, penile structural abnormalities, penile implants, bleeding disorders, active peptic ulcer, coronary artery disease, hypotension or severe hypertension, congenital prolonged QT interval, or severe hepatic or renal disorders.
- Assess baseline status before beginning therapy to determine any potential adverse effects.
- Assess skin and lesions to monitor for adverse reactions to the drug and cardiovascular perfusion.
- Monitor orientation, affect, and reflexes to evaluate CNS changes that might be related to changes in blood pressure and blood flow.
- Assess blood pressure, pulse, respiration, and adventitious sounds to evaluate blood flow and potential changes in cardiovascular function.
- When using alprostadil, perform a local inspection of the penis to assess local reaction to injection and to monitor for potential infection.
- Evaluate laboratory tests for bleeding time and liver function to monitor potential adverse effects on the liver.

Nursing Conclusions

Nursing conclusions related to drug therapy might include the following:

- Altered body image perception related to drug effects and indication
- Impaired comfort related to injection of alprostadil
- Altered tissue perfusion related to hypotension
- Knowledge deficit risk regarding drug therapy

Planning

- The patient will receive the best therapeutic effect from the drug therapy.
- The patient will have limited adverse effects from the drug therapy.
- The patient will have an understanding of the drug therapy, adverse effects to anticipate, and measures to relieve discomfort and improve safety.

Intervention With Rationale

- Assess the cause of dysfunction before beginning therapy to ensure appropriate use of the drug.
- Monitor patients with vascular disease for any sign of exacerbation so that the drug can be discontinued before severe adverse effects occur.
- Instruct the patient in the injection of alprostadil, storage of the drug, filling of the syringe, sterile technique, site rotation, and proper disposal of needles to ensure safe and proper administration of the drug.
- Monitor patients who are taking PDE5 inhibitors for use of nitrates or alpha-blockers to avert potentially serious cardiovascular drug–drug interactions.
- Provide thorough patient teaching, including measures to avoid adverse effects and warning signs of problems, as well as the need for regular evaluation, to enhance patient knowledge about drug therapy and to promote adherence to the drug regimen.

Evaluation

- Monitor patient response to the drug (improvement in penile erection).
- Monitor for adverse effects (dizziness, flushing, local inflammation or infection, fibrosis, diarrhea, dyspepsia, priapism, hypotension, hearing or eyesight impairment).
- Evaluate the effectiveness of the teaching plan (patient can name drug, dosage, adverse effects to watch for, and specific measures to avoid them; patient can demonstrate proper administration of injected drug).
- Monitor the effectiveness of comfort measures and adherence to the regimen.

Key Points

- Penile erectile dysfunction can inhibit erection and male sexual function.
- Alprostadil, a prostaglandin, can be injected into the penis or inserted into the urethra to stimulate erection.
- The PDE5 inhibitors are oral agents that act quickly to promote vascular filling of the corpus cavernosum and promote penile erection. Some of these medications are also indicated to treat pulmonary hypertension in males and females.

SUMMARY

- Androgens are male sex hormones—specifically testosterone or testosteronelike compounds.
- Androgens are responsible for the development and maintenance of male sex characteristics and secondary sex characteristics or androgenic effects.
- Side effects related to androgen use involve excess of the desired effects as well as potentially deadly hepatocellular carcinoma.
- Androgens can be used for replacement therapy or to block other hormone effects, as is seen with their use in the treatment of specific breast cancers and symptoms of endometriosis.
- Anabolic steroids are analogues of testosterone that have been developed to have more anabolic or protein-building effects and fewer androgenic effects.
- Anabolic steroids are sometimes abused to enhance muscle development and athletic performance, but there are dangerous side effects that can be fatal.
- Anabolic steroids are used to increase hematocrit and improve protein anabolism.
- Penile erectile dysfunction can inhibit erection and male sexual function.
- Alprostadil, a prostaglandin, can be injected into the penis or inserted into the urethra to stimulate erection.
- The PDE5 inhibitors are oral agents that act quickly to promote vascular filling of the corpus cavernosum and promote penile erection. They are also used in the treatment of pulmonary arterial hypertension.
- Dangerous cardiovascular effects, including death, have occurred when the PDE5 inhibitors are combined with organic nitrates or alpha-blockers. Careful patient teaching is important to avoid this drug–drug interaction.

CHECK YOUR UNDERSTANDING

Answers to the questions in this chapter can be found in Answers to Check Your Understanding Questions on thePoint®.

MULTIPLE CHOICE

Select the best answer.

1. Testosterone is approved for use in
   a. the treatment of breast cancers.
   b. increasing muscle strength in athletes.
   c. oral contraceptives.
   d. increasing hair distribution in male pattern baldness.

2. Illegal use of large quantities of unprescribed anabolic steroids to enhance athletic performance has been associated with
   a. increased sexual prowess.
   b. muscle rupture from overexpansion.
   c. development of chronic obstructive pulmonary disease.
   d. cardiomyopathy and liver cancers.

3. Anabolic steroids would be indicated for the treatment of
   a. hair loss.
   b. angioedema.
   c. debilitation and severe weight loss.
   d. breast cancers in males.

4. What cause of erectile penile dysfunction is treated with PDE5 inhibitors?
   a. Problems with childhood authority figures preventing a male erection
   b. The corpus cavernosum not filling with blood to allow for penile erection
   c. The sympathetic nervous system failing to function
   d. Past exposure to sexually transmitted infection causing physical damage within the penis

5. A potentially deadly drug–drug interaction can occur if a PDE5 inhibitor (sildenafil, avanafil, tadalafil, or vardenafil) is combined with
   a. corticosteroids.
   b. oral contraceptives.
   c. organic nitrates.
   d. halothane anesthetics.

6. A female may be prescribed an androgen for which diagnosis?
   a. Breast cancer
   b. Infertility
   c. Pain during intercourse
   d. Females are never prescribed androgens

7. Patients taking alprostadil for treatment of erectile dysfunction must
   a. take the drug orally about 1 hour before anticipated intercourse.
   b. arrange for sexual stimulation to promote erection.
   c. learn to inject the drug directly into the penis.
   d. avoid the use of nitrates for cardiovascular disorders.

8. *Viagra* is known to
   a. cause unexpected and enlarged erections.
   b. make a person young and agile.
   c. promote interpersonal relationships between partners.
   d. increase nitrous oxide levels in the corpus cavernosum, causing vascular relaxation and promoting blood flow into the corpus cavernosum.

MULTIPLE RESPONSE

Select all that apply.

1. In assessing a patient for androgenic effects, you would expect to find which conditions?
   a. Hirsutism
   b. Deepening of the voice
   c. Testicular enlargement
   d. Acne
   e. Elevated body temperature
   f. Sudden growth

2. A child treated with anabolic steroids because of anemia associated with renal disease will need
   a. early sex education classes because of the effects of the drug.
   b. x-rays of the long bones every 3 to 6 months so the drug can be stopped when the bone size is appropriate to the child's age.
   c. to learn to shave.
   d. to learn to cope with an altered body image.
   e. regular monitoring of liver function tests.
   f. monitoring for the development of edema.

REFERENCES

Bianchi, V. E. (2017). Testosterone a key factor in gender related metabolic syndrome. *Obesity Reviews, 19*, 557–575. 10.1111/obr.12633

Brunton, L., Hilal-Dandan, R., & Knollman, B. (2018). *Goodman and Gilman's the pharmacological basis of therapeutics* (12th ed.). McGraw-Hill.

Butts, J., Jacobs, B., & Silvis, M. (2017). Creatine use in sports. *SPORTS Health: A Multidisciplinary Approach, 10*(1), 31–34. 10.1177/1941738117737248

Emmelot-Vork, M. H., Verhaar, H. J. J., Nakhai Pour, H. R., Aleman, A., Lock, T. M. T. W., Ruud Bosch, J. L. H., Grobbee, D. E., & van der Schouw, Y. T. (2008). Effect of testosterone supplementation on function, mobility, cognition and other parameters in older men. *Journal of the American Medical Association, 299*(1), 39–52. 10.1001/jama.2007.51

Fried, R. (2014). *Erectile dysfunction as a cardiovascular impairment.* Academic Press.

Hall, J. E., & Hall, M. E. (2021). *Guyton and Hall's textbook of medical physiology* (14th ed.). Saunders.

Khera, M., Adaikan, G., Buvat, J., Carrier, S., El-Meliegy, A., Hatzimouratidis, K., McCullough, A., Morgentaler, A., Torres, L. O., & Salonia, A. (2016). Diagnosis and treatment of testosterone deficiency: Recommendations from the fourth international consultation for sexual medicine (ICSM 2015). *The Journal of Sexual Medicine, 13*, 1787–1804. https://doi.org/10.1016/j.jsxm.2016.10.009

Nieschlag, E. (2010). *Andrology: Male reproductive health and dysfunction* (3rd ed.). Springer.

Roy, C. N., Snyder, P. J., Stephens-Shields, A. J., Artz, A. S., Bhasin, S., Cohen, H. J., Farrar, J. T., Gill, T. M., Zeldow, B., Cella, D., Barrett-Connor, E., Cauley, J. A., Crandall, J. P., Cunningham, G. R., Ensrud, K. E., Lewis, C. E., Matsumoto, A. M., Molitch, M. E., Pahor, M., … Ellenberg, S. S. (2017). Association of testosterone levels with anemia in older men. A controlled clinical trial. *JAMA Internal Medicine, 177*(4), 480–490. 10.1001/jamaintermed.2016.9540

Troiano, G., & Lazzeri, G. (2021). The potential toxic combination of grapefruit juice and sildenafil. *Toxin Reviews, 40*(3), 334–337. https://doi.org/10.1080/15569543.2019.1603163

Vigen, W., O'Donnell, C., Baron, A., Grunwald, G. K., Maddox, T. M., Bradley, S. M., Barqawi, A., Woning, G., Wierman, M. E., Plomondon, M. E., Rumsfeld, J. S., & Michael Ho, P. (2013). Association of testosterone therapy with mortality, myocardial infarction and stroke in men with low testosterone levels. *Journal of the American Medical Association, 310*(17), 1829–1836. 10.1001/jama.2013.280386

Wein, A. J., Kavoussi, L. R., Novick, A. C., Partin, A. W., & Peters, C. A. (Eds.). (2011). *Campbell-Walsh urology* (10th ed.). W.B. Saunders.

PART 8

Drugs Acting on the Cardiovascular System

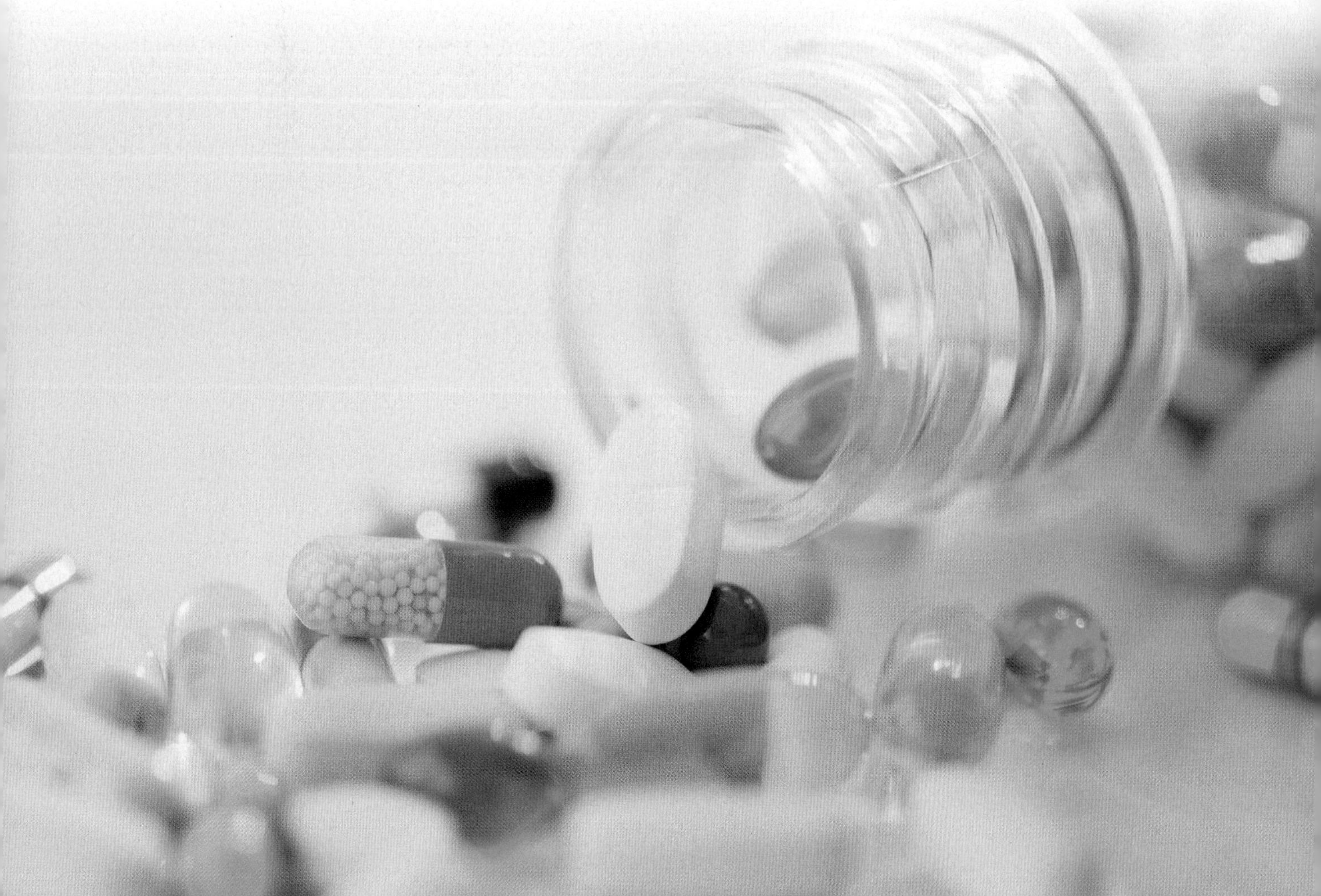

CHAPTER 42

Introduction to the Cardiovascular System

Learning Objectives

Upon completion of this chapter, you will be able to:

1. Label a diagram of the heart, including all chambers, valves, great vessels, coronary vessels, and the conduction system.
2. Describe the flow of blood during the cardiac cycle, including flow to the cardiac muscle.
3. Outline the conduction system of the heart, correlating the normal electrocardiogram (ECG) pattern with the underlying electrical activity in the heart.
4. Discuss four normal controls of blood pressure.
5. Describe the capillary fluid shift, including factors that influence the movement of fluid in clinical situations.

Key Terms

actin: thin filament, a component of a sarcomere, or muscle unit

aldosterone: hormone released from the adrenal cortex that acts in the distal convoluted tubule of the kidney to increase retention of sodium and water

angiotensin: peptide hormone that causes vasoconstriction and stimulates aldosterone and ADH release; part of the renin–angiotensin system

antidiuretic hormone (ADH): hormone released from the posterior pituitary that acts in the distal convoluted tubule of the kidney to increase water retention

arrhythmia: disruption in cardiac rate or rhythm, also called dysrhythmia

arteries: vessels that take blood away from the heart; muscular, resistance vessels

atrium: top chamber of the heart, receives blood from veins

auricle: appendage on the atria of the heart, holds blood to be pumped out with atrial contraction

automaticity: property of heart cells to generate an action potential without an external stimulus

capacitance system: the venous system; distensible, flexible veins that are capable of holding large amounts of blood

capillary: small vessel made up of loosely connected endothelial cells that connect arteries to veins

cardiac cycle: period of cardiac muscle relaxation (diastole) followed by a period of contraction (systole) in the heart

conductivity: property of heart cells to rapidly conduct an action potential of electrical impulse

diastole: resting phase of the heart; blood is returned to the heart during this phase

dysrhythmia: disruption in cardiac rate or rhythm, also called an arrhythmia

ectopic focus: shift in the pacemaker of the heart from the sinoatrial node to some other site

electrocardiogram (ECG): electrical tracing reflecting the conduction of an electrical impulse through the heart muscle; does not reflect mechanical activity

hydrostatic pressure (HP): pushing force of fluid against solid objects

myocardium: muscle of the heart

myosin: thick filament with projections; a component of a sarcomere, or muscle unit

natriuretic peptide: peptide produced by the brain, heart, and vasculature that causes natriuresis, excretion of sodium in the urine; degraded by the enzyme neprilysin

oncotic pressure (OP): pulling pressure of the plasma proteins, responsible for returning fluid to the vascular system at the capillary level

pulse pressure: systolic blood pressure minus the diastolic blood pressure; reflects the filling pressure of the coronary arteries

resistance system: the arteries; the muscles of the arteries provide resistance to the flow of blood, leading to control of blood pressure

sarcomere: functional unit of a muscle cell, composed of actin and myosin molecules arranged in layers to give the unit a striped or striated appearance

sinoatrial (SA) node: normal pacemaker of the heart; composed of primitive cells that constantly generate an action potential

Starling's law of the heart: addresses the contractile properties of the heart: the more the muscle is stretched, the stronger it will react until it is stretched to a point at which it will not react at all

systole: contracting phase of the heart during which blood is pumped out of the heart

troponin: chemical in heart muscle that prevents the reaction between actin and myosin, leading to muscle relaxation; inactivated by calcium during muscle stimulation to allow actin and myosin to react, causing muscle contraction

veins: vessels that return blood to the heart; distensible tubes

ventricle: bottom chamber of the heart, which contracts to pump blood out of the heart

Structure and Function of the Heart

The cardiovascular system is responsible for delivering oxygen and nutrients to all of the cells of the body and for removing waste products for excretion. The cardiovascular system consists of a pump—the heart—and an interconnected series of vessels that continually move blood throughout the body.

The heart is a hollow, muscular organ that is divided into four chambers. The heart may actually be viewed as two joined hearts: a right heart and a left heart, each of which is divided into two parts, an upper part called the **atrium** (literally "porch" or entryway) and a lower part called the **ventricle**.

Attached to each atrium is an appendage called the **auricle**, which collects blood that is then pumped into the ventricles by atrial contraction. The right auricle is quite large; the left auricle is small. The ventricles pump blood out of the heart to the lungs or the body. Between the atria and ventricles are two cardiac valves—thin tissues that are anchored to an annulus, or fibrous ring, which also gives the hollow organ some structure and helps keep the organ open and divided into distinct chambers.

A partition called a septum separates the right half of the heart from the left half. The right half receives deoxygenated blood from everywhere in the body through the **veins** (vessels that carry blood toward the heart) and directs that blood into the lungs through the pulmonary artery. The left half receives the oxygenated blood from the lungs and directs it into the aorta. The aorta delivers blood into the systemic circulation by way of **arteries** (vessels that carry blood away from the heart) (Fig. 42.1). The aorta delivers blood into the systemic circulation by way of arteries. The two semilunar valves, the aortic valve and the pulmonic valve, separate these great vessels from the heart and are also anchored onto two fibrous rings or annuli. These valves, like the atrioventricular (AV) valves, keep the blood flowing in one direction. The circulatory system is composed of about 60,000 miles of interconnecting blood vessels that carry the needed oxygen and nutrients to the cells and carry away the metabolic waste products from the tissues.

Cardiac Cycle

The heart, a muscle that contracts thousands of millions of times in a lifetime, possesses structural and functional properties that are different from those of other muscles. The fibers of the cardiac muscle, or **myocardium**, form two intertwining networks called the atrial and ventricular syncytia. These interlacing structures enable the atria and then the ventricles to contract synchronously when excited by the same stimulus.

Simultaneous contraction is a necessary property for a muscle that acts as a pump. A hollow pumping mechanism must also pause long enough in the pumping cycle to allow the chambers to fill with fluid. The heart muscle relaxes long enough to ensure adequate filling; the more completely it fills, the stronger the subsequent contraction. This occurs because the muscle fibers of the heart, stretched by the increased volume of blood that has returned to them, spring back to normal size. This is similar to the stretching of a rubber band, which returns to its normal size after it is stretched. The further it is stretched, the stronger the spring back to normal until it is stretched to a point at which it will not react at all. This property is **Starling's law of the heart.**

During **diastole**—the period of cardiac muscle relaxation—blood returns to the heart from the systemic and

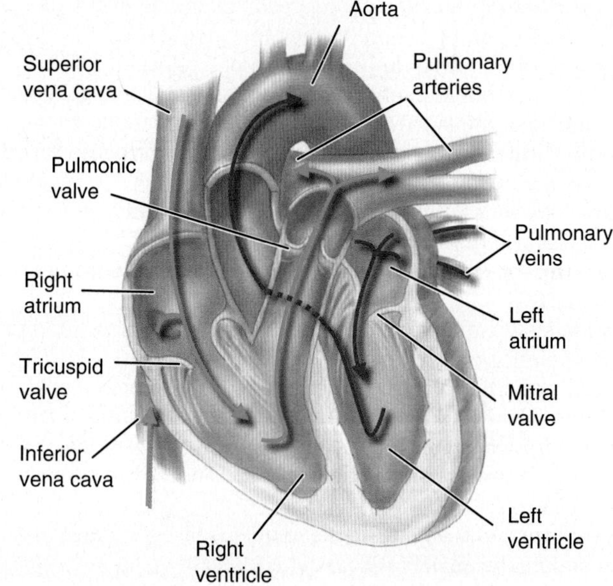

FIGURE 42.1 Blood flow into and out of the heart. Deoxygenated blood enters the right atrium from the great cardiac vein and the superior and inferior venae cavae and flows through the tricuspid valve into the right ventricle, which contracts and sends the blood through the pulmonic valve into the pulmonary artery and to the lungs. Oxygenated blood from the lungs enters the left atrium through the pulmonary veins and passes through the mitral valve into the left ventricle, which contracts and ejects the blood through the aortic valve into the aorta and out to the systemic circulation.

pulmonary veins, flowing into the right and left atria, respectively. When the pressure generated by the blood volume in the atria is greater than the pressure in the ventricles, blood flows through the AV valves into the ventricles. The valve on the right side of the heart is called the tricuspid valve because it is composed of three leaflets or cusps. The valve on the left side of the heart, called the mitral or bicuspid valve, is composed of two leaflets or cusps (see Fig. 42.1). Just before the ventricles are stimulated to contract, the atria contract, pushing about one more tablespoon of blood into each ventricle. The much more powerful ventricles then contract, pumping blood out to the lungs through the pulmonary valve or out to the aorta through the aortic valve and into the systemic circulation. The contraction of the ventricles is referred to as **systole**. Each period of systole followed by a period of diastole is called a **cardiac cycle**. The heart's series of one-way valves keeps the blood flowing in the correct direction as follows:

- *Deoxygenated blood enters* the right atrium, flows through the tricuspid valve to the right ventricle, and flows through the pulmonary valve to the pulmonary arteries and the lungs.
- *Oxygenated blood from the lungs returns* through the pulmonary veins to the left atrium, flows through the mitral valve into the left ventricle, and then flows through the aortic valve to the aorta and the rest of the body.

The AV valves close tightly when the ventricles contract, preventing blood from flowing backward into the atria, thereby keeping blood moving forward through the system. The pulmonary and aortic valves open with the pressure of ventricular contraction and close tightly during diastole, keeping blood from flowing backward into the ventricles. These valves operate much like one-way automatic doors; you can go through in the intended direction, but if you try to go the wrong way, the doors close and stop your movement. The proper functioning of the cardiac valves is important in maintaining the functioning of the cardiovascular system.

Cardiac Conduction

Each cycle of cardiac contraction and relaxation is controlled by impulses that arise spontaneously in certain pacemaker cells of the **sinoatrial (SA) node** of the heart. These impulses are conducted from the pacemaker cells by a specialized conducting system that activates all of the parts of the heart muscle almost simultaneously. These continuous, rhythmic contractions are controlled by the heart itself; the brain does not stimulate the heart to beat. This safety feature allows the heart to beat as long as it has enough nutrients and oxygen to survive regardless of the status of the rest of the body. This property protects the vital cardiovascular function in many disease states; it is the same property that allows the heart to continue functioning in a patient who is "brain dead."

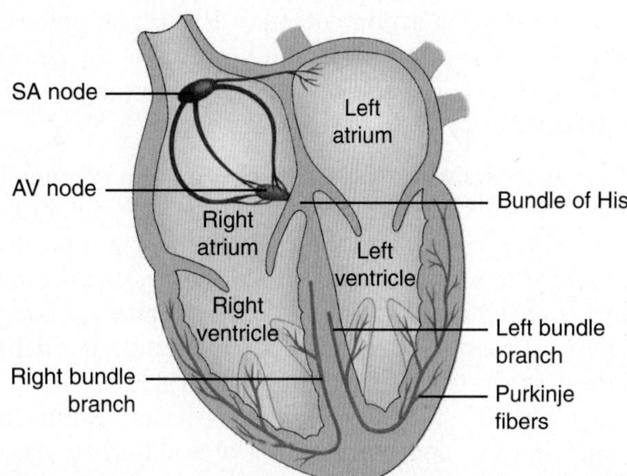

FIGURE 42.2 The conducting system of the heart. Impulses originating in the sinoatrial (SA) node are transmitted through the atrial bundles to the atrioventricular (AV) node and down the bundle of His and the bundle branches by way of the Purkinje fibers through the ventricles.

The conduction system of the heart consists of the SA node, atrial bundles, AV node, bundle of His, bundle branches, and Purkinje fibers (Fig. 42.2). The SA node, which is located near the top of the right atrium and composed of primitive cells that constantly generate an action potential, acts as the normal pacemaker of the heart. Atrial bundles conduct the impulse through the atrial muscle. The AV node, which is located near the bottom of the right atrium, slows the impulse and allows the delay needed for atrial contraction and ventricular filling. The AV node then sends the impulse from the atria into the ventricles by way of the bundle of His, which enters the septum and then divides into three bundle branches. These bundle branches, which conduct the impulse through the ventricles, break into a fine network of conducting fibers called the Purkinje fibers, which deliver the impulse to the ventricular cells and stimulate contraction of the ventricles.

Automaticity

The sinus node is the normal pacemaker. However, ectopic pacemakers (a pacemaker outside of the sinus node) can exist. An ectopic pacemaker can be created when cells in the AV node or Purkinje fibers discharge action potentials at faster rates than the sinus node. In rare occasions, the atrial or ventricular muscle cells develop increased excitability and become ectopic pacemakers. The cells of the impulse-forming and conducting system are rather primitive, uncomplicated cells called pale or P cells. Because of their simple cell membranes, these cells possess a special property that differentiates them from other cells: They can generate action potentials or electrical impulses without being excited to do so by external stimuli. This property is called **automaticity**.

All cardiac cells possess some degree of automaticity. During diastole or rest, these cells undergo a spontaneous depolarization because they decrease the flow of potassium ions out of the cell and probably leak sodium into the cell, causing an action potential. This action potential is basically the same as the action potential of the neuron (see Chapter 19). The action potential of the cardiac muscle cell consists of the following five phases:

- Phase 0 occurs when the cell reaches a point of stimulation. The sodium gates open along the cell membrane, and sodium rushes into the cell, resulting in a positive flow of electrons into the cell—an electrical potential. This is called depolarization. The membrane no longer has a positive side, or pole, and a negative side; it is depolarized, or electrically the same on both sides.
- Phase 1 is the short period when the fast sodium ion channels close and permeability of sodium decreases. There is slight repolarization due to potassium ions beginning to leave the cell.
- Phase 2, or the plateau stage, occurs as the cell membrane becomes less permeable to potassium. Calcium slowly enters the cell, and potassium efflux is very slow. The plateau stage is unique to cardiac muscle and allows for the action potential to last longer than action potentials for skeletal muscle.
- Phase 3 is a period of rapid repolarization as the calcium influx stops, permeability of potassium increases, and potassium rapidly moves out of the cell. At the end of phase 3, the potassium and sodium distributions across the membrane return to their resting states.
- Phase 4 occurs when the cell comes to resting membrane potential. The sodium–potassium pump maintains this state by moving sodium out of the cell in exchange for potassium.

Each area of the heart has an action potential that appears slightly different from the other action potentials, reflecting the complexity of the cells in that particular area. Because of these differences in the action potential, each area of the heart has a slightly different rate of automaticity, and cells have different looking action potentials. The SA node generates an impulse about 90 to 100 times a minute, the AV node about 40 to 50 times a minute, and the complex ventricular muscle cells only about 10 to 20 times a minute (Fig. 42.3).

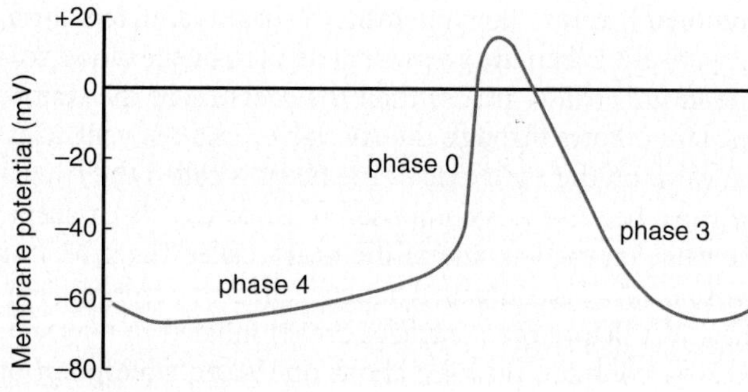

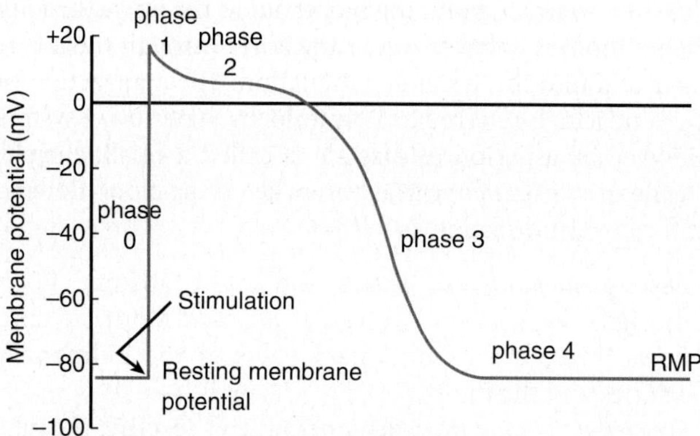

FIGURE 42.3 Action potentials recorded from a cell in the sinoatrial (SA) node (**A**) showing diastolic depolarization in phase 4 and recorded from a ventricular muscle cell (**B**). In phase 0, the cell is stimulated, sodium rushes into the cell, and the cell is depolarized. In phase 1, sodium levels equalize. In phase 2, the plateau phase, calcium enters the cell (the slow current) and potassium and sodium leave. In phase 3, the slow current stops and sodium and potassium leave the cell. In phase 4, the resting membrane potential (RMP) returns and the pacemaker potential begins in the SA node cell.

Conductivity

Normally, the SA node sets the pace for the heart rate because it depolarizes faster than any cell in the heart. However, the other cells in the heart are capable of generating an impulse if anything happens to the SA node, which is another protective feature of the heart. As mentioned earlier, the SA node is said to be the pacemaker of the heart because it acts to stimulate the rest of the cells to depolarize at its rate. When the SA node sets the pace for the heart rate, the person is said to be in sinus rhythm.

The specialized cells of the heart can conduct an impulse rapidly through the system so that the muscle cells of the heart are stimulated at approximately the same time. This property of cardiac cells is called **conductivity**. The conduction velocity, or the speed at which the cells can pass on the impulse, is slowest in the AV node and fastest in the Purkinje fibers.

A delay in conduction at the AV node, between the atria and the ventricles, accounts for the fact that the atria contract a fraction of a second before the ventricles contract. This allows extra time for the ventricles to fill completely before they contract. The almost simultaneous spread of the impulse through the Purkinje fibers permits a simultaneous and powerful contraction of the ventricle muscles, making them an effective pump.

After a cell membrane has conducted an action potential, there is a span of time called the absolute refractory period, in which it is impossible to stimulate that area of membrane. The absolute refractory period is the minimal amount of time that must elapse between two stimuli applied at one site in the heart for each of these stimuli to cause an action potential. This time reflects the responsiveness of the heart cells to stimuli. Cardiac drugs may affect the refractory period of the cells to make the heart more or less responsive.

Autonomic Influences

The heart can generate action potentials on its own and could function without connection to the rest of the body.

However, the autonomic nervous system (see Chapter 29) can influence the heart rate and rhythm and the strength of contraction. The parasympathetic nerves—primarily the vagus or 10th cranial nerve—can slow the rate of sinus node activation and decrease the speed of conduction through the AV node. This allows the heart to rest and conserve its strength. In addition, the parasympathetic influence on the SA node is the dominant influence most of the time, keeping the resting heart rate at 70 to 80 beats/min.

The sympathetic nervous system stimulates the heart to beat faster, speeds conduction through the AV node, and causes the heart muscle to contract harder. This action is important during exercise or stress when the body's cells need to have more oxygen delivered.

These two branches of the autonomic nervous system work together to help the heart meet the body's demands. Drugs that influence either branch can exert autonomic effects on the heart.

Myocardial Contraction

The end result of the electrical stimulation of the heart cells is the unified contraction of the atria and then the ventricles, which moves the blood throughout the vascular system. The basic unit of the cardiac muscle is the **sarcomere**. A sarcomere is made up of two contractile proteins—**actin**, a thin filament, and **myosin**, a thick filament with small projections on it. These proteins are anchored at the Z bands, the outer edges of each sarcomere. The proteins readily react with each other; however, at rest, they are kept apart by the protein **troponin** (Fig. 42.4).

When a cardiac muscle cell is stimulated, calcium enters the cell through channels in the cell membrane and also from storage sites within the cell. This occurs during phase 3 of the action potential and prevents fast repolarization. The calcium reacts with the troponin and inactivates it. This action allows the actin and myosin proteins to react with each other, forming actomyosin bridges. These bridges then break quickly, and the myosin slides along to form new bridges.

As long as calcium is present, the actomyosin bridges continue to form. This action slides the proteins together, shortening or contracting the sarcomere. Cardiac muscle cells are linked together; when one cell is stimulated to contract, they are all stimulated to contract.

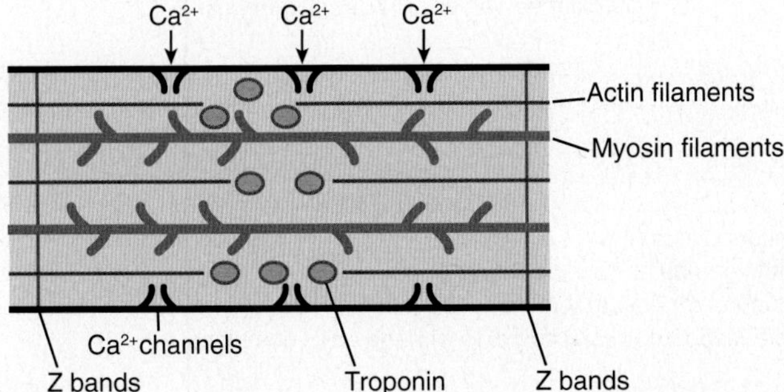

FIGURE 42.4 A sarcomere, the functioning unit of cardiac muscle.

The shortening of numerous sarcomeres causes the contraction and pumping action of the heart muscle. At the end of the plateau portion of the action potential, the influx of calcium stops. Calcium is removed from the muscle cells by a sodium–calcium pump, and calcium released from storage sites within the cells returns to those storage sites. The contraction process requires energy and oxygen for the chemical reaction that allows the formation of the actomyosin bridges; it also requires calcium to allow the bridge formation to occur.

The degree of shortening (the strength of contraction) is determined by the amount of calcium present—the more calcium present, the more bridges will be formed—and by the stretch of the sarcomere before contraction begins. To a certain degree, the further apart the actin and myosin proteins are before the cell is stimulated, the more bridges will be formed and the stronger the contraction will be. This correlates with Starling's law of the heart. The more the cardiac muscle is stretched, the greater the contraction. The more blood that enters the heart, the greater the contraction needed to empty the heart. However, if the actin and myosin molecules are stretched too far apart, less actomyosin bridges can be made, and the force of contraction will be decreased.

Key Points

- The heart, a hollow muscle with four chambers composed of two upper atria and two lower ventricles, pumps oxygenated blood to the body's cells and pumps deoxygenated blood to the lung tissues.
- The two-step process known as the cardiac cycle includes diastole (resting period when the veins carry blood back to the heart) and systole (contraction period when the heart pumps blood out to the arteries for distribution to the body).
- Specialized heart cells are able to generate action potential without neural innervation, but the autonomic nervous system may increase or decrease the rate of action potentials.
- The heart's conduction (or stimulatory) system consists of the SA node, the atrial bundles, the AV node, the bundle of His, the bundle branches, and the Purkinje fibers.

Electrocardiography

Electrocardiography is a process of recording the patterns of electrical impulses as they move through the heart. It is an important diagnostic tool in the care of the cardiac patient. The electrocardiography machine detects the patterns of electrical impulse generation and conduction through the heart and translates that information into a recorded pattern, which is displayed as a waveform on a cardiac monitor or printout on calibrated paper.

An **electrocardiogram** (ECG) is a measure of electrical activity; it provides no information about the mechanical activity of the heart. The important aspect of cardiac output—the degree to which the heart is doing its job of pumping blood out to all of the tissues—requires careful assessment of the patient.

The normal ECG waveform is made up of five main waves: the P wave, which is formed as impulses originating in the SA node or pacemaker pass through the atrial tissues; the QRS complex, which represents depolarization of the bundle of His (Q wave) and the ventricles (R and S waves); and the T wave, which represents repolarization of the ventricles (Fig. 42.5).

The P wave immediately precedes the contraction of the atria. The QRS complex immediately precedes the contraction of the ventricles and then relaxation of the ventricles during the T wave. The repolarization of the atria (the Ta wave) occurs during the QRS complex and is usually not seen on an ECG. In certain conditions of atrial hypertrophy, the Ta wave may appear around the QRS complex.

In addition to the five waves, several areas represent critical points on the ECG. These include the following:

P–R interval: Reflects the normal delay of conduction at the AV node and the beginning of electrical excitation of the atria to the beginning of electrical excitation of the ventricles

Q–T interval: Reflects the critical timing of depolarization and repolarization of the ventricles

S–T segment: Reflects important information about the repolarization of the ventricles

A person with a normal ECG pattern and a heart rate within the normal range for that person's age group is said to be in normal sinus rhythm. However, abnormalities in the shape or timing of each part of an ECG tracing help reveal the presence of particular cardiac disorders.

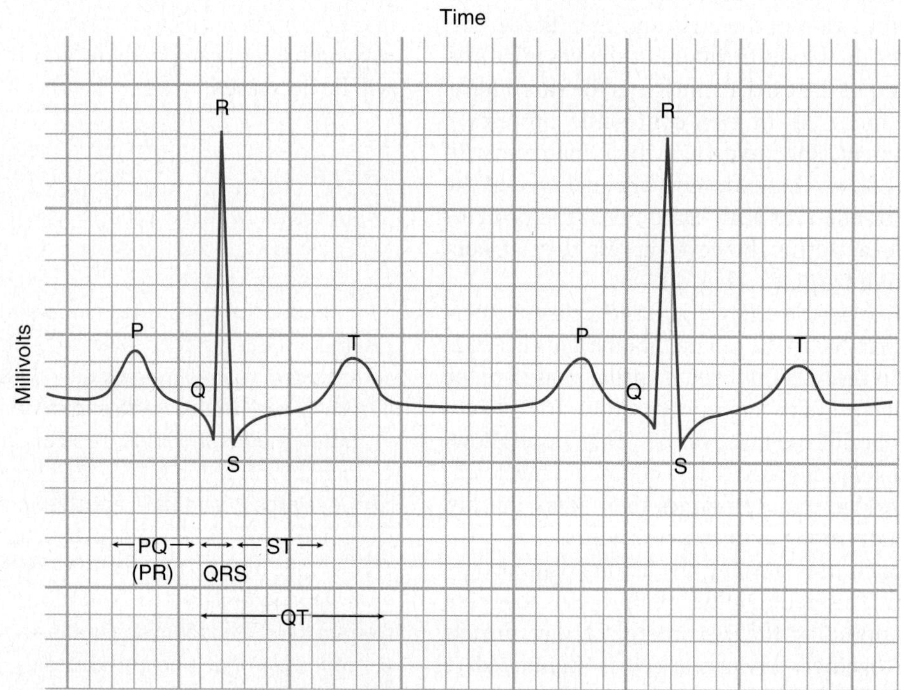

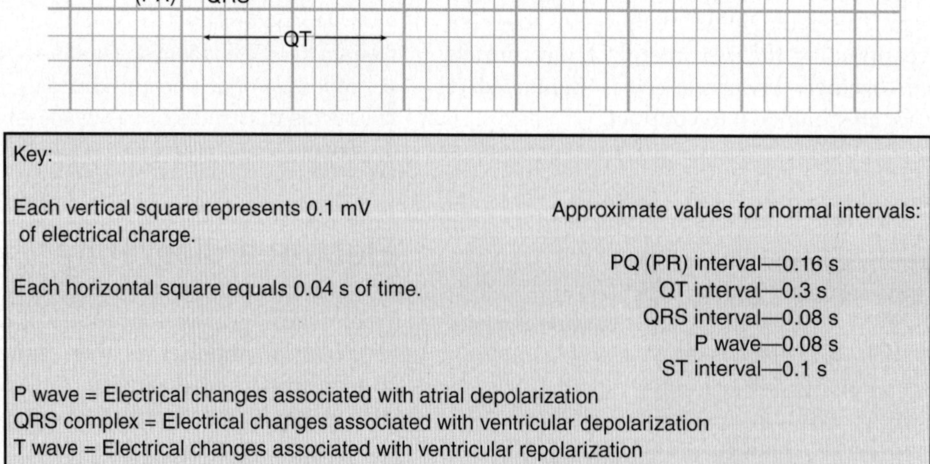
Key:

Each vertical square represents 0.1 mV of electrical charge.

Each horizontal square equals 0.04 s of time.

Approximate values for normal intervals:

PQ (PR) interval—0.16 s
QT interval—0.3 s
QRS interval—0.08 s
P wave—0.08 s
ST interval—0.1 s

P wave = Electrical changes associated with atrial depolarization
QRS complex = Electrical changes associated with ventricular depolarization
T wave = Electrical changes associated with ventricular repolarization
The electrical changes associated with atrial repolarization normally coincide with the QRS complex and are obscured by it.

FIGURE 42.5 The normal electrocardiogram waveform.

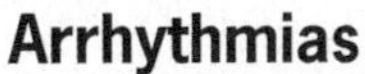

Arrhythmias

A disruption in cardiac rate or rhythm is called an **arrhythmia**, or **dysrhythmia**. Various factors, such as drugs, acidosis, decreased oxygen level, changes in the electrolytes in the area, and buildup of waste products, can change the cardiac rate and rhythm. Arrhythmias can arise because of changes in the automaticity or conductivity of the heart cells. They are significant if they interfere with the work of the heart and can disrupt the cardiac output, which eventually will affect every cell in the body. Several different types of arrhythmias may occur.

Sinus Arrhythmias

The SA node is influenced by the autonomic nervous system to change the rate of firing to meet the body's demands for oxygen. A faster-than-normal heart rate—usually anything faster than 100 beats/min in an adult—with a normal-appearing ECG pattern is called sinus tachycardia. If sinus tachycardia becomes too fast, it can lead to decreased time for cardiac filling and a decrease in cardiac output. Many activities or conditions, such as exercise, fear, or stress, can cause sinus tachycardia. The underlying physical condition of the patient will determine whether this fast heart rate is problematic. Sinus bradycardia is a slower-than-normal heart rate (usually less than 60 beats/min) with a normal-appearing ECG pattern. Sinus bradycardia allows increased time for ventricular filling and decreases the oxygen need for the heart cells. This is often seen in athletes who have a slow heart rate. In other people, this rate might be too slow to adequately perfuse all of the tissues. A sinus pause or sinus arrest is when the SA node does not discharge an action potential and an ectopic pacemaker takes over the pacemaker functions.

Supraventricular Arrhythmias

Arrhythmias that originate above the ventricles but not in the SA node are called supraventricular arrhythmias. These arrhythmias feature an abnormally shaped P wave because the site of origin is not the sinus node. However, they show normal QRS complexes because the ventricles are still conducting impulses normally. Supraventricular arrhythmias include the following:

- *Premature atrial contractions*, which reflect an **ectopic focus** (a shift in the pacemaker of the heart from the SA node to some other site) in the atria that is generating an impulse out of the normal rhythm
- *Paroxysmal atrial tachycardia*, sporadically occurring runs of rapid heart rate originating in the atria
- *Atrial flutter*, characterized by sawtooth-shaped P waves reflecting a single ectopic focus that is generating a regular, fast atrial depolarization
- *Atrial fibrillation*, with irregular P waves representing many ectopic foci firing in an uncoordinated manner through the atria

With atrial flutter, often only one of every two to three impulses is transmitted to the ventricles. The person may have a 2:1 or 3:1 ratio of P waves to QRS complexes. The ventricles beat faster than normal, losing some efficiency. With atrial fibrillation, so many impulses are bombarding the AV node that the number of impulses transmitted to the ventricles becomes unpredictable. The ventricles are stimulated to beat in a fast, irregular, and often inefficient manner.

Atrioventricular Block

Atrioventricular (AV) block, also called heart block, reflects a slowing or lack of conduction at the AV node. This can occur because of structural damage, hypoxia, or injury to the heart muscle. First-degree heart block, in which all of the impulses from the SA node arrive in the ventricles after a longer-than-normal period, is characterized by a lengthening of the P–R interval beyond the normal 0.16 to 0.20 seconds. Each P wave is followed by a QRS complex. In second-degree heart block, some of the impulses are lost and do not get through, resulting in a slow rate of ventricular contraction. With this arrhythmia, a QRS complex may follow one, two, three, or four P waves. In third-degree heart block, or complete heart block, no impulses from the SA node get through to the ventricles, and the much slower ventricular automaticity takes over. The waveform shows a total dissociation of P waves from QRS complexes and T waves. Because the P waves can come at any time, the P–R interval is not constant. The QRS complexes appear at a slow rate and may not be sufficient to meet the body's needs.

Ventricular Arrhythmias

Impulses that originate below the AV node originate from ectopic foci that do not use the normal conduction pathways. The QRS complexes appear wide and prolonged, and the T waves are inverted, reflecting slower conduction across cardiac tissue that is not part of the rapid conduction system. Premature ventricular contractions (PVCs) can arise from a single ectopic focus in the ventricles, with all of them having the same shape, or from many ectopic foci, which produces PVCs with different shapes. Runs or bursts of PVCs from many different foci are more ominous because they can reflect extensive damage or hypoxia in the myocardium. Runs of several PVCs at a rapid rate are called ventricular tachycardia. A particular type of polymorphic ventricular tachycardia is called *torsade de pointes* (twisting or rotating around a point). This type of ventricular tachycardia is more likely to be triggered when there is a long QT interval. It results in a QRS complex in which polarity rotates from positive to negative on the ECG. Long QT syndrome can be an inherited trait or acquired due to electrolyte imbalance, infection, and/or medications. Ventricular fibrillation is seen as an irregular, distorted wave. It is potentially fatal because it reflects a lack of any coordinated stimulation of the ventricles. The ventricles' inability to contract in a coordinated fashion results in no blood being pumped to the body or the brain. Thus, there is a total loss of cardiac output.

Key Points

- The normal ECG waveform is made up of five main waves: the P wave, which is formed as impulses originating in the SA node or pacemaker pass through the atrial tissues; the QRS complex, which represents depolarization of the bundle of His (Q wave) and the ventricles (R and S waves); and the T wave, which represents repolarization of the ventricles.
- A person with a normal ECG pattern and a heart rate within the normal range for that person's age group is considered to be in normal sinus rhythm.
- When the generation of impulses is altered, the result is known as an arrhythmia (or dysrhythmia), which can upset the normal balance of the cardiovascular system. If there is a resulting decrease in cardiac output, all of the cells of the body will be affected.

Circulation

The purpose of the heart's continual pumping action is to keep blood flowing to and from all of the body's tissues and cells. Blood delivers oxygen and much-needed nutrients to the cells for energy production, and it carries away carbon dioxide and other waste products of metabolism. The steady circulation of blood is essential for the proper functioning of all of the body's organs, including the heart.

The circulation of the blood follows two courses:

- *Heart–lung or pulmonary circulation*: The right side of the heart sends blood to the lungs, where carbon dioxide and some waste products are removed from the blood and oxygen is picked up by the red blood cells.
- *Systemic circulation*: The left side of the heart sends oxygenated blood out to all of the cells in the body.

The heart muscle, like any other muscle, requires adequate oxygen and nutrients to function. This is accomplished via coronary circulation.

The blood moves from areas of high pressure to areas of lower pressure. The system is a "closed" system; that is, it has no openings or holes that would allow blood to leak out. The closed nature of the system is what keeps the pressure differences in the proper relationship so that blood always flows in the proper direction (Fig. 42.6).

Pulmonary Circulation

The right atrium is a low-pressure area in the cardiovascular system. All of the deoxygenated blood from the body

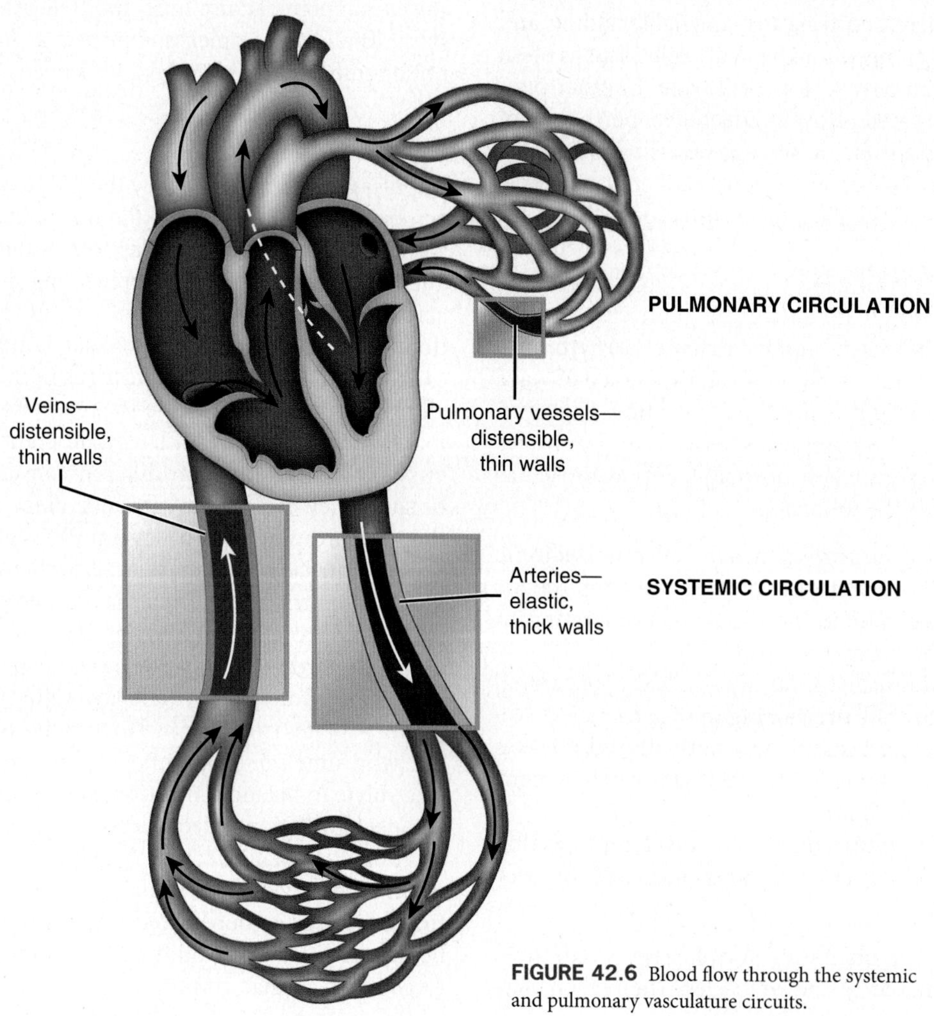

FIGURE 42.6 Blood flow through the systemic and pulmonary vasculature circuits.

flows into the right atrium from the inferior and superior venae cavae (see Fig. 42.1) and from the great cardiac vein, which returns deoxygenated blood to the heart muscle. As the blood flows into the atrium, the pressure increases. When the pressure becomes greater than the pressure in the right ventricle, most of the blood flows into the right ventricle; this is called the rapid-filling phase. At this point in the cardiac cycle, the atrium is stimulated to contract and pushes the remaining blood into the right ventricle. The ventricle is then stimulated to contract; it generates pressure that opens the pulmonic valve (see Fig. 42.1) and sends blood into the pulmonary artery, which takes the blood into the lungs, a low-pressure area. The blood then circulates around the alveoli of the lungs, picking up oxygen and getting rid of carbon dioxide; flows through pulmonary capillaries (the tiny blood vessels that connect arteries and veins) into the pulmonary veins; and then returns to the left atrium.

Systemic Circulation

When the pressure of blood volume in the left atrium is greater than the pressure in the large left ventricle, this oxygenated blood flows into the left ventricle. The left atrium contracts and pushes any remaining blood into the left ventricle, which is stimulated to contract, generating tremendous pressure to push the blood through the aorta, carrying it throughout the body. The aorta and other large arteries have thick, muscular walls. The entire arterial system contains muscles in the walls of the vessels all the way to the terminal branches or arterioles, which consist of fragments of muscle and endothelial cells. These muscles offer resistance to the blood that is sent pumping into the arterial system by the left ventricle, generating pressure. The arterial system is referred to as a **resistance system**. The vessels can either constrict or dilate, respectively increasing or decreasing resistance, based on the needs of the body. The arterioles are able to completely shut off blood flow to some areas of the body; that is, they can shunt blood to another area where it is needed more. The arterioles, because of their ability to increase or decrease resistance in the system, are one of the main regulators of blood pressure.

Blood from the tiny arterioles flows into the **capillary** system, which connects the arterial and venous systems. These microscopic vessels are composed of loosely connected endothelial cells. Oxygen, fluid, and nutrients are able to pass through the arterial end of the capillaries and enter the interstitial area between tissue cells. Fluid at the venous end of the capillary, which contains carbon dioxide and other waste products, is drawn back into the vessel. This shifting of fluid in the capillaries, called the capillary fluid shift, is carefully regulated by a balance between hydrostatic (fluid pressure) forces on the arterial end of the capillary and **oncotic pressure** (OP), the pulling pressure of the large vascular proteins on the venous end of the capillary. Normally, the higher pressure at the arterial end of a capillary forces fluid out of the vessel and into the tissue, and the now-concentrated proteins (which are too large to leave the capillary) exert a pull on the fluid at the venous end of the capillary to pull it back in. A disruption in the **hydrostatic pressure** (HP), which is the pushing force of fluid against solid objects, or in the concentration of proteins in the capillary can lead to fluid being left in the tissue, a condition referred to as edema. The capillaries merge into venules, which merge into veins, the vessels responsible for returning the blood to the heart (Fig. 42.7).

The veins are thin-walled, very elastic, low-pressure vessels that can hold large quantities of blood if necessary. The venous system is referred to as a **capacitance system**

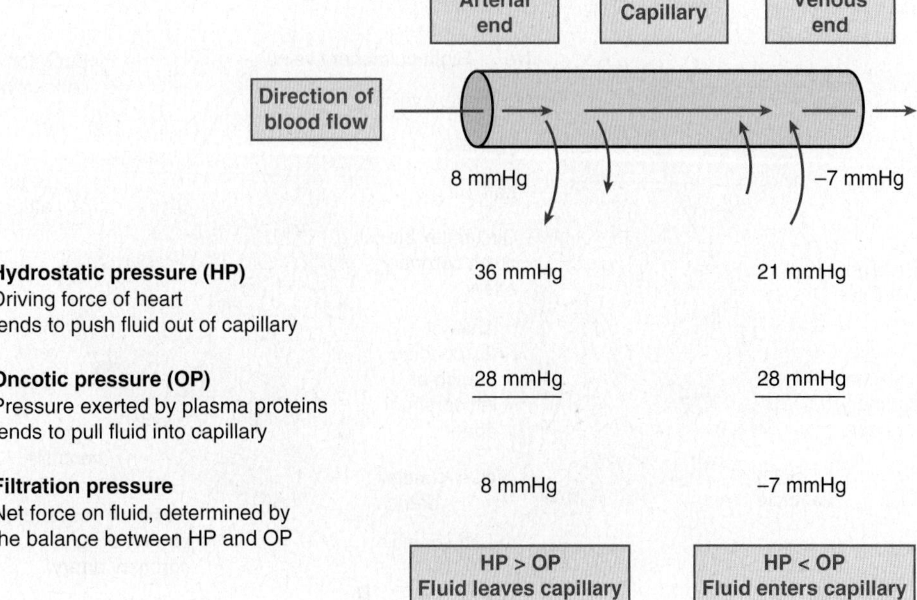

FIGURE 42.7 The net shift of fluid out of and into the capillary is determined by the balance between the hydrostatic pressure (HP) and the oncotic pressure (OP). The HP tends to push fluid out of the capillary, and the OP tends to pull it back into the capillary. At the arterial end of the capillary bed, the blood pressure is higher than at the venous end. At the arterial end, HP exceeds OP and fluid filters out. At the venous end, HP has fallen and is less than OP; fluid is pulled back into the capillary from the surrounding tissue. The lymphatic system also returns fluids and substances from the tissues to the circulation.

because the veins have the capacity to hold large quantities of fluid as they distend with fluid volume. These capacitance vessels have a great deal of influence on the amount of blood that is delivered to the right atrium in the venous return to the heart.

Coronary Circulation

The heart muscle requires a constant supply of oxygenated blood to keep contracting. The myocardium receives its blood through two main coronary arteries that branch off the base of the aorta from an area called the sinuses of Valsalva. These arteries encircle the heart in a pattern resembling a crown, which is why they are called "coronary" arteries.

The left coronary artery arises from the left side of the aorta and bifurcates, or divides, into two large vessels called the left circumflex artery (which travels down the left side of the heart and feeds most of the left lateral wall of the ventricle) and the left anterior descending coronary artery (which travels down the front of the heart and feeds the septum and anterior areas of the left ventricle, including much of the conduction system). The artery arising from the right side of the aorta, called the right coronary artery, supplies most of the right side of the heart, including the SA node.

The coronary arteries receive blood during diastole, when the muscle is at rest and relaxed so that blood can flow freely into the muscle. When the ventricle contracts, it forces the aortic valve open, which in turn causes the leaflets of the valve to cover the openings of the coronary arteries. When the ventricles relax, the blood is no longer pumped forward and starts to flow back toward the ventricle. The blood flowing down the sides of the aorta closes the aortic valve and fills the coronary arteries. The pressure in the coronary arteries is the difference between the systolic (ejection) pressure and the diastolic (resting) pressure. This is called the **pulse pressure** (systolic minus diastolic blood pressure readings). The pulse pressure is monitored clinically to evaluate the filling pressure of the coronary arteries. The oxygenated blood that is fed into the heart by the coronary circulation reaches every cardiac muscle fiber as the vessels divide and subdivide throughout the myocardium (Fig. 42.8).

The heart has a pattern of circulation called end artery circulation. The arteries go into the muscle and end without a great deal of backup or collateral circulation. Normally, this is an efficient system and is able to meet the needs of the heart muscle. The heart's supply of and demand for oxygen are met by changes in the delivery of oxygen through the coronary artery system. Problems can arise, however, when an imbalance develops between the supply of oxygen delivered to the heart muscle and the myocardial demand for oxygen.

The main forces that determine the heart's use of oxygen or oxygen consumption include the following:

- *Heart rate*: The more the heart has to pump, the more oxygen it requires.
- *Preload (amount of blood that is brought back to the heart to be pumped throughout the body)*: The more blood that is returned to the heart, the harder it will have to work to pump the blood. The volume of blood in the system is a determinant of preload. The more blood that is returned, the greater the stretch on the ventricles.
- *Afterload (resistance against which the heart has to beat)*: The higher the resistance in the system, the harder the heart will have to contract to force open the valves and pump the blood. Blood pressure is a measure of afterload.
- *Contractility*: This is increased with more influx of calcium into the heart cell. More calcium allows for more actomyosin bridges and less relaxation of the muscles.

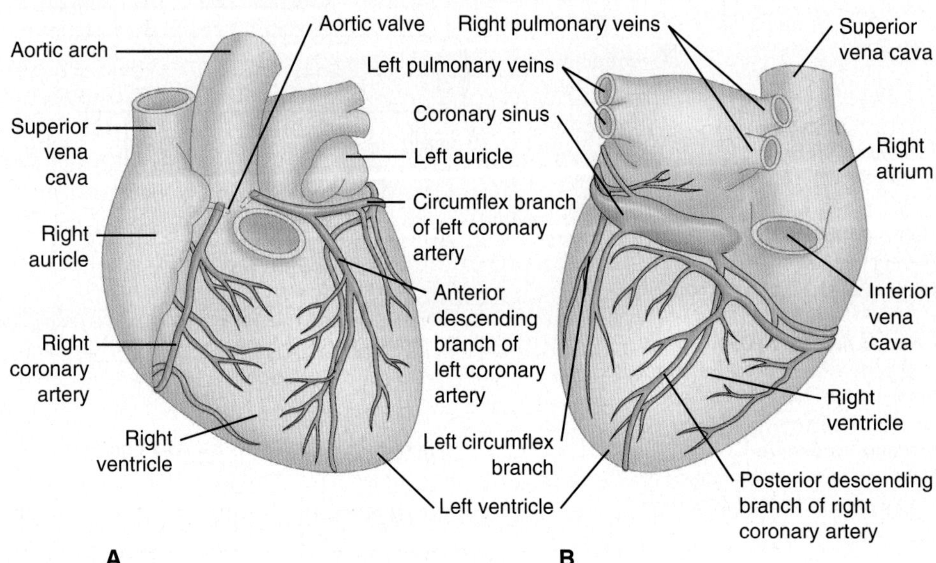

FIGURE 42.8 Coronary arteries and veins. **A.** Anterior view. **B.** Posterior view.

This causes more force of contraction and greater need for oxygen in the heart cells. This will be higher with increased sympathetic nervous system stimulation. The supply of blood to the myocardium can be altered if the heart fails to pump effectively and cannot deliver blood to the coronary arteries. This may happen in HF and cases of hypotension. The supply is most frequently altered, however, when the coronary vessels become narrow and unresponsive to stimuli to dilate and deliver more blood. This happens in atherosclerosis or coronary artery disease. The end result of this narrowing can be total blockage of a coronary artery, leading to hypoxia and eventual death of the cells that depend on that vessel for oxygen. This is called a myocardial infarction or heart attack.

Systemic Arterial Pressure

The contraction of the left ventricle, which sends blood surging out into the aorta, creates pressure that continues to force blood into all of the branches of the aorta. This pressure against arterial walls is greatest during systole (cardiac contraction) and falls to its lowest level during diastole. Measurement of both the systolic and the diastolic pressures indicates both the pumping pressure of the ventricle and the generalized pressure in the system, or the pressure the ventricle has to overcome to pump blood out of the heart.

Hypotension

The pressure of the blood in the arteries needs to remain relatively high to ensure that blood is delivered to every cell in the body and to keep the blood flowing from high-pressure to low-pressure areas. The pressure can fall dramatically—termed hypotension—from loss of blood volume, excessive vasodilation, or from failure of the heart muscle to pump effectively. Severe hypotension can progress to shock and even death as cells are not able to get the oxygen and nutrients they need.

Hypertension

Constant, excessive high blood pressure—called hypertension—can damage the fragile inner lining of blood vessels and cause a disruption of blood flow to the tissues. It also puts a tremendous strain on the heart muscle, increasing myocardial oxygen consumption and putting the heart muscle at risk. Hypertension can be caused by neurostimulation of the blood vessels that causes them to constrict, subsequently raising pressure, or by increased volume in the system. In most cases, the cause of hypertension is not known, and drug therapy to correct it is aimed at changing one or more of the normal reflexes that control vascular resistance or the force of cardiac muscle contraction.

Vasomotor Tone

The smooth muscles in the walls of the arteries receive constant input from nerve fibers of the sympathetic nervous system. These impulses work to dilate the vessels if more blood flow is needed in an area, to constrict vessels if increased pressure is needed in the system, and to maintain muscle tone so that the vessels remain patent and responsive. The nerves work by opening and closing calcium channels. When the calcium channels are open and the calcium can cross the muscle membrane, the smooth muscle contracts and constricts the blood vessel. There are also local chemicals that can influence the vasoconstriction and dilation of blood vessels. For example, nitric oxide released from the endothelium produces smooth muscle relaxation and vasodilation.

The coordination of neural impulses is regulated through the medulla in an area called the cardiovascular center. If increased pressure is needed, this center increases sympathetic flow to the vessels. If pressure becomes too high, it is sensed by baroreceptors or pressure receptors, and the sympathetic flow is decreased. Chapter 43 discusses the drugs that are used to influence the stimulation of vessels to alter blood pressure.

Humoral Mechanisms of Blood Pressure Control

There are chemicals released into the blood that assist with blood pressure regulation. One of the more powerful controls of blood pressure results from chemicals released from the renin–angiotensin–aldosterone system (Fig. 42.9). This system is activated when blood flow to the kidneys is decreased. The juxtaglomerular cells, near the afferent arterioles in the kidney, release an enzyme called renin. Renin is released into the bloodstream and converts the protein angiotensinogen (produced in the liver) to **angiotensin** I. Angiotensin I travels to the lungs, where it is converted by angiotensin-converting enzyme to angiotensin II. Angiotensin II travels through the body and reacts with angiotensin II receptor sites on blood vessels to cause severe vasoconstriction. This increases blood pressure and should increase blood flow to the kidneys to decrease the release of renin. Angiotensin II contributes to longer-term control of blood pressure by stimulating the release of **aldosterone** from the adrenal cortex. Aldosterone acts in the kidneys to retain more sodium and water. This system works constantly, whenever a position change alters flow to the kidney or blood volume or when pressure changes, to help maintain the blood pressure within a range that ensures perfusion (delivery of blood to all of the tissues).

Low blood volume, low blood pressure, and/or high blood osmolality will trigger vasopressin, or **antidiuretic hormone** (**ADH**), to be released from the posterior pituitary. This substance acts in the kidneys to cause more retention of water, which increases blood volume. Increasing blood volume increases blood flow to the kidney and affects the amount of renin that is released.

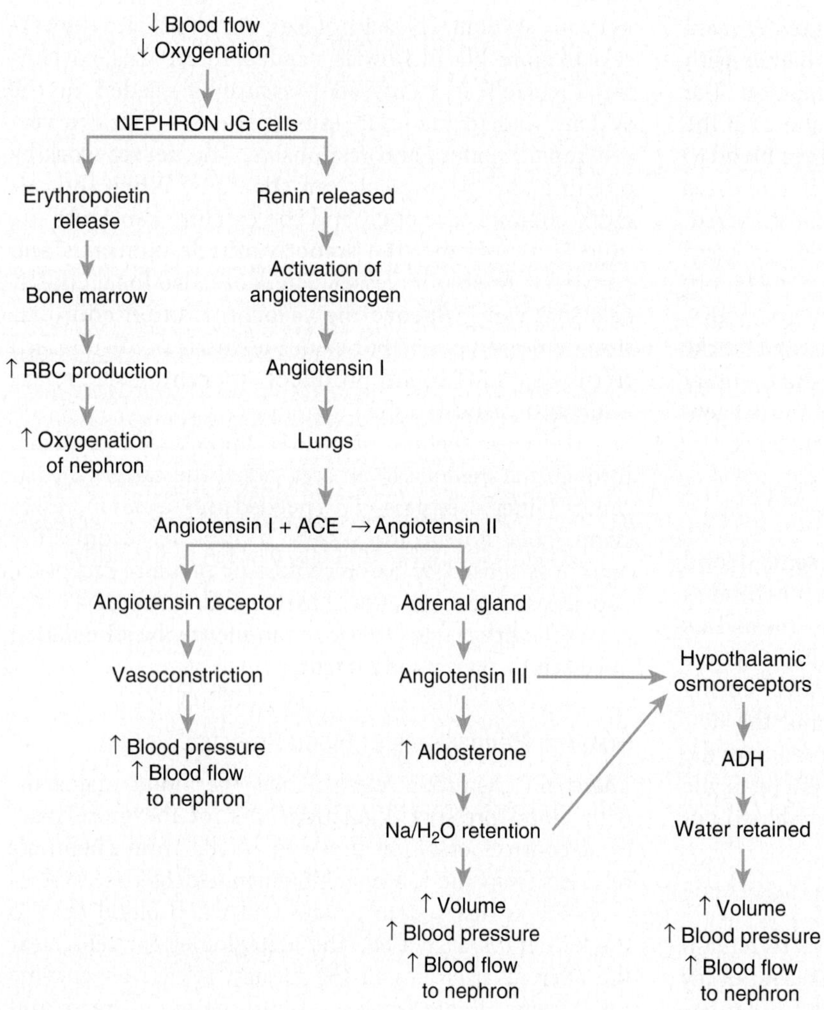

FIGURE 42.9 The renin–angiotensin–aldosterone system for reflex maintenance of blood pressure control.

Natriuretic Peptides

Natriuretic peptides are formed in the atria of the heart, where they are called atrial natriuretic peptides (ANPs), and in the atria and ventricles, where they are called brain natriuretic peptides (BNPs). There are other natriuretic peptides, labeled CNPs (C-type natriuretic peptides), thought to act in the vasculature, and DNPs (dendroaspis natriuretic peptides), thought to be released from the atria, though not as much research is available on these two peptides. The natriuretic peptides act to inhibit the renin–angiotensin–aldosterone system and cause a diuretic, natriuretic, and blood pressure–lowering effect. They are broken down in the body by the enzyme neprilysin. ANP and BNP are released in response to high heart chamber–filling pressure, which is linked to volume overload. Volume overload can result from a weak heart muscle and/or poor kidney function.

Venous Pressure

Blood in the veins also exerts pressure that may sometimes rise above normal. This can happen if the heart is not pumping effectively and is unable to pump out all of the blood that is trying to return to it. This results in a backup or congestion of blood waiting to enter the heart. Pressure rises in the right atrium and then in the veins that are trying to return blood to the heart as they encounter resistance. The venous system begins to back up, or become congested with blood.

Heart Failure

If the heart muscle fails to do its job of effectively pumping blood through the system, blood backs up and the system becomes congested. This is called heart failure (HF). The rise in venous pressure that results from this backup of blood increases the HP in the venous end of the capillaries. The HP pushing fluid out of the capillary is soon higher than the OP that is trying to pull the fluid back into the vessel, causing fluid to be lost into the tissues. This shift of fluid accounts for the edema seen with HF. Pulmonary edema results when the left side of the heart fails. Peripheral, abdominal, and liver edema occurs when the right side of the heart fails.

Other factors, including protein loss and fluid retention, can contribute to a loss of fluid in the tissues. Protein loss can lead to a fall in OP and an inability to pull fluid back into the vascular system. Protein levels fall in renal failure, when protein is lost in the urine, and in liver failure, when the liver is no longer able to produce plasma proteins. Fluid retention, which often is stimulated by aldosterone and ADH as described earlier, can increase the HP so greatly that fluid is pushed out under higher pressure, and the balancing pressure to pull it back into the vessel is not sufficient. Drugs that are used to treat HF may affect the vascular system at any of these areas in an attempt to return a balance to the pressures in the system.

Key Points

- Blood pressure is maintained by stimuli from the sympathetic system and reflex control of blood volume and pressure by the renin–angiotensin system and the aldosterone–ADH system. Alterations in blood pressure (hypotension or hypertension) can upset the balance of the cardiovascular system and lead to problems in blood delivery.
- Fluid shifts out of the blood at the arterial ends of capillaries to deliver oxygen and nutrients to the tissues. It moves out due to the hydrostatic or fluid pressure of the arterial side of the system. Fluid returns to the system at the venous end of the capillaries because of the oncotic pull of proteins in the vessels. Disruptions in these pressures can lead to edema or loss of fluid in the tissues.

SUMMARY

- The heart is a hollow muscle that is divided into a right and a left side by a thick septum and into four chambers—the two upper atria and the two lower ventricles. The right side of the heart receives all of the deoxygenated blood from the body through the veins and directs it into the lungs. The left side of the heart receives oxygenated blood from the lungs and pumps it out to every cell in the body through the arteries.
- The cardiovascular system is responsible for delivering oxygenated blood to every cell in the body and for picking up waste products from the tissues.
- The cardiac cycle consists of a period of rest, or diastole, when blood is returned to the heart by veins, and a period of contraction, or systole, when the blood is pumped out of the heart.
- The heart muscle possesses the properties of automaticity (the ability to generate an action potential in the absence of stimulation) and conductivity (the ability to rapidly transmit an action potential).
- The heart muscle is stimulated to contract by impulses generated in the heart, not by stimuli from the brain or nervous system. However, the autonomic nervous system can affect the heart to increase (sympathetic) or decrease (parasympathetic) activity.
- In normal sinus rhythm, cells in the SA node generate an impulse that is transmitted through the atrial bundles and delayed slightly at the AV node before being sent down the bundle of His into the ventricles. When cardiac muscle cells are stimulated, they contract.
- Alterations in the generation of conduction of impulses in the heart cause arrhythmias (dysrhythmias), which can upset the normal balance in the cardiovascular system and lead to a decrease in cardiac output, affecting all cells of the body.
- Heart muscle contracts by the sliding of actin and myosin filaments in a functioning unit called a sarcomere. Contraction requires energy and calcium to allow the filaments to react with each other and slide together.
- The heart muscle needs a constant supply of blood, which is furnished by the coronary arteries. Increase in demand for oxygen can occur with changes in heart rate, preload, afterload, or contractility of the muscle.
- The cardiovascular system is a closed pressure system that uses arteries (muscular, pressure, or resistance vessels) to carry blood from the heart, veins (flexible, distensible capacitance vessels) to return blood to the heart, and capillaries (which connect arteries to veins) to keep blood flowing from areas of high pressure to areas of low pressure.
- Blood pressure is maintained by stimulus from the sympathetic system and reflex control of blood volume and pressure by the renin–angiotensin system and the aldosterone–ADH system. Alterations in blood pressure (hypotension or hypertension) can upset the balance of the cardiovascular system and lead to problems in blood delivery.
- Fluid shifts out of the blood at the arterial ends of capillaries to deliver oxygen and nutrients to the tissues. It moves out due to the hydrostatic or fluid pressure of the arterial side of the system. Fluid returns to the system at the venous end of the capillaries because of the oncotic pull of proteins in the vessels. Disruptions in these pressures can lead to edema or loss of fluid in the tissues.

CHECK YOUR UNDERSTANDING

Answers to the questions in this chapter can be found in Answers to Check Your Understanding Questions on thePoint®.

MULTIPLE CHOICE

Select the best answer.

1. When describing heart valves to a group of students, which information would the instructor include?
   a. The closing of the AV valves is what is solely responsible for heart sounds.
   b. Small muscles attached to the AV valves are responsible for opening and closing the valves.
   c. The aortic valve opens when the pressure in the left ventricle becomes greater than the aortic pressure.
   d. The valves leading to the great vessels are called the cuspid valves.

2. In the heart, the
   a. ventricles will not contract unless they are stimulated by action potentials arising from the SA node.
   b. fibrillation of the atria will cause blood pressure to fall to zero.
   c. absence of nerve stimulation can cause spontaneous depolarization of the muscle membrane.
   d. muscle can continue to contract for a long period of time in the absence of oxygen.

3. The activity of the heart depends on both the inherent properties of the cardiac muscle cells and the activity of the autonomic nerves to the heart. Therefore,
   a. cutting all of the autonomic nerves to the heart produces a decrease in resting heart rate.
   b. blocking the parasympathetic nerves to the heart decreases the heart rate.
   c. stimulating the sympathetic nerves to the heart increases the time available to fill the ventricles during diastole.
   d. the heart rate will increase in cases of dehydration, which will lead to less filling time.

4. A heart transplantation patient has no nerve connections to the transplanted heart. In such a person, one would expect to find
   a. a slower-than-normal resting heart rate.
   b. atria that contract at a different rate than ventricles.
   c. an increase in heart rate during emotional stress.
   d. inability to exercise because there is no way to increase heart rate.

5. Which is correct regarding the cardiac cycle?
   a. Blood that has a high amount of oxygen enters the left atrium.
   b. Blood that has a high amount of oxygen enters the right ventricle.
   c. The highest pressure is found in the right ventricle of the heart.
   d. The mitral valve allows for bidirectional blood flow.

6. Cardiac cells differ from skeletal muscle cells in that they
   a. contain actin and myosin.
   b. possess automaticity and conductivity.
   c. require calcium for muscle contraction to occur.
   d. do not require oxygen to survive.

7. Clinically, dysrhythmias, or arrhythmias, may cause
   a. altered cardiac output that could affect all cells.
   b. changes in capillary filling pressures.
   c. alterations in osmotic pressure.
   d. valvular dysfunction.

8. A patient is brought to the emergency room with a suspected myocardial infarction. The patient is upset because they had just had an ECG in their provider's office and it was fine. The explanation of this common phenomenon would include the fact that the ECG
   a. only reflects changes in cardiac output.
   b. is not a very accurate test.
   c. only measures the flow of electrical current through the heart.
   d. is not related to the heart problems.

9. Blood flow to the myocardium differs from blood flow to the rest of the cells of the body in that blood
   a. perfuses the myocardium during systole.
   b. flow is determined by many local factors, including buildup of acid.
   c. perfuses the myocardium during diastole.
   d. that is oxygenated flows to the myocardium via veins.

MULTIPLE RESPONSE

Select all that apply.

1. During diastole, which would occur?
   a. Opening of the AV valves
   b. Relaxation of the myocardial muscle
   c. Flow of blood from the atria to the ventricles
   d. Contraction of the ventricles
   e. Closing of the semilunar valves
   f. Filling of the coronary arteries

2. The sympathetic nervous system would be expected to have which effects?
   a. Stimulates the heart to beat faster
   b. Speeds conduction through the AV node
   c. Causes the heart muscle to contract harder
   d. Slows conduction through the AV node
   e. Decreases overall vascular volume
   f. Increases total peripheral resistance

REFERENCES

Barrett, K. E., Barman, S. M., Boitano, S., & Brooks, H. L. (2015). *Ganong's review of medical physiology* (25th ed.). McGraw-Hill.

Bonow, R. O., Mann, D. L., Libby, P., & Zipes, D. P. (Eds.). (2014). *Braunwald's heart disease: A textbook of cardiovascular medicine* (10th ed.). W. B. Saunders.

Brunton, L., Hilal-Dandan, R., & Knollman, B. (2018). *Goodman and Gilman's the pharmacological basis of therapeutics* (13th ed.). McGraw-Hill.

Fuster, V., Alexander, R. W., & Rourke, R. A. (Eds.). (2011). *Hurst's the heart* (13th ed.). McGraw-Hill.

Hall, J. E., & Hall, M. E. (2021). *Guyton and Hall's textbook of medical physiology* (14th ed.). Saunders.

Norris, T. L. (2019). *Porth's pathophysiology concepts of altered health states* (10th ed.). Wolters Kluwer.

CHAPTER 43

Drugs Affecting Blood Pressure

Learning Objectives

Upon completion of this chapter, you will be able to:

1. Outline the normal controls of blood pressure and explain how the various drugs used to treat hypertension or hypotension affect these controls.
2. Discuss the use of drugs that affect blood pressure across the lifespan.
3. Describe the therapeutic actions, indications, pharmacokinetics, contraindications, most common adverse effects, and important drug–drug interactions associated with drugs affecting blood pressure.
4. Compare and contrast the prototype drugs captopril, losartan, diltiazem, nitroprusside, and droxidopa with other agents in their classes and with other agents used to affect blood pressure.
5. Outline the nursing considerations, including important teaching points, for patients receiving drugs used to affect blood pressure.

Key Terms

angiotensin-converting enzyme (ACE) inhibitor: drug that blocks ACE, the enzyme responsible for converting angiotensin I to angiotensin II in the lungs; this blocking reduces the vasoconstriction and aldosterone release related to angiotensin II

angiotensin II receptors: specific receptors found in the vascular smooth muscle of the blood vessels and in the adrenal gland that react with angiotensin II to cause vasoconstriction and release of aldosterone

baroreceptor: pressure receptor; located in the arch of the aorta and in the carotid artery; responds to changes in pressure and influences the medulla to stimulate the sympathetic system to increase or decrease blood pressure

cardiovascular center: area of the medulla at which stimulation will activate the sympathetic nervous system to increase blood pressure and heart rate

essential or primary hypertension: sustained blood pressure above normal limits with no discernible underlying cause

hypotension: sustained blood pressure that is lower than that required to adequately perfuse all of the body's tissues

peripheral resistance (PVR): force that resists the flow of blood through the vessels, mostly determined by the arterioles, which contract to increase resistance; important in determining overall blood pressure

renin–angiotensin–aldosterone system (RAAS): compensatory process that leads to increased blood pressure and blood volume to ensure perfusion of the kidneys; important in the continual regulation of blood pressure

shock: severe hypotension that can lead to accumulation of waste products and cell death

stroke volume: amount of blood pumped out of the ventricle with each beat; important in determining blood pressure

Drug List

ANTIHYPERTENSIVE AGENTS

Drugs Affecting the Renin–Angiotensin–Aldosterone System

Angiotensin-Converting Enzyme Inhibitors

benazepril
(P) captopril
enalapril
enalaprilat
fosinopril
lisinopril
moexipril
perindopril
quinapril
ramipril
trandolapril

Angiotensin II Receptor Blockers

azilsartan
candesartan
irbesartan
(P) losartan
olmesartan
telmisartan
valsartan

Direct Renin Inhibitor
aliskiren

Calcium-Channel Blockers
amlodipine
clevidipine
diltiazem
felodipine
isradipine
levamlodipine
nicardipine
nifedipine
nisoldipine
verapamil

Vasodilators
hydralazine
minoxidil
nitroglycerin
nitroprusside

Vasodilators for Pulmonary Artery Hypertension
ambrisentan
bosentan
epoprostenol
iloprost
sildenafil
tadalafil
treprostinil

Other Antihypertensive Agents

Diuretic Agents

Thiazide and Thiazidelike Diuretics
chlorothiazide
chlorthalidone
hydrochlorothiazide
indapamide
metolazone

Potassium-Sparing Diuretics
amiloride
eplerenone
spironolactone
triamterene

Sympathetic Nervous System Drugs

Beta-Blockers
acebutolol
atenolol
betaxolol
bisoprolol
esmolol
metoprolol
nadolol
nebivolol
pindolol
propranolol
timolol

Alpha- and Beta-Blockers
carvedilol
labetalol

Alpha-Adrenergic Blockers
phenoxybenzamine
phentolamine

$Alpha_1$-Blockers
doxazosin
prazosin
terazosin

$Alpha_2$-Agonists
clonidine
guanfacine
methyldopa

ANTIHYPOTENSIVE AGENTS

Sympathetic Adrenergic Agonists or Vasopressors
dobutamine
dopamine
droxidopa
ephedrine
epinephrine
isoproterenol
midodrine
norepinephrine
phenylephrine
vasopressin

The cardiovascular (CV) system is a closed system of blood vessels that is responsible for delivering oxygenated blood to the tissues and removing waste products from the tissues. The blood in this system flows from areas of higher pressure to areas of lower pressure. The area of highest pressure in the system is typically the left ventricle during systole. The pressure in this area propels the blood out of the aorta and into the system. The lowest pressure is in the right atrium, which collects all of the deoxygenated blood from the body. The maintenance of this pressure system is controlled by specific areas of the brain and various hormones. If the pressure becomes too high, the person is said to be hypertensive. If the pressure becomes too low and blood cannot be delivered effectively, the person is said to be hypotensive. Severe low blood pressure (BP) is called **shock** and is a life-threatening situation. Helping the patient maintain BP within normal limits is the goal of drug therapy.

Review of Blood Pressure Control

The mean arterial pressure (MAP) is the average pressure in the arteries during ventricular contraction and relaxation. The MAP is determined by three elements:

- Heart rate
- **Stroke volume**, or the amount of blood that is pumped out of the ventricle with each heartbeat
- Total **peripheral resistance (PVR)**, or the resistance of the muscular arteries to the blood being pumped through

Cardiac output (CO) is heart rate multiplied by stroke volume. Therefore, the mathematical equation for MAP is: MAP = CO × PVR.

The small arterioles are thought to be the most important factors in determining PVR. Because they have the smallest diameter, they are able to almost stop blood flow into capillary beds when they constrict, building up tremendous pressure in the arteries behind them as they prevent the blood from flowing through. The arterioles are responsive to stimulation from the sympathetic nervous system; they constrict when the sympathetic system is stimulated, increasing total PVR and MAP. The body uses this responsiveness to regulate BP on a constant basis to ensure that there is enough pressure in the system to deliver sufficient blood to the brain.

Autonomic Nervous System

The autonomic nervous system is a powerful regulator of BP. The parasympathetic system primarily lowers BP by decreasing heart rate and contractility. The sympathetic nervous system acts directly on the heart muscle to increase heart rate and contractility. The sympathetic nerve fibers also innervate the arteries to constrict and decrease blood flow to tissues and innervate veins to constrict and decrease the blood volume held within the venous system. The sympathetic and parasympathetic nerve fibers that stimulate the heart and blood vessels are innervated by the vasomotor center located in the medulla and pons area of the brain. The nerves from the higher levels of the brain (cerebral cortex and hypothalamus) are able to excite and inhibit the vasomotor center.

During stressful situations and during exercise, the vasomotor system can increase both the CO and PVR so that the MAP increases. In conjunction with local vasodilation of the skeletal muscle blood vessels, the increase in MAP increases the blood flow that is needed for body movement.

Baroreceptors and Other Reflexes

As the blood leaves the left ventricle through the aorta, it influences specialized cells in the arch of the aorta called **baroreceptors** (pressure receptors). Similar cells are located in the carotid arteries, which deliver blood directly to the brain. If there is sufficient pressure in these vessels, the baroreceptors are stimulated, sending that information to the brain. If the pressure falls, the stimulation of the baroreceptors falls off. That information is also sent to the brain.

The sensory input from the baroreceptors is received in the medulla in an area called the **cardiovascular center** or vasomotor center. If the pressure is high, the medulla stimulates vasodilation and a decrease in cardiac rate and output via the parasympathetic nervous system, causing the pressure in the system to drop. If the pressure is low, the medulla directly stimulates an increase in cardiac rate and output and vasoconstriction via the sympathetic nervous system; this increases total PVR and raises the BP. The medulla mediates these effects through the autonomic nervous system (see Chapter 29).

The baroreceptor reflex functions continually maintain BP within a predetermined range of normal. For example, if you have been lying down flat and suddenly stand up, the blood will rush to your feet (an effect of gravity). You may even feel lightheaded or dizzy for a short time. When you stand and the blood flow drops, the baroreceptors are not stretched. The medulla senses this drop in stimulation of the baroreceptors and stimulates a rise in cardiac output and a generalized vasoconstriction, which increases total PVR and BP. These increases should raise pressure in the system, which restores blood flow to the brain and stimulates the baroreceptors. The stimulation of the baroreceptors leads to a decrease in stimulatory impulses from the medulla, and the BP falls back within normal limits (Fig. 43.1).

Chemoreceptors work very similarly to baroreceptors except they are innervated by low oxygen or high carbon dioxide and hydrogen ion levels. When innervated, the chemoreceptors can excite the vasomotor center to increase arterial pressure back to a normal level. It is more influential when the BP has dropped below 80 mm Hg.

Renin–Angiotensin–Aldosterone System

Another compensatory system is activated when the BP within the kidneys falls. Because the kidneys require constant perfusion to function properly, they have a compensatory mechanism to help ensure blood flow is maintained. This mechanism is called the **renin–angiotensin–aldosterone system** (RAAS).

Low BP or poor oxygenation of a nephron causes the release of renin from the juxtaglomerular cells, a group of cells that monitor BP and flow into the glomerulus. Renin is released into the bloodstream and reacts with angiotensinogen (made in the liver) to produce angiotensin I. Angiotensin I travels in the bloodstream to the lungs, where the metabolic cells of the alveoli use angiotensin-converting enzyme (ACE) to convert angiotensin I to angiotensin II. Angiotensin II reacts with specific angiotensin II receptor sites on blood vessels to cause intense vasoconstriction. This effect raises the total PVR and raises the BP, restoring blood flow to the kidneys and decreasing the release of renin.

Angiotensin II, probably after conversion to angiotensin III, also stimulates the adrenal cortex to release aldosterone. Aldosterone acts on the nephrons to cause the retention of sodium and water. This effect increases blood volume, which should also contribute to increasing BP. The sodium-rich blood stimulates the osmoreceptors in the hypothalamus to cause the release of antidiuretic hormone, which in turn causes retention of water in the nephrons, further increasing the blood volume. This increase in blood volume increases the BP, which should increase blood flow to the kidneys. This should lead to a decrease in the release of renin, thus causing the compensatory mechanisms to stop (Fig. 43.2).

Hypertension

When a person's BP is above the normal limit for a sustained period, a diagnosis of hypertension is made. It is estimated that about 45% of adults in the United States have hypertension, and many are unaware of it. Only about 54% of the patients being treated for hypertension are thought to have it under control. It is also estimated that one in three adults in the United States has what is called prehypertension and could avert or delay hypertension with lifestyle changes.

Of people with hypertension, 90% have what is called **essential or primary hypertension**, or hypertension with no known cause. People with essential hypertension usually have elevated total PVR. Their organs are being perfused effectively, and they usually display no symptoms. A few people develop secondary hypertension, or high BP, resulting from a known cause. For instance, a tumor in the adrenal medulla called a pheochromocytoma can cause hypertension related to the release of large amounts of norepinephrine from tumor cells; the hypertension resolves after the tumor is removed.

The underlying danger of hypertension of any type is body organ damage. Organ damage from chronic hypertension can occur within the heart, kidneys, brain, eyes, blood vessels, and other organs. High intravascular

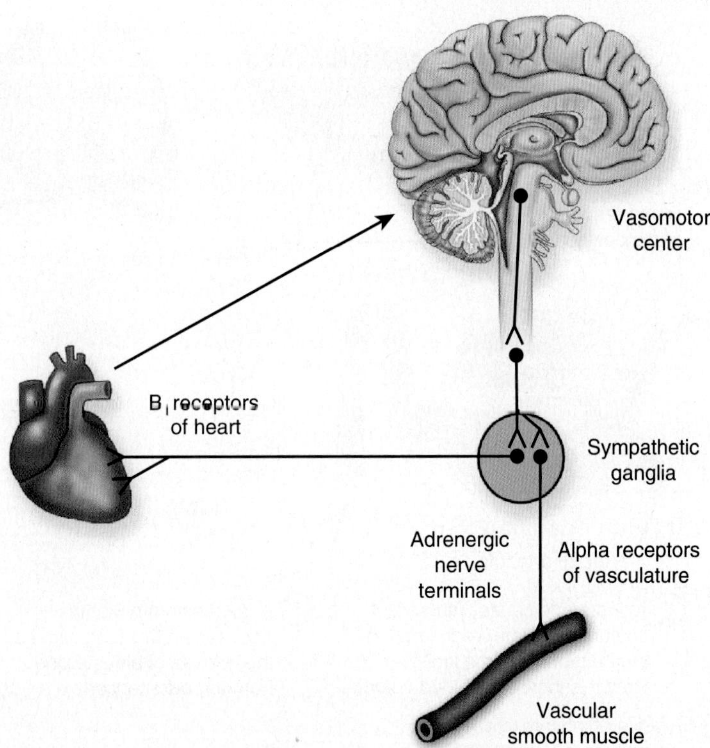

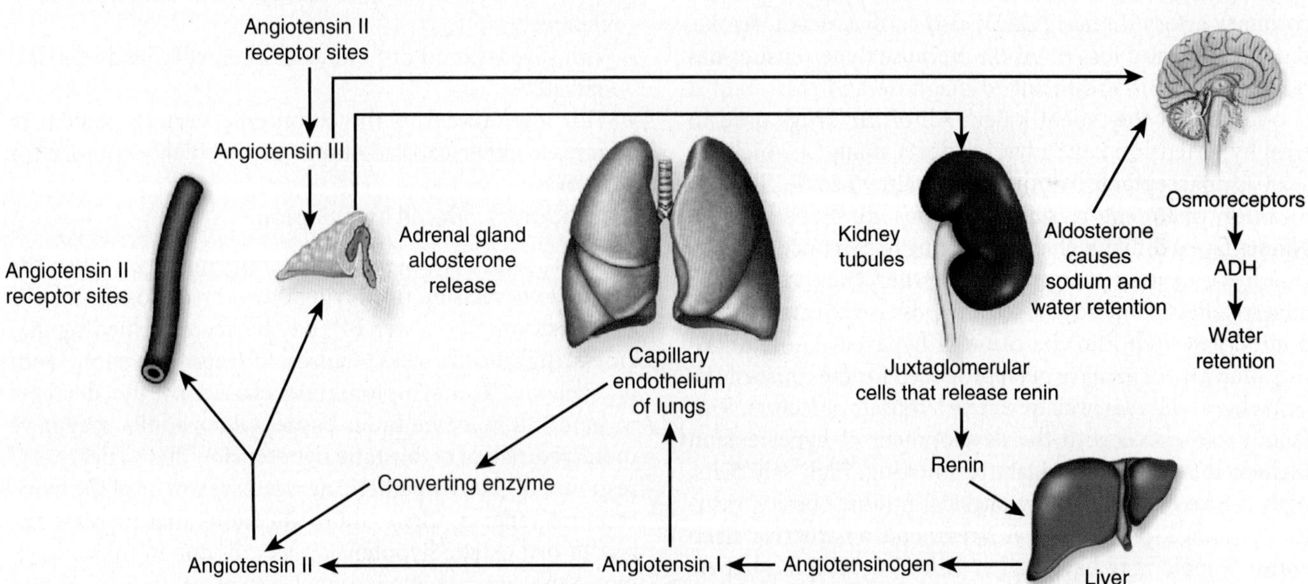

FIGURE 43.1 Control of blood pressure. The vasomotor center in the medulla responds to stimuli from aortic and carotid baroreceptors to cause sympathetic stimulation. The kidneys release renin to activate the renin–angiotensin–aldosterone system, causing vasoconstriction and increased blood volume.

pressure can harm the endothelial lining of the blood vessels, which increases the risk of development of atherosclerotic vascular disease (see Chapter 46). Atherosclerotic vascular disease is the leading cause of ischemic heart and brain disease. Damage to the blood vessels can also cause visual impairment and renal dysfunction. Chronic hypertension can cause the left ventricle to thicken because the muscle must constantly work hard to expel blood at a greater force. The thickening of the heart muscle and the increased pressure that the muscle has to generate every time it contracts increase the workload of the heart and the risk of heart failure. Tiny vessels can be damaged and destroyed, leading to losses of vision (if the vessels are in the retina), kidney function (if the vessels include the glomeruli in the nephrons), or cerebral function (if the vessels are the small and fragile vessels in the brain).

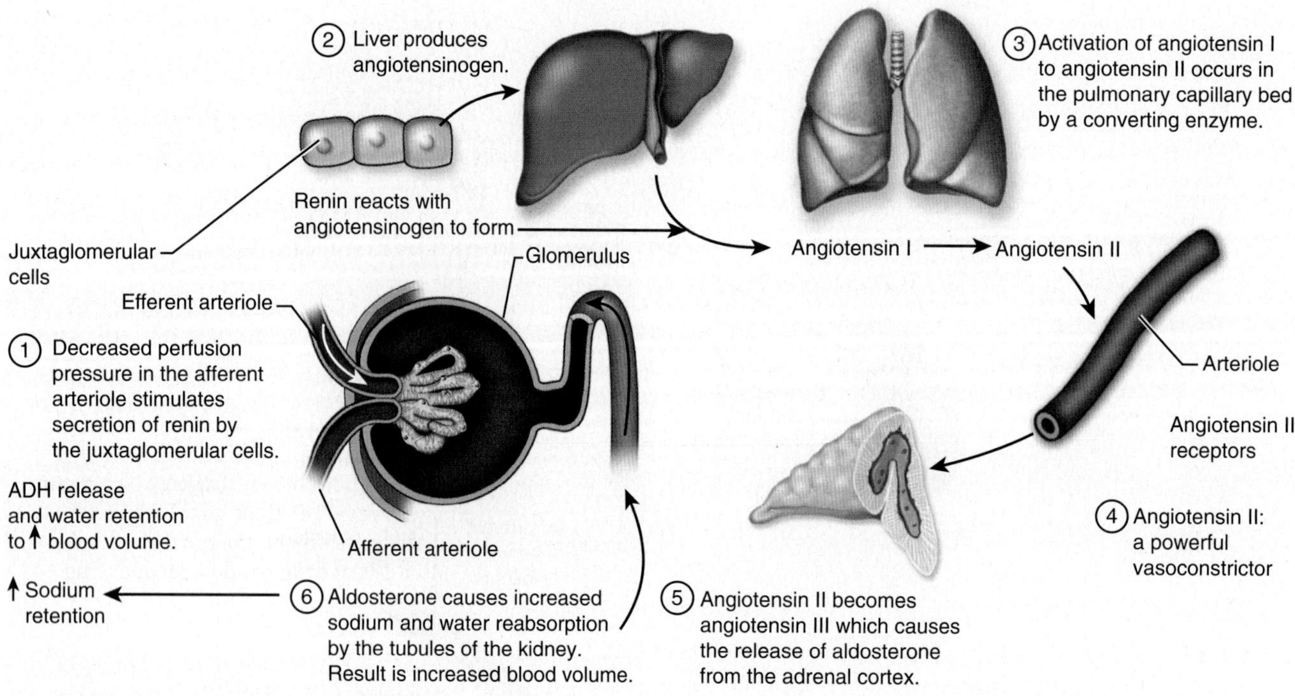

2 Liver produces angiotensinogen.
3 Activation of angiotensin I to angiotensin II occurs in the pulmonary capillary bed by a converting enzyme.
Renin reacts with angiotensinogen to form
Angiotensin I
Angiotensin II
Juxtaglomerular cells
Glomerulus
Efferent arteriole
1 Decreased perfusion pressure in the afferent arteriole stimulates secretion of renin by the juxtaglomerular cells.
Arteriole
Angiotensin II receptors
ADH release and water retention to ↑ blood volume.
Afferent arteriole
4 Angiotensin II: a powerful vasoconstrictor
↑ Sodium retention
6 Aldosterone causes increased sodium and water reabsorption by the tubules of the kidney. Result is increased blood volume.
5 Angiotensin II becomes angiotensin III which causes the release of aldosterone from the adrenal cortex.

FIGURE 43.2 The renin–angiotensin–aldosterone system.

Untreated hypertension increases a person's risk for coronary artery disease (CAD) and cardiac death, stroke, renal failure, and loss of vision. Because hypertension has no symptoms, it is difficult to diagnose and treat, and it is often called the "silent killer." All of the drugs used to treat hypertension have adverse effects, many of which are seen as unacceptable by otherwise healthy people. See Box 43.1 for treatment recommendations for hypertension. Nurses face a difficult challenge trying to convince patients to adhere to their drug regimens when they experience adverse effects and do not see any positive effects on their bodies. Research into the cause of hypertension is ongoing. Many theories have been proposed for the cause of the disorder, and it may well be due to a mosaic of factors. Risk factors associated with the development of hypertension include increased age, cigarette smoking, high salt diets, high intake of alcohol, low physical fitness, obesity, insulin resistance, psychological stress, and obstructive sleep apnea. People may have higher risk of developing hypertension based on their family history. People with chronic kidney disease and diabetes mellitus also have increased risk of developing hypertension (Boxes 43.1 to 43.3).

Hypotension

If BP becomes too low, the vital centers in the brain, as well as the rest of the tissues of the body, may not receive enough oxygenated blood to continue functioning. **Hypotension** can progress to shock, in which the body is in serious jeopardy as waste products accumulate and cells die from lack of oxygen. Hypotensive states can occur in the following situations:

- When the heart muscle is damaged and unable to pump effectively
- With severe blood or fluid loss, when volume drops dramatically
- With impairment of the autonomic nervous system to increase either cardiac output or vascular resistance (or both)
- Medication-induced hypotension

Orthostatic hypotension is a lowering of BP when the person either sits up from lying down or stands from a sitting position. The lower BP may be accompanied by dizziness, lightheadedness, nausea, change in vision, and/or syncope. The symptoms are caused by the decrease in blood flow to the brain tissue. Older adults may have increased risk of orthostatic hypotension due to decreased response of the sympathetic nervous system or of the baroreceptor reflexes. There are medications that increase the risk of orthostatic hypotension as well due to their blocking of the sympathetic nervous system or lowering blood volume.

Key Points

- The CV system depends on pressure changes to circulate blood to the tissues and back to the heart.
- Heart rate, stroke volume, and peripheral vascular resistance are factors that determine BP.
- The overall fluid volume, viscosity of the blood, and constriction and relaxation of the arterioles result in PVR.

BOX 43.1

Treatment Recommendations for Hypertension

Treatment Goals

The treatment guidelines and definitions of HTN have been variable in the last few years. The BP must be based on the average of at least two careful readings obtained on at least two occasions. The most recent guidelines from the AHA/ACC recommend the following definitions.

BP Category	SBP		DBP
Normal	<120 mm Hg	and	<80 mm Hg
Elevated	120–129 mm Hg	and	<80 mm Hg
Hypertension			
Stage 1	130–139 mm Hg	or	80–89 mm Hg
Stage 2	≥140 mm Hg	or	≥90 mm Hg

SBP, systolic blood pressure; DBP, diastolic blood pressure.
Reprinted with permission from Whelton, P. K., Carey, R. M., Aronow, W. S., et al. (2017). 2017 ACC/AHA/AAPA/ABC/ACPM/AGS/APhA/ASH/ASPC/NMA/PCNA guideline for the prevention, detection, evaluation, and management of high blood pressure in adults. *Hypertension, 71*(6), 1269–1324. © 2017 by the American College of Cardiology Foundation and the American Heart Association, Inc. doi: 10.1161/HYP.0000000000000065.

If the patient has stage 1 HTN and has a high CV risk, it is recommended that a medication to treat BP is started. It is recommended that all people with stage 2 HTN be started on medication.

Treatment Guidelines

Patients who are not African American, including diabetic patients, may initiate treatment with a thiazide diuretic, calcium-channel blocker, ACE inhibitor, or ARB.

African American patients, including diabetic patients, may initiate treatment with a thiazide or thiazidelike diuretic or calcium-channel blocker before ACE inhibitor or ARB due to better effectiveness.

Patients 18 years or older with chronic kidney disease should initiate treatment with an ACE inhibitor or ARB.

The main objective of hypertension treatment is to attain and maintain the patient's goal BP. If the goal BP is not reached within a month of treatment, the provider should increase the dose of the initial drug or add a second drug from another recommended classification. The provider should continue to assess BP and adjust the treatment regimen until the goal BP is reached. If the goal BP cannot be reached with two drugs, a third drug from the list provided should be added and titrated. An ACEI and an ARB should not be used together. If the goal BP cannot be reached using only the drugs recommended, if there is a contraindication, or if more than three drugs are needed to reach goal BP, referral to a hypertension specialist may be indicated.

Box 43.2 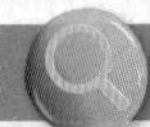 Focus on the Evidence

"WHITE COAT" HYPERTENSION

The diagnosis of hypertension has serious ramifications, such as increased risk for numerous diseases and CV death; the potential need for significant lifestyle changes; and the potential need for drug therapy, which may include many unpleasant adverse effects. Consequently, it is important that a patient be correctly diagnosed before being labeled hypertensive.

Researchers in the 1990s discovered that some patients were hypertensive only when they were in the doctor's office having BP measured. This was correlated to a sympathetic stress reaction (which elevates systolic BP) and a tendency to tighten the muscles (isometric exercise, which elevates diastolic BP), while waiting to be seen and during BP measurement. The researchers labeled this phenomenon "white coat" hypertension.

The American Heart Association has put forth new guidelines for the diagnosis of hypertension. A patient should have at least two consecutive BP readings above normal when taken by a nurse or trained technician over a period of 2 to 3 weeks. Whoever is taking the BP should attempt to have the person relax prior to the assessment. These guidelines point out the importance of using the correct technique when taking a patient's BP, especially because the results can have such a tremendous impact on a patient. It is good practice to periodically review the process for performing this routine task. The nurse should do the following:

- Select a cuff that is the correct size for the patient's arm (a cuff that is too small may give a high reading; a cuff that is too large may give a low reading).
- Try to put the patient at ease; remember that waiting alone in a cold room can be stressful to the body and mind and can increase BP.
- Ensure that the arm that will be used for the cuff is supported.
- Make sure the rest of the patient's muscles are not tensed, while the BP is being taken.
- Place both the cuff and the stethoscope directly on the patient instead of on their clothing.
- Listen carefully and record the first sound heard, the muffling of sounds, and the absence of sound (the actual diastolic pressure is thought to be between these two sounds).

BP machines found in grocery stores and pharmacies often give different readings than those recorded in a health care setting. Patients are encouraged that if they monitor their BP at home, they are to record the day, time, and BP reading to show their health care provider. The American Heart Association offers guidelines for accurate BP measurement. Nurses are the health care providers most likely to be taking and recording patient BP. It is important to always use proper techniques and to make accurate records.

Box 43.3  Focus on **Cultural Considerations**

ANTIHYPERTENSIVE THERAPY

In the United States, African Americans are at highest risk for developing hypertension, with males more likely than females to develop the disease. African Americans have documented differences in response to antihypertensive therapy. For example, African Americans are

- More responsive to diuretics, calcium-channel blockers, and alpha-adrenergic blockers.
- Less responsive to ACE inhibitors, ARBs, renin inhibitors, and beta-blockers.
- Screening for hypertension among African Americans is important for detecting hypertension early and preventing the organ damage that occurs with prolonged hypertension. Because African Americans are more responsive to diuretics and calcium-channel blockers, the treatment approach should include the first-line use of either one of these medications or a combination of both along with diet and other lifestyle changes.

- When there is low pressure on the baroreceptors, the medulla is stimulated to increase the sympathetic nervous system to constrict the blood vessels and increase peripheral vascular resistance.
- A decrease in blood flow to the kidneys triggers the RAAS, by which the blood vessels constrict and water is retained. This activity increases BP and restores blood flow to the kidneys.
- Hypertension is a sustained state of higher-than-normal BP that can lead to blood vessel damage, atherosclerosis, and damage to small vessels in end organs.
- The cause of essential hypertension is unknown; treatment varies among people and is aimed at altering the normal reflex responses that control BP.
- Hypotension can be dangerous when it causes poor oxygen perfusion to the brain and other vital organs.

Antihypertensive Agents

Because the underlying cause of hypertension is usually unknown, altering the body's regulatory mechanisms is the best treatment currently available. Drugs used to treat hypertension work to alter the normal reflexes that control BP. See Figure 43.3 for a review of the sites of action of drugs used to treat hypertension. Treatment for essential hypertension does not cure the disease but is aimed at maintaining the BP within normal limits to prevent the damage that hypertension can cause. Not all patients respond in the same way to antihypertensive drugs because different factors may contribute to each person's hypertension. Patients may have complicating conditions, such as diabetes, renal impairment, or acute myocardial infarction (MI), that may require a change to the type of medication and/or dosage of the medication.

Several different types of drugs that affect different aspects of BP control may need to be used in combination to maintain a patient's BP within normal limits. Trials of drugs and combinations of drugs are often needed to develop an individual regimen that is effective without producing adverse effects that are unacceptable to the patient. Doses are typically started low and slowly titrated higher until BP is maintained at a normal level. Many combination formulations can be prescribed (Box 43.4). Research is ongoing into the treatment of more specific types of hypertension (e.g., pulmonary hypertension). The development of drugs that target specific blood vessel sites and chemicals could lead to a new approach to the treatment of essential hypertension (Box 43.5).

Antihypertensive agents include ACE inhibitors; angiotensin II receptor blockers (ARBs); calcium-channel blockers; vasodilators; and other antihypertensive agents, including diuretic agents, renin inhibitors, and sympathetic nervous system drugs. See Table 43.1 for a complete list of antihypertensive agents. See Box 43.6 for use of these agents across the lifespan.

Stepped Care Approach to Treating Hypertension

The importance of treating hypertension has been proven in numerous research studies. If hypertension is controlled, the patient's risk for CV death and disease is reduced. The risk for developing CV complications is directly related to the patient's degree of hypertension. Lowering the degree of hypertension lowers the risk.

The most recent guidelines for the treatment of hypertension (HTN) are demonstrated in an algorithm in Figure 43.4 and described in both Boxes 43.1 and 43.7.

Hypertensive treatment is further complicated by the presence of other chronic conditions including diabetes or chronic kidney insufficiency. An algorithm for the treatment of HTN with chronic kidney insufficiency is shown in Figure 43.5. With or without other chronic conditions, the goal of treatment should be reduction in BP. There are five main medication classes for which there is evidence showing prevention of CV disease compared with placebo. They are diuretics, ACE inhibitors, ARBs, CCBs, and beta-blockers. There may be evidence supporting the use of the long-acting thiazidelike medication chlorthalidone as first-line medication therapy. It has been shown that many people will require more than one agent to control BP. A patient's response to a given antihypertensive agent is often unique; the drug of choice for one patient may have little to no effect on another patient.

Drugs Affecting the Renin–Angiotensin–Aldosterone System

The RAAS is one of the body's main reflexes for maintaining BP. In the absence of a known cause for hypertension, one approach to lowering BP is to affect the reflexes that

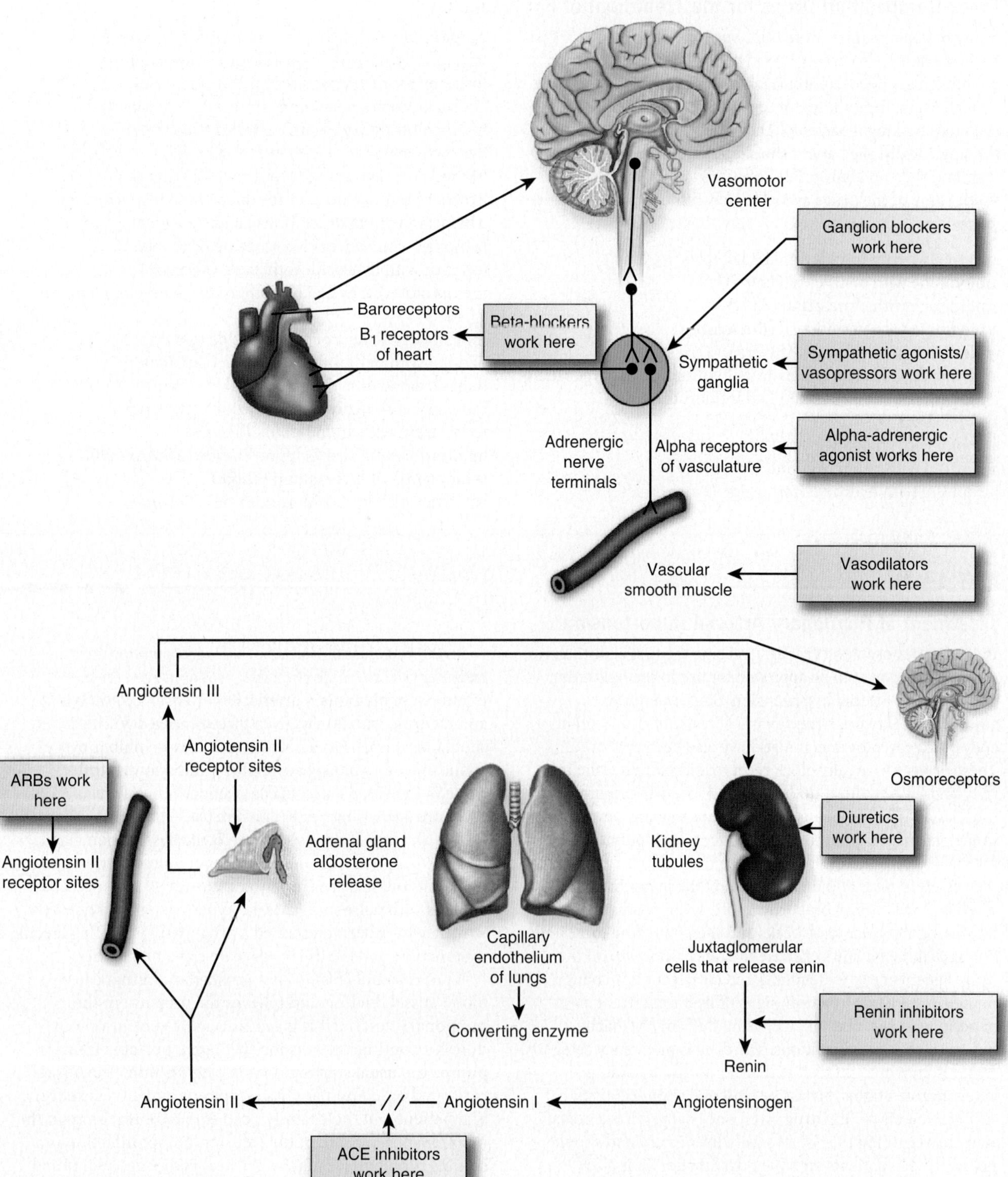

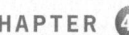

FIGURE 43.3 Sites of action of antihypertensive drugs.

control BP levels. Several classes of drugs alter the RAAS: the **angiotensin-converting enzyme (ACE) inhibitors**, which block the conversion of angiotensin I to angiotensin II; the ARBs, which block the angiotensin receptor site on the blood vessels; and a renin inhibitor, which blocks the reflex at the beginning by inhibiting renin. Medications that are aldosterone antagonists also alter the RAAS; these are covered in Chapter 51 with the other diuretic agents.

Angiotensin-Converting Enzyme Inhibitors

The ACE inhibitors include the following agents: benazepril (*Lotensin*), captopril (generic), enalapril (*Epaned*,

BOX 43.4

Fixed-Combination Drugs for the Treatment of Hypertension

Many patients require more than one type of antihypertensive to achieve good control of their BP. There are now many fixed-combination drugs available for treating hypertension. This allows for fewer tablets or capsules each day, making it easier for the patient to adhere to drug therapy. Ideally, the patient should be stabilized on each drug first, and then an appropriate combination product can be used. Some of the drugs available in combination include the following:

aliskiren with hydrochlorothiazide (*Tekturna HCT*)
amlodipine with benazepril (*Lotrel*)
amlodipine with olmesartan (*Azor*)
amlodipine with perindopril (*Prestalia*)
amlodipine with valsartan (*Exforge*)
amlodipine, valsartan, and hydrochlorothiazide (*Exforge HCT*)
amlodipine, olmesartan, and hydrochlorothiazide (*Tribenzor*)
atenolol with chlorthalidone (*Tenoretic*)
azilsartan with chlorthalidone (*Edarbyclor*)
bisoprolol with hydrochlorothiazide (*Lotensin HCT*)
candesartan with hydrochlorothiazide (*Atacand HCT*)
enalapril with hydrochlorothiazide (*Vaseretic*)
fosinopril with hydrochlorothiazide (generic)
hydrochlorothiazide with benazepril (*Lotensin HCT*)
hydrochlorothiazide with captopril (*Capozide*)
hydrochlorothiazide with hydralazine (*Hydra-Zide*)
hydrochlorothiazide with propranolol (generic)
hydrochlorothiazide with spironolactone (*Aldactazide*)
irbesartan with hydrochlorothiazide (*Avalide*)
lisinopril with hydrochlorothiazide (*Zestoretic*)
losartan with hydrochlorothiazide (*Hyzaar*)
metoprolol with hydrochlorothiazide (*Dutoprol, Lopressor HCT*)
moexipril with hydrochlorothiazide (generic)
nadolol with bendroflumethiazide (*Corzide*)
olmesartan with hydrochlorothiazide (*Benicar HCT*)
quinapril with hydrochlorothiazide (*Accuretic*)
telmisartan with amlodipine (*Twynsta*)
telmisartan with hydrochlorothiazide (*Micardis HCT*)
trandolapril with verapamil (*Tarka*)
valsartan with hydrochlorothiazide (*Diovan HCT*)

BOX 43.5

Treatment of Pulmonary Arterial Hypertension

In late 2001, bosentan (*Tracleer*) became the first endothelin receptor antagonist to be approved for use in the treatment of pulmonary arterial hypertension. Since that time, ambrisentan (*Letairis*), treprostinil (*Remodulin*), and other endothelin receptor antagonists have also been approved. These drugs specifically block receptor sites for endothelin (ET_A and ET_B) in the endothelium and vascular smooth muscles; these endothelins are chemicals that are elevated in the plasma and lung tissues of patients with pulmonary arterial hypertension. Blocking these receptor sites allows the vessels to relax and dilate, relieving the pressure in the arteries. *Tracleer* is an oral drug that is given to adults, initially as 62.5 mg PO b.i.d. for 4 weeks and then increased to 125 mg PO b.i.d. if the patient's exercise tolerance improves on the drug. Patients need to be monitored closely for any change in their respiratory function; signs of liver toxicity; or signs of peripheral vasodilation, including flushing, headache, hypotension, and palpitations. The drug is pregnancy category X and is known to interact with other drugs, including ketoconazole, statins, glyburide, and oral contraceptives. Ambrisentan is an oral drug given once daily. It has a boxed warning regarding the risk of severe liver injury and should not be used in patients with liver dysfunction. It is also pregnancy category X and should not be used in pregnancy.

Treprostinil (*Remodulin*) is administered by continuous subcutaneous infusion. The patient needs to learn how to care for the infusion port and to use the pump. Dosage adjustments are made based on the patient's response and exercise tolerance. Headache and injection site pain are common and may be relieved by the use of analgesics. The drug cannot be discontinued abruptly; it needs to be tapered to prevent a rebound worsening of the condition. Treprostinil (*Orenitram*) is an oral formulation indicated for treatment of pulmonary hypertension, and treprostinil (*Tyvaso*) is an inhaled solution.

In 2005, sildenafil (*Revatio*), a drug known for the treatment of erectile dysfunction, was approved for the treatment of pulmonary arterial hypertension. *Revatio* is an oral drug, with 20 mg given three times a day. The doses should be at least 4 to 6 hours apart. *Revatio* inhibits cyclic guanosine monophosphate (cGMP); this allows nitrous oxide in the blood vessel to cause smooth muscle relaxation, therefore decreasing vessel pressure (see Chapter 41). Tadalafil (*Adcirca*), another drug used for erectile dysfunction, has also been approved for the treatment of pulmonary arterial hypertension. It is given orally at a dose of 40 mg once a day. Patients with pulmonary arterial hypertension may question why they have been prescribed a drug used for treating erectile dysfunction, and the use needs to be explained to them.

Epoprostenol (*Flolan*) is a prostaglandin that causes blood vessel dilation and relieves the pressure in the pulmonary vessels. It is given through a central venous line as a continuous infusion through a portable infusion pump. The usual starting dose is 2 ng/kg/min. The dosage is titrated based on patient's symptoms and adverse effects. The patient and their family need extensive teaching on the maintenance and use of the infusion pump. Infection is a serious problem. Headache, nausea, vomiting, abdominal pain, and muscle aches are the most commonly reported adverse effects.

Iloprost (*Ventavis*) is an inhaled synthetic prostacyclin that directly dilates the pulmonary vascular bed, reducing pressure in the pulmonary vascular system, increasing gas exchange, and easing the signs and symptoms of pulmonary arterial hypertension. It is inhaled using a special delivery device six to nine times a day while awake. Patients report dizziness and syncope after using the drug and are encouraged to change positions slowly. They should not ingest the drug or get it on their skin.

Table 43.1 ***Drugs in Focus:* Antihypertensive Agents**

Drug Name	Usual Dosage	Usual Indications
ACE Inhibitors		
benazepril (*Lotensin*)	*Adult:* 10–40 mg/d PO, reduce dose with renal impairment *Pediatric (6 y and older):* 0.2–0.6 mg/kg/d PO	Treatment of hypertension
captopril (*Capoten*)	Initial dose as low as 6.25; should be titrated up to 25–150 mg PO b.i.d. to t.i.d.; target dosing varies based on individual response and indication; max dose should not exceed 450 mg/d; reduce dose in patients with renal impairment	Treatment of hypertension; adjunct therapy for HF; treatment of left ventricular dysfunction after MI, diabetic nephropathy; for use in adults
enalapril (*Epaned, Vasotec*)	*Adult:* 2.5–40 mg/d PO; dose and frequency varies based on indication; reduce dose in patients with renal impairment *Pediatric (Epaned):* 0.08 mg/kg PO daily, max 5 mg	Treatment of hypertension, HF, left ventricular dysfunction
enalaprilat (generic)	1.25 mg q6h IV over 5 min	Short-term treatment of acute hypertension when oral therapy is not feasible
fosinopril (generic)	10–80 mg/d PO; titrate based on response; reduce dose in patients with renal impairment	Treatment of hypertension and adjunct treatment for heart failure
lisinopril (*Prinivil, Qbrelis, Zestril*)	*Adult:* 2.5–40 mg/d PO; dose varies based on indication; reduce dose for renal impairment *Pediatric:* 0.7 mg/kg PO daily; max dose 5 mg/d	Treatment of hypertension in patients 6 y of age or older, HF; treatment of stable patients within 24 h after acute MI to increase survival
moexipril (generic)	7.5–30 mg/d PO, based on response; reduce dose in patients with renal impairment	Treatment of hypertension in adults
perindopril (generic)	4–16 mg/d PO; reduce dose in patients with renal impairment	Treatment of hypertension, treatment of adults with stable coronary artery disease to reduce risk of CV mortality or MI
quinapril (*Accupril*)	10–80 mg/d PO, dose varies based on response for hypertension; 5–20 mg PO b.i.d. for HF; reduce dose in patients with renal impairment	Treatment of hypertension, adjunctive treatment of HF; for use in adults
ramipril (*Altace*)	2.5–20 mg/d PO for hypertension and CV risk reduction, 5 mg PO b.i.d. for HF; reduce dose in patients with renal impairment	Treatment of hypertension, adjunctive treatment of HF; reduces risk of MI, stroke, or death from CV cause in adults 55 y or older at high risk of developing a major CV event
trandolapril (generic)	1–2 mg PO/d initially and titrate up to 4 mg/d PO or high dose tolerated reduce dose in patients with renal or hepatic impairment	Treatment of hypertension, HF, and after MI; for use in adults
Angiotensin II Receptor Blockers		
azilsartan (*Edarbi*)	80 mg/d PO; reduce dose if patient is taking high doses of diuretics	Used alone or as part of combination therapy for treatment of hypertension in adults
candesartan (*Atacand*)	*Adult:* 4–32 mg/d PO; dose varies based on indication and individual response *Pediatric (1–17 y):* dose varies based on age and weight	Used alone or as part of combination therapy for treatment of hypertension; treatment of heart failure; reduces risk of CV death and HF hospitalization
irbesartan (*Avapro*)	150–300 mg/d PO	Used alone or as part of combination therapy for treatment of hypertension in adults, slows progression of diabetic nephropathy in patients with hypertension and type 2 diabetes
losartan (*Cozaar*)	*Adult:* 25–100 mg/d PO *Pediatric:* 0.7 mg/kg once daily (up to 50 mg)	Used alone or as part of combination therapy for treatment of hypertension, slows progression of diabetic nephropathy with elevated serum creatinine and proteinuria in patients with hypertension and type 2 diabetes; reduces risk of stroke in patients with hypertension and left ventricular hypertrophy

(continues on page 750)

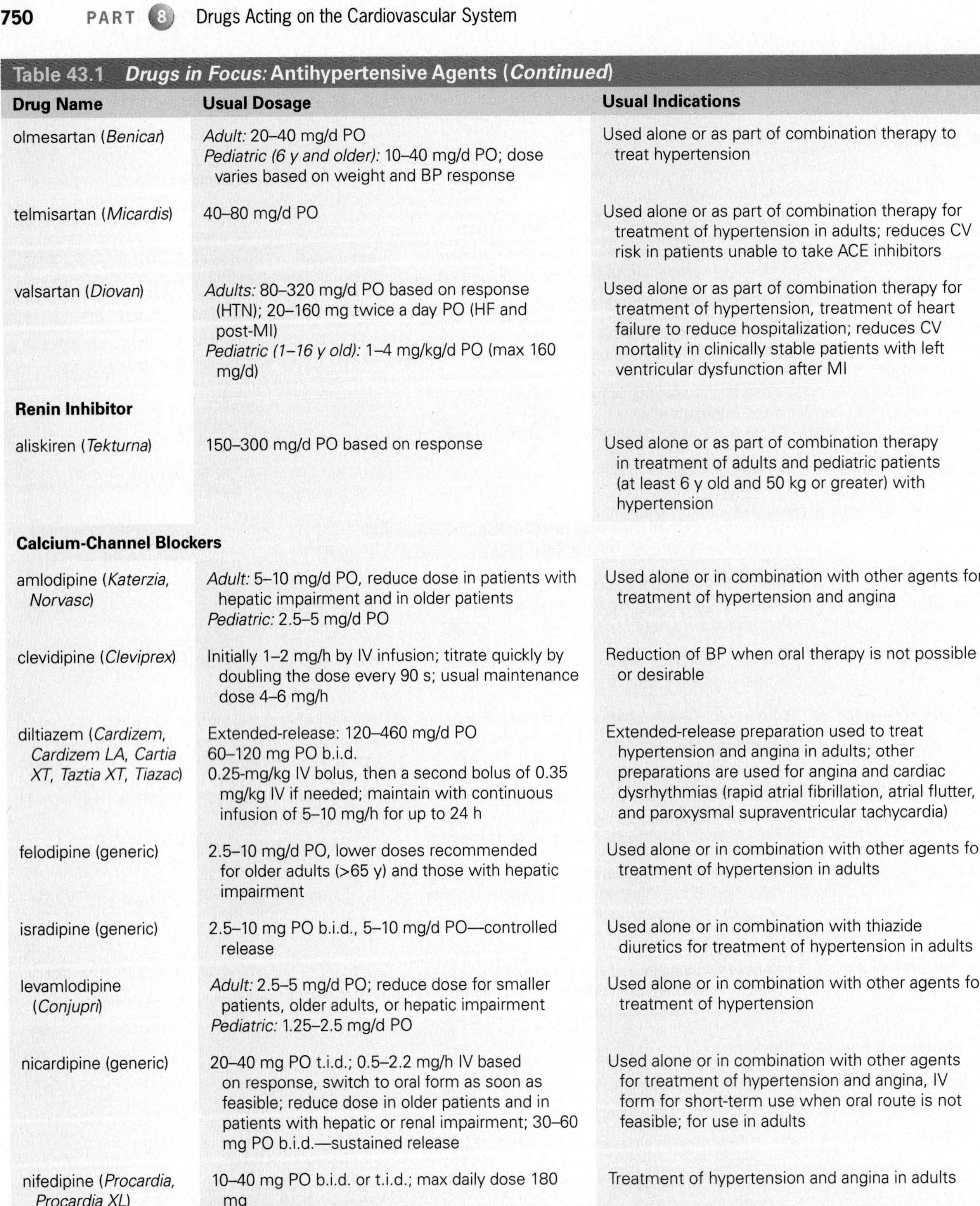

Table 43.1 *Drugs in Focus:* Antihypertensive Agents (*Continued*)

Drug Name	Usual Dosage	Usual Indications
olmesartan (*Benicar*)	*Adult:* 20–40 mg/d PO *Pediatric (6 y and older):* 10–40 mg/d PO; dose varies based on weight and BP response	Used alone or as part of combination therapy to treat hypertension
telmisartan (*Micardis*)	40–80 mg/d PO	Used alone or as part of combination therapy for treatment of hypertension in adults; reduces CV risk in patients unable to take ACE inhibitors
valsartan (*Diovan*)	*Adults:* 80–320 mg/d PO based on response (HTN); 20–160 mg twice a day PO (HF and post-MI) *Pediatric (1–16 y old):* 1–4 mg/kg/d PO (max 160 mg/d)	Used alone or as part of combination therapy for treatment of hypertension, treatment of heart failure to reduce hospitalization; reduces CV mortality in clinically stable patients with left ventricular dysfunction after MI
Renin Inhibitor		
aliskiren (*Tekturna*)	150–300 mg/d PO based on response	Used alone or as part of combination therapy in treatment of adults and pediatric patients (at least 6 y old and 50 kg or greater) with hypertension
Calcium-Channel Blockers		
amlodipine (*Katerzia, Norvasc*)	*Adult:* 5–10 mg/d PO, reduce dose in patients with hepatic impairment and in older patients *Pediatric:* 2.5–5 mg/d PO	Used alone or in combination with other agents for treatment of hypertension and angina
clevidipine (*Cleviprex*)	Initially 1–2 mg/h by IV infusion; titrate quickly by doubling the dose every 90 s; usual maintenance dose 4–6 mg/h	Reduction of BP when oral therapy is not possible or desirable
diltiazem (*Cardizem, Cardizem LA, Cartia XT, Taztia XT, Tiazac*)	Extended-release: 120–460 mg/d PO 60–120 mg PO b.i.d. 0.25-mg/kg IV bolus, then a second bolus of 0.35 mg/kg IV if needed; maintain with continuous infusion of 5–10 mg/h for up to 24 h	Extended-release preparation used to treat hypertension and angina in adults; other preparations are used for angina and cardiac dysrhythmias (rapid atrial fibrillation, atrial flutter, and paroxysmal supraventricular tachycardia)
felodipine (generic)	2.5–10 mg/d PO, lower doses recommended for older adults (>65 y) and those with hepatic impairment	Used alone or in combination with other agents for treatment of hypertension in adults
isradipine (generic)	2.5–10 mg PO b.i.d., 5–10 mg/d PO—controlled release	Used alone or in combination with thiazide diuretics for treatment of hypertension in adults
levamlodipine (*Conjupri*)	*Adult:* 2.5–5 mg/d PO; reduce dose for smaller patients, older adults, or hepatic impairment *Pediatric:* 1.25–2.5 mg/d PO	Used alone or in combination with other agents for treatment of hypertension
nicardipine (generic)	20–40 mg PO t.i.d.; 0.5–2.2 mg/h IV based on response, switch to oral form as soon as feasible; reduce dose in older patients and in patients with hepatic or renal impairment; 30–60 mg PO b.i.d.—sustained release	Used alone or in combination with other agents for treatment of hypertension and angina, IV form for short-term use when oral route is not feasible; for use in adults
nifedipine (*Procardia, Procardia XL*)	10–40 mg PO b.i.d. or t.i.d.; max daily dose 180 mg Extended release: 30–60 mg/d PO, max dose 120 mg/d	Treatment of hypertension and angina in adults
nisoldipine (*Sular*)	8.5–34 mg/d PO; reduce dose in patients 65 y or older and in patients with hepatic impairment	Extended-release tablets used as monotherapy or as part of combination therapy for treatment of hypertension in adults

Table 43.1 *Drugs in Focus:* Antihypertensive Agents (*Continued*)

Drug Name	Usual Dosage	Usual Indications
verapamil (*Calan SR, Verelan, Verelan PM*)	120–240 mg/d PO, reduce dose in the morning; extended-release capsules: 100–300 mg/d PO at bedtime; lower doses may be needed for older adults, low-weight adults, and those with renal and/or hepatic impairment IV *Adult*: 5–10 mg IV over 2 min, may repeat with 10 mg in 30 min if needed IV *Pediatric*: 0.1–0.3 mg/kg IV over 2 min; do not exceed 5 mg per dose, may repeat in 30 min if needed	Extended-release formulations for the treatment of essential hypertension; other preparations are used for angina and treating various arrhythmias (rapid atrial fibrillation, atrial flutter, and paroxysmal supraventricular tachycardia)
Vasodilators		
hydralazine (generic)	*Adult:* 20–40 mg IM or IV repeated as necessary; 10–50 t.i.d. or q.i.d. (max daily dose 300 mg) *Pediatric:* 1.7–3.5 mg/kg per 24 h IV or IM in four to six divided doses	Treatment of severe hypertension (IV, IM) Treatment of hypertension (oral)
minoxidil (generic)	*Adult:* 10–40 mg/d PO in single or divided doses *Pediatric (<12 y):* 0.25–1 mg/kg/d PO as a single dose	Treatment of severe hypertension unresponsive to other therapy
nitroglycerin (generic)	Initial dose 5 mcg/min IV; titrate up q5–10min based on BP response	Treatment of hypertension and angina not responsive to sublingual nitro
nitroprusside (*Nitropress*)	*Adult and pediatric:* 3 mcg/kg/min, do not exceed 10 mcg/kg/min	Treatment of hypertensive crisis, also used to maintain controlled hypotension during surgery
Other Antihypertensive Agents		
Diuretic Agents		
See Chapter 51	See Chapter 51	Treatment of mild hypertension, often first agents used, often used in combination with other agents
Sympathetic Nervous System Blockers		
See Chapter 31	See Chapter 31	

ACE, angiotensin-converting enzyme; HF, heart failure; MI, myocardial infarction; BP, blood pressure; CV, cardiovascular.

Box 43.6 Focus on Drug Therapy Across the Lifespan

DRUGS AFFECTING BLOOD PRESSURE

Children

National standards for determining normal levels of BP in children are quite new. It has been determined that hypertension may start as a childhood disease, and more screening studies are being done to establish normal values for each age group. Children are thought to be more likely to have secondary hypertension caused by renal disease or congenital problems such as coarctation of the aorta.

Treatment of childhood hypertension should be done cautiously because the long-term effects of the antihypertensive agents are not known. Lifestyle changes should be instituted before drug therapy if at all possible. Weight loss and increased activity may bring an elevated BP back to normal in many children.

If drug therapy is used, a diuretic may be tried first, with monitoring of blood glucose and electrolyte levels on a regular basis. Beta-blockers have been used with success in some children; adverse effects may limit their usefulness in others. There are some calcium-channel blockers, ACE inhibitors, and ARBs with approved pediatric doses. Careful follow-up of the growing child is essential to monitor for changes in BP and for adverse effects.

Adults

Adults receiving any of these drugs need to be instructed about adverse reactions that should be reported immediately. They need to be reminded of safety precautions that may be needed in hot weather or with conditions that cause fluid depletion (e.g., diarrhea, vomiting). If they are taking any other drugs, then the interactions of the various drugs should be evaluated. The importance of other measures to help lower BP—weight loss, smoking cessation, and increased activity—should be stressed.

ACE inhibitors, ARBs, and renin inhibitors should not be used during pregnancy, and patients who can become pregnant should be advised to use barrier contraceptives to prevent pregnancy while taking these drugs. Calcium-channel blockers and vasodilators should not be used

(continues on page 752)

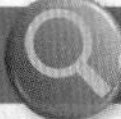

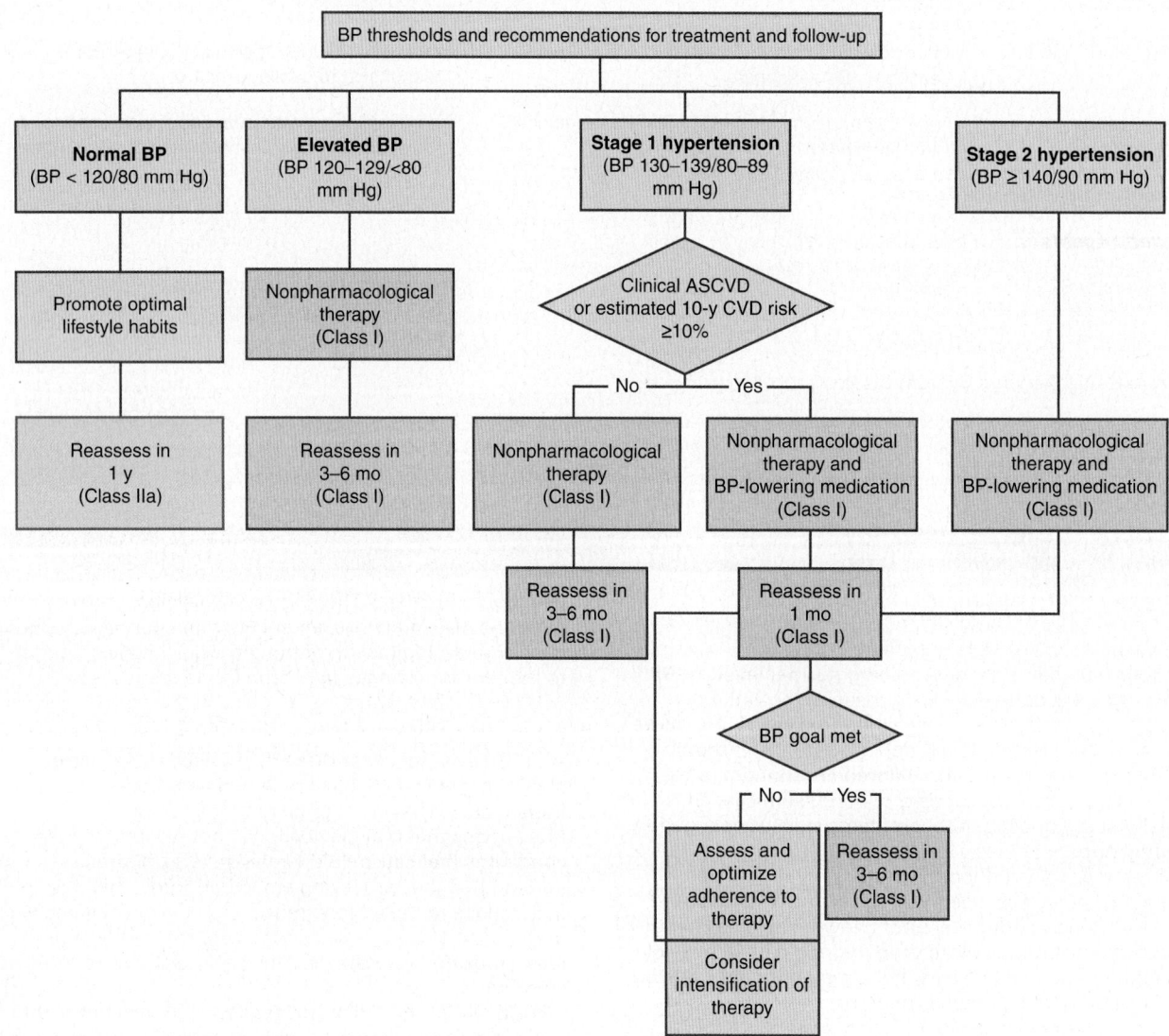

Box 43.6 Focus on Drug Therapy Across the Lifespan (*Continued*)

in pregnancy unless the benefit to the patient clearly outweighs the potential risk to the fetus. The drugs enter human milk and can cause serious adverse effects on the baby. Caution should be used or another method of feeding the baby should be used if one of these drugs is needed during lactation. Labetalol, a beta-blocker, and/or magnesium are often used first when treating HTN during pregnancy.

Older Adults

Older adults frequently are prescribed one or more of these drugs. They are more susceptible to the toxic effects of the drugs and are more likely to have underlying conditions that could interfere with drug metabolism and excretion. Renal or hepatic impairment can lead to accumulation of the drugs in the body. If renal or hepatic dysfunction is present, then the dose should be reduced and the patient monitored closely. The total drug regimen of the older patient should be coordinated with careful attention to interactions among drugs and alternative therapies.

Older adults need to use special caution in any situation that could lead to a reduction in BP, such as loss of fluids from diarrhea or vomiting, lack of fluid intake, or excessive heat with decreased sweating that comes with age. Dizziness, falls, or syncope can occur if BP falls too far in these situations. BP should always be taken immediately before an antihypertensive is administered to an older adult in an institutional setting to avoid excessive lowering of BP.

All patients should be cautioned about sustained-release antihypertensives that cannot be cut, crushed, or chewed to avoid the potential for excessive dosing if these drugs are inappropriately cut.

FIGURE 43.4 Algorithm for the treatment of hypertension. (Reprinted with permission from Whelton, P. K., Carey, R. M., Aronow, W. S., et al. (2017). 2017 ACC/AHA/AAPA/ABC/ACPM/AGS/APhA/ASH/ASPC/NMA/PCNA guideline for the prevention, detection, evaluation, and management of high blood pressure in adults. *Hypertension, 71*(6), 1269–1324. © 2017 by the American College of Cardiology Foundation and the American Heart Association, Inc. doi: 10.1161/HYP.0000000000000065.)

BOX 43.7

Stepped Care Management of Hypertension

Step 1: Lifestyle Modifications
- Weight reduction
- Smoking cessation
- Moderation of alcohol intake
- Reduction of salt in diet
- Increase in aerobic physical activity

Step 2: Inadequate Response
Continue lifestyle modifications. If measures in step 1 are not sufficient to lower BP to an acceptable level, then drug therapy is added:
- Diuretic (decreases serum sodium levels and blood volume)
- ACE inhibitor (blocks the conversion of angiotensin I to angiotensin II)
- Calcium-channel blocker (relaxes muscle contraction) or other autonomic blockers
- Angiotensin II receptor blocker (blocks the effects of angiotensin on the blood vessel)

Step 3: Inadequate Response
Consider change in drug dose or class, or addition of another drug for combined effect. (Note: Fixed-combination drugs should only be used when the patient has been stabilized on each drug separately; see Box 43.4.)

Step 4: Inadequate Response
- All of the above measures are continued.
- A second or third agent or diuretic is added if not already prescribed.

Vasotec), enalaprilat (generic), fosinopril (generic), lisinopril (*Prinivil*, *Zestril*, *Qbrelis*), moexipril (generic), perindopril (generic), quinapril (*Accupril*), ramipril (*Altace*), and trandolapril (generic).

Therapeutic Actions and Indications

ACE inhibitors act in the lungs to prevent ACE from converting angiotensin I to angiotensin II, a powerful vasoconstrictor and stimulator of aldosterone release (see Fig. 43.3). This action leads to a decrease in BP and in aldosterone secretion with a resultant increase in serum potassium and a loss of serum sodium and fluid.

These drugs are indicated for the treatment of hypertension, alone or in combination with other drugs. They are also used in conjunction with other medications for the treatment of heart failure and left ventricular dysfunction. Their therapeutic effect in these cases is thought to be related to a decrease in cardiac workload associated with the decrease in PVR and blood volume. They are also approved for the treatment of diabetic nephropathy. It is thought that the decrease in stimulation of the angiotensin receptors in the renal artery will slow the damage to the renal artery that occurs in diabetes. See Table 43.1 for usual indications for each of these drugs.

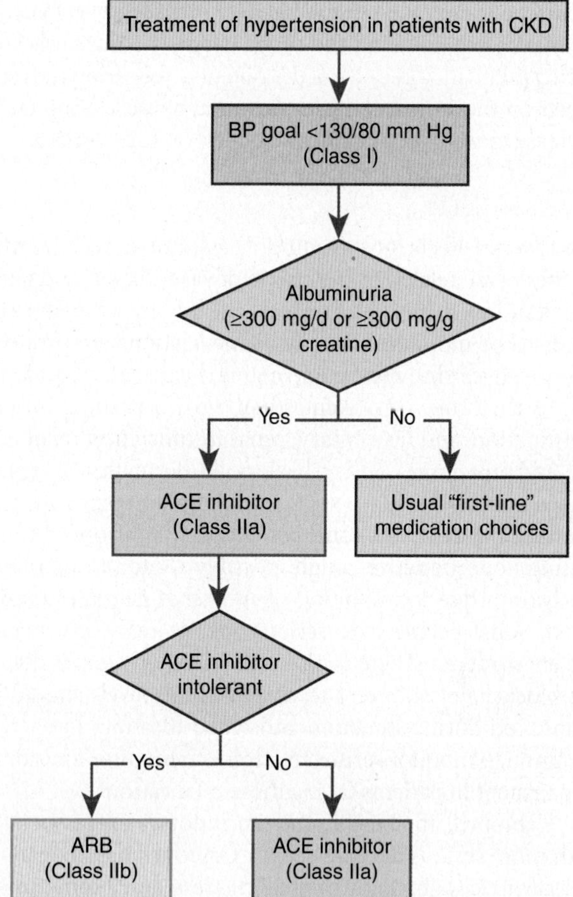

FIGURE 43.5 Treatment of HTN in persons with chronic kidney disease (CKD). (Reprinted with permission from Whelton, P. K., Carey, R. M., Aronow, W. S., et al. (2017). 2017 ACC/AHA/AAPA/ABC/ACPM/AGS/APhA/ASH/ASPC/NMA/PCNA guideline for the prevention, detection, evaluation, and management of high blood pressure in adults. *Hypertension, 71*(6), 1269–1324. © 2017 by the American College of Cardiology Foundation and the American Heart Association, Inc. doi: 10.1161/HYP.0000000000000065.)

Pharmacokinetics

All of the ACE inhibitors are administered orally. Enalapril also has the advantage of parenteral use (enalaprilat) if oral use is not feasible or rapid onset is desirable. These drugs are well absorbed, widely distributed, metabolized in the liver, and excreted in the urine and feces. They have been detected in human milk, are known to cross the placenta, and have been associated with serious fetal abnormalities so they should not be used during pregnancy.

Contraindications and Cautions

ACE inhibitors are contraindicated in people with a history of allergic reaction (including angioedema) to any of the ACE inhibitors and to prevent hypersensitivity reactions. Caution should be used in patients with impaired renal function, which could be exacerbated by the effects of this drug in decreasing renal blood flow; with acute heart failure exacerbation because the change in hemodynamics could be detrimental in some cases; and with salt/volume depletion, which could be exacerbated by the drug effects. Patients who can become pregnant who choose to use one of these drugs should be encouraged to use barrier contraceptives to avoid pregnancy while taking the drug. Usage is contraindicated during pregnancy because of the potential for serious adverse effects on the fetus and during lactation because of potential decrease in milk production and effects on the neonate.

Adverse Effects

The adverse effects most commonly associated with the ACE inhibitors are related to the effects of vasodilation and alterations in blood flow. Such effects include hypotension (BP needs to be monitored closely as medications are titrated), reflex tachycardia, chest pain, angina, heart failure, and cardiac arrhythmias; gastrointestinal (GI) irritation, ulcers, constipation, and liver injury; renal insufficiency, renal failure, and proteinuria; and rash, alopecia, dermatitis, and photosensitivity (Fig. 43.6). ACE inhibitors are generally well tolerated but can cause some patients to suffer from an unrelenting nonproductive cough, possibly related to increased bradykinin due to inhibition of ACE that degrades bradykinin. Some people have serious allergic reactions including angioedema. There is also risk of hyperkalemia due to the blockage of aldosterone, so potassium levels should be monitored during initiation and when titrating doses. It is common to monitor serum creatinine to monitor for kidney impairment in patients taking these medications.

Captopril, moexipril, and perindopril are associated with more serious adverse effects. Captopril has been associated with cough, unpleasant GI distress, and a sometimes-fatal pancytopenia. Moexipril is associated with many unpleasant GI and skin effects, cough, and cardiac arrhythmias; fatal MI and pancytopenia have sometimes been associated with this drug as well. Perindopril and lisinopril are associated with a sometimes-fatal pancytopenia as well as serious-to-fatal airway obstruction. This is found to occur more frequently in African American patients.

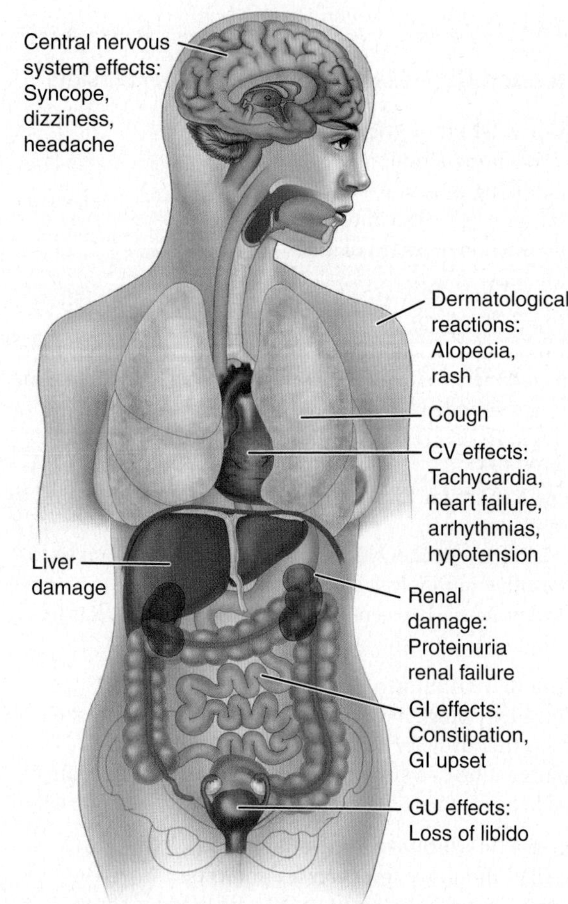

FIGURE 43.6 Variety of adverse effects and toxicities associated with drugs affecting blood pressure.

Clinically Important Drug–Drug Interactions

The risk of hypersensitivity reactions increases if these drugs are taken with allopurinol. There is a risk of decreased antihypertensive effects if taken with nonsteroidal anti-inflammatory drugs, and there are additive antihypertensive effects if taken with diuretics and other antihypertensive medications; patients should be monitored. Potassium supplements and potassium-sparing diuretics increase the risk of hyperkalemia. There is increased risk of lithium toxicity with coadministration, so levels need to be monitored carefully. The combination of drugs used to alter the RAAS is not recommended due to potentially serious adverse effects and should not be combined with other ACE inhibitors, ARBs, or a renin inhibitor.

Clinically Important Drug–Food Interactions

Most ACE inhibitors can be taken with or without food. However, absorption of captopril and moexipril may be altered when ingested with food, so they should be taken at least 1 hour before food.

Prototype Summary: Captopril

Indications: Treatment of hypertension, heart failure, diabetic nephropathy, and left ventricular dysfunction after MI.

Actions: Blocks ACE from converting angiotensin I to angiotensin II, leading to a decrease in BP, a decrease in aldosterone production, and a small increase in serum potassium levels along with sodium and fluid loss.

Pharmacokinetics:

Route	Onset	Peak
Oral	15 min	30–90 min

$T_{1/2}$: 2 hours; excreted in the urine.

Adverse Effects: Allergic reactions, angioedema, neutropenia, hypotension, tachycardia, rash, pruritus, gastric irritation, aphthous ulcers, peptic ulcers, dysgeusia, proteinuria, bone marrow suppression, cough, renal impairment, hyperkalemia.

Nursing Considerations for Patients Receiving Angiotensin-Converting Enzyme Inhibitors

Assessment: History and Examination

- Assess for the following conditions, which could be cautions or contraindications to use of the drug: any known allergies to these drugs to prevent hypersensitivity reactions; impaired kidney function, which could be exacerbated by these drugs; pregnancy or lactation because of the potential adverse effects on the fetus or neonate; and salt/volume depletion and heart failure, which could be exacerbated by these drugs.
- Assess baseline status before beginning therapy to determine any potential adverse effects. This includes body temperature and weight; skin color, lesions, and temperature; pulse, BP, baseline electrocardiogram (ECG), and perfusion; respirations and adventitious breath sounds; bowel sounds and abdominal examination; and renal function tests, complete blood count with differential, and serum electrolytes.

Nursing Conclusions

Nursing conclusions related to drug therapy might include the following:

- Altered tissue perfusion (total body) related to changes in cardiac output
- Altered skin integrity related to dermatological effects
- Impaired comfort related to GI distress and cough
- Electrolyte imbalance risk related to action of RAAS
- Knowledge deficit risk regarding drug therapy

Planning

- The patient will receive the best therapeutic effect from the drug therapy.
- The patient will have limited adverse effects from the drug therapy.
- The patient will understand the drug therapy, adverse effects to anticipate, and measures to relieve discomfort and improve safety.

Intervention With Rationale

- Encourage patient to implement lifestyle changes, including weight loss, smoking cessation, decreased alcohol and salt in the diet, and increased exercise to increase the effectiveness of antihypertensive therapy.
- Administer on an empty stomach 1 hour before or 2 hours after meals to ensure proper absorption of the drug (captopril and moexipril).
- Alert the surgeon and mark the patient's chart prominently if the patient is to undergo surgery to alert medical personnel that the blockage of compensatory angiotensin II could result in hypotension after surgery that would need to be reversed with volume expansion.
- Give the parenteral form of enalapril only if an oral form is not feasible; transfer to an oral form as soon as possible to avoid increased risk for adverse effects.
- Consult with the prescriber to reduce the dose in patients with renal failure to account for their decreased production of renin and lower-than-normal levels of angiotensin II.
- Monitor the patient carefully in any situation that might lead to a drop in fluid volume or change in electrolytes (e.g., excessive sweating, vomiting, diarrhea, dehydration) to detect and treat excessive hypotension or electrolyte imbalance that may occur.
- Provide thorough patient teaching, including the name of the drug, dosage prescribed, measures to avoid adverse effects, warning signs of problems, and the need for periodic monitoring and evaluation, to enhance patient knowledge about drug therapy and to promote adherence.
- Offer support and encouragement to help the patient deal with the diagnosis and the drug regimen.

Evaluation

- Monitor patient response to the drug (maintenance of BP within normal limits).
- Monitor for adverse effects (hypotension, hyperkalemia, cardiac arrhythmias, renal dysfunction, skin reactions, cough, pancytopenia).
- Evaluate the effectiveness of the teaching plan (patient can name drug, dosage, adverse effects to watch for, specific measures to avoid them, and the importance of continued follow-up).
- Monitor the effectiveness of comfort measures and adherence to the treatment regimen.

Angiotensin II Receptor Blockers

The ARBs include the following drugs: azilsartan (*Edarbi*), candesartan (*Atacand*), irbesartan (*Avapro*), losartan (*Cozaar*), olmesartan (*Benicar*), telmisartan (*Micardis*), and valsartan (*Diovan*).

Therapeutic Actions and Indications

The ARBs selectively bind with the **angiotensin II receptors** in the vascular smooth muscle of the blood vessels and in the adrenal cortex to block vasoconstriction and the release of aldosterone. These actions block the BP-raising effects of the RAAS and lower BP. They are indicated to be used alone or in combination therapy for the treatment of hypertension, and some are indicated for the treatment of heart failure and after MI. Recently, some were found to slow the progression of renal disease in patients with hypertension and type

2 diabetes. This action is thought to be related to the effects of blocking angiotensin receptors in the vascular endothelium. There are some ARBs that are indicated for use in children who have hypertension. See Table 43.1 for usual indications for each drug.

Pharmacokinetics

These agents are all given orally. They are well absorbed and undergo metabolism in the liver by the cytochrome P-450 system. They are excreted in the feces and urine. The ARBs cross the placenta. It is not known whether they enter human milk during lactation (see "Contraindications and Cautions").

Contraindications and Cautions

The ARBs are contraindicated in the presence of allergic reaction, including angioedema, to any of these drugs to prevent hypersensitivity reactions. Caution should be used in the presence of hepatic or renal dysfunction, which could alter the metabolism and excretion of these drugs, and with hypovolemia because of the blocking of potentially life-saving compensatory mechanisms. These drugs are also contraindicated during pregnancy because of association with serious fetal abnormalities and even death. Although it is not known whether the ARBs enter human milk during lactation, these drugs should not be used during lactation because of the potential for serious adverse effects on the neonate. Patients who can become pregnant should be advised to use barrier contraceptives to avoid pregnancy; if a pregnancy does occur, the ARB should be discontinued immediately.

Adverse Effects

The adverse effects most commonly associated with ARBs include headache, dizziness, syncope, and weakness, which could be associated with decrease in BP; GI complaints, including diarrhea, abdominal pain, and nausea; dry mouth and tooth pain; symptoms of upper respiratory tract infections and cough; and rash, dry skin, and alopecia. They have also been associated with renal dysfunction in some patients; therefore, it is important to monitor renal function regularly when using these drugs.

Clinically Important Drug–Drug Interactions

ARBs will have increased effect if used with other antihypertensive medications, so BP response should be monitored carefully. There is increased risk of hyperkalemia when administered with potassium supplements or potassium-sparing diuretic medication. There is increased risk of lithium toxicity, so lithium levels should be closely monitored. Coadministration with NSAIDs increases risk of renal impairment and decreases antihypertensive effects.

Prototype Summary: Losartan

Indications: Alone or as part of combination therapy for the treatment of hypertension; treatment of diabetic nephropathy with elevated serum creatinine and proteinuria in patients with type 2 diabetes and hypertension.

Actions: Selectively blocks the binding of angiotensin II to specific tissue receptors found in the vascular smooth muscle and adrenal glands; blocks the vasoconstriction and release of aldosterone associated with the RAAS.

Pharmacokinetics:

Route	Onset	Peak	Duration
Oral	Varies	1–3 h	24 h

$T_{1/2}$: 2 hours, then 6 to 9 hours; metabolized in the liver and excreted in urine and feces.

Adverse Effects: Allergic reactions, angioedema, hypotension, dizziness, headache, diarrhea, abdominal pain, symptoms of upper respiratory tract infection, cough, back pain, fever, muscle weakness, hypotension.

Nursing Considerations for Patients Receiving Angiotensin II Receptor Blockers

Assessment: History and Examination

- Assess for the following conditions, which could be cautions or contraindications to use of the drug: any known allergies to these drugs to prevent hypersensitivity reactions; impaired kidney or liver function, which could be exacerbated by these drugs; pregnancy and lactation because of the potential adverse effects on the fetus and neonate; and hypovolemia, which could potentiate the BP-lowering effects.
- Assess baseline status before beginning therapy to determine any potential adverse effects; this includes body temperature and weight; skin color, lesions, and temperature; pulse, BP, baseline ECG, and perfusion; respirations and adventitious breath sounds; bowel sounds and abdominal examination; and renal and liver function tests.

Nursing Conclusions

Nursing conclusions related to drug therapy might include the following:

- Altered tissue perfusion (total body) related to changes in cardiac output
- Altered skin integrity related to dermatological effects
- Impaired comfort related to GI distress, skin effects, and headache

- Electrolyte imbalance risk related to action of the RAAS
- Knowledge deficit risk regarding drug therapy

Planning

- The patient will receive the best therapeutic effect from the drug therapy.
- The patient will have limited adverse effects from the drug therapy.
- The patient will understand the drug therapy, adverse effects to anticipate, and measures to relieve discomfort and improve safety.

Intervention With Rationale

- Encourage the patient to implement lifestyle changes, including weight loss, smoking cessation, decreased alcohol and salt in the diet, and increased exercise, to increase the effectiveness of antihypertensive therapy.
- Administer without regard to meals; give with food to decrease GI distress if needed.
- Alert the surgeon and mark the patient's chart prominently if the patient is to undergo surgery to notify medical personnel that the blockage of compensatory angiotensin II could result in hypotension after surgery that would need to be reversed with volume expansion.
- Ensure that the patient is not pregnant before beginning therapy and suggest the use of barrier contraceptives while the patient is taking these drugs to avert potential fetal abnormalities and fetal death, which have been associated with these drugs.
- Help the patient find an alternative method of feeding the baby if they are nursing to prevent the potentially dangerous blockade of the RAAS in the neonate.
- Monitor the patient carefully in any situation that might lead to a drop in fluid volume (e.g., excessive sweating, vomiting, diarrhea, dehydration) or electrolyte alterations to detect and treat excessive hypotension and electrolyte imbalances that may occur.
- Provide thorough patient teaching, including the name of the drug, dosage prescribed, measures to avoid adverse effects, warning signs of problems, and the need for periodic monitoring and evaluation, to enhance patient knowledge about drug therapy and to promote adherence.
- Offer support and encouragement to help the patient deal with the diagnosis and the drug regimen.

Evaluation

- Monitor patient response to the drug (maintenance of BP within normal limits).
- Monitor for adverse effects (hypotension, hyperkalemia, edema, GI distress, skin reactions, cough, headache, dizziness).
- Evaluate the effectiveness of the teaching plan (patient can name drug, dosage, adverse effects to watch for; measures to avoid them; and the importance of continued follow-up).
- Monitor the effectiveness of comfort measures and adherence to the regimen.

Renin Inhibitor

In late 2007, a class of drugs for treating hypertension was introduced with the approval of aliskiren (*Tekturna*). Aliskiren directly inhibits renin, leading to decreased plasma renin activity and inhibiting the conversion of angiotensinogen to angiotensin I. This inhibition of the RAAS leads to decreased BP, decreased aldosterone release, and decreased sodium reabsorption. It is poorly and slowly absorbed from the GI tract (high-fat meals decrease absorption) with steady-state blood level reached in 7 to 8 days. It is metabolized in the liver with a half-life of 24 hours and is excreted in the urine. Aliskiren crosses the placenta and enters human milk. It should be avoided in pregnancy because of the potential for serious adverse effects on the fetus. It is suggested that patients who can become pregnant use contraceptive measures while on this drug. Patients who are breast or chestfeeding should find another method of feeding the baby if this drug is needed. Because it blocks the RAAS and aldosterone will not be stimulated to be released, there is a risk of hyperkalemia. Patients should have their potassium levels monitored before and periodically during therapy. If aliskiren is combined with furosemide, there may be a loss of diuretic effect. There is increased effect with other antihypertensive medications. There is increased risk of hyperkalemia when used with ACE inhibitors, ARBs, or potassium-sparing diuretics, so these combinations should almost always be avoided. Although it is generally well tolerated, cases of angioedema with respiratory involvement have been reported in patients using this drug. Patients should be advised to report any difficulty in breathing or swelling of the face, lips, or tongue. There is also risk of renal impairment, so renal function should be closely monitored. The most common side effect is diarrhea.

Calcium-Channel Blockers

Calcium-channel blockers decrease BP, cardiac workload, and myocardial oxygen consumption. The effects of these drugs on cardiac workload also make them effective in the treatment of angina (see Chapter 46). The calcium-channel blockers available in oral formulations include amlodipine (*Katerzia*, *Norvasc*), diltiazem (*Cardizem LA*, *Cartia XT*, and others), felodipine (generic), isradipine (generic), levamlodipine (*Conjupri*), nicardipine (generic), nifedipine (*Procardia XL*), nisoldipine (*Sular*), and verapamil (*Calan SR*). Clevidipine (*Cleviprex*) is only available in intravenous (IV) form for short-term management of hypertension when an oral calcium-channel blocker cannot be used.

Therapeutic Actions and Indications

Calcium-channel blockers inhibit the movement of calcium ions across the membranes of myocardial and arterial muscle cells, altering the action potential and blocking muscle cell contraction. This effect depresses myocardial contractility, slows cardiac impulse formation in the conductive tissues, and relaxes and dilates arteries, causing a fall in BP and a decrease in venous return. The dihydropyridine type of calcium-channel blockers primarily act on blood vessels, so they have less negative inotropic effect on the heart. Diltiazem and verapamil are nondihydropyridine calcium-channel blockers, so they have the benefit of treating some cardiac tachyarrhythmias. However, they also have the potential to cause and/or exacerbate heart failure. See Table 43.1 for usual indications for each of these drugs.

Pharmacokinetics

Most calcium-channel blockers are given orally and are generally well absorbed, metabolized in the liver, and excreted in the urine. These drugs cross the placenta and enter human milk (see "Contraindications and Cautions"). Nicardipine and clevidipine are available in IV form for short-term use when oral administration is not feasible.

Contraindications and Cautions

These drugs are contraindicated in the presence of allergy to any of these drugs to prevent hypersensitivity reactions. Nondihydropyridine calcium-channel blockers are not safe to administer to patients with heart block or sick sinus syndrome, heart failure, or acute MI with pulmonary edema, which could be exacerbated by the conduction-slowing effects of these drugs, and with renal or hepatic dysfunction, which could alter the metabolism and excretion of these drugs. Although there are no well-defined studies about effects during pregnancy, fetal toxicity has been reported in animal studies; therefore, because of the potential for adverse effects on the fetus or neonate, many of these drugs should not be used during pregnancy unless the benefit to the patient clearly outweighs any potential risk to the fetus. In addition, another method of feeding the infant should be used if these drugs are required during lactation. One major exception is that nifedipine is commonly administered during pregnancy to treat high BP. Some medications have special administration rules due to how they are absorbed. See Box 43.8 for more detail.

Adverse Effects

The adverse effects associated with these drugs relate to their effects on cardiac output and on smooth muscle. CNS effects include dizziness, lightheadedness, headache, and fatigue. GI problems include nausea, constipation, and hepatic injury related to direct toxic effects on hepatic cells. CV effects include hypotension, bradycardia, peripheral edema, and heart block. Skin flushing and rash may also occur.

Box 43.8 Focus on Safe Medication Administration

Several drugs that are used to treat hypertension cannot be cut, crushed, or chewed. This is important information to share with patients. Sometimes patients cut tablets in half to facilitate swallowing or to get twice the number of days for any given prescription. Most drugs formulated for extended release or sustained release are delivered in a matrix system that slowly dispenses the drug into the system. If the coating of the matrix is cut, all of the drugs are being released at once, creating a toxic level of the drug. Then the patient receives no drug as the day goes on. Some antihypertensives to be aware of are diltiazem, isradipine, nicardipine, nifedipine, nisoldipine, and verapamil.

Clinically Important Drug–Drug Interactions

Drug–drug interactions vary with each of the calcium-channel blockers used to treat hypertension. A potentially serious effect to note is an increase in serum levels and toxicity of cyclosporine if taken with diltiazem.

Clinically Important Drug–Food Interactions

The calcium-channel blockers are a class of drugs that interact with grapefruit juice. When grapefruit juice is present in the body, the concentrations of calcium-channel blockers increase, sometimes to toxic levels. Advise patients to avoid drinking grapefruit juice if they are taking a calcium-channel blocker. If a patient on a calcium-channel blocker reports toxic effects, ask whether they have been drinking grapefruit juice.

Prototype Summary: Diltiazem

Indications: Treatment of essential hypertension in the extended-release form; angina and tachyarrhythmias.

Actions: Inhibits the movement of calcium ions across the membranes of cardiac and arterial muscle cells, depressing the impulse and leading to slowed conduction, decreased myocardial contractility, and dilation of arterioles, which lowers BP and decreases myocardial oxygen consumption.

Pharmacokinetics:

Route	Onset	Peak	Duration
Oral, extended release	30–60 min	6–11 h	12 h

$T_{1/2}$: 5 to 7 hours; metabolized in the liver and excreted in the urine.

Adverse Effects: Dizziness, lightheadedness, headache, peripheral edema, bradycardia, atrioventricular block, flushing, nausea, hypotension.

Nursing Considerations for Patients Receiving Calcium-Channel Blockers

Calcium-channel blockers are mainly used for the treatment of angina and hypertension. See Chapter 46 for nursing considerations related to calcium-channel blockers. See the "Critical Thinking Scenario" for more on the initiation of antihypertensive therapy using calcium-channel blockers.

CRITICAL THINKING SCENARIO
Initiating Antihypertensive Therapy

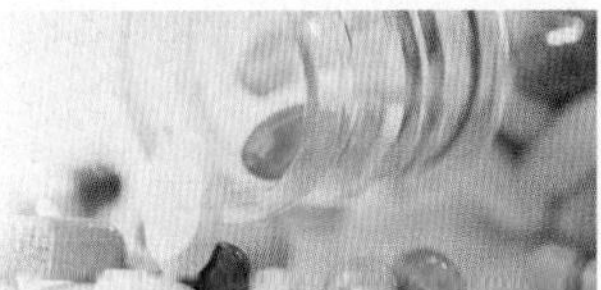

THE SITUATION

B.R., a 46-year-old African American male business executive, was seen for a routine physical examination. The examination was normal except for a BP reading of 164/102 mm Hg. B.R. was also approximately 20 pounds overweight. Urinalysis and blood work results were all within normal limits. B.R. was given a 1,500-calorie-per-day diet to follow and was encouraged to reduce salt and alcohol intake, start exercising, and stop smoking. B.R. was asked to return in 3 weeks for a follow-up appointment (step 1). Three weeks later, B.R. returned with a 7-pound weight loss and an average BP reading (of three readings) of 145/92 mm Hg. Discussion was held about starting B.R. on a diuretic (step 2) in addition to the lifestyle changes that B.R. was undertaking. B.R. was reluctant to take a diuretic and, after much discussion, was prescribed a calcium-channel blocker. B.R. asked for a couple more weeks to try to bring their BP down with lifestyle changes before starting the drug.

CRITICAL THINKING

What nursing interventions should be done at this point? Consider the risk factors that B.R. has for hypertension and the damage that hypertension can cause.

What are the chances that B.R. can bring his BP within a normal range with lifestyle changes alone?

What additional teaching points should be covered with B.R. before a treatment decision is made?

What implication does the diagnosis of hypertension have for B.R.'s insurance and job security?

What effects could diuretic therapy have on B.R.'s busy business daily life?

DISCUSSION

B.R. was asked to change many things in their life over the last 3 weeks. These changes themselves can be stressful and can increase a person's BP. B.R.'s reluctance to take a diuretic is understandable given that they are a business executive who might not want the day interrupted by many bathroom stops. This may have an impact on B.R.'s business and home life. The decision to use a calcium-channel blocker may decrease some of the stress B.R. was feeling about the diuretic.

B.R. should receive a complete teaching program outlining what is known about hypertension and all of the risk factors involved with the disease. The good effects of weight loss, exercise, and other lifestyle changes should be stressed, and B.R. should be praised for their success over the last 3 weeks.

B.R. may benefit from trying for a couple more weeks to make lifestyle changes that will help bring their BP into normal range. B.R. will then feel that they have some control over and input on the situation, and if drug therapy is needed, they may be more willing to comply with the prescribed treatment. The initiation of drug therapy may be delayed for these 2 weeks while B.R. changes their lifestyle. Only two BP measurements are required for the diagnosis of hypertension. Pharmaceutical intervention would be indicated at this time; however, if the patient feels strongly about delaying for 2 weeks, it is important to honor their autonomy. It would be important to monitor carefully and initiate medication treatment if the BP was still elevated after the 2 weeks. The accuracy of the BP measurement is extremely important, since any medication treatment has side effects and costs.

In the past, many insurance companies and some employers viewed hypertension as a hiring and insurability risk. As a business executive, B.R. may be assuming there will be a risk to having this diagnosis on their medical record. They may wish to look into biofeedback for relaxation, a fitness program, smoking cessation programs, and stress reduction. As long as B.R. receives regular follow-up and frequent BP checks, it may be a good idea to allow them to take some control and continue lifestyle changes. If, at the end of the 2 weeks, no further progress has been made or B.R.'s BP has risen, drug therapy should be highly recommended. Teaching should be aimed at helping B.R. incorporate the drug effects into their lifestyle to improve adherence to and tolerance of the therapy.

NURSING CARE GUIDE FOR B.R.: CALCIUM-CHANNEL BLOCKERS

Assessment: History and Examination

Concentrate the health history on allergies to any calcium-channel blocker, renal dysfunction, salt/volume depletion, or heart failure and concurrent use

(continues on page 760)

of barbiturates, hydantoins, erythromycin, cimetidine, ranitidine, antifungal agents, and/or grapefruit juice.

Focus the physical examination on the following:

CV: BP, pulse, perfusion, baseline ECG
CNS: Orientation, affect
Skin: Color, lesions, texture, temperature
Respiratory: Respiration, adventitious sounds
GI: Abdominal examination, bowel sounds
Laboratory tests: Renal function tests, complete blood count, electrolyte levels

Nursing Conclusions

Altered tissue perfusion related to changes in cardiac output
Altered skin integrity related to skin effects
Impaired comfort related to GI effects of drug
Knowledge deficit regarding drug therapy

Planning

The patient will receive the best therapeutic effect from the drug therapy.
The patient will have limited adverse effects from the drug therapy.
The patient will have an understanding of the drug therapy, adverse effects to anticipate, and measures to relieve discomfort and improve safety.

Intervention

Encourage lifestyle changes to increase drug effectiveness.
Do not cut, crush, or chew this tablet.
Give with food if GI upset occurs.
Provide comfort and safety measures.
Reduce dosage if patient has renal failure.
Monitor for any situation that might lead to a drop in BP.
Provide support and reassurance to deal with drug effects.
Provide patient teaching regarding drug, dosage, adverse effects, signs and symptoms of problems to report, and safety precautions.

Evaluation

Evaluate drug effects: Maintenance of BP within normal limits.
Monitor for adverse effects: Nausea, dizziness, hypotension, congestive heart failure, skin reactions.
Monitor for drug–drug interactions as listed.
Evaluate effectiveness of patient teaching program and comfort and safety measures.

PATIENT TEACHING FOR B.R.

- The drug that has been prescribed to treat your hypertension is called a calcium-channel blocker. When used to treat high BP, this drug is called an antihypertensive. High BP is a disorder that may have no symptoms but can cause serious problems, such as heart attack, stroke, or kidney problems if left untreated.
- It is important to take your medication every day as prescribed, even if you feel good without the medication. It is possible that you may feel worse because of the adverse effects associated with the medication when you take it. Even if this happens, it is crucial that you take your medication.
- If you find that the adverse effects of this drug are too uncomfortable, discuss with your health care provider the possibility of taking a different antihypertensive medication.
- This drug should be taken on an empty stomach 1 hour before or 2 hours after meals.
- Common effects of these drugs include the following:
  - *Dizziness, drowsiness, lightheadedness*: These effects often pass after the first few days. Until they do, avoid driving or performing hazardous or delicate tasks that require concentration. If these effects occur, change positions slowly to decrease the lightheadedness.
  - *Nausea, vomiting, change in taste perception*: Small, frequent meals may help ease these effects, which may pass with time. If they persist and become too uncomfortable, consult your health care provider.
  - *Skin rash, mouth sores*: Frequent mouth care may help. Keep the skin dry and use prescribed skin care (lotions, coverings, medication) if needed.
  - Report any of the following to your health care provider: difficulty breathing; mouth sores; swelling of the feet, hands, or face; chest pain; palpitations; sore throat; and fever or chills.
- Do not stop taking this drug for any reason. Consult your health care provider if you have problems taking this medication.
- You should avoid drinking grapefruit juice while you are taking this drug because the combination of grapefruit juice and a calcium-channel blocker may cause toxic effects.
- Tell any doctor, nurse, or others involved in your health care that you are taking this drug.
- Avoid taking over-the-counter medications while you are taking this drug. If you feel that you need one of these, consult with your health care provider for the best choice. Many of these drugs may interfere with the antihypertensive effect that usually occurs with this drug.
- Be extremely careful in any situation that might lead to a drop in BP (e.g., excessive sweating, vomiting, diarrhea, dehydration). If you experience lightheadedness or dizziness in any of these situations, consult your health care provider immediately.
- Keep this drug, and all medications, out of the reach of children.

Vasodilators

If other drug therapies do not achieve the desired reduction in BP, it is sometimes necessary to use a direct vasodilator. Most of the vasodilators are reserved for use in severe hypertension, refractory hypertension, or hypertensive emergencies. These include hydralazine (generic), minoxidil (generic), nitroglycerin (generic), and nitroprusside (*Nitropress*).

Therapeutic Actions and Indications

The vasodilators act directly on vascular smooth muscle to cause muscle relaxation, leading to vasodilation and drop in BP. They do not block the reflex tachycardia that occurs when BP drops. They are indicated for the treatment of severe hypertension that has not responded to other therapy (see Table 43.1).

Pharmacokinetics

Nitroprusside is used IV; hydralazine is available for oral, IV, and intramuscular (IM) use; and minoxidil is available as an oral agent only. Nitroglycerin is administered in a variety of forms (see Chapter 43) and is indicated for both angina and hypertension. These drugs are rapidly absorbed and widely distributed. They are metabolized in the liver and primarily excreted in the urine. They cross the placenta and enter human milk (see "Contraindications and Cautions").

Contraindications and Cautions

The vasodilators are contraindicated in the presence of known allergy to the drug to prevent hypersensitivity reactions and with any condition that could be exacerbated by a sudden fall in BP, such as cerebral insufficiency. Caution should be used in patients with peripheral vascular disease, CAD, heart failure, or tachycardia, all of which could be exacerbated by the fall in BP.

These drugs are also contraindicated with pregnancy unless the benefit to the patient clearly outweighs the potential risk because of the potential for adverse effects on the fetus or neonate. If they are needed by a patient who is breast or chestfeeding, another method of feeding the baby should be selected because of the potential for adverse effects on the baby.

Adverse Effects

The adverse effects most frequently seen with these drugs are related to the changes in BP. These include dizziness, anxiety, and headache; reflex tachycardia, heart failure, chest pain, and edema; skin rash and lesions (abnormal hair growth with minoxidil); and GI upset, nausea, and vomiting. Cyanide toxicity (dyspnea, headache, vomiting, dizziness, ataxia, loss of consciousness, imperceptible pulse, absent reflexes, dilated pupils, pink color, distant heart sounds, and shallow breathing) may occur with nitroprusside, which is metabolized to cyanide and also suppresses iodine uptake and can cause hypothyroidism.

Clinically Important Drug–Drug Interactions

Each of these drugs works differently in the body, so each drug should be checked for potential drug–drug interactions before use.

Prototype Summary: Nitroprusside

Indications: Severe hypertension, maintenance of controlled hypotension during anesthesia, acute heart failure.

Actions: Acts directly on vascular smooth muscle to cause vasodilation and drop of BP; does not inhibit CV reflexes and tachycardia; renin release will occur.

Pharmacokinetics:

Route	Onset	Peak	Duration
IV	1–2 min	Rapid	1–10 min

$T_{1/2}$: 2 minutes; metabolized in the liver and excreted in the urine.

Adverse Effects: Apprehension, headache, retrosternal pressure, palpitations, cyanide toxicity, diaphoresis, nausea, vomiting, abdominal pain, irritation at the injection site, hypotension.

Nursing Considerations for Patients Receiving Vasodilators

Assessment: History and Examination

- Assess for the following conditions, which could be cautions or contraindications to use of the drug: any known allergies to these drugs; impaired kidney or liver function; pregnancy or lactation because of the potential adverse effects on the fetus or neonate; and CV dysfunction, which could be exacerbated by a fall in BP.
- Assess baseline status before beginning therapy to determine any potential adverse effects; this includes body temperature and weight; skin color, lesions, and temperature; pulse, BP, baseline ECG, and perfusion; respirations and adventitious breath sounds; bowel sounds and abdominal examination; renal and liver function tests; and blood glucose.

Nursing Conclusions

Nursing conclusions related to drug therapy might include the following:

- Altered tissue perfusion (total body) related to changes in cardiac output
- Altered skin integrity related to dermatological effects
- Impaired comfort related to GI distress, skin effects, or headache
- Knowledge deficit regarding drug therapy

Planning

- The patient will receive the best therapeutic effect from the drug therapy.

(continues on page 762)

- The patient will have limited adverse effects from the drug therapy.
- The patient will have an understanding of the drug therapy, adverse effects to anticipate, and measures to relieve discomfort and improve safety.

Intervention With Rationale

- Encourage the patient to implement lifestyle changes, including weight loss, smoking cessation, decreased alcohol and salt in the diet, and increased exercise to increase the effectiveness of antihypertensive therapy.
- Monitor BP closely during administration to evaluate for effectiveness and to ensure quick response if BP falls rapidly or too much.
- Monitor heart rate, blood glucose, and serum electrolytes to avoid potentially serious adverse effects.
- Monitor the patient carefully in any situation that might lead to a drop in fluid volume (e.g., excessive sweating, vomiting, diarrhea, dehydration) to detect and treat excessive hypotension that may occur.
- Provide comfort measures to help the patient tolerate drug effects, including small, frequent meals; access to bathroom facilities; safety precautions if CNS effects occur; environmental controls; appropriate skin care as needed; and analgesics as needed.
- Provide thorough patient teaching, including the name of the drug, dosage prescribed, measures to avoid adverse effects, warning signs of problems, and the need for periodic monitoring and evaluation to enhance patient knowledge about drug therapy and to promote adherence.
- Offer support and encouragement to help the patient deal with the diagnosis and the drug regimen.

Evaluation

- Monitor patient response to the drug (maintenance of BP within normal limits).
- Monitor for adverse effects (hypotension, GI distress, skin reactions, tachycardia, headache, dizziness).
- Evaluate the effectiveness of the teaching plan (patient can name drug, dosage, adverse effects to watch for, specific measures to avoid them, and the importance of continued follow-up).
- Monitor the effectiveness of comfort measures and adherence to the regimen.

Other Antihypertensive Agents

Diuretic agents and sympathetic nervous system blocking agents are frequently used to treat HTN.

Diuretic Agents

Diuretics are drugs that increase the excretion of sodium and water from the kidney (see Fig. 43.3). See Chapter 51 for a detailed discussion of these agents. Diuretics are very important for the treatment of hypertension. These drugs are often the first agents tried in mild hypertension; they affect blood sodium levels and blood volume. The use of a thiazide or thiazidelike diuretic is currently considered one of the first-line medications used in the stepped-care management of hypertension. Although these drugs increase urination and can disturb electrolyte and acid–base balances, they are usually tolerated well by most patients. Diuretic agents used to treat hypertension include the following:

- Thiazide and thiazidelike diuretics: chlorothiazide (*Diuril*), hydrochlorothiazide (*HydroDIURIL*), methyclothiazide (generic), chlorthalidone (generic), indapamide (generic), and metolazone (*Zaroxolyn*)
- Potassium-sparing diuretics: amiloride (*Midamor*), spironolactone (*Aldactone*), and triamterene (*Dyrenium*)

Sympathetic Nervous System Blockers

Drugs that block the effects of the sympathetic nervous system are useful in blocking many of the compensatory effects of the sympathetic nervous system (see Fig. 43.3). See Chapter 31 for a detailed discussion of these drugs.

- Beta-blockers block vasoconstriction, decrease heart rate, decrease cardiac muscle contraction, and tend to increase blood flow to the kidneys, leading to a decrease in the release of renin. These drugs have many adverse effects and are not recommended for all people. They are often used as monotherapy in step 2 treatment, and they control BP adequately in some patients. Beta-blockers used to treat hypertension include acebutolol (*Sectral*), atenolol (*Tenormin*), betaxolol (generic), bisoprolol (*Zebeta*), metoprolol (*Lopressor*), nadolol (*Corgard*), nebivolol (*Bystolic*), pindolol (generic), propranolol (*Inderal*), and timolol (generic).
- Alpha- and beta-blockers are useful in conjunction with other agents and tend to be somewhat more powerful, blocking all of the receptors in the sympathetic system. Patients often complain of fatigue, loss of libido, inability to sleep, and GI and genitourinary disturbances, and they may be unwilling to continue taking these drugs. Alpha- and beta-blockers used to treat hypertension include carvedilol (*Coreg*) and labetalol (*Trandate*).
- Alpha-adrenergic blockers inhibit the postsynaptic $alpha_1$-adrenergic receptors, decreasing sympathetic tone in the vasculature and causing vasodilation, which leads to a lowering of BP. However, these drugs also block presynaptic $alpha_2$-receptors, preventing the feedback control of norepinephrine release. The result is an increase in the reflex tachycardia that occurs when BP decreases. These drugs are used to diagnose and manage episodes of pheochromocytoma, but they have limited usefulness in essential hypertension because of the associated adverse effects. Alpha-adrenergic blockers include phenoxybenzamine (*Dibenzyline*) and phentolamine (*Regitine*).

- Alpha$_1$-blockers are used to treat hypertension because of their ability to block the postsynaptic alpha$_1$-receptor sites. This decreases vascular tone and promotes vasodilation, leading to a fall in BP. These drugs do not block the presynaptic alpha$_2$-receptor sites; therefore, the reflex tachycardia that accompanies a fall in BP does not occur. Alpha$_1$-blockers used to treat hypertension include doxazosin (*Cardura*), prazosin (*Minipress*), and terazosin (generic).
- Alpha$_2$-agonists (see Chapter 30) stimulate the alpha$_2$-receptors in the CNS and inhibit the CV centers, leading to a decrease in sympathetic outflow from the CNS and a resultant drop in BP. These drugs are associated with many adverse CNS and GI effects as well as cardiac dysrhythmias. Alpha$_2$-blockers used to treat hypertension include clonidine (*Catapres*), guanfacine (*Tenex*), and methyldopa (generic).

Key Points

- Hypertension is a sustained state of higher-than-normal BP that can lead to blood vessel damage, atherosclerosis, and damage to small vessels in end organs.
- The cause of essential hypertension is unknown; treatment varies among patients.
- Drug treatment of hypertension aims to change one or more of the normal reflexes that control BP.
- Diuretic agents lower BP by various mechanisms, but they all lower blood plasma. ACE inhibitors prevent the conversion of angiotensin I to angiotensin II, leading to a fall in BP.
- ARBs prevent the body from responding to angiotensin II, causing a loss of effectiveness of the RAAS by blocking the angiotensin receptor in blood vessels.
- Renin inhibitors block the whole system by inhibiting the release of renin.
- Calcium-channel blockers interfere with the influx of calcium, decreasing the ability of muscles to contract, which leads to vasodilation, which in turn reduces BP.
- Other drugs used to treat hypertension include various medications that act on the sympathetic nervous system.

Antihypotensive Agents

As mentioned earlier, if BP becomes too low (hypotension), the vital centers in the brain and the rest of the tissues of the body may not receive sufficient oxygenated blood to continue functioning. Severe hypotension or shock puts the body in serious jeopardy; it is often an acute emergency situation requiring treatment to save the patient's life. The first-choice drug for treating shock is usually a sympathomimetic drug. See Figure 43.3 for sites of action of drugs used to treat hypotension. Antihypotensive agents are also discussed in Table 43.2.

Table 43.2 *Drugs in Focus:* Antihypotensive Agents

Drug Name	Usual Dosage	Usual Indications
Drugs for Treating Hypotension		
midodrine (generic)	10 mg PO t.i.d.	Treatment of orthostatic hypotension in adults
droxidopa (*Northera*)	100 mg PO t.i.d.; max 600 mg/d	Treatment of neurogenic hypotension caused by autonomic failure
Sympathetic Adrenergic Agonists or Vasopressors		
See Chapter 30	See Chapter 30	First choice drugs for treatment of hypotension or shock

Sympathetic Adrenergic Agonists or Vasopressors

Sympathomimetic drugs are the first choice for treating severe hypotension or shock. The sympathomimetic drugs are discussed in detail in Chapter 30. Sympathomimetic drugs used to treat shock include dobutamine (generic), dopamine (generic), ephedrine (generic), epinephrine (*Adrenalin*, *Adrenaclick*), isoproterenol (*Isuprel*), norepinephrine (*Levophed*), and phenylephrine (generic).

Therapeutic Actions and Indications

Sympathomimetic drugs react with sympathetic adrenergic receptors to cause the effects of a sympathetic stress response: increased BP, increased blood volume, and increased strength of cardiac muscle contraction. These actions increase BP and may restore balance to the CV system while the underlying cause of the shock (e.g., volume depletion, blood loss) is treated.

Adverse Effects

The adverse effects related to these drugs are the effects of stimulation of the sympathetic system: decreased GI activity with nausea and constipation; increased respiratory rate and changes in BP; headache; and changes in peripheral blood flow with numbness, tingling, and even gangrene in extreme cases. These drugs should be used with caution with any disease that limits blood flow, with tachycardia, or with hypertension.

Clinically Important Drug–Drug Interactions

There is a risk of tachycardia, tachyarrhythmias, and HTN if these drugs are used concurrently with other agents that can increase HR and BP. Patients who are receiving any of these combinations should be monitored carefully for the need for dose adjustment.

Blood Pressure–Raising Agents

Midodrine (generic) is an alpha-specific adrenergic agent used to treat orthostatic hypotension (hypotension that occurs with position change) that interferes with a person's ability to function and has not responded to any other therapy (see Table 43.2).

Therapeutic Actions and Indications

Midodrine activates alpha-receptors in arteries and veins to produce an increase in vascular tone and an increase in BP. It is indicated for the symptomatic treatment of orthostatic hypotension in patients whose lives are impaired by the disorder and who have not had a response to any other therapy.

Pharmacokinetics

Midodrine is rapidly absorbed from the GI tract, reaching peak level within 1 to 2 hours. It is metabolized in the liver and excreted in the urine with a half-life of 3 to 4 hours. It should not be used during pregnancy except in cases in which the benefit to the patient clearly outweighs the potential risk to the fetus. It is not known whether midodrine enters human milk, so caution should be used if the patient is breast or chestfeeding.

Contraindications and Cautions

Midodrine is contraindicated in the presence of supine hypertension or pheochromocytoma because of the risk of precipitating a hypertensive emergency. Caution should be used if patient has severe heart disease, which could be exacerbated by high BP; with acute renal disease, which might interfere with excretion of the drug; with urinary retention because the stimulation of alpha-receptors can exacerbate this problem; and with thyrotoxicosis, which could further increase BP. Caution should be used with pregnancy and lactation because of the potential for adverse effects on the fetus or neonate; with visual problems, which could be exacerbated by vasoconstriction; and with renal or hepatic impairment, which could alter the metabolism and excretion of the drug.

Adverse Effects

The most common adverse effects associated with this drug are related to the stimulation of alpha-receptors and include piloerection, chills, and rash; hypertension and bradycardia; dizziness, vision changes, vertigo, and headache; and problems with urination.

Clinically Important Drug–Drug Interactions

There is a risk of increased effects and toxicity of cardiac glycosides, beta-blockers, alpha-adrenergic agents, and corticosteroids if they are taken with midodrine. Patients who are receiving any of these combinations should be monitored carefully for the need for a dose adjustment.

Droxidopa

Droxidopa (*Northera*) is another BP-raising agent indicated for the treatment of orthostatic dizziness, lightheadedness, or the "about to black out" feeling in adults with symptomatic neurogenic orthostatic hypotension caused by primary autonomic failure, dopamine beta-hydroxylase deficiency, and nondiabetic autonomic neuropathy.

Therapeutic Actions and Indications

Droxidopa is an amino acid analog that is metabolized to norepinephrine by dopa decarboxylase. It is widely distributed throughout the body, and it is thought that its actions on BP are related to the norepinephrine effects causing vasoconstriction.

Pharmacokinetics

This drug is absorbed through the GI tract and reaches peak level in 1 to 4 hours. It is widely distributed and metabolized by the normal catecholamine pathways with excretion through the urine. Droxidopa has a half-life of 2.5 hours.

Contraindications and Cautions

Droxidopa is contraindicated for patients with history of allergy to this drug or its ingredients. Caution should be used with any history of CV issues because the stimulatory effects of norepinephrine can cause exacerbation of these disorders and with renal impairment because this could affect the excretion of the drug. Patients who are breast or chestfeeding should select a different method of feeding the baby because effects on infants have not been studied.

Adverse Effects

The most common adverse effects associated with this drug are related to the sympathetic effects of the drugs and include supine hypertension, headache, dizziness, nausea, and arrhythmias.

Clinically Important Drug–Drug Interactions

There is a risk of increased effects of droxidopa if combined with any dopa decarboxylase inhibitors.

Nursing Considerations for Patients Receiving Antihypotensive Drugs

Assessment: History and Examination

- Assess for the following conditions, which could be contraindications or cautions: any known allergy to the drug to prevent hypersensitivity reactions; impaired kidney or liver function, which could interfere with metabolism and excretion of the drugs; pregnancy or lactation because of the potential adverse effects on the fetus or neonate; CV dysfunction; visual problems; urinary retention; and pheochromocytoma, which could be exacerbated by the effects of the drugs.
- Assess baseline status before beginning therapy to determine any potential adverse effects; this includes body temperature and weight; skin color, lesions, and temperature; pulse, BP, orthostatic BP, and perfusion; respiration and adventitious sounds; bowel sounds and abdominal examination; and renal and liver function tests.

Nursing Conclusions

Nursing conclusions related to drug therapy might include the following:

- Altered tissue perfusion (total body) related to changes in cardiac output
- Altered sensory perception (visual, kinesthetic, tactile) related to CNS effects
- Impaired comfort related to GI distress, piloerection, chills, or headache
- Knowledge deficit regarding drug therapy

Planning

- The patient will receive the best therapeutic effect from the drug therapy.
- The patient will have limited adverse effects from the drug therapy.
- The patient will have an understanding of the drug therapy, adverse effects to anticipate, and measures to relieve discomfort and improve safety.

Intervention With Rationale

- Monitor BP carefully to monitor effectiveness and BP changes.
- Do not administer the drug to patients who are bedridden but only to patients who are up and mobile to ensure therapeutic effects and decrease the risk of severe supine hypertension.
- Monitor heart rate regularly when beginning therapy to monitor for bradycardia, which commonly occurs at the beginning of therapy; if bradycardia persists, it may indicate a need to discontinue the drug.
- Monitor patients with known visual problems carefully to ensure that the drug is discontinued if visual fields change.
- Provide comfort measures to help the patient tolerate drug effects, including small, frequent meals; access to bathroom facilities; safety precautions if CNS effects occur; environmental controls; appropriate skin care as needed; and analgesics as needed.
- Provide thorough patient teaching, including the name of the drug, dosage prescribed, measures to avoid adverse effects, warning signs of problems, and the need for periodic monitoring and evaluation to enhance patient knowledge about drug therapy and to promote adherence.
- Offer support and encouragement to help the patient deal with the diagnosis and the drug regimen.

Evaluation

- Monitor patient response to the drug (maintenance of BP within normal limits).
- Monitor for adverse effects (hypertension, dizziness, visual changes, headache, chills, urinary problems).
- Evaluate the effectiveness of the teaching plan (patient can name drug, dosage, adverse effects to watch for, specific measures to avoid them, and the importance of continued follow-up).
- Monitor the effectiveness of comfort measures and adherence to the regimen.

Key Points

- Severe hypotension, or shock, is treated with sympathomimetic drugs that stimulate the sympathetic system to increase BP.
- Midodrine and droxidopa are oral drugs used to treat people with orthostatic hypotension whose lives are considerably impaired by the fall in BP when they stand.

SUMMARY

The CV system is a closed system that depends on pressure differences to ensure the delivery of blood to the tissues and the return of that blood to the heart.

BP is related to heart rate, stroke volume, and the total PVR against which the heart has to push the blood.

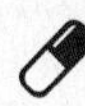
PVR is primarily controlled by constriction or relaxation of the arterioles. Constricted arterioles raise pressure; dilated arterioles lower pressure.

Control of BP involves baroreceptor (pressure receptor) stimulation of the medulla to activate the sympathetic nervous system, which causes vasoconstriction and increased fluid retention when pressure is low in the

aorta and carotid arteries and vasodilation of blood vessels when pressure is too high.

- The kidneys activate the RAAS when blood flow to the kidneys is decreased. Renin activates the conversion of angiotensinogen to angiotensin I in the liver; angiotensin I is converted by ACE to angiotensin II in the lungs; angiotensin II then reacts with specific receptor sites on blood vessels to cause vasoconstriction to raise BP and in the adrenal gland to cause the release of aldosterone, which leads to the retention of fluid and increased blood volume.
- Hypertension is a sustained state of higher-than-normal BP that can lead to damage to blood vessels, increased risk of atherosclerosis, and damage to small vessels in end organs. Because hypertension often has no signs or symptoms, it is called the silent killer.
- Essential hypertension has no underlying cause, and treatment can vary widely from person to person. Treatment approaches include lifestyle changes first followed by careful addition and adjustment of various antihypertensive drugs.
- Drug treatment of hypertension is aimed at altering one or more of the normal reflexes that control BP: Diuretics decrease plasma volume; sympathetic nervous system drugs alter the sympathetic response and lead to vascular dilation and decreased pumping power of the heart; ACE inhibitors prevent the conversion of angiotensin I to angiotensin II; ARBs prevent the body from responding to angiotensin II; renin inhibitors directly block the effects of renin; calcium-channel blockers interfere with the ability of muscles to contract and lead to vasodilation; and vasodilators directly cause the relaxation of vascular smooth muscle.
- Hypotension is a state of lower-than-normal BP that can result in decreased oxygenation of the tissues, cell death, tissue damage, and even death.
- Hypotension is most often treated with sympathomimetic drugs, which stimulate the sympathetic receptor sites to cause vasoconstriction, fluid retention, and return of normal pressure.

Unfolding Patient Stories: Junetta Cooper • Part 2

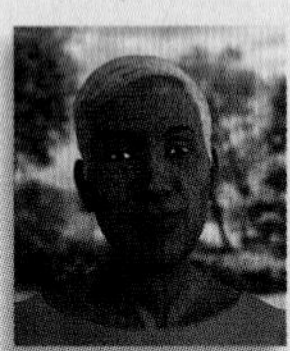

Think back to Junetta Cooper from Chapter 4, a 75-year-old female with coronary artery disease (CAD) and a 20-year history of hypertension controlled with the antihypertensive hydrochlorothiazide. While hospitalized for a cardiac catheterization, her blood pressure is elevated, and the health care team is considering the addition of amlodipine. Describe the mechanisms of action in the drug response that are associated with these different antihypertensive medications. How would the nurse explain why hydrochlorothiazide and amlodipine are selected for Junetta? What patient education should the nurse prepare if both medications are ordered for her?

Care for Junetta and other patients in a realistic virtual environment: ***vSim** for Nursing* (thepoint.lww.com/vSimPharm). Practice documenting these patients' care in DocuCare (thepoint.lww.com/DocuCareEHR).

CHECK YOUR UNDERSTANDING

Answers to the questions in this chapter can be found in Answers to Check Your Understanding Questions on thePoint*.

MULTIPLE CHOICE

Select the best answer.

1. Baroreceptors are the most important factor in controlling fast changes in BP. Baroreceptors
   a. are evenly distributed throughout the body to maintain pressure in the system.
   b. sense pressure and immediately send that information to the medulla in the brain.
   c. sense changes in neurons and are directly connected to the sympathetic nervous system.
   d. sense hemoglobin changes and are as sensitive to oxygen levels as to pressure changes.

2. Essential hypertension is the most commonly diagnosed form of high BP. Essential hypertension is
   a. caused by a tumor in the adrenal gland.
   b. associated with no known cause.
   c. related to renal disease.
   d. caused by liver dysfunction.

3. Hypertension is associated with
   a. loss of vision.
   b. strokes.
   c. atherosclerosis.
   d. all of the above.

4. The stepped-care approach to the treatment of hypertension includes
   a. lifestyle modification, including exercise, diet, and decreased smoking and alcohol intake.
   b. use of a diuretic, beta-blocker, or ACE inhibitor to supplement lifestyle changes.
   c. a combination of antihypertensive drug classes to achieve desired control.
   d. all of the above.

5. ACE inhibitors work on the RAAS to prevent the conversion of angiotensin I to angiotensin II. Because this blocking occurs in the cells in the lung, which is usually the site of this conversion, the use of ACE inhibitors often results in
   a. spontaneous pneumothorax.
   b. pneumonia.
   c. unrelenting cough.
   d. respiratory depression.

6. A patient taking an ACE inhibitor is scheduled for surgery. Because this medication may be dangerous in the setting of general anesthesia, the nurse should
   a. stop the drug without discussing with the providers.
   b. alert the provider caring for the patient and mark the patient's chart prominently.
   c. cancel the surgery and consult with the prescriber.
   d. monitor fluid levels and make sure the fluids are restricted before surgery.

7. A patient who is hypertensive becomes pregnant. Which is the safest medication for this patient?
   a. Angiotensin II receptor blocker
   b. ACE inhibitor
   c. Beta-blocker
   d. Calcium-channel blocker

8. Droxidopa, an antihypotensive drug, should be used
   a. only with patients who are confined to bed.
   b. in the treatment of acute shock.
   c. in patients with known pheochromocytoma.
   d. to treat orthostatic hypotension in patients whose lives are impaired by the disorder.

MULTIPLE RESPONSE

Select all that apply.

1. Pressure within the vascular system is determined by which?
   a. Peripheral resistance
   b. Stroke volume
   c. Sodium load
   d. Heart rate
   e. Total intravascular volume
   f. Rate of erythropoietin release

2. The RAAS is associated with which?
   a. Intense vasoconstriction and BP elevation
   b. Blood flow through the kidneys
   c. Production of surfactant in the lungs
   d. Release of aldosterone from the adrenal cortex
   e. Retention of sodium and water in the kidneys
   f. Liver production of fibrinogen

REFERENCES

American Heart Association. (2021). Heart disease and stroke statistics—2021 update. *Circulation, 143*, e254–e743. doi.org/10.1161/CIR.0000000000000950

Andrews, M., & Boyle, J. (2011). *Transcultural concepts in nursing care* (6th ed.). Lippincott Williams & Wilkins.

Bonow, R. O., Mann, D. L., Zipes, D. P., & Libby, P. (2014). *Braunwald's heart disease: A textbook of cardiovascular medicine* (10th ed.). W. B. Saunders.

Brunton, L., Hilal-Dandan, R., & Knollman, B. (2018). *Goodman and Gilman's: The pharmacological basis of therapeutics* (13th ed.). McGraw-Hill.

Eihorn, P. T., Davis, B. R., Wright, J. T., Rahman, M., Whelton, P. K., & Pressel, S. L. (2010). ALLHAT: Still providing correct answers after seven years. *Hypertension, 53*, 617–623. https://ccct.sph.uth.tmc.edu/allhat/Publications/ALLHAT%20Correct%20Answers%20After%207%20Years.pdf

Hall, J. E., & Hall, M. E. (2021). *Guyton and Hall textbook of medical physiology* (14th ed.). Elsevier.

James, P., Oparil, S., Carter, B., Cushman, W. C., Dennison-Himmelfarb, C., Handler, J., Lackland, D. T., LeFevre, M. L., MacKenzie, T. D., Ogedegbe, O., Smith, S. C., Svetkey, L. P., Taler, S. J., Townsend, R. R., Wright, J. T., Narva, A. S., & Ortiz, E. (2014). Evidence based guideline for the management of high blood pressure in adults: Report from the panel members appointed to the 8th JNC. *Journal of the American Medical Association, 311*(5), 507–520. 10.1001/jama.2013.284427

Matchar, D. B., McCrory, D. C., Orlando, L. A., Patel, M. R., Patel, U. D., Patwardhan, M. B., Powers, B., Samsa, G. P., & Gray, R. N. (2008). Systematic review: Comparative effectiveness of angiotensin-converting enzyme inhibitors and angiotensin II receptor blockers for treating essential hypertension. *Annals of Internal Medicine, 148*, 16–29. 10.7326/0003-4819-148-1-200801010-00189

Norris, T. L. (2019). *Porth's pathophysiology concepts of altered health states* (13th ed.). Wolters Kluwer.

Whelton, P. K., Carey, R. M., Aronow, W. S., Casey, D. E., Collins, K. J., Himmelfarb, C. D., DePalma, S. M., Gidding, S., Jamerson, K. A., Jones, D. W., MacLaughlin, E. J., Muntner, P., Ovbiagele, B., Smith, S. C., Spencer, C. C., Stafford, R. S., Taler, S. J., Thomas, R. J., Williams, K. A., Williamson, J. D., & Wright, J. T. (2017). 2017 ACC/AHA/AAPA/ABC/ACPM/AGS/APhA/ASH/ASPC/NMA/PCNA guideline for the prevention, detection, evaluation, and management of high blood pressure in adults. *Journal of the American College of Cardiology, 71*(19). http://www.onlinejacc.org/content/71/19/e127?_ga=2.5320883.1857899560.1543677415-334429004.1543677415

Williams, S. K., Ravenell, J., Seyedali, S., Nayef, S., & Ogedegbe, G. (2016). Hypertension treatment in blacks: Discussion of the U.S. Clinical practice guidelines. *Progress in Cardiovascular Diseases, 59*(3), 282–288. https://doi.org/10.1016/j.pcad.2016.09.004

CHAPTER 44

Agents for Treating Heart Failure

Learning Objectives

Upon completion of this chapter, you will be able to:

1. Describe the pathophysiologic process of heart failure and the resultant clinical signs.
2. Explain the body's compensatory mechanisms that occur in response to heart failure.
3. Discuss the use of cardiotonic agents across the lifespan.
4. Describe the therapeutic actions, indications, pharmacokinetics, contraindications and cautions, most common adverse effects, and important drug–drug interactions associated with the cardiotonic agents.
5. Compare and contrast the prototype drugs digoxin, ivabradine, and milrinone with other agents for treating heart failure.
6. Outline the nursing considerations including important teaching points for patients receiving cardiotonic agents.

Key Terms

afterload: resistance/pressure against which the heart has to push

cardiac output: volume of blood being pumped by the heart; cardiac output = heart rate × stroke volume

cardiomegaly: enlargement of the heart, commonly seen with chronic hypertension, valvular disease, and heart failure

cardiomyopathy: disease of the heart muscle that leads to a weakened heart and can eventually lead to complete heart muscle failure and death

dyspnea: discomfort with respirations, often with a feeling of anxiety and inability to breathe; seen often with left-sided heart failure

heart failure (HF): condition in which the heart muscle has less ability to adequately pump blood around the cardiovascular system, leading to a backup or congestion of blood in the system

hemoptysis: blood-tinged sputum seen in left-sided heart failure when blood backs up into the lungs and fluid leaks out into the lung tissue

nocturia: getting up to void at night, reflecting increased renal perfusion with fluid shifts in the supine position when a person has gravity-dependent edema related to heart failure or other medical conditions, including urinary tract infection, increasing the need to get up and void

orthopnea: difficulty breathing when lying down, often referred to by the number of pillows required to allow a person to breathe comfortably

positive inotropic: describes an agent that causes an increased force of muscle contraction

preload: amount of blood that is brought back to the heart to be pumped throughout the body; this blood exerts pressure on the heart ventricles

pulmonary edema: increased fluid in the lung tissue that can be due to left-sided heart failure

tachypnea: rapid and shallow respirations that can be seen with left-sided heart failure

Drug List

AGENTS FOR HEART FAILURE

Cardiac Glycoside
Ⓟ digoxin

Phosphodiesterase Inhibitor
Ⓟ milrinone

Hyperpolarization-Activated Cyclic Nucleotide–Gated Channel Blocker
Ⓟ ivabradine

Angiotensin Receptor Neprilysin Inhibitor
Ⓟ sacubitril/valsartan

When weakening of the heart muscle is diagnosed, the first goal of therapy is to look for reversible causes. There are times that weakening of the heart can be reversed and/or the progression of weakening slowed. The medications described in Chapter 43 that lower blood pressure and the medications described in Chapter 46 that are antianginal medications are often used to decrease the workload and oxygen consumption of the heart. Some of these medications have been shown to help slow progression of heart failure by helping to reduce the **preload** (amount of blood that is brought back to the heart to be pumped throughout the body) and **afterload** (resistance/pressure against which the heart has to push) that may stress the heart muscle.

Once the patient is not able to tolerate medications that lower heart rate and/or blood pressure due to weakening of the heart muscle, there are other medications that are used, including cardiotonic agents and a new class introduced in 2015, the hyperpolarization-activated cyclic nucleotide–gated channel blockers (HCN blockers). Cardiotonic agents are drugs used to increase the contractility of the heart muscle for patients experiencing **heart failure (HF)**, a condition in which the heart fails to pump blood around the body effectively. Because the cardiac cycle normally involves a tight balance between the pumping of the right and left sides of the heart, any failure of the muscle to pump blood out of either side of the heart can result in a backup of blood. If this happens, the blood vessels become congested; eventually, the body's cells are deprived of oxygen and nutrients, and waste products build up in the tissues. The new class of drugs approved for treating HF works in the heart's pacemaker, affecting the channels responsible for repolarization leading to a slower heart rate. Slowing the heart rate may help bring balance back into the cardiac cycle.

Heart Failure

HF is a syndrome in which, due to structural and/or functional irregularities in the heart, there is low **cardiac output**, or volume of blood being pumped by the heart, that results in pulmonary and/or systemic congestion of fluid. The American College of Cardiology and American Heart Association (ACC/AHA) have classified HF in four stages:

Stage A: At high risk for HF but without structural heart disease or symptoms of HF
Stage B: Structural heart disease but without signs or symptoms of HF
Stage C: Structural heart disease with prior or current symptoms of HF
Stage D: Refractory HF requiring specialized interventions

The New York Heart Association (NYHA) has defined functional classifications of HF:

Class I: No limitation of physical activity. Ordinary physical activity does not cause symptoms of HF.
Class II: Slight limitation of physical activity. Comfortable at rest, but ordinary physical activity results in symptoms of HF.
Class III: Marked limitation of physical activity. Comfortable at rest, but less than ordinary activity causes symptoms of HF.
Class IV: Unable to perform any physical activity without symptoms of HF, or there are symptoms of HF at rest.

The ACC/AHA and NYHA classifications are helpful when working with patients and assessing the progression of HF and their functional quality of life. Another important classification of HF is systolic versus diastolic dysfunction, which is based on the ventricular ejection fraction. Normal ejection fraction of the left ventricle is about 55% to 70%, which means that about 55% to 70% of the blood is pushed out of the ventricle each time it contracts. Systolic dysfunction is also called HF with reduced ejection fraction (HFrEF). This is when the ejection fraction is ≤40%. Diastolic dysfunction is when the ejection fraction is preserved, but there is abnormal relaxation of the heart muscle that impairs filling the ventricles with blood. Both types of HF can lead to impaired blood flow, decreased perfusion of tissues, and fluid overload. People can also have a mixture of both systolic and diastolic dysfunction.

HF usually involves dysfunction of the cardiac muscle, of which the sarcomere is the basic unit. The sarcomere contains two contractile proteins, actin and myosin, which are highly reactive with each other but at rest are kept apart by the chemical troponin. When a cardiac muscle cell is stimulated, calcium enters the cell and inactivates the troponin, allowing the actin and myosin to form actomyosin bridges. The formation of these bridges allows the muscle fibers to slide together or contract (Fig. 44.1). The formation of these bridges and subsequent contraction require a constant supply of oxygen, glucose, and calcium. (See Chapter 42 for a review of heart muscle contraction processes.)

HF can occur due to genetic, acquired, or mixed etiologies. Some common disorders that damage or overwork the heart muscle and lead to HF are the following:

- Coronary artery disease (CAD) is one of the leading causes of HF (see Chapter 46 for a discussion of CAD). CAD results in an insufficient supply of blood to meet the oxygen demands of the myocardium. Consequently, the muscles become hypoxic and can no longer function efficiently. When CAD evolves into a myocardial infarction (MI), muscle cells die or are damaged, which can lead to an inefficient pumping effort.
- **Cardiomyopathy** (conditions of the heart muscle that can lead to an enlarged heart, **cardiomegaly**, and at times eventually to complete muscle failure and death) can occur as a result of a viral infection, alcoholism, anabolic steroid abuse, genetic mutations, or a collagen disorder. It causes muscle alterations and ineffective contraction and pumping.

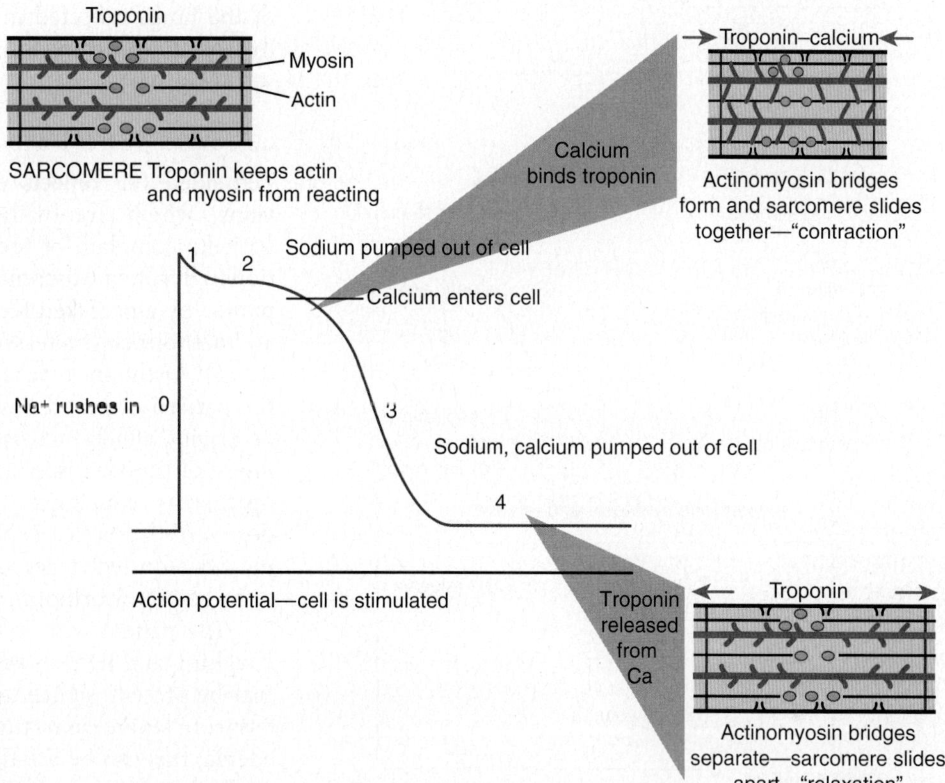

FIGURE 44.1 The sliding filaments of myocardial muscles. Calcium entering the cell deactivates troponin and allows actin and myosin to react, causing contraction. Calcium pumped out of the cell frees troponin to separate actin and myosin; the sarcomere filament slides apart, and the cell relaxes.

- Hypertension eventually leads to an enlarged cardiac muscle because the heart must work harder than normal to pump against the high pressure in the arteries. Hypertension puts constant increased demands for oxygen on the system because the heart is pumping so forcibly.
- Valvular heart disease leads to an overload of the ventricles because either the valves do not close tightly, which allows blood to leak backward into the ventricles, or the valves are stenotic, which increases the pressure against which the ventricles must pump. When blood regurgitates (flows backward), the heart muscle is stretched more than normal. The increased stretch and higher volumes of blood in the ventricles increase the demand for oxygen and energy as the heart muscle must constantly contract harder.

There are many etiologies that can cause the heart muscle to be less effective in pumping blood throughout the vascular system. If the left ventricle pumps inefficiently, blood first backs up into the lungs, causing pulmonary vessel congestion and fluid leakage into the alveoli and lung tissue. In severe cases, **pulmonary edema** (increased fluid in the lung tissue manifested by rales, wheezes, blood-tinged sputum, low oxygenation, and development of a third heart sound [S_3]) can occur. If the right side of the heart is the primary problem, blood backs up in the venous system, leading to the right side of the heart. Liver congestion and edema of the legs and feet reflect right-sided failure. Because the CV system works as a closed system, one-sided failure, if left untreated, eventually leads to failure of both sides, and the signs and symptoms of total HF occur.

Compensatory Mechanisms

Because effective pumping of blood to the cells is essential for life, the body has several compensatory mechanisms that function if the heart muscle begins to fail (Fig. 44.2). Decreased cardiac output stimulates the baroreceptors in the aortic arch and the carotid arteries, causing a sympathetic stimulation (see Chapter 29). This sympathetic stimulation increases the heart rate, blood pressure, and rate and depth of respirations. It also causes a **positive inotropic** effect (increased force of contraction) on the heart and an increase in blood volume (through the release of aldosterone). The decrease in cardiac output also stimulates the release of renin from the kidneys and activates the renin–angiotensin–aldosterone system (RAAS), which further increases blood pressure and blood volume.

If these mechanisms work effectively, compensation is occurring, and the patient may not have signs or symptoms of HF. Over time, however, the compensation mechanisms increase the workload of the heart, contributing to further development of HF. Eventually, the heart muscle overstretches and/or thickens from the increased workload, and the chambers of the heart are not able to effectively pump the blood that the body requires. The hypertrophy (enlargement) of the heart muscle, called cardiomegaly,

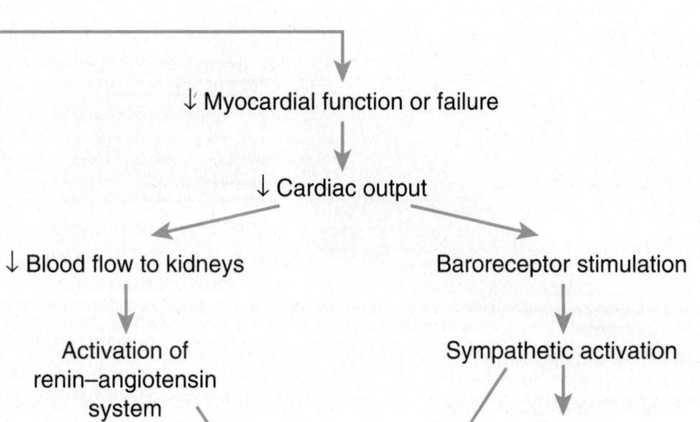

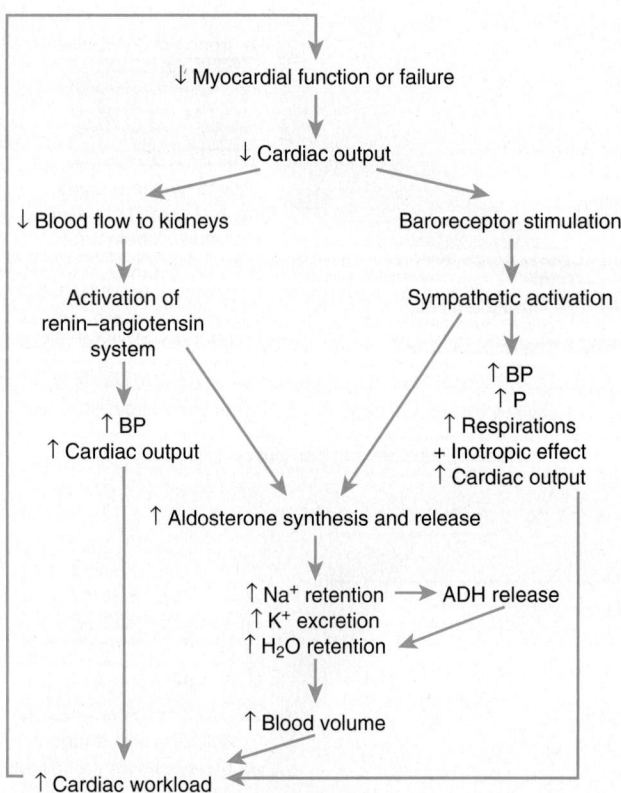

FIGURE 44.2 Compensatory mechanisms in heart failure (HF), which lead to increased cardiac workload and further HF. ADH, antidiuretic hormone; BP, blood pressure; P, pulse.

leads to decreased blood flow to tissue and eventually to increased HF.

Clinical Manifestations

The patient with HF presents a predictable clinical picture that reflects not only the problems with heart pumping but also the compensatory mechanisms that are working to balance the problem. Radiography, electrocardiography (ECG), and echocardiogram (ECHO) are helpful diagnostic tools to detect changes in the heart muscle and function. The heart may look enlarged on a chest x-ray, and the ECG may show signs of ventricular hypertrophy. There are times that the patient may develop atrial flutter or fibrillation as the atrial chambers are stretched and damaged. Anxiety often occurs as the body stimulates the sympathetic stress reaction. Heart murmurs may develop if there is turbulent flow caused by valvular stenosis or regurgitation.

Peripheral congestion and edema occur as the organs and vessels become engorged waiting for blood to be pumped through the heart as a result of pump failure. With right-sided failure, there is an enlarged liver (hepatomegaly), an enlarged spleen (splenomegaly), decreased blood flow to the gastrointestinal (GI) tract causing feelings of nausea and abdominal pain, swelling of the legs and feet, and dependent edema in the coccyx or other dependent areas with decreased peripheral pulses and hypoxia of those tissues. In addition, with left-sided failure, edema of the lungs reflected in engorged vessels and increased hydrostatic pressure throughout the CV system are also seen (Fig. 44.3).

Left-Sided Heart Failure

Left-sided HF reflects engorgement of the pulmonary veins, which eventually leads to difficulty breathing. Patients complain of **tachypnea** (rapid, shallow respirations), **dyspnea** (discomfort with breathing, often accompanied by a panicked feeling of being unable to breathe), and **orthopnea** (increased difficulty breathing when lying down). Orthopnea occurs in the supine position when the pattern of blood flow changes because of the effects of gravity, which increases pressure and perfusion in the lungs. Orthopnea is usually relieved when the patient sits up, thereby reducing the blood flow through the lungs. The degree of orthopnea is often described by the number of pillows required to get relief (e.g., one-pillow, two-pillow, or three-pillow orthopnea).

The patient with left-sided HF may also experience coughing and **hemoptysis** (coughing up of blood). Rales may be present, signaling the presence of fluid in the lung tissue. In severe cases, the patient may develop pulmonary edema; this can be life-threatening because, as the spaces in the lungs fill up with fluid, there is no place for gas exchange to occur.

Right-Sided Heart Failure

Right-sided HF usually occurs as a result of left-sided HF, but it can also be due to chronic obstructive pulmonary disease or other lung diseases that elevate the pulmonary pressure. It often results when the right side of the heart, normally a low-pressure system, must generate more and more force to move the blood into the lungs. Pulmonary hypertension can increase the pressure against which the right heart must pump and cause right-sided HF.

In right-sided HF, venous return to the heart can be decreased because of the increased pressure in the right side of the heart. This causes a congestion and backup of blood in the systemic system. Jugular venous pressure (JVP) rises and can be seen in distended neck veins, reflecting increased central venous pressure. The liver enlarges and becomes congested with blood, which leads initially to pain and tenderness and eventually to liver dysfunction and jaundice.

Dependent areas develop edema or swelling of the tissues as fluid leaves the congested blood vessels and pools in the tissues. Pitting edema in the legs is a common finding, reflecting fluid pooling in the tissues. When the patient with right-sided HF changes position and the legs are no longer dependent, for example, the fluid moves back into circulation to be returned to the heart. This increase in CV volume increases blood flow to the kidneys, causing increased urine output. This is often seen as **nocturia** (excessive voiding during the night) in a person who is up and around during the day and supine at night. The person

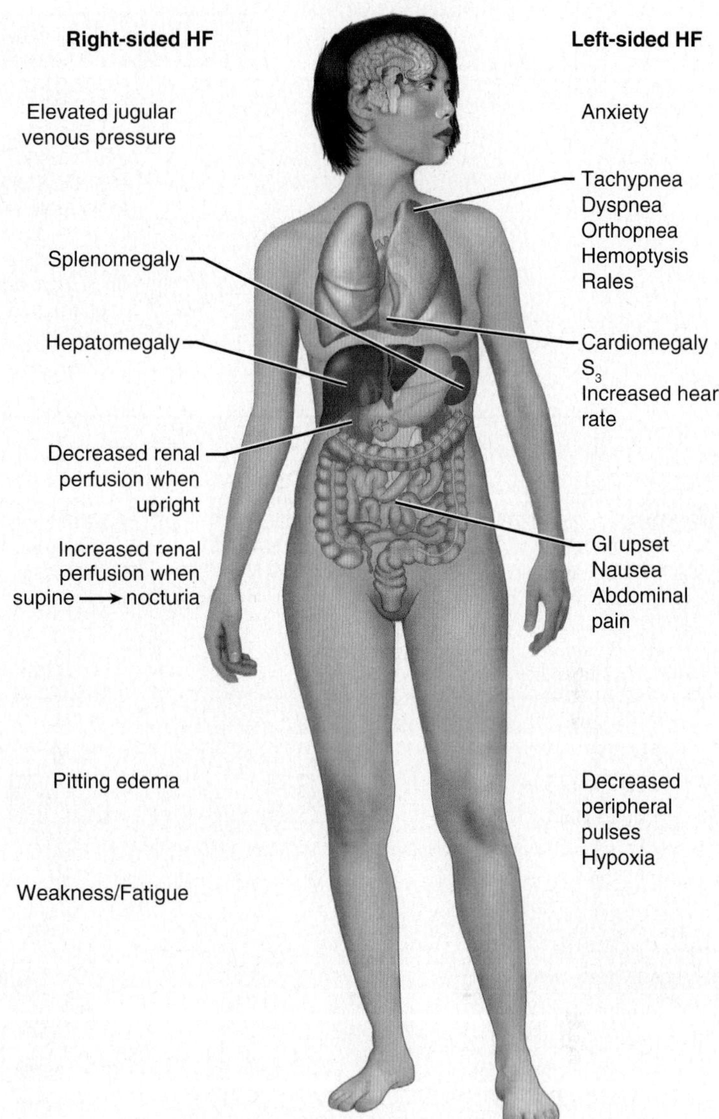

FIGURE 44.3 Signs and symptoms of heart failure (HF).

may need to get up during the night to eliminate all of the urine that has been produced as a result of the fluid shift.

Treatments

The ACC/AHA have published recommendations for treatment of HF. The term "guideline-directed medical therapy" is a description of treatment options that are supported by clinical practice guidelines because they have been shown to reverse and/or slow the progression of the HF disease process. Figure 44.4 shows an algorithm for treatment recommendations for patients with HFrEF. Most of the medications in the algorithm are discussed in other chapters due to their mechanisms of actions. As described in the treatment algorithm in Figure 44.4:

- The first goal is to decrease the work on the heart. An angiotensin receptor-neprilysin inhibitor (ARNI), angiotensin-converting enzyme inhibitor (ACEI) (Chapter 43), or angiotensin receptor blocker (ARB) (Chapter 43) is indicated to block the renin–angiotensin–aldosterone compensatory mechanism. A beta-blocker (Chapter 31) is also indicated to decrease the sympathetic stimulation that can increase the workload of the heart. The three beta-blockers that are approved for treating HF are bisoprolol, carvedilol, and metoprolol succinate (*Toprol XL*).
- An aldosterone antagonist (Chapter 51) should be added to the treatment regimen for most patients with HF as long as their kidney function can tolerate the medication and they are not hyperkalemic.
- People with persistent volume overload will have fewer symptoms with appropriate dosing of a diuretic medication (Chapter 51). Diuretics decrease venous return and blood pressure, resulting in decreased afterload, preload, and cardiac workload.
- Some of the sodium-glucose cotransporter-2 (SGLT2) (Chapter 38) medications have been shown to benefit people with HF and decrease risk of CV death and hospitalization due to HF. Therefore, this is another medication that is indicated for people with HF if the estimated glomerular filtration rate is high enough.

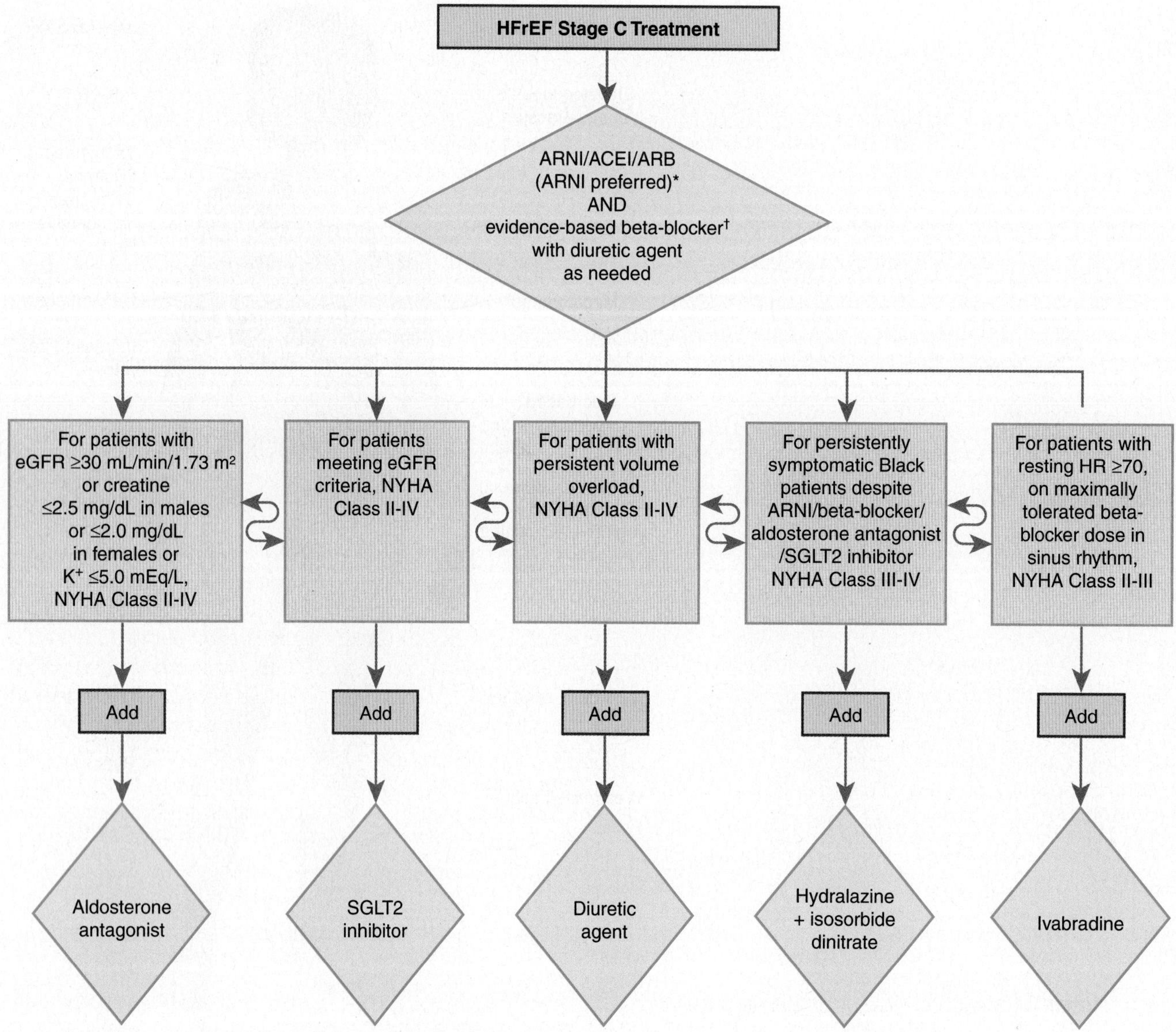

*ACEI/ARB should only be considered in patients with contraindications, intolerance or inaccessibility to ARNI.
†Carvedilol, metoprolol succinate, or bisoprolol.

ACEI = angiotensin-converting enzyme inhibitors; ARNI = angiotensin receptor-neprilysin inhibitors; ARB = angiotensin receptor blocker; eGFR = estimated glomerular filtration rate; HFrEF = heart failure with reduced ejection fraction; HR = heart rate; K^+ = potassium; NYHA = New York Heart Association; SGLT2 = sodium-glucose contrasporter-2.

FIGURE 44.4 Treatment algorithm for guideline-directed medical therapy for heart failure (HF). (Reprinted from JACC 7[6]: Maddox et al. 2021 Update to the 2017 ACC Expert Consensus Decision Pathway for Optimization of Heart Failure Treatment: Answers to 10 Pivotal Issues About Heart Failure With Reduced Ejection Fraction: A Report of the American College of Cardiology Solution Set Oversight Committee, 772-810. © 2021 with permission from the American College of Cardiology Foundation. doi: 10.1016/j.jacc.2020.11.022.)

- Hydralazine (Chapter 43) and isosorbide dinitrate (Chapter 46) have been shown to benefit Black patients who have persistent symptoms despite treatment with ARNI, beta-blocker, and aldosterone antagonist. See Box 44.1 for more info about a combination medication to treat HF.
- Ivabradine is indicated for patients whose heart rates are high despite maximal beta-blocker doses. This medication is described in more detail in this chapter.

These medications are helpful in reversing or slowing the progression of HF due to decreasing the workload of the heart by lowering afterload and to sympathetic stimulation of the heart muscle. However, there are times when a person with HF will have acute decompensation leading to a low heart rate and/or blood pressure and even acute kidney insufficiency. Therefore, the above medications may have to be stopped. The treatment goal would then be to help to increase the cardiac output.

Beta-adrenergic agonists stimulate the beta-receptors in the sympathetic nervous system, increasing calcium flow into the myocardial cells and causing increased contraction, a positive inotropic effect. Other sympathetic

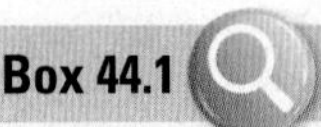

Box 44.1 Focus on Cultural Considerations

DRUGS FOR HEART FAILURE

In 2005, the Food and Drug Administration (FDA) approved a drug for use in a specific racial group for the first time. The approval caused a great deal of debate and controversy because of the implications of having a drug approved only for use in Black patients. The FDA approved the drug for use in self-identified Black patients as an adjunct therapy to standard therapy to improve survival, prolong time to hospitalization for HF, and improve patient-reported functional status. The drug, *BiDil*, is a fixed-combination drug containing isosorbide dinitrate and hydralazine. This combination of a nitrate vasodilator and an arteriolar vasodilator was studied in 1999 in the Vasodilator–Heart Failure Study and was found to be only moderately effective in general but very effective in the subset of Black patients. Further studies were done, and the African American Heart Failure Study (A-HeFT) found that this combination of drugs had a significant impact in decreasing deaths and hospitalizations related to HF in Black patients. Black patients have been found to be less responsive to angiotensin-converting inhibitors, a standard therapy for hypertension and HF; this new combination showed promise for treating this population. It is thought that there are race-related differences in endothelial functioning and responsiveness that could explain these findings. *BiDil* contains 20 mg isosorbide dinitrate and 37.5 mg hydralazine. In this combination, the drugs are rapidly absorbed and reach peak level within 1 hour. They are both metabolized in the liver and have half-lives of 4 hours (hydralazine) and 3 to 6 hours (isosorbide). *BiDil* should not be taken with any of the phosphodiesterase inhibitors (sildenafil, vardenafil, tadalafil) because of the risk of serious hypotension. Adverse effects that occurred commonly with the use of this drug were headache, dizziness, and orthostatic hypotension.

stimulation effects can cause increased HF because the heart's workload is increased by most sympathetic activity. (See Chapter 30 for additional information.)

This chapter focuses on the cardiotonic drugs (also called inotropic drugs), which work to directly increase the force of cardiac muscle contraction; the HCN blockers, which alter the heart's pacemaker and slow heart rate; and the combination medication *Entresto*, an angiotensin receptor neprilysin inhibitor.

Key Points

- In HF, the heart pumps blood so ineffectively that blood builds up, causing congestion in the CV system.
- HF can result from damage to the heart muscle combined with an increased workload related to CAD, hypertension, cardiomyopathy, valvular disease, or congenital heart abnormalities. As the heart pump fails, the muscle cells are less able to contract with adequate force and/or are less effective in relaxing to allow for adequate blood flow to the ventricles.
- Signs and symptoms of HF result from the backup of blood in the vascular system and the loss of fluid in the tissues. Right-sided HF is characterized by edema, liver congestion, elevated JVP, and nocturia, while left-sided HF is marked by tachypnea, dyspnea, orthopnea, hemoptysis, anxiety, and poor oxygenation of the blood.
- Guideline-directed medical therapy is directed at reducing the workload of the heart and decreasing symptoms of fluid overload.
- Cardiotonic (inotropic) agents (to stimulate more effective muscle contractions) and a phosphodiesterase inhibitor may be needed to increase cardiac output as a second-line treatment or for use during HF exacerbations.

Cardiotonic Agents

Cardiotonic (inotropic) drugs affect the intracellular calcium levels in the heart muscle, leading to increased contractility. This increase in contraction strength leads to increased cardiac output, which causes increased renal blood flow and increased urine production. Increased renal blood flow decreases renin release, interfering with the effects of the RAAS, and increases urine output, leading to decreased blood volume. Two types of cardiotonic drugs are used—the classic cardiac glycosides, which have been used for hundreds of years, and the newer phosphodiesterase inhibitors. Table 44.1 presents a complete list of these agents. Box 44.2 summarizes the use of cardiotonic drugs in different age groups.

Cardiac Glycosides

The cardiac glycosides were originally derived from the foxglove or digitalis plant. Digoxin (*Lanoxin*) is the drug in this classification used to treat HF symptoms.

Therapeutic Actions and Indications

Digoxin increases intracellular calcium and allows more calcium to enter myocardial cells during depolarization (Fig. 44.5), causing the following effects:

- Increased force of myocardial contraction (a positive inotropic effect)
- Increased cardiac output and renal perfusion (which has a diuretic effect, increasing urine output and decreasing blood volume while decreasing renin release and activation of the RAAS)
- Slowed heart rate, owing to slowing of the rate of cellular repolarization (a negative chronotropic effect)
- Decreased conduction velocity through the atrioventricular (AV) node

The overall effect is to increase cardiac output, which may relieve symptoms of HF in some people. Digoxin is

Table 44.1 *Drugs in Focus:* HF Treatment Agents

Drug Name	Usual Dosage	Usual Indications
Cardiac Glycoside		
digoxin (*Lanoxin*)	*Adult and pediatric*: Loading and maintenance doses vary based on age, weight, renal function, and ventricular response. Careful monitoring is necessary because toxic levels are only slightly higher than therapeutic levels.	Treatment of mild to moderate HF, control of resting ventricular rate in patients with chronic atrial fibrillation; increasing myocardial contractility in pediatric patients with HF
Phosphodiesterase Inhibitor		
milrinone (generic)	50 mcg/kg IV bolus over 10 min, then 0.375–0.75 mcg/kg/min IV infusion; do not exceed 1.13 mg/kg/d; reduce dose in renal impairment	Short-term management of HF
HCN Blocker		
ivabradine (*Corlanor*)	*Adult and pediatric >40 kg:* 2.5–5 mg PO b.i.d., adjust based on heart rate to maximum 7.5 mg PO b.i.d. *Pediatric patients <40 kg:* Starting dose is 0.05 mg/kg PO b.i.d. with food. Adjust dose based on heart rate to maximum dose of 0.2 mg/kg (for patients 6 mo to <1 y old) or 0.3 mg/kg (for patients 1 y old and older), up to a total of 7.5 mg b.i.d.	Reducing the risk of hospitalization in stable chronic HF patients with ejection factor of 35% or less and heart rate of 70 or more; treatment of stable symptomatic HF due to dilated cardiomyopathy in pediatric patients ages 6 mo and older
Angiotensin Receptor Neprilysin Inhibitor		
sacubitril/valsartan (*Entresto*)	*Adult and pediatric ≥50 kg:* 49/51 mg PO twice a day initially, can titrate up; reduce doses for pediatric patients <50 kg and with moderate liver or severe renal impairment	Decreasing the risk of CV death and hospitalization for HF in adult patients with chronic HF; treatment of symptomatic HF with systemic left ventricular systolic dysfunction in pediatric patients aged 1 y and older

HF, heart failure.

Box 44.2 Focus on Drug Therapy Across the Lifespan

AGENTS TO TREAT HF

Children

Digoxin may be used in children with heart defects and related cardiac problems. The margin of safety for the dosage of the drug is small with children. The dosage needs to be carefully calculated and should be double-checked by another nurse before administration. Children should be monitored closely for any sign of impending digitalis toxicity and should have serum digoxin levels monitored.

Ivabradine is indicated for treatment of stable symptomatic HF due to dilated cardiomyopathy in pediatric patients ages 6 months and older. Dosing is weight based for children less than 40 kg.

Adults

Adults receiving any of these drugs need to be instructed about what adverse effects to report immediately. They should learn to take their own pulse and should be encouraged to keep track of rate and regularity on a calendar. They may be asked to weigh themselves in the same clothing and at the same time of the day to monitor for fluid retention. Any changes in diet, GI activity, or medications should be reported to the health care provider because of the potential for altering serum levels and causing toxic reactions or ineffective dosing.

Safety of the use of these drugs during pregnancy has not been established. They should not be used in pregnancy unless the benefit to the patient clearly outweighs the potential risk to the fetus. The drugs do enter human milk, but they have not been associated with any adverse effects in the neonate. Caution should be exercised, however, if one of these drugs is needed when a patient is breast or chestfeeding.

Older Adults

Older adults are frequently prescribed one of these drugs. Like children at the other end of the life spectrum, older adults are more susceptible to the toxic effects of the drugs and are more likely to have underlying conditions that could interfere with their metabolism and excretion.

Renal impairment can lead to the accumulation of digoxin in the body. If renal dysfunction is present, the dosage needs to be reduced, and the patient is monitored closely for signs of digoxin toxicity. The total drug regimen of the older patient should be coordinated, with careful attention to interacting drugs and/or alternative therapies.

For backup in situations of stress or illness, a significant other should be instructed in how to take the patient's pulse and the adverse effects to watch for, while the patient is taking this drug.

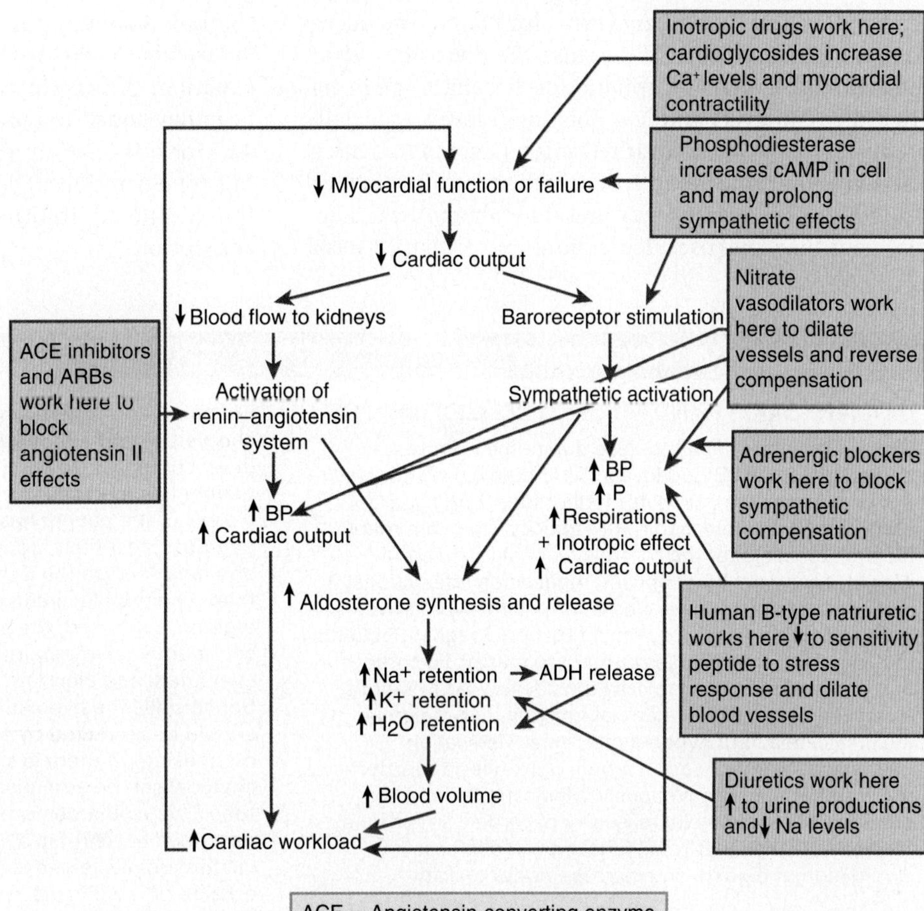

FIGURE 44.5 Sites of action of drugs used to treat heart failure (HF).

indicated for the treatment of HF, atrial flutter, atrial fibrillation, and paroxysmal atrial tachycardia (see Table 44.1). Digoxin has a narrow margin of safety (meaning that the therapeutic dose is close to the toxic dose), so extreme care must be taken when using this drug (see "Adverse Effects" for information on digoxin antidote).

Pharmacokinetics

Digoxin is available for oral and parenteral administration. The drug has a rapid onset of action and rapid absorption (30 to 120 minutes when taken orally, 5 to 30 minutes when given IV). It is widely distributed throughout the body. Digoxin is primarily excreted unchanged in the urine. Because of this, caution should be exercised in the presence of renal impairment because the drug may not be excreted and could accumulate, causing toxicity.

Contraindications and Cautions

Cardiac glycosides are contraindicated in the presence of allergy to any component of the digitalis preparation to prevent hypersensitivity reactions. Digoxin is contraindicated in the following conditions: ventricular tachycardia or fibrillation, which are potentially fatal arrhythmias and should be treated with other drugs; heart block or sick sinus syndrome, which could be made worse by slowing of conduction through the AV node; idiopathic hypertrophic subaortic stenosis (IHSS) because the increase in force of contraction could obstruct the outflow tract to the aorta and cause severe problems; acute MI because the increase in force of contraction could cause more muscle damage and infarct; renal insufficiency because the drug is excreted through the kidneys and toxic levels could develop; and electrolyte abnormalities (e.g., increased calcium, decreased potassium, decreased magnesium), which could alter the action potential and change the effects of the drug.

Digoxin should be used cautiously in patients who are pregnant or lactating because of the potential for adverse effects on the fetus or neonate. It is not known whether digoxin causes fetal toxicity; it should be given during pregnancy only if the benefit to the patient clearly outweighs the risk to the fetus. Digoxin does enter human milk, but it has not been shown to cause problems for the neonate. Caution should be exercised, however, during lactation.

Adverse Effects

The adverse effects most frequently seen with the cardiac glycosides include headache, weakness, drowsiness, and vision changes (a yellow halo around objects is often reported). GI upset and anorexia also commonly occur. Arrhythmias may develop because the glycosides affect the action potential and conduction system of the heart. High digoxin levels and low potassium levels especially predispose a person to dysrhythmias. Digoxin toxicity is a serious syndrome that can occur when the digoxin level is too high. The patient may present with anorexia; nausea; vomiting; malaise; depression; and irregular heart rhythms including heart block, atrial arrhythmias, and ventricular tachycardia. This can be a life-threatening situation. A digoxin antidote, digoxin immune fab, has been developed to rapidly treat digoxin toxicity. See Box 44.3 for information regarding digoxin toxicity and nursing considerations. See the "Critical Thinking Scenario" for additional information about inadequate digoxin absorption.

Box 44.3  **Focus on the Evidence**

DIGOXIN TOXICITY AND NURSING CONSIDERATIONS

Digoxin may be difficult to dose due to the narrow therapeutic index. Blood levels lower than 0.5 ng/mL may not be therapeutic, and levels higher than 2 ng/mL are associated with increased risk of toxicity. There are many factors that can alter the blood level of digoxin: body weight, age, renal function, and medication interactions. It is recommended to lower doses for patients with lower lean body weight and impaired renal function. Pregnant patients may need increased doses during pregnancy. Factors that increase the risk of toxicity include low body weight, advanced age or impaired renal function, hypokalemia, hypercalcemia, and hypomagnesemia. Medication interactions primarily occur when digoxin is administered orally rather than intravenously. Medications that alter potassium levels may increase risk of cardiac arrhythmia. Medications that alter renal function can decrease the elimination of digoxin and increase risk of toxicity.

Signs of Toxicity

Adverse effects are dose dependent and much less likely to occur if levels are within therapeutic range. Toxicity is directly related to the blood level; when the level is over 1.2 ng/mL, there is increased potential for adverse effects. General signs of toxicity include anorexia, nausea, vomiting, visual changes, alteration in color vision, fatigue, weakness, dizziness, and cardiac arrhythmias.

The first sign of toxicity in infants and children is sinus bradycardia or any other cardiac arrhythmia. Any change in cardiac conduction that occurs after the child is taking digoxin should be first suspected to be related to digoxin toxicity. Other common signs in infants and children are weight loss and/or failure to thrive, abdominal pain, drowsiness, and behavioral disturbances.

Most adults with digoxin toxicity will first present with nausea, vomiting, anorexia, and fatigue. Very high levels can cause hyperkalemia, especially if the person has renal impairment. Toxicity has presented with most types of cardiac arrhythmias, including heart blocks, junctional rhythms, atrial tachycardia with A-V nodal block, and others.

It may be difficult to diagnose digoxin toxicity in adults with HF without drawing blood levels due to some of the signs and symptoms being similar to those of HF exacerbation.

Nursing Implications

Assess renal function and electrolytes regularly in patients taking digoxin. Teach patients and caregivers to check heart rate and blood pressure, and instruct them to monitor both daily. If the heart rate is lower than what is normal for the patient or if there are any missed beats, the provider should be notified. Check for any potential medication interactions before administering doses of digoxin. If the patient has medication changes, monitor digoxin levels closely. If the patient has signs or symptoms of digoxin overdose, test their blood digoxin level. Notify the provider and hold medication if the serum level is elevated (greater than 2 ng/mL). In circumstances of chronic overdose, the digoxin is stopped; the patient should be monitored with continuous telemetry, medication interactions should be evaluated, and electrolyte levels should be optimized. Specifically, the hypokalemia and hypomagnesemia should be corrected by administering potassium and magnesium. If there is an acute overdose, activated charcoal can be administered orally or via nasogastric tube. This would be done in addition to the treatments described for chronic overdose. Digoxin is not removed via hemodialysis due to large amounts being distributed outside of the plasma. Symptomatic arrhythmia can be treated with digoxin immune fab, which is very effective in reversing signs and symptoms of digoxin overdose. Atropine may be administered if bradycardia and/or heart block is seen. The patient also may need a temporary pacemaker. Ventricular arrhythmia may be treated with phenytoin or lidocaine.

Digoxin Immune Fab

Digoxin immune fab (*DigiFab*) is an antigen-binding fragment (fab) derived from specific antidigoxin antibodies. These antibodies bind molecules of digoxin, making them unavailable at their site of action. The digoxin antibody–antigen complexes accumulate in the blood and are excreted through the kidney. Digoxin immune fab is used for the treatment of life-threatening digoxin intoxication (serum level greater than 10 ng/mL with serum potassium greater than 5 mEq/L in a setting of digoxin intoxication) and potential life-threatening digoxin overdose.

The amount of digoxin immune fab that is infused IV is determined by the amount of digoxin ingested or by the serum digoxin level if the ingested amount is unknown. The patient's cardiac status should be monitored while the drug is given and for several hours after the infusion is finished. Because there is a risk of hypersensitivity reaction to the infused protein, life support equipment should be on standby.

Serum digoxin levels will be high and unreliable for about 3 days after the digoxin immune fab infusion because of the high levels of digoxin in the blood. The patient should not be redigitalized for several days to 1 week after digoxin immune fab has been used because of the potential for fragments remaining in the blood.

Concept Mastery Alert

Digoxin

Pulse rates/rhythms, serum digoxin levels, potassium levels, and renal function need to be monitored closely when initiating treatment with digoxin.

Clinically Important Drug–Drug Interactions

There is a risk of increased therapeutic effects and toxic effects of digoxin if it is taken with verapamil, amiodarone, quinidine, quinine, erythromycin, tetracycline, or cyclosporine. If digoxin is combined with any of these drugs, it may be necessary to decrease the digoxin dose to prevent toxicity. If one of these drugs has been part of a medical regimen with digoxin and is discontinued, the digoxin dose may need to be increased. The risk of cardiac arrhythmias could increase if these drugs are taken with potassium-losing diuretics. If this combination is used, the patient's potassium level should be checked regularly and appropriate replacement done. Digoxin may be less effective if it is combined with thyroid hormones, metoclopramide, or penicillamine, and increased digoxin dose may be needed.

Absorption of oral digoxin may be decreased if it is taken with cholestyramine, charcoal, colestipol, antacids, bleomycin, cyclophosphamide, or methotrexate. If it is used in combination with any of these agents, the drugs should not be taken at the same time but should be administered 2 to 4 hours apart. Box 44.4 highlights important information about the interactions between digoxin and common herbal remedies.

Box 44.4 Focus on Herbal and Alternative Therapies

St. John's wort and psyllium have been shown to decrease the effectiveness of digoxin; this combination should be avoided. Increased digoxin toxicity has been reported with ginseng, hawthorn, and black licorice. Patients should be advised to avoid these combinations. Licorice acts as a pseudoaldosterone in the body, leading to loss of potassium and retention of sodium and water. This combination can cause serious digoxin toxicity. Patients should be advised to avoid this combination.

CRITICAL THINKING SCENARIO
Inadequate Digoxin Absorption

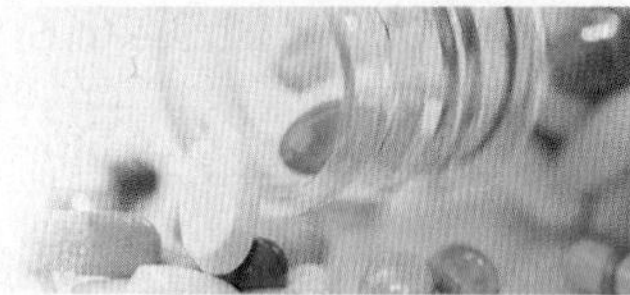

THE SITUATION

G.J. is an 82-year-old White patient with a 50-year history of rheumatic mitral valve disease. G.J. has been stabilized on digoxin for 10 years in a compensated state of HF. G.J. recently moved into an extended care facility because they were having difficulty caring for themself independently. G.J. was examined by the admitting facility physician and was found to be stable. Note was made of an irregular pulse of 76 beats/min with ECG documentation of their chronic atrial fibrillation.

Three weeks after G.J.'s arrival at the nursing home, they began to develop progressive weakness, dyspnea on exertion, two-pillow orthopnea, and peripheral 2+ pitting edema. These signs and symptoms became progressively worse, and 5 days after the first indication that the HF was returning, G.J. was admitted to the hospital with a diagnosis of HF. Physical examination revealed a heart rate of 120 to 140 beats/min with atrial fibrillation, third heart sound, rales, wheezes, 2+ pitting edema bilaterally up to the knees, elevated JVP, cardiomegaly, weak pulses, and poor peripheral perfusion. G.J.'s serum digoxin level was 0.12 ng/mL (therapeutic range, 0.5 to 2 ng/mL). G.J. was treated with diuretics and was loaded with digoxin in the hospital with close cardiac monitoring.

After their condition stabilized, G.J. reported that they knew they had been taking digoxin every day because they recognized the pill. The only difference G.J. could identify was that they were given the pill with some cereal with bran fiber, while at home they always took it on an empty stomach first thing in the morning. The nursing home staff confirmed that G.J. had received the drug daily in the morning with breakfast and that it was the same brand name medication G.J. had used at home.

CRITICAL THINKING

What nursing interventions should be done at this point? Think about the signs and symptoms of HF and how they show its progression.

How could the change in the timing of drug administration be related to the decreased serum digoxin levels noted on G.J.'s admission?

Consider the factors that affect absorption of a drug. What alterations in dosing could be suggested that would prevent this from happening to G.J. again?

What potential problems with trust could develop for G.J. upon their return to the nursing home? Suggest an explanation for what happened to G.J. and possible ways that this problem could have been averted.

DISCUSSION

G.J.'s immediate needs involve trying to alleviate the alteration to cardiac output that occurred when they lost the therapeutic effects of digoxin. Digoxin has a small

(continues on page 780)

margin of safety and requires an adequate serum level to be therapeutic. G.J. was not absorbing enough digoxin to achieve a therapeutic serum level; consequently, their body began to go through the progression of HF related to uncontrolled atrial fibrillation.

NURSING CARE GUIDE FOR G.J.: DIGOXIN

Assessment: History and Examination

- Assess the patient's health history for allergies to any digitalis product, renal dysfunction, IHSS, pregnancy, lactation, arrhythmias, heart block, and electrolyte abnormalities.
- Focus the physical examination on the following areas:
  - *CV:* Blood pressure, pulse, perfusion, electrocardiography
  - *Central nervous system (CNS):* Orientation, affect, reflexes, vision
  - *Skin:* Color, lesions, texture, perfusion
  - *Respiratory system:* Respiratory rate and character, adventitious sounds
  - *GI:* Abdominal examination, bowel sounds
  - *Laboratory tests:* Serum electrolytes, body weight

Nursing Conclusions

- Altered heart rate related to cardiac effect
- Impaired comfort due to GI upset (anorexia, nausea)
- Risk of altered tissue perfusion due to dysrhythmias
- Injury risk due to CNS effects (fatigue, vision changes, weakness)
- Knowledge deficit regarding drug therapy

Planning

- The patient will receive the best therapeutic effect from the drug therapy.
- The patient will have limited adverse effects from the drug therapy.
- The patient will have an understanding of the drug therapy, adverse effects to anticipate, and measures to relieve discomfort and improve safety.

Intervention

- Administer a loading dose to provide rapid therapeutic effects.
- Monitor apical pulse rate and rhythm, and notify the provider if the patient's heart rate is less than 60 beats/min.
- Check dose carefully.
- Administer medication daily at the same time of day.
- If administering IV, infuse over at least 5 minutes and monitor for dysrhythmias.
- Provide support and reassurance to deal with drug effects.
- Provide patient teaching regarding drug, dosage, adverse effects, what to report, and safety precautions.

Evaluation

- Evaluate drug effects: Relief of signs and symptoms of HF, resolution of atrial arrhythmias, serum digoxin levels 0.5 to 2 ng/mL.
- Monitor for adverse effects, including arrhythmias, vision changes (yellow halo), GI upset, headache, and drowsiness.
- Monitor for drug–drug interactions as indicated for each drug.
- Evaluate the effectiveness of the patient teaching program.
- Evaluate the effectiveness of comfort and safety measures.

PATIENT TEACHING FOR G.J.

- Digoxin is a digitalis preparation. Digitalis has many helpful effects on the heart; for example, it helps the heart beat more slowly and efficiently. These effects promote better circulation and should help reduce the swelling in your ankles and legs. It should also increase the amount of urine you produce every day.
- Digoxin is a powerful drug that must be taken exactly as prescribed. It is important to have regular medical checkups to ensure that the dose of the drug is correct for you and that it is having the desired effect on your heart.
- Do not stop taking this drug without consulting your health care provider. Never skip doses, and never try to "catch up" by doubling any missed doses because serious adverse effects could occur.
- Learn to take your pulse. Take it each morning before engaging in any activity. Write your pulse rate on a calendar so you will be aware of any changes and can notify your health care provider if the rate or rhythm of your pulse shows a change. Your normal pulse rate is ________. Notify your provider and do not take the digoxin if your pulse rate is less than ________.
- Try to monitor your weight fairly closely. Weigh yourself every other day at the same time of the day and in the same amount of clothing. Record your weight on your calendar for easy reference. If you gain or lose 3 lb or more between two weigh-ins, it may indicate a problem with your drug. Consult your health care provider.
- Some of the following adverse effects may occur:
  - *Dizziness, drowsiness, headache*: Avoid driving or performing hazardous tasks or delicate tasks that require concentration if these occur. Consult your health care provider for an appropriate analgesic if headaches become a problem.
  - *Nausea, GI upset, loss of appetite*: Small, frequent meals may help; monitor your weight loss; if it becomes severe, consult your health care provider.
  - *Vision changes, "yellow" halos around objects*: These effects may pass with time. Take extra care in your activities for the first few days. If these reactions do not go away after 3 to 4 days, consult your health care provider.
  - Report any of the following to your health care provider: unusually slow or irregular pulse; rapid weight gain; new "yellow vision" or other eyesight changes; unusual tiredness or weakness; skin rash or hives; swelling of the ankles, legs, or fingers; difficulty breathing.

- Tell any doctor, nurse, dentist, or other health care provider that you are taking this drug.
- Keep this drug, and all medications, out of the reach of children.
- Avoid the use of over-the-counter medications while you are taking this drug. If you think that you need one of these, consult your health care provider for the best choice. Many of these drugs contain ingredients that could interfere with your digoxin.
- Consider wearing or carrying some form of medical identification to alert any medical personnel who might take care of you in an emergency that you are taking this drug.
- Schedule regular medical checkups to evaluate the actions of the drug and to adjust the dose if necessary.

Prototype Summary: Digoxin

Indications: Treatment of HF, atrial fibrillation.

Actions: Increases intracellular calcium and allows more calcium to enter the myocardial cell during depolarization; this causes a positive inotropic effect (increased force of contraction), increased renal perfusion with a diuretic effect and decrease in renin release, a negative chronotropic effect (slower heart rate), and slowed conduction through the AV node.

Pharmacokinetics:

Route	Onset	Peak	Duration
Oral	30–120 min	2–6 h	6–8 d
IV	5–30 min	1–5 h	4–5 d

$T_{1/2}$: 30 to 40 hours; largely excreted unchanged in the urine.

Adverse Effects: Headache, weakness, drowsiness, visual disturbances, arrhythmias, GI upset.

Nursing Considerations for Patients Receiving Cardiac Glycosides

Assessment: History and Examination

- Assess for contraindications or cautions: known allergies to any digitalis product to avoid hypersensitivity reactions; impaired kidney function, which could alter the excretion of the drug; ventricular tachycardia or fibrillation, which require treatment with other life-saving drugs; heart block, sick sinus syndrome, or IHSS, which could be exacerbated by the drug; acute MI, which could lead to increased muscle damage and infarction; electrolyte abnormalities (increased calcium, decreased potassium, or decreased magnesium), which could alter the action potential and drug effects; and current status of pregnancy or lactation to evaluate benefits versus potential risk to the fetus when using the drug.
- Perform a physical assessment to establish baseline status before beginning therapy, determine the effectiveness of therapy, and evaluate for any potential adverse effects.
- Obtain the patient's weight, noting any recent increases or decreases to determine the patient's fluid status.
- Assess cardiac status closely, including pulse and blood pressure, to identify changes requiring a change in dosage of the drug or the presence of adverse effects, and auscultate heart sounds, noting any evidence of abnormal sounds to identify conduction problems.
- Inspect the skin and mucous membranes for color, and check nail beds and capillary refill for evidence of perfusion.
- Monitor affect, orientation, and reflexes to evaluate CNS effects of the drug.
- Assess the patient's respiratory rate and auscultate lungs for evidence of adventitious breath sounds to monitor for evidence of left-sided HF.
- Examine the abdomen for distension; auscultate bowel sounds to evaluate GI motility.
- Assess voiding patterns and urinary output to provide a gross indication of renal function.
- Obtain a baseline ECG to identify rate and rhythm and evaluate for possible changes.
- Monitor the results of laboratory tests, including digoxin levels, serum electrolyte levels, and renal function tests to determine the need for possible dose adjustment.

Nursing Conclusions

Nursing conclusions related to drug therapy might include the following:

- Altered heart rate related to cardiac effect
- Impaired comfort due to GI upset (anorexia, nausea)
- Risk of altered tissue perfusion due to dysrhythmias
- Injury risk due to CNS effects (fatigue, vision changes, weakness)
- Knowledge deficit regarding drug therapy

Planning

- The patient will receive the best therapeutic effect from the drug therapy.
- The patient will have limited adverse effects from the drug therapy.
- The patient will have an understanding of the drug therapy, adverse effects to anticipate, and measures to relieve discomfort and improve safety.

(continues on page 782)

Intervention With Rationale

- Consult with the prescriber about the need for a loading dose when beginning therapy to achieve desired results as soon as possible.
- Monitor apical pulse and rhythm before administering the drug to monitor for adverse effects. Hold the dose if the pulse is less than 60 beats/min in an adult, less than 70 beats/min in children, or less than 90 beats/min in an infant; retake the pulse in 1 hour. If the pulse remains low, document it, withhold the drug, and notify the prescriber because the pulse rate could indicate digoxin toxicity (see Table 44.2 for signs and symptoms).
- Monitor the pulse for any change in quality or rhythm to detect arrhythmias or early signs of toxicity.
- Check the dose and preparation carefully because digoxin has a small margin of safety, and inadvertent drug errors can cause serious problems.
- Check the pediatric dose with extreme care because children are more likely to develop digoxin toxicity. Have the dose double-checked by another nurse before administration.
- Follow dilution instructions carefully for IV use; use promptly to avoid drug degradation.
- Administer IV doses slowly over at least 5 minutes to avoid cardiac arrhythmias and adverse effects.
- Avoid IM administration, which could be quite painful.
- Arrange for the patient to be weighed at the same time each day in the same clothes to monitor for fluid retention and HF. Assess dependent areas for edema; note the amount and degree of pitting to evaluate the severity of fluid retention.
- Avoid administering the oral drug with food or antacids to avoid delays in absorption.
- Maintain emergency equipment on standby: potassium salts, lidocaine (for treatment of arrhythmias), phenytoin (for treatment of seizures), atropine (to increase heart rate), and a cardiac monitor in case severe toxicity should occur.
- Obtain digoxin level as ordered; monitor the patient for therapeutic digoxin level (0.5 to 2 ng/mL) to evaluate therapeutic dosing and to monitor for the development of toxicity.
- Provide comfort measures to help the patient tolerate drug effects. These include small, frequent meals to help alleviate GI upset or nausea; access to bathroom facilities if GI upset is severe and to accommodate increased urination related to increased cardiac output; safety precautions to reduce the risk of injury secondary to weakness and drowsiness; adequate lighting to accommodate vision changes if they occur; positioning for comfort; and frequent rest periods to balance supply and demand of oxygen.
- Offer support and encouragement to help the patient deal with the diagnosis and the drug regimen.
- Provide thorough patient teaching, including the name of the drug, dosage prescribed, technique for monitoring pulse and acceptable pulse parameters, dietary measures if appropriate, measures to avoid adverse effects, warning signs of possible toxicity and need to notify health care provider, and the need for periodic monitoring and evaluation, including ECGs and laboratory testing to enhance patient knowledge about the drug therapy and to promote adherence.

Evaluation

- Monitor patient response to the drug (improvement in signs and symptoms of HF, resolution of atrial arrhythmias, serum digoxin level of 0.5 to 2 ng/mL).
- Monitor for adverse effects (vision changes, arrhythmias, HF, headache, dizziness, drowsiness, GI upset, nausea).
- Monitor the effectiveness of comfort measures and adherence to the regimen.
- Evaluate the effectiveness of the teaching plan (patient can name drug, dosage, proper administration, adverse effects to watch for, specific measures to avoid them, and the importance of continued follow-up).

Phosphodiesterase Inhibitors

The phosphodiesterase inhibitors (see Table 44.1) belong to a second class of drugs that act as cardiotonic (inotropic) agents. The only drug currently available in this class is milrinone (generic).

Therapeutic Actions and Indications

The phosphodiesterase inhibitors block the enzyme phosphodiesterase. This blocking effect leads to an increase in myocardial cell cyclic adenosine monophosphate (cAMP), which increases the calcium level in the cell (see Fig. 44.5). Increased cellular calcium causes a stronger contraction and prolongs the effects of sympathetic stimulation, which can lead to vasodilation, increased oxygen consumption, and arrhythmias. Milrinone is indicated for the short-term treatment of HF that has not responded to digoxin or diuretics alone or that has had a poor response to digoxin, diuretics, and vasodilators. See Table 44.1 for usual indications for the drug. Because this drug has been associated with the development of potentially fatal ventricular arrhythmias, its use is limited to severe situations.

Table 44.2 Congestive HF and Response to Cardiac Glycosides

	Response	
Signs and Symptoms[a]	**During Congestive HF**	**With Therapeutic Levels of Digoxin**[b]
Heart rate, rhythm, and size	Heart hypertrophied, dilated; rate rapid, irregular; "palpitations"; auscultation—S_3	Dilation decreased, hypertrophy remains; rate, 70–80 beats/min, may be regular; auscultation—no S_3
Lungs	Dyspnea on exertion; orthopnea; tachypnea; paroxysmal nocturnal dyspnea; wheezing, rales, cough, hemoptysis (pulmonary edema)	Normal rate of respiration; reduction or elimination of wheezes and rales
Peripheral congestion	Pitting edema of dependent parts, hepatomegaly, JVP, cyanosis, oliguria, nocturia	Cardiac output and renal blood flow leads to better urine flow, decreased edema, and fewer signs and symptoms of poor perfusion
Other	Weakness, fatigue, anorexia, insomnia, nausea, vomiting, abdominal pain	Increased appetite, strength, energy

[a]Because the clinical picture in HF varies with the stage and degree of severity, the signs and symptoms may vary considerably in different patients.
[b]Therapeutic levels of digoxin will not overcome similar symptoms when they are caused by conditions other than HF. Overdosage may actually cause symptoms similar to those of HF (e.g., anorexia, nausea, vomiting, cardiac arrhythmias, peripheral congestion).
HF, heart failure; JVP, jugular venous pressure.

Pharmacokinetics

Milrinone is available only for IV use. It is widely distributed after injection. It is metabolized in the liver and excreted primarily in the urine.

Contraindications and Cautions

Phosphodiesterase inhibitors are contraindicated in the presence of allergy to either of these drugs or to bisulfites to avoid hypersensitivity reactions. Caution should be taken administering milrinone in the following conditions: severe aortic or pulmonic valvular disease, which could be exacerbated by increased contraction; acute MI, which could be exacerbated by increased oxygen consumption and increased force of contraction; fluid volume deficit, which could be made worse by increased renal perfusion; and ventricular arrhythmias, which could be exacerbated by this drug.

Caution should be exercised in older adults, who are more likely to develop adverse effects. There are no adequate studies a-bout the effects of these drugs during pregnancy, and use should be reserved for situations in which the benefit to the patient clearly outweighs the potential risk to the fetus. It is not known whether this drug enters human milk, so caution should be exercised if the patient is breast or chestfeeding.

Adverse Effects

The adverse effects most frequently seen with this drug are ventricular arrhythmias (which can progress to fatal ventricular fibrillation), hypotension, and chest pain. GI effects include nausea, vomiting, anorexia, and abdominal pain. Thrombocytopenia can occur with milrinone. Hypersensitivity reactions associated with this drug include vasculitis, pericarditis, pleuritis, and ascites. Burning at the IV injection site is also a frequent adverse effect (Fig. 44.6).

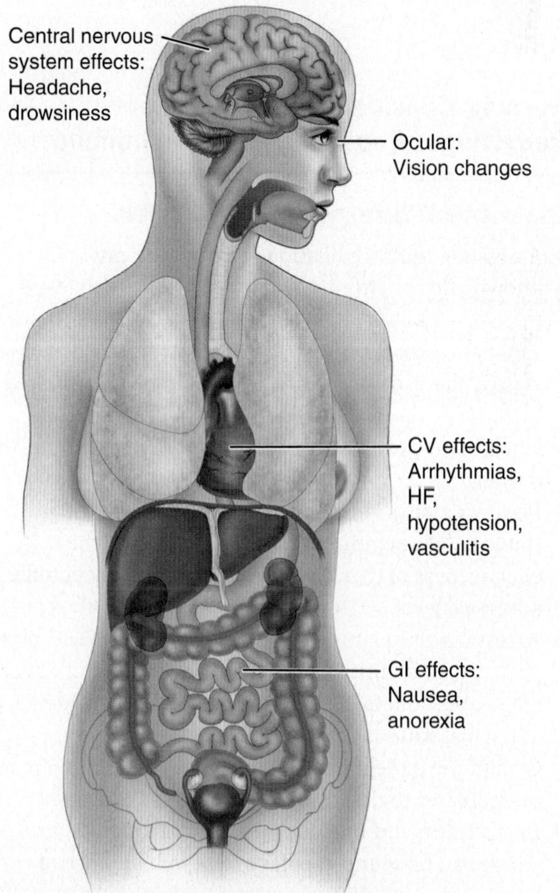

FIGURE 44.6 Variety of adverse effects and toxicities associated with cardiotonic agents.

Clinically Important Drug–Drug Interactions

Precipitates form when milrinone is given in solution with furosemide. Avoid this combination in solution. Use alternate lines if both of these drugs are being given IV.

Prototype Summary: Milrinone

Indications: Short-term treatment of HF in patients who have not responded to digitalis, diuretics, or vasodilators.

Actions: Blocks the enzyme phosphodiesterase, which leads to an increase in myocardial cell cAMP, which increases calcium levels in the cell, causing a stronger contraction and prolonged response to sympathetic stimulation; directly relaxes vascular smooth muscle.

Pharmacokinetics:

Route	Onset	Peak	Duration
IV	Immediate	10 min	8 h

$T_{1/2}$: 2.3 to 3.5 hours, metabolized in the liver and excreted in the urine and feces.

Adverse Effects: Arrhythmias, hypotension, nausea, vomiting, thrombocytopenia, pericarditis, pleuritis, fever, chest pain, burning at injection site.

Nursing Considerations for Patients Receiving a Phosphodiesterase Inhibitor

Assessment: History and Examination

- Assess for contraindications or cautions: any known allergies to this drug or to bisulfites to avoid hypersensitivity reactions; acute aortic or pulmonic valvular disease, acute MI or fluid volume deficit, and ventricular arrhythmias, which could be exacerbated by these drugs; and current status of pregnancy or lactation to prevent potential adverse effects to the fetus or baby.
- Perform a physical assessment to establish baseline status before beginning therapy, determine the effectiveness of therapy, and evaluate for any potential adverse effects.
- Assess cardiac status closely, including pulse and blood pressure, to identify changes or the presence of adverse effects; auscultate heart sounds, noting any evidence of abnormal sounds.
- Obtain the patient's weight, noting any recent increases or decreases to determine the patient's fluid status.
- Inspect skin and mucous membranes for color, and check nail beds and capillary refill for evidence of perfusion.
- Examine the abdomen for distension; auscultate bowel sounds to evaluate GI motility.
- Assess voiding patterns and urinary output to provide a gross indication of renal function.
- Obtain a baseline ECG to identify rate and rhythm and evaluate for possible changes.
- Monitor the results of laboratory tests, including serum electrolyte levels, complete blood count, and renal and hepatic function tests, to determine the need for possible dose adjustment.

Nursing Conclusions

Nursing conclusions related to drug therapy might include the following:

- Altered cardiac output related to development of arrhythmias or hypotension
- Injury risk related to CNS or CV effects
- Altered tissue perfusion (total body) related to hypotension, thrombocytopenia, or arrhythmias
- Knowledge deficit related to drug therapy

Planning

- The patient will receive the best therapeutic effect from the drug therapy.
- The patient will have limited adverse effects from the drug therapy.
- The patient will have an understanding of the drug therapy, adverse effects to anticipate, and measures to relieve discomfort and improve safety.

Intervention With Rationale

- Protect the drug from light to prevent drug degradation.
- Ensure that patient has a patent IV access site available to allow for IV administration of the drug.
- Monitor pulse and blood pressure frequently during administration to monitor for adverse effects so that the dose can be altered if needed to avoid toxicity.
- Monitor input and output and record daily weight to evaluate the resolution of HF.
- Monitor platelet counts before and regularly during therapy to ensure that the dose is appropriate, inspect the skin for bruising or petechiae to detect early signs of thrombocytopenia, and consult with the prescriber about the need to decrease the dose at the first sign of thrombocytopenia.
- Monitor IV injection sites and provide comfort measures if infusion is causing irritation.
- Provide life support equipment on standby in case of severe reaction to the drug or development of ventricular arrhythmias.
- Provide comfort measures to help the patient tolerate drug effects. These include small, frequent meals to alleviate GI upset and anorexia; access to bathroom facilities to provide needed facilities if GI upset is severe and when increased urination occurs secondary to increased cardiac output; safety precautions to protect the patient if visual changes, dizziness, or weakness occurs; and orientation to surroundings to support the patient if CNS changes occur.
- Offer support and encouragement to help the patient deal with the diagnosis and the drug regimen.

- Provide thorough patient teaching, including the name of the drug, dosage prescribed, measures to avoid adverse effects, warning signs of problems, and the need for periodic monitoring and evaluation to enhance patient knowledge about the drug therapy and to promote adherence.

Evaluation

- Monitor patient response to the drug (alleviation of signs and symptoms of HF).
- Monitor for adverse effects (hypotension, cardiac arrhythmias, GI upset, thrombocytopenia).
- Monitor the effectiveness of comfort measures and adherence to the regimen.
- Evaluate the effectiveness of the teaching plan (patient can name drug, dosage, adverse effects to watch for, specific measures to avoid them, and the importance of continued follow-up).

Hyperpolarization-Activated Cyclic Nucleotide–Gated Channel Blockers

In 2015, a new class of drugs was approved for the treatment of patients with chronic HF. The HCN blocker introduced, ivabradine (*Corlanor*), does not affect muscle contraction but does affect the pacemaker of the heart to reduce heart rate.

Therapeutic Actions and Indications

Blocking HCNs slows the heart's pacemaker, the sinus node, in the repolarizing phase of the action potential. This leads to a reduction in heart rate. Slowing the heart rate allows more time for ventricular filling, which may improve cardiac output. The systemic effects seen with beta-blockers are not seen with this class of drug. There are no effects on ventricular repolarization or on ventricular contractility. This action also affects channels in the retina, which may alter the retinal response to bright light and explain some of the adverse effects seen with this drug. Ivabradine is indicated to reduce the risk of hospitalization for worsening HF in patients with stable, symptomatic, chronic HF with a left ventricular ejection fraction of 35% or less, who are in sinus rhythm with a rate of 70 or more and who are on the maximally tolerated dose of beta-blockers or who have a contraindication to the use of beta-blockers. See Table 44.1.

Pharmacokinetics

Ivabradine is rapidly absorbed through the GI tract, reaching peak level in 1 hour. It is metabolized in the liver and intestines and excreted in the feces and bile with a half-life of 2 hours and effective duration of 6 hours.

Contraindications and Cautions

Ivabradine is contraindicated in the presence of allergy to ivabradine or to bisulfites to avoid hypersensitivity reactions. It is also contraindicated in the following conditions: active, decompensated HF; hypotension; sick sinus syndrome of AV block; resting heart rate under 60 beats/min prior to treatment; complete patient dependency on a pacemaker, which could be exacerbated by the drug leading to serious adverse effects; severe hepatic impairment, which could lead to drug accumulation; and concurrent use of strong CYP3A4 inhibitors, which could lead to drug accumulation and toxic effects.

Caution should be exercised with atrial fibrillation or moderate heart block because the drug effects may be unpredictable and not therapeutic. Fetal toxicity has been reported, so use should be discouraged during pregnancy and reserved for situations in which the benefit to the patient clearly outweighs the potential risk to the fetus. Patients who can become pregnant should be encouraged to use contraceptive measures. It is not known whether this drug enters human milk, so it is not recommended to use this drug if breast or chestfeeding.

Adverse Effects

The adverse effects most frequently seen with this drug are bradycardia, hypertension, atrial fibrillation, and luminous phenomena (sudden changes in brightness in parts of the visual field, colored bright lights, image decompensation, and/or multiple images). Safety precautions need to be taken with the visual changes.

Clinically Important Drug–Drug Interactions

Altered plasma concentrations occur with strong CYP3A4 inhibitors or inducers; this combination should be avoided. Severe bradycardia can occur if combined with other negatively chronotropic drugs.

Prototype Summary: Ivabradine

Indications: Treatment of chronic HF in stable patients at maximum beta-blocker doses, to prevent rehospitalizations.

Actions: Blocks HCNs to slow the heart's pacemaker and reduce heart rate with no effect on muscle contraction.

Pharmacokinetics:

Route	Onset	Peak	Duration
PO	Rapid	1 h	6 h

$T_{1/2}$: 2.5 hours; metabolized in the liver and intestines; excreted in the urine and feces.

Adverse Effects: Bradycardia, atrial fibrillation, hypertension, luminous phenomena (visual changes).

Nursing Considerations for Patients Receiving Ivabradine

Assessment: History and Examination

- Assess for contraindications or cautions: any known allergies to this drug to avoid hypersensitivity reactions; AV block, decompensated HF, dependence on a pacemaker, decreased resting heart rate, and hypotension, which could be exacerbated by these drugs; severe hepatic impairment or concurrent use of CYP3A4 inhibitors, which could lead to accumulation of the drug; and current status of pregnancy or lactation to prevent potential adverse effects to the fetus or baby.
- Perform a physical assessment to establish baseline status before beginning therapy, determine the effectiveness of therapy, and evaluate for any potential adverse effects.
- Assess cardiac status closely, including pulse and blood pressure, to identify changes or the presence of adverse effects; auscultate heart sounds, noting any evidence of abnormal sounds.
- Obtain the patient's weight, noting any recent increases or decreases to determine the patient's fluid status.
- Inspect skin and mucous membranes for color, and check nail beds and capillary refill for evidence of perfusion.
- Assess voiding patterns and urinary output to provide a gross indication of renal function.
- Obtain a baseline ECG to identify rate and rhythm and evaluate for possible changes.
- Monitor the results of laboratory tests, including serum electrolyte levels, complete blood count, and renal and hepatic function tests, to determine the need for possible dose adjustment.

Nursing Conclusions

Nursing conclusions related to drug therapy might include the following:

- Altered cardiac output related to development of arrhythmias or hypotension
- Injury risk related to visual or CV effects
- Altered tissue perfusion (total body) related to hypotension or bradycardia
- Knowledge deficit related to drug therapy

Planning

- The patient will receive the best therapeutic effect from the drug therapy.
- The patient will have limited adverse effects from the drug therapy.
- The patient will have an understanding of the drug therapy, adverse effects to anticipate, and measures to relieve discomfort and improve safety.

Intervention With Rationale

- Ensure appropriate use of drug to avoid serious adverse effects.
- Monitor heart rate and blood pressure regularly to evaluate drug effects and intervene as needed.
- Monitor input and output and record daily weight to evaluate the resolution of HF.
- Provide safety measures if visual disturbances occur, including limiting driving and operation of hazardous machinery to ensure patient safety.
- Provide comfort measures to help the patient tolerate drug effects.
- Offer support and encouragement to help the patient deal with the diagnosis and the drug regimen.
- Provide thorough patient teaching, including the name of the drug, dosage prescribed, measures to avoid adverse effects, warning signs of problems, and the need for periodic monitoring and evaluation, to enhance patient knowledge about the drug therapy and to promote adherence.

Evaluation

- Monitor patient response to the drug (alleviation of signs and symptoms of HF).
- Monitor for adverse effects (hypotension, cardiac arrhythmias, visual disturbances).
- Monitor the effectiveness of comfort and safety measures and adherence to the regimen.
- Evaluate the effectiveness of the teaching plan (patient can name drug, dosage, adverse effects to watch for, specific measures to avoid them, and the importance of continued follow-up).

Angiotensin Receptor Neprilysin Inhibitor

In 2015, a combination drug (*Entresto*) was approved for reducing hospitalizations and risk for CV death in patients with chronic HF and a reduced ejection fraction. It is also indicated for treatment of pediatric patients with symptomatic HF due to low left ventricular systolic function. *Entresto* (an ARNI) is a combination of valsartan (an ARB) and sacubitril, a neprilysin inhibitor.

Therapeutic Actions and Indications

Neprilysin is the enzyme that breaks down natriuretic peptides in the body. These peptides are responsible for loss of sodium and resultant water in response to ventricular overload. By blocking their breakdown, their effects last longer and more sodium and water are lost. This effect in combination with blocking the angiotensin II receptors, which inhibits the effects of the RAAS, leads to decreased cardiac workload, lower vascular volume, lower blood pressure, and improved HF symptoms. This medication is indicated to reduce the risk of CV death and hospitalization for HF in adult patients with chronic HF. Benefits are most evident in patients with left ventricular ejection fraction (LVEF) below normal. It is also indicated for the treatment of symptomatic HF with systemic left ventricular systolic dysfunction in pediatric patients aged 1 year and older. *Entresto* reduces NT-proBNP and improves CV outcomes. The ARNI is preferred over treatment with ACEI or ARB if the patient is able to afford the medication and is free of adverse effects. See Table 44.1 for information on *Entresto*.

Pharmacokinetics

After oral administration, *Entresto* dissociates into sacubitril and valsartan. Peak plasma concentration is reached quickly (between 30 minutes and 1.5 hours), and a steady level is reached in about 3 days with twice-a-day dosing. The medication can be administered with or without food. The medication is highly bound to plasma proteins. Sacubitril is mostly metabolized by enzymes called esterases, and valsartan mostly remains unmetabolized. The medication is eliminated in both urine and feces. The half-life is about 10 hours.

Contraindications and Cautions

Entresto is contraindicated in the presence of allergy or history of angioedema related to exposure to ACEI or ARB medication to protect the patient from hypersensitivity reactions. Concurrent use with an ACEI is contraindicated due to increased risk of angioedema. Concurrent use with aliskiren (renin inhibitor) in patients with poor renal function increases risk of severe renal impairment. It cannot be used in pregnancy or during breast or chest-feeding (because of the ARB component) due to evidence of increased risk of fetal harm or fatality.

Adverse Effects

Common side effects include hypotension, hyperkalemia, cough, dizziness, and renal impairment. Patients should be monitored for signs or symptoms of low blood pressure and of angioedema. Renal function and serum potassium levels should be monitored routinely.

Clinically Important Drug–Drug Interactions

Entresto is contraindicated with ACEIs. If the patient is taking an ACEI, it must be discontinued for at least 36 hours prior to initiation of *Entresto*. Patients with a glomerular filtration rate lower than 60 should not take *Entresto* and aliskiren together due to increased risk of renal impairment. Taking *Entresto* with potassium-sparing diuretics increases the risk of hyperkalemia. Concurrent use with lithium increases risk of lithium toxicity. Concurrent use with other nephrotoxic medications increases risk of renal impairment.

Prototype Summary: Sacubitril/Valsartan (*Entresto*)

Indications: Reduces the risk of CV death and hospitalization for HF in adult patients with chronic HF; treatment of pediatric patients with symptomatic HF due to decreased left ventricular function.

Actions: Inhibits neprilysin, which breaks down natriuretic peptides in the body; by blocking the breakdown of the peptides, more sodium and water are lost. This effect in combination with the blocking of the angiotensin II receptors, which inhibits the effects of the RAAS, leads to decreased cardiac workload, lower vascular volume, lower blood pressure, and fewer HF symptoms.

Pharmacokinetics:

Route	Onset	Peak	Duration
PO	30 min	1.5 h	12 h

$T_{1/2}$: 10 hours; Sacubitril is mostly metabolized by enzymes called esterases, and valsartan mostly remains unmetabolized; excreted in the urine and feces.

Adverse Effects: Hypersensitivity, angioedema, hypotension, hyperkalemia, cough, dizziness, and renal impairment.

Nursing Considerations for Patients Receiving *Entresto*

Assessment: History and Examination

- Assess for contraindications or cautions: any known allergies to this drug to avoid hypersensitivity reactions; hypotension, which could be exacerbated by this medication; severe hepatic impairment or concurrent use of CYP3A4 inhibitors, which could lead to accumulation of the drug; and current status of pregnancy or lactation to prevent potential adverse effects to the fetus or baby.
- Perform a physical assessment to establish baseline status before beginning therapy, determine the effectiveness of therapy, and evaluate for any potential adverse effects.
- Assess cardiac status closely, including pulse and blood pressure, to identify changes or the presence of adverse effects; auscultate heart sounds, noting any evidence of abnormal sounds.
- Obtain the patient's weight, noting any recent increases or decreases to determine the patient's fluid status.
- Inspect skin and mucous membranes for color, and check nail beds and capillary refill for evidence of perfusion.
- Assess voiding patterns and urinary output to provide a gross indication of renal function.

(*continues on page 788*)

- Obtain a baseline ECG to identify rate and rhythm and evaluate for possible changes.
- Monitor the results of laboratory tests, including serum electrolyte levels, complete blood count, and renal and hepatic function tests, to determine the need for possible dose adjustment.

Nursing Conclusions

Nursing conclusions related to drug therapy might include the following:

- Altered cardiac output related to development of arrhythmias or hypotension
- Injury risk related to visual or CV effects
- Altered tissue perfusion (total body) related to hypotension or bradycardia
- Knowledge deficit related to drug therapy

Planning

- The patient will receive the best therapeutic effect from the drug therapy.
- The patient will have limited adverse effects from the drug therapy.
- The patient will have an understanding of the drug therapy, adverse effects to anticipate, and measures to relieve discomfort and improve safety.

Intervention With Rationale

- Ensure appropriate use of the drug to avoid serious adverse effects.
- Monitor heart rate and blood pressure regularly to evaluate drug effects and intervene as needed.
- Monitor input and output and record daily weight to evaluate the resolution of HF.
- Provide safety measures if visual disturbances occur, including limiting driving and operation of hazardous machinery to ensure patient safety.
- Provide comfort measures to help the patient tolerate drug effects.
- Offer support and encouragement to help the patient deal with the diagnosis and the drug regimen.
- Provide thorough patient teaching, including the name of the drug, dosage prescribed, measures to avoid adverse effects, warning signs of problems, and the need for periodic monitoring and evaluation, to enhance patient knowledge about the drug therapy and to promote adherence.

Evaluation

- Monitor patient response to the drug (alleviation of signs and symptoms of HF).
- Monitor for adverse effects (hypotension, cardiac arrhythmias, visual disturbances).
- Monitor the effectiveness of comfort and safety measures and adherence to the regimen.
- Evaluate the effectiveness of the teaching plan (patient can name drug, dosage, adverse effects to watch for, specific measures to avoid them, and the importance of continued follow-up).

Key Points

- The cardiac glycoside digoxin increases the movement of calcium into the heart muscle. This results in increased force of contraction, which increases blood flow to the kidneys (causing a diuretic effect), slows the heart rate, and slows conduction through the AV node.
- Phosphodiesterase inhibitors block the breakdown of cAMP in the cardiac muscle. This allows more calcium to enter the cell (inotropic effect on cardiac muscle) and increases the relaxation in vascular muscle (which can lead to vasodilation and lower blood pressure).
- Milrinone, the only phosphodiesterase inhibitor available, is associated with increased risk of dysrhythmias, is only available via IV, and is reserved for use in refractory HF.
- Ivabradine is the first HCN blocker, which is used with stable, chronic HF to slow the pacemaker of the heart, reducing heart rate without the systemic effects that occur with beta-blockers. Slowing the heart rate allows more time for ventricular filling and improves cardiac output without the systemic effects seen with beta-blockers.
- *Entresto* is a combination drug approved for reducing hospitalizations and risk for CV death in patients with chronic HF and a reduced ejection fraction. It is a combination of valsartan (an ARB) and sacubitril, a neprilysin inhibitor (ARNI).

SUMMARY

- HF, a condition in which the heart muscle fails to effectively pump blood through the CV system, can be the result of a damaged heart muscle and increased demand to work harder.
- The sarcomere—the functioning unit of the heart muscle—is made up of protein fibers, thin actin fibers, and thick myosin fibers, which react with each other when calcium is present to inactivate troponin. The fibers slide together, resulting in contraction. Failing cardiac muscle cells lose the ability to effectively use energy to move calcium into the cell, and contractions become weak and ineffective.
- Guideline-directed medical therapy is aimed at reducing the workload of the heart and decreasing symptoms of fluid overload.

- Cardiotonic (inotropic) agents are one class of drugs used in the treatment of HF. These agents directly stimulate the muscle to contract with more force.
- Cardiac glycosides increase the movement of calcium into the heart muscle. This results in increased force of contraction, which increases blood flow to the kidneys (causing a diuretic effect), slows the heart rate, and slows conduction through the AV node.
- Phosphodiesterase inhibitors block the breakdown of cAMP in the cardiac muscle. This allows more calcium to enter the cell (inotropic effect on cardiac muscle) and increases the relaxation of vascular muscle (which can lead to vasodilation and lower blood pressure).
- HCN blockers slow the repolarization of the heart's pacemaker, leading to a slower heart rate. Slowing the heart rate allows more time for filling and improves cardiac output. This class of drugs does not affect ventricular cell activity. The systemic effects seen with the use of beta-blockers do not occur with this class of drugs.
- *Entresto* is a combination drug approved for reducing hospitalizations and risk for CV death in patients with chronic HF and a reduced ejection fraction. It is a combination of valsartan (an ARB) and sacubitril, a neprilysin inhibitor (ARNI).

CHECK YOUR UNDERSTANDING

Answers to the questions in this chapter can be found in Answers to Check Your Understanding Questions on thePoint®.

MULTIPLE CHOICE

Select the best answer.

1. A nurse assessing a patient with HF would expect to find
   a. cardiac arrest.
   b. congestion of blood vessels.
   c. an infection.
   d. a pulmonary embolism.

2. Calcium is needed in the cardiac muscle to
   a. break apart actin–myosin bridges.
   b. activate troponin.
   c. promote contraction via sliding.
   d. maintain the electrical rhythm.

3. When assessing a patient with right-sided HF, the nurse would expect to find edema
   a. in gravity-dependent areas.
   b. in the hands and fingers.
   c. around the eyes.
   d. when the patient is lying down.

4. ACE inhibitors and beta-blockers are used in the treatment of HF to slow the progression of disease. They act to
   a. decrease workload on the heart by lowering contractility, preload, and afterload.
   b. increase arterial pressure and perfusion.
   c. cause pooling of the blood and decreased venous return to the heart.
   d. increase the release of aldosterone and improve fluid balance.

5. A nurse is preparing to administer a prescribed cardiac glycoside to a patient based on the understanding that this group of drugs acts in which way?
   a. They work in the kidneys to increase fluid excretion.
   b. They affect renin release in the renin–angiotensin system.
   c. They block the parasympathetic influence on the heart muscle.
   d. They affect intracellular calcium levels in the heart muscle.

6. A nurse would instruct a patient taking digoxin (*Lanoxin*) for the treatment of HF to take which action?
   a. Make up any missed doses the next day.
   b. Report changes in heart rate.
   c. Avoid exposure to the sun.
   d. Avoid potassium supplements.

7. A nurse is about to administer digoxin (*Lanoxin*) to a patient whose apical pulse is 48 beats/min. The nurse should
   a. administer the drug and notify the prescriber that the heart rate is low.
   b. retake the pulse in 15 minutes and give the drug if the pulse has not changed.
   c. retake the pulse in 1 hour and withhold the drug if the pulse is still less than 60 beats/min.
   d. withhold the drug and notify the prescriber that the heart rate is below 60 beats/min.

8. How does ivabradine (*Corlanor*) work in the body?
   a. Blocks beta-receptors to slow the heart rate
   b. Slows influx of calcium to decrease force of contraction
   c. Slows influx of calcium and relaxes blood vessels
   d. Reduces heart rate by inhibiting action potentials at the SA node

MULTIPLE RESPONSE

Select all that apply.

1. HF occurs when the heart fails to pump effectively. Which could cause HF?
   a. Coronary artery disease
   b. Chronic hypertension
   c. Cardiomyopathy
   d. Fluid overload
   e. Pneumonia
   f. Cirrhosis
2. A patient develops left-sided HF after an MI. Which would the nurse expect to find during the patient assessment?
   a. Orthopnea
   b. Polyuria
   c. Tachypnea
   d. Dyspnea
   e. Blood-tinged sputum
   f. Swollen ankles

REFERENCES

American Heart Association. (2021). Heart disease and stroke statistics—2021 update. *Circulation, 143*, e254–e743. 10.1161/CIR.0000000000000950

Bonow, R. O., Mann, D. L., Libby, P., & Bonow, R. (2014). *Braunwald's heart disease: A textbook of cardiovascular medicine* (10th ed.). W. B. Saunders.

Brunton, L., Hilal-Dandan, R., & Knollman, B. (2018). *Goodman and Gilman's the pharmacological basis of therapeutics* (13th ed.). McGraw-Hill.

Carson, P., Ziesche, S., Johnson, G., & Cohn, J. N. (1999). Racial differences in response therapy for heart failure: Analysis of the vasodilator-heart failure trials. *Journal of Cardiac Failure, 5*(3), 178–187. https://doi.org/10.1016/s1071-9164(99)90001-5

Hall, J. E., & Hall, M. E. (2021). *Guyton and Hall textbook of medical physiology* (14th ed.). Elsevier.

Harkness, K., Spalling, M. A., Currie, K., Strachan, P. H., & Clark, A. M. (2015). A systematic review of patient heart failure self-care strategies. *Journal of Cardiovascular Nursing, 30*(2), 121–135. 10.1097/JCN.0000000000000118

Maddox, T. M., Januzzi, J. L., Allen, L. A., Breathett, K., Butler, J., Davis, L. L., Fonarow, G. C., Ibrahim, N. E., Lindenfeld, J., Masoudi, F. A., Motiwala, S. R., Oliverso, E., Patterson, H., Walsh, M. N., Wasserman, A., Yancy, C. W., & Youmans Q. R. (2021). 2021 update to the 2017 ACC expert consensus decision pathway for optimization of heart failure treatment: Answers to 10 pivotal issues about heart failure with reduced ejection fraction: A report of the American College of Cardiology Solution Set Oversight Committee. *Journal of the American College of Cardiology, 77*(6), 772–810. https://doi.org/10.1016/j.jacc.2020.11.022

Mann, D. (2015). *Heart failure: A companion to Braunwald's heart disease.* W. B. Saunders.

Norris, T. L. (2019). *Porth's pathophysiology concepts of altered health states* (13th ed.). Wolters Kluwer.

Paul, S. (2008). Hospital discharge education for patients with heart failure: What really works and what is the evidence. *Critical Care Nurse, 28*, 66–82. https://www.ghdonline.org/uploads/Paul_2008_Evidence_of_hospital_discharge_Ed_for_HF_patients.pdf

Roubille, F., & Tardif, J.-C. (2013). New therapeutic targets in cardiology: Heart failure and arrhythmia: HCN channels. *Circulation, 127*, 1986–1996. https://doi.org/10.1161/CIRCULATIONAHA.112.000145

Taylor, A. L., Ziesche, S., Yancy, C., Carson, P., D'Agostino, Jr., R., Ferdinand, K., Taylor, M., Adams, K., Sabolinski, M., Worcel, M., & Cohn, J. N. (2004). Combination of isosorbide dinitrate and hydralazine in blacks with heart failure. *The New England Journal of Medicine, 2004*(351), 2049–2057. 10.1056/NEJMoa042934

CHAPTER 45

Antiarrhythmic Agents

Learning Objectives

Upon completion of this chapter, you will be able to:

1. Describe the cardiac action potential and its phases to explain the changes made by each class of antiarrhythmic agents.
2. Discuss the use of antiarrhythmic agents across the lifespan.
3. Describe the therapeutic actions, indications, pharmacokinetics, contraindications and cautions, most common adverse effects, and important drug–drug interactions associated with antiarrhythmic agents.
4. Compare and contrast the prototype antiarrhythmic drugs lidocaine, propranolol, amiodarone, and diltiazem with other agents in their class and with other classes of antiarrhythmics.
5. Outline the nursing considerations, including important teaching points, for patients receiving antiarrhythmic agents.

Key Terms

antiarrhythmics: drugs that affect the action potential of cardiac cells and are used to treat arrhythmias and restore normal rate and rhythm

bradycardia: slower-than-normal heart rate (less than 60 beats/min)

cardiac output: amount of blood the heart can pump per beat (stroke volume) x heart rate

heart blocks: blocks to conduction of an impulse through the cardiac conduction system; can occur at the atrioventricular node, interrupting conduction from the atria into the ventricles, or in the bundle branches within the ventricles, preventing the normal conduction of the impulse

hemodynamics: the forces that move blood throughout the cardiovascular system

premature atrial contraction (PAC): an early contraction caused by an ectopic focus in the atria that stimulates an atrial response

premature ventricular contraction (PVC): an early contraction caused by an ectopic focus in the ventricles that stimulates the cells

proarrhythmic: tending to cause arrhythmias; many of the drugs used to treat arrhythmias have been found to generate them

tachycardia: faster-than-normal heart rate (greater than 100 beats/min)

Drug List

ANTIARRHYTHMIC AGENTS

Class I Antiarrhythmics

Class Ia
disopyramide
procainamide
quinidine

Class Ib
(P) lidocaine
mexiletine

Class Ic
flecainide
propafenone

Class II Antiarrhythmics
acebutolol
adenosine
digoxin
esmolol
(P) propranolol

Class III Antiarrhythmics
(P) amiodarone
dofetilide
dronedarone
ibutilide
sotalol

Class IV Antiarrhythmics
(P) diltiazem
verapamil

Disruptions in impulse formation and in the conduction of impulses through the myocardium are called dysrhythmias, which are similar to arrhythmias (irregular heartbeats). Changes in the flow of action potential and electrical impulses in the heart can be disrupted for several reasons. A unique characteristic of heart cells is that they possess the property of automaticity, which allows for the potential of generating an excitatory impulse. Disruptions in the normal rhythm of the heart can interfere with myocardial contractions and affect the stroke volume, the amount of blood pumped with each beat. Arrhythmias that seriously disrupt **cardiac output**, or the amount of blood the heart can pump per beat (stroke volume) multiplied by heart rate, can be fatal. Drugs used to treat arrhythmias, called antiarrhythmics, suppress automaticity or alter the conductivity of the heart.

Arrhythmias

Arrhythmias involve changes to the automaticity or conductivity of the heart cells. These changes can result from several factors, including electrolyte imbalances that alter the action potential, decreased oxygen delivery to cells that changes their action potential, structural damage that changes the conduction pathway, or acidosis or waste product accumulation that alters the action potential. In some cases, changes to the heart's automaticity or conductivity may result from drugs that alter the action potential or cardiac conduction.

Conductivity

With normal heart function, each cycle of cardiac contraction and relaxation is controlled by impulses arising spontaneously in the sinoatrial (SA) node and transmitted via a specialized conducting system to activate all parts of the heart muscle almost simultaneously (see Chapter 42) (Fig. 45.1). These continuous rhythmic contractions are controlled by the heart itself. This property allows the heart to beat as long as it has enough nutrients and oxygen to survive, regardless of the status of the rest of the body.

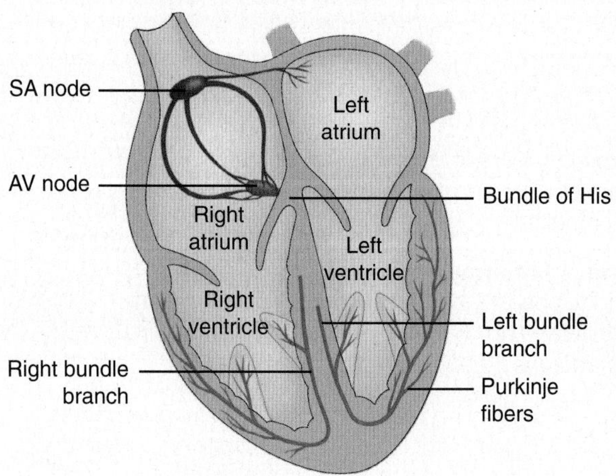

FIGURE 45.1 The conducting system of the heart. Impulses originating in the sinoatrial (SA) node are transmitted through the atrial bundles to the atrioventricular (AV) node and down the bundle of His and the bundle branches by way of the Purkinje fibers through the ventricles.

Automaticity

All cardiac cells possess some degree of automaticity (see Chapter 42) in which the cells undergo a spontaneous depolarization during diastole or rest because they decrease the flow of potassium ions out of the cell and probably leak sodium into the cell, causing an action potential.

The action potential of the cardiac muscle cell consists of the following five phases:

- Phase 0 occurs when the cell reaches a point of stimulation. The sodium gates open along the cell membrane, and sodium rushes into the cell, resulting in a positive flow of electrons into the cell—an electrical potential. This is called depolarization. The membrane no longer has a positive side and a negative side; it is depolarized, or electrically the same on both sides.
- Phase 1 is the short period when the fast sodium ion channels close and there is decreased permeability of sodium. There is slight repolarization due to potassium ions beginning to leave the cell.
- Phase 2, or the plateau stage, occurs as the cell membrane becomes less permeable to potassium. Calcium slowly enters the cell, and potassium efflux is very slow. The plateau stage is unique to cardiac muscle and allows for the action potential to last longer than that for skeletal muscle.
- Phase 3 is a period of rapid repolarization as the calcium influx stops. There is an increase in permeability of potassium, and potassium rapidly moves out of the cell. At the end of phase 3, the potassium and sodium distributions across the membrane are back to resting states.
- Phase 4 occurs when the cell comes to resting membrane potential. The sodium–potassium pump maintains this state by moving sodium out of the cell in exchange for potassium.

Each area of the heart has a slightly different-appearing action potential that reflects the complexity of the cells in that area. Because of these differences in the action potential, each area of the heart has a slightly different rate of rhythmicity. The SA node generates an impulse about 60 to 100 times per minute, the atrioventricular (AV) node about 40 to 50 times per minute, and the complex ventricular muscle cells about 10 to 20 times per minute.

Hemodynamics

The forces that move blood throughout the cardiovascular system are called **hemodynamics**. The ability of the heart to effectively pump blood depends on the coordinated contraction of the atrial and ventricular muscles, which are stimulated to contract via the conduction system. The conduction system is designed so that atrial stimulation is followed by total atrial contraction and ventricular stimulation is followed by total ventricular contraction.

To pump effectively, these muscles need to contract together. If this orderly initiation and conduction of impulses is altered, the result can be a poorly coordinated contraction of the ventricles that is unable to deliver an adequate supply of oxygenated blood to the brain and other organs, including the heart muscle. If these hemodynamic alterations are severe, serious complications can occur. For example, lack of sufficient blood flow to the brain can cause syncope or precipitate stroke; lack of sufficient blood flow to the myocardium can exacerbate atherosclerosis and cause angina or myocardial infarction (MI).

Types of Arrhythmias

Various factors can change the cardiac rate and rhythm, resulting in an arrhythmia. Arrhythmias can be caused by changes in rate (**tachycardia**, which is a faster-than-normal heart rate [greater than 100 beats per minute], or **bradycardia**, which is a slower-than-normal heart rate [less than 60 beats per minute]); by stimulation from an ectopic focus, such as premature atrial contractions (PACs) or premature ventricular contractions (PVCs), atrial flutter, atrial fibrillation (AF) (see Box 45.1), or ventricular

BOX 45.1

Understanding Atrial Fibrillation

AF is a relatively common arrhythmia of the atria. It has been associated with coronary artery disease, myocardial inflammation, valvular disease, cardiomegaly, and rheumatic heart disease. The cells of the atria are connected side to side and top to bottom and are relatively simple cells. In contrast, the cells of the ventricles are connected only from top to bottom, with one cell connected only to one or two other cells. It is much easier, therefore, for an ectopic focus in the atria to spread that impulse throughout the entire atria, setting up a cycle of chaotic depolarization and repolarization. It is more difficult to stimulate fibrillation in the ventricles, because one ectopic site cannot rapidly spread impulses to many other cells, only to the cells connected in its two- or three-cell set.

Fibrillation results in lack of any coordinated pumping action because the muscles are not stimulated to contract and pump out blood. In the ventricles, this is a life-threatening situation. If the ventricles do not pump blood, no blood is delivered to the brain, the tissues of the body, or the heart muscle itself. However, loss of pumping action in the atria on its own does not usually cause much of a problem. The atrial contraction is like an extra kick of blood into the ventricles; it provides a nice backup to the system, but most of the blood will still flow normally without that kick.

Danger of Blood Clots

One of the problems with AF occurs when it persists. The auricles (the appendages hanging on the atria to collect blood; see Chapter 42) fill with blood that is not effectively pumped into the ventricles. Over time, this somewhat stagnant blood tends to clot. Because the auricles are sacks of striated muscle fibers, blood clots form around these fibers. In this situation, if the atria were to contract in a coordinated manner, there is a substantial risk that those clots or emboli would be pumped into the ventricles and then into the lungs (from the right auricle), which could lead to pulmonary emboli, or to the brain or periphery (from the left auricle), which could cause a stroke or occlusion of peripheral vessels.

Treatment Choices

AF is classified as paroxysmal (<7 days), persistent (>7 days), long-standing (>12 months), and permanent. Treatment of AF can be complicated if the length of time the patient has been in AF is not known. The first step is to confirm that the person is in AF with a 12-lead ECG. Then it is beneficial to characterize the AF by defining the person's stroke risk, the symptom burden, and severity. The CHA_2DS_2-VASc score is a way to quantify the stroke risk. The score takes into account the person's age, sex, HF history, hypertension history, stroke or thromboembolism history, vascular disease history, and diabetes history. The higher the score, the higher the risk of stroke. The patient and/or family should be informed of the risks and benefits of anticoagulation therapy based on how high the risk of thromboembolism is.

If a patient goes into AF acutely, drug and/or electrical therapy is available for rapid conversion. For example, amiodarone and ibutilide are often effective when given IV for rapid conversion of the AF. Electrocardioversion, a DC current shock to the chest, may break the cycle of fibrillation and convert a patient to sinus rhythm, after which the rhythm will need to be stabilized with drug therapy.

If the onset of AF is not known and it is suspected that the atria may have been fibrillating for longer than 1 week, the patient needs to be evaluated for potential blood clots in the heart before attempting conversion of the rhythm. Prophylactic oral anticoagulants are given to decrease the risk of clot formation and emboli being pumped into the system. There are several oral anticoagulants available for clot prophylaxis in AF including warfarin (*Coumadin*), dabigatran (*Pradaxa*), apixaban (*Eliquis*), rivaroxaban (*Xarelto*), and edoxaban (*Savaysa*). Each of these drugs has risks and benefits. They are discussed in Chapter 48. Without first ruling out a clot in the heart, conversion could result in potentially life-threatening embolization of the lungs, brain, or other tissues. The medications that can be used for pharmacological cardioversion to sinus rhythm are amiodarone, dofetilide, flecainide, ibutilide, and propafenone. Flecainide and propafenone are not safe to use in patients with structural heart disease.

There are also situations when treatment for AF is based on rate control versus conversion to sinus rhythm. First-line medications for reducing fast rates from AF are beta blockers and nondihydropyridine calcium channel blockers. Digoxin can be used if those drugs are not successful and/or are contraindicated in specific patients.

Implications for Nurses

Careful patient assessment is essential before beginning treatment for AF. If a history cannot be established from patient information and medical records are not available, it is usually recommended that AF not be converted unless a clot in the heart has been ruled out or the patient has been anticoagulated. This can pose a challenge for the nurse in trying to teach patients about why their rapid and irregular heart rate will not be treated and explaining all of the factors involved in the long-term use of oral anticoagulants.

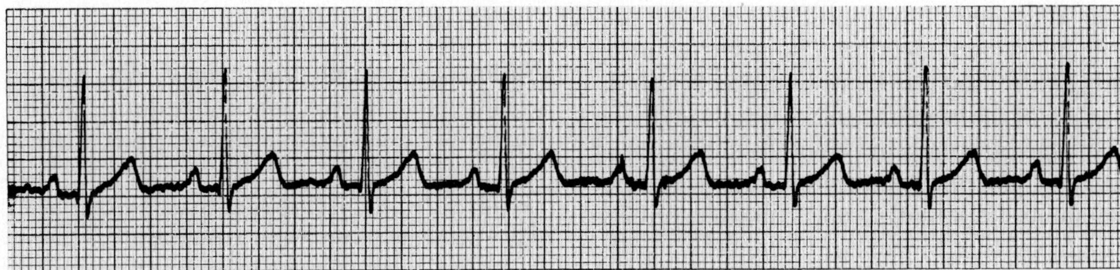

FIGURE 45.2 Normal sinus rhythm. Rhythm: Regular. Rate: 60 to 100 beats/min. P–R interval: 0.12 to 0.20 seconds. QRS: 0.06 to 0.10 seconds.

fibrillation; or by alterations in conduction through the muscle, such as heart blocks and bundle-branch blocks. A **premature atrial contraction** (PAC) is an early contraction caused by an ectopic focus in the atria that stimulates an atrial response. A **premature ventricular contraction** (PVC) is an early contraction caused by an ectopic focus in the ventricles that stimulates the cells. **Heart blocks** occur when there is a disruption in conduction of an impulse through the cardiac conduction system. They can occur at the atrioventricular node, interrupting conduction from the atria into the ventricles, or in the bundle branches within the ventricles, preventing the normal conduction of the impulse. Figure 45.2 displays an electrocardiogram (ECG) strip showing normal sinus rhythm; Figures 45.3 to 45.5 depict various arrhythmias.

Key Points

- Arrhythmias (also called dysrhythmias) are disruptions in the normal rate or rhythm of the heart.
- The cardiac conduction system determines the heart's rate and rhythm. Automaticity is the property by which the cardiac cells generate an action potential internally to stimulate the cardiac muscle without other stimulation.
- Electrolyte disturbances, decreases in the oxygen delivered to the cells, structural damage in the conduction pathway, drug effects, acidosis, or the accumulation of waste products can trigger arrhythmias.
- Changes in the heart rate, uncoordinated heart muscle contractions, or heart blocks that alter the movement of impulses through the system can disrupt heart rhythm.
- Arrhythmias may change the mechanics of blood circulation (hemodynamics), which can interrupt delivery of blood to the brain, other tissues, and the heart.

Antiarrhythmic Agents

Antiarrhythmics affect the action potential of the cardiac cells by altering their automaticity, conductivity, or both. Because of this effect, antiarrhythmic drugs can also produce new arrhythmias; that is, they can be **proarrhythmic**.

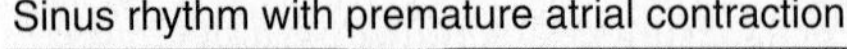

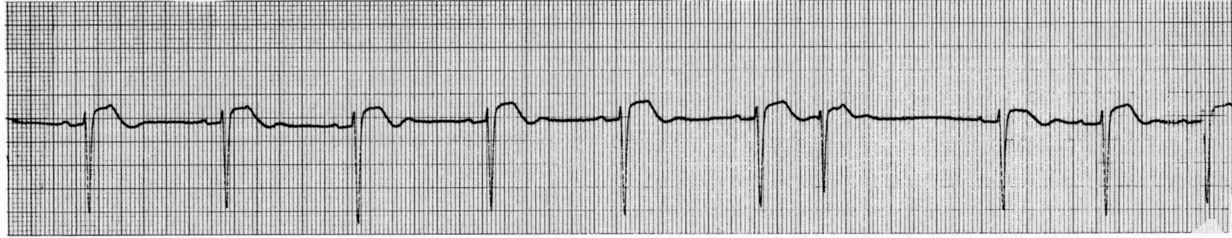

A

Atrial fibrillation

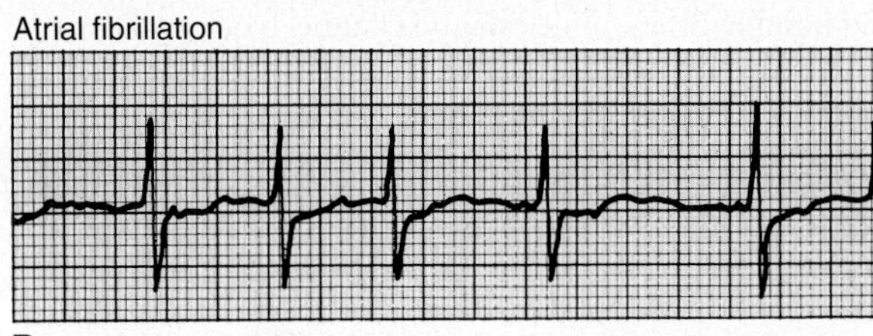

B

FIGURE 45.3 Atrial arrhythmias. **A.** Premature atrial contractions (PACs). Rhythm: Irregular due to the origination of a beat outside the normal conduction system (ectopic). Rate: Normal sinus rate, except for PACs. P–R interval: P wave is abnormal, and interval may be slightly shortened in ectopic beat. QRS: Normal. **B.** Atrial fibrillation. Rhythm: Irregularly irregular. Rate: Variable; usually rapid on initiation of rhythm; decreases when controlled by medication. P–R interval: No P waves are seen, replaced by an irregular wavy baseline. The atria are fibrillating because impulses are arising at a rate greater than 350 per minute. The ventricles respond when the atrioventricular (AV) node is stimulated to threshold and can receive the impulse. QRS: Normal.

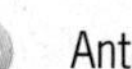

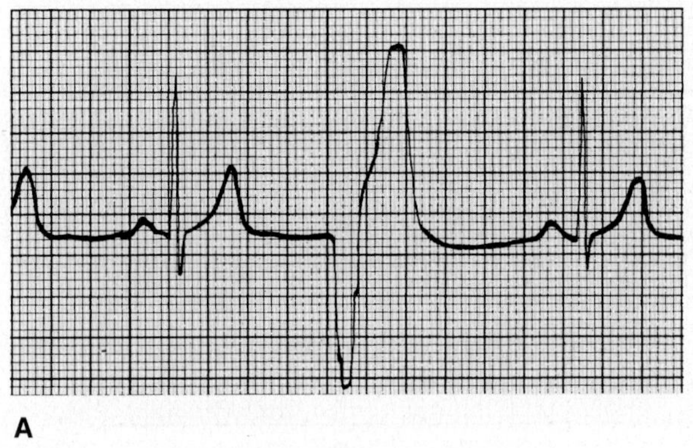

A

Premature ventricular contraction (PVC).

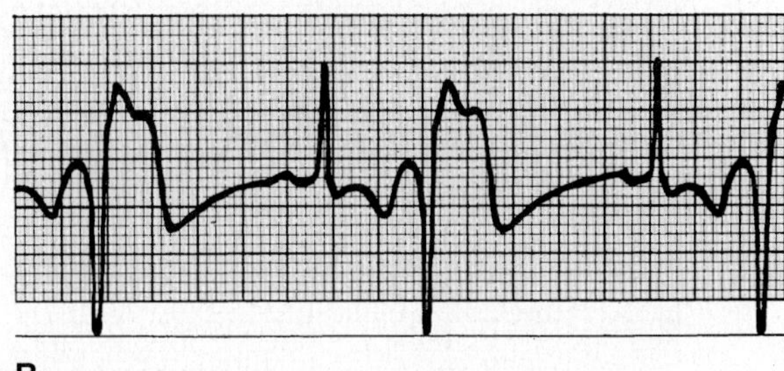

B

Ventricular bigeminy. (Every other beat is a PVC.)

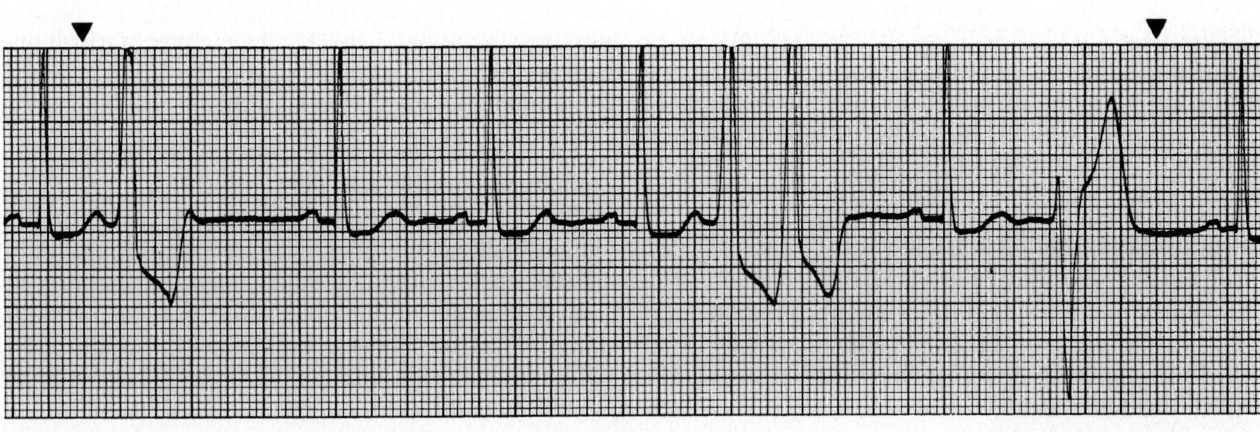

C

Multiformed PVCs.

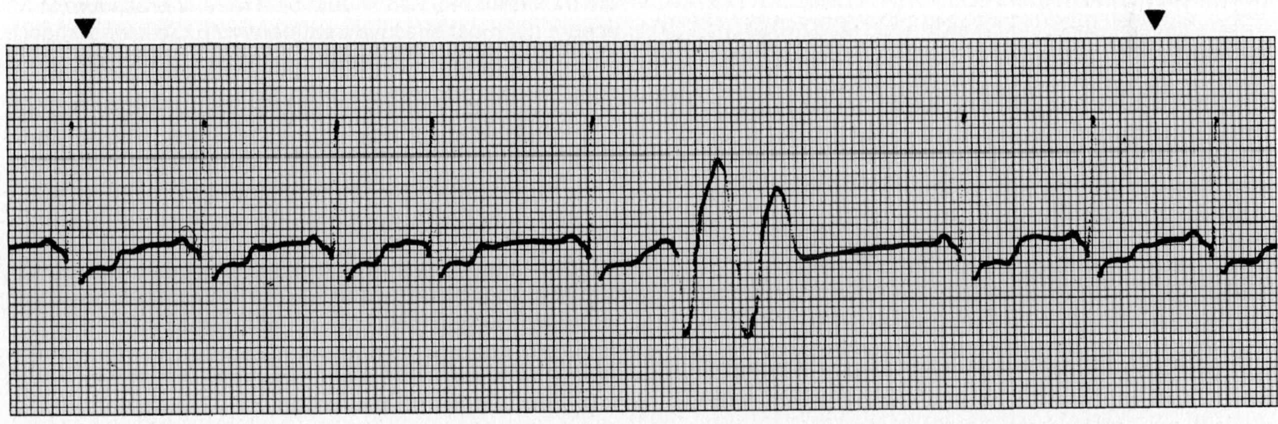

D

Heart block with PVCs.

FIGURE 45.4 A–D. Premature ventricular contractions (PVCs) or ventricular premature beats (VPBs). Rhythm: Irregular. Rate: Variable; only interrupts the cycle of the ectopic, ventricular contraction. P–R interval: Normal in sinus beats, not measurable in PVCs. QRS: Wide, bizarre, >0.12 seconds.

Antiarrhythmics are used in emergency situations when the hemodynamics arising from the patient's arrhythmia are severe and could potentially be fatal. These medications may also be used if the patient's arrhythmia significantly decreases their quality of life or if not treating it puts the person at risk for a worse prognosis. Antiarrhythmic agents are classified based on their mechanisms of action. The class 0 antiarrhythmic is ivabradine (*Corlanor*); it is discussed in Chapter 44 due to its indication to treat patients with heart failure (HF) with reduced left ventricular ejection fraction. Class I antiarrhythmic medications are sodium channel blockers. Class II antiarrhythmic

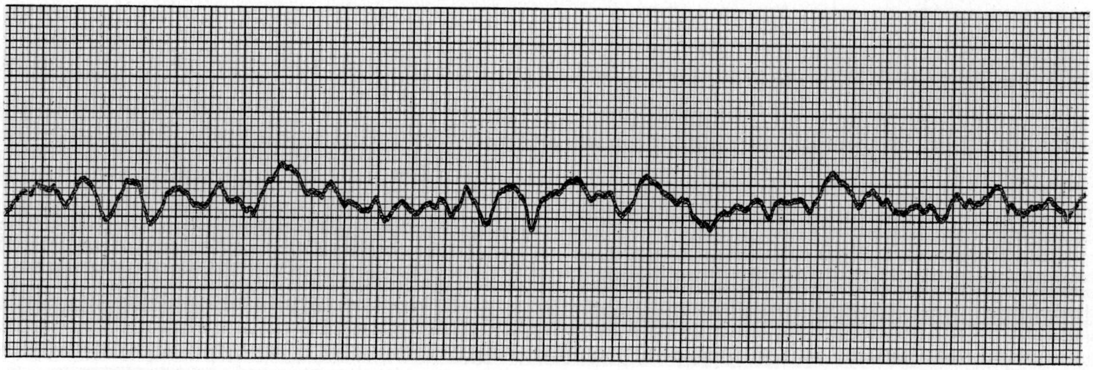

FIGURE 45.5 Ventricular fibrillation. Rhythm: Irregular. Rate: Not measurable. P–R interval: Not measurable. QRS: Not measurable, replaced by an irregular wavy baseline. No coordinated electrical or mechanical activity in the ventricle, no cardiac output.

medications act on autonomic receptors. Class III antiarrhythmic medications act on potassium channels, and the class IV medications modulate calcium channels. Box 45.2 contains information regarding use of antiarrhythmic agents across the lifespan.

Class I Antiarrhythmics

Class I antiarrhythmics (Table 45.1) are drugs that block the sodium channels in the cell membrane during an action potential. These drugs are further broken down into three subclasses, reflecting the manner in which their blockage of sodium channels affects the action potential. These subclasses include the following:

- Class Ia antiarrhythmics: disopyramide (*Norpace*), procainamide (generic), and quinidine (generic)
- Class Ib antiarrhythmics: lidocaine (*Xylocaine*) and mexiletine (generic)
- Class Ic antiarrhythmics: flecainide (generic) and propafenone (*Rythmol*)
- Class Id antiarrhythmics: ranolazine (*Ranexa*), which is discussed in Chapter 46 due to its indication to treat angina

BOX 45.2 Focus on Drug Therapy Across the Lifespan

ANTIARRHYTHMIC AGENTS

Children

Antiarrhythmic agents are not used as often in children as they are in adults. Children who do require these drugs, after cardiac surgery or because of congenital heart problems, need to be monitored closely to deal with the related adverse effects that can occur with these drugs.

Digoxin is approved for use in children to treat arrhythmias and has an established recommended dose. If other antiarrhythmics are used, the dose should be carefully calculated using weight and age and should be double-checked by another nurse before administration.

Adenosine, propranolol, procainamide, and digoxin have been successfully used to treat supraventricular arrhythmias, with propranolol and digoxin being the drugs of choice for long-term management.

Many arrhythmias in children are now treated by ablation techniques to destroy the arrhythmia-producing cells. This has been successful in treating Wolff-Parkinson-White and related syndromes in children. If lidocaine is used for ventricular arrhythmias related to cardiac surgery or digoxin toxicity, serum levels should be monitored regularly to determine the appropriate dose and to avoid the potential for serious proarrhythmias and other adverse effects. The child should receive continuous cardiac monitoring.

Adults

Adults receive these drugs most often as emergency measures. Patient monitoring and careful evaluation of the total drug regimen should be a routine procedure to ensure the most effective treatment with the lowest chance of adverse effects. Frequent monitoring and medical follow-up is important for these patients.

The safety for the use of these drugs during pregnancy has not been established. It is recommended that they are avoided during the first trimester of pregnancy if possible. They should not be used in pregnancy unless the benefit to the patient clearly outweighs the potential risk to the fetus. The drugs enter human milk, and some have been associated with adverse effects on the neonate. Class I, III, and IV agents should not be used when a patient is breast or chestfeeding; if they are needed, another method of feeding the baby should be used. Beta-1 selective blockers (except atenolol) or verapamil are typically first-line recommendations for prevention of SVT in patients who are pregnant.

Older Adults

Older adults are frequently prescribed one of these drugs. Older adults are more likely to have renal and/or hepatic impairment related to underlying medical conditions, which could interfere with the metabolism and excretion of these drugs.

The dose for an older adult may need to be started at a lower level than that recommended for other adults. The patient should be monitored closely and the dose adjusted based on patient response. If other drugs are added to or removed from the drug regimen, appropriate dose adjustments may need to be made.

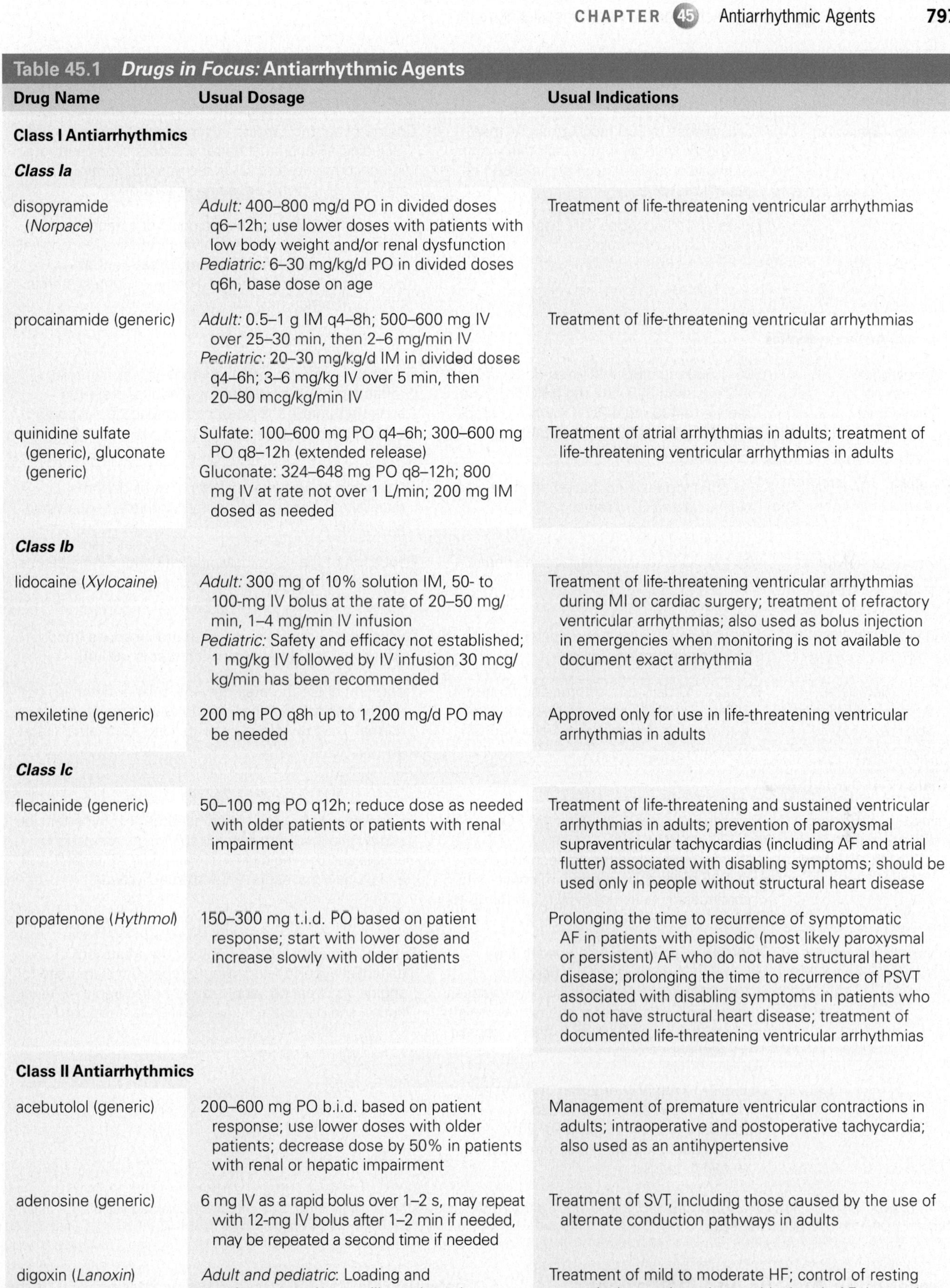

Table 45.1 *Drugs in Focus:* Antiarrhythmic Agents

Drug Name	Usual Dosage	Usual Indications
Class I Antiarrhythmics		
Class Ia		
disopyramide (*Norpace*)	*Adult:* 400–800 mg/d PO in divided doses q6–12h; use lower doses with patients with low body weight and/or renal dysfunction *Pediatric:* 6–30 mg/kg/d PO in divided doses q6h, base dose on age	Treatment of life-threatening ventricular arrhythmias
procainamide (generic)	*Adult:* 0.5–1 g IM q4–8h; 500–600 mg IV over 25–30 min, then 2–6 mg/min IV *Pediatric:* 20–30 mg/kg/d IM in divided doses q4–6h; 3–6 mg/kg IV over 5 min, then 20–80 mcg/kg/min IV	Treatment of life-threatening ventricular arrhythmias
quinidine sulfate (generic), gluconate (generic)	Sulfate: 100–600 mg PO q4–6h; 300–600 mg PO q8–12h (extended release) Gluconate: 324–648 mg PO q8–12h; 800 mg IV at rate not over 1 L/min; 200 mg IM dosed as needed	Treatment of atrial arrhythmias in adults; treatment of life-threatening ventricular arrhythmias in adults
Class Ib		
lidocaine (*Xylocaine*)	*Adult:* 300 mg of 10% solution IM, 50- to 100-mg IV bolus at the rate of 20–50 mg/min, 1–4 mg/min IV infusion *Pediatric:* Safety and efficacy not established; 1 mg/kg IV followed by IV infusion 30 mcg/kg/min has been recommended	Treatment of life-threatening ventricular arrhythmias during MI or cardiac surgery; treatment of refractory ventricular arrhythmias; also used as bolus injection in emergencies when monitoring is not available to document exact arrhythmia
mexiletine (generic)	200 mg PO q8h up to 1,200 mg/d PO may be needed	Approved only for use in life-threatening ventricular arrhythmias in adults
Class Ic		
flecainide (generic)	50–100 mg PO q12h; reduce dose as needed with older patients or patients with renal impairment	Treatment of life-threatening and sustained ventricular arrhythmias in adults; prevention of paroxysmal supraventricular tachycardias (including AF and atrial flutter) associated with disabling symptoms; should be used only in people without structural heart disease
propafenone (*Rythmol*)	150–300 mg t.i.d. PO based on patient response; start with lower dose and increase slowly with older patients	Prolonging the time to recurrence of symptomatic AF in patients with episodic (most likely paroxysmal or persistent) AF who do not have structural heart disease; prolonging the time to recurrence of PSVT associated with disabling symptoms in patients who do not have structural heart disease; treatment of documented life-threatening ventricular arrhythmias
Class II Antiarrhythmics		
acebutolol (generic)	200–600 mg PO b.i.d. based on patient response; use lower doses with older patients; decrease dose by 50% in patients with renal or hepatic impairment	Management of premature ventricular contractions in adults; intraoperative and postoperative tachycardia; also used as an antihypertensive
adenosine (generic)	6 mg IV as a rapid bolus over 1–2 s, may repeat with 12-mg IV bolus after 1–2 min if needed, may be repeated a second time if needed	Treatment of SVT, including those caused by the use of alternate conduction pathways in adults
digoxin (*Lanoxin*)	*Adult and pediatric*: Loading and maintenance doses will vary based on age, weight, renal function, and ventricular response; careful monitoring is necessary based on toxic levels being only slightly higher than therapeutic levels	Treatment of mild to moderate HF; control of resting ventricular rate in patients with chronic AF; increasing myocardial contractility in pediatric patients with HF

(continues on page 798)

Table 45.1 *Drugs in Focus:* Antiarrhythmic Agents *(Continued)*

Drug Name	Usual Dosage	Usual Indications
esmolol (*Brevibloc*)	Loading dose of 500 mcg/kg/min IV, then 50 mcg/kg/min for 4 min, maintain with IV infusion 50–300 mcg/kg/min based on patient response	Control of ventricular rate in supraventricular tachycardia including AF and atrial flutter and control of heart rate in noncompensatory sinus tachycardia; control of perioperative tachycardia and hypertension
propranolol (*Hemangeol, Inderal, Innopran XL*)	Doses and frequencies vary based on indication and formulation	Treatment of SVT caused by digoxin or catecholamines in adults; also used as an antihypertensive, antianginal, and antimigraine headache drug; treatment of proliferating infantile hemangioma requiring systemic therapy (*Hemangeol*)
Class III Antiarrhythmics		
amiodarone (*Pacerone, Nexterone*)	800–1,600 mg/d PO in divided doses for 1–3 wk, then 600–800 mg/d PO for 1 mo; reduce to 400 mg/d PO if rhythm is stable, 1,000 mg IV over 24 h, then 540 mg IV at 0.5 mg/min for 18–96 h	Treatment of life-threatening ventricular arrhythmias refractory to other treatment in adults; preferred antiarrhythmic in the advanced cardiac life support protocol
dofetilide (*Tikosyn*)	125–500 mcg PO b.i.d. based on creatinine clearance and QT interval	Conversion of AF/flutter to normal sinus rhythm; maintenance of normal sinus rhythm after conversion for adults
dronedarone (*Multaq*)	400 mg PO b.i.d. with the morning and evening meals	Reduction of the risk of hospitalization for AF in patients in sinus rhythm with a history of paroxysmal or persistent AF
ibutilide (*Corvert*)	1 mg infused IV over 1 min, may be repeated in 10 min if needed	Conversion of recent-onset AF/flutter in adults (most effective if the duration of AF/flutter is <90 d)
sotalol (*Betapace, Betapace AF, Sorine, Sotylize*)	80 mg/d PO daily or b.i.d., may be titrated to 240–320 mg/d PO; reduce dose in patients with renal impairment and prolonged QT interval	Treatment of life-threatening ventricular arrhythmias not responding to any other drug in adults; maintenance of normal sinus rhythm in patients with AF or atrial flutter
Class IV Antiarrhythmics		
diltiazem (*Cardizem, Cardizem LA, Cartia XT, Taztia XT, Tiazac*)	Extended release: 120–460 mg/d PO 60–120 mg PO b.i.d. 0.25-mg/kg IV bolus, then a second bolus of 0.35 mg/kg IV if needed; maintain with continuous infusion of 5–10 mg/h for up to 24 h	Extended-release preparation used to treat hypertension and angina in adults; other preparations are used for angina and cardiac dysrhythmias (rapid AF, atrial flutter, and paroxysmal supraventricular tachycardia)
verapamil (*Calan SR, Verelan, Verelan PM*)	120–240 mg/d PO, reduce dose in the morning; extended-release capsules: 100–300 mg/d PO at bedtime; lower doses may be needed for older adults, low weight adults, and those with renal and/or hepatic impairment IV *Adult:* 5–10 mg IV over 2 min, may repeat with 10 mg in 30 min if needed *Pediatric:* 0.1–0.3 mg/kg IV over 2 min; do not exceed 5 mg per dose, may repeat in 30 min if needed	Extended-release formulations for the treatment of essential hypertension; other preparations are used for angina and treating various arrhythmias (rapid AF, atrial flutter, and paroxysmal supraventricular tachycardia)

MI, myocardial infarction; PAT, paroxysmal atrial tachycardia; PSVT, paroxysmal supraventricular tachycardia; SVT, supraventricular tachycardia; AF, atrial fibrillation; CAD, coronary artery disease.

Therapeutic Actions and Indications

The class I antiarrhythmics stabilize the cell membrane by binding to sodium channels, depressing phase 0 of the action potential, and changing the duration of the action potential (Fig. 45.6). *Class Ia drugs* depress phase 0 of the action potential and prolong the duration of the action potential. *Class Ib drugs* depress phase 0 somewhat and shorten the duration of the action potential. *Class Ic drugs*

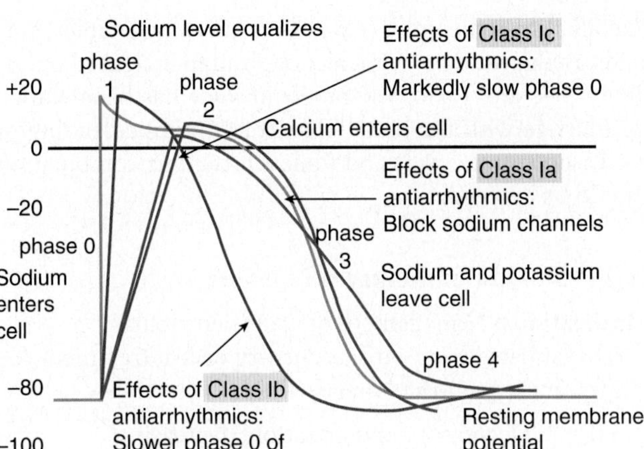

FIGURE 45.6 The cardiac action potentials, showing the effects of class Ia, Ib, and Ic antiarrhythmics.

markedly depress phase 0, with a resultant extreme slowing of conduction, but they have little effect on the duration of the action potential. The *class Id drug* (ranolazine) inhibits the late sodium current after the rapid influx of sodium during an action potential.

These drugs are local anesthetics or membrane-stabilizing agents. They bind more quickly to sodium channels that are open or inactive, ones that have been stimulated and are not yet repolarized. This characteristic makes these drugs preferable in conditions such as tachycardia, in which the sodium gates are open frequently. These drugs are indicated for the treatment of potentially life-threatening ventricular arrhythmias and should not be used to treat ventricular arrhythmias that are not thought to be life threatening, due to the risk of a proarrhythmic effect. Some are also indicated for symptomatic paroxysmal atrial arrhythmias (including AF and atrial flutter) in patients without structural heart disease. See Table 45.1 for usual indications for each class I antiarrhythmic agent.

Pharmacokinetics

These drugs are widely distributed after injection or after rapid absorption through the gastrointestinal (GI) tract. They undergo extensive hepatic metabolism and are excreted in the urine. These drugs cross the placenta and are found in human milk (see "Contraindications and Cautions").

Disopyramide is available in oral form. Procainamide is available in intramuscular (IM) and intravenous (IV) forms. Quinidine is also available for oral, IM, or IV administration and is administered to adults only.

Lidocaine for treatment of arrhythmias is administered by the IM or IV route and can also be given as a bolus injection in emergencies when monitoring is not available to document the exact arrhythmia. Lidocaine can be administered topically when used for analgesia. Mexiletine is an oral drug administered to adults only.

Flecainide and propafenone are available in oral form and should only be administered to patients without structural heart disease.

Contraindications and Cautions

Class I antiarrhythmics are contraindicated in the presence of allergy to any of these drugs to prevent hypersensitivity reactions; with bradycardia or heart block unless an artificial pacemaker is in place because changes in conduction could lead to complete heart block; with HF, hypotension, or shock, which could be exacerbated by effects on the action potential; and with electrolyte disturbances, which could alter the effectiveness of these drugs. Caution should be used in patients with renal or hepatic dysfunction, which could interfere with the biotransformation and excretion of these drugs.

These drugs cross the placenta, and although no specific adverse effects have been associated with their use, it is suggested that they be used in pregnancy only if the benefits to the patient clearly outweigh the potential risks to the fetus. Class I antiarrhythmics enter human milk, and because of the potential for adverse effects on the neonate, they should not be used during lactation. Another method of feeding the baby should be chosen.

Adverse Effects

The adverse effects of the class I antiarrhythmics are associated with their membrane-stabilizing effects and effects on action potentials. Central nervous system (CNS) effects can include dizziness, drowsiness, fatigue, twitching, mouth numbness, slurred speech, vision changes, and tremors that can progress to convulsions. GI symptoms include changes in taste, nausea, and vomiting. Cardiovascular effects include the proarrhythmic effects that lead to the development of arrhythmias (including heart blocks), hypotension, vasodilation, and the potential for cardiac arrest. Respiratory depression progressing to respiratory arrest can also occur (Fig. 45.7). Other adverse effects include rash, hypersensitivity reactions, loss of hair, and potential bone marrow depression. Due to risk of new and perhaps more dangerous arrhythmias with these medications, patients often need close monitoring when first starting the medication.

Procainamide has a boxed warning regarding risk of development of positive antinuclear antibody test, with or without symptoms of systemic lupus syndrome. Symptoms include fever, painful and/or swollen joints, a butterfly-shaped rash on the face, pericarditis, and hepatomegaly. There is also rare but sometimes fatal risk of neutropenia, thrombocytopenia, or hemolytic anemia and liver failure.

Clinically Important Drug–Drug Interactions

Several drug–drug interactions have been reported with these agents, so the possibility of an interaction should

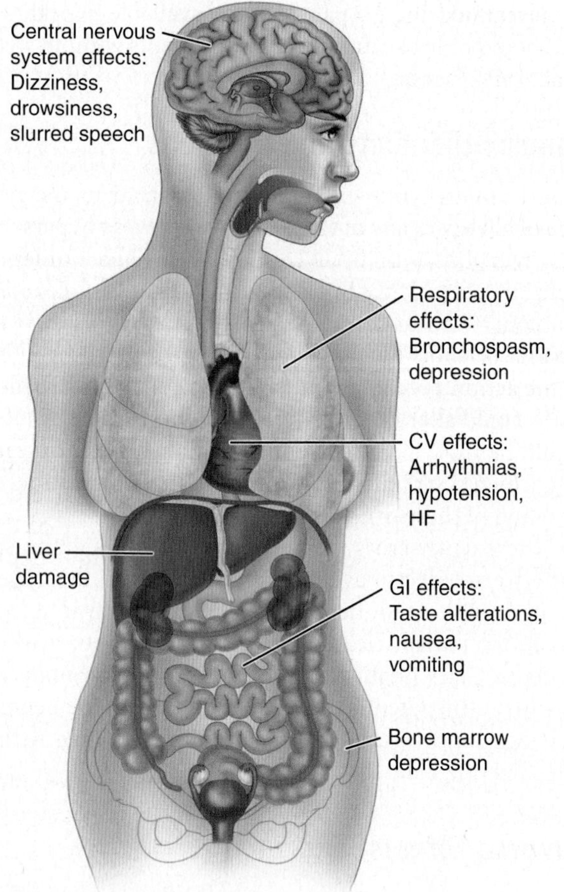

FIGURE 45.7 Variety of adverse effects and toxicities associated with antiarrhythmics.

always be considered before any drug is added to a regimen containing an antiarrhythmic. The risk for arrhythmia increases if these agents are combined with other drugs that are known to cause arrhythmias, such as digoxin and the beta-blockers.

Because quinidine competes for renal transport sites with digoxin, the combination of these two drugs can lead to increased digoxin levels and digoxin toxicity. If these drugs are used in combination, the patient's digoxin level should be monitored and appropriate dose adjustment made. Serum levels and toxicity of the class Ia antiarrhythmics increase if they are combined with cimetidine; extreme caution should be used if patients are receiving this combination.

The risk of bleeding effects of these drugs increases if they are combined with warfarin (*Jantoven, Coumadin*); patients receiving this combination should be monitored closely and have their warfarin dose reduced as needed. Check individual drug monographs for specific interactions associated with each drug.

Clinically Important Drug–Food Interactions

Quinidine requires a slightly acidic urine (normal state) for excretion. Patients receiving quinidine should avoid foods that alkalinize the urine (e.g., citrus juices, vegetables, antacids, milk products), which could lead to increased quinidine levels and toxicity. Grapefruit juice has been shown to interfere with the metabolism of quinidine, leading to increased serum levels and toxic effects; this combination should be avoided.

Prototype Summary: Lidocaine

Indications: Management of acute ventricular arrhythmias during cardiac surgery or MI; treatment of refractory ventricular arrhythmias.

Actions: Decreases depolarization, decreasing automaticity of the ventricular cells; increases ventricular fibrillation threshold.

Pharmacokinetics:

Route	Onset	Peak	Duration
IM	5–10 min	5–15 min	2 h
IV	Immediate	Immediate	10–20 min

$T_{1/2}$: 10 minutes, then 1.5 to 3 hours; metabolized in the liver and excreted in the urine.

Adverse Effects: Dizziness, lightheadedness, fatigue, arrhythmias, cardiac arrest, nausea, vomiting, anaphylactoid reactions, hypotension, vasodilation.

Key Points

- Antiarrhythmics are drugs that alter the action potential of the heart cells and interrupt arrhythmias. There are risks of fatal arrhythmias with these medications, so patients need close monitoring, especially when initiating the medication.
- Class I antiarrhythmics block sodium channels and depress phase 0 of the action potential, often leading to a slowing of conduction and automaticity.
- Class I antiarrhythmics are membrane stabilizers; many of the adverse effects seen are related to the stabilization of cell membranes, including those in the CNS and the GI tract.

Class II Antiarrhythmics

Many of the class II antiarrhythmics are beta-adrenergic blockers that block beta-receptors, causing a depression of phase 4 of the action potential (Fig. 45.8). Chapter 31 has more detail and an entire list of beta-blocker medications. Several beta-adrenergic blockers, such as acebutolol (*Sectral*), esmolol (*Brevibloc*), and propranolol (*Inderal*), are primarily used as antiarrhythmics. Other class II antiarrhythmics also act on the autonomic nervous system. There are muscarinic receptor inhibitors and anticholinergic

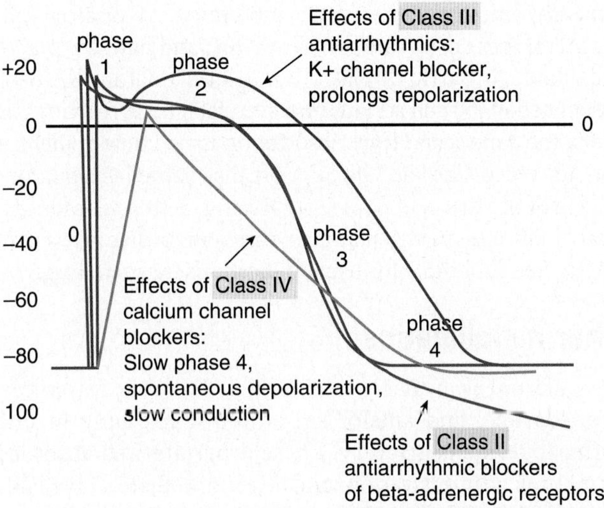

FIGURE 45.8 The cardiac action potentials, showing the effects of class II, III, and IV antiarrhythmics.

agents such as atropine, which are discussed in Chapter 33. Digoxin (see Chapter 44) is also used at times to treat arrhythmias and can act as a muscarinic receptor activator. Adenosine is also a class II antiarrhythmic that activates adenosine receptors in the supraventricular heart tissue.

Therapeutic Actions and Indications

Many of the class II antiarrhythmics competitively block beta-receptor sites in the heart and kidneys. The result is a decrease in heart rate, cardiac excitability, and cardiac output, a slowing of conduction through the AV node, and a decrease in the release of renin. These effects stabilize excitable cardiac tissue and decrease blood pressure, which decreases the heart's workload and may further stabilize hypoxic cardiac tissue. These drugs are indicated for the treatment of rapid AF, atrial flutter, paroxysmal SVTs, hypertension, angina, PVCs, and ventricular tachycardia.

Digoxin slows calcium leaving the cell, prolonging the action potential and slowing conduction through the AV node, and decreases automaticity of the SA node. Digoxin is effective in the treatment of atrial arrhythmias. The drug exerts a positive inotropic effect, leading to increased cardiac output, which may increase perfusion of the coronary arteries and may eliminate the cause of some arrhythmias as hypoxia is resolved and waste products are removed more effectively.

Adenosine is used to convert SVT to sinus rhythm if vagal maneuvers have been ineffective. It is often the drug of choice for terminating SVTs, including those associated with the use of alternative conduction pathways around the AV node (e.g., Wolff-Parkinson-White syndrome), for two reasons: (a) it has a short duration of action (about 15 seconds), after which it is picked up by circulating red blood cells and cleared through the liver, and (b) it is associated with few adverse effects (headache, flushing, and dyspnea of short duration).

See Table 45.1 for usual indications for each drug.

Pharmacokinetics

Acebutolol is an oral drug. Esmolol is administered IV. Propranolol may be administered orally or IV. These drugs are absorbed from the GI tract or have an immediate effect when given IV and undergo hepatic metabolism. They are excreted in the urine. Food has been found to increase the bioavailability of propranolol, though this effect has not been found with other beta-adrenergic blocking agents. Adenosine is given via IV push with continuous telemetry monitoring of the patient. It has an extremely short half-life. Digoxin can be administered IV or orally.

Contraindications and Cautions

The use of these drugs is contraindicated in the presence of sinus bradycardia (rate less than 45 beats/min) and AV block, which could be exacerbated by the effects of these drugs; and with cardiogenic shock or respiratory depression, which could worsen due to blockage of beta-receptors.

Caution should be used in patients with diabetes and thyroid dysfunction, which could be altered by the blockade of the beta-receptors; patients with asthma or COPD, who may have respiratory distress due to reduced ability to dilate bronchi; with pregnancy and lactation because of the potential for adverse effects on the fetus or neonate; and in patients with renal and hepatic dysfunction, which could alter the metabolism and excretion of these drugs.

Since adenosine slows conduction through the AV node, prolongs the refractory period, and decreases automaticity in the AV node, it is contraindicated in patients with second- or third-degree AV block (except in patients with a functioning artificial pacemaker); sinus node disease, such as sick sinus syndrome or symptomatic bradycardia (except in patients with a functioning artificial pacemaker); or known hypersensitivity to adenosine.

Adverse Effects

The adverse effects associated with class II antiarrhythmics are related to the effects of blocking beta-receptors in the sympathetic nervous system. CNS effects include dizziness, insomnia, dreams, and fatigue. Cardiovascular symptoms can include hypotension, bradycardia, AV block, arrhythmias, and alterations in peripheral perfusion. Respiratory effects can include bronchospasm and dyspnea. GI problems frequently include nausea, vomiting, anorexia, constipation, and diarrhea. Other effects to anticipate include a loss of libido, decreased exercise tolerance, and alterations in blood glucose levels.

Adenosine is known to cause flushing, headache, and shortness of breath. Side effects are usually very short term due to the drug's short half-life.

Clinically Important Drug–Drug Interactions

The risk of additive cardiovascular effects increases if these drugs are taken with verapamil or diltiazem; if this combination is used, monitor for necessary dose adjustment.

There is risk of masked hypoglycemic effect when beta blockers are taken with antidiabetic medications. Blood glucose levels should be closely monitored.

Methylxanthines (theophylline and caffeine) block adenosine receptors and decrease therapeutic effect.

Other specific drug interactions may occur with each drug; check a drug reference before combining these drugs with any others.

Prototype Summary: Propranolol

Indications: Treatment of cardiac arrhythmias, especially supraventricular tachycardia; treatment of ventricular tachycardia induced by digitalis or catecholamines; also used as an antihypertensive, antianginal, and antimigraine headache drug.

Actions: Competitively blocks beta-adrenergic receptors in the heart and kidney, has a membrane-stabilizing effect, and decreases the influence of the sympathetic nervous system.

Pharmacokinetics:

Route	Onset	Peak	Duration
Oral	20–30 min	60–90 min	6–12 h
IV	Immediate	1 min	4–6 h

$T_{1/2}$: 3 to 5 hours; metabolized in the liver and excreted in the urine.

Adverse Effects: Bradycardia, heart failure, cardiac arrhythmias, heart blocks, cerebrovascular accident, pulmonary edema, gastric pain, flatulence, nausea, vomiting, diarrhea, impotence, decreased exercise tolerance.

Key Points

- Class II antiarrhythmics are beta-adrenergic receptor blockers that prevent sympathetic stimulation.
- Adverse effects related to class II antiarrhythmics are associated with blocking of the sympathetic response.

Class III Antiarrhythmics

The class III antiarrhythmics include amiodarone (*Pacerone, Nexterone*), dofetilide (*Tikosyn*), dronedarone (*Multaq*), ibutilide (*Corvert*), and sotalol (*Betapace, Betapace AF, Sorine, Sotylize*).

Therapeutic Actions and Indications

The class III antiarrhythmics block potassium channels and slow the outward movement of potassium during phase 3 of the action potential, prolonging it (see Fig. 45.8). They are indicated for treatment of life-threatening ventricular arrhythmias (e.g., ventricular tachycardia) and for maintenance of sinus rhythm in patients with symptomatic AF or atrial flutter. All of these drugs are proarrhythmic and have the potential of inducing arrhythmias. Although amiodarone has been associated with such serious and even fatal toxic reactions, in 2005, the American Heart Association issued new guidelines for Advanced Cardiac Life Support that named amiodarone as one of the drugs of choice for treating ventricular fibrillation or pulseless ventricular tachycardia in cardiac arrest situations. See Table 45.1 for usual indications for each drug.

Pharmacokinetics

Amiodarone is available in an oral or IV form. Dofetilide, dronedarone, and sotalol are administered only in oral form. Ibutilide is given IV. These drugs are well absorbed after oral administration and are immediately available after IV administration and widely distributed. Absorption of sotalol is decreased by the presence of food. They are metabolized in the liver and excreted in the urine.

Contraindications and Cautions

When these drugs are used to treat life-threatening arrhythmias for which no other drug has been effective, there are no contraindications. Ibutilide and dofetilide should not be used in the presence of AV block, which could be exacerbated by the drug. The patient's renal function, electrolytes, and ECG should be monitored closely at the initiation of therapy with both dofetilide and sotalol since there is risk of arrhythmias that could require cardiac resuscitation. Caution should be used with all of these drugs in the presence of shock, hypotension, or respiratory depression; with a prolonged QTc (corrected) interval, which could worsen due to the depressive effects on action potentials; and with renal or hepatic disease, which could alter the biotransformation and excretion of these drugs. Caution should be used with amiodarone in patients with thyroid or pulmonary disease due to risk of thyroid hormone abnormalities and pulmonary toxicity. Dronedarone is contraindicated for patients with permanent AF, decompensated HF requiring hospitalization or class IV HF, second- or third-degree AV block or sick sinus syndrome (unless a functioning pacemaker is in place), liver or lung toxicity, prolonged QT interval (≥500 ms), and bradycardia (<50 bpm). It should never be used during pregnancy because it has been associated with fetal abnormalities.

Adverse Effects

The adverse effects associated with these drugs are related to the changes they cause in action potentials. Nausea, vomiting, and GI distress; weakness and dizziness; and hypotension are common. They may also cause bradycardia or AV block that could progress to heart failure. QT prolongation needs to be monitored carefully when administering dofetilide and sotalol. Amiodarone has been associated with potentially fatal liver toxicity, ocular abnormalities, lung fibrosis, phototoxicity, and the development of serious cardiac arrhythmias. The most common adverse effects seen with dronedarone are HF, prolonged QT interval, nausea, diarrhea, and rash.

Clinically Important Drug–Drug Interactions

These drugs can cause serious toxic effects if they are combined with digoxin or quinidine. There is an increased risk of proarrhythmias if they are combined with antihistamines, phenothiazines, or tricyclic antidepressants. There is an increased risk of serious adverse effects if dofetilide is combined with ketoconazole, cimetidine, verapamil, and others. Many of these combinations should be avoided, and a drug interaction database should be checked before initiation or discontinuation of any medication. Sotalol may lose effectiveness if it is combined with nonsteroidal anti-inflammatory drugs, aspirin, or antacids. With concurrent use with beta blockers, verapamil, or diltiazem, there is increased risk of bradycardia and heart block.

Other specific drug–drug interactions have been reported with individual drugs; a drug reference should always be consulted when adding a new drug to a regimen containing any of these agents.

Prototype Summary: Amiodarone

Indications: Treatment of life-threatening ventricular arrhythmias.

Actions: Acts directly on heart muscle cells to prolong repolarization and the refractory period, increasing the threshold for ventricular fibrillation; also acts on peripheral smooth muscle to decrease peripheral resistance.

Pharmacokinetics:

Route	Onset	Peak	Duration
Oral	2–3 d	3–7 h	Prolonged
IV	Immediate	20 min	Infusion

$T_{1/2}$: 10 days; metabolized in the liver and excreted in the urine; active metabolites and redistribution prolong $t_{1/2}$.

Adverse Effects: Malaise, fatigue, dizziness, heart failure, cardiac arrhythmias, cardiac arrest, constipation, nausea, vomiting, hepatotoxicity, pulmonary toxicity, corneal microdeposits, vision changes, phototoxicity that may cause a blue-gray discoloration of the skin.

Key Points

- Class III antiarrhythmics block potassium channels and prolong phase 3 of the action potential.
- Amiodarone is the drug recommended for use during life support measures. It is associated with serious to potentially fatal hepatotoxicity and lung fibrosis if used long term.

Class IV Antiarrhythmics

Class IV antiarrhythmics include two nondihydropyridine calcium channel blockers (CCBs): diltiazem (*Cardizem, Cardizem LA, Cartia XT, Taztia XT, Tiazac*) and verapamil (*Calan SR, Verelan, Verelan PM*). They have more direct negative inotropic (less heart pumping force) and chronotropic (lower heart rate) effects than the dihydropyridine CCBs. See Chapter 43 for a full list of CCBs. The nondihydropyridine CCBs are better as antiarrhythmics than are dihydropyridine CCBs, but they should be avoided in HF patients due to the potential for decreased heart muscle function.

Therapeutic Actions and Indications

The class IV antiarrhythmics block the movement of calcium ions across the cell membrane in cardiac and vascular smooth muscle cells, depressing the generation of action potentials and delaying phases 1 and 2 of repolarization, which slows automaticity and conduction (see Fig. 45.8). Electrical activity through the SA and AV nodes is partially dependent on the calcium influx, so the medications slow AV conduction and ventricular rate. Both diltiazem and verapamil are used as antihypertensives (see Chapter 43) and to treat angina (see Chapter 46). They are also indicated for treatment of rapid supraventricular dysrhythmias (rapid AF, atrial flutter, and paroxysmal supraventricular tachycardia). Table 45.1 describes the usual indications for each drug.

Pharmacokinetics

Diltiazem and verapamil may be administered in IV or oral forms. These drugs are well absorbed after oral administration. They are highly protein bound, metabolized in the liver, and excreted in the urine. They cross the placenta and enter human milk.

Contraindications and Cautions

These drugs are contraindicated with known allergy to any CCB to avoid hypersensitivity reactions, with sick sinus syndrome or heart block (unless an artificial pacemaker is in place) because the block could be exacerbated by these drugs, and with severe HF or hypotension because of the hypotensive effects of these drugs. Caution should be used in cases of pregnancy or lactation because of the potential for adverse effects on the fetus or neonate; idiopathic hypertrophic subaortic stenosis, which could be exacerbated; or impaired renal or liver function, which could affect the metabolism or excretion of these drugs.

Adverse Effects

The adverse effects associated with these drugs are related to their vasodilation of blood vessels throughout the body, slowing heart rate and causing negative inotropic effects.

CNS effects include dizziness, weakness, fatigue, depression, constipation, and headache. GI upset, nausea, and vomiting can occur. Hypotension, HF, shock, arrhythmias, AV block, and edema have also been reported.

Clinically Important Drug–Drug Interactions

Verapamil has been associated with many drug–drug interactions, including increased risk of cardiac depression with beta-blockers; additive AV slowing with digoxin; increased serum levels and toxicity of digoxin, carbamazepine, prazosin, and quinidine; increased respiratory depression with atracurium, pancuronium, and vecuronium; and decreased effects if combined with calcium products or rifampin.

There is a risk of severe cardiac effects if these drugs are given IV within 48 hours of IV beta-adrenergic drugs.

Diltiazem can increase the serum levels and toxicity of cyclosporine if the drugs are taken concurrently. There is increased risk of hypertension, bradycardia, and heart block when the drug is administered with other antihypertensive and/or negative chronotropic medications. There is increased risk of HF exacerbation if it is given with other negative inotropic medications.

Prototype Summary: Diltiazem

Indications: Extended-release preparation used to treat hypertension and angina in adults; other preparations are used for angina and cardiac dysrhythmias (rapid AF, atrial flutter, and paroxysmal supraventricular tachycardia).

Actions: Blocks the movement of calcium ions across the cell membrane, depressing the generation of action potentials, delaying phases 1 and 2 of repolarization, and slowing conduction through the AV node.

Pharmacokinetics:

Route	Onset	Peak	Duration
Oral	30–60 min	2–3 h	6–8 h
IV	Immediate	2–3 min	Unknown

$T_{1/2}$: 3.5 to 6 hours; metabolized in the liver and excreted in the urine.

Adverse Effects: Dizziness, lightheadedness, headache, asthenia, peripheral edema, bradycardia, AV block, flushing, nausea, hepatic injury.

Nursing Considerations for Patients Receiving Antiarrhythmic Agents

Assessment: History and Examination

- Assess for contraindications or cautions: any known allergies to these drugs to avoid hypersensitivity reactions; impaired liver or kidney function, which could alter the metabolism and excretion of the drug; any condition that could be exacerbated by the depressive effects of the drugs (e.g., heart block, HF, hypotension, shock, respiratory dysfunction, electrolyte disturbances) to avoid exacerbation of these conditions; and current status of pregnancy and lactation to prevent potential adverse effects on the fetus or baby.
- Perform a physical assessment to establish a baseline before beginning therapy and during therapy to determine the effectiveness of therapy and evaluate for any potential adverse effects.
- Assess the patient's neurological status, including level of alertness, speech and vision, and reflexes, to identify possible CNS effects.
- Assess cardiac status closely, including pulse, blood pressure, heart rate, and rhythm, to identify changes requiring a change in the dosage of the drug or the presence of adverse effects; auscultate heart sounds, noting any evidence of abnormal sounds, for early detection of HF; and anticipate cardiac monitoring to evaluate heart rate and rhythm and aid in identifying arrhythmia. Some of the drugs also require monitoring of QT interval.
- Monitor respiratory rate and depth and auscultate lungs for evidence of adventitious sounds to identify respiratory depression and detect changes associated with HF.
- Inspect abdomen for evidence of distention; auscultate bowel sounds to evaluate GI motility.
- Evaluate skin for color, lesions, and temperature to detect adverse reactions and to assess cardiac output.
- Obtain a baseline ECG to evaluate heart rate and rhythm; monitor the results of laboratory tests, including complete blood count, to identify possible bone marrow suppression, and renal and liver function tests to determine the need for possible changes in dose and identify toxic effects.

Nursing Conclusions

Nursing conclusions related to drug therapy might include the following:

- Altered cardiac output related to cardiac effects
- Altered sensory perception (visual, auditory, kinesthetic, gustatory, tactile) related to CNS effects
- Injury risk related to adverse drug effects
- Knowledge deficit regarding drug therapy

Planning

- The patient will receive the best therapeutic effect from the drug therapy.
- The patient will have limited adverse effects from the drug therapy.
- The patient will have an understanding of the drug therapy, adverse effects to anticipate, and measures to relieve discomfort and improve safety.

Intervention With Rationale

- Titrate the dose to the smallest amount needed to achieve control of the arrhythmia to decrease the risk of severe adverse effects.
- Continually monitor cardiac rhythm when initiating or changing dose to detect potentially serious adverse effects and to evaluate drug effectiveness.
- Ensure that emergency life support equipment is readily available to treat severe adverse reactions that might occur.
- Administer parenteral forms as ordered only if the oral form is not feasible; expect to switch to the oral form as soon as possible to decrease the potential for severe adverse effects.
- Consult with the prescriber to reduce the dose in patients with renal or hepatic dysfunction; a reduced dose may be needed to ensure therapeutic effects without increased risk of toxic effects.
- Establish safety precautions, including side rails, lighting, and noise control, if CNS effects occur to ensure patient safety.
- Arrange for periodic monitoring of cardiac rhythm when the patient is receiving long-term therapy to evaluate effects on cardiac status.
- Provide comfort measures to help the patient tolerate drug effects. These include small, frequent meals to minimize nausea and vomiting; access to bathroom facilities; bowel program as needed to deal with nausea, vomiting, and constipation; administration of food with drug if GI upset is severe to alleviate the discomfort; environmental controls, such as temperature regulation, light control, and decreased noise, to alleviate overstimulation if CNS effects occur; and reorientation as needed.
- Offer support and encouragement to help the patient deal with the diagnosis and the drug regimen.
- Provide thorough patient teaching, including the name of the drug, dosage prescribed, measures to avoid adverse effects, warning signs of problems, and the need for periodic monitoring and evaluation, to enhance patient knowledge about drug therapy and to promote adherence.

Evaluation

- Monitor patient response to the drug (stabilization of cardiac rhythm and output).
- Monitor for adverse effects (sedation, hypotension, cardiac arrhythmias, respiratory depression, CNS effects).
- Evaluate the effectiveness of the teaching plan (patient can name drug, dosage, adverse effects to watch for, specific measures to avoid them, and the importance of continued follow-up).
- Monitor the effectiveness of comfort measures and adherence to the regimen.

See the "Critical Thinking Scenario" for information on managing the patient on chronic antiarrhythmic therapy.

Key Points

- Class IV antiarrhythmics are calcium channel blockers that shorten the action potential, disrupting ineffective rhythms and rates.
- Whichever type of antiarrhythmic is used, the patient receiving an antiarrhythmic drug needs to be monitored closely while medication is being initiated and/or titrated to detect the development of arrhythmias or other adverse effects associated with alteration of the action potentials of other muscles or nerves.

CRITICAL THINKING SCENARIO
Managing the Patient on Chronic Antiarrhythmic Therapy

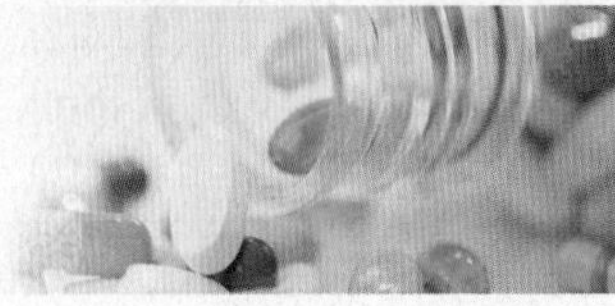

THE SITUATION

R.A., a 63-year-old patient, developed AF 2 years ago, with a rapid drop in blood pressure and a rapid pulse of 160 beats/min, irregularly irregular. They were cardioverted within a few hours of onset to normal sinus rhythm with a heart rate of 74 beats/min. R.A. was started on dofetilide (*Tikosyn*) and remained stable for more than a year. They did well, but during the winter holidays they developed some heartburn. R.A. took cimetidine (*Tagamet*), which they had found as an over-the-counter medication. After a few days, R.A.'s heartburn was relieved, but they felt a severe headache and occasional palpitations, and they had fatigue with shortness of breath. When R.A. went to be evaluated, an ECG demonstrated bradycardia with frequent premature ventricular beats and prolonged QT interval.

CRITICAL THINKING

Based on your knowledge of the drug dofetilide and the symptoms R.A. reported, what do you think happened?

What actions should be taken at this time to make sure that R.A.'s heart rhythm remains stable?

(*continues on page 806*)

What teaching points will be essential to convey to R.A. before they go home?
What other screening should be done at this time to prevent problems in the future?

DISCUSSION

R.A. has the signs and symptoms of increased dofetilide levels: headache and ventricular arrhythmias. Initially, R.A. should be placed on a cardiac monitor, and they should be supported to ensure that the ventricular arrhythmias do not progress. The dofetilide should be stopped until the situation is stabilized. Emergency life support equipment should be readily available in case the situation deteriorates.

R.A. stabilized rapidly, and they were given IV fluids to dilute the drug effects and encourage excretion. R.A.'s PVCs became less and less frequent, and they transitioned to normal sinus rhythm with a normal QT interval. R.A. was questioned about how and when they take the drug and any other drugs they might be taking. R.A. was reminded that concurrent use of *Tikosyn* with many medications can be dangerous, and that any new prescription or over-the-counter medications should be checked by a provider or pharmacist prior to administration. Because R.A. was self-medicating with cimetidine, it is possible that the toxicity that developed was a drug–drug interaction. R.A. was encouraged to maintain regular fluid intake, to eat small meals, and to use a different heartburn medication that is not contraindicated with *Tikosyn*. Before leaving, R.A. should have drug information reviewed to increase its safe use. They should take the drug every 12 hours and not skip any doses. If R.A. does miss a dose, they should not catch up doses but should just resume the regular schedule. R.A. should avoid cimetidine and other antiarrhythmics while on this drug. It is a good idea to keep a complete list of drugs being taken—including over-the-counter drugs and herbal remedies—so the health care provider and/or pharmacist can make sure that there is no potential reaction to be concerned about. R.A. should also be reminded about the importance of regular medical follow-up, which will include an ECG and blood tests, to evaluate the effects of the drug on their body.

While R.A. is within the health care system, it would be a good idea to do a full ECG and to get blood tests to measure their creatinine levels as well as serum electrolytes, which have an effect on cardiac conduction.

NURSING CARE GUIDE FOR R.A.: DOFETILIDE (ANTIARRHYTHMIC AGENTS)

Assessment: History and Examination

Assess the patient's health history for allergies to dofetilide or ibutilide; for any heart block or prolonged QT intervals; history of AF, including onset of last episode; and drug history for use of antihistamines, drugs that could prolong the QT interval, other antiarrhythmics, or tricyclic antidepressants.

Focus the physical examination on the following areas:
CV: Blood pressure, pulse, heart rhythm, perfusion
CNS: Orientation, affect, reflexes
Respiratory system: Respiratory rate and character, adventitious sounds
Laboratory tests: Renal function tests, serum electrolytes, ECG

Nursing Conclusions

Altered cardiac output related to cardiac effects
Altered sensory perception (visual, auditory, kinesthetic, gustatory, tactile) related to CNS effects
Injury risk related to adverse drug effects
Knowledge deficit regarding drug therapy

Planning

The patient will receive the best therapeutic effect from the drug therapy.
The patient will have limited adverse effects from the drug therapy.
The patient will have an understanding of the drug therapy, adverse effects to anticipate, and measures to relieve discomfort and improve safety.

Intervention

Continually monitor cardiac rhythm when initiating or changing dose.
Ensure that emergency life support equipment is readily available.
Establish safety precautions, including side rails, lighting, and noise control, if CNS effects occur.
Arrange for periodic monitoring of cardiac rhythm when the patient is receiving long-term therapy.
Provide comfort measures, including small, frequent meals to minimize nausea and vomiting; access to bathroom facilities; and environmental controls, such as temperature regulation, light control, and decreased noise.
Offer support and encouragement to help the patient deal with the diagnosis and the drug regimen.
Provide patient teaching regarding drug name, dosage, schedule of administration, measures to reduce adverse effects, other drugs to avoid, what to report, and the need for regular, periodic monitoring.

Evaluation

Monitor patient response to the drug (stabilization of cardiac rhythm and output).
Monitor for adverse effects (sedation, hypotension, cardiac arrhythmias, respiratory depression, CNS effects).
Monitor for drug–drug interactions.
Evaluate the effectiveness of the teaching plan (patient can name drug, dosage, adverse effects to watch for, specific measures to avoid them, and the importance of continued follow-up).
Monitor the effectiveness of comfort measures and adherence to the regimen.

PATIENT TEACHING FOR R.A.

- Antiarrhythmic drugs such as dofetilide act to increase the ability of your heart to stay in normal sinus rhythm, helping it to beat more regularly and, therefore, more efficiently.
- When taking dofetilide, you should remember to take it twice a day, every 12 hours. If you miss a dose and it is a more that 3–4 hours late, do not make up the dose, just return to your regular schedule. Never take more than two doses in a day.
- Do not take cimetidine while you are on this drug; this combination can increase the adverse effects, which can be quite serious. There are other drugs that should be avoided; make sure you give your health care provider a complete list of the drugs that you are taking, including over-the-counter drugs and herbal remedies, so the safety of any combinations can be checked.
- Some adverse effects that might occur include the following:
  - *Headache*: Medication may be available to help if this is a problem.
  - *Dizziness, lightheadedness*: Avoid driving a car or operating dangerous machinery until you know how this drug will affect you.
  - *Nausea, diarrhea, flatulence*: Small, frequent meals may help alleviate these problems.
  - Report any of the following to your health care provider: chest pain, difficulty breathing, palpitations, numbness, or tingling.
- Tell any doctor, nurse, or other health care provider involved in your care that you are taking this drug.
- Keep this drug, and all medications, out of the reach of children.
- Schedule regular medical appointments while you are on this drug to evaluate your heart rhythm and your response to the drug and to monitor your blood levels of important electrolytes that affect heart function.
- Do not stop taking this medication without first discussing it with your cardiologist. If you have to stop the medication, contact your health care provider immediately.

SUMMARY

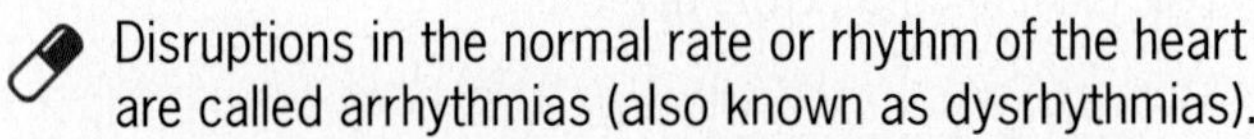

- Disruptions in the normal rate or rhythm of the heart are called arrhythmias (also known as dysrhythmias).

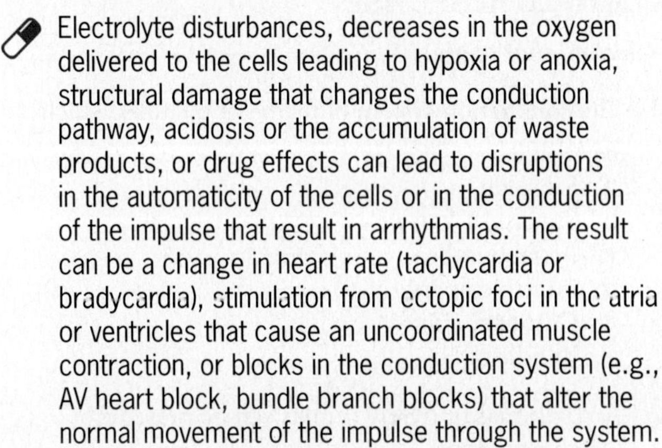

- Electrolyte disturbances, decreases in the oxygen delivered to the cells leading to hypoxia or anoxia, structural damage that changes the conduction pathway, acidosis or the accumulation of waste products, or drug effects can lead to disruptions in the automaticity of the cells or in the conduction of the impulse that result in arrhythmias. The result can be a change in heart rate (tachycardia or bradycardia), stimulation from ectopic foci in the atria or ventricles that cause an uncoordinated muscle contraction, or blocks in the conduction system (e.g., AV heart block, bundle branch blocks) that alter the normal movement of the impulse through the system.
- Arrhythmias cause problems because they alter the hemodynamics of the cardiovascular system. They can cause a decrease in cardiac output related to the uncoordinated pumping action of the irregular rhythm, leading to lack of filling time for the ventricles. Any of these effects can interfere with the delivery of blood to the brain, to other tissues, or to the heart muscle.

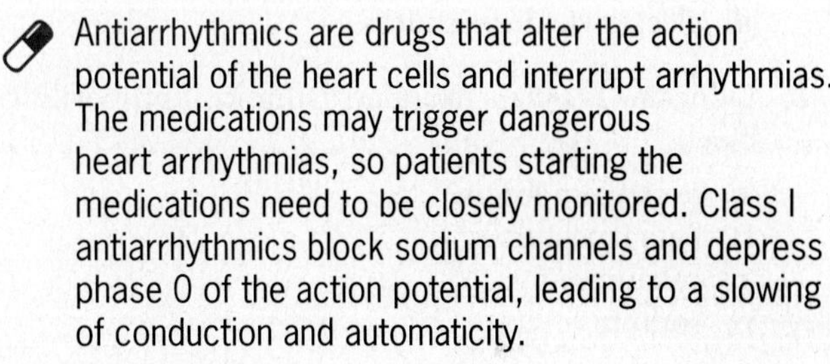

- Antiarrhythmics are drugs that alter the action potential of the heart cells and interrupt arrhythmias. The medications may trigger dangerous heart arrhythmias, so patients starting the medications need to be closely monitored. Class I antiarrhythmics block sodium channels and depress phase 0 of the action potential, leading to a slowing of conduction and automaticity.
- Class II antiarrhythmics are medications that act on the autonomic nervous system; these include the beta-adrenergic receptor blockers that prevent sympathetic stimulation.
- Class III antiarrhythmics block potassium channels and prolong phase 3 of the action potential.
- Class IV antiarrhythmics are calcium channel blockers that shorten the action potential, disrupting ineffective rhythms and rates.
- A patient receiving an antiarrhythmic drug needs to be carefully monitored while medication is initiated and as it is being titrated to detect the development of arrhythmias or other adverse effects associated with alteration of the action potentials of other muscles or nerves.

CHECK YOUR UNDERSTANDING

Answers to the questions in this chapter can be found in Answers to Check Your Understanding Questions on thePoint®.

MULTIPLE CHOICE

Select the best answer.

1. Cardiac contraction and relaxation are controlled by
   a. a specific area in the brain.
   b. the sympathetic nervous system.
   c. the autonomic nervous system.
   d. an action potential and electrical conduction arising within the heart.

2. Antiarrhythmic drugs alter the action potential of the cardiac cells. Because they alter the action potential, antiarrhythmic drugs often cause
   a. HF.
   b. altered blood flow to the kidney.
   c. new arrhythmias.
   d. electrolyte disturbances.

3. Lidocaine is a class Ib antiarrhythmic. It primarily blocks
   a. potassium influx.
   b. beta receptors.
   c. calcium influx.
   d. sodium influx.

4. Ibutilide (*Corvert*) is a class III antiarrhythmic drug that is used for
   a. sedation during electrocardioversion.
   b. conversion of recent-onset AF and flutter.
   c. treatment of life-threatening ventricular arrhythmias.
   d. treatment of arrhythmias complicated by HF.

5. Which of the following is known to have a negative inotropic effect and increase risk of a patient developing heart failure?
   a. Digoxin
   b. Verapamil
   c. Lidocaine
   d. Adenosine

6. A patient who is receiving an antiarrhythmic drug needs
   a. careful cardiac monitoring until stabilized.
   b. frequent blood tests, including drug levels.
   c. an antidepressant to deal with psychological depression.
   d. dietary changes to prevent irritation of the heart muscle.

7. A patient is brought into the emergency room with a potentially life-threatening ventricular arrhythmia. Immediate treatment might include
   a. a loading dose of digoxin.
   b. injection of quinidine.
   c. bolus and titrated doses of lidocaine.
   d. loading dose of propafenone.

8. A patient stabilized on quinidine for the regulation of AF would be cautioned to avoid foods
   a. rich in potassium.
   b. containing tyrosine.
   c. high in sodium.
   d. that alkalinize the urine.

MULTIPLE RESPONSE

Select all that apply.

1. The conduction system of the heart includes which structures?
   a. SA node
   b. Sinuses of Valsalva
   c. Atrial bundles
   d. Purkinje fibers
   e. Coronary sinus
   f. Bundle of His

2. Arrhythmias or dysrhythmias can be caused by which situations?
   a. Lack of oxygen to the heart muscle cells
   b. Acidosis near a cell
   c. Structural damage in the conduction pathway through the heart
   d. Vasodilation in the myocardial vascular bed
   e. Thyroid hormone imbalance
   f. Electrolyte imbalances

REFERENCES

Abhishek, M., Mansour, M., McManus, D., Patel, V. V., Cheng, A., Ruskin, J. N., & Heist, E. K. (2014). Novel therapeutic targets in the management of atrial fibrillation. *American Journal of Cardiovascular Drugs*, *14*(6), 403–421. https://doi.org/10.1007/s40256-014-0085-0

Al-Khatib, A. M., Stevenson, W. G., Ackerman, M. J., Bryant, W. J., Callans, D. J., Curtis, A. B., Deal, B. J., Dickfeld, T., Field, M. E., Fonarow, G. C., Gillis, A. M., Granger, C. B., Hammill, S. C., Hlatky, M. A., Joglar, J. A., Kay, G. N., Matlock, D. D., Myerburg, R. J., & Page, R. L. (2018). 2017 AHA/ACC/HRS guideline for management of patients with ventricular arrhythmias and the prevention of sudden cardiac death. *Journal of the American College of Cardiology*, *72*(14), e91–220. https://doi.org/10.1016/j.jacc2017.10.054

Andrade, J. G., Macle, L., Nattel, S., Verma, A., & Cairns, J. (2017). Contemporary atrial fibrillation management: A comparison of the current AHA/ACC/HRS, CCS, and ESC guidelines. *Canadian Journal of Cardiology*, *33*, 965–976. https://doi.org/10.1016/j.cjca.2017.06.002

Bonow, R. O., Mann, D. L., Libby, P., & Bonow, R. (2014). *Braunwald's heart disease: A textbook of cardiovascular medicine* (10th ed.). W. B. Saunders.

Brugada, J., Katritsis, D. G., Arbelo, E., Arribas, F., Bax, J. J., Blomstro, C., Calkins, H., Corrado, D., Deftereos, S. G., Diller, G., Gomez-Doblas, J. J., Gorenek, B., Grace, A., Ho, S. Y., Kaski, J., Kuck, K., Lambiase, P. D., Sacher, F., Sarquella-Brugada, G., et al. (2020). 2019 ESC guidelines for the management of patients with supraventricular tachycardia. *European Heart Journal*, *41*, 655–720. https://doi.org/10.1093/eurheartj/ehz467

Brunton, L., Hilal-Dandan, R., & Knollman, B. (2018). *Goodman and Gilman's the pharmacological basis of therapeutics* (13th ed.). McGraw-Hill.

Crijns, H. J., Prinzen, F., Lambiase, P. D., Sanders, P., & Brugada, J. (2021). The year in cardiovascular medicine 2020: Arrhythmias. *European Society of Cardiology*, *42*, 499–507. https://doi.org/10.1093/eurheartj/ehaa1091

Epstein, A. E., Hallstrom, A. P., Rogers, W. J., et al. (1993). Mortality following ventricular arrhythmia suppression by encainide, flecainide, and moricizine after myocardial infarction. The original design concept of the Cardiac Arrhythmia Suppression Trial (CAST). *Journal of the American Medical Association*, *270*, 2451–2455.

Fuster, V., Alexander, R. W., & Rourke, R. A. (Eds.). (2011). *Hurst's the heart* (13th ed.). McGraw-Hill.

Gross, A., & Stern, T. A. (2013). The cognitive impact of atrial fibrillation. *The Primary Care Companion for CNS Disorders*, *15*(1), PCC.12f01471. https://doi.org/10.4088/PCC.12f01471

Hall, J. E., & Hall, M. E. (2021). *Guyton and Hall textbook of medical physiology* (14th ed.). Elsevier.

Hazinski, M. F., Nadkarni, V. M., Hickey, R. W., O'Connor, R., Becker, L. B., & Zaritsky, A. (2005). Major changes in the 2005 AHA Guidelines for CPR and ECC. *Circulation*, *112*, IV-206–IV-211. https://doi.org/10.1161/CIRCULATIONAHA.105.170809

January, C. T., Wann, L. S., Alpert, J. S., Calkins, H., Cigarroa, J. E., Cleveland, J. C., Conti, J. B., Ellinor, P. T., Ezekowitz, M. D., Field, M. E., Murray, K. T., Sacco, R. L., Stevenson, W. G., Tchou, P. J., Tracy, C. M., & Yancy, C. W. (2014). 2014 AHA/ACC/HRS guideline for the management of patients with atrial fibrillation. *Circulation*, *130*(23), e199–e267. https://doi.org/10.1161/CIR.0000000000000041

Lei, M., Wu, L., Terrar, D. A., & Huang, C. L. (2018). Modernized classification of cardiac antiarrhythmic drugs. *Circulation*, *138*, 1879–1896. https://doi.org/10.1161/CIRCULATIONAHA.118.035455

McCabe, P. (2010). Psychological distress in patients diagnosed with atrial fibrillation: The state of the science. *Journal of Cardiovascular Nursing*, *25*(1), 40–51. https://doi.org/10.1097/JCN.0b013e3181b7be36

Norris, T. L. (2019). *Porth's pathophysiology concepts of altered health states* (13th ed.). Wolters Kluwer.

Schnabel, R., Aspelund, T., Li, G., Sullivan, L. M., Suchy-Dicey, A., Harris, T. B., Pencina, M. J., D'Agostino, R. B., Levy, D., Kannel, W. B., Wang, T. J., Kronmal, R. A., Wolf, P. A., Burke, G. L., Launer, L. J., Vasan, R. S., Psaty, B. M., Benjamin, E. J., Gudnason, V., & Heckbert, S. R. (2010). Validation of atrial fibrillation risk algorithm in Whites and African Americans. *Archives of Internal Medicine*, *170*, 1909–1917. https://doi.org/10.1001/archinternmed.2010.434

CHAPTER 46

Antianginal Agents

Learning Objectives

Upon completion of this chapter, you will be able to:

1. Describe atherosclerotic cardiovascular disease and coronary artery disease, including identified risk factors and clinical presentation.
2. Discuss the use of antianginal agents across the lifespan.
3. Describe the therapeutic actions, indications, pharmacokinetics, contraindications and cautions, most common adverse reactions, and important drug–drug interactions associated with the nitrates, beta-blockers, and calcium channel blockers used to treat angina.
4. Compare and contrast the prototype drugs nitroglycerin, metoprolol, and diltiazem with other agents used to treat angina.
5. Outline the nursing considerations, including important teaching points, for patients receiving drugs used to treat angina.

Key Terms

angina pectoris: "suffocation of the chest"; pain caused by the imbalance between oxygen being supplied to the heart muscle and demand for oxygen by the heart muscle

atheromas: fatty tumors in the endothelial lining of arteries; contain fats, blood cells, lipids, inflammatory agents, and platelets; lead to narrowing of the lumen of the artery, stiffening of the artery, and loss of distensibility and responsiveness

atherosclerosis: narrowing of the arteries caused by buildup of atheromas, swelling, and accumulation of platelets; leads to a loss of elasticity and responsiveness to normal stimuli

coronary artery disease (CAD): characterized by progressive narrowing of coronary arteries leading to a decreased delivery of oxygen to cardiac muscle cells

myocardial infarction: end result of vessel blockage in the heart; leads to ischemia and then necrosis of the area cut off from the blood supply; dead cells replaced by scar tissue

Prinzmetal angina: drop in blood flow through the coronary arteries caused by a vasospasm in the artery

pulse pressure: the systolic blood pressure minus the diastolic blood pressure; reflects the filling pressure of the coronary arteries

stable angina: pain due to the imbalance of myocardial oxygen supply and demand; the pain is relieved by rest or stoppage of activity

unstable angina: episode of myocardial ischemia with pain due to the imbalance of myocardial oxygen supply and demand when the person is at rest and/or at unpredictable times

Drug List

ANTIANGINAL AGENTS

Nitrates
isosorbide dinitrate
isosorbide mononitrate
(P) nitroglycerin

BETA-BLOCKERS
atenolol
(P) metoprolol
nadolol
propranolol

CALCIUM CHANNEL BLOCKERS
amlodipine
(P) diltiazem
nicardipine
nifedipine
verapamil

PIPERAZINE ACETAMIDE
ranolazine

Antianginal agents are used to help restore the appropriate supply-and-demand ratio in oxygen delivery to the myocardium. An imbalance in this ratio, often manifested by pain, is most commonly due to atherosclerotic cardiovascular disease (ASCVD). ASCVD is caused by an accumulation of cholesterol plaque in arteries and can lead to peripheral arterial disease, myocardial infarction, and ischemic stroke. **Coronary artery disease (CAD)** is a type of ASCVD characterized by progressive narrowing of the coronary arteries leading to decreased delivery of oxygen to cardiac muscle cells. There are multiple risk factors associated with worsening ASCVD: dyslipidemia, diabetes mellitus, obesity, inactive lifestyle, hypertension, smoking, and family history. Heart disease has been the leading cause of death in the United States and worldwide for many years and CAD is a frequently-diagnosed cause of heart disease. Despite strides in understanding the contributing causes of this disease and ways to prevent it, CAD is still a chronic disease that is managed but not curable. The drugs discussed in this chapter are used to prevent myocardial cell death when the coronary vessels are already seriously damaged and are having trouble maintaining the blood flow to the heart muscle. Chapters 47 and 48 discuss drugs that are used to prevent the blocking of the coronary arteries before they become narrowed and damaged or to restore blood flow through narrowed vessels.

Coronary Artery Disease

The myocardium must receive a constant supply of blood to have the oxygen and nutrients needed to maintain a constant pumping action. The myocardium receives all of its blood from two coronary arteries that exit the sinuses of Valsalva at the base of the aorta. These vessels divide and subdivide to form the capillaries that deliver oxygen to heart muscle fibers.

Unlike other tissues in the body, the heart muscle receives its blood supply during diastole, while it is at rest. This is important because when the heart muscle contracts, it becomes tight and clamps the blood vessels closed, rendering them unable to receive blood during systole, which is when all other tissues receive fresh blood. The openings in the sinuses of Valsalva, which are the beginnings of the coronary arteries, are positioned so that they can be filled when the blood flows back against the aortic valve when the heart is at rest. The pressure that fills these vessels is the **pulse pressure** (the systolic pressure minus the diastolic pressure)—the pressure of the column of blood falling back onto the closed aortic valve. The heart has just finished contracting and using energy and oxygen. The acid and carbon dioxide built up in the muscle cause a local vasodilation, and the blood flows freely through the coronary arteries and into the muscle cells.

With CAD, the lumens of the blood vessels become narrowed so that blood is no longer able to flow freely to the muscle cells. The narrowing of the vessels is caused by the development of **atheromas**, or fatty tumors containing fats, blood cells, lipids, inflammatory agents, and platelets in the endothelial lining of arteries, in a process called **atherosclerosis** (Fig. 46.1A). These deposits cause damage to the intimal lining of the vessels, attracting platelets and immune factors and causing swelling and the development of a larger deposit. Over time, these deposits severely decrease the size of the vessel. While the vessel is being narrowed by the deposits in the intima, it is also losing its natural elasticity and becoming unable to respond to the normal stimuli to dilate or constrict to meet the needs of the tissues.

The person with atherosclerosis has a classic supply-and-demand problem. The heart may function without problem until increases in activity or other stresses place a demand on it to beat faster or harder. Normally, the heart would stimulate the vessels to deliver more blood

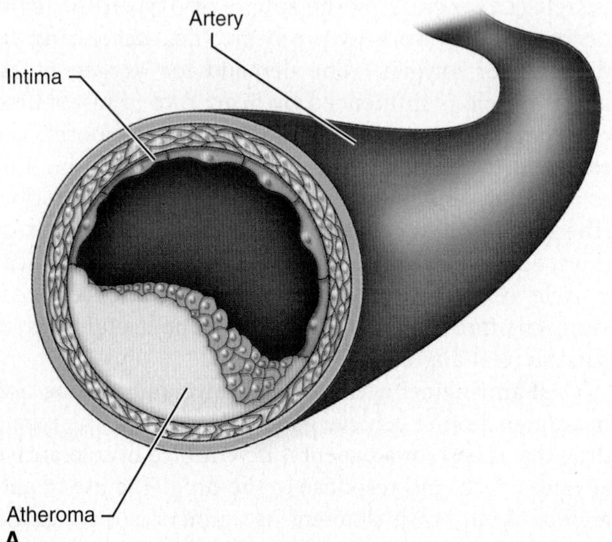

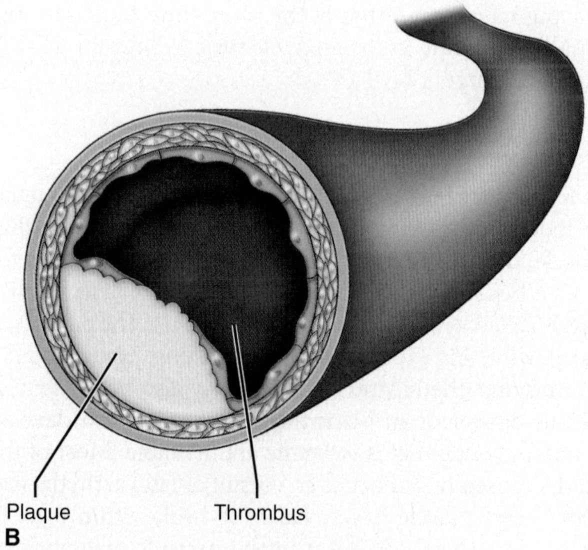

FIGURE 46.1 **A.** Schematic illustration of atheromatous plaque. **B.** Thrombosis of atherosclerotic plaque. It may partially or completely occlude the lumen of the vessel.

when this occurs, but the narrowed vessels are not able to respond and cannot supply the blood needed by the working heart. The heart muscle then becomes hypoxic. This imbalance between oxygen supply and demand is manifested as pain, or **angina pectoris**, which literally means "suffocation of the chest."

Angina

The body's response to a lack of oxygen in the heart muscle is pain, called angina. Although the heart muscle does not have any pain fibers, a substance called substance P is released from ischemic myocardial cells, and pain is felt wherever substance P reacts with a pain receptor. For many people, this is the chest, and for others, it is the left arm; still others have pain in the jaw and teeth. The basic response to this type of pain is to stop whatever one is doing and wait for the pain to go away. In cases of minor limitations to the blood flow through vessels, stopping activity may bring the supply and demand for blood back into balance. This condition is called **stable angina**. There is no damage to the heart muscle, and the basic reflexes surrounding the pain restore blood flow to the heart muscle. This process can go on for a long time with no resultant myocardial infarction (MI). This is called chronic angina, and this condition can severely limit a person's activities and quality of life.

If the narrowing of the coronary arteries becomes more pronounced, the heart may experience episodes of ischemia even when the patient is at rest. This condition is called **unstable angina**. Although no damage to the heart muscle occurs, the person is at increased risk of a complete blockage of blood supply to the heart muscle if the heart needs to work harder or the oxygen demand increases.

Prinzmetal angina, a drop in blood flow through the coronary arteries caused by a vasospasm in the artery, is an unusual form of angina because it seems to be caused by spasm of the blood vessels and not just by vessel narrowing. The person with this type of angina has angina at rest, often at the same time each day, and usually with an associated electrocardiogram (ECG) pattern change.

Acute Myocardial Infarction

If a coronary vessel becomes mostly or completely occluded and is unable to deliver blood to the cardiac muscle, the area of muscle that depends on that vessel for oxygen becomes ischemic and then necrotic (Fig. 46.1B). This is called a **myocardial infarction** (MI). The pain associated with this event can be excruciating. Nausea and a severe sympathetic stress reaction may also be present. A serious danger of an MI is that arrhythmias can develop in nearby tissue that is ischemic and irritable. Most of the deaths caused by MI occur as a result of fatal arrhythmias. If the heart muscle has a chance to heal, within 6 to 10 weeks, scar tissue will form in the necrotic area and the muscle will compensate for the injury. If the area of the muscle that is damaged is large, however, the muscle may not be able to compensate for the loss, and heart failure (HF) and even cardiogenic shock may occur. These conditions can be fatal or can leave a person severely limited by the weakened heart muscle.

Key Points

- CAD involves changes in the coronary vessels that promote atheromas (tumors), which narrow the coronary arteries and decrease their elasticity and responsiveness to normal stimuli.
- Angina pectoris occurs when the narrowed vessels cannot accommodate the myocardial demand for oxygen.
- Stable angina occurs when the heart muscle is perfused adequately except during exertion or increased demand. Unstable angina occurs when the vessels are so narrow that the myocardial cells are deprived of sufficient oxygen even at rest. Prinzmetal angina is a spasm of a coronary vessel that decreases the flow of blood through the narrowed lumen.
- When a coronary vessel is mostly or completely occluded, the cells that depend on that vessel for oxygen become ischemic, then necrotic, and die. The result is known as an MI.

Antianginal Agents

Antianginal drugs (Table 46.1) are used to help restore the appropriate supply-and-demand ratio in oxygen delivery to the myocardium when rest is not enough. These drugs can work to improve blood delivery to the heart muscle in one of two ways: (a) by dilating blood vessels (i.e., increasing the supply of oxygen) or (b) by decreasing the work of the heart (i.e., decreasing the demand for oxygen). The demand for oxygen by the heart muscle is influenced by heart rate (a faster heart rate requires more energy), the preload (the more blood returned to the heart, the more pumping will be done to empty it, which requires more energy), the afterload (the more pressure the heart has to pump against the more energy is required), and contractility of the heart muscle cells. Nitrates, beta-adrenergic blockers, calcium channel blockers, and piperazine acetamides are used to treat angina (Fig. 46.2).

All antianginal agents are effective and may be used in combination to achieve good pain control. The type of drug that is best for a patient is determined by tolerance of adverse effects and response to the drug. The use of antianginal agents with different age groups is discussed in Box 46.1.

Table 46.1 *Drugs in Focus:* Antianginal Agents

Drug Name	Usual Dosage	Usual Indications
Nitrates		
isosorbide dinitrate (*Isordil*)	2.5–5 mg SL; 5-mg chewable tablet; 5–20 mg PO; maintenance 10–40 mg PO q6h or 40–80 mg PO SR q8–12h *Acute prophylaxis:* 5–10 mg SL or chewable tablets q2–3h	Taken before chest pain begins in situations in which exertion or stress can be anticipated for prevention of angina in adults; taken daily for management of chronic angina
isosorbide mononitrate (*Monoket*)	2.5–5 mg SL; 5-mg chewable tablet; 5–20 mg PO; maintenance 10–40 mg PO q6h or 40–80 mg PO SR q8–12h *Acute prophylaxis:* 5–10 mg SL or chewable tablets q2–3h	Taken before chest pain begins in situations in which exertion or stress can be anticipated for prevention of angina in adults; taken daily for management of angina
nitroglycerin (*GoNitro, Nitro-Dur, Nitromist, Nitrostat*, and others)	5 mcg/min via IV infusion pump every 3–5 min; one tablet/packet SL every 5 min for acute attack, up to three tablets/packets in 15 min; 0.4-mg metered dose translingual, up to three doses in 15 min for acute attacks *Prevention:* One tablet (0.3–0.6 mg) sublingually 5–10 min before activities that might precipitate an attack: 2.5–9 mg PO of SR tablet q8–12h; doses as high as 26 mg PO q.i.d. have been used; 0.5 in q8h for topical application, up to 4–5 in. (1 in. = 15 mg) have been used; one pad (60–75 mg) has been used; one pad transdermal system per day; 1 mg q3–5h while awake for transmucosal system	Nitrate of choice for treatment of acute angina attack; prevention of anginal attacks
Beta-Blockers		
atenolol (*Tenormin*)	Initially 50 mg/d PO, may be increased to 100 mg/d; reduce dose with renal impairment	Treatment of MI, chronic angina, and hypertension in adults
metoprolol (*Lopressor, Toprol XL*)	100–400 mg/d PO, based on patient response; XL preparation for treatment of angina: 50–200 mg/d PO based on patient response. *Acute MI:* 3 IV bolus doses of 5 mg each at 2-min intervals; if tolerated, start PO therapy 15 min after last IV dose	Treatment of hypertension; prevention of reinfarction after MI; early acute MI treatment; treatment of stable and symptomatic HF (extended-release preparation only)
nadolol (*Corgard*)	*Angina*: 40–80 mg/d PO *Hypertension*: 40–80 mg/d PO, up to 320 mg/d may be needed; reduce dose in renal impairment	Treatment of hypertension, management of chronic angina in adults
propranolol (*Inderal, Hemangeol, Innopran XL*)	Dose varies widely based on indication; check drug guide for specific information	Treatment of hypertension, angina, idiopathic hypertrophic subaortic stenosis–induced palpitations, angina and syncope, certain cardiac arrhythmias induced by catecholamines or digoxin, and pheochromocytoma; prevention of reinfarction after MI; prophylaxis for migraine headache (which may be caused by vasodilation and is relieved by vasoconstriction, although the exact action is not clearly understood); prevention of manifestations of some anxiety disorders; treatment of essential tremors; treatment of proliferating infantile hemangioma
Calcium Channel Blockers		
amlodipine (*Katerzia, Norvasc*)	*Adult:* 5–10 mg/d PO; reduce dose in patients with hepatic impairment and in older patients *Pediatric:* 2.5–5 mg/d PO	Used alone or in combination with other agents for treatment of hypertension and angina

(*continues on page 814*)

Table 46.1 *Drugs in Focus*: Antianginal Agents (*Continued*)

Drug Name	Usual Dosage	Usual Indications
diltiazem (*Cardizem, Cardizem LA, Cartia XT, Taztia XT, Tiazac)*	Extended-release: 120–460 mg/d PO 60–120 mg PO b.i.d. 0.25-mg/kg IV bolus, then a second bolus of 0.35 mg/kg IV if needed; maintain with continuous infusion of 5–10 mg/h for up to 24 h	Extended-release preparation used to treat hypertension and angina in adults, other preparations are used for angina and cardiac dysrhythmias (rapid atrial fibrillation, atrial flutter, and paroxysmal supraventricular tachycardia)
nicardipine (generic)	20–40 mg PO t.i.d. or 30–60 mg PO b.i.d.; 0.5–2.2 mg/h IV based on response, switch to oral form as soon as feasible; reduce dose in older patients and in patients with hepatic or renal impairment	Used alone or in combination with other agents for treatment of hypertension and angina; IV form for short-term use when oral route is not feasible
nifedipine (*Procardia, Procardia XL*)	10–40 mg PO b.i.d. or t.i.d.; max daily dose 180 mg Extended-release: 30–60 mg/d PO, max dose 120 mg/d	Treatment of hypertension and angina in adults
verapamil (*Calan SR, Verelan, Verelan PM*)	120–240 mg/d PO, reduce dose in the morning Extended-release capsules: 100–300 mg/d PO at bedtime; lower doses may be needed for older adults, low-weight adults and those with renal and/or hepatic impairment IV *Adult:* 5–10 mg IV over 2 min, may repeat with 10 mg in 30 min if needed *Pediatric:* 0.1–0.3 mg/kg IV over 2 min; do not exceed 5 mg per dose, may repeat in 30 min if needed	Extended-release formulations for the treatment of essential hypertension; other preparations used for angina and various arrhythmias (rapid atrial fibrillation, atrial flutter, and paroxysmal supraventricular tachycardia)
Piperazine Acetamide		
ranolazine (*Ranexa*)	500 mg PO b.i.d., to a maximum 1,000 mg PO b.i.d.	Treatment of chronic angina in adults, as primary therapy or in combination with nitrates, amlodipine, or beta-blockers

SL, sublingual; SR, standard release; ER, extended release; MI, myocardial infarction.

Nitrates

Nitrates are drugs that act directly on smooth muscle to cause relaxation and to depress muscle tone. Because the action is direct, these drugs do not influence any nerve or other activity, and the response is usually quite fast. Nitrates include isosorbide dinitrate (*Isordil*), isosorbide mononitrate (*Monoket*), and nitroglycerin (*GoNitro Nitro-Dur, Nitromist, Nitrostat,* and others).

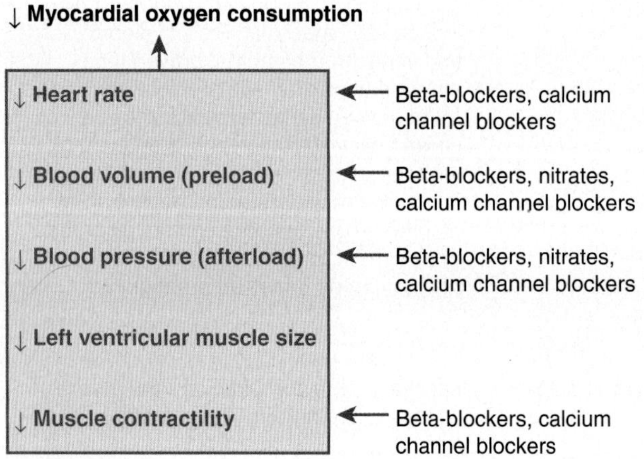

↓ Myocardial oxygen consumption

Factor	Affected by
↓ Heart rate	Beta-blockers, calcium channel blockers
↓ Blood volume (preload)	Beta-blockers, nitrates, calcium channel blockers
↓ Blood pressure (afterload)	Beta-blockers, nitrates, calcium channel blockers
↓ Left ventricular muscle size	
↓ Muscle contractility	Beta-blockers, calcium channel blockers

FIGURE 46.2 Interaction of antianginal agents with factors affecting myocardial oxygen demand.

Therapeutic Actions and Indications

The nitrates relax and dilate veins, arteries, and capillaries, allowing increased blood flow through the vessels and lowering systemic blood pressure because of a drop in resistance. Because CAD causes a stiffening and lack of responsiveness in the coronary arteries, the nitrates probably have little effect on increasing blood flow through these arteries. However, they do increase blood flow through healthy coronary arteries. Therefore, the blood supply through any healthy vessels in the heart increases, possibly helping the heart to compensate somewhat. They are also able to help to decrease vasospasm of arteries.

The main effect of nitrates, however, seems to be related to the drop in blood pressure that occurs. The vasodilation causes blood to pool in veins and capillaries, decreasing preload, while the relaxation of the vessels decreases afterload. The combination of these effects greatly reduces the cardiac workload and the demand for oxygen, thus bringing the supply-and-demand ratio back into balance. Nitrates are indicated for the prevention and treatment of attacks of angina pectoris. See Table 46.1 for usual indications for each of these drugs.

Box 46.1 Focus on Drug Therapy Across the Lifespan

ANTIANGINAL AGENTS

Children

Children are not prescribed antianginal medications to treat CAD. However, some of them are indicated for pediatrics to treat HTN and/or cardiac dysrhythmia. Nitroglycerin would be the most commonly used nitrate for children. The dose of the drug should be determined by considering age and weight. The child should be carefully monitored for adverse reactions, including potentially dangerous changes in blood pressure.

Adults

Adults who receive these drugs should be instructed in their proper administration, particularly if varying forms of nitroglycerin are used. Patients should also be encouraged to determine what activities or situations tend to precipitate an anginal attack so that they can take measures to avoid those circumstances or take an antianginal agent before the event occurs.

With nitroglycerin use, it is important that the patient knows how to use the drug, how to store the drug, how to determine whether it is still effective, and how much to take before seeking emergency medical care.

Patients should know that regular medical follow-up is important and should be instructed in nonpharmacological measures—weight loss, smoking cessation, activity changes, diet changes—that could decrease their risk of CAD and improve the effectiveness of the antianginal therapy.

The safety for the use of these drugs during pregnancy has not been established. There is a significant potential for adverse effects on the fetus related to blood flow changes and direct drug effects when the drugs cross the placenta. The drugs do enter human milk, and it is advised that another method of feeding the baby be used if one of these drugs is prescribed during lactation.

Older Adults

Older adults frequently are prescribed one or more of these drugs. There is a risk of adverse effects which increases if multiple medications are prescribed. Safety measures may be needed if hypotension and/or arrhythmias occur and interfere with the patient's mobility and balance. Patients should be taught how to monitor their blood pressure at home and recommended to change positions slowly.

Older adults are also more likely to have renal and/or hepatic impairment related to underlying medical conditions, which could interfere with the metabolism and excretion of these drugs. For some of the medications, the dose for older adults should be started at a lower level than that recommended for younger adults. The patient should be monitored closely and dose adjusted based on patient response.

If other drugs are added to or removed from the drug regimen, appropriate dose adjustments may need to be made. If the patient is using a different form of nitroglycerin, special care should be taken to make sure that the proper administration, storage, and timing of use are understood.

Figures reprinted with permission from Grundy, S. M., Stone, N. J., Bailey, A. L., Beam, C., Birtcher, K. K., Blumenthal, R. S., Braun, L. T., deFerranti, S., Fajella-Tommasino, J., Forman, D. E., Goldberg, R., Heidenreich, P. A., Hlatky, M. A., Jones, D. W., Lloyd-Jones, D., Lopez-Pajares, N., Ndumele, C. E., Orringer, C. E., Peralta, C. A., Saseen, J. J., Smith, S. C., Sperling, L., Virani, S. S., & Yeboah, J. (2018). AHA/ACC/AACVPR/AAPA/ABC/ACPM/ADA/AGS/APhA/ASPC/NLA/PCNA guideline on the management of blood cholesterol: a report of the American College of Cardiology/American Heart Association Task Force on Clinical Practice Guidelines. *Circulation, 139*, e1082–e1143. pii: S0735-1097(18)39033-8. https://doi.org/10.1161/CIR.0000000000000625

Pharmacokinetics

Nitroglycerin is available as a sublingual tablet, a translingual spray, an intravenous (IV) solution (for bolus injection or infusion), a transdermal patch, a topical ointment or paste, or a transmucosal agent. It can be carried with the patient, who then can use it when the need arises. Slow-release forms are also available for use in preventing anginal attacks. There is also a topical indication for nitroglycerin for treatment of anal fissures (see Chapter 58). There are a variety of forms of administration for nitroglycerin (Box 46.2). Isosorbide dinitrate and isosorbide mononitrate are available in oral form.

Nitrates are rapidly absorbed, metabolized in the liver, and excreted in the urine. They cross the placenta and enter breast milk. Nitroglycerin is available in many forms, and absorption, onset of action, and duration vary with the form used (see "Prototype Summary"). Isosorbide dinitrate and isosorbide mononitrate, when given orally, have onset of action in 14 to 45 minutes, or up to 4 hours if the sustained release (SR) form is used. The drug may have a duration of action of 4 to 6 hours, or 6 to 8 hours if the SR form is used.

Contraindications and Cautions

Nitrates are contraindicated in the presence of any allergy to nitrates to prevent hypersensitivity reactions. These drugs are also contraindicated in the following conditions: severe anemia because the decrease in cardiac output could be detrimental in a patient who already has a decreased ability to deliver oxygen because of a low red blood cell count; head trauma or cerebral hemorrhage because the relaxation of cerebral vessels could cause intracranial bleeding.

Caution should be used in patients with hepatic or renal disease, which could alter the metabolism and excretion of these drugs, and in patients who are pregnant or lactating because of potential adverse effects on the neonate and ineffective blood flow to the fetus. Caution is also required for patients with hypotension, hypovolemia, and conditions that limit cardiac output (e.g., tamponade, low ventricular filling pressure, low pulmonary capillary wedge pressure, aortic stenosis) because these conditions could be exacerbated, resulting in serious adverse effects.

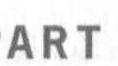

Box 46.2 Focus on Safe Medication Administration

SUBLINGUAL, TRANSBUCCAL, AND TRANSDERMAL ADMINISTRATION OF NITROGLYCERIN

Sublingual/transbuccal administration. Patients often prefer this route of administration, opting to administer the drug themselves even in the institutional setting. Make sure that the drug is given correctly:

- Check under the tongue to make sure there are no lesions or abrasions that could interfere with the absorption of the drug. Have the patient take a sip of water to moisten the mucous membranes so the tablet will dissolve quickly. Have the patient lie down or sit prior to administration of the medication. Then instruct the patient to place the tablet under the tongue or buccal pouch, close the mouth, and wait until the tablet has dissolved.
- Caution the patient not to swallow the tablet; its effectiveness would be lost if the tablet entered the stomach. If the patient uses translingual drugs often, encourage the patient to alternate sides of the tongue, placing it under the left side for one dose and under the right side for the other dose.
- To help in administering sublingual medications to patients who cannot do it themselves or who cannot open their mouths, use a tongue depressor to move the tongue aside and place the tablet, or slide the tablet down through a straw to the underside of the tongue.
- Translingual spray can be substituted for tablets. The spray should be administered against the oral mucosa and not inhaled.

Transdermal administration. Errors have been reported with inappropriate use of nitroglycerin patches and nitroglycerin paste. Make sure to discuss safe administration with the patient:

- It is important to teach patients to remove the old transdermal system and to wash the area before placing a new system to prevent adverse effects such as severe hypotension. There will often need to be a planned nitrate-free interval for the patient for the medication to be effective over longer periods of time and to decrease risk of tolerance to the medication.
- Urge patients who are given tubes of nitroglycerin paste or ointment to label tubes clearly in large letters and to store them safely away from other people in a secure place. This prevents accidental misuse of nitroglycerin paste for hand cream, which can result in a toxic dose of the drug.
- Nitroglycerin ointment may be prescribed for prevention of angina. Nitroglycerin ointment comes with a paper applicator with a ruled line for measuring the dose (in inches). Instruct patients to place the paper on a flat surface and squeeze the prescribed amount of ointment onto the paper. Then the paper is placed on the skin with the ointment side down. The paper can be used to spread the ointment to cover an area of skin at least as large as the applicator, but the ointment should not be rubbed into the skin. The applicator can be taped in and covered with a piece of plastic kitchen wrap to prevent the ointment from staining patients' clothes. Show patients how to apply without getting ointment on fingers. To be cautious, it is recommended that patients wash hands after applying the ointment.
- There is nitroglycerin ointment that can be prescribed for treatment of pain with anal fissures (Chapter 58). This formulation should only be used intra-anally and is not indicated for treatment of angina. Patients need to be taught how to apply this ointment. The patient should use disposable gloves or wrap their finger in plastic wrap to prevent the medication from getting on their hands. Once the finger is covered, the patient can squeeze the ointment on to the finger for the same length as marked on the box by the 1-in. dosing line. Then the patient should gently insert the finger with the ointment into the anal canal, up to the first finger joint. The ointment can be spread around the inside of the anal canal. If this is too painful, patients can apply the ointment directly to the outside of the anus. After administration, the finger covering should be disposed, and the patient should wash their hand with soap and water.

Adverse Effects

The adverse effects associated with these drugs are related to vasodilation and the decrease in blood flow that occurs. Central nervous system (CNS) effects include headache, dizziness, and weakness. Gastrointestinal (GI) side effects include nausea and vomiting. Cardiovascular (CV) problems include hypotension, which can be severe and must be monitored; reflex tachycardia that occurs when blood pressure falls; syncope; and angina, which could be exacerbated by the hypotension and changes in cardiac output (Fig. 46.3). Skin-related effects include flushing, pallor, and increased perspiration. With the transdermal preparation, there is a risk of contact dermatitis and local hypersensitivity reactions. With continual use, tolerance can develop.

Clinically Important Drug–Drug Interactions

There is a risk of hypertension and decreased antianginal effects if these drugs are given with ergot derivatives. There is also a risk of decreased therapeutic effects of heparin if these drugs are given together with heparin; if this combination is used, the patient should be monitored and appropriate dose adjustments made. Patients should not combine nitrates with phosphodiesterase type 5 inhibitors (sildenafil, tadalafil, or vardenafil), drugs used to treat erectile dysfunction, because serious hypotension and CV events could occur. There is risk of increased antihypertensive effect with other medications that can lower BP.

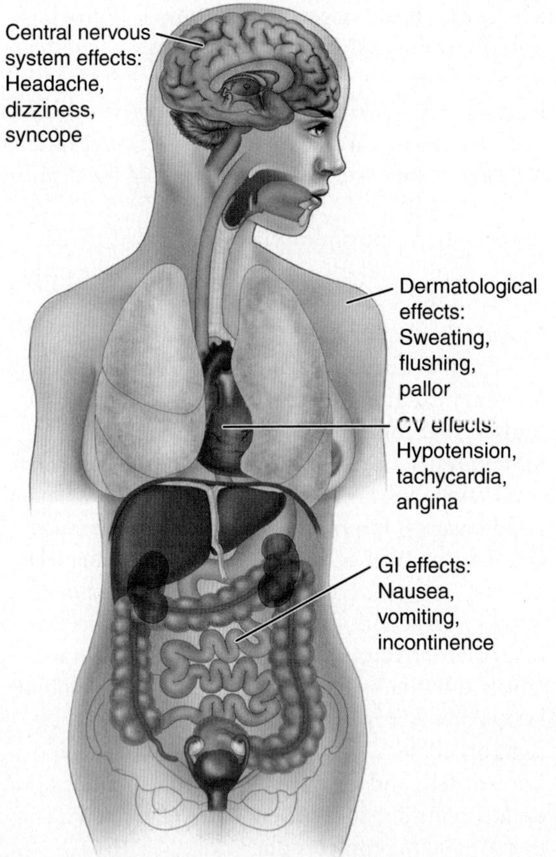

FIGURE 46.3 Variety of adverse effects and toxicities associated with antianginals.

Prototype Summary: Nitroglycerin

Indications: Treatment of acute angina, prophylaxis of angina, IV treatment of angina unresponsive to beta-blockers or organic nitrates, perioperative hypertension, and heart failure associated with acute MI; to produce controlled hypotension during surgery.

Actions: Relaxes vascular smooth muscle with a resultant decrease in venous return and decrease in arterial blood pressure, reducing the left ventricular workload and decreasing myocardial oxygen consumption.

Pharmacokinetics:

Route	Onset	Duration
IV	1–2 min	3–5 min
Sublingual tablet	1–3 min	30–60 min
Translingual spray	2 min	30–60 min
Transmucosal tablet	1–2 min	3–5 min
Oral, SR tablet	20–45 min	8–12 h
Topical ointment	30–60 min	4–8 h
Transdermal	30–60 min	24 h

$T_{1/2}$: 1 to 4 minutes; metabolized in the liver and excreted in the urine.

Adverse Effects: Hypotension, headache, dizziness, reflex tachycardia, rash, flushing, nausea, vomiting, sweating, chest pain.

Nursing Considerations for Patients Receiving Nitrates

Assessment: History and Examination

- Assess for contraindications or cautions: any known allergies to nitrates to avoid hypersensitivity reactions; impaired liver or kidney function, which could alter the metabolism and excretion of the drug; any condition that could be exacerbated by the hypotension and change in blood flow caused by these drugs, such as early MI, head trauma, cerebral hemorrhage, hypotension, hypovolemia, anemia, or low cardiac output states; and current status of pregnancy or lactation because of the potential for adverse effects on the fetus or nursing baby.
- Perform a physical assessment to establish baseline status before beginning therapy and during therapy to determine effectiveness and to evaluate for any potential adverse effects.
- Inspect the skin for color, intactness, and any signs of redness, irritation, or breakdown, especially if the patient is using the transdermal or topical form of the drug, to prevent possible skin reaction and ensure adequate surface for application and absorption of transdermal or topical drug. Also check the patient's oral or buccal mucosa (including the area under the tongue) if sublingual or buccal forms are ordered to reduce the risk of irritation and ensure adequate surface for absorption.
- Assess the patient's complaint of pain, including onset, duration, intensity, location, and measures used to relieve it. Investigate activity level prior to and after the onset of pain to aid in identifying possible contributing factors to the pain and its progression.
- Assess the patient's neurological status, including level of alertness, affect, and reflexes, to evaluate for CNS effects.
- Monitor respirations and auscultate lungs to evaluate changes in cardiac output.
- Assess cardiopulmonary status closely, including pulse rate, blood pressure, heart rate, and rhythm, to determine the effects of therapy and identify any adverse effects.
- Obtain an ECG as ordered to evaluate heart rate and rhythm, which could indicate changes in cardiac perfusion.
- Monitor laboratory test results, including liver and renal function tests, complete blood count, and hemoglobin level, to determine the need for possible dose adjustment.

Nursing Conclusions

Nursing conclusions related to drug therapy might include the following:

- Altered cardiac output related to vasodilation and hypotensive effects
- Injury risk related to CNS or CV effects

(continues on page 818)

- Altered tissue perfusion (total body) related to hypotension or change in cardiac output
- Knowledge deficit regarding drug therapy

Planning

- The patient will receive the best therapeutic effect from the drug therapy.
- The patient will have limited adverse effects to the drug therapy.
- The patient will have an understanding of the drug therapy, adverse effects to anticipate, and measures to relieve discomfort and improve safety.

Intervention With Rationale

- Have the patient lay down or sit down prior to administration. There is a risk of low blood pressure causing the patient to feel light-headed or dizzy and even pass out.
- Give sublingual preparations under the tongue or in the buccal pouch and encourage the patient not to swallow to ensure that therapeutic effectiveness is achieved (see "Pharmacokinetics" for discussion of safe medication administration).
- Ask the patient if the tablet "fizzles" or burns, which indicates potency. Always check the expiration date on the bottle and protect the medication from heat and light because these drugs are volatile and lose their potency.
- Instruct the patient that a sublingual dose may be repeated in 5 minutes if relief is not felt for a total of three doses; if pain persists, the patient should go to an emergency room to ensure proper medical support if an MI should occur.
- Give SR forms with water, and caution the patient not to chew or crush them because these preparations need to reach the GI tract intact.
- Long-acting preparations should be administered with plans for nitrate-free intervals because there is risk of tolerance decreasing effectiveness if given continuously.
- Rotate the sites of topical forms to decrease the risk of skin abrasion and breakdown; monitor for signs of skin breakdown to arrange for appropriate skin care as needed.
- Make sure that translingual spray is used under the tongue and not inhaled to ensure that the therapeutic effects can be achieved.
- Keep a record of the number of sprays used if a translingual spray form is used to prevent running out of medication and episodes of untreated angina.
- Have emergency life support equipment readily available in case of severe reaction to the drug or MI.
- Taper the dose gradually (over 4 to 6 weeks) after long-term therapy because abrupt withdrawal could cause a severe reaction, including MI.
- Provide comfort measures to help the patient tolerate drug effects. These include small, frequent meals to alleviate GI upset; access to bathroom facilities if GI upset is severe or the patient experiences incontinence; environmental controls such as temperature, controlled lighting, and noise reduction to decrease stresses that could aggravate cardiac workload; safety precautions such as lying or sitting down after taking the drug and assistance with ambulation to reduce the risk of injury; reorientation; and appropriate skin care as needed.
- Offer support and encouragement to help the patient deal with the diagnosis and the drug regimen.
- Provide thorough patient teaching, including the name of the drug; dosage prescribed; proper technique for administration (oral, sublingual, transbuccal, transdermal, inhalation spray, or topical); need for removal of transdermal or topical drug before application of the next dose; the importance of having an adequate supply of drug (e.g., teaching the patient to count the number of sprays used for a translingual spray so as not to run short); measures to prevent anginal attacks, and actions to take when an attack occurs; use of medication during an attack (such as the number of tablets and time span that the patient can take sublingual tablets); measures to avoid adverse effects, warning signs of problems, and signs and symptoms to report immediately; and the need for periodic monitoring and evaluation to enhance patient knowledge about drug therapy and to promote adherence.

Evaluation

- Monitor patient response to the drug (alleviation of signs and symptoms of angina, prevention of angina).
- Monitor for adverse effects (hypotension, cardiac arrhythmias, GI upset, skin reactions, headache).
- Evaluate the effectiveness of the teaching plan (patient can name drug, dosage, proper administration, adverse effects to watch for, specific measures to avoid them, and the importance of continued follow-up).
- Monitor the effectiveness of comfort measures and adherence to the regimen.

See the "Critical Thinking Scenario" for measures for handling an angina attack.

Key Points

- Nitrates cause blood vessels to relax and dilate. This results in a drop in peripheral resistance and blood pressure and a decrease in venous return to the heart. These actions will decrease myocardial workload and can restore the appropriate balance in the supply-and-demand ratio in the heart.
- Nitrates are available in many forms that vary in time of onset and duration of action. Fast-acting nitrates are used to treat acute anginal attacks. Slower-acting nitrates are used to prevent anginal attacks from occurring.

CRITICAL THINKING SCENARIO
Handling an Angina Attack

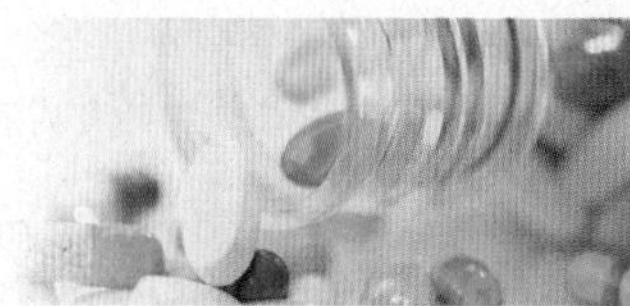

THE SITUATION

S.W. is a 48-year-old patient with a 2-year history of angina pectoris. S.W was given sublingual nitroglycerin to use when they had chest pain. For the past 6 months, S.W. has been stable, experiencing little chest pain. This morning after their exercise class, S.W. had an argument with their teenage child and experienced severe chest pain that was unrelieved by four nitroglycerin tablets taken over a 20-minute period. S.W. was rushed to the hospital, where she was given oxygen through nasal cannula and placed on a cardiac monitor, which showed a sinus tachycardia of 110 beats/min. A 12-lead ECG showed no changes from her previous ECG of 7 months ago.

S.W. did not have elevated troponin levels. The chest pain subsided within 3 minutes after they received another sublingual nitroglycerin. It was decided that S.W. should stay in the emergency department (ED) for a few hours for observation. The diagnosis of an acute angina attack was made.

CRITICAL THINKING

What nursing interventions are appropriate for S.W. while still in the ED? Consider the progression of CAD and the ways in which that progression can be delayed and chest pain avoided.

What teaching points should be stressed with this patient?

What type of guilt may the child experience after the argument with S.W.?

What interventions would be useful in dealing with the family dynamics during this crisis?

Should any further tests or treatments be addressed with S.W. when discussing her heart disease?

DISCUSSION

S.W.'s vital signs should be monitored closely while they are in the ED. If the attack subsides, S.W. will be discharged, and teaching points about CAD will be reviewed with them. It would be a good time to discuss angina with S.W. and their teenage child, explaining the pathophysiology of the disease and ways to avoid disrupting the supply-and-demand ratio in the heart muscle.

Because S.W. took four nitroglycerin tablets with no effect before coming to the ED, it would be important to find out the age and potency of the drug. Review the storage requirements for the drug, ways to tell whether it is potent, and the importance of replacing the pills at least every 6 months.

S.W. and their child should be encouraged to air their feelings about this episode; for example, this scare may have caused guilt or anger. They should have the opportunity to explore other ways of handling their problems, try to pace activities to avoid excessive demand for oxygen, and plan what to do if this happens again. They should both receive support and encouragement to cope with the angina and its implications.

Written information, including drug information, should be given to S.W. Once the condition is stabilized, further studies may be indicated to monitor the progress of disease. The use of dietary interventions, avoidance of smoking as appropriate, blood pressure control, and monitoring of activity should be considered.

NURSING CARE GUIDE FOR S.W.: ANTIANGINAL NITRATES

Assessment: History and Examination

Assess S.W. for allergies to any nitrates, renal or hepatic dysfunction, pregnancy and lactation (if appropriate), early MI, head trauma, hypotension, and hypovolemia.

Focus the physical examination on the following areas:

CV: Blood pressure, pulse, perfusion, ECG
CNS: Orientation, affect, reflexes, vision
Skin: Color, lesions, texture
Respiratory system: Respiratory rate and character, adventitious sounds
GI: Abdominal examination, bowel sounds
Laboratory tests: Liver and renal function tests, complete blood count, hemoglobin

Nursing Conclusions

Altered cardiac output related to hypotension
Injury risk related to CNS and CV effects
Altered tissue perfusion (total body) related to CV effects
Fear and anxiety related to disease
Knowledge deficit regarding drug therapy

Planning

The patient will receive the best therapeutic effect from the drug therapy.

The patient will have limited adverse effects to the drug therapy.

The patient will have an understanding of the drug therapy, adverse effects to anticipate, and measures to relieve discomfort and improve safety.

(continues on page 820)

Intervention

Ensure proper administration of drug, and protect the drug from heat and light.
Provide comfort and safety measures.
Offer environmental control for headaches.
Give drug with food if GI upset occurs.
Provide skin care as needed.
Taper dose after long-term use.
Provide support and reassurance to deal with drug effects.
Provide patient teaching regarding drug, dosage, adverse effects, what to report, and safety precautions.

Evaluation

Evaluate drug effects: relief of signs and symptoms of angina, prevention of angina.
Monitor for adverse effects: headache, dizziness; arrhythmias; GI upset; skin reactions; hypotension; and CV effects.
Monitor for drug–drug interactions as indicated for each drug.
Evaluate the effectiveness of the patient teaching program and comfort and safety measures.

PATIENT TEACHING FOR S.W.

- A nitrate is given to patients with chest pain that occurs because the heart muscle is not receiving enough oxygen. The nitrates act by decreasing the heart's workload and thus its need for oxygen, which it uses for energy. This relieves the pain of angina.
- Besides taking the drug as prescribed, you can also help your heart by decreasing the work that it must do. For example, you can:
  - Reduce weight, if necessary.
  - Decrease or avoid the use of coffee, cigarettes, or alcoholic beverages.
  - Avoid going outside in very cold weather; if this cannot be avoided, dress warmly and avoid exertion while outside.
  - Reduce stress levels. Stress can be high physical exertion or emotional distress (anger, anxiety, fear), and it can strain the heart. Moderate exercise is helpful and can usually be performed safely. Discuss potentially helpful activities with health care providers. Some people may benefit from stress reduction programs to assist with coping with difficult life situations.
- Nitroglycerin tablets are taken sublingually. Be sure to sit or lie down prior to taking a tablet. Place one tablet under your tongue. Do not swallow until the tablet has dissolved. The tablet should burn slightly or "fizzle" under your tongue; if this does not occur, the tablet is not effective and you should get a fresh supply of tablets.
- Sublingual nitroglycerin is an unstable compound. Do not buy large quantities at a time because it does not store well. Keep the drug in a dark, dry place and in a dark-colored glass container, not a plastic bottle, with a tight lid. Leave it in its own bottle. Do not combine it with other drugs.
- Notify your cardiologist if you have pain that requires you to take your nitroglycerin.
- Some of the following adverse effects may occur:
  - *Dizziness, light-headedness:* This often passes as you adjust to the drug. Use great care if you are taking sublingual or transmucosal forms of the drug. Sit or lie down to avoid dizziness or falls. Change position slowly to help decrease the dizziness.
  - *Headache:* This is a common problem. Over-the-counter headache remedies often provide no relief for the pain. Lying down in a cool environment and resting may help alleviate some of the discomfort.
  - *Flushing of the face and neck:* This is usually a minor problem that passes as the drug's effects pass.
  - Report any of the following to your health care provider: *blurred vision, persistent or severe headache, skin rash, more frequent or more severe angina attacks, or fainting.*
- Sublingual nitroglycerin usually relieves chest pain within 3 to 5 minutes. If pain is not relieved within 5 minutes, take another tablet. If pain continues, take another tablet in 5 minutes. A total of _____ tablets may be used, spaced every 5 minutes. If the pain is not relieved after that time, call your health care provider or go to a hospital emergency room as soon as possible.
- Tell any doctor, nurse, or other health care provider involved in your care that you are taking this drug.
- Keep this drug, and all medications, out of the reach of children.
- Avoid taking over-the-counter medications while you are taking this drug. If you feel that you need one of these, consult with your health care provider for the best choice. Many of these drugs can change the effects of this drug and cause problems.
- Avoid alcohol while you are taking this drug because the combination can cause serious problems by lowering your blood pressure.
- If you are taking this drug on a scheduled basis for a prolonged period of time, do not stop taking it suddenly. Your body will need time to adjust to the discontinuation of the drug. The dose must be gradually reduced to prevent serious problems.

Beta-Adrenergic Blockers

As discussed in Chapter 31, beta-adrenergic blockers are used to block the stimulatory effects of the sympathetic nervous system. The beta-blockers recommended for use in angina include atenolol (*Tenormin*), metoprolol (*Lopressor, Toprol XL*), propranolol (*Inderal, Hemangeol, Innopran XL*), and nadolol (*Corgard*).

Therapeutic Actions and Indications

The beta-blockers competitively block beta-adrenergic receptors in the heart and juxtaglomerular apparatus, decreasing the influence of the sympathetic nervous system on these tissues. The result is a decrease in the excitability of the heart, a decrease in cardiac output, a decrease in cardiac oxygen consumption, and a lowering of blood pressure. They are indicated for the long-term management of angina pectoris caused by atherosclerosis. These drugs are sometimes used in combination with nitrates to increase exercise tolerance. See Table 46.1 for usual indications for each of these drugs.

Beta-blockers are not indicated for the treatment of Prinzmetal angina because they could cause peripheral ischemia and may exacerbate vasospasm due to blocking of beta-receptor sites. Propranolol and metoprolol can also be used to prevent reinfarction in stable patients 1 to 4 weeks after an MI. This effect is thought to be caused by the suppression of myocardial oxygen demand for a prolonged period.

Pharmacokinetics

These drugs are absorbed from the GI tract after oral administration and undergo hepatic metabolism. They reach peak levels in 60 to 90 minutes and have varying duration of effects, ranging from 6 to 19 hours. Food has been found to increase the bioavailability of propranolol, but this effect has not been found with other beta-adrenergic blocking agents.

Contraindications and Cautions

The beta-blockers are contraindicated in patients with bradycardia, heart block, and cardiogenic shock because blocking of the sympathetic response could exacerbate these diseases.

Caution should be used in patients with diabetes, peripheral vascular disease, asthma, chronic obstructive pulmonary disease, or thyrotoxicosis because the blockade of the sympathetic response blocks normal reflexes that are necessary for maintaining homeostasis in patients with these diseases. Many patients with these complicating disorders receive beta-blockers, and these patients need to be monitored carefully to avoid serious adverse effects.

Adverse Effects

Beta-blockers have many adverse effects associated with the blockade of the sympathetic nervous system. However, the dose used to prevent angina is lower than doses used to treat hypertension. Therefore, there is a decreased incidence of adverse effects associated with this specific use of beta-blockers.

Adverse effects do occur. CNS effects include dizziness, fatigue, emotional depression, and sleep disturbances. GI problems include gastric pain, nausea, vomiting, colitis, and diarrhea. CV effects can include HF, reduced cardiac output, and arrhythmias. Respiratory effects can include bronchospasm, dyspnea, and cough. Decreased exercise tolerance and malaise are also common complaints.

Clinically Important Drug–Drug Interactions

A decreased antihypertensive effect occurs when beta-blockers are given with nonsteroidal anti-inflammatory drugs; if this combination is used, the patient should be monitored closely and a dose adjustment made.

An initial hypertensive episode followed by bradycardia occurs if these drugs are given with epinephrine, and a possibility of peripheral ischemia exists if beta-blockers are taken in combination with ergot alkaloids.

There is also a potential for masked symptoms of hypoglycemia if these drugs are given with insulin or antidiabetic agents, and the patient will not have the usual signs and symptoms of hypoglycemia or hyperglycemia to alert them to potential problems. If this combination is used, the patient should monitor blood glucose frequently throughout the day and should be alert to new warnings about glucose imbalance.

Prototype Summary: Metoprolol

Indications: Treatment of stable angina pectoris; also used for treatment of hypertension, prevention of reinfarction in MI patients, and treatment of stable, symptomatic HF.

Actions: Competitively blocks beta-adrenergic receptors in the heart and kidneys, decreasing the influence of the sympathetic nervous system on these tissues and the excitability of the heart; decreases cardiac output, which results in a lowered blood pressure and decreased cardiac workload.

Pharmacokinetics:

Route	Onset	Peak	Duration
Oral	15 min	90 min	Formulations will vary
IV	Immediate	60–90 min	15–19 h

$T_{1/2}$: 3 to 4 hours; metabolized in the liver and excreted in the urine.

Adverse Effects: Dizziness, vertigo, HF, arrhythmias, gastric pain, flatulence, diarrhea, vomiting, impotence, decreased exercise tolerance.

Nursing Considerations for Patients Receiving Beta-Blockers

See Chapter 31 for the nursing considerations associated with beta-blockers.

Key Points

- Beta-blockers are used in the treatment of angina to help restore the balance between supply of oxygen and demand for oxygen.
- Beta-blockers prevent the activation of sympathetic receptors, which normally would increase heart rate, increase blood pressure, and increase cardiac contraction. All of these actions would increase the demand for oxygen; blocking these actions decreases the demand for oxygen.

Calcium Channel Blockers

Calcium channel blockers include amlodipine (*Katerzia, Norvasc*), diltiazem (*Cardizem* and others), nicardipine (generic), nifedipine (*Procardia, Procardia XL*), and verapamil (*Calan SR* and others). There are two main types of calcium channel blockers: nondihydropyridine (diltiazem and verapamil) and dihydropyridine (all other calcium channel blockers). The nondihydropyridines have more direct negative inotropic (less heart pumping force) and chronotropic (lower heart rate) effects than the dihydropyridine calcium channel blockers. See Chapter 43 for full list of calcium channel blockers. Both types may be used to treat angina. The nondihydropyridine calcium channel blockers are more dangerous to use for patients with HF due to potentially decreasing heart muscle function.

Therapeutic Actions and Indications

Calcium channel blockers inhibit the movement of calcium ions across the membranes of myocardial and arterial muscle cells, altering the action potential and blocking muscle cell contraction. A loss of smooth muscle tone, vasodilation, and decreased peripheral resistance occur. Subsequently, preload and afterload are decreased, which in turn decreases cardiac workload and oxygen consumption.

Calcium channel blockers are indicated for the treatment of Prinzmetal angina, chronic angina, effort-associated angina, and hypertension. In Prinzmetal angina, these agents relieve coronary artery vasospasm, increasing blood flow to the muscle cells. Research also indicates that these drugs block the proliferation of cells in the endothelial layer of the blood vessel, slowing the progress of atherosclerosis. Verapamil and diltiazem may be used to treat cardiac tachyarrhythmias because they slow conduction more than the other calcium channel blockers do. The drug of choice depends on the patient's diagnosis and ability to tolerate adverse drug effects. See Table 46.1 for usual indications for each of these drugs.

Pharmacokinetics

These drugs are generally well absorbed after oral administration, metabolized in the liver, and excreted in the urine. They have an onset of action of 20 minutes and a duration of action of 2 to 4 hours. These drugs cross the placenta and enter human milk.

Contraindications and Cautions

Calcium channel blockers are contraindicated in the presence of allergy to any of these drugs to avoid hypersensitivity reactions and with pregnancy or lactation because of the potential for adverse effects on the fetus or neonate.

Caution should be used with heart block or sick sinus syndrome, which could be exacerbated by the conduction-slowing effects of these drugs; with renal or hepatic dysfunction, which could alter the metabolism and excretion of these drugs; and with HF, which could be exacerbated by the decrease in cardiac output that could occur.

Adverse Effects

The adverse effects associated with these drugs are related to their effects on cardiac output and on smooth muscle. CNS effects include dizziness, light-headedness, headache, and fatigue. GI effects can include nausea and hepatic injury related to direct toxic effects on hepatic cells. CV effects include hypotension, bradycardia, peripheral edema, and heart block. Skin effects include flushing and rash.

Clinically Important Drug–Drug Interactions

Drug–drug interactions vary with each of the calcium channel blockers. Potentially serious effects to keep in mind include increased serum levels and toxicity of cyclosporine if they are taken with diltiazem, and increased risk of heart block and digoxin toxicity if they are combined with verapamil (because verapamil increases digoxin serum levels). Both verapamil and digoxin depress myocardial conduction. If any combinations of these drugs must be used, the patient should be monitored closely and appropriate dose adjustments made. Verapamil has also been associated with serious respiratory depression when given with general anesthetics or as an adjunct to anesthesia.

Prototype Summary: Diltiazem

Indications: Treatment of Prinzmetal angina, effort-associated angina, and chronic stable angina; also used to treat essential hypertension and paroxysmal supraventricular tachycardia.

Actions: Inhibits the movement of calcium ions across the membranes of myocardial and arterial muscle cells, altering the action potential and blocking muscle cell contraction, which depresses myocardial contractility; slows cardiac impulse formation in the conductive tissues, and relaxes and dilates arteries, causing a fall in blood pressure and a decrease in venous return; decreases the workload of the heart and myocardial oxygen consumption; relieves the vasospasm of the coronary artery, increasing blood flow to the muscle cells (Prinzmetal angina).

Pharmacokinetics:

Route	Onset	Peak
Oral	30–60 min	2–3 h
SR, extended release (ER)	30–60 min	6–11 h
IV	Immediate	2–3 min

$T_{1/2}$: 3.5 to 6 hours SR, 5 to 7 hours ER; metabolized in the liver and excreted in the urine.

Adverse Effects: Dizziness, light-headedness, headache, asthenia, peripheral edema, bradycardia, atrioventricular block, flushing, rash, nausea.

Nursing Considerations for Patients Receiving Calcium Channel Blockers

Assessment: History and Examination

- Assess for contraindications or cautions: known allergies to any of these drugs to avoid hypersensitivity reactions; impaired liver or kidney function, which could alter the metabolism and excretion of the drug; heart block, which could be exacerbated by the conduction depression of these drugs; and current status of pregnancy or lactation because of the risk of adverse effects to the fetus or baby.
- Perform a physical assessment to establish baseline status before beginning therapy and during therapy to determine the effectiveness and evaluate for any potential adverse effects.
- Inspect skin for color and integrity to identify possible adverse skin reactions.
- Assess the patient's complaint of pain, including onset, duration, intensity, and location, and measures used to relieve the pain. Investigate activity level prior to and after the onset of pain to aid in identifying possible contributing factors to the pain and its progression.
- Assess cardiopulmonary status closely, including pulse rate, blood pressure, heart rate, and rhythm, to determine the effects of therapy and identify any adverse effects.
- Obtain an ECG as ordered to evaluate heart rate and rhythm.
- Monitor respirations and auscultate lungs to evaluate changes in cardiac output.
- Monitor laboratory test results, including liver and renal function tests, to determine the need for possible dose adjustment.

Nursing Conclusions

Nursing conclusions related to drug therapy might include the following:

- Altered cardiac output risk related to hypotension and vasodilation
- Injury risk related to CNS or CV effects
- Altered tissue perfusion (total body) related to hypotension or change in cardiac output
- Knowledge deficit regarding drug therapy

Planning

- The patient will receive the best therapeutic effect from the drug therapy.
- The patient will have limited adverse effects to the drug therapy.
- The patient will have an understanding of the drug therapy, adverse effects to anticipate, and measures to relieve discomfort and improve safety.

Intervention With Rationale

- Monitor the patient's blood pressure, cardiac rhythm, and cardiac output closely while the drug is being titrated or dose is being changed to ensure early detection of potentially serious adverse effects.
- If a patient is on long-term therapy, periodically monitor blood pressure and cardiac rhythm while the patient is using these drugs because of the potential for adverse CV effects.
- Provide comfort measures to help the patient tolerate drug effects. These include small, frequent meals to alleviate GI upset; adequate hydration to decrease risk of orthostatic hypotension; and recommending caution when changing position due to risk of dizziness when sitting up or standing quickly.
- Offer support and encouragement to help the patient deal with the diagnosis and the drug regimen.
- Provide thorough patient teaching, including the name of the drug and dosage prescribed; measures to avoid adverse effects and prevent anginal attacks; actions to take when an attack occurs; warning signs of problems, and signs and symptoms to report immediately; and the need for periodic monitoring and evaluation to enhance patient knowledge about drug therapy and to promote adherence.

(continues on page 824)

Evaluation

- Monitor patient response to the drug (alleviation of signs and symptoms of angina, prevention of angina).
- Monitor for adverse effects (hypotension, dizziness, cardiac arrhythmias, GI upset, skin reactions, headache).
- Monitor the effectiveness of comfort measures and adherence to the regimen.
- Evaluate the effectiveness of the teaching plan (patient can name drug, dosage, proper administration, adverse effects to watch for, specific measures to avoid them, and the importance of continued follow-up).

Key Points

- Calcium channel blockers block muscle contraction in smooth muscle and decrease the heart's workload, relax vasospasm in Prinzmetal angina, and possibly block proliferation of the damaged endothelium in coronary vessels.
- Patients on calcium channel blockers need to be monitored for signs of decreased cardiac output and response, including slow heart rate, hypotension, dizziness, and headache.

Piperazine Acetamide Agent

In late 2006, the U.S. Food and Drug Administration approved the first new drug in more than 10 years for the treatment of chronic angina. Since its approval, postmarketing studies have shown that the drug is effective in treating angina and has the added benefits of decreasing blood glucose levels when used in diabetic patients and decreasing the incidence of ventricular fibrillation, atrial fibrillation, and bradycardia in patients with chronic angina. Ranolazine (*Ranexa*) is available in an ER tablet form for oral use. The mechanism of action of the drug is not completely understood. It may inhibit late sodium influx, but it is not clear if this facilitates the antianginal effect. It does prolong the QT interval; it does not necessarily decrease heart rate or blood pressure. There is a decrease in myocardial workload, bringing the supply and demand for oxygen back into balance.

Ranolazine is approved as a first-line treatment for angina or for use in combination with nitrates, beta-blockers, or amlodipine. It is rapidly absorbed, reaching peak level in 2 to 5 hours. It is metabolized in the liver with a half-life of 7 hours and is excreted in the urine and feces. Ranolazine is contraindicated for use with any known sensitivity to the drug; with preexisting prolonged QT interval or in combination with drugs that would prolong QT intervals; and with hepatic impairment and lactation. Caution should be used with pregnancy or renal impairment.

Concurrent use with CYP3A (diltiazem, verapamil, erythromycin) and P-gp inhibitors (cyclosporine) can increase exposure to ranolazine. Combination with strong CYP3A inhibitors/inducers is not recommended. Digoxin levels may become high if the two drugs are combined; if this combination is needed, the digoxin dose will need to be decreased. Tricyclic antidepressants and antipsychotic drug levels may increase if these agents are combined with ranolazine; if they are combined, the dose of these drugs may need to be decreased. Grapefruit juice should be avoided while taking this drug. It is recommended that patient drug regimens be checked for potential medication interactions when initiating treatment. Dizziness, headache, nausea, and constipation are the most commonly experienced adverse effects. Patients must be cautioned not to cut, crush, or chew the tablets, which need to be swallowed whole. Safety precautions may be needed if dizziness is an issue.

SUMMARY

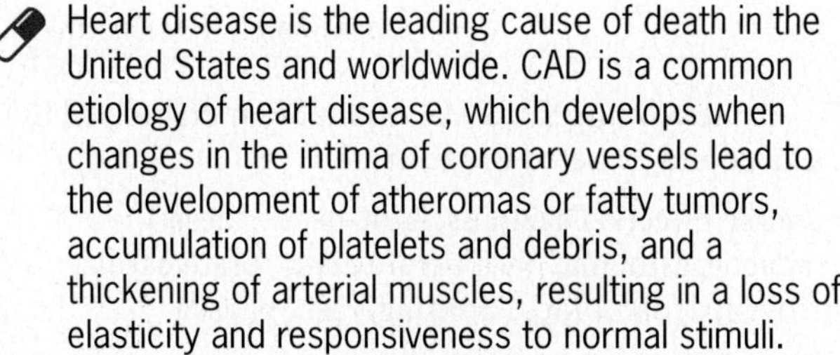

- Heart disease is the leading cause of death in the United States and worldwide. CAD is a common etiology of heart disease, which develops when changes in the intima of coronary vessels lead to the development of atheromas or fatty tumors, accumulation of platelets and debris, and a thickening of arterial muscles, resulting in a loss of elasticity and responsiveness to normal stimuli.
- Narrowing of the coronary arteries secondary to atheroma buildup is called atherosclerosis.
- Narrowed coronary arteries eventually become unable to deliver all the blood that is needed by the myocardial cells, causing a problem of supply and demand.
- Angina pectoris, or "suffocation of the chest," occurs when the myocardial demand for oxygen cannot be met. Pain, anxiety, shortness of breath, and/or fatigue develop when the supply-and-demand ratio is upset. Types of angina include stable, unstable, and Prinzmetal angina.
- MI occurs when a coronary vessel is completely occluded and the cells that depend on that vessel for oxygen become ischemic, then necrotic, and die.
- Angina can be treated by drugs that either increase the supply of oxygen or decrease the heart's workload, which decreases the demand for oxygen.
- Nitrates are used to cause vasodilation and to decrease venous return and arterial resistance—effects that decrease cardiac workload and oxygen consumption.
- Nitroglycerin is the drug of choice for treating an acute anginal attack. It is available in various forms.

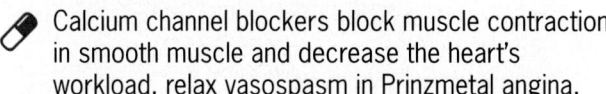

- Beta-blockers prevent the activation of sympathetic receptors, which normally would increase heart rate, increase blood pressure, and increase cardiac contraction. All of these actions would increase the demand for oxygen; blocking these actions decreases the demand for oxygen.
- Calcium channel blockers block muscle contraction in smooth muscle and decrease the heart's workload, relax vasospasm in Prinzmetal angina, and possibly block the proliferation of the damaged endothelium in coronary vessels.
- The newest drug approved for the treatment of angina is the piperazine acetamide agent ranolazine. The mechanism of action of this drug is not completely understood. It prolongs QT intervals, does not slow heart rate or blood pressure, but decreases myocardial oxygen demand.

CHECK YOUR UNDERSTANDING

Answers to the questions in this chapter can be found in Answers to Check Your Understanding Questions on thePoint®.

MULTIPLE CHOICE

Select the best answer.

1. Coronary artery disease results in
   a. an imbalance in cardiac muscle oxygen supply and demand.
   b. delivery of blood to the heart muscle during systole.
   c. increased pulse pressure.
   d. a decreased workload on the heart.
2. Angina
   a. causes death of heart muscle cells.
   b. is pain due to lack of oxygen to myocardial cells.
   c. cannot occur at rest.
   d. is not treatable.
3. Nitrates are commonly used antianginal drugs that act to
   a. increase the preload on the heart.
   b. increase the afterload on the heart.
   c. dilate coronary vessels to increase the delivery of oxygen through those vessels.
   d. decrease venous return to the heart, decreasing the myocardial workload.
4. Calcium channel blockers are effective in treating angina because they
   a. prevent any CV exercise, preventing strain on the heart.
   b. block strong muscle contractions, causing vasodilation.
   c. alter the electrolyte balance of the heart, preventing arrhythmias.
   d. increase the heart rate, making it more efficient.
5. A nurse would recognize that increased monitoring would be recommended if a patient was taking both verapamil and which medication?
   a. Oral contraceptives
   b. Cyclosporine
   c. Digoxin
   d. Barbiturate anesthetics
6. Prinzmetal angina occurs as a result of
   a. electrolyte imbalance.
   b. a spasm of a coronary vessel.
   c. decreased venous return to the heart.
   d. a ventricular arrhythmia.

MULTIPLE RESPONSE

Select all that apply.

1. Treating angina involves modifying factors that could decrease myocardial oxygen consumption. It could be expected that this might include
   a. weight loss.
   b. use of nitrates.
   c. use of angiotensin-converting enzyme inhibitors.
   d. activity modification.
   e. use of a piperazine acetamide agent.
   f. use of a calcium channel blocker.
2. An acute myocardial infarction is usually associated with which conditions?
   a. Permanent injury to the heart muscle
   b. Potentially serious arrhythmias
   c. Pain
   d. The development of hypertension
   e. Loss of consciousness
   f. A feeling of anxiety

3. When describing the action of antianginal drugs to a patient, which would the nurse include?
   a. Decrease the workload on the heart
   b. Increase the supply of oxygen to the heart
   c. Change the metabolic pathway in the heart muscle to remove the need for oxygen
   d. Restore the supply-and-demand balance of oxygen in the heart
   e. Decrease venous return to the heart
   f. Alter the coronary artery filling pathway

4. A client who has nitroglycerin to avert an acute anginal attack would need to be taught to
   a. take five or six tablets and then seek medical help if no relief occurs.
   b. buy the tablets in bulk to decrease the cost.
   c. protect tablets from light and humidity.
   d. store the tablets in a clearly marked, clear container in open view.
   e. use the nitroglycerin before an event or activity that will most likely precipitate an anginal attack.
   f. discard them if they do not fizzle when placed under the tongue.

REFERENCES

Amsterdam, E. A., Wenger, N. K., Brindis, R. G., Casey, D. E., Ganiats, T. G., Holmes, D. R., Jaffe, A. S., Jneid, H., Kelly, R. F., Kontos, M. C., Levine, G. N., Liebson, P. R., Mukherjee, D., Peterson, E. D., Sabatine, M. S., Smalling, R. W., & Zieman, S. J. (2014). ACC/AHA guideline for the management of patients with non–ST-elevation acute coronary syndromes: A report of the American College of Cardiology/American Heart Association Task Force on Practice Guidelines. *Circulation, 130*, e344–e426. https://doi.org/10.1161/CIR.0000000000000134

Brunton, L., Hilal-Dandan, R., & Knollman, B. (2018). *Goodman and Gilman's the pharmacological basis of therapeutics* (13th ed.). McGraw-Hill.

DeVon, H., Hogan, N., Ochs, A., & Shapiro, M. (2010). Time to treatment of acute coronary syndromes: The cost of indecision. *Journal of Cardiovascular Nursing, 25*(2), 106–114. https://doi.org/10.1097/JCN.0b013e3181bb14a0

Fuster, V., Alexander, R. W., & Rourke, R. A. (Eds.). (2011). *Hurst's the heart* (13th ed.). McGraw-Hill.

Hall, J. E., & Hall, M. E. (2021). *Guyton and Hall textbook of medical physiology* (14th ed.). Elsevier.

Jneid, H., Anderson, J. L., Wright, R. S., Adams, C. D., Bridges, C. R., Casey, D. E., Ettinger, S. M., Fesmire, F. M., Ganiats, T. G., Lincoff, A. M., Peterson, E. D., Philippides, G. J., Theroux, P., Wenger, N. K., & Zidar, J. P. (2012). 2012 Focused update of the guideline for the management of patients with unstable angina/non-ST-elevation myocardial infarction. *Circulation, 126*(7), 875–910. https://doi.org/10.1161/CIR.0b013e318256f1e0Circulation

Kloner, R. A., & Chaitman, B. (2017). Angina and its management. *Journal of Cardiovascular Pharmacology and Therapeutics, 22*(3), 199–209. https://doi.org/10.1177/1074248416679733

Mapel, D. W., Schum, M., & Worley, A. (2014). The epidemiology and treatment of anal fissures in a population-based cohort. *BMC Gastroenterology, 14*, 129. https://www.ncbi.nlm.nih.gov/pmc/articles/PMC4109752/

Norris, T. L. (2019). *Porth's pathophysiology concepts of altered health states* (13th ed.). Wolters Kluwer.

CHAPTER 47

Lipid-Lowering Agents

Learning Objectives

Upon completion of this chapter, you will be able to:

1. Outline the mechanisms of fat metabolism in the body and discuss the role of hyperlipidemia as a risk factor for atherosclerotic cardiovascular disease.
2. Discuss the use of drugs that lower lipid levels across the lifespan.
3. Describe the therapeutic actions, indications, pharmacokinetics, contraindications and cautions, most common adverse effects, and important drug–drug interactions associated with bile acid sequestrants, HMG–CoA inhibitors (statins), cholesterol absorption inhibitors, PCSK9 inhibitors, and other agents used to lower lipid levels.
4. Compare and contrast the various drugs used to lower lipid levels.
5. Outline the nursing considerations, including important teaching points, for patients receiving drugs used to lower lipid levels.

Key Terms

antihyperlipidemic agents: general term used for drugs used to lower lipid levels in the blood

bile acids: cholesterol-containing acids found in the bile that act like detergents to break up fats in the small intestine

cholesterol: necessary component of human cells that is produced and processed in the liver and then stored in the bile until stimulus causes the gallbladder to contract and send the bile into the duodenum via the common bile duct; has a steroid nucleus made from fatty acids; essential for the formation of steroid hormones and cell membranes; produced in cells and obtained from dietary sources

chylomicron: carrier for lipids in the bloodstream, consisting of proteins, lipids, cholesterol, and other components

high-density lipoprotein (HDL): loosely packed chylomicron-containing fats, able to absorb fats and fat remnants in the periphery; thought to have a protective effect, decreasing the development of atherosclerotic cardiovascular disease

hydroxymethylglutaryl–coenzyme A (HMG–CoA) reductase: enzyme that regulates the last step in cellular cholesterol synthesis

hyperlipidemia: increased levels of lipids in the serum, associated with increased risk of development of atherosclerotic cardiovascular disease

low-density lipoprotein (LDL): tightly packed fats that are thought to contribute to the development of atherosclerotic cardiovascular disease when remnants left over from the LDL are processed in the arterial lining

metabolic syndrome: collection of factors, including insulin resistance, abdominal obesity, low high-density lipoprotein, high triglyceride levels, hypertension, and proinflammatory and prothrombotic states, that increase the incidence of atherosclerotic cardiovascular disease

phospholipids: type of fat with a phosphate group; important structure to make lipoproteins, blood-clotting components, the myelin sheath, and cell membranes

proprotein convertase subtilisin/kexin type 9 (PCSK9): an enzyme that binds to LDL receptor on liver cells, which causes higher LDL levels in the blood

triglycerides: type of lipid that is also called "neutral fat"; composed of fatty acids and a glycerol molecule; primarily used in the body as a source of energy

Drug List

LIPID-LOWERING AGENTS

Bile Acid Sequestrants

(P) cholestyramine
colesevelam
colestipol

HMG–CoA REDUCTASE INHIBITORS (STATINS)

(P) atorvastatin
fluvastatin
lovastatin
pitavastatin
pravastatin
rosuvastatin
simvastatin

CHOLESTEROL ABSORPTION INHIBITOR

(P) ezetimibe

PCSK9 INHIBITORS

alirocumab
(P) evolocumab

OTHER LIPID-LOWERING AGENTS

Fibrates
fenofibrate
fenofibric acid
gemfibrozil

VITAMIN B_3
niacin

OMEGA-3 FATTY ACIDS
icosapent ethyl
omega-3-acid ethyl esters
omega-3-carboxylic acids

OTHER
bempedoic acid
lomitapide

The drugs discussed in this chapter lower the serum levels of cholesterol and various lipids. These drugs are sometimes called **antihyperlipidemic agents** and are used to treat **hyperlipidemia**—an increase in the level of lipids in the blood. There is mounting evidence that the incidence of atherosclerotic cardiovascular disease (ASCVD), the leading killer of adults in the United States and worldwide, is higher among people with high serum lipid levels. The cause of ASCVD is poorly understood, but some evidence indicates that cholesterol and fat may play a major role in disease development. Lipid and triglyceride levels play a role in metabolic syndrome. **Metabolic syndrome** is a collection of factors including insulin resistance, abdominal obesity, low high-density lipoprotein (HDL), high triglyceride levels, hypertension, and proinflammatory and prothrombotic states. It has been shown to increase the incidence of ASCVD. See Table 47.1.

Atherosclerotic Cardiovascular Disease

As explained in Chapter 46, ASCVD is characterized by the progressive growth of atheromatous plaques, or atheromas, in the coronary arteries. These plaques, which begin as fatty streaks in the endothelium, eventually injure the endothelial lining of the artery, causing an inflammatory reaction. This inflammatory process triggers the development of characteristic foam cells containing fats and white blood cells that further injure the endothelial lining. Over time, platelets, fibrin, other fats, and remnants collect on the injured vessel lining and cause the atheroma to grow, further narrowing the interior of the blood vessel and limiting blood flow.

The injury to the vessel also causes scarring and a thickening of the vessel wall. As the vessel thickens, it becomes less distensible and less reactive to many neurological and chemical stimuli that would ordinarily dilate or constrict it. As a result, the coronary vessels are no longer able to balance the myocardial demand for oxygen with increased blood supply. More recent evidence indicates that the makeup of the core of the atheroma may be a primary determinant of which atheromas might rupture and cause acute blockage of a vessel. The softer, more lipid-filled atheromas appear to be more likely to rupture than the stable, harder cores.

It is important to note that the process of atherosclerosis and blood vessel injury is not isolated to the coronary arteries. This process can damage peripheral and cerebral arteries as well. It is this process that can increase a person's risk for ischemic stroke and peripheral artery disease.

Table 47.1 Clinical Aspects of Metabolic Syndrome

Parameter	Significant Values
Insulin resistance	Fasting blood sugar ≥100 mg/dL
Abdominal obesity	Waist measurement >40 in. in males; >35 in. in females
Lipid abnormalities	HDL < 40 mg/dL in males; <50 mg/dL in females; any triglyceride levels ≥150 mg/dL
Hypertension	Blood pressure ≥130/85 mm Hg
Proinflammatory state	Increased macrophages, increased levels of interleukin-6 and tumor necrosis factor
Prothrombotic state	Increased plasminogen activator levels

HDL, high-density lipoproteins.

Risk Factors

There is evidence that atheroma development occurs more quickly in patients with elevated cholesterol and lipid levels. Patients who consume diets high in saturated fats are more likely to develop high lipid levels. There is evidence that people eating plant-based diets have lower risk of cardiovascular disease and overall mortality. However, patients without increased lipid levels can also develop atheromas leading to ASCVD, so other factors contribute to this process. Although the exact mechanism of atherogenesis (atheroma development) is not understood, certain risk factors increase the likelihood that a person will develop ASCVD. Metabolic syndrome occurs when a patient has several risk factors: increased insulin resistance, high blood pressure, altered lipid levels, and a proinflammatory and prothrombotic state, all of which seem to increase the risk of ASCVD development dramatically. Unmodifiable and modifiable risk factors are presented in Box 47.1. Different racial and ethnic groups also have different risk factors, as discussed in Box 47.2, and risk factors also vary by sex, as discussed in Box 47.3.

BOX 47.1 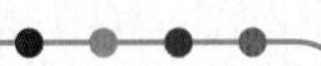

Risk Factors for Atherosclerotic Cardiovascular Disease

Unmodifiable Risk Factors

- *Genetic predispositions*: ASCVD is more likely to occur in people who have a family history of the disease, particularly if the disease occurs in relatives younger than the age of 55 years.
- *Age*: The incidence of ASCVD increases with age. After menopause, a person has a greater risk of ASCVD compared to before menopause.
- *Sex*: Males are more likely than premenopausal females to have ASCVD; however, the incidence is almost equal in males and postmenopausal females, possibly because of a protective effect of estrogens (see Box 47.3).

Modifiable Risk Factors

- *Gout*: Increased uric acid levels seem to injure vessel walls.
- *Cigarette smoking*: The risk of ischemic heart disease is about doubled when compared to a lifetime of not smoking; the risk is related to duration and amount of smoking. Cessation of smoking reduces risk immediately, but it may take 20 years or more to completely reverse the risk.
- *Sedentary lifestyle*: Exercise increases the levels of chemicals that seem to protect the coronary arteries.
- *Unhealthy diet:* Diets high in fat, processed sugar, and red meats tend to increase risk. Plant-based diets are best. Whole grains, fresh fruits, lean meats, and vegetables are thought to be parts of a healthy diet.
- *High stress levels*: Constant sympathetic reactions increase the myocardial oxygen demand while causing vasoconstriction and may contribute to a remodeling of the blood vessel endothelium, leading to increased susceptibility to atheroma development.
- *Hypertension*: High pressure in the arteries causes endothelial injury and increases afterload and myocardial oxygen demand.
- *High blood cholesterol levels:* Reduction in total cholesterol and LDL decreases risk of ASCVD.
- *Obesity*: This may reflect altered fat metabolism and will increase the heart's workload.
- *Diabetes*: Adults with diabetes are two to four times more likely to die from heart disease than adults without diabetes. The development of ASCVD can be delayed by managing blood sugar and other risk factors.
- *Other factors that if untreated may contribute to ASCVD* include bacterial infections (*Chlamydia* infections have been correlated with onset of ASCVD, and treatment with tetracycline and fluororoentgenography has been associated with decreased incidence of ASCVD, indicating a possible bacterial link) and autoimmune processes (some plaques contain antibodies and other products of immune reactions, making autoimmune reactions a possibility).

The American Heart Association and American College of Cardiology have published a calculator for estimating the 10-year risk of developing a first ASCVD event (nonfatal MI, death from coronary heart disease, or stroke). The following risk factors are included in the calculation: sex, age, race, total cholesterol, HDL, systolic blood pressure, treatment for elevated blood pressure, diabetes, and smoking. The ASCVD Risk Estimator Plus is found at https://tools.acc.org/ascvd-risk-estimator-plus/#!/calculate/estimate/. The 10-year risk for ASCVD is categorized as low risk (<5%), borderline risk (5% to 7.4%), intermediate risk (7.5% to 19.9%), and high risk (≥20%).

Box 47.2 Focus on Cultural Considerations

The American College of Cardiology/American Heart Association (ACC/AHA) guidelines discuss some important cultural considerations regarding cholesterol and risk of ASCVD in people of certain races and ethnicities. There is an increased risk of ASCVD in people of South Asian descent. People of East Asian descent may have increased sensitivity to statins. The authors of the guidelines also note that race, ethnicity, and country of origin, together with socioeconomic status and acculturation level, may be more prominent factors in explaining ASCVD risk more precisely among specific Latino ethnic and national identities compared to the broad category of Hispanic/Latino. The authors of the guidelines conclude this is due to evidence that Latino people of differing geographic locations demonstrate dissimilar risk of disease (e.g., ASCVD risk is higher among individuals from Puerto Rico than those from Mexico). High metabolic risk factors and increased risk of diabetes mellitus account for higher risk of ASCVD in Mexican Americans. In addition, Native Americans and Alaskan natives have higher rates of risk factors for ASCVD compared to non-Hispanic Whites.

Box 47.3 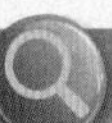 **Focus on Sex Differences**

HEART DISEASE IN FEMALE PATIENTS

Until the late 1990s, heart disease was considered to be a condition that primarily affected males. Because of that belief, females were seldom screened for heart disease, and when they did experience acute cardiac events, they were not treated promptly or adequately. However, recent research has shown that heart disease is the leading cause of death among females, surpassing such diseases as breast and colon cancers. This finding has led to further research, still ongoing, about the relationship between assigned sex and heart disease.

Females enjoy a protective hormone effect against the development of ASCVD until menopause, when estrogen loss seems to rapidly increase the production of atheromas and the development of ASCVD. In several studies, participants who received hormone replacement therapy (HRT) at menopause had a significantly reduced risk of ASCVD and MI in the first few years after the onset of menopause. Research showed, however, that after 5 years of HRT, the incidence of MI and stroke rose sharply, leading to an early closure of the study. Studies have found that female patients experience different symptoms of heart disease than males do, such as jaw and neck pain, fatigue, and insomnia, and that sometimes these symptoms are overlooked.

HRT is not recommended as a means of reducing the risk of heart disease or stroke, though it is still recommended for the treatment of severe menopausal symptoms in the first few years after menopause. Female patients should be advised to reduce other cardiac risk factors by eating a diet low in saturated fats; exercising regularly; not smoking; controlling weight; managing stress; and seeking treatment for gout, hypertension, and diabetes.

Clearly, heart disease is not just a disease affecting males. Research will continue to offer health care professionals new information on preventing and treating heart disease in females.

Treatment

Because an exact cause of ASCVD is not known, successful treatment involves manipulating a number of these risk factors (Table 47.2). Overall treatment and prevention of ASCVD should include decreasing saturated fats (decreasing total fat intake and limiting saturated fats seem to have the most impact on serum lipid levels); decreasing intake of processed foods and refined sugars; losing weight, which helps to decrease insulin resistance and risk of development of type 2 diabetes; eliminating smoking; increasing exercise levels; decreasing stress; and treating hypertension, diabetes, and gout.

Key Points

- ASCVD is the leading cause of death in the United States and worldwide. It is associated with the development of atheromas or plaques in the arterial linings that lead to narrowing of the lumen of the artery and hardening of the artery wall with loss of distensibility and responsiveness to stimuli for contraction or dilation.
- The cause of ASCVD is not completely understood, but many contributing risk factors have been identified, including increasing age, male sex, genetic predisposition, high-fat diet, sedentary lifestyle, smoking, obesity, high stress levels, bacterial infections, diabetes, hypertension, gout, and menopause. The presence of many of these factors constitutes metabolic syndrome.
- Treatment and prevention of ASCVD are aimed at manipulating the known risk factors to decrease development and progression of atherosclerosis.

Fats and Biotransformation (Metabolism)

Lipids, or fats, are primarily classified as triglycerides, phospholipids, and **cholesterol**. **Triglycerides** (also called "neutral fats") are made of three fatty acids and a glycerol molecule. They are primarily metabolized and used for energy. **Phospholipids** are made of fatty acids and have a phosphate group attached. They are structurally important for cell membranes, blood-clotting components, and the myelin sheath. Cholesterol has a steroid nucleus that is made of fatty acids and is an important substance for cell membranes and facilitating needed cellular functions.

Fats are taken into the body as dietary fats and then broken down in the stomach to fatty acids, lipids, and cholesterol (Fig. 47.1). The presence of these products in the duodenum stimulates contraction of the gallbladder and the release of bile. **Bile acids**, which contain high levels of cholesterol, act like a detergent in the small intestine and break up the fats into small units, called micelles, which can be absorbed into the wall of the small intestine. (Imagine dishwashing detergents breaking up the grease and fats in the dishwashing water; bile acids do much the same thing.) The bile acids are then reabsorbed and recycled to the gallbladder, where they remain until the gallbladder is again stimulated to release them to facilitate fat absorption.

Fats and water do not mix and cannot be absorbed directly into the plasma. To allow absorption, micelles are carried in a **chylomicron**, a package of fats and proteins. This packaging is done by brush enzymes in the wall of the small intestine. The chylomicrons pass through the wall of the small intestine, are picked up by the surrounding intestinal lymphatic system, travel through the system to the heart, and then are sent out into circulation. The proteins that are exposed on the chylomicron, called apoproteins,

Table 47.2 Risk Factors for Atherosclerotic Cardiovascular Disease

Unmodifiable Risks	Modifiable Risks	Suggested Modifications
Family history	Sedentary lifestyle	Exercise
Age	High-fat diet; diet high in processed food and/or refined sugar	Heart healthy diet includes fruits and vegetables, lean meats (if any), whole grains, low-fat dairy. Plant-based diets are best that are low in sodium and processed sugars
Sex	Smoking	Smoking cessation
	Obesity	Weight loss
	High stress levels	Stress management
	Bacterial infections	Antibiotic treatment
	Diabetes	Control of blood glucose levels
	Hypertension	Control of blood pressure
	Gout	Control of uric acid levels
	Hyperlipidemia	Take lipid-lowering agents as prescribed
Menopause		

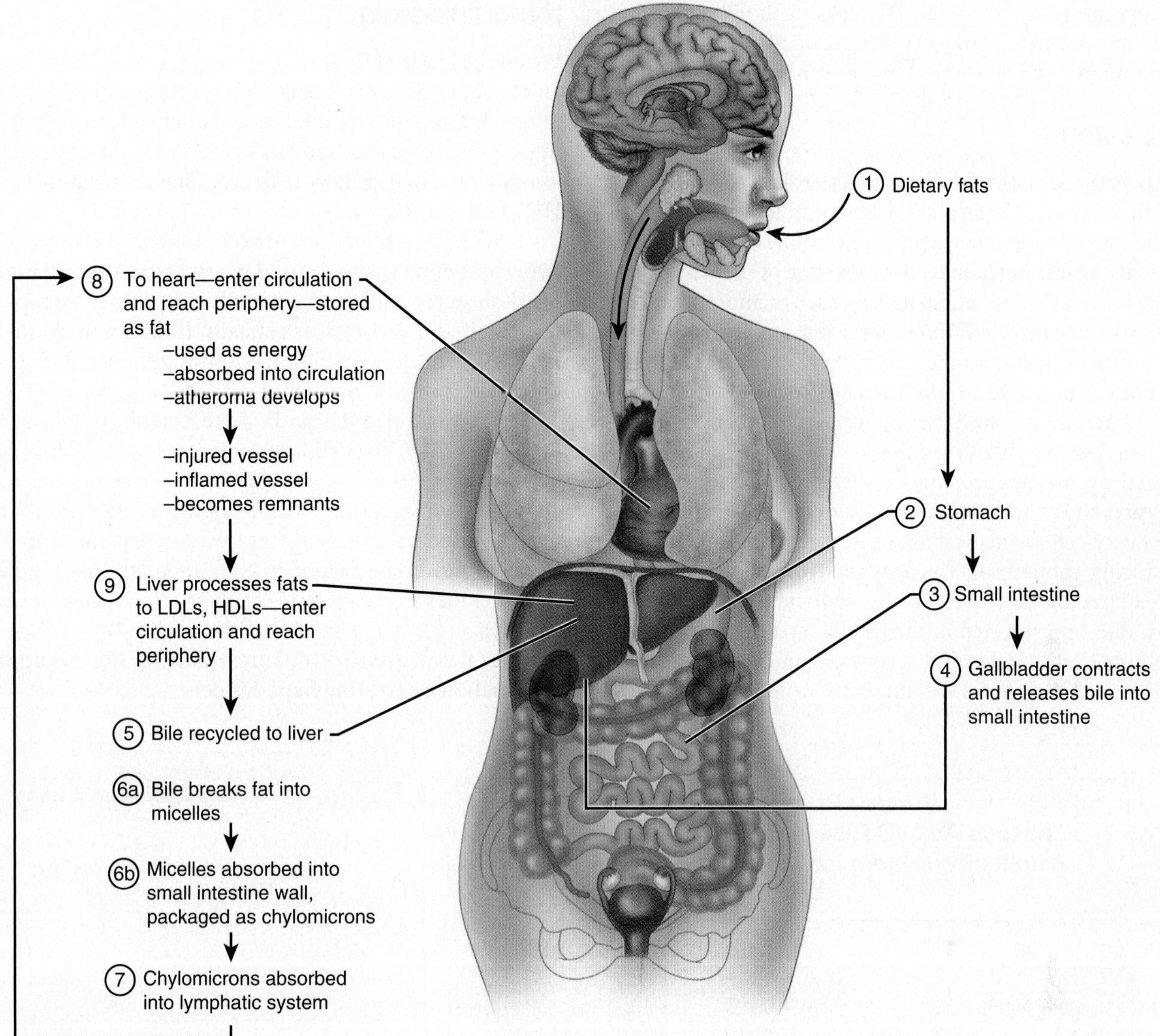

FIGURE 47.1 Metabolism of fats in the body.

determine the fate of the lipids or fats being carried. For example, some of these packages are broken down in the tissues to be used for energy, some are stored in fat deposits for future use as energy, and some continue to the liver, where they are further processed into lipoproteins.

Lipoproteins

There are five classifications of lipoproteins: chylomicrons, very-low-density, intermediate-density, low-density, and high-density. Chylomicrons are made in the small intestine wall. Other lipoproteins are produced in the liver. Very-low-density lipoproteins (VLDLs) have large amounts of triglycerides and low amounts of cholesterol. They carry triglycerides to fat and muscle cells. When the triglycerides are removed, the VLDLs become intermediate-density lipoprotein (IDL). These IDLs travel back to the liver to be converted back to VLDL or into **low-density lipoprotein (LDL)**. LDL is the main molecule that transports cholesterol. The LDL molecule can be taken up by cells (hepatic and others that may need the cholesterol) or can be scavenged by white blood cells in the plasma or arterial wall. It is thought that when macrophages engulf LDL into the arterial wall, the development of atherosclerosis is increased. **High-density lipoprotein (HDL)** transports cholesterol from the tissues to the liver, where the cholesterol can be made into bile and eliminated from the body via feces. HDL is thought to play a protective role against the development of atherosclerosis. It is known that HDL levels increase during exercise, which could explain why people who exercise regularly lower their risk of ASCVD. HDL levels also increase in response to estrogen, which could explain some of the protective effect of estrogen before menopause. A low HDL level is considered a risk for development of metabolic syndrome.

The liver cells have LDL receptors that can be used to decrease the LDL levels in the blood. The **proprotein convertase subtilisin/kexin type 9 (PCSK9)** enzyme binds to this LDL receptor and decreases the ability of the liver to process the LDL, so more LDL stays in the blood. It has been shown that higher expression of PCSK9 results in higher blood LDL levels and higher cardiovascular risk.

Cholesterol

The body needs fats, including cholesterol, to maintain normal function. Cholesterol is the base unit for the formation of the steroid hormones (the sex hormones, as well as the adrenal cortical hormones). It is also one of the basic units in the formation and maintenance of cell membranes. Cholesterol can be provided through the diet and the fat metabolism process just described. If dietary cholesterol falls off, the body is prepared to produce cholesterol to ensure that the cell membranes and the endocrine system are intact.

The liver is able to synthesize cholesterol that is circulated by the lipoproteins. A diet high in saturated fat increases the production of cholesterol in the liver.

Every cell in the body has the metabolic capability of producing cholesterol. The enzyme **hydroxymethylglutaryl–coenzyme A (HMG–CoA) reductase** regulates the early, rate-limiting step in the cellular synthesis of cholesterol. If dietary cholesterol is severely limited, the cellular synthesis of cholesterol will increase.

Hyperlipidemia

When the levels of lipids in the blood increase, hyperlipidemia occurs. This can result from excessive dietary intake of fats or from genetic alterations in fat metabolism, leading to a variety of elevated fats in the blood (e.g., hypercholesterolemia, hypertriglyceridemia, alterations in LDL and HDL concentrations).

Dietary modifications are often successful in treating hyperlipidemia that is caused by excessive dietary intake of cholesterol and/or saturated fats. Drug therapy is needed if the cause is genetically linked alterations in lipid levels or if dietary limits do not decrease the serum lipid levels to an acceptable range. Figures 47.2 and 47.3 give the current standard treatment guidelines for lipid levels. Antihyperlipidemic agents such as bile acid sequestrants, HMG–CoA inhibitors, fibrates, niacin, cholesterol absorption inhibitors, or PCSK9 inhibitors may be used. These drugs are often used in combination and should be part of an overall health care regimen that includes exercise, dietary restrictions, and lifestyle changes.

See the "Critical Thinking Scenario" for additional information on treating hyperlipidemia.

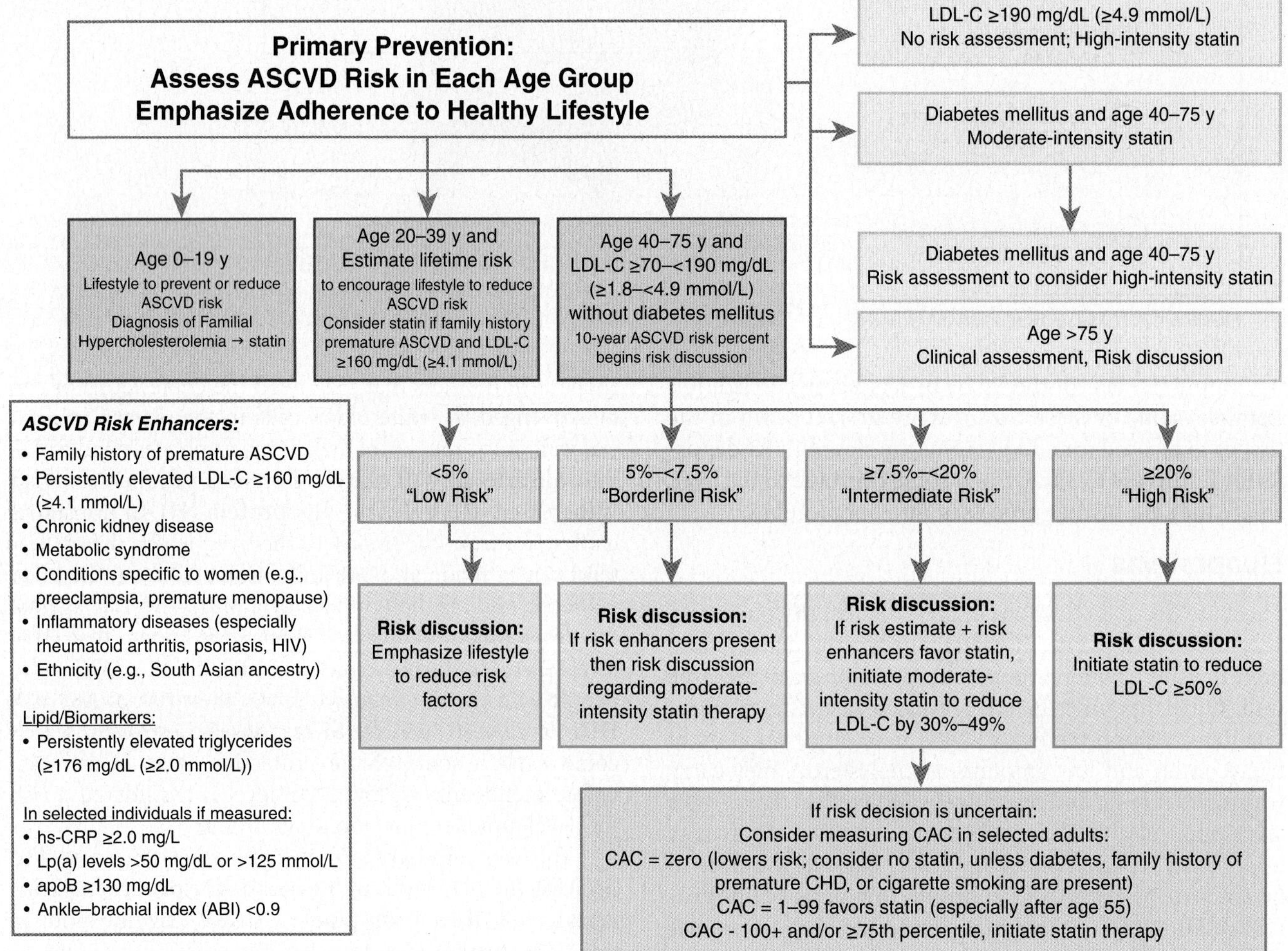

FIGURE 47.2 Primary prevention in patients with clinical ASCVD.

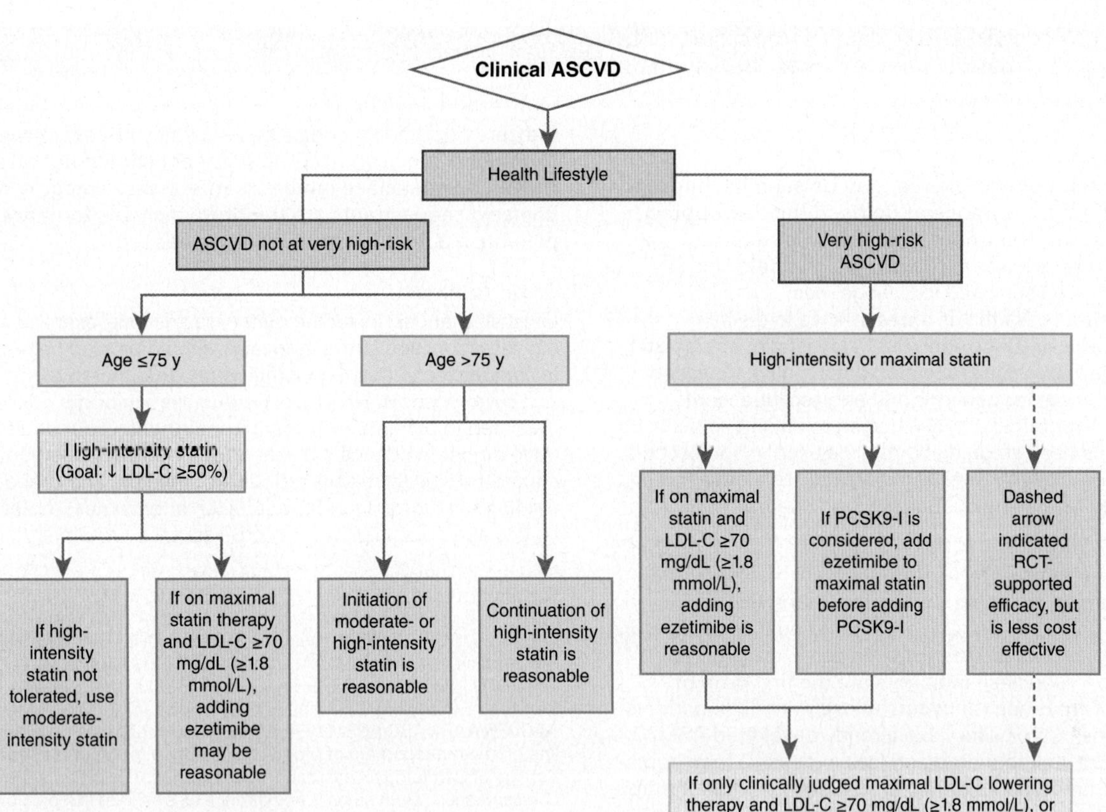

FIGURE 47.3 Secondary prevention in patients with clinical ASCVD.

Key Points

- ASCVD is associated with arterial atheromas or plaques, narrowed arterial lumens, and hardening of the artery wall, all of which lead to impaired contraction and vascular dilation.
- Risk factors for ASCVD include increasing age, male sex, genetic predisposition, high-fat diet, sedentary lifestyle, smoking, obesity, high stress levels, bacterial infections, diabetes, hypertension, gout, and menopause.
- ASCVD prevention and treatment aim at decreasing risk factors to delay disease or decrease its progress.
- Hyperlipidemia refers to an increase in the level of lipids (cholesterol and triglycerides) in the blood. Hyperlipidemia increases a person's risk for the development of ASCVD.
- Fats are taken into the body as dietary fats and then broken down in the stomach to fatty acids, lipids, and cholesterol.
- Bile acids act like detergents to break down or metabolize fats into small molecules called micelles, which are absorbed into the intestinal wall and combined with proteins to become chylomicrons to allow transport throughout the circulatory system.
- Cholesterol is a lipid that is used to make bile acids. The liver and other cells can produce cholesterol, which is the base for steroid hormones and cell membrane structure.
- The enzyme HMG–CoA reductase controls the early rate-limiting step in the production of cellular cholesterol; HMG–CoA is active in every cell.

Lipid-Lowering Agents

Lipid-lowering agents lower the serum levels of cholesterol and various lipids. These include bile acid sequestrants, HMG–CoA reductase inhibitors, a cholesterol absorption inhibitor, and PCSK9 inhibitors. Other drugs that are used to affect lipid levels do not fall into any of the classes but are also approved for use in combination to lower lipid levels with changes in diet and exercise (see "Other Lipid-Lowering Agents"). Box 47.4 summarizes the use of lipid-lowering agents in different age groups.

Bile Acid Sequestrants

Bile acid sequestrants are used to decrease plasma cholesterol levels. Three bile acid sequestrants currently in use are cholestyramine (*Prevalite*), colestipol (*Colestid*), and colesevelam (*Welchol*).

Box 47.4 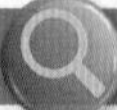 Focus on Drug Therapy Across the Lifespan

LIPID-LOWERING AGENTS

Children

Familial hypercholesterolemia may be seen in children. Because of the importance of lipids in the developing nervous system, treatment is usually restricted to tight dietary restrictions to limit fats and calories.

Fibrates have been used to treat genetic hypercholesterolemia that is unresponsive to dietary restrictions. The HMG–CoA inhibitors lovastatin, pravastatin, rosuvastatin, simvastatin, and atorvastatin have indicated doses appropriate for pediatric and adolescent patients being treated for familial hypercholesterolemia. Evolocumab (*Repatha*) has been studied and may be used in adolescents 13 to 17 years old with familial hypercholesterolemia but is not indicated for patients younger than 13 years.

Adults

Lifestyle changes, including dietary restrictions, exercise, smoking cessation, and stress reduction, should be tried before or in conjunction with any antihyperlipidemic drug therapy.

HMG–CoA reductase inhibitors are the first drug of choice in the treatment of hypercholesterolemia in patients who are at risk for or who have already developed ASCVD. The drugs are well tolerated and less expensive than some of the other antihyperlipidemic drugs. Combination therapy with ezetimibe is recommended first if lipid levels are still high. PCSK9 inhibitors can also be used with the statins, but they are not the first choice because they are expensive.

Patients who can become pregnant should not take HMG–CoA reductase inhibitors (pregnancy category X). Bile acid sequestrants are the drug of choice for these patients if a lipid-lowering agent is needed.

Older Adults

Lifestyle changes, including dietary restrictions, exercise, smoking cessation, and stress reduction, should be tried before and in conjunction with antihyperlipidemic drug therapy.

Lower doses of HMG–CoA reductase inhibitors are often indicated in patients with renal impairment. Older adults have higher incidence of renal impairment, so renal function should be closely monitored. Risk of myalgia and rhabdomyolysis is higher in older adults. Liver enzymes, cholesterol levels, and muscle pain should be assessed routinely.

Figures reprinted with permission from Grundy, S. M., Stone, N. J., Bailey, A. L., Beam, C., Birtcher, K. K., Blumenthal, R. S., Braun, L.T., deFerranti, S., Fajella-Tommasino, J., Forman, D. E., Goldberg, R., Heidenreich, P. A., Hlatky, M. A., Jones, D. W., Lloyd-Jones, D., Lopez-Pajares, N., Ndumele, C. E., Orringer, C. E., Peralta, C. A., Saseen, J. J., Smith, S. C., Sperling, L., Virani, S. S., & Yeboah, J. (2018). AHA/ACC/AACVPR/AAPA/ABC/ACPM/ADA/AGS/APhA/ASPC/NLA/PCNA guideline on the management of blood cholesterol: a report of the American College of Cardiology/American Heart Association Task Force on Clinical Practice Guidelines. *Circulation*, 139, e1082–e1143. pii: S0735-1097(18)39033-8. https://doi.org/10.1161/CIR.0000000000000625

Therapeutic Actions and Indications

Bile acid sequestrants bind with bile acids in the intestine to form an insoluble complex that is then excreted in the feces (Fig. 47.4). Bile acids contain high levels of cholesterol. As a result of the increased bile elimination, the liver must use cholesterol to make more bile acids. The hepatic intracellular cholesterol level falls, leading to increased absorption of cholesterol-containing LDL segments from circulation to replenish the cell's cholesterol. The serum levels of cholesterol and LDL decrease as the circulating cholesterol is used to provide the cholesterol that the liver needs to make bile acids. These drugs are used to reduce serum cholesterol in patients with primary hypercholesterolemia (manifested by high cholesterol and high LDLs) as an adjunct to diet and exercise. Cholestyramine is also used to treat pruritus associated with partial biliary obstruction. See Table 47.3 for the usual indications for each of these drugs.

Pharmacokinetics

Bile acid sequestrants are not absorbed systemically. They act while in the intestine and are excreted directly in the feces. Their action is limited to their effects while they are present in the intestine. Cholestyramine is a powder that must be mixed with liquids and is usually administered once or twice a day but can be taken up to six times a day. Colestipol is available in both powder and tablet form and is taken only four times a day. Colesevelam is available in tablet form and is taken once or twice a day.

Contraindications and Cautions

Bile acid sequestrants are contraindicated in the presence of allergy to any bile acid sequestrant to prevent hypersensitivity reactions. These drugs are also contraindicated with complete biliary obstruction, which would prevent bile from being secreted into the intestine, and with abnormal intestinal function, which could be aggravated by the presence of these drugs. Caution should be taken administering these drugs to patients who are pregnant or lactating because the potential decrease in the absorption of fat and fat-soluble vitamins could have a detrimental effect on the fetus or neonate. However, if a lipid-lowering drug is needed for a pregnant patient, a bile acid sequestrant is probably the least risky choice.

Adverse Effects

Adverse effects associated with the use of these drugs include headache, anxiety, fatigue, and drowsiness, which could be related to changes in serum cholesterol levels. Direct GI irritation, including nausea, constipation that may progress to fecal impaction, and aggravation of hemorrhoids, may occur. Other effects include increased bleeding time related to decreased absorption of vitamin K and consequent decreased production of clotting factors, vitamin A and D deficiencies related to decreased absorption of fat-soluble vitamins, rash, and muscle aches and pains.

Clinically Important Drug–Drug Interactions

Malabsorption of fat-soluble vitamins occurs when they are combined with these drugs. These drugs decrease or

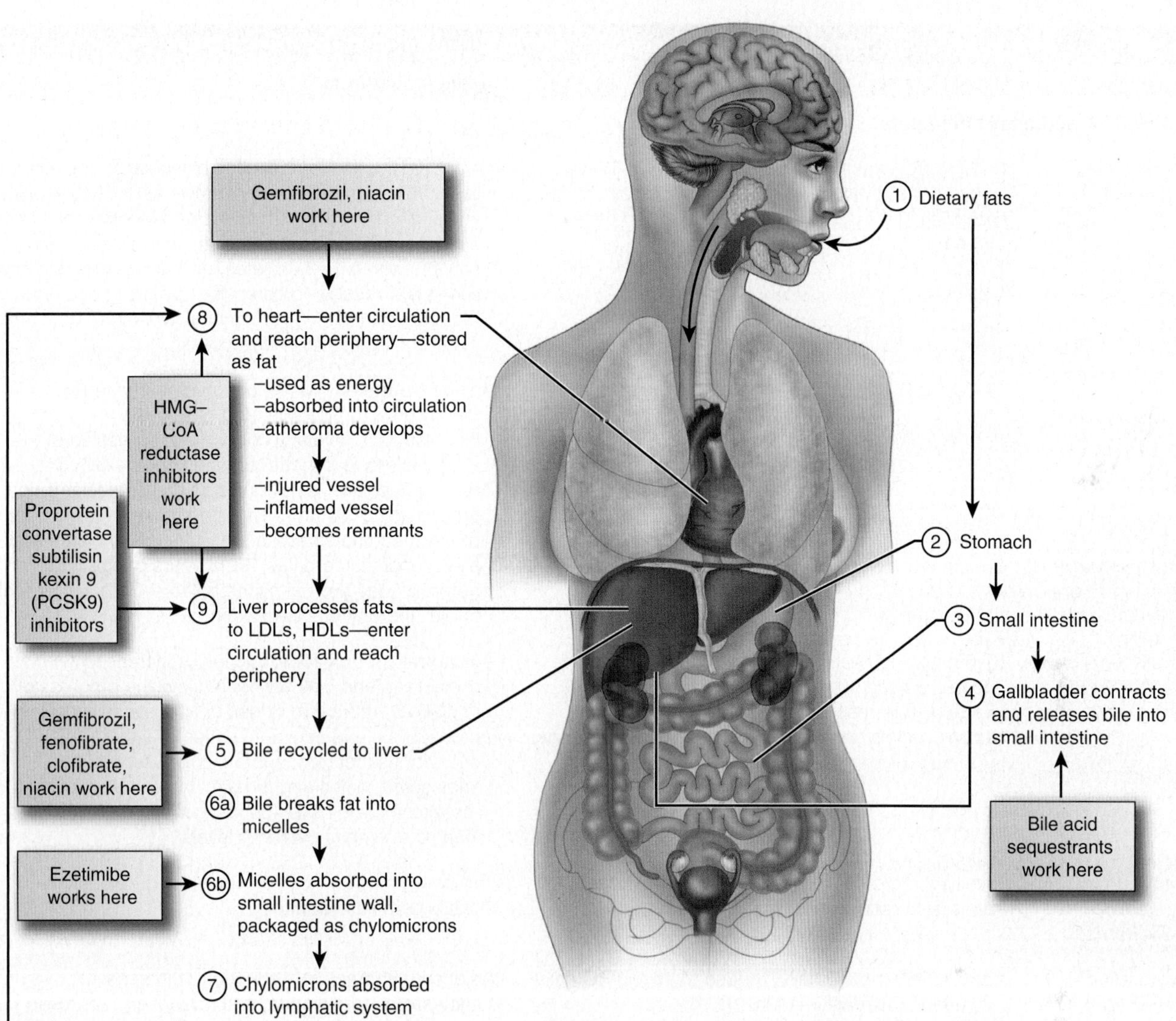

FIGURE 47.4 Sites of action of lipid-lowering agents.

Table 47.3 *Drugs in Focus:* Lipid-Lowering Drugs

Drug Name	Usual Dosage	Usual Indications
Bile Acid Sequestrants		
cholestyramine (*Prevalite*)	4 g PO one to two times per day, maximum dose of 24 g/d; must be mixed with water or other noncarbonated fluid	Adjunctive treatment of primary hypercholesterolemia that has not responded to dietary modifications; treatment of pruritus associated with partial biliary obstruction
colesevelam (*Welchol*)	625-mg tablets taken twice a day with meals or six tablets taken once daily with a meal; or 3.75-g packet once a day with meal	Adjunctive treatment with diet and exercise to reduce LDL in adults; reduction of LDL in pediatric patients with heterozygous familial hypercholesterolemia; improvement of glycemic control in adults with type 2 diabetes mellitus
colestipol (*Colestid*)	*Granule form*: 5–30 g/d PO; may be taken in divided doses; must be mixed in water or other liquid *Tablet form*: 2–16 g/d PO taken once or in divided doses; tablets must not be cut, crushed, or chewed	Adjunctive treatment of primary hypercholesterolemia

(continues on page 836)

Table 47.3 *Drugs in Focus*: Lipid-Lowering Drugs (*Continued*)

Drug Name	Usual Dosage	Usual Indications
HMG–CoA Reductase Inhibitors		
atorvastatin (*Lipitor*)	10 mg/d PO with a possible dose range of 10–80 mg/d; may be taken at any time of the day *Pediatric (10–17 y)*: 10 mg/d PO, maximum dose of 20 mg/d	Adjunctive therapy for reduction of increased cholesterol and LDL levels, triglycerides; prevention of MI, stroke, and angina in adults with multiple risk factors for heart disease, with patients with heart disease, and in patients with type 2 diabetes mellitus; approved to lower cholesterol levels in children 10–17 years of age who meet specific criteria with familial hypercholesterolemia if trial of diet therapy is unsuccessful
fluvastatin (*Lescol XL*)	20–80 mg PO daily	Adjunctive therapy for reduction of increased cholesterol, triglyceride, and LDL levels and to increase HDL levels; to slow the progression of atherosclerosis in patients with known ASCVD; reduction of the risk of undergoing revascularization procedures in patients with heart disease; reduction of elevated cholesterol and LDL levels in males and postmenarchal females 10–16 years of age with heterozygous familial hypercholesterolemia after trial of diet therapy is unsuccessful
lovastatin (*Altoprev*)	20–60 mg/d PO daily; maximum dose of 80 mg/d; do not exceed 20 mg/d if patient is taking immunosuppressives or has renal impairment *Pediatric males, females 1 y postmenarche:* 20 mg/d PO, may increase to 80 mg/d	Adjunctive therapy for reduction of increased cholesterol and LDL levels; to slow the progression of ASCVD; reduction of risk of MI, revascularization procedures, and angina in patients without ASCVD but with risk factors; approved for use with adolescent males and females (at least 1 year past menarche) who have specific genetic disorders leading to high cholesterol levels
pitavastatin (*Livalo, Zypitamag*)	Initially, 2 mg/d PO, range of 1–4 mg/d PO; reduce dose with renal impairment	Treatment of primary hyperlipidemia or mixed dyslipidemias in adults
pravastatin (*Pravachol*)	*Adult:* 40–80 mg PO daily; reduce to 10 mg PO daily if patient has renal impairment *Pediatric (8–13 y)*: 20 mg/d PO *Pediatric (14–18 y)*: 40 mg/d PO	Adjunctive therapy for reduction of increased cholesterol, triglyceride, and LDL levels; approved for use with children >8 years of age with genetically linked hyperlipidemia, as an adjunct to diet and exercise; reduction of risk of MI, revascularization, and cardiovascular mortality in hypercholesterolemic patients without clinically evident CHD; reduction of risk of total mortality by reducing coronary death, MI, revascularization, stroke/TIA, and the progression of coronary atherosclerosis in patients with clinically evident CHD; treatment of primary dysbetalipoproteinemia not responding to diet
rosuvastatin (*Ezallor Sprinkle, Crestor*)	*Adult:* Initial dose 20 mg/d PO; range 5–40 mg/d PO *Pediatric (8–9 years):* 5–10 mg/d PO *Pediatric (10–17 years):* 5–20 mg/d PO *Pediatric (7–17 years) with homozygous familial hypercholesterolemia:* 20 mg/d PO	Adjunctive therapy for reduction of increased cholesterol, triglycerides, and LDL levels and to increase HDL levels; adjunctive therapy with diet to slow the progression of atherosclerosis; reduction of risk of MI, stroke, and arterial revascularization procedures in patients without evident ASCVD but multiple risk factors; reduction of cholesterol in pediatric patients with heterozygous or homozygous familial hypercholesterolemia after trial of diet therapy is unsuccessful
simvastatin (*Flolipid, Zocor*)	5–40 mg/d PO taken once a day in the evening; start with 5 mg/d in older patients and in patients with hepatic or renal impairment *Pediatric (10–17 y)*: 10 mg/d PO, up to 40 mg/d based on response	Adjunctive therapy for reduction of increased cholesterol, triglycerides, and LDL levels and to increase HDL levels; approved to lower cholesterol levels in children 10–17 years of age with heterozygous familial hypercholesterolemia; reduction of risk of total mortality by reducing risk of CHD death; reduction of risk of nonfatal MI, stroke, and the need for revascularization procedures in patients at high risk of coronary events

Table 47.3 *Drugs in Focus*: Lipid-Lowering Drugs (*Continued*)

Drug Name	Usual Dosage	Usual Indications
Cholesterol Absorption Inhibitor		
ezetimibe (*Zetia*)	10 mg/d PO with or without food	Adjunct to diet and exercise to reduce cholesterol as monotherapy or combined with an HMG–CoA inhibitor, fenofibrate, or a bile acid sequestrant; adjunct to diet to reduce elevated sitosterol and campesterol levels in homozygous sitosterolemia (to reduce elevated sitosterol and campesterol levels, the enzymes that are elevated when patients have this rare disorder); used in combination with atorvastatin or simvastatin as treatment for homozygous familial hypercholesterolemia
PCSK9 Inhibitors		
alirocumab (*Praluent*)	75 mg or 150 mg SQ every 2 wk; or 300 mg SQ every 4 wk	Reduction of risk of MI, stroke, and unstable angina requiring hospitalization in adults with established cardiovascular disease; adjunct to diet, alone or in combination with other therapies to lower LDL, in adults with primary hyperlipidemia; adjunct to other therapies to lower LDL in adult patients with homozygous familial hypercholesterolemia (HoFH) to reduce LDL
evolocumab (*Repatha*)	140 mg SQ every 2 wk or 420 mg SQ once monthly injected in the abdomen, thigh, or upper arm; to administer 420 mg, give three injections consecutively within 30 min	Reduction of risk of MI, stroke, and coronary revascularization in adults with cardiovascular disease; adjunct to diet, alone or in combination with other therapies to lower LDL, in adults with primary hyperlipidemia; adjunct to other therapies to lower LDL in patients with homozygous familial hypercholesterolemia (HoFH) to reduce LDL
Other Lipid-Lowering Agents ***Fibrates***		
fenofibrate (*Antara, Fenoglide, Lipofen, Tricor, Triglide*)	Dosing varies per formulation; reduce dose if patient has renal impairment	Adjunctive therapy to diet to reduce triglycerides; therapy to reduce elevated cholesterol and triglycerides and increase HDL in patients with primary hypercholesterolemia or mixed dyslipidemia
fenofibric acid (*Trilipix*)	45–135 mg/d PO; reduce dose if patient has renal impairment	Adjunctive therapy to diet to reduce triglycerides; therapy to reduce elevated cholesterol and triglycerides and increase HDL in patients with primary hypercholesterolemia or mixed dyslipidemia
gemfibrozil (*Lopid*)	1,200 mg/d PO divided into two doses and taken before the morning and evening meals	Treatment of high triglyceride levels in adults with risk of pancreatitis that has not responded to dietary effort; reduction of risk of developing coronary heart disease only in type 2b patients without history of or symptoms of existing coronary heart disease who have had an inadequate response to weight loss, dietary therapy, exercise, and other pharmacologic agents and who have the following triad of lipid abnormalities: low HDL, elevated LDL, elevated triglycerides
Vitamin B_3		
niacin (*Niacor, Niaspan*)	1.5–2 g/d PO in divided doses for tablets; 500–2,000 mg/d PO for ER tablets taken at bedtime	Treatment of hyperlipidemia not responding to diet and weight loss; to slow progression of ASCVD when combined with a bile acid sequestrant; reduction of risk of recurrent nonfatal MI in patients with a history of MI and hyperlipidemia

(continues on page 838)

Table 47.3 *Drugs in Focus*: Lipid-Lowering Drugs (*Continued*)

Drug Name	Usual Dosage	Usual Indications
Omega-3 Fatty Acids		
icosapent ethyl (*Vascepa*)	4 g/d PO	Adjunct to statin therapy to reduce the risk of MI, stroke, coronary revascularization, and unstable angina requiring hospitalization in adult patients with elevated triglycerides (≥150 mg/dL) and either established cardiovascular disease or diabetes mellitus and 2 or more additional risk factors for cardiovascular disease; adjunct to diet to reduce triglycerides in adult patients with severe (≥500 mg/dL) hypertriglyceridemia
omega-3-acid ethyl esters (*Lovaza*)	4 g/d PO	Adjunct to diet to reduce high triglycerides
Other		
bempedoic acid (*Nexletol*)	180 mg/d PO with or without food	Adjunct to diet and statin therapy for the treatment of adults with heterozygous familial hypercholesterolemia or established atherosclerotic cardiovascular disease who require additional lowering of LDL
lomitapide (*Juxtapid*)	Initially 5 mg/d PO; may be slowly titrated up to max dose of 60 mg/d PO; take with water (not food) at least 2 hours after evening meal	Adjunct to a low-fat diet and other lipid-lowering treatments, including LDL apheresis, to reduce cholesterol in patients with homozygous familial hypercholesterolemia

LDL, low-density lipoproteins; HMG–CoA, hydroxymethylglutaryl–coenzyme A; ASCVD, atherosclerotic cardiovascular disease; MI, myocardial infarction; HDL, high-density lipoproteins; ER, extended release; PCSK9, proprotein convertase subtilisin/kexin type 9.

delay the absorption of thiazide diuretics, digoxin, warfarin, thyroid hormones, hormonal contraceptives, and corticosteroids. Consequently, any of these drugs should be taken 1 hour before or 4 to 6 hours after the bile acid sequestrant. Contraceptive methods other than oral medications should be used to prevent pregnancy. If a person is pregnant and taking a bile acid sequestrant, extra fat-soluble vitamins may be indicated.

Prototype Summary: Cholestyramine

Indications: Reduction of elevated serum cholesterol in patients with primary hypercholesterolemia, pruritus associated with partial biliary obstruction.

Actions: Binds with bile acids in the intestine, allowing excretion in the feces instead of reabsorption, causing cholesterol to be oxidized in the liver and serum cholesterol levels to fall.

Pharmacokinetics: Not absorbed systemically.

$T_{1/2}$: Not absorbed systemically, excreted in the feces.

Adverse Effects: Rash, headache, anxiety, vertigo, dizziness, constipation due to fecal impaction, exacerbation of hemorrhoids, cramps, flatulence, nausea, increased bleeding tendencies, vitamin A and D deficiencies, and muscle and joint pain.

Nursing Considerations for Patients Receiving Bile Acid Sequestrants

Assessment: History and Examination

- Assess for contraindications or cautions: known allergies to these drugs to avoid hypersensitivity reactions; impaired intestinal function, which could be exacerbated by these drugs; biliary obstruction, which could block the effectiveness of these drugs; and current status related to pregnancy and lactation because of the potential for adverse effects on the fetus or nursing baby.
- Perform a physical assessment to establish a baseline before beginning therapy and during therapy to determine the effectiveness of therapy and evaluate for any potential adverse effects.
- Weigh the patient to establish a baseline and evaluate for changes reflecting lifestyle changes that accompany drug therapy.
- Inspect the patient's skin for color, bruising, and rash to evaluate for possible adverse effects.
- Assess neurological status, including level of orientation and alertness, to determine any CNS effects.
- Inspect the abdomen for distention and auscultate bowel sounds for changes in GI motility.

- Assess bowel elimination patterns, including frequency of stool passage and stool characteristics, to identify possible constipation and fecal impaction.
- Monitor the results of laboratory tests, including serum cholesterol and lipid levels, to evaluate the effectiveness of drug therapy.

Nursing Conclusions

Nursing conclusions related to drug therapy might include the following:

- Impaired comfort related to headache and GI effects
- Constipation risk related to GI effects
- Injury risk related to CNS changes and potential for bleeding
- Knowledge deficit regarding drug therapy

Planning

- The patient will receive the best therapeutic effect from the drug therapy.
- The patient will have limited adverse effects from the drug therapy.
- The patient will have an understanding of the drug therapy, adverse effects to anticipate, and measures to relieve discomfort and improve safety.

Intervention With Rationale

- Do not administer powdered agents in dry form; these drugs must be mixed in fluids to be effective. Mix with fruit juices, soups, liquids, cereals, or pulpy fruits. Mix colestipol, but not cholestyramine, with carbonated beverages. Stir, and encourage the patient to swallow all of the dose.
- If the patient is taking tablets, ensure that tablets are not cut, chewed, or crushed because they are designed to be broken down in the GI tract; if they are crushed, the active ingredients will not be effective. Urge the patient to swallow tablets whole with plenty of fluid.
- Give the drug before meals to ensure that the drug is in the GI tract with food.
- Administer other oral medications 1 hour before or 4 to 6 hours after the bile sequestrant to avoid drug–drug interactions.
- Arrange for a bowel program as appropriate to effectively deal with constipation if it occurs.
- Provide comfort measures to help the patient tolerate the drug effects. These include small, frequent meals to reduce the risk of nausea; adequate hydration and increased dietary fiber to prevent constipation; safety precautions to prevent injury if bleeding occurs due to decreased vitamin K absorption; replacement of fat-soluble vitamins; and skin care as needed.
- Offer support and encouragement to help the patient deal with the diagnosis and the drug regimen and lifestyle changes that may be necessary.
- Provide thorough patient teaching, including the name of the drug, dosage prescribed, and schedule for administration; method to administer the drug, such as mixing the powder form in fluids or taking tablets whole (without crushing, chewing, or cutting); appropriate fluids for mixing the drug; measures to avoid adverse effects, warning signs of problems, and the need for follow-up laboratory testing to monitor cholesterol and lipid levels; dietary and lifestyle changes for risk reduction; and monitoring and evaluation to enhance patient knowledge about drug therapy and to promote adherence.

Evaluation

- Monitor patient response to the drug as appropriate (reduction in serum cholesterol levels).
- Monitor for adverse effects (headache, vitamin deficiency, increased bleeding times, constipation, nausea, rash).
- Evaluate the effectiveness of the teaching plan (patient can name drug, dosage, adverse effects to watch for, and specific measures to avoid them; patient understands the importance of continued follow-up).
- Monitor the effectiveness of comfort measures and adherence to the regimen.

Key Points

- Bile acid sequestrants prevent the reabsorption of bile salts, which are high in cholesterol. Consequently, the liver will pull cholesterol from the blood to make new bile acids, lowering the serum cholesterol level.
- Patients receiving bile acid sequestrants need to learn how to mix the powders or, if taking the tablet form, the importance of swallowing the tablet whole and not cutting, crushing, or chewing it. Doses should not be taken with other drugs to avoid problems with absorption.
- GI problems, including nausea, bloating, and constipation, are often reported when using bile acid sequestrants.

HMG–CoA Reductase Inhibitors (Statins)

The HMG–CoA reductase inhibitors include atorvastatin (*Lipitor*), fluvastatin (*Lescol XL*), lovastatin (*Altoprev*), pitavastatin (*Livalo, Zypitamag*), pravastatin (*Pravachol*), rosuvastatin (*Ezallor Sprinkle, Crestor*), and simvastatin (*Flolipid, Zocor*).

Therapeutic Actions and Indications

The early rate-limiting step in the synthesis of cellular cholesterol involves the enzyme HMG–CoA reductase. If this enzyme is blocked, serum cholesterol and

LDL levels decrease because more LDLs are absorbed by the cells for processing into cholesterol. In contrast, HDL levels increase slightly with this alteration in fat metabolism. HMG–CoA reductase inhibitors block HMG–CoA reductase from completing the synthesis of cholesterol (see Fig. 47.4). Most of these drugs are chemical modifications of compounds produced by fungi. As a group, they are frequently referred to as "statins." Because these drugs undergo a marked first-pass effect in the liver, most of their effects are seen in the liver (see "Adverse Effects"). These drugs may also have some protective cardiovascular effects on the blood vessels to inhibit the process that generates atheromas in vessel walls. This may be due to an antiinflammatory effect on the blood vessel wall. These drugs are indicated as adjuncts with diet and exercise for the treatment of increased cholesterol, triglyceride, and LDL levels that are unresponsive to dietary restrictions alone.

Many of the statins are indicated to slow progression of ASCVD in patients known to have the disease. The statins are also used to assist with prevention of MI, stroke, and revascularization procedures in patients without known disease but who have multiple ASCVD risk factors. The statin medications are categorized as high-, moderate-, and low-intensity statins based on the exact medication and the dose. When dosed appropriately, atorvastatin and rosuvastatin are currently the only high-intensity statin medications. Table 47.3 discusses usual indications for each of the HMG–CoA reductase inhibitors. Several of the statin drugs have been formulated as combination therapies. Examples of combination therapies are highlighted in Box 47.5.

BOX 47.5

Combination and Other Therapies for Treating Atherosclerotic Cardiovascular Disease

- *Caduet* is a combination of amlodipine and atorvastatin. This medication is indicated for patients who have hypertension and also need treatment with a statin. The combination provides the blood pressure–lowering and antianginal effect of the amlodipine with the lipid-lowering effects of the atorvastatin. The dosing of *Caduet* is based on the patient's response. Blood pressure, angina, and hyperlipidemia should be monitored as doses are titrated.
- *Vytorin* is a combination of ezetimibe and simvastatin that was approved to help lower lipid levels in patients who did not have good results with single-drug therapy. Ezetimibe decreases the absorption of cholesterol, and simvastatin decreases the body's production of cholesterol. The dose should be determined based on lipid levels. There is increased risk of myopathy and rhabdomyolysis with the 10/80 mg dose, so careful monitoring is recommended if this dose is prescribed.
- *Roszet* is a combination of rosuvastatin and ezetimibe. It is indicated for adults as an adjunct to diet for treatment of nonfamilial hyperlipidemia and for patients with homozygous familial hypercholesterolemia. The dose is determined by lipid levels, and a lower dose is indicated in patients who have renal impairment and are not on hemodialysis. *Nexlizet* is a combination of bempedoic acid and ezetimibe. It is indicated as an adjunct to diet and maximally tolerated statin therapy to treat adults with heterozygous familial hypercholesterolemia or established atherosclerotic cardiovascular disease who require additional lowering of LDL. Bempedoic acid works to lower LDL by inhibiting cholesterol synthesis in the liver. This medication may cause an elevation of uric acid, so levels should be monitored regularly. There is a correlation with risk of tendon rupture, so caution should be taken when administering to patients with history of tendon disorders.

Pharmacokinetics

The statins are all absorbed from the GI tract and undergo first-pass metabolism in the liver. They are excreted through the feces and urine. The peak effect of these drugs is usually seen within 2 to 4 weeks. Some of these medications can be taken daily at any time of the day, with or without food. These drugs cross the placenta, and most have been found in human milk.

Contraindications and Cautions

These drugs are contraindicated in the presence of allergy to any of the statins or to fungal byproducts or compounds to avoid hypersensitivity reactions. Statins also are contraindicated in patients with acute liver disease and are used with caution with patients with history of or current chronic liver impairment, due to risk of exacerbation leading to severe liver failure, and with pregnancy or lactation, because of the potential for adverse effects on the fetus or neonate.

Atorvastatin levels are not affected by renal disease, but patients with renal impairment who are taking other statins require close monitoring and reduced doses since rhabdomyolysis, a potential adverse effect associated with these drugs, can be harmful to the kidneys. Caution should be used in patients with impaired endocrine function because of the potential alteration in the formation of steroid hormones.

Adverse Effects

The most common adverse effects associated with these drugs reflect their effects on the GI system: flatulence, abdominal pain, cramps, nausea, vomiting, and constipation. CNS effects can include headache, dizziness, blurred vision, insomnia, and fatigue. Increased concentrations of liver enzymes commonly occur, and the patient must

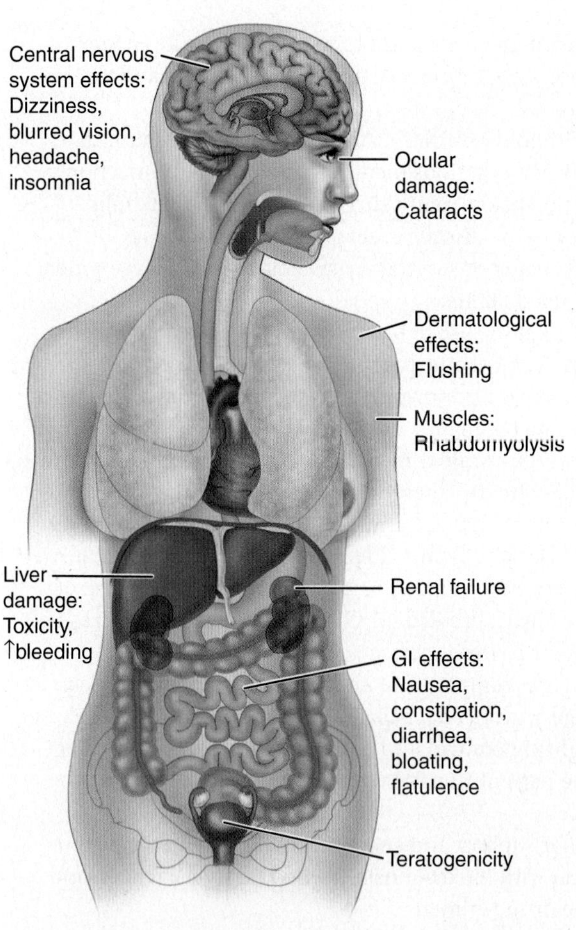

FIGURE 47.5 Variety of adverse effects and toxicities associated with lipid-lowering drugs.

be monitored for hepatotoxicity (Fig. 47.5). Myopathy is a common side effect. Rhabdomyolysis, a breakdown of muscles with waste products that can injure the glomerulus and cause acute renal failure, is not common but is a serious complication of which nurses should be aware. There is increased risk of rhabdomyolysis in older patients, those with low body weight, and those with hypothyroidism.

Clinically Important Drug–Drug Interactions

Medications that suppress CYP3A4 (erythromycin, ketoconazole, HIV protease inhibitors, cyclosporine, and others), fibrates, and ezetimibe can increase levels of statins in the serum and may increase risk of myopathy and liver impairment. If they are used concurrently, monitor the patient carefully. There are multiple medication interactions known with the statins, so nurses are recommended to check for medication interactions for all patients taking a statin.

Serum levels and the risk of toxicity increase if these drugs are combined with grapefruit juice (Box 47.6).

Box 47.6 Focus on Safe Medication Administration

Patients who are taking HMG–CoA inhibitors need to be cautioned to avoid drinking grapefruit juice while taking these drugs. Grapefruit juice alters the metabolism of the drugs, leading to an increased serum level of the drug and increased risk for adverse effects, such as the potentially fatal rhabdomyolysis with renal failure. The metabolism of the components of grapefruit juice takes about 48 hours. Since the effects may last for several days, simply drinking the grapefruit juice at a different time of the day does not protect the patient from risk.

Prototype Summary: Atorvastatin

Indications: Adjunctive therapy for reduction of increased cholesterol, triglyceride, and LDL levels; prevention of MI, stroke, and angina in adults with multiple risk factors for heart disease, in patients with heart disease, and in patients with type 2 diabetes; approved to lower cholesterol levels in children 10 to 17 years of age who meet specific criteria with familial hypercholesterolemia after failing trial of diet therapy.

Actions: Inhibits HMG–CoA, causing a decrease in serum cholesterol, triglyceride, and LDL levels and an increase in HDL levels.

Pharmacokinetics:

Route	Onset	Peak	Duration
Oral	Slow	1–2 h	20–30 h

$T_{1/2}$: 14 hours; metabolized in the liver and cells and excreted in the bile.

Adverse Effects: Headache, flatulence, abdominal pain, cramps, constipation, rhabdomyolysis with acute renal failure, liver impairment, myalgias.

Nursing Considerations for Patients Receiving HMG–CoA Reductase Inhibitors (Statins)

Assessment: History and Examination

- Assess for contraindications and cautions: any known allergies to these drugs or to fungal byproducts to avoid hypersensitivity reactions; active liver disease or history of alcoholic liver disease, which could be exacerbated by the effects of these drugs; current status of pregnancy or lactation because of potential adverse effects on the fetus or neonate; and impaired endocrine function, which could be exacerbated by effects on steroid hormones.

(continues on page 842)

- Perform a physical assessment to establish a baseline before beginning therapy and during therapy to determine its effectiveness and evaluate for any potential adverse effects.
- Weigh the patient to establish a baseline and evaluate for changes reflecting lifestyle changes that accompany drug therapy.
- Assess the patient's neurological status, including level of orientation, affect, and reflexes, which show early changes related to CNS function, to evaluate for possible CNS effects of the drug.
- Inspect the abdomen for distention and auscultate bowel sounds for changes in GI motility.
- Assess bowel elimination patterns, including frequency of stool passage and stool characteristics, to identify possible constipation.
- Monitor the results of laboratory tests, including renal and liver function tests, to identify possible toxicity and serum lipid levels to evaluate the drug's effectiveness.

Nursing Conclusions

Nursing conclusions related to drug therapy might include the following:

- Altered sensory perception (visual, kinesthetic, gustatory) related to CNS effects
- Injury risk related to CNS, liver, and renal effects
- Impaired comfort related to headache, myalgia, and GI effects
- Knowledge deficit regarding drug therapy

Planning

- The patient will receive the best therapeutic effect from the drug therapy.
- The patient will have limited adverse effects from the drug therapy.
- The patient will have an understanding of the drug therapy, adverse effects to anticipate, and measures to relieve discomfort and improve safety.

Intervention With Rationale

- Administer the drug daily with or without food.
- Monitor serum cholesterol and LDL levels before and periodically during therapy to evaluate the effectiveness of this drug.
- Monitor liver function tests before and periodically during therapy to monitor for liver damage; consult with the prescriber to discontinue the drug if the aspartate aminotransferase (AST) or alanine aminotransferase (ALT) level increases to three times higher than normal.
- Ensure that the patient has been educated regarding a cholesterol-lowering diet and exercise program to facilitate the best response to drug therapy.
- Encourage the patient to make the lifestyle changes necessary to decrease the risk for ASCVD and to increase the effectiveness of drug therapy.
- Withhold lovastatin, atorvastatin, or fluvastatin in any acute, serious medical condition (e.g., infection, hypotension, major surgery or trauma, metabolic endocrine disorders, seizures) that might suggest myopathy or serve as a risk factor for the development of renal failure.
- Suggest the use of barrier contraceptives for patients who can become pregnant because there is a risk of severe fetal abnormalities if these drugs are taken during pregnancy.
- Provide comfort measures to help the patient tolerate drug effects. These include small, frequent meals to minimize nausea and vomiting; access to bathroom facilities to ensure adequate bowel evacuation; bowel program as needed to address constipation; use of food with the drug if GI upset is severe to decrease direct irritating effects; environmental controls, such as temperature and lighting controls, to help deal with headaches; and safety precautions, such as lighting control and activity restrictions, to protect the patient if vision changes and muscle effects occur.
- Offer support and encouragement to help the patient deal with the diagnosis, needed lifestyle changes, and the drug regimen.
- Provide thorough patient teaching, including the name of the drug, dosage prescribed, and administration at bedtime for best effectiveness; measures to avoid adverse effects, warning signs of problems, and the need for follow-up laboratory testing to monitor cholesterol and lipid levels; importance of follow-up renal and liver function testing; dietary and lifestyle changes for risk reduction; and monitoring and evaluation, to enhance patient knowledge about drug therapy and to promote adherence.

See the "Critical Thinking Scenario" for discussion of a patient receiving an HMG–CoA inhibitor.

Evaluation

- Monitor patient response to the drug (lowering of serum cholesterol, triglyceride, and LDL levels; prevention of MI, stroke, and revascularization procedures; slowing of progression of ASCVD).
- Monitor for adverse effects (headache, dizziness, blurred vision, GI upset, liver failure, myalgia, rhabdomyolysis).
- Monitor the effectiveness of comfort measures and adherence to the regimen.
- Evaluate the effectiveness of the teaching plan (patient can name drug, dosage, adverse effects to watch for, and specific measures to avoid them; patient understands the importance of continued follow-up).

CRITICAL THINKING SCENARIO
Treating Hyperlipidemia

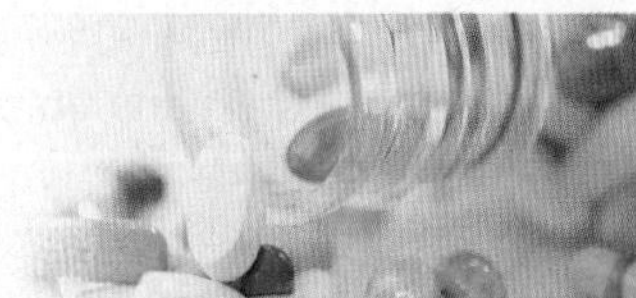

THE SITUATION

M.M., a 55-year-old patient, was seen for a routine physical examination. M.M. was found to be obese and borderline hypertensive, with a nonfasting cholesterol level of 325 mg/dL (very high). M.M. reported smoking two packs of cigarettes a day and noted in their family history that both parents died of heart attacks before age 50. M.M. described themself as a "workaholic" with no time to exercise and a tendency to eat most meals in restaurants. The primary medical regimen suggested for M.M. included ceasing or decreasing smoking, weight loss, dietary changes to decrease consumption of saturated fats, and decreased stress. On a return visit after 4 weeks, M.M. had lost 7 lb and reported a decrease in smoking, but their cholesterol level had not significantly decreased. The use of an antihyperlipidemic drug was discussed. M.M. was started on atorvastatin and advised to continue the diet and exercise program and to return in 3 months for follow-up.

Critical Thinking

What nursing interventions are appropriate at this point? Consider all of the known risk factors for ASCVD; then rank M.M.'s risk based on those factors.

What lifestyle changes can help M.M. reduce their risk of heart disease?

What support services should be consulted to help M.M.?

Should other tests be done before considering any drug therapy for M.M.? Think about the kind of patient teaching that would help M.M. cope with the overwhelming lifestyle changes that have been suggested and remain adherent to their medical regimen.

DISCUSSION

M.M.'s description of themself as a workaholic should alert the nurse to the possibility that they will have trouble adapting to any prescribed lifestyle changes. M.M. should first receive extensive teaching about ASCVD, their risk factors, and the options. The benefits of decreasing or eliminating risk factors should be discussed. Drug therapy is intended as an adjunct to diet and exercise, and the effectiveness of drug therapy improves remarkably when diet and exercise changes are made. M.M. may be more adherent if they exercise some control over the situation, so they should be invited to suggest possible lifestyle changes or adaptations. M.M. should also be encouraged to set short-range goals that are achievable to help them feel successful. M.M. needs to understand that beginning drug therapy does not mean that exercise and diet are no longer important.

M.M. also needs to understand that antihyperlipidemic drugs can cause dizziness, headaches, gastrointestinal (GI) upset, muscle and/or joint pain, and constipation. Because of their busy lifestyle, M.M. may have trouble coping with these adverse effects. M.M.'s health care provider may need to try a variety of different drugs or combinations of drugs to find ones that are effective but do not cause unacceptable adverse effects.

The American Heart Association (AHA) has numerous booklets, diets, support groups, and counselors who can help M.M. as they adapt to the medical regimen. M.M. can contact the AHA online at www.americanheart.org for a quick reference guide and referrals to other sources. M.M. will benefit from having a consistent health care team who can offer encouragement, answer any questions, and allow M.M. to vent their feelings. Often, lifestyle changes are the most difficult part of this medical regimen, so M.M. will need constant support.

NURSING CARE GUIDE FOR M.M.: HMG–COA REDUCTASE INHIBITORS (STATINS)

Assessment: History and Examination

Assess M.M.'s health history for allergies to any HMG–CoA reductase inhibitor or fungal byproducts, hepatic dysfunction, or endocrine disorders.

Focus the physical examination on the following areas:

Cardiovascular (CV): blood pressure, pulse, perfusion
Central nervous system (CNS): orientation, affect, reflexes, vision
Skin: color, lesions, texture
Respiratory system: rate, adventitious sounds
GI: abdominal examination, bowel sounds
Laboratory tests: liver and renal function tests, serum lipids

Nursing Conclusions

Altered sensory perception related to CNS effects
Injury risk related to CNS, liver, and renal effects
Impaired comfort related to headache, myalgia, and GI effects
Knowledge deficit regarding drug therapy

Planning

The patient will receive the best therapeutic effect from the drug therapy.

The patient will have limited adverse effects from the drug therapy.

The patient will have an understanding of the drug therapy, adverse effects to anticipate, and measures to relieve discomfort and improve safety.

(continues on page 844)

Intervention

Administer the drug any time of day with or without food.
Monitor serum lipids prior to therapy and periodically during therapy.
Give the drug with food if GI upset occurs.
Institute bowel program if needed to treat constipation.
Monitor liver function, and arrange to stop the drug if liver impairment occurs.
Provide support and reassurance to deal with drug effects and the need to make lifestyle, diet, and exercise changes.
Provide patient teaching regarding drug, dosage, adverse effects, what to report, and safety precautions.

Evaluation

Evaluate drug effects: Lowering of serum cholesterol and lipid levels, prevention of first myocardial infarction (MI), slowed progression of ASCVD.
Monitor for adverse effects: Sedation, dizziness, headache, cataracts, GI upset; hepatic or renal dysfunction; rhabdomyolysis.
Monitor for drug–drug interactions as indicated for each drug.
Evaluate the effectiveness of the patient teaching program.
Evaluate the effectiveness of comfort and safety measures.

PATIENT TEACHING FOR M.M.

- An HMG–CoA reductase inhibitor, or "statin," is an antihyperlipidemic agent, which means that it works to decrease the levels of certain lipids, or fats, in your blood. An increase in serum lipid levels has been associated with the development of many blood vessel disorders, including ASCVD, which can lead to a heart attack and/or stroke. This drug should be used in conjunction with a low-calorie, low-saturated fat diet and an exercise program.
- Some of the following adverse effects may occur:
  - *Headache, blurred vision, nervousness, insomnia*: Avoid driving or performing hazardous or delicate tasks that require concentration; these effects may pass with time.
  - *Nausea, vomiting, flatulence, constipation*: Small, frequent meals may help. If constipation becomes a problem, consult your health care provider for appropriate interventions. If you experience severe nausea, vomiting, or yellowing of the skin, notify your health care provider immediately.
  - *Muscle aches:* If you have new or worsening muscle and/or joint pain report these symptoms to your health care provider.
  - Report any of the following immediately to your health care provider: severe GI upset, vision changes, unusual bleeding, dark urine or light-colored stools, or sudden muscle pain accompanied by fever.
- You will need to have regular medical examinations to monitor the effectiveness of this drug on your lipid levels and to detect any adverse effects.
- Avoid grapefruit juice while you are taking this drug.
- Tell any doctor, nurse, or other health care provider that you are taking this drug.
- Keep this drug and all medications out of the reach of children.
- To help decrease your risk of ASCVD, follow these guidelines: Adhere to a diet that is low in calories and saturated fat, exercise regularly, stop smoking, and reduce stress.

Key Points

- HMG–CoA reductase inhibitors, or statins, block the enzyme HMG–CoA reductase, resulting in lower serum cholesterol levels, a resultant breakdown of LDLs, and a slight increase in HDLs.
- Patients receiving HMG–CoA reductase inhibitors should avoid pregnancy because of serious fetal adverse effects, should take the drug in the evening to mimic the normal patterns of lipid formation, should have liver function monitored regularly, and should be instructed to report any sudden muscle pain, especially if accompanied by fever.

Cholesterol Absorption Inhibitors

Ezetimibe (*Zetia*) was first approved in 2003. After approval, there was some controversy about how effective the medication was compared to statin therapy alone. However, current guidelines suggest that using ezetimibe as an adjunct with a statin may help lower total and LDL cholesterol. It can also be used as an adjunct with a fenofibrate for familial hyperlipidemia as this assists with lowering both serum cholesterol and triglyceride levels. Ezetimibe is not indicated to reduce morbidity and mortality of cardiovascular disease. It can also be used as monotherapy.

Therapeutic Actions and Indications

Ezetimibe works in the brush border of the small intestine to decrease the absorption of dietary cholesterol from the small intestine. As a result, less dietary cholesterol is delivered to the liver, and the liver increases the clearance of cholesterol from the serum to make up for the drop in dietary cholesterol, causing the total serum cholesterol level to drop. See Table 47.3 for usual indications.

Pharmacokinetics

Ezetimibe is absorbed well after oral administration, reaching peak level in 4 to 6 hours. It is metabolized in the liver and the small intestine, with a half-life of 22 hours. Excretion is through the feces and urine. It is not known whether the drug crosses the placenta or enters human milk.

Contraindications and Cautions

Ezetimibe is contraindicated in patients with an allergy to any component of the drug to avoid hypersensitivity reactions. If it is used in combination with a statin, it should not be used during pregnancy or lactation or with severe liver disease because of the known effects of statins, including possible liver problems and renal failure.

The drug should be used with caution as monotherapy during pregnancy or lactation because the effects on the fetus or neonate are not known and with older adult patients or patients with liver disease because of the potential for adverse reactions.

Adverse Effects

The most common adverse effects associated with ezetimibe are mild abdominal pain and diarrhea. It is not associated with the bloating and flatulence that occurs with the bile acid sequestrants and another class of lipid-lowering drugs called fibrates. Other adverse effects that have been reported include headache, dizziness, fatigue, upper respiratory tract infection, back pain, and muscle aches and pains. In rare cases, it can cause hepatitis.

Clinically Important Drug–Drug Interactions

Administration with bile acid sequestrants interferes with absorption, so ezetimibe should be taken 2 hours before or 4 hours after a bile sequestrant. Concurrent use with statins increase risk of myopathy and liver dysfunction.

The risk of elevated serum levels of ezetimibe increases if it is given with cyclosporine and fibrates. If the drug is administered with fenofibrate and cholelithiasis is suspected, gallbladder studies are indicated, and there should be strong consideration of changing the lipid-lowering therapy. Concurrent use of ezetimibe and fibrates other than fenofibrate is not recommended.

The risk for toxicity also increases if ezetimibe is combined with cyclosporine. If this combination cannot be avoided, the patient should be monitored closely.

If ezetimibe is combined with any fibrate, the risk of cholelithiasis increases. The patient should be monitored closely.

Warfarin levels increase in a patient who is also taking ezetimibe; if this combination is used, the patient should be monitored closely.

Prototype Summary: Ezetimibe

Indications: Adjunct to diet and exercise to lower serum cholesterol levels; in combination with atorvastatin or simvastatin for the treatment of homozygous familial hypercholesterolemia; with diet for the treatment of homozygous sitosterolemia to lower sitosterol and campesterol levels.

Actions: Works in the brush border of the small intestine to inhibit the absorption of cholesterol.

Pharmacokinetics:

Route	Onset	Peak
Oral	Moderate	4–12 h

$T_{1/2}$: 22 hours; metabolized in the liver and small intestine and excreted in the feces and urine.

Adverse Effects: Headache, dizziness, abdominal pain, diarrhea, URI, back pain, myalgia, arthralgia, hepatitis or liver dysfunction.

Nursing Considerations for Patients Receiving Cholesterol Absorption Inhibitors

Assessment: History and Examination

- Assess for contraindications or cautions: any known allergies to any component of the drug to avoid hypersensitivity reactions; liver dysfunction or advanced age because the processing of the drug may differ from the norm; and current status of pregnancy or lactation because the possible effects on the fetus or neonate are not known.
- Perform a physical assessment to establish a baseline before beginning therapy and during therapy to determine its effectiveness and evaluate for any potential adverse effects.
- Monitor orientation and reflexes to detect changes in CNS function, such as dizziness, that could require safety measures.
- Inspect the abdomen for distention, auscultate bowel sounds, and observe for signs of liver dysfunction (nausea, anorexia, vomiting, jaundice) due to risk of liver impairment.
- Assess bowel elimination patterns, including frequency of stool passage and stool characteristics, to identify possible changes that could require intervention.
- Monitor the results of laboratory tests, including serum cholesterol and lipid levels, to evaluate the effectiveness of drug therapy, and liver function studies to monitor for toxic effects.

(continues on page 846)

Nursing Conclusions

Nursing conclusions related to drug therapy may include the following:

- Altered sensory perception (visual, kinesthetic, gustatory) related to CNS effects
- Impaired comfort related to headache, myalgia, and GI effects
- Knowledge deficit regarding drug therapy

Planning

- The patient will receive the best therapeutic effect from the drug therapy.
- The patient will have limited adverse effects from the drug therapy.
- The patient will have an understanding of the drug therapy, adverse effects to anticipate, and measures to relieve discomfort and improve safety.

Intervention With Rationale

- Monitor serum cholesterol, triglyceride, and LDL levels before and periodically during therapy to evaluate the effectiveness of this drug.
- Monitor liver function tests before and periodically during therapy to detect possible liver damage.
- Encourage the patient to make the lifestyle changes necessary to decrease the risk of ASCVD and to increase the effectiveness of drug therapy.
- Suggest the use of barrier contraceptives for patients who can become pregnant if the drug is being used in combination with a statin because there is a risk of severe fetal abnormalities if these drugs are taken during pregnancy.
- Provide comfort measures to help the patient tolerate drug effects. These include readily available access to bathroom facilities to help if the patient has episodes of diarrhea, safety precautions to protect the patient if dizziness is an issue, and analgesics for headache and muscle aches if appropriate.
- Offer support and encouragement to help the patient deal with the diagnosis, needed lifestyle changes, and the drug regimen.
- Provide thorough patient teaching, including the name of the drug, dosage prescribed, and schedule for administration; measures to avoid adverse effects, warning signs of problems, and the need for follow-up laboratory testing to monitor cholesterol and lipid levels; dietary and lifestyle changes for reducing the risk of ASCVD and increasing the effectiveness of drug therapy; and monitoring and evaluation to enhance patient knowledge about drug therapy and to promote adherence.

Evaluation

- Monitor patient response to the drug (lowering of serum cholesterol, triglycerides, and LDL levels, lowering of sitosterol and campesterol levels).
- Monitor for adverse effects (headache, dizziness, GI pain, muscle aches and pains, upper respiratory tract infection).
- Monitor the effectiveness of comfort measures and adherence to the regimen.
- Evaluate the effectiveness of the teaching plan (patient can name drug, dosage, adverse effects to watch for, and specific measures to avoid them; patient understands the importance of continued follow-up).

Key Points

- The cholesterol absorption inhibitor ezetimibe works in the brush border of the small intestine to prevent the absorption of dietary cholesterol, which leads to increased clearance of cholesterol by the liver and a resultant fall in serum cholesterol.
- Change in diet and increased exercise are important parts of the overall treatment of a patient receiving a cholesterol absorption inhibitor.

Proprotein Convertase Subtilisin/Kexin Type 9 (PCSK9) Inhibitors

Alirocumab (*Praluent*) and evolocumab (*Repatha*) are PCSK9 inhibitors, which are indicated for reducing the risk of MI, stroke, and coronary revascularization in adults with cardiovascular disease. They are used to lower LDL in adults with primary hyperlipidemia and in patients with homozygous familial hypercholesterolemia.

Therapeutic Actions and Indications

Alirocumab and evolocumab are monoclonal antibodies that bind to the free PCSK9 enzyme and inhibit the PCSK9 attachment to the LDL receptors on the liver cell. This allows for the liver to process more LDL, which decreases the level of LDL in the blood plasma. See Table 47.3 for usual indications.

Pharmacokinetics

Alirocumab is administered via subcutaneous injection. Bioavailability is 85% after one injection, and steady state is achieved in the blood after two to three doses. It is distributed in the circulatory system and metabolized as a protein. Half-life was found to be 17 to 20 days. It is not known if it is safe for people who are pregnant or whether the drug crosses the placenta or enters human milk.

Evolocumab is administered via subcutaneous injection. Bioavailability after one injection is 72%, and the level peaks in serum after 3 to 4 days. It is distributed via the circulatory system. The half-life is 11 to 17 days. It is not known if it is safe for people who are pregnant or whether it crosses the placenta or enters human milk.

Contraindications and Cautions

Both medications are contraindicated for people with history of serious hypersensitivity reactions to PCSK9 inhibitors.

Adverse Effects

The most common adverse effects associated with these drugs are common to other monoclonal antibodies and include risk of infections such as nasopharyngitis, urinary tract infections, and upper respiratory infections. There can also be injection site reactions. The most dangerous adverse effect is an allergic reaction (serious hypersensitivity) including rash, pruritus, and even vasculitis.

Clinically Important Drug–Drug Interactions

These medications may be administered with other hyperlipidemia medications. There are no dosage adjustments necessary for mild to moderate renal or liver dysfunction. The medications have not been studied with severe renal or hepatic impairment.

Prototype Summary: Evolocumab (*Repatha*)

Indications: Reduction of risk of MI, stroke, and coronary revascularization in adults with cardiovascular disease; adjunct to diet, alone or in combination with other therapies to lower LDL, in adults with primary hyperlipidemia; adjunct to other therapies to lower LDL in patients with homozygous familial hypercholesterolemia (HoFH).

Actions: Bind to free PCSK9 to allow for the liver to decrease the blood LDL levels.

Pharmacokinetics:

Route	Onset	Peak
Subcutaneous	Fast	Maximum enzyme suppression in 4 h

$T_{1/2}$: 11 to 17 days; eliminated via binding to PCSK9 and via lytic process of the protein.

Adverse Effects: Hypersensitivity effects (rash, urticaria), upper respiratory tract infection, nasopharyngitis, influenza, injection site reactions.

Nursing Considerations for Patients Receiving PCSK9 Inhibitors

Assessment: History and Examination

- Assess for contraindications or cautions: any known allergies to any component of the drug to avoid hypersensitivity reactions; current status of pregnancy or lactation because the possible effects on the fetus or neonate are not known.
- Perform a physical assessment to establish a baseline before beginning therapy and during therapy to determine its effectiveness and evaluate for any potential adverse effects.
- Monitor for any infection due to some increased risk of infection with the medications.
- Monitor the results of laboratory tests, including serum cholesterol and lipid levels to evaluate the effectiveness of drug therapy and liver function studies to monitor for toxic effects.

Nursing Conclusions

Nursing conclusions related to drug therapy may include the following:

- Impaired comfort or acute pain from injection
- Infection risk at injection site
- Impaired skin integrity due to injection site
- Knowledge deficit regarding drug therapy

Planning

- The patient will receive the best therapeutic effect from the drug therapy.
- The patient will have limited adverse effects from the drug therapy.
- The patient will have an understanding of the drug therapy, adverse effects to anticipate, and measures to relieve discomfort and improve safety.

Intervention With Rationale

- Monitor serum cholesterol, triglyceride, and LDL levels before and periodically during therapy to evaluate the effectiveness of this drug.
- Encourage the patient to make the lifestyle changes necessary to decrease the risk of ASCVD and to increase the effectiveness of drug therapy.
- Suggest the use of barrier contraceptives for patients who can become pregnant if the drug is being used in combination with a statin because there is a risk of severe fetal abnormalities if these drugs are taken during pregnancy.
- Provide comfort measures to help the patient tolerate drug effects. These include analgesics if needed due to injection site discomfort.
- Offer support and encouragement to help the patient deal with the diagnosis, needed lifestyle changes, and the drug regimen.
- Provide thorough patient teaching, including the name of the drug, dosage prescribed, and schedule for administration; measures to avoid adverse effects, warning signs of problems, and the need for follow-up laboratory testing to monitor cholesterol and lipid levels; dietary and lifestyle changes for reducing the risk of ASCVD and increasing the effectiveness of drug therapy; and monitoring and evaluation to enhance patient knowledge about drug therapy and to promote adherence.

(continues on page 848)

Evaluation

- Monitor patient response to the drug (lowering of serum cholesterol and LDL levels).
- Monitor for adverse effects (hypersensitivity effects including rash, vasculitis, pruritus, and urticaria; upper respiratory tract infection, nasopharyngitis; influenza; and injection site reactions).
- Monitor the effectiveness of comfort measures and adherence to the regimen.
- Evaluate the effectiveness of the teaching plan (patient can name drug, dosage, adverse effects to watch for, and specific measures to avoid them; patient understands the importance of continued follow-up).

Key Points

- The PCSK9 inhibitors are monoclonal antibodies that work by binding to an enzyme that decreases the liver's ability to clear LDL from the blood. The effect of the medications is lower blood LDL levels.
- They are administered subcutaneously every 2 or 4 weeks.

Other Lipid-Lowering Agents

Other drugs that are used to affect lipid levels do not fall into any of the classes discussed previously. They are approved for use in combination with changes in diet and exercise. These include the fibrates (derivatives of fibric acid), omega-3 fatty acids, and the vitamin niacin (see Table 47.3). Other drugs have been approved for treating familial lipid disorders.

Fibrates

The fibrates stimulate the breakdown of lipoproteins from the tissues and their removal from the plasma. They lead to a decrease in lipoprotein and triglyceride synthesis and secretion. The fibrates are absorbed from the GI tract and are metabolized in the liver and excreted in urine. Fibrates in use today include the following:

- Fenofibrate (*Tricor* and others) is a peroxisome proliferator receptor alpha activator. It increases lipolysis and elimination of triglycerides by activating the receptor in the liver. The decrease in triglycerides changes the composition of LDL cholesterol, which makes it more easily eliminated. This medication also increases uric acid secretion. It is indicated for adults with high triglyceride levels as an adjunct to diet modifications. It is also indicated for adjunct treatment to decrease LDL and increase HDL cholesterol. The peak effect is usually seen within 4 weeks, and the patient's serum lipid levels should be reevaluated at that time.
- Gemfibrozil (*Lopid*) inhibits peripheral breakdown of lipids, reduces production of triglycerides and LDLs, and increases HDL concentrations. It is associated with GI and muscle discomfort. This drug should not be combined with statins. There is an increased risk of rhabdomyolysis from 3 weeks to several months after therapy if this combination is used. If this combination cannot be avoided, the patient should be monitored closely.
- Fenofibric acid (*Trilipix*) is also a peroxisome proliferator–activated receptor alpha agonist. This drug works to activate a specific hepatic receptor that results in increased breakdown of lipids, elimination of triglyceride-rich particles from the plasma, and reduction in the production of an enzyme that naturally inhibits lipid breakdown. The result is seen as a decrease in triglyceride levels, changes in LDL production that makes them more easily broken down in the body, and an increase in HDL levels. Fenofibric acid is approved to be used as adjunctive therapy to reduce triglyceride levels, decrease LDL, and increase HDL levels in patients with mixed lipid disorders and primary hypercholesterolemia. Fenofibric acid is slowly absorbed from the GI tract, with peak level occurring in 4 to 5 hours. It is metabolized in the liver, has a half-life of 20 hours, and is excreted in the urine. Caution should be used in patients with renal impairment, and the drug should be avoided in patients with severe renal impairment. The most common adverse effects that have been reported are headache, back pain, nausea, diarrhea, muscle pain, runny nose, and respiratory infections. Gallstones have also been reported with this drug. Patients complaining of gallstone-type pain should be screened carefully. There is an increased risk of muscle breakdown and rhabdomyolysis if taken with a statin, and patients using this combination need to be monitored closely. Caution must be used with warfarin anticoagulants; increased bleeding can occur. The patient should be monitored closely and the dose of the anticoagulant regulated to achieve therapeutic anticoagulation.

Vitamin B_3

Vitamin B_3, known as niacin (*Niacor, Niaspan*) or nicotinic acid, inhibits the release of free fatty acids from adipose tissue, increases the rate of triglyceride removal from plasma, and generally reduces LDL and triglyceride levels and increases HDL levels. It may also decrease the levels of apoproteins needed to form chylomicrons. The initial effect on lipid levels is usually seen within 5 to 7 days, with the maximum effect occurring in 3 to 5 weeks. Niacin is associated with intense cutaneous flushing, nausea, and abdominal pain, making its use somewhat limited. It also increases the serum levels of uric acid and may predispose patients to the development of gout. Niacin is often combined with bile acid sequestrants for increased effect. It is given at bedtime to make maximum use of nighttime cholesterol synthesis, and it must be given 4 to 6 hours after the bile sequestrant to ensure absorption.

Omega-3 Fatty Acids

Omega-3-acid ethyl esters (*Lovaza*) are a combination of omega-3 fatty acids and an activator that inhibits liver enzyme systems to decrease the synthesis of triglycerides, a risk factor in metabolic syndrome, lowering serum triglyceride levels. It is approved to lower triglycerides in adults with high triglyceride levels. It should be combined with appropriate diet and exercise to help keep overall lipid levels lower. It is not recommended in pregnancy or lactation. There is substantial research evidence to support the effects of this drug, unlike research on over-the-counter fish oil products, which do not appear to be effective in lowering lipid levels. This drug may prolong bleeding time so caution must be used with any other drugs that affect bleeding. Diarrhea, nausea, abdominal pain, and discomfort are the most common adverse effects.

Icosapent ethyl (*Vascepa*) is made of the component in omega-3 fatty acids that reduces triglyceride synthesis in the liver (eicosapentaenoic acid). It is indicated to be used as an adjunct with statin therapy to reduce risk of MI, stroke, and other cardiovascular events in patients with high triglyceride levels. It can also be used as an adjunct to diet to reduce triglyceride levels in patients with severe hypertriglyceridemia (≥500 mg/dL). Capsules are to be swallowed whole twice a day. Caution should be taken with people with fish allergy due to risk of allergic reaction. There is evidence of increased risk of development of atrial fibrillation/flutter that could require hospitalization. There is also increased risk of bleeding, especially if taken concurrently with antiplatelet and/or anticoagulant medications.

Other Therapies

Bempedoic acid (*Nexletol*) is indicated as an adjunct to statin therapy and diet for treatment of heterozygous familial hypercholesterolemia or ASCVD in patients who need additional lowering of LDL cholesterol. This medication works by inhibiting an enzyme (adenosine triphosphate-citrate lyase) that is part of the cholesterol biosynthesis pathway. It decreases the amount of LDL made by the liver and released into the blood. It is administered orally daily with or without food. There are cautions regarding potential for hyperuricemia and tendon rupture in some patients.

Lomitapide (*Juxtapid*) is an agent approved as an adjunct to diet, exercise, and other lipid-lowering therapies for treatment of patients with homozygous familial hypercholesterolemia. It has a boxed warning regarding the potential for serious hepatotoxicity; because of this risk, it is available only through a limited-access program. Lomitapide inhibits the triglyceride transfer protein, which is necessary for the liver cells to make LDL. Therefore, synthesis of LDL is prevented and plasma LDL is lowered. Lomitapide will inhibit absorption of fat-soluble vitamins, so supplements are recommended. It is not recommended during pregnancy or lactation due to risk of fetal and/or neonate harm.

Combination Therapy

Frequently, if the patient shows no response to strict dietary modification, exercise, and lifestyle changes with the use of one lipid-lowering agent, combination therapy may be initiated to achieve desirable serum LDL and cholesterol levels. For example, a bile acid sequestrant might be combined with niacin; this combination would decrease the synthesis of LDLs while lowering the serum levels of LDLs. This combination is thought to help slow the progression of ASCVD. Numerous fixed-combination therapies are available. However, care must be taken not to combine agents that increase the risk of rhabdomyolysis. For example, HMG–CoA reductase inhibitors are not usually combined with niacin or gemfibrozil.

Key Points

Other agents used to lower cholesterol include fibrates and niacin. Often, lipid-lowering agents are used in combination to lower the cholesterol at different sites.

SUMMARY

- ASCVD is the leading cause of death in the United States and worldwide. It is often associated with the development of atheromas or plaques in arterial linings that lead to narrowing of the lumen of the artery and hardening of the artery wall with loss of distensibility and responsiveness to stimuli for contraction or dilation.
- The cause of ASCVD is not completely understood, but many contributing risk factors have been identified, including increasing age, male sex, genetic predisposition, high-fat diet, sedentary lifestyle, smoking, obesity, high stress levels, bacterial infections, diabetes, hypertension, gout, and menopause. The presence of many of these factors constitutes metabolic syndrome.
- Treatment and prevention of ASCVD are aimed at manipulating the known risk factors to decrease atherosclerosis development and progression.
- Fats are metabolized with the aid of bile acids, which act as a detergent to break fats into small molecules called micelles. Micelles are absorbed into the intestinal wall and combined with proteins to become chylomicrons, which can be transported throughout the circulatory system.
- Some fats are used immediately for energy or are stored in adipose tissue; others are processed in the liver to LDLs, which are associated with the development of ASCVD. LDLs are broken down in the periphery and leave many remnants (e.g., fats) that must be removed from blood vessels. This process involves the inflammatory reaction and may initiate or contribute to atheroma production.
- Some fats are processed into HDLs, which are able to absorb fats and remnants from the periphery and offer a protective effect against the development of ASCVD.

- Cholesterol is an important fat that is used to make bile acids. It is the base for steroid hormones and provides the necessary structure for cell membranes. All cells can produce cholesterol.
- HMG–CoA reductase is an enzyme that controls the final step in the production of cellular cholesterol.
- Patients taking lipid-lowering drugs need to make diet, exercise, and lifestyle changes to reduce the risk of ASCVD.
- Bile acid sequestrants bind with bile acids in the intestine and lead to their excretion in feces. This results in lower bile acid levels as the liver uses cholesterol to produce more bile acids. The end result is a decrease in serum cholesterol and LDL levels as the liver changes its metabolism of these fats to meet the need for more bile acids.
- HMG–CoA reductase inhibitors, or statins, block the enzyme HMG–CoA reductase, resulting in lower serum cholesterol levels, a resultant breakdown of LDLs, and a slight increase in HDLs.
- The cholesterol absorption inhibitor ezetimibe works in the brush border of the small intestine to prevent the absorption of dietary cholesterol, which leads to increased clearance of cholesterol by the liver and a resultant fall in serum cholesterol.
- The PCSK9 inhibitors are monoclonal antibodies that bind to PCSK9, which increases the liver's ability to clear LDL from the blood.
- Other agents used to lower cholesterol include fibrates, niacin, and omega-3 fatty acids. Often lipid-lowering agents are used in combination to lower the cholesterol at different sites.

CHECK YOUR UNDERSTANDING

Answers to the questions in this chapter can be found in Answers to Check Your Understanding Questions on thePoint®.

MULTIPLE CHOICE

Select the best answer.

1. Which of the following descriptions accurately reflects how the body uses cholesterol?
   a. Production of water-soluble vitamins
   b. Formation of steroid hormones
   c. Mineralization of bones
   d. Development of dental plaques

2. The formation of atheromas in blood vessels precedes the signs and symptoms of
   a. hepatitis.
   b. atherosclerotic cardiovascular disease.
   c. diabetes mellitus.
   d. chronic obstructive pulmonary disease (COPD).

3. Hyperlipidemia is considered to be a
   a. normal finding in adult males.
   b. condition related to stress levels.
   c. treatable ASCVD risk factor.
   d. side effect of cigarette smoking.

4. The bile acid sequestrants
   a. are absorbed into the liver.
   b. take several weeks to show an effect.
   c. have no associated adverse effects.
   d. prevent bile salts from being reabsorbed.

5. HMG–CoA reductase inhibitors work in the
   a. process of bile secretion.
   b. process of cholesterol formation in the cell.
   c. intestinal wall to block fat absorption.
   d. kidney to block fat excretion.

6. When teaching a patient about HMG–CoA reductase inhibitors, the nurse would include that the patient
   a. will not have a heart attack.
   b. will not develop ASCVD.
   c. might develop cataracts as a result.
   d. might stop absorbing fat-soluble vitamins.

7. Which would the nurse expect the health care provider to prescribe for a patient who has high lipid levels and cannot take fibrates or HMG–CoA reductase inhibitors?
   a. Nicotine
   b. Vitamin C
   c. PCSK9 inhibitor
   d. Nitrates

8. Which would alert the nurse to suspect that a patient receiving HMG–CoA reductase inhibitors is developing rhabdomyolysis?
   a. Flatulence and abdominal bloating
   b. Increased bleeding and bruising
   c. Development of cataracts and blurred vision
   d. Muscle pain and weakness

MULTIPLE RESPONSE

Select all that apply.

1. A bile acid sequestrant is the drug of choice for a patient who has which conditions?
   a. High LDL concentration
   b. High triglyceride concentration
   c. Biliary obstruction
   d. Vitamin K deficiency
   e. High HDL concentration
   f. Intolerance to statins

2. Teaching a patient who is prescribed an HMG–CoA reductase inhibitor to treat high cholesterol and high lipid levels should include which information?
   a. The importance of exercise
   b. The need for dietary changes to alter cholesterol levels
   c. That taking a statin will allow a full, unrestricted diet
   d. That drug therapy is always needed when these levels are elevated
   e. The importance of controlling blood pressure and blood glucose levels
   f. That stopping smoking may also help to lower lipid levels

REFERENCES

Aronne, L. J. (2007). Therapeutic options for modifying cardiometabolic risk factors. *American Journal of Medicine, 120*(3, Suppl. 1), S26–S34. https://doi.org/10.1016/j.amjmed.2007.01.005

Bray, G. (2008). *Metabolic syndrome and obesity*. Humana Press.

Brunton, L., Hilal-Dandan, R., & Knollman, B. (2018). *Goodman and Gilman's the pharmacological basis of therapeutics* (13th ed.). McGraw-Hill.

Glynn, R., Koenig, W., Nordestgaard, B., & Ridker, P. M. (2010). Rosuvastatin for primary prevention in older persons with elevated C-reactive protein and low to average low-density lipoprotein cholesterol levels: Exploratory analysis of a randomized trial; secondary analysis of the JUPITER study. *Annals of Internal Medicine, 152*, 488–496. https://doi.org/10.7326/0003-4819-152-8-201004200-00005

Grundy, S. M., Stone, N. J., Bailey, A. L., Beam, C., Birtcher, K. K., Blumenthal, R. S., Braun, L. T., deFerranti, S., Fajella-Tommasino, J., Forman, D. E., Goldberg, R., Heidenreich, P. A., Hlatky, M. A., Jones, D. W., Lloyd-Jones, D., Lopez-Pajares, N., Ndumele, C. E., Orringer, C. E., Peralta, C. A., … Yeboah, J. (2019). 2018 AHA/ACC/AACVPR/AAPA/ABC/ACPM/ADA/AGS/APhA/ASPC/NLA/PCNA guideline on the management of blood cholesterol: A report of the American College of Cardiology/American Heart Association Task Force on Clinical Practice Guidelines. *Circulation, 139*, e1082–e1143. https://doi.org/10.1161/CIR.0000000000000625

Hajar, R. (2017). Risk factors for coronary artery disease. *Heart Views, 18*(3), 109–114. https://doi.org/10.4103/HEARTVIEWS.HEARTVIEWS_106_17

Hall, J. E., & Hall, M. E. (2021). *Guyton and Hall textbook of medical physiology* (14th ed.). Elsevier.

Kastelen, J. J., Adkim, F., Stroes, E. S., Zwinderman, A. H., Bots, M. L., Stalenhoef, A. F. H., Visseren, F. L. J., Sijbrands, E. J. G., Trip, M. D., Stein, E. A., Gaudet, D., Duivenvoorden, R., Veltri, E. P., Marais, A. D., & DeGroot, E. (2008). ENHANCE: Simvastatin with or without ezetimibe in familial hypercholesterolemia. *New England Journal of Medicine, 358*, 1431–1443. https://doi.org/10.1056/NEJMoa0800742

Kim, H., Caulfield, L. E., Garcia-Larsen, V., Steffen, L. M., Coresh, J., & Rebholz, C. M. (2019). Plant-based diets are associated with a lower risk of incident cardiovascular disease, cardiovascular disease mortality and all-cause mortality in a general population of middle-aged adults. *Journal of the American Heart Association, 8*(16), e012865. https://doi.org/10.1161/JAHA.119.012865

Norris, T. L. (2019). *Porth's pathophysiology concepts of altered health states* (13th ed.). Wolters Kluwer.

Spinler, S. A. (2006). Challenges associated with metabolic syndrome. *Pharmacotherapy, 26*, 209S–217S. https://doi.org/10.1592/phco.26.12part2.209S

CHAPTER 48

Drugs Affecting Blood Coagulation

Learning Objectives

Upon completion of this chapter, you will be able to:

1. Outline the mechanisms by which blood clots form and dissolve in the body, correlating this information with the actions of drugs used to affect blood clotting.
2. Discuss the use of drugs that affect blood coagulation across the lifespan.
3. Describe the therapeutic actions, indications, pharmacokinetics, contraindications, most common adverse effects, and important drug–drug interactions associated with drugs affecting blood coagulation.
4. Compare and contrast the prototype drugs aspirin, heparin, alteplase, antihemophilic factor, and aminocaproic acid with other agents used to affect blood coagulation.
5. Outline the nursing considerations, including important teaching points, for patients receiving drugs used to affect blood coagulation.

Key Terms

anticoagulants: drugs that block or inhibit any step of the coagulation process, preventing or slowing clot formation

antiplatelet agents: drugs that interfere with the aggregation or clumping of platelets to form the platelet plug

clotting factors: substances formed in the liver—many requiring vitamin K—that react in a cascading sequence to cause the formation of thrombin from prothrombin; thrombin then breaks down fibrin threads from fibrinogen to form a clot

coagulation: process of blood changing from a fluid state to a solid state to plug injuries to the vascular system

extrinsic pathway: cascade of clotting factors in blood that has escaped the vascular system to form a clot on the outside of the injured vessel

Hageman factor: first factor activated when a blood vessel or cell is injured; starts the cascading reaction of the clotting factors, activates the conversion of plasminogen to plasmin to dissolve clots, and activates the kinin system responsible for activation of the inflammatory response

hemorrhagic disorders: disorders characterized by a lack of clot-forming substances, leading to states of excessive bleeding

hemostatic agents: drugs that stop blood loss, usually by blocking the plasminogen mechanism and preventing clot dissolution

intrinsic pathway: cascade of clotting factors leading to the formation of a clot within an injured vessel

plasminogen: natural clot-dissolving system, converted to plasmin (also called fibrinolysin) by many substances to dissolve clots that have formed and to maintain the patency of injured vessels

platelet aggregation: property of platelets to adhere to an injured surface and then attract other platelets, which clump together or aggregate at the area, plugging up an injury to the vascular system

thromboembolic disorders: disorders characterized by the formation of clots or thrombi on injured blood vessels with potential breaking of the clot to form emboli that can travel to smaller vessels, where they become lodged and occlude the vessel

thrombolytic agents: drugs that lyse, or break down, a clot that has formed; these drugs activate the plasminogen mechanism to dissolve fibrin threads

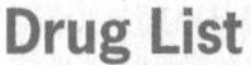

Drug List

DRUGS AFFECTING CLOT FORMATION AND RESOLUTION

Antiplatelet Agents
- abciximab
- anagrelide
- aspirin
- cilostazol
- clopidogrel
- dipyridamole
- eptifibatide
- prasugrel
- ticagrelor
- ticlopidine
- tirofiban
- vorapaxar

Anticoagulants
- antithrombin
- apixaban
- argatroban
- betrixaban
- bivalirudin
- dabigatran
- dalteparin
- desirudin
- edoxaban
- enoxaparin
- fondaparinux
- heparin
- protein C concentrate
- rivaroxaban
- warfarin

Thrombolytic Agents
- alteplase
- reteplase
- tenecteplase

Anticoagulant Adjunctive Therapy
- coagulation factor Xa (recombinant)
- idarucizumab
- protamine sulfate
- prothrombin complex concentrate
- vitamin K

Hemorrheologic Agent
- pentoxifylline

DRUGS USED TO CONTROL BLEEDING

Antihemophilic Agents
- antihemophilic factor
- antihemophilic factor Fc fusion protein
- antihemophilic factor porcine sequence
- antiinhibitor coagulant complex
- coagulation factor VIIa
- factor IX
- factor IX complex
- factor XIII concentrate

Hemostatic Agents

Systemic
- aminocaproic acid

Topical
- absorbable gelatin
- human fibrin sealant
- microfibrillar collagen
- thrombin
- thrombin, recombinant

The cardiovascular (CV) system is a closed system, and blood remains in a fluid state while in it. Because blood is in a closed space, it maintains the difference in pressures required to keep the system moving along. The fluid blood in the CV system moves from areas of higher pressure to those of lower pressure. If the vascular system is injured—from a cut, a puncture, or a capillary destruction—the fluid blood could leak out, causing the system in that area to lose pressure, changing the flow in the system and potentially harming the tissues and organs. There are protective mechanisms to prevent excess blood loss. They are vascular constriction, formation of the platelet plug, activation of coagulation cascade, and formation of a blood clot. The mechanisms work together to create hemostasis (stoppage of blood flow). Two categories of dysfunction of hemostasis are inappropriate clotting (thrombosis) and inability to clot (bleeding).

Hemostasis

People injure blood vessels all the time (e.g., by coughing too hard, by knocking into the corner of a desk when sitting down). Consequently, the vascular system must maintain an intricate balance between the tendency to clot or form a solid state, called **coagulation**, and the need to "unclot," or reverse coagulation, to keep the vessels open and the blood flowing. If a great deal of vascular damage occurs, such as with a major cut or incision, the balance in the area shifts to a procoagulation mode, and a large clot is formed. At the same time, the enzymes in the plasma work to dissolve this clot before blood flow to tissues is lost, which would otherwise lead to hypoxia and potential cell death.

Drugs that affect blood coagulation work at various steps in the blood-clotting and clot-dissolving processes to restore the balance that is needed to maintain the CV system. Box 48.1 discusses the uses of these drugs in various age groups.

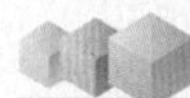

Concept Mastery Alert

Monitoring Anticoagulation Therapy

The treatment to manage a significant episode of bleeding in a patient prescribed an anticoagulant is to apply firm, constant pressure to the bleeding site and to notify the health care provider immediately.

Vasoconstriction

The first reaction to a blood vessel injury is transient local vasoconstriction (Fig. 48.1). If the injury to the blood vessel is small, this vasoconstriction can seal off any break and allow the area to heal. If the injury is large, the vascular spasm could last hours. The causes of the vasoconstriction are multifactorial and include local smooth muscle spasm, neural reflexes, and local chemicals released from endothelium and platelets. In small vessels in particular, the platelets enhance vasoconstriction by releasing thromboxane A_2, a powerful vasoconstricting prostaglandin.

Platelet Aggregation

Injury to a blood vessel exposes blood to the collagen and other substances under the endothelial lining of the vessel. This exposure causes platelets in the circulating blood to change shape and release substances that allow them to become more adhesive to the collagen and the protein von

Box 48.1 Focus on Drug Therapy Across the Lifespan

DRUGS AFFECTING BLOOD COAGULATION

Children

Use of anticoagulants, antiplatelets, and thrombolytics in children is an evolving field in which more research is needed to better guide safe practice. They are needed less frequently in the pediatric population compared to adults and older adults. When they are used, the child needs to be monitored carefully to avoid excessive bleeding related to drug interactions or alterations in GI or liver function. People who interact with the child need to understand the importance of preventing injuries and providing safety precautions and should be aware of what to do if the child is injured and begins to bleed.

Due to guidelines driven by weaker evidence, policies are often written by individual institutions. Low molecular weight heparin is the preferred anticoagulant for children. However, both heparin and warfarin are also frequently used.

Adults

Adults receiving these drugs need to be instructed in ways to prevent injury, such as using an electric razor instead of a straight razor, using a soft-bristled toothbrush to protect the gums, and avoiding contact sports. They also need to be instructed in what to do if bleeding does occur (apply constant firm pressure and contact a health care provider). They should receive a written list of signs of bleeding to watch for and to report to their health care providers.

Because so many drugs and alternative therapies are known to interact with these agents, it is important that these patients be urged to report the use of this drug to any other health care providers and to consult with one before using any over-the-counter drugs or alternative therapies.

It is prudent to advise any patient using one of these drugs in the home setting to carry or wear MedicAlert identification in case of emergency.

The patient also needs to understand the importance of regular, periodic blood tests necessary to evaluate the effects of some of the drugs. The newer oral anticoagulants do not require regular blood testing to demonstrate effectiveness.

Because of the many risks associated with increased bleeding or increased blood clotting during pregnancy, these drugs should not be used during pregnancy unless the benefit to the patient clearly outweighs the potential risk to the fetus and to the patient at delivery. Risks of altered blood clotting in the neonate make these drugs generally inadvisable for use during lactation.

Older Adults

Older adults may have many underlying medical conditions that require the need for drugs that alter blood clotting (e.g., CAD, CVA, peripheral vascular disease, TIAs). Statistically, older adults also take more medications, making them more likely to encounter drug–drug interactions associated with these drugs. The older adult is also more likely to have impaired liver and kidney function, conditions that can alter the metabolism and excretion of these drugs.

The older adult should be carefully evaluated for liver and kidney function, use of other medications, and ability to follow through with regular blood testing and medical evaluation before therapy begins. Therapy should be started at the lowest possible level and adjusted accordingly after the patient response has been noted.

Careful attention needs to be given to the patient's total drug regimen. Starting, stopping, or changing the dose of another drug may alter the body's metabolism of the drug that is being used to affect coagulation, leading to increased risk of bleeding or ineffective anticoagulation.

Willebrand factor that is released into the traumatized tissue. On the surface of the platelets there are specialized glycoproteins (GPIIb/IIIa) that bind to von Willebrand factor in the tissues, to fibrinogen in the tissues, and to other platelets. Once they are bound to the tissue, the platelets release adenosine diphosphate (ADP), platelet-activating factor, serotonin, and other chemicals that attract other platelets, causing them to gather or aggregate and to stick as well. ADP is also a precursor of the prostaglandins, from which thromboxane A_2 is formed. Thromboxane A_2 causes local vasoconstriction and further **platelet aggregation**, the property of platelets to adhere to an injured surface and then attract other platelets, which clump together or aggregate at the area. This series of events forms a platelet plug at the site of the vessel injury. In many injuries, the combination of vasoconstriction and platelet aggregation is enough to seal off the injury and keep the CV system intact (Fig. 48.2).

Coagulation

Conversion of the plasma protein fibrinogen into a fibrin clot is the next mechanism of hemostasis. The intrinsic and extrinsic blood coagulation pathways work together to form a blood clot. Coagulation is a process completed in a specific sequence. Many of the **clotting factors** are inactive in the plasma; they must be activated in order. Most clotting factors are proteins made within the liver, and vitamin K is necessary for synthesis of several of the factors. Calcium is required for activation of many of the clotting factors during this process.

Intrinsic Pathway

As blood comes in contact with the exposed collagen of the injured blood vessel, one of the clotting factors, **Hageman factor** (also called factor XII), a chemical substance that is found circulating in the blood, is activated. (Clotting factors are often known by a name and by a Roman numeral. When one of these factors becomes activated, the lowercase letter "a" is added; e.g., activated Hageman factor is also called factor XIIa.) The activation of Hageman factor starts a number of reactions in the area: The clot formation process is activated, the clot-dissolving process is activated, and the inflammatory response is started (see Chapter 15). The activation of Hageman factor first

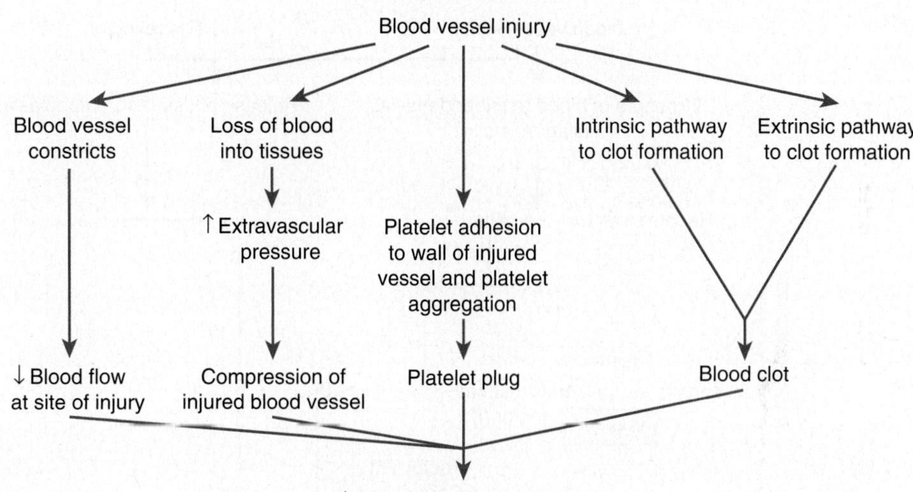

FIGURE 48.1 Process of blood coagulation.

activates clotting factor XI (plasma thromboplastin antecedent) and then activates a cascading series of coagulant substances called the **intrinsic pathway** (Fig. 48.3) that ends with the conversion of prothrombin to thrombin. Activated thrombin breaks down fibrinogen to form insoluble fibrin threads, which form a clot inside the blood vessel. The clot, called a thrombus, acts to plug the injury and seal the system.

Extrinsic Pathway

While the coagulation process is going on inside the blood vessel via the intrinsic pathway, the **extrinsic pathway** causes the blood that has leaked out of the vascular system and into the surrounding tissues to clot. Injured cells release a substance called tissue thromboplastin, which activates clotting factors in the blood and starts the clotting cascade to form a clot on the outside of the blood vessel. The injured vessel is now vasoconstricted and has a platelet plug as well as a clot on both the inside and the outside of the blood vessel in the area of the injury. These actions maintain the closed nature of the CV system (see Fig. 48.3). The extrinsic and intrinsic clotting pathways converge into the common clotting pathway starting at the activation of Stuart factor (X).

Common Clotting Pathway

In the presence of calcium, activated factors X and V, with additional phospholipids in the plasma, combine to form a complex called the prothrombin activator. This complex is able to split the plasma protein prothrombin into a smaller molecule, thrombin. Thrombin acts as an enzyme to convert fibrinogen (another plasma protein) into a mesh of fibrin fibers that combines platelets, blood cells, and plasma to form a clot.

Clot Resolution and Anticlotting Process

Blood plasma also contains anticlotting substances that inhibit clotting reactions that might otherwise lead to an

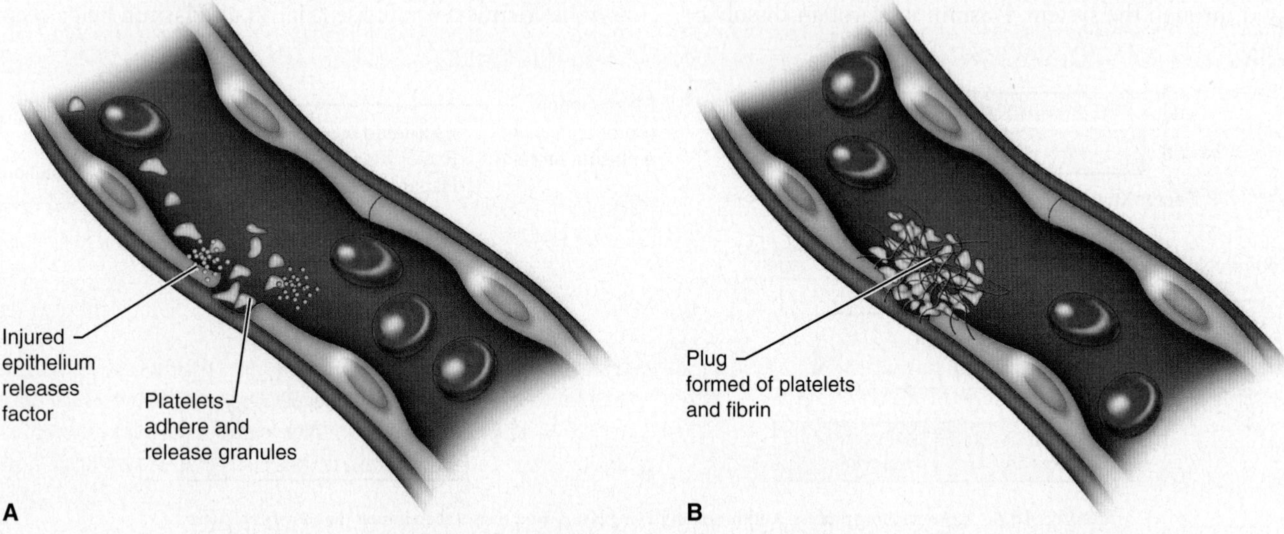

FIGURE 48.2 **A.** Damaged vessel endothelium is a stimulus to circulating platelets, causing platelet adhesion. **B.** Platelets release mediators, and platelet aggregation results.

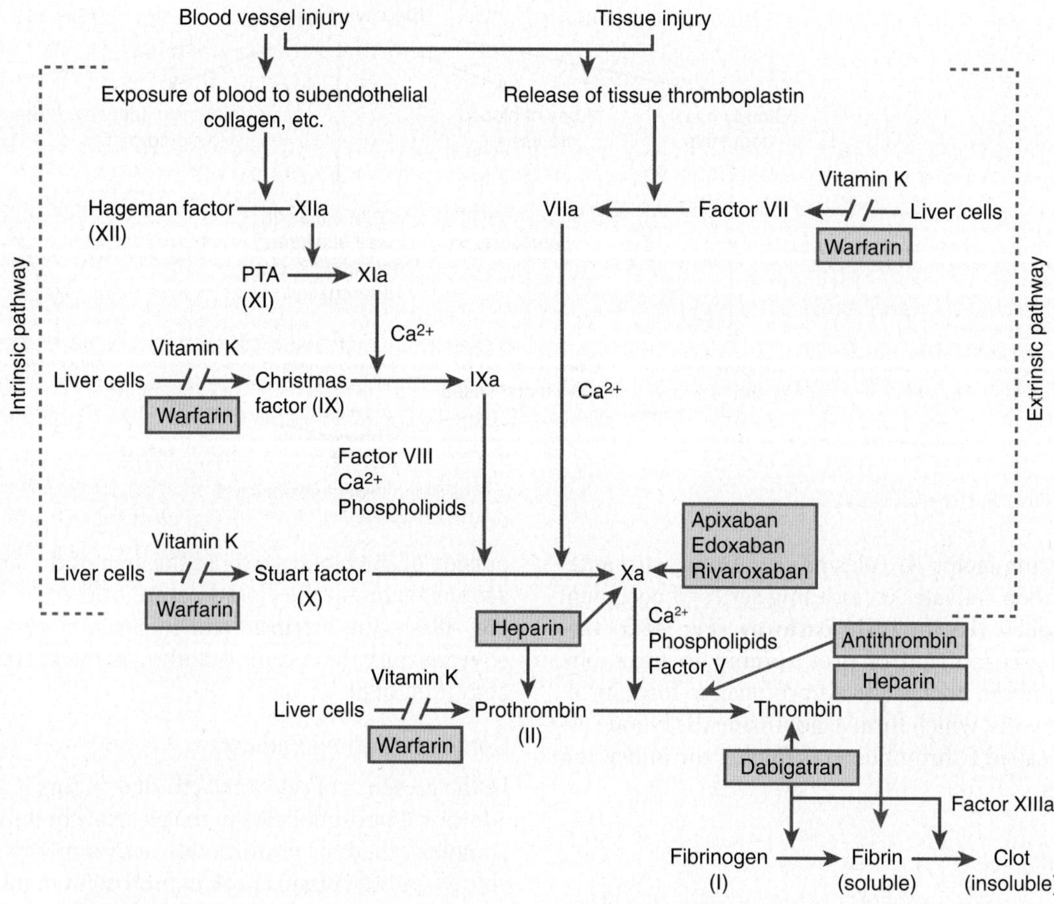

FIGURE 48.3 Details of the intrinsic and extrinsic clotting pathways. The sites of action of some of the drugs that can influence these processes are shown in *red*.

obstruction of blood vessels by blood clots. For example, antithrombin III prevents the formation of thrombin, thus slowing the development of fibrin threads. Plasma proteins C and S work as anticoagulants to inactivate clotting factors V and VIII.

Another substance in the plasma, called plasmin or fibrinolysin, dissolves clots to ensure free movement of blood through the system. Plasmin is a protein-dissolving substance that breaks down the fibrin framework of blood clots and opens up vessels. Its precursor, called **plasminogen**, is made in the liver and is found in the plasma. The conversion of plasminogen to plasmin begins with the activation of Hageman factor and is facilitated by a number of other factors, including antidiuretic hormone, epinephrine, pyrogens, emotional stress, physical activity, and the chemical urokinase (Fig. 48.4). Plasmin helps keep

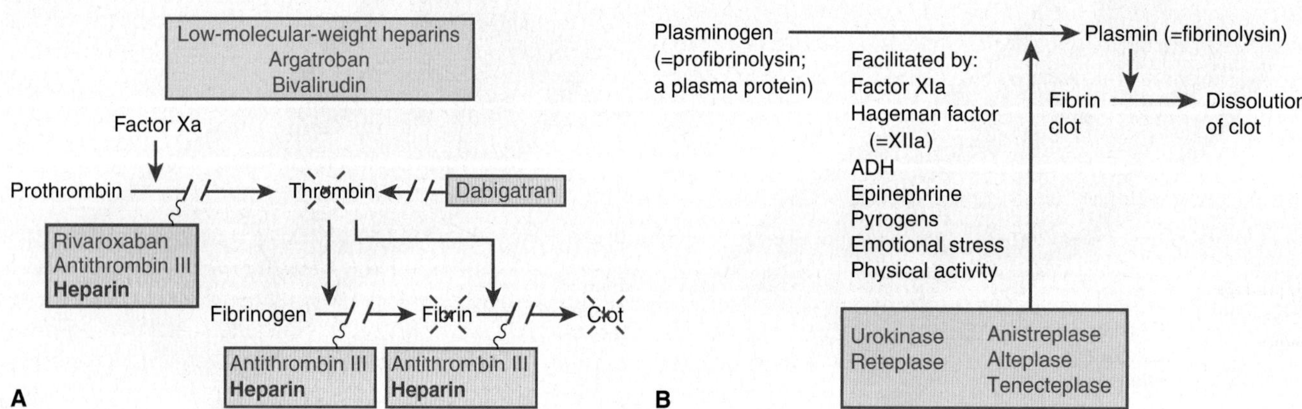

FIGURE 48.4 **A.** Anticlotting process. Antithrombin III (in plasma) and rivaroxaban inhibit the activity of Stuart factor (factor Xa) and thrombin; the drug heparin enhances the activity of antithrombin III. Steps in clot formation that are inhibited by heparin are shown in *red*. Dabigatran directly inhibits thrombin. **B.** Fibrinolytic process: Clots are dissolved. The step that is facilitated by the clot-dissolving drugs and by other agents is shown in *blue*.

blood vessels open and functional. Very high levels of plasmin are found in the lungs (which contain millions of tiny, easily injured capillaries) and in the uterus (which in pregnancy must maintain a constant blood flow for the developing fetus). The action of plasmin is evident in menstrual flow, in that clots do not form rapidly when the lining of the uterus is shed; the blood oozes slowly over a period of days.

Key Points

- Coagulation is the transformation of fluid blood into a solid state to seal breaks in the vascular system.
- The coagulation process involves vasoconstriction, platelet aggregation to form a plug, and intrinsic and extrinsic clot formation to plug any breaks in the system.
- The conversion of prothrombin to thrombin, which results in insoluble fibrin threads, is the final step of clot formation.
- To prevent the occlusion of blood vessels and the denying of blood to the tissues, a formed clot must be dissolved.
- The base of the clot-dissolving system is the conversion of plasminogen to plasmin (fibrinolysin) by several factors, including Hageman factor. Plasmin dissolves fibrin threads and resolves the clot.

Disorders Affecting Blood Coagulation

Disorders that directly affect the coagulation process fall into two main categories: (a) conditions that involve overproduction of clots, or thromboembolic disorders, and (b) conditions in which the clotting process is not working effectively, resulting in risk for excess bleeding or hemorrhagic disorders.

Thromboembolic Disorders

Thromboembolic disorders are medical conditions that involve the formation of thrombi resulting in decreased blood flow through or total occlusion of a blood vessel. These conditions are marked by the signs and symptoms of hypoxia, anoxia, or even necrosis in areas affected by the decreased blood flow. In some of these disorders, pieces of the thrombus, called emboli, can break off and travel through the CV system until they become lodged in a tiny vessel, plugging it up.

Conditions that predispose a person to the formation of clots and emboli are called thromboembolic disorders. Atherosclerotic CV disease is a common cause of damage and narrowing of blood vessels that can precipitate excessive thrombus accumulation. Infection and trauma can also damage the endothelial lining to facilitate more clotting. Blood is more likely to clot when there is slow blood flow or if the blood is especially viscous. There are also inherited conditions that increase clotting activity. For example, factor V Leiden is an inherited condition in which the person is resistant to the anticoagulant protein C. People with antiphospholipid syndrome have increased risk of thrombus due to production of antibodies that bind phospholipids and increase coagulation. These conditions that increase the risk of development of thrombi and emboli are often treated with antiplatelet, anticoagulant, and/or thrombolytic agents.

Hemorrhagic Disorders

Hemorrhagic disorders, in which excess bleeding occurs, are less common than thromboembolic disorders. These disorders include hemophilia, in which there is a genetic lack of clotting factors; liver disease, in which clotting factors and proteins needed for clotting are not produced; and thrombocytopenia, in which there is a low number of platelets in the blood. These disorders are treated with clotting factors and drugs that promote the coagulation process. Bleeding disorders may also need to be treated with blood transfusions.

Key Points

- Disorders that are directly related to the clotting process include thromboembolic disorders, in which too much clotting can lead to emboli and occlusion of blood vessels, and hemorrhagic disorders, including hemophilia, in which lack of efficient clotting can lead to excessive blood loss.

Drugs Affecting Clot Formation and Resolution

Drugs that affect clot formation include antiplatelet drugs, which alter platelet aggregation and the formation of the platelet plug; anticoagulants, which interfere with the clotting cascade and thrombin formation; and thrombolytic agents, which break down the thrombus or clot that has been formed by stimulating the plasmin system (Table 48.1). Box 48.2 discusses the interaction of herbal remedies with these agents.

Antiplatelet Agents

Antiplatelet agents decrease the formation of the platelet plug by decreasing the responsiveness of the platelets to stimuli that would cause them to stick and aggregate on a vessel wall. Antiplatelet agents available for use include abciximab (*ReoPro*), anagrelide (*Agrylin*), aspirin (generic), cilostazol (generic), clopidogrel (*Plavix*), dipyridamole (*Persantine*), eptifibatide (generic), prasugrel (*Effient*), ticagrelor (*Brilinta*), ticlopidine (generic), tirofiban (*Aggrastat*), and vorapaxar (*Zontivity*).

Table 48.1 *Drugs in Focus*: Drugs Affecting Clot Formation and Resolution

Drug Name	Usual Dosage	Usual Indications
Antiplatelet Agents		
abciximab (*ReoPro*)	0.25-mg/kg IV bolus 10–60 min before procedure, then continuous infusion of 10 mcg/kg/min for 12 h *Angina*: 0.25 mg/kg by IV bolus, then 10 mcg/kg/min IV for 18–24 h	Adjunct to percutaneous coronary intervention for the prevention of cardiac ischemic complications in patients undergoing percutaneous coronary intervention or in patients with unstable angina not responding to conventional medical therapy when percutaneous coronary intervention is planned within 24 hours
anagrelide (*Agrylin*)	0.5 mg PO q.i.d. or 1 mg PO b.i.d., may increase by 0.5 mg/d each week; maximum dose 10 mg/d or 2.5 mg as a single dose	Treatment of essential thrombocythemia to reduce elevated platelet count and decrease the risk of thrombosis
aspirin (*Durlaza*, *Vazalore*, and others)	Doses vary based on indication and formulation; administered PO	Reduction of the risk of death and MI in patients with chronic coronary artery disease, such as patients with a history of MI or unstable angina pectoris or with chronic stable angina; reduction of the risk of death and recurrent stroke in patients who have had an ischemic stroke or transient ischemic attack; also indicated for use as analgesic and fever reducer
cilostazol (generic)	100 mg PO b.i.d.	Reduction of symptoms of intermittent claudication, allowing increased walking distance in adults
clopidogrel (*Plavix*)	300-mg PO loading dose followed by 75 mg/d PO	Treatment of patients who are at risk for ischemic events; patients with a history of MI, peripheral artery disease, or ischemic stroke; and patients with acute coronary syndrome
dipyridamole (*Persantine*)	Dosing and route vary based on indication	Prevention of thromboembolism in patients with artificial heart valves when used in combination with warfarin; aids diagnosis of CAD in patients who cannot exercise; used in combination with aspirin to reduce the risk of stroke in patients who have had transient ischemia of the brain or completed ischemic stroke due to thrombosis
eptifibatide (generic)	180-mcg/kg IV bolus over 1–2 min ×1 or 2 times, then 2 mcg/kg/min IV; reduce dose for patients with renal impairment	Treatment of acute coronary syndrome; prevention of ischemic episodes in patients undergoing percutaneous coronary interventions
prasugrel (*Effient*)	60 mg PO loading dose then 10 mg/d PO; reduce dose if the patient weighs <60 kg	Reduction of thrombotic CV events (including stent thrombosis) in patients with acute coronary syndrome who are to be managed with percutaneous coronary intervention
ticagrelor (*Brilinta*)	180-mg PO loading dose then 60 or 90 mg PO b.i.d. with daily aspirin 325-mg loading dose, then 75–100 mg/d; exact dosing based on indication	Reduction of the risk of CV death, MI, and stroke in patients with ACS or a history of MI; of stent thrombosis in patients who have been stented for treatment of ACS; of a first MI or stroke in patients with CAD at high risk for such events; of stroke in patients with acute ischemic stroke (NIH Stroke Scale score ≤5) or high-risk TIA
ticlopidine (generic)	250 mg PO b.i.d.	Reduction of the risk of thrombotic stroke in patients with TIAs or history of stroke who are intolerant of aspirin therapy, and of in-stent stenosis when dosed with antiplatelet doses of aspirin
tirofiban (*Aggrastat*)	25 mcg/kg IV in 5 min followed by 0.15 mcg/kg/min for up to 18 h Modify for renal impairment	Treatment of acute coronary syndrome and prevention of cardiac ischemic events during percutaneous coronary intervention; used in combination with heparin
vorapaxar (*Zontivity*)	2.5 mg/d PO	Reduction of thrombotic CV events in patients with a history of MI or peripheral arterial disease

Table 48.1 ***Drugs in Focus:* Drugs Affecting Clot Formation and Resolution *(Continued)***

Drug Name	Usual Dosage	Usual Indications
Anticoagulants		
antithrombin (*Thrombate III*)	Dose must be calculated using body weight and baseline levels of antithrombin	Replacement in hereditary antithrombin III deficiency; treatment of patients with this deficiency who are to undergo surgery or obstetrical procedures that might put them at risk for thromboembolism
apixaban (*Eliquis*)	2.5–5 mg PO b.i.d.; 10 mg PO b.i.d. for first 7 days for treatment of DVT or PE	Reduction of the risk of stroke and systemic embolism in patients with nonvalvular AF; prevention and treatment of DVT and PE in patients who have undergone hip or knee replacement; treatment of DVT and PE and reduction of risk of recurrent DVT and PE
argatroban (*Acova*)	Dose varies based on indication and body weight	Treatment of thrombosis in HIT; anticoagulant in adult patients with or at risk for HIT undergoing percutaneous coronary intervention
betrixaban (*Bevyxxa*)	160-mg PO loading dose once, then 80 mg/d for 35–42 d	Prevention of venous thromboembolism in patients hospitalized and at risk for clotting
bivalirudin (*Angiomax*)	0.75-mg/kg IV bolus, then 1.75 mg/kg/h IV for duration of procedure and up to 4 h for some patients; 0.3-mg/kg additional bolus may be given based on ACT measured 5 min after initial bolus	Prevention of ischemic events in patients undergoing transluminal coronary angioplasty when used in combination with aspirin
dabigatran (*Pradaxa*)	150 mg PO b.i.d.; reduce dose if patient has renal impairment	Reduction of the risk of stroke and systemic embolism in patients with nonvalvular AF; prevention and treatment of DVT and PE
dalteparin (*Fragmin*)	Subcutaneous injections; dosing varies based on age and indication	Prophylaxis of ischemic complications of unstable angina and non—wave MI; prophylaxis of DVT in abdominal surgery, hip replacement surgery, or medical patients with severely restricted mobility during acute illness; treatment of symptomatic VTE to reduce the recurrence in adult patients with cancer; treatment of symptomatic VTE to reduce the recurrence in pediatric patients 1 month of age and older
desirudin (*Iprivask*)	15 mg by subcutaneous injection q12h beginning 5–15 min before surgery and continuing for 9–12 d	Prevention of DVT in patients undergoing elective hip replacement
edoxaban (*Savaysa*)	60 mg/d PO; 30 mg/d PO with renal impairment	Reduction of the risk of stroke and systemic embolism in patients with nonvalvular AF; treatment of DVT and PE
enoxaparin (*Lovenox*)	Subcutaneous injections; dosing varies based on indication and renal function	Prophylaxis of DVT in abdominal surgery, hip replacement surgery, knee replacement surgery, or medical patients with severely restricted mobility during acute illness; inpatient treatment of acute DVT with or without PE; outpatient treatment of acute DVT without PE; prophylaxis of ischemic complications of unstable angina and non–Q-wave MI; treatment of acute STEMI managed medically or with subsequent percutaneous coronary intervention
fondaparinux (*Arixtra*)	*Prevention:* 2.5 mg/d by subcutaneous injection starting 6–8 h after surgical closure and continuing for 5–9 d *Treatment:* 5–10 mg/d by subcutaneous injections for 5–9 d until INR 2–3	Prevention and treatment of venous thromboembolic events following surgery for hip fracture, hip replacement, or knee replacement; treatment of DVT or PE when used with warfarin
heparin (generic)	*Adult and pediatric*: Dose varies based on weight and indication	Prevention and treatment of venous thrombosis, PE, and AF with embolization; prevention of clotting in blood samples, dialysis, and venous tubing; treatment of DIC (see Box 48.3); adjunct in the treatment of MI and stroke

(continues on page 860)

Table 48.1 *Drugs in Focus:* **Drugs Affecting Clot Formation and Resolution** *(Continued)*

Drug Name	Usual Dosage	Usual Indications
protein C concentrate (*Ceprotin*)	100–120 IU/kg IV injection, then 60–80 IU/kg IV q6h for three doses *Maintenance:* 45–60 IU/kg IV q6–12h	Replacement therapy for congenital protein C deficiency for prevention and treatment of venous thrombosis and purpura fulminans
rivaroxaban (*Xarelto*)	Oral dosing; dose and frequency vary based on indication	Prevention of DVTs that may lead to PE in patients undergoing knee or hip replacement surgery; reduction of risk of recurrent DVT or PE; reduction of the risk of stroke and systemic embolism in nonvalvular atrial fibrillation; treatment of DVT and PE; reduction of the risk of major CV events in patients with chronic CAD or PAD
warfarin (*Jantoven*)	PO dosing based on INR, individualized per patient and indication	Treatment of patients with AF, artificial heart valves, or valvular damage that makes the patient susceptible to thrombus and embolus formation; prevention and treatment of venous thrombosis, PE, embolus with AF, and systemic emboli after MI
Thrombolytic Agents		
alteplase (*Activase*)	IV administration; dosing varies based on indication	Treatment of MI, acute PE, and acute ischemic stroke; restoration of function in occluded central venous access devices
reteplase (*Retavase*)	10 IU + 10 IU double-bolus IV, each over 2 min, 30 min apart	Treatment of coronary artery thrombosis associated with an acute MI
tenecteplase (*TNKase*)	30–50 mg IV over 5 s; based on patient weight	Reduction of mortality associated with acute MI
Anticoagulant Adjunctive Therapy		
coagulation factor Xa (recombinant) (*Andexxa*)	IV dosing based on dose of oral anticoagulant and timing of last dose; dosed as IV bolus and then continuous infusion for up to 2 hours	Reversal of anticoagulation due to life-threatening or uncontrolled bleeding in patients treated with rivaroxaban or apixaban
idarucizumab (*Praxbind*)	5 g IV	Reversal of the anticoagulant effects of dabigatran as needed due to emergency surgery/urgent procedures and/or life-threatening or uncontrolled bleeding in patients treated with *Pradaxa*
protamine sulfate (generic)	1 mg IV neutralized 90–115 USP units of heparin; dose based on specific overdose	Treatment of heparin overdose
prothrombin complex concentrate (*Kcentra*)	25–50 units/kg IV based on INR	Treatment of warfarin-related bleeding
vitamin K (generic)	2.5–10 mg orally or IV; may be repeated in 6–8 h based on INR	Treatment of anticoagulant-induced prothrombin deficiency
Hemorrheologic Agent		
pentoxifylline (generic)	400 mg PO t.i.d. with meals	Treatment of intermittent claudication to improve function and reduce symptoms; improve blood flow in vascular diseases

MI, myocardial infarction; CV, cardiovascular; ACS, acute coronary syndrome; TIA, transient ischemic attack; CAD, coronary artery disease; AF, atrial fibrillation; DVT, deep vein thrombosis; PE, pulmonary embolism; HIT, heparin-induced thrombocytopenia; VTE, venous thromboembolism; STEMI, heparin-induced thrombocytopenia; DIC, disseminated intravascular coagulation; PAD, peripheral artery disease; INR, international normalized ratio.

Box 48.2 Focus on Herbal and Alternative Therapies

Many herbal therapies can cause problems when used with drugs that affect blood coagulation. Patients taking these drugs should be cautioned to avoid angelica, cat's claw, chamomile, chondroitin, feverfew, garlic, ginkgo, goldenseal, grape seed extract, green leaf tea, horse chestnut seed, psyllium, and turmeric. If a patient who is taking an anticoagulant presents with increased bleeding and no other interaction or cause is found, question the patient about the possibility of use of herbal therapies.

Therapeutic Actions and Indications

Antiplatelet agents inhibit platelet adhesion and aggregation by blocking receptor sites on the platelet membrane, preventing platelet–platelet interaction or the interaction of platelets with other clotting chemicals. One drug, anagrelide, blocks the production of platelets in the bone marrow. These agents are used effectively to treat CV diseases that are prone to producing occluded vessels, for the maintenance of venous and arterial grafts, to prevent cerebrovascular occlusion, for treatment of peripheral arterial disease, and as adjuncts to thrombolytic therapy in the treatment of myocardial infarction (MI) and the prevention of reinfarction after MI. The prescriber's choice of drug depends on the intended use and the patient's tolerance of the associated adverse effects. See Table 48.1 for usual indications for each of these agents.

Pharmacokinetics

Abciximab, eptifibatide, and tirofiban are administered intravenously (IV). Antiplatelet agents that are administered orally include anagrelide, aspirin, cilostazol, clopidogrel, prasugrel, ticagrelor, ticlopidine, and vorapaxar. Dipyridamole is used orally or as an IV agent.

These drugs are generally well absorbed and highly bound to plasma proteins. They are metabolized in the liver and excreted in the urine, and they tend to enter human milk (see "Contraindications and Cautions").

Contraindications and Cautions

Antiplatelet agents are contraindicated in the presence of allergy to the specific drug to avoid hypersensitivity reactions. Caution should be used in the presence of any known bleeding disorder or active bleeding because of the risk of excessive blood loss, recent surgery because of the risk of increased bleeding in unhealed vessels, and closed head injuries because of the risk of bleeding in the brain.

The safety evidence for these medications when used during pregnancy varies. They all increase risk of bleeding; however, for some indications (like acute MI or ischemic stroke), the maternal and fetal benefit can be greater than the risks. Due to lack of evidence of exact risks for most of these medications, caution should be used during pregnancy and lactation.

Anagrelide should be used with caution with any history of thrombocytopenia because it decreases the production of platelets in the bone marrow. Platelet levels should be checked regularly to monitor for thrombocytopenia if a patient is on this drug.

Clopidogrel (*Plavix*) has a boxed warning for people who poorly metabolize the liver enzyme CYP2C19. The effectiveness of the medication is dependent on the conversion to an active form by the cytochrome P450 system in the liver but primarily the enzyme CYP2C19. Therefore, people who poorly metabolize CYP2C19 may not benefit from the effect of clopidogrel. It is recommended that a different antiplatelet medication be used in this population of people.

There is a boxed warning discouraging use of vorapaxar in patients with a history of stroke, transient ischemic attack (TIA), intracranial bleeding, or other active bleeding. Caution should be used with ticlopidine due to risk of life-threatening hematological adverse reactions like neutropenia/agranulocytosis, thrombotic thrombocytopenic purpura, and aplastic anemia. Patients should be monitored for at least the first 3 months of therapy.

Ticagrelor has a boxed warning regarding risk of fatal bleeding. It should not be used in patients with active bleeding or history of intracranial hemorrhage. It should not be started in patients who will undergo coronary artery bypass graft surgery. Abrupt stopping of the medication can increase the risk of CV events, so when possible minor adverse effects or bleeding should be managed while the patient continues the medication.

Prasugrel has a boxed warning regarding the risk of significant, even fatal, bleeding. It should not be used in patients with active bleeding or history of ischemic stroke or transient ischemic stroke. It should not be used in patients who are undergoing coronary artery bypass graft surgery. There should be extreme caution if used in patients aged 75 years or older or of low body weight (<60 kg) due to increased risk of bleeding. Abrupt discontinuation of prasugrel increases risk of CV events, so caution should be used when discontinuing the medication.

Adverse Effects

The most common adverse effect seen with these drugs is bleeding, which often occurs as increased bruising and bleeding while brushing the teeth. Other common problems include headache, dizziness, and weakness; the cause of these reactions is not understood (Fig. 48.5). Nausea and gastrointestinal (GI) distress may occur because of the direct irritating effects of the oral drug on the GI tract. Skin rash, another common effect, may be related to direct drug effects on the dermis. Aspirin is associated with GI irritation and increased risk of ulcers; in high doses, it can cause tinnitus.

Clinically Important Drug–Drug Interactions

The risk of excessive bleeding increases if any of these drugs is combined with another drug that affects blood clotting.

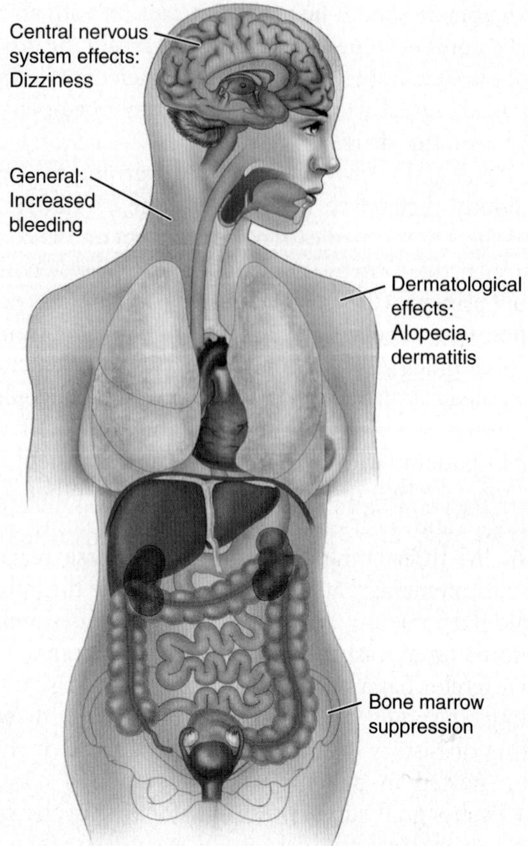

FIGURE 48.5 Variety of adverse effects and toxicities associated with drugs affecting blood coagulation.

Prototype Summary: Aspirin

Indications: Reduction of the risk of death and MI in patients with chronic coronary artery disease, such as patients with a history of MI or unstable angina pectoris or with chronic stable angina; reduction of the risk of death and recurrent stroke in patients who have had an ischemic stroke or transient ischemic attack; also indicated for use as analgesic and fever reducer.

Actions: Inhibits prostaglandin synthesis resulting in inhibition of platelet aggregation. Inhibits platelet aggregation by inactivating cyclooxygenase-1 (COX-1), which prevents conversion of arachidonic acid to thromboxane A2. The lack of thromboxane A2 inhibits platelet aggregation.

Pharmacokinetics:

Route	Onset	Peak	Duration
Oral	5–30 min	0.25–2 h	3–6 h

$T_{1/2}$: 15 minutes to 12 hours, metabolized in the liver and excreted in the urine.

Adverse Effects: Acute aspirin toxicity with hyperpnea, possibly leading to fever, coma, and CV collapse; nausea; dyspepsia; heartburn; epigastric discomfort; GI bleeding; occult blood loss; dizziness; tinnitus; difficulty hearing; and anaphylactoid reaction.

Nursing Considerations for Patients Receiving Antiplatelet Agents

Assessment: History and Examination

- Assess for the following conditions, which could be cautions or contraindications to use of the drug: any known allergies to these drugs because of the risk of hypersensitivity reactions; pregnancy or lactation because of the unknown adverse effects on the patient, fetus, or neonate; bleeding disorders, recent surgery, or closed head injury because of the potential for excessive bleeding; and use of other drugs or herbs that could affect bleeding because of the risk of excessive bleeding.
- Assess baseline status before beginning therapy to determine any potential adverse effects. This includes body temperature; skin color, lesions, and temperature; affect, orientation, and reflexes; pulse, blood pressure, and perfusion; respirations and adventitious sounds; complete blood count (CBC); and clotting studies (Table 48.2).

Nursing Conclusions

Nursing conclusions related to drug therapy might include the following:

- Injury risk related to bleeding effects or central nervous system (CNS) effects
- Impaired comfort related to GI or CNS effects
- Knowledge deficit regarding drug therapy

Planning

- The patient will receive the best therapeutic effect from the drug therapy.
- The patient will have limited adverse effects from the drug therapy.
- The patient will have an understanding of the drug therapy, adverse effects to anticipate, and measures to relieve discomfort and improve safety.

Intervention With Rationale

- Provide small, frequent meals to relieve GI discomfort if GI upset is a problem.
- Provide comfort measures and analgesia for headache to relieve pain and improve patient adherence to the drug regimen.
- Suggest safety measures, including the use of an electric razor and avoidance of contact sports, to decrease the risk of bleeding.
- Monitor platelet count if the patient is using anagrelide to detect thrombocytopenia and increased risk of bleeding.
- Provide increased precautions against bleeding during invasive procedures; use pressure dressings and ice to decrease excessive blood loss caused by anticoagulation.

- Mark the chart of any patient receiving this drug to alert medical staff that there is a potential for increased bleeding.
- Provide thorough patient teaching, including the name of the drug, dosage prescribed, measures to avoid adverse effects, warning signs of problems, the need for periodic monitoring and evaluation, and the need to wear or carry MedicAlert identification, to enhance patient knowledge about drug therapy and to promote adherence to the drug regimen.
- Offer support and encouragement to help the patient deal with the diagnosis and the drug regimen.

Evaluation

- Monitor patient response to the drug (increased bleeding time, prevention of occlusive events).
- Monitor for adverse effects (bleeding, GI upset, dizziness, headache).
- Evaluate the effectiveness of the teaching plan (patient can name drug, dosage, adverse effects to watch for, and specific measures to avoid them; patient understands the importance of continued follow-up).
- Monitor the effectiveness of comfort measures and adherence to the regimen.

Anticoagulants

Anticoagulants are drugs that interfere with the normal coagulation process by interfering with the clotting cascade and thrombin formation. Drugs in this class include antithrombin III (*Thrombate III*); argatroban (generic); bivalirudin (*Angiomax*); dalteparin (*Fragmin*), desirudin (*Iprivask*); enoxaparin (*Lovenox*), fondaparinux (*Arixtra*); heparin (generic); warfarin (*Jantoven*); the direct acting oral anticoagulants dabigatran (*Pradaxa*), rivaroxaban (*Xarelto*), apixaban (*Eliquis*), betrixaban (*Bevyxxa*), and edoxaban (*Savaysa*); and protein C concentrate (*Ceprotin*).

Therapeutic Actions and Indications

Anticoagulants interfere with the normal cascade of events involved in the clotting process. Warfarin causes a decrease in the production of vitamin K–dependent clotting factors in the liver. The eventual effect is a depletion of these clotting factors and an extension of clotting time. It is used to maintain a state of anticoagulation in situations in which the patient is susceptible to potentially dangerous clot formation (see Table 48.1 for usual indications for warfarin). See the "Critical Thinking Scenario" for additional nursing care for the patient taking warfarin.

Newer oral drugs include betrixaban, dabigatran, rivaroxaban, apixaban, and edoxaban. Dabigatran (*Pradaxa*) directly inhibits thrombin, which blocks the last step to clot formation. It is approved to reduce the risk of stroke and systemic embolism in patients with nonvalvular atrial fibrillation (AF), for the treatment of deep vein thrombosis (DVT) and pulmonary embolism (PE) in patients treated with a parenteral anticoagulant for 5 to 10 days, and for the prevention of recurrence of DVT and PE. Rivaroxaban (*Xarelto*), apixaban (*Eliquis*), and edoxaban (*Savaysa*) are factor Xa inhibitors that stop the coagulation cascade at this early step. They are approved for prevention of DVT (which might lead to PE), in patients undergoing knee or hip replacement surgery, for prevention of stroke in patients with nonvalvular AF, and for the prevention and treatment of DVT and PE.

Betrixaban (*Bevyxxa*) is a factor Xa inhibitor that is indicated for prevention of venous thromboembolism in hospitalized patients at risk for clotting.

Heparin, argatroban, desirudin, and bivalirudin block the formation of thrombin from prothrombin. The usual indications for heparin include acute treatment and prevention of venous thrombosis and PE, treatment of AF with embolization, prevention of clotting in blood samples and in dialysis and venous tubing, and diagnosis and treatment of disseminated intravascular coagulation (DIC) (Box 48.3). Because heparin must be injected, it is often not the drug of choice for outpatients, who would be responsible for injecting the drug several times during the day. Patients may be started on heparin in an acute situation and then switched to an oral anticoagulant.

Table 48.2 Review of Clotting Studies

Test	Measure	Therapeutic Range	Uses
aPPT PTT	Activity of intrinsic pathway of coagulation	1.5–2.5 times baseline	Dose adjustment for heparin, low molecular weight heparins, desirudin, argatroban, bivalirudin, dabigatran, rivaroxaban
INR	Standardized measure of prothrombin levels	2–3.5	Warfarin dose adjustment, fondaparinux dose adjustment
PT	Time required for clotting to occur; extrinsic pathway activity	1.3–1.5	No longer used clinically

aPPT, activated partial thromboplastin time; PPT, partial thromboplastin time; INR, international normalized ratio; PT, prothrombin time.

BOX 48.3

Understanding Disseminated Intravascular Coagulation

Disseminated intravascular coagulation (DIC) is a syndrome in which bleeding and thrombosis are found together. It can occur as a complication of many problems, including severe infection with septic shock, traumatic childbirth or abortion, and massive injuries. In these disorders, local tissue damage causes the release of coagulation-stimulating substances into the circulation. These substances then stimulate the coagulation process, causing fibrin clot formation in small vessels in the lungs, kidneys, brain, and other organs. This continuing reaction consumes excessive amounts of fibrinogen, other clotting factors, and platelets. The end result is increased bleeding. In essence, the patient clots too much, resulting in the possibility of bleeding to death.

The first step in treating this disorder is to control the problem that initially precipitated it. For example, treating the infection, performing dilation and curettage to clear the uterus, or stabilizing injuries can help stop this continuing process. Whole-blood infusions or the infusion of fibrinogen may be used to buy some time until the patient is stable and can form clotting factors again. There are associated problems with giving whole blood (e.g., development of antibodies and having transfusion reactions), and there is a risk that fibrinogen may set off further intravascular clotting. Paradoxically, the treatment of choice for DIC is the anticoagulant heparin. Heparin prevents the clotting phase from being completed, thus inhibiting the breakdown of fibrinogen. It may also help avoid hemorrhage by preventing the body from depleting its entire store of coagulation factors.

Because heparin is usually administered to prevent blood clotting and the adverse effects that are monitored with heparin therapy include signs of bleeding, it can be challenging for the nursing staff to feel comfortable administering heparin to a patient who is bleeding to death. Understanding the disease process can help alleviate any doubts about the treatment.

Dalteparin and enoxaparin are low molecular weight heparins. These drugs inhibit thrombus and clot formation by blocking factors Xa and IIa. Because of the size and nature of the molecules, these drugs do not greatly affect thrombin, clotting, or PT; therefore, they cause fewer systemic adverse effects. They also have been found to block angiogenesis, the process that allows cancer cells to develop new blood vessels. These drugs are indicated for specific uses in the prevention of clots and emboli formation after certain surgeries or prolonged bed rest.

Antithrombin and protein C concentrate are blood products that are used for replacement in specific genetic deficiencies. Antithrombin interferes with the formation of thrombin from prothrombin; it is a naturally occurring anticoagulant and a natural safety feature in the clotting system. Fondaparinux inhibits factor Xa and blocks the clotting cascade to prevent clot formation. It is supplied in prefilled syringes, making it more convenient for patients who self-administer the drug at home. Many of the parenteral medications can be used concurrently with warfarin while the patient's INR is subtherapeutic.

Pharmacokinetics

Heparin is injected IV or subcutaneously and has an almost immediate onset of action. It is excreted in the urine. The low molecular weight heparins (dalteparin and enoxaparin) are administered by subcutaneous injection. Warfarin, dabigatran, apixaban, edoxaban, betrixaban, and rivaroxaban are available as oral formulations. Warfarin can also be administered IV. All other drugs in this class are given parenterally. Warfarin is readily absorbed through the GI tract, metabolized in the liver, and excreted in the urine and feces. Warfarin's onset of action is about 3 days; its effects last for 4 to 5 days. Because of the time delay, warfarin is not the drug of choice in an acute situation, but it is convenient and useful for prolonged effects. Apixaban, betrixaban, dabigatran, edoxaban, and rivaroxaban are all well absorbed orally and have a rapid onset of action. These medications are metabolized through the liver and kidneys to varying degrees. They have relatively short half-lives, which is beneficial for patients undergoing procedures.

Because antithrombin and protein C concentrate are exogenous forms of naturally occurring anticoagulants, the body handles them in the same way that it handles the naturally occurring products. Argatroban is given as a continuous IV infusion. Desirudin and fondaparinux are absorbed quickly from subcutaneous sites and metabolized and excreted by the kidneys. Bivalirudin is given IV and is excreted through the kidneys.

Contraindications and Cautions

The anticoagulants are contraindicated in the presence of known allergy to the drugs to avoid hypersensitivity reactions. They also should not be used with any conditions that could be compromised by increased bleeding tendencies, including hemorrhagic disorders, recent trauma, spinal puncture (some of the oral anticoagulants have boxed warnings of the risk of hemorrhage with spinal puncture or neuraxial anesthesia), GI ulcers, recent surgery, intrauterine device placement, tuberculosis, presence of indwelling catheters, and threatened abortion. Warfarin is contraindicated for patients who are pregnant unless they need anticoagulation due to artificial heart valve. Heparin and the low molecular weight heparins are generally safer for anticoagulation in pregnant patients. Caution should be used with administering anticoagulants to patients with renal or hepatic disease, which could interfere with the metabolism and effectiveness of these drugs.

CRITICAL THINKING SCENARIO
Oral Anticoagulant Therapy

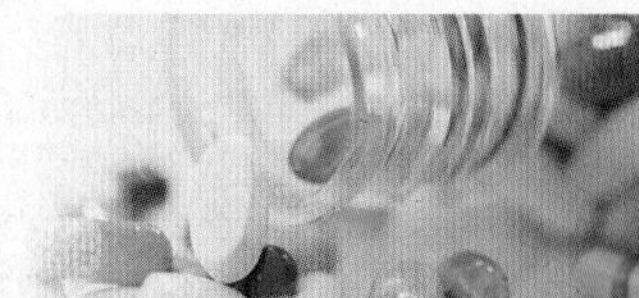

THE SITUATION

G.R. is a 68-year-old patient with a history of severe mitral valve disease who had a prosthetic mitral valve replacement 5 years ago. For the last several years following the surgery, G.R. has been doing well. However, on a recent visit to their physician, G.R. disclosed that they had been experiencing periods of breathlessness, palpitations, and dizziness. Tests showed that G.R. was having frequent periods of AF with a heart rate of up to 140 beats/min. Because of the danger of emboli as a result of G.R.'s valve disease and the bouts of AF, warfarin therapy was initiated.

CRITICAL THINKING

What nursing interventions should be done at this point? Think about why emboli form when the atria fibrillate.
Stabilizing G.R. on warfarin may take several weeks of blood tests and dose adjustments.
How can this process be made easier?
What patient teaching points should be covered with G.R. to ensure that they are protected from emboli and do not experience excessive bleeding?

DISCUSSION

G.R.'s situation is complex. They have a progressive degenerative valve disease that without surgery usually leads to heart failure (HF) and frequently to other complications. Since G.R. has developed new AF, the valve function should be evaluated with an echocardiogram. G.R. may be experiencing this new AF because of irritation to the atrial cells caused by the damaged mitral valve and associated swelling and scarring. If this is the case, an anticoagulant will help protect G.R. against emboli, which form in the auricles when blood pools there while the atria are fibrillating. There is less chance of emboli formation if clotting is slowed.

G.R. will need extensive teaching about warfarin, including the need for frequent blood tests, the list of potential drug–drug interactions, the importance of being alert to the many factors that can affect dose needs (including illness and diet), and how to monitor for subtle blood loss. G.R. may need teaching about the reason that this oral anticoagulant was selected. Media campaigns and advertising widely urge the use of the other oral agents. This can also be a good opportunity to review teaching about valvular disease and HF and to answer any questions that G.R. might have about how all of these things interrelate. If possible, it would be useful to teach G.R. or a responsible caregiver how to take a pulse so that G.R. can be alerted to potential arrhythmias and avert problems before they begin. It also would be a good idea to check on support services for G.R. to ensure that their blood tests can be done and that their response to the drug is monitored carefully.

NURSING CARE GUIDE FOR G.R.: WARFARIN

Assessment: History and Examination

Assess G.R.'s health history for allergies to warfarin, subacute bacterial endocarditis, hemorrhagic disorders, renal or hepatic dysfunction, gastric ulcers, or severe trauma. Also, assess concurrent use of numerous drugs and herbal therapies due to a variety of interactions.
Focus the physical examination on the following areas:
CV: blood pressure, pulse, perfusion, and baseline electrocardiogram (ECG)
CNS: orientation, affect, reflexes, and vision
Skin: color, lesions, and texture
Respiratory system: respiratory rate and character and adventitious sounds
GI: abdominal examination and guaiac stool test results (for occult blood)
Laboratory tests: liver and renal function tests, CBC, prothrombin time (PT), and international normalized ratio (INR)

Nursing Conclusions

Altered tissue perfusion (total body) related to change in homeostasis
Injury risk related to anticoagulant effects
Knowledge deficit regarding drug therapy

Planning

The patient will receive the best therapeutic effect from the drug therapy.
The patient will have limited adverse effects from the drug therapy.
The patient will have an understanding of the drug therapy, adverse effects to anticipate, and measures to relieve discomfort and improve safety.

Intervention

Ensure proper administration of the drug.
Provide comfort and safety measures, protection from injury during invasive and other procedures, standby antidotes (e.g., vitamin K), and careful skin care.
Provide support and reassurance to deal with drug effects.
Provide patient teaching regarding drug, dosage, adverse effects, what to report, and safety precautions.

(continues on page 866)

Evaluation

Evaluate drug effects: increased bleeding times or INR 2 to 3.

Monitor for adverse effects: bleeding, alopecia, rash, GI upset, and excessive bleeding.

Monitor for drug–drug interactions (numerous).

Evaluate the effectiveness of the patient teaching program and comfort and safety measures.

PATIENT TEACHING FOR G.R.

- An anticoagulant slows the body's normal blood-clotting processes to prevent harmful blood clots from forming. This type of drug is often called a "blood thinner"; however, it cannot dissolve any clots that have already formed and does not make your blood thin.
- *Never* change any medication that you are taking—such as adding or stopping another drug, taking a new over-the-counter medication or herbal agent, or stopping one that you have been taking regularly—without consulting your health care provider. Many other drugs and herbs affect the way that your anticoagulant works; starting or stopping another drug can cause excessive bleeding or interfere with the desired effects of the drug.
  - The most common and concerning adverse effect is increased risk of bleeding. Do not engage in contact sports/activities. It is recommended that you use an electric razor to decrease risk of cuts. Monitor for GI bleeding by noting if your stool is dark black or has bloody streaks. If you have a cut, apply constant firm pressure; the wound will bleed/ooze longer when taking this medication.
- Report any of the following to your health care provider: unusual bleeding (e.g., when brushing your teeth, excessive bleeding from an injury, excessive bruising); black or tarry stools; cloudy or dark urine; sore throat, fever, or chills; and severe headache or dizziness.
- Tell any doctor, nurse, or other health care provider involved in your care that you are taking this drug. You should carry or wear medical identification stating that you are taking this drug to alert emergency medical personnel that you are at increased risk for bleeding.
- Avoid situations in which you could be easily injured—for example, engaging in contact sports or games with children or using a straight razor.
- Keep this drug, and all medications, out of the reach of children.
- Avoid the use of over-the-counter medications and herbal agents while you are taking this drug. If you feel that you need one of these, consult your health care provider for the best choice. Many of these drugs and herbs can interfere with your anticoagulant.
- Schedule regular, periodic blood tests while you are taking this drug to monitor the effects of the drug on your body and adjust your dose as needed.

Adverse Effects

The most commonly encountered adverse effect of anticoagulants is bleeding, ranging from bleeding gums with tooth brushing to severe internal hemorrhage. Patients need teaching about administration routes and frequencies, disposal of syringes (if applicable), and signs of bleeding to watch for. Periodic blood tests may be needed to assess the effects of the drug on the body. With many of these medications, clotting times are monitored frequently in the acute setting. INR levels are monitored regularly in patients taking warfarin. There are times when the effects of warfarin must be reversed quickly. Box 48.4 discusses vitamin K and prothrombin complex concentrate. The other oral anticoagulants do not have required monitoring. Table 48.2 reviews clotting studies that should be monitored. The newer oral anticoagulants are not indicated for use in patients with artificial heart valves, which can become obstructed, due to lack of research on these medications in this patient population. Several of the newer oral anticoagulants have a boxed warning of the risk for rebound thromboembolic events when the drugs are suddenly stopped. This is a concern if a patient forgets to get a refill of the drug, is traveling and runs out of the drug, or is instructed to stop the medication for a

Box 48.4 Focus on Safe Medication Administration

Injectable and oral vitamin K are used to reverse the effects of warfarin. Vitamin K promotes the liver synthesis of several clotting factors. When these pathways have been inhibited by warfarin, clotting time is increased. If an increased level of vitamin K is provided, more of these factors are produced, and the clotting time can be brought back within a normal range. Because of the way in which vitamin K exerts its effects on clotting, there is a delay of up to 24 hours from the time the drug is given until some change can be seen. This occurs because there is no direct effect on the warfarin but rather an increased stimulation of the liver, which must then produce the clotting factors. The usual dose for the treatment of anticoagulant-induced prothrombin deficiency is 2.5 to 10 mg orally or IV. Ab INR response within 6 to 8 hours after parenteral doses or 12 to 48 hours after oral doses will determine the need for a repeat dose. If a response is not seen and the patient is bleeding excessively, fresh frozen plasma or an infusion of whole blood may be needed. In 2014, a quick reversal agent was approved for warfarin overdose. Prothrombin complex concentrate (*Kcentra*), a blood product, is infused IV to supply the clotting factors needed to restore hemostatic balance. The IV dosing is based on the patient's INR.

Box 48.5 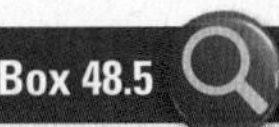 **Focus on Safe Medication Administration**

In cases of a heparin overdose, the antidote is protamine sulfate (generic). This strongly basic protein drug forms stable salts with heparin as soon as the two drugs come in contact, immediately reversing heparin's anticoagulant effects. Paradoxically, if protamine is given to a patient who has not received heparin, it has anticoagulant effects. The dose is determined by the amount of heparin that was given and the time that elapsed since then. A dose of 1-mg IV protamine neutralizes 90 units of heparin derived from lung tissue or 110 USP of heparin derived from the intestinal mucosa. The drug must be administered slowly, not to exceed 50 mg IV in any 10-minute period. Care must be taken to calculate the amount of heparin that has been given to the patient. Potentially, fatal anaphylactic reactions have been reported with the use of protamine sulfate, so life support equipment should be readily available when it is used.

planned procedure. Patient selection must be done carefully, and teaching needs to be explicit. These drugs also have a boxed warning about the risk for spinal and epidural hematoma if used during spinal anesthesia or spinal puncture; permanent paralysis has occurred. Heparin-induced thrombocytopenia (antibody-included low platelet counts and increased development of thrombi) is an important side effect for which to monitor in patients taking heparin products. Box 48.5 discusses the treatment of heparin overdose.

Clinically Important Drug–Drug Interactions

Increased bleeding can occur if anticoagulants are combined and/or administered with other medications or substances that increase bleeding risk.

Warfarin has documented drug–drug interactions with a vast number of other drugs. It is a wise practice to never add or take away a drug from the regimen of a patient receiving warfarin without careful patient monitoring and adjustment of the warfarin dose to prevent serious adverse effects. Because of the many factors that can affect the therapeutic levels of warfarin, it is often difficult to reach a stable level and maintain that level. When starting therapy and with new medication changes, the INR needs to be monitored regularly. The warfarin dose can be changed based on the INR.

Dabigatran, edoxaban, apixaban, and rivaroxaban must be used with caution with antifungals, erythromycin, ritonavir, phenytoin, and rifampin because of alterations in metabolism. P-glycoprotein inhibitors like amiodarone, azithromycin, verapamil, ketoconazole, and clarithromycin can result in higher plasma levels of betrixaban. All of these drugs should be used with caution if combined with any other drugs or herbs known to increase or decrease clotting effects. It is always important to check for drug–drug interactions with any of these anticoagulant medications.

P Prototype Summary: Heparin

Indications: Prevention and treatment of venous thrombosis and PE, treatment of AF with embolization, treatment of DIC, prevention of clotting in blood samples and heparin lock sets, adjunct in the treatment of MI and stroke.

Actions: Inhibits thrombus and clot production by blocking the conversion of prothrombin to thrombin and fibrinogen to fibrin.

Pharmacokinetics:

Route	Onset	Peak	Duration
IV	Immediate	Minutes	2–6 h
Subcutaneous	20–60 min	2–4 h	8–12 h

$T_{1/2}$: 30 to 180 minutes, metabolized in the cells and excreted in the urine.

Adverse Effects: Bleeding, epidural or spinal hematoma, heparin-induced thrombocytopenia, hypersensitivity reactions, loss of hair, bruising, chills, fever, osteoporosis, suppression of renal function (with long-term use).

Nursing Considerations for Patients Receiving Anticoagulants

Assessment: History and Examination

- Assess for any known allergies to these drugs to avoid potential hypersensitivity reactions. Screen for conditions that could be exacerbated by increased bleeding tendencies, including hemorrhagic disorders, recent trauma, spinal puncture, GI ulcers, recent surgery, intrauterine device placement, tuberculosis, presence of indwelling catheters, and threatened abortion. Also, screen for pregnancy and ensure that benefits outweigh any potential risks (contraindicated with warfarin unless the patient has a mechanical heart valve); lactation because of the potential for risks to the baby (the use of heparin is suggested if an anticoagulant is needed during lactation); renal or hepatic disease, which could interfere with the metabolism, excretion, and effectiveness of these drugs; HF; thyrotoxicosis; senility or psychosis because of the potential for unexpected effects; and diarrhea or fever, which could alter the normal clotting process.
- Assess baseline status before beginning therapy to determine any potential adverse effects. This includes body temperature; skin color, lesions, and temperature; affect, orientation, and reflexes; pulse, blood pressure, and perfusion; respirations and adventitious sounds; clotting studies, renal and hepatic function tests, CBC, and stool guaiac; and ECG, if appropriate.

(continues on page 868)

Nursing Conclusions

Nursing conclusions related to drug therapy might include the following:

- Injury risk related to bleeding effects and bone marrow depression
- Altered tissue perfusion (total body) related to blood loss if bleeding
- Knowledge deficit regarding drug therapy

Planning

- The patient will receive the best therapeutic effect from the drug therapy.
- The patient will have limited adverse effects from the drug therapy.
- The patient will have an understanding of the drug therapy, adverse effects to anticipate, and measures to relieve discomfort and improve safety.

Intervention With Rationale

- Evaluate for therapeutic effects of warfarin—often INR of 2 to 3 but may vary based on indication.
- Evaluate for therapeutic effects of heparin—often whole-blood clotting time (WBCT) of 2.5 to 3 times the control value or activated partial thromboplastin time (APTT) of 1.5 to 3 times the control value—to evaluate the effectiveness of the drug dose.
- Evaluate the patient regularly for any sign of blood loss (petechiae, bleeding gums, bruises, dark-colored stools, dark-colored urine) to evaluate the safety of the drug dose and to determine the need to consult with the prescriber if bleeding becomes apparent.
- Establish safety precautions to protect the patient from injury.
- Provide safety measures, such as the use of an electric razor and avoidance of contact sports, to decrease the risk of bleeding.
- Provide increased precautions against bleeding during invasive procedures; use pressure dressings; avoid IM injections if possible; and do not rub subcutaneous injection sites because the state of anticoagulation increases the risk of blood loss.
- Maintain antidotes on standby (protamine sulfate for heparin, vitamin K or prothrombin complex concentrate for warfarin) in case of overdose or significant bleeding.
- Monitor for clotting if apixaban, edoxaban, dabigatran, or rivaroxaban is stopped suddenly for any reason other than pathological bleeding because of the risk of thromboembolic events.
- Monitor the patient carefully when any drug or herb is added to or withdrawn from the drug regimen of a patient taking warfarin because of the risk of drug–drug interactions that would change the effectiveness of the anticoagulant.
- Make sure that the patient receives regular follow-up and monitoring, including measurement of clotting times (when applicable), to ensure maximum therapeutic effects.
- Provide thorough patient teaching, including the name of the drug, dosage prescribed, measures to avoid adverse effects, warning signs of problems, the need for periodic monitoring and evaluation, and the need to wear or carry MedicAlert identification, to enhance patient knowledge about drug therapy and to promote adherence to the drug regimen.
- Offer support and encouragement to help the patient deal with the diagnosis and the drug regimen.

Evaluation

- Monitor patient response to the drug: increased bleeding time (warfarin, INR of 2 to 3; heparin, WBCT of 2.5 to 3 times the control value or APTT of 1.5 to 3 times the control value).
- Monitor for adverse effects (bleeding, low platelet counts, alopecia, GI upset, rash).
- Evaluate the effectiveness of the teaching plan (patient can name drug, dosage, adverse effects to watch for, and specific measures to avoid them; the patient understands the importance of continued follow-up).
- Monitor the effectiveness of comfort measures and adherence to the regimen.

Thrombolytic Agents

Thrombolytic agents break down the thrombus that has been formed by stimulating the plasmin system. This process is called clot resolution. Thrombolytic agents include alteplase (*Activase*), reteplase (*Retavase*), and tenecteplase (*TNKase*).

Therapeutic Actions and Indications

If a thrombus has already formed in a vessel (e.g., during an acute MI, ischemic stroke, or PE), it may be necessary to dissolve that clot to open the vessel and restore blood flow to the dependent tissue. All of the drugs that are available for this purpose work to activate the natural anticlotting system—conversion of plasminogen to plasmin. They are tissue plasminogen activators. The activation of this system breaks down fibrin threads and dissolves any formed clot. The thrombolytics are effective only if the patient has plasminogen in the plasma. See Table 48.1 for usual indications for each of these agents.

Pharmacokinetics

These drugs are given IV and are cleared from the body after liver metabolism. They cross the placenta, but it is not known whether they enter human milk (see "Contraindications and Cautions").

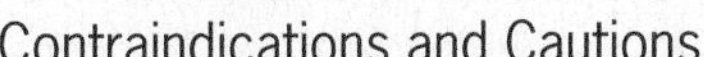

Contraindications and Cautions

The use of thrombolytic agents is contraindicated in the presence of allergy to any of these drugs to prevent hypersensitivity reactions. Also, they should be used with extreme caution with any condition that could be worsened by the dissolution of clots, including recent surgery, active internal bleeding, cerebrovascular accident (CVA) within the last 3 months unless symptoms started within the last few hours, aneurysm, obstetrical delivery, organ biopsy, recent serious GI bleeding, rupture of a noncompressible blood vessel, recent major trauma (including cardiopulmonary resuscitation), known blood-clotting defects, cerebrovascular disease, uncontrolled hypertension, and liver disease, which could affect normal clotting factors and the production of plasminogen.

These drugs should only be used during pregnancy and lactation if the benefit to the patient clearly outweighs the potential risks to the fetus. There is risk to the fetus if maternal bleeding occurs.

Adverse Effects

The most common adverse effect associated with the use of thrombolytic agents is bleeding. Hemoglobin and hematocrit should be monitored. Patients should be monitored closely for the occurrence of cardiac arrhythmias, hypotension, mental status changes, and GI bleeding. Hypersensitivity reactions are not uncommon; they range from rash and flushing to bronchospasm and anaphylactic reaction.

Clinically Important Drug–Drug Interactions

The risk of hemorrhage increases if thrombolytic agents are used with any anticoagulant or antiplatelet drug.

Prototype Summary: Alteplase

Indications: Treatment of MI, acute PE, and acute ischemic stroke; restoration of function in occluded central venous access devices.

Actions: Acts as an enzyme to convert endogenous plasminogen to plasmin, which breaks down fibrin clots, fibrinogen, and other plasma proteins; lyses thrombi and emboli.

Pharmacokinetics:

Route	Onset	Peak	Duration
IV	Immediate	End of injection	Unknown

$T_{1/2}$: 72 minutes; metabolized in the plasma; excretion method unknown.

Adverse Effects: Bleeding, hypersensitivity.

Nursing Considerations for Patients Receiving Thrombolytic Agents

Assessment: History and Examination

- Assess for any known allergies to these drugs to prevent hypersensitivity reactions. Also, screen for any conditions that could be worsened by the dissolution of clots, including recent surgery, active internal bleeding, CVA within the last 3 months, aneurysm, obstetrical delivery, organ biopsy, recent serious GI bleeding, rupture of a noncompressible blood vessel, recent major trauma (including cardiopulmonary resuscitation), known blood-clotting defects, cerebrovascular disease, and uncontrolled hypertension; liver disease, which could affect normal clotting factors and the production of plasminogen; and pregnancy or lactation because of the possible adverse effects on the neonate.
- Assess baseline status before beginning therapy to determine any potential adverse effects.
- Assess body temperature; skin color, lesions, and temperature; affect, orientation, and reflexes; pulse, blood pressure, and perfusion; respirations and adventitious sounds; and clotting studies, renal and hepatic function tests, CBC, guaiac test for occult blood in stool, and ECG.

Nursing Conclusions

Nursing conclusions related to drug therapy might include the following:

- Injury risk related to clot-dissolving effects
- Altered tissue perfusion (total body) related to possible blood loss
- Altered cardiac output related to bleeding and arrhythmias
- Knowledge deficit regarding drug therapy

Planning

- The patient will receive the best therapeutic effect from the drug therapy.
- The patient will have limited adverse effects from the drug therapy.
- The patient will have an understanding of the drug therapy, adverse effects to anticipate, and measures to relieve discomfort and improve safety.

Intervention With Rationale

- Arrange to administer tissue plasminogen activators to reduce mortality associated with acute MI or ischemic stroke as soon as possible after the onset of symptoms because the timing for the administration of these drugs is critical to resolving the clot before permanent damage occurs to the myocardial or nerve cells.

(continues on page 870)

- Discontinue heparin if it is being given before administration of a thrombolytic agent unless specifically ordered for coronary artery infusion to prevent excessive loss of blood.
- Evaluate the patient regularly for any sign of blood loss (petechiae, bleeding gums, bruises, dark-colored stools, dark-colored urine) to evaluate drug effectiveness and for the need to consult with the prescriber if blood loss becomes apparent.
- Monitor coagulation studies regularly; consult with the prescriber to adjust the drug dose appropriately.
- Arrange to type and crossmatch blood in case of serious blood loss that requires whole-blood transfusion.
- Monitor cardiac rhythm continuously if the drug is being given for acute MI because of the risk of alteration in cardiac function; have life support equipment on standby as needed.
- Provide increased precautions against bleeding during invasive procedures, use pressure dressings and ice, avoid IM injections, and do not rub subcutaneous injection sites because of the risk of increased blood loss in the anticoagulated state.
- Mark the chart of any patient receiving this drug to alert medical staff that there is a potential for increased bleeding.
- Provide thorough patient teaching, including the name of the drug, dosage prescribed, measures to avoid adverse effects, warning signs of problems, and the need for periodic monitoring and evaluation, to enhance patient knowledge about drug therapy and to promote adherence to the drug regimen.
- Offer support and encouragement to help the patient deal with the diagnosis and the drug regimen.

Evaluation

- Monitor patient response to the drug (dissolution of the clot and return of blood flow to the area).
- Monitor for adverse effects (bleeding, arrhythmias, hypotension, hypersensitivity reaction).
- Evaluate the effectiveness of the teaching plan (patient can name drug, adverse effects to watch for, and specific measures to avoid them).
- Monitor the effectiveness of comfort measures and adherence to the regimen.

Other Drugs Affecting Clot Formation

Other drugs that affect clot formation are also effective in preventing thromboembolic episodes. These drugs include the adjunctive agents used to help alleviate adverse reactions to these drugs and one hemorrheologic agent.

Anticoagulant Adjunctive Therapy

Agents used in anticoagulant adjunctive therapy include coagulation factor Xa (*Andexxa*), idarucizumab (*Praxbind*), protamine sulfate, prothrombin complex concentrate, and vitamin K. Boxes 48.4 and 48.5 provide additional information about vitamin K and protamine sulfate. See also Table 48.1 for additional information for each of these agents.

Coagulation factor Xa (recombinant) was modified from the human factor Xa protein. It is for patients taking rivaroxaban or apixaban who require acute reversal of anticoagulation due to uncontrollable bleeding or life-threatening bleeding. There is a boxed warning regarding risk of thromboembolic events that include MI and ischemic stroke that could lead to cardiac arrest and fatality. It is to be administered IV bolus and then continuous infusion for up to 120 minutes. Dosing of coagulation factor Xa is based on the oral anticoagulant dose and timing.

Idarucizumab (*Praxbind*) is a monoclonal antibody that is indicated to treat patients who are taking dabigatran and require acute reversal due to emergent surgery/procedures or life-threatening or uncontrollable bleeding. It is administered IV as bolus administration. The risks include hypersensitivity reactions and thromboembolic events.

Hemorrheologic Agent

Pentoxifylline (generic) is known as a hemorrheologic agent or a drug that can induce hemorrhage. It is a xanthine that, like caffeine and theophylline, decreases platelet aggregation and decreases the fibrinogen concentration in the blood. These effects can decrease blood clot formation and increase blood flow through narrowed or damaged vessels. The mechanism of action by which pentoxifylline does these things is not known. It is one of the few drugs found to be effective in treating intermittent claudication, a painful vascular problem of the legs.

Because pentoxifylline is a xanthine, it is associated with many CV stimulatory effects; patients with underlying CV problems need to be monitored carefully when taking this drug. Pentoxifylline can also cause headache, dizziness, nausea, and upset stomach. It is taken orally three times a day for at least 8 weeks to evaluate its effectiveness. See Table 48.1 for additional information about this drug.

Key Points

- To keep blood from coagulating, anticoagulants block blood aggregates or interfere with the mechanisms that cause blood to clot.
- Thrombolytic drugs activate the plasminogen system to dissolve clots naturally.

Drugs Used to Control Bleeding

On the other end of the spectrum of coagulation problems are various bleeding disorders. These include the following:

- *Hemophilia*, in which there is a genetic lack of clotting factors that leaves the patient vulnerable to excessive bleeding with any injury

- *Liver disease,* in which clotting factors and proteins needed for clotting are not produced
- *Bone marrow disorders,* in which platelets are not formed in sufficient quantity to be effective

Bleeding disorders are treated with clotting factors and drugs that promote the coagulation process. These include antihemophilic agents and hemostatic agents (systemic and topical) (see Table 48.3).

Table 48.3 *Drugs in Focus:* Drugs Used to Control Bleeding

Drug Name	Usual Dosage	Usual Indications
Antihemophilic Agents		
antihemophilic factor (recombinant) (*Kovaltry, ReFacto, Eloctate, Obizur,* and others)	IV dose based on level of antihemophilic factor, weight, and patient response	Treatment of hemophilia A; to correct or prevent bleeding episodes or to allow necessary surgery; routine prophylaxis to reduce frequency of bleeding episodes
antiinhibitor coagulant complex (*Feiba*)	50–100 units/kg IV at intervals determined by indication for use and type of bleeding	Control and prevention of bleeding episodes in hemophilia A and B patients with inhibitors; perioperative management; routine prophylaxis to prevent or reduce the frequency of bleeding episodes
coagulation factor VIIa (*NovoSeven*)	90 mcg/kg IV q2h until hemostasis is achieved	Treatment of bleeding episodes in patients with hemophilia A or B
factor IX (*Profilnine SD*)	IV dose based on weight and levels of factor IX	Prevention and control of bleeding in patients with factor IX deficiencies
factor IX complex (*BeneFix* and others)	IV dose based on factor levels, weight, and desired response	Treatment or prevention of hemophilia B (Christmas disease, a deficiency of factor IX); treatment of bleeding episodes in patients with factor VII and factor VIII deficiencies; controls bleeding episodes in patients with hemophilia A
factor XIII (*Corifact*)	40 units/kg IV, subsequent dosing based on patient response	Prevention of bleeding in patients with congenital factor XIII deficiencies
Hemostatic Agents		
Systemic		
aminocaproic acid (*Amicar*)	5 g PO or IV, then 1–1.25 g/h; not to exceed 30 g in 24 h	Treatment of excessive bleeding in hyperfibrinolytic states; prevention of recurrence of bleeding with subarachnoid hemorrhage; sometimes used for treatment of attacks of hereditary angioedema
Topical		
absorbable gelatin (*Gelfoam*)	Smear or press onto surface; do not remove, will be absorbed	Controls bleeding from surface cuts or injury
human fibrin sealant (*Artiss*)	Spray a thin layer on prepared graft bed	Adheres autologous skin grafts to surgically prepared wound beds resulting from burns in adults and children
human fibrin sealant (*Evicel*)	Spray or drip solution onto site to produce a thin, even layer	Adjunct to hemostasis in liver or vascular surgery when control of bleeding by standard surgical techniques is ineffective
microfibrillar collagen (*Avitene*)	Use when dry (do not moisten); apply to area and apply pressure for 3–5 min	Controls bleeding from surface cuts or injury
thrombin (*Thrombinar*)	100–1,000 units/mL freely mixed with blood	Controls bleeding from surface cuts or injury
thrombin, recombinant (*Recothrom*)	Apply solution directly to bleeding site in conjunction with absorbable gelatin sponge	Adjunct to hemostasis whenever oozing blood and minor bleeding from capillaries and small venules are accessible and control of bleeding by standard surgical techniques is ineffective or impractical; decreases possibility for allergic reactions associated with bovine thrombin

Antihemophilic Agents

The drugs used to treat hemophilia are replacement factors for the specific clotting factors that are genetically missing in that particular type of hemophilia. These drugs include antihemophilic factor (*Eloctate, Obizur, ReFacto,* and others), coagulation factor VIIa (*NovoSeven*), factor IX (*BeneFix, Profilnine SD,* and others), factor IX complex (*Bebulin VH, Profilnine SD*), antiinhibitor coagulant complex (*Feiba NA*), and factor XIII (*Corifact*).

Therapeutic Actions and Indications

The antihemophilic drugs replace clotting factors that are either genetically missing or low in a particular type of hemophilia. The drug of choice depends on the particular hemophilia that is being treated. Antihemophilic factor is factor VIII, the clotting factor that is missing in classic hemophilia (hemophilia A). This agent is used to correct or prevent bleeding episodes or to allow necessary surgery.

Coagulation factor VIIa and factor IX complex are used for patients with hemophilia A or B (see Table 48.3 for usual indications for each of these agents). Factor IX complex contains plasma fractions of many of the clotting factors and increases blood levels of factors II, VII, IX, and X. Factor XIII replaces factor XIII in patients with a congenital deficiency. Antiinhibitor coagulant complex is used to control spontaneous bleeding or to cover surgical procedures in patients with hemophilia A and B with inhibitors. Antihemophilic factor Fc fusion protein is used to prevent and control bleeding episodes in adults and children with hemophilia A (factor VIII deficiency), and antihemophilic factor porcine sequence is used for treating bleeding episodes in adults with acquired hemophilia A. The drug of choice for any given patient is determined by their particular coagulation abnormalities.

Pharmacokinetics

These agents replace normal clotting factors and are processed as such by the body. They must be given IV and are processed by the body in the same way that naturally occurring clotting factors are processed in the plasma, usually with a half-life of 24 to 36 hours.

Contraindications and Cautions

Antihemophilic factor is contraindicated in the presence of known allergy to prevent hypersensitivity reactions. Factor IX is contraindicated in the presence of liver disease with signs of intravascular coagulation or fibrinolysis to prevent serious aggravation of these disorders. Coagulation factor VIIa is contraindicated with known allergies to prevent hypersensitivity reactions. These drugs are not recommended for use during lactation, and caution should be used during pregnancy because of the potential for adverse effects on the baby or fetus. They should be used during pregnancy only if the benefit to the patient clearly outweighs the potential risk to the fetus. It is recommended that another method of feeding the baby be used if these drugs are needed during lactation. Because these drugs are used to prevent serious bleeding problems or to treat bleeding episodes, there are few contraindications to their use.

Adverse Effects

The most common adverse effects associated with antihemophilic agents involve risks associated with the use of blood products. Headache, flushing, chills, fever, and lethargy may occur as a reaction to the injection of a foreign protein. Nausea and vomiting may also occur, as may stinging, itching, and burning at the site of the injection.

Prototype Summary: Antihemophilic Factor

Indications: Treatment of classic hemophilia to provide temporary replacement of clotting factors to correct or prevent bleeding episodes or to allow necessary surgery.

Actions: Normal plasma protein that is needed for the transformation of prothrombin to thrombin, the final step in the clotting pathway.

Pharmacokinetics:

Route	Onset	Peak	Duration
IV	Immediate	Unknown	Unknown

$T_{1/2}$: 12 hours, cleared from the body by normal protein metabolism.

Adverse Effects: Allergic reaction, stinging at injection site, headache, rash, chills, nausea.

Nursing Considerations for Patients Receiving Antihemophilic Agents

Assessment: History and Examination

- Assess for any known allergies to these drugs and for liver disease, which could be cautions or contraindications to use of the drug.
- Assess baseline status of weight, factor levels, and bleeding risk before beginning therapy to determine initial dosing.
- Assess body temperature; skin color, lesions, and temperature; affect, orientation, and reflexes; pulse, blood pressure, and perfusion; respirations and adventitious sounds; clotting studies; and hepatic function tests.

Nursing Conclusions

Nursing conclusions related to drug therapy might include the following:

- Altered tissue perfusion (total body) related to changes in coagulation
- Impaired comfort related to GI, CNS, or skin effects
- Anxiety or fear related to the diagnosis and use of blood-related products
- Knowledge deficit regarding drug therapy

Planning

- The patient will receive the best therapeutic effect from the drug therapy.
- The patient will have limited adverse effects from the drug therapy.
- The patient will have an understanding of the drug therapy, adverse effects to anticipate, and measures to relieve discomfort and improve safety.

Intervention With Rationale

- Ensure that appropriate clotting factor is being used for the patient to ensure therapeutic effectiveness and prevent inappropriate increase in other clotting factors.
- Administer by the IV route only to ensure therapeutic effectiveness.
- Monitor clinical response and clotting factor levels regularly to arrange to adjust dose as needed.
- Monitor the patient for any sign of thrombosis to determine need for comfort and support measures (e.g., support hose, positioning, ambulation, exercise).
- Decrease the rate of infusion if headache, chills, fever, or tingling occurs to prevent severe drug reaction; in some people, the drug will need to be discontinued.
- Arrange to type and crossmatch blood in case of serious blood loss that will require whole-blood transfusion.
- Provide thorough patient teaching, including the name of the drug, dosage prescribed, measures to avoid adverse effects, warning signs of problems, and the need for periodic monitoring and evaluation, to enhance patient knowledge about drug therapy and to promote adherence to the drug regimen.
- Offer support and encouragement to help the patient deal with the diagnosis and the drug regimen.

Evaluation

- Monitor patient response to the drug (control of bleeding episodes, prevention of bleeding episodes).
- Monitor for adverse effects (thrombosis, CNS effects, nausea, hypersensitivity reaction).
- Evaluate the effectiveness of the teaching plan (patient can name drug, dosage of drug, adverse effects to watch for, specific measures to avoid them, and warning signs to report).
- Monitor the effectiveness of comfort measures and adherence to the regimen.

Hemostatic Agents

Some situations result in a fibrinolytic state with excessive plasminogen activity and risk of bleeding from clot dissolution. For example, patients undergoing repeat coronary artery bypass graft (CABG) surgery are especially prone to excessive bleeding and may require blood transfusion. **Hemostatic agents** are used to stop bleeding. Hemostatic drugs may be either systemic or topical.

The hemostatic drug that is used systemically is aminocaproic acid (*Amicar*). Topical hemostatic agents include absorbable gelatin (*Gelfoam*), human fibrin sealant (*Artiss*, *Evicel*), microfibrillar collagen (*Avitene*), thrombin (*Evithrom*, *Thrombostat*), and thrombin recombinant (*Recothrom*).

Therapeutic Actions and Indications

Systemic Hemostatic Agents

The systemic hemostatic agents are used to prevent body-wide or systemic clot breakdown, thus preventing blood loss in situations in which serious systemic bleeding could occur, or hyperfibrinolysis. There is only one systemic hemostatic agent available for use in the United States.

Aminocaproic acid inhibits plasminogen-activating substances and has some antiplasmin activity. When taking the oral form of aminocaproic acid, the patient may need to take 10 tablets in the first hour and then continue taking the drug around the clock. See Table 48.3 for usual indications for aminocaproic acid.

Topical Hemostatic Agents

Some surface injuries involve so much damage to the small vessels in the area that clotting does not occur and blood is slowly and continually lost. For these situations, topical or local hemostatic agents are often used. The use of these drugs is also incorporated into the care of wounds or decubitus ulcers as adjunctive therapy. The drug of choice depends on the nature of the injury and the prescriber's preference. The newest topical hemostatic agent is human fibrin sealant. Thrombin recombinant is the first topical hemostatic agent approved to be made using recombinant DNA technology (this will decrease many of the potential allergic reactions associated with bovine thrombin; see "Contraindications and Cautions"). See Table 48.3 for additional information about these agents.

Pharmacokinetics

Systemic Hemostatic Agents

Aminocaproic acid is available in oral and IV forms. It is rapidly absorbed and widely distributed throughout the body. It is excreted largely unchanged in urine, with a half-life of 2 hours.

Topical Hemostatic Agents

Absorbable gelatin and microfibrillar collagen are available in sponge form and are applied directly to the injured area until the bleeding stops.

Human fibrin sealant (*Artiss*) is available in spray form and applied in a thin layer onto the graft bed. *Evicel* is sprayed directly onto any active bleeding site.

Thrombin, which is derived from bovine sources, is a solution that is applied topically and mixed in with the blood. Thrombin recombinant is also a solution and is applied directly to the bleeding site surface in conjunction with absorbable gelatin sponge; the amount needed varies with the area of tissue to be treated.

Contraindications and Cautions

Systemic Hemostatic Agents

Aminocaproic acid is contraindicated in the presence of allergy to the drug to prevent hypersensitivity reactions and with acute DIC because of the risk of tissue necrosis. Caution should be used in cardiac disease because of the risk of arrhythmias and in renal and hepatic dysfunction, which could alter the excretion of this drug and the normal clotting processes. Although the safety for use of this drug during pregnancy has not been established, it should be used only if the benefits to the patient clearly outweigh the potential risks to the neonate because of the potential for adverse effects on the fetus. It is recommended that patients who are breast or chestfeeding use a different method for feeding the baby if this drug is used because of the potential for adverse effects on the baby.

Topical Hemostatic Agents

Use thrombin with caution for those patients who are allergic to bovine products. Because thrombin comes from animal sources, it may precipitate an allergic response; the patient needs to be carefully monitored for such a reaction. Many of the potential allergic reactions associated with bovine thrombin will be decreased as a result of approval for thrombin recombinant to be made using recombinant DNA technology. Safety for use of thrombin recombinant in children has not been established.

Adverse Effects

Systemic Hemostatic Agents

The most common adverse effect associated with systemic hemostatic agents is excessive clotting. CNS effects of aminocaproic acid can include hallucinations, drowsiness, dizziness, headache, and psychotic states, all of which could be related to changes in cerebral blood flow associated with changes in clot dissolution. GI effects, including nausea, cramps, and diarrhea, may be related to excessive clotting in the GI tract, causing reflex GI stimulation. Weakness, fatigue, malaise, and muscle pain can occur as small clots build up in muscles. Intrarenal obstruction and renal dysfunction have also been reported.

Topical Hemostatic Agents

The use of absorbable gelatin and microfibrillar collagen can pose a risk of infection because bacteria can become trapped in the vascular area when the sponge is applied. Immediate removal of the sponge and cleaning of the area can help to decrease this risk.

Clinically Important Drug–Drug Interactions

Systemic Hemostatic Agents

Aminocaproic acid is associated with the development of hypercoagulation states if it is combined with oral contraceptives or estrogens. The risk of bleeding increases if it is given with heparin.

Topical Hemostatic Agents

There are no reported drug–drug interactions with the topically applied hemostatic agents.

P Prototype Summary: Aminocaproic Acid

Indications: Treatment of excessive bleeding resulting from hyperfibrinolysis; also used to prevent the recurrence of subarachnoid hemorrhage, for management of megakaryocytic thrombocytopenia, to decrease the need for platelet administration, and to abort and treat attacks of hereditary angioneurotic edema.

Actions: Inhibits plasminogen activator substances and has antiplasmin activity that inhibits fibrinolysis and prevents the breakdown of clots.

Pharmacokinetics:

Route	Onset	Peak	Duration
Oral	Rapid	2 h	Unknown
IV	Immediate	Minutes	2–3 h

$T_{1/2}$: 2 hours; excreted unchanged in the urine.

Adverse Effects: Dizziness, tinnitus, headache, weakness, hypotension, nausea, cramps, diarrhea, fertility problems, malaise, and elevated serum creatine phosphokinase.

Nursing Considerations for Patients Receiving Systemic Hemostatic Agents

Nursing considerations for a patient receiving topical hemostatic agents are similar to those with the use of any topical drug (see Appendix B). However, the considerations for patients receiving systemic hemostatic agents are different than the topical agents (see below).

Assessment: History and Examination

- Assess for the following conditions, which could be cautions or contraindications to the use of systemic hemostatic agents: any known allergies to any component of the drug to prevent hypersensitivity reactions; acute disseminated intravascular coagulation because of the risk of tissue necrosis; renal and hepatic dysfunction, which could alter the excretion of these drugs and the normal clotting processes; and lactation because of the potential for adverse effects on the neonate.
- Assess body temperature; skin color, lesions, and temperature; affect, orientation, and reflexes; pulse, blood pressure, and perfusion; respirations and adventitious sounds; bowel sounds and normal output; urinalysis and clotting studies; and renal and hepatic function tests.

Nursing Conclusions

Nursing conclusions related to drug therapy might include the following:

- Altered sensory perception related to CNS effects
- Impaired comfort related to GI, CNS, or muscle effects
- Injury risk related to CNS or blood-clotting effects
- Knowledge deficit regarding drug therapy

Planning

- The patient will receive the best therapeutic effect from the drug therapy.
- The patient will have limited adverse effects from the drug therapy.
- The patient will have an understanding of the drug therapy, adverse effects to anticipate, and measures to relieve discomfort and improve safety.

Intervention With Rationale

- Monitor clinical response and clotting factor levels regularly to arrange to adjust dose as needed.
- Monitor the patient for any sign of thrombosis to determine need for comfort and support measures (e.g., support hose, positioning, ambulation, exercise).
- Orient the patient and offer support and safety measures if hallucinations or psychoses occur to prevent patient injury.
- Offer comfort measures to help the patient deal with the effects of the drug, including small, frequent meals, mouth care, environmental controls, and safety measures.
- Provide thorough patient teaching, including the name of the drug, dosage prescribed, measures to avoid adverse effects, warning signs of problems, and the need for periodic monitoring and evaluation, to enhance patient knowledge about drug therapy and to promote adherence to the drug regimen.
- Offer support and encouragement to help the patient deal with the diagnosis and the drug regimen.

Evaluation

- Monitor patient response to the drug (control of bleeding episodes).
- Monitor for adverse effects (thrombosis, CNS effects, nausea, hypersensitivity reaction).
- Evaluate the effectiveness of the teaching plan (patient can name drug, dosage of drug, adverse effects to watch for, specific measures to avoid them, and warning signs to report).
- Monitor the effectiveness of comfort measures and adherence to the regimen.

Key Points

- Hemostatic agents are used to stop bleeding from occurring. They are used in situations that result in a fibrinolytic state with excessive plasminogen activity and the risk of bleeding from clot dissolution. For example, patients undergoing repeat CABG surgery are especially prone to excessive bleeding and may require blood transfusion.
- Aminocaproic acid is a systemic hemostatic agent used to treat conditions resulting from systemic hyperfibrinolysis. Several topical agents are also available for local use on active bleeding sites, often during surgery or with severe injury.

SUMMARY

- Coagulation is the transformation of fluid blood into a solid state to plug up breaks in the vascular system.
- Coagulation involves several processes, including vasoconstriction, platelet aggregation to form a plug, and intrinsic and extrinsic clot formation initiated by Hageman factor to plug any breaks in the system.
- The final step of clot formation is the conversion of prothrombin to thrombin, which breaks down fibrinogen to form insoluble fibrin threads.
- Once a clot is formed, it must be dissolved to prevent the occlusion of blood vessels and loss of blood supply to tissues.
- Plasminogen is the basis of the clot-dissolving system. It is converted to plasmin (fibrinolysin) by several factors, including Hageman factor. Plasmin dissolves fibrin threads and resolves the clot.

- Anticoagulants block blood coagulation by interfering with one or more of the steps involved, such as blocking platelet aggregation or inhibiting the intrinsic or extrinsic pathways to clot formation.
- Thrombolytic drugs dissolve clots or thrombi that have formed. They activate the plasminogen system to stimulate natural clot dissolution.
- Hemostatic drugs are used to stop bleeding. They may replace missing clotting factors or prevent the plasminogen system from dissolving formed clots.
- Hemophilia, a genetic lack of essential clotting factors, results in excessive bleeding. It is treated by replacing missing clotting factors.

Unfolding Patient Stories: Rachel Heidebrink • Part 2

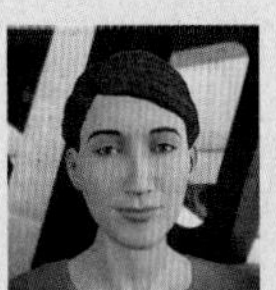

Think back to Chapter 40, where you met Rachel Heidebrink, who underwent a right hemiarthroplasty for a fracture to the right greater trochanter sustained in a motorcycle accident. She is diagnosed with a pulmonary embolism (PE) on postoperative day 1. How would the nurse explain the effect of heparin for the management of a PE and why the route of administration begins with an intravenous loading dose followed by a continuous infusion? What nursing assessments and interventions ensure the safe administration of intravenous heparin? How would the nurse explain the combination of oral and intravenous anticoagulant therapy?

Care for Rachel and other patients in a realistic virtual environment: ***vSim** for Nursing* (thepoint.lww.com/vSimPharm). Practice documenting these patients' care in DocuCare (thepoint.lww.com/DocuCareEHR).

CHECK YOUR UNDERSTANDING

Answers to the questions in this chapter can be found in Answers to Check Your Understanding Questions on thePoint®.

MULTIPLE CHOICE

Select the best answer.

1. Blood coagulation is a complex reaction that involves
   a. vasoconstriction, platelet aggregation, and plasminogen action.
   b. vasodilation, platelet aggregation, and activation of the clotting cascade.
   c. vasoconstriction, platelet aggregation, and conversion of prothrombin to thrombin.
   d. vasodilation, platelet inhibition, and action of the intrinsic and extrinsic clotting cascades.
2. Warfarin, an oral anticoagulant, acts
   a. to directly prevent the conversion of prothrombin to thrombin.
   b. to decrease the production of vitamin K clotting factors in the liver.
   c. as a catalyst in the conversion of plasminogen to plasmin.
   d. immediately, so it is the drug of choice in emergency situations.
3. Heparin reacts to prevent the conversion of prothrombin to thrombin. Heparin
   a. is available in oral and parenteral forms.
   b. takes about 72 hours to have a therapeutic effect.
   c. has its effects reversed with the administration of protamine sulfate.
   d. has its effects reversed with the injection of vitamin K.
4. The low molecular weight heparin of choice for preventing DVT after hip replacement therapy is
   a. heparin.
   b. betrixaban.
   c. fondaparinux.
   d. enoxaparin.
5. A thrombolytic agent would be most indicated for which circumstance?
   a. CVA within the last 2 months
   b. Acute MI within the last 3 hours
   c. Recent, serious GI bleeding
   d. Obstetric delivery

6. Which is true of warfarin?
   a. Side effects include increased risk of clotting.
   b. Therapy may take multiple days of dosing to become therapeutic.
   c. It works by inhibiting activation of factor X.
   d. It is only administered IV.

MULTIPLE RESPONSE

Select all that apply.

1. Hageman factor is known to activate which?
   a. The clotting cascade
   b. The anticlotting process
   c. The inflammatory response
   d. Platelet aggregation
   e. Thromboxane A_2
   f. Troponin coupling
2. Plasminogen is converted to plasmin, a clot-dissolving substance, by which?
   a. Nicotine
   b. Hageman factor
   c. Tenecteplase
   d. Pyrogens
   e. Thrombin
   f. Christmas factor
3. Antiplatelet drugs block the aggregation of platelets and keep vessels open. These drugs would be useful in which circumstances?
   a. Maintaining the patency of grafts
   b. Decreasing the risk of fatal MI
   c. Preventing reinfarction after MI
   d. Dissolving a PE and improving oxygenation
   e. Decreasing damage in a subarachnoid bleed
   f. Preventing thromboembolic strokes
4. Evaluating a patient who is taking an anticoagulant for blood loss would usually include assessing for which conditions?
   a. Presence of petechiae
   b. Bleeding gums while brushing the teeth
   c. Dark-colored urine
   d. Yellow color to the sclera or skin
   e. Presence of ecchymotic areas
   f. Loss of hair

REFERENCES

Adam, S. S., McDuffie, J. R., Ortel, T. L., & Williams, J. W. (2012). Comparative effectiveness of warfarin and new oral anticoagulants for the management of atrial fibrillation and venous thromboembolism: A systematic review. *Annals of Internal Medicine, 157*(11), 796–807. https://doi.org/10.7326/0003-4819-157-10-201211200-00532

Brunton, L., Hilal-Dandan, R., & Knollman, B. (2018). *Goodman and Gilman's the pharmacological basis of therapeutics* (13th ed.). McGraw-Hill.

Hall, J. E., & Hall, M. E. (2021). *Guyton and Hall textbook of medical physiology* (14th ed.). Elsevier.

Law, C., & Raffini, L. (2015). A guide to the use of anticoagulant drugs in children. *Pediatric Drugs, 17,* 105–114. https://doi.org/10.1007/s40272-015-0120-x

Mannucci, P. M. (2004). Treatment of von Willebrand's disease. *New England Journal of Medicine, 351,* 683–694. https://doi.org/10.1056/NEJMra040403

Norris, T. L. (2019). *Porth's pathophysiology concepts of altered health states* (13th ed.). Wolters Kluwer.

Shimol, V., & Gage, B. (2011). Cost-effectiveness of dabigatran for stroke prophylaxis in atrial fibrillation. *Circulation, 123,* 2562–2570. https://doi.org/10.1161/CIRCULATIONAHA.110.985655

Streiff, M., & Haut, E. (2009). The CMS ruling on venous thromboembolism after total knee or hip arthroplasty: Weighing risks and benefits. *Journal of the American Medical Association, 301*(10), 1063–1065. https://doi.org/10.1001/jama.301.10.1063

Williams, M. D. (2009). Thrombolysis in children. *British Journal of Haematology, 148*(1), 26–36. https://doi.org/10.1111/j.1365-2141.2009.07914.x

CHAPTER 49

Drugs Used to Treat Anemias

Learning Objectives

Upon completion of this chapter, you will be able to:

1. Explain the process of erythropoiesis and its correlation with the development of different types of anemias.
2. Discuss the use of drugs used to treat anemias across the lifespan.
3. Describe the therapeutic actions, indications, pharmacokinetics, contraindications and cautions, most common adverse effects, and important drug–drug interactions associated with drugs used to treat anemias.
4. Compare and contrast the prototype drugs epoetin alfa, ferrous sulfate, folic acid, and hydroxocobalamin with other agents in their class.
5. Outline the nursing considerations, including important teaching points, for patients receiving drugs used to treat anemias.

Key Terms

anemia: disorder involving too few red blood cells (RBCs) or ineffective RBCs that can alter the blood's ability to carry oxygen

aplastic anemia: disorder of the bone marrow cells that decreases production of RBCs, white blood cells, and platelets

erythrocytes: RBCs, responsible for carrying oxygen to the tissues and removing carbon dioxide; they have no nucleus and live approximately 120 days

erythropoiesis: process of RBC production and life cycle; hematopoietic stem cells are induced to differentiate into erythroblasts by erythropoietin, and as they are produced, hemoglobin is synthesized; folic acid and vitamin B_{12} are required to make mature RBCs; RBCs circulate in the vascular system for about 120 days and then are lysed and some of their parts are recycled

erythropoietin: glycoprotein produced by the kidneys, released in response to decreased blood flow or low oxygen tension in the kidney; stimulates RBC production in the bone marrow

hemolytic anemia: inherited or acquired states of early destruction of RBCs

iron deficiency anemia: low RBC count with low iron availability because of high demand, poor diet, or poor absorption; treated with iron replacement

megaloblastic anemia: anemia usually caused by lack of vitamin B_{12} and/or folic acid, in which RBCs are fewer in number and have a weak stroma and a short lifespan; treated by replacement of folic acid and vitamin B_{12}

pernicious anemia: type of megaloblastic anemia characterized by lack of vitamin B_{12} secondary to low production of intrinsic factor by gastric cells; vitamin B_{12} must be replaced by intramuscular (IM) injection or nasal spray because it cannot be absorbed through the gastrointestinal tract

plasma: liquid part of the blood; consists mostly of water and plasma proteins, glucose, and electrolytes

reticulocyte: RBC that has lost its nucleus and entered circulation just recently; it is not yet fully matured

sickle cell anemia: type of inherited hemolytic anemia; autosomal recessive disorder that causes abnormalities in the hemoglobin in the RBCs causing them to change into a sickle shape, which is more likely to become stuck in and occlude blood vessels, causing damage to the blood vessels and obstructing blood flow to other tissues and organs

thalassemia: inherited disorders that can cause decreased synthesis of α or β-globin chains of hemoglobin in the RBCs; severity varies but these disorders generally lead to a hypochromic, microcytic hemolytic anemia

Drug List

ERYTHROPOIESIS-STIMULATING AGENTS
darbepoetin alfa
(P) epoetin alfa
methoxy polyethylene glycol-epoetin beta

AGENTS USED FOR IRON DEFICIENCY ANEMIA
ferrous fumarate
ferrous gluconate
(P) ferrous sulfate
ferrous sulfate exsiccated
ferumoxytol
iron dextran
iron sucrose
sodium ferric gluconate complex

AGENTS USED FOR OTHER ANEMIAS

Agents for Megaloblastic Anemias

Folic Acid Derivatives
(P) folic acid
leucovorin
levoleucovorin

vitamin B_{12}
cyanocobalamin
(P) hydroxocobalamin

AGENTS FOR SICKLE CELL ANEMIA
crizanlizumab
(P) hydroxyurea
voxelotor

Agent for *Beta* Thalassemia
luspatercept-aamt

Agent for Aplastic Anemia
eltrombopag

Blood is essential for cell survival because it carries oxygen and nutrients and removes waste products that could be toxic to the tissues. It also contains clotting factors that help maintain the vascular system and keep it intact. In addition, blood contains the important components of the immune and inflammatory systems that protect the body from infection.

Blood is composed of liquid and formed elements. The liquid part of blood is called **plasma**. Plasma is mostly water, but it also contains proteins that are essential for the immune response and for blood clotting. The formed elements of the blood include leukocytes (white blood cells), which are an important part of the immune system (see Chapter 15); **erythrocytes** (red blood cells [RBCs]), which carry oxygen to the tissues and remove carbon dioxide for delivery to the lungs; and platelets, which play an important role in coagulation (see Chapter 48). This chapter discusses drugs that are used to treat anemias, which are disorders that involve too few RBCs or ineffective RBCs and can alter the blood's ability to carry oxygen.

Anemia

Anemia is a disorder in which there are low levels of RBCs, hemoglobin, or both. **Erythropoiesis** is the process of RBC production and life cycle. **Erythropoietin** induces hematopoietic stem cells in the bone marrow to differentiate into erythroblasts. Erythropoietin is released from the kidneys in response to decreased blood flow or decreased oxygen tension in the kidneys and will stimulate a faster rate of RBC production in the bone marrow. Under the influence of erythropoietin, an undifferentiated cell in the bone marrow becomes a hemocytoblast. This cell uses certain amino acids, lipids, carbohydrates, vitamin B_{12}, folic acid, and iron to become an immature RBC. In the last phase of RBC production, the cell loses its nucleus and enters circulation. This cell, called a **reticulocyte**, finishes its maturing process in circulation (Fig. 49.1).

As the RBCs are produced, hemoglobin is synthesized. Hemoglobin is a structure that has different types of polypeptide chains (*alpha, beta, gamma, delta*). Each hemoglobin molecule is made with four chains, and each chain has a structure with an iron molecule that can loosely bind to one molecule of oxygen. The types of chains have varying binding affinity to oxygen. Adults most commonly have high amounts of hemoglobin A, which has 2 *alpha* chains and 2 *beta* chains.

Although the mature RBC has no nucleus, it does have a vast surface area to improve its ability to transport oxygen and carbon dioxide. Because it lacks a nucleus, the RBC cannot reproduce or maintain itself, so it will eventually wear out. The average lifespan of an RBC is about

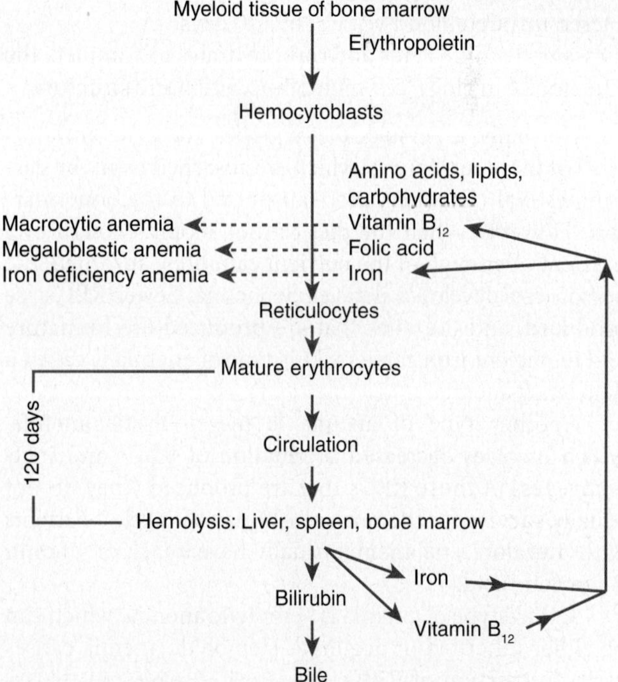

FIGURE 49.1 Erythropoiesis. Red blood cells are produced in the myeloid tissue of the bone marrow in response to the hormone erythropoietin. The hemocytoblasts require various essential factors to produce mature erythrocytes. A lack of any one of these can result in an anemia of the type indicated opposite each factor. Mature erythrocytes survive for about 120 days and are then lysed in the liver, spleen, or bone marrow.

120 days. At that time, the RBC is lysed in the liver, spleen, or bone marrow. Some of the building blocks of the RBC (e.g., iron, vitamin B_{12}) are then recycled and returned to the bone marrow for the production of new RBCs. One part of the RBC that cannot be recycled is the toxic pigment bilirubin, which is conjugated in the liver, passed into the bile, and excreted from the body in the feces or the urine. Bilirubin is what gives color to both of these excretions. Erythropoiesis is a constant process by which about 1% of the body's RBCs are destroyed and replaced each day in normal circumstances.

Etiology of Anemia

Anemia can result from four different etiologies: Bleeding can increase the loss of RBCs, hemolysis can destroy RBCs, RBC production can be ineffective, and there can be bone marrow failure. One of the causes of ineffective RBC production is low erythropoietin levels. This is seen in renal failure, when the kidneys are no longer able to produce erythropoietin. Ineffective RBC production can also occur if the body does not have enough of the building blocks necessary to form RBCs or if a person has genetic predisposition to forming abnormal RBCs, as in sickle cell anemia. To produce healthy RBCs, the bone marrow must have the following:

- Adequate amounts of iron, which is used in forming hemoglobin rings to carry the oxygen
- Minute amounts of vitamin B_{12} and folic acid to form a strong supporting structure that can survive being battered through blood vessels for 120 days
- Essential amino acids and carbohydrates to complete the hemoglobin rings, cell membrane, and basic structure

Normally, a person's diet supplies adequate amounts of all of these substances, which are absorbed from the gastrointestinal (GI) tract and transported to the bone marrow. However, when the diet cannot supply enough of a nutrient or enough of the nutrient cannot be absorbed, the person can develop a deficiency anemia. Fewer RBCs are produced, and the ones that are produced are immature and inefficient iron carriers. This type of anemia is called a deficiency anemia.

Another type of anemia is megaloblastic anemia, which involves decreased production of RBCs and ineffectiveness of those RBCs that are produced (they do not usually survive for the normal 120-day life cycle). Patients with megaloblastic anemia usually have a lack of vitamin B_{12} or folic acid.

A third type of anemia is hemolytic anemia, which can be either inherited or acquired. Hemolytic anemia causes early destruction of RBCs. Sickle cell disease and thalassemia are causes of inherited hemolytic anemia. RBC hemolysis by medications, antibodies, or infections are examples of acquired hemolytic anemia.

Aplastic anemia is a disorder of the bone marrow cells that decreases production of RBCs, white blood cells, and platelets. High doses of radiation, complications of infection, and chemotherapy that suppresses bone marrow cells are potential causes of aplastic anemia.

Iron Deficiency Anemia

All cells in the body require some amount of iron, but high amounts of iron can be toxic to cells, especially neurons. To maintain the necessary iron levels and avoid toxic levels, the body has developed a system for controlling the amount of iron that can enter the body through intestinal absorption. Only enough iron is absorbed to replace the amount of iron that is needed. Once iron is absorbed, it is carried by a plasma protein called transferrin, a beta globulin. This protein carries iron to various tissues to be stored and transports iron from RBC lysis back to the bone marrow for recycling.

Only about 1 mg of iron is actually lost each day in sweat, in sloughed skin, and from the GI and urinary tract linings. Because of the body's efficient iron recycling, very little iron is usually needed in the diet, and most diets adequately replace the iron that is lost. However, in situations in which blood is being lost, a negative iron balance might occur, and the patient could develop **iron deficiency anemia**. This can occur in certain rare GI diseases in which the patient is unable to absorb iron from the GI tract, but iron deficiency anemia is also a relatively common problem in certain groups, including:

- Menstruating people, who lose RBCs monthly
- Pregnant and lactating people, who have increased demands for iron
- Rapidly growing adolescents, especially those who do not have a nutritious diet
- Persons with GI bleeding, including people with slow bleeding associated with use of nonsteroidal antiinflammatory drugs

The person with this type of anemia may complain of being tired because there is insufficient oxygen delivery to the tissues. These conditions are usually treated with iron replacement therapy (see "Agents Used for Iron Deficiency Anemia").

Megaloblastic Anemia

Megaloblastic anemia usually results from insufficient amounts of folic acid or vitamin B_{12} to adequately create the stromal structure needed in a healthy RBC. With these deficiencies, there is a slowing of nuclear DNA synthesis that results in larger immature cells. This effect occurs in rapidly dividing cells such as the bone marrow. The bone marrow contains a large number of megaloblasts, or large, immature RBCs. Because these RBCs are so large, they become crowded in the bone marrow and fewer RBCs are produced, increasing the number of immature cells in circulation. Cells in the GI tract are additional examples of cells that are often affected. When the GI tract is involved, this can result in the appearance of a characteristic red and glossy tongue and diarrhea.

Folic Acid Deficiency

Folic acid is essential for cell division in all types of tissue. Deficiencies in folic acid are noticed first in rapidly growing cells, such as those in cancerous tissues, in the GI tract, and in the bone marrow. Folic acid is important for the developing fetus, a site of rapidly growing cells. Pregnant patients are urged to take folic acid supplements to help prevent fetal abnormalities, particularly neural tube defects. Most people can get all the folic acid they need from their diets. For example, folic acid is found in green leafy vegetables, milk, eggs, and liver. Deficiency in folic acid may occur in certain malabsorption states, such as sprue and celiac diseases. Malnutrition that accompanies alcoholism is also a common cause of folic acid deficiency. Repeated pregnancies and extended treatment with certain antiepileptic medications can also contribute to folic acid deficiency. Folic acid deficiency is treated by the administration of folic acid or folate.

Vitamin B_{12} Deficiency

Vitamin B_{12} is used in minute amounts by the body and is stored for use if dietary intake falls. It is necessary not only for the health of the RBCs but also for the formation and maintenance of the myelin sheath in the central nervous system (CNS). It is found in the diet in meats, seafood, eggs, and cheese. Strict vegetarians who eat only vegetables may develop vitamin B_{12} deficiency; they typically respond to vitamin B_{12} replacement therapy to reverse the anemia.

The most common cause of this deficiency, however, is inability of the GI tract to absorb the necessary amounts of the vitamin. Gastric mucosal cells produce a substance called intrinsic factor, which is necessary for the absorption of vitamin B_{12} by the upper intestine.

Pernicious anemia occurs when the gastric mucosa cannot produce intrinsic factor and vitamin B_{12} cannot be absorbed. The person with pernicious anemia will complain of fatigue and lethargy and will also have CNS effects because of damage to the myelin sheath. Patients will also complain of numbness, tingling, and eventually lack of coordination and motor activity. Pernicious anemia was once a fatal disease, but it is now treated with parenteral or nasal vitamin B_{12} to replace the amount that can no longer be absorbed.

Hemolytic Anemia

Hemolytic anemia can be either inherited or acquired. Two types of inherited hemolytic anemias that warrant further discussion are from sickle cell disease and thalassemia.

Sickle Cell Disease

Sickle cell disease is an inherited disorder that causes abnormal hemoglobin due to a mutation in the *beta* hemoglobin chain. It is characterized by a genetically inherited hemoglobin S, which gives the RBCs sickle-shaped appearance. The patient with sickle cell disease produces fewer than normal RBCs, and the RBCs that are produced are unable to carry oxygen efficiently, which results in **sickle cell anemia**. The sickle-shaped RBCs can become lodged in tiny blood vessels, where they stack up on one another and occlude the vessel. This occlusion leads to anoxia and infarction of the tissue in that area, which is characterized by severe pain and an acute inflammatory reaction—a condition often called a sickle cell crisis (the patient may even have ulcers on the extremities as a result of such occlusions). Severe, acute episodes of sickling with vessel occlusion may be associated with acute infections and the body's reactions to the immune and inflammatory responses. In the past, sickle cell anemia was treated only with pain medication and support for the patient. Now there are several medications that are indicated for treatment or prevention of acute exacerbations of sickle cell disease.

Thalassemia

Thalassemia is a group of inherited disorders that can cause decreased synthesis of *alpha* (α) or *beta* (β)-globin chains of hemoglobin in the RBC. The severity varies depending on whether the person is heterozygous or homozygous for the genetic trait. These disorders generally lead to a hypochromic, microcytic hemolytic anemia in which ineffective maturation of the RBC leads to early lysis.

Key Points

- RBCs are produced in the bone marrow in a process called erythropoiesis, the rate of which is controlled by the glycoprotein erythropoietin produced in the kidneys. The bone marrow uses iron, amino acids, carbohydrates, folic acid, and vitamin B_{12} to produce healthy, efficient RBCs.
- Anemia is a state of too few RBCs or ineffective RBCs. Anemia can be caused by a lack of erythropoietin or a lack of the components needed to produce RBCs.
- Anemia can be categorized as aplastic, iron deficiency, megaloblastic (folic acid or vitamin B_{12} deficiency), or hemolytic (sickle cell or thalassemia).

Erythropoiesis-Stimulating Agents

Patients who are no longer able to produce enough erythropoietin in the kidneys may benefit from treatment with exogenous erythropoietin, which is available as the drugs epoetin alfa (*Epogen/Procrit, Retacrit*), darbepoetin alfa (*Aranesp*), and methoxy polyethylene glycol-epoetin beta (*Mircera*). When agents are used to stimulate the bone marrow to make more RBCs, it is important to ensure that the patient has adequate levels of the components required to make RBCs, including adequate iron. See Table 49.1 for additional information about each of these agents. Box 49.1 highlights important considerations for different age groups when this group of drugs and other drugs used to treat anemia are administered. There are boxed warnings associated with the erythropoiesis-stimulating agents noting increased risk of death, myocardial infarction, stroke, venous thromboembolism, thrombosis of vascular access, and tumor progression or recurrence.

Table 49.1 ***Drugs in Focus*: Erythropoiesis-Stimulating Agents**

Drug Name	Usual Dosage	Usual Indications
darbepoetin alfa (*Aranesp*)	*Chronic kidney disease*: Initially 0.45 mcg/kg IV or subcutaneously once per wk or 0.75 mcg/kg IV or subcutaneously every 2 wk *Chemotherapy*: Initially 2.25 mcg/kg/wk subcutaneously or 500 mcg subcutaneously every 3 wk	Treatment of anemia associated with chronic renal failure, including in dialysis patients; treatment of chemotherapy-induced anemia
epoetin alfa (*Epogen/Procrit, Retacrit*)	IV or subcutaneous: Dosing varies based on indication and individual response	Treatment of anemia associated with renal failure and in patients on dialysis; reduction in need for transfusions in surgical patients; treatment of anemia associated with AIDS therapy; treatment of anemia associated with cancer chemotherapy
methoxy polyethylene glycol-epoetin beta (*Mircera*)	*Initial*: 0.6 mcg/kg IV or subcutaneously every 2 wk *Pediatric and/or when conversion from another erythropoiesis-stimulating agent*: Dose q2–4 wk and based on other agent at the time of dosing	Treatment of anemia associated with chronic kidney disease for adults on or off dialysis and for pediatric patients 5–17 y on hemodialysis who are converting from another erythropoiesis-stimulating agent

Therapeutic Actions and Indications

Epoetin alfa acts like the natural glycoprotein erythropoietin to stimulate the production of RBCs in the bone marrow (Fig. 49.2). This drug is indicated in the treatment of anemia associated with chronic kidney disease, medication therapy for clients with human immunodeficiency virus, and cancer chemotherapy that suppresses the bone marrow. It may also be used to reduce the number of required red blood cell transfusions in clients undergoing surgery. It is not approved to treat other anemias and is not a replacement for whole blood in the emergency treatment of anemia. See Table 49.1 for additional indications.

Darbepoetin alfa is an erythropoietin-like protein produced in Chinese hamster ovary cells with the use of recombinant DNA technology. This drug has the advantage of once-weekly administration, compared with two

Box 49.1 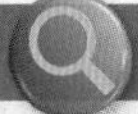 **Focus on Drug Therapy Across the Lifespan**

DRUGS USED TO TREAT ANEMIAS

Children

Proper nutrition should be established for children to provide the essential elements needed for the formation of RBCs. The cause of the anemia should be determined to avoid prolonged problems.

Iron doses for replacement therapy are determined by age. If a liquid solution is being used, the child should drink it through a straw to avoid staining of the teeth. Periodic blood counts should be performed; it may take 4 to 6 months of oral therapy to reverse an iron deficiency. Remember that iron can be toxic to children, and iron supplements should be kept out of their reach and administration monitored.

Maintenance doses for folic acid have been established for children based on age. Nutritional means should be used to establish folic acid levels whenever possible.

Children with pernicious anemia require a monthly injection of vitamin B_{12}; the nasal form has not been approved for use with children.

Adults

The underlying cause of the anemia should be established and appropriate steps should be taken to reverse the cause if possible. Adults receiving epoetin alfa or darbepoetin alfa should be monitored closely for response, for the need for iron or other RBC building blocks, and for the possibility of development of pure red cell aplasia.

Adults receiving iron replacement may experience GI upset and frequently experience constipation. Appropriate measures to maintain bowel function may be needed. Adults also need to know that periodic blood tests will be needed to evaluate response.

Adults being treated for pernicious anemia may opt for nasal vitamin B_{12}. These patients need to receive careful instructions about the proper administration of the drug and should have nasal mucous membranes evaluated periodically.

Proper nutrition during pregnancy and lactation is often still not an adequate way to meet the increased demands of those states. Prenatal vitamins contain iron and folic acid and are usually prescribed for pregnant patients. Folic acid is known to be important for the development of the neural tube, and often people who are considering becoming pregnant are encouraged to take folic acid to build up levels for the planned pregnancy. Use of epoetin alfa or darbepoetin alfa is not recommended during pregnancy or lactation because of the potential for adverse effects on the fetus or baby. Iron replacement is frequently needed postpartum to provide the iron lost during delivery. The new parent should be reminded to keep the drug out of the reach of children and not to combine prescribed iron with an OTC preparation containing high levels of iron.

Patients maintained on vitamin B_{12} before pregnancy should continue the treatment during pregnancy. Increased doses may be needed due to changes associated with the pregnancy.

Older Adults

Older adults may have decreased absorption of iron and may suffer from anemia associated with chronic illness.

Replacement therapy in the older adult can cause the same adverse effects as are seen in the younger person. A bowel regimen may be needed to prevent severe constipation.

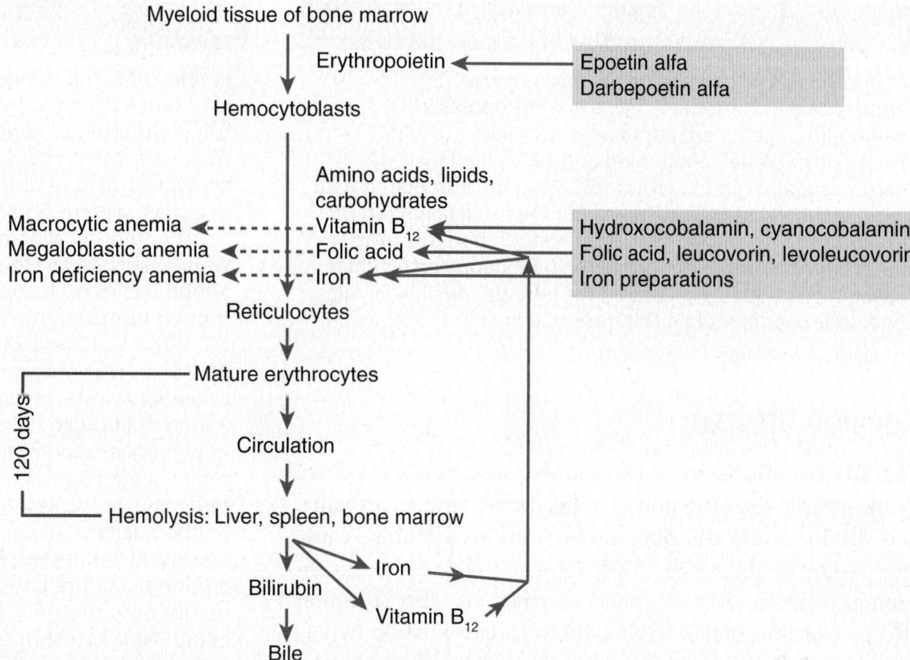

FIGURE 49.2 Sites of action of drugs used to treat anemia.

to three times a week administration for epoetin. Darbepoetin alfa is approved to treat anemias associated with chronic renal failure, including patients receiving dialysis. Darbepoetin alfa is also used for treatment of anemia induced by cancer chemotherapy. (See also Table 49.1.)

Methoxy polyethylene glycol-epoetin beta is an injection indicated to stimulate erythropoiesis in people with chronic renal disease. Adults may be on or off dialysis treatments. It is also indicated for pediatric patients 5 to 17 years of age on hemodialysis when converting from another stimulating agent. It is not indicated for patients with anemia due to cancer chemotherapy.

Pharmacokinetics

These drugs can be given intravenously (IV) or by subcutaneous injection. The substances are metabolized and excreted similarly to the endogenous erythropoietin. Epoetin alfa has a slow onset and peaks in 5 to 24 hours, and its duration of effect is usually 24 hours. It has a half-life of 4 to 13 hours and is excreted in the urine. Darbepoetin alfa has a half-life of 21 hours after IV administration or 49 hours after subcutaneous administration. It reaches peak effect in 14 hours (if given IV) or 34 hours (subcutaneously). Duration of effects is 24 to 72 hours, and excretion is through the urine. It is not known whether epoetin alfa enters human milk. Methoxy polyethylene glycol-epoetin beta has a long half-life: 119 hours (IV) and 124 hours (subcutaneous). The onset of hemoglobin increase after administration is 7 to 15 days after the first dose. Steady-state levels are achieved with dosing every 2 weeks.

Contraindications and Cautions

These drugs are contraindicated in the presence of uncontrolled hypertension because of the risk of worsening hypertension when RBC numbers increase and the pressure within the vascular system increases, and with known hypersensitivity to any component of the drug to avoid hypersensitivity reactions. There are no adequate studies in pregnancy or lactation, so use should be limited to those situations in which the benefit to the patient clearly outweighs the potential risk to the fetus or baby.

Use caution when administering any of these drugs to patients with some cancers due to increased risk of tumor progression, in patients with normal renal functioning and adequate levels of erythropoietin because of the rebound decrease in erythropoietin that will occur, and when administering them to a patient with anemia and normal renal function because this can cause more severe anemia (Fig. 49.3; Box 49.2).

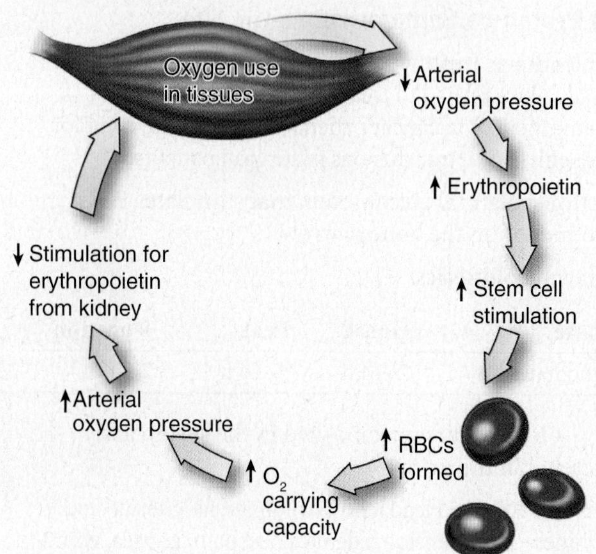

FIGURE 49.3 Erythropoiesis controls the rate of blood cell production.

Box 49.2 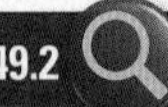 **Focus on Safe Medication Administration**

There is a risk of decreasing the endogenous erythropoietin from the kidneys if erythropoiesis-stimulating agents are administered to patients who have normal renal functioning and adequate levels of erythropoietin. High levels of RBCs that are stimulated with exogenous substance decrease the renal cell secretion of endogenous erythropoietin. Administration of this drug to an anemic patient with normal renal function can actually cause a more severe anemia if the endogenous levels fall and no longer stimulate RBC production.

Adverse Effects

The adverse effects most commonly associated with these drugs include the CNS effects of headache, fatigue, asthenia, and dizziness and the potential for serious seizures. These effects may be the result of a cellular response to the glycoprotein. Nausea, vomiting, and diarrhea are also common effects. Cardiovascular (CV) symptoms can include hypertension, edema, and possible chest pain, all of which may be related to the increase in RBC numbers changing the balance within the CV system. Serious CV effects and increased risk for deep vein thrombosis have been seen when the hemoglobin is higher than 11 g/dL. Patients receiving IV administration must also be monitored for possible clotting of the access line related to direct cellular effects of the drug. Rapid growth of cancer is seen when hemoglobin becomes higher than 11 g/dL. Postmarketing studies showed that pure red cell aplasia associated with erythropoietin-neutralizing antibodies could occur with all of these products. In 2008, after analyses of several postmarketing studies, boxed warnings were required on the drugs' prescribing information (Box 49.3).

Clinically Important Drug–Drug Interactions

These drugs should never be mixed in solution with any other drugs because of a risk of interactions in the solution.

Prototype Summary: Epoetin Alfa

Indications: Treatment of anemia associated with chronic renal failure related to treatment of HIV infection or to chemotherapy in cancer patients; to reduce the need for allogenic blood transfusions in surgical patients.

Actions: Natural glycoprotein that stimulates RBC production in the bone marrow.

Pharmacokinetics:

Route	Onset	Peak	Duration
Subcutaneous	7–14 d	5–24 h	24 h

$T_{1/2}$: 4 to 13 hours; metabolized in the serum and excreted in the urine.

Adverse Effects: Headache, arthralgias, fatigue, asthenia, dizziness, hypertension, edema, chest pain, nausea, vomiting, diarrhea, deep vein thrombosis, thrombotic events.

Box 49.3 **Focus on Safe Medication Administration**

In late 2005, the makers of epoetin and darbepoetin sent out warning letters to health care professionals to bring attention to serious adverse effects that had been noted in postmarketing studies. Cases of pure red cell aplasia (defective or insufficient production) and severe anemias, with or without cytopenias (decreased levels of other blood cells), had been reported. These cases were associated with the development of neutralizing antibodies to erythropoietin. Use of any therapeutic protein brings with it the risk of antibody production. All of the erythropoietic proteins (*Aranesp, Epogen, Mircera, Procrit*) now carry a warning about the potential for this problem. If a patient is being treated with one of these drugs and develops a sudden loss of response, accompanied by severe anemia and low reticulocyte count, the patient should be assessed for the possible causes. Assays for binding and neutralizing antibodies should be done. If an antibody-mediated anemia is confirmed, the drug should be permanently stopped, and the patient should not be switched to another erythropoietic protein because cross-reaction could occur. Most of the patients in the reported cases had chronic renal failure and were being treated with subcutaneous injections. It is now recommended that patients on hemodialysis receive the drug IV rather than subcutaneously. If the drug is started and there is no response or if a patient fails to maintain a response, the dose should not be increased, and red blood cell aplasia should be suspected. The patient should be evaluated with the appropriate tests and supported.

In recent years, the U.S. Food and Drug Administration alerted providers to the importance of a target hemoglobin of no more than 11 g/dL when using these drugs. Higher levels have been associated with CV events, including death, and increased rates of tumor progression death in cancer patients in whom the drug was being used to treat anemia associated with toxic drug therapy. Monitoring the hemoglobin levels is critical for safe and therapeutic use of the erythropoiesis-stimulating agents. An increase in tumor growth was also found in cancer patients treated with these drugs when hemoglobin levels were not kept within the guidelines of no more than 11 g/dL. This has been added to the boxed warnings for these drugs to alert caregivers to carefully monitor hemoglobin levels to assure patient safety.

Nursing Considerations for Patients Receiving Erythropoiesis-Stimulating Agents

Assessment: History and Examination

- Assess for contraindications or cautions: any known allergies to any component of the drug to avoid hypersensitivity reactions; severe hypertension, which could be exacerbated; and lactation because of potential adverse effects on the neonate. These drugs should be used with caution in patients with anemia and normal renal function to prevent rebound decrease in normal erythropoietin production and in patients with cancer receiving the drugs to increase hematocrit after antineoplastic chemotherapy because of the risk

of rapid tumor progression if hemoglobin levels exceed guidelines.
- Perform a physical assessment to establish a baseline before beginning therapy and during therapy to determine drug effectiveness and evaluate any potential adverse effects.
- Assess neurological status, including affect, orientation, and muscle strength, to identify possible adverse CNS effects.
- Monitor vital signs, including pulse and blood pressure, for changes, and assess CV status to identify possible CV effects; inspect lower extremities for evidence of edema, which could indicate a change in CV function.
- Assess respirations and auscultate lung sounds for adventitious breath sounds for early detection of changes in CV function.
- Monitor the results of laboratory tests, including renal function tests, complete blood count, hematocrit, iron concentration, transferrin, and electrolyte levels, to evaluate the effectiveness of therapy and to ensure that the hemoglobin level does not exceed 11 g/dL.

Nursing Conclusions

Nursing conclusions related to drug therapy might include the following:
- Nausea related to adverse GI effects
- Diarrhea related to GI effects
- Injury risk related to CNS effects
- Altered fluid volume related to CV effects
- Knowledge deficit regarding drug therapy

Planning

- The patient will receive the best therapeutic effect from the drug therapy.
- The patient will have limited adverse effects from the drug therapy.
- The patient will have an understanding of the drug therapy, adverse effects to anticipate, and measures to relieve discomfort and improve safety.

Intervention With Rationale

- Confirm the chronic, renal nature of the patient's anemia before administering the drug to treat renal failure anemia to ensure proper use of the drug.
- Give epoetin alfa as prescribed, either IV or subcutaneously, to achieve appropriate therapeutic drug levels. Administer darbepoetin alfa as prescribed, subcutaneously or IV.
- Provide the patient with a calendar of marked days to aid in remembering dates for injection and promote increased adherence to the drug regimen.
- Do not mix with any other drug solution, to avoid potential incompatibilities.
- Monitor access lines for clotting and arrange to clear line as needed.
- Ensure that prescribed laboratory testing, such as hematocrit levels, is completed before drug administration to determine correct dose. If the patient does not respond within 8 weeks, reevaluate the cause of anemia. Anticipate a target hemoglobin of 11 g/dL.
- Evaluate iron stores before and periodically during therapy because supplemental iron may be needed as the patient makes more RBCs.
- Monitor blood pressure due to risk for hypertension.
- Maintain seizure precautions on standby in case seizures occur as a reaction to the drug.
- Provide comfort measures to help the patient tolerate the drug effects. These include small, frequent meals to help minimize nausea and vomiting, readily available access to bathroom facilities should diarrhea occur, and analgesia for headache or arthralgia.
- Offer support and encouragement to help the patient deal with the diagnosis and the drug regimen.
- Provide thorough patient teaching, including the name of the drug, dosage prescribed, administration technique and frequency of administration, measures to avoid adverse effects, warning signs of problems and need to notify health care provider, and the need for follow-up laboratory testing, to enhance patient knowledge about drug therapy and to promote adherence.

Evaluation

- Monitor patient response to the drug (alleviation of anemia).
- Monitor for adverse effects (headache, hypertension, nausea, vomiting, seizures, dizziness).
- Monitor the effectiveness of comfort measures and adherence to the regimen.
- Evaluate the effectiveness of the teaching plan (patient can name drug, dosage, adverse effects to watch for, and specific measures to avoid them; patient understands the importance of continued follow-up).

Key Points

- Erythropoiesis-stimulating drugs are used to act like erythropoietin and stimulate the bone marrow to produce more RBCs.
- These drugs must be given IV or by subcutaneous injection. Patients must have an adequate supply of the other components of RBCs, including iron, for these drugs to be effective.
- Erythropoiesis-stimulating drugs should be used with a target hemoglobin level of no more than 11 g/dL. Higher levels are associated with an increased risk for CV events and increased tumor growth in cancer patients.

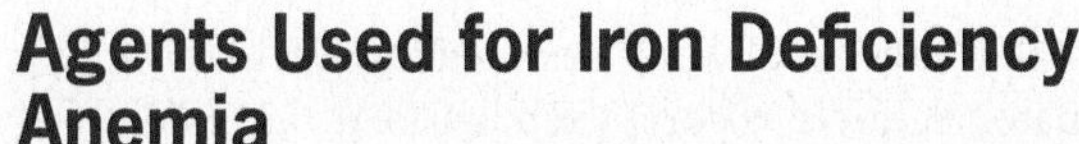

Agents Used for Iron Deficiency Anemia

Although most people get all of the iron they need through diet, in some situations, diet alone may not be adequate. The iron preparations that are available include ferrous fumarate (*Feostat*), ferrous gluconate (*Fergon*), ferrous sulfate (*Feosol*), ferrous sulfate exsiccated (*Ferralyn Lanacaps, Slow FE*), ferumoxytol (*Feraheme*), iron dextran (*InFeD*), iron sucrose (*Venofer*), and sodium ferric gluconate complex (*Ferrlecit*). See Table 49.2.

Therapeutic Actions and Indications

Iron preparations elevate the serum iron concentration. The iron molecules are then either converted to hemoglobin or stored for later use. Oral iron preparations are often used to help these patients regain a positive iron balance; these preparations should be supplemented with adequate dietary intake of iron. These agents are indicated for the treatment of iron deficiency anemias and may also be used as adjunctive therapy in patients receiving an erythropoiesis-stimulating drug. The drug of choice depends on the prescriber's personal preference and experience and the amount of elemental iron in each salt form. See Table 49.2 for usual indications.

Pharmacokinetics

Ferrous fumarate, ferrous gluconate, ferrous sulfate, ferrous sulfate exsiccated, and others are available for oral administration. Multiple preparations of iron are available in a parenteral form given either by IV or intramuscular (IM) injection. If given by IM injection, the Z-track method (Box 49.4) is recommended to avoid injecting into the subcutaneous tissue. The parenteral forms of iron replacement are primarily to be administered when oral replacement is either not tolerated or insufficient to replace stores. There may be increased benefit to IV iron in adults who have chronic kidney disease.

Table 49.2 *Drugs in Focus*: Agents Used for Iron Deficiency Anemia

Drug Name	Dosage/Route	Usual Indications
ferrous fumarate (*Feostat*)	100–200 mg/d PO *Pediatric 2–12 y*: 50–100 mg/d PO *Pediatric 6 mo to 2 y*: 6 mg/kg/d PO *Infants*: 10–25 mg/d PO	Treatment of iron deficiency anemia
ferrous gluconate (*Fergon*)	100–200 mg/d PO *Pediatric 2–12 y*: 50–100 mg/d PO *Pediatric 6 mo to 2 y*: 6 mg/kg/d PO *Infants*: 10–25 mg/d PO	Treatment of iron deficiency anemia
ferrous sulfate (*Feosol*)	100–200 mg/d PO *Pediatric 2–12 y*: 50–100 mg/d PO *Pediatric 6 mo to 2 y*: 6 mg/kg/d PO *Infants*: 10–25 mg/d PO	Treatment of iron deficiency anemia
ferrous sulfate exsiccated (*Ferralyn Lanacaps, Slow FE*)	100–200 mg/d PO *Pediatric 2–12 y*: 50–100 mg/d PO *Pediatric 6 mo to 2 y*: 6 mg/kg/d PO *Infants*: 10–25 mg/d PO	Treatment of iron deficiency anemia
ferumoxytol (*Feraheme*)	510 mg IV followed 3–8 d later with 510 mg IV, depending on patient response	Treatment of iron deficiency anemia in adults with chronic renal failure or in patients who have intolerance or unsatisfactory response to oral iron
iron dextran (*InFeD*)	IV: Dose varies based on weight and individual response	Treatment of iron deficiency anemia (parenteral)
iron sucrose (*Venofer*)	IV: Dose and frequency varies based on type of dialysis; pediatric dosing based on patient weight	Treatment of iron deficiency in patients with chronic kidney disease
sodium ferric gluconate complex (*Ferrlecit*)	*Adult:* 10 mL (125 mg of elemental iron) diluted in 100 mL of 0.9% sodium chloride administered IV over 1 hr per dialysis session or undiluted as a slow IV injection (at a rate of up to 12.5 mg/min) per dialysis session. *Pediatric:* 0.12 mL/kg (1.5 mg/kg of elemental iron) diluted in 25 mL 0.9% sodium chloride and administered by IV infusion over 1 hr per dialysis session.	Treatment of iron deficiency in patients 6 years and older undergoing chronic hemodialysis who are also receiving supplemental erythropoietin therapy

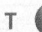

Box 49.4 Focus on Safe Medication Administration

Z-TRACK INJECTIONS

The Z-track method is used when injecting iron to reduce the risk of subcutaneous staining and irritation. It is a good idea to review the method of giving Z-track injections before giving one. Prep the area that will be injected. Place your gloved finger on the skin surface and pull the skin and the subcutaneous layers out of alignment with the muscle lying beneath. Try to move the skin about 1 cm, or 1/2 in. Insert the needle at a 90-degree angle at the point where you originally placed your finger. Inject the drug and then withdraw the needle. Remove your finger from the skin, which will allow the layers to slide back into their normal position. The track that the needle made when inserting into the muscle is now broken by the layers, and the drug is trapped in the muscle (Fig. 49.4).

Patients should be switched to the oral or IV form if at all possible because of the pain associated with IM administration of iron. Iron sucrose, ferumoxytol, and sodium ferric gluconate complex are given IV for patients who are undergoing chronic hemodialysis or who are in renal failure and not on dialysis but are receiving supplemental erythropoietin therapy and for patients with intolerance to oral replacement.

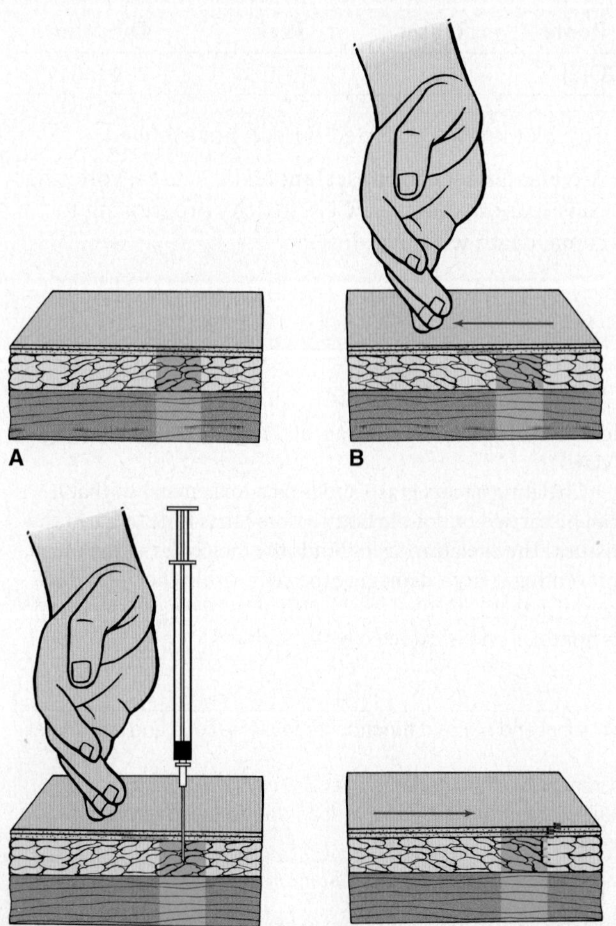

FIGURE 49.4 Use of the Z-track, or zigzag, technique for injections. **A.** Normal skin and tissues. **B.** Move the skin to one side. **C.** Insert the needle at a 90-degree angle and aspirate for blood. **D.** Withdraw the needle, and allow the displaced tissue to return to normal position, thereby keeping the solution from leaving the muscle tissue.

Iron is primarily absorbed from the small intestine by an active transport system. It is transported in the blood, bound to transferrin. Small amounts are lost daily in the sweat, urine, sloughing of the skin and mucosal cells, and sloughing of intestinal cells, as well as in menstrual flow. Most of the oral drug that is taken is lost in the feces, but some is absorbed slowly into the intestine and transported to the bone marrow. It can take 2 to 3 weeks to see improvement and up to 6 to 10 months for a return to a stable iron level once a deficiency exists. It is used during pregnancy and lactation to help the pregnant patient meet the increased demands for iron that occur at those times.

Contraindications and Cautions

These drugs are contraindicated for patients with known allergy to any of these preparations because severe hypersensitivity reactions have been associated with the parenteral form of iron. They also are contraindicated with hemochromatosis (excessive iron); anemias that are not iron deficiency anemias, which may increase serum iron levels and cause toxicity; normal iron balance because the drug will not be absorbed and will just pass through the body; and peptic ulcer, colitis, or regional enteritis because the drug can be directly irritating to these tissues and can cause exacerbation of diseases.

Adverse Effects

The most common adverse effects associated with oral iron are related to direct GI irritation; these include GI upset, anorexia, nausea, vomiting, diarrhea, dark stools, and constipation (Fig. 49.5). With increasing serum levels, iron can be directly toxic to the CNS, causing coma and even death. Box 49.5 discusses iron toxicity and drugs that are used to counteract this effect. Parenteral iron is associated with severe anaphylactic reactions, local irritation, staining of the tissues, and phlebitis. Ferumoxytol is a supermagnetic iron oxide that can alter magnetic resonance imaging (MRI) images and interpretation for up to 3 months after administration; patients should be aware that they have been given this drug and cautioned to report it before undergoing any medical testing. See the "Critical Thinking Scenario" for additional information about iron preparations and toxicity.

Clinically Important Drug–Drug Interactions

Iron absorption decreases if iron preparations are taken with antacids, substances with calcium and magnesium (all divalent cations), tetracyclines, or cimetidine; if these drugs must be used, they should be spaced at least 2 hours apart.

Antiinfective response to fluoroquinolones or tetracyclines can decrease if these drugs are taken with iron because of a decrease in absorption; they should also be administered at least 2 hours apart.

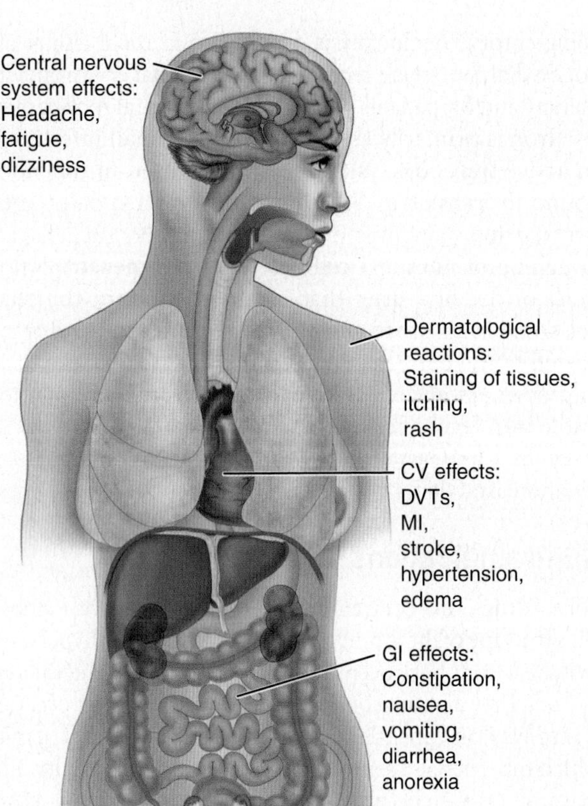

FIGURE 49.5 Variety of adverse effects and toxicities associated with drugs used to treat anemias.

Increased iron levels occur if iron preparations are taken with chloramphenicol; patients receiving this combination should be monitored closely for any sign of iron toxicity. The effects of levodopa may decrease if it is taken with iron preparations; patients receiving both of these drugs should take them at least 2 hours apart.

Clinically Important Drug–Food Interactions

Iron is not absorbed well if taken with antacids, eggs, milk, other calcium-containing substances, coffee, or tea. These substances should not be administered concurrently. Vitamin C may enhance the absorption of iron but also may increase the GI side effects.

Prototype Summary: Ferrous Sulfate

Indications: Prevention and treatment of iron deficiency anemia; dietary supplement for iron.

Actions: Elevates the serum iron concentration and is then converted into hemoglobin or stored for eventual conversion to a usable form of iron.

Pharmacokinetics:

Route	Onset	Peak	Duration
Oral	4 d	7–10 d	2–4 mo

$T_{1/2}$: Not known; recycled for use; not excreted.

Adverse Effects: GI upset, anorexia, nausea, vomiting, constipation, diarrhea, CNS toxicity progressing to coma, death with overdose.

BOX 49.5

Chelating Agents

Heavy metals, including iron, lead, arsenic, mercury, copper, and gold, can cause toxicity in the body with their ability to tie up in living tissue chemicals that need to be free in order for the cell to function normally. When these vital substances (thiols, sulfurs, carboxyls, and phosphoryls) are bound to the metal, certain cellular enzyme systems become deactivated, resulting in failure of cellular function and eventual cell death. Drugs that have been developed to counteract metal toxicity are called chelating agents (from the Greek word for "claw").

Chelating agents grasp and hold a toxic metal so that it can be carried out of the body before it has time to harm the tissues. The chelating agent binds the molecules of the metal, preventing it from damaging the cells within the body. The complex that is formed by the chelating agent and the metal is nontoxic and is excreted by the kidneys.

Chelating Agent	Toxic Metal	Notes
calcium disodium edetate	Lead	Given IM or IV; monitor renal and hepatic function because serious and even fatal toxicity can occur
deferasirox (*Exjade, Jadenu*)	Iron	Oral agent for chronic iron overload in patients over 2 y
deferiprone (*Ferriprox*)	Iron	Oral agent for treatment of transfusional iron overload due to thalassemia syndrome, sickle cell disease, or other anemias
deferoxamine mesylate (*Desferal*)	Iron	Given IM, subcutaneous, or IV; treatment of acute iron intoxication and of chronic iron overload due to transfusion-dependent anemias
dimercaprol (*BAL*)	Arsenic, gold, mercury	Given IM only for treatment of arsenic, gold, and mercury poisoning; treatment of acute lead poisoning when used concomitantly with edetate calcium disodium injection
penicillamine (*Cuprimine, Depen*)	Copper	Oral agent to reduce excess copper in patients with Wilson disease; used to suppress rheumatoid arthritis symptoms and decrease cystine excretion in cystinuria
succimer (*Chemet*)	Lead	Oral lead chelator that can be administered to pediatric patients
trientine (*Syprine*)	Copper	Oral agent to reduce excess copper in patients with Wilson disease

CRITICAL THINKING SCENARIO
Iron Preparations and Toxicity

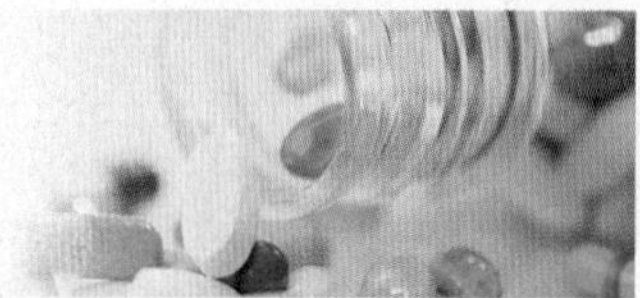

THE SITUATION

L.L., a 28-year-old patient, suffered a miscarriage 6 weeks ago. L.L. lost a great deal of blood during the miscarriage and underwent a dilation and curettage to control the bleeding. During the 6-week routine follow-up visit, L.L. was found to have recovered physically from the event but was still depressed over the loss. L.L.'s hematocrit was 31%, and they admitted feeling tired and weak. L.L. was offered emotional support and given a supply of ferrous sulfate tablets with instructions to take one tablet three times a day.

At home, L.L. transferred the pills to a decorative bottle that had once held vitamins and left it on the kitchen table as a reminder to take the tablets. The next day, L.L. discovered their 3-year-old child eating the tablets and punished the child for getting into them. About 1 hour later, the child complained of a really bad "tummy ache" and started vomiting. The child then became lethargic, and L.L. called the pediatrician, who told them to go immediately to the emergency department and bring the remaining tablets with them. The child was found to have a weak, rapid pulse (156 beats/min); rapid, shallow respirations (32/min); and a low blood pressure (60/42 mmHg). When a diagnosis of acute iron toxicity was made, L.L. became distraught. L.L. said they had no idea that iron could be dangerous because it can be bought over the counter (OTC) in so many preparations. L.L. had not read the written information given to them because it was "just iron."

CRITICAL THINKING

What nursing interventions should be done at this point?

What sort of crisis intervention would be most appropriate for L.L.? Think about the combined depression from the miscarriage, fear and anxiety related to this crisis, and L.L.'s iron-depleted state.

What kind of reserve does L.L. have for dealing with this crisis? Which measures would be appropriate for helping the parent cope with this crisis and for treating the child?

DISCUSSION

The first priority is to support and detoxify the child suffering from iron toxicity. In cases of acute iron toxicity, IV fluids should be administered to treat low blood volume and hypoperfusion. Deferoxamine is a medication that can bind to and assist with removal of iron from tissues. Whole-bowel irrigation and gastric lavage may be helpful treatments if there is unabsorbed iron still in the stomach. Patients who are symptomatic and have signs of instability in their vital signs should be admitted to a hospital for treatment. Supportive measures to deal with shock, dehydration, and GI damage will be necessary.

During this crisis, L.L. will need a great deal of support, including a responsible partner, relative, friend, or other person who can stay with L.L. They also will need reassurance and a place to rest. After the situation is stabilized, L.L. will need teaching and additional support. For example, they should be reassured that many people do not take OTC drugs as seriously as prescription medication, and many do not even read the labels. However, the nurse can use this opportunity to stress the importance of reading all of the labels and following the directions that come with OTC drugs. L.L. should also be commended for calling the pediatrician and getting medical care for the child quickly. Finally, L.L. should receive a review of the teaching information and be encouraged to ask questions.

This case is a good example for a staff in-service program, stressing not only the dangers of iron toxicity but also the vital importance of providing good patient education before sending a patient home with a new drug. Simply giving a patient written information is often not enough. The nursing care guide and teaching guidelines for L.L. when they were given the iron supplement should have been more thorough.

NURSING CARE GUIDE FOR L.L.: IRON PREPARATIONS

Assessment: History and Examination

Assess L.L.'s health history for allergies to any iron preparation, colitis, enteritis, hepatic dysfunction, or peptic ulcer.

Then, focus the physical examination on:

CV: Blood pressure, pulse, perfusion

CNS: Orientation, affect, reflexes, vision

Skin: Color, lesions, gums, teeth

Respiratory system: Respiratory rate and character, adventitious sounds

GI: Abdominal examination, bowel sounds

Laboratory tests: Complete blood count, hemoglobin, hematocrit, serum ferritin assays

Nursing Conclusions

Impaired comfort related to GI and CNS effects

Injury risk related to CNS effects

Knowledge deficit regarding drug therapy

Planning

The patient will receive the best therapeutic effect from the drug therapy.

The patient will have limited adverse effects from the drug therapy.

The patient will have an understanding of the drug therapy, adverse effects to anticipate, and measures to relieve discomfort and improve safety.

(continues on page 890)

Intervention

Confirm iron deficiency anemia before administering the drug.

Provide comfort and safety measures; for example, give small meals, ensure access to bathroom facilities, give the drug with food if GI upset occurs, and institute a bowel program as needed.

Arrange for the treatment of the underlying cause of anemia.

Provide support and reassurance to deal with drug effects.

Provide patient teaching regarding drug, dosage, adverse effects, what to report, and safety precautions.

Evaluation

Evaluate drug effects (relief of signs and symptoms of anemia, hematocrit within normal limits).

Monitor for adverse effects: GI upset, CNS toxicity, coma.

Monitor hematocrit and hemoglobin periodically.

Monitor for drug–drug interactions as indicated for each drug.

Evaluate the effectiveness of the patient teaching program and comfort and safety measures.

PATIENT TEACHING FOR L.L.

- Iron is a naturally occurring mineral found in many foods. It is used by the body to make RBCs, which carry oxygen to all parts of the body. Supplemental iron needs to be taken when the body does not have enough iron available to make healthy RBCs, a condition called anemia.
- Iron is a toxic substance if too much is taken. You must avoid self-medicating with OTC preparations containing iron while you are taking this drug.
- You will need to return for regular medical checkups while taking this drug to determine its effectiveness.
- Take your medication as follows, depending on the specific iron preparation that has been prescribed:
  - Dissolve ferrous salts in orange juice to improve the taste.
  - Take liquid iron preparations with a straw to prevent the iron from staining the teeth.
  - Place iron drops on the back of the tongue to prevent staining of the teeth.
- Some of the following adverse effects may occur:
  - *Dark, tarry, or green stools*: The iron preparations stain the stools; the color remains as long as you are taking the drug and should not cause concern.
  - *Constipation*: This is a common problem; if it becomes too uncomfortable, consult your health care provider for an appropriate remedy.
  - *Nausea, indigestion, and vomiting*: These problems can often be solved by taking the drug with food, making sure to avoid eggs, milk, coffee, and tea.
  - Report any of the following to your health care provider: severe diarrhea, severe abdominal pain or cramping, unusual tiredness or weakness, or bluish tint to the lips or fingernail beds.
- Tell any doctor, nurse, or other health care provider that you are taking this drug.
- Keep this drug and all medications out of the reach of children. Because iron can be toxic, seek emergency medical help immediately if you suspect that a child has taken this preparation unsupervised.
- Because iron can interfere with the absorption of some drugs, do not take iron at the same time as quinolones, tetracycline, or antacids. These drugs must be taken during intervals when iron is not in the stomach.

Nursing Considerations for Patients Receiving Iron Preparations

Assessment: History and Examination

- Assess for contraindications or cautions: any known allergies to this drug to avoid hypersensitivity reactions; hyperchromatosis to avoid increasing already increased iron levels; colitis, enteritis, or peptic ulcer, which could lead to increased GI irritation from the drug and exacerbation of the disorder; and hemolytic anemias, which could increase serum iron levels and lead to toxicity.
- Perform a physical assessment to establish a baseline before beginning therapy and during therapy to determine drug effectiveness and to evaluate for any potential adverse effects.
- Inspect the color and integrity of the skin and mucous membranes to identify potential signs and symptoms associated with anemia and evaluate for possible adverse effects of the parenteral form.
- Assess the patient's neurological status, including level of orientation, affect, and reflexes, to identify possible CNS effects and early signs of possible toxicity.
- Monitor pulse, blood pressure, perfusion, respirations, and adventitious sounds to check CV function and detect early signs of toxicity.
- Inspect the abdomen for distention and auscultate bowel sounds to evaluate GI motility.
- Inspect the skin integrity of the intended parenteral administration site to ensure intactness and evaluate for possible staining.
- Monitor the results of laboratory tests, including complete blood count, hematocrit, hemoglobin, and serum ferritin assays, to determine drug effectiveness and identify toxic levels.

Nursing Conclusions

Nursing conclusions related to drug therapy might include the following:

- Impaired comfort related to CNS or GI effects or parenteral administration

- Nausea related to adverse GI effects
- Constipation related to adverse GI effects
- Altered body image related to drug staining of the skin from parenteral injection
- Injury risk related to CNS effects
- Knowledge deficit regarding drug therapy

Planning

- The patient will receive the best therapeutic effect from the drug therapy.
- The patient will have limited adverse effects from the drug therapy.
- The patient will have an understanding of the drug therapy, adverse effects to anticipate, and measures to relieve discomfort and improve safety.

Intervention With Rationale

- Ensure that iron deficiency anemia is confirmed before administering drugs to ensure proper use of the drug.
- Consult with the health care provider to arrange for the treatment of the underlying cause of anemia if possible because iron replacement will not correct the cause of the iron loss.
- Administer the oral form with meals that do not include eggs, milk, coffee, and tea to relieve GI irritation and nausea if GI upset is severe and to prevent drug–food interactions; have the patient drink oral solutions through a straw to prevent staining of the teeth.
- Caution the patient that stools may be dark or green to prevent undue alarm if this occurs.
- Take measures to help alleviate constipation to prevent discomfort and the adverse effects of severe constipation.
- Administer IM only by the Z-track technique to ensure proper administration and to avoid brown staining of the tissues. Warn the patient that the injection can be painful.
- Arrange for hematocrit and hemoglobin measurements before administration and periodically during therapy to monitor drug effectiveness.
- Provide comfort measures to help the patient tolerate drug effects. These include small, frequent meals to minimize nausea, readily available access to bathroom facilities should constipation occur, and increased fiber and fluid intake and increased exercise to help alleviate constipation.
- Offer support and encouragement to help the patient deal with the diagnosis and the drug regimen.
- Provide thorough patient teaching, including the drug name, dosage, and route of administration; administration technique, such as parenteral Z-track injection or oral solution through a straw, and frequency of administration; foods and fluids to avoid and to include to ensure proper absorption; need for increased fluids and fiber foods in diet and increased exercise to prevent constipation; notification of change in stool color and consistency; potential for pain at site and staining of the skin with parenteral administration; measures to avoid adverse effects; warning signs of problems and need to notify health care provider; and the need for follow-up laboratory testing, to enhance patient knowledge about drug therapy and to promote adherence.

Evaluation

- Monitor patient response to the drug (alleviation of anemia).
- Monitor for adverse effects (GI upset and reaction, CNS toxicity, coma).
- Monitor the effectiveness of comfort measures and adherence to the regimen.
- Evaluate the effectiveness of the teaching plan (patient can name drug, dosage, adverse effects to watch for, and specific measures to avoid them; patient understands the importance of continued follow-up).

Key Points

- Iron products are used to replace iron in cases of iron deficiency anemia, which can occur because of deficient iron intake or because of blood loss leading to lower iron levels.
- Iron products commonly cause constipation, nausea, dark stools, and GI upset.
- Iron toxicity can cause severe CNS toxicity, coma, and even death because high iron levels are toxic to nerve cell membranes.

Agents Used for Other Anemias

The following section discusses treatment for megaloblastic hemolytic and aplastic anemia. Table 49.3 provides a complete list of agents.

Agents for Megaloblastic Anemias

Megaloblastic anemia is treated with folic acid and vitamin B_{12}. Folate deficiencies usually occur secondary to increased demand (as in pregnancy or growth spurts), as a result of absorption problems in the small intestine, because of drugs that cause folate deficiencies, or secondary to the malnutrition of alcoholism. Vitamin B_{12} deficiencies can result from poor diet or increased demand but can also be due to a lack of intrinsic factor in the stomach, which is necessary for absorption. Folic acid derivatives include folic acid (generic), leucovorin (generic), and levoleucovorin (*Fusilev, Khapzory*). Vitamin B_{12} includes hydroxocobalamin (generic) and cyanocobalamin (*Calomist, Nascobal, Vibisone*).

Table 49.3 *Drugs in Focus*: Agents Used for Other Anemias

Drug Name	Dosage/Route	Usual Indications
Agents for Megaloblastic Anemias		
Folic Acid Derivatives		
folic acid (generic)	1 mg/d PO, IM, subcutaneously, or IV	Replacement therapy and treatment of megaloblastic anemia due to folate deficiency; prevention of neural tube defects; supplement for malabsorption syndromes and alcohol use disorder
leucovorin (generic)	IM, IV, and PO dosing; amount varies based on formulation and indication	Treatment after high-dose methotrexate therapy or toxicity; treatment of megaloblastic anemias due to folic acid deficiency; used in combination with 5-fluorouracil to prolong survival in the palliative treatment of patients with advanced colorectal cancer
levoleucovorin (*Fusilev, Khapzory*)	PO and IV dosing; varies based on indication	Replacement therapy and treatment of megaloblastic anemia; used as "leucovorin rescue" after chemotherapy, allowing noncancerous cells to survive the chemotherapy; used with fluorouracil for palliative treatment of colorectal cancer; lowers toxicity and counteracts the effects of impaired methotrexate elimination and of inadvertent overdose of folic acid antagonists after high-dose methotrexate therapy in osteosarcoma
Vitamin B_{12}		
cyanocobalamin (*Calomist, Nascobal, Vibisone*)	Nasal spray, oral, sublingual, IM, subcutaneous injection; dose varies based on formulation	Replacement therapy; treatment of megaloblastic anemia due to lack of vitamin B_{12}
hydroxocobalamin (generic)	30 mcg/d IM for 5–10 d and then 100–200 mcg/mo IM *Pediatric*: 1–5 mg IM over ≥2 wk and then 30–50 mcg IM every 4 wk	Replacement therapy; treatment of megaloblastic anemia, pernicious anemia
Agents for Sickle Cell Anemia		
crizanlizumab-tmca (*Adakveo*)	5 mg/kg IV over 30 min on wk 0, 2, and every 4 wk after	Reduction of the frequency of vasoocclusive crises in patients with sickle cell disease
hydroxyurea (Droxia, Hydrea, Siklos)	PO dosing varies based on formulation and individual response; reduce dose with renal impairment	Reduction of frequency of painful crises and to decrease the need for blood transfusions in adults with sickle cell anemia
voxelotor (Oxbryta)	1,500 mg PO daily; reduce dose with severe hepatic impairment	Treatment of sickle cell disease in adults and pediatric patients 12 years and older
Agent for Beta Thalassemia		
luspatercept-aamt (*Reblozyl*)	1 mg/kg subcutaneous every 3 wk	Treatment of anemia in adult patients with beta thalassemia who require RBC transfusions; anemia failing an erythropoiesis-stimulating agent and requiring 2 or more RBC units over 8 weeks in adult patients with very low- to intermediate-risk myelodysplastic syndromes
Agent for Aplastic Anemia		
eltrombopag (*Promacta*)	PO dosing varies per indication; reduce dose with hepatic impairment and for patients with Asian ancestry	Treatment of thrombocytopenia in adult and pediatric patients 1 year and older with persistent or chronic ITP who have had an insufficient response to corticosteroids, immunoglobulins, or splenectomy; treatment of thrombocytopenia in patients with chronic hepatitis C to allow the initiation and maintenance of interferon-based therapy; combination with standard immunosuppressive therapy for first-line treatment of adult and pediatric patients 2 years and older with severe aplastic anemia; treatment of patients with severe aplastic anemia who have had an insufficient response to immunosuppressive therapy

Therapeutic Actions and Indications

Folic acid and vitamin B_{12} are essential for cell growth and division and for the production of a strong stroma in RBCs (see Fig. 49.3). Folic acid is necessary for the production of DNA, RBC, WBC, and platelets. Vitamin B_{12} is also necessary for maintenance of the myelin sheath in nerve tissue. Both are given as replacement therapy for dietary deficiencies, as replacement in high-demand states such as pregnancy and lactation, and to treat megaloblastic anemia. Folic acid is used as a rescue drug for cells exposed to some toxic chemotherapeutic agents. Leucovorin is used as a rescue drug following methotrexate therapy to decrease the toxicity of methotrexate caused by decreased elimination or overdose of folic acid antagonists such as trimethoprim and for the treatment of various megaloblastic anemias. Levoleucovorin is the newest drug in this class and is approved to decrease the toxicity of methotrexate caused by decreased elimination or overdose of folic acid antagonists in the treatment of osteosarcomas. See Table 49.3 for usual indications for each of these agents.

Pharmacokinetics

Folic acid can be given in oral, IM, IV, and subcutaneous forms. Parenteral drugs are preferred for patients with potential absorption problems; all other patients should be given the oral form if at all possible. Leucovorin is a reduced form of folic acid that is available for oral, IM, and IV use. Levoleucovorin is only available in an IV form.

Hydroxocobalamin must be given IM every day for 5 to 10 days to build up levels and then once a month for life. It cannot be taken orally because the problem with pernicious anemia is the inability to absorb vitamin B_{12} secondary to low levels of intrinsic factor. It can be used in states of increased demand (e.g., pregnancy, growth spurts) or dietary deficiency, but oral vitamins are preferred in most of those cases. Cyanocobalamin is not as tightly bound to proteins and does not last in the body as long as hydroxocobalamin. This drug is primarily stored in the liver and slowly released as needed for metabolic functions. It is available in oral and sublingual forms, as an intranasal gel that allows vitamin B_{12} absorption directly through the nasal mucosa, and as injectable medication.

Folic acid and vitamin B_{12} are well absorbed after injection, metabolized mainly in the liver, and excreted in the urine. These vitamins are considered essential during pregnancy and lactation because of the increased demands of the pregnant person's metabolism. Folate deficiency during pregnancy can cause neural tube defects.

Contraindications and Cautions

These drugs are contraindicated in the presence of known allergies to these drugs or to their components to avoid hypersensitivity reactions. Nasal cyanocobalamin should be used with caution in the presence of nasal erosion or ulcers, which could alter absorption of the drug.

Adverse Effects

These drugs have relatively few adverse effects because they are used as replacements for required chemicals. Hydroxocobalamin has been associated with itching, rash, and signs of excessive vitamin B levels, which can also include peripheral edema and heart failure. Mild diarrhea has been reported with these drugs. Pain and discomfort can occur at injection sites. Nasal irritation can occur with the use of intranasal spray.

Prototype Summary: Folic Acid

Indications: Treatment of megaloblastic anemia due to folate deficiency, malabsorption, or nutritional deficiency; prevention of neural tube defects.

Actions: Reduced form of folic acid, required for nucleoprotein synthesis and maintenance of normal erythropoiesis.

Pharmacokinetics:

Route	Onset	Peak
Oral, IM, subcutaneous, IV	Varies	30–60 min

$T_{1/2}$: Unknown; metabolized in the liver and excreted in the urine.

Adverse Effects: Allergic reactions, pain and discomfort at injection site.

Prototype Summary: Hydroxocobalamin

Indications: Treatment of vitamin B_{12} deficiency; to meet increased vitamin B_{12} requirements related to disease, pregnancy, or blood loss; treatment of pernicious anemia.

Actions: Essential for nucleic acid and protein synthesis; used for growth, cell reproduction, hematopoiesis, and nucleoprotein and myelin synthesis.

Pharmacokinetics:

Route	Onset	Peak
IM	Intermediate	60 min

$T_{1/2}$: 24 to 36 hours; metabolized in the liver and excreted in the urine.

Adverse Effects: Itching, transitory exanthema, mild diarrhea, anaphylactic reaction, heart failure, pulmonary edema, hypokalemia, pain at injection site.

Nursing Considerations for Patients Receiving Folic Acid Derivatives or Vitamin B_{12}

Assessment: History and Examination

- Assess for contraindications or cautions: any known allergies to these drugs or drug components, other anemias, and nasal erosion.
- Assess baseline status before beginning therapy to determine any potential adverse effects and effectiveness of supplements. This includes affect, orientation, and reflexes; pulse, blood pressure, and perfusion; respirations and adventitious sounds; signs of vitamin B_{12} deficiency (beefy red tongue, pallor, neuropathy); and complete blood count, hematocrit, vitamin B_{12}, folate, and iron levels.

Nursing Conclusions

Nursing conclusions related to drug therapy might include the following:

- Impaired comfort related to injection or nasal irritation
- Risk for fluid volume imbalance related to CV effects
- Knowledge deficit regarding drug therapy

Planning

- The patient will receive the best therapeutic effect from the drug therapy.
- The patient will have limited adverse effects from the drug therapy.
- The patient will have an understanding of the drug therapy, adverse effects to anticipate, and measures to relieve discomfort and improve safety.

Intervention With Rationale

- Confirm the nature of the megaloblastic anemia to ensure that the proper drug regimen is being used.
- Give both types of drugs in cases of pernicious anemia to ensure therapeutic effectiveness.
- Give parenteral vitamin B_{12} IM each day for 5 to 10 days and then once a month for life if used to treat pernicious anemia.
- Arrange for nutritional consultation to ensure a well-balanced diet.
- Monitor for the possibility of hypersensitivity reactions; have life support equipment on standby in case reactions occur.
- Arrange for hematocrit readings before and periodically during therapy to monitor drug effectiveness.
- Provide comfort measures to help the patient tolerate drug effects. These include small, frequent meals; access to bathroom facilities; and analgesia for muscle or nasal pain.
- Provide thorough patient teaching, including the name of the drug, dosage prescribed, measures to avoid adverse effects, warning signs of problems, and the need for periodic monitoring and evaluation, to enhance patient knowledge about drug therapy and to promote adherence to the drug regimen.
- Offer support and encouragement to help the patient deal with the diagnosis and the drug regimen.

Evaluation

- Monitor patient response to the drug (alleviation of anemia).
- Monitor for adverse effects (nasal irritation, pain at injection site, nausea).
- Evaluate the effectiveness of the teaching plan (patient can name drug, dosage, adverse effects to watch for, and specific measures to avoid them; patient understands the importance of continued follow-up).
- Monitor the effectiveness of comfort measures and adherence to the regimen.

Agents for Hemolytic and Aplastic Anemias

Two types of inherited hemolytic anemia result from sickle cell disease and thalassemia. Some patients with sickle cell anemia are treated with antibiotics to help fight the infections that can occur when blood flow is decreased to any area and with pain-relieving activities to help alleviate the pain associated with the anoxia to tissues, which can range from heat applied to the area to OTC pain medications to prescription opioids. There are also some prescription medications indicated for patients with sickle cell disease. They include crizanlizumab-tmca (*Adakveo*), hydroxyurea (*Droxia, Hydrea, Siklos*), and voxelotor (*Oxbryta*). Hydroxyurea is a cytotoxic antineoplastic drug that is also used to treat leukemia, ovarian cancer, and melanoma (see Chapter 14). Luspatercept-aamt (*Reblozyl*) is an erythroid maturation agent indicated for the treatment of anemia in patients with beta thalassemia and some myelodysplastic syndromes.

Aplastic anemia is a disease caused by damage to the bone marrow and the bone marrow stem cells. The damage can be caused by drugs, radiation exposure, infection, immune pancytopenia disorders, and sometimes genetics. There are deficiencies in all of the blood components formed in the bone marrow; this is called pancytopenia. Low RBC count (anemia), low white blood cell count (leukopenia), and low platelet count (thrombocytopenia) are characteristic of pancytopenia. In addition, the stem cell count in the bone marrow becomes low and that area of the bone marrow is often replaced by fat deposits. The patient with this situation is at high risk for bleeding (loss of platelets) and infection (loss of white cells) and is often tired and pale (loss of red cells). Treatment may involve the use of immunosuppressant drugs, corticosteroids, or replacement elements in critical situations; bone marrow transplant is often an option. Eltrombopag (*Promacta*) is an oral drug that is now approved for use in treating aplastic anemia and immune thrombocytopenia (ITP).

Therapeutic Actions and Indications

Hydroxyurea, taken for several months, increases the amount of fetal hemoglobin produced in the bone marrow and dilutes the formation of the abnormal hemoglobin S in adults who have sickle cell anemia. This results in less clogging of small vessels and the painful, anoxic effects associated with RBC sickling or stacking. Crizanlizumab-tmca is a monoclonal antibody that binds to P-selectin and inhibits the interactions between endothelium and platelets, RBCs, and leukocytes. Inhibiting the attachment of blood cells to the endothelium is helpful in reducing the frequency of vasoocclusive crises in adults and pediatric patients aged 16 years and older with sickle cell disease. Voxelotor is a hemoglobin S polymerization inhibitor indicated for the treatment of sickle cell disease in adults and pediatric patients 12 years of age and older. It reduces the hemoglobin S polymerization and RBC sickling. This may decrease symptoms by improving RBC deformability and reducing whole blood viscosity.

Luspatercept-aamt (*Reblozyl*) is an agent administered subcutaneously every few weeks to patients who require RBC transfusions due to anemia associated with beta thalassemia and some myelodysplastic syndromes.

Eltrombopag is a thrombopoietin receptor agonist that initiates signaling cascades in the bone marrow leading to proliferation and differentiation of the bone marrow progenitor cells, leading to increased production of blood components. See Table 49.3 for usual indications.

Pharmacokinetics

Crizanlizumab-tmca is administered intravenously. It is metabolized into small peptides. It is eliminated slowly with a terminal half-life of about 10 days.

Given orally, hydroxyurea is absorbed well from the GI tract, reaching peak level in 1 to 4 hours. It is metabolized in the liver and excreted in the urine with a half-life of 3 to 4 hours. It is known to cross the placenta and to enter human milk.

Voxelotor is absorbed after oral administration, reaching peak concentration in 6 to 18 hours. It binds to the hemoglobin on RBCs. It is metabolized in the liver primarily by CYP3A4; the dose should be lowered if the patient has severe liver impairment. It is eliminated in urine and feces. The half-life is about 35 hours.

Luspatercept-aamt is slowly absorbed after subcutaneous injection over about 7 days. Its half-life is about 11 days, and it is metabolized by tissues to be changed into amino acids.

Eltrombopag is absorbed from the GI tract and reaches peak level in 2 to 6 hours; after hepatic metabolism, it is excreted primarily in the feces with a half-life of 21 to 32 hours.

Contraindications and Cautions

Hydroxyurea is contraindicated with known allergy to any component of the drug to prevent hypersensitivity reactions and with severe anemia or leukopenia because it can cause further bone marrow suppression. It should be used with caution in the presence of impaired liver or renal function, which could interfere with metabolism and excretion of the drug, and it should only be used in pregnancy and lactation if the benefit to the patient clearly outweighs the potential risk to the fetus or baby because this drug crosses the placenta and enters human milk and could cause serious adverse effects in the fetus or baby.

Caution should be taken when administering crizanlizumab-tmca and luspatercept-aamt during pregnancy due to animal studies showing potential for fetal harm. These drugs are not recommended during lactation. There is no significant human evidence of harm or safety of voxelotor being administered during pregnancy, so individual risks and benefits should be examined.

Eltrombopag has a boxed warning about the risk of severe hepatic impairment if used in patients with chronic hepatitis C, though it is approved for the treatment of thrombocytopenia in patients with chronic hepatitis C to allow for interferon treatment. These patients must be monitored closely. It also has a boxed warning that the dose needs to be reduced when used in patients of eastern Asian heritage because the drug level will be higher.

Adverse Effects

Hydroxyurea is cytotoxic and is associated with adverse effects associated with the death of cells, especially in cells that are rapidly turning over. GI effects include anorexia, nausea, vomiting, stomatitis, diarrhea, or constipation; dermatological effects include rash or erythema; and bone marrow suppression usually occurs. Headache, dizziness, disorientation, fever, chills, and malaise have been reported, possibly related to the effects of cell death in the body. As with other cytotoxic drugs, there is increased risk of cancer development.

The most common side effects of crizanlizumab-tmca are nausea, joint and back pain, abdominal pain, and pyrexia. It should be discontinued if there are signs of infusion reactions that include pain and/or respiratory distress. Voxelotor can cause headache, diarrhea, abdominal pain, nausea, fatigue, rash, and pyrexia. Signs of hypersensitivity reactions should be monitored, as well.

Luspatercept-aamt is associated with increased risk of thrombosis, hypertension, fatigue, headache, muscle/joint pain, dizziness/vertigo, nausea, diarrhea, abdominal pain, and shortness of breath. Eltrombopag is associated with hepatotoxicity, thrombosis, nausea, cough, fatigue, headache, and diarrhea.

Clinically Important Drug–Drug Interactions

There is an increased risk of increased uric acid levels if hydroxyurea is combined with any uricosuric agents; if this combination must be used, dose adjustments will be needed for the uricosuric agent. Concurrent use of cytotoxic medication or antivirals can increase the adverse effects. Due to its metabolism, coadministration of voxelotor and other medications that either inhibit or induce the CYP3A4 enzymes will affect the plasma concentration of voxelotor. Therefore, either avoidance of coadministration or titration of the dose is recommended.

Prototype Summary: Hydroxyurea

Indications: Reduction of frequency of painful crisis and need for blood transfusions in adult patients with sickle cell anemia.

Actions: Increases fetal hemoglobin production in the bone marrow and dilutes the formation of abnormal hemoglobin S.

Pharmacokinetics:

Route	Onset	Peak	Duration
Oral	Varied	1–4 h	18–20 h

$T_{1/2}$: 3 to 4 hours; metabolized in the liver and excreted in the urine.

Adverse Effects: Dizziness, headache, rash, erythema, anorexia, nausea, vomiting, stomatitis, bone marrow depression, cancer.

Key Points

- Megaloblastic anemia is treated with folic acid and vitamin B_{12}. There are multiple routes of administration for these supplements, but if the patient lacks intrinsic factor, vitamin B_{12} will not be effective if administered orally.
- Sickle cell disease and thalassemia can cause hemolytic anemia.
- Hydroxyurea, an antineoplastic drug, is useful in reducing the painful crises and need for blood transfusions in adults with sickle cell anemia. It is associated with many adverse effects because it is a cytotoxic drug.
- Aplastic anemia can be treated with eltrombopag, a thrombopoietin receptor agonist that stimulates the bone marrow to make more blood cells.

SUMMARY

- Blood is composed of liquid plasma and formed elements (white blood cells, RBCs, and platelets) and contains oxygen and nutrients that are essential for cell survival; it delivers these to the cells and removes waste products from the tissues.
- RBCs are produced in the bone marrow in a process called erythropoiesis, which is controlled by the glycoprotein erythropoietin, produced by the kidneys.
- RBCs do not have a nucleus, and their lifespan is about 120 days, at which time they are lysed and their building blocks are recycled to make new RBCs.
- The bone marrow uses iron, amino acids, carbohydrates, folic acid, and vitamin B_{12} to produce healthy, efficient RBCs.
- An insufficient number or immaturity of RBCs results in low oxygen levels in the tissues, with tiredness, fatigue, and loss of reserve.
- Anemia is a state of too few RBCs or ineffective RBCs. Anemia can be caused by a lack of erythropoietin or by a lack of the components needed to produce RBCs.
- Iron deficiency anemia occurs when there is inadequate iron intake in the diet or an inability to absorb iron from the GI tract. Iron is needed to produce hemoglobin, which carries oxygen. Iron deficiency anemia is treated with iron replacement.
- Iron is a toxic mineral at high levels. The body controls the absorption of iron and carefully regulates its storage and movement in the body.
- Folic acid and vitamin B_{12} are needed to produce a strong supporting structure in the RBC so that it can survive 120 days of being propelled through the vascular system. Both folic acid and vitamin B_{12} are usually found in adequate amounts in the diet. Deficiencies that cause megaloblastic anemia are treated with folic acid and vitamin B_{12} replacement.
- Pernicious anemia is a lack of intrinsic factor that is required for absorption of vitamin B_{12}.
- Sickle cell disease and thalassemia can cause hemolytic anemia.
- Hydroxyurea, an antineoplastic drug, is useful in reducing the painful crises and need for blood transfusions in adults with sickle cell anemia. It is associated with many adverse effects because it is a cytotoxic drug.
- Aplastic anemia can be treated with eltrombopag, a thrombopoietin receptor agonist that stimulates the bone marrow to make more blood cells.

CHECK YOUR UNDERSTANDING

Answers to the questions in this chapter can be found in Answers to Check Your Understanding Questions on thePoint®.

MULTIPLE CHOICE

Select the best answer.

1. After teaching a group of students about RBC production, the instructor determines that the teaching was effective when the group states that the rate of RBC production is controlled by
   a. iron.
   b. folic acid.
   c. erythropoietin.
   d. vitamin B_{12}.

2. RBCs must be continually produced by the body because they
   a. contain iron that wears out and must be replaced.
   b. cannot maintain themselves and wear out.
   c. are continuously entering and being lost from the GI tract.
   d. are processed into bile salts and must be replaced.

3. Which would the nurse include in the teaching plan when describing all types of anemia to a patient?
   a. Decreased number of or abnormal RBCs
   b. Lack of iron in the body
   c. Lack of vitamin B_{12} in the body
   d. Excessive number of platelets

4. Megaloblastic anemia is a result of insufficient folic acid or vitamin B_{12}, affecting which?
   a. White blood cell production
   b. Vegetarians
   c. Rapid cell turnover
   d. Slow-growing cells

5. The nurse would expect the provider to prescribe epoetin alfa (*Epogen*) for
   a. acute blood loss during surgery.
   b. replacement of blood after a traumatic injury.
   c. treatment of anemia during lactation.
   d. treatment of anemia associated with renal failure.

6. A patient with aplastic anemia may be prescribed which medication?
   a. Eltrombopag
   b. Luspatercept
   c. Vitamin B_{12}
   d. Folic acid

7. To ensure maximum absorption, a nurse instructs a patient receiving oral iron therapy to avoid taking the iron with
   a. protein.
   b. many antibiotics.
   c. fats.
   d. antiplatelet medications.

8. After teaching a patient with pernicious anemia about vitamin B_{12} therapy, which patient statement would indicate that the teaching was successful?
   a. "I can take this pill with breakfast."
   b. "I should take this pill at bedtime."
   c. "I need to inject this drug subcutaneously every day."
   d. "I need to inject this drug IM every 5 to 10 days."

MULTIPLE RESPONSE

Select all that apply.

1. Instructions for a patient prescribed iron pills should include which of the following?
   a. Taking the drug with milk to avoid GI problems
   b. The potential for constipation
   c. Keeping these potentially toxic pills away from children
   d. Taking the drug with antacids to alleviate GI upset
   e. Having periodic blood tests to evaluate the drug effect
   f. Being aware that stools may be green in color

2. In a healthy person, little iron is needed on a daily basis. Loss of iron is associated with which conditions?
   a. Heavy menstrual flow
   b. Bile duct obstruction
   c. Internal bleeding
   d. Penetrating traumatic injury
   e. Bone marrow suppression
   f. Alcoholic cirrhosis

REFERENCES

Balducci, L., Ershlor, W., & Bennett, J. (2007). *Anemia in the elderly.* Springer Science.

Bennett, C. L., Silver, S. M., Djulbegovic, B., Samaras, A. T., Blau, C. A., Gleason, K. J., Barnato, S. E., Elverman, K. M., Courtney, D. M., McKoy, J. M., Edwards, B. J., Tigue, C. C., Raisch, D. W., Yarnold, P. R., Dorr, D. A., Kuzel, T. M., Tallman, M. S., Trifilio, S. M., West, D. P., … Henke, M. (2008). Venous thromboembolism and mortality associated with recombinant erythropoietin and darbepoetin administration for the treatment of cancer-associated anemia. *Journal of the American Medical Association, 299*, 914–924. http://doi.org/10.1001/jama.299.8.914

Brookhart, M., Schneeweiss, S., Ahorn, J., Bradbury, B. D., Liu, J., & Winkelmayer, W. C. (2010). Comparative mortality risk of anemia management practices in incident hemodialysis patients. *Journal of the American Medical Association, 303*(9), 857–864. http://doi.org/10.1001/jama.2010.206

Brunton, L., Hilal-Dandan, R., & Knollman, B. (2018). *Goodman and Gilman's the pharmacological basis of therapeutics* (13th ed.). McGraw-Hill.

Hall, J. E., & Hall, M. E. (2021). *Guyton and Hall textbook of medical physiology* (14th ed.). Elsevier.

Norris, T. L. (2019). *Porth's pathophysiology concepts of altered health states* (13th ed.). Wolters Kluwer.

Yawn, B., Buchanan, G., Afenyi-annan, A., Ballas, S. K., Hassell, K. L., James, A. H., Jordan, L., Lanzkron, S. M., Lottenberg, R., Savage, W. J., Tanabe, P. J., Ware, R. E., Murad, M. H., Goldsmith, J. C., Ortiz, E., Fulwood, R., Horton, A., & John-Sowah, J. (2014). Management of sickle cell disease: Summary of the 2014 evidence-based report by expert panel members. *Journal of the American Medical Association, 312*(10), 1033–1048. http://doi.org/10.1001/jama.2014.10517

Yuen, H., & Becker W. (2021). *Iron toxicity*. StatPearls Publishing. https://www.ncbi.nlm.nih.gov/books/NBK459224/

PART 9

Drugs Acting on the Renal System

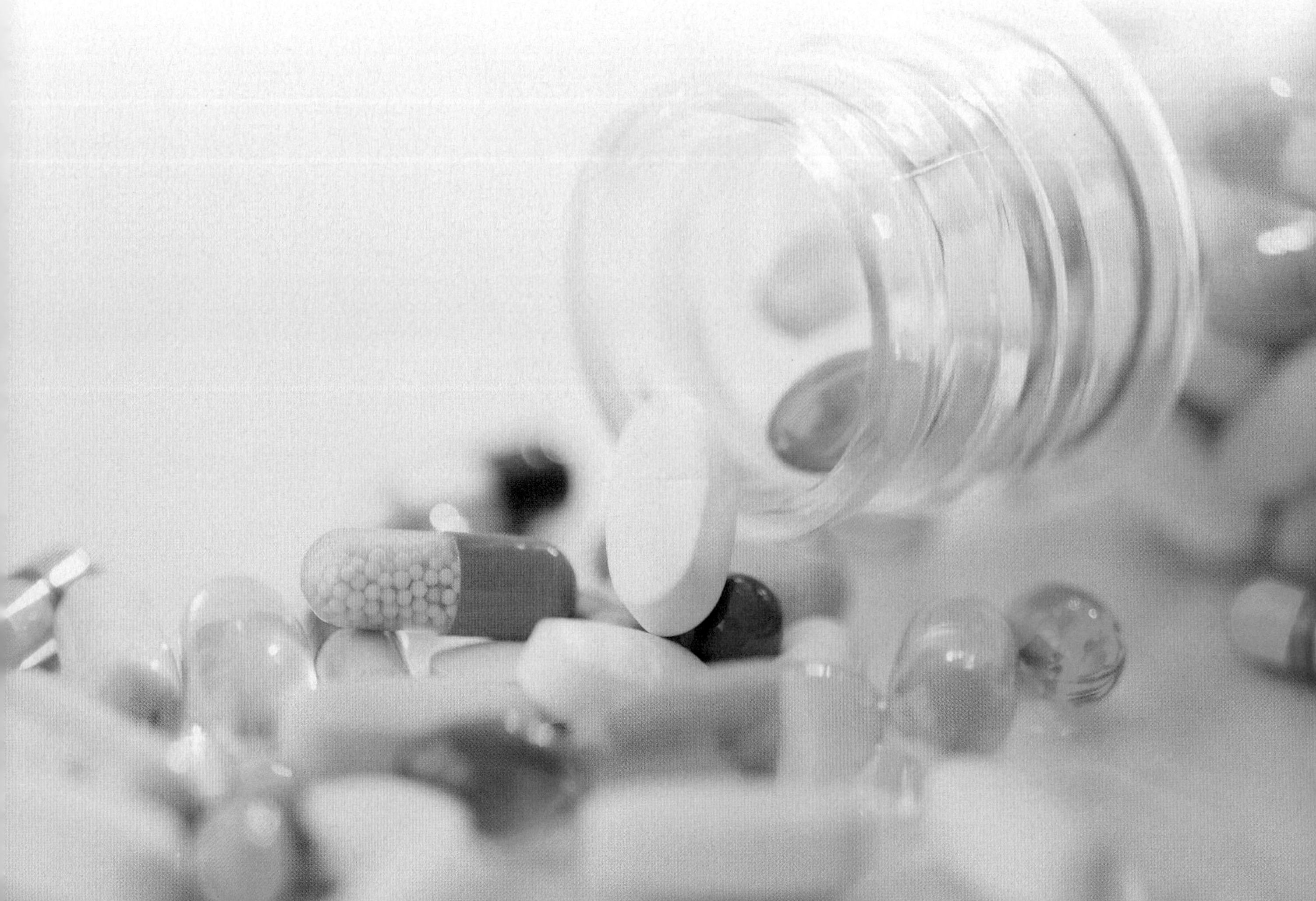

CHAPTER 50

Introduction to the Renal System

Learning Objectives

Upon completion of this chapter, you will be able to:

1. Review the anatomy of the kidney, including the structure of the nephron.
2. Explain the basic processes of the kidney and where these processes occur.
3. Explain the control of sodium, chloride, potassium, and calcium in the nephron.
4. Discuss the countercurrent mechanism and the control of urine concentration and dilution, applying these effects to various clinical scenarios.
5. Describe the renin–angiotensin–aldosterone system, including controls and clinical situations in which this system is active.
6. Discuss the role of the kidney in acid–base balance, calcium regulation, and red blood cell production, integrating this information to explain the clinical manifestations of renal failure.
7. Describe anatomy of the urinary tract.

Key Terms

aldosterone: hormone produced by the adrenal gland that causes the distal tubule to retain sodium, and therefore water, while losing potassium into the urine

antidiuretic hormone (ADH): hormone produced by the hypothalamus and stored in the posterior pituitary gland; important in maintaining fluid balance; causes the distal tubules and collecting ducts of the kidney to become permeable to water, leading to an antidiuretic effect and fluid retention

carbonic anhydrase: catalyst that speeds up the chemical reaction combining water and carbon dioxide, which react to form carbonic acid and immediately dissociate to form sodium bicarbonate and a free hydrogen ion

countercurrent mechanism: process used by medullary nephrons to concentrate or dilute the urine in response to body stimuli to maintain fluid and electrolyte balance

filtration: passage of fluid and small components of the blood through the glomerulus into the nephron tubule

glomerulus: a membrane composed of several layers that function to provide a size-dependent diffusion barrier in which small molecules are able to be filtered into the nephron, but large proteins and blood cells typically are kept outside the nephron

nephron: functional unit of the kidney; composed of Bowman's capsule, the proximal and distal convoluted tubules, and the collecting duct

prostate gland: gland located around the urethra; responsible for producing an acidic fluid that maintains sperm and lubricates the urinary tract

reabsorption: movement of substances from the renal tubule back into the vascular system

renin–angiotensin–aldosterone system (RAAS): compensatory process that leads to increased blood pressure and blood volume to ensure perfusion of the kidneys; important in the continual regulation of blood pressure

secretion: active movement of substances from the blood into the renal tubule for excretion

The renal system is composed of the kidneys and the structures of the urinary tract: the ureters, the urinary bladder, and the urethra. This system has four major functions in the body:

- Maintaining the volume and composition of body fluids within normal ranges, including the following functions:
  - Clearing nitrogenous wastes from protein metabolism
  - Maintaining acid–base balance and electrolyte levels
  - Excreting various drugs and drug metabolites
- Regulating vitamin D activation, which helps maintain and regulate calcium levels
- Regulating blood pressure through the renin–angiotensin–aldosterone system
- Regulating red blood cell production through the production and secretion of erythropoietin

The Kidneys

The kidneys are two small organs that make up about 0.5% of total body weight but receive about 25% of the cardiac output. Approximately 180 L of blood is filtered by the nephrons each day. Most of the fluid that is filtered out by the kidneys is returned to the body, and the waste products that remain are excreted in a relatively small amount of water as urine.

Structure

The kidneys are located outside the peritoneal cavity in the posterior upper abdomen at the level between the 12th thoracic and 3rd lumbar vertebrae. They have protective layers including the renal capsule (a fibrous layer) and fatty connective tissue. The capsule contains pain fibers, which are stimulated if the capsule is stretched secondary to an inflammatory process.

The kidneys have three identifiable regions: the outer cortex, the inner medulla, and the renal pelvises. The renal pelvises drain the urine into the ureters. The ureters are muscular tubes that lead into the urinary bladder, where urine is stored until it is excreted (Fig. 50.1).

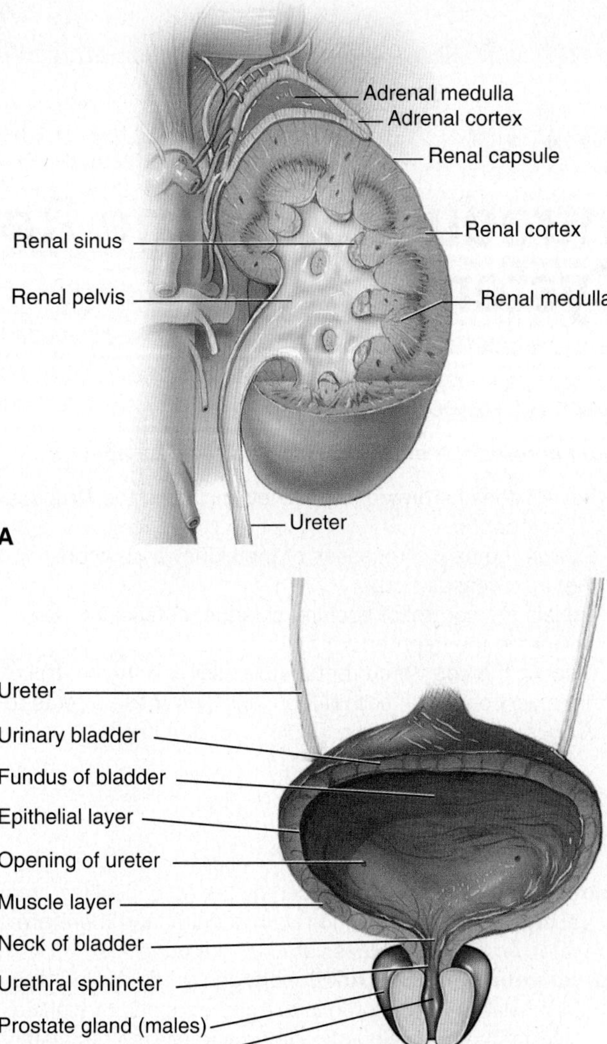

FIGURE 50.1 The kidney (**A**) and organs of the urinary tract (**B**).

Nephron

The functional unit of the kidneys is called the **nephron**. There are approximately 2 million nephrons in a young adult. Humans are not able to make new nephrons, and the number of nephrons decreases after the age of 40. There are two main types of nephrons. The cortical nephrons are in the cortex of the kidney, and the juxtamedullary nephrons that have longer loops of Henle extend deep into the renal medulla. All of the nephrons filter fluid and make urine, but the juxtamedullary nephrons can concentrate or dilute urine. It is estimated that only about 25% of the total number of nephrons are necessary to maintain healthy renal function. That means that the renal system is well protected from failure with a large backup system. However, it also means that by the time a patient manifests signs and symptoms suggesting failure of the kidneys, extensive kidney damage has already occurred.

The nephron is a tube that begins at Bowman's capsule and becomes the proximal and then distal convoluted tubule (Fig. 50.2). Bowman's capsule is a structure that surrounds the glomerulus, a high-pressure capillary system that brings blood to the nephron to be filtered. The tube exits the capsule, curling around in a section called the proximal convoluted tubule. From there, it narrows to form the descending and ascending loop of Henle. It widens as the distal convoluted tubule and then flows into the collecting ducts, which meet at the renal pelvises. Each section of the tubule functions in a slightly different manner to maintain fluid and electrolyte balance in the body.

Blood Supply

The blood flow to the nephron is unique. The renal arteries come directly off the aorta and enter each kidney at a deep medial fissure called the hilus as segmental arteries. Segmental arteries divide further into lobular and then interlobar arteries. These become smaller arcuate (bowed) arteries and then afferent arterioles. The afferent arterioles branch to form the glomerulus inside Bowman's capsule. The **glomerulus** membrane has three layers (capillary endothelial layer, basement membrane, and single-celled capsular epithelial layer). The layers of the glomerulus function to provide a size-dependent diffusion barrier in which small molecules are able to be filtered into the nephron, but large proteins and blood cells typically are not. The efferent arteriole exits from the glomerulus and branches into the peritubular capillary system, which contains concentrated blood and returns fluid and electrolytes that have been reabsorbed from the tubules to the bloodstream. These capillaries flow into the vasa recta (capillary network that runs along the loop of Henle in the nephron), which flows into intralobar veins, which in turn drain into the inferior vena cava. The two arterioles around the glomerulus work together to closely regulate the flow of fluid into the glomerulus, increasing or decreasing pressure on either side of the glomerulus as needed.

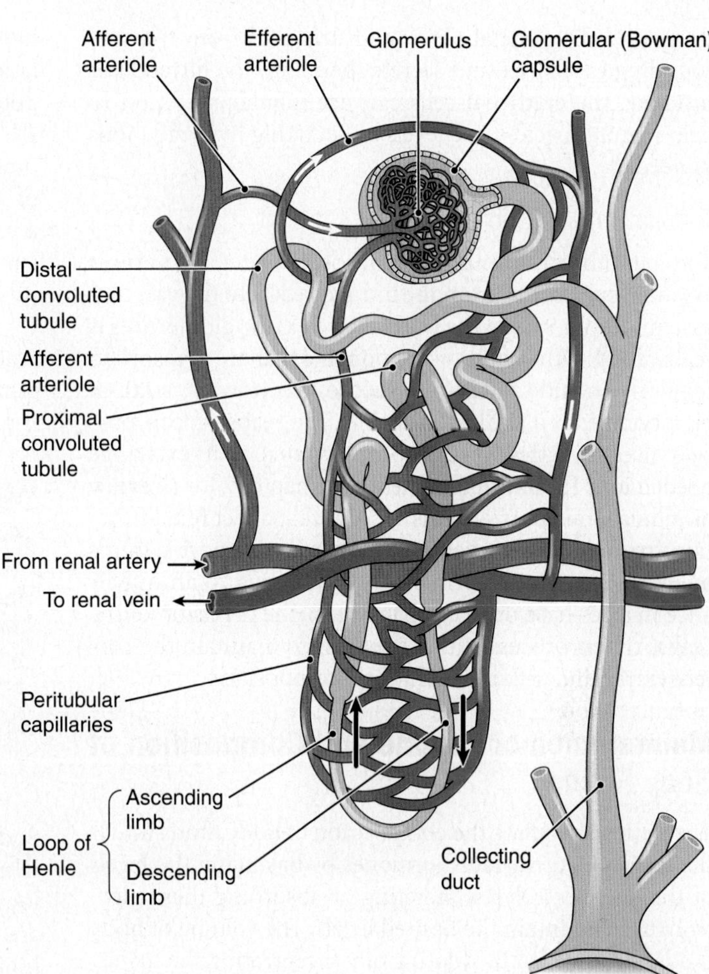

FIGURE 50.2 The nephron—the functional unit of the kidneys. Secretion and reabsorption of water, electrolytes, and other solutes in the various segments of the renal tubule, the loop of Henle, and the collecting duct can be influenced by diuretics, other drugs, and endogenous substances, including certain hormones. In the kidneys, the distal convoluted tubule wraps around and is actually next to the afferent arteriole.

Other Structures

A small group of cells called the juxtaglomerular apparatus help to control the rate of glomerular filtration (passage of fluid and small components of the blood through the glomerulus into the nephron tubule). The juxtaglomerular cells are in the walls of the afferent and efferent arterioles, and they are able to secrete renin. After a series of chemical conversions, renin is able to increase constriction of arterioles and increase the glomerular hydrostatic pressure, which increases filtration rate. Specialized endothelial cells in the distal tubule, called the macula densa, sense low sodium concentration. If sodium levels are low in the distal tubule, the macula densa will signal for the afferent arterioles to decrease resistance and for the juxtaglomerular cells to increase release of renin. Both of these actions are designed to enhance blood flow to the kidneys and increase the glomerular filtration rate.

Nephron Function

The nephrons function by using three basic processes: glomerular **filtration** (passage of fluid and small components of the blood through the glomerulus into the nephron tubule), tubular **secretion** (movement of substances from the blood into the renal tubule), and tubular **reabsorption** (movement of substances from the renal tubule back into the vascular system).

Glomerular Filtration

The glomerulus acts as an ultrafine filter for all of the blood that flows into it. The semipermeable membrane keeps blood cells, proteins, and lipids inside the vessel, while hydrostatic pressure from the blood pushes water and smaller components of the plasma into the tubule. The resulting fluid is called the filtrate. Scarring or swelling of or damage to the semipermeable membrane leads to the escape of larger plasma components, such as blood cells or protein, into the filtrate. The large size of these components prevents them from being reabsorbed by the tubule, and they are lost in the urine. Thus, a clinical sign of renal damage is the presence of blood cells or protein in the urine.

Approximately 125 mL of fluid is filtered out each minute, or 180 L/d. About 99% of the filtered fluid is returned to the bloodstream as the filtrate continues its movement through the renal tubule. Approximately 1% of the filtrate—less than 2 L of fluid—is excreted each day in the form of urine.

Tubular Secretion

The epithelial cells that line the renal tubule can secrete substances from the blood into the tubular fluid. Most of the time secretion is an energy-using process that allows active transport systems to remove electrolytes, some drugs and drug metabolites, and uric acid from the surrounding capillaries and secrete them into the filtrate. For instance, the epithelial cells can use tubular secretion to help maintain acid–base levels by secreting hydrogen ions as needed.

Tubular Reabsorption

The cells lining the renal tubule reabsorb water and various essential substances from the filtrate back into the vascular system. About 99% of the water filtered at the glomerulus is reabsorbed. Other filtrate components that are reabsorbed regularly include vitamins, glucose, electrolytes, sodium bicarbonate, and sodium chloride. The reabsorption process uses a series of transport systems that exchange needed ions for unwanted ones (see Chapter 7 for a review of cellular transport systems). Drugs that affect renal function frequently overwhelm one of these transport systems or interfere with its normal activity, leading to an imbalance in acid–base or electrolyte levels. The precision of the reabsorption process allows the body to maintain the correct extracellular fluid volume and composition.

Maintenance of Volume and Composition of Body Fluids

The kidneys regulate the composition of body fluids under the influence of various hormones by balancing the levels of the key electrolytes, secreting or absorbing these electrolytes to maintain the desired levels. The volume of body fluids is controlled by diluting or concentrating the urine.

Sodium Regulation

Sodium is one of the body's major cations (positively charged ions). It filters through the glomerulus and enters the renal tubule; then, it is actively reabsorbed in the proximal convoluted tubule to the peritubular capillaries. As sodium is actively moved out of the filtrate, it takes chloride ions and water with it. This occurs by passive diffusion as the body maintains the osmotic and electrical balances on both sides of the tubule.

Sodium ions are also reabsorbed via a transport system that functions under the influence of the catalyst **carbonic anhydrase**. This enzyme speeds the combining of carbon dioxide and water to form carbonic acid. The carbonic acid immediately dissociates to form sodium bicarbonate, using a sodium ion from the renal tubule and a free hydrogen ion (an acid). The hydrogen ion remains in the filtrate, causing the urine to be slightly acidic. The bicarbonate is stored in the renal tubule as the body's alkaline reserve for use when the body becomes too acidic and a buffer is needed.

The distal convoluted tubule acts to further adjust the sodium levels in the filtrate under the influence of **aldosterone** (a hormone produced by the adrenal gland) and natriuretic hormone (probably produced by the hypothalamus). Aldosterone is released into the circulation as part of the diurnal rhythm in response to high potassium levels, sympathetic stimulation, or angiotensin III. Aldosterone stimulates a sodium–potassium exchange pump in the cells of the distal tubule, causing reabsorption of sodium in exchange for potassium (see Chapter 7 for a review of the sodium pump). As a result of aldosterone stimulation, sodium is reabsorbed into the system and potassium is lost in the filtrate.

Natriuretic hormone causes a decrease in sodium reabsorption from the distal tubules with a resultant diluted urine or increased volume. Natriuretic hormone is released in response to fluid overload or hemodilution.

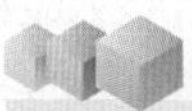
Concept Mastery Alert

Acid–Base Balance in the Urinary System

The kidneys return bicarbonate to the body's circulation; the bicarbonate is stored in the renal tubule as the body's alkaline reserve for use when the body becomes too acidic and a buffer is needed, helping to maintain the body's acid–base balance.

Countercurrent Mechanism

Sodium is further regulated in the medullary nephrons in what is known as the **countercurrent mechanism** in the loop of Henle. In the descending loop of Henle, the cells are freely permeable to water; water will flow out into the high osmolar tissue surrounding the nephron. Sodium is actively reabsorbed into the surrounding peritubular tissue in most areas of the nephron, except the descending limb of the loop of Henle, which is less permeable to sodium. The filtrate at the end of the descending loop of Henle is concentrated in comparison to the rest of the filtrate.

In contrast, the ascending loop of Henle is impermeable to water, and so water that remains in the tubule is trapped there. Sodium, potassium, and chloride are actively transported out of the tubule using energy in a process that is referred to as the sodium/potassium/chloride cotransport system. As a result, the fluid in the ascending loop of Henle becomes hypotonic in comparison to the hypertonic situation in the peritubular tissue.

Antidiuretic hormone (ADH), which is produced by the hypothalamus and stored in the posterior pituitary gland, is important in maintaining fluid balance. ADH is released in response to falling blood volume, sympathetic stimulation, or rising sodium levels (a concentration that is sensed by the osmotic cells of the hypothalamus).

If ADH is present at the distal convoluted tubule and the collecting duct, the permeability of the membrane to water is increased. Consequently, the water remaining in the tubule rapidly flows into the hypertonic tissue surrounding the loop of Henle, where it either is absorbed by the peritubular capillaries or reenters the descending loop

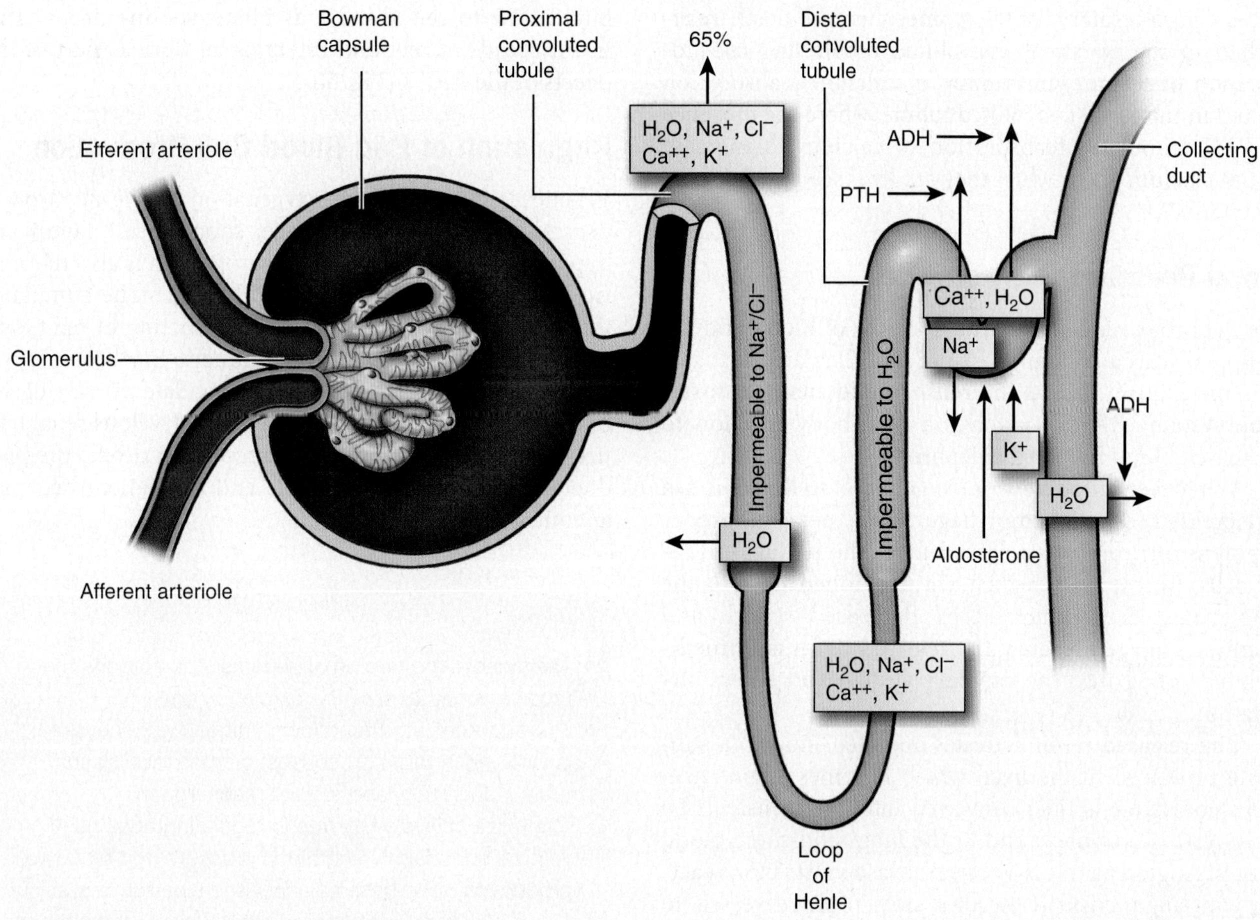

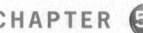

FIGURE 50.3 Nephron and points of regulation of sodium, chloride, potassium, calcium, and water. ADH, antidiuretic hormone; PTH, parathyroid hormone.

of Henle in a countercurrent style. The resulting urine is hypertonic and of small volume. If ADH is not present, the tubule remains impermeable to water. The water that has been trapped in the ascending loop of Henle passes into the collection duct, resulting in hypotonic urine of greater volume. This countercurrent mechanism and the influence of the hypothalamus and ADH release allow the body to finely regulate fluid volume by regulating the control of sodium and water (Fig. 50.3).

Chloride Regulation

Chloride is an important negatively charged ion that helps maintain electrical neutrality with the movement of cations across the cell membrane. Chloride is reabsorbed at the second half of the proximal convoluted tubule. Chloride is actively reabsorbed in the loop of Henle and distal convoluted tubule, where it promotes the movement of sodium out of the nephron.

Potassium Regulation

Potassium is another cation that is vital to proper functioning of the nervous system, muscles, and cell membranes. About 65% of the potassium that is filtered at the glomerulus is reabsorbed at Bowman's capsule and the proximal convoluted tubule. Another 25% to 30% is reabsorbed in the ascending loop of Henle. The fine tuning of potassium levels occurs in the distal convoluted tubule, where aldosterone activates sodium–potassium exchange, leading to a loss of potassium. If potassium levels are very high, the retention of sodium in exchange for potassium also leads to a retention of water and a dilution of blood volume, which further decreases the potassium concentration (see Fig. 50.3).

Calcium Regulation

Calcium is important in muscle function, blood clotting, bone formation, contraction of cell membranes, and muscle movement and is another important cation that is regulated by the kidneys. The absorption of calcium from the gastrointestinal (GI) tract is regulated by vitamin D ingested as part of the diet. The vitamin then must be activated in the kidneys to a form that will promote calcium absorption. Once absorbed from the GI tract, calcium levels are maintained within a tight range by the activity of parathyroid hormone (PTH) and calcitonin.

Calcium is filtered at the glomerulus and mostly reabsorbed in the proximal convoluted tubule and ascending loop of Henle. Fine tuning of calcium reabsorption occurs in the distal convoluted tubule, where the presence of PTH stimulates reabsorption of calcium to increase serum calcium levels when they are low (see Fig. 50.3 and Chapter 37).

Blood Pressure Control

The nephrons require a constant supply of blood and are equipped with a system to ensure that they are perfused. This mechanism, called the **renin–angiotensin–aldosterone system (RAAS)**, involves a total body reaction to decreased blood flow to the nephrons.

Whenever blood flow or oxygenation to the nephron is decreased (due to hemorrhage, shock, heart failure, or hypotension), renin is released from the juxtaglomerular cells. (These cells, which are positioned next to the glomerulus, are stimulated by decreased stretch and decreased oxygen levels.) The released renin is immediately absorbed into the capillary system and enters circulation.

The released renin activates angiotensinogen, a substrate produced in the liver, which becomes angiotensin I. Angiotensin I is then converted into angiotensin II by a converting enzyme found in the lungs and some blood vessels. Angiotensin II is a powerful vasoconstrictor, reacting with angiotensin II receptor sites in blood vessels to cause vasoconstriction. This powerful vasoconstriction raises blood pressure and should increase blood flow to the kidneys.

Angiotensin II is converted in the adrenal gland to angiotensin III, which stimulates the release of aldosterone from the adrenal gland. Aldosterone acts on the distal convoluted tubules to retain sodium and therefore water. This increases blood volume and further increases blood pressure, which should increase blood flow to the kidneys. The osmotic center in the brain senses the increased sodium levels and releases ADH, leading to a further retention of water and a further increase in blood volume and pressure, which should again increase blood flow to the kidneys.

The RAAS constantly works to maintain blood flow to the kidneys. For example, a person rising from a lying position experiences a drop in blood flow to the kidneys as blood pools in the legs because of gravity. This causes a massive release of renin and activation of this system to ensure that blood pressure is maintained and the kidneys are perfused. Blood loss from injury or during surgery also activates this system to increase blood flow through the kidneys.

Drugs that interfere with any aspect of this system will cause a reflex response. For instance, taking a drug such as a diuretic to decrease fluid volume can lead to decreased blood flow to the kidneys as blood volume drops. This in turn leads to rebound retention of fluid as part of the effects of the RAAS (Fig. 50.4).

Regulation of Red Blood Cell Production

Whenever blood flow or oxygenation to the nephron is decreased (due to hemorrhage, shock, heart failure, or hypotension), the hormone erythropoietin is also released from the juxtaglomerular cells. This hormone stimulates the bone marrow to increase the production of red blood cells, which bring oxygen to the kidneys. Erythropoietin is the only known hormone that can regulate the rate of red blood cell production. When a patient develops renal failure and the production of erythropoietin drops, the production of red blood cells falls and the patient becomes anemic.

Key Points

- The kidneys are two small, bean-shaped organs that receive about 25% of the cardiac output.
- The nephron is the functional unit of the kidneys and is involved in three processes: glomerular filtration, tubular secretion, and tubular reabsorption.
- The kidney plays a key role in regulating body fluid volume and maintaining blood pressure, red blood cell production, acid–base balance, and electrolyte stability.
- The RAAS is activated when blood flow to the nephron is decreased and renin is released. The end results are increased vasoconstriction and increased blood pressure and sodium and water retention, which increase blood volume and pressure.
- Red blood cell production is controlled by erythropoietin released from the juxtaglomerular apparatus when oxygen delivery to the nephron is decreased. Erythropoietin stimulates the bone marrow to produce red blood cells to increase oxygen delivery to the nephrons.

The Urinary Tract

As noted previously, the urinary tract is composed of the ureters, urinary bladder, and urethra (see Fig. 50.1).

Ureters

One ureter exits each kidney, draining the filtrate from the collecting ducts. The ureters have a smooth endothelial lining and circular muscular layers. Urine entering the ureter stimulates a peristaltic wave that pushes the urine down toward the urinary bladder.

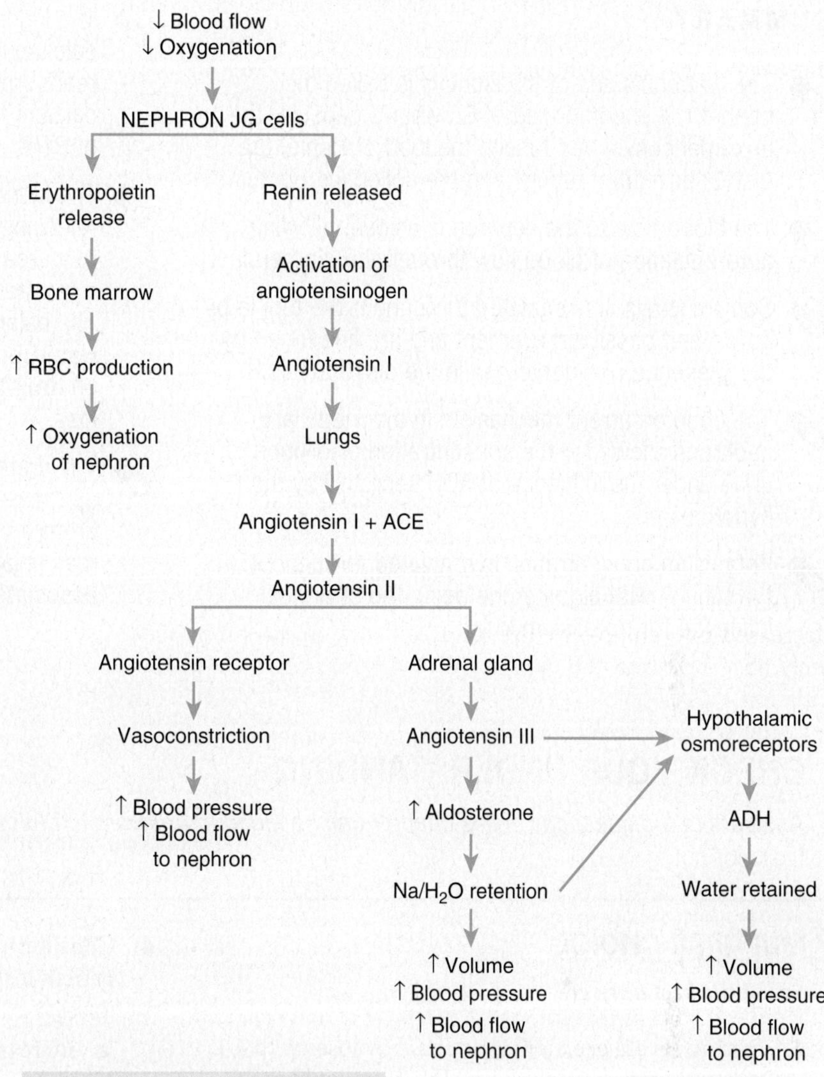

FIGURE 50.4 The renin–angiotensin–aldosterone system for reflex maintenance of blood pressure control.

Urinary Bladder

The urinary bladder is a muscular pouch that stretches and holds the urine until it is excreted from the body. Urine is usually a slightly acidic fluid; this acidity helps to maintain the normal transport systems and to destroy bacteria that may enter the bladder. Control of bladder emptying is learned control over the external urethral sphincter. Both the sympathetic and parasympathetic nervous systems innervate the bladder muscle and sphincters.

Urethra

The female urethra is a short tube that leads from the bladder to an area populated by normal flora, including *Escherichia coli*, which can cause bladder infections or cystitis. The male urethra is much longer and passes through the **prostate gland**, a small gland that produces an alkaline fluid that is important in maintaining the sperm and lubricating the tract. Enlargement and infection in the prostate gland are often problems in older males.

Key Points

- The ureters, urinary bladder, and urethra make up the rest of the urinary tract.
- The shorter female urethra leads from the urinary bladder to the outer body into an area rich in gram-negative bacteria. Cystitis, or infection of the urinary bladder, is a common problem for females.
- The longer male urethra passes through the prostate gland, which may enlarge or become infected, a problem often associated with advancing age.

SUMMARY

- The functional unit of the kidneys is called the nephron; it is composed of Bowman's capsule, the proximal convoluted tubule, the loop of Henle, the distal convoluted tubule, and the collecting duct.
- The blood flow to the nephron is unique, allowing autoregulation of blood flow through the glomerulus.
- Sodium levels are regulated throughout the tubule by active and passive movement and are fine tuned by the presence of aldosterone in the distal tubule.
- The countercurrent mechanism in the medullary nephrons allows for the concentration or dilution of urine under the influence of ADH secreted by the hypothalamus.
- Potassium concentration is regulated throughout the tubule, with aldosterone being the strongest influence for potassium loss.
- The kidneys play a key role in the regulation of calcium by activating vitamin D to allow GI calcium reabsorption and by reabsorbing or excreting calcium from the tubule under the influence of PTH.
- The kidneys influence blood pressure control, releasing renin to activate the RAAS, which leads to increased blood pressure and volume and a resultant increased blood flow to the kidney. The balance of this reflex system can lead to water retention or excretion and has an impact on drug therapy that promotes water or sodium loss.
- The ureters, urinary bladder, and urethra make up the rest of the urinary tract. The longer male urethra passes through the prostate gland, which may enlarge or become infected, a problem often associated with advancing age.

CHECK YOUR UNDERSTANDING

Answers to the questions in this chapter can be found in Answers to Check Your Understanding Questions on thePoint®.

MULTIPLE CHOICE

Select the best answer.

1. During severe exertion, a person may lose up to 4 L of hypotonic sweat per hour. This loss would result in
   a. decreased plasma volume.
   b. decreased plasma osmolarity.
   c. decreased circulating levels of ADH until ingestion of 100 mL of water.
   d. return of body fluid balance to normal after ingestion of 100 mL of water.

2. Urine passes through the ureter by
   a. osmosis.
   b. air pressure.
   c. filtration.
   d. peristalsis.

3. When describing renal reabsorption to a group of students, the instructor would identify it as the movement of which?
   a. Substances from the renal tubule into the blood
   b. Substances from the blood into the renal tubule
   c. Water that is increased in the absence of ADH
   d. Sodium occurring only in the proximal tubule

4. Considering the functions of the kidney, if a patient lost kidney function, a nurse would expect to see
   a. increased red blood cell count.
   b. decreased fluid volume.
   c. low blood potassium.
   d. variability in control of blood pressure.

5. Blood flow to the nephron differs from blood flow to other tissues in that
   a. the venous system is not involved in blood flow around the nephron.
   b. there are no capillaries in the nephron allowing direct flow from the artery to the vein.
   c. efferent and afferent arterioles allow for autoregulation of blood flow.
   d. the capillary bed has a fenestrated membrane to allow passage of fluid and small particles.

6. Concentration and dilution of urine are controlled by
   a. afferent arterioles.
   b. the renin–angiotensin–aldosterone system.
   c. aldosterone release.
   d. the countercurrent mechanism.

7. Females tend to have more problems with bladder infections than males because
   a. females have *Escherichia coli* in the urinary tract.
   b. the female urethra is short, making access to the bladder easier for bacteria.
   c. the prostate gland secretes a substance that protects males from bladder infections.
   d. females' urine is more acidic, encouraging the growth of bladder bacteria.

MULTIPLE RESPONSE

Select all that apply.

1. Considering the metabolic functions of the kidneys, renal failure would be expected to cause which conditions?
   a. Anemia
   b. Loss of calcium regulation
   c. Urea buildup on the skin
   d. Respiratory alkalosis
   e. Metabolic acidosis
   f. Changes in the function of blood cells

2. During severe diarrhea, there is a loss of water, bicarbonate, and sodium from the GI tract. Physiological compensation for this would probably include which conditions?
   a. Increased alveolar ventilation
   b. Decreased hydrogen ion secretion by the renal tubules
   c. Decreased urinary excretion of sodium and water
   d. Increased renin secretion
   e. Increased hydrogen ion secretion by the renal tubules
   f. Increased ADH levels

3. Maintenance of blood pressure is important in maintaining the fragile nephrons. Reflex systems that work to ensure blood flow to the kidneys include which of the following?
   a. The RAAS causing vasoconstriction
   b. Baroreceptor monitoring of the renal artery
   c. Aldosterone release secondary to angiotensin stimulation
   d. ADH release in response to decreased blood volume with increased osmolarity
   e. Release of erythropoietin
   f. Local response of the afferent arterioles

REFERENCES

Barrett, K., Barman, S., Brooks, H. L., & Yuan, J. (2019). *Ganong's review of medical physiology* (26th ed.). McGraw-Hill.

Brunton, L., Hilal-Dandan, R., & Knollman, B. (2018). *Goodman and Gilman's the pharmacological basis of therapeutics* (13th ed.). McGraw-Hill.

Eaton, D. C., & Pooler, J. P. (2013). *Vander's renal physiology* (8th ed.). McGraw-Hill.

Hall, J. E., & Hall, M. E. (2021). *Guyton and Hall textbook of medical physiology* (14th ed.). Elsevier.

Norris, T. L. (2019). *Porth's pathophysiology concepts of altered health states* (13th ed.). Wolters Kluwer.

Rennke, H. G., & Denker, B. M. (2019). *Renal pathophysiology: The essentials* (5th ed.). Wolters Kluwer.

CHAPTER 51

Diuretic Agents

Learning Objectives

Upon completion of this chapter, you will be able to:

1. Define the term diuretic and list the five classes of diuretics.
2. Discuss the use of diuretic agents across the lifespan.
3. Describe the therapeutic actions, indications, pharmacokinetics, contraindications and cautions, most common adverse reactions, and important drug–drug interactions associated with the various classes of diuretic drugs.
4. Compare and contrast the prototype drugs of each class of diuretic drugs with other agents in their class.
5. Outline the nursing considerations, including important teaching points, for patients receiving diuretic agents.

Key Terms

alkalosis: a rise in serum pH to an alkaline state

edema: increased movement of fluid into the interstitial spaces from the blood vessels

fluid rebound: reflex reaction of the body to the loss of fluid or sodium; the hypothalamus causes the release of antidiuretic hormone, which promotes water retention, and stress related to fluid loss combines with decreased blood flow to the kidneys to activate the renin–angiotensin–aldosterone system, leading to further water and sodium retention

high-ceiling diuretics: powerful diuretics that work in the loop of Henle to inhibit the reabsorption of sodium and chloride, leading to a sodium-rich diuresis

hyperaldosteronism: excessive output of aldosterone from the adrenal gland, leading to increased sodium and water retention and loss of potassium

hypokalemia: low potassium in the blood, which may occur with some diuretic treatment; characterized by weakness, muscle cramps, trembling, nausea, vomiting, diarrhea, and cardiac arrhythmias

osmotic pull: drawing force of large molecules on water, pulling it into a tubule or capillary essential for maintaining normal fluid balance within the body; used to draw out excess fluid into the vascular system or the renal tubule

Drug List

DIURETICS

Thiazide Diuretics and Thiazide-Like Diuretics

Thiazide Diuretics
chlorothiazide
(P) hydrochlorothiazide

Thiazide-Like Diuretics
chlorthalidone
indapamide
metolazone

LOOP DIURETICS
bumetanide
ethacrynic acid
(P) furosemide
torsemide

CARBONIC ANHYDRASE INHIBITORS
(P) acetazolamide
dichlorphenamide
methazolamide

POTASSIUM-SPARING DIURETICS
amiloride
eplerenone
(P) spironolactone
triamterene

OSMOTIC DIURETICS
(P) mannitol

Diuretic agents are commonly thought of simply as drugs that increase the amount of urine produced by the kidneys. Most diuretics do increase the volume of urine produced to some extent, but the greater clinical significance of diuretics is their ability to increase sodium excretion.

Most diuretics prevent the cells lining the renal tubules from reabsorbing an excessive proportion of the sodium ions in the glomerular filtrate. As a result, sodium and other ions (and the water in which they are dissolved) are lost in the urine instead of being returned to the blood, where they would cause increased intravascular volume and therefore increased hydrostatic pressure, which could result in leaking of fluids at the capillary level.

Diuretics are indicated for the treatment of edema associated with heart failure (HF), acute pulmonary edema, liver disease (including cirrhosis), and renal disease and for the treatment of hypertension. **Edema** occurs when there is increased movement of fluid into the interstitial spaces from the blood vessels. Diuretics are also used to decrease fluid pressure in the eye (intraocular pressure [IOP]), which is useful in treating glaucoma. Diuretics that decrease potassium levels may also be indicated in the treatment of conditions that cause hyperkalemia.

HF can cause edema as a result of several factors. The failing heart muscle does not pump sufficient blood to the kidneys, causing activation of the renin–angiotensin–aldosterone system and resulting in increases in blood volume and sodium retention. Because the failing heart muscle cannot respond to the usual reflex stimulation, the increased volume is slowly pushed out into the capillary level as venous pressure increases because the blood is not being pumped effectively (see Chapter 44).

Pulmonary edema, often due to left-sided HF, develops when the increased volume of fluids backs up into the lungs. The fluid pushed out into the capillaries in the lungs interferes with gas exchange. If this condition develops rapidly, it can be life-threatening.

Patients with liver failure and cirrhosis often present with edema and ascites. This is caused by (a) reduced plasma protein production, which results in less oncotic pull in the vascular system and fluid loss at the capillary level, and (b) obstructed blood flow through the portal system, which is caused by increased pressure from congested hepatic vessels.

Renal disease produces edema because of the loss of plasma proteins into the urine when there is damage to the glomerular basement membrane. Other types of renal disease produce edema because of activation of the renin–angiotensin–aldosterone system as a result of decreasing volume (associated with the loss of fluid into the urine), which causes a drop in blood pressure, or because of failure of the renal tubules to regulate electrolytes effectively.

Hypertension is predominantly an idiopathic disorder; in other words, the underlying pathology is not known. Treatment of hypertension is aimed at reducing the higher-than-normal blood pressure, which can damage end organs and lead to serious cardiovascular (CV) disorders. Diuretics are often key in the treatment of hypertension. The goal is to decrease volume and sodium, which would then decrease pressure in the system. There are several other classes of drugs, including angiotensin-converting enzyme inhibitors, angiotensin receptor blockers, beta-blockers, and calcium channel blockers that are also available for hypertension treatment. See Chapter 43 for discussion of medications that assist with blood pressure control.

Glaucoma is an eye disease characterized by increased pressure in the eye—known as IOP—which can cause optic nerve atrophy and blindness. Some diuretics are used to provide **osmotic pull**, a drawing force of large molecules on water. Osmotic pull is used to draw out excess fluid into the vascular system or the renal tubule; diuretics used for this purpose remove some of the fluid from the eye, which decreases the IOP. These drugs are also used as adjunctive therapy to reduce fluid volume and pressure in the CV system, which also decreases pressure in the eye somewhat.

Diuretics

There are five classes of diuretics, each working at a slightly different site in the nephron or using a different mechanism. Diuretic classes include the thiazide and thiazide-like diuretics, loop diuretics, carbonic anhydrase inhibitors, potassium-sparing diuretics, and osmotic diuretics (Table 51.1). For the most part, the overall nursing care of a patient receiving any diuretic is similar, though there are specific differences. Adverse effects associated with diuretics are also specific to the particular class used. For details, see "Adverse Effects" for each class of diuretics discussed in this chapter and refer to Table 51.2. The most common adverse effects seen with diuretics include gastrointestinal (GI) upset, fluid and electrolyte imbalances, hypotension, and electrolyte disturbances.

Box 51.1 highlights important considerations related to diuretic use across the lifespan. Box 51.2 describes the process of "fluid rebound" that can occur with diuretic use.

Key Points

- Many diuretics increase sodium excretion and therefore water excretion from the kidneys.
- Diuretics help relieve edema associated with HF and pulmonary edema, liver failure and cirrhosis, and various types of renal disease. They are also used in treating hypertension.

Thiazide and Thiazide-Like Diuretics

The thiazide and thiazide-like diuretics have slightly different chemical structure but work similarly and have identical indications for use. Thiazide diuretics include chlorothiazide (*Diuril*) and hydrochlorothiazide (generic). Thiazide-like diuretics include chlorthalidone (generic), indapamide (generic), and metolazone (*Zaroxolyn*). Thiazide and thiazide-like diuretics are among the most frequently used diuretics.

Table 51.1 *Drugs in Focus:* Diuretics

Drug Name	Usual Dosage	Usual Indications
Thiazide Diuretics and Thiazide-Like Diuretics		
Thiazide Diuretics		
chlorothiazide (*Diuril*)	*Adult:* 0.5–2 g PO or IV, daily to b.i.d. for edema; 0.5–2 g/d PO for hypertension *Pediatric (<6 mo):* up to 33 mg/kg/d PO in two doses *Pediatric (>6 mo to 2 y):* 125–325 mg PO in two divided doses *Pediatric (2–12 y):* 375 mg to 1 g PO in two divided doses	Treatment of edema caused by HF, liver disease, or renal disease; monotherapy or as adjunctive treatment of hypertension
hydrochlorothiazide (generic)	*Adult:* 25–100 mg/d PO or intermittently, up to 200 mg/d maximum for edema; 25–100 mg/d PO for hypertension *Pediatric (<6 mo):* up to 3 mg/kg/d PO in two divided doses *Pediatric (6 mo to 2 y):* 12.5–37.5 mg/d PO in two divided doses *Pediatric (2–12 y):* 37.6–100 mg/d PO in two divided doses	Treatment of edema caused by HF, liver disease, or renal disease; monotherapy or as adjunctive treatment of hypertension
Thiazide-Like Diuretics		
chlorthalidone (generic)	50–100 mg/d PO for edema; 25–100 mg/d PO for hypertension	Treatment of edema caused by HF or by liver or renal disease; adjunctive treatment of hypertension
indapamide (generic)	1.25–5 mg/d PO for edema or hypertension, based on patient response	Treatment of edema caused by HF or by liver or renal disease; adjunctive treatment of hypertension
metolazone (*Zaroxolyn*)	2.5–5 mg/d PO for hypertension; 5–20 mg/d PO for edema, based on patient response	Treatment of edema caused by HF or by liver or renal disease; adjunctive treatment of hypertension
Loop Diuretics		
bumetanide (*Bumex*)	0.5–2 mg/d PO as a single dose repeated to a maximum of 10 mg; 0.5–1 mg IM or IV given over 1–2 min, may be repeated in 2–3 h, not to exceed 10 mg/d *Older or renal-impaired patient:* 12 mg by continuous IV infusion over 12 h may be most effective and least toxic	Treatment of acute HF, acute pulmonary edema, hypertension, and edema of HF, renal disease, or liver disease
ethacrynic acid/sodium (*Edecrin*)	*Adult:* 50–200 mg/d PO based on patient response; 0.5–1 mg/kg IV slowly *Pediatric:* 25 mg PO with slow titration up as needed	Treatment of acute HF, acute pulmonary edema, hypertension, and edema of HF, renal disease, ascites due to malignancy, lymphedema, or liver disease; indicated for treatment of edema when an agent with greater diuretic potential than those commonly employed is required *Special consideration:* not for use in infants
furosemide (*Lasix*)	*Adult:* 20–80 mg/d PO, up to 600 mg/d may be given; 20–40 mg IM or IV given slowly; 40 mg IV over 1–2 min for acute pulmonary edema, increase to 80 mg after 1 h if response is not adequate; 40 mg PO b.i.d. for hypertension *Older or renal-impaired patient:* 2–2.5 g/d PO *Pediatric:* 2 mg/kg/d PO for hypertension, not to exceed 6 mg/kg/d; 1 mg/kg IV or IM for edema, increased by 1 mg/kg as needed; not to exceed 6 mg/kg	Treatment of acute HF, acute pulmonary edema, hypertension, and edema of HF, renal disease, or liver disease
torsemide (*Soaanz*)	5–20 mg/d PO initially based on indication; titration to max of 200 mg/d PO based on individual response	Treatment of acute HF, acute pulmonary edema, hypertension, and edema of HF, renal disease, or liver disease

Table 51.1 *Drugs in Focus:* Diuretics (*Continued*)

Drug Name	Usual Dosage	Usual Indications
Carbonic Anhydrase Inhibitors		
acetazolamide (generic)	PO or IV dosing; dosages vary per indication and acuity of the situation	Treatment of edema, chronic simple (open-angle) and secondary glaucoma; adjunctive treatment of edema due to heart failure, centrencephalic epilepsy, altitude sickness, preoperative acute angle-closure glaucoma to lower intraocular pressure if need to delay surgery
dichlorphenamide (*Keveyis*)	50 mg once or twice daily; titrate based on individual response, max dose of 200 mg/d	Treatment of primary hyperkalemic paralysis
methazolamide (generic)	50–100 mg PO b.i.d. to t.i.d.	Treatment of glaucoma
Potassium-Sparing Diuretics		
amiloride (*Midamor*)	5–20 mg/d PO with monitoring of electrolytes	Adjunctive treatment of edema caused by HF, liver disease, or renal disease; hypertension; hypokalemia; and hyperaldosteronism *Special consideration:* not for use in children
eplerenone (*Inspra*)	25–50 mg PO daily for HF patients; 50 mg PO daily or 50 mg twice a day for HTN	Improve survival for patients with HF with reduced ejection fraction after acute MI; treatment for hypertension
spironolactone (*Aldactone, CaroSpir*)	PO dosing will vary per indication and medication formulation	Adjunctive treatment of edema caused by HF, liver disease, or renal disease; hypertension; hypokalemia; and hyperaldosteronism; increases survival, and decreases need of hospitalization for patients with HF with reduced ejection fraction
triamterene (*Dyrenium*)	100 mg/d PO b.i.d., max of 300 mg/d for edema; 25–100 mg/d PO for hypertension	Adjunctive treatment of edema caused by HF, liver disease, or renal disease; hypertension; hyperkalemia; and hyperaldosteronism *Special consideration:* not for use in children
Osmotic Diuretics		
mannitol (*Osmitrol*)	50–100 g IV for oliguria; 1.5–2 g/kg IV to reduce intracranial pressure; dose not established for children <12 y	Treatment of elevated intracranial pressure, acute renal failure, acute glaucoma; also used to decrease intracranial pressure, to prevent oliguric phase of renal failure, and to promote movement of toxic substances through the kidneys

HF, heart failure.

Therapeutic Actions and Indications

Thiazide and thiazide-like diuretics act to block the chloride pump. Chloride is actively pumped out of the tubule by cells lining the ascending limb of the loop of Henle and the distal tubule. Sodium passively moves with the chloride to maintain electrical neutrality. (Chloride is a negative ion, and sodium is a positive ion.) Blocking of the chloride pump keeps the chloride and the sodium in the tubule to be excreted in the urine, thus preventing the reabsorption of both chloride and sodium in the vascular system (Fig. 51.1). Because these segments of the tubule are impermeable to water, there is little increase in the volume of urine produced, but it will be sodium-rich, a natriuretic effect. It is common for there to be some loss of potassium and bicarbonate as well. Thiazides are considered to be mild diuretics compared with the more potent loop diuretics.

Table 51.2 Comparison of Diuretics

Diuretic Class	Major Site of Action	Usual Indications	Major Adverse Effects
Thiazide, thiazide-like	Distal convoluted tubule	Edema of HF, renal, and liver disease	GI upset, CNS complications, hypovolemia, electrolyte alterations, hyperglycemia, hyperuricemia
Loop	Loop of Henle	Acute HF; acute pulmonary edema; hypertension; edema of HF, liver, and renal disease	Hypokalemia and other electrolyte alterations, volume depletion, hypotension, CNS effects, GI upset, hyperglycemia, ototoxicity, hyperuricemia
Carbonic anhydrase inhibitors	Proximal tubule	Glaucoma, diuresis in HF, mountain sickness, epilepsy	GI upset, urinary frequency
Potassium-sparing	Distal tubule and collecting duct	Adjunct for edema of HF, liver, and renal disease; treatment of hypokalemia; adjunct for hypertension; hyperaldosteronism	Hyperkalemia, CNS effects, diarrhea
Osmotic	Glomerulus, tubule	Reduction of intracranial pressure, prevention of oliguric phase of renal failure, reduction of IOP, renal clearance of toxic substances	Hypotension, GI upset, fluid and electrolyte imbalances

GI, gastrointestinal; CNS, central nervous system; HF, heart failure; IOP, intraocular pressure.

Box 51.1 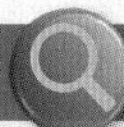 **Focus on Drug Therapy Across the Lifespan**

DIURETIC AGENTS

Children

Diuretics are often used in children to treat edema associated with heart defects, to control hypertension, and to treat edema associated with renal and pulmonary disorders.

Hydrochlorothiazide and chlorothiazide have established pediatric dosing guidelines. Furosemide is often used when a stronger diuretic is needed; care should be taken to not exceed 6 mg/kg/d when using this drug. Ethacrynic acid may be used orally in some situations but should not be used in infants. Spironolactone is the only potassium-sparing diuretic that is recommended for use in children, but as with adults, it should not be used in the presence of severe renal impairment.

Because of the size and rapid metabolism of children, the effects of diuretics may be rapid and adverse effects may occur suddenly. The child receiving a diuretic should be monitored for serum electrolyte changes; for evidence of fluid volume changes; for rapid weight gain or loss, which could reflect fluid volume; and for signs of ototoxicity.

Adults

Adults may be taking diuretics for prolonged periods and need to be aware of the signs and symptoms of fluid imbalance to report to the health care provider. Adults receiving chronic diuretic therapy should weigh themselves on the same scale, in the same clothes, and at the same time each day to monitor for fluid retention or sudden fluid loss. They should be alerted to situations that could aggravate fluid loss, such as diarrhea, vomiting, or excessive heat and sweating, which could change their need for the diuretic. They should also be urged to maintain their fluid intake to help balance their bodies' compensatory mechanisms and to prevent fluid rebound (Box 51.2).

Patients taking potassium-losing diuretics should be encouraged to be consistent with their potassium intake and have their serum potassium levels checked periodically. Some patients with low potassium levels may need to take potassium supplements. Patients taking potassium-sparing diuretics should be cautioned to avoid eating too much potassium if their blood levels are high.

The use of diuretics to change the fluid shifts associated with pregnancy is not appropriate. Pregnant patients maintained on these drugs for underlying medical reasons should not stop taking them, but they need to be aware of the potential for adverse effects on the fetus. Patients who are nursing and need a diuretic should find another method of feeding the baby because of the potential for adverse effects on the baby as well as the lactating patient.

Older Adults

Older adults often have conditions that are treated with diuretics. They are also more likely to have renal or hepatic impairment, which requires cautious use of these drugs.

Frequent serum electrolyte measurements should be done to monitor for adverse reactions.

The intake and activity level of the patient can alter the effectiveness and need for the diuretic. High-salt diets and inactivity can aggravate conditions that lead to edema, and patients should be encouraged to follow activity and dietary guidelines if possible.

Box 51.2 Focus on Safe Medication Administration

EXPLAINING FLUID REBOUND

Care must be taken when using diuretics to avoid **fluid rebound**, which is a reflex reaction of the body to the loss of fluid or sodium. If a patient stops taking in water and takes the diuretic, the result will be a concentrated plasma of smaller volume. The decreased volume is sensed by the nephrons, which activate the renin–angiotensin–aldosterone cycle. When the concentrated blood is sensed by the osmotic center in the brain, the hypothalamus will release more antidiuretic hormone (ADH) to retain water and dilute the blood. The result can be "rebound" edema as fluid is retained.

Many patients who are taking a diuretic markedly decrease fluid intake in order to decrease the number of trips to the bathroom. The result is a rebound of water retention after the diuretic effect. This effect can also be seen in many diets that promise "immediate results"; they frequently contain a key provision to increase fluid intake to 8 to 10 full glasses of water daily. The reflex result of diluting the system with so much water is a drop in ADH release and fluid loss. Some people can lose 5 lb in a few days by doing this. However, the body's reflexes soon kick in, causing rebound retention of fluid to reestablish fluid and electrolyte balance. Most people get frustrated at this point and give up the fad diet. It is important to be able to explain this effect. Teaching patients about balancing the desired diuretic effect with the actions of the normal reflexes is a clinical skill.

These drugs are the first-line drugs used to manage essential hypertension when drug therapy is needed. See Table 51.2 for usual indications for these agents.

Pharmacokinetics

These drugs are well absorbed from the GI tract after oral administration, with onset of action ranging from 1 to 3 hours. Most have peak effects within 4 to 6 hours and duration of effects of 6 to 12 hours. They are metabolized in the liver and excreted in the urine. These diuretics cross the placenta and enter human milk. Hydrochlorothiazide, the most frequently used of the thiazide diuretics and the prototype of this class, can be used in small doses because it is more potent than chlorothiazide, the oldest drug of this class. Chlorothiazide is also available for intravenous (IV) infusion. It also has a longer duration of action (up to 72 hours).

Contraindications and Cautions

Thiazide and thiazide-like diuretics are contraindicated with allergy to thiazides or sulfonamides to prevent hypersensitivity reactions; hypovolemia, which can be worsened by these diuretics; and severe renal disease, which can increase risk of azotemia (increased blood urea nitrogen and serum creatinine).

Caution should be used with systemic lupus erythematosus (SLE), which frequently causes glomerular changes

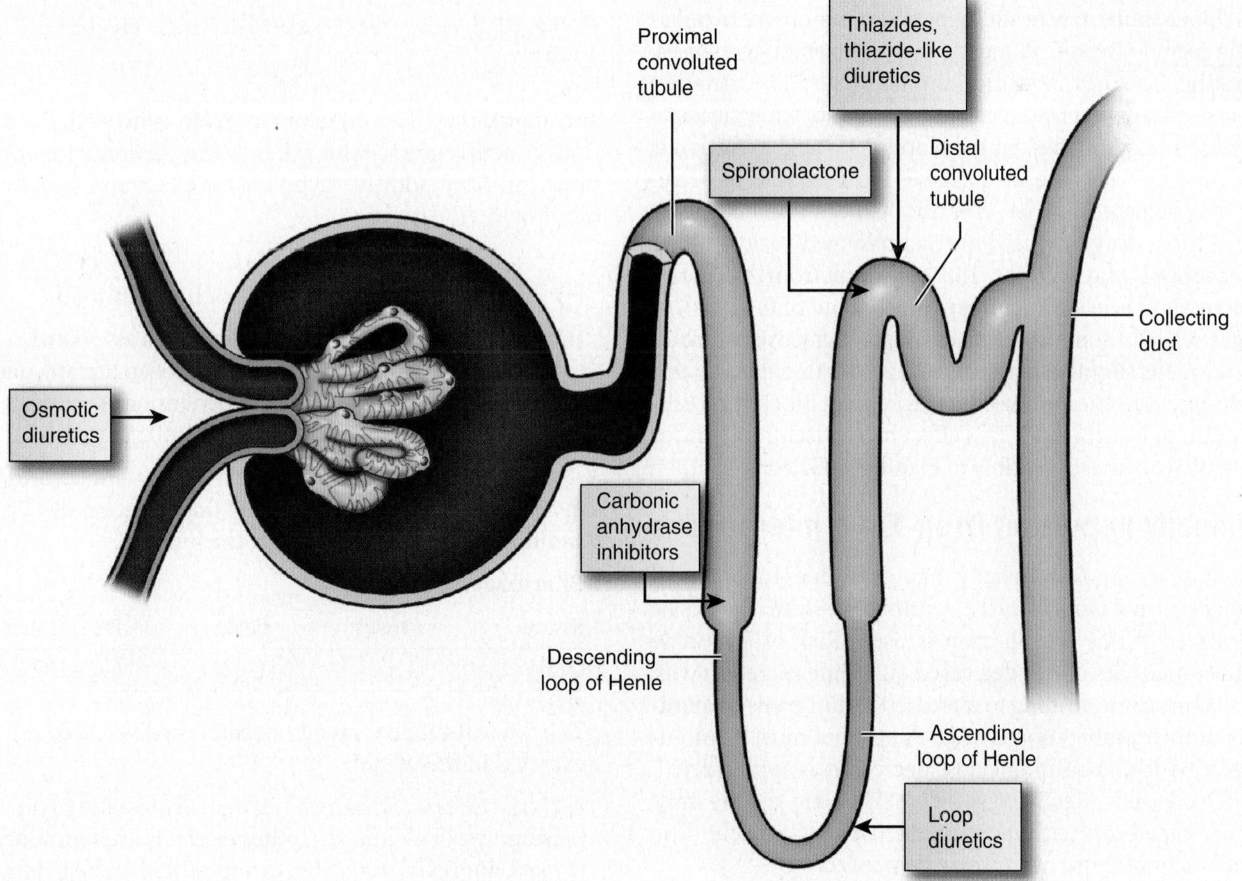

FIGURE 51.1 Sites of action of diuretics in the nephron.

and renal dysfunction that could precipitate renal failure in some cases; glucose tolerance abnormalities or diabetes mellitus, which is worsened by the glucose-elevating effects of many diuretics; gout, which reflects an abnormality in normal tubule reabsorption and secretion; liver disease, which could interfere with the normal metabolism of the drugs, leading to an accumulation of the drug or toxicity; hyperparathyroidism, which could be exacerbated by the renal effects of these drugs; and bipolar disorder, which could be exacerbated by the changes in calcium levels that occur with these drugs. Routine use during pregnancy is not appropriate; these drugs should be reserved for situations in which the pregnant patient has pathological reasons for use, not pregnancy manifestations or complications, and only if the benefit to the patient clearly outweighs the risk to the fetus. If one of these drugs is needed during lactation, another method of feeding the baby should be used because of the potential for adverse effects on fluid and electrolyte changes in the fetus and the baby.

Adverse Effects

The most common adverse effects associated with diuretic agents include GI upset, fluid and electrolyte imbalances, and hypotension. Adverse effects associated with the use of thiazide and thiazide-like diuretics are related to interference with the normal regulatory mechanisms of the nephron. Potassium is lost at the distal tubule because of the actions on the pumping mechanism, and **hypokalemia** (low blood levels of potassium) may result. Signs and symptoms of hypokalemia include weakness, muscle cramps, trembling, nausea, vomiting, diarrhea, and arrhythmias (Fig. 51.2). Another adverse effect is decreased calcium excretion, which leads to increased calcium levels in the blood. Uric acid excretion is also decreased because the thiazides interfere with its secretory mechanism. High levels of uric acid can result in gout.

If these drugs are used over a prolonged period, blood glucose levels may increase. This may result from the change in potassium levels (which keeps glucose out of the cells), or it may relate to some other mechanism of glucose control.

Urine is slightly alkalinized when the thiazides or thiazide-like diuretics are used because they block the reabsorption of bicarbonate. This effect can cause problems for patients who are susceptible to bladder infections.

Clinically Important Drug–Drug Interactions

The risk of digoxin toxicity increases due to potential changes in potassium levels; serum potassium should be monitored if this combination is used. Risk of quinidine toxicity increases due to decreased quinidine excretion with an alkaline urine, leading to increased serum levels of quinidine. If this combination is used, the patient must be monitored closely and quinidine dose decreased as appropriate.

Decreased effectiveness of antidiabetic agents may occur related to the changes in glucose metabolism; dose adjustment of those agents may be needed.

The risk of lithium toxicity may increase if these drugs are combined. Serum lithium levels should be monitored and appropriate dose adjustment made as needed. In addition, concurrent use with other antihypertensive medications can have additive hypotensive effect and should be monitored.

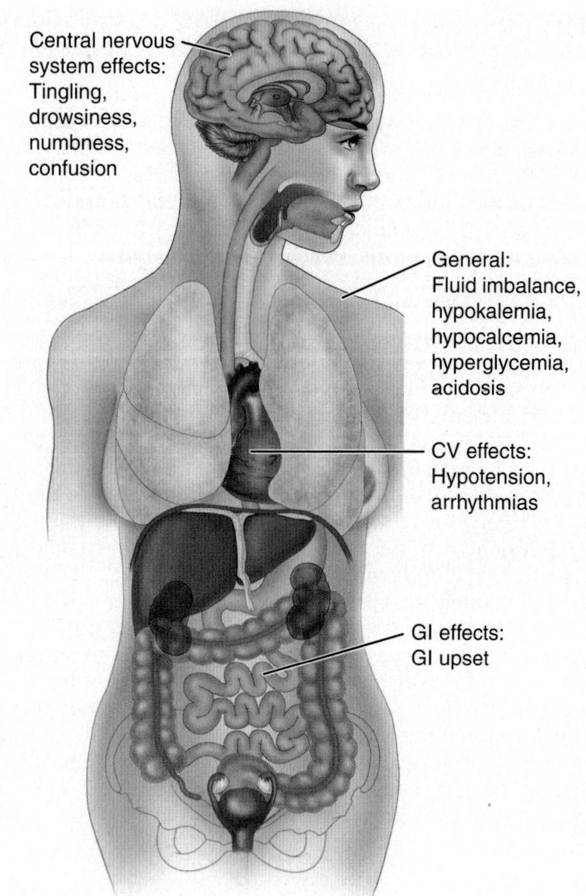

FIGURE 51.2 Variety of adverse effects and toxicities associated with diuretics.

Prototype Summary: Hydrochlorothiazide

Indications: Adjunctive therapy for edema associated with HF, cirrhosis, corticosteroid or estrogen therapy, and renal dysfunction; treatment of hypertension as monotherapy or in combination with other antihypertensives.

Actions: Inhibits reabsorption of sodium and chloride in distal renal tubules, increasing the excretion of sodium, chloride, and water by the kidneys.

Pharmacokinetics:

Route	Onset	Peak	Duration
Oral	2 h	4–6 h	6–12 h

$T_{1/2}$: 5.6 to 14 hours; metabolized in the liver and excreted in the urine.

Adverse Effects: Dizziness, vertigo, orthostatic hypotension, hypokalemia and other electrolyte alterations, nausea, anorexia, vomiting, dry mouth, diarrhea, dehydration, polyuria, nocturia, muscle cramps, or spasms.

Loop Diuretics

Loop diuretics are so named because they work in the loop of Henle. Loop diuretics are also referred to as **high-ceiling diuretics** because they cause a greater degree of diuresis than other diuretics. Four loop diuretics are available: ethacrynic acid (*Edecrin*), the first loop diuretic introduced, bumetanide (*Bumex*), furosemide (*Lasix*), and torsemide (*Soaanz*) (Box 51.3).

Box 51.3 Focus on Safe Medication Administration

Name confusion has been reported between furosemide and torsemide; the dose and strength of effect of these two drugs are different. Use extreme caution to make sure you are using the prescribed drug and dose.

Therapeutic Actions and Indications

Loop diuretics block the chloride pump in the ascending loop of Henle, where 30% of all filtered sodium is normally reabsorbed. This action decreases the reabsorption of sodium and chloride. The loop diuretics have a similar effect in the descending loop of Henle and in the distal convoluted tubule, resulting in the production of a copious amount of sodium-rich urine. These drugs work even in the presence of acid–base disturbances, renal insufficiency, electrolyte imbalances, or nitrogen retention.

Because in acute settings with high doses they can produce a loss of fluid of up to 20 lb per day, loop diuretics are the drugs of choice when a rapid and extensive diuresis is needed. In cases of severe edema or acute pulmonary edema, it is important to remember that these drugs can have an effect only on the blood that reaches the nephrons. If a person is not able to perfuse the kidney because of HF or vascular disease, these drugs will not have an effect. A rapid diuresis occurs, producing a more hypertonic intravascular fluid. In pulmonary edema, this fluid then circulates back to the lungs, pulls fluid out of the interstitial spaces by its oncotic pull, and delivers this fluid to the kid neys, where the water is pulled out, completing the cycle. In the treatment of pulmonary edema, it can sometimes take hours or days to move all of the fluid out of the lungs because the fluid must be pulled out of the interstitial spaces in the lungs before it can be circulated to the kidneys for removal. Remembering how the drugs work and the way in which fluid moves in the vascular system will make it easier to understand the effects to anticipate.

Loop diuretics are commonly indicated for the treatment of acute HF, acute pulmonary edema, edema associated with HF or with renal or liver disease, and hypertension. See Table 51.1 for usual indications for each of these agents. See the "Critical Thinking Scenario" for additional information about using furosemide with HF.

CRITICAL THINKING SCENARIO
Using Furosemide (*Lasix*) in Heart Failure

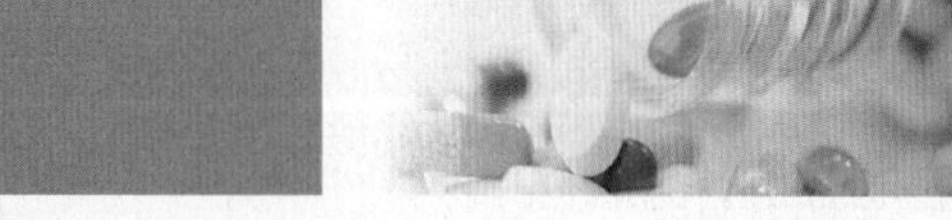

THE SITUATION

M.R. is a 68-year-old patient with rheumatic mitral valve heart disease. They have refused any surgical intervention and have developed progressively worsening HF. Recently, furosemide (*Lasix*), 40 mg/d PO, was prescribed for them along with digoxin. After 10 days with the new prescription, M.R. calls to tell you that they are allergic to the new medicine and cannot take it anymore. They report extensive ankle swelling and difficulty breathing. You refer them to a cardiologist for immediate review.

CRITICAL THINKING

Think about the physiology of mitral valve disease and the progression of HF in this patient. How does furosemide work in the body?

What additional activities will be important to help maintain some balance in this patient's cardiac status?

What is the nature of M.R.'s reported allergy, and what other options could be tried?

DISCUSSION

Over time, an incompetent mitral valve leads to an enlarged and overworked left ventricle as the backup of blood "waiting to be pumped" continues to progress. Drug therapy for a patient with this disorder is usually aimed at decreasing the workload of the heart as much as possible to maintain cardiac output. Digoxin increases the contractility of the heart muscle, which should lead to better perfusion of the kidneys. Furosemide, a loop diuretic, acts on the loop of Henle to block the reabsorption of sodium and water and lead to a diuresis, which decreases the volume of blood the heart needs to pump and makes the blood that is pumped more efficient. This blood then has an oncotic pull to move fluid from the tissue into circulation, where it can be acted on by the kidneys, leading to further diuresis.

M.R. should be encouraged to maintain fluid intake and to engage in activity as much as possible but to take frequent rest periods. Their potassium level should be monitored regularly (this is especially important because they are also taking digoxin, which is sensitive

(continues on page 918)

to potassium levels), their edematous limbs should be elevated periodically during the day, they can wear compression stockings to assist with venous return, they should monitor their weight daily and report changes of ±3 lb in a day and ±5 lb in a week, and they should limit their sodium intake. Their symptoms of shortness of breath and increased swelling are indications that their furosemide dose is not high enough.

When M.R. was questioned about their reported allergy, it was discovered that their "allergic reaction" was actually increased urination (a therapeutic effect). M.R. needs to learn about the actions of the drug. They also need information about the timing of administration so that the resultant diuresis will not interfere with rest or with daily activities. HF is a progressive, incurable disease, so patient education is an important part of the overall management regimen.

NURSING CARE GUIDE FOR M.R.: DIURETIC AGENTS

Assessment: History and Examination

Assess M.R.'s health history, including allergies to diuretics, fluid or electrolyte disturbances, gout, glucose tolerance abnormalities, liver disease, systemic lupus erythematosus, and pregnancy and lactation status.

Focus the physical examination on the following areas:

Neurological: orientation, reflexes, strength

Skin: color, texture, edema

CV: blood pressure, pulse, cardiac auscultation

GI: liver evaluation

Genitourinary (GU): urinary output

Laboratory tests: hematology; serum electrolytes, glucose, uric acid; liver function tests

Nursing Conclusions

Hypovolemia risk related to diuretic effect

Electrolyte imbalance risk related to loss of sodium, potassium, and chloride.

Knowledge deficit risk regarding drug therapy

Planning

The patient will receive the best therapeutic effect from the drug therapy.

The patient will have limited adverse effects to the drug therapy.

The patient will have an understanding of the drug therapy, adverse effects to anticipate, and measures to relieve discomfort and improve safety.

Intervention

Obtain daily weight and monitor urine output.

Provide comfort and safety measures: sugarless lozenges, mouth care, safety precautions, skin care, and nutrition.

Administer the drug with food early in the day.

Provide support and reassurance to deal with drug effects and lifestyle changes.

Provide patient teaching regarding drug name, dosage, side effects, precautions, warnings to report, daily weighing, and recording dietary changes as needed.

Evaluation

Evaluate drug effects: urinary output, weight changes, status of edema, blood pressure changes.

Monitor for adverse effects: hypotension, hypokalemia, hyponatremia, hypocalcemia, hyperglycemia, increased uric acid levels.

Monitor for drug–drug interactions as indicated.

Evaluate the effectiveness of the patient teaching program and comfort and safety measures.

PATIENT TEACHING FOR M.R.

- A diuretic, or "water pill," such as furosemide (*Lasix*), will help reduce the amount of fluid that is in your body by causing the kidneys to pass larger amounts of water and salt into your urine. By removing this fluid, the diuretic helps decrease the work of the heart, lower blood pressure, and get rid of edema, or swelling in your tissues.
- This drug can be taken with food, which may eliminate possible stomach upset. When taking a diuretic, you should maintain your usual fluid intake and try to avoid excessive intake of salt.
- Furosemide is a diuretic that may cause potassium loss. Your potassium will need to be monitored.
- Weigh yourself each day at the same time of the day and in the same clothing. Record these weights on a calendar. Report any loss or gain of 3 lb or more in a day or 5 lb change in a week.
- Common effects of this drug include the following:
  - *Increased volume and frequency of urination:* Have ready access to bathroom facilities. Once you are used to the drug, you will know how long the effects last for you.
  - *Dizziness, feeling faint on arising, drowsiness:* Loss of fluid can lower blood pressure and cause these feelings. Change positions slowly; if you feel drowsy, avoid driving or other dangerous activities. These feelings are often increased if alcohol is consumed; avoid this combination or take special precautions if you combine them.
  - *Increased thirst:* As fluid is lost, you may experience a feeling of thirst. Sucking on sugarless lozenges and frequent mouth care might help to alleviate this feeling. Do not drink an excessive amount of fluid while taking a diuretic. Try to maintain your usual fluid intake.
  - Report any of the following to your health care provider: muscle cramps or pain, loss or gain of more than 3 lb in a day or 5 lb in a week, swelling in your fingers or ankles, nausea or vomiting, unusual bleeding or bruising, trembling, or weakness.
- Avoid the use of any over-the-counter (OTC) medication without first checking with your health care provider. Several OTC medications can interfere with the effectiveness of this drug.
- Tell any doctor, nurse, or other health care provider involved in your care that you are taking this drug.
- Keep this drug and all medications out of the reach of children.

Pharmacokinetics

Loop diuretics are available for oral or IV use. Furosemide may also be given intramuscularly (IM). They reach peak levels in 60 to 120 minutes (orally) or 30 minutes (parenterally). Their metabolism and excretion vary based on medication.

Contraindications and Cautions

Among the contraindications to these drugs are allergy to a loop diuretic to prevent hypersensitivity reactions; electrolyte depletion, which could be aggravated by the electrolyte effects of these drugs; anuria—severe renal failure—which may prevent the diuretic from working or precipitate a crisis stage due to the blood flow changes brought about by the diuretic; and hepatic encephalopathy, which could be exacerbated by the fluid shifts associated with drug use. Routine use during pregnancy is not appropriate; these drugs should be reserved for situations in which the pregnant patient has pathological reasons for use, not pregnancy manifestations or complications, and only if the benefit to the patient clearly outweighs the risk to the fetus.

Caution should be used with the following conditions: SLE, which frequently causes glomerular changes and renal dysfunction that could precipitate renal failure in some cases; glucose tolerance abnormalities or diabetes mellitus, which is worsened by the glucose-elevating effects of many diuretics; and gout, which reflects an abnormality in normal tubule reabsorption and secretion.

Adverse Effects

Adverse effects are related to the imbalance in electrolytes and fluid that these drugs cause. Hypokalemia is a common adverse effect because potassium is lost when the transport systems in the tubule try to save some of the sodium being lost. **Alkalosis**, or a rise in serum pH to an alkaline state, may occur if more chloride is excreted in the urine compared to bicarbonate. Calcium is also lost in the tubules along with the bicarbonate, which may result in hypocalcemia and tetany. The rapid loss of fluid can result in hypotension and dizziness if it causes a rapid imbalance in fluid levels. Long-term use of these drugs may also result in hyperglycemia because of the diuretic effect on blood glucose levels, so susceptible patients need to be monitored for this effect. Ototoxicity and even deafness have been reported with too rapid IV pushing of these drugs, but the loss of hearing is usually reversible after the drug is stopped. This may be an effect of electrolyte changes on the conduction of fragile nerves in the central nervous system. Hyperuricemia and hypomagnesemia are also common findings.

Clinically Important Drug–Drug Interactions

The risk of ototoxicity increases if loop diuretics are combined with aminoglycosides or cisplatin. Anticoagulation effects may increase if these drugs are given with anticoagulants. There may also be a decreased loss of sodium and decreased antihypertensive effects if these drugs are combined with indomethacin, ibuprofen, salicylates, or other nonsteroidal antiinflammatory agents; a patient receiving this combination should be monitored closely, and appropriate dose adjustments should be made. There is increased risk of digoxin toxicity if medication administration causes hypokalemia. Concurrent use of lithium should be monitored carefully, since hyponatremia could cause increase in lithium levels.

P Prototype Summary: Furosemide

Indications: Treatment of edema associated with HF, acute pulmonary edema, hypertension.

Actions: Inhibits the reabsorption of sodium and chloride from the distal renal tubules and the loop of Henle, leading to a sodium-rich diuresis.

Pharmacokinetics:

Route	Onset	Peak	Duration
Oral	60 min	60–120 min	6–8 h
IV, IM	5 min	30 min	2 h

$T_{1/2}$: 120 minutes; metabolized in the liver and excreted in the urine.

Adverse Effects: Dizziness, vertigo, paresthesia, orthostatic hypotension, rash, urticaria, nausea, anorexia, vomiting, hyperglycemia, hyperuricemia, urinary bladder spasm, ototoxicity, dehydration, electrolyte alterations.

Carbonic Anhydrase Inhibitors

The carbonic anhydrase inhibitors are relatively mild diuretics. Available agents include acetazolamide (generic), dichlorphenamide (*Keveyis*), and methazolamide (generic).

Therapeutic Actions and Indications

The enzyme carbonic anhydrase is a catalyst for the formation of sodium bicarbonate, which is stored as the alkaline reserve in the renal tubule, and for the excretion of hydrogen, which results in a slightly acidic urine. Diuretics that block the effects of carbonic anhydrase slow down the movement of hydrogen ions; as a result, more sodium and bicarbonate are lost in the urine. These drugs are used as adjuncts to other diuretics when a more intense diuresis is needed. Most often, carbonic anhydrase inhibitors are used to treat glaucoma because the inhibition of carbonic anhydrase results in decreased secretion of aqueous humor of the eye. See Table 51.1 for usual indications for each of these agents.

Pharmacokinetics

These drugs are rapidly absorbed and widely distributed. Acetazolamide is available orally and for IV use. These drugs peak in 2 to 4 hours (15 minutes if given IV) and have a 6- to 12-hour duration. They are excreted in urine. Some of these agents have been associated with fetal abnormalities in animals, and they should not be used during pregnancy in most circumstances. Because of the potential for adverse effects on the baby, another method of feeding the infant should be used if one of these drugs is needed during lactation.

Contraindications and Cautions

Carbonic anhydrase inhibitors are contraindicated in patients with allergy to the drug or to antibacterial sulfonamides or thiazides to prevent hypersensitivity reactions or in patients with chronic noncongestive angle-closure glaucoma, which could mask warning symptoms that the glaucoma is worsening. Routine use during pregnancy is not appropriate; these drugs should be reserved for situations in which the pregnant patient has pathological reasons for use, not pregnancy manifestations or complications, and only if the benefit to the patient clearly outweighs the risk to the fetus.

Cautious use is recommended in patients who have fluid or electrolyte imbalances, renal or hepatic disease, adrenocortical insufficiency, respiratory acidosis, or chronic obstructive pulmonary disease, which could be exacerbated by the fluid and electrolyte changes caused by these drugs.

Adverse Effects

Adverse effects of carbonic anhydrase inhibitors are related to the disturbances in acid–base and electrolyte balances. Metabolic acidosis is a relatively common and potentially dangerous effect that occurs when bicarbonate is lost. Hypokalemia is also common because potassium excretion is increased as the tubule loses potassium in an attempt to retain some of the sodium that is being excreted. Patients also report paresthesia (tingling) of the extremities, confusion, and drowsiness, all of which are probably related to the neural effect of the electrolyte changes.

Clinically Important Drug–Drug Interactions

There is higher risk of salicylate toxicity with these medications due to the potential of metabolic acidosis. Therefore, high-dose aspirin is contraindicated, and patients taking low-dose aspirin should be monitored carefully. Any medication with the potential of causing metabolic acidosis could have an additive effect with these medications. Concurrent administration with medications that lower potassium should also be monitored carefully. The excretion of other medications may either be increased or decreased with administration of these medications, so medication interactions should be checked and dosage adjustments made as needed.

Prototype Summary: Acetazolamide

Indications: Adjunctive treatment of open-angle glaucoma, secondary glaucoma; preoperative use in acute angle-closure glaucoma when delay of surgery is indicated; edema caused by heart failure; and drug-induced edema; prevention or treatment of symptoms of acute mountain sickness.

Actions: Inhibits carbonic anhydrase, which decreases aqueous humor formation in the eye, intraocular pressure, and hydrogen secretion by the renal tubules.

Pharmacokinetics:

Route	Onset	Peak	Duration
Oral	1 h	2–4 h	6–12 h
Sustained-release oral	2 h	8–12 h	18–24 h
IV	1–2 min	15–18 min	4–5 h

$T_{1/2}$: 5 to 6 hours; excreted unchanged in the urine.

Adverse Effects: Weakness, fatigue, rash, anorexia, nausea, urinary frequency, renal calculi, bone marrow suppression, weight loss, metabolic acidosis, hypersensitivity reactions, liver impairment, hypokalemia, hyponatremia, paresthesia, tinnitus.

Potassium-Sparing Diuretics

The potassium-sparing diuretics are not as powerful as the loop diuretics, but they retain potassium instead of wasting it. Drugs include amiloride (*Midamor*), eplerenone (*Inspra*), spironolactone (*Aldactone, Carospir*), and triamterene (*Dyrenium*). These diuretics are used for patients who are at high risk for hypokalemia associated with diuretic use (e.g., patients receiving digitalis or patients with cardiac arrhythmias) and adjunctive treatment of edema. Some are indicated to improve survival for patients with HF.

Therapeutic Actions and Indications

Potassium-sparing diuretics cause a loss of sodium while promoting the retention of potassium. Spironolactone and eplerenone are aldosterone antagonists, blocking the actions of aldosterone in the distal tubule. Amiloride and triamterene block potassium secretion through the tubule. The diuretic effect of these drugs comes from the balance achieved in losing sodium to offset the potassium retained.

Potassium-sparing diuretics are often used as adjuncts with thiazide or loop diuretics or in patients who are especially at risk if hypokalemia develops, such as patients taking certain antiarrhythmics or digoxin and those who have particular neurological conditions. Spironolactone, the most frequently prescribed of these drugs, is the drug of choice for treating **hyperaldosteronism**, a condition seen in cirrhosis of the liver and nephrotic syndrome of excessive output of aldosterone from the adrenal gland, leading to increased sodium and water retention and loss of potassium (see Table 51.1). Eplerenone and spironolactone are indicated to improve survival and reduce hospitalizations in patients with HF with reduced left ventricular ejection fraction.

Pharmacokinetics

These drugs are well absorbed after oral administration, are protein-bound, and are widely distributed. They are metabolized in the liver and primarily excreted in the urine. These diuretics cross the placenta and enter human milk. Peak plasma concentrations of spironolactone and its active metabolite are between 2.5 and 4 hours, and the elimination half-lives of the metabolites are about 15 hours. It is eliminated in urine and bile. Amiloride and triamterene reach peak effects in 6 to 10 hours and have a duration of effect of 16 to 24 hours. Peak plasma concentrations of eplerenone are seen in 1.5 to 2 hours and the half-life is estimated at 3 to 6 hours.

Contraindications and Cautions

These drugs are contraindicated for use in patients with allergy to the drug to prevent hypersensitivity reactions and hyperkalemia, severe renal disease, or anuria, which could be exacerbated by the effects of these drugs. Routine use during pregnancy is not appropriate; these drugs should be reserved for situations in which the pregnant patient has pathological reasons for use, not pregnancy manifestations or complications, and only if the benefit to the patient clearly outweighs the risk to the fetus.

Adverse Effects

The most common adverse effect of potassium-sparing diuretics is hyperkalemia, which can cause lethargy, confusion, ataxia, muscle cramps, and cardiac arrhythmias. Patients taking these drugs need to be evaluated regularly for signs of increased potassium and informed about the signs and symptoms to watch for. They also should be advised to be cautious about eating foods that are high in potassium (Box 51.4). Because spironolactone blocks androgen production and alters the testosterone–estrogen ratio, it is associated with various hormonal changes including decreased libido, hirsutism, gynecomastia, breast tenderness, deepening of the voice, and irregular menses. Eplerenone does not cause the hormonal side effects due to its increased selectivity for the aldosterone receptors over steroid receptors.

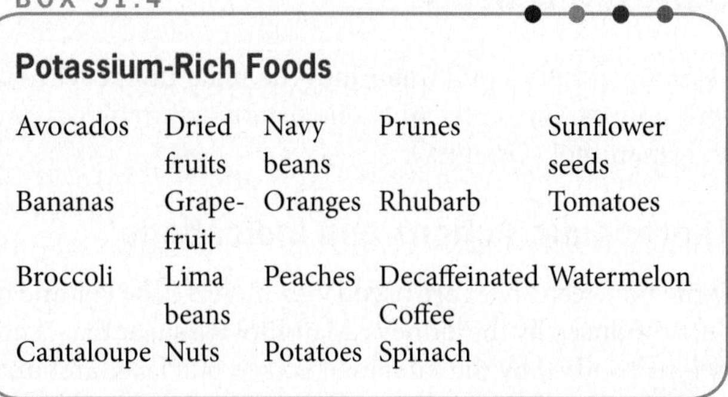

BOX 51.4

Potassium-Rich Foods

Avocados	Dried fruits	Navy beans	Prunes	Sunflower seeds
Bananas	Grapefruit	Oranges	Rhubarb	Tomatoes
Broccoli	Lima beans	Peaches	Decaffeinated Coffee	Watermelon
Cantaloupe	Nuts	Potatoes	Spinach	

Clinically Important Drug–Drug Interactions

The diuretic effect decreases if potassium-sparing diuretics are combined with salicylates. There is increased risk of hypotension when concurrently used with other antihypertensives. There is increased risk of hyperkalemia when used with other medications that block the renin–angiotensin–aldosterone pathway.

Prototype Summary: Spironolactone

Indications: Primary hyperaldosteronism, adjunctive therapy in the treatment of edema associated with HF, nephrotic syndrome, ascites associated with cirrhosis; treatment of hypokalemia or prevention of hypokalemia in patients at high risk if hypokalemia occurs; essential hypertension; increases survival, and decreases need of hospitalization for patients with HF with reduced ejection fraction.

Actions: Competitively blocks the effects of aldosterone in the renal tubule, causing loss of sodium and water and retention of potassium.

Pharmacokinetics:

Route	Onset	Peak in Plasma	Duration
Oral	Unknown	2.5–4 h	48–72 h

$T_{1/2}$: 1.4 hours for drug; about 15 hours for active metabolites; metabolized in the liver and excreted in the urine.

Adverse Effects: Dizziness, headache, drowsiness, rash, cramping, diarrhea, hyperkalemia, hirsutism, gynecomastia, deepening of the voice, irregular menses.

Osmotic Diuretics

Osmotic diuretics pull water into the renal tubule without sodium loss. Currently, only one osmotic diuretic is available, mannitol (*Osmitrol*).

Therapeutic Actions and Indications

Some nonelectrolytes are used IV to increase the volume of fluid produced by the kidneys. Mannitol is a sugar that is not well reabsorbed by the tubules; it acts to pull large amounts of fluid into the urine due to the osmotic pull exerted by the large sugar molecule. Because the tubule is not able to reabsorb all of the sugar pulled into it, large amounts of fluid are lost in the urine. The effects of this osmotic drug are not limited to the kidneys because the injected substance pulls fluid into the vascular system from extravascular spaces, including the aqueous humor. Therefore, mannitol is often used in acute situations when it is necessary to decrease IOP before eye surgery or during acute attacks of glaucoma. It is also the diuretic of choice in cases of increased cranial pressure or acute renal failure due to shock, drug overdose, or trauma. See Table 51.1 for usual indications for mannitol.

Pharmacokinetics

Mannitol is only available for IV use. It is freely filtered at the renal glomerulus, poorly reabsorbed by the renal tubule, not secreted by the tubule, and resistant to metabolism. Action depends on the concentration of osmotic activity in the solution. It is not known whether this drug can cause fetal harm. In addition, the effects during lactation are not well understood.

Contraindications and Cautions

Mannitol is contraindicated in patients with renal disease and anuria from severe renal disease, pulmonary congestion, intracranial bleeding, dehydration, and HF, which could be exacerbated by the large shifts in fluid related to use of these drugs. Routine use during pregnancy is not appropriate; it should be reserved for situations in which the pregnant patient has pathological reasons for use, not pregnancy manifestations or complications, and only if the benefit to the patient clearly outweighs the risk to the fetus.

Adverse Effects

The most common and potentially dangerous adverse effect related to an osmotic diuretic are the fluid shifts. If fluid is pulled from extravascular spaces into the vascular system, it may cause HF and pulmonary edema. Its diuretic effect can cause hypotension and dehydration. Patients should be monitored for new or worsening renal function, hypersensitivity reactions, and central nervous system toxicity (confusion, lethargy, coma). Other common side effects include nausea, vomiting, hypotension, lightheadedness, electrolyte imbalances, infusion site reactions, and headache.

Prototype Summary: Mannitol

Indications: Prevention and treatment of the oliguric phase of renal failure, reduction of intracranial pressure and treatment of cerebral edema, reduction of elevated IOP, promotion of urinary excretion of toxic substances, diagnostic use for measurement of glomerular filtration rate; also available as an irrigant in transurethral prostatic resection and other transurethral procedures.

Actions: Elevates the osmolarity of the glomerular filtrate, leading to a loss of water, sodium, and chloride; creates an osmotic gradient in the eye, reducing IOP; creates an osmotic effect that decreases swelling after transurethral surgery.

Pharmacokinetics:

Route	Onset	Peak	Duration
IV	20–40 min	1 h	6–8 h
Irrigant	Rapid	Rapid	Short

$T_{1/2}$: 15 to 100 minutes; excreted unchanged in the urine.

Adverse Effects: Dizziness, headache, hypotension, rash, nausea, anorexia, dry mouth, thirst, diuresis, fluid and electrolyte imbalances, hypersensitivity reactions, injection site reactions.

Nursing Considerations for Patients Receiving Diuretics

Assessment: History and Examination

- Assess for contraindication or cautions: any known allergies to substances in the medications to prevent hypersensitivity reactions; fluid or electrolyte disturbances, which could be exacerbated by the diuretic; gout, which could be exacerbated if the medication increases uric acid in the blood; glucose tolerance abnormalities, which may be exacerbated by the glucose-elevating effects; liver disease, which could alter the metabolism of the drug, leading to toxic levels; systemic lupus erythematosus, which frequently affects the glomerulus and could be exacerbated by the use of a thiazide or thiazide-like diuretic; renal function, which could be worsened with medication administration; and current status of pregnancy or lactation because of the potential for adverse effects on the fetus or baby.
- Perform a physical assessment to establish baseline data before beginning therapy to determine the effectiveness of therapy and to evaluate for occurrence of any adverse effects associated with drug therapy.
- Inspect the skin carefully for signs and symptoms of edema; note the extent and degree of edema, including evidence of pitting, to provide a baseline as a reference

for drug effectiveness; check skin turgor to determine hydration status.
- Assess cardiopulmonary status, including blood pressure and pulse, and auscultate heart and lung sounds for abnormalities to evaluate fluid movement and state of hydration and monitor the effects on the heart and lungs.
- Obtain an accurate body weight to provide a baseline to monitor fluid balance.
- Monitor intake and output and assess voiding patterns to evaluate fluid balance and renal function.
- Monitor the results of laboratory tests, including serum electrolyte levels, especially potassium and calcium, uric acid, and glucose levels, to determine the drug's effect, and renal and liver function tests to identify the need for possible dose adjustment and toxic effects.

Nursing Conclusions

Nursing conclusions related to drug therapy may include the following:
- Risk of alterations in fluid volume related to drug effect
- Risk of electrolyte disturbances related to drug effect
- Hypotension risk related to decreased fluid volume. Knowledge deficit risk regarding drug therapy

Planning

- The patient will receive the best therapeutic effect from the drug therapy.
- The patient will have limited adverse effects to the drug therapy.
- The patient will have an understanding of the drug therapy, adverse effects to anticipate, and measures to relieve discomfort and improve safety.

Intervention With Rationale

- Administer oral drug with food or milk to buffer the drug effect on the stomach lining if GI upset is a problem.
- IV diuretics and high doses of diuretics administered orally can cause symptomatic changes in fluid and electrolytes, and patients should be carefully monitored.
- Monitor urinary output, cardiac response, and heart rhythm of patients receiving IV diuretics to monitor for rapid fluid shifts and potential electrolyte disturbances, leading to cardiac arrhythmia. Switch to the oral form as soon as possible as appropriate.
- Administer diuretics early in the day so that increased urination will not interfere with sleep.
- Monitor the dose carefully and reduce the dose of one or both drugs if patient becomes hypotensive; loss of fluid volume can precipitate hypotension.
- Monitor the patient response to the drug (e.g., blood pressure, urinary output, weight, serum electrolytes, hydration, periodic blood glucose monitoring) to evaluate the effectiveness of the drug and monitor for adverse effects.
- Assess weight daily to evaluate fluid balance.
- Check skin turgor to evaluate for possible fluid volume deficit, and assess edematous areas for changes, including a decrease in amount or degree of pitting.
- Provide comfort measures, including skin care and nutrition consultation, to increase adherence with drug therapy and decrease the severity of adverse effects; provide safety measures if dizziness and weakness are a problem to prevent injury.
- Provide a potassium-rich or low-potassium diet as appropriate to maintain electrolyte balance and replace lost potassium or prevent hyperkalemia.
- Provide thorough patient teaching, including the name of the drug and dosage prescribed, to enhance patient knowledge about drug therapy and to promote adherence. Additional patient teaching includes the following:
  - Importance of taking the diuretic early in the day to avoid interference with sleep
  - Administration of the drug with food or meals if GI upset occurs
  - Need to weigh oneself daily and report any increase in weight of 3 lb or more in 1 day or 5 lb or more in a week
  - Importance of maintaining an adequate fluid intake to prevent fluid rebound (see "Safe Medication Administration" in this chapter's introduction to diuretic agents)
  - Need to have readily available access to bathroom facilities after taking the prescribed dose
  - Signs and symptoms of adverse effects, and when they need to notify the health care provider
  - Safety measures, such as moving slowly if dizziness is an issue and avoiding hot environments and other situations potentially, leading to extra loss of fluid
  - Dietary sources of foods high in potassium, with an emphasis on the need for appropriate intake of nutrients
  - Need for adherence with therapy to achieve intended results
  - Importance of continued follow-up and monitoring, including laboratory testing to determine the effectiveness of therapy

Evaluation

- Monitor patient response to the drug (weight, urinary output, edema changes, blood pressure).
- Monitor for adverse effects (electrolyte imbalance, orthostatic hypotension, rebound edema, hyperglycemia, increased uric acid levels, acid–base disturbances, dizziness).
- Monitor the effectiveness of comfort measures and adherence with the regimen.
- Evaluate the effectiveness of the teaching plan (patient can name drug, dosage, adverse effects to watch for, and specific measures to avoid them).

SUMMARY

- Diuretics—drugs that increase the excretion water from the kidneys—are used in the treatment of edema associated with HF and pulmonary edema, liver failure and cirrhosis, and various types of renal disease and as agents to treat hypertension.
- Classes of diuretics differ in their sites of action, mechanisms, and intensity of effects. Thiazide diuretics work to block the chloride pump in the distal convoluted tubule. This effect leads to a loss of sodium and potassium and a minor loss of water. Thiazides are frequently used alone or in combination with other drugs to treat hypertension. They are considered to be less potent diuretics.
- Loop diuretics work in the loop of Henle and by blocking the chloride pumps and have a powerful diuretic effect, leading to the loss of water, sodium, and potassium. These drugs are the most potent diuretics and are used in acute situations, as well as in chronic conditions not responsive to less potent diuretics.
- Carbonic anhydrase inhibitors work to block the formation of carbonic acid and bicarbonate in the renal tubule. These drugs can cause an alkaline urine and loss of the bicarbonate buffer. Carbonic anhydrase inhibitors are used in combination with other diuretics when additional diuresis is needed, and they are indicated to be used to treat glaucoma because they decrease the amount of aqueous humor produced in the eye.
- Potassium-sparing diuretics are mild diuretics that act to spare potassium in exchange for the loss of sodium and water in the urine. Patients can become hyperkalemic while taking these drugs.
- The osmotic diuretic mannitol uses hypertonic pull to remove fluid from the intravascular spaces and to deliver large amounts of water into the renal tubule. There is a danger of sudden change of fluid volume and massive fluid loss with this drug. This drug is used to decrease intracranial pressure and is also indicated to reduce elevated intraocular pressure.

CHECK YOUR UNDERSTANDING

Answers to the questions in this chapter can be found in Answers to Check Your Understanding Questions on thePoint®.

MULTIPLE CHOICE

Select the best answer.

1. Most diuretics act in the body to cause
   a. loss of calcium.
   b. loss of sodium.
   c. retention of potassium.
   d. retention of chloride.

2. Diuretics cause a loss of fluid volume in the body. The drop in volume activates compensatory mechanisms to restore the volume, including
   a. suppression of ADH release and stimulation of the countercurrent mechanism.
   b. suppression of aldosterone release and increased ADH release.
   c. activation of the renin–angiotensin–aldosterone system with increased ADH and aldosterone.
   d. stimulation of the countercurrent mechanism with reflex drop in renin release.

3. Thiazide diuretics are considered less potent diuretics because they
   a. block the sodium pump in the loop of Henle.
   b. cause loss of sodium and chloride but little water.
   c. do not cause fluid rebound when they work in the kidneys.
   d. have little or no effect on electrolyte levels.

4. The nurse would anticipate an order for a loop diuretic as the drug of choice for a patient with
   a. hypertension.
   b. septic shock.
   c. pulmonary edema.
   d. fluid retention of pregnancy.

5. When providing care to a patient who is receiving a loop diuretic, which would the nurse typically need to monitor regularly?
   a. Calorie intake
   b. Bone marrow function
   c. Blood pressure
   d. Protein levels

6. When developing the plan of care for a patient with hyperaldosteronism, the nurse would expect the physician to prescribe which agent?
   a. Spironolactone
   b. Furosemide
   c. Hydrochlorothiazide
   d. Acetazolamide

7. A patient with severe glaucoma who is about to undergo eye surgery would benefit from a decrease in intraocular fluid. This is often best accomplished by giving the patient a(n)
   a. loop diuretic.
   b. thiazide diuretic.
   c. carbonic anhydrase inhibitor.
   d. osmotic diuretic.

8. The nurse would instruct a patient receiving a loop diuretic to report
   a. yellow vision.
   b. weight loss of 1 lb/d.
   c. muscle cramping.
   d. increased urination.

MULTIPLE RESPONSE

Select all that apply.

1. Diuretics are currently recommended for the treatment of which conditions?
   a. Hypertension
   b. Renal disease
   c. Obesity
   d. Severe liver disease
   e. Fluid retention of pregnancy
   f. Heart failure

2. Routine nursing care of a client receiving a diuretic would include which interventions?
   a. Daily weighing
   b. Tight fluid restrictions
   c. Periodic electrolyte evaluations
   d. Monitoring of urinary output
   e. Regular IOP testing
   f. Teaching the patient to report muscle cramping

REFERENCES

Brunton, L., Hilal-Dandan, R., & Knollman, B. (2018). *Goodman and Gilman's the pharmacological basis of therapeutics* (13th ed.). McGraw-Hill.

Einhorn, P. T., Davis, B. R., Wright, J. T., Rahman, M., Whelton, P. K., & Pressel, S. L. (2010). ALLHAT: Still providing correct answers after 7 years. *Current Opinion in Cardiology, 25*, 355–365. https://doi.org/10.1097/HCO.0b013e32833a8828

Fuster, V., Alexander, R. W., & Rourke, R. A. (Eds.). (2011). *Hurst's the heart* (13th ed.). McGraw-Hill.

Hall, J. E., & Hall, M. E. (2021). *Guyton and Hall textbook of medical physiology* (14th ed.). Elsevier.

Mosenkis, A., & Townsend, R. R. (2007). Gynecomastia and antihypertensive therapy. *Journal of Clinical Hypertension, 6*(8), 469–470. https://doi.org/10.1111/j.1524-6175.2004.3735.x

Norris, T. L. (2019). *Porth's pathophysiology concepts of altered health states* (13th ed.). Wolters Kluwer.

Shafi, T., Appel, L. J., Miller, E. R., Klag, M. J., & Parekh, R. S. (2008). Changes in serum potassium mediate thiazide-induced diabetes. *Hypertension, 52*, 1002–1029. https://doi.org/10.1161/HYPERTENSIONAHA.108.119438

Stafford, R. S., Bartholomew, L. K., Cushman, W. C., Cutler, J. A., Davis, B. R., Dawson, G., Einhorn, P. T., Furberg, C. D., Piller, L. B., Pressel, S. L., Whelton, P. K., & ALLHAT Collaborative Research Group. (2010). Impact of the ALLHAT/JNC7 dissemination project on thiazide-type diuretic use. *Archives of Internal Medicine, 170*, 851–858. https://doi.org/10.1001/archinternmed.2010.130

CHAPTER 52

Drugs Affecting the Urinary Tract and the Bladder

Learning Objectives

Upon completion of this chapter, you will be able to:

1. Describe four common problems associated with the urinary tract, including the clinical manifestations of these problems.
2. Discuss the use of drugs affecting the urinary tract and bladder across the lifespan.
3. Describe the therapeutic actions, indications, pharmacokinetics, contraindications and cautions, most common adverse effects, and important drug–drug interactions associated with urinary tract antiinfectives, antispasmodics, analgesics, the bladder protectant, and drugs used to treat benign prostatic hyperplasia (BPH).
4. Compare and contrast the prototype drugs fosfomycin, oxybutynin, phenazopyridine, pentosan polysulfate sodium, doxazosin, and finasteride with other agents in their class.
5. Outline the nursing considerations, including important teaching points, for patients receiving drugs affecting the urinary tract and bladder.

Key Terms

acidification: process of increasing the acid level; used to treat bladder infections, making the bladder an undesirable place for bacteria

antispasmodics: agents that block muscle spasm associated with irritation or neurological stimulation

benign prostatic hyperplasia (BPH): enlargement of the prostate gland, associated with age and inflammation; also called benign prostatic hypertrophy

cystitis: inflammation of the bladder caused by infection or irritation

dysuria: painful urination

interstitial cystitis: chronic inflammation of the interstitial connective tissue of the bladder; may extend into deeper tissue

nocturia: getting up to void at night, reflecting increased renal perfusion with fluid shifts in the supine position; can occur when a person has gravity-dependent edema that could be related to heart failure; other medical conditions, including urinary tract infection, increase the need to get up and void

pyelonephritis: inflammation of the structures of the kidney, frequently caused by backward flow problems or by bacteria ascending the ureter from the bladder

urgency: the feeling that one needs to void immediately; often associated with infection and inflammation in the urinary tract

urinary frequency: the need to void often; usually seen in response to irritation of the bladder, age, and inflammation

Drug List

URINARY TRACT ANTIINFECTIVES

- (P) fosfomycin
- methenamine
- nitrofurantoin
- trimethoprim
- trimethoprim–sulfamethoxazole

URINARY TRACT ANTISPASMODICS

Anticholinergics

- darifenacin
- fesoterodine
- flavoxate
- (P) oxybutynin
- solifenacin
- tolterodine
- trospium

Beta-Agonists

- mirabegron
- vibegron

OTHER DRUGS USED THAT AFFECT THE URINARY TRACT AND BLADDER

Urinary Tract Analgesic

- (P) phenazopyridine

Bladder Protectant

- (P) pentosan polysulfate sodium

DRUGS FOR TREATING BENIGN PROSTATIC HYPERPLASIA

Alpha-Adrenergic Blockers

- alfuzosin
- (P) doxazosin
- silodosin
- tamsulosin
- terazosin

DRUGS THAT BLOCK TESTOSTERONE PRODUCTION

- dutasteride
- (P) finasteride

Conditions affecting the urinary tract and bladder are common problems. These conditions include acute urinary tract infections (UTIs), bladder spasms, bladder pain, and benign prostatic hyperplasia (BPH).

Acute UTIs occur second in frequency only to respiratory tract infections in the U.S. population. People with shorter female urethras are particularly vulnerable to repeated urinary tract, bladder, and even kidney infections. Children may also have frequent urinary tract problems. Patients with indwelling catheters or intermittent catheterizations often develop bladder infections or **cystitis** (inflammation of the bladder, often due to infection), which can result from bacteria introduced into the bladder by these devices. Blockage anywhere in the urinary tract can lead to backflow problems and the spread of bladder infections into the kidney to cause inflammation in the kidney (**pyelonephritis**).

The signs and symptoms of a UTI are uncomfortable and include **urinary frequency** (the need to void often), **urgency** (the feeling that one needs to void immediately), burning on urination (associated with cystitis), chills, fever, flank pain, and tenderness (associated with acute pyelonephritis). Some may suffer from **nocturia** (increased frequency in voiding at night) that can be triggered by UTI or fluid shifts when the person is in supine positions. In older adults, the only presentation may be confusion, disorientation, and other central nervous system (CNS) effects. To treat these infections, providers often prescribe specific urinary tract antiinfectives. There is a lot of variability around the world regarding which agents to use first for UTI infections. In the United States, most agree that nitrofurantoin, trimethoprim-sulfamethoxazole, and fosfomycin are appropriate first-line agents. Some guidelines refer to the fluoroquinolones (Chapter 9) as first-line treatment as well; however, their adverse effect profile limits their use.

Drugs are also available to block spasms of the urinary tract muscles, decrease urinary tract pain, protect the cells

Table 52.1 Drugs Used to Treat Urinary Tract and Bladder Problems

Urinary Tract Problem	Potential Medications
Infection	*Urinary tract antiinfectives*: fosfomycin, methenamine, nitrofurantoin, trimethoprim, trimethoprim–sulfamethoxazole
Overactive bladder	*Beta-3-adrenergic agonists*: mirabegron (*Myrbetriq*), vibegron (*Gemtesa*)
Spasm	*Antispasmodics*: flavoxate, oxybutynin, tolterodine, trospium
Pain	*Urinary tract analgesic*: phenazopyridine *Bladder protectant for interstitial cystitis*: pentosan
BPH	*Alpha-adrenergic blockers*: doxazosin, tamsulosin, terazosin, alfuzosin *Testosterone inhibitors*: finasteride, dutasteride

BPH, benign prostatic hyperplasia.

BOX 52.1 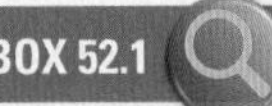 **Focus on Drug Therapy Across the Lifespan**

URINARY TRACT AGENTS

Children

Children may develop UTIs, including cystitis, and need to be treated with a urinary tract antiinfective. Some children, because of congenital problems, neurogenic disorders, or indwelling catheters, require other urinary tract agents such as urinary tract analgesics or antispasmodics. Some of the antiinfectives have established pediatric guidelines (see Table 52.2). A child with repeated UTIs should be evaluated for potential sexual abuse or congenital structural abnormalities.

Children need to be instructed in proper hygiene and should not be given bubble baths if UTIs occur. They should be encouraged to avoid alkaline ash juices such as orange or grapefruit juice and urged to drink lots of water.

If an antispasmodic is needed, oxybutynin is indicated for children older than 5 years of age, and flavoxate can be used in children older than 12 years of age. Phenazopyridine is indicated as a urinary tract analgesic for children 6 to 12 years of age. The child should be cautioned about the change in urine color that might occur with phenazopyridine because it might be frightening if the child is not expecting it.

Adults

Adults need to be cautioned about the various measures that can be used to decrease the likelihood of UTIs. They should be encouraged to drink plenty of fluids to maintain urinary tract health.

If they are taking an anticholinergic to block spasms, adult patients need to be advised of other precautions to take when the parasympathetic system is blocked.

Adults being treated for BPH need to be aware of the possibility of decreased sexual function, as well as fatigue, lethargy, and the potential for dizziness, which could interfere with working or activities of daily living.

The use of urinary tract agents during pregnancy should be approached with caution. If an antibiotic is needed, it is important to note the specific trimester of pregnancy. Some of the mediations have safer profiles at certain times of the pregnancy. Patients who are breast or chestfeeding should use these agents with caution because of the potential for adverse effects on the baby, or they should find another method of feeding the baby.

Older Adults

Older adults often have conditions that are treated with urinary tract agents. They are also more likely to have renal or hepatic impairment, which requires caution in the use of these drugs. Older adults should be started on the lowest possible dose of the drug, and it should be titrated slowly based on patient response. Special precautions to monitor cardiac function, intraocular pressure, blood pressure, and bladder emptying need to be taken when using alpha-adrenergic blockers with these patients. Older patients may have a difficult time maintaining fluid intake and might benefit from extra encouragement to drink fluids, including cranberry juice, and to avoid alkaline ash drinks. Some of these agents have anticholinergic effects that tend to cause more adverse effect in older adults. Chapter 33 provides more details about the effects of anticholinergic agents in older adults.

of the bladder from irritation, and treat enlargement of the prostate gland. Table 52.1 summarizes urinary tract problems and the drugs used to treat them. Box 52.1 highlights important considerations related to urinary tract drugs based on the patient's age.

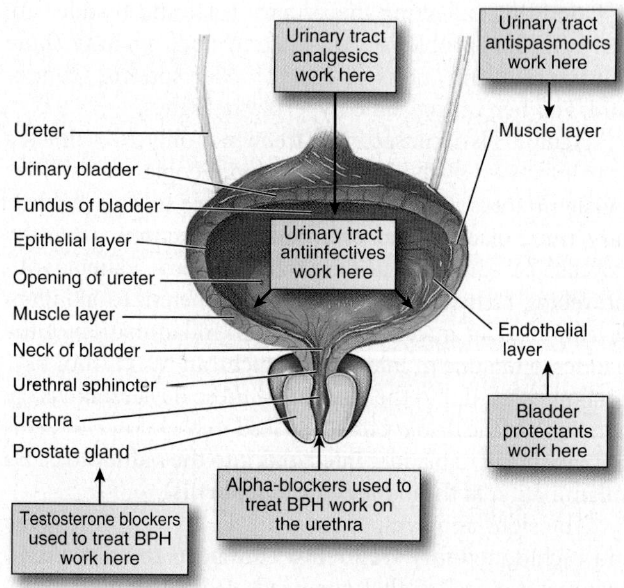

FIGURE 52.1 Sites of action of drugs acting on the urinary tract.

Urinary Tract Antiinfectives

There are two types of urinary tract antiinfectives (Table 52.2). One type is the antibiotics, which have been shown to be effective against many of the pathogens that cause UTIs. The antibiotics used specifically to treat UTIs include fosfomycin (*Monurol*), nitrofurantoin (*Furadantin*), and trimethoprim (generic). Ciprofloxacin (*Cipro*), ofloxacin (*Floxin*), levofloxacin (*Levaquin*), and cefixime (*Suprax*) are also used frequently to treat UTIs but are not specific to UTIs and are also used for treating other infections (see Chapter 9). The combination medication trimethoprim–sulfamethoxazole (*Bactrim, Septra*) is often administered to treat UTIs, shigellosis, and otitis media. The other type of urinary tract antiinfective works to acidify the urine, killing bacteria that might be in the bladder. This group includes methenamine (*Urex*).

Therapeutic Actions and Indications

Some of the urinary tract antiinfectives act specifically within the urinary tract to destroy bacteria, either through a direct antibiotic effect or through **acidification** of the urine, which is the process of increasing the acid level, producing an environment that is not conducive to bacterial survival and leading to bacterial cell death. If they are acting locally in the urinary tract, they do not have an antibiotic effect systemically (Fig. 52.1). Trimethoprim is an antiinfective that works systemically; it is active against *Staphylococcus saprophyticus* (a common pathogen that causes UTIs). Nitrofurantoin and fosfomycin are used to treat susceptible gram-positive and gram-negative pathogens. Those that cause acidification of the urine are used to treat chronic UTIs, as adjunctive therapy in acute cystitis and pyelonephritis, and as prophylaxis with urinary tract anatomic abnormalities and residual urine disorders. See the "Critical Thinking Scenario" for additional information regarding teaching the patient about treatment for cystitis. Table 52.2 discusses usual indications for each of the urinary tract antiinfectives.

Table 52.2 *Drugs in Focus*: Urinary Tract Antiinfectives

Drug Name	Usual Dosage	Usual Indications for Urinary Tract/Bladder
fosfomycin (*Monurol*)	One packet (3 g) dissolved in water PO	Treatment of UTIs caused by susceptible bacteria (one-dose drug) in patients >12 y
methenamine (*Urex*)	*Adult*: 1 g b.i.d. or q.i.d. and HS PO *Pediatric (6–12 y)*: 0.5–1 g PO b.i.d. to q.i.d. *Pediatric (<6 y)*: 50 mg/kg/d PO in three divided doses	Suppression or prevention of bacteriuria associated with recurrent UTIs and anatomic abnormalities
nitrofurantoin (*Furadantin, Macrobid, Macrodantin*)	*Adult*: 50–100 mg PO q.i.d. for 10–14 d or 100 mg PO b.i.d. for 7 d (*Macrobid*); 50–100 mg PO at bedtime for chronic suppressive therapy *Pediatric*: 5–7 mg/kg/d in four divided doses; 1 mg/kg/d PO in one to two doses or chronic suppressive therapy	Treatment of UTIs caused by susceptible bacteria
trimethoprim (*Primsol*)	100 mg PO q12h or 200 mg PO daily for 10 d; reduce dose with renal impairment	Treatment of UTIs
trimethoprim–sulfamethoxazole (*Bactrim, Bactrim DS, Septra, Septra DS*)	*Adult*: 160 mg TMP/800 mg SMZ q12h for 10 d *Child 2 mo and older:* 8 mg/kg TMP 40 mg/kg SMZ given in two divided doses q12h for 10 d	Treatment of UTIs, shigellosis, and otitis media

UTI, urinary tract infection.

Pharmacokinetics

Fosfomycin, taken orally, has the convenience of a one-time dose. It is not recommended for children younger than 12 years of age. It is rapidly absorbed, undergoes slow hepatic metabolism, and is excreted in the urine and feces. Unpleasant GI effects limit its usefulness in some patients. The dose does not need to be changed in cases of renal impairment.

Nitrofurantoin is also administered orally. The absorption is enhanced when taken with food. It has been successfully used to treat acute uncomplicated cystitis but due to lack of broad tissue distribution is not indicated for pyelonephritis, and patients should be monitored for recurrent infection. It is well absorbed when taken orally, metabolized in the liver, and excreted in the urine. No dose adjustment is needed with renal impairment.

CRITICAL THINKING SCENARIO
Teaching About Cystitis Treatment

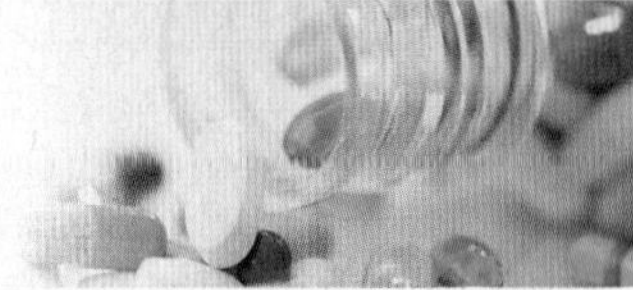

THE SITUATION

J.K. is a 6-year-old patient assigned female at birth who has a history of repeated UTIs. J.K. was screened for potential sexual abuse, which may present as repeated UTIs, and was found to have no evidence of sexual abuse. J.K. is also going to have imaging performed to evaluate for any anatomic abnormalities that could increase risk of UTIs. J.K. is seen today after being treated with *Bactrim* for 10 days. J.K. denies complaints of **dysuria** (painful urination), frequency, urgency, or fever. J.K.'s parents are very concerned about a recurrent UTI since the treatments have only worked for a few weeks at a time. A urine sample is sent for urinalysis and culture and sensitivity testing. The physician prescribes methenamine (*Urex*), 500 mg q.i.d., and refers J.K. and their parents to the nurse for teaching.

CRITICAL THINKING

What is the best approach for this patient?

What key teaching points (at least five) should be emphasized to assist the pharmacological therapy in treating this infection? Think about what the drug is doing, how it works, and how it works best.

DISCUSSION

Cystitis can be difficult to treat in young patients and can become a chronic problem. Patient and parent education is important for blocking the growth of bacteria and curing the infection. Teaching points should emphasize activities that will decrease the number of bacteria introduced into the bladder, acidify the urine to make the bladder an inhospitable environment for bacterial growth, and flush the bladder to prevent stagnant urine from encouraging bacterial growth.

To decrease the number of bacteria introduced into the bladder, patient education should cover the following hygiene measures: Always wipe from front to back and never from back to front to avoid the introduction of intestinal bacteria into the urethra; avoid baths, particularly bubble baths, which can be more irritating to the vaginal mucosa; and wear dry cotton underwear to discourage bacterial growth.

Patient education should also stress the importance of avoiding alkaline ash foods (e.g., citrus fruits, certain vegetables) and antacids and encouraging foods that acidify the urine. Cranberry juice is often recommended as a choice for fruit juice because it helps prevent the bacteria from adhering to the bladder wall, helping to prevent infection. Fluid intake, especially water, should be encouraged as much as possible to keep the bladder flushed. Finally, the patient should be encouraged to complete the full course of medication prescribed and to not stop taking the drug when symptoms disappear. See Box 52.2, "Focus on the Evidence: Cranberry for UTIs?"

PATIENT TEACHING FOR J.K.: URINARY TRACT ANTIINFECTIVE METHENAMINE

Assessment: History and Examination

Assess J.K.'s health history, particularly any allergies to antibacterial medications, and liver or renal dysfunction. (If J.K. were of childbearing age, you would assess pregnancy and lactation status.)

Focus the physical examination on the following areas:

CNS: orientation, reflexes, strength

Skin: color, texture, edema

Gastrointestinal (GI): liver evaluation

Genitourinary (GU): urinary output

Laboratory tests: liver function tests, urinalysis, urine culture, and sensitivity testing

Nursing Conclusions

Impaired comfort related to GI, CNS, and skin effects of the drug

Altered sensory perception related to CNS effects

Knowledge deficit regarding drug therapy

Planning

The patient will receive the best therapeutic effect from the drug therapy.

The patient will have limited adverse effects from the drug therapy.

The patient will have an understanding of the drug therapy, adverse effects to anticipate, and measures to relieve discomfort and improve safety.

(continues on page 930)

Intervention

Obtain urine sample for urinalysis and culture and sensitivity test.
Provide comfort and safety measures: safety precautions, skin care, and nutrition.
Encourage eating acidifying foods and drinking lots of fluids.
Teach hygiene measures.
Administer medication with food if GI upset is a problem.
Provide support and reassurance to deal with drug effects and lifestyle changes.
Provide patient teaching to J.K. and their parents or caregivers regarding drug name, dosage, adverse effects, precautions, warnings to report, hygiene measures, and dietary changes as needed.

Evaluation

Evaluate drug effects: relief of symptoms and resolution of infection.
Monitor for adverse effects: GI upset, headache, dizziness, confusion, dysuria, pruritus, and urticaria.
Monitor for drug–drug interactions as indicated, especially use of antacids.
Evaluate the effectiveness of patient teaching program and comfort and safety measures.

PATIENT TEACHING FOR J.K.

- A urinary tract antiinfective such as methenamine treats UTIs by making the urine more acidic, which produces an environment that is not conducive to bacterial growth.
- If this drug causes stomach upset, it can be taken with food. It is important to avoid foods that alkalinize the urine, such as citrus fruits and milk, because they decrease the effectiveness of the drug. Cranberry juice and/or tablets may also acidify the urine. As much fluid as possible (eight to ten 8-oz glasses of water a day) should be taken to help flush out the bacteria and treat the infection.
- Avoid using any over-the-counter (OTC) medication that might contain sodium bicarbonate (e.g., antacids, baking soda) because these drugs alkalinize the urine and interfere with the ability of methenamine to treat the infection. If you question the use of any OTC drug, check with your health care provider.
- Take the full course of your prescription. Do not use this drug to self-treat any other infection.
- Common adverse effects of this drug may include the following:
  - Stomach upset, nausea: Taking the drug with food or eating small, frequent meals may help.
  - Painful urination: If this occurs, report it to your health care provider. A dose adjustment may be needed.
  - Report any of the following to your health care provider: skin rash or itching, severe GI upset, GI upset that prevents adequate fluid intake, and very painful urination (and pregnancy in patients who are able to become pregnant).
- The following can help to decrease UTIs:
  - Avoid bubble baths if they irritate the mucosal lining.
  - Void whenever you feel the urge; try not to wait.
  - Always wipe from front to back, never from back to front.
  - Limit alkaline ash foods, such as citrus juices, and avoid the use of antacids.
  - Hydrate well to avoid dehydration and potential irritation of the urinary anatomy.
  - Tell any doctor, nurse, or other health care provider involved in your care that you are taking this drug.

Methenamine, taken orally, is well absorbed. It is hydrolyzed in the kidneys, where it is active, and then excreted in the urine. Methenamine has established dose guidelines for children and comes in a suspension form.

Treatment of UTIs during pregnancy can differ based on the trimester. Nitrofurantoin and trimethoprim–sulfamethoxazole are to be avoided in the first trimester due to possible risk of congenital anomalies, but they can usually

Box 52.2 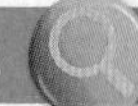 Focus on the Evidence: Cranberry for UTIs?

Cranberry juice and cranberries have long been accepted as a good choice for treating and preventing UTIs. In the past, it was thought that the compounds in the cranberry caused acidic urine and that was what made them effective. Evidence-based research did not support that claim, finding that patients could not consume the amount of juice necessary to make the urine acidic enough to kill bacteria. Studies did show, however, that compounds in cranberries, A-type proanthocyanidins, inhibited *Escherichia coli* bacteria from adhering to the bladder wall and prevented infections from occurring. Research studies showed no efficacy in the use of cranberry to treat UTIs. Research studies vary widely, however, on supporting or not supporting the use of cranberry in preventing UTIs. In 2011, a study showed no difference between placebo and cranberry products in UTI prevention (Barbosa-Cesnik et al., 2011). A systemic review published in 2017 showed cranberry products may have a protective role in preventing UTIs, but the authors pointed out that larger high-quality studies would be helpful (Fu et al., 2017). The bottom line is that patients with UTIs should drink six to eight glasses of fluids a day. Alkaline fluids should be avoided, so adding a juice that is not alkaline ash may be a good idea and that may help the situation. Nurses need to be aware that there is a lot of sugar in regular cranberry juice, so patients who need to limit sugar intake should be cautious. Many cranberry products are also relatively expensive, a problem that could be an issue for patients on fixed incomes or with other financial issues. An older patient with diabetes on a fixed income may not be a candidate, and making sure that the patient drinks enough water every day may or may not be just as effective. Research continues.

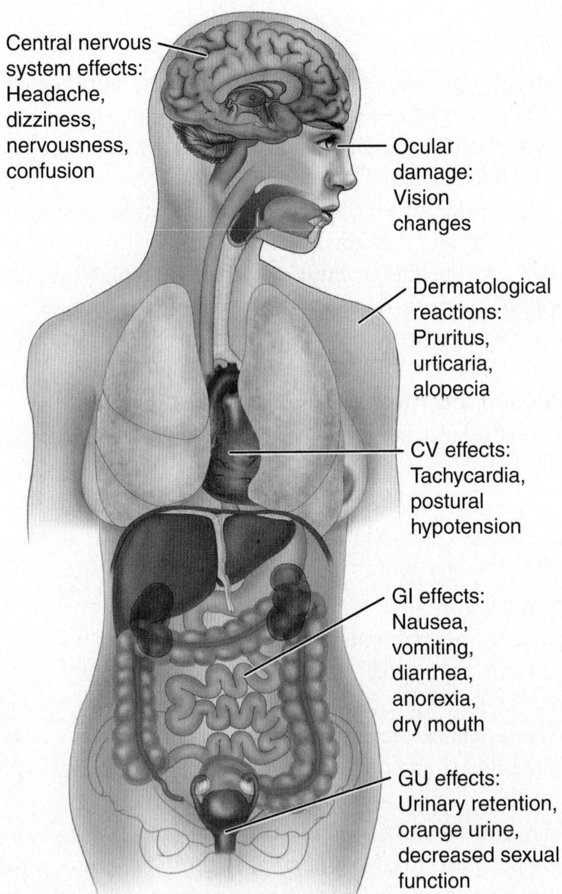

FIGURE 52.2 Variety of adverse effects and toxicities associated with drugs affecting the urinary tract and bladder.

be given safely in the 2nd and 3rd trimesters. Nitrofurantoin may also have the risk of causing hemolytic anemia in some neonates if given at term. Trimethoprim–sulfamethoxazole may increase the risk of jaundice in newborns if given close to term. Fosfomycin and some beta-lactam antibiotics may be administered to treat UTI during pregnancy as well.

Contraindications and Cautions

These drugs are contraindicated in the presence of any known allergy to any of these drugs to prevent hypersensitivity reactions. They should be used with caution in the presence of renal dysfunction, which could interfere with the excretion and action of these drugs, and with pregnancy and lactation because of the potential for adverse effects on the fetus or neonate.

Adverse Effects

Adverse effects associated with these drugs include nausea, vomiting, diarrhea, anorexia, bladder irritation, and dysuria (Fig. 52.2). Infrequent symptoms include blood dyscrasias, pruritus, urticaria, headache, dizziness, nervousness, and confusion. These effects may result from GI irritation caused by the agent, which may be somewhat alleviated if the drug is taken with food, or from a systemic reaction to urinary tract irritation. Fosfomycin is associated with unpleasant GI effects, which limits its usefulness in some patients.

Clinically Important Drug–Drug Interactions

Because these drugs are from several different chemical classes, the drug–drug interactions that can occur are specific to the drug being used. Consult a nursing drug guide for specific interactions.

Prototype Summary: Fosfomycin

Indications: Treatment of acute uncomplicated UTIs caused by susceptible strains of bacteria.

Actions: Interferes with cell wall formation of gram-negative bacteria, leading to cell death.

Pharmacokinetics:

Route	Onset	Peak	Duration
Oral	Varies	2 h	12 h

$T_{1/2}$: 5.7 to 9.5 hours; excreted unchanged in the urine.

Adverse Effects: Headache, dizziness, nausea, diarrhea, vaginitis.

Nursing Considerations for Patients Receiving Urinary Tract Antiinfectives

Assessment: History and Examination

- Assess for contraindications or cautions: any history of allergy to antibiotics or antiinfectives to avoid hypersensitivity reactions; liver or renal dysfunction that might interfere with the drug's metabolism and excretion; and current status of pregnancy and lactation, which require cautious use of the drug.
- Perform a physical assessment before therapy to establish baseline data and during therapy to determine the effectiveness of the drug and any adverse effects associated with drug therapy.
- Inspect the skin to evaluate for the development of rash or hypersensitivity reactions.
- Assess level of consciousness and monitor orientation and reflexes to evaluate any CNS effects of the drug.
- Assess urinary elimination patterns, including amount and episode frequency, and for complaints of frequency, urgency, pain, or difficulty voiding to determine the effectiveness of therapy.
- Monitor laboratory test results, including urinalysis and urine culture and sensitivity, to evaluate effectiveness and appropriateness of drug choice and renal and hepatic function tests to determine the need for possible dose adjustment and to identify possible toxicity.

(continues on page 932)

Nursing Conclusions

Nursing conclusions related to drug therapy might include the following:

- Impaired comfort related to GI, CNS, or skin effects of drug
- Altered sensory perception (kinesthetic, tactile, visual) related to CNS effects
- Impaired urinary elimination related to the underlying problem necessitating drug therapy
- Injury risk related to possible CNS effects
- Knowledge deficit regarding drug therapy

Planning

- The patient will receive the best therapeutic effect from the drug therapy.
- The patient will have limited adverse effects from the drug therapy.
- The patient will have an understanding of the drug therapy, adverse effects to anticipate, and measures to relieve discomfort and improve safety.

Intervention With Rationale

- Ensure that culture and sensitivity tests are performed before therapy begins and are repeated if the response is not as expected to ensure appropriate treatment of the infection.
- Administer the drugs with food to decrease GI adverse effects if they occur.
- Institute safety precautions if the patient experiences CNS effects to prevent patient injury.
- Advise the patient to continue the full course of the drug ordered and to not stop taking it as soon as the uncomfortable signs and symptoms pass to ensure eradication of the infection and prevent the emergence of resistant strains of bacteria.
- Encourage the patient to drink lots of fluids (unless contraindicated by other conditions) to promote flushing of the bladder and prevent urinary stasis and to avoid citrus juices and antacids, which promote an alkaline urine and provide opportunity for bacteria growth.
- Provide or assist with perineal hygiene as indicated to reduce the risk of reinfection or prevent transmission of infection.
- Educate the patient with chronic UTIs about additional activities that can facilitate acidic urine to increase the effectiveness of urinary tract antiinfectives.
- Provide thorough patient teaching, including drug name, dosage, intended effect, and schedule for administration; measures to prevent or alleviate adverse effects; the need to avoid alkaline ash foods that produce alkaline urine (e.g., citrus juices, antacids); the need to take the drug with food or meals to reduce GI effects; the importance of increasing fluid intake, including the use of cranberry juice; measures to prevent the recurrence of UTIs; and the need for periodic monitoring and laboratory testing, such as urinalysis and urine culture and sensitivity, to enhance patient knowledge about drug therapy and to promote adherence.

Evaluation

- Monitor patient response to the drug (resolution of UTI and relief of signs and symptoms); repeat culture and sensitivity tests as recommended for evaluation of the effectiveness of all of these drugs.
- Monitor for adverse effects (skin evaluation, orientation and reflexes, GI effects).
- Evaluate the effectiveness of the teaching plan (patient can name drug, dosage, adverse effects to watch for, specific measures to avoid them, and measures to take to increase the effectiveness of the drug).
- Monitor the effectiveness of comfort and safety measures and adherence to the therapeutic regimen.

Key Points

- Urinary tract antiinfectives destroy bacteria in the urinary tract that could be causing infections.
- Urinary tract–specific antibiotics prevent bacterial reproduction and cause bacterial cell death.
- Some urinary tract antiinfectives kill urinary tract bacteria by acidifying the urine, making the tract a poor host for bacterial growth, or by killing the bacteria outright.
- Hygiene measures, proper diet, and extra hydration are activities that help decrease harmful bacteria in the urinary tract, which promotes the effect of urinary tract antiinfective agents.

Urinary Tract Antispasmodics

Urinary tract **antispasmodics** (Table 52.3) block the spasms of urinary tract muscles caused by various conditions. The antispasmodics that are available include the anticholinergics flavoxate (generic), oxybutynin (*Ditropan XL* and others), tolterodine (*Detrol*), fesoterodine (*Toviaz*), darifenacin (*Enablex*), solifenacin (*VESIcare*), and trospium (generic), and the beta-agonists mirabegron (*Myrbetriq*) and vibegron (*Gemtesa*).

Therapeutic Actions and Indications

Inflammation in the urinary tract, such as cystitis, prostatitis, urethritis, and urethrocystitis/urethrotrigonitis, causes smooth muscle spasms along the urinary tract. Irritation of the urinary tract leading to muscle spasm also occurs in patients with neurogenic bladder. These spasms lead to the uncomfortable effects of dysuria (pain or discomfort with urination), urgency, incontinence, nocturia (frequent nighttime urination), and suprapubic pain. There are also disorders of the brain and/or spinal cord that can cause neurogenic detrusor overactivity, which can cause bladder spasms. Most of the urinary tract antispasmodics

Table 52.3 *Drugs in Focus*: Urinary Tract Antispasmodics

Drug Name	Usual Dosage	Usual Indications
Anticholinergics		
darifenacin (*Enablex*)	7.5 mg/d PO; may be increased to 15 mg/d	Treatment of overactive bladder in patients with urinary urgency, incontinence, or frequency
fesoterodine (*Toviaz*)	*Adult and pediatric*: Initial dose 4 mg/d PO, may be increased to 8 mg/d if needed	Treatment of overactive bladder with symptoms of urgency, incontinence, and frequency; treatment of neurogenic detrusor overactivity in pediatric patients 6 y and older
flavoxate (generic)	100–200 mg PO t.i.d. to q.i.d.; reduce dose when patient improves	Symptomatic relief of urinary bladder spasm in patients >12 y
oxybutynin (*Ditropan XL, Oxytrol, Gelnique*)	*ER tablets*: 5 mg/d PO up to a maximum 30 mg/d, 5 mg PO in divided doses *Transdermal patch*: Apply to dry, intact skin q3–4d. *Gel*: Apply 1 mL to the thigh, abdomen, or upper arm once q24h. *Pediatric (>5 y)*: 5 mg PO b.i.d., up to a maximum 5 mg PO t.i.d. *Pediatric (>6 y)*: ER tablets 5 mg/d PO	Symptomatic relief of urinary bladder spasm; treatment of overactive bladder; treatment of neurogenic detrusor overactivity in pediatric patients 6 years and older
solifenacin (*VESIcare, VESIcare LS*)	*Adult:* 5–10 mg/d PO swallowed whole with water *Pediatric:* 2–10 mg/d PO; based on weight Reduce dose with renal impairment and hepatic impairment	Treatment of overactive bladder in patients with urinary urgency, incontinence, or frequency; treatment of neurogenic detrusor overactivity in pediatric patients aged 2 y and older
tolterodine (*Detrol, Detrol LA*)	1–2 mg PO b.i.d.; ER capsules 2–4 mg/d; reduce dose in patients with hepatic impairment to 1 mg PO b.i.d.	Treatment of overactive bladder in patients with urinary urgency, frequency, or incontinence
trospium (generic)	20 mg PO b.i.d. at least 1 h before meals or 60-mg ER tablet PO daily; reduce dose in patients with renal or hepatic impairment	Symptomatic relief of overactive bladder with symptoms of urinary incontinence, urgency, and urinary frequency
Beta-Agonist		
mirabegron (*Myrbetriq, Myrbetriq granules*)	*Adult and pediatric ≥35 kg or more:* 25–50 mg/d PO *Pediatric:* 24–64 mg/d PO; dose based on weight	Treatment of overactive bladder with symptoms of urinary incontinence, frequency, and urgency; treatment of NDO in pediatric patients aged ≥3 years and weighing ≥35 kg
vibegron (*Gemtesa*)	*Adult:* 75 mg/d PO	Treatment of overactive bladder with symptoms of urgency, urinary incontinence, and urinary frequency

ER, extended release; NDO, neurogenic detrusor overactivity.

relieve these spasms by blocking parasympathetic activity, thus suppressing overactivity, which leads to relaxation of the detrusor and other urinary tract muscles (see Fig. 52.1). Because the parasympathetic system uses acetylcholine to cause its effects, these drugs are called anticholinergic drugs.

Trospium specifically blocks muscarinic receptors and reduces the muscle tone of the bladder. It is specifically indicated for the treatment of overactive bladder with symptoms of urinary incontinence, urgency, and urinary frequency.

Mirabegron (*Myrbetriq*) and vibegron (*Gemtesa*) are drugs for treating overactive bladder and incontinence that work differently than the anticholinergic medications. They are beta^3-agonists and stimulate the sympathetic nerves in the bladder, which leads to detrusor muscle relaxation. This effect allows for more urine to accumulate in the bladder, helping to increase muscle pressure and urine flow rate. They do not have the anticholinergic effects seen with the other drugs but do have stimulatory sympathetic effects that may cause an increase in blood pressure, heart rate, etc. See Table 52.3 for usual indications of other urinary tract antispasmodics.

Pharmacokinetics

All of these agents are administered orally with the exception of oxybutynin, which is administered not only orally but also as a dermal patch and a topical gel. These drugs are rapidly absorbed, have a slow onset of action, and have a duration of action of 6 to 12 hours. Oxybutynin, when given by the transdermal patch, has a duration of action of 96 hours. The system has to be replaced every 3 to 4 days.

These drugs are metabolized in the liver and excreted in the urine. They cross the placenta and are found in human milk. Mirabegron is absorbed from the GI tract with peak levels in 3.5 hours. After hepatic metabolism, it is excreted in the urine with a half-life of approximately 50 hours.

Contraindications and Cautions

These drugs are contraindicated in the presence of known allergy to the drugs to avoid hypersensitivity reactions; with pyloric or duodenal obstruction or recent surgery because the anticholinergic effects can cause serious complications; with obstructive urinary tract problems, which could be further aggravated by the blocking of muscle activity or relaxation of the bladder; and with glaucoma, myasthenia gravis, or acute hemorrhage, which could all be exacerbated by the anticholinergic effects of these drugs. Caution should be used in patients with renal or hepatic dysfunction, which could alter the metabolism and excretion of the drugs, and in pregnant and lactating patients because of potential adverse effects on the fetus or neonate secondary to the anticholinergic effects of the drugs. Mirabegron should be used with caution in the presence of hypertension because this could be aggravated by the drug effects.

Adverse Effects

Adverse effects of the anticholinergic urinary tract antispasmodics are related to the blocking of the parasympathetic system and include nausea, vomiting, dry mouth, nervousness, tachycardia, and vision changes. Flavoxate is associated with CNS effects (blurred vision, dizziness, confusion) that make it less desirable to use in certain patients, such as the older adults or patients with neurological problems. Oxybutynin has numerous anticholinergic effects, making it undesirable with certain conditions or situations that might be aggravated by decreased sweating, urinary retention, tachycardia, and changes in GI activity. Mirabegron stimulates the sympathetic system and may cause hypertension and urinary retention.

Clinically Important Drug–Drug Interactions

Decreased effectiveness of phenothiazines and haloperidol has been associated with the combination of these drugs with oxybutynin. If any such combinations must be used, the patient should be monitored closely and appropriate dose adjustments made. If darifenacin or fesoterodine is combined with antifungals or antiviral agents, there is a risk of toxic effects. The dose of darifenacin or fesoterodine must be reduced. There is a risk of increased QT interval and serious cardiac arrhythmias if solifenacin is combined with other drugs that prolong the QT interval (antihistamines, antipsychotics); the patient must be monitored closely if this combination is used. There is also a risk of increased serum levels and toxic effects if solifenacin is combined with ketoconazole or other cytochrome P-450 (CYP) 3A4 inhibitors; the dose of solifenacin must be reduced and the patient followed closely. Tolterodine levels and toxicity can increase if it is taken with CYP2D6 inhibitors (fluoxetine); the dose of tolterodine must be reduced if this combination is used. Trospium can interfere with the excretion of drugs by tubular secretion, leading to increased serum levels of those drugs, such as digoxin, morphine, metformin, and tenofovir. The patient needs close monitoring and appropriate dose adjustments if necessary. Mirabegron should not be combined with drugs that are metabolized by the CYP2D6 system as it inhibits that system. Digoxin should be started at a lower dose in patients taking mirabegron, and the patient should be monitored closely.

Prototype Summary: Oxybutynin

Indications: Relief of symptoms of bladder instability associated with uninhibited neurogenic and reflex neurogenic bladder; treatment of signs and symptoms of overactive bladder; treatment of pediatric patients aged 6 years and older with symptoms of detrusor overactivity associated with a neurological condition (e.g., spina bifida).

Actions: Acts directly to relax smooth muscle in the bladder; inhibits the effects of acetylcholine at muscarinic receptors.

Pharmacokinetics:

Route	Onset	Peak	Duration
Oral	30–60 min	3–6 h	6–10 h
Transdermal system	Varies	6–8 h	96 h

$T_{1/2}$: Unknown; metabolized in the liver and excreted in the urine.

Adverse Effects: Drowsiness, dizziness, blurred vision, tachycardia, dry mouth, nausea, urinary hesitancy, decreased sweating, angioedema.

Nursing Considerations for Patients Receiving Urinary Tract Antispasmodics

Assessment: History and Examination

- Assess for contraindications or cautions: any history of allergy to these drugs to prevent hypersensitivity reactions; pyloric or duodenal obstruction or other GI lesions or obstructions of the lower urinary tract (e.g., prostate hypertrophy), which could be dangerously exacerbated by these drugs and cause GI adverse reactions and/or urinary retention; glaucoma, which could increase intraocular pressure due to blockage of the parasympathetic nervous system; and current status of pregnancy or lactation, which would require cautious use.

- Perform a physical assessment before therapy to establish baseline data and during therapy to determine the effectiveness of the drug and any adverse effects associated with drug therapy.
- Inspect the skin to evaluate for the development of rash or hypersensitivity reactions.
- Assess level of consciousness, orientation, and reflexes to evaluate for any CNS effects of the drug.
- Assess urinary elimination pattern, including amount and frequency of episodes, and for any complaints of frequency, urgency, pain, or difficulty voiding to monitor for excessive parasympathetic blockade or development of underlying UTI.
- Arrange for ophthalmological examination, including intraocular pressure, to assess for any developing glaucoma.
- Assess vital signs, including pulse, to establish a baseline for evaluating the extent of parasympathetic blockade.
- Monitor the results of laboratory tests, such as urinalysis and urine culture and sensitivity, to evaluate the effectiveness if UTI is the problem, and renal and hepatic function tests to determine the need for possible dose adjustment and to evaluate for possible toxicity.

Nursing Conclusions

Nursing conclusions related to drug therapy might include the following:

- Impaired comfort related to GI, CNS, or ophthalmological effects of drug
- Altered sensory perception (visual) related to CNS or ophthalmological effects
- Knowledge deficit regarding drug therapy
- Risk of impaired urinary elimination related to parasympathetic blocking

Planning

- The patient will receive the best therapeutic effect from the drug therapy.
- The patient will have limited adverse effects from the drug therapy.
- The patient will have an understanding of the drug therapy, adverse effects to anticipate, and measures to relieve discomfort and improve safety.

Intervention With Rationale

- Arrange for the appropriate treatment of any underlying UTI or neurological disease that may be causing the spasm.
- Arrange for an ophthalmological examination at the beginning of therapy and periodically during long-term treatment to evaluate drug effects on intraocular pressure so that the drug can be stopped if intraocular pressure increases.
- Administer the drug with food if GI upset occurs to alleviate GI discomfort.
- Encourage fluid intake to maintain urinary flow, flush the bladder, and prevent urinary stasis.
- Offer frequent sips of water or use of sugarless hard candy to alleviate dry mouth.
- Monitor urinary output to ensure adequate renal function and bladder emptying.
- Institute safety precautions if the patient experiences CNS effects to prevent patient injury.
- Encourage the patient to continue treatment for the underlying cause of the spasm to treat the cause and prevent the return of the signs and symptoms.
- Offer support and encouragement to help the patient deal with the discomfort of the drug therapy.
- Provide thorough patient teaching, including drug name and dosage, rationale for use, and schedule for administration; signs and symptoms of adverse effects; measures to alleviate or prevent adverse effects; use of fluids and sugarless hard candy to combat dry mouth; danger signs and symptoms to report immediately; appropriate perineal hygiene measures to reduce the risk of infection if that is the underlying cause; and the importance of periodic monitoring, including laboratory testing and evaluation, to enhance patient knowledge about drug therapy and to promote adherence.

Evaluation

- Monitor patient response to the drug (resolution of urinary tract spasms and relief of signs and symptoms).
- Monitor for adverse effects (skin evaluation, orientation and reflexes, intraocular pressure, hypertension with mirabegron).
- Monitor the effectiveness of comfort and safety measures and adherence to the regimen.
- Evaluate the effectiveness of the teaching plan (patient can name drug, dosage, adverse effects to watch for, and specific measures to avoid them).

Key Points

- Smooth muscle spasms affecting the urinary tract may be caused by inflammation and irritation or may be due to neurological disorders that cause detrusor muscle overactivity. The effects of the spasms include dysuria, urinary urgency, incontinence, nocturia, and suprapubic pain.
- Many antispasmodics block parasympathetic activity, thereby relaxing detrusor and other urinary tract muscles. Mirabegron is a beta-agonist and causes the detrusor muscle to relax, allowing increased urine storage and improved muscle pressure and urine outflow.

Other Drugs Affecting the Urinary Tract and Bladder

Two other types of drugs are frequently used to alleviate problems in the urinary tract and bladder. Urinary tract analgesics are used to decrease pain, and the bladder protectant pentosan is used to prevent irritation to the bladder wall. See Table 52.4 for a summary of these agents.

Urinary Tract Analgesics

Pain involving the urinary tract can be uncomfortable and lead to urinary retention and increased risk of infection. The agent phenazopyridine (*Azo-Standard, Baridium*, and others) is a dye that is used to relieve urinary tract pain (see Table 52.4).

Therapeutic Actions and Indications

Phenazopyridine exerts a direct, topical analgesic effect on the urinary tract mucosa (see Fig. 52.1). It is used to relieve symptoms (burning, urgency, frequency, pain, discomfort) related to urinary tract irritation from infection, trauma, or surgery.

Pharmacokinetics

Phenazopyridine is available for oral use and has a rapid onset of action. It is widely distributed, crossing the placenta and entering human milk. It is metabolized in the liver and excreted in the urine.

Contraindications and Cautions

Phenazopyridine is contraindicated in the presence of known allergy to the drug to prevent hypersensitivity reactions and with severe renal or liver dysfunction, which would interfere with the metabolism and excretion of the drug. Caution should be taken if administered during pregnancy due to lack of human studies. Lactation should be discontinued temporarily if this medication is needed.

Table 52.4 *Drugs in Focus*: Other Drugs Affecting the Urinary Tract and Bladder

Drug Name	Usual Dosage	Usual Indications
Urinary Tract Analgesic		
phenazopyridine (*Azo-Standard, Baridium, Pyridium*)	100–200 mg PO t.i.d. after meals for up to 2 d *Pediatric (6–12 y)*: 12 mg/kg/d *or* 350 mg/m²/d PO, divided into three doses; do not exceed 2 d	Symptomatic relief of the discomforts associated with urinary tract trauma or infection
Bladder Protectant		
pentosan polysulfate sodium (*Elmiron*)	100 mg PO t.i.d. on empty stomach	Relief of bladder pain or discomfort associated with interstitial cystitis

Adverse Effects

Adverse effects associated with this drug include GI upset, headache, rash, a reddish-orange coloring of the urine, and staining of contact lenses, all of which are related to the drug's chemical actions in the system. There is also a potential for renal or hepatic toxicity. Use of this drug for longer than 2 days is not recommended due to lack of evidence of effectiveness after 2 days of treatment with antibacterial medication.

Clinically Important Drug–Drug Interactions

There are no known drug–drug interactions with this medication. Due to its properties as an azo dye, phenazopyridine HCl may interfere with urinalysis using spectrometry or color reactions.

Prototype Summary: Phenazopyridine

Indications: Symptomatic relief of pain, urgency, burning, frequency, and discomfort related to lower urinary tract irritation caused by infection, trauma, surgery, or various procedures.

Actions: Has a direct, topical analgesic effect on the urinary tract mucosa; exact mechanism of action is not known.

Pharmacokinetics:

Route	Onset	Peak
Oral	Rapid	Unknown

$T_{1/2}$: Unknown; metabolized in the liver and excreted in the urine.

Adverse Effects: Headache; rash; yellowish tinge to skin, sclera, and urine; reddish-orange coloring of the urine; staining of contact lenses; GI disturbances.

Nursing Considerations for Patients Receiving a Urinary Tract Analgesic

Assessment: History and Examination

- Assess for contraindications or cautions: history of allergy to these drugs to prevent hypersensitivity reactions; renal insufficiency, which could interfere with the excretion and effectiveness of the drug; and current status of pregnancy or lactation because of the potential for adverse effects on the fetus or baby.

- Perform a physical assessment before therapy to establish baseline data and during therapy to determine the effectiveness of the drug and any adverse effects associated with drug therapy.
- Inspect the skin to evaluate for the development of rash or hypersensitivity reactions; check the sclera for evidence of possible jaundice.
- Assess GI and hepatic function, including auscultating bowel sounds, to establish baseline data to assess adverse effects of the drug.
- Assess urinary elimination patterns, including color, amount, frequency, dysuria, or difficulty voiding, to identify possible underlying infection and evaluate the effectiveness of the drug.
- Monitor the results of laboratory tests, including urinalysis and urine culture and sensitivity, to identify possible underlying conditions such as infection or renal dysfunction, and renal and hepatic function tests, to determine the need for possible dose adjustment or to determine the possible risk for toxic effects.

Nursing Conclusions

Nursing conclusions related to drug therapy might include the following:

- Impaired comfort related to GI effects of drug and headache
- Impaired urinary elimination related to the underlying condition necessitating drug therapy
- Knowledge deficit regarding drug therapy

Planning

- The patient will receive the best therapeutic effect from the drug therapy.
- The patient will have limited adverse effects from the drug therapy.
- The patient will have an understanding of the drug therapy, adverse effects to anticipate, and measures to relieve discomfort and improve safety.

Intervention With Rationale

- Arrange for appropriate treatment of any underlying UTI that may be causing the pain.
- Caution the patient that since this drug is a dye, their urine may be reddish-orange and the drug may stain fabrics and contact lenses to prevent undue anxiety when this adverse effect occurs.
- Administer the drug with food to alleviate GI irritation if GI upset is a problem.
- Urge the patient to discontinue use of the drug and contact their health care provider if the sclera or skin becomes yellowish, a sign of drug accumulation in the body and a possible sign of hepatic toxicity.
- Provide thorough patient teaching, including drug name, dosage, rationale for use, and schedule for administration; signs and symptoms of adverse effects; measures to alleviate or prevent adverse effects; possible discoloration of urine (reddish-orange); measures to prevent or reduce the risk of recurring underlying problems such as UTI; and importance of periodic monitoring, including laboratory testing and evaluation, to enhance patient knowledge about drug therapy and to promote adherence.

Evaluation

- Monitor patient response to the drug (resolution of urinary tract pain).
- Monitor for adverse effects (skin evaluation, GI upset and complaints, headache).
- Evaluate the effectiveness of the teaching plan (patient can name drug, dosage, adverse effects to watch for, and specific measures to avoid them).
- Monitor the effectiveness of comfort measures and adherence to the regimen.

Bladder Protectant

The bladder protectant pentosan polysulfate sodium (*Elmiron*) is used to coat or adhere to the bladder mucosal wall and protect it from irritation related to solutes in urine.

Therapeutic Actions and Indications

Pentosan polysulfate sodium, available for oral administration, is a heparinlike compound that has anticoagulant and fibrinolytic effects. This drug adheres to the bladder wall mucosal membrane and acts as a buffer to control cell permeability, preventing irritating solutes in the urine from reaching the bladder wall cells (see Fig. 52.1). It is used specifically to decrease the pain and discomfort associated with **interstitial cystitis**, which is chronic inflammation of the interstitial connective tissue of the bladder that may extend into deeper tissue. See Table 52.4.

Pharmacokinetics

After oral administration, little of this drug is absorbed (3%). It is distributed to the GI tract, liver, spleen, skin, bone marrow, and periosteum. It undergoes metabolism in the liver and spleen and is excreted in the urine and feces. It has a half-life of about 20 hours. It is not known whether the drug crosses the placenta or enters human milk due to the lack of adequate studies of the effects of the drug during pregnancy or lactation; caution should be used if the drug is needed during pregnancy or lactation.

Contraindications and Cautions

Pentosan should not be used with any condition that involves an increased risk of bleeding (surgery, pregnancy, anticoagulation, hemophilia) because of its heparinlike

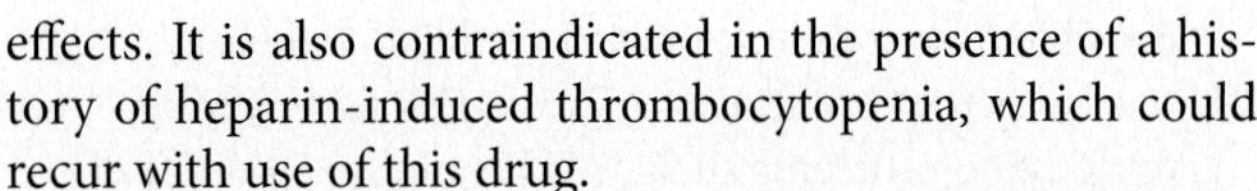

effects. It is also contraindicated in the presence of a history of heparin-induced thrombocytopenia, which could recur with use of this drug.

Caution should be used in patients with hepatic or splenic dysfunction, which could be affected by the heparinlike actions of the drug, and in pregnant or lactating patients because it is unknown if there is potential for adverse effects on the fetus or neonate.

Adverse Effects

Adverse effects associated with pentosan use include bleeding that may progress to hemorrhage (related to the drug's heparin effects), headache, alopecia (seen with heparin-type drugs), and GI disturbances related to local irritation of the GI tract with administration.

Clinically Important Drug–Drug Interactions

There is a potential for increased bleeding risks if this drug is combined with anticoagulants, aspirin, or nonsteroidal antiinflammatory drugs (NSAIDs). If such a combination is used, the patient should be monitored closely for any signs of bleeding, and appropriate dose adjustments should be made to the anticoagulant, aspirin, or NSAID.

Prototype Summary: Pentosan Polysulfate Sodium

Indications: Relief of bladder pain associated with interstitial cystitis.

Actions: Adheres to the bladder wall mucosal membrane and acts as a buffer to control cell permeability, preventing irritating solutes in the urine from reaching the bladder wall cells.

Pharmacokinetics:

Route	Onset	Peak
Oral	Varies	2 hr

$T_{1/2}$: 20 to 27 hours; metabolized in the liver and spleen and excreted in the urine and feces.

Adverse Effects: Bleeding, headache, alopecia, and GI disturbances.

Nursing Considerations for Patients Receiving a Bladder Protectant

Assessment: History and Examination

- Assess for contraindications or cautions: history of allergy to these drugs to prevent hypersensitivity reactions; renal insufficiency, which could interfere with excretion of the drug; history of bleeding abnormalities, splenic disorders, or hepatic dysfunction, which could be exacerbated by the heparinlike effects; and current status of pregnancy and lactation, which require cautious use of this drug.
- Perform a physical assessment before therapy to establish baseline data and during therapy to determine the effectiveness of the drug and any adverse effects associated with drug therapy.
- Inspect the skin for color and note any evidence of petechiae or bruising that may suggest coagulation problems and possible hypersensitivity reactions.
- Assess vital signs for changes to provide early evidence of bleeding.
- Assess the urinary elimination pattern to evaluate the effects of the underlying condition and the effectiveness of therapy.
- Monitor laboratory test results, including liver function tests and coagulation studies, to establish a baseline for monitoring safe use of the drug and the occurrence of adverse effects.

Nursing Conclusions

Nursing conclusions related to drug therapy may include the following:

- Altered tissue perfusion related to bleeding secondary to heparinlike effects of the drug
- Impaired comfort related to headache and GI effects of the drug
- Alteration in body image related to alopecia
- Injury risk related to bleeding
- Knowledge deficit regarding drug therapy

Planning

- The patient will receive the best therapeutic effect from the drug therapy.
- The patient will have limited adverse effects from the drug therapy.
- The patient will have an understanding of the drug therapy, adverse effects to anticipate, and measures to relieve discomfort and improve safety.

Intervention With Rationale

- Assist with establishing the presence of interstitial cystitis by biopsy or cystoscopy before beginning therapy to ensure that appropriate therapy is being used.
- Administer the drug on an empty stomach, 1 hour before or 2 hours after meals, to relieve GI discomfort and improve absorption.
- Obtain specimens for coagulation studies as ordered to assess for excessive heparinlike effect.
- Monitor urinary elimination for amount and characteristics and patient's complaints of pain or difficulty voiding to evaluate the effectiveness of therapy.
- Arrange for a wig or appropriate head covering if alopecia develops as a result of drug therapy.

- Inspect the skin frequently for evidence of petechiae, bruising, or oozing from insertion sites to identify increased risk for bleeding.
- Institute safety precautions such as minimizing invasive procedures and protection from injury to minimize the patient's risk for injury.
- Provide thorough patient teaching, including drug name, dosage, rationale for use, and schedule for administration; signs and symptoms of adverse effects; measures to alleviate or prevent adverse effects; danger signs and symptoms to report immediately; comfort measures, such as taking the drug on an empty stomach, use of a wig if alopecia occurs, and analgesics for headache; measures to prevent or reduce the risk of recurrent interstitial cystitis; and the importance of periodic monitoring, including laboratory testing and evaluation, to enhance patient knowledge about drug therapy and to promote adherence.

Evaluation

- Monitor patient response to the drug (relief of bladder pain and discomfort).
- Monitor for adverse effects (skin evaluation, GI upset and complaints, headache, coagulation studies).
- Evaluate the effectiveness of the teaching plan (patient can name drug, dosage, adverse effects to watch for, and specific measures to avoid them).
- Monitor the effectiveness of comfort measures and adherence to the regimen.

Key Points

- Phenazopyridine is a urinary tract analgesic that is used to decrease bladder pain that could result in changes in bladder function and emptying. This drug is a dye, and patients need to be warned about changes in the color of urine and potential for staining skin and clothing.
- Pentosan is a bladder protectant. It is a heparinlike drug that protects the inner lining of the bladder from irritation by solutes in the urine. Because it is a heparinlike drug, the risk of bleeding must be considered.

Drugs for Treating Benign Prostatic Hyperplasia

Benign prostatic hyperplasia (BPH), also called benign prostatic hypertrophy or enlarged prostate, is a common problem in males that increases in incidence with age. The prostate completely encircles the urethra. The enlargement of the gland surrounding the urethra leads to discomfort, difficulty in initiating a stream of urine, feelings of bloating, urinary retention, and an increased incidence of cystitis.

Box 52.3 Focus on Herbal and Alternative Therapies

Saw palmetto is an herbal therapy that has been used successfully for the relief of symptoms associated with BPH. It may act similarly to the 5α-reductase inhibitors (dutasteride and finasteride). It has been shown to decrease prostate enlargement. Patients with BPH should be cautioned not to combine saw palmetto with finasteride because serious toxicity can occur. Patients should also be cautioned that random studies of various saw palmetto products have shown great variation in contents and activity of the tablets. If patients choose to use this alternative therapy, they should be cautioned to check products carefully and to avoid switching products once they have success with one.

Two types of drugs are used to relieve the symptoms of BPH. These drugs include the alpha-adrenergic blockers doxazosin (*Cardura*), tamsulosin (*Flomax*), alfuzosin (*Uroxatral*), silodosin (*Rapaflo*), and terazosin (generic). Finasteride (*Proscar*) and dutasteride (*Avodart*) are drugs that block the conversion of testosterone to 5α-dihydrotestosterone (DHT), an androgen that increases enlargement of the prostate gland. There is also a combination medication, *Jalyn*, that contains tamsulosin and dutasteride. Box 52.3 discusses an alternative therapy used to treat BPH.

Therapeutic Actions and Indications

Before any of these drugs are used, it is important to make sure that the prostate enlargement is benign and not caused by cancer, infection, stricture, or hypotonic bladder, which would require a different treatment. Patients receiving long-term therapy need to be reassessed periodically to make sure that they have not developed a serious underlying problem like prostate cancer. Alpha-adrenergic blockers block postsynaptic $alpha_1$-adrenergic receptors, which results in a dilation of arterioles and veins and a relaxation of sympathetic effects on the bladder and urinary tract. In addition to treating BPH, most of these drugs are also indicated for treating hypertension (see Chapter 43).

Drugs that block testosterone conversion—dutasteride and finasteride—inhibit the intracellular enzyme that converts testosterone to the potent androgen dihydrotestosterone (DHT), on which the prostate gland depends for its development and maintenance (see Fig. 52.1). In 2011, postmarketing studies found that the use of these drugs was associated with the development of an aggressive form of prostate cancer. The incidence was small, but it led to the recommendation that this information be considered when selecting an appropriate drug to treat BPH.

See Table 52.5 for usual indications for alpha-adrenergic blockers and drugs that block testosterone conversion. See the "Critical Thinking Scenario" for additional information about treating a patient with BPH.

Table 52.5 ***Drugs in Focus*: Drugs for Treating Benign Prostatic Hyperplasia**

Drug Name	Usual Dosage	Usual Indications
Alpha-Adrenergic Blockers		
alfuzosin (*Uroxatral*)	10 mg/d PO, take after the same meal each day	Relief of symptoms of BPH
doxazosin (*Cardura, Cardura XL*)	1 mg PO daily with titration up to 8 mg/d (16 mg/d for HTN) if needed; or ER tablets 4 or 8 mg PO daily at breakfast; not for use in children	Relief of symptoms of BPH; hypertension (not *Cardura XL*)
silodosin (*Rapaflo*)	8 mg/d PO with a meal; reduce dose with moderate renal impairment	Relief of symptoms of BPH
tamsulosin (*Flomax*)	0.4–0.8 mg/d PO, 30 min after the same meal each day	Treatment of BPH
terazosin (generic)	Initial dose 1 mg PO at bedtime; 1–20 mg/d PO titrated based on patient response	Relief of symptoms of BPH; hypertension
Drugs That Block Testosterone Production		
dutasteride (*Avodart*)	0.5 mg/d PO	Long-term treatment of symptomatic BPH to shrink the prostate and relieve symptoms of hyperplasia
finasteride (*Proscar, Propecia*)	5 mg/d PO for BPH, 1 mg/d PO for male-pattern baldness (*Propecia*)	Long-term treatment of symptomatic BPH to shrink the prostate and relieve symptoms of hyperplasia; prevention of male-pattern baldness in patients with strong family history (*Propecia*)

BPH, benign prostatic hyperplasia.

CRITICAL THINKING SCENARIO
Dealing With Benign Prostatic Hyperplasia

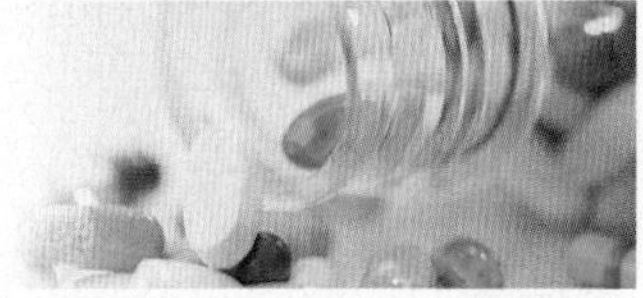

THE SITUATION

P.F. is a 72-year-old male patient who has been having difficulty urinating. It has become so uncomfortable to start a stream that P.F. has come into the clinic to be evaluated. P.F. has a history of angina and uses sublingual nitroglycerin as needed. P.F. also has a history of erectile dysfunction. P.F. tells you that they do use sildenafil (*Viagra*) when needed but never combines it with nitroglycerin, per physician orders. P.F. is diagnosed with BPH and wants to learn various treatment options.

CRITICAL THINKING

What is the best approach for this patient?

What important drug interactions need to be considered when talking about drug treatment? Think about the following points: what the drug is doing, how it works, and how it works best.

What nondrug actions can the patient take to help with the problem and to make drug therapy more effective?

DISCUSSION

BPH is a common problem caused by enlargement of the prostate gland. The gland responds to testosterone and slowly grows over time. Since the gland encircles the urethra, much like an inner tube, as it grows, it compresses the urethra and eventually it becomes difficult to start urine moving into the urethra (just like blowing up an inner tube makes the opening in the middle smaller and smaller). Since the growth of the prostate is a normal process that occurs over time, most patients are not aware of it until they become older and the gland is compressing the urethra enough to cause urinary symptoms. This is not a cancer. However, the possibility of prostate cancer will need to be discussed and the prostate evaluated.

Two classes of drugs are available for treating BPH. Alpha-adrenergic blockers cause a relaxation of the muscles in the urethra and the vessels in the area; this may be enough to allow easier urine flow. This class of drugs must be used with caution with any other drugs that lower blood pressure, as the relaxation of muscle in the blood vessels occurs throughout the body. Since P.F. uses nitroglycerin on occasion and erectile dysfunction drugs, both of which cause vasodilation and drop in blood pressure, this class of drugs may not be the best for them. The other class of drugs blocks testosterone, so the prostate loses the hormone influence to grow and be maintained; over time, this could cause a shrinking of the gland to allow urine flow. The patient needs to know that they should use contraceptives with any partners who can become pregnant, they should not donate blood during use of the drug and for 6 months following use, and that anyone who can become pregnant should not touch the tablet. P.F. felt this class of drugs could fit better with their life situation. P.F. needs to be cautioned to avoid saw palmetto while on this drug.

P.F. can be encouraged to make some lifestyle changes that have been shown to help with BPH symptoms. Limiting fluid intake to about 2 qt per day, limiting use of or avoiding alcohol and caffeine, limiting drinking fluids after dinner and before bed, trying to urinate every 3 hours, and staying active and warm have all been shown to help.

In severe cases, the prostate may be removed surgically or with ablation. There are many nerves in the area; therefore, this surgery always comes with some risk of loss of sexual function or bladder control.

NURSING CARE GUIDE FOR P.F.: BENIGN PROSTATIC HYPERPLASIA DRUG ANDROGEN HORMONE INHIBITOR

Assessment: History and Examination

Assess P.F.'s health history, particularly any allergies to finasteride or any components of the tablet, and liver dysfunction.

Focus the physical examination on:

GI: abdominal examination, liver evaluation

GU: prostate examination, urinary output

Laboratory tests: renal function tests, prostate-specific antigen (PSA) level

Nursing Conclusions

Altered self-image related to breast enlargement/tenderness and/or loss of libido

Depression risk related to age-related changes, sexual dysfunction

Knowledge deficit regarding drug therapy

Planning

The patient will receive the best therapeutic effect from the drug therapy.

The patient will have limited adverse effects from the drug therapy.

The patient will have an understanding of the drug therapy, adverse effects to anticipate, and measures to relieve discomfort and improve safety.

Intervention

Ensure that diagnosis of BPH is accurate (rule out prostate cancer, infections, hypotonic bladder).

Administer without regard to meals.

Monitor urine flow and symptoms.

Encourage lifestyle changes to improve BPH symptoms: avoidance of alcohol and caffeine, frequent bladder emptying, limiting excessive fluid intake, and timing of regular fluid intake.

Provide support and reassurance to deal with drug effects and lifestyle changes.

Provide patient teaching regarding drug name and dosage, adverse effects, precautions, warnings to report, using contraceptives and avoiding blood donation during use of the drug and for 6 months after stopping, warning people who can become pregnant to avoid touching the tablet, and avoiding the use of saw palmetto.

Evaluation

Evaluate drug effects: relief of symptoms and improvement in urine flow.

Monitor for adverse effects: abdominal upset, gynecomastia, and loss of libido.

Monitor for drug–drug interactions with saw palmetto.

Evaluate the effectiveness of patient teaching program and comfort and safety measures.

PATIENT TEACHING FOR J.K.

- This drug is an androgen blocker that will stop the stimulation of prostrate growth and may shrink the prostate, which will help with urine flow.
- Take this tablet once a day without regard to food. It may take some time to see the improvement in symptoms.
- Avoid using saw palmetto while you are on this drug. This herb is often advertised to treat BPH. Combining it with this drug can lead to adverse effects.
- Take the full course of your prescription. Do not use this drug to self-treat any other infection.
- Be aware that you will not be able to donate blood and should use contraceptives during use of the drug and for 6 months after stopping this drug because of the adverse effects it could have on a fetus. People who can become pregnant should not touch the tablets because the drug can be absorbed through the skin.
- Common adverse effects of this drug may include the following:
  - *Impotence, loss of libido, and decreased volume of ejaculate*: This effect usually resolves over time and will stop when the drug is stopped.
  - *Breast enlargement or tenderness*: This effect is related to the hormonal effects of the drug; consult with your health care provider if this becomes too uncomfortable.
  - Report any of the following to your health care provider: inability to pass urine, groin pain, fever, and weakness.
- The following can help to decrease the symptoms of BPH:
  - Limit fluid intake to about 2 qt a day.
  - Avoid or limit alcohol and caffeine.
  - Empty your bladder at least every 3 hours.
  - Limit fluids in the evening before bed; this works best if you avoid fluid after your evening meal.
  - Stay active and warm. Cold and inactivity tend to make the problem worse.
  - Tell any doctor, nurse, or other health care provider involved in your care that you are taking this drug.

Pharmacokinetics

The alpha$_1$-selective adrenergic blocking agents are well absorbed after oral administration, reaching peak level in 2 to 8 hours, and they undergo extensive hepatic metabolism. They are excreted in the urine. Finasteride and dutasteride are rapidly absorbed from the GI tract after oral administration, undergo hepatic metabolism, and are excreted in the feces and urine.

Contraindications and Cautions

Both groups of drugs are contraindicated in patients who are allergic to the drugs to prevent hypersensitivity reactions. Caution should be used in patients with hepatic or renal dysfunction, which could alter the metabolism and excretion of the drugs. The adrenergic blockers should be used with caution in patients with heart failure or known coronary disease, which could be aggravated by the drop in blood pressure or tachycardia. Finasteride and dutasteride have no indications for female patients and are contraindicated because of androgen effects. Family members or caregivers must be cautioned not to touch finasteride or dutasteride tablets because of the risk of absorption through the skin.

Adverse Effects

Adverse effects of alpha-adrenergic blockers include headache, fatigue, dizziness, postural dizziness, lethargy, tachycardia, hypotension, GI upset, and sexual dysfunction, all of which are effects seen with blockade of the alpha-receptors. There is risk of floppy iris syndrome (small pupil syndrome) during cataract surgery if there is concurrent use with alpha-adrenergic blockers, so these medications should be held before cataract surgery. Finasteride and dutasteride are associated with decreased libido, impotence, and sexual dysfunction, all of which are related to decreased levels of DHT. Patients using either finasteride or dutasteride cannot donate blood for 6 months after the last dose to protect potential blood recipients from exposure to the testosterone-blocking effects. Patients should use contraceptives during and for 6 months following treatment and will not be able to donate blood during that same time period because of the risk of exposing the fetus or blood recipients to the drug.

Clinically Important Drug–Drug Interactions

There is a possibility of increased antihypertensive effects if the alpha-adrenergic blockers are combined with any other antihypertensives, nitrates, or erectile dysfunction drugs, all of which can cause lower blood pressure. The patient should be monitored and appropriate dose adjustments made to the antihypertensive agent if this combination is used; patients should be advised not to use with nitrates or erectile dysfunction drugs. The testosterone blockers should not be used with saw palmetto, an herb often used to treat BPH, as toxic adverse effects can occur.

Prototype Summary: Doxazosin

Indications: Treatment of BPH.

Actions: Blocks postsynaptic alpha$_1$-adrenergic receptors, which results in a dilation of arterioles and veins and a relaxation of sympathetic effects on the bladder and urinary tract.

Pharmacokinetics:

Route	Onset	Peak
Oral	Varies	2–3 h

$T_{1/2}$: 22 hours; metabolized in the liver and excreted in the urine, bile, and feces.

Adverse Effects: Headache, fatigue, dizziness, postural dizziness, lethargy, vertigo, tachycardia, palpitations, nausea, dyspepsia, diarrhea, sexual dysfunction, rash.

Prototype Summary: Finasteride

Indications: Treatment of BPH.

Actions: Inhibits the intracellular enzyme that converts testosterone to a potent androgen that the prostate depends on for its development and maintenance.

Pharmacokinetics:

Route	Onset	Peak
Oral	Rapid	8 h

$T_{1/2}$: 6 hours; metabolized in the liver and excreted in the urine, bile, and feces.

Adverse Effects: Impotence, decreased libido, abdominal upset, breast enlargement/tenderness, gynecomastia.

Nursing Considerations for Patients Receiving Drugs to Treat Benign Prostatic Hypertrophy

Assessment: History and Examination

- Assess for contraindications or cautions: history of allergy to the drug to prevent hypersensitivity reaction; renal or hepatic failure, which could alter the metabolism and excretion of the drug; or history of heart failure or coronary heart disease (with alpha-adrenergic blockers), which could be exacerbated by the effects of the alpha-adrenergic blockers.
- Perform a physical assessment before therapy to establish baseline data and during therapy to determine the effectiveness of the drug and any adverse effects associated with drug therapy.

- Inspect the skin to evaluate for the development of rash or hypersensitivity reactions.
- Assess cardiopulmonary status; including vital signs, especially blood pressure and pulse rate; and auscultate heart sounds and assess tissue perfusion; to determine possible cardiovascular effects of alpha-adrenergic blockade.
- Assess urinary elimination pattern and renal function to assure adequate kidney function and evaluate for potential changes in drug excretion.
- Assist with prostate examination and palpation to establish hyperplasia and rule out other potential medical problems.
- Monitor laboratory test results, including urinalysis, to evaluate for possible changes; renal and hepatic function tests to determine the need for dose adjustment; and PSA levels to eliminate the diagnosis of prostate cancer.

Nursing Conclusions

Nursing conclusions related to drug therapy might include the following:

- Impaired sexual function related to drug effects
- Impaired comfort related to headache, CNS effects, and GI effects of the drug
- Injury risk related to blockage of alpha-receptors and potential for hypotension
- Knowledge deficit regarding drug therapy

Planning

- The patient will receive the best therapeutic effect from the drug therapy.
- The patient will have limited adverse effects from the drug therapy.
- The patient will have an understanding of the drug therapy, adverse effects to anticipate, and measures to relieve discomfort and improve safety.

Intervention With Rationale

- Determine the presence of BPH and periodically evaluate through prostate examination and measurement of PSA levels to reconfirm that no other problem is occurring.
- Administer the drug without regard to meals, but administer with meals if GI upset is a problem.
- Arrange for analgesics if needed for headache.
- Encourage the patient to change positions slowly and to sit at the edge of the bed or chair for a few minutes before rising if low blood pressure becomes a problem.
- Offer support and encouragement and refer for counseling if appropriate to help the patient cope with potential decreases in sexual functioning.
- Provide thorough patient teaching, including drug name and dosage, rationale for use, and schedule for administration; signs and symptoms of adverse effects; measures to alleviate or prevent adverse effects, such as changing positions slowly and taking drug with food if GI upset occurs; and the importance of periodic monitoring, including laboratory testing and evaluation, to enhance patient knowledge about drug therapy and to promote adherence.

Evaluation

- Monitor patient response to the drug (relief of signs and symptoms of BPH, improved urine flow, decrease in discomfort).
- Monitor for adverse effects (skin evaluation, GI upset and complaints, headache, cardiovascular effects, changes in sexual functioning).
- Monitor the effectiveness of comfort measures and adherence to the regimen.
- Evaluate the effectiveness of the teaching plan (patient can name drug, dosage, adverse effects to watch for, and specific measures to avoid them).

Key Points

- BPH is a common enlargement of the prostate gland in older males.
- Drugs frequently used to relieve the signs and symptoms of prostate enlargement include alpha-adrenergic blockers, which relax the sympathetic effects on the bladder and sphincters, and finasteride and dutasteride, which block the body's production of a powerful androgen. The prostate is dependent on testosterone for its maintenance and development; blocking androgen leads to shrinkage of the gland and relief of symptoms.

SUMMARY

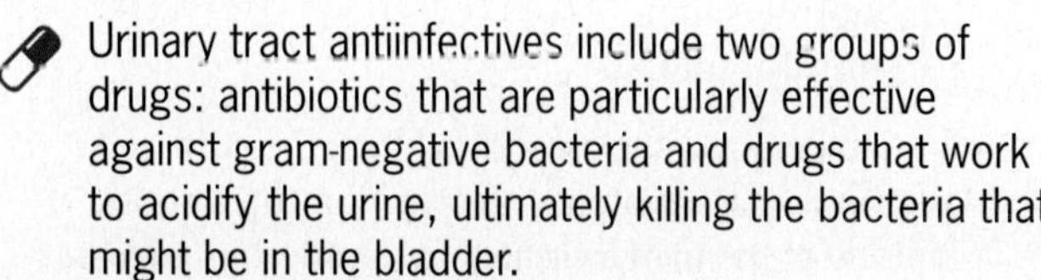

- Urinary tract antiinfectives include two groups of drugs: antibiotics that are particularly effective against gram-negative bacteria and drugs that work to acidify the urine, ultimately killing the bacteria that might be in the bladder.
- Many activities are necessary to help decrease the bacteria in the urinary tract (e.g., hygiene measures, proper diet, forcing fluids) to facilitate the treatment of UTIs and help the urinary tract antiinfectives be more effective.
- Inflammation and irritation of the urinary tract can cause smooth muscle spasms along the urinary tract. Neurogenic disorders can cause detrusor muscle overactivity, causing spasms. These spasms lead to the uncomfortable effects of dysuria, urgency, incontinence, nocturia, and suprapubic pain.
- Many of the urinary tract antispasmodics act to relieve spasms of the urinary tract muscles by blocking parasympathetic activity and relaxing the detrusor and other urinary tract muscles.

- The urinary tract analgesic phenazopyridine is used to provide relief of symptoms (burning, urgency, frequency, pain, discomfort) related to urinary tract irritation resulting from infection, trauma, or surgery.
- Pentosan polysulfate sodium is a heparinlike compound that has anticoagulant and fibrinolytic effects and adheres to the bladder wall mucosal membrane to act as a buffer to control cell permeability. This action prevents irritating solutes in the urine from reaching the cells of the bladder wall. It is used specifically to decrease the pain and discomfort associated with interstitial cystitis.
- BPH is a common enlargement of the prostate gland in older males.
- Drugs frequently used to relieve the signs and symptoms of prostate enlargement include alpha-adrenergic blockers, which relax the sympathetic effects on the bladder and sphincters, and finasteride and dutasteride, which block the body's production of a powerful androgen DHT. The prostate is dependent on DHT for its maintenance and development; blocking androgen leads to shrinkage of the gland and relief of symptoms.

CHECK YOUR UNDERSTANDING

Answers to the questions in this chapter can be found in Answers to Check Your Understanding Questions on thePoint®.

MULTIPLE CHOICE

Select the best answer.

1. Trimethoprim–sulfamethoxazole and nitrofurantoin are indicated to treat
   a. pyelonephritis.
   b. benign prostate hypertrophy (BPH).
   c. bladder spasms.
   d. acute uncomplicated cystitis.
2. The antibiotic of choice for a patient with cystitis who has great difficulty following medical regimens is
   a. penicillin.
   b. fosfomycin.
   c. ciprofloxacin.
   d. nitrofurantoin.
3. Urinary tract antispasmodics block the pain and discomfort associated with spasm in the smooth muscle of the urinary tract. The numerous adverse effects associated with these drugs are related to their
   a. blockade of sympathetic beta-receptors.
   b. stimulation of cholinergic receptors.
   c. stimulation of sympathetic receptors.
   d. blockade of cholinergic receptors.
4. When planning the care for an older patient diagnosed with BPH, which two types of drugs would the nurse most likely expect the physician to prescribe?
   a. Alpha-adrenergic blockers and anticholinergic drugs
   b. Alpha-adrenergic blockers and testosterone production blockers
   c. Anticholinergic drugs and alpha-adrenergic stimulators
   d. Testosterone production stimulators and adrenal androgens
5. The drug of choice for treatment of BPH in a patient with known hypertension might be
   a. doxazosin.
   b. dutasteride.
   c. finasteride.
   d. propranolol.
6. Before administering a drug for the treatment of BPH, the nurse should ensure that the patient
   a. has had a prostate examination, including measurement of the PSA level.
   b. has not had a vasectomy.
   c. is still sexually active.
   d. is hypertensive.
7. A patient being treated for BPH who is concerned about hair loss might prefer treatment with
   a. doxazosin.
   b. finasteride.
   c. tamsulosin.
   d. terazosin.
8. After bladder surgery, many patients experience burning, urgency, frequency, and pain related to urinary tract irritation. Such patients would benefit from treatment with
   a. methylene blue.
   b. fosfomycin.
   c. phenazopyridine.
   d. flavoxate.

MULTIPLE RESPONSE

Select all that apply.

1. In evaluating a patient for the presence of a bladder infection, one would expect to find reports of which conditions?
   a. Frequency of urination
   b. Painful urination
   c. Edema of the fingers and hands
   d. Urgency of urination
   e. Feelings of abdominal bloating
   f. Itching, scaly skin

2. Important educational points for patients with cystitis include which information?
   a. Avoidance of bubble baths
   b. Voiding immediately after sexual intercourse
   c. Always wiping from back to front
   d. Avoidance of foods high in alkaline ash
   e. Tight fluid restriction
   f. Always wiping from front to back

REFERENCES

Barbosa-Cesnik, C., Brown, M. B., Buxton, M., Zhang, L., BeBusscher, J., & Foxman, B. (2011). Cranberry juice fails to prevent recurrent urinary tract infection: Results from a randomized placebo-controlled trial. *Clinical Infectious Diseases, 52*(1), 23–30. https://doi.org/10.1093/cid/ciq073

Brunton, L., Hilal-Dandan, R., & Knollman, B. (2018). *Goodman and Gilman's the pharmacological basis of therapeutics* (13th ed.). McGraw-Hill.

Chu, C. M., & Lowder, J. L. (2018). Diagnosis and treatment of urinary tract infections across age groups. *American Journal of Obstetrics and Gynecology, 1*, 40–51. https://doi.org/10.1016/j.ajog.2017.12.231

Fu, Z., Liska, D., Talan, D., & Chung, M. (2017). Cranberry reduces the risk of urinary tract infection recurrence in otherwise healthy women: A systemic review and meta-analysis. *The Journal of Nutrition, 147*(12), 2282–2288. https://doi.org/10.3945/jn.117.254961

Gilchrist, K. (2004). Benign prostatic hyperplasia: Is it a precursor to prostate cancer? *Nurse Practitioner, 29*(6), 30–37. https://doi.org/10.1097/00006205-200406000-00006.

Hall, J. E., & Hall, M. E. (2021). *Guyton and Hall textbook of medical physiology* (14th ed.). Elsevier.

Knezevich, E., Knezevich, J., & Spangler, M. (2011). Benign prostatic hyperplasia and the medication management of associated lower urinary tract symptoms. *U.S. Pharmacist, 36*(6), 20–24. https://www.uspharmacist.com/article/benign-prostatic-hyperplasia-and-the-medication-management-of-associated-lower-urinary-tract-symptoms

Malmros, K., Huttner, B. D., McNulty, C., Rodriguez-Bano, J., Pulcini, C., & Tangden, T. (2019). Comparison of antibiotic treatment guidelines for urinary tract infections in 15 European countries: Results of an online survey. *International Journal of Antimicrobial Agents, 54*(4), 478–486. https://doi.org/10.1016/j.ijantimicag.2019.06.015

Markowitz, M. A., Wood, L. N., Raz, S., Miller, L. G., Haake, D. A., & Kim, J. (2019). Lack of uniformity among United States recommendations for diagnosis and management of acute, uncomplicated cystitis. *International Urogynecology Journal, 30*, 1187–1194. https://doi.org/10.1007/s00192-018-3750-z

McMurdo, M. E., Bissett, L. Y., Price, R. J., Price, R. J. G., Phillips, G., & Crombie, I. K. (2005). Does ingestion of cranberry juice reduce symptomatic urinary tract infections in older people in the hospital? A double-blind, placebo-controlled trial. *Age and Ageing, 34*(3), 256–261. https://doi.org/10.1093/ageing/afi101

Mehnert-Kay, S. A. (2005). Diagnosis and management of uncomplicated urinary tract infections. *American Family Physician, 72*, 451–456. https://www.aafp.org/afp/2005/0801/p451.html

Norris, T. L. (2019). *Porth's pathophysiology concepts of altered health states* (13th ed.). Wolters Kluwer.

Sudeep, H. V., Thomas, J. V., & Shyamprasad, K. (2020). A double blind, placebo-controlled randomized comparative study on the efficacy of phytosterol-enriched and conventional saw palmetto oil in mitigating benign prostate hyperplasia and androgen deficiency. *BMC Urology, 20*, 86. https://bmcurol.biomedcentral.com/articles/10.1186/s12894-020-00648-9

Wang, C., Fang, C., Chen, N., Liu, S. S., Yu, P., Wu, T., Chen, W., Lee, C., & Chen, S. (2012). Cranberry-containing products for prevention of urinary tract infections in susceptible populations: A systematic review and meta-analysis of randomized controlled trials. *Archives of Internal Medicine, 172*(13), 988–996. https://doi.org/10.1001/archinternmed.2012.3004

PART 10

Drugs Acting on the Respiratory System

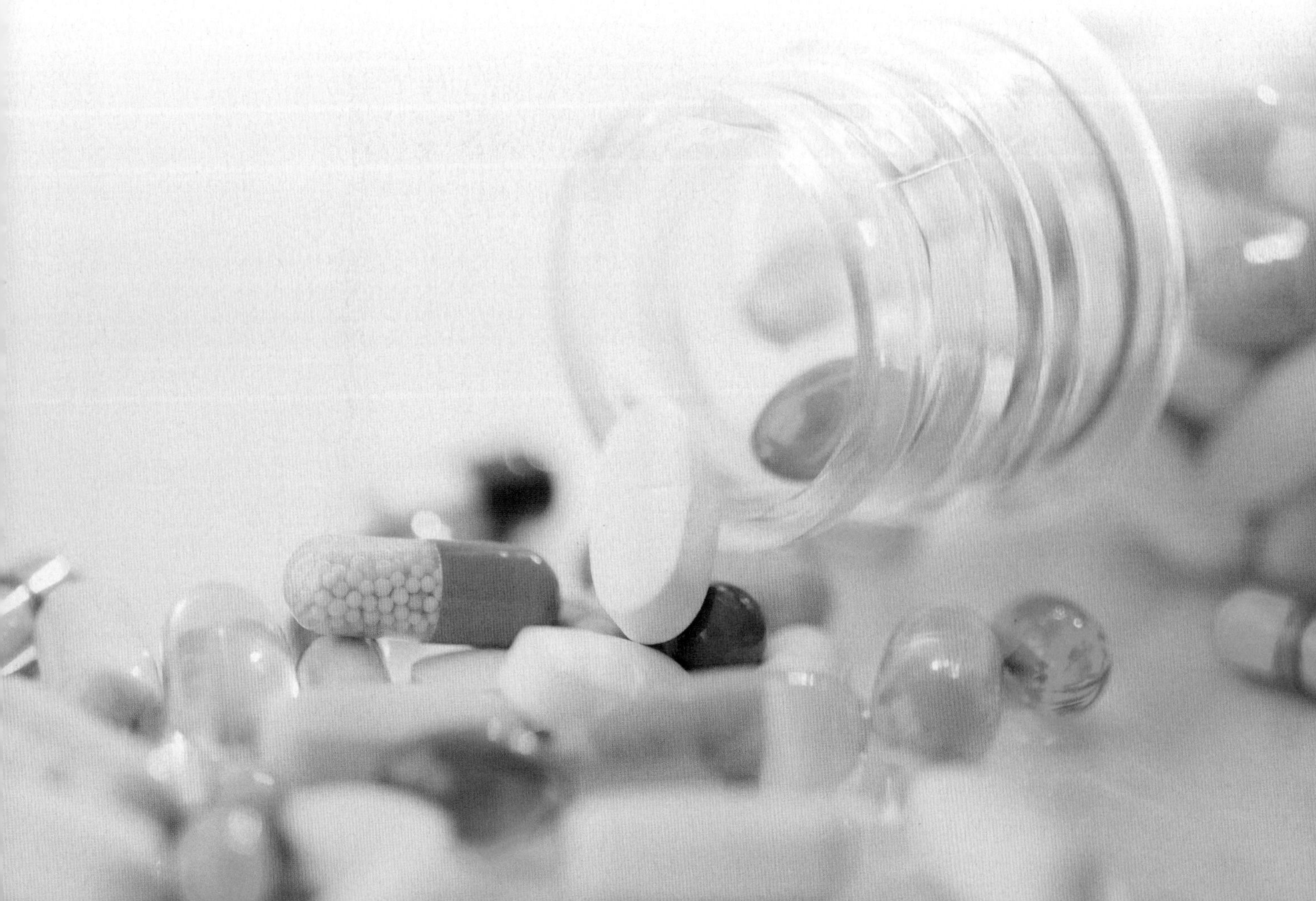

CHAPTER 53

Introduction to the Respiratory System

Learning Objectives

Upon completion of this chapter, you will be able to:

1. Describe the major structures of the respiratory system, including the role of each in respiration.
2. Describe the process of respiration, with clinical examples of problems that can arise with alterations in the respiratory membrane.
3. Differentiate the common respiratory tract infections.
4. Discuss the processes involved in ventilation and gas exchange disorders.

Key Terms

acute respiratory distress syndrome (ARDS): progressive loss of lung compliance and increasing hypoxia typically due to a severe insult to the body, such as cardiovascular collapse, major burns, severe trauma, or rapid depressurization

alveoli: respiratory sacs, the smallest units of the lungs, where gas exchange occurs

asthma: disorder characterized by recurrent and reversible episodes of bronchospasm (i.e., bronchial muscle spasm leading to narrowed or obstructed airways)

atelectasis: incomplete expansion of alveoli

bronchial tree: the conducting airways leading into the alveoli; they branch smaller and smaller, appearing much like a tree

chronic obstructive pulmonary disease (COPD): chronic condition that occurs over time; often the result of chronic bronchitis, emphysema, and/or refractory asthma; obstruction is not fully reversible

cilia: microscopic, hairlike projections of the epithelial cell membrane lining the upper respiratory tract; they are constantly moving and directing the mucus and any trapped substance toward the throat

common cold: viral infection of the upper respiratory tract that initiates the release of histamine and prostaglandins and causes an inflammatory response

conducting airways: parts of the respiratory system composed of the upper respiratory tract (nose, mouth, pharynx, larynx, trachea), and bronchi; primary purpose is to move air in and out of the lung tissues

cough: reflex response to irritation in the conducting airways, results in expelling of forced air through the mouth

cystic fibrosis: hereditary disease that results in the accumulation of copious amounts of thick secretions in the lungs, which will eventually lead to obstruction of the airways and destruction of the lung tissue

larynx: the vocal chords and the epiglottis, which close during swallowing to protect the lower respiratory tract from any foreign particles

pharynx: the membrane-lined cavity that is behind the mouth and nose and before the esophagus and larynx

pneumonia: inflammation of the lungs that can be caused by bacterial or viral invasion of the tissue or by aspiration of foreign substances

pneumothorax: air in the pleural space exerting high pressure against the alveoli

respiration: exchange of oxygen and carbon dioxide at the alveoli and capillary

respiratory airways: portions of the respiratory tract responsible for gas exchange; composed of the lobules of the lungs that include a bronchiole, arteriole, pulmonary capillaries, veins, and alveolar sacs; the bronchi and lobules of the lungs can be categorized as the lower respiratory tract

respiratory distress syndrome (RDS): disorder found in premature neonates whose lungs have not had time to mature and who are lacking sufficient surfactant to maintain open airways to allow for respiration

respiratory membrane: area through which gas exchange must be made; made up of the capillary endothelium, the capillary basement membrane, the interstitial space, the alveolar basement membrane, the alveolar endothelium, and the surfactant layer

seasonal rhinitis: inflammation of the nasal cavity, commonly called hay fever; caused by reaction to a specific antigen

sinuses: air-filled passages through the skull that open into the nasal passage

sinusitis: inflammation of the epithelial lining of the sinus cavities

sneeze: reflex response to irritation of receptors in the nares, resulting in expulsion of forced air through the nose

surfactant: lipoprotein that reduces surface tension in the alveoli, allowing them to stay open to allow gas exchange

trachea: main conducting airway leading into the lungs

ventilation: movement of gases in and out of the lungs

The respiratory system is essential for survival. It brings oxygen into the body, allows for the exchange of gases, and leads to the expulsion of carbon dioxide and other waste products. The normal functioning of the respiratory system depends on an intricate balance of the nervous, cardiovascular, and musculoskeletal systems. Numerous conditions can affect the respiratory tract and interfere with the body's ability to ensure adequate oxygenation and gas exchange.

Structure and Function of the Respiratory System

The respiratory system (Fig. 53.1) consists of two major components: the conducting airways and the respiratory airways. The **conducting airways** are composed of the upper respiratory tract (nose, mouth, pharynx, larynx, trachea) and bronchi that move air in and out of the lung tissues. The **respiratory airways** are responsible for gas exchange. The lobules of the lungs consist of a bronchiole and arteriole, pulmonary capillaries, and veins. Alveolar sacs are small pouches at the ends of the bronchioles where gas is exchanged between air and blood. The bronchi and lobules of the lungs can be categorized as the lower respiratory tract.

The Conducting Airways

The conducting airways are primarily involved in **ventilation**, the movement of air in and out of the body. These airways also change the quality of the atmospheric air. It is warmed, filtered, and moistened prior to reaching the alveoli. Air usually moves into the body through the nose and into the nasal cavity. The nasal hairs catch and filter foreign substances that may be present in the inhaled air. The air is warmed and humidified as it passes by blood vessels close to the surface of the epithelial lining in the nasal cavity. Oxygen moves more efficiently when in warm and humid air, making respiration easier. The epithelial lining contains goblet cells that produce mucus. This mucus traps dust, microorganisms, pollen, and any other foreign substances. The epithelial cells of the lining also contain **cilia**—microscopic, hairlike projections of the cell membrane—which are constantly moving and directing the mucus and any trapped substances down toward the throat (Fig. 53.2). The action of the goblet cells and cilia is commonly called the mucociliary escalator or blanket.

Pairs of **sinuses** (air-filled passages through the skull) open into the nasal cavity. Because the epithelial lining of the nasal passage is continuous with the lining of the sinuses, the mucus produced in the sinuses drains into the nasal cavity. From there, the mucus drains into the throat

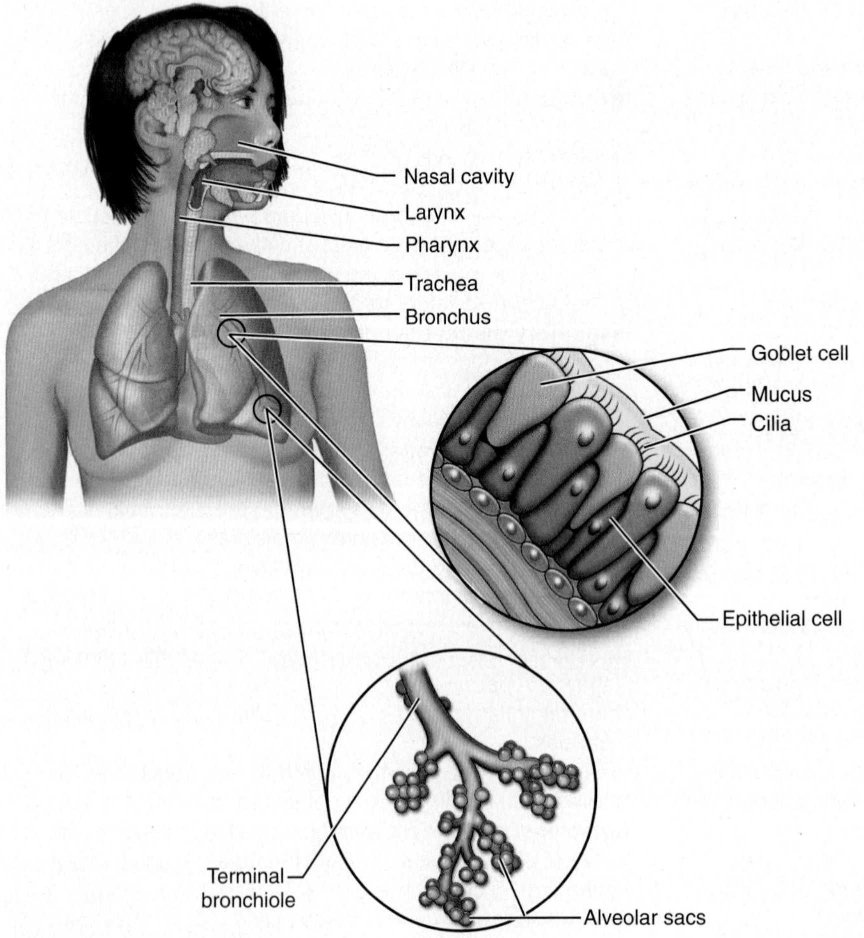

FIGURE 53.1 The respiratory system.

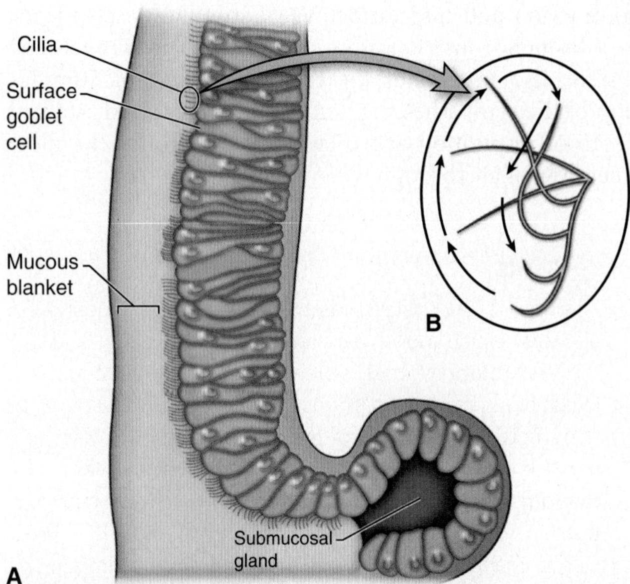

FIGURE 53.2 A. The mucociliary escalator. B. Conceptual scheme of ciliary movement, which allows forward motion to move the viscous gel layer and backward motion to occur entirely within the less viscous layer of the mucous blanket.

and is swallowed into the gastrointestinal tract, where stomach acid destroys foreign materials.

Air moves from the nasal cavity into the pharynx and larynx. The **pharynx** is the membrane-lined cavity that is behind the mouth and nose and before the esophagus and larynx. The **larynx** contains the vocal chords and the epiglottis, which closes during swallowing to protect the lower respiratory tract from any foreign particles. From the larynx, air proceeds to the **trachea**, the main conducting airway into the lungs. The trachea bifurcates, or divides, into two main bronchi, which further divide into smaller and smaller branches. All of these tubes contain mucous-producing goblet cells and cilia to entrap any particles that may have escaped the upper protective mechanisms. The cilia in these tubes move the mucus up the trachea and into the throat, where again it can be swallowed or coughed into the oral cavity.

The walls of the trachea and conducting bronchi are highly sensitive to irritation. When receptors in the walls are stimulated, a central nervous system (CNS) reflex is initiated and a **cough** results. The cough causes air to be pushed through the bronchial tree under tremendous pressure, cleaning out any foreign irritant. This reflex, along with the similar **sneeze** reflex (which is initiated by receptors in the nasal cavity), forces foreign materials directly out of the system, opening it for more efficient flow of gas.

Throughout the airways, many macrophage scavengers move freely about the epithelium and destroy invaders. Mast cells are present in abundance and release histamine, serotonin, adenosine triphosphate, and other chemicals to ensure a rapid and intense inflammatory reaction to any cell injury. The end result of these various defense mechanisms is that the lower respiratory tract is kept as free as possible from pathogens that can cause respiratory infection, which could interfere with essential gas exchange.

The Respiratory Airways

The lower respiratory tract (i.e., the respiratory airways) is composed of the lobules and alveoli (see Fig. 53.1). The lobules include the smallest bronchioles, an arteriole, pulmonary capillaries, and veins. The bronchial tubes are composed of three layers: cartilage, smooth muscle, and epithelial cells. The cartilage keeps the tube open, but it becomes progressively less abundant as the bronchi divide and get smaller. The smooth muscles are able to contract and narrow the airways. The muscles in the bronchi become smaller and less abundant as the bronchi divide, with only a few muscle fibers remaining in the terminal bronchi and alveoli. The epithelial cells are similar in structure and function to the epithelial cells in the nasal passage. The **alveoli**, or respiratory sacs, at the end of the bronchioles form the respiratory membrane. The alveoli are the smallest units of the lung. These structures are the functional units of the lungs where gas exchange occurs.

The lungs are two spongy organs that fill the chest cavity. They are separated by the mediastinum, which contains the heart, esophagus, thymus gland, and various blood vessels and nerves. The lungs are made up of the **bronchial tree** (the conducting airways that branch smaller and smaller, appearing much like a tree), the alveoli, the blood supply to the lungs, the blood coming from the right ventricle to the alveoli for gas exchange, and elastic tissue, which is important in allowing the expansion and recoil of the lungs to allow ventilation. The left lung is composed of two lobes or sections, and the right lung is composed of three lobes. The lung tissue receives its blood supply from the bronchial artery, which branches directly off the aorta. The alveoli receive unoxygenated blood from the right ventricle via the pulmonary artery. The delivery of this blood to the alveoli is referred to as pulmonary perfusion.

Gas Exchange

Gas exchange occurs in the alveoli. In this process, carbon dioxide diffuses from the blood and oxygen is transferred to the blood. The exchange of gases at the alveolar level is called **respiration**. The alveolar sac holds the gas, allowing needed oxygen to diffuse across the respiratory membrane into the capillary while carbon dioxide, which is more abundant in the capillary blood, diffuses across the membrane and enters the alveolar sac to be expired. Type I alveolar cells are extremely thin cells that occupy most of the surface area of the alveoli.

The **respiratory membrane** is where gas exchange occurs. It is made up of the capillary endothelium, the capillary basement membrane, the interstitial space, the alveolar basement membrane, the alveolar epithelium, and the **surfactant** layer (Fig. 53.3). The sac is able to stay open because the surface tension of the cells is decreased by the

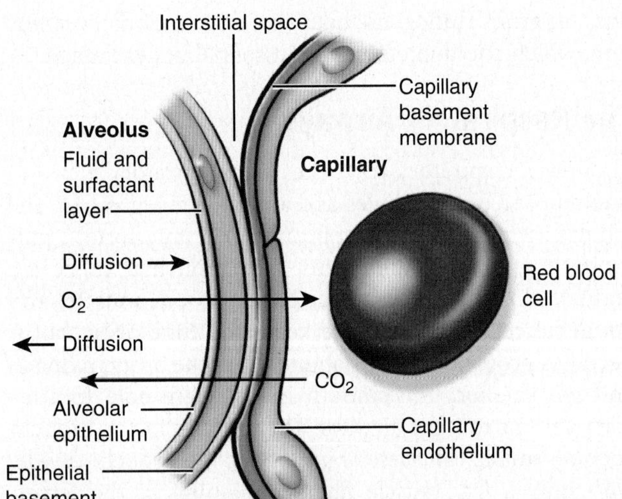

FIGURE 53.3 The respiratory membrane.

lipoprotein surfactant. Absence of surfactant leads to alveolar collapse. Surfactant is produced by the type II cells in the alveoli. These cells have other metabolic functions, including the conversion of angiotensin I to angiotensin II by angiotensin-converting enzyme, the degradation of serotonin, and possibly the metabolism of various hormones.

The oxygenated blood is returned to the left atrium via the pulmonary veins; from there, it is pumped throughout the body to deliver oxygen to the cells and to pick up waste products. The carbon dioxide that diffuses into the alveoli is moved back out into the atmosphere in the process of ventilation.

Ventilation

Ventilation, or the act of breathing to allow gas exchange, is controlled by the CNS. The inspiratory muscles—diaphragm, external intercostals, and abdominal muscles—are stimulated to contract by the respiratory center in the brain that include neurons in the pons and the medulla. The respiratory center receives input from chemoreceptors (neuroreceptors sensitive to carbon dioxide, oxygen, and acid levels) and lung receptors. The rate and/or depth of breathing can be increased quickly if the chemoreceptors note higher acid levels or carbon dioxide levels. Low oxygen levels will also trigger breathing, but this is a secondary or back-up system in people who do not have chronically high carbon dioxide levels. The lung receptors consist of stretch and irritant receptors. If the stretch receptors are stimulated, expiration will be triggered. Irritant receptors can protect airways from noxious stimuli (e.g., dust, cigarette smoke, cold air) by stimulating airway constriction. People can have voluntary control of breathing as well. For example, people are able to temporarily suspend breathing and regulate the timing of breathing when talking or singing.

The vagus nerve, a predominantly parasympathetic nerve, plays a key role in stimulating diaphragm contraction and inspiration. Vagal stimulation also leads to a bronchoconstriction or tightening. The sympathetic system also innervates the respiratory system. Stimulation of the sympathetic system leads to increased rate and depth of respiration and dilation of the bronchi to allow freer flow of air through the system.

Key Points

- The respiratory system has two parts: the conducting airways, which moves air in and out of the lungs, and the respiratory airways, where gas exchange occurs.
- Nasal hairs, mucous-producing goblet cells, cilia, the superficial blood supply of the upper respiratory tract, and the cough and sneeze reflexes all work to keep foreign substances from entering the lower respiratory tract.
- Gas exchange occurs across the respiratory membrane in the alveolar sac. The type II cells of the alveoli produce surfactant, which reduces surface tension to keep the alveoli open for gas exchange.
- The CNS controls ventilation, which depends on a functioning muscular system and a balance between the sympathetic and parasympathetic systems.

Respiratory Pathophysiology

Several conditions or disorders of the conducting and respiratory airways can interfere with the functioning of the respiratory system. These problems can range from generalized discomfort to life-threatening changes in gas exchange. Having a basic understanding of the processes at work will facilitate the understanding of the drugs that are used to treat these disorders.

Respiratory Tract Infections

The most common conditions that affect the conducting airways involve the inflammatory response and its effects on the mucosal layer of the conducting airways. Common triggers for the inflammatory responses are due to infection. Pathogens causing infection will also stimulate the immune cells to act.

The Common Cold

A number of viruses cause the **common cold**. These viruses invade the tissues of the upper respiratory tract, initiating the release of histamine and prostaglandins and causing an inflammatory response. As a result of the inflammatory response, the mucous membranes become engorged with blood, the tissues swell, and the goblet cells increase the production of mucus. These effects cause the person with a common cold to complain of sinus pain, nasal congestion, runny nose, sneezing, watery eyes, scratchy throat, and headache. In susceptible people, this swelling can block the outlet of the eustachian tube, which drains the inner ear and equalizes pressure across the tympanic membrane. If this outlet becomes blocked, feelings of ear stuffiness and pain can occur, and the person is more likely to develop an ear infection (otitis media).

Seasonal Rhinitis

A similar condition that afflicts many people is allergic or **seasonal rhinitis** (an inflammation of the nasal cavity), commonly called hay fever. This condition occurs when the upper airways respond to a specific antigen (e.g., pollen, mold, dust) with a vigorous inflammatory response, resulting in nasal congestion, sneezing, stuffiness, and watery eyes.

Sinusitis

Other areas of the upper respiratory tract can become irritated or infected, with a resultant inflammation of that particular area. **Sinusitis** occurs when the epithelial lining of the sinus cavities becomes inflamed. The resultant swelling often causes severe pain due to pressure against the bone, which cannot stretch, leading to blockage of the sinus passage. The danger of a sinus infection is that if it is left untreated, microorganisms can travel up the sinus passages and into brain tissue or affect eyesight.

Pharyngitis, Laryngitis, and Bronchitis

Pharyngitis, laryngitis, and bronchitis are inflammations of the pharynx, larynx, and bronchi, respectively. The inflammation is commonly caused by either viral or bacterial infections. Pharyngitis and laryngitis are frequently seen with influenza, which is caused by a variety of different viruses and produces uncomfortable respiratory symptoms or other inflammations along with fever, muscle aches and pains, and malaise. Acute bronchitis is most often caused by viral infection. Chronic bronchitis is commonly caused by irritation from noxious stimuli (e.g., cigarette smoke) in conjunction with recurrent infections.

Pneumonia

Pneumonia is inflammation of the lungs caused either by bacterial or viral invasion of the tissue or by aspiration of foreign substances into the lower respiratory tract. The rapid inflammatory response to any foreign presence in the lower respiratory tract leads to localized swelling, engorgement, and exudation of protective sera. The respiratory membrane is affected, resulting in decreased gas exchange. Patients complain of difficulty breathing and fatigue, and they may present with fever, noisy breath sounds, and poor oxygenation.

Tuberculosis

Tuberculosis is caused by *Mycobacterium tuberculosis* that is slow to replicate but also more resistant to destruction than other pathogens. Tuberculosis and medications to treat this disease are discussed in Chapter 9. It is spread via respiratory droplets, so even though many parts of the body can be infected by *M. tuberculosis*, the most common infection involves the lung tissue. Some people are asymptomatic after exposure, but others who may be immunocompromised may have lung tissue destroyed by the mycobacterium and the immune system response. Symptoms can include cough (often bloody tinged), fatigue, shortness of breath, fever, chills, weight loss, and night sweats.

Ventilation and Gas Exchange Disorders

A number of disorders affect the lower respiratory tract, including atelectasis, bronchiectasis, asthma, chronic obstructive pulmonary disease (COPD), cystic fibrosis (CF), and respiratory distress syndrome (RDS). All of these disorders involve an alteration in the ability to move gases in and out of the lungs to some degree, and they all have the potential to hinder gas exchange.

Atelectasis

Atelectasis, the incomplete expansion of alveoli, can occur as a result of outside pressure against the alveoli—for example, from a pulmonary tumor, **pneumothorax** (air in the pleural space exerting high pressure against the alveoli), or pleural effusion. Atelectasis can commonly occur as a result of airway blockage, which prevents air from entering the alveoli, keeping the lung expanded. This occurs when a mucous plug, edema of the bronchioles, or a collection of pus or secretions occludes the airway and prevents the movement of air. Patients may experience atelectasis after surgery, when the effects of anesthesia, pain, and decreased coughing reflexes can lead to a decreased tidal volume and accumulation of secretions in the lower airways. Finally, atelectasis can occur when the lung does not have enough surfactant, so the surface tension increases the lung's elasticity. Patients may present with crackles, dyspnea, fever, cough, hypoxia, and changes in chest wall movement. Treatment may involve clearing the airways, delivering oxygen, and assisting ventilation. In the case of pneumothorax, treatment also involves the insertion of a chest tube to restore the negative pressure to the space between the pleura.

Bronchiectasis

Bronchiectasis is a chronic disease that involves the bronchi and bronchioles. It is characterized by dilation of the bronchial tree and chronic infection and inflammation of the bronchial passages. With chronic inflammation, the bronchial epithelial cells are replaced by a fibrous scar tissue. The loss of the protective mucus and ciliary movement of the epithelial cell membranes combined with the dilation of the bronchial tree leads to chronic infections in the now-unprotected lower areas of the lung tissue. Patients with bronchiectasis often have an underlying medical

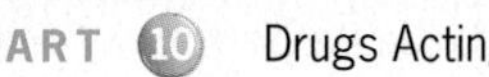

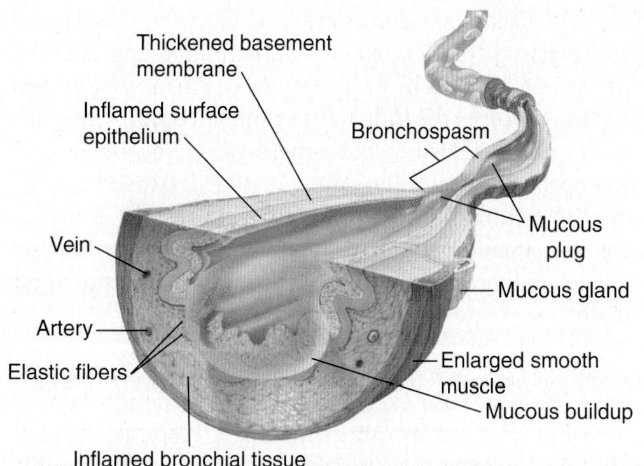

FIGURE 53.4 Asthma. The bronchiole is obstructed on expiration, particularly by muscle spasm, edema of the mucosa, and thick secretions.

condition that makes them more susceptible to infections (e.g., immune suppression, CF, chronic inflammatory conditions). Patients present with the signs and symptoms of acute infection, including fever, malaise, myalgia, arthralgia, and a purulent, productive cough.

Asthma

Asthma is characterized by reversible bronchospasm, inflammation, and hyperactive airways (Fig. 53.4). The hyperactivity is triggered by allergens, nonallergic inhaled irritants, infections, or factors such as exercise and emotions. The trigger causes inflammation mediated by eosinophils, lymphocytes, and mast cells. Cytokine-mediated inflammation, mucous production, and edema contributing to obstruction are important factors in the chronic inflammatory response. The inflammatory processes are able to cause recurrent episodes of airway obstruction. Symptoms can include wheezing, shortness of breath, chest tightness, and/or cough. Appropriate treatment includes preventing asthma episodes when possible, antiinflammatory medications, and bronchodilators. The extreme case of asthma is called status asthmaticus; this is a life-threatening bronchospasm that does not respond to usual treatment and occludes airflow into the lungs.

Chronic Obstructive Pulmonary Disease

Chronic obstructive pulmonary disease (COPD) is a progressive and not completely reversible chronic obstruction of airways, often related to cigarette smoking or other noxious stimuli. It is characterized by two related disorders—emphysema and chronic bronchitis—both of which result in airflow obstruction on expiration as well as increased inflation of the lungs and poor gas exchange. Emphysema is characterized by loss of the elastic tissue of the lungs, destruction of alveolar walls, and a resultant alveolar hyperinflation with a tendency to collapse with expiration. Chronic bronchitis is diagnosed when there is long-term (at least 3 months in the past 2 years) inflammation of the airways with mucous secretion, edema, and other signs and symptoms of inflammation. The characteristics of both disorders are often present in a person with COPD (Fig. 53.5). COPD is diagnosed with spirometry, a breathing test that can measure volumes and flow rates of air. A low peak flow rate of expired air in conjunction with shortness of breath and/or productive cough is key to a COPD diagnosis.

Cystic Fibrosis

Cystic fibrosis (CF) is a hereditary disease involving the epithelial lining of the respiratory, gastrointestinal, and reproductive tracts. There is a defective gene on chromosome 7 that make the epithelial membrane more impermeable to chloride. The alteration in chloride transport decreases the amount of sodium and water excreted in sweat and into the respiratory tract. CF results in the accumulation of copious amounts of thick secretions in the lungs. These thick secretions can obstruct the airways, leading to recurrent infections and potential destruction of

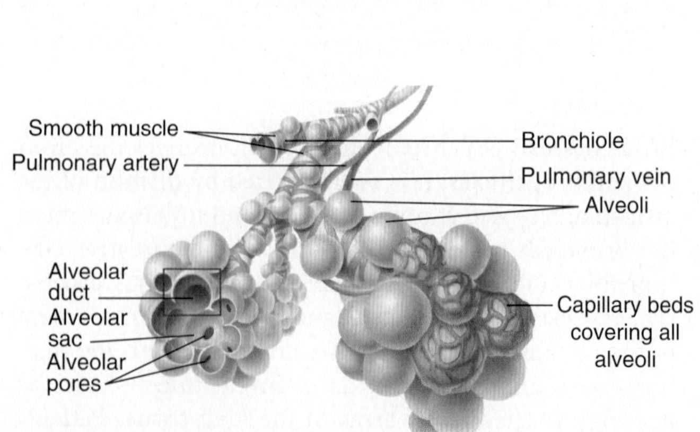

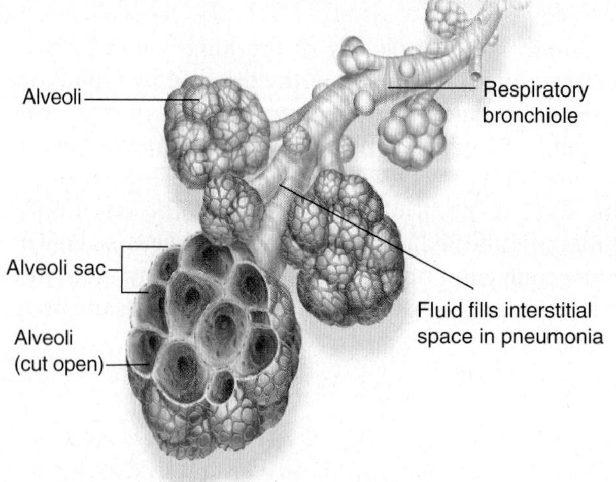

FIGURE 53.5 Normal alveoli versus distended and destroyed alveoli.

the lung tissue. Treatment includes preventing and treating infections, chest physical therapy, and nutritional therapy.

Respiratory Distress Syndrome and Acute Respiratory Distress Syndrome

Respiratory distress syndrome (RDS) causes obstruction at the alveolar level. It is frequently seen in premature infants who are delivered before their lungs have fully developed and while surfactant levels are still low. Surfactant is necessary for lowering the surface tension in the alveoli so that they can stay open to allow the flow of gases. If surfactant levels are low, the alveoli do not expand and cannot receive air, leading to decreased gas exchange, low oxygen levels, and generalized distress throughout the body as cells do not receive the oxygen that they need to survive. Treatment is aimed at instilling surfactant to prevent atelectasis and to allow the lungs to expand.

Acute respiratory distress syndrome (ARDS) is characterized by progressive loss of lung compliance and increasing hypoxia. This syndrome typically results from a severe insult to the body, such as cardiovascular collapse, major burns, severe trauma, or rapid depressurization. There is extensive epithelial cell damage and increased permeability in the alveolar–capillary membrane that allows for more fluid, proteins, and blood cells to move from the blood to the lung tissue and alveoli. Treatment of ARDS involves reversal of the underlying cause of the problem combined with supportive care including mechanical ventilation.

Key Points

- Infections and inflammation of the respiratory tract can range from irritating but mild to serious life-threatening disorders that interfere with gas exchange.
- There are multiple ventilation and gas exchange disorders that can affect people of all ages, including asthma, COPD, CF, and RDS.

SUMMARY

- The respiratory system is composed of the conducting airways, which are responsible for moving air in and out of the lung tissues, and the respiratory airways, which are where gas exchange occurs.
- The respiratory system is essential for survival; it brings oxygen into the body, allows for the exchange of gases, and expels carbon dioxide and other waste products.
- The upper airways have many features to protect the fragile alveoli: hairs filter the air; goblet cells produce mucus to trap foreign material; cilia move the trapped material toward the throat for swallowing; the blood supply close to the surface warms the air and adds humidity to improve gas movement and gas exchange; and the cough and sneeze reflexes clear the airways.
- The alveolar sac is where gas exchange occurs across the respiratory membrane. The alveoli produce surfactant to decrease surface tension within the sac and facilitate diffusion.
- Ventilation is controlled through the respiratory center in the CNS and depends on a balance between the sympathetic and parasympathetic systems and a functioning muscular system.
- Infections and inflammation of the respiratory tract can range from irritating but mild to serious life-threatening disorders that interfere with gas exchange.
- There are multiple ventilation and gas exchange disorders that can affect people of all ages, including asthma, COPD, CF, and RDS.

CHECK YOUR UNDERSTANDING

Answers to the questions in this chapter can be found in Answers to Check Your Understanding Questions on thePoint®.

MULTIPLE CHOICE

Select the best answer.

1. The nurse emphasizes the need to take sinusitis seriously because
   a. it can cause a loss of sleep and exhaustion.
   b. it can lead to a painful otitis media.
   c. if it is left untreated, microorganisms can travel to brain tissue.
   d. drainage from infected sinus membranes often leads to pneumonia.

2. Diffusion of CO_2 from the tissues into the capillary blood
   a. occurs if the tissue concentration of CO_2 is greater than that in the blood.
   b. decreases as blood acidity increases.
   c. increases in the absence of carbonic anhydrase.
   d. is accompanied by a decrease in plasma bicarbonate.

3. The type II cells of the walls of the alveoli function to
   a. replace mucus in the alveoli.
   b. produce serotonin.
   c. secrete surfactant.
   d. protect the lungs from bacterial invasion.

4. A patient who coughs is experiencing a reflex caused by
   a. inflammation irritating the sinuses in the skull.
   b. irritants affecting receptor sites in the nasal cavity.
   c. pressure against the eustachian tube.
   d. irritation to receptors in the trachea and conducting airways.

5. Which is most critical to trigger ventilation?
   a. Low levels of oxygen
   b. Low levels of CO_2
   c. Functioning inspiratory muscles
   d. An actively functioning autonomic system

6. After teaching a community group about the common cold, the instructor determines that the teaching was successful when the group states which as the cause?
   a. Bacteria that grow best in the cold
   b. Allergens in the environment
   c. Irritation of the delicate mucous membrane
   d. A number of different viruses

7. A patient with COPD would be expected to have
   a. an acute viral infection of the respiratory tract.
   b. loss of protective respiratory mechanisms due to prolonged irritation or damage.
   c. localized swelling and inflammation within the lungs.
   d. inflammation or swelling of the sinus membranes over a prolonged period.

MULTIPLE RESPONSE

Select all that apply.

1. What would a nurse expect to assess if a patient has inflammation of the upper respiratory tract?
   a. Runny nose
   b. Laryngitis
   c. Sneezing
   d. Hypoxia
   e. Rales
   f. Wheezing

2. For gas exchange to occur in the lungs, oxygen must pass through which structures?
   a. Conducting airways
   b. Alveolar epithelium
   c. Pleural fluid
   d. Interstitial alveolar wall
   e. Capillary basement membrane
   f. Interstitial space

3. The nose performs which functions in the respiratory system?
   a. Serves as a passageway for air movement
   b. Warms and humidifies the air
   c. Cleanses the air using hair fibers
   d. Stimulates surfactant release from the alveoli
   e. Initiates the cough reflex
   f. Initiates the sneeze reflex

REFERENCES

Barrett, K., Barman, S., Yuan, J., & Brooks, H. (2019). *Ganong's review of medical physiology* (26th ed.). McGraw-Hill.

Brunton, L., Hilal-Dandan, R., & Knollman, B. (2018). *Goodman and Gilman's the pharmacological basis of therapeutics* (13th ed.). McGraw-Hill.

George, R. B., Light, R. W., Matthay, M. A., & Matthay, R. A. (2006). *Chest medicine: Essentials of pulmonary and critical care medicine* (5th ed.). Lippincott Williams & Wilkins.

Hall, J. E., & Hall, M. E. (2021). *Guyton and Hall textbook of medical physiology* (14th ed.). Elsevier.

Levitzky, M. G. (2018). *Pulmonary pathophysiology* (9th ed.). McGraw-Hill.

Norris, T. L. (2019). *Porth's pathophysiology concepts of altered health states* (13th ed.). Wolters Kluwer.

CHAPTER 54

Drugs Acting on the Upper Respiratory Tract

Learning Objectives

Upon completion of this chapter, you will be able to:

1. Outline the underlying physiological events that occur with upper respiratory disorders.
2. Discuss the use of drugs that act on the upper respiratory tract across the lifespan.
3. Describe the therapeutic actions, indications, pharmacokinetics, contraindications, most common adverse effects, and important drug–drug interactions associated with drugs acting on the upper respiratory tract.
4. Compare and contrast the prototype drugs with other agents in their class and with other classes of drugs that act on the upper respiratory tract.
5. Outline the nursing considerations, including important teaching points, for patients receiving drugs acting on the upper respiratory tract.

Key Terms

antihistamines: drugs that block the release or action of histamine, a chemical released during inflammation that increases secretions and narrows airways

antitussives: drugs that block the cough reflex

decongestants: drugs that decrease the blood flow to the upper respiratory tract and decrease the production of secretions

expectorants: drugs that increase productive cough to clear the airways

mucolytics: drugs that increase or liquefy respiratory secretions to aid the clearing of the airways

rebound congestion: process that occurs when the nasal passages become congested as the effect of a decongestant drug wears off; patients tend to use more drug to decrease the congestion, and a vicious circle of congestion, drug, and congestion develops, leading to abuse of the decongestant; also called rhinitis medicamentosa

rhinitis medicamentosa: reflex reaction to vasoconstriction caused by decongestants; a rebound vasodilation that often leads to prolonged overuse of decongestants; also called rebound congestion

Drug List

ANTITUSSIVES
benzonatate
codeine
(P) dextromethorphan
hydrocodone

DECONGESTANTS

Topical Nasal Decongestants
naphazoline
oxymetazoline
phenylephrine
(P) tetrahydrozoline
xylometazoline

Oral Decongestants
phenylephrine
(P) pseudoephedrine

Steroid Nasal Decongestants
beclomethasone
budesonide
(P) flunisolide
fluticasone
triamcinolone

ANTIHISTAMINES

First Generation
brompheniramine
carbinoxamine
chlorpheniramine
clemastine
cyproheptadine
dexchlorpheniramine
dimenhydrinate
(P) diphenhydramine
hydroxyzine
meclizine
promethazine
triprolidine

Second Generation (Nonsedating)
azelastine
cetirizine
desloratadine
fexofenadine
levocetirizine
loratadine

EXPECTORANT
(P) guaifenesin

MUCOLYTICS
(P) acetylcysteine
dornase alfa

The drugs that are described in this chapter affect the respiratory system to treat symptoms of allergic or nonallergic rhinitis as well as cough and other symptoms from the common cold, influenza, and other respiratory disorders. They are designed for symptom relief and to keep the respiratory airways patent. They are not designed to treat or cure infection. Figure 54.1 displays the sites of action of these drugs. Figure 54.2 shows the structures of the upper respiratory tract.

Antitussives

Antitussives are drugs that suppress the cough reflex (Table 54.1). Many disorders of the respiratory tract, including the common cold, sinusitis, pharyngitis, and pneumonia, are accompanied by an uncomfortable, unproductive cough. Persistent coughing can be exhausting and can cause muscle strain and further irritation of the respiratory tract. A cough that occurs without the presence of any active disease process or persists after treatment may be a symptom of another disease process and should be investigated before any medication is given to alleviate it. Box 54.1 discusses the use of antitussives and other drugs acting on the upper respiratory tract in various age groups.

Therapeutic Actions and Indications

The traditional antitussives include codeine (generic), hydrocodone (generic), and dextromethorphan (generic), which act directly on the medullary cough center of the brain to depress the cough reflex. Because they are centrally acting, they are not the drugs of choice for anyone who has a head injury or who could be impaired by central nervous system (CNS) depression. Codeine and hydrocodone are opioid agonists that are primarily indicated for pain relief (see Chapter 26). They are used as cough suppressant medications in several combination formulations (*Tuxarin ER*, *Hycodan*, and others). They are controlled substances, designated schedule II when used alone and schedule V when used in combination and low amounts.

Other antitussives have a direct effect on the respiratory tract. Benzonatate (*Tessalon*) acts as a local anesthetic on the respiratory passages, lungs, and pleurae, blocking the effectiveness of the stretch receptors that stimulate a cough reflex.

Pharmacokinetics

Codeine, hydrocodone, and dextromethorphan are rapidly absorbed, metabolized in the liver, and excreted in the urine. They cross the placenta and enter human milk.

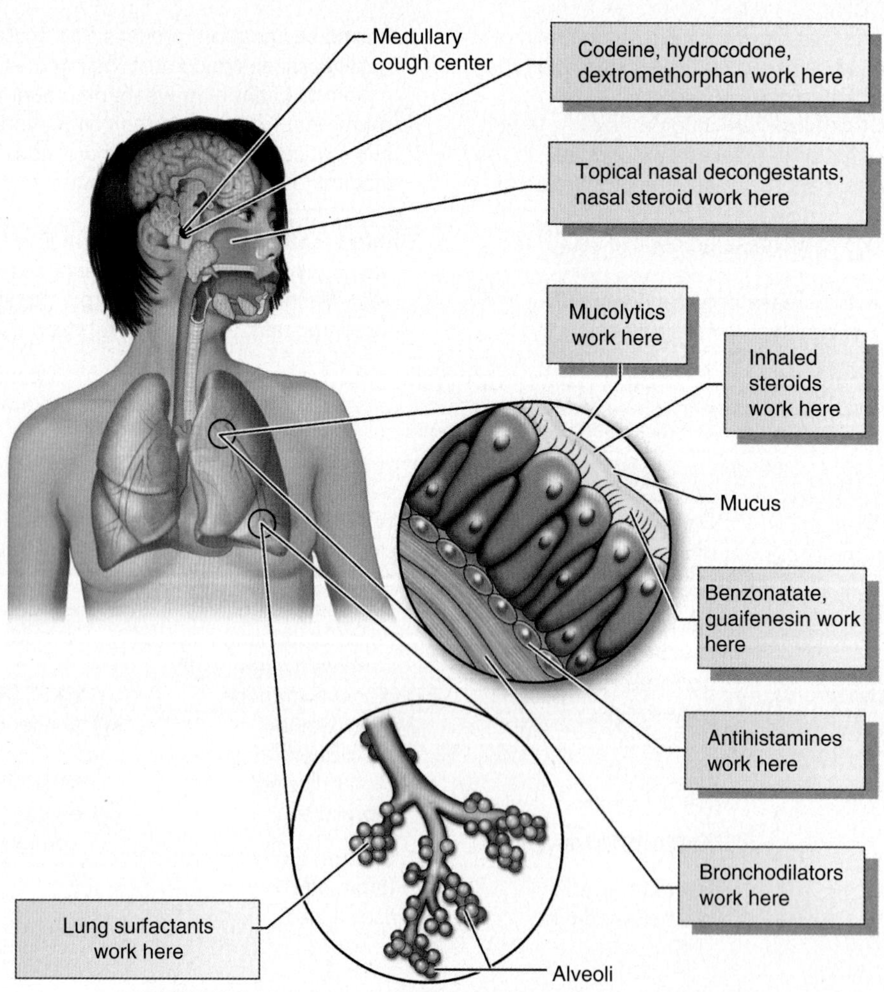

FIGURE 54.1 Sites of action of drugs acting on the upper respiratory tract.

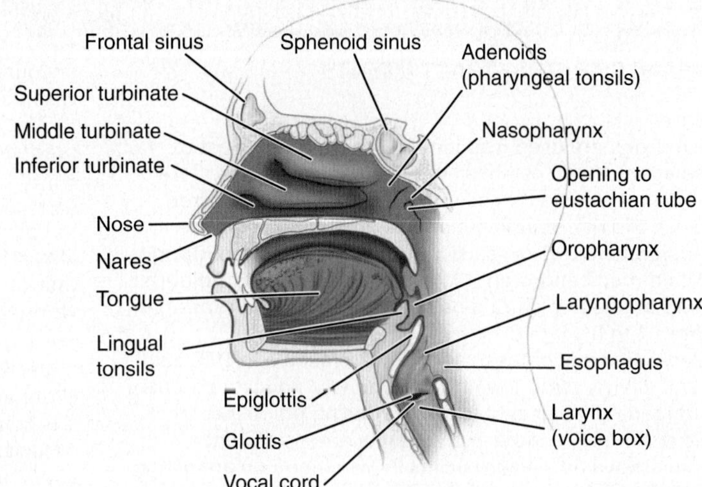

FIGURE 54.2 Structures of the upper respiratory tract.

Benzonatate is metabolized in the liver and excreted in the urine. These drugs should not be used during pregnancy and lactation (see "Contraindications and Cautions").

Contraindications and Cautions

Antitussives are contraindicated in patients who need to cough to maintain the airways (e.g., postoperative patients and those who have undergone abdominal or thoracic surgery) to avoid respiratory distress. Careful use is recommended for patients with asthma and emphysema because cough suppression in these patients could lead to an accumulation of secretions and a loss of respiratory reserve. Caution should also be used in patients who are hypersensitive to or have a history of addiction to narcotics (codeine, hydrocodone). Codeine and hydrocodone are narcotics and have addiction potential. Patients who need to drive or be alert should use codeine, hydrocodone, and dextromethorphan with extreme caution because these drugs can cause sedation and drowsiness. These drugs should not be used during pregnancy and lactation because of the potential for adverse effects on the fetus or baby, including sedation and CNS depression.

Adverse Effects

Traditional antitussives have a drying effect on the mucous membranes and can increase the viscosity of respiratory tract secretions. Because they affect centers in the brain, these antitussives are associated with CNS adverse effects, including respiratory depression, drowsiness, and sedation. Other common side effects are nausea, vomiting, and constipation (Fig. 54.3). There is risk of addiction and dependence with the opioid substances. Locally acting antitussives are associated with gastrointestinal (GI) upset, headache, feelings of congestion, and sometimes dizziness. However, when taken at recommended doses, the adverse effects are generally mild.

Clinically Important Drug–Drug Interactions

Dextromethorphan should not be used with monoamine oxidase (MAO) inhibitors; hypotension, fever, nausea, myoclonic jerks, and coma could occur. Concurrent use of the opioid medications with other medications or substances (like alcohol) can increase the risk of respiratory depression, sedation, coma, and even death.

Table 54.1 ***Drugs in Focus*: Antitussives**

Drug Name	Usual Dosage	Usual Indications
benzonatate (*Tessalon*)	*Adult and pediatric (> 10 y)*: 100–200 mg PO t.i.d.	Symptomatic relief of cough
codeine (generic)	*Adult*: 10–20 mg PO q4–6h *Pediatric (6–12 y)*: 5–10 mg PO q4–6h *Pediatric (2–6 y)*: 2.5–5 mg PO q4–6h	Symptomatic relief of cough
dextromethorphan (generic)	*Adult*: 10–30 mg PO q4–8h; 60 mg PO b.i.d. for sustained action *Pediatric (6–12 y)*: 5–10 mg PO q4h; 30 mg PO b.i.d. for sustained action *Pediatric (2–6 y)*: 2.5–7.5 mg PO q4–8h; 15 mg PO b.i.d. for sustained action	Symptomatic relief of cough
hydrocodone (generic)	*Adult*: 5–10 mg PO q4–6h *Pediatric (2–12 y)*: 1.25–5 mg PO q4–6h	Symptomatic relief of cough

Box 54.1 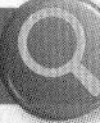 Focus on **Drug Therapy Across the Lifespan**

UPPER RESPIRATORY TRACT AGENTS

Children

These drugs are used frequently with children. Most of these agents have established pediatric guidelines. Care must be taken when these drugs are used with children because the risk of adverse effects, including sedation, confusion, and dizziness, is common with children. Cough and cold medications should not be used in children under 4 years of age and should be used with extreme caution in children 4 to 6 years of age.

Because many of these agents are available in OTC cold, flu, and allergy remedies, it is important to educate parents about reading labels and following dosing guidelines to avoid potentially serious accidental overdose. Parents should always be asked specifically whether they are giving the child an OTC or herbal remedy.

Parents should also be encouraged to implement nondrug measures to help the child cope with the upper respiratory problem—drinking plenty of fluids, using a humidifier, avoiding smoke-filled areas and contact with known allergens or irritants, and washing hands frequently during cold and flu season.

Adults

Adults may inadvertently overdose on these agents when taking multiple OTC preparations to help them get through a cold or flu. They need to be questioned specifically about the use of OTC or herbal remedies before any of these drugs are advised or administered. Adults can also be encouraged to use nondrug measures to help them cope with the signs and symptoms.

The safety for the use of many of these drugs during pregnancy and lactation has not been established. There is a potential for adverse effects on the fetus related to blood flow changes and direct drug effects when the drugs cross the placenta. The drugs may enter human milk and may also alter fluid balance and milk production. It is advised that caution be used if one of these drugs is prescribed when the patient is breast or chestfeeding.

Older Adults

Older adults are frequently prescribed one of these drugs. It is common for older adults to develop adverse effects associated with the use of these drugs, including sedation, confusion, and dizziness. Safety measures may be needed if these effects interfere with the patient's mobility and balance.

Older adults also are more likely to have renal and/or hepatic impairment related to underlying medical conditions, which could interfere with the metabolism and excretion of these drugs. The dose for older adults may need to be started at a lower level if there is renal and/or hepatic impairment. The patient should be monitored closely, and dose adjustment should be based on the patient's response.

These patients also need to be alerted to the potential for medication interactions when using OTC preparations and should be advised to check with their health care provider before beginning any OTC drug regimen.

Central nervous system effects: Restlessness, headache, drowsiness, sedation
Nasal: Dryness, local stinging
CV effects: Tachycardia, hypertension, arrhythmias
GI effects: Upset, nausea
GU effects: Dysuria, hesitancy

FIGURE 54.3 Variety of adverse effects and toxicities associated with drugs affecting the upper respiratory tract.

Prototype Summary: Dextromethorphan

Indications: Reduce symptoms of cough.

Actions: Depresses the cough center in the medulla to control cough spasms.

Pharmacokinetics:

Route	Onset	Peak	Duration
Oral	25–30 min	2 h	3–6 h

$T_{1/2}$: 2 to 4 hours; metabolized in the liver and excreted in the urine.

Adverse Effects: Dizziness, respiratory depression, nausea, dry mouth.

Nursing Considerations for Patients Receiving Antitussives

Assessment: History and Examination

- Assess for possible contraindications or cautions: any history of allergy to any component of the drug or drug vehicle to avoid allergic reactions; cough that persists longer than 1 week or is accompanied by other signs and symptoms, which could indicate a serious underlying medical condition that should be addressed before suppressing symptoms; and pregnancy or lactation because of the potential for adverse effects on the fetus or baby.

- Perform a physical examination to establish baseline data for assessing the effectiveness of the drug and the occurrence of any adverse effects associated with drug therapy.
- Monitor temperature to evaluate for possible underlying infection.
- Assess respirations and adventitious sounds to assess drug effectiveness and to monitor for accumulation of secretions.
- Evaluate orientation and affect to monitor for CNS effects of the drug.

Nursing Conclusions

Nursing conclusions related to drug therapy might include

- Ineffective airway clearance related to suppression of the cough reflex
- Altered sensory perception related to CNS effects
- Knowledge deficit regarding drug therapy

Planning

- The patient will receive the best therapeutic effect from the drug therapy.
- The patient will have limited adverse effects from the drug therapy.
- The patient will have an understanding of the drug therapy, adverse effects to anticipate, and measures to relieve discomfort and improve safety.

Intervention With Rationale

- Ensure that the drug is not taken any longer than recommended to prevent serious adverse effects and increased respiratory tract problems.
- Arrange for further medical evaluation for coughs that persist or are accompanied by high fever, rash, or excessive secretions to detect the underlying cause of the cough and to arrange for appropriate treatment of the underlying problem.
- Provide other measures to help relieve cough (e.g., humidity, cool temperatures, fluids, use of topical lozenges) as appropriate.
- Provide thorough patient teaching, including the drug name and prescribed dosage, measures to help avoid adverse effects, warning signs that may indicate problems, and the need for periodic monitoring and evaluation, to enhance patient knowledge about drug therapy and to promote adherence.
- Offer support and encouragement to help the patient cope with the disease and the drug regimen.

Evaluation

- Monitor patient response to the drug (control of nonproductive cough).
- Monitor for adverse effects (respiratory depression, dizziness, sedation, GI symptoms).
- Evaluate the effectiveness of the teaching plan (patient can name drug, dosage, adverse effects to watch for and specific measures to avoid them, and measures to take to increase the effectiveness of the drug).
- Monitor the effectiveness of other measures to relieve cough.

Key Points

- Antitussive drugs suppress the cough reflex by acting centrally to suppress the respiratory cough center or locally as an anesthetic or to increase secretion and buffer irritation.
- Antitussive drugs can cause CNS depression, including drowsiness and sedation.
- Antitussive drugs should be used with caution in any situation in which coughing could be important for clearing the airways.

Decongestants

Decongestants decrease the overproduction of secretions by causing local vasoconstriction to the upper respiratory tract (Table 54.2). This vasoconstriction leads to a shrinking of swollen mucous membranes and tends to open clogged nasal passages, providing relief from the discomfort of a blocked nose and promoting drainage of secretions and improved airflow. An adverse effect that accompanies frequent or prolonged use of these drugs is a rebound congestion, technically called rhinitis medicamentosa. The reflex reaction to vasoconstriction is a rebound vasodilation, which often leads to prolonged overuse of decongestants.

Decongestants are usually adrenergics or sympathomimetics (see Chapter 30). Topical steroids are also used as decongestants, though they take several weeks to become effective and are more often used in cases of chronic rhinitis.

Topical Nasal Decongestants

Topical nasal decongestants include naphazoline (*Privine*), oxymetazoline (*Afrin* and others), phenylephrine (*Coricidin* and many others), tetrahydrozoline (*Tyzine*), and xylometazoline (*Otrivin*). Many of these are available as over-the-counter (OTC) preparations. The choice of a topical nasal decongestant varies among people. Some patients may have no response to one and respond well to another.

Table 54.2 *Drugs in Focus*: Decongestants

Drug Name	Usual Dosage	Usual Indications
Topical Nasal Decongestants		
naphazoline (*Privine*)	*Adult and pediatric (>12 y):* 1–2 sprays into nostrils every 6 h as needed	Relieves discomfort of nasal congestion associated with the common cold, sinusitis, and allergic rhinitis
oxymetazoline (*Afrin*)	*Adult and pediatric (>6 y)*: 2–3 sprays or drops in each nostril b.i.d. *Pediatric (2–5 y)*: 2–3 drops of 0.05% solution in each nostril b.i.d.	Relieves discomfort of nasal congestion associated with the common cold, sinusitis, and allergic rhinitis
phenylephrine (*Coricidin*)	*Adult and pediatric (>6 y)*: 1–2 sprays in each nostril q3–4h *Pediatric (2–6 y)*: 2–3 drops of 0.125% solution in each nostril q4h as needed	Relieves discomfort of nasal congestion associated with the common cold, sinusitis, and allergic rhinitis
tetrahydrozoline (*Tyzine*)	*Adult and pediatric (>6 y)*: 2–4 drops in each nostril t.i.d. to q.i.d. *Pediatric (2–6 y)*: 2–3 drops of 0.05% solution in each nostril q4–6h	Relieves discomfort of nasal congestion associated with the common cold, sinusitis, and allergic rhinitis; relieves pressure of otitis media
xylometazoline (*Otrivin*)	*Adult*: 2–3 sprays or 2–3 drops in each nostril q8–10h (0.17% solution) *Pediatric (2–12 y)*: 2–3 drops of 0.05% solution q8–12h	Relieves discomfort of nasal congestion associated with the common cold, sinusitis, and allergic rhinitis; relieves pressure of otitis media
Oral Decongestant		
phenylephrine (*Neo-Synephrine Nasal*)	*Adult and pediatric:* Dose varies based on age and combination product	Decreases nasal congestion associated with the common cold, and allergic rhinitis; relieves pain and congestion of otitis media
pseudoephedrine (*Sudafed*)	*Adult*: 60 mg PO q4–6h *Pediatric (6–12 y)*: 30 mg PO q4–6h *Pediatric (2–5 y)*: 15 mg PO q4–6h *Pediatric (1–2 y)*: 0.02 mL/kg PO q4–6h *Pediatric (3–12 mo)*: 3 drops/kg PO q4–6h	Decreases nasal congestion associated with the common cold, and allergic rhinitis; relieves pain and congestion of otitis media
Steroid Nasal Decongestants		
beclomethasone (*Beconase AQ, Qnasl*)	*Adult and pediatric*: 1-2 inhalations in each nostril q.d. or b.i.d.	Relieves symptoms of seasonal or perennial allergic and nonallergic (vasomotor) rhinitis; relieves inflammation following removal of nasal polyps
budesonide (*Rhinocort*)	*Adult and pediatric (>6 y)*: 1 spray in each nostril daily	Relieves symptoms of seasonal or perennial allergic and nonallergic (vasomotor) rhinitis; relieves inflammation following removal of nasal polyps
flunisolide (generic)	*Adult*: 2 sprays in each nostril b.i.d. *Pediatric (6–14 y)*: 1 spray in each nostril t.i.d. to two sprays in each nostril b.i.d.	Relieves symptoms of seasonal or perennial allergic and nonallergic (vasomotor) rhinitis; relieves inflammation following removal of nasal polyps
fluticasone (*Flonase Allergy Relief*)	*Adult and pediatric (4–11 y)*: 2 sprays in each nostril daily	Relieves symptoms of seasonal or perennial allergic and nonallergic (vasomotor) rhinitis; relieves inflammation following removal of nasal polyps
triamcinolone (*Nasacort Allergy 24 Hour*)	*Adult*: 2 sprays in each nostril every day *Pediatric*: 1 spray in each nostril daily	Relieves symptoms of seasonal or perennial allergic and nonallergic (vasomotor) rhinitis; relieves inflammation following removal of nasal polyps

Therapeutic Actions and Indications

Topical decongestants are sympathomimetics, meaning they imitate the effects of the sympathetic nervous system to cause vasoconstriction, leading to decreased edema and inflammation of the nasal membranes. They are available as nasal sprays that are used to relieve the discomfort of nasal congestion that accompanies the common cold, sinusitis, and allergic rhinitis. These drugs can also be used when dilation of the nares is desired to facilitate medical

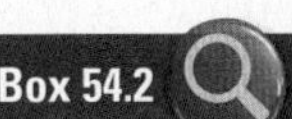

Focus on Patient and Family Teaching

ADMINISTERING NASAL MEDICATIONS

Proper administration technique is important for assuring that drugs given nasally have the desired therapeutic effect. It is important to periodically check the nares for any signs of erosion or lesions, which could allow systemic absorption of the drug. Most patients prefer to self-administer nasal drugs, so patient teaching is important. Explain the technique, and then observe the patient using the technique.

Nasal Spray

Teach the patient to sit upright and press a finger over one naris to close it. Hold the spray bottle upright and place the tip of the bottle about half an inch into the open naris. Firmly squeeze the bottle to deliver the drug. Repeat with the other naris. The patient should be encouraged to refrain from blowing their nose soon after administration so as not to expel the medication.

examination or to relieve the pain and congestion of otitis media. Opening the nasal passage allows better drainage of the eustachian tube, relieving pressure in the middle ear. See Table 54.2 for usual indications for each of these agents.

Pharmacokinetics

Because these drugs are applied topically, the onset of action is almost immediate and there is less chance of systemic effects. Although they are not generally absorbed systemically, any portion of these topical decongestants that is absorbed is metabolized in the liver and excreted in the urine. See Box 54.2 for tips on how to teach patients to use these medications.

Contraindications and Cautions

Caution should be used when there is any lesion or erosion in the mucous membranes that could lead to systemic absorption. Caution should also be used in patients with any condition that might be exacerbated by sympathetic activity, such as glaucoma, hypertension, diabetes, thyroid disease, coronary disease, or prostate problems, because these agents have adrenergic properties. Because there are no studies regarding the effects of these topical drugs in pregnancy or lactation, if used during pregnancy or lactation, caution is advised.

Adverse Effects

Adverse effects associated with topical decongestants include local stinging and burning, which may occur the first few times the drug is used. If the sensation does not pass, use should be discontinued because it may indicate lesions or erosion of the mucous membranes. Use for longer than 3 to 5 days can lead to a **rebound congestion** (also called **rhinitis medicamentosa**), which occurs when the nasal passages become congested as the drug effect wears off. As a result, patients tend to use more drug to decrease the congestion, thus initiating a cycle of congestion–drug–congestion, which leads to abuse of the decongestant. Sympathomimetic effects (e.g., increased pulse and blood pressure; urinary retention) should be monitored because some systemic absorption may occur, though these effects are less likely with topical administration than with other routes.

Clinically Important Drug–Drug Interactions

The use of topical nasal decongestants with other medications that affect the sympathetic nervous system should be monitored carefully.

Prototype Summary: Tetrahydrozoline

Indications: Symptomatic relief of nasal and nasopharyngeal mucosal congestion due to the common cold, hay fever, or other respiratory allergies.

Actions: Sympathomimetic effects, partly due to release of norepinephrine from nerve terminals; vasoconstriction leads to decreased edema and inflammation of the nasal membranes.

Pharmacokinetics:

Route	Peak	Duration
Topical (nasal spray)	5–10 min	6–10 h

$T_{1/2}$: Unknown; metabolized in the liver and excreted in the urine; little is usually absorbed for systemic metabolism.

Adverse Effects: Disorientation, confusion, lightheadedness, nausea, vomiting, fever, dyspnea, and rebound congestion.

Nursing Considerations for Patients Receiving Topical Nasal Decongestants

Assessment: History and Examination

- Assess for possible contraindications or cautions: any history of allergy to the drug or a component of the drug vehicle; glaucoma, hypertension, diabetes, thyroid disease, coronary disease, and prostate problems, all of which could be exacerbated by the sympathomimetic effects; and pregnancy or lactation, which require cautious use of the drug.
- Perform a physical examination to establish baseline data for assessing the effectiveness of the drug and the occurrence of any adverse effects associated with drug therapy.
- Assess skin color and temperature to assess sympathetic response.

(continues on page 964)

- Evaluate orientation and reflexes to evaluate CNS effects of the drug.
- Monitor pulse, blood pressure, and cardiac auscultation to assess cardiovascular (CV) and sympathomimetic effects.
- Evaluate respirations and adventitious breath sounds to assess the effectiveness of the drug and potential excess effect.
- Monitor urinary output to evaluate for urinary retention.
- Evaluate nasal mucous membrane to monitor for lesions that could lead to systemic absorption and to evaluate decongestant effect.

Nursing Conclusions

Nursing conclusions related to drug therapy might include

- Impaired comfort related to GI, CNS, or local effects of drug
- Altered sensory perception (kinesthetic) related to CNS effects (less likely with this route of administration)
- Knowledge deficit regarding drug therapy

Planning

- The patient will receive the best therapeutic effect from the drug therapy.
- The patient will have limited adverse effects from the drug therapy.
- The patient will have an understanding of the drug therapy, adverse effects to anticipate, and measures to relieve discomfort and improve safety.

Intervention With Rationale

- Teach the patient the proper administration of the drug to ensure therapeutic effect (see Box 54.2). The patient should be instructed to clear the nasal passages before use. Some formulations are administered with the head upright; for others, the patient should tilt their head slightly forward. The medication should be sprayed into the open nostril. The patient should breathe in through their nose. It is recommended that the patient refrain from blowing their nose for several minutes after administration.
- Caution the patient not to use the drug for longer than 5 days and to seek medical care if signs and symptoms persist after that time to facilitate detection of underlying medical conditions that may require treatment.
- Caution the patient that these drugs are found in many OTC preparations and that care should be taken not to inadvertently combine drugs with the same ingredients, which could lead to overdose.
- Provide safety measures if dizziness or sedation occurs as a result of drug therapy, to prevent patient injury.
- Institute other measures to help relieve the discomfort of congestion (e.g., use of a humidifier, increased fluid intake, cool environment, avoidance of smoke-filled areas) as appropriate.
- Provide thorough patient teaching, including the drug name and prescribed dosage, measures to help avoid adverse effects, warning signs that may indicate problems, and the need for periodic monitoring and evaluation, to enhance patient knowledge about drug therapy and to promote adherence.
- Offer support and encouragement to help the patient cope with the disease and the drug regimen.

Evaluation

- Monitor patient response to the drug (relief of nasal congestion).
- Monitor for adverse effects (local burning and stinging; adrenergic effects such as increased pulse, blood pressure, urinary retention, cool and clammy skin).
- Evaluate the effectiveness of the teaching plan (patient can name drug, dosage, adverse effects to watch for and specific measures to avoid them, measures to take to increase the effectiveness of the drug, proper administration technique).
- Monitor the effectiveness of comfort and safety measures and adherence to the regimen.

Oral Decongestants

The oral decongestants currently available for use are pseudoephedrine and phenylephrine (*Sudafed* and many combination products) (see Table 54.2).

Therapeutic Actions and Indications

Oral decongestants are drugs that are taken orally to decrease nasal congestion related to the common cold, sinusitis, and allergic rhinitis. They are also used to relieve the pain and congestion of otitis media. Opening of the nasal passage allows better drainage of the eustachian tube, relieving pressure in the middle ear.

Oral decongestants shrink the nasal mucous membrane by stimulating the alpha-adrenergic receptors in the nasal mucous membranes. This shrinkage results in a decrease in membrane size, promoting drainage of the sinuses and improving airflow.

Pharmacokinetics

Pseudoephedrine is generally well absorbed and reaches its peak level quickly, in 20 to 45 minutes. It is widely distributed in the body, metabolized in the liver, and primarily excreted in the urine. Phenylephrine is available in a nasal spray and combination products.

Contraindications and Cautions

Because these medications have adrenergic properties, caution should be used in patients with any condition that

Box 54.3 Focus on Safe Medication Administration

The ingredient pseudoephedrine has been used to make methamphetamine, so there are federal and state laws restricting sales amounts. Medications with pseudoephedrine are designated "behind-the-counter" instead of OTC. To procure a behind-the-counter medication, a patient does not need a prescription. However, the medications are sold in limited quantities and a pharmacist must allow access. This policy helps to limit the amount of pseudoephedrine that a person can buy. There are many cough and allergy OTC products that contain a combination of medications, so patients need to be able to read labels to be cautious when treating these symptoms without assistance from a provider and/or pharmacist.

might be exacerbated by sympathetic activity, such as glaucoma, hypertension, diabetes, thyroid disease, coronary disease, and prostate problems. Because there are no adequate studies about use during pregnancy and lactation, such use should be reserved for situations in which the benefit to the patient outweighs any potential risk to the fetus or neonate.

Adverse Effects

Adverse effects associated with these decongestants include rebound congestion. Because these drugs may be taken systemically, adverse effects related to the sympathomimetic effects are more likely to occur, including feelings of anxiety, tenseness, restlessness, tremors, hypertension, arrhythmias, sweating, and pallor. Pseudoephedrine is found in many "behind-the-counter" cold and flu preparations, and phenylephrine is OTC, so care must be taken to avoid inadvertent overdose when more than one such drug is used. There are safety measures in place limiting access to pseudoephedrine (Box 54.3).

Clinically Important Drug–Drug Interactions

Many behind-the-counter and OTC products, including cold remedies, allergy medications, and flu remedies, may contain pseudoephedrine or phenylephrine. Taking such products concurrently can cause serious adverse effects. Teach patients to read the labels to avoid inadvertent overdose.

Prototype Summary: Pseudoephedrine

Indications: Temporary relief of nasal congestion caused by the common cold, hay fever, and sinusitis; promotion of nasal and sinus drainage; relief of eustachian tube congestion.

Actions: Sympathomimetic effects; causes vasoconstriction in mucous membranes of nasal passages resulting in their shrinkage, which promotes drainage and improvement in ventilation.

Pharmacokinetics:

Route	Onset	Duration
Oral	30 min	4–6 h

$T_{1/2}$: 7 hours; metabolized in the liver and excreted in the urine.

Adverse Effects: Anxiety, restlessness, headache, dizziness, drowsiness, vision changes, seizures, hypertension, arrhythmias, pallor, nausea, vomiting, urinary retention, respiratory difficulty.

Nursing Considerations for Patients Receiving an Oral Decongestant

Assessment: History and Examination

- Assess for possible contraindications or cautions: any history of allergy to the drug and pregnancy or lactation, which are contraindications to drug use; hypertension or coronary artery disease, which require cautious use; and hyperthyroidism, diabetes mellitus, or prostate enlargement, all of which could be exacerbated by these drugs.
- Perform a physical examination to establish baseline data for assessing the effectiveness of the drug and the occurrence of any adverse effects associated with drug therapy.
- Assess skin color and lesions to monitor for adverse reactions.
- Evaluate orientation, reflexes, and affect to monitor CNS effects of the drug.
- Monitor blood pressure, pulse, and auscultation to assess CV stimulations.
- Evaluate respiration and adventitious sounds to monitor drug effectiveness.
- Monitor urinary output to evaluate for urinary retention.

Nursing Conclusions

Nursing conclusions related to drug therapy might include

- Impaired comfort related to GI, CNS, or skin effects of the drug
- Altered tissue perfusion related to sympathomimetic actions of the drug
- Altered sensory perception (kinesthetic) related to CNS effects
- Knowledge deficit regarding drug therapy

Planning

- The patient will receive the best therapeutic effect from the drug therapy.
- The patient will have limited adverse effects from the drug therapy.

(continues on page 966)

- The patient will have an understanding of the drug therapy, adverse effects to anticipate, and measures to relieve discomfort and improve safety.

Intervention With Rationale

- Note that these drugs are found in many behind-the-counter and OTC products, especially combination cold and allergy preparations; care should be taken to prevent inadvertent overdose or excessive adverse effects.
- Provide safety measures as needed if CNS effects occur, to prevent patient injury.
- Monitor pulse, blood pressure, and cardiac response to the drug, especially in patients who are at risk for adverse effects with sympathetic stimulation, to detect adverse effects early and arrange to reduce dose or discontinue the drug.
- Encourage the patient not to use these drugs for longer than 1 week and to seek medical evaluation if symptoms persist after that time to encourage the detection of underlying medical conditions that could be causing these symptoms and to arrange for appropriate treatment.
- Provide thorough patient teaching, including the drug name and prescribed dosage, measures to help avoid adverse effects, warning signs that may indicate problems, and the need for periodic monitoring and evaluation, to enhance patient knowledge about drug therapy and to promote adherence.
- Offer support and encouragement to help the patient cope with the disease and the drug regimen.

Evaluation

- Monitor patient response to the drug (improvement in nasal congestion).
- Monitor for adverse effects (sympathomimetic reactions, including increased pulse, blood pressure, pallor, sweating, arrhythmias, feelings of anxiety, tension, urinary retention, constipation).
- Evaluate the effectiveness of the teaching plan (patient can name drug, dosage, adverse effects to watch for and specific measures to avoid them, and measures to take to increase the effectiveness of the drug).
- Monitor the effectiveness of comfort and safety measures and adherence to the regimen.

Steroid Nasal Decongestants

Topical nasal steroid decongestants (see Table 54.2) include beclomethasone (*Beconase AQ* and others), budesonide (*Rhinocort*), flunisolide (generic), fluticasone (*Flonase Allergy Relief*), and triamcinolone (*Nasacort Allergy 24 Hour*).

Therapeutic Actions and Indications

Topical nasal steroid decongestants are used for the treatment of allergic rhinitis and to relieve inflammation after the removal of nasal polyps. They are first-line medications for nasal congestion. The exact mechanism of action of topical steroids is not known. Their anti-inflammatory action results from their ability to produce a direct local effect that blocks many of the complex reactions responsible for the inflammatory response.

Pharmacokinetics

The onset of action is not immediate, and these drugs may actually require up to 1 week to cause any changes. If no effects are seen after 3 weeks, the drug should be discontinued. Because these drugs are not generally absorbed systemically, their pharmacokinetics are not reported. If they were to be absorbed systemically, they would have the same pharmacokinetics as other steroids (see Chapter 36).

Contraindications and Cautions

Because nasal steroids block the inflammatory response, their use is contraindicated in the presence of acute infections. Increased incidence of *Candida albicans* infection has been reported with their use related to the anti-inflammatory and anti-immune activities associated with steroids. Caution should be used in any patient who has an active infection, including tuberculosis, because systemic absorption would interfere with the inflammatory and immune responses. Patients using nasal steroids should avoid exposure to any airborne infection, such as chickenpox or measles. As with all drugs, caution should always be used when taking these drugs during pregnancy or lactation, but because the systemic absorption of these drugs is minimal, they are often used during pregnancy and lactation.

Adverse Effects

Because they are applied topically, there is less chance of systemic absorption and associated adverse effects. The most common adverse effects are local burning, irritation, stinging, dryness of the mucosa, and headache. Because healing is suppressed by steroids, patients who have recently experienced nasal surgery or trauma should be monitored closely until healing has occurred.

Clinically Important Drug–Drug Interactions

The steroid nasal decongestants are applied topically and thus do not typically interact with other systemic medications. However, concurrent nasal medications should not be administered without discussion with a health care provider.

Prototype Summary: Flunisolide

Indications: Relief of the symptoms of seasonal or perennial allergic and nonallergic (vasomotor) rhinitis; relief of inflammation following removal of nasal polyps.

Actions: Anti-inflammatory action, which results from the ability to produce a direct local effect that blocks many of the complex reactions responsible for the inflammatory response.

Pharmacokinetics:

Route	Onset	Peak	Duration
Topical (nasal spray)	Fast <30 min	10–30 min	4–6 h

$T_{1/2}$: Not generally absorbed systemically.

Adverse Effects: Local burning, irritation, stinging, dryness of the mucosa, headache, increased risk of infection.

Nursing Considerations for Patients Receiving Steroid Nasal Decongestants

Assessment: History and Examination

- Assess for possible contraindications or cautions: any history of allergy to steroid drugs or any components of the drug, which would be a contraindication, and acute infection, which would require cautious use.
- Perform a physical examination to establish baseline data for assessing the effectiveness of the drug and the occurrence of any adverse effects associated with drug therapy.
- Perform an intranasal examination to determine the presence of any lesions that would increase the risk of systemic absorption of the drug.
- Monitor temperature to monitor for the possibility of acute infection.

Nursing Conclusions

Nursing conclusions related to drug therapy might include

- Impaired comfort related to local effects of the drug
- Infection risk related to suppression of inflammatory reaction
- Knowledge deficit regarding drug therapy

Planning

- The patient will receive the best therapeutic effect from the drug therapy.
- The patient will have limited adverse effects from the drug therapy.
- The patient will have an understanding of the drug therapy, adverse effects to anticipate, and measures to relieve discomfort and improve safety.

Intervention With Rationale

- Teach the patient how to administer these drugs properly, which is important to ensure effectiveness and prevent systemic effects. A variety of preparations are available, including sprays and aerosols. Advise the patient about the proper administration technique for whichever preparation is recommended.
- Have the patient clear the nasal passages before using the drug to improve its effectiveness.
- Encourage the patient to continue using the drug regularly, even if results are not seen immediately, because benefits may take 2 to 3 weeks to appear.
- Monitor the patient for the development of acute infection that would require medical intervention. Encourage the patient to avoid areas where airborne infections could be a problem because steroid use decreases the effectiveness of the immune and inflammatory responses.
- Provide thorough patient teaching, including the drug name and prescribed dosage, measures to help avoid adverse effects, warning signs that may indicate problems, and the need for periodic monitoring and evaluation, to enhance patient knowledge about drug therapy and to promote adherence.
- Offer support and encouragement to help the patient cope with the disease and the drug regimen.

Evaluation

- Monitor patient response to the drug (relief of nasal congestion).
- Monitor for adverse effects (local burning and stinging).
- Evaluate the effectiveness of the teaching plan (patient can name drug, dosage, adverse effects to watch for and specific measures to avoid them, and measures to take to increase the effectiveness of the drug).
- Monitor the effectiveness of comfort and safety measures and adherence to the regimen.

Key Points

- Decongestants cause local vasoconstriction, thereby reducing blood flow to the mucous membranes of the nasal passages and sinus cavities.
- Rebound vasodilation (rhinitis medicamentosa) is an adverse effect of excessive or long-term decongestant use.
- Topical nasal decongestants are preferred for patients who need to avoid the systemic adrenergic effects associated with oral decongestants.
- Topical nasal steroid decongestants block the inflammatory response and are preferred for patients with allergic rhinitis.

Antihistamines

Antihistamines (Table 54.3) block the release or action of histamine, a chemical released during inflammation that increases secretions and narrows airways. Antihistamines

Table 54.3 *Drugs in Focus:* Antihistamines

Drug Name	Usual Dosage	Usual Indications
First Generation		
brompheniramine (*BroveX, J-Tan, Lo-Hist 12, Respa-AR*)	*Adult and pediatric*: Oral dosing varies based on formulation	Relieves symptoms of common cold, sinusitis, and seasonal and perennial allergic rhinitis
carbinoxamine (*Karbinal ER*)	*Adults and pediatric (>12 y)*: 6–16 mg PO q12h *Pediatric (6–11 y)*: 6–12 mg PO q12h *Pediatric (4–5 y)*: 3–8 mg PO q12h *Pediatric (2–3 y)*: 3–4 mg PO q12h	Relieves nasal and nonnasal symptoms of seasonal and perennial rhinitis, vasomotor rhinitis, allergic conjunctivitis, and mild allergic skin reactions; therapy for anaphylactic reactions adjunctive to epinephrine and other standard measures after acute manifestations have been controlled
chlorpheniramine (*Aller-Chlor*, others)	*Adult and pediatric (>12 y)*: 4 mg PO q4–6h; 8–12 mg at bedtime for sustained release; use caution in older patients *Pediatric (6–12 y)*: 2 mg PO q4–6h *Pediatric (2–5 y)*: 1 mg PO q4–6h (sustained release) *Pediatric (6–12 y)*: 8 mg PO at bedtime *Pediatric (<6 y)*: Not recommended	Relieves symptoms of seasonal and perennial allergic rhinitis, allergic conjunctivitis, uncomplicated urticaria, and angioedema; amelioration of allergic reactions; relieves discomfort associated with dermographism; used as adjunctive therapy in anaphylactic reactions
clemastine (*Dayhist Allergy*)	*Adult and pediatric (>12 y)*: 1.34 mg PO b.i.d.; use caution with older patients *Pediatric (6–12 y)*: 0.67 mg PO b.i.d. *Pediatric (<6 y)*: Not recommended	Relieves symptoms of seasonal and perennial allergic rhinitis, allergic conjunctivitis, uncomplicated urticaria, and angioedema; amelioration of allergic reactions; relieves discomfort associated with dermographism; used as adjunctive therapy in anaphylactic reactions
cyproheptadine (generic)	*Adult*: 4–20 mg/d PO in divided doses *Pediatric (7–14 y)*: 4 mg PO b.i.d. to t.i.d. *Pediatric (2–6 y)*: 2 mg PO b.i.d. to t.i.d.	Relieves symptoms of seasonal and perennial allergic rhinitis, allergic conjunctivitis, uncomplicated urticaria, and angioedema; amelioration of allergic reactions; relieves discomfort associated with dermographism; used as adjunctive therapy in anaphylactic reactions
dexchlorpheniramine (generic)	*Adult and pediatric (>12 y)*: 4–6 mg PO at bedtime or q8–10h during the day *Pediatric (6–12 y)*: 4 mg/d PO at bedtime	Relieves symptoms of seasonal and perennial allergic rhinitis, allergic conjunctivitis, uncomplicated urticaria, and angioedema; amelioration of allergic reactions; relieves discomfort associated with dermographism; used as adjunctive therapy in anaphylactic reactions
dimenhydrinate (*Dimentabs*, others)	*Adult and pediatric (>12 y)*: 50–100 mg PO q4–6h or 50 mg IM as needed *Pediatric (<2 y)*: 1.25 mg/kg IM q.i.d. *Pediatric (2–6 y)*: 25 mg PO q6–8h *Pediatric (6–12 y)*: 25–50 mg PO q6–8h	Relieves nausea and vomiting associated with motion sickness
diphenhydramine (*Benadryl*, others)	*Adult*: 25–50 mg PO q4–6h or 10–50 mg IM or IV; use caution with older patients *Pediatric*: 12.5–25 mg PO t.i.d. to q.i.d. or 5 mg/kg/d IM or IV	Relieves symptoms of seasonal and perennial allergic rhinitis, allergic conjunctivitis, uncomplicated urticaria, and angioedema; amelioration of allergic reactions; relieves discomfort associated with dermographism; also used as adjunctive therapy in anaphylactic reactions, as a sleeping aid, and for parkinsonism
hydroxyzine (*Vistaril*, others)	*Adult*: 25–100 mg PO t.i.d. to q.i.d. or 25–100 mg IM q4–6h *Pediatric (>6 y)*: 50–100 mg/d PO in divided doses *Pediatric (<6 y)*: 50 mg/d PO in divided doses or 1.1 mg/kg per dose IM	Relieves symptoms of seasonal and perennial allergic rhinitis, allergic conjunctivitis, uncomplicated urticaria, and angioedema; amelioration of allergic reactions; relieves discomfort associated with dermographism; used as adjunctive therapy in anaphylactic reactions; also used for sedation

Table 54.3 *Drugs in Focus:* Antihistamines *(Continued)*

Drug Name	Usual Dosage	Usual Indications
meclizine (*Antivert*)	*Adult and pediatric (>12 y)*: 25–100 mg/d PO; use caution with older patients	Relieves nausea and vomiting associated with motion sickness
promethazine (*Phenergan*)	*Adult*: 25 mg PO, PR, IM, or IV *Pediatric*: 6.25–25 mg PO or PR	Relieves symptoms of seasonal and perennial allergic rhinitis, allergic conjunctivitis, uncomplicated urticaria, and angioedema; ameliorates allergic reactions; relieves discomfort associated with dermographism; used as adjunctive therapy in anaphylactic reactions; also used for sedation
triprolidine (generic)	*Adults and pediatric (≥12 y)*: 10 mL PO q4–6h *Pediatric (6–12 y)*: 5 mL PO q4–6h *Pediatric (4–6 y)*: 3.75 mL PO q4–6h *Pediatric (2–4 y)*: 2.5 mL PO q4–6h *Pediatric (4 mo–2 y)*: 1.25 mL PO q4–6h	Relieves signs and symptoms of seasonal and perennial allergic rhinitis
Second Generation (Nonsedating)		
azelastine (*Astelin, Astepro*)	*Adult and pediatric (>12 y)*: 1–2 sprays per nostril b.i.d. *Pediatric (5–11 y)*: 1 spray per nostril b.i.d. *Pediatric (6 m–11 y)*: 1 spray per nostril b.i.d. (*Astepro*)	Relieves symptoms of seasonal and perennial allergic rhinitis
cetirizine (*Zyrtec* and others)	*Adult and pediatric (>12 y)*: 10 mg/d PO or 5 mg PO b.i.d.; use 5 mg/d with hepatic or renal impairment *Pediatric (6–11 y)*: 5 or 10 mg/d PO *Pediatric (6 mo–5 y)*: 2.5 mg PO q12h *or* 5 mg/d PO	Relieves symptoms of seasonal and perennial allergic rhinitis; management of chronic urticaria
desloratadine (*Clarinex*)	*Adult and pediatric (>12 y)*: 5 mg/d PO *Pediatric (6–11 y)*: 1 tsp, 2.5 mg/5 mL/d PO *Pediatric (12 mo–5 y)*: 1/2 tsp, 1.25 mg/2.5 mL/d PO *Pediatric (6–11 mo)*: 1 mg/d PO *Hepatic or renal impairment*: 5 mg PO every other day	Relieves symptoms of seasonal allergic rhinitis and chronic idiopathic urticaria
fexofenadine (*Allegra Allergy*)	*Adult and pediatric (>12 y)*: 60 mg PO b.i.d. or 180 mg PO daily *Pediatric (6–11 y)*: 30 mg PO b.i.d. or 5-mL suspension b.i.d. *Pediatric (2–12 y)*: 5-mL suspension b.i.d. *Older or renal-impaired patient*: 60 mg PO every day	Relieves symptoms of seasonal and perennial allergic rhinitis
levocetirizine (*Xyzal Allergy 24 hour*)	*Adults and pediatric (≥12 y)*: 5 mg PO, once daily in the evening *Pediatric (6–11 y)*: 2.5 mg PO once daily in the evening *Pediatric (6 mo–5 y)*: 1.25-mg oral solution PO once daily in the evening	Relieves symptoms of seasonal and perennial allergic rhinitis; chronic idiopathic urticaria
loratadine (*Alavert, Claritin*)	*Adult and pediatric (>6 y)*: 10 mg/d PO; 1 tablet daily (*Alavert*) *Pediatric (2–5 y)*: 5 mg/d PO (syrup) *Older or hepatic-impaired patient*: 10 mg PO every other day	Relieves symptoms of seasonal and perennial allergic rhinitis, allergic conjunctivitis, uncomplicated urticaria, and angioedema; amelioration of allergic reactions; relieves discomfort associated with dermographism; used as adjunctive therapy in anaphylactic reactions
olopatadine (*Patanase*)	*Adults and pediatric (≥12 y)*: 2 sprays per nostril twice daily *Pediatric (6–11 y)*: 1 spray per nostril twice daily	Relieves symptoms of seasonal allergic rhinitis

are found in multiple OTC preparations that are designed to relieve respiratory symptoms and to treat symptoms of allergies. When choosing an antihistamine, the individual patient's reaction to the drug is usually the governing factor. Because first-generation antihistamines have greater anticholinergic effects with resultant drowsiness, a person who needs to be alert should be given one of the second-generation, less-sedating antihistamines. In some people, the second-generation antihistamines are also sedating, so care must be taken until the patient knows what response will occur. Because of their OTC availability, these drugs are often misused to treat colds and influenza (Box 54.4).

First-generation antihistamines include brompheniramine (*J-Tan* and others), carbinoxamine (*Karbinal ER*), chlorpheniramine (*Aller-Chlor* and others), clemastine (*Dayhist Allergy*), cyproheptadine (generic), dexchlorpheniramine (generic), dimenhydrinate (*Dimentabs* and others), diphenhydramine (*Benadryl* and others), hydroxyzine (*Vistaril* and others), meclizine (*Antivert*), promethazine (*Phenergan*), and triprolidine (generic).

Second-generation antihistamines include azelastine (*Astelin, Astepro*), cetirizine (*Zyrtec*), desloratadine (*Clarinex*), fexofenadine (*Allegra*), levocetirizine (*Xyzal*), loratadine (*Claritin*), and olopatadine (*Patanase*).

Therapeutic Actions and Indications

Antihistamines selectively block the effects of histamine at the histamine-1 receptor sites, decreasing the allergic response. They also have anticholinergic and antipruritic effects. Antihistamines are used for the relief of symptoms associated with seasonal and perennial allergic rhinitis, allergic conjunctivitis, uncomplicated urticaria, and angioedema. They are also used for the amelioration of allergic reactions to blood or blood products, for relief of discomfort associated with dermographism, and as adjunctive therapy in anaphylactic reactions. They are most effective for symptoms of itching, sneezing, and rhinorrhea. Some can be used to treat or prevent motion sickness and insomnia. See Table 54.3 for usual indications for each of these agents. Other uses that are being explored include relief of exercise- and hyperventilation-induced asthma and histamine-induced bronchoconstriction in asthmatics. They are most effective if used before the onset of symptoms.

Pharmacokinetics

Antihistamines are well absorbed orally with an onset of action ranging from 1 to 3 hours. They are generally metabolized in the liver, with excretion in the feces and urine. These drugs cross the placenta and enter human milk (see "Contraindications and Cautions").

Contraindications and Cautions

Antihistamines are contraindicated during pregnancy or lactation unless the benefit to the patient clearly outweighs the potential risk to the fetus or baby. Some of the medications have higher safety profiles than others, so medication labels should be evaluated to determine risk of use during pregnancy and/or lactation. Some should be used with caution, and there may need to be dosage adjustment for patients with renal or hepatic impairment, which could alter the metabolism and excretion of the drug. Special care should be taken when some of the first-generation antihis-

Box 54.4 Focus on Patient and Family Teaching

Following reports of serious and even fatal adverse effects when OTC cough and cold medicines were used in children under the age of 2 years, the FDA held meetings to evaluate the safety and efficacy of the use of these products in young children. The evidence continues to be evaluated, and current recommendations include the following:

- Do not give OTC cough and cold products to children younger than 2 years of age unless specifically instructed to do so by a health care provider.
- Cough medications that contain the opioids codeine and hydrocodone are not recommended for children younger than 18 years of age.
- Do not give your child OTC cough and cold medicines made for adults; look for children's, infant's, or pediatric use on the label.
- Always check the active ingredients on the drug label.
- Be careful if you are giving your child more than one cough and cold medicine; many contain the same active ingredients, and overdose can occur.
- Carefully follow the directions in the "Drug Facts" section of the label and follow the directions for how often you can give the drug.
- Use the measuring spoons or cups that come with the medicine; do not use household spoons, which can vary widely in the amount of medicine they hold.
- Use OTC cough and cold medicines with child-proof caps and keep them out of the reach of children to avoid possible overdose.
- Consult your health care provider; these drugs only treat signs and symptoms and do not cure any disease; contact your health care provider if the symptoms get worse.
- Do not use these products to make your child sleepy.
- Tell any health care provider taking care of your child the names of any OTC products that you are giving your child.
- Nondrug approaches to handling the symptoms of a cold include using a humidifier, making sure the child drinks plenty of fluids, use of a bulb syringe aspirator in younger children, use of saline nasal spray or drops to help with congestion, appropriate use of analgesics to help with any pain or discomfort, and positioning to promote drainage of fluids. If your child does not improve or continues to have a fever, consult your health care provider.

tamines are used by a patient with a history of arrhythmias or prolonged QT intervals because fatal cardiac arrhythmias have been associated with the use of certain antihistamines and drugs that increase QT intervals, including erythromycin. Box 54.4 presents topics for patient education in the use of these OTC products.

Adverse Effects

The adverse effects most often seen with antihistamine use are drowsiness and sedation (see "Critical Thinking Scenario" for additional information), though second-generation antihistamines are less sedating in many people. The anticholinergic effects that can be anticipated include drying of the respiratory and GI mucous membranes, GI upset and nausea, arrhythmias, dysuria, urinary hesitancy, and skin eruption and itching associated with dryness.

Clinically Important Drug–Drug Interactions

Drug–drug interactions vary among the antihistamines; for example, anticholinergic effects may be prolonged if

CRITICAL THINKING SCENARIO
Dangers of Self-Medicating for Seasonal Rhinitis

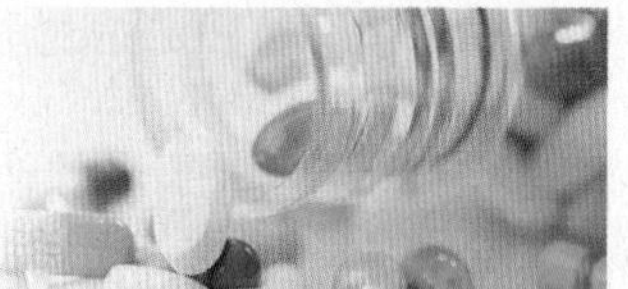

THE SITUATION

K.E. is a 46-year-old patient who has been self-treating for seasonal rhinitis and a cold. Their spouse calls the physician's office, concerned that K.E. is dizzy, has lost their balance several times, and is very drowsy. K.E. is unable to drive to work or to stay awake. K.E.'s spouse wants to take K.E. to the emergency department of the local hospital.

CRITICAL THINKING

What is the best approach for this patient?
What crucial patient history questions should you ask before proceeding any further?
If you do not know this patient, given their presenting story, what medical conditions would need to be ruled out before proceeding?
If K.E. is self-medicating for the signs and symptoms of seasonal rhinitis, what could be causing the drowsiness and dizziness?
What teaching points should be emphasized with this patient and their spouse?

DISCUSSION

The first impression of K.E.'s condition is that it is a neurological disorder. K.E. should be evaluated by a health care provider to rule out significant neurological problems. However, after a careful patient history and physical examination, K.E.'s condition seemed to be related to high levels of OTC medications.

There are a multitude of OTC cold and allergy remedies, most of which contain the same ingredients in varying proportions. A patient may be taking one to stop their nasal drip, another to help their cough, another to relieve congestion, and so on. By combining OTC medications like this, a patient is at great risk for inadvertently overdosing or at least allowing the medication to reach toxic levels.

In this situation, the first thing to determine is exactly what medications are being taken and how often. K.E. seems to have suffered from adverse reactions to the antihistamines, decongestants, or other upper respiratory tract agents. The nurse should encourage K.E.—and all patients—to check the labels of any OTC medications being taken and to check with the health care provider if there are any questions. K.E. and their spouse should receive written information about the drugs that K.E. is taking. They also should be shown how to read OTC bottles or boxes for information on the contents of various preparations. In addition, they should be encouraged to use alternative methods to relieve the discomfort of seasonal rhinitis (e.g., using a humidifier, drinking lots of liquids, and avoiding smoky areas) to allay the belief that many OTC drugs are needed. Finally, K.E. and their spouse should be advised to check with their health care provider if they have any questions about OTC or prescription drugs or if they have continued problems coping with seasonal allergic reactions. Other prescription medication may prove more effective.

NURSING CARE GUIDE FOR K.E.: ANTIHISTAMINES

Assessment: History and Examination

Assess K.E.'s health history for allergies and GI stenosis or obstruction, bladder obstruction, narrow-angle glaucoma, benign prostatic hypertrophy, and concurrent use of MAO inhibitors and OTC allergy or cold products.

Focus the physical examination on

CNS: Orientation, reflexes, affect, coordination
Skin: Lesions
CV: Blood pressure, pulse, peripheral perfusion
GI: Bowel sounds, abdominal exam
Hematological: Complete blood count
Respiratory: Respiratory rate and character, nares, adventitious sounds
Genitourinary (GU): Urinary output

Nursing Conclusions

Impaired comfort related to GI effects or dry mouth
Altered sensory perception (kinesthetic)

(continues on page 972)

Safety risk due to dizziness and/or sedation
Knowledge deficit regarding drug therapy

Planning

The patient will receive the best therapeutic effect from the drug therapy.
The patient will have limited adverse effects from the drug therapy.
The patient will have an understanding of the drug therapy, adverse effects to anticipate, and measures to relieve discomfort and improve safety.

Intervention

Provide comfort and safety measures (e.g., reduce risk of falls and GI discomfort); teach about mouth care; increase humidity.
Provide support and reassurance to deal with drug effects and allergy.
Provide patient teaching regarding drug name, dosage, adverse effects, precautions, and warning signs to report.

Evaluation

Evaluate drug effects (relief of respiratory symptoms).
Monitor for adverse effects: CNS effects, thickening of secretions, urinary retention, constipation, sedation, dizziness, glaucoma.
Monitor for drug–drug interactions as indicated.
Evaluate the effectiveness of support and encouragement strategies, patient teaching program, and comfort and safety measures.

PATIENT TEACHING FOR K.E.

- Antihistamines are commonly used to treat the signs and symptoms of various allergic reactions. Because these drugs work throughout the body, their use can cause many systemic effects (e.g., dry mouth, dizziness, drowsiness, constipation).
- Some of the antihistamines have less risk for adverse effects compared to others.
- Take this drug only as prescribed. Do not increase the dose if symptoms are not relieved. Instead, consult your health care provider.
- Common effects of this drug include
  - *Drowsiness, dizziness*: Do not drive or operate dangerous machinery if this occurs. Use caution to prevent injury.
  - *GI upset, nausea, vomiting, heartburn*: Taking the drug with food may help this problem.
  - *Dry mouth*: Frequent mouth care and sucking sugarless lozenges may help.
  - *Thickening of the mucus, difficulty coughing, tightening of the chest*: Use a humidifier, or if you do not have one, place pans of water throughout the house to increase the humidity of the room air; avoid smoke-filled areas; drink plenty of fluids.
  - Report any of the following to your health care provider: difficulty breathing, rash, hives, difficulty voiding, abdominal pain, visual changes, and disorientation or confusion.
- Avoid the use of alcoholic beverages while you are taking this drug. Serious drowsiness or sedation can occur if these are combined.
- Avoid the use of any OTC medication without first checking with your health care provider. Several of these medications contain drugs that can interfere with the effectiveness of this drug, or they can contain similar drugs and you could experience toxic effects.
- Tell any doctor, nurse, or other health care provider involved in your care that you are taking this drug.
- Take this drug only as prescribed. Do not give this drug to anyone else, and do not take similar preparations that have been prescribed for someone else. Keep this drug and all medications out of the reach of children.

---

diphenhydramine is taken with an MAO inhibitor, and the interaction of fexofenadine with ketoconazole or erythromycin may raise fexofenadine concentrations to toxic levels. Concurrent use with other CNS depressants can increase the sedative effect of the antihistamines. For more information, consult a nursing drug handbook or package insert for individual details.

Prototype Summary: Diphenhydramine

Indications: Symptomatic relief of perennial and seasonal rhinitis, vasomotor rhinitis, allergic conjunctivitis, urticaria, and angioedema; also used for treating motion sickness and parkinsonism and as a nighttime sleep aid and to suppress coughs.

Actions: Competitively blocks the effects of histamine at histamine-1 receptor sites; has atropinelike antipruritic and sedative effects.

Pharmacokinetics:

Route	Onset	Peak	Duration
Oral	15–30 min	1–4 h	4–7 h
IM	20–30 min	1–4 h	4–8 h
IV	Rapid	30–60 min	4–8 h

$T_{1/2}$: 2.5 to 7 hours; metabolized in the liver and excreted in the urine.

Adverse Effects: Drowsiness, sedation, dizziness, epigastric distress, thickening of bronchial secretions, urinary retention, rash, bradycardia.

Nursing Considerations for Patients Receiving Antihistamines

Assessment: History and Examination

- Assess for possible contraindications or cautions: any history of allergy to antihistamines, pregnancy or lactation, or prolonged QT interval, which are contraindications or cautions to the use of the drugs; and renal or hepatic impairment, which may require cautious use of the drug.
- Perform a physical examination to establish baseline data for assessing the effectiveness of the drug and the occurrence of any adverse effects associated with drug therapy.
- Assess the skin color, texture, and lesions to monitor for anticholinergic effects or allergy.
- Evaluate orientation, affect, and reflexes to monitor for changes due to CNS effects.
- Assess respirations and adventitious sounds to monitor for drug effects.
- Evaluate liver and renal function tests to monitor for factors that could affect the metabolism or excretion of the drug.

Nursing Conclusions

Nursing conclusions related to drug therapy might include

- Impaired comfort related to GI, CNS, or skin effects of the drug
- Altered sensory perception (kinesthetic) related to CNS effects
- Safety risk due to dizziness and/or sedation
- Knowledge deficit regarding drug therapy

Planning

- The patient will receive the best therapeutic effect from the drug therapy.
- The patient will have limited adverse effects from the drug therapy.
- The patient will have an understanding of the drug therapy, adverse effects to anticipate, and measures to relieve discomfort and improve safety.

Intervention With Rationale

- Administer the drug on an empty stomach 1 hour before or 2 hours after meals to increase the absorption of the drug; the drug may be given with meals if GI upset is a problem.
- Note that the patient may have poor response to one of these agents but an effective response to another; the prescriber may need to try several different agents to find the one that is most effective.
- Because of the drying nature of antihistamines, patients often experience dry mouth; suggest sugarless candies or lozenges to relieve some of this discomfort.
- Provide safety measures as appropriate if CNS effects occur to prevent patient injury.
- Increase humidity and hydration to decrease the problem of thickened secretions and dry nasal mucosa.
- Provide skin care as needed if skin dryness and lesions become a problem to prevent skin breakdown.
- Caution the patient to avoid an excessive dose and to check OTC drugs for the presence of antihistamines, which are found in many OTC preparations and could cause toxicity.
- Caution the patient to avoid alcohol and other CNS depressants while taking these drugs because concurrent use can increase sedation.
- Provide thorough patient teaching, including the drug name and prescribed dosage, measures to help avoid adverse effects, warning signs that may indicate problems, and the need for periodic monitoring and evaluation, to enhance patient knowledge about drug therapy and to promote adherence.
- Offer support and encouragement to help the patient cope with the disease and the drug regimen.

Evaluation

- Monitor patient response to the drug (relief of the symptoms of allergic rhinitis).
- Monitor for adverse effects (skin dryness, GI upset, sedation and drowsiness, constipation, thickened secretions, glaucoma).
- Evaluate the effectiveness of the teaching plan (patient can name drug, dosage, adverse effects to watch for and specific measures to avoid them, and measures to take to increase the effectiveness of the drug).
- Monitor the effectiveness of comfort and safety measures and adherence to the regimen.

Key Points

- Antihistamines selectively block the effects of histamine at the histamine-1 receptor sites, decreasing the allergic response. Antihistamines are used for the relief of symptoms associated with seasonal and perennial allergic rhinitis, allergic conjunctivitis, uncomplicated urticaria, and angioedema.
- Patients taking antihistamines may have dryness of the skin and mucous membranes. The nurse should encourage them to drink plenty of fluids, use a humidifier if possible, avoid smoke-filled rooms, and use good skin care and moisturizers.
- Some first-generation antihistamines should be avoided with any patient who has a prolonged QT interval because serious cardiac complications and even death have occurred.

Table 54.4 *Drugs in Focus*: Expectorant

Drug Name	Usual Dosage	Usual Indications
guaifenesin (*Mucinex*)	*Adult and pediatric (>12 y)*: 200–400 mg PO q4h or 600–1,200 mg PO ER tablets q12h *Pediatric (6–12 y)*: 100–200 mg PO q4h or 600 mg PO ER tablets q12h *Pediatric (2–6 y)*: 50–100 mg PO q4h	Relieves symptoms of respiratory conditions

Expectorants

Expectorants (Table 54.4) increase productive cough to clear the airways. They liquefy lower respiratory tract secretions, reducing the viscosity of these secretions and making it easier for the patient to cough them up. Expectorants are available in many OTC combination preparations, making them widely available to the patient without advice from a health care provider. Currently, the only available expectorant sold outside of the combination formulations is guaifenesin (*Mucinex*).

Therapeutic Actions and Indications

Guaifenesin enhances the output of respiratory tract fluids by reducing the adhesiveness and surface tension of these fluids, allowing easier movement of the less viscous secretions. The results of this thinning of secretions are a more productive cough and enhanced patency of the respiratory airways. See Table 54.4 for usual indications.

Pharmacokinetics

Guaifenesin is rapidly absorbed with an onset of 30 minutes and a duration of 4 to 6 hours. Sites of metabolism and excretion have not been reported.

Contraindications and Cautions

This drug should not be used in patients with a known allergy to the drug to prevent hypersensitivity reactions, and it should be used with caution in pregnancy and lactation because of the potential for adverse effects on the fetus or baby and with persistent coughs, which could be indicative of underlying medical problems.

Adverse Effects

The most common adverse effects associated with expectorants are GI symptoms (e.g., nausea, vomiting, anorexia). Some patients experience headache, dizziness, or both. A rash may be a sign of an allergic reaction. The most important consideration in the use of these drugs is diagnosing the cause of the underlying cough. Prolonged use of OTC preparations could result in the masking of important symptoms of a serious underlying disorder. These drugs should not be used for more than 1 week; if the cough persists, encourage the patient to seek health care.

Clinically Important Drug–Drug Interactions

There are no known significant drug interactions with guaifenesin. However, patients should be cautioned that there may be drug interactions with other medications that guaifenesin is combined with in OTC formulations.

Prototype Summary: Guaifenesin

Indications: Symptomatic relief of respiratory conditions by thinning mucous secretions, promoting ability to expel mucous and decrease respiratory congestion.

Actions: Enhances the output of respiratory tract fluid by reducing the adhesiveness and surface tension of the fluid, facilitating the removal of viscous mucus.

Pharmacokinetics:

Route	Onset	Peak	Duration
Oral	30 min	Unknown	4–6 h

$T_{1/2}$: Unknown; metabolism and excretion are also unknown.

Adverse Effects: Nausea, vomiting, headache, dizziness, rash.

Nursing Considerations for Patients Receiving Expectorants

Assessment: History and Examination

- Assess for possible contraindications or cautions: any history of allergy to the drug; persistent cough due to smoking, asthma, or emphysema, which would be cautions to the use of the drug; and productive cough lasting more than a week, which would indicate an underlying problem that should be evaluated.
- Perform a physical examination to establish baseline data for assessing the effectiveness of the drug and the occurrence of any adverse effects associated with drug therapy.
- Assess the skin for the presence of rash to monitor for any sign of allergic reaction.
- Monitor temperature to assess for an underlying infection.

- Assess respirations and adventitious sounds to evaluate the respiratory response to the drug effects.
- Monitor orientation and affect to monitor CNS effects of the drug.

Nursing Conclusions

Nursing conclusions related to drug therapy might include

- Impaired comfort related to GI, CNS, or skin effects of the drug
- Altered sensory perception (kinesthetic) related to CNS effects
- Knowledge deficit regarding drug therapy

Planning

- The patient will receive the best therapeutic effect from the drug therapy.
- The patient will have limited adverse effects from the drug therapy.
- The patient will have an understanding of the drug therapy, adverse effects to anticipate, and measures to relieve discomfort and improve safety.

Intervention With Rationale

- Caution the patient not to use these drugs for longer than 1 week and to seek medical attention if the cough persists after that time to evaluate for any underlying medical condition and to arrange for appropriate treatment.
- Advise the patient to take small, frequent meals to alleviate some of the GI discomfort associated with these drugs.
- Advise the patient to avoid driving or performing dangerous tasks if dizziness and drowsiness occur, to prevent patient injury.
- Alert the patient that these drugs may be found in OTC preparations and that care should be taken to avoid excessive doses.
- Provide thorough patient teaching, including the drug name and prescribed dosage, measures to help avoid adverse effects, warning signs that may indicate problems, and the need for periodic monitoring and evaluation, to enhance patient knowledge about drug therapy and to promote adherence.
- Offer support and encouragement to help the patient cope with the disease and the drug regimen.

Evaluation

- Monitor patient response to the drug (improved effectiveness of cough).
- Monitor for adverse effects (skin rash, GI upset, CNS effects).
- Evaluate the effectiveness of the teaching plan (patient can name drug, dosage, adverse effects to watch for and specific measures to avoid them, and measures to take to increase the effectiveness of the drug).
- Monitor the effectiveness of comfort and safety measures and adherence to the regimen.

Key Points

- Expectorants are drugs that liquefy respiratory tract secretions. They are used for the symptomatic relief of respiratory conditions in which thick mucus exacerbates cough and decreases airway patency.
- Guaifenesin is the only expectorant currently available. Care should be taken to avoid inadvertent overdose when using OTC and/or combination products that contain this drug.

Mucolytics

Mucolytics (Table 54.5) increase or liquefy respiratory secretions to aid the clearing of the airways in high-risk respiratory patients who are coughing up thick, tenacious secretions. Patients may be suffering from conditions such as chronic obstructive pulmonary disease (COPD), cystic fibrosis, pneumonia, or tuberculosis. Mucolytics include acetylcysteine (generic) and dornase alfa (*Pulmozyme*).

Therapeutic Actions and Indications

Acetylcysteine is used orally or intravenously to protect liver cells from being damaged during episodes of acetaminophen toxicity because it normalizes hepatic glutathione levels and binds with a reactive hepatotoxic metabolite of acetaminophen. Acetylcysteine affects the mucoproteins in the respiratory secretions by splitting apart disulfide bonds that are responsible for holding the mucus material together. The result is a decrease in the tenacity and viscosity of the secretions. See Table 54.5 for usual indications.

Dornase alfa is a mucolytic prepared by recombinant DNA techniques that selectively break down respiratory tract mucus by separating extracellular DNA from proteins. It is used in cystic fibrosis, which is characterized by thick, tenacious mucous production. See Table 54.5 for usual indications. See Box 54.5 for information about targeted treatment of cystic fibrosis.

Pharmacokinetics

The medication may be administered by nebulization or by direct instillation into the trachea via an endotracheal tube or tracheostomy.

Acetylcysteine is metabolized in the liver and excreted somewhat in the urine. It is not known whether it crosses the placenta or enters human milk. Dornase alfa is metabolized by proteases, and its half-life is 3 to 4 hours.

Contraindications and Cautions

The medications are contraindicated in patients who have history of hypersensitivity reactions to the medications or components in the medications. Caution should be used with patients who have asthma due to potential for bronchospasm. There are no adequate human studies to

Table 54.5 *Drugs in Focus*: Mucolytics

Drug Name	Usual Dosage	Usual Indications
acetylcysteine (generic)	By nebulization, 2–20 mL of 10% solution q2–6h; by direct instillation, 1–2 mL of 10%–20% solution q1–4h; 300 mg/kg given intravenously as 3 separate doses for treatment of acetaminophen overdose	Liquefaction of secretions in high-risk respiratory patients who have difficulty moving secretions, including postoperative patients (e.g., patients with tracheostomies to facilitate airway clearance and suctioning); clearing of secretions for diagnostic tests (e.g., diagnostic bronchoscopy); used orally to protect the liver from acetaminophen toxicity; treatment of atelectasis from thick mucus secretions
dornase alfa (*Pulmozyme*)	2.5 mg inhaled through nebulizer, may increase to 2.5 mg b.i.d. if needed	Relieves buildup of secretions in high-risk respiratory patients who have difficulty moving secretions, including postoperative patients (e.g., patients with tracheostomies to facilitate airway clearance and suctioning); clearing of secretions for diagnostic tests (e.g., diagnostic bronchoscopy); treatment of atelectasis from thick mucus secretions as in cystic fibrosis

evaluate risk during pregnancy or lactation, but there has been no evidence of fetal harm in animal studies.

Adverse Effects

Adverse effects most commonly associated with mucolytic drugs include GI upset, stomatitis, rhinorrhea, bronchospasm, and occasionally a rash.

Clinically Important Drug–Drug Interactions

There are no known drug interactions with acetylcysteine or dornase alfa.

BOX 54.5

Targeted Treatment of Cystic Fibrosis

Between 2012 and 2019, several medications were approved by the FDA for treatment of cystic fibrosis. Ivacaftor (*Kalydeco*) and combination medications that include ivacaftor (*Orkambi*, *Symdeko*, and *Trikafta*) are designed as targeted treatment for patients with cystic fibrosis. Ivacaftor is a cystic fibrosis transmembrane conductance regulator (CFTR) that facilitates increased chloride transport at the surface of epithelial cells in multiple organs. In cystic fibrosis patients taking this drug, the end result was improved lung function. Ivacaftor is approved for patients 4 months of age and older who have a type of CFTR gene mutation that is responsive to ivacaftor. If the patient's genotype is not known, tests should be run to attempt to detect a CFTR mutation. The FDA has approved a cystic fibrosis mutation test that can be used to determine the appropriateness of this drug. It is an oral agent and needs to be used with caution in patients with liver impairment or those also using CYP3A inhibitors. The most common adverse effects include abdominal pain, rash, nausea, dizziness, headache, and sore throat. A serious but rare effect can be the development of noncongenital lens opacities/cataracts in pediatric patients.

Prototype Summary: Acetylcysteine

Indications: Mucolytic adjunctive therapy for abnormal, viscid, or inspissated mucous secretions in acute and chronic bronchopulmonary disorders; to lessen hepatic injury in cases of acetaminophen toxicity.

Actions: Splits links in the mucoproteins contained in the respiratory mucus secretions, decreasing the viscosity of the secretions; protects liver cells from acetaminophen effects.

Pharmacokinetics:

Route	Onset	Peak	Duration
Instillation, inhalation	1 min	5–10 min	2–3 h
Oral	30–60 min	1–2 h	Unknown

$T_{1/2}$: 6.25 hours; metabolized in the liver and excreted in the urine.

Adverse Effects: Nausea, stomatitis, urticaria, bronchospasm, rhinorrhea.

Nursing Considerations for Patients Receiving Mucolytics

Assessment: History and Examination

- Assess for possible contraindications or cautions: any history of allergy to the drugs and the presence of acute bronchospasm, which are contraindications to the use of these drugs.
- Perform a physical examination to establish baseline data for assessing the effectiveness of the drug and the occurrence of any adverse effects associated with drug therapy.

- Assess skin color and lesions to monitor for adverse reactions.
- Monitor blood pressure and pulse to evaluate cardiac response to drug treatment.
- Evaluate respirations and adventitious sounds to monitor drug effectiveness.

Nursing Conclusions

Nursing conclusions related to drug therapy might include

- Impaired comfort related to GI, CNS, or skin effects of the drug
- Altered sensory perception (kinesthetic) related to CNS effects
- Ineffective airway clearance related to bronchospasm
- Knowledge deficit regarding drug therapy

Planning

- The patient will receive the best therapeutic effect from the drug therapy.
- The patient will have limited adverse effects from the drug therapy.
- The patient will have an understanding of the drug therapy, adverse effects to anticipate, and measures to relieve discomfort and improve safety.

Intervention With Rationale

- Avoid combining with other drugs in the nebulizer to avoid the formation of precipitates and the potential loss of effectiveness of either drug.
- Dilute the concentrate with sterile water for injection if buildup becomes a problem that could impede drug delivery.
- Note that patients receiving acetylcysteine by face mask should have the residue wiped off the face mask and off the face with plain water to prevent skin breakdown.
- Review use of the nebulizer with patients receiving dornase alfa at home to ensure the most effective use of the drug. Patients should be cautioned to store the drug in the refrigerator, protected from light.
- Caution cystic fibrosis patients receiving dornase alfa about the need to continue all therapies for their cystic fibrosis because dornase alfa is only a palliative therapy that improves respiratory symptoms and other therapies are still needed.
- Provide thorough patient teaching, including the drug name and prescribed dosage, measures to help avoid adverse effects, warning signs that may indicate problems, and the need for periodic monitoring and evaluation, to enhance patient knowledge about drug therapy and to promote adherence.
- Offer support and encouragement to help the patient cope with the disease and the drug regimen.

Evaluation

- Monitor patient response to the drug (improvement of respiratory symptoms and loosening of secretions).
- Monitor for adverse effects (CNS effects, skin rash, bronchospasm, and GI upset).
- Evaluate the effectiveness of the teaching plan (patient can name drug, dosage, adverse effects to watch for and specific measures to avoid them, and measures to take to increase the effectiveness of the drug).
- Monitor the effectiveness of comfort and safety measures and adherence to the regimen.

Key Points

- Mucolytics work to break down mucus to aid high-risk respiratory patients in coughing up thick, tenacious secretions.
- Dornase alfa is specific for the treatment of patients with cystic fibrosis, which is characterized by a thick, tenacious mucus production that can block airways.

SUMMARY

- Antitussives are drugs that suppress the cough reflex. They can act centrally to suppress the respiratory cough center or locally to increase secretion and buffer irritation or to act as local anesthetics. These drugs should not be used longer than 1 week; patients with persistent cough after that time should seek medical evaluation.
- Decongestants are drugs that cause local vasoconstriction and, therefore, decrease the blood flow to the irritated and dilated capillaries of the mucous membranes lining the nasal passages and sinus cavities.
- An adverse effect that may accompany frequent or prolonged use of topical decongestants is rebound vasodilation, called rhinitis medicamentosa. The reflex reaction to vasoconstriction is a rebound vasodilation, which can lead to prolonged overuse of decongestants.
- Topical nasal decongestants are preferable in patients who need to avoid systemic adrenergic effects. Oral decongestants are associated with more systemic adrenergic effects and require caution in patients with CV disease, hyperthyroidism, or diabetes mellitus.
- Nasal steroid decongestants block the inflammatory response from occurring. These drugs, which take several days to weeks to reach complete effectiveness, are preferred therapy for patients with allergic rhinitis.

- The antihistamines selectively block the effects of histamine at the histamine-1 receptor sites, decreasing the allergic response. Antihistamines are used for the relief of symptoms associated with seasonal and perennial allergic rhinitis, allergic conjunctivitis, uncomplicated urticaria, or angioedema.
- Patients taking antihistamines may react to dryness of the skin and mucous membranes. The nurse should encourage them to drink plenty of fluids, use a humidifier if possible, avoid smoke-filled rooms, and use good skin care and moisturizers.
- Some first-generation antihistamines should be avoided with any patient who has a prolonged QT interval because serious cardiac complications and even death have occurred.
- Expectorants are drugs that liquefy lower respiratory tract secretions. They are used for the symptomatic relief of respiratory conditions characterized by cough in conjunction with thick viscous mucus.
- Mucolytics work to break down mucus to aid high-risk respiratory patients in coughing up thick, tenacious secretions.
- Many of the drugs that act on the upper respiratory tract are found in various OTC cough and allergy preparations. Many of these preparations are a combination of medications. Patients need to be advised to always read the labels carefully to avoid inadvertent overdose and toxicity.

Unfolding Patient Stories: Yoa Li • Part 2

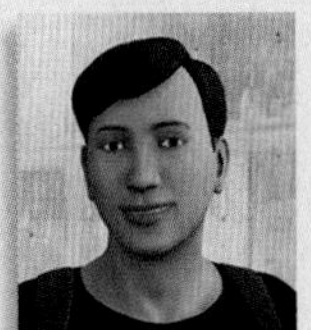

Recall Yoa Li, a 26-year-old male with a strangulated groin hernia from Chapter 26. He arrived on the medical–surgical unit following surgical repair of the hernia. What are the desired outcomes for postoperative pain management? What assessments should the nurse perform when administering morphine intravenously and evaluating Yoa's response?

Care for Yoa and other patients in a realistic virtual environment: ***vSim** for Nursing* (thepoint.lww.com/vSimPharm). Practice documenting these patients' care in DocuCare (thepoint.lww.com/DocuCareEHR).

CHECK YOUR UNDERSTANDING

Answers to the questions in this chapter can be found in Answers to Check Your Understanding Questions on thePoint®.

MULTIPLE CHOICE

Select the best answer.

1. A patient with sinus pressure and pain related to seasonal rhinitis would benefit from taking a(n)
   a. antitussive.
   b. expectorant.
   c. mucolytic.
   d. decongestant.
2. Antitussives are useful in blocking the cough reflex and preserving the energy associated with prolonged, nonproductive coughing. Antitussives are best used with
   a. postoperative patients.
   b. asthma patients.
   c. patients with a dry, irritating cough.
   d. COPD patients who tire easily.
3. Patients with seasonal rhinitis experience irritation and inflammation of the nasal passages and passages of the upper airways. Treatment for these patients might include
   a. systemic corticosteroids.
   b. mucolytic agents.
   c. an expectorant.
   d. topical nasal steroids.
4. A patient taking a behind-the-counter cold medication and a behind-the-counter allergy medicine is found to be taking double doses of pseudoephedrine. As a result, the patient might exhibit
   a. ear pain and eye redness.
   b. restlessness and palpitations.
   c. sinus pressure and ear pain.
   d. an irritating cough and nasal drainage.

5. Common adverse effects that can occur in patients taking antihistamines include
   a. sedation and anticholinergic effects.
   b. bacterial and fungal infections.
   c. diarrhea and insomnia.
   d. cough and fever.

6. A patient is not getting a response to the antihistamine that was prescribed. Appropriate action might include
   a. switching to a decongestant.
   b. stopping the drug and increasing fluids.
   c. trying a different antihistamine.
   d. switching to a corticosteroid.

7. Dornase alfa (*Pulmozyme*), because of its mechanism of action, is reserved for use in
   a. clearing secretions before diagnostic tests.
   b. facilitating the removal of secretions postoperatively.
   c. protecting the liver from acetaminophen toxicity.
   d. relieving the buildup of secretions in cystic fibrosis.

MULTIPLE RESPONSE

Select all that apply.

1. Common adverse effects associated with the use of topical nasal steroids would include which conditions?
   a. Local burning and stinging
   b. Dryness of the mucosa
   c. Headache
   d. Constipation and urinary retention
   e. Fungal infections
   f. Osteonecrosis

2. An antihistamine would be the drug of choice for treating which conditions?
   a. Itchy eyes
   b. Irritating cough
   c. Nasal congestion
   d. Runny nose
   e. Idiopathic urticaria
   f. Thick, tenacious secretions

3. Additional nursing interventions for patients receiving antihistamines would probably include which recommendations?
   a. Using a humidifier
   b. Advising the patient to suck sugarless lozenges to help relieve dry mouth
   c. Limiting fluid intake to decrease swelling
   d. Providing safety measures to prevent falls or injury
   e. Encouraging pushing fluids, if allowed
   f. Placing bowls of water around the house to increase humidity

REFERENCES

Brunton, L., Hilal-dandan, R., & Knollman, B. (2018). *Goodman and Gilman's the pharmacological basis of therapeutics* (13th ed.). McGraw-Hill.

Dykewicz, M. (2011). Management of rhinitis: Guidelines, evidence basis and systematic clinical approach. *Immunology and Allergy Clinics of North America, 31*(3), 619–634. 10.1016/j.iac.2011.05.002

Irwin, R. S., Baumann, M. H., Bolser, D. C., Boulet, L., Braman, S. S., Brightling, C. E., Brown, K. K., Canning, B. J., Chang, A. B., Dicpinigaitis, P. V., Eccles, R., Glomb, W. B., Goldstein, L. B., Graham, L. M., Hargreave, F. E., Kvale, P. A., Lewis, S. Z., McCool, F. D., McCrory, D. C., … Tarlo, S. M. (2006). Diagnosis and management of cough executive summary: ACCP evidence-based clinical practice guidelines. *Chest, 129*(1 Suppl), 1S–23S. 10.1378/chest.129.1_suppl.1S

Nguyen, P., Vickery, J., & Blaiss, M. (2011). Management of rhinitis: Allergic and non-allergic. *Allergy, Asthma and Immunology Research, 3*(3), 148–156. 10.4168/aair.2011.3.3.148

Tharpe, C., & Kemp, S. (2015). Pediatric allergic rhinitis. *Immunology and Allergy Clinics of North America, 35*(1), 185–198. 10.1016/j.iac.2014.09.003

CHAPTER 55

Drugs Acting on the Lower Respiratory Tract

Learning Objectives

Upon completion of this chapter, you will be able to:

1. Describe the underlying pathophysiology involved in obstructive pulmonary disease and correlate this information with the presenting signs and symptoms.
2. Discuss the use of drugs used to treat obstructive pulmonary disorders across the lifespan.
3. Describe the therapeutic actions, indications, pharmacokinetics, contraindications, most common adverse effects, and important drug–drug interactions associated with drugs used to treat lower respiratory tract disorders.
4. Compare and contrast the prototype drugs used to treat obstructive pulmonary disorders with other agents in their classes and with other classes of drugs used to treat obstructive pulmonary disorders.
5. Outline the nursing considerations, including important teaching points, for patients receiving drugs used to treat obstructive pulmonary disorders.

Key Terms

bronchodilator: medication used to facilitate respirations by dilating the airways; helpful in symptomatic relief or prevention of bronchial asthma and bronchospasm associated with chronic obstructive pulmonary disease (COPD)

Cheyne-Stokes respiration: abnormal pattern of breathing characterized by apneic periods followed by periods of tachypnea; may reflect delayed blood flow through the brain

leukotriene receptor antagonists: drugs that selectively and competitively block or antagonize receptors for the production of leukotrienes D_4 and E_4, components of slow-reacting substance of anaphylaxis (SRSA)

mast cell stabilizer: drug that prevents the release of inflammatory and bronchoconstricting substances from mast cells

sympathomimetics: drugs that mimic the effects of the sympathetic nervous system

xanthines: naturally occurring substances, including caffeine and theophylline, that have a direct effect on the smooth muscle of the respiratory tract, both in the bronchi and in the blood vessels

Drug List

BRONCHODILATORS/ ANTIASTHMATICS

Xanthines
aminophylline
caffeine
(P) theophylline

Sympathomimetics
(P) albuterol
arformoterol
ephedrine
epinephrine
formoterol
indacaterol
isoproterenol
levalbuterol
metaproterenol
olodaterol
salmeterol
terbutaline

Anticholinergics
aclidinium
glycopyrrolate
(P) ipratropium
revefenacin
tiotropium
umeclidinium

DRUGS AFFECTING INFLAMMATION

Inhaled Steroids
beclomethasone
(P) budesonide
ciclesonide
fluticasone
triamcinolone

LEUKOTRIENE RECEPTOR ANTAGONISTS
montelukast
(P) zafirlukast
zileuton

Immune Modulators
benralizumab
dupilumab
mepolizumab
(P) omalizumab
reslizumab

LUNG SURFACTANTS
(P) beractant
calfactant
poractant

DRUGS FOR PULMONARY FIBROSIS
nintedanib
pirfenidone

The lower respiratory tract includes the bronchial tree and the alveoli, where gas exchange occurs (Fig. 55.1). Disorders of the lower respiratory tract can have a direct impact on gas exchange and oxygenation and can include infections such as bronchiectasis, bronchitis, and pneumonia and obstructive disorders that directly interfere with airflow to the alveoli.

Pulmonary obstructive diseases include asthma and chronic obstructive pulmonary disease (COPD), which irreversibly decreases airflow rates and often is a combination of emphysema and chronic bronchitis. (See Chapter 53 for detailed pathophysiology.) The obstruction of asthma and COPD can be related to inflammation that results in narrowing of the interior of the airway and to muscular constriction that results in narrowing of the conducting tube (Fig. 55.2). Asthma is associated with the development of immunoglobulin E (IgE) antibodies to specific antigens that, when activated, cause the immediate release of inflammatory chemicals from mast cells. The reaction to the chemicals causes rapid swelling of the inner lining of the airways and a narrowing of the conducting tubes. COPD is most often caused by chronic exposure to irritants that cause a chronic inflammation and swelling in the airway. Inhalation of cigarette smoke is the leading cause of COPD. With chronic inflammation, muscular and cilial action is lost, and complications related to the loss of these protective processes can occur, such as infections, pneumonia, and movement of inhaled substances deep into the respiratory system. In severe COPD, air is trapped in the lower respiratory tract, the alveoli degenerate and fuse together, and the exchange of gases is greatly impaired. See Box 55.1 for information on reducing COPD exacerbations.

The first step for treatment includes reducing environmental exposure to irritants such as stopping smoking, filtering allergens from the air, and avoiding exposure to known irritants and allergens. Pharmacological treatment is aimed at opening the conducting airways through muscular bronchodilation and decreasing the effects of inflammation on the lining of the airway. See Box 55.2 for guidelines for maintenance treatment of asthma.

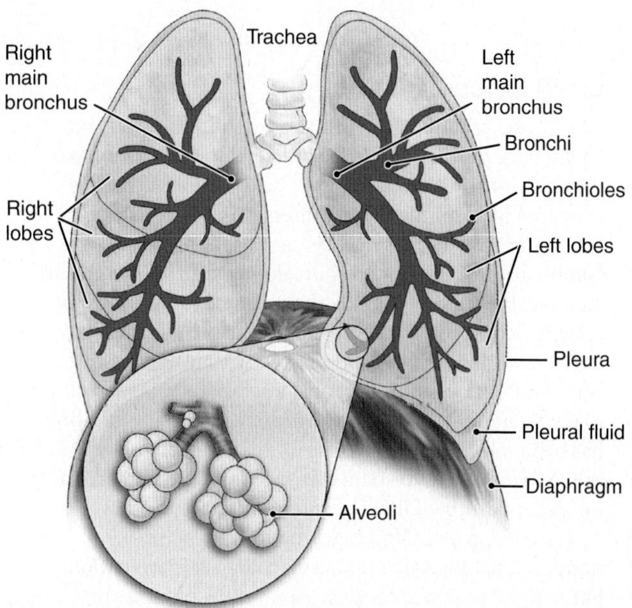

FIGURE 55.1 The lower respiratory tract.

Additional obstructive pulmonary diseases are respiratory distress syndrome (RDS), which causes obstruction at the alveolar level and is seen in neonates, and adult respiratory distress syndrome (ARDS), which is characterized by progressive loss of lung compliance and increasing hypoxia. This syndrome occurs as a result of a severe insult to the body, such as cardiovascular (CV) collapse, major burns, severe trauma, and rapid depressurization. The obstruction of RDS in the neonate is related to a lack of the lipoprotein surfactant, which leads to an inability to maintain an open alveolus. Surfactant is essential in decreasing the surface tension in the tiny alveolus, allowing it to expand and remain open. If surfactant is lacking, the alveoli collapse and gas exchange cannot occur. Pharmacological therapy for RDS involves instilling surfactant into the alveoli. The treatment of ARDS involves reversal of the

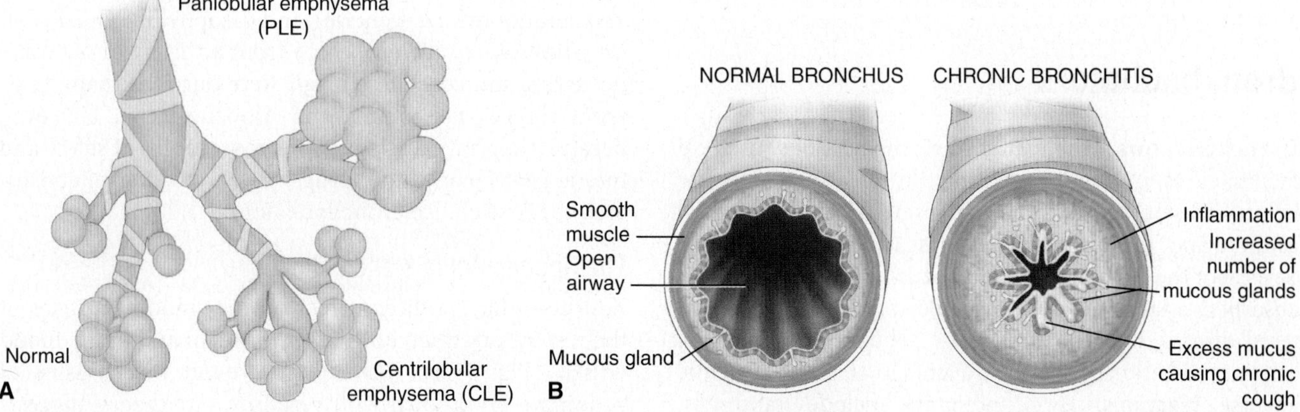

FIGURE 55.2 Changes in the airways with chronic obstructive pulmonary disease (COPD). **A.** Example of alveolar changes in COPD. **B.** Airway changes in bronchitis.

BOX 55.1

COPD Exacerbation

COPD exacerbations can range from mild to severe, but all are demonstrated by worsening respiratory symptoms that require additional therapy. Exacerbations are often triggered by respiratory tract infections. Short-acting inhaled beta2-agonists may be used as monotherapy or combination therapy with short-acting anticholinergics to facilitate bronchodilation. A short course (5 to 7 days) of systemic corticosteroids should be considered since they have been shown to decrease recovery time and hospital stay. Antibiotics should be considered if there is suspicion of bacterial infection. Noninvasive mechanical ventilation has been found to improve gas exchange, decrease work of breathing, shorten hospital stay, and improve survival rate for patients with COPD in acute respiratory distress.

Prevention of COPD exacerbations includes nonpharmacological and pharmacological interventions. Smoking cessation is the best way to slow progression and decrease exacerbations for COPD. Influenza and pneumococcal vaccination may decrease risk of exacerbations by lowering infection frequency.

Roflumilast (*Daliresp*) is available to reduce exacerbation risk in patients with COPD. It is a phosphodiesterase 4 inhibitor, which leads to an accumulation of intracellular cyclic adenosine monophosphate (AMP) in lung tissues. This effect, though the action is not completely understood, causes a reduction in sputum neutrophils and eosinophils and improved lung function. It is not a bronchodilator and cannot be used for acute bronchospasm. It is an oral agent, reaching peak level in 0.5 to 1 hour. It is metabolized in the liver and excreted in the urine with a half-life of 17 to 30 hours. It is contraindicated with liver impairment. It has been associated with acute bronchospasm and CNS changes including suicidality and weight loss. It should be avoided with the concurrent use of strong CYP450 inducers, which can increase serum levels and toxicity.

BOX 55.2

Maintenance Treatment of Asthma

Asthma treatment guidelines are provided by the Global Initiative for Asthma. They have published treatment management strategies for children and adults with asthma. The strategies include a stepwise approach to pharmacological management. For every step, there are recommended "controller" and "reliever" medications. The controller medications are designed to be taken on a regular basis to decrease asthma exacerbations. The reliever medications are prescribed on an as-needed basis when symptoms need to be suppressed and/or if the patient is having an acute exacerbation. If the patient's symptoms are not controlled at a lower "step," the dose of the medication can be increased and/or different medications can be added. Low-dose inhaled corticosteroid medications are prescribed as the preferred controller medications. The 2021 Global Initiative for Asthma recommendations for reliever medications are an as-needed low-dose inhaled corticosteroid–formoterol combination or an inhaled short-acting beta2-agonist. There is evidence that the corticosteroid–formoterol combination may be better at reducing severe exacerbations compared with the beta2-agonist.

Asthma exacerbations can be decreased by nonpharmacological strategies. People with asthma need to be taught how to monitor any symptoms and have a written action plan for when symptoms occur. The action plan should have the list of the patient's medications, when each medication should be used, and when the patient should call a medical center for help. It is important for people with asthma to avoid cigarette smoke and other noxious pulmonary stimuli. Some patients suffer from allergens that trigger asthma attacks. If a patient has known allergies, they need to be careful to avoid those substances. Some people have exercise-induced asthma. They are recommended to use their prescribed medication before exercise to prevent asthma symptoms.

underlying cause of the problem combined with ventilatory support. See Box 55.3 for the use of lower respiratory tract agents with different age groups.

Bronchodilators

Bronchodilators (Table 55.1) are medications used to facilitate respiration by dilating the airways. They are helpful in symptomatic relief or prevention of bronchial asthma and for bronchospasm associated with COPD. Several of the bronchodilators are administered orally and absorbed systemically. Other medications are administered directly into the airways by nebulizers or inhalers. These medications have the advantage of fewer systemic adverse reactions. Bronchodilators include xanthines, sympathomimetics, and anticholinergics. A different type of drug used to treat alpha$_1$-protease deficiency, *Zemaira*, is discussed in Box 55.4.

Xanthines

Xanthines, including caffeine (*Cafcit*, *Caffedrine*, and others), aminophylline (generic), and theophylline (*Elixophyllin*, *Theo-24*, *Theochron*), come from a variety of naturally occurring sources. These drugs were once the main treatment choices for asthma and bronchospasm. However, because they have a relatively narrow margin of safety and interact with many other drugs, they are no longer considered the first-choice bronchodilators.

Therapeutic Actions and Indications

Xanthines have a direct effect on the smooth muscles of the respiratory tract, both in the bronchi and in the blood vessels (Fig. 55.3). Although the exact mechanisms of action are not known with certainty, one theory suggests that xanthines work by directly affecting the mobilization of calcium within the cell to enhance force of contractions of muscles. Bronchodilation is probably due to

Box 55.3  Focus on Drug Therapy Across the Lifespan

LOWER RESPIRATORY TRACT AGENTS

Children

Antiasthmatics are frequently used in children. The starting treatment is often a daily inhaled corticosteroid medication with a short-acting beta2-agonist taken as needed. Leukotriene receptor antagonists are another option for maintenance therapy.

Parents need to be encouraged to take measures to prevent acute attacks, including avoidance of known allergens, smoke-filled rooms, and crowded or dusty areas. Parents should be cautioned about the proper way to measure liquid preparations to avoid inadvertent toxic doses or lack of therapeutic effects.

Theophylline has been used in children, but because of its many adverse effects and the better control afforded by newer agents, its use is rare.

As the child grows and matures, the disease will need to be reevaluated and dose adjustments made to meet the needs of the growing child. Puberty brings the impact of many new hormones on the body, and this frequently will change the presentation of asthma and prompt readjustment of treatment. Teenagers need to learn the proper administration and use of inhaled steroids for prevention of exercise-induced asthma.

The parents of premature babies undergoing surfactant therapy will require consistent support and education to help them to cope with the stress of this event.

Adults

Adults may be able to manage their asthma quite well with the use of inhalers and avoidance of aggravating situations. Periodic review of the proper use of the various inhalers should be part of routine evaluation of these patients. Periodic spirometry readings should be done to evaluate the effectiveness of the therapy, and review of triggers and ways to avoid triggers should be included in each visit.

The safety of these drugs during pregnancy and lactation is variable. Patients who can become pregnant should be instructed to discuss with their health care provider if they are thinking about becoming or are pregnant so medications can be optimized. The drugs may enter human milk and also may alter fluid balance and milk production. It is advised that caution be used if one of these drugs is prescribed during lactation.

Older Adults

Older adults are also more likely to have renal and/or hepatic impairment related to underlying medical conditions, which could interfere with the metabolism and excretion of these drugs. Patients should be monitored closely, with dose adjustment made based on patient response.

These patients also need to be alerted to the potential for toxic effects when using OTC preparations and should be advised to check with their health care provider before beginning any OTC drug regimen. Older adults with progressive COPD may be taking many combined drugs to help them maintain effective respirations. These patients should have an overall treatment plan involving complex pulmonary hygiene, positioning, fluids, nutrition, humidified air, rest, and activity plans, as well as a complicated drug regimen to deal with the impact of this disease.

Table 55.1 *Drugs in Focus:* Bronchodilators

Drug Name	Usual Dosage	Usual Indications
Xanthines		
Aminophylline (generic)	*Adult and pediatric:* IV loading dose to serum concentration 10–15 mcg/mL and then IV infusion based on age; dose adjusted based on serum levels	Adjunct to inhaled beta-2 selective agonists and systemically administered corticosteroids for the treatment of acute exacerbations of the symptoms and reversible airflow obstruction associated with asthma and other chronic lung diseases, for example, emphysema and chronic bronchitis
caffeine (*Caffedrine, Cafcit,* and others)	*Adult and pediatric:* oral, IV, and IM formulations; dosage varies based on age and formulation	Relief of symptoms or prevention of bronchial asthma and reversal of bronchospasm associated with COPD; supportive treatment for respiratory depression
theophylline (*Elixophyllin, Theo-24, Theochron*)	Dosage varies widely based on preparation and patient response	Relief of symptoms or prevention of bronchial asthma and reversal of bronchospasm associated with COPD

(continues on page 984)

Table 55.1 *Drugs in Focus:* Bronchodilators (*Continued*)

Drug Name	Usual Dosage	Usual Indications
Sympathomimetics		
albuterol (*Accuneb, Proair HFA, Proventil HFA*)	*Adult:* 2–4 mg PO t.i.d. to q.i.d. or two inhalations q4–6h or two inhalations 15 min before exercise or 2.5 mg oral inhalation nebulizer t.i.d. or q.i.d. *Pediatric (>12 y):* Adult dose *Pediatric (6–12 y):* 2 mg t.i.d. to q.i.d. oral tablets *Pediatric (6–14 y):* 2 mg t.i.d. to q.i.d. PO oral syrup *Pediatric (2–6 y):* 0.1 mg/kg PO t.i.d. oral syrup *Pediatric (2–12 y [inhalation]):* 1.25–2.5 mg; for prevention of exercise-induced bronchospasm, 200-mcg capsule inhaled 15 min before exercise	Treatment and prophylaxis of bronchospasm and prevention of exercise-induced bronchospasm
arformoterol (*Brovana*)	*Adult:* 15 mcg b.i.d. by nebulization	Long-term maintenance treatment of bronchoconstriction in COPD
ephedrine (generic)	*Adult:* 25–50 mg IM, subcutaneous, or IV; 12–25 mg PO q4h *Pediatric:* 0.5 mg/kg IM or subcutaneous divided into four to six doses	Treatment of acute bronchospasm in adults and children, though epinephrine is the drug of choice
epinephrine (*Adrenaclick, Adrenalin, EpiPen*, and others)	*Adult:* 0.1–0.3 mL subcutaneous q20min for 4 h as needed; may also be given by aerosol inhalation or nebulization *Pediatric:* 0.01–0.3 mL/m² subcutaneous q20min for 4 h as needed	Drug of choice for treatment of acute bronchospasm; emergency treatment of allergic reactions including anaphylaxis
formoterol (*Foradil, Perforomist*)	*Adult and pediatric (≥5 y for asthma maintenance):* 12-mcg capsule q12h, inhaled using the *Aerolizer inhaler* *Adult and pediatric (≥12 y):* 12-mcg capsule inhaled using the *Aerolizer* inhaler, at least 15 min before exercising *Adult for COPD treatment:* One 20-mcg/2 mL vial every 12 h	Maintenance treatment of asthma and prevention of bronchospasm in patients ≥5 y of age with reversible obstructive airway disease, prevention of exercise-induced bronchospasm in patients ≥12 y of age; maintenance treatment of bronchoconstriction in patients with COPD (*Perforomist*)
isoproterenol (*Isuprel*)	*Adult:* 0.01–0.02 mg IV during anesthesia; 1:200 solution with 5–15 deep inhalations for acute bronchial asthma or 5–15 inhalations using nebulizer for COPD-related bronchospasm *Pediatric:* 0.25 mL or the 1:200 solution for each 10–15 min of nebulization	Treatment of bronchospasm during anesthesia; prophylaxis of bronchospasm (when used as inhalant) in adults and children
levalbuterol (*Xopenex HFA*)	*Adult and pediatric (>12 y):* 0.63 mg q6–8h by nebulization *Pediatric (6–11 y):* 0.31 mg t.i.d. by nebulizer	Treatment and prevention of bronchospasm in patients ≥6 y of age who have reversible obstructive pulmonary disease
metaproterenol (generic)	*Adult:* 20 mg PO t.i.d. to q.i.d.; two to three inhalations q3–4h; use caution if patient is >60 y *Pediatric (>12 y):* inhalation and oral doses, same as adult *Pediatric (6–12 y):* nebulizer, 0.1–0.2 mL in saline *Pediatric (6–9 y):* 10 mg PO t.i.d. to q.i.d.	Treatment and prophylaxis of bronchospasm and acute asthma attacks in children ≥6 y of age
olodaterol (*Striverdi Respimat*)	*Adult:* Two inhalations (5 mcg/d) once a day at the same time each day	LABA for treatment of airflow obstruction in patients with COPD
salmeterol (*Serevent*)	*Adult and pediatric (≥4 y):* One inhalation (50 mcg) q12h or one inhalation 30 min before exercise	Prevention of exercise-induced asthma; treatment of asthma in patients ≥4 y of age with an inhaled corticosteroid; maintenance treatment of bronchospasm for patients with COPD
terbutaline (generic)	*Adult and pediatric (>15 y):* 2.5–5 mg PO q6h while awake; 0.25 mg subcutaneous, repeat in 15 min as needed; two inhalations separated by 60 s q4–6h *Pediatric (12–15 y):* 2.5 mg PO t.i.d.; two inhalations separated by 60 s q4–6h as needed	Treatment and prophylaxis of bronchospasm in patients ≥12 y of age

Table 55.1 *Drugs in Focus:* Bronchodilators (*Continued*)

Drug Name	Usual Dosage	Usual Indications
Anticholinergics		
aclidinium (*Tudorza Pressair*)	400 mcg b.i.d. by oral inhalation using provided device	Long-term maintenance and treatment of bronchospasm for adults with COPD
ipratropium (*Atrovent HFA*)	*Adult and pediatric (12 y and older):* oral inhalation t.i.d. or q.i.d. or via nebulizer 6–8 h apart *Nasal spray:* Two sprays per nostril t.i.d. to q.i.d.	Maintenance and treatment of bronchospasm for adults with COPD; nasal spray for rhinorrhea associated with seasonal and perennial rhinitis or the common cold
glycopyrrolate (*Lonhala Magnair*)	One vial inhaled twice a day	Long-term maintenance and treatment of adults with COPD
revefenacin (*Yupelri*)	One oral inhalation once daily	Maintenance treatment of patients with COPD
tiotropium (*Spiriva*)	*Adult:* 18 mcg/d (one capsule) using the *HandiHaler* inhalation device *Adult and pediatric (≥6 y):* 1.25 mcg/d as two inhalations daily	Long-term, once-daily maintenance and treatment of bronchospasm associated with COPD in adults and asthma
umeclidinium (*Incruse Ellipta*)	62.5 mcg/d for oral inhalation using device provided	Long-term, once-daily maintenance and treatment of airflow obstruction associated with COPD in adults

COPD, chronic obstructive pulmonary disease; LABA, long-acting beta-agonist.

phosphodiesterase inhibition, which can lead to increased cyclic-AMP since phosphodiesterase is the enzyme that degrades the second messenger molecule bonds. Caffeine is also a central nervous system (CNS) stimulant, has positive inotropic and chronotropic effects on the heart, constricts blood vessels in the brain, increases force of contraction of skeletal muscle, increases gastric acid secretion, increases renal blood flow, and dilates peripheral blood vessels. Xanthines also inhibit the release of slow-reacting substance of anaphylaxis and histamine, decreasing the bronchial swelling and narrowing that occurs as a result of these two chemicals. See Table 55.1 for usual indications for these drugs.

Unlabeled uses include stimulation of respirations in **Cheyne-Stokes respiration**, an abnormal pattern of breathing characterized by apneic periods followed by periods of tachypnea that may reflect delayed blood flow through the brain, and the treatment of apnea and bradycardia in premature infants. Because xanthines are associated with many adverse effects and management can be difficult, they are not the drug of choice when starting to treat patients with obstructive pulmonary disease. There are still some prescribers, however, who use them. Xanthines are still used in the intensive care unit when acute asthma attacks have progressed to a critical situation.

BOX 55.4

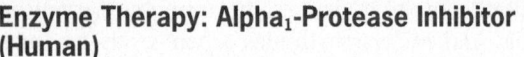

Enzyme Therapy: Alpha$_1$-Protease Inhibitor (Human)

An alpha$_1$-protease inhibitor, *Zemaira*, was approved in 2003 for the treatment of alpha$_1$-protease deficiency, a chronic, hereditary, autosomal-dominant disorder that presents as progressive, severe emphysema, usually during a person's 30s or 40s. Alpha$_1$-protease inhibitor is normally present in the lungs and acts to neutralize neutrophil elastase, which is increased by smoking or lung infection. Patients who do not produce enough alpha$_1$-protease inhibitor are at risk for progressive lung tissue destruction with smoking or lung infection. This type of emphysema and COPD does not respond well to the drug therapy usually associated with COPD. *Zemaira* is infused during a period of 15 minutes once each week at a dose of 60 mg/kg and provides protection from tissue destruction.

Pharmacokinetics

The xanthines are rapidly absorbed from the gastrointestinal (GI) tract when given orally, reaching peak level within 2 hours. They are also given intravenously (IV), reaching peak effect within minutes. They are widely distributed and metabolized in the liver and excreted in the urine. Xanthines cross the placenta and enter human milk (see "Contraindications and Cautions").

Contraindications and Cautions

Caution should be taken with any patient with GI problems, coronary disease, respiratory dysfunction, renal or

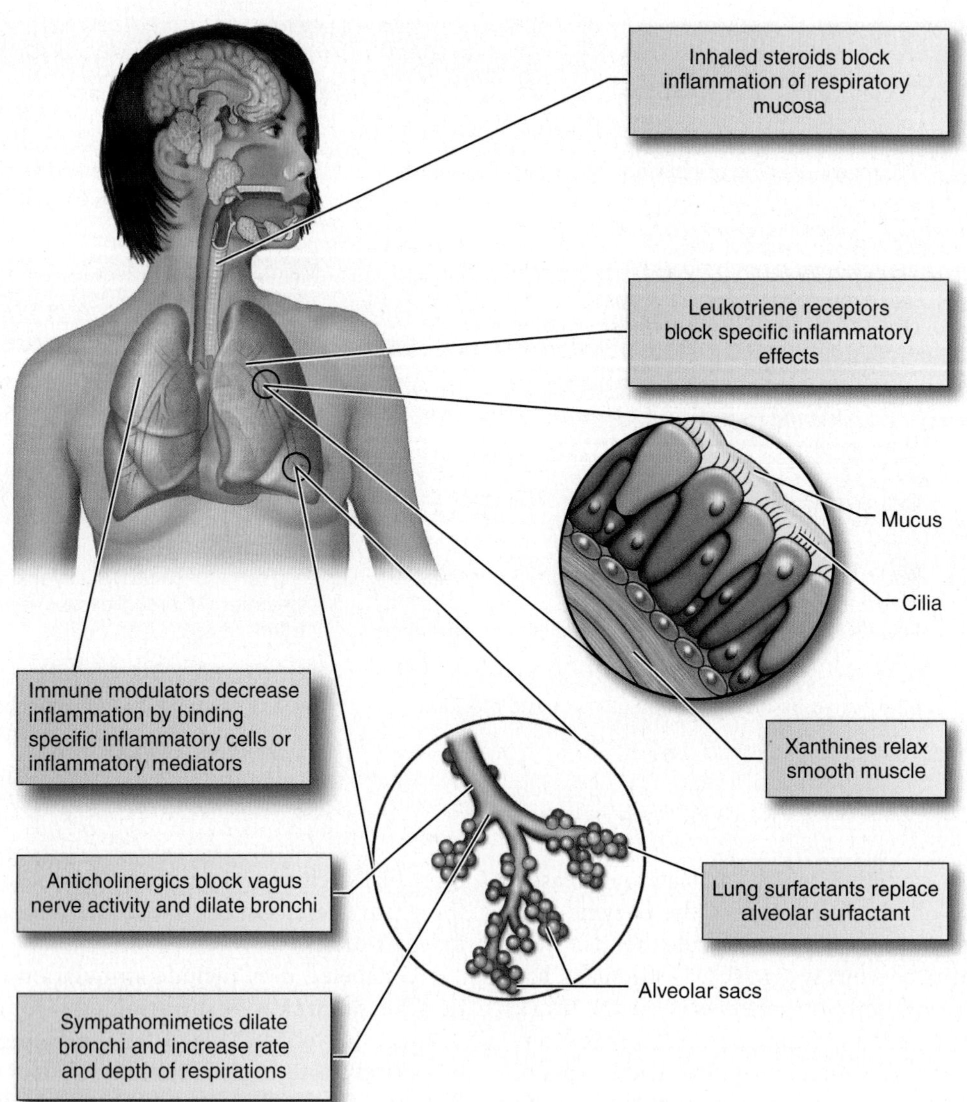

FIGURE 55.3 Sites of action of drugs used to treat obstructive pulmonary disorders.

hepatic disease, alcoholism, or hyperthyroidism because these conditions can be exacerbated by the systemic effects of xanthines. Xanthines are available for oral and parenteral use; the parenteral drug should be switched to the oral form as soon as possible because the parenteral forms are only indicated for acute or emergency situations.

Although no studies are available of xanthine effects on human pregnancy, they have been associated with fetal abnormalities and breathing difficulties at birth in animal studies, so use should be limited to situations in which the benefit to the patient clearly outweighs the potential risk to the fetus. Because the xanthines enter human milk and could affect the baby, another method of feeding the baby should be selected if these drugs are needed during lactation.

Adverse Effects

Adverse effects associated with theophylline are related to levels in the blood (see the "Critical Thinking Scenario" for additional information on toxic reaction to theophylline). Therapeutic theophylline levels are from 10 to 20 mcg/mL. Patients may have adverse effects with therapeutic levels. However, there are increased chances of side effects including nausea, vomiting, irritability, tremors, nervousness, insomnia, and tachyarrhythmias when levels are higher than 20 mcg/mL. Symptoms of severe toxicity include seizures, life-threatening arrhythmias, hypotension, and coma.

Clinically Important Drug–Drug Interactions

Because of the mechanism of xanthine metabolism in the liver, many drugs interact with xanthines. The list of interacting drugs should be checked any time a drug is added to or removed from a drug regimen. Concurrent use of caffeine and theophylline increases the risk of adverse effects.

Substances in cigarettes increase the metabolism of xanthines in the liver; the xanthine dose must be increased in patients who continue to smoke while using xanthines. In addition, the dose should be reduced if the patient decides to decrease or discontinue smoking, otherwise severe xanthine toxicity can occur.

CRITICAL THINKING SCENARIO
Toxic Reaction to Theophylline

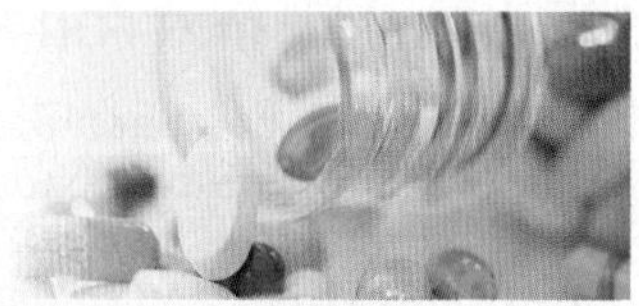

THE SITUATION

R.P. is a 50-year-old patient with a medical history of asthma, hypertension, and obesity. R.P. has been stabilized on theophylline for many years; whenever their provider has recommended switching to newer and safer medications, R.P. has refused. R.P. has been labeled as nonadherent to medical advice because they continue to smoke cigarettes (one pack per day) despite knowing that smoking can exacerbate asthma symptoms. R.P. presented to the emergency department with complaints of nasal congestion, cough, myalgia, fatigue, fever, shortness of breath, and chest tightness. R.P. was diagnosed with influenza A and discharged with oseltamivir. They returned to the emergency department 48 hours later due to symptoms of shortness of breath, chest pain, palpitations, headache, tremors, nausea, and vomiting. R.P.'s heart rate was 140 beats/min and their blood pressure was 85/50. Their theophylline level was found to be 32 mcg/mL. R.P. reported that the only change was the oseltamivir and that they have not had a cigarette for 72 hours.

CRITICAL THINKING

What probably happened to R.P.?
What information would be helpful for the patient to know concerning theophylline toxicity?
How could that information have been included in the patient teaching program?
What would be the best approach for this patient now?

DISCUSSION

R.P. stopped smoking, perhaps due to the influenza A infection. However, R.P. was not aware that cigarette smoking increases the metabolism of theophylline and that they had been stabilized on a dose that took that information into account. When R.P. cut down on smoking, theophylline was not metabolized as quickly and began to accumulate. The other change for R.P. was that they were prescribed oseltamivir. Oseltamivir may inhibit the metabolism of theophylline. This situation is a difficult challenge since a healthy behavior (stopping smoking) resulted in R.P. feeling worse and having to return to the emergency room. A careful teaching approach will be necessary to encourage R.P. to continue abstaining from cigarette smoking. It would be safest if R.P. also agreed to change from theophylline to an inhaled corticosteroid to control their asthma symptoms. However, if R.P. is continued on theophylline, careful monitoring of their levels will be necessary during their acute infection.

NURSING CARE GUIDE FOR R.P.: XANTHINES

Assessment: History and Examination

Assessment parameters include a health history focused particularly on allergies, peptic ulcer, gastritis, renal or hepatic dysfunction, coronary disease, cigarette use, pregnancy and lactation, and concurrent use of caffeine. All drug interactions should be checked whenever a patient is taking theophylline.

Focus the physical examination on

CNS: Orientation, reflexes, affect, coordination
Respiratory: Respiratory rate and character, adventitious sounds
Skin: Color, lesions
CV: Blood pressure, pulse, peripheral perfusion, baseline electrocardiogram
GI: Bowel sounds, abdominal exam
Laboratory tests: Serum theophylline levels, renal and hepatic function tests

Nursing Conclusions

Impaired comfort related to GI effects or dry mouth
Altered heart rate and blood pressure
Altered sensory perception (kinesthetic, visual)
Knowledge deficit regarding drug therapy

Planning

The patient will receive the best therapeutic effect from the drug therapy.
The patient will have limited adverse effects from the drug therapy.
The patient will have an understanding of the drug therapy, adverse effects to anticipate, and measures to relieve discomfort and improve safety.

Intervention

Provide supportive care with comfort and safety measures.
Ensure dietary control of caffeine.
Provide reassurance to deal with drug effects and lifestyle changes.
Provide patient teaching regarding drug name, dosage, adverse effects, precautions, warnings to report, dietary cautions, and need for follow-up.

Evaluation

Evaluate drug effects: relief of respiratory difficulty, improvement of air movement.
Monitor for adverse effects: GI upset, CNS effects, cardiac arrhythmias.
Monitor for drug–drug interactions as appropriate.
Evaluate the effectiveness of the patient teaching program and comfort and safety measures.

(continues on page 988)

PATIENT TEACHING FOR R.P.

- The drug that has been prescribed for you, theophylline, is a bronchodilator. Bronchodilators work by relaxing the airways, helping to make breathing easier and to decrease wheezes and shortness of breath. To be effective, this drug must be taken exactly as prescribed.
- This drug can be taken with or without food. Do not chew the enteric-coated or time-release capsules or tablets since it may lead to a rapid release of the medication and resulting toxicity. If the tablet you are prescribed is scored, you may cut it in half.
- Common effects of this drug include
  - *GI upset, nausea, vomiting, heartburn*: Taking the drug with food may help with these problems.
  - *Restlessness, nervousness, difficulty in sleeping*: The body often adjusts to these effects over time. Avoiding other stimulants, such as caffeine, may help decrease some of these symptoms.
  - *Headache*: This often goes away with time. If headaches persist or become worse, notify your health care provider.
- Report any of the following to your health care provider: vomiting, severe abdominal pain, pounding or fast heartbeat, confusion, unusual tiredness, muscle twitching, skin rash, or hives.
- Many foods can change the way that your drug works; if you decide to change your diet, consult your health care provider.
- Adverse effects of the drug can be avoided by avoiding foods that contain caffeine or other xanthine derivatives (coffee, cola, chocolate, tea) or by using them in moderate amounts. This is especially important if you experience nervousness, restlessness, or sleeplessness.
- Cigarette smoking affects the way your body uses this drug. If you decide to change your smoking habits, such as increasing or decreasing the number of cigarettes you smoke each day, consult your health care provider regarding the possible need to adjust your dose.
- Avoid the use of any over-the-counter (OTC) medication without first checking with your health care provider. Several of these medications can interfere with the effectiveness of this drug.
- Tell any doctor, nurse, or other health care provider involved in your care that you are taking this drug.
- Keep this drug and all medications out of the reach of children.

Prototype Summary: Theophylline

Indications: Symptomatic relief or prevention of bronchial asthma and reversible bronchospasm associated with chronic bronchitis and emphysema.

Actions: Directly relaxes bronchial smooth muscle, causing bronchodilation and increasing vital capacity; increases force of diaphragmatic muscle.

Pharmacokinetics:

Route	Onset	Peak	Duration
Oral	1–6 h	4–8 h	6–8 h
IV	Immediate	30 min	4–8 h

$T_{1/2}$: About 8 hours for oral but may vary per patient and type of formulation.

Adverse Effects: Irritability, restlessness, dizziness, palpitations, life-threatening arrhythmias, loss of appetite, proteinuria, respiratory arrest, fever, flushing.

Nursing Considerations for Patients Receiving Xanthines

Assessment: History and Examination

- Assess for possible contraindications or cautions: any known allergies to prevent hypersensitivity reactions; cigarette use, which affects the metabolism of the drug; peptic ulcer, gastritis, renal or hepatic dysfunction, and coronary disease, all of which could be exacerbated and require cautious use; and pregnancy and lactation, for which the medications should be used with caution because of the potential for adverse effects on the fetus or nursing baby.
- Perform a physical examination to establish baseline data for assessing the effectiveness of the drug and the occurrence of any adverse effects associated with drug therapy.
- Perform a skin examination, including color and the presence of lesions, to provide a baseline as a reference for drug hypersensitivity reactions.
- Monitor blood pressure, pulse, cardiac auscultation, peripheral perfusion, and baseline electrocardiogram to provide a baseline for effects on the CV system.
- Assess bowel sounds, do a liver evaluation, and monitor liver and renal function tests to provide a baseline for renal and hepatic function tests.
- Evaluate serum theophylline levels to assist in keeping medication in the therapeutic range and to avoid toxicity.

Nursing Conclusions

Nursing conclusions related to drug therapy might include

- Impaired comfort related to headache and GI upset
- Altered sensory perception (kinesthetic, visual) related to CNS effects
- Knowledge deficit regarding drug therapy

Planning

- The patient will receive the best therapeutic effect from the drug therapy.

- The patient will have limited adverse effects from the drug therapy.
- The patient will have an understanding of the drug therapy, adverse effects to anticipate, and measures to relieve discomfort and improve safety.

Intervention With Rationale

- Administer oral drug with food or milk to relieve GI irritation if GI upset is a problem.
- Monitor patient response to the drug (e.g., relief of respiratory difficulty, improved airflow) to determine the effectiveness of the drug dose and to adjust dose as needed.
- Provide comfort measures, including rest periods, quiet environment, dietary control of caffeine, and headache therapy as needed to help the patient cope with the effects of drug therapy.
- Provide periodic follow-up, including blood tests, to monitor serum theophylline levels.
- Provide thorough patient teaching, including the drug name and prescribed dosage, measures to help avoid adverse effects, warning signs that may indicate problems, and the need for periodic monitoring and evaluation, to enhance patient knowledge about drug therapy and to promote adherence.

Evaluation

- Monitor patient response to the drug (improved airflow, ease of respirations).
- Monitor for adverse effects (CNS effects, cardiac arrhythmias, GI upset, local irritation).
- Monitor for potential drug–drug interactions; consult with the prescriber to adjust doses as appropriate.
- Evaluate the effectiveness of the teaching plan (patient can name drug, dosage, adverse effects to watch for, and specific measures to avoid adverse effects).
- Monitor the effectiveness of comfort measures and adherence to the regimen.

Sympathomimetics

Sympathomimetics are drugs that mimic the effects of the sympathetic nervous system. One of the actions of the sympathetic nervous system is dilation of thebronchi with increased rate and depth of respiration. This is the desired effect when selecting a sympathomimetic as a bronchodilator. Sympathomimetics used as bronchodilators include albuterol (*Proventil HFA* and others), arformoterol (*Brovana*), ephedrine (generic), epinephrine (*EpiPen* and others), formoterol (*Foradil* and others), isoproterenol (*Isuprel* and others), levalbuterol (*Xopenex HFA*), metaproterenol (generic), olodaterol (*Striverdi*), salmeterol (*Serevent*), and terbutaline (generic).

Therapeutic Actions and Indications

Most of the sympathomimetics used as bronchodilators are beta$_2$-selective adrenergic agonists. That means that at therapeutic levels, their actions are specific to the beta$_2$-receptors found in the bronchi (see Chapter 30). This specificity is lost at higher levels. Other systemic effects of sympathomimetics include increased blood pressure, increased heart rate, and decreased renal and GI blood flow—all actions of the sympathetic nervous system. These overall effects limit the systemic usefulness of these drugs in certain patients.

Some of the bronchodilators are indicated for short-term and/or emergency use to reverse bronchospasm during an allergic reaction or asthma attack. Others are longer acting and are taken on a scheduled basis to decrease symptoms of COPD or asthma.

See Table 55.1 for usual indications for each of these agents.

Pharmacokinetics

Sympathomimetics available as inhalants include arformoterol, formoterol, levalbuterol, olodaterol, and salmeterol. Other sympathomimetics are available in various forms. Albuterol and metaproterenol are available in inhaled and oral forms. Terbutaline can be used as an inhalant and as an oral and parenteral agent. Isoproterenol is available for IV use. Ephedrine is used orally and in parenteral form (for IV, intramuscular [IM], and subcutaneous use). Epinephrine is administered IV, subcutaneously, and via inhalation. The sympathomimetics vary in their duration of action; long-acting beta-adrenergics have longer half-lives than the shorter-acting medications.

These drugs are rapidly distributed after injection; they are transformed in the liver to metabolites that are excreted in the urine. They are known to cross the placenta and to enter human milk (see "Contraindications and Cautions"). The inhaled drugs are rapidly absorbed into the lung tissue. Although less of the drug is absorbed systemically when administered via inhalation, any absorbed drug will still be metabolized in the liver and excreted in the urine.

Contraindications and Cautions

These drugs are contraindicated or should be used with caution, depending on the severity of the underlying condition in conditions that would be aggravated by the sympathetic stimulation, including cardiac disease, vascular disease, arrhythmias, diabetes, and hyperthyroidism. These drugs should be used during pregnancy and lactation only if the benefits to the patient clearly outweigh potential risks to the fetus or neonate. The long-acting beta-agonists (LABAs) have a boxed warning about the increased risk of asthma-related deaths when patients use these drugs as monotherapy without inhaled corticosteroid. They are only recommended as part of combination treatment for patients with asthma.

Adverse Effects

Adverse effects of these drugs, which can be attributed to sympathomimetic stimulation, include CNS stimulation, GI upset, cardiac arrhythmias, hypertension, angina, sweating, pallor, and flushing (Fig. 55.4). Life-threatening paradoxical bronchospasm is a rare but dangerous side effect. Patients should also be monitored for hypersensitivity reactions.

Clinically Important Drug–Drug Interactions

Special precautions should be taken to avoid the combination of sympathomimetic bronchodilators with the general anesthetics cyclopropane and halogenated hydrocarbons. Because these drugs sensitize the myocardium to catecholamines, serious cardiac complications could occur. If taken concurrently with other medications that can increase heart rate and blood pressure, the patient should be monitored carefully. Beta-blocking medications can decrease the effect of the sympathomimetic medication if both are administered systemically.

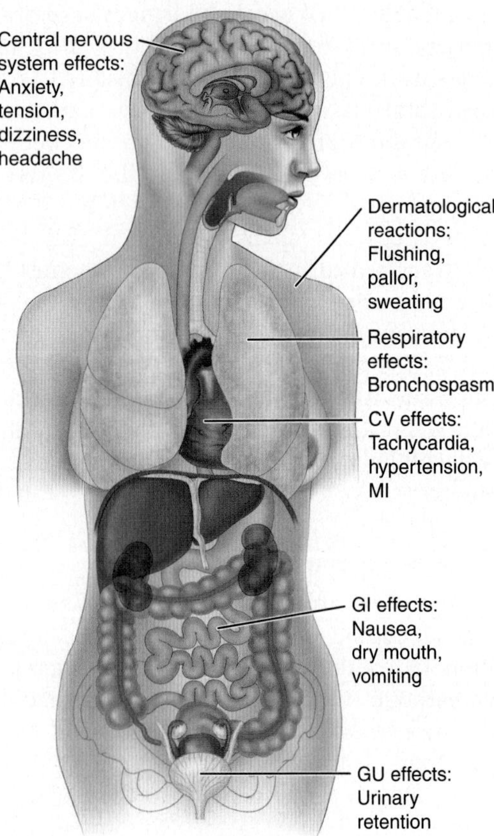

FIGURE 55.4 Variety of adverse effects and toxicities associated with drugs acting on the lower respiratory tract.

Prototype Summary: Albuterol

Indications: Treatment and prophylaxis of bronchospasm and prevention of exercise-induced bronchospasm.

Actions: Reacts as an agonist at beta-receptor sites in the sympathetic nervous system to cause bronchodilation via smooth muscle relaxation, increased heart rate, increased respiratory rate, and increased blood pressure.

Pharmacokinetics:

Route	Onset	Peak	Duration
Oral	Rapid	2 h	6–8 h
Inhalation	3–5 min	20 min	1–3 h

$T_{1/2}$: About 6 hours for inhalation; metabolized by enzymes; eliminated primarily by kidneys.

Adverse Effects: Fear, anxiety, restlessness, headache, sore throat, dizziness, nausea, palpitation, tachycardia, paradoxical bronchospasm, hypersensitivity reactions.

Nursing Considerations for Patients Receiving Sympathomimetics

Assessment: History and Examination

- Assess for possible contraindications or cautions: any known allergies to any sympathomimetic or drug components to prevent hypersensitivity reactions; cigarette use, which affects the metabolism of the drug; pregnancy or lactation, which require cautious use of the drug; cardiac disease, vascular disease, arrhythmias, diabetes, and hyperthyroidism, which may be exacerbated by sympathomimetic effects; and use of the general anesthetics cyclopropane and halogenated hydrocarbons, which sensitize the myocardium to catecholamines and could cause serious cardiac complications if used with these drugs.
- Perform a physical examination to establish baseline data for assessing the effectiveness of the drug and the occurrence of any adverse effects associated with drug therapy.
- Assess reflexes and orientation to evaluate CNS effects of the drug.
- Monitor respirations and adventitious sounds to establish a baseline for drug effectiveness and possible adverse effects.
- Evaluate pulse, blood pressure, and, in certain cases, a baseline electrocardiogram to monitor the CV effects of sympathetic stimulation.

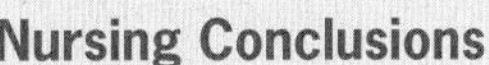

Nursing Conclusions

Nursing conclusions related to drug therapy might include

- Altered tissue perfusion related to sympathomimetic effects
- Impaired comfort related to CNS, GI, or cardiac effects of the drug
- Anxiety or restlessness related to CNS effects
- Knowledge deficit related to drug therapy

Planning

- The patient will receive the best therapeutic effect from the drug therapy.
- The patient will have limited adverse effects from the drug therapy.
- The patient will have an understanding of the drug therapy, adverse effects to anticipate, and measures to relieve discomfort and improve safety.

Intervention With Rationale

- Reassure the patient that the drug of choice will vary with each person. The different sympathomimetics are slightly different chemicals and are prepared in a variety of delivery systems. A patient may need to try several different sympathomimetics before the most effective one is found.
- Advise the patient who is prescribed a short-acting medication to use the minimal amount needed for the shortest period necessary, to prevent adverse effects.
- Teach patients who use one of these drugs for exercise-induced asthma to use it 30 to 60 minutes before exercising to ensure peak therapeutic effects when they are needed.
- Provide safety measures as needed if CNS effects become a problem, to prevent patient injury.
- Provide thorough patient teaching, including the drug name and prescribed dosage, measures to help avoid adverse effects, warning signs that may indicate problems, and the need for periodic monitoring and evaluation, to enhance patient knowledge about drug therapy and to promote adherence. Carefully teach the patient about proper use of the prescribed delivery system. Review that procedure periodically because improper use may result in ineffective therapy (Box 55.5).
- Offer support and encouragement to help the patient cope with the disease and the drug regimen.

Evaluation

- Monitor patient response to the drug (improved breathing, absence of wheezing, decreased asthma exacerbations).
- Monitor for adverse effects (CNS effects, increased pulse and blood pressure, GI upset).
- Evaluate the effectiveness of the teaching plan (patient can name drug, dosage, adverse effects to watch for and specific measures to avoid them, and measures to take to increase the effectiveness of the drug).
- Monitor the effectiveness of other measures to ease breathing.

Anticholinergics

The anticholinergic drugs ipratropium (*Atrovent*), tiotropium (*Spiriva*), aclidinium (*Tudorza Pressair*), glycopyrrolate (*Lonhala Magnair*), revefenacin (*Yupelri*), and umeclidinium (*Incruse Ellipta*) can be used to treat bronchospasm in patients with COPD. These drugs are not as fast acting as the sympathomimetics but can provide maintenance treatment with the potential of having fewer adverse effects. Other anticholinergic medications that do not act on the respiratory system are described in Chapter 33.

Therapeutic Actions and Indications

The anticholinergics are used as bronchodilators due to their effect on the vagus nerve. They can block or antagonize the action of the neurotransmitter acetylcholine at vagal-mediated receptor sites (see Fig. 55.3). Normally, vagal stimulation results in a stimulating effect on smooth muscle, causing contraction. By blocking the vagal effect, relaxation of smooth muscle in the bronchi occurs, leading to bronchodilation. See Table 55.1 for usual indications for these drugs.

Pharmacokinetics

These drugs are available for inhalation using an inhaler device. Ipratropium is also available as a nasal spray for seasonal rhinitis. When inhaled, most of the medication is not absorbed. Metabolism, excretion, and half-lives can vary. Some have shorter half-lives and need more frequent dosing. Most are partially excreted unchanged in the urine.

Contraindications and Cautions

Caution should be used in any condition that would be aggravated by the anticholinergic or atropinelike effects of the drug, such as narrow-angle glaucoma (drainage of the vitreous humor can be blocked by smooth muscle relaxation), bladder neck obstruction or prostatic hypertrophy (relaxed muscle causes decreased bladder tone), and conditions aggravated by dry mouth and throat. The use of an anticholinergic is contraindicated in the presence of known allergy to the drug or to components in the medication. These medications are not indicated for acute episodes of bronchospasm that require rapid reversal, and patients should be monitored for paradoxical bronchoconstriction. High amounts of these medications are not usually absorbed systemically, but as with all drugs, caution should be used in pregnancy and lactation because of the potential for adverse effects on the fetus or nursing baby.

Adverse Effects

Local adverse effects include dry mouth and/or hoarse throat. Adverse effects are related to the anticholinergic effects of the drug if it is absorbed systemically. These effects include dizziness, headache, fatigue, nervousness, eyesight changes, palpitations, and urinary retention. There have been reported events of hypersensitivity and paradoxical bronchospasm.

Box 55.5 Focus on Patient and Family Teaching

TEACHING PATIENTS TO SELF-ADMINISTER MEDICATION

It is important to deliver inhaled drugs into the lungs to achieve a rapid reaction and decrease the occurrence of systemic adverse effects. Patients who are self-administering inhaled drugs may be using an inhaler or a nebulizer.

INHALERS

An inhaler is a device that allows a canister containing the drug to be inserted into a metered dose device that will deliver a specific amount of the drug when the patient compresses the canister. The inhaler has a mouthpiece and may also have a spacer, which is used to hold the dose of the drug while the patient inhales. This is advantageous if the patient has difficulty compressing the canister and inhaling at the same time or if inhaling is difficult. If a powder for inhalation is being administered, a spacer is not used.

Each inhaler or nasal spray has specific instructions for medication administration. Some inhalers need to be shaken; others do not. Some require "priming" (i.e., being sprayed away from the body) before use. The patient should be cautioned to avoid spraying the medication in the eyes. It is recommended that patients have written and verbal instructions prior to use. It is also recommended that providers demonstrate and watch the patient perform correct administration technique.

NEBULIZERS

A nebulizer uses compressed air to change a liquid drug into a fine mist for inhalation. If a patient is using a handheld device or a mask, they should sit upright or in a semi-Fowler position and place the correct amount of liquid (drug dose) in the nebulizer chamber, which is attached to a compressed gas system. The patient should breathe slowly and deeply during the treatment. After the liquid is gone, the patient should rinse their mouth and clean the mask or device.

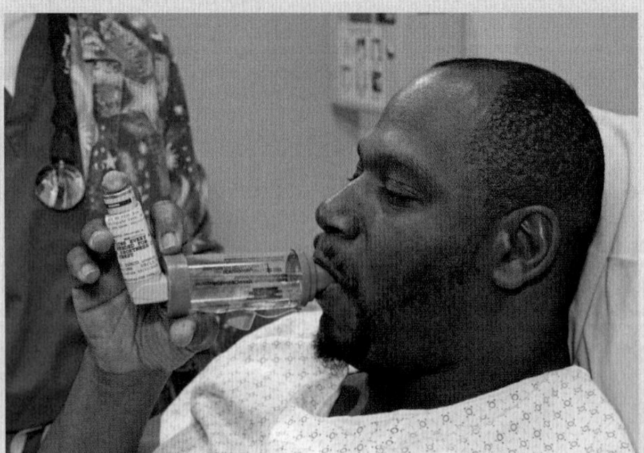

Patients may use these devices for several years. It is important to check patients' administration techniques periodically to ensure that they are getting a therapeutic dose of the drug.

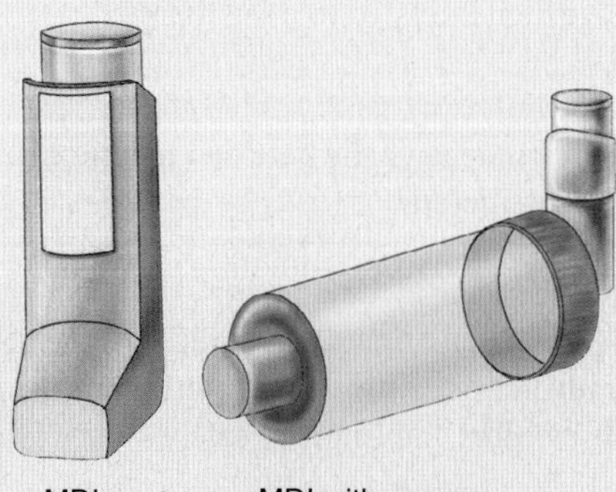

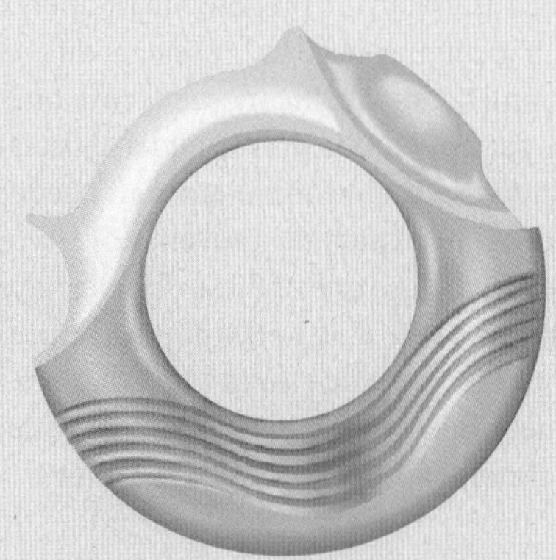

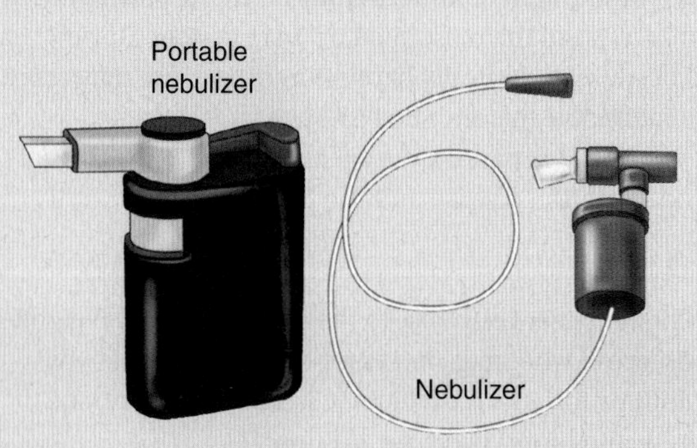

Clinically Important Drug–Drug Interactions

There is an increased risk of adverse effects if these drugs are combined with any other anticholinergics.

Prototype Summary: Ipratropium

Indications: Maintenance treatment of bronchospasm associated with COPD; as a nasal spray, treatment of seasonal allergic rhinitis.

Actions: Anticholinergic that blocks vagally mediated reflexes by antagonizing the action of acetylcholine; blocks muscarinic receptors in the bronchi causing smooth muscle relaxation and bronchodilation.

Pharmacokinetics:

Route	Onset	Peak	Duration
Inhalation	15 min	1–2 h	about 6 h

$T_{1/2}$: 2 to 4 hours; most not absorbed systemically.

Adverse Effects: Nervousness, dizziness, headache, nausea, cough, palpitations, ocular changes, hypersensitivity, urinary retention, paradoxical bronchospasm.

Nursing Considerations for Patients Receiving an Anticholinergic

Assessment: History and Examination

- Assess for possible contraindications or cautions: allergy to anticholinergics or any component of the drug to prevent hypersensitivity reactions; acute bronchospasm, which would be a contraindication; narrow-angle glaucoma (drainage of the vitreous humor can be blocked by smooth muscle relaxation), bladder neck obstruction or prostatic hypertrophy (relaxed muscle causes decreased bladder tone), and conditions aggravated by dry mouth and throat, all of which could be exacerbated by the use of this drug; and pregnancy and lactation, which would require cautious use.
- Perform a physical examination to establish baseline data for assessing the effectiveness of the drug and the occurrence of any adverse effects associated with drug therapy.
- Assess the skin color and lesions for dryness or allergic reaction and to evaluate oxygenation.
- Evaluate orientation, affect, and reflexes to evaluate CNS effects.
- Assess pulse and blood pressure to monitor CV effects of the drug.
- Evaluate respirations and adventitious sounds to monitor drug effectiveness and possible adverse effects.
- Evaluate urinary output if appropriate to monitor anticholinergic effects.

Nursing Conclusions

Nursing conclusions related to drug therapy might include

- Impaired comfort related to CNS, GI, or respiratory effects of the drug
- Altered breathing pattern due to patient diagnosis of COPD
- Knowledge deficit regarding drug therapy

Planning

- The patient will receive the best therapeutic effect from the drug therapy.
- The patient will have limited adverse effects from the drug therapy.
- The patient will have an understanding of the drug therapy, adverse effects to anticipate, and measures to relieve discomfort and improve safety.

Intervention With Rationale

- Ensure adequate hydration and provide environmental controls, such as the use of a humidifier, to make the patient more comfortable if dry mouth occurs.
- Encourage the patient to report any change in voiding due to potential for urinary retention related to drug effects.
- Provide safety measures if CNS effects occur, to prevent patient injury.
- Provide small, frequent meals and sugarless lozenges to relieve dry mouth and GI upset.
- Advise the patient not to drive or use hazardous machinery if nervousness, dizziness, and drowsiness occur with this drug to prevent injury.
- Provide thorough patient teaching, including the drug name and prescribed dosage, measures to help avoid adverse effects, warning signs that may indicate problems, and the need for periodic monitoring and evaluation, to enhance patient knowledge about drug therapy and to promote adherence.
- Review the use of the inhalator with the patient; caution the patient not to exceed the number of inhalations indicated, to prevent serious adverse effects.
- Offer support and encouragement to help the patient cope with the disease and the drug regimen.

Evaluation

- Monitor patient response to the drug (improved breathing).
- Monitor for adverse effects (hypersensitivity reactions, paradoxical bronchospasm, CNS effects, increased pulse or blood pressure, GI upset, dry skin, and mucous membranes).
- Evaluate the effectiveness of the teaching plan (patient can name drug, dosage, adverse effects to watch for and specific measures to avoid them, and measures to take to increase the effectiveness of the drug).
- Monitor the effectiveness of other measures to ease breathing.

Key Points

- Asthma, COPD, and RDS are pulmonary obstructive diseases. Asthma and COPD involve obstruction of the major airways; RDS obstructs the alveoli.
- Drug treatment for asthma and COPD aims to relieve inflammation and promote bronchial dilation.
- Xanthine-derived drugs affect the smooth muscles of the respiratory tract—both in the bronchi and in the blood vessels. The effects of theophylline are directly related to blood levels of theophylline. Excessive or toxic levels can lead to coma and death. This drug is not used as often as in the past since safer drugs have been approved.
- Sympathomimetics replicate the effects of the sympathetic nervous system; they dilate the bronchi and increase the rate and depth of respiration.
- Anticholinergics relax bronchial smooth muscle, thereby promoting bronchodilation.

Drugs Affecting Inflammation

Bronchodilation is important in opening the airway to allow air to flow into the alveoli. The second component of treating obstructive pulmonary disorders is to alter the inflammatory process that leads to swelling, excessive mucous, and more airway narrowing. Effective treatment of asthma and COPD targets both components. The drugs used to affect inflammation are the inhaled steroids, the leukotriene receptors, the immune modulators, and a mast cell stabilizer (only one OTC product is available), which can affect both bronchodilation and inflammation (Table 55.2).

Inhaled Steroids

Inhaled steroids have been found to be an effective treatment for prevention and treatment of inflammation. Agents approved for this use include beclomethasone (*QVAR Redihaler*), budesonide (*Pulmicort Respules, Pulmicort Flexhaler*), ciclesonide (*Alvesco*), fluticasone (*Flovent Diskus, Flovent HFA*), and triamcinolone (generic). The drug of choice depends on the individual patient's response; a patient may have little response to one agent but do well on another. It is usually useful to try another preparation if one is not effective within 2 to 3 weeks. Some of these medications are also available as nasal sprays to decrease symptoms of allergic rhinitis. Corticosteroids that are administered systemically are discussed in more detail in Chapter 36.

Fixed-combination drugs are also available using some of these drugs (Box 55.6).

Therapeutic Actions and Indications

Inhaled steroids are used to decrease the inflammatory response in the airway. In an airway that is swollen and narrowed by mucosal secretions and swelling, this action will increase airflow and facilitate respiration. Inhaling the steroid tends to decrease the numerous systemic effects that are associated with steroid use. When administered into the lungs by inhalation, steroids decrease the effectiveness of the inflammatory cells. This has two effects: decreased swelling associated with inflammation and promotion of beta-adrenergic receptor activity, which may promote smooth muscle relaxation and inhibit bronchoconstriction (see Fig. 55.2). See Table 55.2 for usual indications.

Table 55.2 *Drugs in Focus:* Drugs Affecting Inflammation

Drug Name	Usual Dosage	Usual Indications
Inhaled Steroids		
beclomethasone (*Qvar Redihaler*)	*Adult and pediatric ≥12 y:* 40–160 mcg inhalation b.i.d. and titrate for response *Pediatric (5–11 y):* 40 mcg b.i.d.	Prevention and treatment of asthma; treatment of chronic steroid-dependent bronchial asthma; used as adjunctive therapy for asthma patients who do not respond to traditional bronchodilators
budesonide (*Pulmicort Respules, Pulmicort Flexhaler*)	*Adult and pediatric (≥12 y):* 360 mcg inhalation b.i.d. and titrate for response; maximum dose 720 mcg b.i.d. *Pediatric (5–11 y):* 180 mcg inhaled b.i.d.; max 360 mcg inhaled daily	Prevention and treatment of asthma; treatment of chronic steroid-dependent bronchial asthma; used as adjunctive therapy for asthma patients who do not respond to traditional bronchodilators
ciclesonide (*Alvesco*)	*Adult and pediatric (≥12 y):* 80–320 mcg b.i.d. by inhalation	Prevention and treatment of asthma; treatment of chronic steroid-dependent bronchial asthma; used as adjunctive therapy for asthma patients who do not respond to traditional bronchodilators

Table 55.2 ***Drugs in Focus:*** **Drugs Affecting Inflammation (*Continued*)**

Drug Name	Usual Dosage	Usual Indications
fluticasone (*Flovent Discus, Flovent HFA*)	*Adult and pediatric (≥12 y):* One inhalation daily or b.i.d. (COPD); starting dose based on severity *Pediatric (4–11 y):* One inhalation b.i.d.	Prevention and treatment of asthma; treatment of chronic steroid-dependent bronchial asthma; used as adjunctive therapy for asthma patients who do not respond to traditional bronchodilators; maintenance treatment of COPD
Leukotriene Receptor Antagonists		
montelukast (*Singulair*)	*Adult and pediatric (>15 y):* 10 mg PO daily in the evening *Pediatric (6–23 mo):* 4-mg granules PO in the evening *Pediatric (2–5 y):* 4-mg chewable tablet PO in the evening *Pediatric (6–14 y):* 5-mg chewable tablet PO in the evening	Prophylaxis and treatment of asthma in adults and children; relief of symptoms from allergic rhinitis
zafirlukast (*Accolate*)	*Adult and pediatric (>12 y):* 20 mg PO b.i.d. *Pediatric (5–11 y):* 10 mg PO b.i.d.	Prophylaxis and treatment of chronic bronchial asthma in adults and in children ≥5 y of age
zileuton (*Zyflo*)	*Adult and pediatric (≥12 y):* 1,200 mg PO b.i.d. 1 h after a.m. and p.m. meals for a total of 2,400 mg/d	Prophylaxis and treatment of chronic bronchial asthma in patients ≥12 y of age
Immune Modulators		
benralizumab (*Fasenra*)	*Adult and pediatric (≥12 y):* 30 mg subcutaneous every 4 wk for 3 doses and then every 8 wk	Add-on maintenance treatment of patients with severe asthma with an eosinophilic phenotype
dupilumab (*Dupixent*)	*Adult and pediatric:* subcutaneous injections; exact dose and frequency varies based on indication and body weight	Treatment of patients ≥6 y of age with moderate to severe atopic dermatitis whose disease is not adequately controlled with topical prescription therapies; add-on maintenance treatment in patients with moderate-to-severe asthma ≥12 y of age with an eosinophilic phenotype or with oral corticosteroid dependent asthma; add-on maintenance treatment in adult patients with inadequately controlled chronic rhinosinusitis with nasal polyposis
mepolizumab (*Nucala*)	*Adult and pediatric (≥12 y) for asthma:* 100 mg administered subcutaneously once every 4 wk *Pediatric (6–11 y) for asthma:* 40 mg administered subcutaneously once every 4 wk *Adult for EGPA and adult and pediatric (≥12 y) for HES* : 300 mg as 3 separate 100-mg injections administered subcutaneously once every 4 wk	Add-on maintenance treatment of patients ≥6 y of age with severe asthma and with an eosinophilic phenotype; treatment of adult patients with EGPA; treatment of adult and pediatric patients aged 12 years and older with HES for ≥6 months without an identifiable nonhematologic secondary cause
omalizumab (*Xolair*)	*Adult and pediatric:* subcutaneous dosing every 2–4 wk; dose varies based on indication and body weight	Treatment of moderate to severe persistent asthma in adults and pediatric patients ≥6 y of age with a positive skin test or in vitro reactivity to a perennial aeroallergen and symptoms that are inadequately controlled with inhaled corticosteroids; add-on maintenance therapy for nasal polyps in adult patients ≥18 y of age with inadequate response to nasal corticosteroids, as add-on maintenance treatment; chronic idiopathic urticaria in adults and pediatric patients ≥12 y of age who remain symptomatic despite H1 antihistamine treatment
Reslizumab (*Cinqair*)	*Adult:* 3 mg/kg once every 4 wk by IV infusion over 20–50 min	Add-on maintenance treatment of patients ≥128 y of age with severe asthma and with an eosinophilic phenotype

COPD, chronic obstructive pulmonary disease; EGPA, eosinophilic granulomatosis with polyangiitis; HES, hypereosinophilic syndrome.

BOX 55.6

Fixed-Combination Respiratory Drugs

The benefit of combining different classes of drugs for the treatment of asthma and COPD has resulted in the development of fixed-combination drugs. Some of the combination medications available are as follows:

- *Advair Diskus* and *Advair HFA*: fluticasone (a steroid) and salmeterol (a long-acting beta2-adrenergic agonist (an LABA)
- *Combivent Respimat*: ipratropium (an anticholinergic agent) and albuterol (a beta2-adrenergic agonist)
- *Symbicort*: budesonide (a corticosteroid) and formoterol (an LABA)
- *Anoro Ellipta*: umeclidinium (an anticholinergic) and vilanterol (an LABA)
- *Breo Ellipta*: fluticasone (a corticosteroid) and vilanterol (an LABA)
- *Breztri Aerosphere*: budesonide (corticosteroid), glycopyrrolate (an anticholinergic), and formoterol fumarate (an LABA)
- *Bevespi Aerosphere*: glycopyrrolate (an anticholinergic) and formoterol fumarate (an LABA)
- *Duaklir Pressair*: aclidinium bromide (an anticholinergic) and formoterol fumarate (an LABA)
- *Dulera*: mometasone (a corticosteroid) and formoterol (an LABA)
- *Trelegy Ellipta*: fluticasone (a corticosteroid), umeclidinium (an anticholinergic), and vilanterol (an LABA)
- *Airduo Respiclick*: fluticasone (a corticosteroid) and salmeterol (an LABA)

Pharmacokinetics

These drugs are rapidly absorbed from the respiratory tract, but they take from 2 to 3 weeks to reach effective levels, and so patients must be encouraged to continue taking them to reach and then maintain the effective levels. They are metabolized mostly within the liver and are excreted in the urine. The glucocorticoids are known to cross the placenta and to enter human milk (see "Contraindications and Cautions").

Contraindications and Cautions

Inhaled steroids are not for emergency use and not for use during an acute asthma attack or status asthmaticus. They should not be used during pregnancy or lactation unless the benefit to the patient clearly outweighs any potential risk to the fetus or nursing baby. These preparations should be used with caution in any patient who has an active infection of the respiratory system because depression of the inflammatory response could result in serious illness.

Adverse Effects

There are usually fewer adverse effects when steroids are inhaled compared to oral or parenteral administration. Sore throat, hoarseness, coughing, dry mouth, and pharyngeal and laryngeal fungal infections are the most common adverse effects. Hypersensitivity reactions can occur. There is risk of growth impairment in pediatric patients. In patients taking a steroid long term, there is risk of glaucoma, cataracts, and decreased bone mineral density.

Clinically Important Drug–Drug Interactions

There are no known drug interactions with any of the medications in this classification. However, coadministration of fluticasone with ritonavir is not recommended due to evidence that coadministration increases fluticasone plasma levels.

P Prototype Summary: Budesonide

Indications: Prevention and treatment of asthma; to treat chronic steroid-dependent bronchial asthma; as adjunct therapy for patients whose asthma is not controlled by traditional bronchodilators.

Actions: Decreases the inflammatory response in the airway; this action will increase airflow and facilitate respiration in an airway narrowed by inflammation.

Pharmacokinetics:

Route	Onset	Peak	Duration
Inhalation	Slow	Rapid to absorb, but unrelated to clinical response since clinical response can be slow	8–12 h

$T_{1/2}$: 2 to 3 hours; metabolized in the liver and excreted in the urine.

Adverse Effects: Irritability, headache, rebound congestion, hypersensitivity, local infection.

Nursing Considerations for Patients Receiving Inhaled Steroids

Assessment: History and Examination

- Assess for possible contraindications or cautions: acute asthmatic attacks and allergy to the drugs, which are contraindications, and systemic infections, pregnancy, or lactation, which require cautious use.
- Perform a physical examination to establish baseline data for assessing the effectiveness of the drug and the occurrence of any adverse effects associated with drug therapy.
- Assess temperature to monitor for possible infections.
- Assess respirations and adventitious sounds to monitor drug effectiveness.
- Examine the mouth and throat to evaluate for potential local infections.

Nursing Conclusions

Nursing conclusions related to drug therapy might include

- Infection risk related to immunosuppression
- Impaired comfort related to local effects of the drug
- Knowledge deficit regarding drug therapy

Planning

- The patient will receive the best therapeutic effect from the drug therapy.
- The patient will have limited adverse effects from the drug therapy.
- The patient will have an understanding of the drug therapy, adverse effects to anticipate, and measures to relieve discomfort and improve safety.

Intervention With Rationale

- Do not administer the drug to treat an acute asthma attack or status asthmaticus because these drugs are not intended for treatment of acute attack and will not provide the immediate relief that is needed.
- Taper systemic steroids carefully during the transfer to inhaled steroids; deaths have occurred from adrenal insufficiency with sudden withdrawal.
- Have the patient rinse their mouth with water after using the inhaler because this will help reduce the risk of oral thrush.
- Monitor the patient for any sign of respiratory infection; continued use of steroids during an acute infection can lead to serious complications related to the depression of the inflammatory and immune responses.
- Provide thorough patient teaching, including the drug name and prescribed dosage, measures to help avoid adverse effects, warning signs that may indicate problems, and the need for periodic monitoring and evaluation, to enhance patient knowledge about drug therapy and to promote adherence.
- Instruct the patient to continue taking the drug to reach and then maintain effective levels. (The drug takes 2 to 3 weeks to reach effective levels.)
- Offer support and encouragement to help the patient cope with the disease and the drug regimen.

Evaluation

- Monitor patient response to the drug (improved breathing).
- Monitor for adverse effects (mouth and throat irritation or infection, fever, GI upset).
- Evaluate the effectiveness of the teaching plan (patient can name drug, dosage, adverse effects to watch for and specific measures to avoid them, and measures to take to increase the effectiveness of the drug).
- Monitor the effectiveness of other measures to ease breathing.

Leukotriene Receptor Antagonists

Leukotriene receptor antagonists were developed to act more specifically at the site of the problem associated with asthma. Zafirlukast (*Accolate*) was the first drug of this class to be developed. Montelukast (*Singulair*) and zileuton (*Zyflo*) are the other drugs currently available in this class.

Therapeutic Actions and Indications

Leukotriene receptor antagonists selectively and competitively block (zafirlukast, montelukast) or antagonize (zileuton) receptors for the production of leukotrienes. As a result, these drugs block many of the signs and symptoms of asthma, such as neutrophil and eosinophil migration, neutrophil and monocyte aggregation, leukocyte adhesion, airway edema, increased capillary permeability, and smooth muscle contraction. These factors contribute to the inflammation, edema, mucus secretion, and bronchoconstriction seen in patients with asthma. See Table 55.2 for usual indications of these drugs. They do not have immediate effects on the airways and are not indicated for treating acute asthma attacks.

Pharmacokinetics

These drugs are given orally. They are rapidly absorbed from the GI tract. Zafirlukast and montelukast are extensively metabolized in the liver by the cytochrome P-450 system and are primarily excreted in the feces. Zileuton is metabolized and cleared through the liver. These drugs cross the placenta and enter human milk (see "Contraindications and Cautions").

Contraindications and Cautions

Zeleuton and zafirlukast should be used cautiously in patients with hepatic impairment because there is risk of further liver injury with these medications. These drugs should be used during pregnancy only if the benefit to the patient outweighs the potential risks to the fetus; studies in humans have not shown high risk to the fetus when taken during pregnancy. No adequate studies have been done on the effects on the baby if these drugs are used during lactation; caution should be used.

These drugs are not indicated for the treatment of acute asthmatic attacks because they do not provide any immediate effects on the airways. Patients need to be cautioned that they should not rely on these drugs for relief from an acute asthmatic attack.

Adverse Effects

Adverse effects associated with leukotriene receptor antagonists include upper respiratory infection, pharyngitis, cough, headache, dizziness, nausea, diarrhea, abdominal pain, elevated liver enzyme concentrations, vomiting, generalized pain, fever, and myalgia. Serious neuropsychiatric events (including depression, suicide, hallucinations, and aggressive behavior) have been reported in patients taking leukotriene receptor antagonists. Montelukast has a boxed warning regarding the risk of neuropsychiatric events.

Clinically Important Drug–Drug Interactions

There are multiple potential drug–drug interactions with these medications, including concurrent use with warfarin, theophylline, phenytoin, aspirin, and others. Check for interactions before administering these medications.

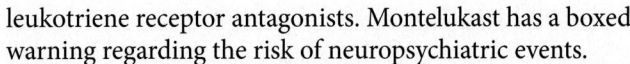

Prototype Summary: Zafirlukast

Indications: Prevention and long-term treatment of asthma in adults and children 5 years of age or older.

Actions: Specifically blocks receptors for leukotrienes, which are components of slow-reacting substance of anaphylaxis, blocking airway edema and processes of inflammation in the airway.

Pharmacokinetics:

Route	Onset	Peak	Duration
Oral	Rapid	3 h	Unknown

$T_{1/2}$: 10 hours; metabolized in the liver and excreted in the urine and feces.

Adverse Effects: Headache, dizziness, nausea, generalized pain and fever, infection, hepatotoxicity, rash, neuropsychiatric events.

Nursing Considerations for Patients Receiving Leukotriene Receptor Antagonists

Assessment: History and Examination

- Assess for possible contraindications or cautions: allergy to the drug, and acute bronchospasm or asthmatic attack, all of which would be contraindications to the use of the drug; impaired hepatic function, which could increase risk of liver dysfunction; and pregnancy or lactation, which require cautious use.
- Perform a physical examination to establish baseline data for assessing the effectiveness of the drug and the occurrence of any adverse effects associated with drug therapy.
- Evaluate temperature to monitor for underlying infection.
- Assess orientation, behavior changes, and affect to monitor for possible neuropsychiatric effects of the drug.
- Evaluate respirations and adventitious breath sounds to monitor the effectiveness of the drug.
- Perform an abdominal evaluation to monitor GI effects of the drug.

Nursing Conclusions

Nursing conclusions related to drug therapy might include

- Impaired comfort related to headache, GI upset, or myalgia
- Risk for injury related to neuropsychiatric effects
- Knowledge deficit regarding drug therapy

Planning

- The patient will receive the best therapeutic effect from the drug therapy.
- The patient will have limited adverse effects from the drug therapy.
- The patient will have an understanding of the drug therapy, adverse effects to anticipate, and measures to relieve discomfort and improve safety.

Intervention With Rationale

- Administer drug per prescribing instructions. The bioavailability is increased if zafirlukast is taken on an empty stomach or 1 hour before or 2 hours after meals; however, this is not true for the other medications.
- Caution the patient that these drugs are not to be used during an acute asthmatic attack or bronchospasm; instead, regular emergency measures will be needed.
- Caution the patient to take the drug continuously and not to stop the medication during symptom-free periods to ensure that therapeutic levels are maintained.
- Provide appropriate safety measures if neuropsychiatric events occur to prevent patient injury.
- Provide teaching regarding specific medication interactions for each patient, which might interfere with the effectiveness and/or safety of these drugs.
- Provide thorough patient teaching, including the drug name and prescribed dosage, measures to help avoid adverse effects, warning signs that may indicate problems, and the need for periodic monitoring and evaluation, to enhance patient knowledge about drug therapy and to promote adherence.
- Offer support and encouragement to help the patient cope with the disease and the drug regimen.

Evaluation

- Monitor patient response to the drug (improved breathing).
- Monitor for adverse effects (depression or other behavior changes, headache, abdominal pain, myalgia).
- Evaluate the effectiveness of the teaching plan (patient can name drug, dosage, adverse effects to watch for and specific measures to avoid them, and measures to take to increase the effectiveness of the drug).
- Monitor the effectiveness of other measures to ease breathing.

Immune Modulators

There are several immune modulators that are indicated for add-on maintenance therapy for patients with moderate to severe asthma. They include benralizumab (*Fasenra*), dupilumab (*Dupixent*), mepolizumab (*Nucala*), omalizumab (*Xolair*), and reslizumab (*Cinqair*).

Therapeutic Actions and Indications

The immune modulators that are indicated for treatment of asthma are antibodies. Benralizumab is a monoclonal antibody that binds to the interleukin-5 receptor expressed on eosinophils and basophils. The binding leads to apoptosis (regulated cell death) of eosinophils and basophils, which reduces inflammation from those cells. Omalizumab is an antibody that binds to IgE receptors on mast cells, basophils, and dendritic cells. The binding decreases the IgE-mediated inflammation that is increased by these cells. Mepolizumab and reslizumab are also antibodies. They bind to and inhibit interleukin-5, which is a cytokine that facilitates growth and activation of the eosinophils. Dupilumab binds to cells that have a receptor shared by interleukin-4 and interleukin-13. There are multiple cells that have this receptor, and several chemicals bind to it to induce inflammatory responses; by binding to the receptor, the medication probably decreases the inflammation reactions.

See Table 55.2 for usual indications of these drugs. They do not have immediate effects on the airways and are not indicated for treating acute asthma attacks.

Pharmacokinetics

Most of the medications are administered subcutaneously and absorbed slowly over several days. Reslizumab is administered IV, and peak absorption occurs at the end of the infusion. The monoclonal antibodies are thought to be primarily metabolized by proteolytic enzymes in the liver and other tissues. The half-lives are 15 to 26 days. Most of the medications have pregnancy registries to gather information about any effects of the medications on pregnancy outcomes. The medications are shown to cross the placenta but have not yet demonstrated any increased risk of adverse effects on the fetus or baby.

Contraindications and Cautions

These drugs are not indicated for the treatment of acute asthmatic attacks because they do not provide any immediate effects on the airways. Patients need to be cautioned that they should not rely on these drugs for relief from an acute asthmatic attack. All of the medications are contraindicated in patients who have hypersensitivity reactions to components of the medications.

There is a boxed warning for omalizumab and reslizumab regarding the potential for anaphylaxis. These medications must be administered in a health care setting in which the patient can be cared for appropriately if they have a hypersensitivity reaction.

Adverse Effects

There are a variety of adverse effects associated with these medications. Patients may demonstrate signs of upper respiratory infection, headaches, fever, injection site reactions, hypersensitivity reactions, and myalgia or arthralgia. Parasitic infections may be more difficult to treat if the patient is taking benralizumab or dupilumab. There may be increased risk of herpes infection and malignancies with some of the medications. There is risk of eosinophilic reactions manifested by vasculitic rash, pulmonary and/or cardiac complications, or neuropathy.

Clinically Important Drug–Drug Interactions

Corticosteroid treatment should not be abruptly discontinued when administering these medications due to risk of masked systemic withdrawal symptoms and increased risk of eosinophilic reactions. Corticosteroids should be titrated slowly if they need to be discontinued.

Prototype Summary: Omalizumab

Indications: Treatment of moderate to severe persistent asthma in adults and pediatric patients 6 years of age and older with a positive skin test or in vitro reactivity to a perennial aeroallergen and symptoms that are inadequately controlled with inhaled corticosteroids; add-on maintenance therapy for nasal polyps in adult patients 18 years of age and older with inadequate response to nasal corticosteroids; treatment of chronic idiopathic urticaria in adults and adolescents 12 years of age and older who remain symptomatic despite H1 antihistamine treatment.

Actions: Omalizumab is an antibody that binds to IgE receptors on mast cells, basophils, and dendritic cells. The binding decreases the IgE-mediated inflammation that is increased by these cells.

Pharmacokinetics:

Route	Onset	Peak	Duration
SQ	Unknown	7–8 d	Unknown

$T_{1/2}$: 24 to 26 days; excreted by liver and in bile.

Adverse Effects: Arthralgia, myalgia, fatigue, dizziness, rash, headache, upper respiratory infection, injection site reactions, hypersensitivity, anaphylaxis.

Nursing Considerations for Patients Receiving Immune Modulators

Assessment: History and Examination

- Assess for possible contraindications or cautions: allergy to the drug and acute bronchospasm or asthmatic attack, all of which would be contraindications to the use of the drug; and pregnancy or lactation, which require cautious use.

(continues on page 1000)

- Perform a physical examination to establish baseline data for assessing the effectiveness of the drug and the occurrence of any adverse effects associated with drug therapy.
- Evaluate temperature to monitor for underlying infection.
- Evaluate respirations and adventitious breath sounds to monitor the effectiveness of the drug.

Nursing Conclusions

Nursing conclusions related to drug therapy might include

- Impaired comfort related to headache, GI upset, or myalgia/arthralgia
- Risk for infection related to immune modulating effects
- Knowledge deficit regarding drug therapy

Planning

- The patient will receive the best therapeutic effect from the drug therapy.
- The patient will have limited adverse effects from the drug therapy.
- The patient will have an understanding of the drug therapy, adverse effects to anticipate, and measures to relieve discomfort and improve safety.

Intervention With Rationale

- Administer drug per instructions; some may need to be administered in a health care facility, where the patient can be monitored for potential hypersensitivity and anaphylaxis reaction.
- Caution the patient that these drugs are not to be used during an acute asthmatic attack or bronchospasm; instead, regular emergency measures will be needed.
- Provide thorough patient teaching, including the drug name and prescribed dosage, measures to help avoid adverse effects, warning signs that may indicate problems, and the need for periodic monitoring and evaluation, to enhance patient knowledge about drug therapy and to promote adherence.
- Offer support and encouragement to help the patient cope with the disease and the drug regimen.

Evaluation

- Monitor patient response to the drug (improved breathing).
- Monitor for adverse effects (hypersensitivity, rash, headache, arthralgia, myalgia, upper respiratory infection).
- Evaluate the effectiveness of the teaching plan (patient can name drug, dosage, adverse effects to watch for and specific measures to avoid them, and measures to take to increase the effectiveness of the drug).
- Monitor the effectiveness of other measures to ease breathing.

Mast Cell Stabilizer

A **mast cell stabilizer** prevents the release of inflammatory and bronchoconstricting substances (like histamine) when the mast cells are stimulated to release these substances because of irritation or the presence of an antigen. Cromolyn (generic) is the only drug still available in this class. It is no longer considered part of the treatment standards because of the availability of more specific and safer drugs.

Key Points

- Corticosteroids decrease the inflammatory response. The inhalable form is associated with many fewer systemic effects than are the other corticosteroid formulations.
- To block various signs and symptoms of asthma, leukotriene receptor antagonists block or antagonize receptors for the production of leukotrienes D_4 and E_4.
- Immune modulating antibodies have been developed as add-on maintenance therapy for patients with severe asthma.

Lung Surfactants

Lung surfactants are naturally occurring compounds or lipoproteins containing lipids and apoproteins that reduce the surface tension within the alveoli, allowing expansion of the alveoli for gas exchange. Lung surfactants available for use are beractant (*Survanta*), calfactant (*Infasurf*), and poractant (*Curosurf*).

Therapeutic Actions and Indications

These drugs are used to replace the surfactant that is missing in the lungs of neonates with RDS (see Fig. 55.2). See Table 55.3 for usual indications.

Pharmacokinetics

These drugs are instilled directly into the trachea and begin to act immediately on instillation. They are metabolized in the lungs by the normal surfactant metabolic pathways.

Contraindications and Cautions

Because lung surfactants are used as emergency drugs in the newborn, there are no contraindications.

Adverse Effects

Adverse effects that are associated with the use of lung surfactants include patent ductus arteriosus, bradycardia, hypotension, intraventricular hemorrhage, pneumothorax, pulmonary air leak, hyperbilirubinemia, and sepsis. These effects may be related to the immaturity of the patient, the invasive procedures used, or reactions to the lipoprotein.

Table 55.3 *Drugs in Focus:* Lung Surfactants

Drug Name	Usual Dosage	Usual Indications
beractant (*Survanta*)	4 mL/kg birth weight, instilled intratracheally; may repeat up to four times in 48 h	Rescue treatment of infants who have RDS; prophylactic treatment of infants at high risk for development of RDS (birth weight of <1,350 g; birth weight >1,350 g with evidence of respiratory immaturity)
calfactant (*Infasurf*)	3 mg/kg birth weight, as soon as possible for prophylaxis; 3 mg/kg birth weight, divided into two doses, repeat up to a total of three doses 12 h apart, for rescue; instilled into the trachea	Rescue treatment of infants who have RDS; prophylactic treatment of infants at high risk for RDS (see prior entry for risks)
poractant (*Curosurf*)	2.5 mL/kg birth weight, intratracheally, half in each bronchus, may repeat with up to two 1.25-mL/kg doses at 12-h intervals; max dose 5 mL/kg	Rescue treatment of infants who have RDS

RDS, respiratory distress syndrome.

Clinically Important Drug–Drug Interactions

Drug interactions are not expected with this classification of medications since they are instilled in the trachea.

Prototype Summary: Beractant

Indications: Prophylactic treatment of infants at high risk for developing RDS; rescue treatment of infants who have developed RDS.

Actions: Natural bovine compound of lipoproteins that reduce the surface tension and allow expansion of the alveoli; replaces the surfactant that is missing in infants with RDS.

Pharmacokinetics:

Route	Onset	Peak
Intratracheal	Immediate	Hours

$T_{1/2}$: Unknown; metabolized by surfactant pathways.

Adverse Effects: Patent ductus arteriosus, intraventricular hemorrhage, hypotension, bradycardia, pneumothorax, pulmonary air leak, pulmonary hemorrhage, apnea, sepsis, infection.

Nursing Considerations for Patients Receiving Lung Surfactants

Assessment: History and Examination

- Assess for possible contraindications or cautions: screen for time of birth and exact weight to determine appropriate dose. Because this drug is used as an emergency treatment, there are no contraindications.
- Perform a physical examination to establish baseline data for assessing the effectiveness of the drug and the occurrence of any adverse effects associated with drug therapy.
- Assess the skin temperature and color to evaluate perfusion.
- Monitor respirations, adventitious sounds, endotracheal tube placement and patency, and chest movements to evaluate the effectiveness of the drug and drug delivery.
- Evaluate blood pressure, pulse, and arterial pressure to monitor the status of the infant.
- Evaluate blood gases and oxygen saturation to monitor drug effectiveness.
- Assess temperature and complete blood count to monitor for sepsis.

Nursing Conclusions

Nursing conclusions related to drug therapy might include

- Decreased cardiac output related to CV and respiratory effects of the drug
- Injury risk related to prematurity and risk of infection
- Ineffective airway clearance related to the possibility of mucus plugs
- Knowledge deficit regarding drug therapy (for parents)

Planning

- The patient will receive the best therapeutic effect from the drug therapy.
- The patient will have limited adverse effects from the drug therapy.
- The patient's parents will have an understanding of the drug therapy, adverse effects to anticipate, and measures to relieve discomfort and improve safety.

Intervention With Rationale

- Monitor the patient continuously during administration and until stable to provide life support measures as needed.

(continues on page 1002)

- Ensure proper placement of the endotracheal tube with bilateral chest movement and lung sounds to provide adequate delivery of the drug.
- Have staff view the manufacturer's teaching video before regular use to review the specific technical aspects of administration.
- Suction the infant immediately before administration, but do not suction for 2 hours after administration unless clinically necessary, to allow the drug time to work.
- Provide support and encouragement to parents of the patient, explaining the use of the drug in the teaching program, to help them cope with the diagnosis and treatment of their infant.
- Continue other supportive measures related to the immaturity of the infant because this is only one aspect of medical care needed for premature infants.

Evaluation

- Monitor patient response to the drug (improved breathing, alveolar expansion).
- Monitor for adverse effects (pneumothorax, patent ductus arteriosus, bradycardia, sepsis).
- Evaluate the effectiveness of the teaching plan and support parents as appropriate.
- Monitor the effectiveness of other measures to support breathing and stabilize the patient.
- Evaluate the effectiveness of other supportive measures related to the immaturity of the infant.

Key Points

- Lung surfactants are naturally occurring compounds that reduce the surface tension in the alveoli, allowing them to expand. They are injected directly into the trachea of infants who have RDS.
- Administration of lung surfactants requires proper placement of the endotracheal tube, suctioning of the infant before administration (but not for 2 hours after administration unless necessary), and careful monitoring and support of the infant to ensure lung expansion and proper oxygenation.

Other Drugs Used to Treat Lower Respiratory Tract Disorders

The other major pathophysiology that can affect the lower respiratory tract is infection. Infection can manifest as bronchitis or pneumonia. These infections occur when pathogens are able to enter the normally well-protected airways and surrounding tissue. Stress, age, and concurrent respiratory dysfunction all increase the opportunities for these pathogens to invade the respiratory tract and cause problems. These infections can be viral, bacterial, fungal, or protozoal in origin. They are treated using the appropriate agents to affect the specific pathogen that is involved. See Chapter 9 for drugs used to treat bacterial infections, Chapter 10 for drugs used to treat viral infections, Chapter 11 for drugs used to treat fungal infection, and Chapter 12 for drugs used to treat protozoal infections. Patients with infections of the respiratory tract may have difficulty breathing, decreased oxygenation leading to fatigue, and changes in ability to carry on the activities of daily living, including eating. These patients require assistance to maintain function, help with nutrition, and support to deal with the uncomfortable feeling of not being able to breathe.

See Box 55.7 for information about two drugs approved for treatment of idiopathic pulmonary fibrosis (IPF).

BOX 55.7

Drugs for Idiopathic Pulmonary Fibrosis

In 2014, the first drugs for the treatment of IPF were approved. IPF is a disease of progressive lung scarring and decline in lung function with no known cause or treatment. Two drugs offer treatment options to these patients. Pirfenidone (*Esbriet*), a pyridine, and nintedanib (*Ofev*), a kinase inhibitor, are both approved for the treatment of IPF. Nintedanib is a small molecule that inhibits numerous kinase receptors including ones associated with proliferation, migration, and formation of fibroblasts that are implicated in the development of IPF. It is also indicated for treating lung fibrosis due to interstitial lung diseases. It should be used with caution with hepatic impairment and can cause embryo or fetal toxicity. Nintedanib can cause severe GI problems, leading to dehydration as well as thromboembolic events including myocardial infarction (MI). Bleeding in patients with known bleeding risks and GI perforation when used after GI surgery have been reported. Pirfenidone has been shown to improve lung function in patients with IPF, but the mechanism of action is not known. It is an oral agent taken three times a day. The drug needs to be tapered to reach the desired therapeutic dosing. It has also been associated with liver toxicity and GI issues. Rash and photosensitivity have also been reported. It should be used with caution with renal impairment, liver impairment, and use of CYP1A2 inhibitors.

SUMMARY

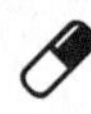
Pulmonary obstructive diseases include asthma and COPD, which includes emphysema and chronic bronchitis (which cause obstruction of the major airways), and RDS, which causes obstruction at the alveolar level.

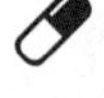
Drugs used to treat asthma and COPD include drugs to decrease inflammation and drugs to dilate bronchi.

- The xanthine derivatives have a direct effect on the smooth muscle of the respiratory tract, both in the bronchi and in the blood vessels.
- The adverse effects of theophylline are directly related to the theophylline concentration in the blood and can progress to coma and death.
- Sympathomimetics are drugs that mimic the effects of the sympathetic nervous system; they are used for dilation of the bronchi and to increase the rate and depth of respiration.
- Anticholinergics can be used as bronchodilators because of their effect on the vagus nerve, resulting in relaxation of smooth muscle in the bronchi, which leads to bronchodilation.
- Steroids are used to decrease the inflammatory response in the airway. Inhaling the steroid tends to decrease the numerous systemic effects that are associated with oral and parenteral steroid administration.
- Leukotriene receptor antagonists block or antagonize receptors for the production of leukotrienes, thus blocking many of the signs and symptoms of asthma.
- Lung surfactants are instilled into the respiratory system of premature infants who do not have enough surfactant to ensure alveolar expansion.

Unfolding Patient Stories: Toua Xiong • Part 2

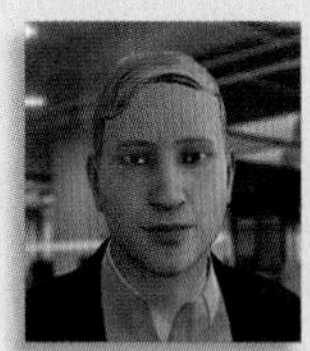

Think back to Toua Xiong, a 64-year-old male with emphysema from Chapter 3. He presents to the clinic with left ear pain and fever following an upper respiratory infection. The provider prescribes amoxicillin for acute otitis media. What patient education would the nurse provide on amoxicillin and the treatment options for fever and pain relief? How would the nurse differentiate a hypersensitivity reaction to amoxicillin from worsening respiratory symptoms associated with an acute exacerbation of emphysema?

Care for Toua and other patients in a realistic virtual environment: ***vSim** for Nursing* (thepoint.lww.com/vSimPharm). Practice documenting these patients' care in DocuCare (thepoint.lww.com/DocuCareEHR).

CHECK YOUR UNDERSTANDING

Answers to the questions in this chapter can be found in Answers to Check Your Understanding Questions on thePoint®.

MULTIPLE CHOICE

Select the best answer.

1. Treatment of obstructive pulmonary disorders is aimed at
   a. opening the conducting airways or decreasing the effects of inflammation.
   b. blocking the autonomic reflexes that alter respirations.
   c. blocking the effects of the immune and inflammatory systems.
   d. altering the respiratory membrane to increase the flow of oxygen and carbon dioxide.

2. You are teaching a patient who has been newly prescribed budesonide. Which instructions would be the most appropriate for this patient?
   a. "Be careful to limit your fluid intake when on this medication."
   b. "It is important to get plenty of iron in your diet when taking this medication."
   c. "You can take this medication only on days when you feel short of breath."
   d. "Rinse your mouth out with water after taking the medication."

3. Your patient has been maintained on theophylline for many years and has recently taken up smoking. The theophylline levels in this patient would be expected to
   a. rise because nicotine prevents the breakdown of theophylline.
   b. stay the same because smoking has no effect on theophylline.
   c. fall because substances in cigarettes stimulate liver metabolism of theophylline.
   d. rapidly reach toxic levels.

4. A person with hypertension and known heart disease has frequent bronchospasms and COPD exacerbations that are most responsive to sympathomimetic drugs. This patient might be best treated with
   a. an inhaled sympathomimetic to decrease systemic effects.
   b. a xanthine.
   c. no sympathomimetics because they would be contraindicated.
   d. an anticholinergic.

5. A patient with many adverse reactions to drugs is tried on an inhaled steroid for treatment of bronchospasm. For the first 3 days, the patient does not notice any improvement. You should anticipate that the provider will
   a. switch the patient to a xanthine.
   b. encourage the patient to continue the drug for 2 to 3 weeks.
   c. switch the patient to a sympathomimetic.
   d. try the patient on a surfactant.

6. Leukotriene receptor antagonists act to block production of a component of slow-reacting substance of anaphylaxis. They are most beneficial in treating
   a. seasonal rhinitis.
   b. pneumonia.
   c. COPD.
   d. asthma.

7. Respiratory distress syndrome occurs in babies
   a. with frequent colds.
   b. with genetic allergies.
   c. who are premature or of low birth weight.
   d. who are stressed during the pregnancy.

8. Lung surfactants used therapeutically are
   a. injected into a developed muscle.
   b. instilled via a nasogastric tube.
   c. injected into the umbilical artery.
   d. instilled into an endotracheal tube properly placed in the baby's lungs.

MULTIPLE RESPONSE

Select all that apply.

1. Patients who are using inhalers require careful teaching about which information?
   a. Avoiding food 1 hour before and 2 hours after dosing
   b. Storage of the drug
   c. Administration techniques to promote therapeutic effects and avoid adverse effects
   d. Lying flat for as long as 2 hours after dosing
   e. Timing of administration
   f. The difference between rescue treatment and prophylaxis

2. A child with repeated asthma attacks may be treated with which drugs?
   a. A leukotriene receptor antagonist
   b. A beta-blocker
   c. An inhaled corticosteroid
   d. An inhaled beta-agonist
   e. A surfactant
   f. A mast cell stabilizer

REFERENCES

Bauldoff, G. (2012). When breathing is a burden: How to help patients with COPD. *American Nurse Today, 7*(8). https://www.myamericannurse.com/when-breathing-is-a-burden-how-to-help-patients-with-copd-2/

Berger, W. (2009). *Asthma*. Oxford University Press.

Brunton, L., Hilal-dandan, R., & Knollman, B. (2018). *Goodman and Gilman's the pharmacological basis of therapeutics* (13th ed.). McGraw-Hill.

Cobridge, S., & Cobridge, T. (2010). Asthma in adolescents and adults. *American Journal of Nursing, 110*(5), 28–38. https://doi.org/10.1097/01.NAJ.0000372069.78392.79

Global Initiative for Asthma. (2021). *Pocket guide for asthma management and prevention.* https://ginasthma.org/wp-content/uploads/2021/05/GINA-Pocket-Guide-2021-V2-WMS.pdf

Global Initiative for Chronic Obstructive Lung Disease. (2021). *Global strategy for the diagnosis, management, and prevention of chronic obstructive pulmonary disease.* https://goldcopd.org/wp-content/uploads/2020/11/GOLD-REPORT-2021-v1.1-25Nov20_WMV.pdf

Hall, J. E., & Hall, M. E. (2021). *Guyton and Hall textbook of medical physiology* (14th ed.). Elsevier.

Khan, Z., & Khan, M. S. (2019). Rare case of theophylline toxicity due to influenza A infection in an adult with asthma. *American Journal of Therapeutics, 26*(4), e553–e555. https://journals.lww.com/americantherapeutics/Fulltext/2019/08000/Rare_Case_of_Theophylline_Toxicity_due_to.30.aspx

Norris, T. L. (2019). *Porth's pathophysiology concepts of altered health states* (13th ed.). Wolters Kluwer.

PART 11

Drugs Acting on the Gastrointestinal System

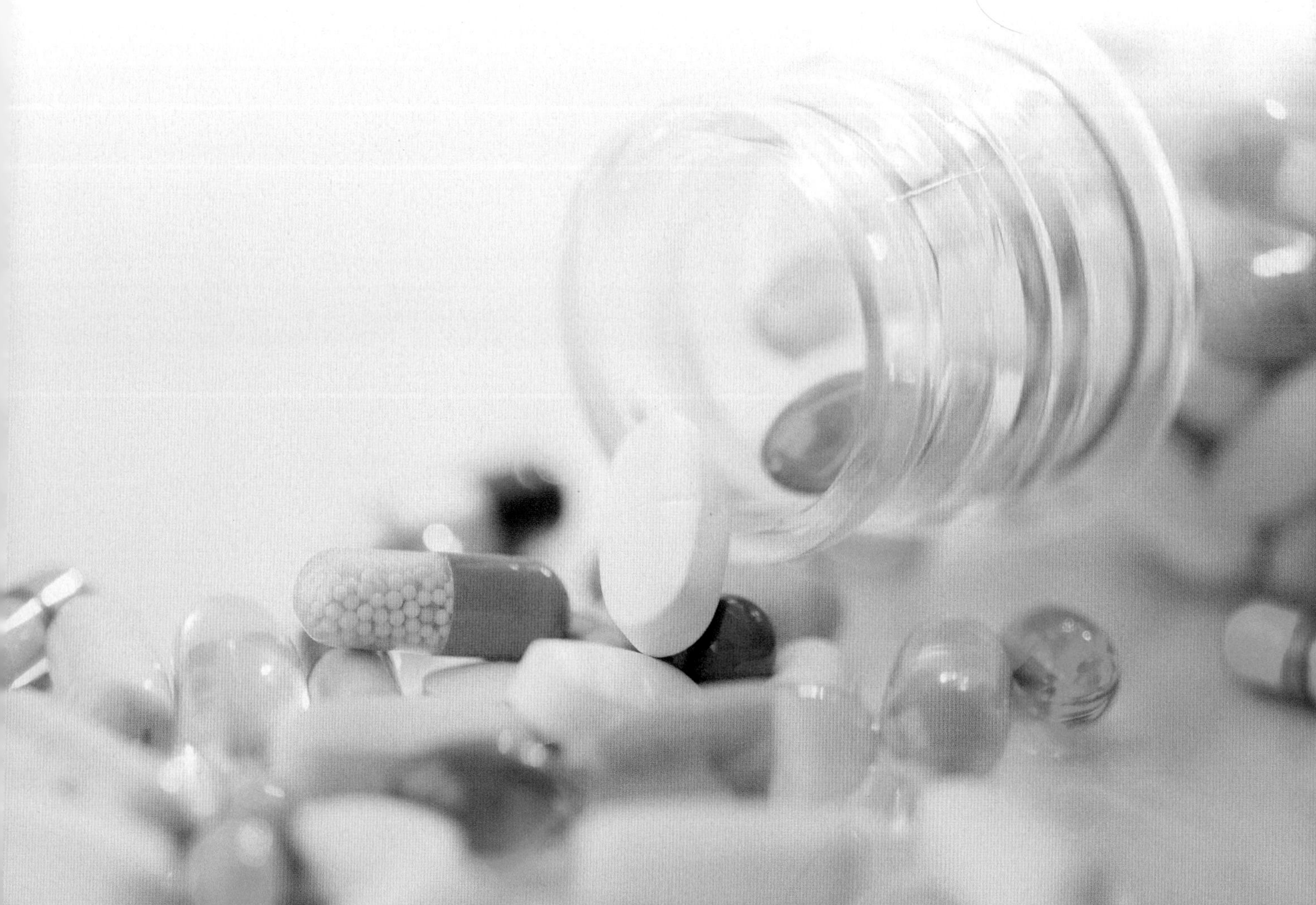

CHAPTER 56

Introduction to the Gastrointestinal System

Learning Objectives

Upon completion of this chapter, you will be able to:

1. Label the parts of the gastrointestinal (GI) tract on a diagram, describing the secretions, absorption, digestion, and type of motility that occurs in each part.
2. Discuss the nervous system control of the GI tract, including influences of the autonomic nervous system on GI activity.
3. List the local GI reflexes, and describe the clinical application of each.
4. Describe the steps involved in swallowing, including factors that can influence this reflex.
5. Discuss the vomiting reflex, addressing factors that can stimulate the reflex.

Key Terms

bile: fluid produced in the liver and stored in the gallbladder; contains cholesterol and bile salts; essential for the proper breakdown and absorption of fats

chyme: contents of the stomach containing ingested food and secreted enzymes, water, and mucus

gallstones: hard crystals formed in the gallbladder when the bile containing many crystalline substances is concentrated

gastrin: substance secreted by the stomach in response to many stimuli; stimulates the release of hydrochloric acid from the parietal cells and pepsin from the chief cells; causes histamine release at histamine-2 receptors to effect the release of acid

histamine-2 (H_2) receptors: sites near the parietal cells of the stomach that, when stimulated, cause the release of hydrochloric acid into the lumen of the stomach; also found near cardiac cells

hydrochloric acid: acid released by the parietal cells of the stomach in response to gastrin release or parasympathetic stimulation; makes the stomach contents more acidic to aid digestion and breakdown of food products

local gastrointestinal reflex: reflex response to various stimuli that allows the GI tract local control of its secretions and movements based on the contents or activity of the whole GI system

nerve plexus: network of nerve fibers running through the wall of the GI tract that allows local reflexes and control

pancreatic enzymes: digestive enzymes secreted by the exocrine pancreas, including pancreatin and pancrelipase, which are needed for the proper digestion of fats, proteins, and carbohydrates

peristalsis: type of GI movement that moves a food bolus forward; characterized by a progressive wave of muscle contraction

saliva: fluid produced by the salivary glands in the mouth in response to tactile stimuli and cerebral stimulation; contains enzymes to begin digestion, as well as water and mucus to make the food bolus slippery and easier to swallow

segmentation: GI movement characterized by contraction of one segment of the small intestine while the next segment is relaxed; the contracted segment then relaxes, and the relaxed segment contracts; exposes the chyme to a vast surface area to increase absorption

swallowing: complex reflex response to a bolus in the back of the throat; allows passage of the bolus into the esophagus and movement of ingested contents into the GI tract

vomiting: complex reflex mediated through the medulla after stimulation of the chemoreceptor trigger zone; protective reflex to remove possibly toxic substances from the stomach

The gastrointestinal (GI) system is a system in the body that is open to the external environment. It begins at the mouth and ends at the anus. The GI system is responsible for only a small part of waste excretion. The kidneys and lungs are responsible for excreting most of the waste products of normal metabolism.

Structure and Function of the Gastrointestinal System

The GI system is composed of one continuous tube that begins at the mouth; progresses through the esophagus, stomach, and small and large intestines; and ends at the anus. The pancreas, liver, and gallbladder are accessory organs that support the functions of the GI system (Fig. 56.1).

Structures

The tube that comprises the GI tract is continuous with the external environment, opening at the mouth and again at the anus. Because of this, the GI tract contains many foreign agents and bacteria that are not found in the rest of the body. These bacteria, the normal flora of the GI tract, have a role in digestion and in protecting the body from other bacteria that might be ingested. The tube begins in the mouth, which has salivary glands that secrete digestive enzymes and lubricants to facilitate swallowing. The mouth leads to the esophagus, which produces mucus to help facilitate movement. The esophagus connects to the stomach, which is responsible for mechanical and chemical breakdown of foods into usable nutrients. The stomach empties into the small intestine, where absorption of nutrients occurs. The pancreas deposits digestive enzymes and sodium bicarbonate into the beginning of the small intestine to neutralize the acid from the stomach and to further facilitate digestion. The liver produces **bile**, which is stored in the gallbladder. Bile is important in the digestion of fats and is deposited into the small intestine when the gallbladder is stimulated to contract by the presence of fats. All of the nutrients absorbed from the small intestine pass into the liver, which is responsible for processing, storing, or clearing them from the system. The small intestine leads to the large intestine, which is responsible for excreting any waste products that are in the GI system. The excretion occurs through the rectum and is an activity that one learns to control.

The peritoneum lines the abdominal wall and also the viscera, with a small "free space" between the two layers. It helps keep the GI tract in place and prevents a buildup of friction with movement. The greater and lesser omenta

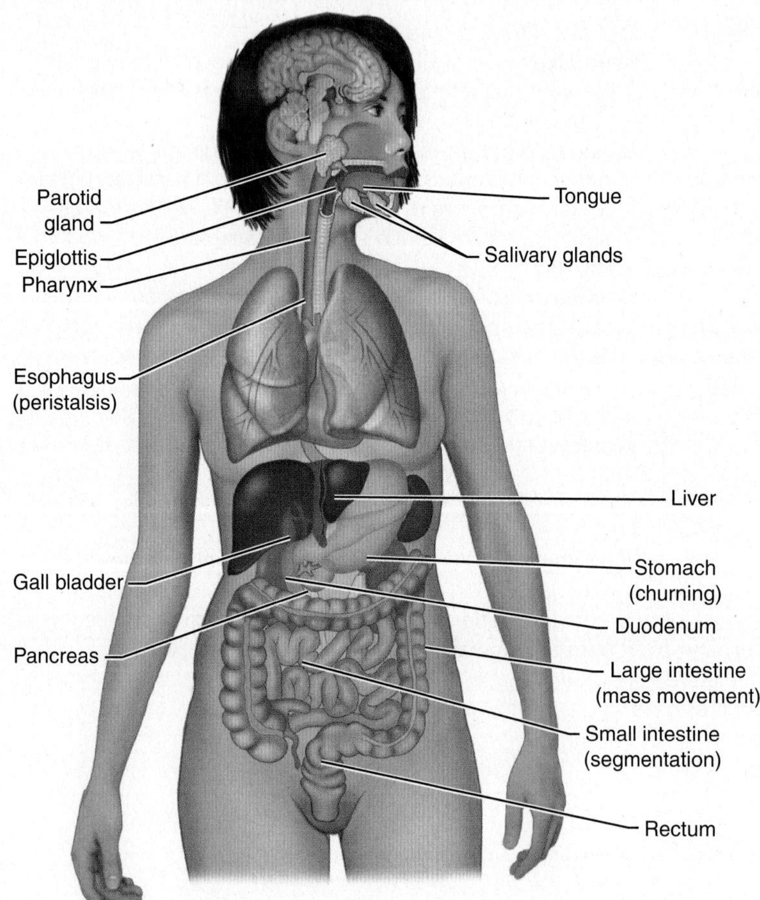

FIGURE 56.1 The gastrointestinal tract.

hang from the stomach over the lower GI tract and are full of lymph nodes, lymphocytes, monocytes, and other components of the immune and inflammatory systems. This barrier provides rapid protection for the rest of the body if any of the bacteria or other foreign agents in the GI tract should be absorbed into the body.

Layers of the GI Tract

The GI tube is composed of four layers. The layers of the tube contain an epithelial lining, smooth muscle, connective tissue, and networks of nerves (Fig. 56.2).

Mucosal Layer

The innermost layer is the mucosal layer, which provides the inner lining of the GI tract. It can be seen in the mouth and is fairly consistent throughout the tube. It is important to remember when assessing a patient that if the mouth is dry or full of lesions, it is a reflection of the state of the entire GI tract and may indicate that the patient has difficulty digesting or absorbing nutrients. The mucosal layer has epithelial cells that reproduce quickly and smooth muscle cells that can contract and change the surface area of the GI tube. The mucosal layer makes mucus that can moisten and act as a barrier protectant, secretes digestive enzymes, and absorbs nutrients.

Submucosal Layer

The submucosal layer surrounds the mucosal layer. It consists of connective tissue, blood vessels, and glands that can secrete substances into the GI tube. There is also a nerve network called the submucosal plexus, which facilitates secretions, absorption, and contraction of GI tract segments.

Muscularis Externa Layer

The muscularis externa layer is made up of muscles. Most of the GI tract has two muscle layers. One layer runs circularly around the tube, helping keep the tube open and squeezing the tube to aid digestion and motility. The other layer runs longitudinally, which helps propel the GI contents down the tract. The myenteric plexus of nerves is between the circular and longitudinal muscles. It facilitates motility of contents down the GI tract. The stomach has a third layer of muscle, which runs obliquely and gives the stomach the ability to move contents in a churning motion.

Serosal Layer

The outermost layer of the GI tract, the serosal layer, is a membrane made of epithelium and connective tissue. This layer is also known as the visceral peritoneum. The peritoneum and mesenteries are connective tissue that encase and attach to the GI tract to keep it in place.

Enteric Nervous System

The enteric nervous system consists of the nerve tracks in the submucosal and muscularis external layers. These nerves allow the GI tract local control over movement, secretions, and digestion. The nerves respond to local stimuli and act on the contents of the GI tract accordingly. The smooth muscle in the GI tract has some pacemaker cells

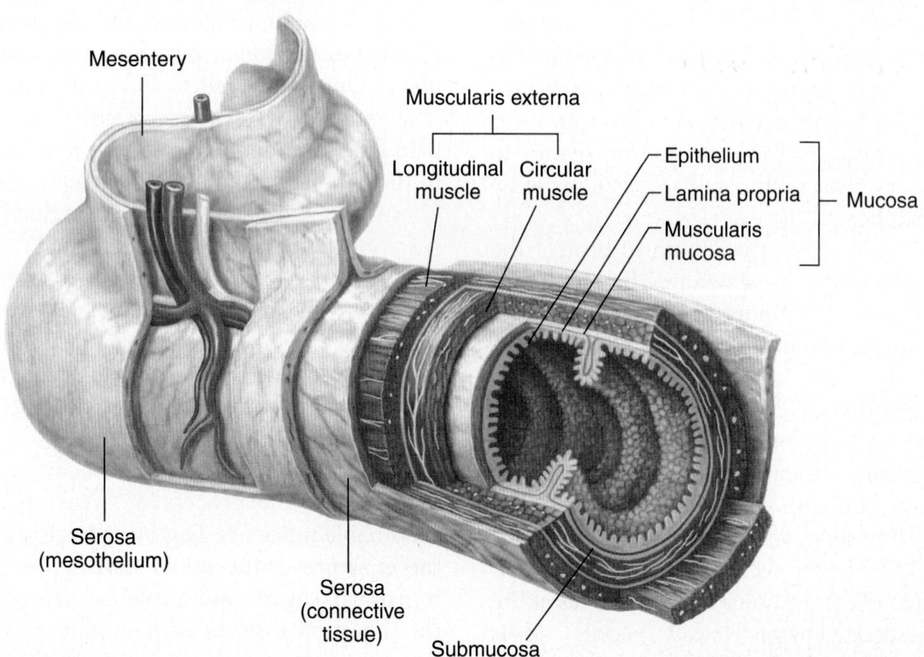

FIGURE 56.2 The gastrointestinal tract is composed of epithelial lining, smooth muscle, connective tissue, and networks of nerve layers. (Reprinted with permission from Norris, T. L. (2019). *Porth's pathophysiology: Concepts of altered health states* (10th ed.). Wolters Kluwer.)

that can initiate action potentials that are slow, rhythmic waves of electrical activity. The amplitude and frequency of these slow waves can be modulated by the enteric nervous system.

The GI tract is also innervated by the sympathetic and parasympathetic nervous systems. These systems can slow down or speed up the activity in the GI tract but cannot initiate local activity. The sympathetic system is stimulated during times of stress ("fight-or-flight" response) when digestion is not a priority. To slow the GI tract, the sympathetic system decreases muscle tone, secretions, and contractions and increases sphincter tone. By slowing down GI activity, the body saves energy for other activities. In contrast, the parasympathetic system ("rest-and-digest" response) stimulates the GI tract, increasing muscle tone, secretions, and contractions and decreasing sphincter tone, allowing easy movement.

Gastrointestinal Activities

The GI system has four major activities:

- *Secretion* of enzymes, acid, bicarbonate, and mucus
- *Digestion* of food into usable and absorbable components
- *Absorption* of water and almost all of the essential nutrients needed by the body
- *Motility* (movement) of food and secretions through the system (what is not used is excreted in the form of feces)

These functions are discussed in detail in the following sections.

Secretion

The GI tract secretes various compounds to aid the movement of the food bolus through the GI tube, to protect the inner layer of the GI tract from injury, and to facilitate the digestion and absorption of nutrients (see Fig. 56.1). Secretions begin in the mouth. **Saliva**, which contains water and digestive enzymes, is secreted from the salivary glands to begin the digestive process and to facilitate swallowing by making the bolus slippery.

Mucus is also produced in the mouth to protect the epithelial lining and to aid in swallowing. The esophagus produces mucus to protect the inner lining of the GI tract and to further facilitate the movement of the bolus down the tube.

The stomach produces acid and digestive enzymes. In addition, it generates a large amount of mucus to protect the stomach lining from the acid and the enzymes. In the stomach, secretion begins with what is called the cephalic phase of digestion. The sight, smell, or taste of food stimulates the stomach to begin secreting before any food reaches the stomach. Once the bolus of food arrives at the stomach, **gastrin** is secreted by gastrin cells (G cells); this is one of the stimulators of acid release. The gastric chief cells will release pepsinogen that can be activated to the enzyme pepsin that breaks down proteins. The parietal cells are responsible for releasing **hydrochloric acid**. More acid is released with parasympathetic stimulation of the vagal nerve that will secrete acetylcholine. Gastrin from the G cells also stimulates acid release. There are specialized cells called enterochromaffin-like cells (ECL) that secrete gastric histamine. These cells are near the parietal cells, and the histamine that is secreted will diffuse and react with **histamine-2 (H_2) receptors** on the parietal cells, causing the parietal cells to release hydrochloric acid into the lumen of the stomach. Proteins, calcium, alcohol, and caffeine in the stomach increase gastrin secretion. High levels of acid decrease the secretion of gastrin. Epithelial cells are able to secrete mucus to protect the lining of the stomach. Peptic ulcers can develop when there is a decrease in the protective mucosal layer or an increase in acid production.

Ghrelin is another substance that is made and secreted by the stomach. It is a peptide hormone that is secreted more after a time of fasting and when growth hormone levels are low. It is thought to prepare the body for digestion of a meal and to stimulate more secretion of growth hormone.

The now-acidic bolus leaves the stomach and enters the small intestine. Secretin is released, which stimulates the pancreas to secrete large amounts of sodium bicarbonate (to neutralize the acid bolus) and decreases gastric acid secretion by inhibiting gastrin. The **pancreatic enzymes** chymotrypsin and trypsin break down proteins to smaller amino acids, other lipases break down fat, and amylases break down sugars. These enzymes are delivered to the GI tract through the common bile duct, which is shared with the gallbladder.

If fat is present in the bolus, the gallbladder contracts and releases bile into the small intestine. Bile contains a detergent-like substance that breaks apart fat molecules so that they can be processed and absorbed. The bile in the gallbladder is produced by the liver during normal metabolism. Once delivered to the gallbladder for storage, it is concentrated; water is removed by the walls of the gallbladder. Some people are prone to developing **gallstones** in the gallbladder when the concentrated bile crystallizes. These stones can move down the duct and cause severe pain or even blockage of the bile duct.

In response to the presence of food, the small and large intestines may secrete various endocrine hormones, including growth hormone, aldosterone, and glucagon. They also secrete large amounts of mucus to facilitate the movement of the bolus through the rest of the GI tract.

Digestion

Digestion is the process of breaking food into usable, absorbable nutrients. Digestion begins in the mouth, with the enzymes in the saliva starting the process of breaking down sugars and proteins. The stomach continues the digestion process with muscular churning, breaking down some foodstuffs while mixing them thoroughly with hydrochloric acid and enzymes. The acid and enzymes further break down sugars and proteins into building blocks and separate vitamins, electrolytes, minerals, and other nutrients from ingested food for absorption. The beginning of the small intestine introduces bile to the food bolus, which is now called **chyme**. Bile breaks down fat molecules for processing and absorption into the bloodstream, and the pancreatic enzymes continue the digestion of sugars, proteins, and fats. Digestion is finished at this point, and absorption of the nutrients begins.

Absorption

Absorption is the active process of removing water, nutrients, and other elements from the GI tract and delivering them to the bloodstream for use by the body. The portal system drains all of the lower GI tract, where absorption occurs, and delivers what is absorbed into the venous system directly to the liver. The liver filters, clears, and further processes most of what is absorbed before it is delivered to the body (see Fig. 56.1). Some absorption (most commonly absorption of water and alcohol) occurs in the lower end of the stomach. Most absorption occurs in the small intestine. Absorption in the small intestine is about 8,500 mL/d, including nutrients, drugs, and anything that is taken into the GI tract, as well as any secretions. The small intestine mucosal layer is specially designed to facilitate this absorption with long villi on the epithelial layer providing a vast surface area for absorption. The large intestine absorbs approximately 350 mL/d, mostly sodium and water.

Motility

The GI tract depends on an inherent motility to keep things moving through the system. The **nerve plexus** (a network of nerve fibers running through the wall of the GI tract) maintains a basic electrical rhythm (BER), much like the pacemaker rhythm in the heart. The cells within the plexus are somewhat unstable and leak electrolytes, leading to the regular firing of an action potential. This rhythm maintains the tone of the GI tract muscles and protects the lining of the GI tract from digestive enzymes and other toxins and is affected by local or autonomic stimuli to increase or decrease the rate of firing.

The basic movement seen in the esophagus is **peristalsis**, a constant wave of contraction that moves from the top to the bottom of the esophagus. The act of swallowing, a response to a food bolus in the back of the throat, stimulates the peristaltic movement that directs the food bolus into the stomach. The stomach uses its three muscle layers to produce a churning action. This action mixes the digestive enzymes and acid with the food to increase digestion. A contraction of the lower end of the stomach sends the chyme into the small intestine.

The small intestine uses a process of **segmentation** with an occasional peristaltic wave to clear the segment. Segmentation involves contraction of one segment of the small intestine while the next segment is relaxed. The contracted segment then relaxes, and the relaxed segment contracts. This action exposes the chyme to a vast surface area to increase absorption. The small intestine maintains a BER of 11 contractions per minute. This regular movement is assessed when listening for bowel sounds.

The large intestine uses a process of mass movement with an occasional peristaltic wave. When the beginning segment of the large intestine is stimulated, it contracts and sends a massive peristaltic movement throughout the entire large intestine. The end result of the mass movement is usually excretion of waste products.

Rectal distention after mass movement stimulates a defecation reflex that causes relaxation of the external and internal sphincters. Control of the external sphincter is a learned behavior. The receptors in the external sphincter adapt relatively quickly and will stretch and require more and more distention to stimulate the reflex if the reflex is ignored.

Key Points

- The GI system begins at the mouth and ends at the anus; a long tube extends between them and is composed of the esophagus, the stomach, the small intestine, and the large intestine. Essential functions are digestion and absorption of nutrients.
- The GI tract is composed of four layers: the mucosa, the muscularis mucosa, the nerve plexus, and the adventitia.
- The GI tract has four major functions: secretion, absorption, digestion, and motility.
- The GI system secretes enzymes, acid, bicarbonate, and mucus to facilitate the digestion and absorption of nutrients.
- The small intestine is the section of the GI tract where most absorption occurs. The veins of the small intestine carry the absorbed products to the liver for filtering, cleaning, and metabolism or the breaking down of absorbed products into usable substances.
- The nerve plexus controls the GI system by maintaining electrical rhythm and responding to local stimuli (increasing or decreasing activity). The autonomic nervous system influences GI activity, with the sympathetic system slowing and the parasympathetic system increasing activity.

Gastrointestinal Reflexes

To function effectively, several local and central reflexes occur. **Local gastrointestinal reflexes** involve stimulation of the nerves in the GI tract and cause movement and secretion. Central reflexes, which include swallowing and vomiting, are controlled by the medulla.

Local Reflexes

Stimulation of local nerves within the GI tract causes increased or decreased movement within the system, maintaining homeostasis. Loss of reflexes or stimulation can result in constipation and the lack of movement of the bolus along the GI tract or diarrhea with increased motility and excretion. The longer a fecal bolus remains in the large intestine, the more sodium and water are absorbed from it and the harder and less mobile it can become. There are many local gastrointestinal reflexes. Some knowledge of how these reflexes operate makes it easier to understand what happens when the reflexes are blocked or overstimulated and how therapeutic measures are often used to cause reflex activity.

- *Gastroenteric reflex*: Stimulation of the stomach by stretching, the presence of food, or cephalic stimulation (the body's response to smelling, seeing, tasting, or thinking about food) causes an increase in activity in the small intestine. It is thought that this prepares the small intestine for the coming chyme.
- *Gastrocolic reflex*: Stimulation of the stomach also causes increased activity in the colon, again preparing it to empty any contents to provide space for the new chyme.
- *Duodenal–colic reflex*: The presence of food or stretching in the duodenum stimulates colon activity and mass movement, again to empty the colon for the new chyme.

It is important to remember the gastroenteric, gastrocolic, and duodenal–colic reflexes when helping patients maintain GI movement. Taking advantage of stomach stimulation (e.g., having the patient drink prune juice or hot water or eat bran) and providing the opportunity of time and privacy for a bowel movement after eating in the morning encourage normal reflexes to keep things in control.

Other local GI reflexes include:

- *Ileogastric reflex*: The introduction of chyme or stretch to the large intestine slows stomach activity, as does the introduction of chyme into the small and large intestine, allowing time for absorption. In part, this reflex explains why patients who are constipated often have no appetite: The continued stretch on the ileum that comes with constipation continues to slow stomach activity and makes the introduction of new food into the stomach undesirable.
- *Intestinal–intestinal reflex*: Excessive irritation to one section of the small intestine causes a cessation of activity above that section to prevent further irritation and an increase in activity below that section, which leads to a flushing of the irritant. This reflex is active in traveler's diarrhea: Local irritation of the intestine causes increased secretions and movement below that section, resulting in watery diarrhea and a cessation of movement above that section. Loss of appetite or even nausea may occur. An extreme reaction to this reflex can be seen after abdominal surgery, when the handling of the intestines causes intense irritation and the reflex can cause the entire intestinal system to cease activity, leading to a paralytic ileus.
- *Peritoneointestinal reflex*: Irritation of the peritoneum as a result of inflammation or injury leads to a cessation of GI activity, preventing continued movement of the GI tract and thus further irritation of the peritoneum.
- *Renointestinal reflex*: Irritation or swelling of the renal capsule causes a cessation of movement in the GI tract, again preventing further irritation to the capsule.
- *Vesicointestinal reflex*: Irritation or overstretching of the bladder can cause a reflex cessation of movement in the GI tract, again preventing further irritation to the bladder from GI movement. Many patients with cystitis or overstretched bladders from occupational constraints or neurological problems complain of constipation, which can be attributable to this reflex.
- *Somatointestinal reflex*: Taut stretching of the skin and muscles over the abdomen irritates the nerve plexus and causes a slowing or cessation of GI activity preventing further irritation. This reflex was often seen in people who wore tight girdles when they were in fashion; constipation was a serious problem for many people who wore the constraining garments. Tight-fitting jeans or other clothing can have the same effect. Patients who complain of chronic constipation may be suffering from overactivity of the somatointestinal reflex.

Central Reflexes

Two centrally mediated reflexes—swallowing and vomiting—are important to the functioning of the GI tract.

Swallowing

The **swallowing** reflex is stimulated whenever a food bolus stimulates pressure receptors in the back of the throat and pharynx. These receptors send impulses to the medulla, which stimulates a series of nerves that cause the following actions: The soft palate elevates and seals off the nasal cavity, respirations cease in order to protect the lungs, the larynx rises and the glottis closes to seal off the airway, and the pharyngeal constrictor muscles contract and force the food bolus into the top of the esophagus, where pairs of muscles contract in turn to move the bolus down the esophagus into the stomach. This reflex is complex, involving more than 25 pairs of muscles.

This reflex can be facilitated in a number of ways if swallowing (food or medication) is a problem. Icing the tongue by sucking on a Popsicle or an ice cube blocks external nerve impulses and allows this more basic reflex to respond. Icing the sternal notch or the back of the neck, though not as appealing, has also proved effective in stimulating the swallowing reflex. In addition, keeping the head straight (not turned to one side) allows the muscle pairs to work together and helps the process. Providing stimulation of the receptors in the mouth through temperature variations and textured foods helps initiate the reflex. Patients who do not produce their own saliva can be given artificial saliva to increase digestion and to lubricate the food bolus, which also helps the swallowing reflex.

Vomiting

The **vomiting** reflex is another basic reflex that is centrally mediated and important in protecting the system from unwanted irritants. The vomiting reflex is stimulated by two centers in the medulla. The more primitive center is called the emetic zone. When stimulated, it initiates projectile vomiting. This type of intense reaction is seen in young children and whenever increased pressure in the brain or brain damage allows the more primitive center to override the more mature chemoreceptor trigger zone (CTZ). The emetic zone is also stimulated by hypoxia. The CTZ is stimulated in several ways:

- Tactile stimulation of the back of the throat, a reflex to get rid of something that is too big or too irritating to be swallowed
- Excessive stomach distention or gastrointestinal inflammation
- Increasing intracranial pressure by direct stimulation
- Stimulation of the vestibular receptors in the inner ear (a reaction often seen with dizziness after "wild" rides in amusement parks)
- Stimulation of stretch receptors in the uterus and bladder (a possible explanation for vomiting in early pregnancy and before delivery)
- Intense pain fiber stimulation
- Direct stimulation by various chemicals, including fumes, certain drugs, and debris from cellular death (a reason for vomiting after chemotherapy or radiation therapy that results in cell death)

There are several neurotransmitters that are thought to influence the vomiting centers in the brain. Dopamine, serotonin, opioids, and acetylcholine may increase risk of nausea and vomiting. Norepinephrine may decrease nausea, especially that caused by motion sickness.

Once the CTZ is stimulated, a series of reflexes occurs. Salivation increases, and there is a large increase in the production of mucus in the upper GI tract, which is accompanied by a decrease in gastric acid production. This action protects the lining of the GI tract from potential damage by the acidic stomach contents. (Nauseated patients who start swallowing repeatedly or complain about secretions in their throat are in the process of preparing for vomiting.) The sympathetic system is stimulated, with a resultant increase in sweating, increased heart rate, deeper respirations, and nausea. This prepares the body for fight-or-flight and the insult of vomiting. The esophagus then relaxes and becomes distended, and the gastric sphincter relaxes. The patient takes one deep respiration, the glottis closes, and the palate rises, trapping the air in the lungs and sealing off entry to the lungs. The abdominal and thoracic muscles contract, increasing intra-abdominal pressure. The stomach then relaxes, and the lower section of the stomach contracts in waves, approximately six times per minute. With nothing in the stomach, this movement is known as retching, and it can be quite tiring and uncomfortable. This action causes a backward peristalsis and movement of stomach contents up the esophagus and out the mouth. The body thus rids itself of offending irritants.

The vomiting reflex is complex and protective, but it can be undesirable in certain clinical situations, when the stimulant is not something that can be vomited or when the various components of the vomiting reflex could be detrimental to a patient's health status.

Key Points

- Stimulation of local nerves via the local reflexes in the GI tract causes increased or decreased movement within the system maintaining homeostasis.
- Swallowing, a centrally mediated reflex important in delivering food to the GI tract for processing, is controlled by the medulla. It involves a complex series of timed reflexes.
- Vomiting is controlled by the CTZ in the medulla or by the emetic zone in immature or injured brains. The CTZ is stimulated by several different processes and initiates a complex series of responses that first prepare the system for vomiting and then cause a strong backward peristalsis to rid the stomach of its contents.

SUMMARY

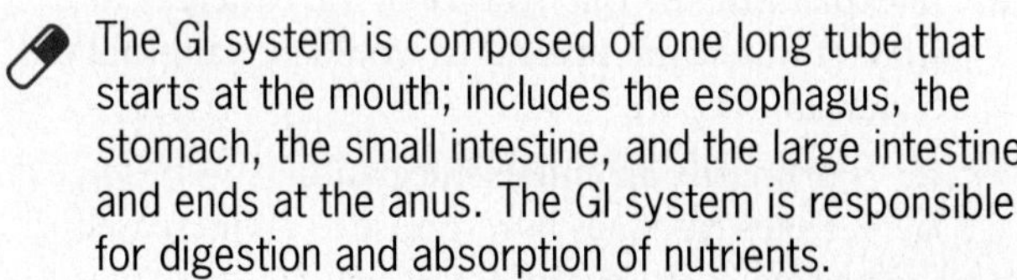

- The GI system is composed of one long tube that starts at the mouth; includes the esophagus, the stomach, the small intestine, and the large intestine; and ends at the anus. The GI system is responsible for digestion and absorption of nutrients.

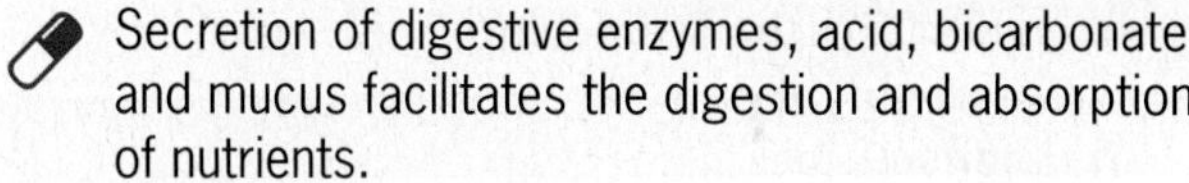

- Secretion of digestive enzymes, acid, bicarbonate, and mucus facilitates the digestion and absorption of nutrients.
- The GI system is controlled by a nerve plexus, which maintains a BER and responds to local stimuli to increase or decrease activity. The sympathetic nervous system, if stimulated, slows GI activity; stimulation of the parasympathetic nervous system increases activity. Initiation of activity depends on local reflexes.
- A series of local reflexes within the GI tract helps maintain homeostasis within the system. A change of any of these reflexes may result in a disruption of homeostasis—constipation (underactivity) or diarrhea (overactivity).
- Swallowing, a centrally mediated reflex important in delivering food to the GI tract for processing, is controlled by the medulla. It involves a complex series of timed reflexes.
- Vomiting is controlled by the CTZ in the medulla or by the emetic zone in immature or injured brains. The CTZ is stimulated by several different processes and initiates a complex series of responses that first prepare the system for vomiting and then cause a strong backward peristalsis to rid the stomach of its contents.

CHECK YOUR UNDERSTANDING

Answers to the questions in this chapter can be found in Answers to Check Your Understanding Questions on thePoint®.

MULTIPLE CHOICE

Select the best answer.

1. After teaching a group of students about GI activity and constipation, the instructor determines that the teaching was successful when the students state that constipation
   a. results from increased peristaltic activity in the intestinal tract.
   b. occurs primarily when a person does not have a daily bowel movement.
   c. leads to decreased salt and water absorption from the large intestine.
   d. can be artificially induced by increasing the volume of the large intestine.

2. In explaining the importance of the pancreas to a student nurse, the instructor would explain that the pancreas
   a. is primarily an endocrine gland.
   b. secretes enzymes in response to an increased plasma glucose concentration.
   c. neutralizes the hydrochloric acid secreted by the stomach.
   d. produces bile.

3. Gastrin
   a. stimulates acid secretion in the stomach.
   b. secretion is blocked by the products of protein digestion in the stomach.
   c. secretion is stimulated by acid in the duodenum.
   d. is responsible for the chemical or gastric phase of intestinal secretion.

4. When explaining the control of the activities of the GI tract—movement and secretion—the nurse would be most accurate to state that the GI is basically controlled by the
   a. sympathetic nervous system.
   b. parasympathetic nervous system.
   c. local nerve reflexes of the GI nerve plexus.
   d. medulla in the brainstem.

5. The presence of fat in the duodenum causes
   a. acid indigestion.
   b. decreased acid production.
   c. increased gastrin release.
   d. contraction of the gallbladder.

6. The basic type of movement that occurs in the small intestine is
   a. peristalsis.
   b. mass movement.
   c. churning.
   d. segmentation.

7. Most of the nutrients absorbed from the GI tract pass immediately into the portal venous system and are processed by the liver. This is possible because almost all absorption occurs through the
   a. lower section of the stomach.
   b. top section of the large intestine.
   c. small intestine.
   d. ileum.

MULTIPLE RESPONSE

Select all that apply.

1. The CTZ in the brain is activated by which processes?
   a. Stretch of the uterus
   b. Stretch of the bladder
   c. Decreased GI activity
   d. Radiation
   e. Cell death
   f. Extreme pain

2. Acid production in the stomach is stimulated by which factors?
   a. Protein in the stomach
   b. Calcium products in the stomach
   c. High levels of acid in the stomach
   d. Alcohol in the stomach
   e. Low levels of acid in the stomach
   f. H_2 stimulation

3. When describing the action of pancreatic digestive enzymes in breaking down substances, which substances would the instructor include?
   a. Gastric acid
   b. Fats
   c. Proteins
   d. Sugars
   e. Bile
   f. Lipids

REFERENCES

Barrett, K., Barman, S. B., Boitano, S., & Brooks, H. (2015). *Ganong's review of medical physiology* (25th ed.). McGraw-Hill.

Brunton, L., Hilal-dandan, R., & Knollman, B. (2018). *Goodman and Gilman's the pharmacological basis of therapeutics* (13th ed.). McGraw-Hill.

Hall, J. E., & Hall, M. E. (2021). *Guyton and Hall textbook of medical physiology* (14th ed.). Elsevier.

Johnson, L. R., & Ghishan, F. K. (2012). *Physiology of the gastrointestinal tract* (5th ed.). Academic Press.

Norris, T. L. (2019). *Porth's pathophysiology concepts of altered health states* (13th ed.). Wolters Kluwer.

Parkman, H., & Fisher, R. S. (2006). *The clinician's guide to acid/peptic disorders and motility disorders of the GI tract.* Slack.

Rhoades, R. A., & Bell, D. R. (2012). *Medical physiology: Principles of clinical medicine.* Lippincott Williams & Wilkins.

Seidel, E. (2006). *Crash course: GI system.* Mosby.

Seifter, J., Rafnon, A., & Sloane, D. (2005). *Concepts in medical physiology.* Lippincott Williams & Wilkins.

CHAPTER 57

Drugs Affecting Gastrointestinal Secretions

Learning Objectives

Upon completion of this chapter, you will be able to:

1. Describe the current theories on the pathophysiological process responsible for the signs and symptoms of peptic ulcer disease.
2. Discuss the drugs used to affect GI secretions across the lifespan.
3. Describe the therapeutic actions, indications, pharmacokinetics, contraindications and cautions, most common adverse effects, and important drug–drug interactions associated with drugs used to affect gastrointestinal (GI) secretions.
4. Compare and contrast the prototype drugs used to affect GI secretions with other agents in their classes and with other classes of drugs used to affect GI secretions.
5. Outline the nursing considerations, including important teaching points, for patients receiving drugs used to affect GI secretions.

Key Terms

acid rebound: condition in which the stomach increases acid release in response to low acid (high pH); this can occur in response to using antacids that decrease acid

antacids: group of inorganic chemicals that neutralize stomach acid

digestive enzymes: enzymes produced in the gastrointestinal tract to break down foods into usable nutrients

gastroesophageal reflux disease (GERD): backward movement of gastric contents into the esophagus that causes mucosal lining damage and/or heartburn symptoms

gastrointestinal protectant: drug that coats any injured area in the stomach to prevent further injury from acid or pepsin

histamine-2 (H_2) antagonist: drug that blocks the H_2 receptor sites; used to decrease acid production in the stomach (H_2 sites are stimulated to cause the release of acid from the parietal cells in response to gastrin or parasympathetic stimulation)

peptic ulcer: erosion of the lining of the stomach or duodenum; results from imbalance between acid produced and the mucous protection of the gastrointestinal lining or possibly from infection by *Helicobacter pylori* bacteria

prostaglandin: any one of numerous tissue hormones that have local effects on various systems and organs of the body, including vasoconstriction, vasodilation, increased or decreased GI activity, and increased or decreased pancreatic enzyme release

proton pump inhibitor: drug that blocks the H^+, K^+–ATPase enzyme system on the secretory surface of the gastric parietal cells, thus interfering with the final step of acid production and lowering acid levels in the stomach

Drug List

DRUGS USED TO TREAT GASTROESOPHAGEAL REFLUX DISEASE AND ULCER DISEASE

Histamine-2 Antagonists

- (P) cimetidine
- famotidine
- nizatidine
- ranitidine

Antacids

- aluminum salts
- calcium salts
- magnesium salts
- (P) sodium bicarbonate

Proton Pump Inhibitors

- dexlansoprazole
- esomeprazole
- lansoprazole
- (P) omeprazole
- pantoprazole
- rabeprazole

Gastrointestinal Protectant

- (P) sucralfate

Prostaglandin

- (P) misoprostol

DRUGS USED TO TREAT DIGESTIVE ENZYME DYSFUNCTION

- (P) pancrelipase
- saliva substitute

Gastrointestinal (GI) disorders are among the more common complaints seen in clinical practice. Many products are available for the self-treatment of upset stomach or heartburn. (See Box 57.1 for a list of some of the over-the-counter [OTC] drugs.) The underlying causes of these disorders can vary from dietary excess, stress, hiatal hernia, gastroesophageal reflux disease (GERD), peptic ulcer disease, and adverse drug effects. This chapter addresses the common classifications of medications that are used to treat symptoms by affecting gastrointestinal secretions. Some of the conditions that can be treated with these medications are described in Box 57.2.

Drugs Used to Treat Gastroesophageal Reflux Disease and Ulcer Disease

Drugs typically used to affect GI secretions in treating GERD, peptic ulcer disease, and disorders involving increased GI acid work to decrease GI secretory activity, block the action of GI secretions, or form protective coverings on the GI lining to prevent erosion from GI secretions. Studies have examined the risks of lowering acid levels. There is evidence of greater risk with long-term use of some of the medications compared to short-term use (Box 57.3).

The drugs used to treat GERD and ulcer disease include histamine-2 (H_2) antagonists, which block the release of hydrochloric acid in response to gastrin; **antacids**, which interact with acids at the chemical level to neutralize them; proton pump inhibitors, which suppress the secretion of hydrochloric acid into the lumen of the stomach; gastrointestinal protectants, which coat any injured area in the stomach to prevent further injury from acid; and prostaglandins, which inhibit the secretion of gastrin and increase the secretion of the mucous lining of the stomach, providing a buffer.

Figure 57.1 depicts the sites of actions of these drugs used to treat GERD and ulcer disease. Box 57.4 highlights important considerations related to the use of these drugs across the lifespan.

BOX 57.1

Over-the-Counter Drugs Affecting Gastrointestinal Secretions

aluminum hydroxide (*Amphojel*)
aluminum–magnesium combinations (*Maalox*, *Mylanta*, and others)
calcium carbonate (*Tums* and others)
cimetidine (*Tagamet HB*)
esomeprazole (*Nexium 24HR*)
famotidine (*Pepcid AC*, *Pepcid Complete*)
lansoprazole (*Prevacid 24 HR*)
magnesium salts (*Phillips Milk of Magnesia* and others)
nizatidine (*Axid AR*)
omeprazole (*Prilosec OTC*)
omeprazole with sodium bicarbonate (*Zegerid OTC*)
sodium bicarbonate (baking soda, *Bell-ans*)

Histamine-2 Antagonists

H_2 antagonists (Table 57.1) block the release of hydrochloric acid in response to gastrin. These drugs include cimetidine (*Tagamet HB*), famotidine (*Pepcid AC*), and nizatidine (*Axid AR*). Oral formulations of these medications are available as OTC medications. Ranitidine (*Zantac*) was available until recently when the U.S. Food and Drug Administration recalled it from the market. It was withdrawn due to ongoing investigation of a contaminant (*N*-nitrosodimethylamine) that is a probable human carcinogen that may increase in levels as the ranitidine is stored.

Therapeutic Actions and Indications

The H_2 antagonists selectively block H_2 receptors located on the parietal cells. Blocking these receptors prevents about 70% of the hydrochloric acid release from the parietal cells. This action also decreases pepsin production by the chief cells. H_2 receptor sites are also found in the heart, and high levels of these drugs can produce cardiac arrhythmias (see "Adverse Effects").

These drugs are used in the following conditions:

- Short-term treatment of active duodenal ulcer or benign gastric ulcer (reduction in the overall acid level can promote healing and decrease discomfort).
- Treatment of pathological hypersecretory conditions such as Zollinger-Ellison syndrome (blocking the overproduction of hydrochloric acid that is associated with these conditions).
- Prophylaxis of ulcers induced by stress or nonsteroidal anti-inflammatory drug (NSAID) use and acute upper GI bleeding in critical patients (blocking the production of acid protects the stomach lining, which is at risk because of decreased mucus production associated with extreme stress). See Box 57.5 for examples of combination medications.
- Treatment of erosive gastroesophageal reflux (decreasing the acid being regurgitated into the esophagus will promote healing and decrease pain).
- Treatment of ulcers caused by *H. pylori* in conjunction with antibiotics.
- Relief of symptoms of heartburn and indigestion.

See the "Critical Thinking Scenario" for additional information on H_2 antagonists.

BOX 57.2

Conditions Involving Gastrointestinal Secretions

Gastroesophageal Reflux Disease

Gastroesophageal reflux disease (GERD) is caused by acid from the stomach moving back into the esophagus. It is often due to a weakened esophageal sphincter that does not stop the contents from moving backward. Common symptoms are heartburn, regurgitation, belching, and even chest pain. The severity of the symptoms does not directly correlate with the amount of mucosal injury. Mucosal injury from the acidic contents can include inflammation, edema, strictures, and narrowing of the esophagus. Barrett esophagus, an abnormal adaption of the mucosal lining to resemble the lining of the stomach, can also occur. Treatment involves avoidance of large meals and substances that reduce esophageal sphincter tone (smoking, caffeine, alcohol). It is also recommended that people stay upright several hours post meals and sleep with the head of the bed elevated. If a person is overweight, symptoms may be relieved with weight loss. Pharmacological treatment includes antiacids, histamine-2 receptor blockers, and proton pump inhibitors.

Ulcer Disease

Erosions in the upper GI tract are called **peptic ulcers**. Ulcer patients present with a predictable description of gnawing, burning pain often occurring a few hours after meals. Many of the drugs that are used to affect GI secretions are designed to prevent, treat, or aid in the healing of these ulcers. The cause of chronic peptic ulcers is not completely understood. For many years, it was believed that ulcers were caused by excessive acid production, and treatment was aimed at neutralizing acid or blocking the parasympathetic system to decrease normal GI activity and secretions. Further research led many to believe that because acid production was often normal in ulcer patients, ulcers were caused by a defect in the mucous lining that coats the inner lumen of the stomach to protect it from digestive enzymes.

The leading cause of peptic ulcers in the United States is the use of nonsteroidal anti-inflammatory drugs (NSAIDs). NSAIDs inhibit cyclooxygenase receptors, and one of the functions of these sites is the production of the mucous lining in the stomach. A thinner protective coat is more susceptible to the erosive action of acid. Treatment is now aimed at improving the balance between the acid produced and the mucous layer that protects the stomach lining. Currently, it is believed that chronic ulcers may be the result of impaired mucous lining and infection by *Helicobacter pylori* bacteria. The combination of antibiotics with proton pump inhibitors has been found to be quite effective in treating some patients with chronic ulcers.

Acute ulcers, or "stress ulcers," are often seen in situations that involve acute physiological stress, such as trauma, burns, or prolonged illness. The activity of the sympathetic nervous system during stress decreases blood flow to the GI tract, leading to less blood flow to the inner layer of the GI tract and weakening of the mucosal layer of the stomach and erosion by acid in the stomach. Many of the drugs available for treating various peptic ulcers act to alter the acid-producing activities of the stomach to decrease the erosive action.

Digestive Enzyme Dysfunction

Some patients require a supplement to the production of digestive enzymes. Patients with strokes, salivary gland disorders, or extreme surgery of the head and neck may not be able to produce saliva. Saliva is important in beginning the digestion of sugars and proteins and is essential in initiating the swallowing reflex. Artificial saliva may be necessary for these patients. Patients with common bile duct problems, pancreatic disease, or cystic fibrosis may not be able to produce or secrete pancreatic enzymes. These enzymes may need to be administered to allow normal digestion and absorption of nutrients.

Box 57.3 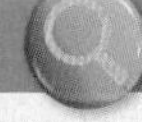 Focus on the Evidence

DRUGS THAT DECREASE ACID MAY AFFECT MORE THAN ACID LEVELS

Many of the medications that can alter acid levels are available as both prescription and over-the-counter medications. Most are designed for short-term use to alleviate GI discomfort. However, some people have taken acid reducing agents for months and/or years. There is a large body of research examining side effects of medications that lower acid levels. There is evidence that patients taking proton pump inhibitors (PPI) or histamine-2 antagonists have increased risk of *C. difficile* infection. Drugs that lower acid levels change the normal environment of the GI tract, perhaps allowing bacteria to thrive that would normally be destroyed by the acid.

Prolonged use of acid reducing medication may have increased risks compared to short-term use. There is some evidence that long-term use of PPI increases risk of osteoporosis-related bone fractures. Continuous use of a PPI for a year or more has been associated with a rare but dangerous occurrence of magnesium deficiency. Other researchers have shown a positive relationship between increased infections and PPI use. In addition, there is potential for reduction of vitamin B_{12} absorption with reduced acid levels. This may cause the association of long-term PPI use and increased risk of dementia that has been reported by some researchers.

Despite years of clinical research, there is much that is not understood regarding modulation of acid levels and long-term effects. It is recommended that if a medication is required for acid reduction for prolonged use, it should be monitored by a health care provider. The patient should also be evaluated for reversible causes of the GI symptoms to ensure the best treatment plan.

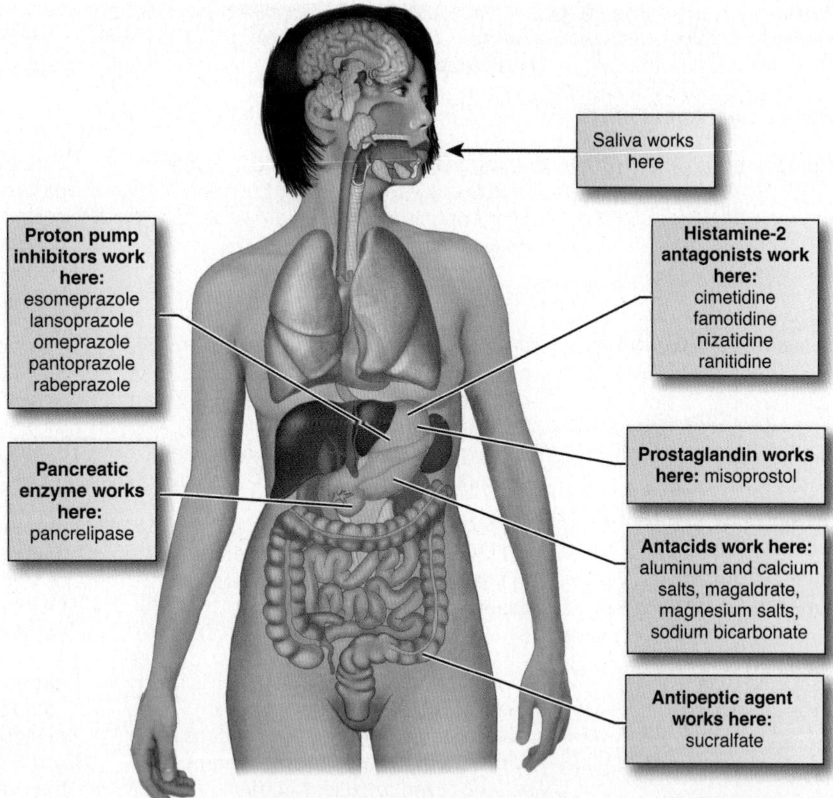

FIGURE 57.1 Sites of action of drugs affecting gastrointestinal secretions.

Box 57.4 Focus on Drug Therapy Across the Lifespan

AGENTS THAT AFFECT GASTROINTESTINAL SECRETIONS

Children

Several of the H_2 antagonists and proton pump inhibitors are approved for use in children. They have been successfully used to decrease ulcer formation related to stress or drug therapy. Dose should be determined by the age and weight of the child and formulation that is being administered.

Antacids may be used in children who complain of upset stomach or who are receiving therapy known to increase acid production.

Special caution should be used with any of these agents to prevent electrolyte disturbances or any interference with nutrition, which could be especially detrimental to children.

Adults

Adults should be cautioned not to overuse any of these agents and to check with a health care provider if GI discomfort continues after repeated use of any of these drugs. Patients should be monitored for any electrolyte disturbances or interference with the absorption or action of other drugs. If antacids are used, they should be spaced 1 to 2 hours before or after the use of other drugs. All patients should be cautioned that prolonged use may increase risk of side effects and nutritional deficiencies. Patients should be cautioned to limit the use of these drugs and to seek medical help for persistent symptoms.

The risk of taking these drugs during pregnancy and lactation has not been extensively studied. Patients who are pregnant or breast or chestfeeding should discuss with a health care provider before taking any of the acid-reducing agents.

Misoprostol acts as an endogenous prostaglandin that can reduce risk of gastric ulcers caused by NSAID use. This medication can induce labor and has the risk of uterine rupture. Patients who can become pregnant should be counseled and provided information in writing regarding the actions of this medication. It is recommended that if it is used off label for obstetric diagnosis that the patient be monitored in a hospital setting. Patients who can become pregnant and who use misoprostol should be advised to use contraceptives to prevent pregnancy.

Older Adults

Older adults are frequently prescribed one or more of these drugs. It is especially important to be aware of the long-term risks of the medications since some of the GI complaints of older adults may require more persistent therapy.

Older adults are also more likely to have renal and/or hepatic impairment related to underlying medical conditions, which could interfere with the metabolism and excretion of these drugs. Some of the medications have recommended dosing adjustments if there is renal or hepatic impairment.

These patients also need to be alerted to the potential for toxic effects when using OTC preparations that may contain the same ingredients as many of these agents. They should be advised to check with their health care providers before beginning any OTC drug regimen.

Table 57.1 ***Drugs in Focus:*** **Drugs Used to Treat Gastroesophageal Reflux Disease and Ulcer Disease**

Drug Name	Usual Dosage	Usual Indications
Histamine-2 Antagonists		
cimetidine (*Tagamet HB*)	300 mg PO q.i.d. at meals and at bedtime or 800 mg PO at bedtime; 200 mg PO for heartburn; reduce dose with patients with renal impairment	Treatment of duodenal ulcer, benign gastric ulcer, pathological hypersecretory syndrome, GERD; prophylaxis of stress ulcers; relief of symptoms of heartburn, acid indigestion, sour stomach *Special considerations:* FDA does not recommend for children <12 y; up to provider judgment
famotidine (*Pepcid AC*)	20–40 mg PO or IV at bedtime or 20 mg PO b.i.d., 10 mg PO for prevention or relief of heartburn; reduce dose with patients with renal impairment *Pediatric:* dosing varies based on age and indication	Treatment of duodenal ulcer, benign gastric ulcer, pathological hypersecretory syndrome, GERD; relief of symptoms of heartburn, acid indigestion
nizatidine (*Axid AR*)	150–300 mg PO at bedtime or 150 mg PO b.i.d., 75 mg PO 30 min before food to prevent heartburn; reduce dose with patients with renal impairment	Treatment of duodenal ulcer, benign gastric ulcer, pathological hypersecretory syndrome, GERD; relief of symptoms of heartburn, acid indigestion *Special considerations:* Not recommended for use in children <12 years old
ranitidine (*Zantac*)	150 mg daily to b.i.d. PO, 300 mg PO at bedtime, or 50 mg IM or IV q6–8h; 75 mg PO as needed for heartburn; reduce dose with patients with renal impairment *Pediatric (1 mo to 16 y)*: 2–4 mg/kg PO b.i.d. for daily maintenance treatment	Treatment of duodenal ulcer, benign gastric ulcer, pathological hypersecretory syndrome, GERD; relief of symptoms of heartburn, acid indigestion **Note:** Recalled by FDA in 2020 and not available in the United States.
Antacids		
aluminum salts (*AlternaGEL* and others)	*Adult:* 500–1,500 mg three to six times per day between meals and at bedtime *Pediatric:* 50–150 mg/kg PO q24h in divided doses q4–6h	Symptomatic relief of GI hyperacidity, treatment of hyperphosphatemia, prevention of formation of phosphate urinary stones
calcium salts (*Oystercal*, *Tums* and others)	0.5–2 g PO as needed as an antacid	Symptomatic relief of GI hyperacidity, treatment of calcium deficiency, prevention of hypocalcemia
magnesium salts (*Milk of Magnesia*, others)	280–1,500 mg PO q.i.d., dose based on salt used *Pediatric:* one-half of the adult dose	Symptomatic relief of GI hyperacidity, prophylaxis of stress ulcers, relief of constipation
sodium bicarbonate (generic)	*Adult:* 300–2,000 mg PO daily to q.i.d.	Symptomatic relief of GI hyperacidity, minimization of uric acid crystalluria, adjunctive treatment in severe diarrhea
Proton Pump Inhibitors		
dexlansoprazole (*Dexilant*)	30–60 mg/d PO for 4–8 wk	Treatment and maintenance of erosive esophagitis, treatment of heartburn associated with GERD
esomeprazole (*Nexium*)	*Acute:* 20–40 mg/d PO daily *Pediatric:* dosing varies based on age and indication	Treatment of GERD, severe erosive esophagitis, duodenal ulcers, and pathological hypersecretory conditions, decreases risk of NSAID-associated gastric ulcers; treatment of *H. pylori* with antibiotics
lansoprazole (*Prevacid*)	15–30 mg/d PO based on condition and response, 30 mg IV over 30 min for up to 7 d *Pediatric:* dosing varies based on age, weight, and indication	Treatment of gastric and duodenal ulcers, GERD, pathological hypersecretory syndromes; maintenance therapy for healing duodenal ulcers and esophagitis; in combination therapy with antibiotics for the eradication of *Helicobacter pylori* infection; reduction of risk and treatment of NSAID-associated ulcers; approved for use in children for treatment of GERD, erosive esophagitis, peptic ulcer, and Zollinger-Ellison syndrome

Table 57.1 *Drugs in Focus:* Drugs Used to Treat Gastroesophageal Reflux Disease and Ulcer Disease *(Continued)*

Drug Name	Usual Dosage	Usual Indications
omeprazole (*Prilosec*)	20–60 mg/d PO for 4–8 wk based on condition and response *Pediatric:* dosing varies based on age and indication	Treatment of gastric and duodenal ulcers, GERD, pathological hypersecretory syndromes; maintenance therapy for healing duodenal ulcers and esophagitis; in combination therapy with antibiotics for the eradication of *H. pylori* infection
pantoprazole (*Protonix*)	40 mg PO daily to b.i.d. *or* 40–240 (max) mg/d IV or 40 mg/d IV for 7–10 d *Pediatric:* dosing varies based on age and weight	Treatment of GERD in adults, healing of erosive esophagitis, treatment of hypersecretory syndromes
rabeprazole (*Aciphex*)	*Adult and pediatric > 12 y:* 20–60 mg/d PO based on condition and response *Pediatric 1–11 y and > 15 kg:* 10 mg/d PO *Pediatric < 15 kg:* 5 mg/d PO	Treatment and maintenance of GERD; treatment of duodenal ulcers, pathological hypersecretory conditions; used as combination therapy for the eradication of *H. pylori* infection
GI Protectant		
sucralfate (*Carafate*)	1 g PO b.i.d. to q.i.d. on empty stomach	Short-term treatment of duodenal ulcers; maintenance of duodenal ulcers (at reduced dose) after healing in adults; treatment of oral and esophageal ulcers due to radiation, chemotherapy, or sclerotherapy
Prostaglandin		
misoprostol (*Cytotec*)	100–200 mcg PO q.i.d. with meals and at bedtime	Prevention of NSAID-induced ulcers in adults at high risk for development of these gastric ulcers, off-label use includes inducing labor and medical termination of pregnancy

GERD, gastroesophageal reflux disease; GI, gastrointestinal; OTC, over the counter; NSAID, nonsteroidal anti-inflammatory drug; FDA, Food and Drug Administration.

BOX 57.5

Combination Medications for Analgesia and Prevention of Gastrointestinal (GI) Ulceration

With many patients taking NSAIDs over a long term for a variety of conditions, including arthritis and cancers, the incidence of GI ulceration and bleeding could increase. There are some combination medications available that combine an analgesic with a substance to decrease risk of GI ulcers. *Duexis* is a combination of the NSAID ibuprofen and the histamine H_2-receptor antagonist famotidine. It is indicated for the relief of signs and symptoms of rheumatoid arthritis and osteoarthritis and to decrease the risk of developing upper gastrointestinal ulcers. *Arthrotec* is a combination of diclofenac sodium, an NSAID, and misoprostol, a prostaglandin-1 (PGE1) analog. It is indicated for the treatment of signs and symptoms of osteoarthritis or rheumatoid arthritis in patients at high risk of developing NSAID-induced gastric and duodenal ulcers. *Vimovo* is a combination of naproxen, an NSAID, and esomeprazole, a proton pump inhibitor. It is indicated for symptomatic relief of arthritis while reducing the risk of developing NSAID-associated gastric ulcers.

Pharmacokinetics

Famotidine is available in oral and parenteral forms. Nizatidine and cimetidine are available only in oral form. Cimetidine was the first drug in this class to be developed. It has been associated with antiandrogenic effects, including gynecomastia and galactorrhea. It reaches peak level in 1 to 1.5 hours and is metabolized mainly in the liver. It can slow the metabolism of many other drugs that use the same metabolizing enzyme system. It is excreted in the urine. It has a half-life of 2 hours and is known to cross the placenta and enter human milk.

Famotidine reaches peak effect in 1 to 3 hours and has a duration of 6 to 15 hours. Famotidine is metabolized in the liver and excreted in the urine with a half-life of 2.5 to 3.5 hours. Famotidine crosses the placenta and enters human milk. Famotidine is approved for use in children aged 1 to 16 years old.

Nizatidine, the newest drug in this class, differs from the other drugs in that it is eliminated by the kidneys with no first-pass metabolism in the liver. It is the drug of choice for patients with liver dysfunction and for those who are taking other drugs whose metabolism is slowed by the hepatic activity of the other H_2 antagonists. It reaches peak effect in 0.5 to 3 hours and has a half-life of 1 to 2 hours. Like the other drugs, it crosses the placenta and enters human milk.

CRITICAL THINKING SCENARIO
Histamine-2 Antagonists

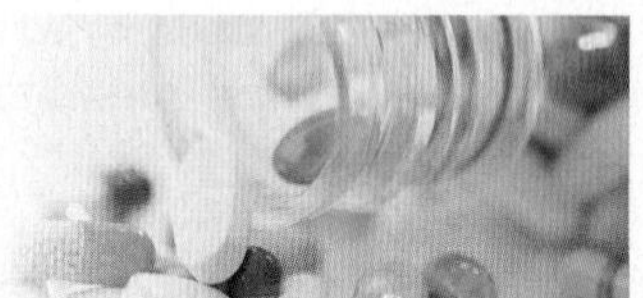

THE SITUATION

W.T., a 48-year-old traveling salesperson, had experienced increasing epigastric discomfort during a 7-month period. When W.T. finally sought medical care, the diagnosis was a peptic ulcer. W.T. began taking calcium carbonate (*Tums*) for relief of immediate discomfort, as well as famotidine (*Pepcid*) 40 mg once daily. W.T. was referred to the nurse for patient teaching and given an appointment for a follow-up visit in 3 weeks.

CRITICAL THINKING

Think about the physiology of duodenal ulcers and the various factors that can contribute to aggravating the problem. What patient teaching points should be covered with this patient regarding diet, stress factors, and use of alcohol and tobacco?

What adverse effects of the drugs should this patient be aware of?

What lifestyle changes may be necessary to ensure ulcer healing, and how can W.T. be assisted in making these changes fit into the demands of their job?

DISCUSSION

Further examination indicated that W.T. is relatively healthy except for the ulcer. W.T. reports taking a daily aspirin because they heard this prevents heart disease. W.T. also admits to smoking cigarettes, drinking alcohol regularly at business lunches and dinners, eating a great deal of fast food, and drinking a lot of coffee when they are on the road. W.T. states that their job has become increasingly stressful and that they worry about the economy. Because W.T. is basically healthy and does not seek medical care unless very uncomfortable (7 months of pain), they may find it difficult to comply with the drug therapy and any suggested lifestyle changes.

W.T. needs patient education, which should preferably be with the same nurse in order to build trust. The instruction should include information on duodenal ulcer disease, ways to decrease acid production (such as avoiding cigarettes, acid-stimulating foods, alcohol, and caffeine), and ways to improve the protective mucous layer of the stomach by decreasing stress and anxiety-causing situations. Aspirin and the other NSAIDS have also been found to increase risk of ulcers due to inhibiting a prostaglandin that facilitates mucus production. In addition, patient education should stress safe frequency and dosing of the famotidine and antacid doses. W.T. should be encouraged to avoid OTC medications and self-medication without discussing potential interactions with a pharmacist or provider because several of these products contain ingredients that could aggravate the ulcer or interfere with the effectiveness of the drugs that have been prescribed. W.T. should be encouraged to return for regular medical evaluation of the drug therapy and their underlying condition.

Finally, W.T. should feel that they have some control over this situation. Because W.T. does not routinely seek medical care, they may be more comfortable with a medical regimen that they have participated in planning. Allow W.T. to suggest ways to decrease stress without interfering with the demands of the job, ways to cut down on smoking or the use of alcohol, and the best times in their schedule to take the drugs. W.T. should be offered nicotine replacement products to assist with smoking cessation. They will learn in time which foods and situations irritate their condition. Research has not shown that bland or restrictive diets are particularly effective in decreasing ulcer pain or spread, and they may actually increase patient anxiety. W.T. should be encouraged to jot down the situations or times of the day that seem to cause them the most problems. This information can help to provide a guide for adjusting lifestyle and/or dietary patterns to aid ulcer healing and prevent further development of ulcers.

NURSING CARE GUIDE FOR W.T.: HISTAMINE-2 ANTAGONISTS

Assessment: History and Examination

Assess W.T.'s health history for allergies to any of these drugs, renal or hepatic failure, and other drugs that may interact.

Focus the physical examination on the following areas:

CNS: Orientation, affect

Skin: Color, lesions

Cardiovascular (CV): Pulse, cardiac auscultation

GI: Liver evaluation

Laboratory tests: Complete blood count, liver, renal function tests

Nursing Conclusions

Impaired comfort related to GI or CNS effects

Altered sensory perception (kinesthetic, auditory) related to CNS effects

Altered tissue perfusion risk related to cardiac effects

Knowledge deficit regarding drug therapy

Planning

The patient will receive the best therapeutic effect from the drug therapy.

The patient will have limited adverse effects from the drug therapy.

The patient will have an understanding of the drug therapy, adverse effects to anticipate, and measures to relieve discomfort and improve safety.

Intervention

Administer with meals and at bedtime.
Provide comfort and safety measures.
Arrange for decreased dose in renal/hepatic disease.
Provide support and reassurance to deal with drug effects and lifestyle changes.
Provide patient teaching regarding drug name, dosage, adverse effects, precautions, and warnings to report.

Evaluation

Evaluate drug effects: relief of GI symptoms, ulcer healing, and prevention of ulcer progression.
Monitor for adverse effects: headache, dizziness, insomnia, gynecomastia, arrhythmias, and GI alterations.
Monitor for drug–drug interactions as listed.
Evaluate the effectiveness of the patient teaching program.
Evaluate the effectiveness of comfort and safety measures.

PATIENT TEACHING FOR W.T.

- The drug that has been prescribed for you, famotidine, is called an H_2 antagonist. An H_2 antagonist decreases the amount of acid that is produced in the stomach. It is used to treat conditions that are aggravated by excess acid.
- Some of the following adverse effects may occur with this drug:
  - *Diarrhea:* Have ready access to bathroom facilities. This usually becomes less severe over time.
  - *Dizziness and headache:* These usually lessen as your body adjusts to the drug. Change positions slowly. If you feel drowsy, avoid driving or dangerous activities.
  - Report any of the following to your health care provider: sore throat, unusual bleeding or bruising, confusion, muscle or joint pain, and tarry stools.
- Avoid taking any new medication without first checking with your health care provider. There are several medications that interact with famotidine.
- If an antacid has been ordered for you, take it exactly as prescribed, spaced apart from your famotidine.
- Tell any physician, nurse, or other health care provider involved in your care that you are taking this drug.
- If you are taking any other medications, do not vary the drug schedules. Consult with your primary health care provider if anything should happen to change any of these drugs or your scheduled doses.
- It is important to have regular medical follow-up while you are taking this drug to evaluate your response to the drug and any possible underlying problems.
- Keep this drug, and all other medications, out of the reach of children.

Contraindications and Cautions

The H_2 antagonists should not be used with known allergy to any drugs of this class to prevent hypersensitivity reactions. Caution should be used during pregnancy or lactation because of the potential for adverse effects on the fetus or nursing baby and with hepatic or renal dysfunction, which could interfere with drug metabolism and excretion. (Hepatic dysfunction is not as much of a problem with nizatidine.) Care should also be taken if prolonged or continual use of these drugs is necessary because they may be masking serious underlying conditions.

Adverse Effects

The adverse effects most commonly associated with H_2 antagonists include GI effects of diarrhea or constipation; CNS effects of dizziness, headache, somnolence, confusion, or even hallucinations (thought to be related to possible H_2 receptor effects in the CNS); cardiac arrhythmias and hypotension (related to H_2 cardiac receptor blocking, more commonly seen with IV or IM administration or with prolonged use); and gynecomastia (with long-term use of cimetidine) and impotence.

Clinically Important Drug–Drug Interactions

Cimetidine can slow the metabolism of the following drugs, leading to increased serum levels and possible toxic reactions: warfarin anticoagulants, phenytoin, beta-adrenergic blockers, alcohol, quinidine, lidocaine, theophylline, chloroquine, benzodiazepines, nifedipine, pentoxifylline, tricyclic antidepressants (TCAs), procainamide, and carbamazepine. There is a risk of increased salicylate levels if nizatidine is taken with aspirin.

Prototype Summary: Cimetidine

Indications: Short-term treatment of active duodenal or benign gastric ulcers; treatment of pathological hypersecretory conditions; prophylaxis of stress-induced ulcers; treatment of erosive gastroesophageal reflux; relief of symptoms of heartburn and acid indigestion.

Actions: Inhibits the actions of histamine at H_2 receptor sites of the stomach, inhibiting gastric acid secretion and reducing total pepsin output.

Pharmacokinetics:

Route	Onset	Peak	Duration
Oral	Varies	1–1.5	4–5 h

$T_{1/2}$: 2 hours, metabolized in the liver and excreted in the urine.

Adverse Effects: Dizziness, confusion, headache, somnolence, cardiac arrhythmias, cardiac arrest, diarrhea, impotence, gynecomastia, rash.

Nursing Considerations for Patients Receiving Histamine-2 Antagonists

Assessment: History and Examination

- Assess for possible contraindications or cautions: history of allergy to any H_2 antagonists to prevent potential allergic reactions; impaired renal or hepatic function, which could affect metabolism and excretion of the drug; a detailed description of the GI problem, including length of time of the disorder and medical evaluation, to evaluate appropriate use of the drug and possibility of underlying medical problems; and current status of pregnancy or lactation because of the potential for adverse effects on the fetus or newborn.
- Perform a physical examination to establish baseline data before beginning therapy, determine effectiveness of the therapy, and evaluate for any adverse effects associated with drug therapy.
- Inspect the skin for evidence of lesions or rash to monitor for adverse reactions.
- Evaluate neurological status, including orientation and affect, to assess CNS effects of the drug and to plan for protective measures.
- Assess cardiopulmonary status, including pulse, blood pressure, and electrocardiogram (if IV use is needed), to evaluate the cardiac effects of the drug.
- Perform abdominal examination, including assessment of the liver, to establish a baseline and rule out underlying medical problems.
- Monitor the results of laboratory tests, including liver and renal function tests, to predict changes in metabolism or excretion of the drug that might require dose adjustment.

Nursing Conclusions

Nursing conclusions related to drug therapy might include the following:

- Impaired comfort related to CNS and GI effects
- Altered sensory perception (kinesthetic, auditory) related to CNS effects
- Injury risk related to CNS effects
- Altered tissue perfusion risk related to cardiac arrhythmias
- Knowledge deficit regarding drug therapy

Planning

- The patient will receive the best therapeutic effect from the drug therapy.
- The patient will have limited adverse effects from the drug therapy.
- The patient will have an understanding of the drug therapy, adverse effects to anticipate, and measures to relieve discomfort and improve safety.

Intervention With Rationale

- Administer oral drug with or before meals or at bedtime (exact timing varies with product) to ensure therapeutic levels when the drug is most needed.
- Arrange for decreased dose in cases of hepatic or renal dysfunction to prevent serious toxicity.
- Assess the patient carefully for any potential drug–drug interactions if administering cimetidine because of the drug's effects on liver enzyme systems.
- Provide comfort, including analgesics, ready access to bathroom facilities, and assistance with ambulation, to minimize possible adverse effects.
- Periodically reorient the patient and institute safety measures if CNS effects occur to ensure patient safety and improve patient tolerance of the drug and drug effects.
- Arrange for regular follow-up to evaluate drug effects and the underlying problem.
- Offer support and encouragement to help patients cope with the disease and the drug regimen.
- Provide patient teaching regarding drug name, dosage, and schedule for administration; importance of spacing administration appropriately as ordered; need for readily available access to bathroom; signs and symptoms of adverse effects and measures to minimize or prevent them; danger signs that necessitate notifying the health care provider immediately; safety measures, such as avoiding driving and asking for assistance when ambulating, to deal with possible effects of dizziness, somnolence, or confusion; the need for adherence to therapy to achieve the intended results; and the importance of periodic monitoring and evaluation, including laboratory testing, to determine drug effectiveness and to enhance patient knowledge about drug therapy and to promote adherence.

Evaluation

- Monitor patient response to the drug (relief of GI symptoms, ulcer healing, prevention of progression of ulcer).
- Monitor for adverse effects (dizziness, confusion, hallucinations, GI alterations, cardiac arrhythmias, hypotension, gynecomastia).
- Evaluate the effectiveness of the teaching plan (patient can name drug, dosage, and adverse effects to watch for and specific measures to avoid them).
- Monitor the effectiveness of comfort measures and adherence to the regimen.

Key Points

- Agents affecting GI secretion include H_2 antagonists, antacids, proton pump inhibitors, GI protectants, and prostaglandins.
- GI symptoms are among the most common complaints addressed in clinical practice.
- Increased acid production, decrease in the protective mucous lining of the stomach, infection with *Helicobacter pylori* bacteria, or a combination of these is the likely cause of peptic ulcers.
- H_2 antagonists block the release of acid in response to gastrin or parasympathetic release; adverse effects can include dizziness, confusion, cardiac arrhythmias, and galactorrhea.

Antacids

Antacids (see Table 57.1) are a group of inorganic chemicals that neutralize stomach acid. Antacids are available OTC, and many patients use them to self-treat a variety of GI symptoms. There is no one perfect antacid (see "Adverse Effects"). The choice of an antacid depends on adverse effects and absorption factors. Available agents are sodium bicarbonate (generic), calcium carbonate (*Oyster-cal*, *Tums*, and others), magnesium salts (*Milk of Magnesia* and others), and aluminum salts (*Amphojel* and others). These medications are often used in combination with other acid-reducing agents.

Therapeutic Actions and Indications

Antacids neutralize stomach acid by direct chemical reaction (see Fig. 57.1). They are recommended for the symptomatic relief of upset stomach associated with hyperacidity, as well as the hyperacidity associated with peptic ulcer, gastritis, peptic esophagitis, gastric hyperacidity, and hiatal hernia. See Table 57.1 for usual indications for each antacid.

Pharmacokinetics

Sodium bicarbonate, the oldest drug in this group, is available in many preparations, including baking soda powder, tablets, solutions, and as an injectable for treating systemic acidosis. This drug is widely distributed when absorbed orally, reaching peak level in 1 to 3 hours. It crosses the placenta and enters human milk. It is excreted in the urine and can cause serious electrolyte imbalance in people with renal impairment.

Calcium carbonate is actually precipitated chalk and is available in tablet and powder forms. The main drawbacks to this agent are constipation and **acid rebound**, in which the stomach increases acid release in response to low acid (high pH). Acid rebound can occur in response to using antacids that decrease acid. It has an onset of action in about 3 to 5 minutes. It can be absorbed systemically and cause calcium imbalance. When absorbed, it is metabolized in the liver and excreted in the urine and feces with a half-life of 1 to 3 hours. Calcium carbonate is known to cross the placenta and enter human milk.

Magnesium salts are effective in buffering acid in the stomach but have been known to cause diarrhea; they are sometimes used as laxatives. They are available as tablets, chewable tablets, capsules, and liquid. Although these agents are not generally absorbed systemically and are excreted in the feces, magnesium can lead to nerve damage and even coma if absorbed. It is excreted in the urine.

Aluminum salts, available as tablets, capsules, suspensions, and liquid, do not cause acid rebound but are not very effective in neutralizing acid. They are bound in the feces for excretion. They have been related to severe constipation. Aluminum binds dietary phosphates, and overuse can cause hypophosphatemia, which can then cause calcium imbalance throughout the system.

Many of these antacids are available in combination forms to take advantage of the acid-neutralizing effect and block adverse effects. For example, a combination of calcium and aluminum salts (*Maalox*) buffers acid and produces neither constipation nor diarrhea.

Contraindications and Cautions

Antacids are contraindicated in the presence of any known allergy to antacid products or any component of the drug to prevent hypersensitivity reactions. Caution should be used in the following instances: any condition that can be exacerbated by electrolyte or acid–base imbalance, to prevent exacerbations and serious adverse effects; any electrolyte imbalance, which could be exacerbated by the electrolyte-changing effects of these drugs; GI obstruction, which could cause systemic absorption of the drugs and increased adverse effects; renal dysfunction, which could lead to electrolyte disturbance if any absorbed antacid is not neutralized properly; and pregnancy and lactation because of the potential for adverse effects on the fetus or neonate.

Adverse Effects

The adverse effects associated with these drugs relate to their effects on acid–base and electrolyte balance. Administering an antacid frequently causes acid rebound, in which the stomach produces more acid in response to the alkaline environment. Neutralizing the stomach contents to an alkaline level stimulates gastrin production to cause an increase in acid production and return the stomach to its normal acidic state. In many cases, acid rebound causes an increase in symptoms, which results in an increased intake of the antacid. This leads to more acid production and an ongoing cycle. When more and more antacid is used, the risk for systemic effects rises. Alkalosis with resultant metabolic changes (nausea, vomiting, neuromuscular changes, headache, irritability, muscle twitching, and even coma) may occur. The use of calcium salts may lead to hypercalcemia and milk–alkali syndrome (seen as alkalosis, renal calcium deposits, or severe electrolyte disorders). Constipation or diarrhea may result, depending on the antacid being used. Hypophosphatemia can occur with the use of aluminum salts. Finally, fluid retention and heart failure can occur with sodium bicarbonate because of its high sodium content.

Clinically Important Drug–Drug Interactions

Antacids can greatly affect the absorption of drugs from the GI tract. Most drugs are prepared for an acidic environment, and an alkaline environment can prevent them from being broken down for absorption or can actually neutralize them so that they cannot be absorbed. Patients taking antacids should be advised to be aware of drug interactions. Some of these medications also have the potential to bind to medications and interfere with the absorption process, so they may need to be taken at different times than their other medications. Drug interactions should be checked carefully for each patient.

If the pH of urine is affected by large doses of antacids, the levels of drugs such as quinidine may increase and the levels of salicylates may decrease.

Prototype Summary: Sodium Bicarbonate

Indications: Symptomatic relief of upset stomach from hyperacidity; prophylaxis for GI bleeding and stress ulcers; adjunctive treatment of severe diarrhea; also used for treatment of metabolic acidosis; may also be used to treat certain drug intoxications to minimize uric acid crystallization.

Actions: Neutralizes or reduces gastric acidity, resulting in an increase in gastric pH, which inhibits the proteolytic activity of pepsin.

Pharmacokinetics:

Route	Onset	Peak	Duration
Oral	Rapid	30 min	1–3 h
IV	Immediate	Rapid	Unknown

$T_{1/2}$: Unknown; excreted unchanged in the urine.

Adverse Effects: Gastric rupture, systemic alkalosis (headache, nausea, irritability, weakness, tetany, confusion), hypokalemia (secondary to intracellular shifting of potassium), gastric acid rebound.

Nursing Considerations for Patients Receiving Antacids

Assessment: History and Examination

- Assess for possible contraindications or cautions: any history of allergy to antacids to prevent hypersensitivity reactions; renal dysfunction, which might interfere with the drug's excretion; electrolyte disturbances, which could be exacerbated by the effects of the drug; and current status of pregnancy or lactation due to possible effects on the fetus or newborn.
- Perform a physical examination to establish baseline data before beginning therapy, determine the effectiveness of the therapy, and evaluate for any potential adverse effects associated with drug therapy.
- Inspect the abdomen. Auscultate bowel sounds to ensure GI motility.
- Assess mucous membrane status to evaluate potential problems with absorption and hydration.
- Monitor laboratory test results, including serum electrolyte levels and renal function tests, to monitor for adverse effects of the drug and potential alterations in excretion that may necessitate dose adjustment.

Nursing Conclusions

Nursing conclusions related to drug therapy might include the following:

- Altered GI motility related to GI effects
- Electrolyte and/or fluid imbalance risks related to medication effects
- Knowledge deficit regarding drug therapy

Planning

- The patient will receive the best therapeutic effect from the drug therapy.
- The patient will have limited adverse effects from the drug therapy.
- The patient will have an understanding of the drug therapy, adverse effects to anticipate, and measures to relieve discomfort and improve safety.

Intervention With Rationale

- Administer the drug apart from any other oral medications approximately 1 hour before or 2 hours after to ensure adequate absorption of the other medications.
- Have the patient take medications as instructed on label. Some tablets need to be chewed thoroughly and followed with water to ensure that therapeutic levels reach the stomach to decrease acidity.
- Assess the patient for any signs of acid–base or electrolyte imbalance to ensure early detection and prompt interventions.

- Monitor the patient for diarrhea or constipation to institute a bowel program before severe effects occur.
- Monitor the patient's nutritional status if diarrhea is severe or constipation leads to decreased food intake, to ensure adequate fluid and nutritional intake and promote healing and GI stability.
- Offer support and encouragement to help the patient cope with the disease and the drug regimen.
- Provide thorough patient teaching, including the drug name and prescribed dosage, schedule for administration, signs and symptoms of adverse effects and measures to minimize or prevent them, warning signs that may indicate possible problems and the need to notify the health care provider immediately, the importance of maintaining fluid and nutritional intake if diarrhea or constipation occurs, possible bowel training programs to deal with constipation or diarrhea if severe, cautions related to prolonged chronic use of drug and increased risk for acid rebound, the importance of checking with the health care provider before using any OTC medications, differences associated with the various OTC antacid formulations, and the need for periodic monitoring and evaluation to enhance patient knowledge about drug therapy and to promote adherence.

Evaluation

- Monitor patient response to the drug (relief of GI symptoms caused by hyperacidity).
- Monitor for adverse effects (GI effects, imbalances in serum electrolytes, and acid–base status).
- Evaluate the effectiveness of the teaching plan (patient can name the drug and dosage as well as describe adverse effects to watch for, specific measures to avoid them, and measures to take to increase the effectiveness of the drug).
- Monitor the effectiveness of comfort measures and adherence to the regimen.

Key Points

- Antacids are used to chemically react with and neutralize acid in the stomach. They can provide rapid relief from increased acid levels. They are known to cause GI alterations such as diarrhea or constipation and can alter the absorption of many drugs.
- Acid rebound occurs when the stomach produces more gastrin and more acid in response to lowered acid levels in the stomach, which commonly occurs with the use of antacids. Balancing the reduction of the stomach acid without increasing acid production is a clinical challenge.

Proton Pump Inhibitors

Proton pump inhibitors (see Table 57.1) suppress the secretion of hydrochloric acid into the lumen of the stomach. Six proton pump inhibitors are available: omeprazole (*Prilosec*), esomeprazole (*Nexium*), lansoprazole (*Prevacid*), dexlansoprazole (*Dexilant*), pantoprazole (*Protonix*), and rabeprazole (*Aciphex*).

Therapeutic Actions and Indications

The gastric acid pump or proton pump inhibitors suppress gastric acid secretion by specifically inhibiting the hydrogen–potassium adenosine triphosphatase (H^+, K^+–ATPase) enzyme system on the secretory surface of gastric parietal cells. This action blocks the final step of acid production, lowering the acid levels in the stomach (see Fig. 57.1). They are recommended for the short-term treatment of active duodenal ulcers, GERD, erosive esophagitis, and benign active gastric ulcer; for the long-term treatment of pathological hypersecretory conditions; as maintenance therapy for healing of erosive esophagitis and ulcers; and in combination with amoxicillin and clarithromycin for the treatment of *Helicobacter pylori* infection. See Table 57.1 for usual indications for each of these agents.

Pharmacokinetics

Esomeprazole, lansoprazole, and pantoprazole are available in delayed-release oral forms and as IV preparations. Rabeprazole, dexlansoprazole, and omeprazole are available only in delayed-release oral forms.

These drugs are acid-labile and are rapidly absorbed from the GI tract, reaching peak level in 3 to 5 hours. They undergo extensive metabolism in the liver and are excreted in the urine. Omeprazole is faster acting and more quickly excreted than the other proton pump inhibitors. It has a half-life of 30 to 60 minutes. Esomeprazole is a longer-acting drug; it has a half-life of 60 to 90 minutes and a duration of 17 hours. It is not broken down as rapidly in the liver as the parent drug omeprazole. Lansoprazole has a half-life of 2 hours and a duration of 12 hours.

Pantoprazole and rabeprazole have half-lives of 90 minutes and durations of 12 to 14 hours. Dexlansoprazole is available in a delayed capsule that offers two releases, having peak effect in 1 to 2 hours and then 4 to 5 hours, offering longer protection throughout the day. There are no adequate studies about whether these drugs cross the placenta or enter human milk.

Contraindications and Cautions

These drugs are contraindicated in the presence of known allergy to either the drug or the drug components to prevent hypersensitivity reactions. They are also contraindicated to be used concurrently with medications containing rilpivirine. Caution should be used in pregnant or lactating patients because of the potential for adverse effects on the fetus or neonate.

Adverse Effects

The adverse effects associated with these drugs are related to their effects on the H^+, K^+–ATPase pump on the parietal and other cells. CNS effects of dizziness and headache are occasionally seen; asthenia (loss of strength), vertigo, insomnia, apathy, and dream abnormalities may also be observed. GI effects can include diarrhea, abdominal pain, nausea, vomiting, dry mouth, and tongue atrophy. Upper respiratory tract symptoms, including cough, stuffy nose, hoarseness, and epistaxis, are frequently seen (Fig. 57.2). Other less common adverse effects include rash, alopecia, pruritus, dry skin, back pain, and fever. In preclinical studies, long-term effects of proton pump inhibitors included the development of gastric cancer. Recent studies show an increase in bone loss and decreased calcium levels, decreased magnesium levels leading to hypertension, and increased incidence of *Clostridium difficile* diarrhea and pneumonia in patients using these drugs long term. These effects are thought to be related to changing the normal acidity in the stomach that changes the environment for absorbing calcium or magnesium and the environment of normal flora bacteria, which can lead to infection from those previously friendly bacteria.

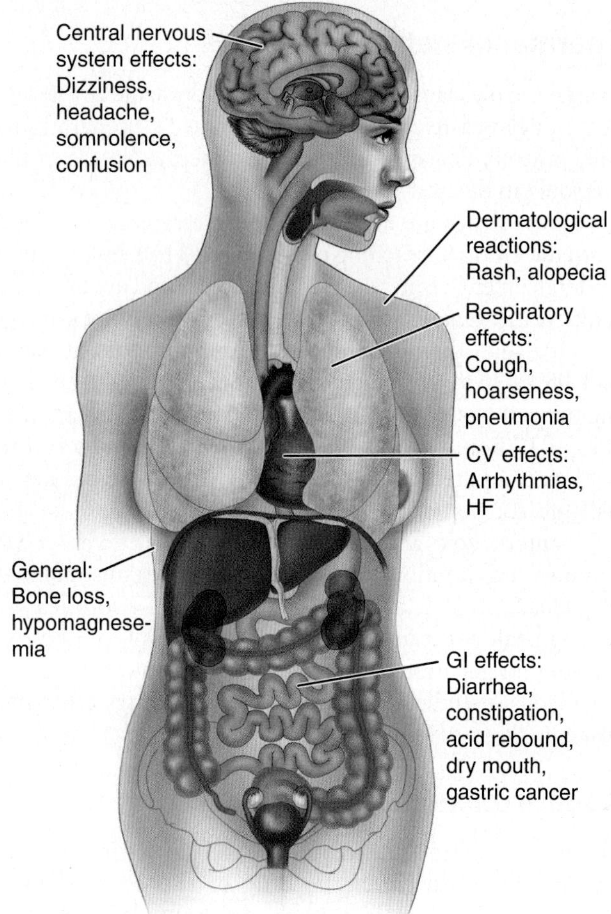

FIGURE 57.2 Variety of adverse effects and toxicities associated with drugs affecting gastrointestinal secretions.

Clinically Important Drug–Drug Interactions

There is a risk of increased serum levels and increased toxicity of benzodiazepines, phenytoin, and warfarin if these are combined with these drugs; patients should be monitored closely. Decreased levels of ketoconazole and theophylline have been reported when combined with these drugs, leading to loss of effectiveness. Concurrent use with some antiretroviral medications, such as rilpivirine, atazanavir, nelfinavir, and saquinavir, is contraindicated because interactions can increase or decrease exposure to the antiviral medications.

Prototype Summary: Omeprazole

Indications: Short-term treatment of active duodenal ulcer or active benign gastric ulcer; treatment of heartburn or symptoms of gastroesophageal reflux; treatment of pathological hypersecretory syndromes; eradication of *Helicobacter pylori* infection as part of combination therapy.

Actions: Specifically inhibits the H^+, K^+–ATPase enzyme system on the secretory surface of gastric parietal cells, blocking the final step in acid production and decreasing gastric acid levels.

Pharmacokinetics:

Route	Onset	Peak	Duration
Oral	Varies	0.5–3.5 h	Varies

$T_{1/2}$: 30 to 60 minutes; metabolized in the liver and excreted in the urine and bile.

Adverse Effects: Headache, dizziness, vertigo, insomnia, rash, diarrhea, abdominal pain, nausea, vomiting, upper respiratory infection symptoms, cough.

Nursing Considerations for Patients Receiving Proton Pump Inhibitors

Assessment: History and Examination

- Assess for possible contraindications or cautions: history of allergy to a proton pump inhibitor, to reduce the risk of hypersensitivity reaction; and current status of pregnancy or lactation, because of the potential for adverse effects on the fetus or nursing baby.

- Perform a physical examination to establish baseline data before beginning therapy, to determine the effectiveness of the therapy, and to evaluate for the occurrence of any adverse effects associated with drug therapy.
- Inspect the skin for lesions, rash, pruritus, and dryness to identify possible adverse effects.
- Assess neurological status, including level of orientation, affect, and reflexes, to evaluate for CNS effects of the drug.
- Inspect and palpate the abdomen to determine potential underlying medical conditions; assess for changes in bowel elimination and GI upset to identify possible adverse effects.
- Assess respiratory status, including respiratory rate and rhythm; note evidence of cough, hoarseness, and epistaxis to monitor for potential adverse effects of the drug.

Planning

- The patient will receive the best therapeutic effect from the drug therapy.
- The patient will have limited adverse effects from the drug therapy.
- The patient will have an understanding of the drug therapy, adverse effects to anticipate, and measures to relieve discomfort and improve safety.

Nursing Conclusions

Nursing conclusions related to drug therapy might include the following:

- Altered GI motility risk related to GI effects
- Imbalanced nutrition risk related to potential for medication to alter absorption of nutrients
- Altered sensory perception (kinesthetic, auditory) related to CNS effects
- Injury risk related to CNS effects
- Knowledge deficit risk regarding drug therapy

Intervention With Rationale

- Administer drug as prescribed. Ensure that the patient does not open, chew, or crush capsules; they should be swallowed whole to ensure the therapeutic effectiveness of the drug.
- Provide appropriate safety and comfort measures if CNS effects occur to prevent patient injury.
- Monitor the patient for diarrhea or constipation to institute an appropriate bowel program as needed.
- Monitor the patient's nutritional status; if GI upset is a problem, the use of small, frequent meals may be helpful.
- Arrange for medical follow-up if symptoms are not resolved after 4 to 8 weeks of therapy because serious underlying conditions could be causing the symptoms.
- Offer support and encouragement to help the patient cope with the disease and the drug regimen.
- Provide thorough patient teaching, including the drug name and prescribed dosage; the importance of taking the drug whole without opening, chewing, or crushing it; signs and symptoms of possible adverse effects and measures to minimize or prevent them; danger signs that need to be reported to the health care provider immediately; nutritional measures, such as small, frequent meals; safety measures, such as avoiding driving and getting assistance with ambulation as needed; methods for dealing with constipation or diarrhea; and the need for periodic monitoring and evaluation, to enhance patient knowledge about drug therapy and to promote adherence.

Evaluation

- Monitor patient response to the drug (relief of GI symptoms caused by hyperacidity, healing of erosive GI lesions).
- Monitor for adverse effects (GI effects, CNS changes, dermatological effects, respiratory effects).
- Monitor the effectiveness of comfort and safety measures and adherence to the regimen.
- Evaluate the effectiveness of the teaching plan (patient can name the drug and dosage and describe adverse effects to watch for, specific measures to avoid them, and measures to take to increase the effectiveness of the drug).

Key Points

- The gastric acid pump or proton pump inhibitors suppress gastric acid secretion by specifically inhibiting the H^+, K^+–ATPase enzyme system on the secretory surface of the gastric parietal cells. This action blocks the final step of acid production, lowering the acid levels in the stomach.
- Proton pump inhibitors are indicated for the short-term treatment of active duodenal ulcer or active benign gastric ulcer, treatment of heartburn or symptoms of gastroesophageal reflux, treatment of pathological hypersecretory syndromes, and eradication of *Helicobacter pylori* infection as part of combination therapy.

Gastrointestinal Protectant

Gastrointestinal protectants (see Table 57.1) coat any injured area in the stomach to prevent further injury from acid. Sucralfate (*Carafate*) is the only GI protectant currently available.

Therapeutic Actions and Indications

Sucralfate forms an ulcer-adherent complex at duodenal ulcer sites, protecting the sites against acid, pepsin, and bile salts. This action prevents further breakdown of the area and promotes ulcer healing. The drug also inhibits pepsin activity in gastric juices, preventing further breakdown of proteins in the stomach, including the protein wall of the stomach (see Fig. 57.1). See Table 57.1 for usual indications.

Pharmacokinetics

Sucralfate is only minimally absorbed after oral administration. Most is excreted via the feces. The small amount that is absorbed is excreted in urine. There is no evidence of harm during pregnancy in animal studies, but there are no adequate human studies to ensure lack of risk. It is unknown if it is excreted in human milk.

Contraindications and Cautions

Sucralfate should not be given to any person with known allergy to the drug or any of its components to prevent hypersensitivity reactions. It should not be given to patients with renal failure or undergoing dialysis because a buildup of aluminum may occur if it is used with aluminum-containing products. Caution should be used in patients who are pregnant or lactating because of lack of evidence regarding risk to the fetus or neonate.

Adverse Effects

The adverse effects associated with sucralfate are primarily related to its GI effects. Constipation is the most frequently seen adverse effect. Diarrhea, nausea, indigestion, gastric discomfort, and dry mouth may also occur. Other adverse effects that have been reported with this drug include dizziness, sleepiness, vertigo, skin rash, and back pain.

Clinically Important Drug–Drug Interactions

If aluminum salts are combined with sucralfate, there is a risk of high aluminum levels and aluminum toxicity. Extreme care should be taken if this combination is used.

In addition, if phenytoin, digoxin, warfarin, fluoroquinolone antibiotics (e.g., ciprofloxacin, norfloxacin), or penicillamine are combined with sucralfate, decreased serum levels and drug effectiveness may result. In such combinations, the individual agents should be administered separately with at least 2 hours between drugs.

Prototype Summary: Sucralfate

Indications: Short-term treatment and maintenance treatment of active duodenal ulcer; treatment of oral and esophageal ulcers due to radiation, chemotherapy, or sclerotherapy.

Actions: Forms an ulcer-adherent complex at the duodenal ulcer site, protecting the sites from acid, bile salts, and pepsin, promoting healing of the ulcer; also inhibits pepsin activity in gastric juices.

Pharmacokinetics:

Route	Onset	Duration
Oral	30 min	5 h

$T_{1/2}$: 6 to 20 hours; mostly excreted in the feces.

Adverse Effects: Sleeplessness, dizziness, vertigo, insomnia, rash, constipation, diarrhea, nausea, indigestion, dry mouth, back pain.

Nursing Considerations for Patients Receiving a Gastrointestinal Protectant

Assessment: History and Examination

- Assess for possible contraindications or cautions: any history of allergy to sucralfate to prevent hypersensitivity reactions; renal dysfunction or dialysis, which can lead to a buildup of aluminum; and current status of pregnancy or lactation.
- Perform a physical examination to establish baseline data before beginning therapy, to determine the effectiveness of therapy, and to evaluate for any adverse effects associated with drug therapy.
- Inspect the skin for color and evidence of lesions or rash that might indicate adverse drug effects.
- Assess the patient's neurological status, including level of orientation, affect, and reflexes, to monitor for CNS effects of the drug.
- Examine the abdomen; auscultate bowel sounds to evaluate GI motility; evaluate bowel elimination pattern or changes that could suggest possible adverse effects.
- Monitor the results of laboratory tests such as renal function studies to identify the need for possible dose adjustments and toxic effects.

Nursing Conclusions

Nursing conclusions related to drug therapy might include the following:

- Altered GI motility related to medication effects
- Imbalanced nutrition risk: less than body requirements related to GI effects

- Altered sensory perception (kinesthetic) related to CNS effects
- Knowledge deficit regarding drug therapy

Planning

- The patient will receive the best therapeutic effect from the drug therapy.
- The patient will have limited adverse effects from the drug therapy.
- The patient will have an understanding of the drug therapy, adverse effects to anticipate, and measures to relieve discomfort and improve safety.

Intervention With Rationale

- Administer the drug on an empty stomach 1 hour before or 2 hours after meals and at bedtime to ensure the therapeutic effectiveness of the drug.
- Monitor the patient for GI discomfort, and arrange to administer antacids to relieve pain if needed.
- Administer antacids or antibiotics, if ordered, between doses of sucralfate, not within 30 minutes of a sucralfate dose, because sucralfate may interfere with absorption of medications.
- Provide comfort and safety measures if CNS effects occur, to prevent patient injury.
- Provide frequent mouth care including sugarless lozenges to suck to alleviate dry mouth.
- Ensure ready access to bathroom facilities if diarrhea occurs, institute bowel training as needed, and provide small, frequent meals if GI effects are uncomfortable.
- Offer support and encouragement to help the patient cope with the disease and the drug regimen.
- Provide thorough patient teaching, including the drug name and prescribed dosage; schedule for administration; importance of taking the drug on an empty stomach; use of antacids if ordered and the need to separate doses by at least 2 hours; signs and symptoms of possible adverse effects and measures to minimize or prevent their occurrence; dietary measures such as small, frequent meals to minimize diarrhea and help with GI upset; increased fluid and fiber in the diet to reduce the risk of constipation; comfort measures such as mouth care and use of sugarless lozenges to alleviate dry mouth; the importance of adherence to therapy to achieve the intended effects; measures to help avoid adverse effects; warning signs that may indicate problems; and the need for periodic monitoring and evaluation to evaluate the effectiveness of therapy, enhance patient knowledge about therapy, and promote adherence.

Evaluation

- Monitor the patient response to the drug (relief of GI symptoms, healing of erosive GI lesions).
- Monitor for adverse effects (GI effects, CNS changes, dermatological effects).
- Monitor the effectiveness of comfort and safety measures and adherence to the regimen.
- Evaluate the effectiveness of the teaching plan (patient can name drug and dosage and describe the adverse effects to watch for, specific measures to avoid them, and measures to take to increase the effectiveness of the drug).

Key Points

- The GI protectant sucralfate forms a protective coating over the eroded stomach lining to protect it from acid and digestive enzymes to aid healing.
- Constipation is a common occurrence with this drug.

Prostaglandins

Prostaglandins are used to protect the stomach lining. The prostaglandin available for this use is the synthetic prostaglandin E_1 analog misoprostol (*Cytotec*).

Therapeutic Actions and Indications

Prostaglandin E_1 inhibits gastric acid secretion and increases bicarbonate and mucus production in the stomach, thus protecting the stomach lining (see Fig. 57.1). Misoprostol is primarily used to prevent NSAID-induced gastric ulcers in patients who are at high risk for complications from a gastric ulcer (e.g., older patients or debilitated patients, patients with a past history of ulcer). See Table 57.1 for more information and usual indications about this drug.

Pharmacokinetics

Misoprostol is given orally. It is rapidly absorbed from the GI tract, metabolized in the liver, and excreted in the urine. Misoprostol crosses the placenta and enters human milk.

Contraindications and Cautions

Misoprostol is contraindicated with allergy to any part of the drug to prevent hypersensitivity reactions. This drug is also contraindicated during pregnancy because it can induce labor and may cause uterine rupture. Patients who can become pregnant should be advised to have a negative serum pregnancy test within 2 weeks of beginning treatment, and they should begin the drug on the 2nd or 3rd day of their next menstrual cycle. In addition, they should be instructed to use contraceptives during therapy. It is recommended to only be used in hospital setting if administered for off-label uses like cervical ripening, induction of labor, or treatment of postpartum hemorrhage. Caution should be used during lactation because of the potential for adverse effects on the newborn. Caution is also necessary in patients with hepatic or renal impairment, which could interfere with the effective metabolism and excretion of the drug.

Adverse Effects

The adverse effects associated with this drug are primarily related to its GI effects—nausea, diarrhea, abdominal pain, flatulence, vomiting, dyspepsia, and constipation. Genitourinary effects, which are related to the actions of prostaglandins on the uterus, include miscarriages, excessive bleeding, spotting, cramping, hypermenorrhea, dysmenorrhea, and other menstrual disorders. People who menstruate or can become pregnant while taking this drug should be notified both in writing and verbally of these potential effects of this drug.

Prototype Summary: Misoprostol

Indications: Prevention of NSAID-induced ulcers in adults at high risk for development of these gastric ulcers; off-label uses include inducing labor and medical termination of pregnancy.

Actions: Inhibits gastric acid secretion and increases bicarbonate and mucous production, protecting the lining of the stomach; increases stimulatory effects in the uterus.

Pharmacokinetics:

Route	Onset	Peak
Oral	Rapid	12–15 min

$T_{1/2}$: 20 to 40 minutes; metabolized in the liver and excreted in the urine.

Adverse Effects: Nausea, diarrhea, abdominal pain, flatulence, vomiting, excessive bleeding or spotting, hypermenorrhea, dysmenorrhea, miscarriage.

Nursing Considerations for Patients Receiving Prostaglandin

Assessment: History and Examination

- Assess for possible contraindications or cautions: any history of allergy to misoprostol, to prevent hypersensitivity reactions; and current status of pregnancy or lactation, because of the potential for adverse effects on the fetus or nursing baby.
- Perform a physical examination to establish baseline data before beginning therapy and during therapy, to determine the effectiveness of the drug, and to evaluate for the occurrence of any adverse effects associated with drug therapy.
- Examine the abdomen for possible changes to rule out medical conditions.
- Perform a pregnancy test and assess normal menstrual activity to make sure that the patient is not pregnant.
- Monitor the results of laboratory tests, including renal and hepatic function tests, to determine the need for possible dose adjustment and identify toxic effects.

Nursing Conclusions

Nursing conclusions related to drug therapy might include the following:

- Impaired comfort related to diarrhea or other GI effects
- Imbalanced nutrition: less than body requirements related to GI effects
- Knowledge deficit risk regarding drug therapy

Planning

- The patient will receive the best therapeutic effect from the drug therapy.
- The patient will have limited adverse effects from the drug therapy.
- The patient will have an understanding of the drug therapy, adverse effects to anticipate, and measures to relieve discomfort and improve safety.

Intervention With Rationale

- Administer to patients at high risk for NSAID-induced ulcers during the full course of NSAID therapy to prevent the development of gastric ulcers. Administer four times a day, with meals and at bedtime, to ensure maximum benefit of the drug.
- For patients who can become pregnant, arrange for a serum pregnancy test within 2 weeks before beginning treatment and begin therapy on the 2nd or 3rd day of the menstrual period to ensure that the patient is not pregnant and to prevent harm to the fetus.
- Provide the patient with both written and oral information regarding the associated risks of pregnancy to ensure that the patient understands the risks involved; advise the use of contraceptives during therapy to ensure the prevention of pregnancy.
- Evaluate nutritional status if GI effects are severe to arrange for appropriate measures to relieve discomfort and ensure nutrition, such as small, frequent meals, and increased fluid intake if appropriate.
- Explain the risk of menstrual disorders and pain, miscarriage, and excessive bleeding related to the drug effects on prostaglandin activity in the uterus.
- Offer support and encouragement to help the patient cope with the disease and the drug regimen.
- Provide thorough patient teaching, including the drug name and prescribed dosage; schedule for administration; the need to take the drug with meals and at bedtime; signs and symptoms of adverse effects and measures to minimize or prevent them;

the importance of avoiding pregnancy while taking drug; the use of contraceptives to prevent pregnancy; dietary measures such as small, frequent meals and increased fluid intake to alleviate or minimize adverse GI effects; danger signs to report to the health care provider immediately; support to deal with changes in sexuality patterns that may occur; and the importance of periodic monitoring and evaluation to enhance patient knowledge about drug therapy and to promote adherence.

Evaluation

- Monitor the patient response to the drug (prevention of GI ulcers related to NSAIDs).
- Monitor for adverse effects (GI, genitourinary).
- Monitor the effectiveness of comfort and safety measures and adherence to the regimen.
- Evaluate the effectiveness of the teaching plan (patient can name drug and dosage and describe adverse effects to watch for, specific measures to avoid them, and measures to take to increase the effectiveness of the drug).

Key Points

- The prostaglandin misoprostol is used to inhibit gastric acid secretion and increase bicarbonate and mucus production in the stomach; this action will protect the lining of the stomach.
- This drug increases prostaglandin effects in the uterus, causing increased contractions, excessive bleeding, and cramping. Use of this drug has potential risk of induction of labor and/or uterine rupture.

Digestive Enzymes

Digestive enzymes (Table 57.2) are substances produced in the GI tract to break down foods into usable nutrients. Some patients—those who have suffered strokes, salivary gland disorders, or extreme surgery of the head and neck and those with cystic fibrosis or pancreatic dysfunction—may require a supplement to the production of digestive enzymes. Two digestive enzymes are available for replacement in conditions that result in lower-than-normal levels of these enzymes: saliva substitute (*Aquoral, Moi-Stir, Mouth Kote, Salivart,* and others) and pancrelipase (*Creon, Pancreaze, Pertzye, Viokace, Zenpep*).

Box 57.6 describes a peptide that is indicated for use as part of the treatment regimen for patients diagnosed with short bowel syndrome who are dependent on parenteral support.

BOX 57.6

Glucagon-Like Peptide-2 (GLP-2) Analog to Treat Short Bowel Syndrome (SBS)

Teduglutide (*Gattex*) is a GLP-2 analog indicated for the treatment of adults and pediatric patients with SBS who are dependent on parenteral support. SBS is associated with extreme loss of absorption that prohibits the person from maintaining fluid and nutrient balance. It can occur due to obstruction, surgery, or congenital defects. The GLP-2 peptide is normally secreted by the small intestine. It acts to increase blood flow to the intestine and liver and to inhibit gastric acid secretion. Teduglutide binds to the receptors for this glucagon peptide and causes the release of many mediators including insulin-like growth factor, nitric oxide, and keratinocyte growth factor. Its actions increase intestinal absorption through increased blood flow and decreased acid secretion. It is given by subcutaneous injection once daily. Teduglutide is associated with neoplastic growth, intestinal obstruction, biliary and pancreatic disorders, and fluid overload. It is important to differentiate this drug and its actions from the GLP-1 agonists that are used to maintain glycemic control.

Therapeutic Actions and Indications

Saliva substitute contains electrolytes and carboxymethylcellulose to act as a thickening agent in dry mouth conditions. This makes the food bolus easier to swallow and begins the early digestion process. Saliva substitute helps

Table 57.2 ***Drugs in Focus:*** **Drugs Used to Treat Digestive Enzyme Dysfunction**

Drug Name	Usual Dosage	Usual Indications
Digestive Enzymes		
pancrelipase (*Creon, Pancreaze, Pertzye, Viokace, Zenpep*)	*Adult and pediatric:* PO dosing based on weight with each meal and snacks; dosing can vary based on formulation	Aids digestion and absorption of fats, proteins, and carbohydrates in conditions that result in a lack of this enzyme; used as replacement therapy in patients with cystic fibrosis, chronic ductal obstruction, pancreatic insufficiency, steatorrhea, or malabsorption syndrome and after pancreatectomy or gastrectomy
saliva substitute (*Aquoral, Moi-Stir, Mouth Kote, Salivart,* and others)	Spray, disintegrating tablets or lozenges, gel, liquid to be applied to oral mucosa	Aids in conditions resulting in dry mouth—stroke, radiation therapy, chemotherapy, and other illnesses

in conditions that result in dry mouth—stroke, radiation therapy, chemotherapy, and other illnesses. Pancreatic enzymes are replacement enzymes that help the digestion and absorption of fats, proteins, and carbohydrates (see Fig. 57.1). See Table 57.2 for usual indications for each agent.

Pharmacokinetics

Saliva substitute is available as a solution, in lozenge form, and on swab sticks for oral administration. It is not generally absorbed systemically. It works when applied to the mouth. Pancrelipase, which is available in capsules, delayed-release capsules, powder, and tablets, is thought to be processed through normal metabolic systems in the body. It is designed to withstand the gastric acid and release enzymes in the higher pH of the small intestine.

Contraindications and Cautions

Saliva substitute is contraindicated in the presence of known allergy to parabens or any component of the drug to prevent hypersensitivity reactions. It should be used cautiously in patients with heart failure, hypertension, or renal failure because there may be an abnormal absorption of electrolytes, including sodium, leading to increased CV load. Pancreatic enzymes should not be used with known allergy to the product or to pork products to prevent hypersensitivity reactions.

Adverse Effects

The adverse effects most commonly seen with saliva substitute involve complications from abnormal electrolyte absorption, such as increased levels of magnesium, sodium, or potassium. The adverse effects that most often occur with pancreatic enzymes are related to GI irritation and include nausea, abdominal cramps, and diarrhea.

Prototype Summary: Pancrelipase

Indications: Replacement therapy in patients with deficient exocrine pancreatic secretions.

Actions: Replaces pancreatic enzymes to aid in the digestion and absorption of fats, proteins, and carbohydrates.

Pharmacokinetics: Enteric-coated tablets designed to stay intact in the high-acid environment of the stomach. Releases enzymes in higher pH environment. Most of the medication is not absorbed from gastrointestinal tract.

$T_{1/2}$: Generally not absorbed systemically.

Adverse Effects: Nausea, abdominal cramps, diarrhea, hyperuricosuria.

Nursing Considerations for Patients Receiving Digestive Enzymes

Assessment: History and Examination

- Assess for possible contraindications or cautions: any history of allergy to any of the drugs or to pork products (pancreatic enzymes) to prevent hypersensitivity reactions; any history of heart failure or hypertension (saliva substitute) because there may be an abnormal absorption of electrolytes including sodium, leading to increased CV load.
- Perform a physical examination to establish baseline data before beginning therapy and during therapy, to evaluate the effectiveness of the drug, and to determine the occurrence of any adverse effects associated with drug therapy.
- Perform an abdominal examination to rule out underlying medical conditions and assess for adverse effects of the drug; auscultate bowel sounds to evaluate GI motility.
- Monitor mucous membranes to assess for their condition and for any indication of the need for saliva substitute.
- Assess cardiopulmonary status, including blood pressure and cardiac rate and rhythm, to identify changes that may indicate electrolyte imbalances.

Nursing Conclusions

Nursing conclusions related to drug therapy might include the following:

- Impaired comfort related to GI effects
- Imbalanced nutrition: less than body requirements related to GI effects
- Knowledge deficit risk regarding drug therapy

Planning

- The patient will receive the best therapeutic effect from the drug therapy.
- The patient will have limited adverse effects from the drug therapy.
- The patient will have an understanding of the drug therapy, adverse effects to anticipate, and measures to relieve discomfort and improve safety.

Intervention With Rationale

- Administer saliva substitute as prescribed to coat the mouth and ensure therapeutic effectiveness of the drug. It should not be swallowed.
- Monitor swallowing because it may be impaired due to the underlying medical conditions or decrease in lubricating effects related to low saliva levels, and additional therapy may be needed.
- Administer pancreatic enzymes with meals and snacks so that enzyme is available when it is needed.

- Assess nutritional status if there are GI effects and arrange for appropriate measures to relieve discomfort and ensure nutrition, such as small, frequent meals.
- Obtain laboratory specimens as indicated to evaluate electrolyte levels and pancreatic enzyme levels.
- Offer support and encouragement to help the patient cope with the disease and the drug regimen.
- Provide thorough patient teaching, including the drug name and prescribed dosage; schedule for administration; the technique for using saliva substitute; the importance of taking pancreatic enzymes with meals and snacks; dietary measures to follow; signs and symptoms of adverse effects and measures to minimize or prevent them; danger signs that need to be reported to the health care provider immediately; the need for periodic monitoring, including laboratory tests to evaluate electrolyte levels (with saliva substitute) to evaluate the effectiveness of therapy; and the importance of complying with therapy and follow-up to enhance patient knowledge about drug therapy and to promote adherence.

Evaluation

- Monitor the patient response to the drug (e.g., relief of dry mouth and throat; digestion of fats, proteins, and carbohydrates).
- Monitor for adverse effects (e.g., electrolyte imbalance, GI effects).
- Monitor the effectiveness of comfort and safety measures and adherence to the regimen.
- Evaluate the effectiveness of the teaching plan (patient can name the drug and dosage and describe adverse effects to watch for, specific measures to avoid them, and measures to take to increase the effectiveness of the drug).

Key Points

- Digestive enzymes such as substitute saliva and pancreatic enzymes may be needed if normal enzyme levels are very low and proper digestion cannot take place.
- Patients receiving replacement enzymes will need to be monitored to ensure that the dose is correct for their particular situation to avoid adverse effects.

SUMMARY

- GI complaints are some of the most common symptoms seen in clinical practice.
- Peptic ulcers may result from increased acid production, decrease in the protective mucous lining of the stomach, infection with *Helicobacter pylori* bacteria, or a combination of these.
- Agents used to decrease the acid content of the stomach include H_2 antagonists, which block the release of acid in response to gastrin or parasympathetic release; antacids, which chemically react with the acid to neutralize it; proton pump inhibitors, which block the last step of acid production to prevent release; and prostaglandins, which block gastric acid secretion and increase bicarbonate production.
- Acid rebound occurs when the stomach produces more gastrin and more acid in response to lowered acid levels in the stomach, which commonly occurs with the use of antacids. Balancing the reduction of the stomach acid without increasing acid production is a clinical challenge.
- The GI protectant sucralfate forms a protective coating over the eroded stomach lining to protect it from acid and digestive enzymes to aid healing.
- The prostaglandin misoprostol blocks gastric acid secretion while increasing the production of bicarbonate and mucous lining in the stomach.
- Digestive enzymes such as substitute saliva and pancreatic enzymes may be needed if normal enzyme levels are low and proper digestion cannot take place.

Unfolding Patient Stories: Suzanne Morris • Part 2

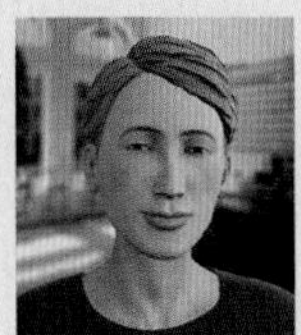

Think back to Suzanne Morris, the 43-year-old female from Chapter 37 who is treated for peptic ulcer disease (PUD) with amoxicillin, clarithromycin, and pantoprazole. During the clinic visit, she expresses concern about a family history of osteoporosis. What patient education should the nurse provide on factors that can influence the development of osteoporosis? If Suzanne's diet is insufficient, what oral supplements would the nurse consider for osteoporosis prevention? What are the nursing implications when administering oral supplements for osteoporosis prevention with her current medications for PUD?

Care for Suzanne and other patients in a realistic virtual environment: ***vSim** for Nursing* (thepoint.lww.com/vSimPharm). Practice documenting these patients' care in DocuCare (thepoint.lww.com/DocuCareEHR).

CHECK YOUR UNDERSTANDING

Answers to the questions in this chapter can be found in Answers to Check Your Understanding Questions on thePoint®.

MULTIPLE CHOICE

Select the best answer.

1. Which would a nurse include when describing the action of H_2 antagonists to a patient?
   a. They block the release of gastrin and pepsin, leading to a decrease in protein digestion.
   b. They selectively block histamine receptors, reducing swelling and inflammation at numerous sites.
   c. They selectively block specific histamine receptor sites, leading to a reduction in gastric acid secretion.
   d. They are effective primarily for long-term use because of their slow onset of action.

2. H_2 receptors are found throughout the body, including in the
   a. nasal passages, upper airways, and stomach.
   b. CNS and upper airways.
   c. respiratory tract and the heart.
   d. heart, CNS, and stomach.

3. A patient has been taking an H_2 antagonist. Which symptom would the nurse expect to be relieved if the medication was effective?
   a. Diarrhea
   b. Flatulence
   c. Heartburn
   d. Headache

4. Which of the following has NOT been considered a risk of taking proton pump inhibitors for long durations?
   a. Loss of bone
   b. Pneumonia
   c. Gastric cancer
   d. Constipation

5. Acid rebound is a condition that occurs when
   a. lowering gastric acid to an alkaline level stimulates the release of gastric acid.
   b. raising gastric acid levels causes heartburn.
   c. combining protein, calcium, and smoking greatly elevates gastric acid levels.
   d. eating citrus fruit neutralizes gastric acid.

6. A nurse taking care of a patient who is receiving a proton pump inhibitor should teach the patient to
   a. take the drug after every meal.
   b. chew or crush tablets to increase their absorption.
   c. swallow tablets or capsules whole.
   d. stop taking the drug after 3 weeks of therapy.

7. Misoprostol (*Cytotec*) is a prostaglandin that is used to
   a. prevent uterine contractions.
   b. prevent NSAID-related gastric ulcers in patients at high risk.
   c. decrease hyperacidity with meals and at bedtime.
   d. relieve the burning associated with hiatal hernia at night.

8. A nurse caring for a patient receiving pancreatic enzymes as replacement therapy should be assessing the patient for
   a. hypertension.
   b. cardiac arrhythmias.
   c. excessive weight gain.
   d. signs of GI irritation.

MULTIPLE RESPONSE

Select all that apply.

1. Patients who use antacids frequently can be expected to experience which adverse effects?
   a. Systemic alkalosis
   b. Electrolyte imbalances
   c. Hypokalemia
   d. Metabolic acidosis
   e. Constipation or diarrhea
   f. Muscular weakness

2. Saliva substitute (*Moi-Stir*) may be useful in which circumstances?
   a. Cancer radiation therapy
   b. Stroke
   c. Parkinson's disease
   d. Brain injury
   e. Situational anxiety
   f. Hypertension

REFERENCES

Broeren, M., Geerdink, E., Vader, H., & van den Wall Bake, A. W. (2009). Hypomagnesemia induced by several proton-pump inhibitors. *Annals of Internal Medicine, 151*, 755–756. https://doi.org/10.7326/0003-4819-151-10-200911170-00016

Brunton, L., Hilal-dandan, R., & Knollman, B. (2018). *Goodman and Gilman's the pharmacological basis of therapeutics* (13th ed.). McGraw-Hill.

Chan, F. (2009). *Peptic ulcer disease, an issue of gastroenterology clinics*. W. B. Saunders.

Hall, J. E., & Hall, M. E. (2021). *Guyton and Hall textbook of medical physiology* (14th ed.). Elsevier.

Khalli, H., Huang, E., Jacobson, B., Camargo, C. A., Feskanich, D., & Chan, A. T. (2012). Proton pump inhibitors and risk of hip fracture in relation to dietary and life style factors: A prospective cohort study. *British Medical Journal, 344*, e372. https://doi.org/10.1136/bmj.e372

Lam, J., Schneider, J., Zhao, W., & Corley, D. A. (2013). Proton pump inhibitor and histamine 2 receptor antagonist use and vitamin B_{12} deficiency. *Journal of the American Medical Association, 310*(16), 1765–1774. https://doi.org/10.1001/jama.2013.280490

Norris, T. L. (2019). *Porth's pathophysiology concepts of altered health states* (13th ed.). Wolters Kluwer.

Novotny, M., Klimova, B., & Valis, M. (2019). PPI long term use: Risk of neurological adverse events. *Frontiers in Neuology, 9*, 1142. https://doi.org/10.3389/fneur.2018.01142

O'Keefe, S. J. D., Buchman, A. L., Fishbein, T. M., Jeejeebhoy, K. N., Jeppesen, P. B., & Shaffer, J. (2006). Short bowel syndrome and intestinal failure: Consensus definitions and overview. *Clinical Gastroenterology and Hepatology, 4*(1), 6–10. https://doi.org/10.1016/j.cgh.2005.10.002

Trujillo, S., Desai, A., Dalal, S., & Sandhu, D. (2020). Proton pump inhibitor therapy and risk of *Clostridium difficile* infection (CDI): A nationwide cohort study. *The American Journal of Gastroenterology, 115*(S68). https://doi.org/10.14309/01.ajg.0000702976.57255.60

Voelker, R. (2010). Proton pump inhibitors linked to fracture risk. *Journal of the American Medical Association, 304*(1), 29. https://doi.org/10.1001/jama.2010.862

Yu-Xiao, Y., Lewis, S. D., Epstein, S., & Metz, D. C. (2007). Long term proton pump inhibitor therapy and risk of hip fracture. *Journal of the American Medical Association, 296*, 2947–2953. https://doi.org/10.1001/jama.296.24.2947

CHAPTER 58

Drugs Affecting Gastrointestinal Motility

Learning Objectives

Upon completion of this chapter, you will be able to:

1. Describe the underlying processes in diarrhea and constipation and correlate them with the types of drugs used to treat these conditions.
2. Discuss the use of laxatives and antidiarrheal agents across the lifespan.
3. Describe the therapeutic actions, indications, pharmacokinetics, contraindications and cautions, most common adverse effects, and important drug–drug interactions associated with laxatives and antidiarrheal drugs.
4. Compare and contrast the prototype laxatives and antidiarrheals with other agents in their class and with other classes of laxatives and antidiarrheals.
5. Outline the nursing considerations, including important teaching points, for patients receiving laxatives and antidiarrheal agents.

Key Terms

antidiarrheal: drug that blocks the stimulation of the gastrointestinal (GI) tract, leading to decreased activity and increased time for absorption of needed nutrients and water

bulk-forming laxatives: agent that increases in bulk, frequently by osmotic pull of fluid into the feces; the increased bulk stretches the GI wall, causing stimulation and increased GI movement

cathartic dependence: overuse of laxatives that can lead to the need for strong stimuli to initiate movement in the intestines; local reflexes become resistant to normal stimuli after prolonged use of harsher stimulants, leading to further laxative use

chemical stimulant: agent that stimulates the normal GI reflexes by chemically irritating the lining of the GI wall, leading to increased activity in the GI tract

constipation: slower-than-normal evacuation of the large intestine, which can result in increased water absorption from the feces and can lead to impaction

diarrhea: more-frequent-than-normal bowel movements, often characterized as fluid-like and watery because not enough time for absorption is allowed during the passage of food through the intestines

lubricant: agent that increases the viscosity of the feces, making it difficult to absorb water from the bolus and easing movement of the bolus through the intestines

Drug List

LAXATIVES

Chemical Stimulants
bisacodyl
castor oil
(P) senna

Bulk-Forming Laxatives
methylcellulose
polycarbophil
(P) psyllium

Osmotic Laxatives
lactitol
lactulose
(P) magnesium citrate
magnesium hydroxide
magnesium sulfate
polyethylene glycol
polyethylene glycol electrolyte solution
sodium picosulfate with magnesium oxide

Lubricants
(P) docusate
glycerin
mineral oil

Opioid Antagonists
alvimopan
(P) methylnaltrexone bromide
naloxegol
naldemedine

Gastrointestinal Stimulants
(P) metoclopramide

ANTIDIARRHEALS
bismuth subsalicylate
crofelemer
(P) loperamide
opium derivatives

OTHER MOTILITY DRUGS
(P) alosetron
eluxadoline
linaclotide
lubiprostone
plecanatide
prucalopride
tegaserod

Drugs used to affect the motor activity or motility of the gastrointestinal (GI) tract can do so in several different ways. They can be used to speed up or improve the movement of intestinal contents along the GI tract when movement becomes too slow or sluggish to allow for proper excretion of wastes, as in **constipation**. Drugs are also used to increase the tone of the GI tract and to stimulate motility throughout the system. They can also be used to decrease movement along the GI tract when rapid movement decreases the time for the absorption of nutrients, leading to a loss of water and nutrients and the discomfort of **diarrhea**. This chapter addresses categories of medications that affect GI motility. See Figure 58.1 for sites of action of these drugs on GI motility. Box 58.1 highlights important considerations related to laxatives and other drugs affecting GI motility based on the patient's age.

Laxatives

Laxative, or cathartic, drugs (Table 58.1) are indicated for the short-term relief of constipation, to prevent straining when it is clinically undesirable (such as after surgery, myocardial infarction [MI], or obstetrical delivery) to evacuate the bowel for diagnostic procedures, to remove ingested poisons from the lower GI tract, and as an adjunct in anthelmintic therapy when it is desirable to flush helminths from the GI tract (see Fig. 58.1). Most laxatives are available in over-the-counter (OTC) preparations, and they have the potential for overuse so that people become dependent on them for stimulation of GI movement. Such people may develop chronic intestinal disorders as a result. Measures such as instituting proper diet and exercise, adequate fluid intake, and taking advantage of the actions of the intestinal reflexes can decrease the need for laxatives in many situations.

Kinds of laxatives include stimulants (which chemically irritate the lining of the GI tract), bulk-forming agents (which cause fecal matter to increase in bulk), osmotic laxatives (which pull more solute and/or water into the GI tract), and lubricants (which help the intestinal contents stay softer and more slippery). Newer laxatives are available for specific needs and alter sodium absorption or affect opioid receptors in the GI tract.

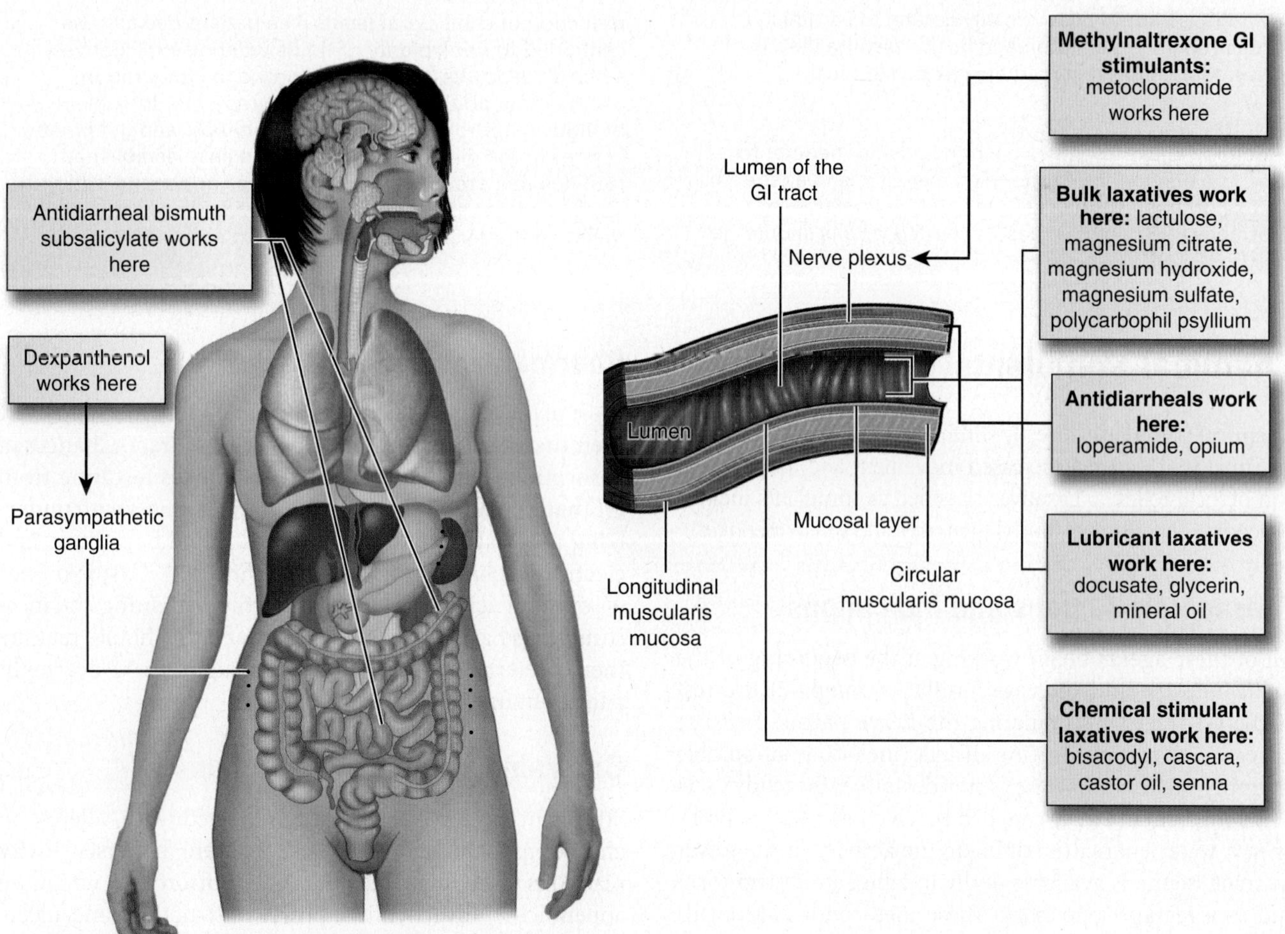

FIGURE 58.1 Sites of action of drugs affecting gastrointestinal motility.

Box 58.1 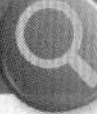 **Focus on Drug Therapy Across the Lifespan**

LAXATIVES AND ANTIDIARRHEAL AGENTS

Children

Laxatives should not be used routinely in children. Proper diet including dietary fiber and plenty of fluids, timed toileting, and exercise should be tried first if a child has a tendency to become constipated. If a laxative is needed, glycerin suppositories are the best choice for infants and young children. Lubricants can be used in older children; harsh stimulants should be avoided. Children with encopresis, however, are often given senna preparations or mineral oil to help them to evacuate the massive stool.

Children receiving these agents should use them for only a short period and should be evaluated for potential underlying medical or nutritional problems if they are not able to return to normal function.

Loperamide may be the antidiarrheal of choice in children older than 2 years of age if such a drug is needed. Special precautions need to be taken to monitor for electrolyte and fluid disturbances and supportive measures taken as needed. Bismuth subsalicylate should not be administered to febrile children or teenagers due to risk of Reye's syndrome. Reye's syndrome is a rare but serious condition that can occur in children recovering from a viral infection who have taken aspirin or other salicylates. It can cause confusion, swelling in the brain, and liver damage.

Many of these medications are available OTC. Guardians should be especially careful to administer proper dosing to children and not to assume that the dosing for children and adults will be identical.

Adults

Adults who use laxatives need to be cautioned not to become dependent. Proper diet, exercise, and adequate intake of fluids should keep the GI tract functioning normally. If an antidiarrheal is needed, adults should be carefully instructed in the proper dosing of the drug and monitoring of their total use to avoid excessive dose.

The safety of using many of these drugs during pregnancy and lactation has not been established. Use should be reserved for those situations in which the benefit to the patient outweighs the potential risk to the fetus. A stool softener is often used after delivery. The drugs may enter human milk and also may affect GI activity in the neonate. It is advised that caution be used if one of these drugs is prescribed during lactation.

Older Adults

Older adults are more likely to develop adverse effects associated with the use of these drugs, including sedation, confusion, dizziness, electrolyte disturbances, fluid imbalance, and cardiovascular effects. Safety measures may be needed if these effects occur and interfere with the patient's mobility and balance.

Older patients may also be taking other drugs that are associated with constipation and may need help to prevent severe problems from developing.

Older adults are more likely to have renal and/or hepatic impairment related to underlying medical conditions, which could interfere with the metabolism and excretion of the antidiarrheal drugs. The dose for patients with renal and/or hepatic impairment may require adjustment.

A psyllium product is often the agent of choice with older adults because there may be potential benefit of reduction of cholesterol levels. The patient needs to be cautioned to drink plenty of fluids when using laxatives, since older adults can be more prone to dehydration.

The older adult should be encouraged to drink plenty of fluids if appropriate, exercise every day, and get plenty of fiber in the diet. Many older adults have established routines that are disrupted with illness or hospitalization. These patients should be encouraged and helped to try to maintain their usual protocol as much as possible.

Chemical Stimulants

Chemical stimulants directly stimulate the nerve plexus in the intestinal wall, causing increased movement and the stimulation of local reflexes. Laxatives classified as stimulants include bisacodyl (*Dulcolax*), castor oil (generic), and senna (*Senokot*).

Therapeutic Actions and Indications

All of these agents begin working at the beginning of the small intestine and increase motility throughout the rest of the GI tract by stimulating the nerve plexus. Because castor oil blocks absorption of fats (including fat-soluble vitamins), its frequent use is not desirable. Bisacodyl acts in a similar manner. It can also be given as a suppository or in a water enema to stimulate the activity in the lower GI tract. Senna is available orally in tablet and syrup form and as a rectal suppository. These medications are available as OTC preparations. There are warnings about taking these medications for longer than a week without discussion with one's health care provider.

Pharmacokinetics

Most of these agents are only minimally absorbed and exert their therapeutic effects directly in the GI tract. Changes in absorption, water balance, and electrolytes resulting from GI changes can have adverse effects on patients with underlying medical conditions that are affected by volume and electrolyte changes (see "Adverse Effects"). Castor oil has an onset of action of 2 to 6 hours; the remaining chemical stimulants have an onset of action of 6 to 8 hours, making them preferable if one wants the drug to work overnight and result in effects in the morning.

Contraindications and Cautions

Stimulant laxatives are contraindicated with allergy to any component of the drug to prevent hypersensitivity reactions and in acute abdominal disorders, including appendicitis, diverticulitis, bowel obstruction, and ulcerative colitis, when increased motility could lead to rupture or further exacerbation of the inflammation. Laxatives should be used with caution in heart block, coronary artery

Table 58.1 *Drugs in Focus:* Laxatives

Drug Name	Usual Dosage	Usual Indications
Chemical Stimulants		
bisacodyl (*Dulcolax*)	5–15 mg PO or 2.5 g in water via enema	Emptying of the GI tract before some surgeries or diagnostic tests (e.g., barium enema); prevention of constipation and straining after GI surgery, MI, and obstetrical delivery; short-term treatment of constipation
castor oil (generic)	15–30 mL PO	Emptying of the GI tract for diagnostic testing, short-term treatment of constipation
senna (*Senokot*)	One to eight tablets per day at bedtime or 10–30 mL of syrup	Short-term treatment of constipation, treatment of encopresis, found in many OTC preparations
Bulk-Forming Laxatives		
methylcellulose (*Citrucel*)	2–6 g/d taken with full glass of water	Treatment of constipation
polycarbophil (*FiberCon*)	1 g PO, one to four times per day as needed; do not exceed 6 g/d for adults or 3 g/d for children	Treatment of constipation
psyllium (*Metamucil*)	1 tsp or packet in cold water, one to three times per day; 1/2 packet for children; also available in capsule form	Treatment of constipation; may lower blood cholesterol in combination with exercise and a diet low in saturated fat
Osmotic Laxatives		
lactitol (*Pizensy*)	10–20 g PO daily with a meal	Treatment of chronic idiopathic constipation
lactulose (*Constilac*)	15–30 mL PO	Short-term treatment of constipation, alternative choice for patients with cardiovascular disorders
magnesium citrate (*Citrate of Magnesia*)	One glassful, 1/2 glass for pediatric patients	Stimulates bowel evacuation before GI diagnostic tests and examinations
magnesium hydroxide (*Milk of Magnesia*)	15–30 mL PO	Short-term treatment of constipation, prevention of straining after GI surgery, obstetrical delivery, MI
magnesium sulfate (*Epsom* salts)	5–10 mL PO; 2.5–5 mL for pediatric patients, rake with full glass of water	Very potent laxative used for total, rapid evacuation of the GI tract (e.g., for treatment of GI poisoning)
polyethylene glycol (*MiraLAX*)	17 g PO in 8 oz water daily, for up to 2 wk	Short-term treatment of constipation (mild laxative)
polyethylene glycol electrolyte solution (*GoLYTELY* and others)	4 L of oral solution at a rate of 240 mL every 10 min	Stimulates bowel evacuation prior to GI examination (e.g., colonoscopy, sigmoidoscopy)
sodium picosulfate/magnesium oxide/anhydrous citric acid (*Clenpiq*)	2 doses PO; one the evening before and one the day of the procedure	Stimulates bowel evacuation prior to colonoscopy
Lubricants		
docusate (*Colace* and others)	50–300 mg PO	Prophylaxis for patients who should not strain (such as after surgery, MI, or obstetrical delivery); short-term treatment of constipation
glycerin (*Sani-Supp*)	4 mL of liquid suppository	Short-term treatment of constipation
mineral oil (*Agoral Liquid*)	5–45 mL PO	Short-term treatment of constipation
Opioid Antagonists		
alvimopan (*Entereg*)	12 mg PO administered 30 min to 5 h prior to surgery followed by 12 mg PO twice daily beginning the day after surgery until discharge for a maximum of 7 d; max is 15 total doses	Speeds gastrointestinal recovery following surgeries that include partial bowel resection with primary anastomosis

(continues on page 1042)

Table 58.1 *Drugs in Focus:* Laxatives *(Continued)*

Drug Name	Usual Dosage	Usual Indications
methylnaltrexone bromide (*Relistor*)	450 mg PO once daily in the morning; 8–12 mg subcutaneously once daily or every other day; reduce dose with renal and/or hepatic impairment	Treatment of opioid-induced constipation in adults with chronic noncancer pain
naloxegol (*Movantik*)	12.5 or 25 mg PO daily	Treatment of opioid-induced constipation in adults with chronic noncancer pain
naldemedine (*Symproic*)	0.2 mg PO daily	Treatment of opioid-induced constipation in adult patients with chronic noncancer pain

GI, gastrointestinal; MI, myocardial infarction; OTC, over the counter.

disease (CAD), or debilitation, which could be affected by the decrease in absorption and changes in electrolyte levels that can occur. Caution with use is encouraged if patient is experiencing acute abdominal pain, nausea, or vomiting, and patients are recommended to discuss with their health care provider prior to use. Patients who are pregnant or breast or chestfeeding should discuss with their health care provider prior to taking these medications.

Castor oil should not be used during pregnancy because its irritant effect has been associated with induction of premature labor.

Adverse Effects

The adverse effects most commonly associated with chemical stimulant laxatives are GI effects such as diarrhea, abdominal cramping, and nausea. Central nervous system (CNS) effects, including dizziness, headache, and weakness, are not uncommon and may relate to loss of fluid and electrolyte imbalances that may accompany laxative use. Sweating, palpitations, flushing, and even fainting have been reported after laxative use. These effects may be related to a sympathetic stress reaction to intense neurostimulation of the GI tract or to the loss of fluid and electrolyte imbalance.

An adverse effect that is seen with frequent laxative use or laxative abuse is **cathartic dependence**. This reaction occurs when patients use laxatives over a long period of time and the GI tract becomes dependent on vigorous stimulation of the laxative. Without this stimulation, the GI tract does not move for a period of time (i.e., several days), which could lead to constipation, drying of the stool, and ultimately impaction.

Castor oil blocks absorption of fats (including fat-soluble vitamins) and may lead to malnutrition if used chronically.

Clinically Important Drug–Drug Interactions

Because laxatives increase the motility of the GI tract and some interfere with the timing or process of absorption, it is advisable to not take laxatives with other prescribed medications.

Prototype Summary: Senna

Indications: Short-term treatment of constipation; treatment of encopresis.

Actions: Directly stimulates the nerve plexus in the intestinal wall, causing increased movement and the stimulation of local reflexes.

Pharmacokinetics: Mostly not absorbed.

$T_{1/2}$: Mostly not absorbed.

Adverse Effects: Diarrhea, abdominal cramps, perianal irritation, dizziness, cathartic dependence.

Bulk-Forming Laxatives

Bulk-forming laxatives cause the fecal matter to increase in bulk. They increase the motility of the GI tract by increasing the size of fecal matter, which helps to pull more fluid in the intestinal contents. This will stimulate local stretch receptors and activate local activity. Available bulk-forming laxatives include methylcellulose (*Citrucel*), polycarbophil (*FiberCon*), and psyllium (*Metamucil*).

Therapeutic Actions and Indications

Bulk-forming laxatives act in a manner similar to dietary fiber. Due to their action on fecal matter, they can be used to decrease diarrhea in patients with diverticulosis or irritable bowel syndrome (IBS) and modulate stool discharge for patients with ileostomy or colostomy. Patients should be instructed to take these with at least 8 ounces of water or other hydrating fluid.

Methylcellulose is a wheat starch bulk-forming fiber that can increase the size of fecal material in the GI tract.

Polycarbophil is a natural substance that forms a gelatin-like bulk out of the intestinal contents. This agent stimulates local activity. It is considered milder and less irritating than many other bulk stimulants.

Psyllium, another gelatin-like bulk stimulant, is similar to polycarbophil in action and effect.

See Table 58.1 for usual indications for each of these agents.

Pharmacokinetics

These drugs are all taken orally. They are directly effective within the GI tract and are not generally absorbed systemically. They can act rapidly, causing effects as they pass through the GI tract. However, some people may not have relief of constipation for a few days with these agents.

Contraindications and Cautions

Bulk-forming laxatives are contraindicated with allergy to any component of the drug to prevent hypersensitivity reactions and in acute abdominal disorders, including appendicitis, or with acute infections, when increased motility could lead to rupture or further exacerbation of the inflammation. These medications should not be taken by patients who have intestinal obstruction, perforation, rectal bleeding, or healing from acute abdominal surgery.

Adverse Effects

The adverse effects most commonly associated with bulk-forming laxatives are GI effects such as diarrhea, abdominal cramping, and nausea (Fig. 58.2). CNS effects, including dizziness, headache, and weakness, may occur due to loss of fluid and electrolyte imbalances that may accompany laxative use. Sweating, palpitations, flushing, and even fainting have been reported after laxative use. These effects may be related to a sympathetic stress reaction to intense neurostimulation of the GI tract or to the loss of fluid and electrolyte imbalance. Patients must use caution and take bulk-forming laxatives with plenty of water (at least 8 oz) to improve effectiveness of the medication and decrease risk of fluid and electrolyte imbalances. If taken with inadequate fluid, bulk-forming laxatives can consolidate in the GI tract, worsening constipation.

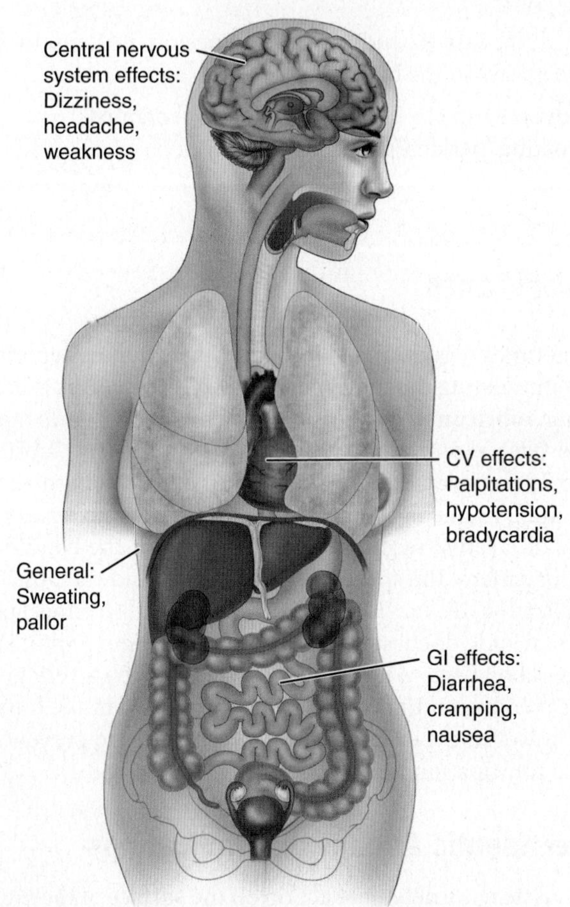

FIGURE 58.2 Variety of adverse effects and toxicities associated with drugs affecting gastric motility.

Clinically Important Drug–Drug Interactions

Bulk-forming laxatives modulate the motility of the GI tract, and some interfere with the timing or process of absorption. It is advisable to not take laxatives with other prescribed medications. It is recommended that the administration of bulk-forming laxatives and other medications be separated by 2 hours.

Prototype Summary: Psyllium

Indications: Short-term relief of occasional constipation; may lower blood cholesterol in combination with exercise and diet low in saturated fat.

Actions: Increases the motility of the GI tract by increasing the bulk of the intestinal contents, which pulls more fluid, stimulates local stretch receptors, and activates local activity.

Pharmacokinetics: Not absorbed systemically.

$T_{1/2}$: Not absorbed systemically.

Adverse Effects: Diarrhea, abdominal cramps, bloating, perianal irritation, dizziness.

Osmotic Laxatives

Osmotic laxatives are medications that have solutes that increase osmotic pull of fluid into the GI tract. This will increase the pressure in the GI tract and stimulate more intestinal motility. The following agents are osmotic laxatives: magnesium sulfate (*Epsom salts*), magnesium citrate (*Citrate of Magnesia*), magnesium hydroxide (*Milk of Magnesia*), lactulose (*Constilac, Cholac*), lactitol (*Pizensy*), polyethylene glycol (*MiraLAX*), polyethylene glycol electrolyte solution (*GoLYTELY*), and sodium picosulfate with magnesium oxide and citric acid (*Clenpiq*).

Therapeutic Actions and Indications

These laxatives draw more water into the GI tract and stimulate increased GI motility.

Lactulose is a saltless osmotic laxative that pulls fluid out of the venous system and into the lumen of the small intestine.

Magnesium citrate works by a saline pull, bringing fluids into the lumen of the GI tract.

Magnesium hydroxide also works by a saline pull, bringing fluids into the lumen of the GI tract.

Magnesium sulfate acts by exerting a hypertonic pull against the mucosal wall, drawing fluid into the intestinal contents.

Polyethylene glycol and polyethylene glycol electrolyte solution are hypertonic fluids containing many electrolytes that pull fluid out of the intestinal wall to increase the bulk of the intestinal contents.

Sodium picosulfate with magnesium oxide provides a combination stimulant laxative with a bulk-forming laxative. It is used to cleanse the colon in adults before colonoscopy procedures.

Pharmacokinetics

These medications can be administered in several ways. Some have both oral and suppository formulations. Others are oral and IV preparations. The IV preparations are not used to treat constipation. The rates of action will vary based on formulation and route of administration.

Contraindications and Cautions

Laxatives are contraindicated in patients with acute surgical abdomen, fecal impaction, or intestinal obstruction. Lactulose is a disaccharide and so should be used with caution in patients with diabetes. It is also contraindicated in patients who have appendicitis.

The substances with magnesium are absorbed systemically. Magnesium is cleared easily via the renal system, but caution is indicated for patients with renal insufficiency.

Polyethylene glycol electrolyte solution should be used with caution in any patient with a history of seizures because of the risk of electrolyte wasting causing neuronal instability and precipitating seizures.

Adverse Effects

The adverse effects most commonly associated with osmotic laxatives are GI effects (diarrhea, abdominal cramping, abdominal bloating, and nausea) and symptoms of dehydration (dry mouth, dizziness, light-headedness). CNS effects, including dizziness, headache, and weakness, are not uncommon and may relate to loss of fluid and electrolyte imbalances that may accompany laxative use. Sweating, palpitations, flushing, and even fainting have been reported after laxative use. These effects may be related to a sympathetic stress reaction to intense neurostimulation of the GI tract or to the loss of fluid and electrolyte imbalance. Medications that are given as suppositories may have the added adverse effect of rectal irritation.

Clinically Important Drug–Drug Interactions

Osmotic laxatives increase the motility of the GI tract, and some interfere with the timing or process of absorption. Some of the laxatives should not be taken at the same time as other medications. Administration instructions should be read carefully for each medication. Milk of magnesia has antacid properties and so may interfere with absorption of medications that require an acidic environment.

There is an increased risk of neuromuscular blockade when using nondepolarizing neuromuscular junction blockers with magnesium salts; if this combination is used, the patient must be closely monitored and appropriate life support provided.

Prototype Summary: Magnesium Citrate

Indications: Short-term relief of constipation; to prevent straining when it is clinically undesirable; to evacuate the bowel for diagnostic procedures; to remove ingested poisons from the lower GI tract; as an adjunct in anthelmintic therapy when it is desirable to flush helminths from the GI tract.

Actions: Increases the motility of the GI tract by increasing the fluid in the intestinal contents, which enlarges bulk, stimulates local stretch receptors, and activates local activity.

Pharmacokinetics: Onset 30 minutes to 4 hours, absorption varies with type of magnesium substance, highly bound to plasma proteins, excreted by kidneys and feces.

$T_{1/2}$: Not easy to study due to magnesium isotopes that are always in the body.

Adverse Effects: Diarrhea, abdominal cramps, bloating, perianal irritation, dizziness.

Lubricants

Sometimes it is desirable to make defecation easier without stimulating the movement of the GI tract. This is done using **lubricants**. Patients with hemorrhoids and those who have recently had rectal surgery may need lubrication of the stool. Some patients who could be harmed by straining might also benefit from this type of laxative. The type of laxative recommended depends on the condition of the patient, the speed of relief needed, and the possible implication of various adverse effects. Lubricating laxatives include docusate (*Colace*), glycerin (*Sani-Supp*), and mineral oil (*Agoral* liquid). Docusate has been a very popular medication to prescribe and administer in the hospital; however, the evidence of its effectiveness to prevent or treat constipation is not very strong (see Box 58.2).

Therapeutic Actions and Indications

Docusate has a detergent action on the surface of the intestinal bolus, increasing the admixture of fat and water and making a softer stool.

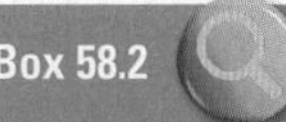

Box 58.2 Focus on the Evidence: Evidence Lacking for Efficacy of Docusate

Docusate has been prescribed for decades to prevent and treat constipation based on the thought that the medication would facilitate passage of bowel movements by softening the stool. However, in several randomized control trials performed from 1968 to 2013, docusate has not demonstrated effectiveness to improve frequency or quality of stool in comparison to placebo. Fakheri and Volpicelli (2019) describe the research that has been performed, and based on the evidence, recommend that docusate not be prescribed. They state that even if docusate is thought to be "benign" due to lack of significant side effects, the costs to the health care system are significant. Furthermore, prescribing medications that lack effectiveness have the risk of decreasing patient experience and quality of care.

Glycerin is a hyperosmolar laxative that is used in suppository form to gently evacuate the rectum without systemic effects higher in the GI tract.

Mineral oil is the oldest of these laxatives. It is not absorbed and forms a slippery coat on the contents of the intestinal tract. When the intestinal bolus is coated with mineral oil, less water is absorbed out of the bolus, and the bolus is less likely to become hard or impacted.

Pharmacokinetics

These drugs are not absorbed systemically and are excreted in the feces. Docusate and mineral oil are given orally. Glycerin is available as a rectal suppository or as a liquid for rectal retention.

Contraindications and Cautions

These laxatives are contraindicated with allergy to any component of the drug to prevent hypersensitivity reactions. A health care provider should be consulted prior to taking the laxative if the patient has any abdominal disorders, including nausea, vomiting, rectal bleeding, or abdominal pain. Caution should be used during pregnancy and lactation, and a health care provider should be consulted prior to use.

Adverse Effects

The adverse effects most commonly associated with lubricant laxatives are GI effects such as diarrhea, abdominal cramping, and nausea. In addition, leakage and staining may be a problem when mineral oil is used and the stool cannot be retained by the external sphincter. CNS effects, including dizziness, headache, and weakness, are uncommon and may relate to loss of fluid and electrolyte imbalances that may accompany laxative use. Sweating, palpitations, flushing, and even fainting have been reported after laxative use. These effects are less likely to happen with the lubricant laxatives than with the chemical or mechanical stimulants.

Clinically Important Drug–Drug Interactions

Frequent use of mineral oil can interfere with absorption of the fat-soluble vitamins A, D, E, and K.

Prototype Summary: Docusate

Indications: Prophylaxis for patients who should not strain (such as after surgery, MI, or obstetrical delivery); short-term treatment of constipation.

Actions: Forms a slippery coat on the contents of the intestinal tract; less water is absorbed out of the bolus, and the bolus is less likely to become hard or impacted.

Pharmacokinetics: Not absorbed systemically.

$T_{1/2}$: Not absorbed systemically.

Adverse Effects: Diarrhea; abdominal cramps; bloating; perianal irritation; dizziness; leakage of stool and staining.

Opioid Antagonists

Opioid antagonists may be used to relieve constipation in specific situations. The medications in this classification include alvimopan (*Entereg*), methylnaltrexone bromide (*Relistor*), naloxegol (*Movantik*), and naldemedine (*Symproic*) (see Table 58.1).

Therapeutic Actions and Indications

Methylnaltrexone bromide, naloxegol, and naldemedine are indicated for the treatment of opioid-induced constipation in adults with chronic noncancer pain whose pain medication is not being titrated frequently. Alvimopan has a very specific narrow therapeutic indication. It is used to hasten the time to gastrointestinal recovery following surgeries that include partial bowel resection with primary anastomosis. These medications are designed to block the effects of opioids on the GI tract by selectively binding to peripheral opioid receptors. Blocking the opioid effects on the GI tract can help to maintain normal motility and secretions while the patient is getting opioid treatment for pain.

Pharmacokinetics

All of the medications may be administered orally, but methylnaltrexone can also be administered subcutaneously. Peak levels when administered orally are reached in 0.75 to 2 hours. Peak level is seen in 30 minutes when methylnaltrexone is administered subcutaneously. Subcutaneous administration will also facilitate higher concentration of medication since it does not undergo the first-pass effect. All but alvimopan are metabolized in the liver; alvimopan is mostly changed to metabolites in the GI tract. The half-lives vary from 6 to 18 hours. They are eliminated partially by the kidneys and partially in the feces.

Contraindications and Cautions

The medications are contraindicated in patients with bowel obstruction due to risk of gastrointestinal perforation. More than 15 doses of alvimopan are contraindicated due to risk of MI. Caution should be taken in patients with hepatic and/or renal function in most of the medications due to increased risk of adverse effects. These medications are not generally recommended for patients who are pregnant or breast or chestfeeding due to risk of opioid withdrawal symptoms in the fetus or neonate.

Adverse Effects

Common adverse effects include abdominal pain, diarrhea, nausea, vomiting, dizziness, flatulence, and headache. Patients should be monitored for opioid withdrawal symptoms including chills, anxiety, irritability, and yawning. Patients who have severe abdominal pain and/or diarrhea may need reduced doses or discontinuation. Patients should be monitored for GI perforation if abdominal pain is severe.

Clinically Important Drug–Drug Interactions

These medications should not be used concurrently with other opioid antagonists due to increased risk of opioid withdrawal. Concurrent use of naloxegol and naldemedine with CYP3A inducers or CYP3A4 inhibitors is not recommended due to decreased and increased concentrations of the medications, respectively.

Prototype Summary: Methylnaltrexone Bromide

Indications: Treatment of opioid-induced constipation in adults with chronic noncancer pain.

Pharmacokinetics: Peak concentration is reached in about 1.5 hours when administered orally and in about 30 minutes when administered subcutaneously. It is metabolized in the liver. The subcutaneous dosing eliminates the first-pass effect of the mediation. It is excreted in urine and feces.

$T_{1/2}$: 15 hours

Adverse Effects: Abdominal pain, diarrhea, headache, abdominal distention, vomiting, hyperhidrosis, anxiety, muscle spasms, rhinorrhea, hot flush, tremor, flatulence, chills.

Nursing Considerations for Patients Receiving Laxatives

Assessment: History and Examination

- Assess for possible contraindications or cautions: history of allergy to laxatives to prevent hypersensitivity reaction; fecal impaction or intestinal obstruction, which could be exacerbated by increased GI activity; acute abdominal pain, nausea, or vomiting, which could represent an underlying medical condition; and current status of pregnancy or lactation, which could be contraindications or require cautious use.
- Perform a physical examination to establish baseline data before beginning therapy and during therapy to determine the effectiveness of the drug and to evaluate for any adverse effects.
- Inspect the skin for rash to monitor for adverse reactions.
- Assess the patient's neurological status, including level of orientation and affect, to evaluate any CNS effects of the drug.
- Obtain a baseline pulse rate to assess for any cardiovascular effects of the drug.
- Assess bowel elimination patterns, including the patient's perception of normal frequency, actual frequency, and stool characteristics, to determine the need for therapy.
- Investigate the patient's nutritional intake, including fluid intake and ingestion of fiber-containing foods, to evaluate for possible contributing factors related to the need for the drug.
- Assess the patient's level of activity to determine possible contributing factors for decreased bowel motility.
- Perform an abdominal examination, including inspecting the abdomen for distension, palpating for masses, and auscultating for bowel sounds, to establish adequate bowel function, rule out underlying medical conditions, and assess the effectiveness of the drug.
- Monitor results of laboratory tests including serum electrolyte levels to detect any changes related to increased excretion.

Nursing Conclusions

Nursing conclusions related to drug therapy may include the following:

- Impaired comfort related to CNS and GI effects
- Diarrhea risk related to drug effects
- Knowledge deficit regarding drug therapy

Planning

- The patient will receive the best therapeutic effect from the drug therapy.

- The patient will have limited adverse effects from the drug therapy.
- The patient will have an understanding of the drug therapy, adverse effects to anticipate, and measures to relieve discomfort and improve safety.

Intervention With Rationale

- Administer a laxative only as a temporary measure to prevent the development of cathartic dependence.
- Arrange for appropriate dietary measures, exercise, and environmental controls to encourage the return of normal bowel function.
- Administer the bulk-forming and osmotic laxatives with a full glass of water. Caution the patient not to chew tablets to ensure that the laxative reaches the GI tract to allow for therapeutic effects. Encourage fluid intake throughout the day as appropriate to maintain fluid balance and improve GI movement.
- Insert rectal suppositories high into the rectum; encourage patients to retain enemas or rectal solution as long as possible to improve effectiveness.
- Do not administer in the presence of acute abdominal pain, nausea, or vomiting, which might indicate a serious underlying medical problem that could be exacerbated by laxative use.
- Monitor bowel function to evaluate drug effectiveness. If diarrhea or cramping occurs, discontinue the drug to relieve discomfort and to prevent serious fluid and electrolyte imbalance.
- Provide comfort and safety measures to improve patient adherence and to ensure patient safety, including ready access to bathroom facilities, assistance with ambulation, and periodic orientation if CNS effects occur.
- Offer support and encouragement to help the patient deal with the discomfort of the condition and drug therapy.
- Offer support and encouragement to help the patient deal with the diagnosis and the drug regimen.
- Provide thorough patient teaching, including the drug name, dosage, and schedule for administration; method of administration, such as ensuring proper hydration, thoroughly mixing the powdered or granular form with water or juice to ensure complete dissolution, inserting the suppository form, or using and retaining an enema; approximate time for achievement of results and importance of having bathroom facilities readily available; safety measures, such as changing positions slowly and using assistance with ambulation if dizziness or weakness occurs; signs and symptoms of possible adverse effects and measures to minimize or prevent them; possible leakage and staining when mineral oil is used and the stool cannot be retained by the external sphincter; danger signs and symptoms to be reported to a health care provider immediately; the importance of daily activity to promote bowel function; the need for the ingestion of high-fiber foods and adequate fluids to stimulate GI motility; the importance of avoiding the overuse of laxatives to prevent chronic or long-term problems with elimination; a bowel training program if indicated to prevent dependence on laxatives; and importance of periodic monitoring and evaluation to evaluate the effectiveness of therapy, enhance patient knowledge about drug therapy, and promote adherence.

Evaluation

- Monitor patient response to the drug (relief of GI symptoms, absence of straining, evacuation of GI tract).
- Monitor for adverse effects (dizziness, confusion, GI alterations, sweating, electrolyte imbalance, cathartic dependence).
- Monitor the effectiveness of comfort measures and adherence to the regimen.
- Evaluate the effectiveness of the teaching plan (patient can name the drug and dosage and describe adverse effects to watch for and specific measures to use to avoid them).

Key Points

- Laxative drugs stimulate GI motility and assist in bowel elimination.
- Types of laxatives include chemical, bulk-forming, osmotic, lubricant, and opioid antagonist.
- In many cases, implementing diet and exercise strategies and promoting natural intestinal reflexes have decreased the need to use laxatives.
- Chronic use of laxatives can lead to dependence on them and on external stimuli for normal GI function.

Gastrointestinal Stimulants

Some drugs are available for more generalized GI stimulation that results in an overall increase in GI activity and secretions (Table 58.2). These drugs stimulate parasympathetic activity or make the GI tissues more sensitive to parasympathetic activity. Metoclopramide (*Reglan*) is a gastrointestinal stimulant.

Therapeutic Actions and Indications

By stimulating parasympathetic activity within the GI tract, metoclopramide increases GI secretions and motility on a

Table 58.2 *Drugs in Focus:* Gastrointestinal Stimulants

Drug Name	Usual Dosage	Usual Indications
metoclopramide (*Gimoti, Reglan*)	IM, IV, nasal spray, or PO. Doses vary based on formulation and patient age. Reduce dose with renal or hepatic impairment.	Relief of symptoms of gastroesophageal reflux disease, prevention of nausea and vomiting after emetogenic chemotherapy or postoperatively, relief of symptoms of diabetic gastroparesis, promotion of GI movement during small bowel intubation or promotion of rapid movement of barium

GI, gastrointestinal.

general level throughout the tract (see Fig. 58.1). It does not have the local effects of laxatives to increase activity only in the intestines. It is indicated when more rapid movement of GI contents is desirable. Metoclopramide works by blocking dopamine receptors and making the GI cells more sensitive to acetylcholine, which leads to increased GI activity and rapid movement of food through the upper GI tract. See Table 58.2 for usual indications for metoclopramide.

Pharmacokinetics

Metoclopramide is given orally, by IM injection, by nasal spray, or by intravenous (IV) infusion and has a peak effect by all routes in 60 to 90 minutes. It is metabolized in the liver and excreted in the feces and urine. Metoclopramide crosses the placenta and enters human milk.

Contraindications and Cautions

GI stimulants should not be used in patients with a history of allergy to any of these drugs to prevent hypersensitivity reactions or with any GI obstruction or perforation, which could be exacerbated by the GI stimulation. They should be used with caution during pregnancy or lactation and only if the benefit to the patient clearly outweighs the potential risk to the fetus or neonate. Caution should be used administering metoclopramide to patients with a history of tardive dyskinesia, seizures, or depression due to potential for development of these with medication use.

Adverse Effects

The most common adverse effects seen with GI stimulants include nausea, vomiting, diarrhea, intestinal spasm, and cramping. Other adverse effects, such as declining blood pressure and heart rate, weakness, and fatigue, may be related to parasympathetic stimulation, extrapyramidal effects, seizures, and Parkinson-like syndrome. Metoclopramide has a boxed warning regarding risk of causing tardive dyskinesia. The risk increases with longer duration and cumulative dosage.

Clinically Important Drug–Drug Interactions

Increased risk of sedation and seizures can occur if metoclopramide is combined with alcohol or other CNS sedative drugs. There is increased risk of tardive dyskinesia when used concurrently with antipsychotic medications. Concurrent use with MAO inhibitors increases risk of hypertension. Concurrent use with strong CYP2D6 inhibitors may increase plasma concentration of metoclopramide.

Prototype Summary: Metoclopramide

Indications: Relief of symptoms of gastroesophageal reflux disease, prevention of nausea and vomiting after emetogenic chemotherapy or postoperatively, relief of symptoms of diabetic gastroparesis, promotion of GI movement during small bowel intubation, promotion of rapid movement of barium.

Actions: Stimulates movement of the upper GI tract without stimulating gastric, pancreatic, or biliary secretions; appears to sensitize tissues to the effects of acetylcholine.

Pharmacokinetics:

Route	Onset	Peak	Duration
Oral	30–60 min	60–90 min	1–2 h
IM	10–15 min	60–90 min	1–2 h
IV	1–5 min	60–90 min	1–2 h

$T_{1/2}$: 5 to 6 hours; metabolized in the liver and excreted in the urine.

Adverse Effects: Restlessness, drowsiness, fatigue, extrapyramidal effects, Parkinson-like reactions, seizures, nausea, diarrhea.

Nursing Considerations for Patients Receiving Gastrointestinal Stimulants

Assessment: History and Examination

- Assess for possible contraindications or cautions: any history of allergy to these drugs to prevent hypersensitivity reactions; intestinal obstruction, bleeding, or perforation, which could be exacerbated by stimulating the GI tract; seizure disorder, due to increased risk of seizure activity, and current status of pregnancy or lactation, which require cautious use.

- Perform a physical examination to establish baseline data before beginning therapy and during therapy to determine the effectiveness of the drug and to evaluate any adverse effects.
- Perform an abdominal examination, including inspecting for distension, palpating for masses, and checking bowel sounds, to ensure adequate GI function and motility.
- Assess cardiopulmonary status, including pulse and blood pressure, to monitor for possible cardiovascular adverse effects.
- Inspect the skin for color and evidence of lesions or rash to assess for hypersensitivity reactions.

Nursing Conclusions

Nursing conclusions related to drug therapy may include the following:

- Diarrhea related to drug effects
- Impaired comfort related to GI effects
- Fall risk related to increased risk of seizures and tardive dyskinesia side effects
- Knowledge deficit regarding drug therapy

Planning

- The patient will receive the best therapeutic effect from the drug therapy.
- The patient will have limited adverse effects from the drug therapy.
- The patient will have an understanding of the drug therapy, adverse effects to anticipate, and measures to relieve discomfort and improve safety.

Intervention With Rationale

- Monitor blood pressure carefully if giving the drug IV to detect changes in blood pressure indicating the need to consult with the prescriber.
- Monitor for any extrapyramidal symptoms, seizures, or sedation to determine if the medication needs to be discontinued.
- Monitor diabetic patients, who will have increased speed of transit through the GI tract, which could alter absorption and glucose levels, to arrange for alteration in insulin dose or timing as appropriate.
- Offer support and encouragement to help the patient deal with the diagnosis and the drug regimen, including the discomfort of cramping and pain.
- Provide thorough patient teaching, including the drug name and prescribed dosage, measures to help avoid adverse effects, warning signs that may indicate problems, and the need for periodic monitoring and evaluation, to enhance patient knowledge about drug therapy and to promote adherence.
- Provide thorough patient teaching, including the drug name, prescribed dosage, and schedule for administration; method for oral administration; signs and symptoms of adverse effects and measures to minimize or prevent them; danger signs that need to be reported to the health care provider immediately; importance of avoiding alcohol or other CNS depressants; safety measures, such as avoiding driving and obtaining assistance with ambulation as needed; and the importance of periodic monitoring and evaluation to enhance patient knowledge about drug therapy and to promote adherence.

Evaluation

- Monitor patient response to the drug (increased tone and movement of GI tract).
- Monitor for adverse effects (GI effects, parasympathetic activity, tardive dyskinesia, seizures).
- Monitor the effectiveness of comfort measures and adherence to the regimen.
- Evaluate the effectiveness of the teaching plan (patient can name the drug and dosage, as well as describe adverse effects to watch for and specific measures to take to avoid them and to increase the effectiveness of the drug).

Key Points

- GI stimulants act to increase parasympathetic stimulation in the GI tract and to increase tone and general movement throughout the GI system.
- Patients receiving GI stimulants should be monitored for generalized increases in parasympathetic activity.

Antidiarrheals

Antidiarrheals block stimulation of the GI tract for symptomatic relief from diarrhea. Available agents include bismuth subsalicylate (*Pepto-Bismol*), crofelemer (*Mytesi*), loperamide (*Imodium A-D*), and opium derivatives (*Paregoric*). There are some anticholinergic medications that are indicated to decrease GI motility and/or secretions. Anticholinergic medications are discussed in Chapter 33. Several antidiarrheal products are available in combination (Box 58.3). There is also a drug approved strictly for use in treating traveler's diarrhea (Box 58.4).

Therapeutic Actions and Indications

Antidiarrheal agents slow the motility of the GI tract through direct action on the lining of the GI tract to inhibit local reflexes (bismuth subsalicylate), through direct action on the muscles of the GI tract to slow activity (loperamide), or through action on CNS centers that cause GI spasm and slowing (opium derivatives; see

BOX 58.3

Combination Antidiarrheal Products

Two popular antidiarrheal agents combine atropine with a meperidine-like compound. Meperidine (*Demerol*) has a local effect on the GI wall, causing a slowing of intestinal motility. Difenoxin and diphenoxylate are chemically related to meperidine and are used at doses that decrease GI activity without having analgesic or respiratory effects. These drugs, which are controlled substances—difenoxin is category C-IV and diphenoxylate is category C-V—are combined with atropine to discourage deliberate use of excessive doses to get the euphoric effects associated with meperidine.

Difenoxin with atropine (*Motofen*)	*Adult:* Two tablets PO, then one tablet after each loose stool; do not exceed eight tablets in 24 h *Pediatric:* Not recommended for use in children <12 y; contraindicated in children <2 y
Diphenoxylate with atropine (*Lomotil*)	*Adult:* 5 mg PO q.i.d. *Pediatric 2–12 y:* Use liquid form only, start with 0.3–0.4 mg/kg/d PO in four divided doses

BOX 58.4

Treating Traveler's Diarrhea: Rifamycin

Rifaximin (*Xifaxan*) was the first antibiotic approved by the U.S. Food and Drug Administration (FDA) specifically for treating traveler's diarrhea. Rifaximin acts locally in the GI tract against noninvasive strains of *Escherichia coli*, the most common cause of traveler's diarrhea. About 80% to 90% of the drug is delivered to the intestines without being absorbed through the GI tract.

Rifaximin acts locally in the GI tract to kill the *E. coli* that causes the signs and symptoms associated with traveler's diarrhea. The drug is taken in 200-mg tablets three times a day for 3 days once the signs and symptoms of the disorder occur. It should not be used if the patient has bloody diarrhea or if diarrhea persists more than 48 hours or worsens during treatment with the drug. Killing the causative organisms will relieve the GI symptoms of diarrhea, nausea, and anorexia. Prevention remains the best intervention for traveler's diarrhea.

Because of its local effect in the GI tract and impact on GI bacteria that produce ammonia, rifaximin has been found to be effective in reducing the risk of overt hepatic encephalopathy recurrence in patients 18 years and older with hepatic cirrhosis. Hepatic encephalopathy is associated with high ammonia levels. For this use, the drug is given orally twice a day.

Fig. 58.1). These drugs are indicated for the relief of symptoms of acute and chronic diarrhea, reduction of volume of discharge from ileostomies, and prevention and treatment of traveler's diarrhea (Table 58.3; see Box 58.4). Bismuth subsalicylate has been found to be helpful in treating diarrhea (see the "Critical Thinking Scenario" for additional information) and in treating GI symptoms associated with dietary excess and some viral infections. Crofelemer works in the inner lining of the GI tract to block specific chloride channels leading to less water loss as diarrhea and return to more balance between water and chloride and sodium in the cells. This drug is specifically for symptomatic relief of noninfectious diarrhea in adult patients on HIV/AIDS antiretroviral therapy.

Table 58.3 *Drugs in Focus:* Antidiarrheals

Drug Name	Usual Dosage	Usual Indications
bismuth subsalicylate (*Pepto-Bismol*)	*Adult and pediatric (12 y and older):* Two tablets or 30 mL (524 mg) PO q30–60 min as needed, up to eight doses per day *Pediatric (9–11 y):* One tablet or 15 mL PO *Pediatric (6–8 y):* 2/3 tablet or 10 mL PO *Pediatric (3–5 y):* 1/3 tablet or 5 mL PO	Treatment of diarrhea, treatment of GI distress associated with dietary excess and some viral infections
crofelemer (*Mytesi*)	*Adult:* One 125-mg tablet PO b.i.d.	Symptomatic relief of noninfectious diarrhea in adults on HIV/AIDS antiretroviral medication
loperamide (*Imodium A-D*)	*Adult:* 4 mg PO, then 2 mg PO after each loose stool *Pediatric (2–12 y and > 13 kg):* 1–2 mg PO t.i.d. *Pediatric (<2 y):* Not recommended	Short-term treatment of diarrhea associated with dietary problems, viral infections
opium derivatives (*Paregoric*)	*Adult:* 5–10 mL PO once to four times daily *Pediatric:* 0.25–0.5 mL/kg PO once to four times daily as needed	Short-term treatment of cramping and diarrhea

Pharmacokinetics

Bismuth subsalicylate is absorbed from the GI tract after oral administration, metabolized in the liver, and excreted in the urine. It crosses the placenta, but it is not known whether it enters human milk. Loperamide is slowly absorbed after oral administration, metabolized in the liver, and excreted in the urine and feces. It may cross the placenta and enter human milk. Opium derivative (*Paregoric*), a category C-III controlled substance, is readily absorbed after oral administration, metabolized in the liver, and excreted in the urine. It crosses the placenta and enters human milk. Crofelemer is minimally absorbed, and its half-life, metabolism, and excretion are unknown.

CRITICAL THINKING SCENARIO
Traveler's Diarrhea

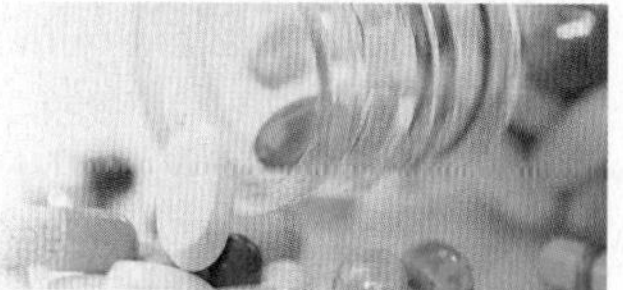

THE SITUATION

P.F. received an all-expenses-paid trip to Mexico to celebrate their graduation from college. P.F. was excited about getting away for a week of sun and fun and arranged to stay in the same hotel as two college friends who were also celebrating. The three friends had a wonderful time visiting the beaches, bars, and nightclubs in the area. On the 3rd day of the trip, P.F. began experiencing nausea, some vomiting, and a low-grade fever. Several hours later, P.F. began experiencing intense cramping and diarrhea. For the next 2 days, P.F. felt so ill they were unable to leave the hotel room. The next morning, they arranged for an emergency trip home.

CRITICAL THINKING

What is probably happening to P.F.? Think about the GI reflexes and explain the underlying cause for their signs and symptoms.

What treatment should be started now?

What could have been done to prevent this problem from occurring?

What possible drug therapy might have been helpful for P.F.?

DISCUSSION

P.F. is probably experiencing the common disorder called traveler's diarrhea. This disorder occurs when a person ingests pathogens found in the food and water of an environment foreign to that person. (Because these pathogens are commonly found in the environment, they do not normally cause problems for the people who live in the area.) When the pathogen, usually a strain of *E. coli*, enters a host who is not accustomed to the bacteria, it releases enterotoxins and sets off an intestinal–intestinal reaction in the host.

The intestinal–intestinal reaction results in a reduction of activity above the point of irritation (which causes nausea and, in some cases, vomiting) and an increase in activity below the point of irritation. The body is trying to flush the invader from the body. A low-grade fever may occur as a reaction to the toxins released by the bacteria. Muscle aches and pains, malaise, and fatigue are often common symptoms. It is important at this stage of the disease to maintain fluid intake to prevent dehydration from occurring.

P.F. may want to return home, but with intense cramping and diarrhea, it might not be a good idea. Bismuth subsalicylate (*Pepto-Bismol*) taken four times a day has been effective in preventing traveler's diarrhea and associated problems. It is available OTC and readily accessible for travelers. Taken during a course of traveler's diarrhea, it may relieve the stomach upset and nausea and some of the discomfort of the diarrhea. Some patients respond to the antibiotics *Bactrim* and *Septra*, combinations of trimethoprim and sulfamethoxazole that are often prescribed as prophylactic measures for patients who are traveling to areas known to be associated with traveler's diarrhea and for those who are known to be susceptible to the disorder. However, it is not recommended that people use antibiotic prophylaxis unless they are at very high risk because of the increasing development of resistant strains of bacteria. Once traveler's diarrhea is diagnosed, rifaximin (*Xifaxan*) or rifamycin (*Aemcolo*) could be prescribed. Antidiarrheals, like loperamide, have been used to help patients with traveler's diarrhea. The Centers for Disease Control and Prevention (CDC) has recommendations for both prevention and treatment of traveler's diarrhea.

The best course of action, however, is prevention. Several measures can be taken to avoid ingestion of the local bacteria including drinking only bottled or mineral water; avoiding fresh fruits and vegetables that may have been washed in the local water unless they are peeled; avoiding ice cubes in drinks because the ice cubes are made from the local water; avoiding any food that might be undercooked or rare, including shellfish; and even being cautious about using water to brush the teeth or gargle. People who have suffered a bout of traveler's diarrhea are cautious about exposure to local bacteria when they travel again; they often combine prophylactic drug therapy with careful avoidance of local pathogens.

(continues on page 1052)

P.F. can be reassured that in a few days, the diarrhea and associated signs and symptoms should pass, and they will regain their strength and energy.

NURSING CARE GUIDE FOR P.F.: ANTIDIARRHEALS

Assessment: History and Examination

Assess the patient's health history for allergies to any of these drugs, acute abdominal pain, concurrent use of medications that could interact with the antidiarrheal therapy.

Focus the physical examination on the following:

CNS: Orientation, reflexes

GI: Abdominal evaluation, bowel sounds

Respiratory: Respiratory rate and depth

Laboratory tests: Serum electrolyte levels

Other: Temperature

Nursing Conclusions

Nursing conclusions related to drug therapy may include the following:

Impaired comfort related to GI and CNS effects

Altered GI motility related to disease process and/or medication therapy

Knowledge deficit regarding drug therapy

Planning

The patient will receive the best therapeutic effect from the drug therapy.

The patient will have limited adverse effects from the drug therapy.

The patient will have an understanding of the drug therapy, adverse effects to anticipate, and measures to relieve discomfort and improve safety.

Intervention

Administer an antidiarrheal agent only as a temporary measure.

Provide comfort and safety measures, including assistance, access to bathroom, and safety precautions if necessary.

Monitor bowel function.

Provide support and reassurance for coping with drug effects and discomfort.

Provide patient teaching regarding drug name and dosage, adverse effects and precautions, and warning signs of serious adverse effects to report.

Evaluation

Evaluate drug effects: relief of GI symptoms.

Monitor for adverse effects: GI alterations, dizziness, confusion, and salicylate toxicity.

Monitor for drug–drug interactions as indicated.

Evaluate the effectiveness of patient teaching program and comfort and safety measures.

PATIENT TEACHING FOR P.F.

- The drug you are taking is called bismuth subsalicylate (*Pepto-Bismol*). This drug is an antidiarrheal agent. It forms a protective coating over the inner lining of the intestine and soothes the irritated areas.
- Take this drug exactly as indicated. Shake the bottle well before using the liquid preparation. If you are using tablets, make sure that you chew them thoroughly; do not swallow them whole.
- Common effects of this drug include the following:
  - *Darkening of the stools:* Do not become concerned; this is a normal effect that will go away when you stop taking the drug.
  - *Ringing in the ears and rapid respirations:* This is more likely to occur if you are taking other products that contain aspirin, which is also a salicylate.
- Report any of the following conditions to your health care provider: diarrhea that does not stop within 2 days, ringing in the ears, rapid respirations, fever, and/or intense abdominal pain.
- Stay away from any food or beverage that may be contaminated with bacteria. Use bottled water for drinking as well as for brushing your teeth. Do not wash fruit or vegetables with water from the local supply.
- Do not use any other medication that contains aspirin; inadvertent overdose may occur.
- Tell any doctor, nurse, or other health care provider involved in your care that you are taking this drug.
- Keep this drug and all medications out of the reach of children.

Contraindications and Cautions

Antidiarrheal drugs should not be given to anyone with known allergy to the drug or any of its components to prevent hypersensitivity reactions. Caution should be used in pregnancy and lactation because of the potential adverse effects to the fetus or baby. Care should also be taken in patients with any history of GI obstruction; with acute abdominal conditions, which could be exacerbated by the effects of the drugs, or diarrhea due to poisonings, which could be worsened by slowing of the GI tract, allowing increased time for absorption of the poison; or with hepatic impairment, which could alter the metabolism of the drugs.

Adverse Effects

The adverse effects associated with antidiarrheal drugs, such as constipation, distension, abdominal discomfort, nausea, vomiting, dry mouth, and even toxic megacolon, are related to their effects on the GI tract. Other adverse effects that have been reported include fatigue, weakness, dizziness, and skin rash. Opium derivatives are also associated with light-headedness, sedation, euphoria, hallucinations, and respiratory depression related to effect on the opioid receptors.

Clinically Important Drug–Drug Interactions

Drug interactions vary depending on the antidiarrheal agent. Consult the drug package insert for specific interactions.

Prototype Summary: Loperamide

Indications: Control and symptomatic relief of acute, nonspecific diarrhea and chronic diarrhea associated with IBS; reduction of volume of discharge from ileostomies.

Actions: Inhibits intestinal peristalsis through direct effects on the longitudinal and circular muscles of the intestinal wall, slowing motility and movement of water and electrolytes.

Pharmacokinetics:

Route	Onset	Peak
Oral (capsule)	Varies	5 h

$T_{1/2}$: 10.8 hours; metabolized in the liver and excreted in the urine and feces.

Adverse Effects: Abdominal pain, distension, or discomfort; dry mouth; nausea; constipation; dizziness; tiredness; drowsiness.

Nursing Considerations for Patients Receiving Antidiarrheals

Assessment: History and Examination

- Assess for possible contraindications or cautions: any history of allergy to these drugs to prevent hypersensitivity reactions; acute abdominal conditions, which could be exacerbated by these drugs; poisoning, which is a contraindication to slowing GI activity; hepatic impairment, which could alter the metabolism of the drug; and current status of pregnancy or lactation, which require cautious use.
- Perform a physical examination to establish baseline data before beginning therapy and during therapy to determine the effectiveness of the drug and to evaluate for any adverse effects.
- Inspect the skin for color and evidence of lesions or rash to monitor for potential hypersensitivity reactions.
- Perform an abdominal examination, including inspecting for distension, palpating for masses, and auscultating bowel sounds, to evaluate GI function and to rule out potential underlying medical conditions.
- Assess bowel elimination pattern, including frequency and characteristics of stool, to assist in determining appropriateness for drug therapy.
- Assess the patient's neurological status, including level of orientation and affect, to monitor for CNS effects of the drug.

Nursing Conclusions

Nursing conclusions related to drug therapy may include the following:

- Altered GI motility related to disease process or medication effects
- Impaired comfort related to GI effects
- Altered sensory perception (kinesthetic, gustatory) related to CNS effects
- Knowledge deficit regarding drug therapy

Planning

- The patient will receive the best therapeutic effect from the drug therapy.
- The patient will have limited adverse effects from the drug therapy.
- The patient will have an understanding of the drug therapy, adverse effects to anticipate, and measures to relieve discomfort and improve safety.

Intervention With Rationale

- Administer the drug as prescribed or recommended per the package insert to facilitate therapeutic effectiveness. Keep track of the exact amount given to ensure that the dose does not exceed the recommended daily maximum dose. If using crofelemer, the drug is taken twice a day to maintain effectiveness against diarrhea caused by antiretroviral medication.
- Monitor the response carefully; note the frequency and characteristics of the stool. If no response is seen within 48 hours, the diarrhea could be related to an underlying medical condition. Arrange to discontinue the drug and arrange for medical evaluation to allow for the diagnosis of underlying medical conditions.
- Provide appropriate safety and comfort measures if CNS effects occur to prevent patient injury.
- Offer support and encouragement to help the patient deal with the diagnosis and the drug regimen.
- Provide thorough patient teaching, including the drug name and prescribed dosage; schedule for administration; use of drug after each loose stool; recommended daily maximum dose and the need not to exceed it; signs and symptoms of adverse effects, including measures to minimize or prevent them; safety measures, such as avoiding driving and obtaining assistance with ambulation as needed to reduce the risk of injury due to weakness or dizziness; danger signs

(continues on page 1054)

and symptoms that need to be reported immediately; the importance of notifying the health care provider if diarrhea is not controlled within 48 hours; and the need for follow-up to enhance patient knowledge about drug therapy and to promote adherence.

Evaluation

- Monitor the patient response to the drug (relief of diarrhea).
- Monitor for adverse effects (GI effects, CNS changes, dermatological effects).
- Monitor the effectiveness of comfort and safety measures and adherence to the regimen.
- Evaluate the effectiveness of the teaching plan (patient can name the drug and dosage, as well as describe adverse effects to watch for, specific measures to use to avoid them, and measures to take to increase the effectiveness of the drug).

Key Points

- Antidiarrheal drugs are used to soothe irritation to the intestinal wall, block GI muscle activity to decrease movement, or affect CNS activity to cause GI spasm and stop movement.
- Antidiarrheal drugs can cause GI discomfort and constipation.

Irritable Bowel Syndrome and Chronic Constipation Drugs

IBS is a common disorder. It affects three times as many females as males and reportedly accounts for half of all referrals to GI specialists. The disorder is characterized by abdominal distress, bouts of diarrhea or constipation, bloating, nausea, flatulence, headache, fatigue, depression, and anxiety. No inflammatory cause has been found for this disorder. Underlying causes might be stress and/or dysregulation of the autonomic nervous system. Patients with this disorder have often suffered for years, not enjoying meals or activities because of their GI pain and discomfort. Medications that can be used to treat IBS symptoms include alosetron (*Lotronex*), eluxadoline (*Viberzi*), linaclotide (*Linzess*), lubiprostone (*Amitiza*), plecanatide (*Trulance*), and tegaserod (*Zelnorm*). Prucalopride (*Motegrity*) is indicated to treat chronic constipation. These medications are listed in Table 58.4. Hyoscyamine is an anticholinergic medication that has also been used for patients with IBS. This medication is discussed in Chapter 33.

Therapeutic Actions and Indications

Alosetron (*Lotronex*) is a serotonin 5-HT antagonist that blocks specific serotonin receptors in the enteric nervous system of the GI tract, which leads to decreased perception of abdominal pain and discomfort, decreased GI motility, and increased colon transit time. Eluxadoline (*Viberzi*)

Table 58.4 *Drugs in Focus:* Other Motility Drugs

Drug Name	Usual Dosage	Usual Indications
alosetron (*Lotronex*)	*Adult female:* 0.5 mg PO b.i.d. as initial dose; may be increased to 1 mg PO b.i.d. after 4 wk if well tolerated	Treatment of severe diarrhea-predominant IBS in patients who have chronic IBS symptoms (generally lasting 6 mo or longer), had anatomic or biochemical abnormalities of the gastrointestinal tract excluded, and did not respond adequately to conventional therapy
eluxadoline (*Viberzi*)	*Adult:* 100-mg tablet PO b.i.d.; reduce dose if not well tolerated or with hepatic/renal impairment	Treatment of IBS with diarrhea
linaclotide (*Linzess*)	*Adult:* 72–290 mcg PO daily 30 minutes before first meal of the day on an empty stomach	Treatment of IBS with constipation and CIC
lubiprostone (*Amitiza*)	*Adult (IBS):* 8 mcg PO b.i.d. *Adult (chronic or opioid-induced constipation)*: 24 mcg PO b.i.d.	Treatment of CIC; opioid-induced constipation in patients with chronic, noncancer pain; and IBS with constipation in females ≥18 y
plecanatide (*Trulance*)	*Adult:* 3 mg PO daily	Treatment of CIC and IBS with constipation
prucalopride (*Motegrity*)	*Adult:* 2 mg PO daily; reduce dose if severe renal impairment	Treatment of CIC
tegaserod (*Zelnorm*)	*Adult female:* 6 mg PO twice daily at least 30 min before meals	Treatment of adult females (<65 y) with IBS with constipation

IBS, irritable bowel syndrome; CIC, chronic idiopathic constipation.

is approved for the treatment of adults with IBS with diarrhea. It is a mu–opioid receptor agonist and a controlled substance (schedule IV). Lubiprostone (*Amitiza*) is a locally acting chloride channel activator that increases the secretion of a chloride-rich intestinal fluid without changing sodium or potassium levels. Increasing the intestinal fluid leads to increased motility. Lubiprostone (*Amitiza*) is approved for the treatment of chronic, idiopathic constipation; opioid-induced constipation; and IBS with constipation in adult females. Prucalopride (*Motegrity*) and tegaserod (*Zelnorm*) act as selective serotonin type 4 receptor agonists that can treat chronic constipation. Tegaserod is specifically indicated for females younger than 65 years of age who suffer from constipation due to IBS. Linaclotide (*Linzess*) and plecanatide (*Trulance*) are guanylate cyclase-C agonists that act in the intestines to increase the secretion of chloride and bicarbonate into the intestinal lumens. They are indicated to treat chronic constipation and constipation type IBS. See Table 58.3 for usual indications for each of these agents.

Pharmacokinetics

These medications are administered orally, and most are absorbed quickly. Linaclotide and plecanatide are only minimally absorbed. Their location and extent of metabolism varies. The half-lives range from 1.5 to 24 hours. Alosetron, prucalopride, and lubiprostone are primarily eliminated in urine; eluxadoline, linaclotide, and tegaserod are primarily eliminated in feces.

Contraindications and Cautions

These medications should not be used in patients with a history of allergy to any of these drugs to prevent hypersensitivity reactions. Medications that treat constipation should not be used in patients with mechanical gastrointestinal obstructions due to risk of perforation.

Alosetron has a boxed warning regarding risk of dangerous GI adverse reactions including constipation and ischemic colitis requiring hospitalization and surgical intervention, so medication should be discontinued if there are any sign of constipation.

Eluxadoline is contraindicated in patients without a gallbladder or with biliary duct obstruction, sphincter of Oddi disease, alcohol use of greater than 3 drinks/day, or history of pancreatitis due to increased risk of pancreatitis.

Lubiprostone and prucalopride are contraindicated with any GI obstruction or perforation, which could be exacerbated by the GI stimulation.

Linaclotide and plecanatide are only indicated for adult patients. They both have warnings based on causing death from dehydration in studies done with neonatal mice.

Tegaserod is contraindicated in patients who experience MI, stroke, transient ischemic attack, or angina during treatment. It is associated with increased cardiovascular risk. It is also contraindicated in patients with ischemic colitis or other forms of intestinal ischemia. Patients with severe renal or moderate to severe hepatic impairment should not use this medication. Patients should be monitored for any worsening of depression and/or emergence of suicidal thoughts or behaviors. If depression worsens, the medication should be discontinued.

The drugs should be used with caution during pregnancy or lactation and only if the benefit to the patient clearly outweighs the potential risk to the fetus or neonate. Lubiprostone may cause fetal harm based on animal studies.

Adverse Effects

The most common adverse effects include GI symptoms such as nausea, abdominal pain, diarrhea, or constipation. Alosetron has the rare but serious risk of causing ischemic colitis, so patients should be instructed to discontinue the medication and notify a provider if any constipation, severe abdominal pain, or bloody diarrhea occurs. There is risk of pancreatitis with eluxadoline. New onset of depression and self-harm behaviors have been associated with prucalopride and tegaserod.

Clinically Important Drug–Drug Interactions

Medications that slow GI motility can increase the risk of constipation if taken concurrently with alosetron or eluxadoline. Concurrent use of alosetron and CYP1A2 inhibitors can increase exposure to alosetron; use with fluvoxamine is contraindicated.

Prototype Summary: Alosetron

Indications: Treatment of severe diarrhea-predominant IBS in patients who have chronic IBS symptoms (generally lasting 6 months or longer), had anatomic or biochemical abnormalities of the gastrointestinal tract excluded, and did not respond adequately to conventional therapy.

Actions: Selective 5-HT3 receptor antagonist for receptors in the GI tract. By blocking these receptors, the medication is able to modulate pain and slow motility and GI secretions.

Pharmacokinetics:

Route	Onset	Peak	Duration
Oral	Unknown	60 min	Unknown

$T_{1/2}$: 1.5 hours; metabolized in the liver and excreted via the kidneys.

Adverse Effects: Constipation, abdominal discomfort and pain, nausea, ischemic colitis.

Nursing Considerations for Patients Receiving Medications for IBS

Assessment: History and Examination

- Assess for possible contraindications or cautions: any history of allergy to these drugs to prevent hypersensitivity reactions; intestinal obstruction, bleeding, or perforation, which could be exacerbated by stimulating the GI tract; and current status of pregnancy or lactation, which require cautious use.
- Perform a physical examination to establish baseline data before beginning therapy and during therapy to determine the effectiveness of the drug and to evaluate for any adverse effects.
- Perform an abdominal examination, including inspecting for distension, palpating for masses, and checking bowel sounds, to ensure adequate GI function and motility.
- Inspect the skin for color and evidence of lesions or rash to assess for hypersensitivity reactions.

Nursing Conclusions

Nursing conclusions related to drug therapy may include the following:

- Altered GI motility related to IBS and drug effects
- Impaired comfort related to GI effects
- Knowledge deficit regarding drug therapy

Planning

- The patient will receive the best therapeutic effect from the drug therapy.
- The patient will have limited adverse effects from the drug therapy.
- The patient will have an understanding of the drug therapy, adverse effects to anticipate, and measures to relieve discomfort and improve safety.

Intervention With Rationale

- Offer support and encouragement to help the patient deal with the diagnosis and the drug regimen, including the abdominal discomfort and altered GI motility.
- Provide thorough patient teaching, including the drug name and prescribed dosage, measures to help avoid adverse effects, warning signs that may indicate problems, and the need for periodic monitoring and evaluation, to enhance patient knowledge about drug therapy and to promote adherence.
- Provide thorough patient teaching, including the drug name, prescribed dosage, and schedule for administration; method for oral administration; signs and symptoms of adverse effects and measures to minimize or prevent them; danger signs that need to be reported to the health care provider immediately; importance of avoiding substances that can interact and/or increase adverse effects; and the importance of periodic monitoring and evaluation to enhance patient knowledge about drug therapy and to promote adherence.

Evaluation

- Monitor patient response to the drug (increased tone and movement of GI tract).
- Monitor for adverse effects (GI effects, parasympathetic activity, tardive dyskinesia, seizures).
- Monitor the effectiveness of comfort measures and adherence to the regimen.
- Evaluate the effectiveness of the teaching plan (patient can name the drug and dosage, as well as describe adverse effects to watch for and specific measures to take to avoid them and to increase the effectiveness of the drug).

Key Points

- IBS is a common disorder that can cause a variety of symptoms including abdominal distress, bouts of diarrhea or constipation, bloating, nausea, flatulence, headache, fatigue, depression, and anxiety.
- Alosetron and eluxadoline may be used to treat diarrhea associated with IBS. Lubiprostone can be prescribed to treat constipation related to IBS.

SUMMARY

- Laxatives are drugs used to stimulate motility of the GI tract and to aid bowel evacuation. They may be used to prevent or treat constipation.
- Laxatives can be chemical stimulants, which directly irritate the local nerve plexus; bulk-forming agents and osmotic stimulants, which increase the size of the food bolus or contents of the GI tract and stimulate stretch receptors in the wall of the intestine; lubricants, which facilitate movement of the bolus through the intestines; or opioid antagonists, which decrease constipation induced by opioid use.
- Using proper diet and exercise, as well as taking advantage of the actions of the intestinal reflexes, has eliminated the need for laxatives in many situations.
- Cathartic dependence can occur with the chronic use of laxatives, leading to a need for external stimuli for normal functioning of the GI tract.

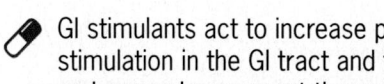

- GI stimulants act to increase parasympathetic stimulation in the GI tract and to increase tone and general movement throughout the GI system.
- Antidiarrheal drugs are used to soothe irritation to the intestinal wall, block GI muscle activity to decrease movement, or affect CNS activity to cause GI spasm and stop movement.
- Drugs used to treat IBS are specific for the main underlying complaint, either diarrhea or constipation, and patient selection must be carefully matched to the effect of the drug.

CHECK YOUR UNDERSTANDING

Answers to the questions in this chapter can be found in Answers to Check Your Understanding Questions on thePoint*.

MULTIPLE CHOICE

Select the best answer.

1. Laxatives are drugs that are used to increase the
   a. quantity of wastes excreted.
   b. speed of passage of the intestinal contents through the GI tract.
   c. digestion of intestinal contents.
   d. water content of the intestinal contents.

2. The laxative of choice when mild stimulation is needed to prevent straining is
   a. senna.
   b. castor oil.
   c. bisacodyl.
   d. magnesium citrate.

3. Cathartic dependence can occur when patients
   a. do not use laxatives routinely and experience severe bouts of constipation.
   b. engage in chronic laxative use leading to reliance on the intense stimulation of laxatives.
   c. maintain a nutritious high-fiber diet.
   d. start an exercise program to promote bowel elimination.

4. Which medication would best be used to treat nausea due to diabetic gastroparesis?
   a. Lubiprostone
   b. Bisacodyl
   c. Metoclopramide
   d. Loperamide

5. The drug of choice for treating and/or preventing traveler's diarrhea is
   a. loperamide.
   b. opium.
   c. rifaximin.
   d. bisacodyl.

MULTIPLE RESPONSE

Select all that apply.

1. A nurse is preparing a teaching plan for a patient who has been prescribed a laxative. The teaching plan should include which information?
   a. The importance of proper diet and fluid intake
   b. The need to take the drug for several weeks to get the full effect
   c. The importance of exercise
   d. The need to take advantage of natural reflexes by providing privacy and time to allow them to work
   e. The need to limit fluids
   f. The importance of limiting the duration of laxative use

2. A nurse might expect an order for mineral oil for which patients?
   a. A debilitated patient low on nutrients
   b. A patient with hemorrhoids
   c. A patient with recent rectal surgery
   d. A child with encopresis
   e. A postpartum patient
   f. A patient with Crohn's disease

3. When explaining the actions of laxatives to a patient, the nurse would state that they can work by
   a. acting as chemical stimulants.
   b. acting as lubricants of the intestinal bolus.
   c. acting to increase bulk of the intestinal bolus and stimulate movement.
   d. stimulating CNS centers in the medulla to cause GI movement.
   e. blocking the parasympathetic nervous system.
   f. causing CNS depression.

REFERENCES

Arcangelo, V. P., Peterson, A. M., Wilbur, V., & Reinhold, J. A. (2017). *Pharmacotherapeutics for advanced practice: A practical approach* (4th ed.). Wolters Kluwer.

Baker, D. E. (2007). Lubiprostone: A new drug for the treatment of idiopathic chronic constipation. *Reviews in Gastroenterological Disorders, 7*(4), 214–222. https://www.researchgate.net/publication/5658507

Brunton, L., Hilal-dandan, R., & Knollman, B. (2018). *Goodman and Gilman's the pharmacological basis of therapeutics* (13th ed.). McGraw-Hill.

Fakheri, R. J., & Volpicelli, F. M. (2019). Things we do for no reason: Prescribing docusate for constipation in hospitalized adults. *Journal of Hospitalized Medicine, 14*(2), 110–113. https://doi.org/10.12788/jhm.3124

Hall, J. E., & Hall, M. E. (2021). *Guyton and Hall textbook of medical physiology* (14th ed.). Elsevier.

Leung, L., Riutta, T., Kotecha, J., & Rosser, W. (2011). Chronic constipation: An evidence-based review. *Journal of the American Board of Family Medicine, 24*(4), 436–451. https://doi.org/10.3122/jabfm.2011.04.100272

Norris, T. L. (2019). *Porth's pathophysiology concepts of altered health states* (13th ed.). Wolters Kluwer.

Shah, S. B., & Hanauer, S. B. (2007). Treatment of diarrhea in patients with inflammatory bowel disease: Concepts and cautions. *Reviews in Gastroenterological Disorders, 7*(Suppl 3), S3–S10. http://medreviews.com/sites/default/files/2016-11/RIGD_7Suppl3_S3_0.pdf

Steffen, R., Hill, D., & DuPont, H. (2015). Travelers diarrhea: A clinical review. *Journal of the American Medical Association, 313*(1), 71–80. https://doi.org/10.1001/jama.2014.17006

Thomas, J., Karver, S., Cooney, G. A., Chamberlain, B. H, Watt, C. K., Slatkin, N. E., Stambler, N., Kremer, A. B., & Israel, R. J. (2008). Methylnaltrexone for opioid-induced constipation in advanced illness. *New England Journal of Medicine, 358*, 2332–2343. https://doi.org/10.1056/NEJMoa0707377

Tobias, N., Mason, D., Lutkenhoff, M., Stoops, M., & Ferguson, D. (2008). Management and principles of organic causes of childhood constipation. *Journal of Pediatric Health Care, 22*(1), 12–23. https://doi.org/10.1016/j.pedhc.2007.01.001

CHAPTER 59

Antiemetic Agents

Learning Objectives

Upon completion of this chapter, you will be able to:

1. Explain the vomiting reflex, including factors that stimulate it and mechanisms for measures used to block it.
2. Discuss the use of antiemetics across the lifespan.
3. Describe the therapeutic actions, indications, pharmacokinetics, contraindications and cautions, most common adverse effects, and important drug–drug interactions associated with each of the classes of antiemetic agents.
4. Compare and contrast the prototype antiemetics with other agents in their classes and with other classes of antiemetics.
5. Outline the nursing considerations, including important teaching points, for patients receiving antiemetics.

Key Terms

antiemetic: agent that blocks innervation of the vomiting center to decrease the symptoms of nausea and vomiting

emetic: agent used to induce vomiting to rid the stomach of toxins or drugs

intractable hiccough: repetitive stimulation of the diaphragm that leads to hiccough, a diaphragmatic spasm that persists over time

Drug List

ANTIEMETIC AGENTS

Phenothiazines
chlorpromazine
perphenazine
(P) prochlorperazine

Nonphenothiazine
(P) metoclopramide

5-HT_3 Receptor Blockers
dolasetron
granisetron
(P) ondansetron
palonosetron

Substance P/Neurokinin 1 Receptor Antagonist
(P) aprepitant
fosaprepitant dimeglumine
rolapitant

Miscellaneous Agents
dexamethasone
dimenhydrinate
dronabinol
hydroxyzine
meclizine
nabilone
scopolamine
trimethobenzamide

One of the more common and uncomfortable complaints encountered in clinical practice is that of nausea and vomiting. Vomiting is a complex reflex reaction to various stimuli (see Chapter 56). When nausea and vomiting are due to stimulation of the vestibular receptors in the inner ear, dizziness or vertigo often accompanies the feelings of nausea. In these situations, antihistamines (see Chapter 54) and anticholinergics (see Chapter 33) are often given for relief of symptoms. In some cases of overdose or poisoning, it may be desirable to induce vomiting to rapidly rid the body of a toxin. This can be accomplished by physical stimuli, often to the back of the throat. In some cases, gastric lavage is used to clear the contents of the stomach. **Emetics**, or drugs that block innervation of the vomiting center to decrease the symptoms of nausea and vomiting, are no longer recommended for at-home poison control (Box 59.1).

In many clinical conditions, the reflex reaction of vomiting is not beneficial in ridding the body of any toxins but is uncomfortable and even clinically hazardous to the patient's condition. In such cases, an antiemetic is used to decrease or prevent nausea and vomiting. Antiemetic agents can be centrally acting or locally acting, and they have varying degrees of effectiveness. See Figure 59.1 for sites of action of antiemetics. Box 59.2 highlights important considerations related to the use of antiemetics across the lifespan.

Box 59.1 Focus on the Evidence

RECOMMENDATIONS AFTER SUSPECTED OVERDOSE OR POISONING

In the past, emetics like ipecac syrup were recommended to ingest after suspected overdose or poison ingestion because it would induce vomiting. However, after the evidence was evaluated, these emetic substances were found to have more risk than benefit for the patient. The American Academy of Pediatrics, U.S. Food and Drug Administration, and the American Association of Poison Control Centers (AAPCC) recommend that experts be consulted in cases of overdose or poisoning. According to the 2019 annual report from the AAPCC, there is still a significant number of mortalities in the United States related to both unintentional and intentional overdoses or poison exposures. The AAPCC has over 50 centers that are staffed by expert health care professionals to answer questions and give recommendations to people calling due to suspected overdose or poisoning. They have also designed an interactive website (PoisonHelp.org) that can be accessed by computer or mobile device and can provide triage and recommendations to people concerned about harmful exposures.

Strategies to decrease risk of unintentional overdose include the following:

- Keep potential poisons/toxins and medications out of sight and out of reach of children.
- Always return any childproof caps to the locked position after they are used.
- Never transfer a substance to a different container; it is important to have the information on the original container in case of emergency.
- Safely dispose of all unused or no longer needed medication.
- Never refer to medications as candy or a treat.

Post the telephone number of the poison control center near the phone. If a local poison control center is not available, post 1-800-222-1222.

Antiemetic Agents

Drugs used in managing nausea and vomiting are called **antiemetics** (Table 59.1). All of them work by reducing the hyperactivity of the vomiting reflex in one of two ways: locally, to decrease the local response to stimuli that are being sent to the medulla to induce vomiting, or centrally, to block the chemoreceptor trigger zone (CTZ) or suppress the vomiting center directly. Locally acting antiemetics may be antacids, local anesthetics, adsorbents, protective drugs that coat the gastrointestinal (GI) mucosa, or drugs that prevent distention and stretch stimulation of the GI tract.

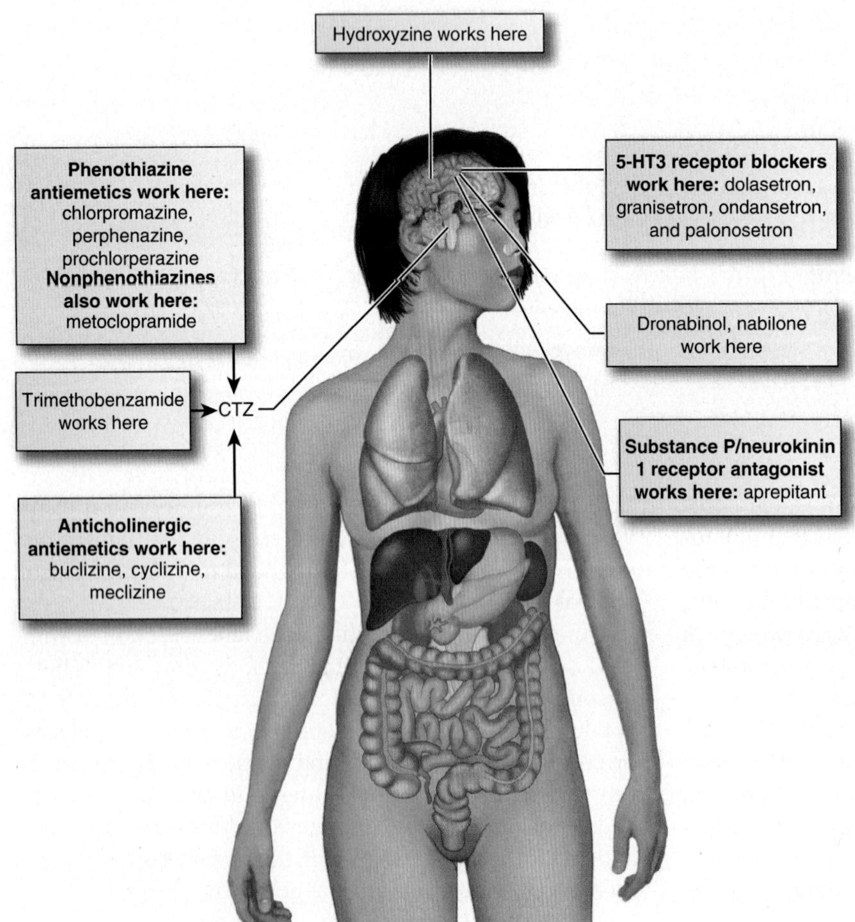

FIGURE 59.1 Sites of action of emetics/antiemetics. CTZ, chemoreceptor trigger zone.

Box 59.2 Focus on Drug Therapy Across the Lifespan

ANTIEMETIC AGENTS

Children

Parents should be taught to call a health care provider or a local poison control center if their children ingest potentially toxic substances. The professionals will advise them of the best treatment in each individual case.

Antiemetics should be used with caution in children who are at higher risk for adverse effects, including CNS effects and fluid and electrolyte disturbances. Targeting the trigger causing the nausea and vomiting may be the best treatment strategy in many instances. However, there are antiemetic medications indicated for children undergoing chemotherapy and/or suffering from nausea and vomiting due to anesthesia.

Adults

Antiemetics are often used after surgery or chemotherapy, and precautions should be used to ensure that CNS effects do not interfere with mobility or other activities.

The safety of these drugs during pregnancy and lactation has not been established. Use should be reserved for those situations in which the benefit to the patient outweighs the potential risk to the fetus. The drugs may enter human milk and also may cause fluid imbalance that could interfere with milk production. It is advised that caution be used if one of these drugs is prescribed during lactation.

Older Adults

Older adults are more likely to develop adverse effects associated with the use of these drugs, including sedation, confusion, dizziness, fluid imbalance, and CV effects. Safety measures may be needed if these effects occur and interfere with the patient's mobility and balance.

Older adults are also more likely to have renal and/or hepatic impairment related to underlying medical conditions, which could interfere with the metabolism and excretion of these drugs. The dose for older adults should be started at a lower level than that recommended for young adults. The patient should be monitored closely, and dose adjustment should be made based on patient response.

Table 59.1 ***Drugs in Focus:* Antiemetic Agents**

Drug Name	Usual Dosage	Usual Indications
Phenothiazines		
chlorpromazine (generic)	*Adult:* 10–25 mg PO q4–6h *or* 50–100 mg PR *or* 25 mg IM *Pediatric:* 0.5 mg/kg PO q4–6h, 1.1 mg/kg PR q6–8h *or* 0.5 mg/kg IM q6–8h	Treatment of nausea and vomiting, including that specifically associated with anesthesia; treatment of intractable hiccoughs; treatment of schizophrenia and other psychoses, mania, and hypomania; treatment of anxiety psychomotor agitation excitement and violent or dangerously impulsive behavior
perphenazine (generic)	8–16 mg/d PO in divided doses; 5–10 mg IM for rapid control; 5 mg IV in divided doses, slowly	Treatment of severe nausea and vomiting, intractable hiccoughs in patients >12 y; management of psychiatric symptoms
prochlorperazine (*Compro, Procomp*)	*Adult:* 5–10 mg PO t.i.d. to q.i.d.; 25 mg PR b.i.d.; 5–10 mg IM q3–4h, up to 40 mg/d; 5–10 mg IM 1–2 h before, during, or after anesthesia, may repeat in 30 min *Pediatric (9.1–13.2 kg):* 2.5 mg PO or PR daily to b.i.d., do not exceed 7.5 mg/d *Pediatric (13.6–17.7 kg):* 2.5 mg PO or PR b.i.d. to t.i.d., do not exceed 10 mg/d *Pediatric (18.2–38.6 kg):* 2.5 mg PO or PR t.i.d. to 5 mg b.i.d., do not exceed 15 mg/d *or* 0.132 mg/kg IM as a single dose	Treatment of severe nausea and vomiting, including that specifically associated with anesthesia; treatment of schizophrenia and nonpsychotic anxiety
promethazine (generic)	*Adult:* 12.5–0 mg PO, PR, IV *Pediatric (>2 y):* 12.5–25 mg PO, PR, IV Frequency varies based on indication	Treatment and prevention of nausea, vomiting, and motion sickness; treatment of allergic and vasomotor rhinitis, allergic conjunctivitis, mild allergic skin manifestations; procedural sedation
Nonphenothiazine		
metoclopramide (*Gimoti, Reglan*)	IM, IV, nasal spray, or PO Doses vary based on formulation and patient age; reduce dose with renal or hepatic impairment	Relief of symptoms of GERD; prevention of nausea and vomiting after emetogenic chemotherapy or postoperatively; relief of symptoms of diabetic gastroparesis, promotion of GI movement during small-bowel intubation or promotion of rapid movement of barium

(continues on page

Table 59.1 *Drugs in Focus:* Antiemetic Agents *(Continued)*

Drug Name	Usual Dosage	Usual Indications
5-HT_3 Receptor Blockers		
granisetron (*Sancuso, Sustol*)	*Adult and pediatric (>2 y):* 10 mcg/kg IV over 5 min starting within 30 min of chemotherapy or 1 mg PO b.i.d. beginning up to 1 h before chemotherapy and giving the second dose 12 h after, use only on days of chemotherapy *Adult:* 1 patch on the skin 24–48 h prior to chemotherapy and keep at least 24 h after chemotherapy or 10 mg sq ER injection 30 min before chemo	Treatment of nausea and vomiting associated with emetogenic chemotherapy
ondansetron (*Zofran*)	*Adult:* 8 mg PO t.i.d. or 24 mg PO 30 min before chemotherapy; three 0.15-mg/kg doses IV over 15 min beginning before chemotherapy or one 32-mg dose infused over 30 min, given 30 min before chemotherapy; 4 mg IV or IM or 16 mg PO 1 h before surgery to prevent postoperative vomiting *Pediatric (4–11 y):* 4 mg PO t.i.d., use same IV dose as adults *Pediatric (6 mo to 18 y):* 0.15 mg/kg IV 30 min before chemotherapy, then 4 and 8 h following chemotherapy	Treatment of severe nausea and vomiting associated with emetogenic chemotherapy, radiation therapy, and postoperative situations
palonosetron (generic)	*Adult:* 0.25 mg IV as a single dose over 30 s given 30 min before the start of chemotherapy, do not repeat dose for 7 d *Pediatric (1 mo to <17 y):* 20 mcg/kg IV over 15 min given 30 min before the start of chemotherapy *Surgery:* 0.075 mg IV once immediately before the induction of anesthesia	Treatment of acute and delayed vomiting associated with highly emetogenic chemotherapy; prevention of postoperative nausea and vomiting for up to 24 h following surgery
Substance P/Neurokinin 1 Receptor Antagonist		
aprepitant and fosaprepitant dimeglumine (*Cinvanti, Emend*)	*Adult and pediatric*: Oral and IV administration; dosing varies per age and formulation	Prevention of acute and delayed nausea and vomiting associated with highly emetogenic cancer chemotherapy
rolapitant (*Varubi*)	180 mg PO, 1–2 h before start of chemotherapy with dexamethasone and any 5-HT_3 receptor inhibitor	Prevention of delayed nausea and vomiting associated with emetogenic cancer chemotherapy
Miscellaneous Agents		
dexamethasone (*Decadron*)	Dosing varies based on indication	Treatment of nausea and vomiting
dimenhydrinate (*Dramamine*)	PO, IM, and IV dosing varies based on formulation	Relief of nausea and vomiting associated with motion sickness
dronabinol (*Marinol*)	PO dosing and frequency varies based on indication	Management of nausea and vomiting associated with cancer chemotherapy in adults; management of anorexia associated with weight loss in patients with AIDS
hydroxyzine (*Vistaril*)	*Adult and pediatric:* PO and IM dosing varies based on formulation	Treatment of prepartum, postpartum, and postoperative nausea and vomiting
meclizine (*Antivert, Bonine*)	*Adult and pediatric:* 25–100 mg/PO	Relief of nausea and vomiting associated with motion sickness
nabilone (*Cesamet*)	1–2 mg PO b.i.d.; initial dose given 1–3 h before chemotherapy begins, continue through chemotherapy and for 48 h after last dose	Treatment of nausea and vomiting associated with cancer chemotherapy in adults
scopolamine (*Transderm Scop*)	1 mg transdermal patch used over 3 d	Prevention of nausea and vomiting associated with motion sickness; treatment of postoperative nausea and vomiting
trimethobenzamide (*Tigan*)	*Adult:* 300 mg PO t.i.d. to q.i.d., 200 mg PR t.i.d. to q.i.d., 200 mg IM t.i.d. to q.i.d. *Pediatric (≥30 lb):* 100–200 mg PO or PR t.i.d. to q.i.d. *Pediatric (<30 lb):* 100 mg PR t.i.d. to q.i.d.	Treatment of nausea and vomiting associated with anesthesia and gastroenteritis

GERD, gastroesophageal reflux disease; AIDS, acquired immunodeficiency syndrome; CTZ, chemoreceptor trigger zone; 5-HT_3, serotonin.

BOX 59.3

Combination Drugs for Nausea/Vomiting

Diclegis is a combination of doxylamine succinate (an antihistamine) and pyridoxine (vitamin B_6 analog). It is approved for the treatment of nausea and vomiting of pregnancy in patients who do not respond to nondrug management. This is the only drug approved for this use. Two tablets are taken at bedtime; if the nausea persists, one additional tablet can be taken in the morning and another in the afternoon (a total of four a day).

Akynzeo is a combination of netupitant, a substance P/NK1 antagonist, and palonosetron, a serotonin-3 antagonist. It is approved for prevention of acute and delayed nausea and vomiting associated with initial and repeat courses of cancer chemotherapy. The palonosetron prevents the nausea and vomiting during the acute phase, while netupitant prevents the nausea and vomiting during the acute and delayed phase. This agent may be administered orally an hour before chemotherapy or via injection 30 minutes before the start of chemotherapy.

These agents are often reserved for use in mild nausea. Many of these drugs are discussed in Chapter 57. See Box 59.3 for information about combination drugs used to treat nausea and vomiting.

Centrally acting antiemetics can be classified into several groups: phenothiazines, nonphenothiazines, serotonin (5-HT_3) receptor blockers, substance P/neurokinin 1 (NK1) receptor antagonist, and a miscellaneous group.

Phenothiazines

There are several medications in the phenothiazine category. Chlorpromazine (generic), perphenazine (generic), and prochlorperazine (*Compro, Procomp*) are also discussed in Chapter 22 due to their psychotherapeutic indications. Promet hazine (generic) is also a phenothiazine derivative. (See the "Critical Thinking Scenario" for additional information about nursing care of a patient taking prochlorperazine.)

CRITICAL THINKING SCENARIO
Handling Postoperative Nausea and Vomiting

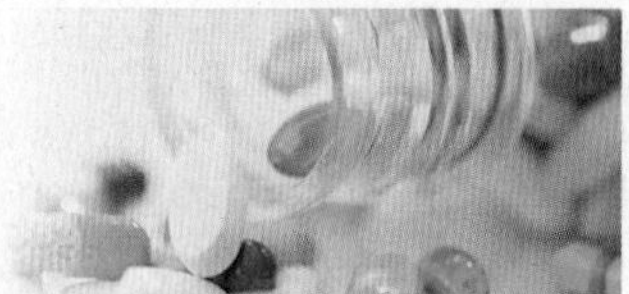

THE SITUATION

A.J. is a 16-year-old patient who has undergone reconstructive knee surgery after a football injury. After the surgery, A.J. complains of nausea and vomits three times in 2 hours. A.J. says that the hospital smells "awful." A.J. becomes increasingly agitated. Rectal prochlorperazine (generic) is ordered to relieve the nausea to be followed by an oral order when tolerated. The prochlorperazine is somewhat helpful in relieving the nausea, but A.J. expresses a desire to try cannabis, which they have read is good for the relief of nausea.

CRITICAL THINKING

What are the important nursing implications in this case?

What other measures could be taken to relieve A.J.'s nausea?

What explanation could be given to the request for cannabis?

DISCUSSION

It is often impossible to pinpoint an exact cause of a patient's nausea and vomiting in a hospital setting. For example, the underlying cause may be related to the pain, a reaction to the pain medication being given, or a response to what A.J. described as the "awful" hospital smell. A combination of factors should be considered when dealing with nausea and vomiting. A.J., as a teenager, may become increasingly agitated by the discomfort and possible embarrassment of vomiting. The administration of rectal prochlorperazine may "take the edge off" the nausea. A.J. will have to be reminded that the drug they are being given may make them dizzy, weak, or drowsy and that they should ask for assistance if they need to move.

Once the nausea and vomiting diminish somewhat, it will be possible to try other interventions to help stop the vomiting reflex. One such intervention is removing the offending odor that A.J. described, if possible, because doing so may relieve a chemical stimulus to the CTZ. Administration of pain medication, as prescribed, may relieve the CTZ stimulus that comes with intense pain. Other interventions include providing a serene, quiet environment and encouraging A.J. to take slow, deep breaths, which stimulate the parasympathetic system (vagus nerve) and partially override the sympathetic activity stimulated by the CTZ to activate vomiting. For many patients, mouth care, ice chips, or small sips of water may also help relieve the discomfort and ease the sensation of nausea.

After A.J. has relaxed a bit and the nausea has abated, the use of cannabis for treating nausea can be discussed. This may be a good opportunity to explain the many effects of cannabis to A.J. The drug does relieve nausea and vomiting, especially in patients undergoing chemotherapy. It also decreases activity in the respiratory tract, affects the development of sperm in males, and alters thinking patterns and brain chemistry. The U.S. Food and Drug Administration has approved

(continues on page 1

the use of the active ingredient in cannabis, delta-9-tetrahydrocannabinol, in an oral form—dronabinol (*Marinol*) and nabilone (*Cesamet*)—for the relief of nausea and vomiting in cancer patients who have not responded to other therapies and for the treatment of anorexia associated with acquired immunodeficiency syndrome (AIDS). It is not approved for use in the postoperative setting.

NURSING CARE GUIDE FOR A.J.: ANTIEMETICS

Assessment: History and Examination

Assess A.J.'s health history for allergies to any antiemetic; coma; CNS depression; severe hypotension; liver dysfunction; bone marrow depression; epilepsy; and concurrent use of alcohol, anticholinergic drugs, or barbiturate anesthetics. Determine the type and amount of anesthesia used.

Focus the physical examination on:

CNS: Orientation, affect

Skin: Color, lesions

CV: Pulse, blood pressure, orthostatic blood pressure

GI: Abdominal and liver evaluation

Laboratory tests: Hematological, complete blood count, liver function tests

Nursing Conclusions

Impaired comfort related to GI, skin, and CNS effects

Injury risk related to CNS and CV effects

Knowledge deficit regarding drug therapy

Planning

The patient will receive the best therapeutic effect from the drug therapy.

The patient will have limited adverse effects from the drug therapy.

The patient will have an understanding of the drug therapy, adverse effects to anticipate, and measures to relieve discomfort and improve safety.

Intervention

Administer antiemetics only as a temporary measure.

Provide comfort and safety measures, including assistance with mobility, access to bathroom, safety precautions, mouth care, and ice chips.

Monitor A.J. for dehydration and provide remedial measures as needed.

Provide support and reassurance for coping with drug effects and discomfort.

Provide patient teaching regarding drug name, dosage, adverse effects, precautions, and warning to report.

Evaluation

Evaluate drug effects (e.g., relief of nausea and vomiting).

Monitor for adverse effects, including GI alterations, orthostatic hypotension, dizziness, confusion, sensitivity to sunlight, and dehydration.

Monitor for drug–drug interactions as appropriate.

Evaluate the effectiveness of the patient teaching program and comfort and safety measures.

PATIENT TEACHING FOR A.J.

- The drug that has been prescribed for you is called prochlorperazine. It belongs to a class of drugs called antiemetics. An antiemetic helps prevent nausea and vomiting and the discomfort they cause.
- Common effects of this drug include the following:
  - *Dizziness, weakness, sedation*: Change positions slowly. If you feel drowsy, avoid driving or dangerous activities for at least 24 hours after the last dose of this drug (such as the use of heavy machinery or tasks requiring coordination).
  - *Dehydration, dry mouth, urinary retention*: Avoid excessive heat exposure; notify the nurse or provider if you have any change in urinary frequency; sips of fluids and/or lozenges may help with dry mouth.
- Report any of the following conditions to your health care provider: fever, rash, yellowing of the eyes or skin, dark urine, pale stools, easy bruising, rash, restlessness, anxiety, muscle spasms, or vision changes.
- Avoid over-the-counter (OTC) medications. If you feel that you need one, check with your health care provider first.
- Tell any doctor, nurse, or other health care provider that you are taking this drug.
- Keep this drug and all medications out of the reach of children.

Therapeutic Actions and Indications

Phenothiazines are centrally acting antiemetics that change the responsiveness or stimulation of the CTZ in the medulla (see Fig. 59.1). Most work as dopamine antagonists which can be used for treatment of some psychiatric diagnoses. However, promethazine is a histamine receptor blocker and has dopaminergic effects. The phenothiazines are recommended for the treatment of nausea and vomiting, including that specifically associated with anesthesia, severe vomiting, and **intractable hiccoughs,** which occur with repetitive stimulation of the diaphragm and lead to persistent diaphragm spasm. See Table 59.1 for usual indications for each of these agents.

Pharmacokinetics

These drugs are available as tablets or as syrup for oral administration, as rectal suppositories, and as solution for intramuscular (IM) or intravenous (IV) use. The route of choice is determined by the patient's condition. They have a rapid onset of action of 5 to 20 minutes and a duration of action of 3 to 12 hours, depending on the route of administration. They are metabolized in the liver and excreted in

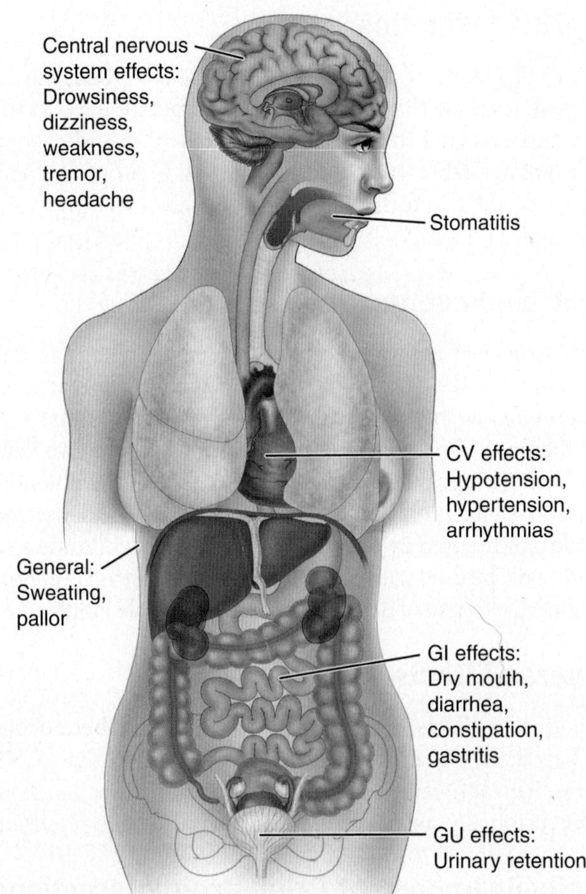

FIGURE 59.2 Variety of adverse effects and toxicities associated with antiemetic agents.

the urine. They are known to cross the placenta and enter human milk.

Contraindications and Cautions

In general, antiemetics should not be used in patients with coma or severe central nervous system (CNS) depression or in those who have experienced brain damage or injury because of the risk of further CNS depression. Other contraindications include severe hypotension or hypertension and severe liver dysfunction, which might interfere with the metabolism of the drug. Caution should be used in patients with renal dysfunction, moderate liver impairment, and active peptic ulcer, or during pregnancy and lactation because of the potential for adverse effects on the fetus or baby. Promethazine is contraindicated in pediatric patients younger than 2 years and should only be used with great caution with any pediatric patients due to risk of severe respiratory depression.

Adverse Effects

Adverse effects associated with antiemetics are linked to their interference with normal CNS stimulation or response. Drowsiness, dizziness, weakness, tremor, and headache are common adverse effects. Other common adverse effects include hypotension and cardiac arrhythmias. Autonomic effects such as dry mouth, nasal congestion, anorexia, pallor, sweating, and urinary retention often occur with phenothiazines (Fig. 59.2). Due to their action to block dopamine, there is risk of extrapyramidal symptoms including restlessness, tardive dyskinesia, tremors, and muscle spasms. Neuroleptic malignant syndrome is a rare but dangerous side effect that can occur with the phenothiazines that are dopamine antagonists. Patients should be cautioned that their urine may be tinged pink to red-brown. This is a normal drug effect but can cause concern if the patient is not expecting it. Endocrine effects such as menstrual disorders, galactorrhea, and gynecomastia have been reported with phenothiazine use. Photosensitivity (increased sensitivity to the sun and ultraviolet light) is a common adverse effect of these antiemetics. Patients should be advised to use sunscreens and protective garments if exposure cannot be avoided, as photosensitivity can lead to severe skin rash and lesions. It can also lead to damage to the eye. There is risk of severe tissue injury (including gangrene) with promethazine, and subcutaneous injection is contraindicated.

Clinically Important Drug–Drug Interactions

Additive CNS depression and hypotension can be seen with any of the antiemetics if they are combined with other CNS depressants (including alcohol) or antihypertensives. Patients should be advised to avoid this combination and any over-the-counter (OTC) preparation unless they check with their health care provider. Other drug–drug interactions are specific to each drug (refer to a nursing drug guide).

Prototype Summary: Prochlorperazine

Indications: Treatment of severe nausea and vomiting, including that specifically associated with anesthesia; treatment of schizophrenia and nonpsychotic anxiety.

Actions: Mechanism of action not completely understood; depresses various areas of the CNS, including the CTZ in the medulla; acts as a dopamine receptor antagonist.

Pharmacokinetics:

Route	Onset	Peak	Duration
Oral	30–40 min	Unknown	3–4 h
Rectal	60–90 min	Unknown	3–4 h
IM	10–20 min	10–30 min	3–4 h
IV	Immediate	10–30 min	3–4 h

$T_{1/2}$: Unknown; metabolized in the liver and excreted in the urine.

Adverse Effects: Drowsiness, dystonia, photophobia, blurred vision, urine discolored pink to red-brown, extrapyramidal symptoms, hypotension, neuroleptic malignant syndrome.

Nonphenothiazine

The only nonphenothiazine currently available for use as an antiemetic is metoclopramide (*Reglan*), which acts by blocking dopamine receptors and making the GI cells more sensitive to acetylcholine. This leads to increased GI activity and rapid movement of food through the upper GI tract. Chapter 58 discusses metoclopramide, which is also commonly used to treat gastroparesis, in greater detail.

Prototype Summary: Metoclopramide

Indications: Relief of symptoms of gastroesophageal reflux disease, prevention of nausea and vomiting after emetogenic chemotherapy or postoperatively, relief of symptoms of diabetic gastroparesis, promotion of GI movement during small bowel intubation or promotion of rapid movement of barium.

Actions: Metoclopramide works by blocking dopamine receptors and making the GI cells more sensitive to acetylcholine, which leads to increased GI activity and rapid movement of food through the upper GI tract.

Pharmacokinetics:

Route	Onset	Peak	Duration
Oral/nasal spray	30–60 min	60–90 min	1–2 h
IM	10–15 min	60–90 min	1–2 h
IV	1–3 min	60–90 min	1–2 h

$T_{1/2}$: 5 to 8 hours; metabolized in the liver and excreted in the urine.

Adverse Effects: Drowsiness, fatigue, restlessness, extrapyramidal symptoms, Parkinson-like reactions, seizures, nausea, diarrhea.

5-HT_3 Receptor Blockers

The 5-HT_3 receptor blockers block those receptors associated with nausea and vomiting in the CTZ and locally. These drugs include granisetron (*Sancuso, Sustol*), ondansetron (*Zofran*), and palonosetron (generic).

Therapeutic Actions and Indications

The 5-HT_3 receptor blockers have proven especially helpful in treating the nausea and vomiting associated with antineoplastic chemotherapy and radiation therapy and postoperative nausea and vomiting. They are specific for the treatment of nausea and vomiting associated with emetogenic chemotherapy. They are approved for use in children and adults.

Pharmacokinetics

The 5-HT_3 receptor blockers are rapidly absorbed, reaching peak levels within 1 hour. They are metabolized in the liver and excreted in the urine. Ondansetron and granisetron are available in oral and IV forms. Granisetron also has a transdermal formulation. Palonosetron is only available in an IV form.

Contraindications and Cautions

These drugs are contraindicated with known allergy to any component of the drug to prevent hypersensitivity reactions. Caution should be used with patients after abdominal surgery because of risk of masking of signs of progressive ileus and during pregnancy and lactation because of the potential for adverse effects on the fetus or nursing baby. Ondansetron should not be used in patients with long QT syndrome and should only be used with caution if there are electrolyte abnormalities due to risk of development of Torsade de Pointes.

Adverse Effects

The adverse effects most frequently seen with these drugs are headache, dizziness, and myalgia related to their CNS effects. Pain at the injection site, rash, constipation, diarrhea, hypotension, and urinary retention have also been reported.

Clinically Important Drug–Drug Interactions

Concurrent use with serotonergic medications can increase risk of serotonin syndrome. Use of ondansetron with other QT-prolonging medications can increase risk of torsade de pointes.

Prototype Summary: Ondansetron

Indications: Control of severe nausea and vomiting associated with emetogenic cancer chemotherapy, radiation therapy; treatment of postoperative nausea and vomiting.

Actions: Blocks specific receptor sites associated with nausea and vomiting, peripherally and in the CTZ.

Pharmacokinetics:

Route	Onset	Peak	Duration
Oral	30–60 min	60–90 min	1.7–2.2 h
IV	Immediate	60–90 min	Duration of infusion

$T_{1/2}$: 3.5 to 6 hours; metabolized in the liver and excreted in the urine.

Adverse Effects: Headache, dizziness, drowsiness, myalgia, urinary retention, constipation, diarrhea, pain at injection site.

Substance P/Neurokinin 1 Receptor Antagonist

The first drug in the newest class of drugs for treating nausea and vomiting is the substance P/NK1 receptor antagonist aprepitant (*Cinvanti, Emend*). Fosaprepitant dimeglumine (*Emend*) and rolapitant (*Varubi*) are also medications in this classification.

Therapeutic Actions and Indications

These drugs act directly in the CNS to block receptors associated with nausea and vomiting with little to no effect on serotonin, dopamine, or corticosteroid receptors. They have been found to work synergistically with serotonin antagonists and dexamethasone to prevent nausea and vomiting associated with chemotherapy. Aprepitant is approved for use in treating the nausea and vomiting associated with highly emetogenic antineoplastic chemotherapy, including cisplatin therapy. It is given orally in combination with dexamethasone. Fosaprepitant is a prodrug of aprepitant, so the effects are due to the actions of aprepitant. It is indicated for treatment of acute and delayed nausea and vomiting associated with cancer chemotherapy. Rolapitant is used in combination with other antiemetics for prevention of delayed nausea and vomiting associated with emetogenic antineoplastic chemotherapy.

Pharmacokinetics

These drugs are metabolized in the liver and excreted in the urine and feces. These drugs are known to cross the placenta and to enter human milk.

Contraindications and Cautions

There are no sufficient data to inform the risk if used during pregnancy and lactation. The medications should not be used if known allergy to any component of the drug to prevent hypersensitivity reactions. Rolapitant cannot be combined with thioridazine or pimozide. Aprepitant and fosaprepitant should not be used with pimozide.

Adverse Effects

The common adverse effects associated with these drugs include GI effects of diarrhea, constipation, and gastritis; nausea; anorexia; headache; and fatigue. There can also be neutropenia, anemia, and leukopenia.

Clinically Important Drug–Drug Interactions

There is a risk of serious increase in serum levels of pimozide if these drugs are used together; this combination should be avoided. There is a decrease in effectiveness of warfarin if it is combined with aprepitant or fosaprepitant, and the patient must be monitored closely and adjustments made in the warfarin dose if this combination must be used. There is a decrease in the effectiveness of hormonal contraceptives if they are taken concurrently with aprepitant and fosaprepitant; the use of a barrier contraceptive should be suggested.

Prototype Summary: Aprepitant

Indications: In combination with other agents for the prevention of acute and delayed nausea and vomiting associated with severely emetogenic cancer chemotherapy.

Actions: Selectively blocks human substance P/NK1 receptors in the CNS, blocking the nausea and vomiting caused by highly emetogenic chemotherapeutic agents.

Pharmacokinetics:

Route	Onset	Peak
Oral	Rapid	4 h
IV	Immediate	End of infusion

$T_{1/2}$: 9 to 13 hours; metabolized in the liver and excreted primarily via metabolism.

Adverse Effects: Anorexia, fatigue, constipation, diarrhea, liver enzyme elevations, dehydration.

Miscellaneous Agents

There are several miscellaneous agents that encompass a variety of medication classifications. See Table 59.1 for these agents and their typical indications. Dexamethasone is a glucocorticoid that can be used as an antiemetic. The mech anism of action as an antiemetic is not completely understood. It can be used in conjunction with other medications to treat chemotherapy-induced nausea and vomiting.

Dimenhydrinate, hydroxyzine, and meclizine are antihistamines that can be used to treat nausea and vomiting, especially associated with motion sickness. They help to block the muscarinic and histaminergic receptors in nerve pathways between the inner ear and vomiting center of the brain. Antihistamines are discussed in more detail in Chapter 54. They may cause sedation and anticholinergic effects (dry mouth, urinary retention, and constipation).

Dronabinol (*Marinol*) and nabilone (*Cesamet*) are cannabinoids that are indicated to treat nausea and vomiting associated with chemotherapy. Dronabinol is also used as an appetite stimulant for patients with AIDS and weight loss. Dronabinol is a category C-III controlled substance, and nabilone is a category C-II substance due to their potential to cause abuse and/or dependency. Patients should be monitored for potential of altered mental and physical states.

Scopolamine (*Transderm Scop*) is an anticholinergic medication that can be used to treat nausea and vomiting associated with motion sickness. Its mechanism of action includes blocking muscarinic receptors and cholinergic nerve communication from the inner ear to the vomiting center. Side effects include sedation and anticholinergic effects (blurred vision, dry mouth, urinary retention, and constipation). Anticholinergic medications are also discussed in Chapter 33.

Trimethobenzamide (*Tigan*) is indicated to treat nausea and vomiting due to surgical anesthesia or gastroenteritis. It is thought to decrease the nerve signals in the vomiting center in the medulla.

Nursing Considerations for Patients Receiving an Antiemetic Agent

Assessment: History and Examination

- Assess for possible contraindications or cautions: history of allergy to antiemetics to avoid potential hypersensitivity reactions; impaired renal or hepatic function, which could interfere with the metabolism or excretion of the drug; coma or semiconscious state, CNS depression, or CNS injury, which could be exacerbated by the CNS-depressing effects of the drug; hypotension or hypertension, which could be affected by the CNS effects of the drug; and current status of pregnancy and lactation because of the potential for adverse effects on the fetus or nursing baby.
- Perform a physical examination to establish baseline data before beginning therapy and during therapy to determine the effectiveness of the drug and evaluate for any adverse effects.
- Assess the patient's neurological status, including level of orientation, affect, and reflexes, to monitor for CNS effects and to rule out underlying CNS problems that could be a contraindication.
- Assess cardiopulmonary status, including baseline pulse and blood pressure, to evaluate effects on the CV system.
- Inspect the skin for color and evidence of lesion or rash to evaluate for photosensitivity and adverse effects of the drug.
- Examine the abdomen, including the liver, and auscultate bowel sounds to evaluate GI function and motility, rule out underlying medical problems, and identify possible adverse drug effects.
- Assess complaints of nausea and evaluate emesis; note color, amount, and frequency of vomiting episodes to determine the need for therapy.
- Monitor laboratory test results, including liver and renal function tests, to monitor for potential problems with metabolism or excretion.

Nursing Conclusions

Nursing conclusions related to drug therapy might include the following:

- Impaired comfort related to CNS, skin, and GI effects
- Injury risk related to CNS effects
- Altered cardiac output related to cardiac effects
- Knowledge deficit regarding drug therapy

Planning

- The patient will receive the best therapeutic effect from the drug therapy.
- The patient will have limited adverse effects from the drug therapy.
- The patient will have an understanding of the drug therapy, adverse effects to anticipate, and measures to relieve discomfort and improve safety.

Intervention With Rationale

- Assure that the route of administration is appropriate for each patient to ensure therapeutic effects and decrease adverse effects. Timing and administration will vary based on indication and formulation of the medications. Often these medications are used before nausea, and vomiting occur in patients undergoing chemotherapy treatments or with patients with risk of motion illness.
- Assess the patient carefully for any potential drug–drug interactions if giving antiemetics in combination with other drugs to avert potentially serious drug–drug interactions.
- Provide comfort and safety measures, including mouth care, ready access to bathroom facilities, assistance with ambulation and periodic orientation if there are adverse CNS effects, ice chips or lozenges if dry mouth occurs, protection from sun exposure, and remedial measures to treat dehydration if it occurs.
- Provide support and encouragement, as well as other measures (quiet environment, carbonated drinks, deep breathing), to help the patient cope with the discomfort of nausea and vomiting and drug effects.
- Provide thorough patient teaching, including the drug name and prescribed dosage; the schedule and method for administration; the need to avoid alcohol and other CNS depressants (if the patient is not hospitalized); signs and symptoms of adverse effects and measures to minimize or prevent them; the use of sunscreen and protective clothing when outside; comfort measures to reduce feelings of nausea, such as adequate ventilation, deep breathing, and a quiet environment; the importance of fluid intake and signs and symptoms of dehydration that should be reported to the health care provider; safety measures, such as assistance with ambulation and gradual position changes; the need to notify the health care provider

before using any OTC medications; and the importance of periodic monitoring and evaluation to enhance patient knowledge about drug therapy and to promote adherence.

Evaluation

- Monitor the patient response to the drug (relief of nausea and vomiting).
- Monitor for adverse effects (these can vary based on the medication).
- Monitor the effectiveness of comfort measures and adherence to the regimen.
- Evaluate the effectiveness of the teaching plan (patient can name the drug and dosage as well as describe adverse effects to watch for and specific measures to avoid them).

Key Points

- Antiemetics are used to manage nausea and vomiting in situations in which these actions are not beneficial and could cause harm to the patient.
- Antiemetics act by depressing the hyperactive vomiting reflex, either locally or through alteration of CNS actions.
- The choice of an antiemetic depends on the cause of the nausea and vomiting and the expected actions of the drug.
- Antiemetics include the phenothiazines and centrally acting nonphenothiazine metoclopramide, the anticholinergic/antihistamines, the 5-HT_3 receptor blockers, and the substance P/NK1 antagonists.
- There are also miscellaneous medications from other classifications that can be used to prevent and/or treat nausea and vomiting.

SUMMARY

- Phenothiazines and the nonphenothiazine metoclopramide are used as antiemetics to depress the CNS, including the CTZ. Patients must be monitored for CNS depression. Photosensitivity and pink to red-brown color of the urine are common adverse effects of these drugs.
- The 5-HT_3 blockers are newer antiemetics that directly block specific receptors in the CTZ to prevent nausea and vomiting. They are used in cases of nausea and vomiting associated with antineoplastic chemotherapy and radiation therapy and postoperative nausea and vomiting.
- Most antiemetics cause some CNS depression, with resultant dizziness, drowsiness, and weakness. Care must be taken to protect the patient; advise them to avoid dangerous situations.
- Side effects can vary greatly based on the specific medication administered. Many of the antiemetics are administered prior to onset of nausea to prevent nausea and vomiting in high-risk situations.

CHECK YOUR UNDERSTANDING

Answers to the questions in this chapter can be found in Answers to Check Your Understanding Questions on thePoint®.

MULTIPLE CHOICE

Select the best answer.

1. The nurse anticipates prochlorperazine would be the antiemetic of choice for which condition?
   a. Nausea and vomiting after anesthesia
   b. Nausea and vomiting due to cancer chemotherapy
   c. Motion sickness
   d. Intractable hiccoughs

2. Most antiemetics work with the CNS to decrease the activity of the
   a. cerebellum.
   b. chemoreceptor trigger zone.
   c. respiratory center.
   d. sympathetic nervous system.

3. Which instruction would be most appropriate to give to a patient to reduce the risk of photosensitivity related to the use of antiemetic agents?
   a. Avoid having your picture taken.
   b. Cover your head at extremes of temperature.
   c. Take extra precautions to avoid heat stroke.
   d. Wear protective clothing when in the sun.

4. The 5-HT_3 receptor blockers, including ondansetron (*Zofran*), are particularly effective in decreasing the nausea and vomiting associated with
   a. vestibular problems.
   b. cancer chemotherapy.
   c. pregnancy.
   d. severe pain.

5. A nurse has been asked to administer ondansetron (*Zofran*) to a patient. Of which dangerous side effect should the nurse be aware?
   a. Torsades de pointes
   b. Intracranial bleeding
   c. Ischemic stroke
   d. Acute angle glaucoma

MULTIPLE RESPONSE

Select all that apply.

1. Nursing interventions for the patient receiving an antiemetic drug would include which?
   a. Frequent mouth care
   b. Bowel program to deal with constipation
   c. Protection from falls or injury
   d. Fluids to guard against dehydration
   e. Protection from sun exposure
   f. Quiet environment and temperature control

2. Palonosetron would be the drug of choice for a patient with which problems?
   a. Nausea and vomiting associated with cancer chemotherapy
   b. A prolonged QT interval
   c. Delayed nausea and vomiting associated with antineoplastic chemotherapy
   d. Difficulty swallowing
   e. Hypokalemia
   f. Hypomagnesemia

REFERENCES

Arcangelo, V. P., Peterson, A. M., Wilbur, V., & Reinhold, J. A. (2017). *Pharmacotherapeutics for advanced practice: A practical approach* (4th ed.). Wolters Kluwer.

Brunton, L., Hilal-Dandan, R., & Knollman, B. (2018). *Goodman and Gilman's the pharmacological basis of therapeutics* (13th ed.). McGraw-Hill.

Forbes, D., & Fairbrother, S. (2008). Cyclic nausea and vomiting in childhood. *Australian Family Physician, 27*(1/2), 33–36. https://www.racgp.org.au/afpbackissues/2008/200801/200801forbes.pdf

Gummin, D. D., Mowry, J. B., Beuhler, M. C., Spyker, D. A., Brooks, D. E., Dibert, K. W., Rivers, L. J., Pham, N. P. T., & Ryan, M. L. (2020). 2019 Annual report of the American Association of Poison Control Centers' National Poison Data System (NPDS): 37th annual report. *Clinical Toxicology, 58*(12):1360–1541. https://piper.filecamp.com/uniq/9ZN62pw4DkShNNNS.pdf

Hall, J. E., & Hall, M. E. (2021). *Guyton and Hall textbook of medical physiology* (14th ed.). Elsevier.

Norris, T. L. (2019). *Porth's pathophysiology concepts of altered health states* (13th ed.). Wolters Kluwer.

Ware, M., Daeninck, P., & Maida, V. (2008). A review of nabilone in the treatment of chemotherapy-induced nausea and vomiting. *Therapeutics and Clinical Risk Management, 4*(1), 99–107. 10.2147/tcrm.s1132

CHAPTER 60

Vitamins, Minerals, and Complementary/ Alternative Medications

Learning Objectives

Upon completion of this chapter, you will be able to:

1. Define the terms vitamins and minerals.
2. Describe the therapeutic actions, indications, interactions, and cautions associated with various vitamins and minerals.
3. Discuss the use of alternative and complementary therapies.
4. Describe the therapeutic actions, indications, interactions, and cautions associated with various alternative supplements.
5. Outline the nursing considerations, including important teaching points, for patients receiving vitamins, minerals, alternative medications, and complementary therapies.

Key Terms

alternative medicine: products and practices for promoting health used in place of conventional medical care

complementary medicine: products and practices for promoting health used together with conventional medicine

integrative health: encourages multimodal interventions that include both conventional and complementary approaches; focuses on improvement of health as opposed to treatment of disease

mineral: naturally occurring inorganic substance; examples that are needed for health include calcium, phosphorus, potassium, sodium, chloride, magnesium, iron, zinc, iodine, chromium, copper, and fluoride

probiotic supplements: live bacteria and yeast preparations that are part of the normal environment of the gastrointestinal tract

vitamin: organic substance that is needed for growth and nutrition; typically not made by the body and therefore must be consumed in the diet

Health promotion and disease prevention include healthy nutrition. A nutritious diet includes adequate amounts of vitamins and minerals. There are times when people may need additional vitamin and/or mineral supplements due to lack of substances in the diet or increased metabolic need. In this chapter, recommended dietary guidelines are discussed. A table of the therapeutic uses and food sources of many vitamins and minerals is also included.

Alternative and complementary therapies are practices outside of standard or traditional medical practices that are used for enhancing health. Nurses need to be aware of common alternative/complementary therapies to adequately care for the diverse population of clients. Some of the therapies can be used very safely with traditional medications. Some have not been well studied so that less is known about the safety profile. Common substances used as alternative/complementary therapies are described in conjunction with any known cautions.

Vitamins and Minerals

The U.S. Department of Agriculture and U.S. Department of Health and Human Services work together to publish dietary guidelines for Americans. The guidelines that were published in 2020 can be found by searching online for "Dietary Guidelines for Americans, 2020-2025." These guidelines include four general recommendations for healthy eating. First, follow a healthy dietary pattern at every life stage, meaning that it is never too early or too late to begin eating healthy foods. Second, enjoy nutrient-dense foods and beverages that align with cultural traditions and budgetary constraints. Nutrient-dense foods are those that have vitamins, minerals, and other contents to promote health and lack added sugars, saturated fats, and sodium. Third, stay within calorie limits by eating foods that are nutrient dense to meet all food group requirements. Finally, limit or abstain from food and beverages with added sugars, saturated fat, high sodium, and alcohol. The guidelines consist of detailed information for healthy eating for each age group. The National Institutes of Health publish dietary reference reports and tables that have specific recommended amounts of nutrients for each age group and sex. These reports and tables can be found by searching the National Institutes of Health for "Nutrient Recommendations: Dietary Reference Intakes."

Vitamins are organic substances that the body requires to carry out essential metabolic reactions. The body cannot synthesize enough vitamins to meet all of its needs; therefore, they must be obtained from animal and vegetable tissues taken in as food. Most vitamins are needed only in small amounts because they function as coenzymes that activate the protein portions of enzymes, which catalyze a great deal of biochemical activity. Vitamins are either water soluble and excreted in the urine or fat soluble and capable of being stored in adipose tissue in the body.

Minerals are naturally occurring inorganic substances; many are also important for normal functioning of the human body. These substances are also taken in via diet. Some of the minerals needed are also electrolytes (minerals that when dissolved in fluid carry an electrical charge). Vitamin and mineral deficiencies can increase risk of health problems including anemias, osteoporosis, and heart arrhythmias. However, many of the vitamins and minerals can be harmful if their levels are too high in the body. Most of the time, these substances can be ingested via a normal healthy diet. However, there are times when supplements are needed to decrease risk of deficiency. The vitamins and minerals specific to treating anemia (iron, vitamin B, folic acid) are discussed in Chapter 49.

Therapeutic Actions and Indications

Vitamins and minerals have many roles to facilitate the functioning of the human body. They are used to build bones, make hormones, regulate fluid volume, generate nerve action potentials, and produce red blood cells. As dietary supplements, they are indicated for the treatment of deficiencies when a person's normal diet does not meet their body's needs. Prenatal vitamins are encouraged before and during pregnancy due to the need to maintain adequate vitamin levels during pregnancy and lactation. Table 60.1 lists specific vitamins and their therapeutic uses. Table 60.2 lists a few select electrolytes that are often recommended or prescribed for supplementation.

Contraindications and Cautions

These dietary supplements are contraindicated in the presence of any known allergy to the colorants, additives, or

Table 60.1 Vitamins

Vitamin	Solubility Type	Therapeutic Uses/Special Considerations	Food Sources
A (*Aquasol A*)	Fat	*Severe deficiency:* 500,000 IU/d for 3 d, then 50,000 IU/d for 2 wk given IM or PO; protect IM vial from light. Hypervitaminosis A can occur, including cirrhotic-like liver syndrome with CNS effects, GI drying, rash, and liver changes; treat by discontinuing the vitamin and giving saline, prednisone, and calcitonin IV; liver damage may be permanent	Liver, fish, dairy, egg yolks, dark green leafy vegetables, yellow-orange vegetables and fruits
Ascorbic acid (*Dull C, Vita-C, N'Ice*)	Water	May be given PO, IM, slow IV, or SC. *Treatment of scurvy:* 300–1,000 mg/d *Enhanced wound healing:* 300–500 mg/d for 7–10 d *Burns:* 1–2 g/d Also being studied for treatment of common cold, asthma, CAD, cancer, and schizophrenia; may be toxic at high doses	Broccoli, green peppers, spinach, Brussels sprouts, citrus fruits, tomatoes, potatoes, strawberries, cabbage, liver
Biotin (B_7)	Water	Involved with carbohydrate and fat metabolism; can be synthesized by intestinal bacteria. Deficiency extremely rare	Meat, egg yolk, nuts, cereals, many vegetables
Calcifediol (D_3) (*Calderol*)	Fat	*Management of metabolic bone disease or hypocalcemia in patients receiving chronic renal dialysis:* 300–350 mcg/wk daily or on alternate days; discontinue if hypercalcemia occurs	Dairy, fortified cereals and orange juice, liver, fish liver oils, saltwater fish, butter, eggs
Cholecalciferol (D_3) (*Delta-D*)	Fat	*Vitamin D deficiency:* 400–1,000 IU/d may be useful for treatment of hypocalcemic tetany and hypoparathyroidism	Dairy, fortified cereals and orange juice, liver, fish liver oils, saltwater fish, butter, eggs

Table 60.1 Vitamins (*Continued*)

Vitamin	Solubility Type	Therapeutic Uses/Special Considerations	Food Sources
Cyanocobalamin (B_{12}) (*Big Shot B_{12}, Twelve Resin-K*)	Water	*Deficiency:* 25–250 mcg/d *Pernicious anemia:* 100 mcg IM each month for life; given with folic acid; nasal route is preferable. **Note**: oral route is not for the treatment of pernicious anemia	Liver, kidney, shellfish, poultry, fish, eggs, milk, blue cheese, fortified cereals
D	Fat	*Vitamin D deficiency:* 400–1,000 IU/d may be useful for the treatment of hypocalcemic tetany and hypoparathyroidism; encourage balanced diet and exposure to sunlight; do not use with mineral oil	Dairy, fortified cereals and orange juice, liver, fish liver oils, saltwater fish, butter, eggs
E (*Aquavit-E, Vita-Plus E Softgels*)	Fat	Used in certain premature infants to reduce the toxic effects of oxygen on the lung and retina; do not give IV; report fatigue, weakness, nausea, or headache	Fish, egg yolks, meats, vegetable oils, nuts, fruits, wheat germ, grains, fortified cereals
Ergocalciferol (D_2) (*Calciferol, Drisdol Drops*)	Fat	Give IM in GI, biliary, or liver disease. *Refractory rickets:* 12,000–500,000 IU/d *Hypoparathyroidism:* 50,000–2,000,000 IU/d *Familial hypophosphatemia:* 10,000–80,000 IU/d plus 1–2 g phosphorus	Dairy, fortified cereals and orange juice, liver, fish liver oils, saltwater fish, butter, eggs
Folate; folic acid (B_9)	Water	Red blood cell formation and cell growth; deficiency during pregnancy can result in neural tube defects, so supplementation is recommended for all patients who can become pregnant	Liver, kidney beans, fresh green vegetable, fortified grains
Niacin (B_3) (*Niacor, Nicotinic Acid, Nicotinex, Slo-Niacin, Niaspan*)	Water	*Prevention and treatment of pellagra:* up to 500 mg/d *Niacin deficiency:* up to 100 mg/d Also used for the treatment of hyperlipidemia if no response to diet and exercise: 1–2 g t.i.d.; do not exceed 6 g/d; feelings of warmth or flushing may occur with administration but usually pass within 2 h	Liver, turkey, tuna, peanuts, beans, yeast, enriched whole grains and cereals, wheat germ
Nicotinamide (B_3) (*Niacinamide*)	Water	*Prevention and treatment of pellagra:* up to 50 mg, 3–10 times per day	Liver, turkey, tuna, peanuts, beans, yeast, enriched whole grains and cereals, wheat germ
Pantothenic acid (B_5)	Water	Needed for fatty acid synthesis and degradation, transfer of acetyl and acyl groups, and other anabolic and catabolic processes	Eggs, liver, salmon, yeast, cauliflower, broccoli, lean beef, potatoes, tomatoes
Phytonadione (K) (*Mephyton*)	Fat	*Hypoprothrombinemia due to anticoagulant use:* 2.5–10 mg PO, IM. *Hemorrhagic disease of the newborn:* 0.5–1 mg IM within 1 h of birth; 1–5 mg IM may be given to the birthing parent before delivery. *Hypoprothrombinemia in adult:* 2.5–25 mg PO or IM	Cheese, spinach, broccoli, Brussels sprouts, kale, cabbage, turnip greens, soybean oil
Pyridoxine HCl (B_6) (*Aminoxin*)	Water	*Deficiency:* 10–20 mg/d PO or IM for 3 wk *Vitamin B_6 deficiency syndrome:* up to 600 mg/d for life *Isoniazid poisoning* (give an equal amount of pyridoxine): 4 g IV followed by 1 g IM q30min Reduces the effectiveness of levodopa and leads to serious toxic effects—avoid this combination	Organ meats, poultry, fish, eggs, peanuts, whole grains, vegetables, nuts, wheat germ, bananas, fortified cereals
Riboflavin (B_2)	Water	*Deficiency:* 5–15 mg/d May cause a yellow or orange discoloration of the urine	Milk, cheddar and cottage cheese, meat, eggs, green leafy vegetables
Thiamine HCl (B_1) (*Thiamilate*)	Water	*Treatment of wet beriberi:* 10–30 mg IV t.i.d. *Treatment of beriberi:* 10–20 mg IM t.i.d. for 2 wk with multivitamin containing 5–10 mg/d for 1 mo Do not mix in alkaline solutions; it is used orally as a mosquito repellant and alters body sweat composition; feeling of warmth and flushing may occur with administration but usually passes within 2 h	Meat, poultry, fish, egg yolk, dried beans, whole grain and cereal, peanuts

CNS, central nervous system; GI, gastrointestinal; CAD, coronary artery disease.

Table 60.2 Select Electrolyte Supplements

Mineral (Electrolyte)	Form of Administration	Therapeutic Uses/Special Considerations	Food Sources
Calcium carbonate; calcium acetate; calcium chloride, calcium gluconate	Oral, IV	Adequate calcium levels required for musculoskeletal, nerve, and cardiovascular function. Used for treatment of calcium deficiency; reducing risk of osteoporosis; treatment deficiencies of parathyroid hormone. Often used in conjunction with vitamin D to increase absorption of calcium.	Dairy, fortified cereals and orange juice, sardines, salmon
Magnesium sulfate, magnesium hydroxide, magnesium oxide, magnesium citrate	Oral, IV	Activation of many intracellular enzymes; helps to regulate skeletal and cardiac muscle contractility. Used as antacid and laxative; to decrease uterine contractions and prevent seizures in patients with preeclampsia. High levels may suppress AV node conduction and cause muscle weakness, respiratory depression, and diarrhea. Calcium gluconate is an antidote for magnesium toxicity.	Meats, seafood, milk, cheese, yogurt, green leafy vegetables, bran cereal, nuts
Phosphorus	Oral	Important for regulation of acid–base balance, bone formation, energy production and storage, and hormone activation; may prevent some kidney stone formation.	Milk, yogurt, cheese, peas, meat, fish, eggs
Potassium chloride, potassium gluconate, potassium phosphate, potassium bicarbonate	Oral, IV	Necessary for regulating acid–base balance, nerve action potentials, and electrical excitability of muscles. Prolonged PR interval and peaked T waves on EKG can indicate hyperkalemia.	Beans, dairy products, fruits, clams, salmon, tomato products, sweet potatoes, potatoes, beet greens, spinach
Sodium	Oral, IV	Helps with regulation of water balance, action potentials of nerves, and acid–base balance. May need to be restricted in people with potential for fluid retention. Often combined with chloride.	Most foods have moderate amounts, often high in processed and canned foods

preservatives used in the supplement. Dietary supplements are also contraindicated when levels are normal or high in the body; this is due to risk of toxicity with many of the substances.

Adverse Effects

The adverse effects primarily associated with these supplements are related to gastrointestinal (GI) upset and irritation, which is caused by direct GI contact with the supplements.

Clinically Important Drug–Drug Interactions

Pyridoxine—vitamin B_6—interferes with the effectiveness of levodopa. Fat-soluble vitamins may not be absorbed if given concurrently with mineral oil, cholestyramine, or colestipol. Some of the minerals (magnesium and calcium) have potential for interfering with absorption of tetracyclines and other antibiotics and with iron. Concurrent use of potassium supplements with potassium-sparing diuretics or other medications that can increase potassium levels increases the risk of hyperkalemia.

Nursing Considerations for Patients Taking Vitamins or Minerals

Assessment: History and Examination

- Obtain a nutritional assessment. Ensure that the patient has an actual vitamin deficiency. Screen for any medical conditions and drugs being taken and for any known allergies.
- Evaluate skin and mucous membranes, as well as pulse, respirations, and blood pressure. For specific vitamins, complete blood count (CBC) and clotting times may need to be evaluated. Basic metabolic panel and magnesium levels may be needed to evaluate sodium, potassium, and magnesium levels.

Nursing Conclusions

Nursing conclusions related to drug therapy might include the following:

- Impaired comfort related to GI discomfort
- Malnutrition risk related to replacement therapy
- Knowledge deficit regarding drug therapy

Planning

- The patient will receive the best therapeutic effect from the therapy.
- The patient will have limited adverse effects from the therapy.
- The patient will have an understanding of the therapy, adverse effects to anticipate, and measures to relieve discomfort and improve safety.

Intervention With Rationale

- Assess the patient's general physical condition before beginning tests to decrease the potential for adverse effects and ensure need for the supplement.
- Advise the patient to avoid the use of over-the-counter preparations that contain the same vitamins and/or minerals to prevent inadvertent overdose.
- Provide comfort measures to help the patient tolerate supplement effects (e.g., take the supplement with meals to alleviate GI distress).
- Include information about potential length of therapy, adverse effects, medication interactions, and follow-up tests that may be needed to monitor levels to enhance patient knowledge about the therapy and promote adherence to the supplement regimen.

Evaluation

- Monitor patient response to the supplement (adequate vitamin and/or mineral levels).
- Monitor for adverse effects (primarily GI upset).
- Evaluate the effectiveness of the teaching plan (patient can name adverse effects to watch for and specific measures to avoid them; patient understands the importance of follow-up that will be needed).
- Monitor the effectiveness of comfort measures and adherence to the regimen.

Key Points

- Health promotion and disease prevention include good nutrition that involves adequate amounts of both vitamins and minerals.
- Vitamins are substances required for normal metabolic reactions and need to be ingested via food or administered in supplemental forms.
- Minerals are naturally occurring inorganic substances needed for normal functioning of the human body.
- Vitamins and minerals may be obtained in foods and also can be administered as supplements.

Alternative and Complementary Therapies

Alternative and complementary therapies are practices outside of standard or traditional medical practices that are used for enhancing health. **Alternative medicine** refers to therapies used in place of conventional medical care, and **complementary medicine** refers to the therapies that are used together with conventional medical care. The term **integrative health** describes a philosophy that encourages health care professionals to facilitate multimodal interventions that include both conventional and complementary approaches. This approach focuses on wellness and improvement of health as opposed to treatment of disease.

Complementary therapies can be classified as nutritional, psychological, physical, and combinations of psychological and physical (Fig. 60.1). Uses of these therapies include treatment of pain, neuropathy, depression, anxiety, insomnia, heart disease, and prostrate hyperplasia. These supplements and practices can often be used in conjunction with more traditional medications and therapies. However, there are sometimes dangerous

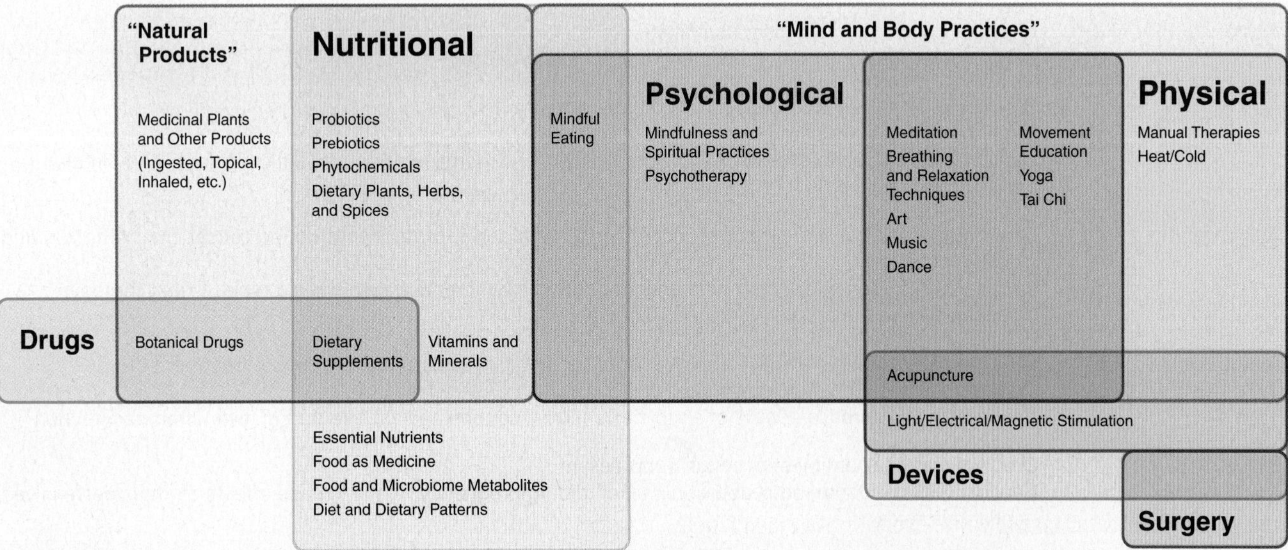

FIGURE 60.1 Examples of complementary health approaches that fall within the categories of psychological, physical, and nutritional.

interactions that need to be avoided. Natural and herbal therapies fall into these categories. These products are often labeled as dietary supplements. Compared to prescribed medications, dietary supplements are not as strictly regulated by the Food and Drug Administration (FDA). The dosages and ingredients are not as precise. Labels for dietary supplements must include the following disclaimer: "This product is not intended to diagnose, treat, cure, or prevent any disease." Some examples of herbal supplements are aloe vera, black cohosh, echinacea, ginkgo biloba, and St. John's wort. **Probiotic supplements**, which are preparations of live bacteria and yeast that are part of the normal environment of the gastrointestinal tract, also fall into this category. These supplements are promoted by manufacturers to support nutrient absorption, facilitate food metabolism, and decrease diarrhea caused by a variety of diagnoses (ulcerative colitis, inflammatory bowel syndrome, *Clostridium difficile* infection, and rotavirus). Alternative therapies can also include health-enhancing practices like imagery, meditation, acupuncture, and relaxation. To decrease risk of any medication interactions or toxicities, clinicians should encourage patients to discuss all of their health practices and provide lists of all dietary supplements. A coordinated treatment plan with both traditional and complementary therapies helps to facilitate a holistic and patient-based approach to health. Table 60.3 lists alternative and complementary therapies.

Table 60.3 Alternative and Complementary Therapies

Substance	Reported Uses and Possible Risks
Alfalfa	*Topical:* Healing ointment, relief of arthritis pain *Oral:* Treatment of arthritis, hot flashes; increased strength; reduction of cholesterol level *Caution:* Increased risk of bleeding with warfarin; increased photosensitivity with chlorpromazine; increased risk of hypoglycemia with antidiabetic drugs; loss of effectiveness with hormonal contraceptives or hormone replacement
Allspice	*Topical:* Anesthetic for teeth and gums; soothes sore joints and muscles *Oral:* Treatment of indigestion, flatulence, diarrhea, fatigue *Caution:* Risk of seizures with excessive use; decreased iron absorption
Aloe leaves, aloe vera	*Topical:* Treatment of burns, wound healing, soothes pain, softens skin *Oral:* Treatment of chronic constipation *Caution:* Check for medication interactions if using oral preparation; oral use may cause serious hypokalemia and fluid imbalances; there is risk of spontaneous abortion if used in third trimester
Androstenedione	*Oral, spray:* Anabolic steroid to increase muscle mass and strength *Caution:* May increase risk of cardiovascular disease and certain cancers
Angelica	*Oral:* "Cure-all" for gynecologic problems, headaches, backaches, loss of appetite, and gastrointestinal spasms; increases circulation in the periphery *Caution:* Risk of bleeding if combined with anticoagulants
Anise	*Oral:* Relief of dry cough, treatment of flatulence *Caution:* May increase *iron* absorption and cause toxicity
Apple	*Oral:* Control of blood glucose, constipation *Caution:* May interfere with antidiabetic drugs, fexofenadine
Arnica	*Topical:* Relief of pain from muscle or soft tissue injury *Oral:* Immune system stimulant *Caution:* May decrease effects of antihypertensives and increase effects of anticoagulants and platelet drugs; toxic to children
Ashwagandha	*Oral:* Improve mental and physical functioning; general tonic; protect cells during cancer chemotherapy and radiation therapy *Caution:* May increase bleeding with anticoagulants; may interfere with thyroid replacement therapy; discourage use during pregnancy and lactation
Astragalus	*Oral:* Increase stamina, energy; improve immune function, resistance to disease; treatment of upper respiratory tract infection, common cold *Caution:* It may increase effects of antihypertensives; caution against use during fever or acute infection
Barberry	*Oral:* Antidiarrheal, antipyretic, cough suppressant *Caution:* Risk of spontaneous abortion if taken during pregnancy; may increase effects of antihypertensives, antiarrhythmics
Basil	*Oral:* Analgesic, antiinflammatory, hypoglycemic *Caution:* Risk of increased hypoglycemic effects of antidiabetic drugs

Table 60.3 Alternative and Complementary Therapies (*Continued*)

Substance	Reported Uses and Possible Risks
Bayberry	*Topical:* Promote wound healing *Oral:* Stimulant, emetic, antidiarrheal *Caution:* May block effects of antihypertensives
Bee pollen	*Oral:* Treatment of allergies, asthma, impotence, prostatitis; suggested use to decrease cholesterol levels *Caution:* Risk of hyperglycemia; discourage use by diabetic patients or with antidiabetic drugs; may cause allergic reaction in patients allergic to bees
Betel palm	*Oral:* Mild stimulant, digestive aid *Caution:* Increased risk of hypertensive crisis with *monoamine* oxidase inhibitors (MAOIs); blocks heart rate reduction of beta-blockers, digoxin; alters effects of antiglaucoma drugs
Bilberry	*Oral:* Treatment of diabetes; cardiovascular problems; lowers cholesterol and triglycerides; treatment of diabetic retinopathy; treatment of cataracts, night blindness *Caution:* Increased risk of bleeding with anticoagulants; disulfiram-like reaction with alcohol
Birch bark	*Topical:* Treatment of infected wounds or cuts *Oral:* As tea for relief of stomach ache *Caution:* Topical form is toxic to children
Blackberry	*Oral:* As tea for generalized healing; treatment of diabetes *Caution:* Risk of interaction with antidiabetic drugs
Black cohosh root	*Oral:* Contains estrogen-like components; treatment of PMS, menopausal disorders, rheumatoid arthritis *Caution:* Caution against use with hormone replacement therapy or hormonal contraceptives; discourage use during pregnancy and lactation; may lower blood pressure with sedatives, antihypertensives, anesthetics; increased risk of fungal infection with immunosuppressants; increased risk of hypoglycemia with concurrent use with other medications that lower blood glucose
Bromelain	*Oral:* Treatment of inflammation, sports injuries, upper respiratory tract infection, PMS; adjunctive therapy in cancer treatment *Caution:* May cause nausea, vomiting, diarrhea, menstrual disorders
Burdock	*Oral:* Treatment of diabetes; uterine stimulant *Caution:* May increase hypoglycemic effects of antidiabetic drugs; atropine-like adverse effects
Butterbur (*Petasites hybridus*)	*Oral:* Treatment of migraine headaches, allergies, and asthma due to antiinflammatory, antispasmodic, and vasodilatory effects *Caution:* Interacts with drugs and supplements that induce CYP3A4 isoenzymes
Capsicum	*Topical:* External analgesic *Oral:* Treatment of bowel disorders, chronic laryngitis, peripheral vascular disease *Caution:* May increase bleeding with warfarin, aspirin; increases cough with *angiotensin*-converting enzyme inhibitors (ACEIs); increases toxicity with MAOIs; increases sedation with *sedatives*
Cascara sagrada	*Oral:* Treatment of constipation *Caution:* Long-term use risk of dehydration, electrolyte alterations
Catnip leaves	*Oral:* Treatment of bronchitis, diarrhea
Cat's claw	*Oral:* Treatment of allergies, arthritis; adjunct in treatment of cancers and AIDS *Caution:* Discourage use during pregnancy and lactation and use by transplant recipients; increased risk of bleeding episodes if taken with oral anticoagulants; increased hypotension with antihypertensives
Cayenne pepper	*Topical:* Treatment of burns, wounds; relief of toothache
Celery	*Oral:* Lowers blood glucose, acts as a diuretic *Caution:* May interact with antidiabetic drugs; may cause potassium depletion
Chamomile	*Topical:* Treatment of wounds, ulcer, conjunctivitis *Oral:* Treatment of migraines, gastric cramps, relief of anxiety *Caution:* Contains coumarin—closely monitor patients taking anticoagulants; may cause depression; monitor patients on antidepressants; cross-reaction with ragweed allergies may occur; discourage use during pregnancy and lactation
Chaste tree berry	*Oral:* Progesterone-like effects; used to treat PMS and menopausal problems and to stimulate lactation *Caution:* Advise caution when taken with hormone replacement therapy and hormonal contraceptives

(continues on page 1078)

Table 60.3 Alternative and Complementary Therapies (*Continued*)	
Substance	**Reported Uses and Possible Risks**
Chicken soup	*Oral:* Breaks up respiratory secretions, bronchodilator, relieves anxiety
Chicory	*Oral:* Treatment of digestive tract problems, gout; stimulates bile secretions
Chinese angelica (dong quai)	*Oral:* General tonic; treatment of anemias, PMS, menopause; antihypertensive; laxative *Caution:* Use caution with the flu and hemorrhagic diseases; monitor patients on antihypertensives, vasodilators, or anticoagulants for toxic effects; advise caution when taken with hormone replacement therapy
Chondroitin	*Oral:* Treatment of osteoarthritis and related disorders (usually combined with glucosamine) *Caution:* Risk of increased bleeding if combined with anticoagulants
Chong cao fungi	*Oral:* Antioxidant; promotes stamina, sexual function *Caution:* Discourage use by children
Coenzyme Q-10	*Oral:* Antioxidant used to treat heart failure, muscle injury from HMG-CoA reductase inhibitors (statins) *Caution:* Safety not established for people who are pregnant or breast or chestfeeding; may produce GI disturbances; may antagonize warfarin effects
Coleus forskohlii	*Oral:* Treatment of asthma, hypertension, eczema *Caution:* Urge caution when taken with antihypertensives or antihistamines; severe additive effects can occur; discourage use if patient has hypotension or peptic ulcer
Comfrey	*Topical:* Treatment of wounds, cuts, ulcers *Oral:* Gargle for tonsillitis *Caution:* Warn against using with *eucalyptus*; oral use may cause severe liver damage
Coriander	*Oral:* Weight loss, lowers blood glucose *Caution:* Advise caution when taken with antidiabetic drugs
Cranberry	*Oral:* Prevention of urinary tract infections; may reduce odor of urine *Caution:* May increase risk of bleeding if taking warfarin
Creatine monohydrate	*Oral:* Enhancement of athletic performance *Caution:* Warn against using with insulin; do not use with *caffeine*
Dandelion root	*Oral:* Treatment of liver and kidney problems; decreases lactation (after delivery or with weaning); lowers blood glucose *Caution:* Advise caution when taken with antidiabetic drugs, antihypertensives, and quinolone antibiotics
DHEA (dehydroepiandrosterone)	*Oral:* Slows aging, improves vigor ("Fountain of Youth"); androgenic side effects *Caution:* Risk of interactions with alprazolam, calcium channel blockers, and antidiabetic drugs; screen patients older than 40 y for hormonally sensitive cancers before use
Di Huang	*Oral:* Treatment of diabetes mellitus *Caution:* Risk of hypoglycemia with antidiabetic drugs
Dried root bark of *Lycium chinense* Miller	*Oral:* Lowers cholesterol, lowers blood glucose *Caution:* Advise caution with antidiabetic drugs
Echinacea (cone flower)	*Oral:* Treatment of colds, flu, skin disorders; stimulates the immune system but decreases inflammation, possibly treats viruses *Caution:* May be liver toxic; discourage use longer than 12 wk; caution against taking with liver toxic drugs or immunosuppressants. Discourage use with antifungals; serious liver injury could occur; advise against use by patients with systemic lupus erythematosus, tuberculosis, and AIDS
Elder bark and flowers	*Topical:* Gargle for tonsillitis, pharyngitis *Oral:* Treatment of fever, chills
Ephedra	*Oral:* Increases energy, relieves fatigue *Caution:* May cause serious complications, including death; increased risk of hypertension, stroke, myocardial infarction; interacts with many drugs; banned by the U.S. Food and Drug Administration
Ergot	*Oral:* Treatment of migraine headaches, treatment of menstrual problems, hemorrhage *Caution:* Monitor patients who take ergot with antihypertensives
Eucalyptus	*Topical:* Treatment of wounds *Oral:* Decreases respiratory secretions; suppresses cough *Caution:* Warn against using with comfrey; toxic in children

Table 60.3 Alternative and Complementary Therapies (*Continued*)

Substance	Reported Uses and Possible Risks
Evening primrose	*Oral:* Treatment of PMS, menopause, rheumatoid arthritis, diabetic neuropathy *Caution:* Discourage use with phenothiazines, antidepressants, including SSRIs—increases risk of seizures; discourage use by those with epilepsy, schizophrenia
False unicorn root	*Oral:* Treatment of menstrual and uterine problems *Caution:* Advise against use during pregnancy and lactation
Fennel	*Oral:* Treatment of colic, gout, flatulence; enhances lactation *Caution:* Significantly decreases levels of ciprofloxacin
Fenugreek	*Oral:* Lowers cholesterol level; reduces blood glucose; aids in healing *Caution:* Advise caution when taken with antidiabetic drugs, anticoagulants
Feverfew	*Oral:* Treatment of arthritis, fever, migraine; may block platelet aggregation *Caution:* Advise caution when taken with anticoagulants; may increase bleeding; discourage use before or immediately after surgery because of bleeding risk
Fish oil	*Oral:* Treatment of coronary diseases, arthritis, colitis, depression, aggression, attention-deficit disorder
Flaxseed	*Oral:* Treatment of constipation and dyslipidemia (lowers total cholesterol and low-density lipoprotein); decrease hot flashes during menopause *Caution:* May cause bloating, flatulence, and abdominal discomfort since it is a dietary fiber; may reduce absorption of medications so should not be taken within 2 hours of other medications
Garlic	*Oral:* Treatment of colds; diuretic; prevention of coronary artery disease; lowers low-density lipoprotein and triglycerides and increases high-density lipoprotein; intestinal antiseptic; lowers blood glucose; antiplatelet effects; decreases blood pressure *Caution:* Advise caution if patient has diabetes or takes oral anticoagulants or antidiabetic agents; known to affect blood clotting; anemia reported with long-term use
Ginger	*Oral:* Treatment of nausea, motion sickness, postoperative nausea; increases gastric mucous production; suppresses platelet aggregation; decrease pain from rheumatoid arthritis *Caution:* Affects blood clotting; warn against use with anticoagulants. May cause uterine contractions
Ginkgo biloba	*Oral:* Vascular dilation; increases blood flow to the brain, improving cognitive function; used in treating Alzheimer's disease; antioxidant; decreases platelet aggregation; decreases bronchospasm *Caution:* Seizures reported with high doses; warn against use with anticoagulants, aspirin, or NSAIDs; can interact with phenytoin, carbamazepine, phenobarbital, tricyclic antidepressants, MAOIs, and antidiabetic drugs; advise caution
Ginseng	*Oral:* Aphrodisiac, mood elevator, tonic; antihypertensive; decreases cholesterol levels; lowers blood glucose; adjunct in cancer chemotherapy and radiation therapy *Caution:* May cause irritability if combined with caffeine; inhibits clotting; warn against use with anticoagulants, aspirin, NSAIDs; warn against use for longer than 3 mo; may cause headaches, manic episodes if used with phenelzine, MAOIs; additive effects of estrogens and corticosteroids; may also interfere with cardiac effects of digoxin; monitor patient closely if they take these drugs or an antidiabetic drug
Glucosamine	*Oral:* Treatment of osteoarthritis and joint diseases, usually combined with chondroitin *Caution:* Increased risk of bleeding if taken concurrently with medications that also increase bleeding. Use with caution in patients with shellfish allergy
Goldenrod leaves	*Oral:* Treatment of renal disease, rheumatism, sore throat, eczema *Caution:* May decrease effects of diuretics by increasing sodium retention; advise caution if patient has a history of allergies
Goldenseal	*Oral:* Lowers blood glucose, aids healing; treatment of bronchitis, colds, flu-like symptoms, cystitis *Caution:* May cause false-negative test results in those who use such drugs as marijuana and cocaine; large amounts may cause paralysis; affects blood clotting; warn against use with anticoagulants; may interfere with antihypertensives, acid blockers, barbiturates; may increase effects of sedatives; death can result from overdose
Gotu kola	*Topical:* Treatment of chronic venous insufficiency *Caution:* Warn against using with antidiabetic drugs, cholesterol-lowering drugs, and sedatives
Grape seed extract	*Oral:* Treatment of allergies, asthma; improves circulation; decreases platelet aggregation *Caution:* Advise caution with oral anticoagulants; may increase bleeding

(continues on page 1080)

Table 60.3 Alternative and Complementary Therapies (*Continued*)

Substance	Reported Uses and Possible Risks
Green tea leaf	*Oral:* Antioxidant, prevention of cancer and cardiovascular disease; increase cognitive function (caffeine effects) *Caution:* Advise caution with oral anticoagulants; may increase bleeding; may increase blood pressure; caution against using with milk
Guarana	*Oral:* Decreases appetite, promotes weight loss *Caution:* Increases blood pressure, risk of cardiovascular events
Guayusa	*Oral:* Lowers blood glucose; promotes weight loss *Caution:* Advise caution with antihypertensives; decreases absorption of iron; may decrease clearance of lithium
Hawthorn	*Oral:* Treatment of angina, arrhythmias, blood pressure problems; decreases cholesterol *Caution:* Advise caution with digoxin, ACEIs, CNS depressants; may potentiate effects
Hops	*Oral:* Sedative; aids healing; alters blood glucose *Caution:* Discourage use with CNS depressants and antipsychotics
Horehound	*Oral:* Expectorant; treatment of respiratory problems, gastrointestinal disorders *Caution:* Use caution with antidiabetic drugs and antihypertensives
Horse chestnut seed	*Oral:* Treatment of varicose veins, hemorrhoids *Caution:* Advise caution with oral anticoagulants; may increase bleeding
Hyssop	*Topical:* Treatment of cold sores, genital herpes, burns, wounds *Oral:* Treatment of coughs, colds, indigestion, and flatulence *Caution:* Warn against use by pregnant patients and those with seizures; toxic in children and pets
Jambolana	*Oral:* Treatment of diarrhea, dysentery; lowers blood glucose *Caution:* Use caution with CNS depressants and Java plum
Java plum	*Oral:* Treatment of diabetes mellitus *Caution:* Advise caution with antidiabetic drugs
Jojoba	*Topical:* Promotion of hair growth, relief of skin problems *Caution:* Toxic if ingested
Juniper berries	*Oral:* Increases appetite, aids digestion; diuretic; urinary tract disinfectant; lowers blood glucose level *Caution:* Advise caution when taken with antidiabetic drugs; not for use in pregnancy
Kava	*Oral:* Treatment of nervous anxiety, stress, restlessness; tranquilizer *Caution:* Warn against use with CNS depressants; may cause coma; advise against use with Parkinson's disease or history of stroke; discourage use with St. John's wort, anxiolytics, alcohol; there is risk of serious liver toxicity
Kudzu	*Oral:* Reduces cravings for alcohol; being researched for use with alcoholics *Caution:* Interacts with anticoagulants, aspirin, antidiabetic drugs, cardiovascular drugs
Lavender	*Topical:* Astringent for minor cuts, burns *Oral:* Treatment of insomnia, restlessness *Caution:* Advise caution with CNS depressants; oil is potentially poisonous
Ledum tincture	*Topical:* Treatment of insect bites, puncture wounds; dissolves some blood clots and bruises
Licorice (black)	*Oral:* Prevents thirst, soothes coughs; treats "incurable" chronic fatigue syndrome; treatment of duodenal ulcer *Caution:* Acts like aldosterone; blocks spironolactone effects; can lead to digoxin toxicity because of effects of lowering aldosterone, advise extreme caution; contraindicated with renal or liver disease, hypertension, coronary artery disease, pregnancy, lactation; warn against taking with thyroid drugs, antihypertensives, and hormonal contraceptives
Ma huang	*Oral:* Treatment of colds, nasal congestion, asthma *Caution:* Contains ephedrine that has been associated with stroke, myocardial infarction, and death; warn against use with antihypertensives, antidiabetic drugs, MAOIs, digoxin; serious adverse effects could occur
Mandrake root	*Oral:* Treatment of fertility problems
Marigold leaves and flowers	*Oral:* Relief of muscle tension, increases wound healing *Caution:* Advise against use during pregnancy and breast or chestfeeding
Melatonin	*Oral:* Relief of jet lag; treatment of insomnia *Caution:* Advise caution with antihypertensives, benzodiazepines, beta-blockers, and methamphetamine

Table 60.3 Alternative and Complementary Therapies (*Continued*)

Substance	Reported Uses and Possible Risks
Milk thistle	*Oral:* Treatment of hepatitis, cirrhosis, fatty liver caused by alcohol or drug use *Caution:* May affect metabolism and increase toxicity of drugs using cytochrome P-450 (CYP450), CYP3A4, and CYP2C9 systems
Milk vetch	*Oral:* Improves resistance to disease; adjunct therapy in cancer chemotherapy and radiation therapy
Mistletoe leaves	*Oral:* Promotes weight loss; relief of signs and symptoms of diabetes *Caution:* Advise caution with antihypertensives, CNS depressants, and immunosuppressants
Momordica charantia (karela)	*Oral:* Blocks intestinal absorption of glucose; lowers blood glucose; weight loss *Caution:* Advise caution when taken with antidiabetic drugs
Nettle	*Topical:* Stimulation of hair growth, treatment of bleeding *Oral:* Treatment of rheumatism, allergic rhinitis; antispasmodic; expectorant *Caution:* Advise against use during pregnancy and breast or chestfeeding; increases effects of diuretics
Nightshade leaves and roots	*Oral:* Stimulates circulatory system; treatment of eye disorders
Octacosanol	*Oral:* Treatment of parkinsonism, enhancement of athletic performance *Caution:* Advise against use during pregnancy and lactation; avoid use with carbidopa–levodopa
Parsley seeds and leaves	*Oral:* Treatment of jaundice, asthma, menstrual difficulties, urinary infections, conjunctivitis *Caution:* Risk of serotonin syndrome with SSRIs, lithium, opioids; increased hypotension with antihypertensives
Passionflower vine	*Oral:* Sedative and hypnotic *Caution:* May increase sedation with other CNS depressants, MAOIs; advise against drinking alcohol while taking this herb; advise patient not to use with anticoagulants
Peppermint leaves	*Oral:* Treatment of nervousness, insomnia, dizziness, cramps, coughs *Topical:* Rubbed on forehead to relieve tension headaches
Probiotics	*Oral:* Replace normal flora of GI tract; prevention or treatment of uncomplicated diarrhea *Caution:* May cause flatulence and/or bloating; should not be administered within 2 h of antibiotics or antifungal medications
Psyllium	*Oral:* Treatment of constipation; lowers cholesterol *Caution:* Can cause severe gas and stomach pain; may interfere with nutrient absorption; avoid use with warfarin, digoxin, lithium; absorption of oral drugs may be blocked; do not combine with laxatives
Raspberry	*Oral:* Healing of minor wounds; control and treatment of diabetes, gastrointestinal disorders, upper respiratory disorders *Caution:* Advise caution with antidiabetic drugs; disulfiram-like reaction with alcohol
Red clover	*Oral:* Estrogen replacement in menopause; suppresses whooping cough, asthma *Caution:* Risk of bleeding with anticoagulants, antiplatelets; discourage use in pregnancy
Red yeast rice	*Oral:* Cholesterol-lowering agent *Caution:* Increased risk of rhabdomyolysis with cyclosporine, fibric acid, niacin, lovastatin, grapefruit juice
Resveratrol	*Oral:* Antioxidant used for antiaging effects and prevention of chronic illness *Caution:* Antiplatelet effects may increase risk of bleeding; mimics effects of estrogen so is not recommended for patients with estrogen-dependent breast cancer; may increase insulin sensitivity
Rose hips	*Oral:* Laxative; boosts the immune system and prevents illness *Caution:* Advise caution with estrogens, iron, and warfarin
Rosemary	*Topical:* Relief of rheumatism, sprains, wounds, bruises, eczema *Oral:* Gastric stimulation, relief of flatulence; stimulation of bile release; relief of colic *Caution:* Disulfiram-like reaction with alcohol
Rue extract	*Topical:* Relief of pain associated with sprains, groin pulls, whiplash *Caution:* Advise caution with antihypertensive drugs, digoxin, and warfarin
Saffron	*Oral:* Treatment of menstrual problems; abortifacient
Sage	*Oral:* Lowers blood pressure; lowers blood glucose *Caution:* Advise caution with antidiabetic drugs, anticonvulsants, and alcohol

(continues on page 1082)

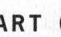

Table 60.3 Alternative and Complementary Therapies (*Continued*)

Substance	Reported Uses and Possible Risks
SAM-e (*AdoMet*)	*Oral:* Promotion of general well-being and health *Caution:* May cause frequent gastrointestinal complaints and headache; risk of serotonin syndrome with antidepressants
Sarsaparilla	*Oral:* Treatment of skin disorders, rheumatism *Caution:* Advise caution with anticonvulsants
Sassafras	*Topical:* Treatment of local pain, skin eruptions *Oral:* Enhancement of athletic performance, "cure" for syphilis *Caution:* Oil may be toxic to fetus, children, and adults when ingested; it interacts with many drugs
Saw palmetto	*Oral:* Treatment of benign prostatic hyperplasia *Caution:* Warn against use with estrogen replacement or hormonal contraceptives, may greatly increase adverse effects; may decrease iron absorption; advise against use with finasteride, toxicity could occur
Schisandra	*Oral:* Health tonic, liver protectant; adjunct in cancer chemotherapy and radiation therapy *Caution:* Warn against use during pregnancy; causes uterine stimulation; advise caution with all drugs metabolized in the liver
Soy	*Oral:* Prevention of breast cancer; treatment of hot flashes caused by menopause *Caution:* Structurally similar to estrogen so should not be used concurrently with medications that block estrogen
Squaw vine	*Oral:* Diuretic; tonic; aid in labor and childbirth; treatment of menstrual problems *Caution:* May cause liver toxicity; increased toxicity of *digoxin*; disulfiram-like reaction with alcohol
St. John's wort	*Oral:* Treatment of depression; analgesic and antiinflammatory; antiviral *Topical:* Treatment of puncture wounds, insect bites, crushed fingers or toes *Caution:* Discourage tyramine-containing foods; hypertensive crisis is possible; thrombocytopenia has been reported; can increase sensitivity to light, advise against taking with drugs that cause photosensitivity, severe photosensitivity can occur in light-skinned people; serious interactions have been reported with SSRIs, MAOIs, kava, digoxin, theophylline, antiviral drugs, sympathomimetics, antineoplastics, hormonal contraceptives, so advise against these combinations
Sweet violet flowers	*Oral:* Treatment of respiratory disorders; emetic *Caution:* Increases effects of laxatives
Tarragon	*Oral:* Weight loss; prevents cancer; lowers blood glucose *Caution:* Advise caution with antidiabetic drugs
Tea tree oil	*Topical:* Antifungal, antibacterial; used to treat burns, insect bites, irritated skin, acne; used as a mouthwash
Thyme	*Topical:* As liniment, gargle; to treat wounds *Oral:* Antidiarrheal; relief of bronchitis, laryngitis *Caution:* May increase sensitivity to light; warn against combining with photosensitivity-causing drugs; also warn against combining with MAOIs or SSRIs; may cause serious adverse effects
Turmeric	*Oral:* Antioxidant, antiinflammatory; used to treat arthritis *Caution:* May cause gastrointestinal distress; warn against use with known biliary obstruction; may cause increased bleeding with oral anticoagulants, NSAIDs; advise caution with immunosuppressants
Valerian	*Oral:* Sedative and hypnotic; reduces anxiety, relaxes muscles *Caution:* Rare cases of liver damage; warn against use with barbiturates, alcohol, CNS depressants, or antihistamines; can cause serious sedation
Went rice	*Oral:* Cholesterol- and triglyceride-lowering effects *Caution:* Warn against use in pregnancy or with liver disease, alcoholism, or acute infection
White willow bark	*Oral:* Treatment of fevers *Caution:* Advise caution with anticoagulants, NSAIDs, and diuretics
Xuan shen	*Oral:* Lowers blood glucose; slows heart rate; treatment of heart failure; treatment of erectile dysfunction *Caution:* Advise caution when taken with antidiabetic drugs; can affect blood pressure; CNS stimulant; has cardiac effects; manic episodes have been reported in psychiatric patients; warn against use with SSRIs and tyramine-containing foods; advise caution with tricyclic antidepressants

PMS, premenstrual syndrome; SSRI, selective serotonin reuptake inhibitor; NSAID, nonsteroidal antiinflammatory drug; MAOI, monoamine oxidase inhibitor; CNS, central nervous system.

Key Points

- Alternative and complementary therapies are practices outside of standard or traditional medical practices that are used for enhancing health.
- The term integrative health describes a philosophy that encourages health care professionals to facilitate multimodal interventions that include both conventional and complementary approaches. This approach focuses on wellness and improvement of health as opposed to treatment of disease.
- Herbal and probiotic supplements are complementary therapies that are labeled as dietary supplements.

SUMMARY

 Vitamins and minerals are required for normal human functioning and are normally consumed via diet. However, there are times when supplements are required to treat deficiencies. Many can be toxic if levels are too high.

 Herbal or alternative therapies are considered to be dietary supplements and are not tightly regulated by the FDA. They can have positive effects on health, but many have the potential to interact with other medications.

 Patients should be encouraged to discuss all alternative therapies with their health care provider to facilitate a holistic and patient-based health care plan.

CHECK YOUR UNDERSTANDING

Answers to the questions in this chapter can be found in Answers to Check Your Understanding Questions on thePoint®.

MULTIPLE CHOICE

Select the best answer.

1. You are caring for a patient who has newly elevated liver enzymes. When you review their list of herbal supplements, which of the following is most likely the cause of liver damage?
   a. Glucosamine
   b. Kava
   c. Saw palmetto
   d. Garlic

2. Which of the following would be helpful instruction from the nurse to a patient who is taking feverfew?
   a. "Due to increased risk of bleeding, you should stop this supplement at least 2 weeks prior to elective surgery."
   b. "This supplement is known to interact with antiviral medications."
   c. "Feverfew can be used to treat burns."
   d. "This supplement may increase risk of migraines."

3. Which of the following is not a common use for ginkgo biloba?
   a. Increasing vasodilation
   b. Decreasing platelet aggregation
   c. Increasing blood flow to the brain
   d. Treating vertigo

4. A patient might be taking a calcium supplement for which of the following diagnoses?
   a. Hypertension
   b. Septic shock
   c. Osteoporosis
   d. Preeclampsia

5. Which of the following is an antidote for magnesium toxicity?
   a. Calcium gluconate
   b. Cyanocobalamin
   c. Iron
   d. Potassium chloride

6. Which of the following nursing interventions would be important when administering potassium via IV to a patient?
   a. Ensure laxatives were ordered.
   b. Place the patient on fall precautions.
   c. Administer the potassium with vitamin D.
   d. Implement cardiac monitoring.

MULTIPLE RESPONSE

Select all that apply.

1. Which of the following are correct regarding vitamins?
   a. Some are water soluble.
   b. They are required for normal human functioning.
   c. Some are fat soluble.
   d. They are only available as prescription medications.
   e. Since they are over-the-counter, it is impossible for people to overdose.
   f. Most can be obtained through a healthy diet.
2. Which of the following are indications for magnesium supplementation?
   a. Diarrhea
   b. Constipation
   c. Facilitation of uterine contractions
   d. Bradycardia
   e. Heartburn
   f. Hypomagnesemia

REFERENCES

Burchum, J. R., & Rosenthal, L. D. (2019). *Lehne's pharmacology of nursing care* (10th ed.). Elsevier.

Kerry, R. G., Patra, J. K., Gouda, S., Park, Y., Shin, H., & Das, G. (2018). Benefaction of probiotics for human health: A review. *Journal of Food and Drug Analysis, 26*, 927–939. https://doi.org/10.1016/j.jfda.2018.01.002

Lopresti, A. L., Smith, S. J., & Drummond, P. D. (2020). Herbal treatments for migraine: A systematic review of randomized-controlled studies. *Phytotherapy Research, 34*(10), 2493–2517. https://doi.org/10.1002/ptr.6701

National Center for Complementary and Integrative Health. (2021). *Complementary, alternative, or integrative: What's in a name?* https://www.nccih.nih.gov/health/complementary-alternative-or-integrative-health-whats-in-a-name

National Institutes of Health. (2021). *Nutrient recommendations: Dietary reference intakes*. https://ods.od.nih.gov/HealthInformation/Dietary_Reference_Intakes.aspx

Plaza-Diaz, J., Ruiz-Ojeda, F. J., Gil-Campos, M., & Gil, A. (2019). Mechanisms of action of probiotics. *Advances in Nutrition (Bethesda, MD), 10*, S49–S66. https://doi.org/10.1093/advances/nmy063

Tucker, R. (2021). *2020 Lippincott pocket drug guide for nurses*. Wolters Kluwer.

U.S. Department of Agriculture and U.S. Department of Health and Human Services. (2020). *Dietary guidelines for Americans, 2020–2025* (9th ed.). https://www.dietaryguidelines.gov/sites/default/files/2021-03/Dietary_Guidelines_for_Americans-2020-2025.pdf

Wojcikowski, K., Vigar, V, & Oliver, C. (2020). New concepts of chronic pain and the potential role of complementary therapies. *Alternative Therapies in Health and Medicine, 26*(S1), 18–31. http://www.alternative-therapies.com/openaccess/ATHM_Wojcikowski_5525.pdf

Wu, B., Liu, C., Su, Y., Chen, S., Chen, Y., & Tsai, M. (2019). A review of complementary therapies with medicinal plants for chemotherapy-induced neuropathy. *Complementary Therapies in Medicine, 42*, 226–232. https://doi.org/10.1016/j.ctim.2018.11.022

Fluids, Electrolytes, and Other Parenteral Agents

Parenteral preparations are fluids, powders, or gels that are made for injection or infusion into the human body. Common routes of administration for parenteral preparations include subcutaneous, intravenous (IV), intramuscular, and intradermal. Fluids, electrolytes, and nutritional substances are often administered IV if the individual is unable to have adequate intake orally. IV access can be via peripheral or central line. Examples of fluids, electrolytes, and other parenteral agents are shown in Table A.

Therapeutic Actions and Indications

Parenteral agents are used for the following purposes: to provide replacement fluids, sugars, electrolytes, medications, and nutrients to patients who are unable to take them in orally; to provide ready access for administration of drugs in an emergency situation; to provide rehydration; and to restore electrolyte balance. The composition of the IV fluids needed for a patient depends on the patient's fluid and electrolyte status. The advantages of parenteral

Table A Fluids, Electrolytes, and Other Parenteral Agents

Solution	Caloric Content (cal/L)	Osmolarity (mOsm/L)	Usual Indications
In Solutions			
Dextrose Solutions			
2.5% (25 g/L)	85	126	Provides calories and fluid
5% (50 g/L)	170	253	Provides calories and fluid, keeps vein open for administration of IV drugs; frequent choice for dilution of IV drugs
10% (100 g/L)	340	505	Hypertonic solution used after admixture with other fluids; provides calories and fluid
20% (200 g/L)	680	1,010	Hypertonic solution used after admixture with other fluids; provides calories and fluid
25% (250 g/L)	850	1,330	Hypertonic solution used after admixture with other fluids; provides calories and fluid; treatment of acute hypoglycemic episodes in infants to restore glucose levels and suppress symptoms; sclerosing agent for varicose veins
30% (300 g/L)	1,020	1,515	Hypertonic solution used after admixture with other fluids; provides calories and fluid
40% (400 g/L)	1,360	2,020	Hypertonic solution used after admixture with other fluids; provides calories and fluid
50% (500 g/L)	1,700	2,525	Hypertonic solution used after admixture with other fluids; provides calories and fluid; treatment of hypoglycemia; sclerosing agent for varicose veins
60% (600 g/L)	2,040	3,030	Hypertonic solution used after admixture with other fluids; provides calories and fluid
70% (700 g/L)	2,380	3,535	Hypertonic solution used after admixture with other fluids; provides calories and fluid

(continues on page 1086)

Table A Fluids, Electrolytes, and Other Parenteral Agents *(Continued)*

Solution	Sodium Content (mEq/L)	Chloride Content (mEq/L)	Osmolarity (mOsm/L)	Usual Indications
Saline Solutions				
0.45% (1/2 normal saline)	77	77	155	Hydrating solution; may be used to evaluate kidney function; treatment of hyperosmolar diabetes
0.9% (normal saline)	154	154	310	Replacement of fluid, sodium, and chloride; flushing lines and catheters; dilution of IV medications; priming of dialysis machines; neonate blood transfusions

Solution	Caloric Content (cal/L)	Osmolarity (mOsm/L)	Usual Indications	
Saline Solutions				
3%	513	513	1,030	Hypertonic solution to treat sodium and chloride depletion; emergency treatment of water intoxication or severe salt depletion
5%	855	855	1,710	Hypertonic solution to treat sodium and chloride depletion; emergency treatment of water intoxication or severe salt depletion

Commonly Used Combination Fluids[a]

Solution	Na Content (mEq/L)	K Content (mEq/L)	Cl Content (mEq/L)	Ca Content (mEq/L)	Mg Content (mEq/L)	Lactate (mEq/L)	Acetate (mEq/L)	Osmolarity (mOsm/L)
Plasma-Lyte-56	40	13	40	–	3	–	18	111
Plasma-Lyte 148	140	5	98	–	3	–	27	294
Ringer's Injection	147	4	156	4	–	–	–	310
Lactated Ringer's	130	4	109	3	–	28	–	273
Normosol-R	140	5	96	–	3	–	27	295

Typical Central Parenteral Nutrition Solution[a,b]—1 L

Component	Purpose	Special Considerations
10% Amino acids	Provides 50-g protein for growth and healing	Monitor blood pressure, cardiac output, blood chemistries, and urine to determine the effect of intravascular protein pull.
50% Dextrose	Provides 850 cal for energy	Monitor blood sugar; evaluate injection site for any sign of infection, irritation.
20% Fat emulsion	Provides 500 fat calories, ready energy	Monitor for any sign of emboli (e.g., shortness of breath, chest pain, deep leg pain, neurological changes); carefully monitor patients for any sign of increased vascular workload, especially very young and geriatric patients.
Sodium chloride	Provides sodium and chloride needed for various chemical reactions within the body	Monitor cardiac rhythm and serum electrolytes.
Calcium gluconate	Provides essential calcium for muscle contraction, blood clotting, numerous chemical reactions	Monitor cardiac rhythm, muscle strength, and serum electrolytes.
Magnesium sulfate	Provides magnesium for various chemical reactions within the body	Monitor blood pressure, deep tendon reflexes, and serum electrolytes.

Table A Fluids, Electrolytes, and Other Parenteral Agents *(Continued)*

Typical Central Parenteral Nutrition Solution[a,b]—1 L

Component	Purpose	Special Considerations
Potassium phosphate	Provides needed potassium for nerve functioning, muscle contractions, etc.	Monitor pulse, including rhythm, muscle function, and serum electrolytes.
Multivitamins	Provide a combination of essential vitamins to maintain cell integrity, promote healing.	Monitor for signs of vitamin deficiency or toxicity.
Trace elements	Provide small amounts of elements essential for numerous chemical reactions in the body and maintenance of cell integrity and healing. Elements often include zinc, copper, manganese, chromium, and selenium.	Periodically monitor blood chemistries to determine adequacy of replacement.

Total nonprotein calories: 1,350
Total volume of solution: 1,250 mL
Dextrose concentration: 25%
Amino acid concentration: 5%
Osmolarity: 1,900 mOsm/L

Typical Peripheral Parenteral Nutrition Solution[a,b,c]—1 L

Component	Purpose	Special Considerations
8.5% Amino acids	Provides 41-g protein for growth and healing	Monitor blood pressure, cardiac output, blood chemistries, urine to determine effect of intravascular protein pull.
20% Dextrose	Provides 340 cal for energy	Monitor blood sugar; evaluate injection site for any sign of infection or irritation.
20% Fat emulsion	Provides 500 fat calories, ready energy	Monitor for any sign of emboli (e.g., shortness of breath, chest pain, deep leg pain, neurological changes); carefully monitor patients for any sign of increased vascular workload, especially very young and geriatric patients.
Sodium chloride	Provides sodium and chloride needed for various chemical reactions within the body	Monitor cardiac rhythm and serum electrolytes.
Calcium gluconate	Provides essential calcium for muscle contraction, blood clotting, numerous chemical reactions	Monitor cardiac rhythm, muscle strength, and serum electrolytes.
Magnesium sulfate	Provides magnesium for various chemical reactions within the body	Monitor blood pressure, deep tendon reflexes, and serum electrolytes.
Potassium phosphate	Provides needed potassium for nerve functioning, muscle contractions, etc.	Monitor pulse, including rhythm, muscle function, and serum electrolytes.
Multivitamins	Provide a combination of essential vitamins to maintain cell integrity, promote healing, etc.	Monitor for signs of vitamin deficiency or toxicity.

Typical Peripheral Parenteral Nutrition Solution[a,b,c]—1 L

Component	Purpose	Special Considerations
Trace elements	Provide small amounts of elements essential for numerous chemical reactions in the body and maintenance of cell integrity and healing. Elements often include zinc, copper, manganese, chromium, and selenium.	Periodically monitor blood chemistries to determine adequacy of replacement.

Total nonprotein calories: 840
Total volume of solution: 1,250 mL
Dextrose concentration: 10%
Amino acid concentration: 4.25%
Osmolarity: 900 mOsm/L

[a]Multiple combination preparations are available commercially. Each preparation varies in the concentration of one or more components and should be checked carefully before hanging.
[b]Actual concentration of solution and components of any particular solution will be determined by assessment of the patient's current status and nutritional needs.
[c]Solutions used for peripheral therapy are usually less concentrated and less irritating to the vessel.

administration are more rapid effects and larger volumes of fluids can be administered. If administered IV versus subcutaneously or intramuscularly, there is usually less irritation to connective tissue and less discomfort after the initial insertion of the IV line.

Parenteral nutrition (PN) is the administration of essential proteins, amino acids, carbohydrates, vitamins, minerals, trace elements, lipids, and fluids intravenously. PN is used to improve or stabilize the nutritional status of cachectic or debilitated patients who cannot take in or absorb oral nutrition to the extent required to maintain their nutritional status. The exact composition and dosing of the PN solution is determined after a nutritional assessment and must take into account the patient's current health status, age, and metabolic needs.

Contraindications and Cautions

PN is contraindicated in anyone with known allergies to any component of the solution. Multiple combination products are available, so a suitable solution may be found *to avoid adverse reactions*. PN and parenteral fluid and electrolyte preparations should be used with caution in patients with unstable cardiovascular status because of the change in fluid volume that might occur and the resultant increased workload on the heart. These preparations should also be used with caution in patients with unstable fluid and electrolyte status, who could react adversely to sudden changes in fluids and electrolytes.

Adverse Effects

Adverse effects associated with the use of PN and IV fluids and electrolytes include irritation to the veins that have been accessed, extravasation of the fluid into the tissues, infection of the insertion site, fluid volume overload, vascular problems related to fluid shifts, and potential electrolyte imbalance. PN and IV administration are also associated with mechanical problems related to insertion of the line, such as pneumothorax, infections, or air emboli; emboli related to protein or lipid aggregation; infections related to nutrient-rich solution and invasive administration; metabolic imbalances related to the composition of the solution; gallstone development (especially in children); and nausea (especially related to the administration of lipids).

Clinically Important Drug–Drug Interactions

Some IV drugs can be diluted only with particular IV solutions to avoid precipitation or inactivation of the drug. IV medications should not be administered through the same tubing as blood, blood produce, or PN products. A drug guide should be checked before diluting any IV drug in solution and compatibility of different IV solutions should always be verified.

Nursing Considerations

Assessment: History and Examination

- Obtain a nutritional assessment. Screen for any medical conditions and drugs being taken.
- Evaluate the insertion site; skin hydration; fluid status, orientation and affect; height and weight; pulse, blood pressure, and respirations; and blood chemistries, complete blood count with differential, and glucose levels.

Nursing Diagnoses

The patient receiving a parenteral agent might have the following nursing diagnoses related to drug therapy:

- Acute pain related to insertion of IV or PN line
- Infection risk related to invasive delivery system
- Malnutrition risk related to inadequacy of oral intake
- Fluid or electrolyte imbalance risk related to fluid compositions and amounts
- Knowledge deficit regarding drug therapy

Planning

- The patient will receive the best therapeutic effect from the parenteral therapy.
- The patient will have limited adverse effects to the parenteral therapy.
- The patient will have an understanding of the parenteral therapy, adverse effects to anticipate, and measures to relieve discomfort and improve safety.

Implementation

- Assess the patient's general physical condition before beginning infusion to decrease the potential for adverse effects.
- Monitor the IV insertion site or central line and regularly consult with the prescriber to discontinue the site of infusion and treat any infection or extravasation as soon as it occurs.
- Follow these administration guidelines to provide the most therapeutic use of parenteral agents with the fewest adverse effects:
  - If directed by pharmacist, refrigerate solutions until ready to use.
  - Check contents before hanging to ensure that no precipitates are present.
  - Ensure IV line is patent prior to administration.

- Use infusion pump to regulate rates whenever possible and follow institution's policy for when to change IV bags and tubing.
- Do not administer two different substances in same IV tubing unless substances have been proven to be compatible with each other.
- Some IV solutions require a filter to be attached to the tubing.

- Discontinue PN only after an alternative source of nutrition has been established to ensure continued nutrition for the patient; taper and titrate slowly to avoid severe reactions.
- If infiltration or extravasation occurs, stop infusion and notify provider.
- Provide comfort measures to help the patient tolerate drug effects (e.g., provide proper skin care as needed, analgesics, appropriate management of extravasation sites).
- Include information about the solution being used (e.g., what to expect, adverse effects that may occur, follow-up tests that may be needed) to enhance patient knowledge about parenteral therapy and promote compliance with the treatment.

Evaluation

- Monitor patient response to the parenteral therapy (stabilization of nutritional state, fluid and electrolyte balance, laboratory values).
- Monitor for adverse effects (local irritation, infection, fluid and electrolyte imbalance).
- Evaluate the effectiveness of the teaching plan (patient can name adverse effects to watch for and specific measures to avoid them; patient understands the importance of follow-up that will be needed).
- Monitor the effectiveness of comfort measures and compliance with the regimen.

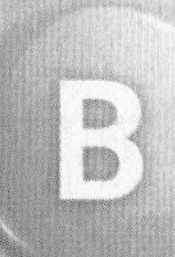

Topical Agents

Topical agents are intended for administration on skin or mucous membranes. The absorption is often slow. Actions of the medication may be primarily for the local area, but some topical medications are absorbed into the blood stream and work systemically. These substances are not typically designed for ingestion or injection. Medications can be in multiple forms: suppositories, sprays, creams, ointments, pastes, lotions, and powders. These drugs may also be prepared as transdermal patches (e.g., nitroglycerin, estrogens, nicotine), which are designed to provide a slow release of the drug from the patch. Drugs prepared for this type of administration are discussed with the specific drug in the text and are not addressed in this appendix.

Therapeutic Actions and Indications

Topical agents are used to treat a variety of disorders. They are often designed to target a problem in a localized area of the body. Table B describes the usual uses for the many different types of topical agents. Because these drugs are designed for topical application, if they are absorbed systemically, absorption is typically slow.

Contraindications and Cautions

The use of topical agents is contraindicated in cases of allergy to the drugs and in the presence of open wounds or abrasions (unless specifically indicated for treatment of open wounds), which could lead to inappropriate and/or dangerous systemic absorption of the drugs. Caution should be used during pregnancy if there is any possibility that the agent might be absorbed systemically and effect the fetus. Caution should also be used in the presence of any known allergy to the vehicles of preparation (creams, lotions). Caution is advised with applying heat (using hot tubs, taking hot baths, or applying heating pads) with use of medication patches since it may change the release of medication. Some patches may contain metal and would need to be removed prior to MRI procedures. Occluding the skin after application of some cream/lotions may increase absorption and risk of side effects.

Adverse Effects

Adverse effects usually associated with topical agents are local effects, including local irritation, stinging, burning, or dermatitis. Toxic effects can be associated with inappropriate and/or excessive systemic absorption.

Nursing Considerations

Assessment: History and Examination

- Screen for the presence of any known allergy to the drug, which would be a contraindication to its use.
- Include screening for baseline status before beginning therapy and for any potential adverse effects. Assess the condition of area to be treated.

Nursing Diagnoses

The patient receiving a topical agent might have the following nursing diagnoses related to drug therapy:

- Injury risk related to toxic effects associated with inappropriate or excessive absorption
- Impaired comfort related to local effects of the drug
- Knowledge deficit regarding drug therapy

Planning

- The patient will receive the best therapeutic effect from the drug therapy.
- The patient will have limited adverse effects to the drug therapy.
- The patient will have an understanding of the drug therapy, adverse effects to anticipate, and measures to relieve discomfort and improve safety.

Implementation

- Ensure proper administration of the drug to provide best therapeutic effect and least adverse effects as follows:
  - Apply sparingly. Some preparations come with applicators, some should be applied while wearing protective gloves, and others are dropped onto the site with no direct contact. Consult information regarding the individual drug being used for specific procedures.
  - Do not use with open wounds or broken skin (unless medication is specifically indicated for open wounds), which could lead to inappropriate or excessive systemic absorption and toxic effects.
  - Avoid contact with the eyes, which could be injured by the drug.
  - Do not use with occlusive dressings, which could increase the risk of systemic absorption.
- Monitor the area being treated to evaluate drug effects on the condition being treated.
- Provide comfort measures to help the patient tolerate drug effects (e.g., analgesia as needed for local pain, itching).
- Provide patient teaching to enhance patient knowledge about drug therapy and promote compliance with the drug regimen:
  - Teach the patient the proper administration technique for the topical agent ordered.
  - Caution the patient that transient stinging or burning may occur.
  - Instruct the patient to report severe irritation, allergic reaction, or worsening of the condition being treated.

Evaluation

- Monitor patient response to the drug (improvement in condition being treated).
- Monitor for adverse effects (local stinging or inflammation).
- Evaluate the effectiveness of the teaching plan (patient can name drug, dosage, adverse effects to watch for, and specific measures to avoid them; patient understands the importance of continued follow-up).
- Monitor the effectiveness of comfort measures and compliance with the regimen.

Table B Topical Agents

Drug	Brand Name	Dosage	Usual Indications/Special Considerations
Emollients			
dexpanthenol	*Panthoderm*	Apply once or twice daily as needed.	Relieves itching and aids in healing for mild skin irritations
urea	*Aquacare, Carmol, Gordon's Urea, Nutraplus, Ureacin*	Apply b.i.d. to q.i.d. to area affected.	Rub in completely; it is used to restore nails—cover with plastic wrap; keep dry and remove in 3, 7, or 14 d
vitamins A and D	generic	Apply locally with gentle massage b.i.d. to q.i.d.	Relieves minor burns, chafing, skin irritations; consult health care provider if not improved within 7 d
zinc oxide	*Borofax Skin Protectant*	Apply as needed.	Relieves burns, abrasion, diaper rash
Eczema Drug			
crisaborole	*Eucrisa*	Apply thin layer to affected area twice a day.	Treatment of mild to moderate eczema
Growth Factor			
becaplermin	*Regranex*	Apply to diabetic foot ulcers b.i.d. to q.i.d.	Increases the incidence of healing of diabetic foot ulcers as adjunctive therapy; must have an adequate blood supply
Lotions and Solutions			
Burow's solution aluminum acetate	*Domeboro Powder*	Dissolve one packet in a pint of water; apply q15–30min for 4–8 h.	Astringent wet dressing for relief of inflammatory conditions, insect bites, athlete's foot, bruises, sores; do not use occlusive dressing

(continues on page 1092)

Table B Topical Agents (*Continued*)

Drug	Brand Name	Dosage	Usual Indications/Special Considerations
calamine lotion	generic	Apply to affected area t.i.d. to q.i.d.	Relieves itching, pain of poison ivy, poison sumac, and poison oak, insect bites, and minor skin irritations
Hamamelis water	*Witch Hazel, A.E.R.*	Apply locally up to six times per day.	Relieves itching and irritation of vaginal infection, hemorrhoids, postepisiotomy discomfort, posthemorrhoidectomy care
Antiseptics			
benzalkonium chloride	*Benza, Mycocide NS, Zephiran*	Mix in solution as needed; spray for preoperative use.	Thoroughly rinse detergents and soaps from skin before use; add antirust tablets for instruments stored in solution; dilute solution as indicated for use.
chlorhexidine gluconate	*BactoShield, Dyna-Hex, Exidine, Hibistat, Hibiclens*	Scrub or rinse; leave on for 15 s; for surgical scrub—3 min.	Use for surgical scrub, preoperative skin preparation, wound cleansing, and preoperative bathing and showering
hexachlorophene	*Pre-Op*	Apply as wash.	Surgical wash, scrub; do not use with burns or on mucous membranes; rinse thoroughly
iodine	generic	Wash affected area.	Highly toxic; avoid occlusive dressings; stains skin and clothing; iodine allergy is common.
povidone–iodine	*Betadine, GRx Dyne, GRx Dyne Scrub, Povidex, Povidex Peri*	Apply as needed.	Treated areas may be bandaged; HIV is inactivated in this solution; causes less irritation than iodine; less toxic
sodium hypochlorite	*Dakin's*	Apply as antiseptic.	Caution—chemical burns can occur
Antibiotics			
ciprofloxacin/ dexamethasone	*Ciprodex*	Apply drops to ears or outer ear canal.	Treatment of acute otitis media with tympanostomy tubes; acute otitis externa
ciprofloxacin/ hydrocortisone	*Cipro-HC Otic drops*	Apply drops to ears or outer ear canal.	Treatment of acute otitis media with tympanostomy tubes; acute otitis externa
gentamicin	generic	Small amount to be applied topically three or four times a day	Treatment of skin infections
mupirocin	*Bactroban, Centany*	Apply small amount to affected area t.i.d.	Used to treat impetigo caused by *Staphylococcus aureus*, *Streptococcus* pathogens; may be covered with a gauze pad; monitor for signs of superinfection, reevaluate if no clinical response in 3–5 d
mupirocin calcium	*Bactroban Nasal*	Apply one-half of the single-use ointment tube between nostrils b.i.d. for 5 d.	Eradication of nasal colonization or methicillin-resistant *Staphylococcus aureus*
neomycin	*Myciguent*	Apply contents to surface of affected area one to three times a day	Prevention of infection in minor cuts, scrapes, and burns
ozenoxacin	*Xepi*	Apply thin layer twice a day for 5 d.	Treatment of impetigo due to *Staphylococcus aureus* or *Streptococcus pyogenes*
retapamulin	*Altabax*	Apply thin layer of ointment to affected area b.i.d. for 5 d for patients ≥9 mo.	Treatment of impetigo

Table B Topical Agents (*Continued*)

Drug	Brand Name	Dosage	Usual Indications/Special Considerations
Antivirals			
acyclovir	*Zovirax*	Apply 0.5-in ribbon to affected area six times per day for 7 d.	Treatment of herpes simplex cold sores and fever blisters (cream); initial herpes simplex virus genital infections (ointment)
acyclovir/ hydrocortisone	*Xerese*	Apply five times a day for 5 d; begin as soon as cold sore becomes apparent.	Treatment of herpes simplex cold sores in patients aged 6 y and older
docosanol	*Abreva*	Apply daily to b.i.d.	Used for treatment of oral and facial herpes simplex cold sores and fever blisters; caution patient not to overuse
penciclovir	*Denavir*	Apply thin layer to affected area q2h while awake for 4 d.	Treatment of cold sores in healthy patients: begin use at first sign of cold sore; reserve use for herpes labialis on lips and face; avoid mucous membranes
Antipsoriatics			
anthralin	*Dritho-Scalp, Micanol, Psoriatec, Zithranol*	Apply daily only to psoriatic lesions.	May stain fabrics, skin, hair, fingernails; use protective dressing
betamethasone	*Sernivo*	Apply to affected skin twice a day for up to 4 wk	Treatment of psoriatic lesions
calcipotriene	*Dovonex*	Apply thin layer twice a day.	Monitor serum calcium levels with extended use; use only for disorder prescribed; it may cause local irritation; is a synthetic vitamin D_3
calcipotriene/ betamethasone	*Taclonex, Taclonex Scalp*	Apply once daily for up to 4 wk.	Monitor serum calcium levels and check for endocrine imbalance.
Antiseborrheics			
selenium sulfide	*Selsun Blue*	Massage 5–10 mL into scalp; rest 2–3 min, rinse.	It may damage jewelry, remove before use; discontinue if local irritation occurs.
Antifungals			
butenafine HCl	*Mentax*	Apply to affected area once a day for 4 wk.	Treatment of athlete's foot (interdigital pedis), tinea corporis, ringworm, tinea cruris
ciclopirox	*Loprox, Penlac, Penlac Nail Lacquer*	Apply directly to affected fingernails or toenails.	Treatment of onychomycosis of the fingernails and toenails in immunocompromised patients
clotrimazole	*Cruex, Desenex, Lotrimin, Mycelex*	Gently massage into affected area b.i.d.	Cleanse area before applying; use for up to 4 wk; discontinue if irritation or worsening of condition occurs.
econazole nitrate	generic	Apply locally daily to b.i.d.	Treatment of athlete's foot (interdigital pedis), tinea corporis, ringworm, tinea cruris: cleanse area before applying; treat for 2–4 wk; for athlete's foot, change socks and shoes at least once a day.
efinaconazole	*Jublia*	Apply daily for 48 wk using flow brush applicator.	Topical treatment of onychomycosis of the toenails
gentian violet	generic	Apply locally b.i.d.	May stain skin and clothing; do not apply to active lesions
ketoconazole	*Extina, Nizoral, Xolegel*	Shampoo daily.	Reduction of scaling due to dandruff; burning may occur

(continues on page 1094)

Table B Topical Agents (*Continued*)

Drug	Brand Name	Dosage	Usual Indications/Special Considerations
luliconazole	*Luzu*	Apply locally once a day for 1 wk, 2 wk for tinea pedis.	Treatment of athlete's foot (interdigital pedis), tinea corporis
naftifine HCl	*Naftin*	Gently massage into affected area b.i.d.	Avoid occlusive dressings; wash hands thoroughly after application; do not use longer than 4 wk
oxiconazole	*Oxistat*	Apply daily to b.i.d.	May be needed for up to 1 mo
sertaconazole nitrate	*Ertaczo*	Apply to affected areas and surrounding tissue b.i.d. for 4 wk.	Treatment of tinea pedis
terbinafine	*Lamisil*	Apply to area b.i.d. until clinical signs are improved; 1–4 wk.	Do not use occlusive dressings; report local irritation; discontinue if local irritation occurs
tolnaftate	*Absorbine Aftate, Genaspor, Quinsana Plus, Tinactin, Ting*	Apply small amount b.i.d. for 2–3 wk; 4–6 wk may be needed if skin is very thick.	Cleanse skin with soap and water before applying drug, dry thoroughly; wear loose, well-fitting shoes; change socks at least q.i.d.
Pediculicides/Scabicides			
benzyl alcohol	generic	Apply to scalp or hair near scalp.	Single application is usually sufficient, for treatment of head lice in patients 6 mo and older
crotamiton	*Crotan, Eurax*	Thoroughly massage into skin over entire body, repeat in 24 h; patient should take a cleansing bath or shower 48 h after last application.	Change all bed linens and clothing the next day; contaminated clothing can be dry cleaned or washed in hot water; shake well before using
ivermectin	*Sklice*	Apply once to head for 10 min, no need for nit picking.	Treatment of head lice in patients 6 mo and older
lindane	generic	Apply thin layer to entire body; leave on 8–12 h; wash thoroughly; shampoo 1–2 oz into dry hair and leave in place for 4 min.	Single application is usually sufficient; reapply after 7 d at signs of live lice; teach hygiene and prevention; treat all contacts; advise parents that this is a readily communicable disease.
malathion	*Ovide Lotion*	Apply to dry hair and leave on for 8–12 h; repeat in 7–9 d.	Avoid use with open lesions; change bed linens and clothing daily; treat all contacts
permethrin	*Nix*	Thoroughly massage into all skin areas; wash off after 8–14 h; shampoo into freshly washed, rinsed, and towel-dried hair, leave on for 10 min, rinse.	Single application is usually curative; notify health care provider if rash or itch becomes worse; it is approved for prophylactic use during head lice epidemics
spinosad	*Natroba*	Apply to dry scalp and hair, leave on for 10 min, rinse; may be repeated every 7 d as needed.	Treatment of head lice in patients 4 y and older
Keratolytics			
podophyllum resin	*Podocon-25, Podofin*	Applied only by physician	Do not use if wart is inflamed or irritated; very toxic; use minimum amount possible to avoid absorption
podofilox	*Condylox*	Apply q12h for 3 consecutive days.	Allow to dry before using area; dispose of used applicator; it may cause burning and discomfort

Table B Topical Agents (*Continued*)

Drug	Brand Name	Dosage	Usual Indications/Special Considerations
Topical Hemostatics			
absorbable gelatin	*Gelfoam*	Smear or press to cut surface; when bleeding stops, remove excess; apply sponge and allow to remain in place; will be absorbed.	Prepare paste by adding 3–4 mL of sterile saline to contents of jar; apply sponge dry or saturated with saline; assess for signs of infection; do not use in presence of infection
absorbable fibrin sealant	*TachoSil*	Apply yellow side of patches directly to bleeding area.	For cardiovascular surgery when usual techniques to control bleeding are ineffective
human fibrin sealant	*Evicel, Artiss*	Spray or drop onto tissue in short bursts to produce a thin layer.	Adjunct used to reduce bleeding in vascular and liver surgery; used to adhere autologous skin grafts
microfibrillar collagen	*Hemopad, Hemostat, Hemotene*	Use dry; apply directly to source of bleeding, apply pressure for 3–5 min; discard leftover product.	Monitor for infection; remove any excess material once bleeding has stopped
thrombin	*Evithrom, Thrombinar, Thrombostat*	Prepare in sterile distilled water; mix freely with blood on the surface of the injury.	Contraindicated in the presence of any bovine allergies; watch for severe allergic reactions in sensitive individuals
thrombin, recombinant	*Recothrom*	Apply solution directly to bleeding site with absorbable gelatin sponge.	Control of minor bleeding and oozing: do not use with allergy to hamster or snake proteins
Pain Relief			
capsaicin	*Axsain, Capsin, Pain Doctor, Pain-X, Qutenza, Zostrix*	Do not apply more than three to four times per day.	It provides temporary relief from the pain of osteoarthritis, rheumatoid arthritis, neuralgias; do not bandage tightly; stop use and seek medical help if condition worsens or persists after 14–28 d.
Burn Preparations			
mafenide	*Sulfamylon*	Apply to a clean, debrided wound, one to two times per day; cover burns at all times with drug; reapply as needed.	Bathe patient in a whirlpool daily to debride wound; continue debridement with a gloved hand; cover; continue until healing occurs. Monitor for infection and toxicity, especially acidosis; may cause severe discomfort requiring premedication before application
silver sulfadiazine	*Silvadene, SSD Cream, Thermazene*	Apply daily to b.i.d. to a clean, debrided wound; use 1/16-in thickness.	Bathe patient in a whirlpool to aid debridement; dressings are not necessary but may be used; reapply when necessary; monitor for fungal infections
Estrogens			
estradiol hemihydrate	*Vagifem*	Insert one tablet intravaginally daily for 2 wk, then one tablet intravaginally two times per week.	Treatment of atrophic vaginitis; attempt to taper every 3–6 mo
Acne, Rosacea, and Melasma Products			
adapalene	*Differin*	Apply a thin film to affected area after washing.	Do not use near cuts or open wounds; avoid sun-burned areas; do not combine with other products; limit exposure to the sun; it is less drying than most acne products
adapalene/benzyl peroxide	*Epiduo*	Apply gel as thin film once a day to affected area on face and/or trunk after washing.	Avoid use on sunburned skin, w/other products, sun exposure

(*continues on page 1096*)

Table B Topical Agents (*Continued*)

Drug	Brand Name	Dosage	Usual Indications/Special Considerations
alitretinoin	*Panretin*	1% gel; apply as needed to cover lesion b.i.d.	Treatment of lesions of Kaposi sarcoma; inflammation, peeling, redness may occur
aminolevulinic acid hydrochloride	*Ameluz*	10% gel; administered only by health care professional.	Treatment of mild to moderate actinic keratosis on face and scalp. Risk of eye injury, photosensitivity, bleeding, ophthalmic adverse reactions, mucous membrane irritation
azelaic acid	*Azelex, Finevin (20%)*	Wash and dry skin; massage thin layer into skin b.i.d.	Wash hands thoroughly after application; improvement usually seen within 4 wk; initial irritation usually passes with time
brimonidine	*Mirvaso*	Apply pea size to forehead, chin, cheeks daily.	Risk of vascular insufficiency; for treatment of persistent facial erythema of rosacea in adults
clindamycin	*Clindesse, Evoclin*	Wash and dry area; massage into area morning and evening.	Do not use occlusive dressings; it may cause transient burning
clindamycin with benzoyl peroxide	*Acanya, BenzaClin*	Apply to affected area b.i.d.	Wash and pat dry area before application
clindamycin with tretinoin	*Ziana, Veltin*	Rub pea-sized amount over entire face once daily at bedtime.	Do not use in patients with colitis
dapsone	*Aczone Gel*	Apply thin layer to affected areas b.i.d.	Follow hemoglobin and reticulocyte counts; do not use with patients with glucose-6-phosphate dehydrogenase deficiencies
erythromycin with benzoyl peroxide	*Benzamycin*	Apply to clean and dry skin b.i.d.	Topical treatment of acne vulgaris; avoid contact with eyes and mucous membranes
fluocinolone, hydroquinone, tretinoin	*Triluma*	Apply to depigmented area of melasma once each evening at least 30 min before bed.	Treatment of melasma; not for use in pregnancy; skin peeling can occur; wear protective clothing when outside
hydrogen peroxide	*Eskata*	Solution 40%	Treatment of seborrheic keratosis. Given by health care provider
ingenol mebutate	*Picato*	Apply gel once a day to face/scalp for 5 d; to trunk for 2 d.	Treatment of acne
ivermectin	*Soolantra*	Apply to affected areas daily.	Treatment of rosacea
metronidazole	*MetroGel, MetroLotion, Noritate*	Apply cream to affected area.	Treatment of rosacea
oxymetazoline hydrochloride	*Rhofade*	Apply thin film to affected areas once daily; cream 1%.	Treatment of rosacea
sodium sulfacetamide	*Klaron*	Apply a thin film b.i.d.	Wash affected area with mild soap and water, pat dry; avoid use in denuded or abraded areas
tazarotene	*Avage, Arazlo, Fabior, Tazorac*	Apply thin film daily in the evening.	Avoid use in pregnancy; drying, causes photosensitivity; do not use with products containing alcohol
tretinoin, 0.025% cream	*Avita*	Apply thin layer daily.	Discomfort, peeling, redness, and worsening of acne may occur for first 2–4 wk
tretinoin, 0.05% cream	*Renova*	Apply thin coat in evening.	Use for the removal of fine wrinkles

Table B Topical Agents (*Continued*)

Drug	Brand Name	Dosage	Usual Indications/Special Considerations
tretinoin, gel	*Retin-A-Micro*	Apply to cover daily, after cleansing.	Exacerbation of inflammation may occur at first; therapeutic effects usually seen in first 2 wk
trifarotene	*Aklief*	Apply think layer to affected areas daily.	Avoid contact with eyes, lips, paranasal creases and mucous membranes
Antihistamine			
azelastine HCl	*Astelin, Astepro, Dymista*	Two sprays per nostril b.i.d.	Avoid use of alcohol and OTC antihistamines; dizziness and sedation may occur
Hair Removal			
eflornithine	*Vaniqa*	Apply to unwanted facial hair b.i.d. for up to 24 wk.	Approved for use in women only
Immune Modulator			
imiquimod	*Aldara*	Apply thin layer to warts and rub in three times per week at bedtime for 16 wk.	For treatment of genital warts and perianal warts; treatment of actinic keratosis; treatment of superficial basal cell carcinoma; remove with soap and water after 6–10 h
imiquimod	*Zyclara*	Apply daily at bedtime for 2 wk, may repeat after a 2-wk break.	Treatment of genital, perianal warts in patients 12 and older
pimecrolimus	*Elidel*	Apply locally b.i.d.	Treatment of mild to moderate atopic dermatitis in nonimmunosuppressed patients over 2 year old
kunecatechins (sinecatechins)	*Veregen*	Apply thin layer to each wart t.i.d. for up to 16 wk.	Antioxidant treatment of external and perianal warts in immune competent patients older than 18 y
Antidiaper Rash Drug			
miconazole/ zinc oxide, petrolatum	*Vusion*	Apply gently for 7 d.	Adjunctive treatment of diaper rash when complicated with candidiasis
Local Anesthetics			
lidocaine/ tetracaine	*Synera*	Apply one patch to intact skin 20–30 min before procedure.	Dermal analgesia for superficial venous access, dermatological procedures
Topical Corticosteroids			
These drugs enter cells and bind to cytoplasmic receptors, initiating complex reactions that are responsible for the antiinflammatory, antipruritic, and antiproliferative effects of these drugs. They are used to relieve the inflammation and pruritic manifestations of corticosteroid-sensitive dermatoses and for temporary relief of minor skin irritations and rashes. These agents should not be applied on open sores or lesions because of the risk of systemic corticosteroid effects if absorbed systemically. Occlusive dressings and tight coverings should be avoided. Prolonged use should also be avoided because of the risk of systemic effects and local irritation and breakdown. These agents are applied topically two to three times daily.			
alclometasone dipropionate	generic	Ointment, cream: 0.05% concentration	Occlusive dressings may be used for the management of refractory lesions of psoriasis and deep-seated dermatoses
beclomethasone	*Beconase AQ, Qnasl*	Nasal spray	Treatment of rhinitis
betamethasone dipropionate	generic	Ointment, cream, lotion, aerosol: 0.05% concentration	
betamethasone dipropionate, augmented	*Diprolene*	Ointment, cream, lotion: 0.05% concentration	

(continues on page 1098)

Table B Topical Agents (*Continued*)

Drug	Brand Name	Dosage	Usual Indications/Special Considerations
betamethasone valerate	*Beta-Val, Luxiq, Valisone*	Ointment, cream, lotion: 0.01% concentration	
ciclesonide	*Alvesco, Omnaris, Zetonna*	Inhalation: 80 mcg, 160 mcg per actuation	
clobetasol propionate	*Cormax, Temovate, Olux*	Ointment, cream: 0.05% concentration	
	Clobex	Spray 0.05%	
clocortolone pivalate	*Cloderm*	Cream: 0.1% concentration	
desonide	*DesOwen, Verdeso*	Ointment, cream: 0.05% concentration	
desoximetasone	*Topicort*	Ointment, cream: 0.25% concentration	
		Gel: 0.05% concentration	
dexamethasone	*Aeroseb-Dex*	Gel: 0.1% concentration	
		Aerosol: 0.01%, 0.04% concentration	
diflorasone diacetate	generic	Ointment, cream: 0.05% concentration	
		Cream: 0.5% concentration	
fluocinolone acetonide	*Synalar*	Ointment: 0.025% concentration	
		Cream: 0.01% concentration	
fluocinonide	*Lidex*	Ointment: 0.05% concentration	
	Fluonex, Lidex	Cream: 0.05% concentration	
	Lidex, Vanos	Solution, gel: 0.05% concentration	
		Cream: 0.1%	
fluticasone fumarate	*Veramyst*	35 mcg/spray, nasal spray	
fluticasone propionate	*Cutivate*	Cream: 0.05% concentration	
	Flonase, Flovent Diskus, Flovent HFA	Ointment: 0.005% concentration Nasal spray; 88–220 mcg b.i.d. using nasal inhalation	
halcinonide	*Halog*	Ointment, cream, solution: 0.1% concentration	
halobetasol propionate	*Ultravate*	Ointment, cream: 0.05% concentration	

Table B Topical Agents (*Continued*)

Drug	Brand Name	Dosage	Usual Indications/Special Considerations
hydrocortisone	*Bactine, Hydrocortisone, Cort-Dome, Dermolate, Dermtex HC, Cortizone 10, Hycort, Tegrin-HC*	Lotion: 0.25% concentration Cream, lotion, ointment, aerosol: 0.5%, 1% concentration	
	Hytone	Cream, lotion, ointment, solution: 1% concentration	
hydrocortisone acetate	*Cortaid, Lanacort 5*	Ointment: 0.5% concentration (OTC preparations)	
	Gynecort, Lanacort 5	Cream: 0.5% concentration (OTC preparations)	
	Anusol-HC	Cream: 1% concentration	
	Cortaid with Aloe	Cream: 0.5%, 1% concentration (OTC preparations)	
hydrocortisone buteprate	generic	Cream: 0.1% concentration	
hydrocortisone butyrate	*Locoid*	Ointment, cream: 0.1% concentration	
hydrocortisone probutate	*Pandel*	Ointment cream: 0.1%	
hydrocortisone valerate	*Westcort*	Ointment, cream: 0.2% concentration	
mometasone furoate	*Elocon*	Ointment, cream, lotion: 0.1% concentration	
	Nasonex	Nasal spray: 0.2% concentration	
	Asmanex Twisthaler	Solution for inhalation: 220 mcg/actuation	
prednicarbate	*Dermatop*	Cream: 0.1% concentration (preservative free)	
triamcinolone	generic	Nasal spray	Treatment of nasal symptoms from allergies
triamcinolone acetonide	*Triacet, Triderm*	Cream: 0.025%, 0.5% concentration Cream: 0.1% concentration Lotion: 0.025%, 0.1% concentration	
triamcinolone acetonide/ nystatin	*Mykacet*	Cream: 100,000 unit/gm; 0/1% cream	

OTC, over-the-counter.

Ophthalmic Agents

Ophthalmic agents are drugs that are intended for direct administration into the conjunctiva of the eye. These drugs are used to treat glaucoma (miotics constrict the pupil and decrease the resistance to aqueous flow); to aid in the diagnosis of eye problems (mydriatics dilate the pupil for examination of the retina; cycloplegics paralyze the muscles that control the lens to aid refraction); to treat local ophthalmic infections or inflammation; and to provide relief from the signs and symptoms of allergic reactions. Table C lists some ophthalmic agents and their indications.

These drugs are not generally absorbed systemically because of their method of administration.

Contraindications and Cautions

These drugs are contraindicated in the presence of allergy to the specific drug or to any component of the product being used. Although they are seldom absorbed systemically, caution should be used in any patient who would have problems with the systemic effects of the drugs if they were absorbed systemically.

Adverse Effects

Adverse effects of these drugs include local irritation, stinging, burning, blurring of vision (prolonged when using ointments), tearing, and headache.

Clinically Important Drug–Drug Interactions

Because of their actions on the eye or because of the components of the drug, many of these drugs cannot be given at the same time but should be spaced 1 to 2 hours apart. Check the specific drug being used for details.

Dosage

The usual dosage for any of these drugs is one to two drops in each eye or in the affected eye two to four times daily, or 0.25 to 0.5 in of ointment in the affected eye or eyes.

Nursing Considerations

Assessment

- Screen for the following: allergy to the specific drug or components of the preparation; underlying medical conditions that would be affected if the drug were absorbed systemically.
- Evaluate eye, conjunctival color; note any lesions. A vision examination may be appropriate.

Nursing Diagnoses

The patient receiving an ophthalmic agent may have the following nursing diagnoses related to drug therapy:

- Impaired comfort related to administration of the drug
- Injury risk related to changes in vision
- Knowledge deficit regarding drug therapy

Planning

- The patient will receive the best therapeutic effect from the drug therapy.
- The patient will have limited adverse effects to the drug therapy.
- The patient will have an understanding of the drug therapy, adverse effects to anticipate, and measures to relieve discomfort and improve safety.

Implementation

- Assess the patient's general physical condition before beginning the test to decrease the potential for adverse effects.

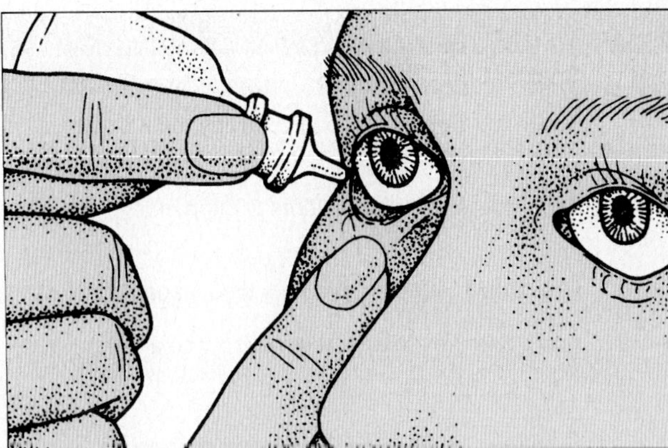

FIGURE C.1 Administration of ophthalmic drops.

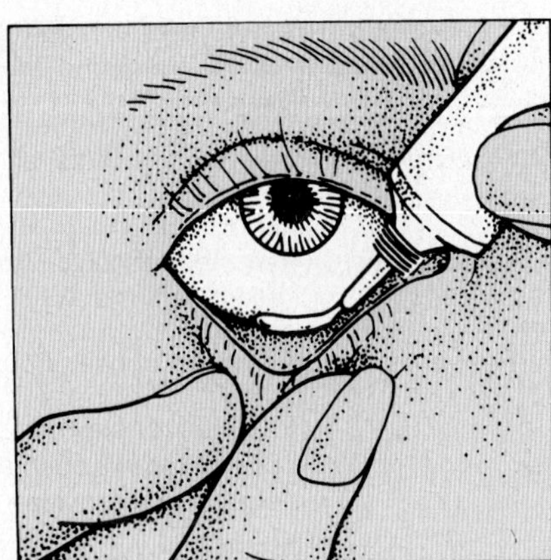

FIGURE C.2 Administration of ophthalmic ointment.

- Follow these administration guidelines to provide the most therapeutic use of the drug with the fewest adverse effects:
  - *Solution or drops*: Wash hands thoroughly before administering; do not touch the dropper to the patient's eye or to any other surface. Have the patient tilt the head backward or lie down, and have the patient stare upward. Gently grasp the lower eyelid and pull the eyelid away from the eyeball; instill drops into the pouch formed by the eyelid. Release the lid slowly; have the patient close the eye and look downward. Apply gentle pressure to the inside corner of the eye for 30 to 60 seconds. Do not rub the eyes; do not rinse the eyedropper. Do not use eye drops that have changed color; if more than one type of eye drop is used, wait at least 5 minutes between administrations. See Figure C.1.
  - *Ointment*: Wash hands thoroughly before administering; hold the tube between the hands for several minutes to warm the ointment. Tilt the patient's head backward or have the patient lie down and stare upward. Gently pull out the lower lid to form a pouch; place 0.25 to 0.5 in of ointment inside the lower lid. Have the patient close the eye for 1 to 2 minutes and roll the eyeball in all directions; remove any excess ointment from around the eye. If using more than one kind of ointment, wait at least 10 minutes between administrations. See Figure C.2.
- Provide comfort measures to help the patient tolerate drug effects (e.g., control light, administer analgesics as needed).
- Include the following information—in addition to the proper administration technique for the drug—in the teaching program for the patient to improve compliance and provide safety and comfort measures as necessary: Safety measures may need to be taken if blurring of vision should occur; burning and stinging may occur on administration but should pass quickly; the pupils will dilate with mydriatic agents, and the eyes may become very sensitive to light (the use of sunglasses is recommended); any severe eye discomfort, palpitations, nausea, or headache should be reported to the health care provider.

Evaluation

- Monitor patient response to the drug (changes in pupil size, relief of pressure of glaucoma, relief of itching and tearing related to allergic reaction).
- Monitor for adverse effects (local irritation, blurring of vision, headache).
- Evaluate the effectiveness of the teaching plan (patient can name adverse effects to watch for and specific measures to avoid them; the patient understands the importance of the follow-up that will be needed).
- Monitor the effectiveness of comfort measures and compliance with the regimen.

Table C Ophthalmic Agents

Drug	Usage	Special Considerations
alcaftadine (*Lastacaft*)	Prevention of itching associated with allergic conjunctivitis	One drop in each eye daily; remove contacts; not for treatment of contact lens irritation.
apraclonidine (*Iopidine*)	To control or prevent postsurgical elevations of IOP after argon laser eye surgery	Monitor for the possibility of vasovagal attack; do not give to patients with allergy to clonidine.
azelastine HCl (generic)	Treatment of ocular itching associated with allergic conjunctivitis	Antihistamine, mast cell stabilizer; dosage (≥3 y): one drop b.i.d.; rapid onset, 8-h duration

(continues on page 1102)

Table C Ophthalmic Agents (*Continued*)

Drug	Usage	Special Considerations
azithromycin (*AzaSite*)	Treatment of bacterial conjunctivitis	Treatment of bacterial conjunctivitis, one drop b.i.d. 8–12 h apart for 2 d, then once a day for 5 d
bepotastine HCl (*Bepreve*)	Treatment of ocular itching associated with allergic rhinitis	Apply twice daily for patients 2 y and older.
besifloxacin (*Besivance*)	Treatment of bacterial conjunctivitis (pink eye)	One drop in affected eye t.i.d. (6–8 h apart) for 7 d
betaxolol hydrochloride (*Betoptic S*)	Treatment of elevated intraocular pressure due to chronic open-angle glaucoma or ocular hypertension	Apply one drop in affected eye/s twice a day
bimatoprost (*Durysta, Latisse, Lumigan*)	Reduction of IOP in patients with open-angle glaucoma or ocular hypertension	Used for patients who are intolerant to other IOP-lowering drugs or who have failed to achieve optimum IOP with other IOP-lowering medications
brimonidine tartrate (*Alphagan P, Lumify, Qoliana*)	Treatment of open-angle glaucoma and ocular hypertension	Selective $alpha_2$-antagonist; minimal effects on cardiovascular and pulmonary systems; do not use with MAOIs; dosage: 1 drop t.i.d.
brimonidine/brinzolamide (*Simbrinza*)	Treatment of increased intraocular pressure in patients with open-angle glaucoma or ocular hypertension	Combination of carbonic anhydrase inhibitor and alpha 2 adrenergic receptor agonist. 1 drop in affected eye(s) t.i.d.
brimonidine with timolol (*Combigan*)	Treatment of IOP	One drop to the affected eye q12h; do not use with contact lenses.
brinzolamide (*Azopt*)	To decrease IOP in open-angle glaucoma	May be given with other agents; dosage: one drop t.i.d.; give 10 min apart from any other agents.
bromfenac (*Bromsite, Prolensa*)	Treatment of postoperative inflammation following cataract surgery	One drop in affected eye b.i.d. starting 24 h after surgery for 2 wk.
carbachol (*Miostat*)	Direct-acting miotic; for treatment of glaucoma; miosis during surgery	Surgical dose: a one-use-only portion; for glaucoma: one to two drops up to t.i.d. as needed.
carteolol (generic)	Reduction of IOP in chronic open-angle glaucoma	One drop in affected eye(s) b.i.d.
cetirizine (0.24%) (*Zerviate*)	Treatment of ocular itching associated with allergic conjunctivitis	1 drop in each affected eye b.i.d. Avoid touching eyelids/surrounding areas w/dropper tip.
ciprofloxacin (*Ciloxan*)	Treatment of ocular infections, conjunctivitis	Apply ¼-inch ribbon to eye sac t.i.d. for 2 d, then b.i.d. for 5 d, or 1–2 drops q2h while awake for 2 d, then q4h for 5 d.
cyclopentolate (*Cyclomydril, Cyclogyl, Pentolair*)	Mydriasis/cycloplegia in diagnostic procedures	Individuals with dark-pigmented irises may require higher doses; compress lacrimal sac for 1–2 min after administration to decrease any systemic absorption.
cyclosporine emulsion (*Cequa, Restasis*)	Increases tear production in patients with decreased tear production related to inflammation or keratoconjunctivitis sicca	One drop in each eye b.i.d., ~12 h apart; remove contact lenses during use.
dexamethasone intravitreal (*Ozurdex*)	Treatment of macular edema following branch retinal artery occlusion or central retinal artery occlusion	Monitor for infection and retinal detachment following injection; use caution with a history of ocular herpes simplex.
diclofenac sodium (*Voltaren Ophthalmic*)	Treatment of photophobia in patients undergoing incisional refractive surgery	Apply one drop q.i.d. beginning 24 h after cataract surgery; continue through the first 2 wk after surgery.
difluprednate (*Durezol*)	Treatment of photophobia in patients undergoing incisional refractory surgery	Administer one drop into the affected eye q.i.d., beginning 2 wk before surgery and continuing for 2 wk after surgery.

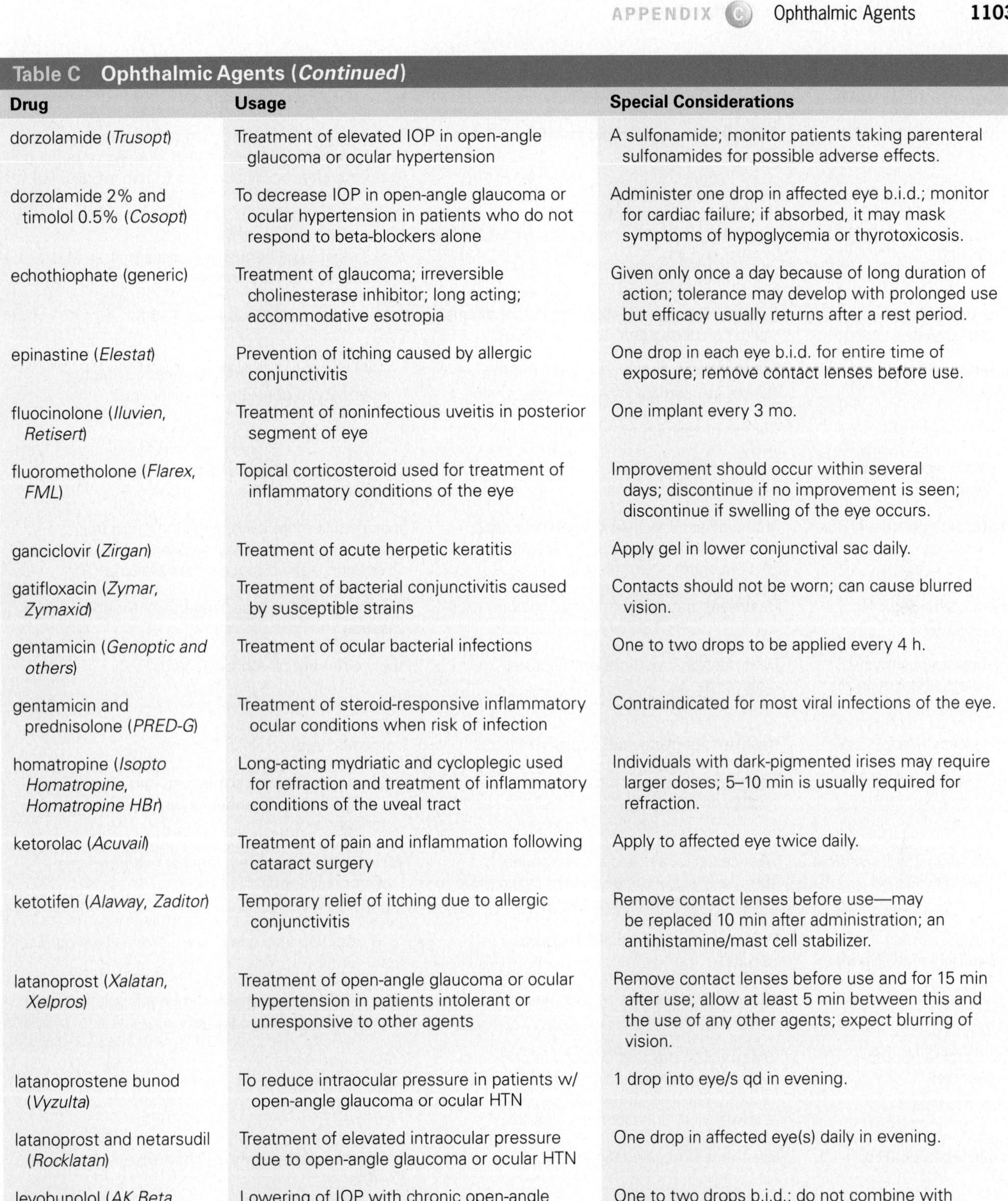

Table C Ophthalmic Agents (*Continued*)

Drug	Usage	Special Considerations
dorzolamide (*Trusopt*)	Treatment of elevated IOP in open-angle glaucoma or ocular hypertension	A sulfonamide; monitor patients taking parenteral sulfonamides for possible adverse effects.
dorzolamide 2% and timolol 0.5% (*Cosopt*)	To decrease IOP in open-angle glaucoma or ocular hypertension in patients who do not respond to beta-blockers alone	Administer one drop in affected eye b.i.d.; monitor for cardiac failure; if absorbed, it may mask symptoms of hypoglycemia or thyrotoxicosis.
echothiophate (generic)	Treatment of glaucoma; irreversible cholinesterase inhibitor; long acting; accommodative esotropia	Given only once a day because of long duration of action; tolerance may develop with prolonged use but efficacy usually returns after a rest period.
epinastine (*Elestat*)	Prevention of itching caused by allergic conjunctivitis	One drop in each eye b.i.d. for entire time of exposure; remove contact lenses before use.
fluocinolone (*Iluvien, Retisert*)	Treatment of noninfectious uveitis in posterior segment of eye	One implant every 3 mo.
fluorometholone (*Flarex, FML*)	Topical corticosteroid used for treatment of inflammatory conditions of the eye	Improvement should occur within several days; discontinue if no improvement is seen; discontinue if swelling of the eye occurs.
ganciclovir (*Zirgan*)	Treatment of acute herpetic keratitis	Apply gel in lower conjunctival sac daily.
gatifloxacin (*Zymar, Zymaxid*)	Treatment of bacterial conjunctivitis caused by susceptible strains	Contacts should not be worn; can cause blurred vision.
gentamicin (*Genoptic and others*)	Treatment of ocular bacterial infections	One to two drops to be applied every 4 h.
gentamicin and prednisolone (*PRED-G*)	Treatment of steroid-responsive inflammatory ocular conditions when risk of infection	Contraindicated for most viral infections of the eye.
homatropine (*Isopto Homatropine, Homatropine HBr*)	Long-acting mydriatic and cycloplegic used for refraction and treatment of inflammatory conditions of the uveal tract	Individuals with dark-pigmented irises may require larger doses; 5–10 min is usually required for refraction.
ketorolac (*Acuvail*)	Treatment of pain and inflammation following cataract surgery	Apply to affected eye twice daily.
ketotifen (*Alaway, Zaditor*)	Temporary relief of itching due to allergic conjunctivitis	Remove contact lenses before use—may be replaced 10 min after administration; an antihistamine/mast cell stabilizer.
latanoprost (*Xalatan, Xelpros*)	Treatment of open-angle glaucoma or ocular hypertension in patients intolerant or unresponsive to other agents	Remove contact lenses before use and for 15 min after use; allow at least 5 min between this and the use of any other agents; expect blurring of vision.
latanoprostene bunod (*Vyzulta*)	To reduce intraocular pressure in patients w/ open-angle glaucoma or ocular HTN	1 drop into eye/s qd in evening.
latanoprost and netarsudil (*Rocklatan*)	Treatment of elevated intraocular pressure due to open-angle glaucoma or ocular HTN	One drop in affected eye(s) daily in evening.
levobunolol (*AK Beta, Betagan Liquifilm*)	Lowering of IOP with chronic open-angle glaucoma, ocular hypertension	One to two drops b.i.d.; do not combine with beta-blockers.
levofloxacin (generic)	Treatment of bacterial conjunctivitis caused by susceptible bacteria	One to two drops per day in affected eye.
lifitegrast (*Xiidra*)	Treatment of signs and symptoms of dry eye	1 drop b.i.d. in each eye (dose 12 h apart). Monitor for visual acuity changes.

(continues on page 1104)

Table C Ophthalmic Agents (*Continued*)

Drug	Usage	Special Considerations
lodoxamide (*Alomide*)	Treatment of vernal conjunctivitis and keratitis	Patients should not wear contact lenses while using this drug; discontinue if stinging or burning persists after instillation; one to two drops q.i.d.
loteprednol etabonate (*Lotemax* [0.5%]), (*Alrex* [0.2%])	Treatment of steroid-resistant ocular disease Treatment of postoperative inflammation after ocular surgery	One to two drops q.i.d. beginning 24 h after surgery and continuing for 2 wk Shake vigorously before use; discard after 14 d; prolonged use may cause nerve or eye damage.
loteprednol with tobramycin (*Zylet*)	Treatment of inflammatory ocular conditions with risk of bacterial ocular infection	Apply one to two drops every 4–6 h.
metipranolol (*OptiPranolol*)	Beta-blocker; used in treating chronic open-angle glaucoma and ocular hypertension	Concomitant therapy may be needed; caution patient about possible vision changes.
mitomycin-C (*Mitosol*)	Control of scarring following trabeculotomy	Applied topically intraoperatively
moxifloxacin (*Moxeza, Vigamox*)	Treatment of bacterial conjunctivitis caused by susceptible strains	Contact lenses should not be worn; can cause blurred vision.
natamycin (*Natacyn*)	Antibiotic used to treat fungal blepharitis, conjunctivitis, and keratitis; drug of choice for *Fusarium solani* keratitis	Shake well before each use; store at room temperature; failure to improve in 7–10 d suggests a nonsusceptible organism; reevaluate.
nedocromil (*Alocril*)	Treatment of itching of allergic conjunctivitis	One to two drops in each eye b.i.d. for entire allergy season.
neomycin/polymyxin B sulfates/bacitracin zinc (*Neosporin*)	Treatment of superficial eye bacterial infections	Apply ointment q3–4h for 7–10 d.
netarsudil (*Rhopressa*)	Treatment of glaucoma, ocular HTN	1 drop into eye/s daily in evening.
ocriplasmin (*Jetrea*)	Treatment of symptomatic vitreomacular adhesion	0.125 mg by intravitreal injection into affected eye as single dose. Potential for lens subluxation. Monitor vision.
olopatadine hydrochloride (*Pataday, Pazeo*)	Mast cell stabilizer and antihistamine; provides fast onset of relief of itching due to conjunctivitis and has prolonged action	Not for use with contact lenses; headache is a common side effect.
oxymetazoline hydrochloride (*Upneeq*)	Treatment of acquired blepharoptosis in adults	Instill one drop into one or both ptotic eye/s once a day.
phenylephrine/ketorolac (*Omidria*)	Prevent intraoperative miosis; pain relief with cataract surgery	4 mL in 500 mL ophthalmic irrigating solution used when needed during surgery.
pilocarpine (*Isopto Carpine*)	Treatment of elevated intraocular pressure with open-angle glaucoma or ocular HTN, acute glaucoma; pretention of postoperative elevated IOP; induction of miosis	1 drop up to 4 x/d.
sulfacetamide (*Bleph-10*)	Treatment of ocular infections	One to two drops every 2–3 h; gradually taper over 7–10 d.
tafluprost (*Zioptan*)	Reduction of IOP in patients with open-angle glaucoma or ocular hypertension	One drop in affected eye(s) once daily in the evening.
timolol (*Timoptic-XE*)	Treatment of elevated IOP in ocular hypertension or open-angle glaucoma	One drop in affected eye(s) each day in the morning.
travoprost (*Travatan Z*)	Reduction of IOP in patients with open-angle glaucoma or ocular hypertension	Reserve for patients who are intolerant of other IOP-lowering medications or who have failed to achieve optimum IOP with other IOP-lowering medications.

Table C Ophthalmic Agents (*Continued*)

Drug	Usage	Special Considerations
trifluridine (*Viroptic*)	Antiviral; used to treat primary keratoconjunctivitis and recurrent epithelial keratitis due to herpes simplex virus types 1 and 2	Transient burning or stinging may occur; reconsider drug choice if improvement is not seen within 7 d; do not administer longer than 21 d at a time.
tropicamide (*Mydriacyl, Tropicacyl*)	Mydriatic and cycloplegic for refraction	One to two drops, repeat in 5 min; may repeat in 30 min for prolonged effects.
tropicamide and hydroxyamphetamine (*Paremyd*)	Mydriasis in routine diagnostic procedures where need short term pupil dilation	1–2 drops
voretigene neparvovec (*Luxturna*)	Treatment of vision loss due to biallelic *RPE65*-mediated inherited retinal disease	0.3 mL injected subretinally in each eye on separate days but no fewer than 6 d apart. Systemic oral corticosteroids administered concomitantly.

IOP, intraocular pressure; MAOI, monoamine oxidase inhibitor.

APPENDIX D

Ear Medications

Optic agents are drugs that are intended for direct administration into the ear. These drugs are used to treat otitis externa. Otitis externa (swimmer's ear) is due to a bacterial infection in the external auditory canal. Growth of bacteria in the external ear canal is more common if there has been any abrasion and/or conditions causing excessive moisture. Avoidance of manual removal of cerumen refraining from putting foreign objects in the ear canal can decrease risk of abrasions. Teach swimmers to decrease risk of otitis externa by encouraging drying the ear canal using a towel and tilting his/her head to remove water as soon as swimming is completed. These medications can also be used to soften and facilitate removal of excess earwax or water inside the ear canal. Ear medications are listed in Table D.

These drugs are not generally absorbed systemically because of their method of administration.

Contraindications and Cautions

These drugs are contraindicated in the presence of allergy to the specific drug or to any component of the product being used. They are contraindicated if there is perforation of the tympanic membrane.

Adverse Effects

Adverse effects of these drugs include local irritation, rash, and central nervous system effects (dizziness, lightheadedness). Much more likely to cause dizziness if solution is cold.

Clinically Important Drug–Drug Interactions

Due to being instilled in the ear canal, there are not clinical drug–drug interactions.

Dosage

The recommended number of drops can vary per medication and indication. Often 3 to 5 drops should be instilled 2 to 4 times a day.

Nursing Considerations

Assessment

- Screen for the following: allergy to the specific drug or components of the preparation to reduce risk of allergic reaction.
- Evaluate ear; note any lesions. A hearing examination may be appropriate.

Nursing Diagnoses

The patient receiving an optic agent may have the following nursing diagnoses related to drug therapy:

- Impaired comfort related to administration of the drug
- Injury risk related to possible central nervous system adverse effects
- Knowledge deficit regarding drug therapy

Planning

- The patient will receive the best therapeutic effect from the drug therapy.
- The patient will have limited adverse effects to the drug therapy.
- The patient will have an understanding of the drug therapy, adverse effects to anticipate, and measures to relieve discomfort and improve safety.

Implementation

- Assess the patient's general physical condition before beginning the test to decrease the potential for adverse effects.

- Follow these administration guidelines to provide the most therapeutic use of the drug with the fewest adverse effects:
  - *Solution or drops:* Clients can be positioned sitting upright or laying on their side. Ensure that the medication is at room temperature or warmer since cold solutions have increased risk of causing dizziness. Pull auricle of ear up and out (adults) (see Fig. D.1) and back (kids less than 3 years) (see Fig. D.2) to straighten the ear canal. Hold the medication dropper about 1 cm from ear canal to instill the medication. Gently press on tragus of ear unless this causes the patient pain. If possible, instruct the patient to continue to lay in side position for 2 to 5 minutes after administration. If needed a cotton ball can be placed in the outermost part of the ear canal but should not be packed in deeply.
- Provide comfort measures to help the patient tolerate drug effects (e.g., warm solution to room temperature, administer analgesics as needed).
- Include the following information—in addition to the proper administration technique for the drug—in the teaching program for the patient to improve compliance and provide safety and comfort measures as necessary: Safety measures may need to be taken if patient becomes dizzy and prone to falling.

Evaluation

- Monitor patient response to the drug (changes in ear pain, relief of ear pressure, relief of itching within ear canal, hearing changes).
- Monitor for adverse effects (local irritation, blurring of vision, headache).
- Evaluate the effectiveness of the teaching plan (patient can name adverse effects to watch for and specific measures to avoid them; the patient understands the importance of the follow-up that will be needed).
- Monitor the effectiveness of comfort measures and compliance with the regimen.

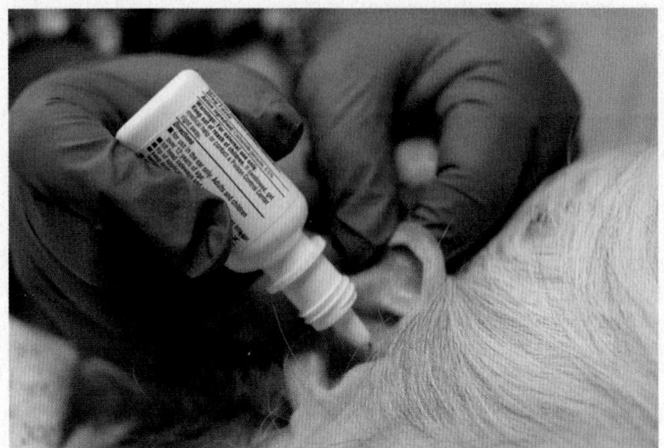

FIGURE D.1 Pulling the pinna up and back and placing dropper tip above auditory canal to administer ear medication to adults and kids older than 3 years old.

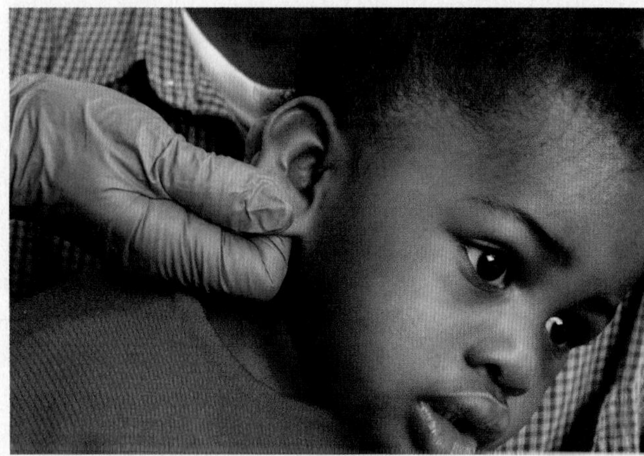

FIGURE D.2 Pulling pinna down and back for an infant or child younger than 3 years.

Table D Ear Medications

Drug	Usage	Special Considerations
acetic acid (*Vosol*)	Treatment of superficial infections of external auditory canal	Contraindicated if perforated tympanic membrane. Insert cotton saturation with medication and apply 3–5 drops every 4–6 hours. Cotton can be removed after 24 hours, and drops can be applied to ear canal as prescribed.
acetic acid and hydrocortisone (*Vosol HC*)	Treatment of superficial infections of external auditory canal	Contraindicated if perforated tympanic membrane. Insert cotton saturation with medication and apply 3–5 drops every 4–6 hours. Cotton can be removed after 24 hours, and drops can be applied to ear canal as prescribed.
carbamide peroxide (*Debrox, Murine, Mollifene* and others)	To soften, loosen, and remove excessive earwax	Place 5–10 drops in affected ear twice a day for up to 4 days. Provider should be consulted before use if ear drainage, ear pain, or recent ear injury/surgery.
chloroxylenol, hydrocortisone, pramoxine (*Cyotic, Exotic-HC, Cortic-ND, Cortane B, Aero Otic HC*)	Treat infections in outer ear canal; relieve minor ear pain and itching	Warm and instill prescribed number of drops in affected ear/s twice a day.
ciprofloxacin (*Cetraxal, Otiprio*)	Treatment of otitis externa and bilateral otitis media with effusion undergoing tympanostomy tube placement	Should be administered only by health care professional.
ciprofloxacin, dexamethasone (*Ciprodex*)	Treatment of infections that cause otitis media in pediatric patients with tympanostomy tubes and acute otitis externa	Place 4 drops in affected ear/s twice a day for 7 days.
ciprofloxacin, fluocinolone (*Otovel*)	Treatment of acute otitis media with tympanostomy tubes in pediatric patients	Instill single-dose vial into affected ear canal twice a day for 7 days.
ciprofloxacin, hydrocortisone (*Cipro HC*)	Treatment of otitis externa	Shake and warm before instilling in ear. Instill 3 drops in affected ear/s twice a day for 7 days.
colistin sulfate, neomycin sulfate, thonzonium bromide, hydrocortisone acetate (*Cortisporin-TC, Coly-Mycin S*)	Treatment of superficial bacterial infections of the external auditory canal; should not be used for viral infections	Shake well before use. Instill 4–5 drops in affected ear/s 3–4 times a day for no more than 10 days.
hydrocortisone, neomycin, polymyxin (*Oticair*)	Treat ear infections caused by bacteria	Apply drops to affected ear/s 3–4 times a day for prescribed duration.
hydrocortisone, neomycin, polymyxin b (*Cortomycin, Cort-Biotic, Casporyn HC*)	Treat infections of ear canal and relieves redness and discomfort in ear canal	Shake bottle before instilling medication in ear canal of affected ears. Instill prescribed number of drops at the prescribed frequency.
fluocinolone (*DermOtic*)	Treatment of chronic eczematous external otitis	5 drops twice a day in affected ear/s for 7–14 days. Product contains refined peanut oil.
isopropyl alcohol (*Auro-Dri*)	Dries water in ears and relieves water filled ears	Apply 4–5 drops in each affected ear. Provider should be consulted before use if ear drainage, ear pain, or recent ear injury/surgery.
ofloxacin (generic)	Treatment of otitis externa, chronic otitis media and acute otitis media	Apply drops in affected ears as prescribed. Frequency and duration varies per indication.

Blood and Blood Products

Blood and blood products are indicated to increase intravascular volume; replace blood lost due to trauma, surgery, or other types of bleeding; and replace clotting factors. Figure E.1 illustrates an example of blood administration. Table E lists several blood products including whole blood, packed red blood cells (pRBCs), platelets, fresh frozen plasma, apheresed granulocytes, and albumin. ABO typing is required prior to blood product administration except for autologous transfusions. If blood products with red blood cells are to be transfused, the patient must also be tested for Rh antigens and have cross-matching performed to check for antibodies that could react to the donor's blood.

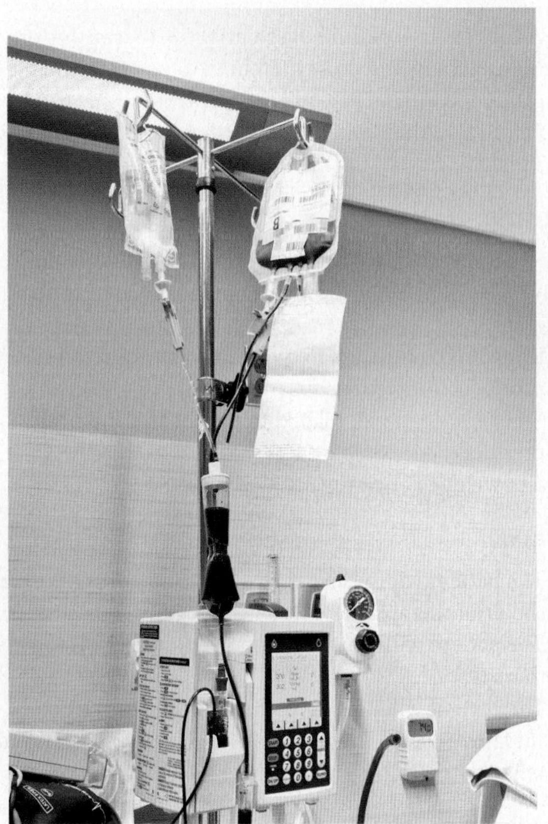

FIGURE E.1 An example of blood administration.

Contraindications and Cautions

These products are contraindicated in patients who hypersensitivity reactions. Caution should be taken in patients with risk of fluid overload. Some patients may have objection to blood products due to cultural and/or religious values.

Adverse Effects

Adverse effects of these drugs include acute hemolytic reactions, febrile nonhemolytic reactions, anaphylactic reactions, mild allergic reactions, fluid overload, sepsis, hyperkalemia due to blood cell lysis, and transfusion-associated graft versus host disease. Immune hemolytic transfusion reactions occur when the donor RBC are lysed by antibodies in the patient getting the transfusion. Nonimmune hemolytic transfusion reactions can be due to mechanical stress, improper storage, infusion with incompatible substances, temperature extremes, or chemical reactions. Signs and symptoms that a patient is having an acute hemolytic reaction include fever, chills, low back pain, tachycardia, tachypnea, and hypotension. Febrile nonhemolytic reactions are fairly common and may be caused by cytokines that are generated during storage of the blood products. A patient may present with chills, headache, flushing, anxiety, muscle pains, and fever when suffering from a febrile nonhemolytic reaction. Allergic reactions can range from mild to severe (anaphylactic). Signs and symptoms of a mild reaction include flushing, itching, and rash/hives. Anaphylactic reactions can also present with hives in addition to wheezing, bronchospasm, shock, and can progress to cardiac arrest. Fluid overload occurs when the blood volume administered is higher than what the patients' circulation system is able to handle. Patients with heart failure and renal failure are at higher risk. Signs and symptoms include cough, shortness of breath, lung sounds with crackles, tachycardia, distended neck veins, hypertension, and pulmonary edema demonstrated on chest x-ray. Transfusion-associated graft versus host disease is a rare posttransfusion reaction in

Table E Blood and Blood Products

Drug	Usage	Special Considerations
Albumin	Treatment of hypovolemia, hypoalbuminemia, burns, and other situations requiring increased circulatory blood volume	Risk of fluid volume excess and subsequent pulmonary edema.
Apheresed granulocytes	Treatment of severe neutropenia, life-threatening infection not responding to antibiotics, neonatal sepsis, neutrophil dysfunction	Adverse reactions include acute hemolytic reaction, febrile nonhemolytic reaction, anaphylactic reactions, circulatory overload, and sepsis
Fresh frozen plasma	Treatment of active bleeding, extensive burns, shock, disseminated intravascular coagulation, emergent reversal of warfarin, and antithrombin III deficiency. Replacement therapy for coagulation factors II, V, VII, IX, X, and XI	Adverse reactions include acute hemolytic reaction, febrile nonhemolytic reaction, anaphylactic reactions, circulatory overload, and sepsis
Packed red blood cells	Treatment of severe anemia, hemolytic anemia of the fetus, hemoglobinopathies	Adverse reactions include acute hemolytic reaction, febrile nonhemolytic reaction, anaphylactic reactions, circulatory overload, hyperkalemia, transfusion-associated graft versus host disease, and sepsis
Platelet concentrate	Treatment of thrombocytopenia and/or active bleeding when low platelet count	Adverse reactions include febrile nonhemolytic reaction, mild allergic reactions, and sepsis
Whole blood	Replacement for acute blood loss due to trauma or surgery and for volume expansion for patients with extensive burns, dehydration, and/or shock	Adverse reactions include acute hemolytic reaction, febrile nonhemolytic reaction, anaphylactic reactions, circulatory overload, hyperkalemia, transfusion-associated graft versus host disease, and sepsis

which the donor's white blood cells attack the recipient's tissues. Signs and symptoms typically present 1 to 2 weeks after the transfusion and include nausea, vomiting, liver dysfunction, and pancytopenia.

Clinically Important Drug–Drug Interactions

The products are administered intravenously and should not be combined in the IV tubing with other products.

Dosage

Dosage will vary based on patient needs and deficiencies.

Nursing Considerations

Assessment

- Screen for the following: allergy to the components of the preparation to reduce risk of allergic reaction.
- Assess if baseline lab values (hemoglobin, hematocrit, platelet counts, total protein, albumin levels, prothrombin, fibrinogen, and potassium) are indicated prior to administration of product.
- Assess for risk of fluid overload prior to transfusion.
- Blood typing and cross matching to be performed if product contains RBCs.
- Prior to administration ensure that the patient has signed a consent for the transfusion.

Nursing Diagnoses

The patient receiving blood or blood products may have the following nursing diagnoses related to drug therapy:

- Impaired comfort related to administration of the products intravenously
- Fluid overload risk related to administration of the product
- Knowledge deficit regarding drug therapy

Planning

- The patient will receive the best therapeutic effect from the drug therapy.
- The patient will have limited adverse effects to the drug therapy.
- The patient will have an understanding of the drug therapy, adverse effects to anticipate, and measures to relieve discomfort and improve safety.

Implementation

- Assess IV patency and ensure IV at least 20-gauge or larger.

- Follow these administration guidelines to provide the most therapeutic use of the drug with the fewest adverse effects:
  - Perform safety checks per institution policy to ensure the correct product is administered to correct patient.
  - Monitor vital signs per facility policy (typically pretransfusion, 15 to 30 minutes poststart of infusion, and at least every hour until completed infusion).
  - Prime tubing with 0.9% sodium chloride. Use correct IV tubing per institution policy and available supply.
  - Document blood product type, total volume infused, time of start and end, vital signs, and any adverse effects.
  - Observe universal precautions when handling and performing the transfusion.
- Stop transfusion and notify provider if signs/symptoms of transfusion reaction.
  - Monitor patient, vital signs, and urinary output.
  - If normal saline is indicated administer via new tubing.
  - Document timing of signs/symptoms and amount of product that had been infused.
  - Notify blood bank and return blood bag and IV tubing for analysis.

Evaluation

- Monitor patient response to the transfusion (resolution of fluid and/or product deficiencies, anemia).
- Monitor for adverse effects (vital sign changes, rash, difficulty breathing, flank pain, changes in urine output).
- Evaluate the effectiveness of the teaching plan (patient can name adverse effects to watch for and specific measures to avoid them; the patient understands the importance of the follow-up that will be needed).
- Monitor the effectiveness of comfort measures and compliance with the regimen.

REFERENCE

Sharma, S., Sharma, P., & Tyler, L. N. (2011). Transfusion of blood and blood products: Indications and complications. *American Family Physician, 83*(6), 719–724. https://www.aafp.org/afp/2011/0315/afp20110315p719.pdf

APPENDIX F

Diagnostic Agents

Some pharmacological agents are used solely to diagnose particular conditions. Diagnostic tests that use these agents include the following:

- In vitro tests, which are done outside the body to measure the presence of particular elements (e.g., proteins, blood glucose, bacteria)
- In vivo tests, which introduce drugs into the body to evaluate specific physiological functions (e.g., cardiac output, intestinal absorption, gastric acid secretion)

Diagnostic agents are listed in Table F.

Therapeutic Actions and Indications

In vitro tests are often performed as part of the nursing evaluation of a patient, or they may be done at home by the patient as part of a medical regimen. These drugs can include reagents that react with specific substances within the body, such as glucose, blood, or human chorionic gonadotropin (HCG). Drugs used for in vivo tests may stimulate or suppress normal body reactions, such as a glucose challenge to evaluate insulin release or thyroid suppression tests to evaluate thyroid response. Specific tests of blood, urine, or other bodily fluids are often needed to evaluate the body's response to these drugs and to make a diagnosis. Drugs given as part of in vivo tests are administered under the supervision of medical personnel who are either conducting the test or making the diagnosis. They are usually given only once or used over a short period of time. Their use is part of an overall diagnostic plan to determine the underlying source of a particular problem.

Contraindications and Cautions

The use of any of the in vivo drugs is contraindicated in cases of allergy to the drugs themselves or to the colorants or preservatives used in them. Specific agents may be contraindicated in conditions that could be exacerbated by the stimulation of particular body responses. These drugs should be used cautiously during pregnancy or lactation.

Adverse Effects

The adverse effects seen with diagnostic agents are usually associated with the suppression or stimulation of the response they are being used to test. Because these drugs are given as only part of a test, the adverse effects usually last for a short period and can be tolerated by the patient.

Clinically Important Drug–Drug Interactions

Drug interactions vary with the particular agent that is being used. Consult a drug guide for specific information before giving any diagnostic agent.

Clinically Important Drug–Food Interactions

Because these tests are designed to elicit specific responses, there is often the possibility that food will interfere with the actions or sensitivity of the test. Consult a drug guide for specific information about drug–food interactions before giving any diagnostic agent.

Nursing Considerations

Assessment: History and Examination

- Screen for the following conditions, which could be contraindications to use of the agent: presence of known allergy to any of these drugs or to the colorants or preservatives used in these drugs.
- Include screening for baseline status before beginning therapy and for any potential adverse effects. Assess the following: skin and mucous membrane condition; orientation, affect, and reflexes; pulse, blood pressure, and respirations; abdominal examination; bowel sounds; and blood and urine tests required for the particular test being performed.

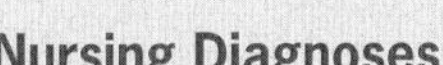

Nursing Diagnoses

The patient receiving a diagnostic agent might have the following nursing diagnoses related to drug therapy:

- Impaired comfort related to effects of the drugs
- Risk of anxiety related to the test being done and possible test results
- Altered body image related to testing procedure and related tests that must be done
- Knowledge deficit regarding drug therapy

Planning

- The patient will receive the best therapeutic effect from the drug therapy.
- The patient will have limited adverse effects to the drug therapy.
- The patient will have an understanding of the drug therapy, adverse effects to anticipate, and measures to relieve discomfort and improve safety.

Implementation

- Assess the patient's general physical condition before beginning the test to decrease the potential for adverse effects.
- Provide comfort measures to help patient tolerate drug effects (e.g., give the drug with food to decrease gastrointestinal upset, provide proper skin care as needed, administer analgesics for headache as appropriate, provide privacy for the collection and storage of urine samples).
- Include information about the drug being used in a test (e.g., what to expect, adverse effects that may occur, follow-up tests that may be needed) to enhance patient knowledge about drug therapy and promote compliance with the drug regimen.

Evaluation

- Monitor patient response to the drug (adverse reactions, collection of diagnostic information).
- Monitor for adverse effects (neurological effects, gastrointestinal upset, skin reaction, hypoglycemia, constipation).
- Evaluate the effectiveness of teaching plan (patient can name adverse effects to watch for and specific measures to avoid them; patient understands importance of follow-up that will be needed).
- Monitor the effectiveness of comfort measures and compliance with the regimen.

Table F Diagnostic Agents

Test Object	Brand Names	Usual Indications	Special Considerations
In Vitro Tests			
Acetone	*Acetest*	Test for ketones in urine, blood, serum, or plasma	Most frequently used to test urine; *Acetest* is the only product that is also used for blood products.
Albumin	*Albustix, Chemstrip Micral*	At-home urine test for the presence of proteins	Advise patient to follow product storage instructions.
Urine bacteria	*Azo Test Strips, Microstix-3, Uricult, Isocult for Bacteriuria*	Test for urine nitrates, uropathogens, gram-negative bacteria	Most accurate if used with a clean-catch urine sample
Bilirubin	*Ictotest*	Test for urine bilirubin levels	Most accurate if used with a clean-catch urine sample
Blood urea nitrogen (BUN)	*Azostix*	Estimate of BUN	Used as a reagent strip with whole blood
Candida tests	*Isocult for Candida*	Culture paddles or reagent slides for testing vaginal smears	Rapid test for the presence of *Candida* with vaginal examination
Chlamydia trachomatis	*Amplicor, Chlamydiazyme, MicroTrak for Chlamydia, Surecell Chlamydia, Clearview Chlamydia, LetsGetChecked*	Kits and slides for testing urogenital, rectal, conjunctival, and nasopharyngeal specimens for the presence of *Chlamydia*	Kits are specific for testing specimens.

(continues on page 1114)

Table F Diagnostic Agents (*Continued*)

Test Object	Brand Names	Usual Indications	Special Considerations
Cholesterol	*Advanced Care Cholesterol Test, Cholestrak Total Home Testing Kit, CardioChek Analyzer Starter Cholesterol Kit, KPI Blood Total Cholesterol Test Kit, SELFCheck Cholesterol Test Kit, and others*	At-home cholesterol test	Kit includes audio instructions; patient should be cautioned to seek medical care and advice.
COVID-19	*BinaxNOW, Ellume, LetsGetChecked, Pixel, and others*	Test kits for COVID-19 antigen	Most are nasal swabs.
Glucose, blood	*Glucostix Glucometer Elite, Accu-Chek, Advantage*, and others	At-home testing of blood glucose levels	Patient should be taught how to calibrate the machine, proper blood-drawing technique, and importance of seeking follow-up medical care.
Glucose, urine	*Diastix, Keto-Diastix*	At-home testing of urine glucose, ketones	Used as reagent strip for urine; discard after 6 mo.
Gonorrhea	*Biocult-GC, Isocult for Neisseria gonorrhoeae, LetsGetChecked*	Kits and culture paddles for the detection of *N. gonorrhoeae* on endocervical, rectal, urethral, and oropharyngeal specimens	Test kits containing reagents, preservatives as needed for detection of *N. gonorrhoeae* during physical examination
Hepatitis B and C	*LetsGetChecked, iCare and others*	Kits to detect hepatitis B and C	May get kits for one or both.
Mononucleosis	*Mono-Plus, Mono-Diff, Mono-Spot*, and others	Kits, reagents, and slides for the testing of serum and blood for mononucleosis	Rapid tests for suspected cases of mononucleosis; all necessary reagents and preservatives are included in the kit.
Occult blood	*EZ Detect, Hemoccult II*, and others	Kits and slides for the testing of fecal swabs for the presence of occult blood	Card forms can be used by patient at home in routine screening programs.
Ovulation	*Answer*, Clearblue Digital Ovulation Predictor Kit, PREGMATE Ovulation and pregnancy test Strips, *OvuQuick Self-Test, First Response Ovulation Predictor*, and others	Kits to determine the levels of luteinizing hormone in the urine as a predictor of ovulation	Used at home by patient as part of fertility program; patient may need instruction
Pregnancy	*Advance, First Response, Pregnosis*, and others	Kits or urine strips to detect the presence of HCG as a predictor of pregnancy	These may be used at home; patient may need instruction and should be advised to seek follow-up medical care.
Rheumatoid factor and biomarkers for rheumatoid arthritis	*Imaware, Rheumatoid Factor Test, Rheumaton*	Slide tests for the presence of rheumatoid factor in blood, serum, or synovial fluid; some products also test for citrullinated peptide antibody	An aid in the diagnosis of autoimmune diseases
Sickle cell	*Sickledex*	Kit for the testing of blood for the presence of hemoglobin S	Diagnostic for sickle cell anemia
Streptococci	*Sure Cell Streptococci, Culturette 10 Minute Group A Strep ID, Bactigen B Streptococcus*, and others	Kits, slides, and culture paddles for the identification of streptococcal infection in blood, serum, urine, throat, and cerebrospinal fluid	Early detection of streptococcal infection to facilitate beginning of treatment before culture and sensitivity results are known
Urinalysis	*Chemstrip, Diagnox Urinox, QTEST*	May be able to detect acidity, pH, leukocytes, protein, glucose, ketones, bilirubin, blood, and other substances in urine	Strip types vary in what information will be available

Table F Diagnostic Agents (*Continued*)

Test Object	Brand Names	Usual Indications	Special Considerations
In Vivo Tests			
Arginine	*R-Gene 10*	Diagnostic aid to assess pituitary reserve of growth hormone	IV infusion, followed by blood tests to monitor response
Benzylpenicilloyl polylysine	*Pre-Pen*	Skin test to evaluate sensitivity to penicillin and safety of administering penicillin in potentially sensitive individuals	Intradermal or scratch test is used; positive reaction is usually seen within 10–15 min
Indocyanine green	Generic	Determining cardiac output, hepatic function, and liver blood flow; also used for ophthalmic angiography	Use caution in patient with known allergy to dyes
Methacholine chloride	*Provocholine*	Diagnosis of bronchial airway hypersensitivity in patients without documented asthma	Inhaled with pulmonary function test immediately; may cause hypotension, chest pain, or gastrointestinal upset
Secretin	Generic	Diagnosis of pancreatic exocrine disease; diagnosis of gastrinoma	Requires a 12- to 15-h fast; passing of a radiopaque tube for pancreatic function or repeated blood samples for gastrinoma diagnosis
Sincalide	*Kinevac*	Stimulation of gallbladder contractions, pancreatic secretion to evaluate for stones, enzyme activity	*Gallbladder:* Given IV over 30–60 s *Pancreatic function:* Given IV over 60 min
Sodium iodide	*Sodium Iodide I-123*	Diagnosis of thyroid function or morphology	Handle with care; oral capsules are radioactive, dispose of properly; thyroid can be evaluated for radiation content within 6 h of dose
Thyrotropin alpha	*Thyrogen*	Differentiation of thyroid function to estimate thyroid reserve	Given IM every 24 h for two doses; follow with radioactive iodine and thyroid scan.

APPENDIX G

Tables of Normal Values

Values and units of measurement listed in these tables (Tables G.1 to G.4) are derived from several resources. Substantial variation exists in the ranges quoted as "normal" and may vary depending on the assay used by different laboratories. Therefore, these tables should be considered as directional only. Some values (e.g., hormones) vary by sex, age, time of day, and condition (e.g., pregnancy), so a text on endocrinology should be consulted for complete data. Where possible, Canadian sources are used; globalrph.com was used to provide non-SI unit conversions.

Abbreviations: CCS, Canadian Cardiovascular Society; HDL, high-density lipoprotein; LDL, low-density lipoprotein; MCC, Medical Council of Canada; PSA, prostate-specific antigen; TIBC, total iron-binding capacity.

Table G.1 Vital Signs and Body Mass Index

Parameter	Normal Values
Blood Pressure (Systolic/Diastolic)	
Hypertension	
Normal	<120/80 mm Hg
Elevated	<130/80 mm Hg
Hypertension	>130/80 mm Hg
Heart Rate (HR) or Pulse	
Bradycardia	<60 beats/min
Normal	60–100 beats/min
Tachycardia	>100 beats/min
Respiration Rate (RR)	
Bradypnea	<12 breaths/min
Normal (eupnea)	12–18 breaths/min
Tachypnea	>18 breaths/min
Body Temperature	
Fever	>37.5°C
Normal	36.5°C–37.5°C (approximate)
Hypothermia	<35.0°C
Body Mass Index (BMI)	
Underweight	<18.5 kg/m^2
Normal	18.5–24.9 kg/m^2 (Caucasian)
Overweight	25.0–29.9 kg/m^2
Obese	30.0 and > kg/m^2

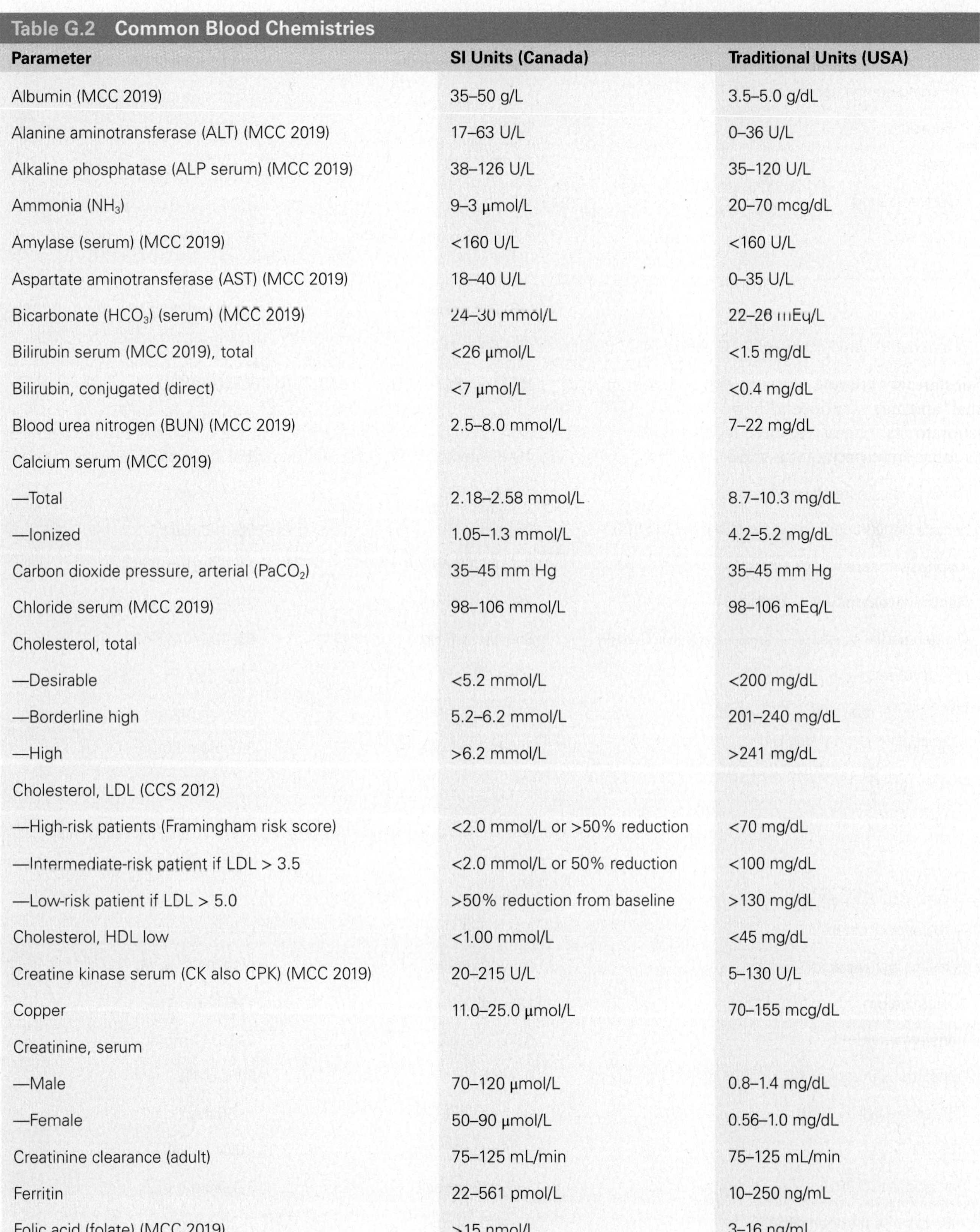

Table G.2 Common Blood Chemistries

Parameter	SI Units (Canada)	Traditional Units (USA)
Albumin (MCC 2019)	35–50 g/L	3.5–5.0 g/dL
Alanine aminotransferase (ALT) (MCC 2019)	17–63 U/L	0–36 U/L
Alkaline phosphatase (ALP serum) (MCC 2019)	38–126 U/L	35–120 U/L
Ammonia (NH_3)	9–3 µmol/L	20–70 mcg/dL
Amylase (serum) (MCC 2019)	<160 U/L	<160 U/L
Aspartate aminotransferase (AST) (MCC 2019)	18–40 U/L	0–35 U/L
Bicarbonate (HCO_3) (serum) (MCC 2019)	24–30 mmol/L	22–28 mEq/L
Bilirubin serum (MCC 2019), total	<26 µmol/L	<1.5 mg/dL
Bilirubin, conjugated (direct)	<7 µmol/L	<0.4 mg/dL
Blood urea nitrogen (BUN) (MCC 2019)	2.5–8.0 mmol/L	7–22 mg/dL
Calcium serum (MCC 2019)		
—Total	2.18–2.58 mmol/L	8.7–10.3 mg/dL
—Ionized	1.05–1.3 mmol/L	4.2–5.2 mg/dL
Carbon dioxide pressure, arterial ($PaCO_2$)	35–45 mm Hg	35–45 mm Hg
Chloride serum (MCC 2019)	98–106 mmol/L	98–106 mEq/L
Cholesterol, total		
—Desirable	<5.2 mmol/L	<200 mg/dL
—Borderline high	5.2–6.2 mmol/L	201–240 mg/dL
—High	>6.2 mmol/L	>241 mg/dL
Cholesterol, LDL (CCS 2012)		
—High-risk patients (Framingham risk score)	<2.0 mmol/L or >50% reduction	<70 mg/dL
—Intermediate-risk patient if LDL > 3.5	<2.0 mmol/L or 50% reduction	<100 mg/dL
—Low-risk patient if LDL > 5.0	>50% reduction from baseline	>130 mg/dL
Cholesterol, HDL low	<1.00 mmol/L	<45 mg/dL
Creatine kinase serum (CK also CPK) (MCC 2019)	20–215 U/L	5–130 U/L
Copper	11.0–25.0 µmol/L	70–155 mcg/dL
Creatinine, serum		
—Male	70–120 µmol/L	0.8–1.4 mg/dL
—Female	50–90 µmol/L	0.56–1.0 mg/dL
Creatinine clearance (adult)	75–125 mL/min	75–125 mL/min
Ferritin	22–561 pmol/L	10–250 ng/mL
Folic acid (folate) (MCC 2019)	>15 nmol/L	3–16 ng/mL

(continues on page 1118)

Table G.2 Common Blood Chemistries (*Contiuned*)

Parameter	SI Units (Canada)	Traditional Units (USA)
Gamma glutamyl transferase (GGT)		
—Female	10–30 U/L	5–36 U/L
—Male	10–48 U/L	8–61 U/L
Glucose, fasting		
—Normal	3.3–5.8 mmol/L	59–105 mg/dL
Glucose, postprandial		
—Normal	3.8–11.1 mmol/L	<120 mg/dL
Glycosylated hemoglobin—HbA1C normal (MCC 2019)	4%–6%	4%–5.7%
Beta-hydroxybutyrate	<270 μmol/L	<2.8 mg/dL
Iron (MCC 2019)	11–32 μmol/L	60–178 pg/dL
Iron-binding capacity, total—TIBC	45–82 μmol/L	251–460 pg/dL
Lactic acid (lactate plasma venous)	1–1.8 mmol/L	9–16 mg/dL
Lactate dehydrogenase serum (LDH) (MCC 2019)	95–195 U/L	95–195 IU/L
Magnesium serum	0.75–0.95 mmol/L	1.82–2.31 mg/dL
Osmolality serum (MCC 2019)	280–300 mmol/kg	280–300 mOsm/kg
Oxygen partial pressure, arterial—PaO_2 (MCC 2019)	85–105 mm Hg	85–105 mm Hg
pH—arterial	7.35–7.45 pH	7.35–7.45 pH
Phosphorus, inorganic (MCC 2019)	0.80–1.50 mmol/L	2.5–4.5 mg/dL
Potassium	3.5–5.0 mmol/L	3.5–5.0 mEq/L
Protein, total		
—Plasma	60–80 g/L	6.0–8.0 g/dL
—Urine	<0.15 g/d	<150 mg/24 h
PSA serum (MCC 2019)		
—40 years or older	0–4 mcg/L	0–4 mcg/L
Pyruvate (pyruvic acid)	31–102 μmol/L	0.30–0.90 mg/dL
Sodium serum	135–145 mmol/L	135–145 mEq/L
Transferrin serum	1.88–3.41 g/L	188–341 mg/dL
Transferrin saturation	0.2–0.5	20%–50%
Triglyceride (MCC 2019)	<1.7 mmol/L	<150 mg/dL
Troponin T	<0.01 mg/L	<0.01 mcg/L
Uric acid (MCC 2019)	180–420 μmol/L	3.0–7.0 mg/dL
—Blood urea nitrogen (BUN)	2.5–8.0 mmol/L	7–22.4 mg/dL
Vitamin B_{12} (*Cyanocobalamin*)	133–674 pmol/L	100–700 pg/mL
Zinc	9.2–19.9 μmol/L	60–130 mcg/dL

Table G.3 Hematological Parameters

Parameter	SI Units (Canada)	Traditional Units (USA)
Red Blood Cells		
Erythrocytes (RBC) (MCC 2019)		
—Female	4.0–5.2 × 10^{12}/L	4.0–5.2 × 10^6/mm^3
—Male	4.4–5.7 × 10^{12}/L	4.4–5.7 × 10^6/mm^3
Reticulocyte count (MCC 2019)	20–84 × 10^9/L	0.5%–2.5%
Hematocrit (MCC 2019)		
—Female	0.370–0.460 g/L	37%–46%
—Male	0.420–0.520 g/L	42%–52%
Hemoglobin		
—Female	123–157 g/L	12.3–15.7 g/dL
—Male	130–170 g/L	14.0–17.4 g/dL
Erythrocyte sedimentation rate (ESR Westergren) (MCC 2019)		
—Female	<10 mm/h	<10 mm/h
—Male	<6 mm/h	<6 mm/h
White Blood Cells (WBCs)		
White blood cell count	4.0–10.0 × 10^9/L	4.0–10.0 × 10^3/mm^3
WBC differential (MCC 2019)		
—Segmented neutrophils	2–7 × 10^9/L	45%–75%
—Lymphocytes	1.5–3.4 × 10^9/L	16%–46%
—Monocytes	0.14–0.86 × 10^9/L	4%–11%
—Band neutrophils	<0.7 × 10^9/L	0%–5%
—Eosinophils	<0.45 × 10^9/L	0%–8%
—Basophils	<0.10 × 10^9/L	0%–3%
Coagulation		
Bleeding time (Ivy) (MCC 2019)	<9 min	<9 min
Clotting time	5–15 min	5–15 min
Fibrinogen	5.1–11.8 μmol/L	175–400 mg/dL
International normalized ratio (INR) (MCC 2019)	0.9–1.2	0.9–1.2
Plasminogen	75%–140%	75%–140%
Platelet count (thrombocytes) (MCC 2019)	130–400 × 10^9/L	130–400 × 10^3/mm^3
Prothrombin time (PT) (MCC 2019)	10–13 s	10–13 s
Partial thromboplastin time (PTT) (MCC 2019)	28–38 s	28–38 s
Thrombin time	14–16 s	14–16 s

Table G.4 Hormones

Parameter	SI Units (Canada)	Traditional Units (USA)
Adrenocorticotropin (ACTH)	1.3–16.7 pmol/L	6.0–76.0 pg/mL
Aldosterone (normal sodium diet adult)	0.52–0.94 nmol/L	19–34 ng/dL
Calcitonin		
—Female	<6.4 ng/L	<6.4 pg/mL
—Male	<13.8 ng/L	<13.8 pg/mL
Cortisol serum		
—Time: a.m.	110–607 nmol/L	5–25 mcg/dL
—Time: p.m.	83–469 nmol/L	3.1–16.7 mcg/dL
Estrogens (such as estradiol)		
—Female (premenopausal)	185–1,625 pmol/L	50–450 pg/mL
—Male	<200	<55
Follicle-stimulating hormone (FSH)		
—Female (premenopausal)	2–12 IU/L	2–12 IU/L
—Male	1–12	1–12
Glucagon	50–200 ng/L	50–200 pg/mL
Growth hormone	<8 mcg/L	<8 ng/mL
Insulin	36–179 pmol/L	5–25 μU/L
Luteinizing hormone (LH)		
—Female (premenopausal)	0.0–76 IU/L	0.0–76 IU/L
—Male	1.5–9.3 IU/L	1.5–9.3 IU/L
Parathyroid hormone (PTH)	1.2–5.8 pmol/L	11–54 pg/mL
Progesterone		
—Female (midluteal phase)	14.3–64 nmol/L	4.5–25.2 ng/mL
—Male	0.95–3.18 nmol/L	0.3–1.0 ng/mL
Prolactin	<1.29 nmol/L	<30 ng/mL
Renin activity		
—Normal sodium diet	0.5–4.0 ng/mL/h	0.5–4.0 ng/mL/h
—Thyroxine (T4 free serum)	8.5–15.2 pmol/L	0.66–1.18 ng/dL
—Triiodothyronine (T3 free serum) (MCC 2019 for SI units)	3.5–6.5 pmol/L	227–422 ng/dL
Testosterone		
—Female	<2.1 nmol/L	<62 ng/dL
—Male	6.7–28.9 nmol/L	300–1,000 ng/dL
Thyroid-stimulating hormone (TSH) (MCC 2019)	0.4–5.0 μU/mL	0.4–5.0 μU/mL
Vitamin D_3	60–105 nmol/L	24–40 ng/mL
—Cholecalciferol		
—25-Hydroxycholecalciferol	25–137 nmol/L	10–55 ng/mL
—1,25-Dihydroxycholecalciferol	58–156 pmol/L	24–65 pg/mL

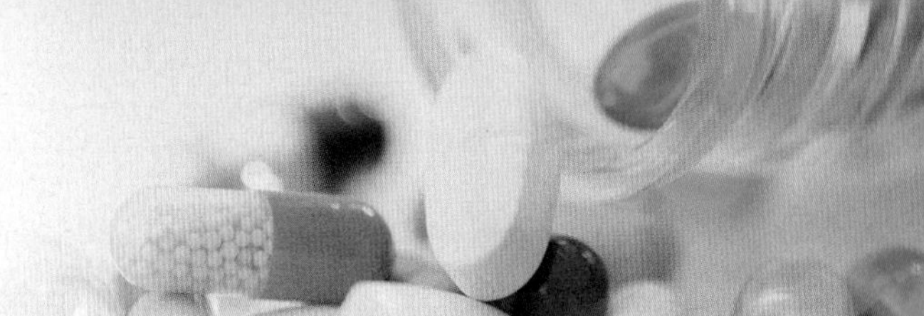

INDEX

Note: Page numbers followed by *f* indicate figures; page numbers followed by *b* indicate boxes; page numbers followed by *t* indicate tables.

B

E

H

M

S

U

V

W